CLINICAL ONCOLOGY

Consultant Editors

Joseph D. Rosenblatt, MD
Department of Hematology/Oncology

Paul Okunieff, MD
Department of Radiation Oncology

James V. Sitzmann, MD
Department of Surgery

University of Rochester Cancer Center
School of Medicine and Dentistry
Rochester, New York

Technical Editors

Amy K. Huser, MA
Taimi Marple

CLINICAL ONCOLOGY

A Multidisciplinary Approach for Physicians and Students

8th Edition

Editor

Philip Rubin, MD
Professor
Department of Radiation Oncology

Associate Editor

Jacqueline P. Williams, PhD
Assistant Professor
Department of Radiation Oncology

University of Rochester Cancer Center
School of Medicine and Dentistry
Rochester, New York

W.B. SAUNDERS COMPANY
A Harcourt Health Sciences Company
Philadelphia London New York St. Louis Sydney Toronto

W.B. SAUNDERS COMPANY
A Harcourt Health Sciences Company

The Curtis Center
Independence Square West
Philadelphia, Pennsylvania 19106

Library of Congress Cataloging-in-Publication Data

Clinical oncology: a multidisciplinary approach for physicians and students / Philip Rubin.—8th ed.

p. cm.

Includes bibliographical references and index.

ISBN 0–7216–7496–8

1. Cancer. 2. Oncology. I. Rubin, Philip.
[DNLM: 1. Neoplasms. 2. Medical Oncology—methods. QZ 200 C641 2001]
RC261. C652 2001
616.99′4—dc21 00–058852

Editor-in-Chief: Richard Zorab
Acquisitions Editor: Richard Zorab
Manuscript Editor: Robin E. Davis
Production Manager: Frank Polizzano
Illustration Specialist: Walt Verbitski

CLINICAL ONCOLOGY: A MULTIDISCIPLINARY APPROACH FOR PHYSICIANS AND STUDENTS ISBN 0–7216–7496–8

Some material in this work was previously published by the American Cancer Society in *Clinical Oncology for Medical Students and Physicians.*

Printed in the United States of America.

Last digit is the print number: 9 8 7 6 5 4 3 2 1

Dedication

IF THE PAST IS THE PROLOGUE TO THE FUTURE . . . On the occasion of the 150th anniversary of the University of Rochester and the 75th anniversary of the University of Rochester School of Medicine and Dentistry—

To the **James P. Wilmot Cancer Center Directors** for weaving the multi- and interdisciplinary fabric for us to wear and share proudly.

Thomas Hall	for the inspiration
Robert Cooper	for the implementation of the vision
Richard Borch	for maintaining the vision
Edward Messing	for reaffirming the role model of clinician-scientist
George Abraham	for navigating us into the new millennium

To the **James P. Wilmot Cancer Center Associate Directors** for representing their specialties while synergizing their disciplinary parts into a greater whole.

Brad Patterson	Surgical Oncology
John Bennett	Medical Oncology
Richard Bakemeier	Medical Oncology
Robert Sutherland	Cancer Biology

For their unselfish devotion to:
- Clinical care
- Translational research
- Clinical trials investigations
- Education
- Community outreach

To the **Deans of the University of Rochester School of Medicine and Dentistry** who created a more dynamic medical institution by allowing for the transition and a metamorphosis beyond the rigid departmental structure into a more interactive matrix model of multiple faculty appointments in more than one discipline.

Lowell Orbison	for his thoughtfulness and foresight
Frank Young	for his optimism and willingness to take risks
Robert Joynt	for his buoyant human and annealing abilities
Marshall Lichtman	for his scientific and academic astuteness and conception of centers of excellence
Lowell Goldsmith	for his humanity and recruitment of a new generation

Many of the individuals to whom this volume is dedicated have contributed to *Clinical Oncology* in past and present editions.

Contributors

Richard F. Bakemeier, MD, FACP
Professor of Medicine (Medical Oncology), University of Colorado School of Medicine; University of Colorado Hospital, Denver, CO
Basic Concepts of Cancer Chemotherapy and Principles of Medical Oncology

Jack Basil, MD
Assistant Professor of Obstetrics and Gynecology, Emory University School of Medicine; Emory University Hospital, Atlanta, GA
Gynecologic Tumors

James B. Benton, MD
Assistant Professor of Radiation Oncology, Emory University School of Medicine; Emory University Hospital, Atlanta, GA
Oncologic Emergencies

Luther W. Brady, MD
Hilda Cohn/American Cancer Society Professor of Clinical Oncology; Professor, Department of Radiation Oncology, MCP-Hahnemann University, Philadelphia, PA
Skin Cancer

David G. Bragg, MD, FACR
Emeritus Professor of Radiology, University of Utah, Salt Lake City, UT
Principles of Oncologic Imaging and Tumor Imaging Strategies

Ralph A. Brasacchio, MD
Assistant Professor of Radiation Oncology, University of Rochester School of Medicine and Dentistry; University of Rochester Cancer Center, Rochester, NY
Central Nervous System Tumors

William Breitbart, MD
Professor of Psychiatry, Weill Medical College of Cornell University; Chief, Psychiatry Service, Department of Psychiatry and Behavioral Sciences, Memorial Sloan-Kettering Cancer Center, New York, NY
Principles of Psychosocial Oncology

Patrick Burch, MD
Assistant Professor of Oncology, Mayo Medical School; Consultant in Medical Oncology, Mayo Clinic, Rochester, MN
Alimentary Cancer

Peter Carroll, MD
Professor and Chair of Urology, University of California, San Francisco, San Francisco, CA
Urologic and Male Genital Cancers

Philippe Chanson, MD
Professor of Endocrinology, Paris-Sud University; Professor, Endocrinology and Reproductive Medicine, University Hospital of Bicetre, Le Kremlin-Bicetre, France
Cancer of the Endocrine Glands

K.S. Clifford Chao, MD
Assistant Professor of Radiation Oncology, Washington University School of Medicine; Assistant Professor, Mallinckrodt Institute of Radiology, St. Louis, MO
Gynecologic Tumors

Frances Collichio, MD
Clinical Assistant Professor of Hematology/Oncology, University of North Carolina, Chapel Hill, NC
Basic Concepts in Drug Development and Clinical Trials

Marc D. Coltrera, MD
Associate Professor of Otolaryngology/Head and Neck Surgery, University of Washington; University of Washington Medical Center, Seattle, WA
Tumors of the Head and Neck

Louis S. Constine III, MD
Professor of Radiation Oncology and Pediatrics, University of Rochester School of Medicine and Dentistry; Associate Chair of Radiation Oncology, University of Rochester Cancer Center, Rochester, NY
Hodgkin's Disease and the Lymphomas; Pediatric Solid Tumors

Jay S. Cooper, MD
Professor of Radiation Oncology, New York University; Attending, Tisch and Bellevue Hospitals, New York, NY
HIV-Associated Malignancies

Robert Dinapoli, MD
Associate Professor of Neurology, Mayo Medical School; Consultant in Neuro-Oncology, Mayo Clinic, Rochester, MN
Central Nervous System Tumors

P. Anthony di Sant'Agnese, MD
Professor of Pathology and Laboratory Medicine, University of Rochester School of Medicine and Dentistry; Attending Pathologist, University of Rochester Medical Center, Rochester, NY
The Pathology of Cancer

Bernadine R. Donahue, MD
Associate Professor of Radiation Oncology, New York University; Attending, Tisch and Bellevue Hospitals, New York University Medical Center, New York, NY
HIV-Associated Malignancies

John Donohue, MD
Professor of Surgery, Mayo Medical School; Consultant in General Surgery, Mayo Clinic, Rochester, MN
Alimentary Cancer

Howard J. Federoff, MD
Professor of Neurology, University of Rochester School of Medicine and Dentistry; Director, Neurology Center on Aging and Developmental Biology, University of Rochester Medical Center, Rochester, NY
Gene Therapy for Cancer

Robert J. Ginsberg, MD
Chief of Thoracic Surgery, Memorial Sloan-Kettering Cancer Center, New York, NY
Principles of Surgical Oncology

Richard Goldberg, MD
Associate Professor of Oncology, Mayo Medical School; Consultant in Medical Oncology, Mayo Clinic, Rochester, MN
Alimentary Cancer

Jennifer Griggs, MD, MPH
Assistant Professor of Medical Oncology, University of Rochester School of Medicine and Dentistry; University of Rochester Cancer Center, Rochester, NY
Basic Concepts in Drug Development and Clinical Trials

Perry W. Grigsby, MD
Professor of Radiation Oncology, Washington University School of Medicine; Professor, Mallinckrodt Institute of Radiology, St. Louis, MO
Gynecologic Tumors

Leonard L. Gunderson, MD
Professor of Oncology, Mayo Medical School; Chair of Oncology and Consultant in Radiation Oncology, Mayo Clinic, Rochester, MN
Alimentary Cancer

Michael G. Haddock, MD
Assistant Professor of Oncology, Mayo Medical School; Consultant in Radiation Oncology, Mayo Clinic, Rochester, MN
Alimentary Cancer

Richard P. Hill, PhD
Professor of Medical Biophysics, University of Toronto; Senior Scientist, Princess Margaret Hospital/Ontario Cancer Institute, Toronto, Ontario, Canada
The Biology of Cancer

Richard T. Hoppe, MD
Henry S. Kaplan–Harry Lebeson Professor of Cancer Biology; Chair of Radiation Oncology, Stanford University, Stanford, CA
Hodgkin's Disease and the Lymphomas

Karen J. Hunt, MD
Staff Physician, Glacier Oncology, Kalispell, MT
Tumors of the Head and Neck

James Dirk Iglehart, MD
Richard Wilson Professor of Surgery, Brigham and Women's Hospital; Charles Dana Investigator in Genetics, Dana-Farber Cancer Institute, Harvard Medical School, Boston, MA
Breast Cancer

Robert B. Jenkins, MD, PhD
Professor of Laboratory Medicine, Mayo Medical School; Consultant, Mayo Clinic, Rochester, MN
Central Nervous System Tumors

James W. Keller, MD
Professor and Clinical Director of Radiation Oncology, Emory University School of Medicine; Emory University Hospital, Atlanta, GA
Oncologic Emergencies

Peter Keng, PhD
Professor of Radiation Oncology and Tumor Biology, University of Rochester School of Medicine and Dentistry, Rochester, NY
Basic Principles of Radiobiology

David N. Korones, MD
Associate Professor of Pediatrics and Oncology, University of Rochester School of Medicine and Dentistry; University of Rochester Cancer Center, Rochester, NY
Pediatric Solid Tumors; Central Nervous System Tumors

George E. Laramore, MD, PhD
Professor and Chair of Radiation Oncology, University of Washington; University of Washington Medical Center, Seattle, WA
Tumors of the Head and Neck

Edith Lord, PhD
Professor of Immunology, University of Rochester School of Medicine and Dentistry, Rochester, NY
Basic Concepts of Tumor Immunology and Principles of Immunotherapy

Calvin R. Maurer Jr, PhD
Director of Image-Guided Surgery Research Lab, University of Rochester School of Medicine and Dentistry; Assistant Professor of Neurosurgery, University of Rochester Medical Center, Rochester, NY
Radiation Physics as Applied to Clinical Radiation Oncology

Sandra McDonald, MD
Clinical Associate Professor of Radiation Oncology, University of Rochester Cancer Center; Chief Radiologist, The Genesee Hospital, Rochester, NY
Lung Cancer

David G. Mutch, MD
Professor of Obstetrics and Gynecology, Washington University School of Medicine; Director, Division of Gynecologic Oncology, Barnes-Jewish Hospital, St. Louis, MO
Gynecologic Tumors

Vesna Najfeld, PhD
Associate Professor of Medicine, The Mount Sinai School of Medicine, New York University; Director, The Tumor Cytogenetics and Oncology-Molecular Detection Laboratory, Mount Sinai NYU Health, New York, NY
The Leukemias

Diana F. Nelson, MD
Professor of Oncology, Mayo Medical School; Consultant in Radiation Oncology, Mayo Clinic, Rochester, MN
Central Nervous System Tumors

Heidi Nelson, MD
Professor of Surgery; Chair, Division of Colon and Rectal Surgery, Mayo Medical School; Chair of Colorectal Surgery and Consultant in Colorectal Surgery, Mayo Clinic, Rochester, MN
Alimentary Cancer

Regis J. O'Keefe, MD, PhD
Professor of Orthopaedic Oncology/Metabolic Bone Disease, University of Rochester School of Medicine and Dentistry; Professor of Orthopaedics, University of Rochester Medical Center, Rochester, NY
Bone Tumors

Paul Okunieff, MD
Professor and Chair of Radiation Oncology, University of Rochester School of Medicine and Dentistry; University of Rochester Cancer Center, Rochester, NY
Statement of the Clinical Oncologic Problem

Stanley E. Order, MD, FACR
Professor of Molecular Oncology, State University of New York, Stony Brook, Long Island, NY; Director, Center for Molecular Medicine, Garden City, NY
Basic Concepts of Tumor Immunology and Principles of Immunotherapy

Robert D. Ornitz, MD
Chair of Radiation Oncology, Rex Healthcare, Raleigh, NC
Metastases and Disseminated Disease

Charles Paidas, MD
Associate Professor of Pediatric Surgery, The Johns Hopkins University Medical Center, Baltimore, MD
Pediatric Solid Tumors

Richard B. Patt, MD
Associate Professor of Anesthesiology, Baylor College of Medicine; President and Chief Medical Officer, The Patt Center for Cancer Pain and Wellness, Houston, TX
Cancer Pain Management: An Essential Component of Comprehensive Cancer Care

James L. Peacock, MD
Associate Professor of Surgery, University of Rochester Medical Center, Rochester, NY
Cancer of the Major Digestive Glands

Carlos A. Perez, MD
Professor of Radiology, Washington University School of Medicine; Radiation Oncologist-in-Chief, Radiation Oncology Center, Barnes-Jewish Hospital, St. Louis, MO
Gynecologic Tumors

Leonard R. Prosnitz, MD, FACR
Professor of Radiation Oncology, Duke University Medical Center, Durham, NC
Breast Cancer

Raman Qazi, MD, FACP
Associate Professor of Medical Oncology, Highland Hospital, Rochester, NY
Basic Concepts of Cancer Chemotherapy and Principles of Medical Oncology; Hodgkin's Disease and the Lymphomas

Corey Raffel, MD
Professor of Neurosurgery, Mayo Medical School; Consultant in Neurosurgery, Mayo Clinic, Rochester, MN
Central Nervous System Tumors

David M. Reese, MD
Assistant Clinical Professor of Medicine, UCSF Comprehensive Cancer Center, San Francisco, CA
Urologic and Male Genital Cancers

John A. Ridge, MD, PhD, FACS
Chief of Head and Neck Surgery, Fox Chase Cancer Center, Philadelphia, PA
Principles of Surgical Oncology

Mack Roach III, MD
Professor of Radiation Oncology, Medical Oncology and Urology, University of California, San Francisco, San Francisco, CA
Urologic and Male Genital Cancers

Joseph D. Rosenblatt, MD
Samuel E. Durand Professor of Medicine, Microbiology and Immunology, University of Rochester School of Medicine and Dentistry; Interim Director, University of Rochester Cancer Center, Rochester, NY
Statement of the Clinical Oncologic Problem; Basic Concepts in Drug Development and Clinical Trials; Gene Therapy for Cancer

Randy N. Rosier, MD, PhD
Professor of Orthopaedic Oncology/Metabolic Bone Disease, University of Rochester School of Medicine and Dentistry; Professor and Chair of Orthopaedics, University of Rochester Medical Center, Rochester, NY
Soft Tissue Sarcoma; Bone Tumors

Andrew J. Roth, MD
Assistant Professor of Psychiatry, Weill Medical College of Cornell University; Assistant Attending Psychiatrist, Department of Psychiatry and Behavioral Sciences, Memorial Sloan-Kettering Cancer Center, New York, NY
Principles of Psychosocial Oncology

Philip Rubin, MD, FACR, FACRO
Emeritus Professor of Radiation Oncology, University of Rochester School of Medicine and Dentistry; University of Rochester Cancer Center, Rochester, NY
Statement of the Clinical Oncologic Problem; Principles of Radiation Oncology and Cancer Radiotherapy; Principles of Oncologic Imaging and Tumor Imaging Strategies; Late Effects of Cancer Treatment: Radiation and Chemotherapy Toxicity

Deepak M. Sahasrabudhe, MD
Associate Professor of Medicine, University of Rochester School of Medicine and Dentistry, University of Rochester Cancer Center, Rochester, NY
Soft Tissue Sarcoma; Bone Tumors

Omar M. Salazar, MD, FACR, FACRO
Chief Radiologist, Oakwood Hospital, Dearborn, MI
Lung Cancer

Ajay Sandhu, MD
Assistant Professor of Radiation Oncology, University of Rochester School of Medicine and Dentistry; University of Rochester Cancer Center, Rochester, NY
Cancer of the Major Digestive Glands

Charles W. Scarantino, MD, PhD
Professor of Radiation Oncology, Rex Healthcare Cancer Center, Raleigh, NC
Metastases and Disseminated Disease

Gilbert Schaison, MD
Professor of Endocrinology, Paris-Sud University; Head, Endocrinology and Reproductive Medicine, University Hospital of Bicetre, Le Kremlin-Bicetre, France
Cancer of the Endocrine Glands

Bernd W. Scheithauer, MD
Professor of Pathology, Mayo Medical School; Consultant in Pathology, Mayo Clinic, Rochester, MN
Central Nervous System Tumors

Michael C. Schell, PhD
Associate Professor of Radiation Oncology, University of Rochester School of Medicine and Dentistry; Director of Medical Physics, University of Rochester Cancer Center, Rochester, NY
Radiation Physics as Applied to Clinical Radiation Oncology

Steven E. Schild, MD
Associate Professor of Oncology, Mayo Medical School; Consultant in Radiation Oncology, Mayo Clinic, Rochester, MN
Central Nervous System Tumors

Martin Schlumberger, MD
Professor of Oncology, Paris-Sud University; Head, Nuclear Medicine and Endocrine Tumors, Institut Gustave-Roussy, Paris, France
Cancer of the Endocrine Glands

Cindy L. Schwartz, MD
Associate Professor of Pediatrics; Clinical Director, The Johns Hopkins University Medical Center, Baltimore, MD
Pediatric Solid Tumors

Eileen Scigliano, MD
Assistant Clinical Professor of Medicine, The Mount Sinai School of Medicine; Assistant Clinical Professor of Medicine, Mount Sinai NYU Health, New York, NY
The Leukemias

J. Anthony Seibert, PhD
Professor of Radiology, School of Medicine, University of California, Davis, Davis, CA
Radiation Physics as Applied to Clinical Radiation Oncology

Brenda Shank, MD, PhD
Clinical Professor of Radiation Oncology, University of California, San Francisco; Medical Director, JC Robinson MD Regional Cancer Center, Doctors Medical Center, San Pablo, CA
The Leukemias

Elin R. Sigurdson, MD, PhD
Attending Surgeon of Surgical Oncology, Fox Chase Cancer Center, Philadelphia, PA
Principles of Surgical Oncology

James V. Sitzmann, MD
Professor and Chair of Surgery, University of Rochester Medical Center, Rochester, NY
Statement of the Clinical Oncologic Problem

Frank T. Slovick, MD
Heartland Hematology-Oncology Associates, Kansas City, MO
Late Effects of Cancer Treatment: Radiation and Chemotherapy Toxicity

Eric Small, MD
Associate Clinical Professor of Medicine and Urology, UCSF Comprehensive Cancer Center, San Francisco, CA
Urologic and Male Genital Cancers

Julia L. Smith, MD
Associate Professor of Medicine, The Genesee Hospital, Rochester, NY
Cancer of the Major Digestive Glands

Merrill J. Solan, MD
Assistant Professor of Radiation Oncology, Thomas Jefferson University, Philadelphia; Medical Director, Jefferson Radiation Oncology, Riddle Memorial Hospital, Media, PA
Skin Cancer

Ira J. Spiro, MD, PhD
Associate Professor of Radiation Oncology, Harvard Medical School; Associate Radiation Oncologist, Massachusetts General Hospital, Boston, MA
Soft Tissue Sarcoma

Patrice F. Spitalnik, MD
Senior Instructor of Pathology and Laboratory Medicine, University of Rochester School of Medicine and Dentistry, Rochester, NY
The Pathology of Cancer

Porter Storey, MD, FACP
Clinical Associate Professor of Medicine, Baylor College of Medicine; Adjunct Assistant Professor in Symptom Control and Palliative Care, University of Texas MD Anderson Cancer Center; Medical Director/Vice-President, The Hospice at the Texas Medical Center, Houston, TX
Palliative Care

Herman D. Suit, MD, DPhil
Andres Soriano Professor of Radiation Oncology, Harvard Medical School; Radiation Oncologist, Massachusetts General Hospital, Boston, MA
Soft Tissue Sarcoma

Robert M. Sutherland, PhD
Consultant Professor of Radiation Oncology, Stanford University, Stanford, CA; President, Varian Biosynergy, Mountain View, CA
Basic Principles of Radiobiology

Khaled A. Tolba, MD
Senior Instructor of Hematology-Oncology Division, University of Rochester School of Medicine and Dentistry; Staff Physician, University of Rochester Cancer Center, Rochester, NY
Gene Therapy for Cancer

Victor Trastek, MD
Professor and Chair of Surgery, Mayo Medical School, Rochester, MN; Consultant in Thoracic Surgery, Mayo Clinic Scottsdale, Scottsdale, AZ
Alimentary Cancer

Maurice Tubiana, MD
Emeritus Professor, Paris-Sud University; Honorary Director, Institut Gustave-Roussy, Paris, France
Cancer of the Endocrine Glands

Paul Van Houtte, MD
Professor and Chief Radiologist, Institut Jules Bordet-Centre des Tumeurs de l'Université Libré de Bruxelles, Brussels, Belgium
Lung Cancer

Adrianna Vlachos, MD
Assistant Professor of Medicine, Albert Einstein College of Medicine; Assistant Professor of Medicine, Schneider Children's Hospital, North Shore–Long Island Jewish Health System, New Hyde Park, NY
The Leukemias

James C. Wernz, MD
Associate Professor of Clinical Medicine, New York University; Attending, Division of Medical Oncology, Tisch and Bellevue Hospitals, New York, NY
HIV-Associated Malignancies

Jacqueline P. Williams, PhD
Assistant Professor of Radiation Oncology, University of Rochester School of Medicine and Dentistry, Rochester, NY
Statement of the Clinical Oncologic Problem; Basic Principles of Radiobiology; Principles of Radiation Oncology and Cancer Radiotherapy; Basic Concepts of Tumor Immunology and Principles of Immunotherapy; Late Effects of Cancer Treatment: Radiation and Chemotherapy Toxicity

Eric P. Winer, MD
Associate Professor of Medicine, Harvard Medical School; Director, Breast Oncology Center, Dana-Farber Institute, Boston, MA
Breast Cancer

Sabra A. Woodard, MD
Staff Radiologist and Medical Director of Nuclear Medicine, Rex Hospital, Raleigh, NC
Metastases and Disseminated Disease

Fang-Fang Yin, PhD
Division Head of Medical Physics, Department of Radiation Oncology, Henry Ford Health System, Detroit, MI
Radiation Physics as Applied to Clinical Radiation Oncology

Alex Yuang-Chi Chang, MD
Oncology Program Director and Consultant Oncologist; Johns Hopkins Singapore, Singapore
Lung Cancer

Preface

Major "paradigm shifts" have occurred and will continue to occur on the pathway to curing cancer as we enter into the new millennium. The National Cancer Institute's goal of a 50% survival rate for all cancer patients by the year 2000 has, in general, been reached. Indeed, in the decades since the introduction of a multidisciplinary approach to cancer management, this survival rate has been exceeded for many specific sites, with clear evidence of a decrease in mortality rates. With each passing decade there have been incremental gains, with an associated paradigm shift:

- In the *1950s,* there were advances in each modality: in surgery, with better anesthesia, antibiotics, and blood replacement products; in radiation oncology, perhaps most dramatically, with the introduction of megavoltage irradiation using telecobalt units and linear accelerators; and in chemotherapy, with the introduction of numerous new agents. For the most part, the treatment plans and sequences were in the pattern of a relay race, with the surgeon passing the baton to the radiation oncologist, then on to the chemotherapist.
- In the *1960s,* a multidisciplinary approach to cancer was initiated as oncologists from surgery, radiation, medicine, gynecology, and pediatrics began to work together. National cooperative oncology groups, initially devoted to one disease and dominated by one discipline—for example, the Breast Surgical Adjuvant Group (BSAG), Eastern Chemotherapy Oncology Group (ECOG), and Radiation Therapy Oncology Group (RTOG)—merged and, over the decade, became multidisciplinary. The preplanning of protocols by all participating investigators and disciplines was a major shift away from the physician as a clinician only toward the physician as a clinician-scientist.
- In the *1970s,* The National Cancer Institute (NCI) declared a "War on Cancer," increasing funding to laboratory researchers and clinical protocol cooperative group and cancer center investigators. Pharmaceutical companies and the NCI, in its extramural screening of agents, spent millions searching for the "magic bullet" that would "blast" the malignancy. In particular, pediatric cooperative groups initiated intergroup studies and entered virtually the entire eligible pediatric cancer population on to studies, thereby setting the pace for the adult groups. These intergroup studies demonstrated that *less* treatment frequently was *more* and *better,* seen most dramatically in patients with Wilms' tumor. Organ structure preservation was emphasized and, indeed, treatment successes were so sufficiently dramatic that late effects in survivors became of increasing concern.
- In the *1980s,* there was an apparent stage migration, when an early diagnosis of breast cancer became possible through the wide utilization of the screening mammogram. This led to a "terrain" analogy: that well-coordinated and synchronized attacks by two or more conservative modalities could modify or avoid the need for aggressive, often mutilating surgery with a more conservative approach.
- In the *1990s,* use of molecular biomarkers—notably prostate specific antigen (PSA)—led to an apparent dramatic increase in the incidence of some cancers, with the incidence of prostate cancer almost doubling early in the decade. However, following the identification of an increasc in observed prostate cancer incidence rate were a striking overall increase in the survival rate and a decrease in mortality rate by the end of the decade. In addition, the use of a single modality was found to be sufficient—for example, either nerve-sparing prostatectomy, three-dimensional conformal external megavoltage, or prostate radioactive seed implants. The end point of treatment then became a biologic one—that is, the monitoring and elimination of serum PSA—with any further elevation leading to the use of other modalities for salvage.

If past achievements are the prologue to innovations ahead, the vision of the continued curability of cancer rests on two emerging concepts. The first concept is that the multistage process leading to carcinogenesis can be viewed through a molecular biologic window; that is, the activation (or suppression) of intrinsic cellular oncogenes (or growth suppressor genes) can lead to dysregulation of the cell cycle, cell proliferation, or differentiation through gene expression. This process can lead to transformation of cells from a normal to a premalignant state and, ultimately, to malignancy and metastatic growth. However, evidence from epidemiologic studies indicates that only 20% of neoplasms are hereditary, suggesting that although intrinsic genetic factors are important, most cancers do not follow one slow recognizable pattern of inheritance. This optimistic message suggests that extrinsic environmental factors are causal and that the majority of cancers are not brought about by inherent factors as a consequence of aging; therefore, a high incidence of cancer is not an inevitable condition of being human.

The second concept involves the ongoing revolution in imaging, including the powerful new techniques of low-dose, spiral computed tomography and the merging of magnetic resonance imaging and magnetic resonance spectroscopy with fusion techniques. These techniques are akin to *in vivo,* noninvasive biopsy, allowing for anatomic spatial resolution and a histologic/chemical analysis at the cellular level. Both advances in molecular biologic understanding and the latest innovations in imaging techniques are described for each major cancer site.

Each site-specific chapter in this, the eighth edition of *Clinical Oncology*, begins with clear and concise data regarding *Epidemiology and Etiology*. Imaging procedures are described in the *Detection and Diagnosis* section. In the *Classification and Staging* section, there is a brief description of the histopathology of the cancer, and the updated staging figures and tables will assist physicians in defining the cancer in its various extentions and spread patterns. Once the histopathologic type of cancer is known and the staging procedure is complete, the process moves towards multidisciplinary decision making, described in the *Principles of Treatment* section. The *Results* section gives the current status of clinical trials, and it is supported by an extensive and updated bibliography.

In addition to the site-specific chapters, there is a series of general introductory chapters on basic concepts in the oncologic sciences of cancer biology, pathology, radiation biology, physics, and gene therapy. The clinical science of oncology is presented in the chapters on the principles of surgery, radiation oncology, medical oncology, psychosocial oncology, and oncologic emergencies. Concluding chapters cover metastases, pain, palliation, and late effects.

As in the past edition, we emphasize the increased curability of cancer and the optimization of combining modalities to reduce morbidity, to decrease complications, and to preserve vital structures. Because past achievements are indeed the prologue to the future, I predict that cancer will be eliminated through continued translational research in the multiple disciplines involved in the science of oncology, through the interaction of the participating clinicians and scientists, and through the synergism of their ideas.

Philip Rubin, MD

Acknowledgments

In the early 1960s, I had the privilege of publishing a textbook devoted to managing cancer patients in the University of Rochester Medical School entitled *Clinical Oncology for Medical Students*; this book had an emphasis on radiation therapy, with the first two editions appearing in 1963 and 1965. In 1967, the title was changed to *Clinical Oncology for Medical Students: A Multidisciplinary Approach*, with updates appearing in 1970 and 1971. These first three editions had contributions from faculties of clinical departments and provided a multidisciplinary syllabus with an interdepartmental editorial board. *Clinical Oncology for Medical Students and Physicians* represented the 1974, 1978, and 1983 editions, which were sponsored by the American Cancer Society. These editions reflected the University of Rochester Cancer Center faculty and environment that created a spirit of cooperation arising in the oncologic departments and divisions in our medical center.

Clinical Oncology: A Multidisciplinary Approach for Physicians and Students has been published by W.B. Saunders for the last two editions, nominally the seventh and eighth, although in reality the ninth and tenth editions. Unique to this eighth edition is the authorship, which is not only multidisciplinary but also multi-institutional. The contributing authors are outstanding leaders in the field of oncologic specialization. With this expansion in authorship, we hope to establish this volume as a long-lasting textbook devoted to the multidisciplinary approach to cancer. Furthermore, it will be the most comprehensive textbook, including both a hard copy and a CD-ROM version.

Therefore, my first and foremost acknowledgment must go to the contributors, not only of the current edition but also of all past editions of this book over the preceding 40 years. The current expanded, multi-institutional authorship, both national and international, provides a comprehensive understanding in each field of oncologic expertise. I am very appreciative of all the authors, who are leaders in oncologic practice, investigation, and research and who have given considerable effort and time out of their busy schedules to assist in the production of the chapters during the long publishing process.

Special thanks and my deepest gratitude go to my hardworking Associate Editor, Jacky Williams, for her assistance in the completion of this book. Her abilities and dedication, combined with her acute insights and scholarship, are truly remarkable and are evident throughout the book. This project could not have been completed without her work. Assisting her was Amy Huser, whose meticulous organizational, literary, research, and editing skills deserve special mention. They both assumed the responsibility of seeing the book through to its completion, working with the authors to check overall accuracy, and fine-tuning the figures and tables. Amy's background in journalism has contributed to the clear and concise text presented in this volume.

Because this edition has been in progress for 4 years, the efforts of other editorial assistants need to be mentioned: Taimi Marple worked on the first round of the book with the many authors; Koren Bakkegard assisted in the editorial process and also spent hours diligently tracking down permission requests for tables and figures in this book. The artwork in the updated staging figures is that of Glen Hintz, Chair of Art Studies at Rochester Institute of Technology; he produced the beautiful graphic displays of the cancer staging systems in the T, N, and M categories.

Finally, I wish to thank the publisher, W.B. Saunders, and especially Richard Zorab, Editor-in-Chief, Medicine, for their vision in realizing the continued need to publish this book. The future of cancer patient treatment rests with the accurate transfer of past and current experience in the field of oncology—its science and clinical investigations—to the next generations of medical students and physicians.

Contents

1 Statement of the Clinical Oncologic Problem

PHILIP RUBIN, MD, Radiation Oncology
JACQUELINE P. WILLIAMS, PhD, Radiation Oncology
PAUL OKUNIEFF, MD, Radiation Oncology
JOSEPH D. ROSENBLATT, MD, Medical Oncology
JAMES V. SITZMANN, MD, Surgical Oncology

The analysis of many a success or failure (in cancer management) often reveals the important role played by the physician or physicians who dealt with the case in its inception and their decisive influence on the eventual result. Where temporizing guesswork, amateurish approaches, and defeatist attitudes may fail, intelligent understanding, prompt skillful treatment, and a hopeful, compassionate attitude may succeed.

ACKERMAN AND DEL REGATO[1]

Perspective

Cancer is viewed as a genetic disease resulting in the abnormal proliferation of a clone of cells. The Human Genome Project, begun in 1990, has as its objective the mapping and sequencing of the entire haploid human chromosome number by the year 2005.[7] This international effort, under the rubric *Human Genome Organization*, is being organized to store DNA and protein sequences into linkage maps of genetic markers in microsatellite sequences of nucleotides; this will provide a scaffold upon which to construct a physical map of the human genome. The first nucleotide sequence was published in 1965; to date, biologists have published over 100 million base pairs of sequence data. When the project is completed, following a complete mapping of the estimated 100,000 human genes, the result will form the platform for molecular medicine and molecular oncology. The completed map will be able to act as a source for identifying the gene or genes responsible for a neoplasm or an associated chromosomal aberration in a specific cancer. Once the human genome is deciphered, the vision is to develop new molecular screening and diagnostic tools as well as innovative gene transfer–based therapeutic strategies.

Carcinogenesis is recognized as a multistep process in which a series of genetic alterations occurs within a cell and, through processes of promotion and progression, leads to malignancy. Delineating the genetic mechanisms of carcinogenesis may provide the key to early detection and genetic approaches to prevention of neoplastic transformation. In addition, a marriage of specific tumor cell genotyping and gene therapy will be an important element for success in clinical trials. It should be no surprise that of the hundreds of Recombinant DNA Advisory Committee–approved gene therapy protocols, the largest number of current clinical trials are in the field of cancer gene therapy (Fig. 1–1).[8] Therefore, each chapter in this textbook, where appropriate, will have a section providing this genetic vision of the importance and impact of advances in molecular biology. Although still in their infancy, genetic approaches will likely see increased use as the genetic "profiling" of tumors accelerates.

Currently, cancer is curable and preventable with available multidisciplinary approaches. This dread disease, which at one time was synonymous with death, has yielded to advances in modern screening, detection, and diagnosis, as well as to progress in developing multimodal treatment. This has been demonstrated by our increased understanding from work in basic science research and in gains made in the number of clinical trial investigations. Compared with decades ago, seemingly incurable and devastating cancers are currently being detected early in their noninvasive or insidious phase, prior to metastatic dissemination. In their localized or advancing stages, many cancers are being ablated by a combined-modality approach that includes surgery, radiation therapy, and chemotherapy, as illustrated by the successful outcomes in all stages and anatomic disease sites. An analysis of trends in survival in both adults and children, respectively (Table 1–1 and Fig. 1–2), based upon analysis of the U.S. Bureau of the Census and the National Cancer Institute's Surveillance, Epidemiology and End Results (SEER) program, shows a significant improvement for 5-year survival rates by decade, from 39% in the 1960s, to 43% in the 1970s, to 50% in the 1980s, and to 60% in the 1990s. This gain in survival has occurred at 15 to 20 sites, most of which have reached

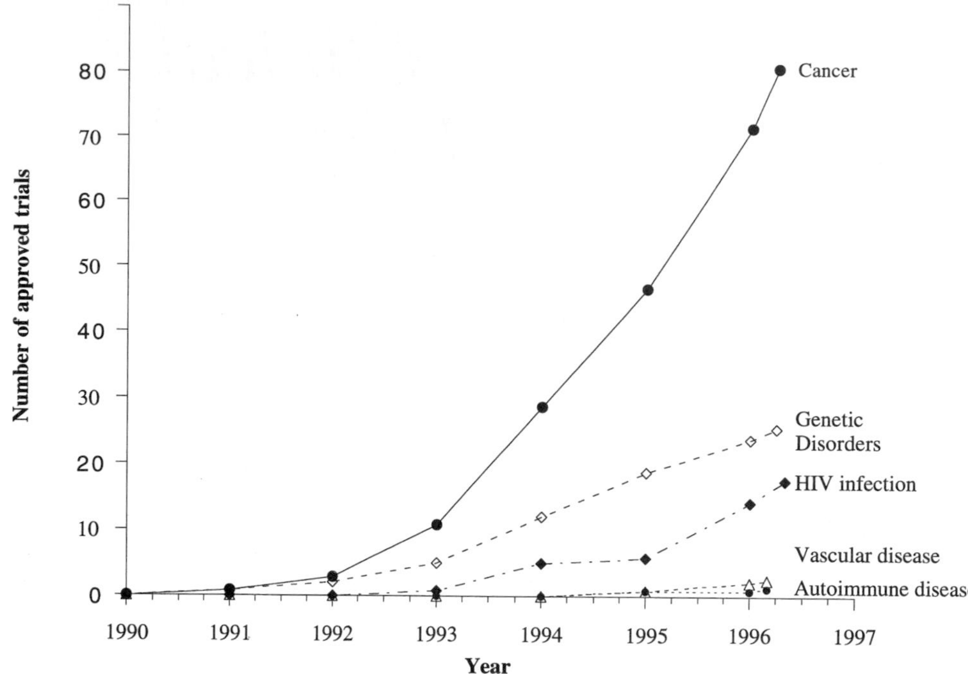

Figure 1–1. Growth in the number of Recombinant DNA Advisory Committee (RAC)—approved gene therapy protocols. (From Culver KW: Gene Therapy. A Primer for Physicians, 2nd ed. Larchmont, Mary Ann Liebert Inc, 1996, with permission.)

TABLE 1–1. **Trends in Survival (%) by Site of Cancer and Cases Diagnosed**

Site	1960–1963		1970–1973		1974–1976		1980–1982		1986–1993	
	White	*Black*	*White*	*Black*	*White*	*Black*	*White*	*Black*	*White*	*Black*
All Sites	39	27	43	31	50	39	52	40	60*	44*
Thyroid	83	NA	86	NA	92	88	94	95	96*	89
Testis	63	NA	72	NA	79	76†	92	90†	95*	86
Endometrium (uterus)	73	31	81	44	89	61	83	54	86*	55
Melanoma-skin	60	NA	68	NA	80	66†	83	60†	88*	67†
Urinary bladder	53	24	61	36	74	47	79	58	83*	61
Breast (female)	63	46	68	51	75	63	77	66	86*	70*
Hodgkin's disease	40	NA	67	NA	72	69	75	72	82*	74
Prostate	50	35	63	55	68	58	75	65	90*	75*
Larynx	53	NA	62	NA	67	58	69	59	69	54
Cervix (uterus)	58	47	64	61	70	64	68	61	71	57*
Colon	43	34	49	37	50	46	56	49	63*	53*
Oral cavity	45	NA	43	NA	55	36	55	31	55	34
Rectum	38	27	45	30	49	42	53	38	61*	52
Kidney and renal pelvis	37	38	46	44	52	49	51	56	60*	55*
Non-Hodgkin's lymphoma	31	NA	41	NA	48	48	52	51	52*	44
Ovary	32	32	36	32	36	40	39	38	47*	42
Leukemia	14	NA	22	NA	35	31	39	33	43*	33
Multiple myeloma	12	NA	19	NA	24	27	28	29	28*	30
Brain and other CNS	18	19	20	19	22	27	25	31	29*	35
Stomach	11	8	13	13	15	17	16	19	19*	20
Lung and bronchus	8	5	10	7	12	11	14	12	14*	11
Esophagus	4	1	4	4	5	4	8	5	12*	8*
Liver	NA	NA	NA	NA	4	1	4	2	6*	4*
Pancreas	1	1	2	2	3	3	3	5	4*	5*

Note: All sites exclude basal and squamous cell skin cancers and *in situ* carcinomas except urinary bladder.
CNS = central nervous system; NA = valid survival rate cannot be calculated.
*The difference in rates between 1974–1976 and 1986–1993 is statistically significant ($p<0.05$).
†The standard error of the survival rate is more than 5 percentage points.
Data sources are the End Results Group, 1960–1973 and the NCI Surveillance, Epidemiology, and End Results Program, 1997. From Landis SH, Murray T, Bolden S, et al: Cancer statistics, 1998. CA Cancer J Clin 1998; 48:6, with permission.

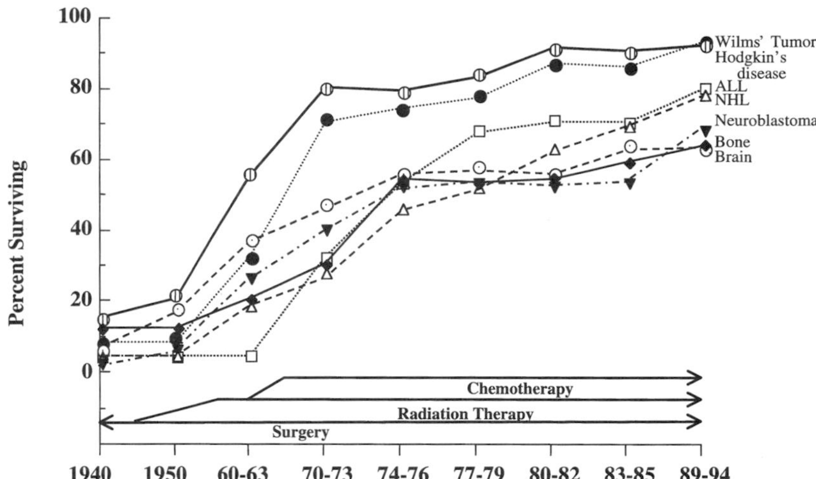

Figure 1–2. Advances in pediatric tumor curability. Includes data from Landis and associates,[10] the United States Bureau of the Census,[11, 12] SEER Cancer Statistics Review,[13, 14] and Simone and Lyons.[15]

significant levels. The National Cancer Institute goal for the decade beginning in 2000 is to reduce the cancer mortality by one half. In fact, this goal is already being reached and promises to be exceeded, inasmuch as numerous innovations have occurred and newer therapeutic modalities, such as monoclonal antibodies or immunotherapy, biologic response modifiers, hyperthermia, chemoprevention, new imaging modalities, and molecular biology diagnosis and gene therapy techniques, are becoming increasingly effective.

The size and scope of the cancer problem are best appreciated with numbers. Almost 60 million Americans now living will be diagnosed as cancer patients—one in every four, according to present rates; it is likely that a family member or friend within your acquaintance will be so affected. By the year 2001, more than one million people will have been diagnosed annually as having cancer[9]; this figure does not include basal and squamous skin cancer (approximately 1 million patients), and other carcinomas *in situ*, such as 39,900 cases of breast cancer *in situ* and 21,100 cases of melanoma *in situ*, which represent underreported populations of thousands of patients. American Cancer Society (ACS) statistics from 1998, for the first time in the twentieth century, reported a reduction in the total number of new cancer cases and declining cancer death rates while, as noted earlier, 5-year survival rates improved for most cancers.[16] Furthermore, there was an estimated 3% decrease in the number of estimated new cases of cancer from 1997 to 2000, from 1,257,800 to 1,220,100.[9, 17] SEER data also confirm decreases for lung cancer, prostate, and breast cancers, as well as gastrointestinal cancers.[18]

Epidemiology and Etiology

Epidemiology

More than one million new cases of cancer were estimated for the United States in 2000.[9] Patterns of incidence and death rates of malignant disease (Fig. 1–3) vary with age, sex, race, and geographic location[19]: males are showing a more favorable decline in mortality rates, exceeding females by 4.3% compared with 1.1%.[16] Improvements in diagnosis and therapy have occurred at many sites, although in women, lung cancer mortality rates have surpassed those for breast cancer and have continued to rise.[13] In pediatric tumors, this improving trend is even more evident (see Fig. 1–2). Neoplasms considered incurable decades ago, such as Wilms' tumor, Hodgkin's disease, acute lymphocytic leukemia, and neuroblastoma, now have become highly curable through multimodal therapy. The trend toward decreasing numbers of cancer deaths results from a variety of factors and should be viewed as evidence that we are achieving the goals of the national cancer program. However, there is a continued counterbalance in that there are increasing cancer deaths resulting from the overall aging of the population, improved diagnosis, more complete reporting, and greater incidence because of carcinogenic exposures.

Age and Sex

Cancer deaths for all adult age groups rank either first or second among the leading causes for mortality for either gender (see Fig. 1–3A). The cancer problem in children, however, is growing. Except for accidents, cancer has been the leading cause of death for children of both sexes aged 1 to 14 years and for young females aged 19 to 39.[10] From age 39, cancer vies with heart disease for the number one position. For females, cancer leads from ages 40 to 79, but drops to second place after age 79. In males, heart disease exceeds cancer for ages 40 to 80+, when mortality rates are highest. In males, lung cancer accounts for the highest mortality by far (156,900 deaths annually, estimated for 2000),[9] followed by digestive tract cancers (69,300 deaths annually) and prostate cancer (31,900 deaths annually) (Fig. 1–4). In females, the order is similar, with breast cancer being in third place—lung is highest (67,600 deaths annually), then digestive tract cancers (60,500 deaths annually), followed by breast (40,800 deaths annually) (Fig. 1–5). Colon cancer is the leading digestive tract cancer, with a combined mortality rate of 47,700 deaths annually for both sexes. The age-adjusted death rate shows a steady increase from ages 40 to 70 for both sexes; however, the good news is that the number of deaths from the majority of sites noted is in general decline. The one dissident note,

Prostate 29%
Lung & bronchus 14%
Colon & rectum 10%
Urinary bladder 6%
Non-Hodgkin's lymphoma 5%
Melanoma of skin 4%
Oral cavity & pharynx 3%
Kidney & renal pelvis 3%
Leukemia 3%
Pancreas 2%
All other sites 19%

30% Breast
12% Lung & bronchus
11% Colon & rectum
6% Uterine corpus
4% Ovary
4% Non-Hodgkin's lymphoma
3% Melanoma of skin
2% Urinary bladder
2% Pancreas
2% Thyroid
22% All other sites

A

† These two cancers both received a ranking of 10;
they have the same number of deaths and contribute the same percentage

B

Figure 1–3. (A) Estimated new cancer cases and (B) estimated cancer deaths, excluding basal and squamous cell skin cancers and *in situ* carcinomas except urinary bladder. Ten leading sites by sex, United States, 1999. (Modified from Landis SH, Murray T, Bolden S, et al: Cancer statistics, 1999. CA Cancer J Clin 1999; 49:8, with permission.)

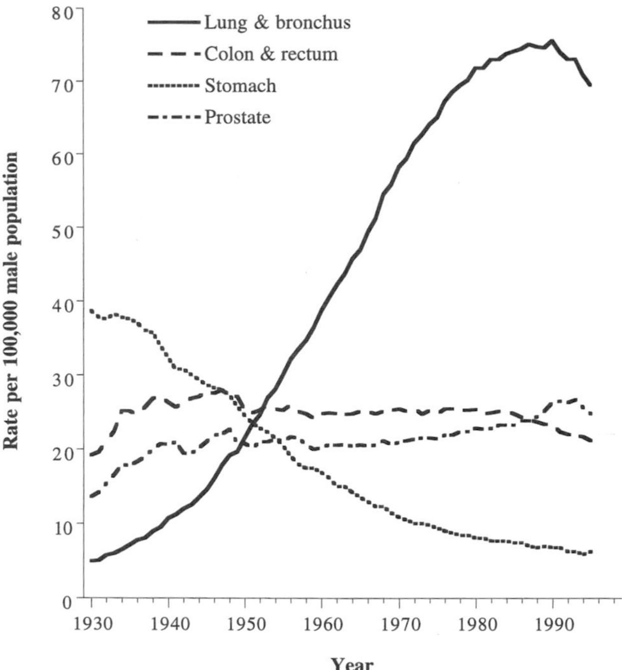

Figure 1–4. Age-adjusted cancer death rates[10] for the male population by site, United States, 1930–1995. Rates are per 100,000 population and are age-adjusted to the 1970 U.S. standard population. Data source is the National Center for Health Statistics.[20] (Modified from Landis SH, Murray T, Bolden S, et al: Cancer statistics, 1999. CA Cancer J Clin 1999; 49:8, with permission.)

observed earlier, is that as lung cancer death rates have decreased in males, they continue to increase in females. ACS and SEER data should be interpreted with caution when used for projecting trends because data are at least 4 years old when published, although by 2000, rates appeared to be undergoing change for the first time in the twentieth century.

Race and Ethnicity

There has been interest in the issues raised by cancer statistics reported by race and ethnicity, particularly the perception that black males were dying more frequently than white males. A SEER publication, entitled *Racial/Ethnic Patterns of Cancer in the United States 1988–1992,*[21] has been analyzed by Parker and associates,[22] and the following conclusions were made (Figs. 1–6 and 1–7):

- For men, cancer incidence rates were highest among blacks and whites, as compared with Asians, and lowest among American Indians and Hispanics from Mexico.
- Among men and women, blacks, Inuit, and whites experienced mortality rates that were at least 40% higher than Asians and other groups.
- Black men have the highest incidence rates of colon and rectum, lung and bronchus, and prostate cancer; they are 34% more likely to die of cancer than are whites and two times more likely than are Asians, Hispanics, or American Indians.
- Asian women had lowest rates of Papanicolaou (Pap) test screening, mammography, and clinical breast examination of any racial or ethnic group.
- Hispanic men and women are 2½ times less likely to have a health care plan, which may impact on screening frequency and adequacy of diagnostic treatment.
- For every racial and ethnic group, overall cancer incidence rates and mortality rates for women were lower than those for men.
- Recently reported Radiation Therapy Oncology Group studies, particularly in nonmetastatic prostate cancer, have shown higher prostate-specific antigen (PSA) serum differences in aggressiveness and advancement of stages in blacks than whites on presentation.[23] However, prostate cancer local control and survival with radiation therapy, as used in Radiation Therapy Oncology Group clinical trials, are comparable in both populations. Furthermore, comparisons between SEER and U.S. census data show that blacks are proportionately well represented in cancer clinical trials.[24]

Etiology

It is conceptually appealing to envision a network of coordinated gene expression where the target of various carcinogenic stimuli would be the cellular DNA encoding for the regulation of oncogene/suppressor gene products. Thus lesions, produced by radiation, viruses, or spontaneous random mutation, would activate or inactivate portions of this regulatory network, ultimately producing a malignancy.[25–28] Chromosomal and somatic changes appearing during cancer progression in the genome and in clinical cancer are diverse in nature, both genetic and epigenetic, as shown in Table 1–2.[29–41]

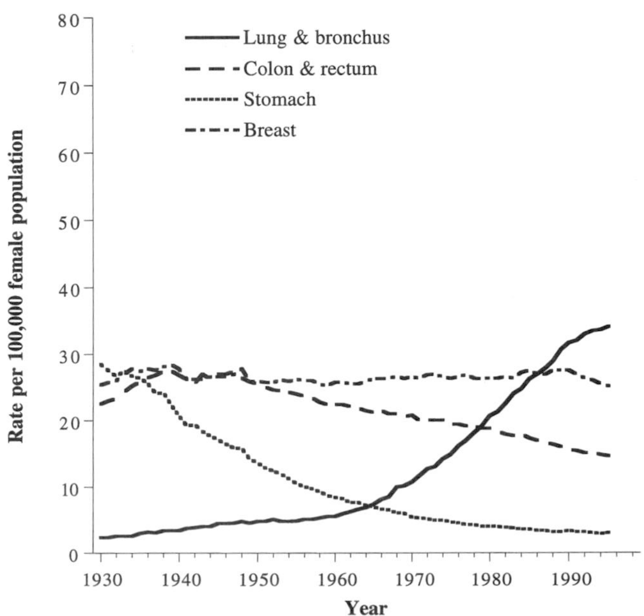

Figure 1–5. Age-adjusted cancer death rates for the female population by site, United States, 1930–1995. Rates are per 100,000 population and are age-adjusted to the U.S. standard population. Data source is the National Center for Health Statistics.[20] (Modified from Landis SH, Murray T, Bolden S, et al: Cancer statistics, 1999. CA Cancer J Clin 1999; 49:8, with permission.)

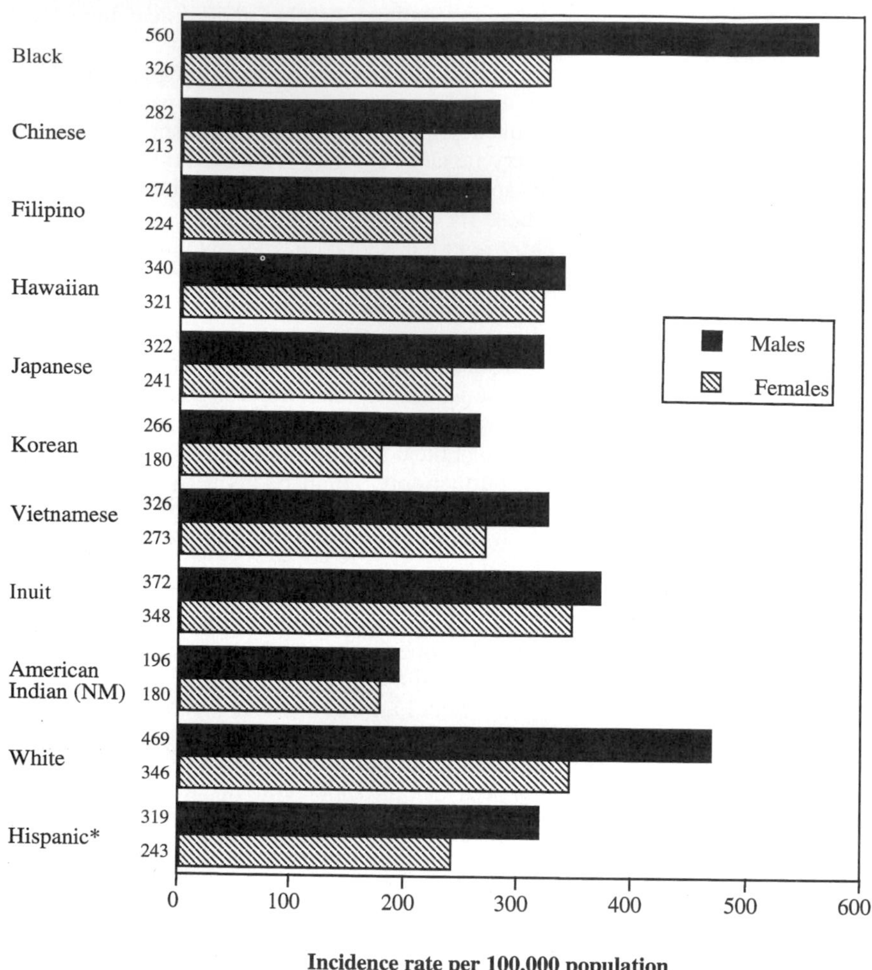

Figure 1–6. Cancer incidence rates for all sites combined by race, ethnicity, and sex, 1988–1992. *Persons of Hispanic origin may be of any race. Data source is Miller and colleagues.[21] (From Parker SL, Johnston Davis K, Wingo PA, et al: Cancer statistics by race and ethnicity. CA Cancer J Clin 1998; 48:31, with permission.)

TABLE 1–2. **Examples of Genetic and Epigenetic Changes in Carcinogenesis**

Heritable Alteration	Gene(s) Affected	Consequences	Cancer Type
Translocation[30]	*BCL* and *ABL*	Fusion protein is an activated oncogene	Chronic myelogenous leukemia
Homozygous deletion[31]	*NFI*	Deregulated $p21^{RAS}$	Neurofibrosarcoma, pheochromocytoma, astrocytoma
Frameshift mutation ± 1–5 bases[32, 33]	*APC*	Null tumor suppressor gene	Colorectal carcinoma
Gene amplification[34]	*EGFR*	Autocrine activation by receptor tyrosine kinase overexpression	Glioma
Single base substitution[35]	*TP53*	Loss of checkpoint control	Numerous
Simple repeat polymorphisms and hypermutability[36, 37]	*hMSH2* and *hMLH1*	Genetic instability	Colorectal carcinoma, Muir-Torre syndrome, small cell lung cancer
Minisatellite polymorphisms[38]	*HRAS*	Cancer predisposition	Numerous
Telomere reduction[39]	Numerous	Chromosomal deletions and/or loss	Colorectal carcinoma
Loss of genetic imprinting (parental allele-specific expression)[40]	*IGF2* and *H19*	Gene dosage effects	Beckwith-Wiedemann syndrome and Wilms' renal tumor
Loss/gain of methylation[41]	Numerous	Altered gene expression, chromatin structure, replication timing(?)	Colorectal carcinoma

From Weinstein IB, Carothers AM, Santella RM, et al: Molecular mechanisms of mutagenesis and multistage carcinogenesis. In: Mendelsohn J, Howley PM, Israel MA, et al (eds): The Molecular Basis of Cancer, p 59. Philadelphia, W.B. Saunders Co., 1995, with permission.

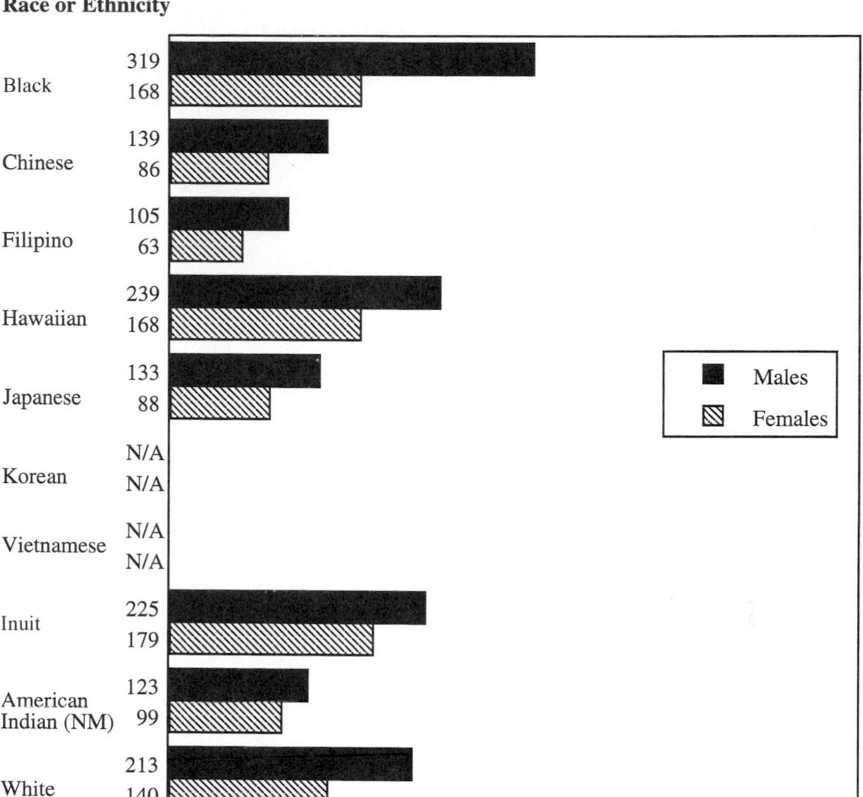

Figure 1–7. Cancer mortality rates for all sites combined by race, ethnicity, and sex, 1988–1992. *Persons of Hispanic origin may be of any race. Data source is Miller and colleagues. (From Parker SL, Johnston Davis K, Wingo PA, et al: Cancer statistics by race and ethnicity. CA Cancer J Clin 1998; 48:31, with permission.)

Thus, *carcinogenesis is a multistage process*[42, 43] in which normal cells are initiated and then promoted into cancer by creating a clonogenic population of transformed neoplastic cells. In current molecular oncologic thinking, intrinsic cellular oncogenes, growth suppressor genes and the dysregulation of steps that control cell cycle, cell proliferation, and differentiation through gene expression play interactive roles that transform normal cells into a premalignant state and, ultimately, into frank malignancy. One of the best studied models for analysis of genetic events is the pathogenesis of colon cancer, in which colonic epithelium changes to a hyperproliferative phase, adenomas form, and, with further growth, progression into overt colorectal cancer is evident (Fig. 1–8). At the end of the aforementioned phases of evolution, specific genetic changes are associated with particular neoplastic phenotypes undergoing malignant metamorphosis.

- Mutation of *APC* (adenomatosis polyposis coli) suppressor gene leads to hyperproliferation.
- Mutations of the *KRAS* gene allow adenomas to progress into carcinomatous foci.
- Mutations in the *DCC* (deleted in colon cancer) gene and *TP53*, the tumor suppressor gene, finally result in frank colorectal cancer.[44]
- More mutations result in changes leading to metastases (see Fig. 1–8).

Evidence from epidemiologic studies suggests that the major percentage of human cancers (50% to 80%) is caused by environmental conditions[45–47] based on time trends in cancer incidence and mortality, geographic variations and migration effects, identification of specific lifestyle features, dietary factors and occupational/environmental chemicals. Although intrinsic genetic factors are important in determining individual susceptibility, the fact is that the majority of human cancers do not follow or show simple patterns of inheritance. This is an optimistic message because it means that the development of several cancers is not an inherent consequence of the aging process per se and a high incidence of cancer is not an inevitable condition of being human.[29] In principle, this means the vast majority of cancers are preventable if the external causative factors can be identified. Therefore, basic research into cancer causation will be a powerful determinant of interventions in the transformation process, reinforcing the need for developing effective molecular tumor biomarkers for early detection of malignant evolution in tissues or organs.

A concise discussion of known external cancer causation factors follows and includes (1) chemical (environmental)

Normal cell

↓ An abnormality develops in the *APC* tumor suppressor gene

Increased cell growth

↓ DNA loses methyl groups

Development of adenoma I

↓ Mutation in the *KRAS* oncogene

Progression to adenoma II

↓ *DCC* tumor suppressor gene loss from chromosome 18

Progression of adenoma III

↓ *TP53* tumor suppressor gene loss from chromosome 17

Development of carcinoma

↓ Other chromosomal losses

Metastatic spread of the carcinoma

Figure 1–8. A proposed model for the genetic basis of oncogenesis in colon cancer. Cancer is thought to be a series of genetic abnormalities that accumulate within a cell. The study of colon cancers has suggested a model for the sequence of genetic defects and their associated histologic and clinical changes. (From Culver KW: Gene Therapy. A Primer for Physicians, 2nd ed. Larchmont, Mary Ann Liebert Inc, 1996, with permission.)

and industrial carcinogens, (2) medical drug–induced cancers, (3) radiation carcinogenesis, and (4) viral mechanisms and lifestyle.

Environmental and Industrial Chemical Carcinogens

Substantial lists of environmental and occupational agents have been identified by the International Agency for Research on Cancer, the National Institute for Occupational Safety and Health, the U.S. Environmental Protection Agency, and the U.S. National Toxicology Program. Table 1–3, adapted from International Agency for Research on Cancer recommendations,[48–50] reviews some of the agents and factors relating to specific cancers. At present, known carcinogenic chemical agents appear to play a decreasing role in the United States and other developed countries as their risk is identified and exposure is reduced.[48] For instance, the polycyclic aromatic hydrocarbons have been studied intensively in animals as inducers of neoplasia; they also have been documented as a factor in skin cancers among petroleum product industrial workers.[51, 52] Ethylene oxide, a widely used agent for sterilization of animal cages, has shown to be associated with leukemia.[53] Haloethers—especially chlorinated ethers and bis (chloromethyl) ether in particular—are highly carcinogenic and have been found to cause lung cancers.[54] Similarly, exposures to arsenic and asbestos, agents known to cause lung cancer and mesotheliomas, respectively,[55, 56] have been reduced as a result of awareness and removal of these products from the workplace. Bladder cancers, caused by dyes used by hairdressers and in the rubber industry (e.g., 2-naphthylamine, benzidene, and 4-aminopiprenyl), have decreased due to proper handling of these agents.[57] With the increasing concern over environmental factors, urban air pollution, water contaminants, food processing (including use of nitrites and nitrosamines for meat-curing processes) and saccharin all are being carefully watched as potential carcinogenic factors.

Medical Drug–Induced Cancers

Medical drug–induced cancers (Table 1–4) are of particular concern to the oncologist because the induction of a treatment-related second neoplasm after curing the first is very frustrating. The use of some systemic agents for secondary or nonrelated conditions has been shown to have carcinogenic properties. For instance, hormonal agents such as estrogen-containing compounds (e.g., the "pill" in younger women) have been implicated in vaginal adenocarcinomas, endometrial cancer, and questionably in breast and ovarian

TABLE 1–3. **Occupational Agents Generally Recognized as Carcinogenic to Humans**

Substance or Process	Site of Cancer
Acrylonite	Lung
4-Aminobiphenyl	Urinary bladder
Arsenic and certain arsenic compounds	Lung, skin
Asbestos	Pleura, peritoneum (lungs when combined with cigarette smoking)
Benzene	Lymphoid tissue
Benzidene	Urinary bladder
Beryllium and beryllium compounds	Lung
Bis (chloromethyl) ether and chloromethyl ether	Lung, respiratory tract
Boot and shoe manufacture and repair	Nasal cavity
1,3-Butadiene	Hematopoietic system
Cadmium and cadmium compounds	Lung
Chromium and certain chromium compounds	Lung
Coal tars and pitches	Skin
Coke production	Lung
Ethylene oxide	Hematopoietic system
Formaldehyde	Nose and nasopharynx
Hairdressing (occupational)	Uninary bladder
Mineral oils, treated and mildly treated	Skin
Mustard gas	Pharynx, lung
2-Naphthylamine	Urinary bladder
Nickel and nickel compounds	Lungs, nose, and nasal sinus
Nonarsenical pesticides, spraying	Lung
Petroleum refining (occupational)	Skin, hematopoietic system
Polychlorinated biphenyls	Liver, skin
Radon	Lung
Shale oils	Skin
Silica	Lung
Soots	Skin
Sulfuric acid, mist	Nasal cavity, larynx, lung
Talc containing asbestiform fibers	Lung
Vinyl chloride	Liver mesenchyma
Wood dust	Nasal cavity

Data from Trichopoulos,[48] IARC,[49] and Miller and Miller.[50]

Modified from Trichopoulos D, Lipworth L, Petridou E, et al: Epidemiology of cancer. In: DeVita VT Jr, Hellman S, Rosenberg SA (eds): Cancer: Principles & Practice of Oncology, 5th ed, p 231. Philadelphia, Lippincott-Raven Publishers, 1997, with permission.

TABLE 1–4. **Medical Agents Recognized as Carcinogenic to Humans**

Agent	Site of Cancer
Immunosuppressive drugs (e.g. azathioprine)	Reticuloendothelial system
Exogenous hormones	
Menopausal estrogens	Endometrium, breast
Transplacental (diethylstilbestrol)	Vagina, cervix uteri
Anabolic steroids	Liver
Oral contraceptives	Liver
Tamoxifen	Endometrium
Phenacetin analgesics	Kidney, pelvis
Inorganic arsenic compounds	Skin
Cancer chemotherapeutic agents	
Melphalan	Lymphoid tissue
Cyclophosphamide	Urinary bladder
MOPP	Bone marrow
Busulphan	Bone marrow

MOPP = mechlorethamine, Oncovin (vincristine), procarbazine, and prednisone.

Data from Trichopoulos,[48] and IARC.[58, 59]

Modified from Trichopoulos D, Lipworth L, Petridou E, et al: Epidemiology of cancer. In: DeVita VT Jr, Hellman S, Rosenberg SA (eds): Cancer: Principles & Practice of Oncology, 5th ed, p 231. Philadelphia, Lippincott-Raven Publishers, 1997, with permission.

cancers.[60, 61] Immunosuppressive agents, such as azathioprine and cyclosporine, have an association with lymphomas, skin cancer, and soft tissue sarcomas.[62, 63] With respect to cancer treatment, the use of alkylating agents such as melphalan and cyclophosphamide has been known to induce leukemias and bladder cancers.[64–66] Increasingly, the clinician needs to assess the benefits and risks of prolonged drug administration with both the patient and the patient's family. For example, the MOPP (*m*echlorethamine, *O*ncovin [vincristine], *p*rocarbazine, and *p*rednisone) chemotherapy program in Hodgkin's disease remains among the most curative treatments available. MOPP, however, is associated with second malignancies, particularly when combined with radiation therapy.[64] Similar multiagent chemotherapies, with or without radiation, used in treating a variety of cancers, have resulted in secondary leukemias.[67, 68]

Radiation Carcinogenesis

The concern about radiation exposure is high because of its known carcinogenic action; however, a small fraction—less than 1%—of all cancers are attributable to this cause. Nonetheless, this small incidence has led to ongoing efforts to minimize population exposure.[28] Radiation is known to be carcinogenic to a variety of organs and tissues.[69, 70] Breast, thyroid, bone marrow, and bone tissue appear vulnerable, whereas kidney, bladder, and ovary are more resistant to radiation carcinogenesis. Leukemia is the most radiogenic tumor; the highest incidence occurs 2 to 4 years following exposure and decreases over a period of 25 years. Interestingly, chronic lymphocytic leukemias are rare after irradiation.

Quantitation of radiation-induced cancer is difficult to accurately assess. Current thinking estimates that carcinogenesis from irradiation by x-rays is approximately linear with dose at low radiation exposures (Fig. 1–9) and reported estimates are 10^{-2} cancers/Sv (sievert) at 20 years. Clinically, however, this model does not accurately predict oncogenesis after therapeutic irradiation.[71] For instance, long-term follow-up studies of cervix cancers after high-dose radiation have not yielded a high incidence of pelvic malignancies, whereas modest sterilizing doses of radiation to the ovary seem to be related to an increase in expected cases of pelvic cancers.

Viral and Immunologic Mechanisms

Many viruses, such as adenoviruses, are capable of transforming normal cells to malignant cells in the laboratory (Table 1–5), but to date the majority of viruses have not been found to be associated with human tumors. In fact, the initial speculation following intensive studies in avian and murine malignancies indicating that a viral etiology could have a parallel in humans has not been realized. Nonetheless, considerable data and knowledge about DNA and RNA viruses have resulted, and at least 15% of human malignancies caused by an infection with human tumor viruses have been identified.[25, 73, 74] For instance, the human retrovirus HTLV-I (human T-cell leukemia virus type I) has been convincingly linked to the pathogenesis of adult T-cell leukemias and lymphomas.[75, 76]

The Epstein-Barr virus (EBV)[77, 78] and hepatitis B and C viruses[79, 80] are agents that chronically infect humans and are associated with neoplasms. Burkitt's discovery[81] of an African lymphoma based on its geographic distribution led to identification of a transmissible agent, that is, EBV, and the association between nasopharyngeal cancers and EBV has been studied extensively.[82, 83] EBV has been clearly

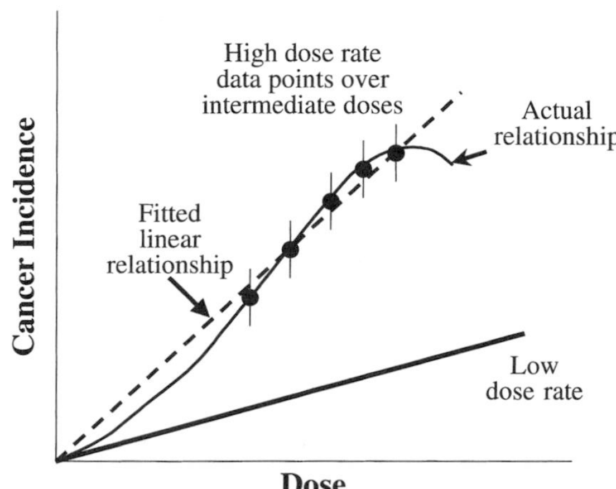

Figure 1–9. The data points for excess solid cancers in a human population exposed to an acute dose of high dose rate linear energy transfer (LET) radiation are frequently fitted by a linear dose function. However, these data are usually poor and cover a limited dose range. The actual dose relationship is, in all probability, more complex; excess cancer incidence rises as a linear-quadratic function of dose but bends over at higher doses as cell killing becomes more important. For low dose rate exposures, excess cancer incidence approximates a linear function of dose, which is a continuation of the linear low-dose component of the high dose rate relationship. (From Hall EJ: Etiology of cancer: Physical factors. In: DeVita VT Jr, Hellman S, Rosenberg SA [eds]: Cancer: Principles & Practice of Oncology, 5th ed, p 203. Philadelphia, Lippincott-Raven Publishers, 1997, with permission.)

TABLE 1–5. **Viral and Immunologic Agents Judged as Involved in Human Carcinogenesis**

Agent	Site of Cancer
Aflatoxin-producing fungal strains	Liver (hepatocellular)
Hepatitis B (HBV) virus	Liver (hepatocellular)
Hepatitis C (HCV) virus	Liver (hepatocellular)
Helicobacter pylori	Stomach, gastric lymphoma
Schistosoma haematobium	Urinary bladder
Opisthorchis viverrini	Liver
HTLV-I	Adult T-cell leukemia or lymphoma
HPV-16, -18, -33, -39	Uterine cervix, anogenital cancer, some upper airway cancers
HPV-5, -8, -17	Skin
Epstein-Barr virus (EBV)	Burkitt's lymphoma, nasopharynx, Hodgkin's disease
HHV-8	Body cavity lymphomas, Kaposi's sarcoma
SV40	Mesothelioma

HTLV-I = human T-cell leukemia virus type I; HPV = human papillomavirus; HHV = human herpesvirus; SV = simian virus.

Data from Trichopoulos,[48] and Howley.[72]

Modified from Trichopoulos D, Lipworth L, Petridou E, et al: Epidemiology of cancer. In: DeVita VT Jr, Hellman S, Rosenberg SA (eds): Cancer: Principles & Practice of Oncology, 5th ed, p 231. Philadelphia, Lippincott-Raven Publishers, 1997, with permission.

linked to the pathogenesis of lymphomas, especially those of the central nervous system, in the setting of immunosuppression seen in acquired immunodeficiency syndrome (AIDS) patients or patients undergoing organ transplantation.[84, 85] The association between primary hepatocarcinogenesis and hepatitis B viral infection, a common worldwide malignancy, has similarly undergone intensive study.[86, 87] Recently, other herpesviruses, for example, human herpesvirus–8 (HHV-8), have been linked to the pathogenesis of unusual body cavity lymphomas and Kaposi's sarcoma in patients with human immunodeficiency virus–1 infection.[88]

Perhaps one of the most important human viral carcinogen groups is the human papillomavirus group, numbering about 77 types.[89, 90] Cervical cancer is most common in young multiparous women with many, and uncircumcised, partners, and human papillomavirus types are the most common viral infections associated with its oncogenesis.[91, 92] It is believed that the proteins E6 and E7, encoded by these viruses, interfere with *TP53* activity and prevent apoptosis, therefore promoting proliferation of genetically abnormal cells.[93] In addition, a strong association has been observed between simian virus 40 (SV40) and malignant mesothelioma, similarly thought to be due to interactions between the SV40 antigen and the retinoblastoma and *TP53* tumor suppressor genes.[94] In this case, an interesting interaction between environmental (e.g., asbestos) and viral (SV40) factors has been postulated.[95]

Lifestyle

Tobacco and alcohol consumption (Table 1–6) are high on the list for causing lung cancer and upper aerodigestive tract malignancies.[97–100] Cigarette smoking has come under continual attack since it was implicated as a major causal factor in lung cancer, and use of tobacco has been associated with oral cavity, oropharyngeal and laryngeal cancers, esophageal cancers, and bladder cancer. In addition, betel nut and tobacco quid chewers are at risk for buccal cavity cancers.[99] Recently implicated is environmental secondhand smoking, leading to public policy changes that have resulted in smoke-free environments at hospitals, offices, airplanes, and restaurants. Diet is under investigation, with evidence that vegetables and fruits prevent cancer at several sites, whereas red meat and saturated fat perhaps increase the risk for large bowel cancer and prostate cancer.[101–103]

Detection and Diagnosis

Molecular Tumor Biomarkers

With new molecular biology technologies and tools, the concept of early detection of cancer is undergoing dramatic transformation. Early clinical detection of asymptomatic cancer, stage T1,N0 or stage I, without evidence of nodal or hematogenous spread, is increasingly common. The ACS has recommended that screening tests for early detection of cancer in asymptomatic individuals include a variety of standard diagnostic procedures such as chest radiographs, sigmoidoscopy, digital rectal examination, pelvic and breast examination in women, as well as Pap test and mammography, as indicated in Table 1–7. These tests are performed on a regular basis and are age adjusted. Currently, with molecular oncology concepts, the search is to identify the cancer in its *in situ* or preinvasive stage (T0,N0), when no lymphatic or vascular seeding has occurred. At this stage, conservation surgery, usually an excisional biopsy with or without adjuvant radiation or chemotherapy, provides the best preservation of organ or structure and most optimal circumstance for long-term survival.

The most vivid illustration of an excellent serum tumor antigen or biomarker is PSA. The impact of this test has been profound in early disease detection, quantitative determination of disease response, and documentation of subclinical disease. Use of PSA levels has even changed our understanding of the incidence of prostate cancer. The most

TABLE 1–6. **Lifestyle Factors Judged as Affecting Human Carcinogenesis**

Factor	Site of Cancer
Tobacco smoking	Lung, bladder, esophagus, mouth, larynx, liver, others
Tobacco products, smokeless	Oral cavity
Environmental tobacco smoke	Lung
Betel quid with tobacco (chewing)	Oral cavity, buccal mucosa
Alcoholic beverages	Esophagus, oral, pharynx, larynx, liver
Ultraviolet radiation (sunlight)	Melanoma and nonmelanocytic skin cancer

Data from Trichopoulos[48] and Ames and Gold.[96]

Modified from Trichopoulos D, Lipworth L, Petridou E, et al: Epidemiology of cancer. In: DeVita VT Jr, Hellman S, Rosenberg SA (eds): Cancer: Principles & Practice of Oncology, 5th ed, p 231. Philadelphia, Lippincott-Raven Publishers, 1997, with permission.

TABLE 1–7. **Protocol for Early Detection of Cancer in Asymptomatic Persons**

	Recommendations		
	Population		
	Sex	*Age/Risk*	**Frequency**
Chest x-ray		Not recommended	
Sputum cytology		Not recommended	
Sigmoidoscopy	M & F	Over 50	Every 3–5 years
Stool blood test	M & F	Over 50	Every year
Digital rectal exam	M & F*	Over 40	Every year
Papanicolaou and pelvic exam	F	Women who are sexually active, or are 18 or older	Every year; after 3+ normal consecutive exams, frequency may be reduced
Endometrial tissue sample	F	At menopause; women at high risk†	At menopause
Breast self-exam	F	Age 20 and older	Every month
Breast clinical exam	F	20–39	Every 2–3 years
		Age 40 and older	Every year
Mammography	F	35–39	Baseline
		40–49	Every 1 to 2 years
		Age 50 and older	Every year
Health counseling and cancer check-up‡	M & F	20–40	Every 3 years
		Age 40 and older	Every year

*In men, this should include palpation of the prostate.
†History of infertility, obesity, failure to ovulate, abnormal uterine bleeding, or estrogen therapy.
‡To include examination for cancer of the thyroid, testicles, prostate, ovaries, lymph nodes, oral region, and skin.

dramatic changes have occurred in analysis of prostate cancer incidence, which appeared to show a striking increase (85%) between 1987 and 1992, reflecting the use of PSA as a screening test, followed by a decline between 1992 and 1995. Many newly screened cases added to the rise, but values are expected to decline further as early treatment improves.[10] Cancer of the prostate is the second commonest cancer by organ site, exceeded only by breast cancer.[9] PSA has revolutionized the staging of cancer as well as the evaluation of response to treatment by either surgery or radiation, and it allows for early recognition of subclinical recurrence or microscopic metastases with the ability to introduce salvage therapy.

A wide variety of tumor-associated antigens are being pursued through the development of targeted monoclonal antibodies against the antigens, which fall into several classes (Table 1–8).[104]

- Oncofetal proteins are seen during an indeterminate period of normal embryonic or fetal life. However, they do not entirely disappear in the adult and may reappear in association with certain malignancies, for example, carcinoembryonic antigen,[105] alpha-fetoprotein,[106] and tumor-associated glycoprotein 72.[107] Antibodies against these have been widely used to identify advanced stages of gastrointestinal and other carcinomas and to predict outcomes.[108, 109]
- CALLA,[110] the *c*ommon *a*cute *l*ymphoblastic *l*eukemia *a*ntigen, represents another class of tumor-associated antigens that are expressed on cells at a given state of differentiation; another example is the CD20 antigen, which is widely expressed on B-cells and B-cell–derived lymphomas.[111]
- The expansion in our understanding of the role played by growth factor receptors in tumorigenesis has led to the development of monoclonal antibodies directed against, for example, receptors for transferrin,[112] epidermal growth factor,[113] and several B-cell and T-cell growth factors such as interleukin 2.[114]
- Similarly, monoclonal antibodies against cell surface oncogene products, such as HER2-NEU (or *ERBB2* gene), have been shown not only to have some prognostic value in breast cancer but also to have an effect on tumor cell proliferation.[115, 116] Antibodies against HER2-NEU and the epidermal growth factor receptor may have direct antitumor effects *in vivo*, as well as synergistic effects when used in combination with chemotherapy.[117]
- Specific and unique antigenic determinants of malignant T-cells and B-cells (the idiotype) provide a highly tumor specific marker. Certain anti-idiotypic antibodies against the lymphoma idiotype have been used for diagnostic or therapeutic purposes, or for both.[118, 119]
- Clusters of differentiation (CD) markers to describe surface components on leukocytes and lymphocytes have been avidly investigated. Analysis of at least 1500 antibodies by multiple laboratories has yielded more than 150 new CD clusters and subclusters in addition to the 14 previously established CDs, as defined in an international workshop (Fifth International Workshop on Human Leukocyte Differentiation Antigens, November 1993). Many of these markers have now been cloned and are being molecularly characterized.
- Cytokines are another class of soluble proteins commonly produced by mononuclear cells of the immune system that have regulatory actions on immune cells and on their target cells in immune reactions. Cytokines have been demonstrated to have both powerful beneficial and deleterious effects, particularly when these are produced by tumors.[120]

TABLE 1–8. **Monoclonal Antibody–Defined Tumor-Associated Antigens Utilized as Markers or Targets in Clinical Trials**

Tumor Type	Tumor-Associated Antigen	Clinical Application
Pancarcinoma	TAG-72	Immunoscintigraphy
	HMW glycoprotein, Le^y	Passive immunotherapy
Gastrointestinal tract	38-kD glycoprotein	Passive immunotherapy, active specific immunotherapy
	Gp72	Active specific immunotherapy
	HMW glycoprotein	Immunoscintigraphy
	Carcinoembryonic antigen	Immunoscintigraphy
Lung	Epidermal growth factor receptor	Immunoscintigraphy
Ovary	38–40-kD glycoprotein	Immunoscintigraphy, passive immunotherapy
	CA125	Immunodiagnosis
Prostate	PSA	Immunodiagnosis
Melanoma	Gp100	Immunodiagnosis
	p97, HMW-MAA	Immunoscintigraphy, passive immunotherapy, active specific immunotherapy
	GD_3 ganglioside	Passive immunotherapy, active specific immunotherapy
	GD_2 ganglioside	Passive immunotherapy

TAG = Tumor-associated glycoprotein; HMW = high-molecular-weight; Gp = glycoprotein; CA = carcinoma antigen; PSA = prostate-specific antigen; MAA = melanoma-associated antigen.

From Ferrone S, Chu T, Hellstrom KE: Tumor antigens recognized by monoclonal antibodies. In: DeVita VT Jr, Hellman S, Rosenberg SA (eds): Biologic Therapy of Cancer, 2nd ed, p 77. Philadelphia, Lippincott-Raven Publishers, 1995, with permission.

In summary, molecular tumor biomarkers are still in their early phases of development and investigative clinical trials. In addition, as yet no simple test is available with sufficient sensitivity and specificity to detect the presence of a cancer before metastasis.[121] Most current tumor markers are in the class of immunologic products; however, to date, serum tumor markers have proved more useful for monitoring patient response and detecting recurrence than as a definitive diagnostic tool in screening for early cancer.[109]

Typical Clinical Presentations

Changes in normal physiologic functions that persist—alterations in eating habits, loss of appetite, difficulty in swallowing, increased constipation or diarrhea, or both—require study. Typical presentations that demand examination and explanation (Table 1–9) are a lump or nodule in any site, particularly if it is painless and increasing in size; the appearance of bleeding from orifices; unexplained recurrent pain; unexplained recurrent fevers; steady weight loss; and repeated infections that may or may not clear with antibiotics. These early signs of cancer have been stressed for different sites and in popular programs for the public, but the fear of the diagnosis of cancer can be an element that delays the patient from seeking medical advice. Each physician must learn to screen patients, particularly those older than 40 years of age, for localized lesions in the skin, uterus, mouth, breast, lungs, rectum, prostate, and thyroid. The best available screening methods, such as mammography, PSA, and rectal examination, should be diligently and conscientiously applied. Only through constant awareness will the asymptomatic patient's occult, localized cancer be found at a stage in which therapy can most often prove successful.

TABLE 1–9. **Cancer's Seven Warning Signs**

Change in bowel or bladder habits
A sore that does not heal
Unusual bleeding or discharge
Thickening of lump in breast or elsewhere
Indigestion or difficulty in swallowing
Obvious change in wart or mole
Nagging cough or hoarseness

Early Clinical Detection

Early clinical detection means the cancer is localized and has not developed regional extensions or distant spread to nodes and viscera. It is essential to listen carefully for new complaints, some of which the patient may think are unimportant. A complete physical examination for high-risk organ systems and key anatomic sites for cancer development can, in most instances, be performed in a short period. If one adds the simple and inexpensive tests recommended, such as the Pap smear, Hemoccult slides, urinalysis, and blood count, most malignancies detectable by early diagnosis will be evident (see Table 1–7). A well-directed history, a well-planned physical examination, and some readily available office procedures will identify early most cancers for which people are at risk.

Screening Procedures

For early detection, it is important to focus on the occult phase, when the lesion is asymptomatic. At some sites, effective screening is possible, such as cytology for cervix cancer; however, this cytologic screening does not apply as readily in many other sites, such as lung, prostate, or bladder. Screening procedures, such as gastric camera and fiberoptic endoscopy, are highly effective for early detection of stomach cancer; however, they are too costly to use in other than specific high-risk groups. Lack of methods and the inaccessibility of some sites often make early recognition impossible. There are two points to remember: first, it is hoped that early clinical detection means the cancer is localized; second, localized small cancers (≤ 2 cm) are often highly curable by current treatment methods.

The literature that attempts to define the role of mammography as a screen for breast cancer[122, 123] best emphasizes the controversy and cost/benefits of screening procedures.

The ACS protocols for early detection of cancer in asymptomatic individuals include a variety of standard diagnostic procedures, such as chest radiographs, sigmoidoscopy, digital rectal examination, pelvic and breast examinations in women along with Pap screening and mammography, as described in Table 1–7, and are usually performed on an annual basis. A brief review of the common cancer screening procedures follows and will be amplified in chapters dealing with specific sites.

Lung Cancer. The results of a Mayo Clinic project[124] in which chest films and sputum cytology were performed every 4 months in chronic smokers and compared with a cohort of randomly assigned patients did not show a decrease in mortality as compared with unscreened controls. Some benefits were seen for squamous cell cancer and adenocarcinomas, but not small or large cell cancers. However, the two curves spread apart at 4 years, with screened patients surviving at a higher rate. This was not statistically significant, and therefore diagnostic films should only be taken on patients with symptoms.

Uterine Cancer. Identification of high-risk groups for cytologic studies is possible. Cancer of the cervix occurs more frequently in those who start intercourse in their teens, have multiple sex partners, and have many children. In contrast, cancer of the endometrium is a disease of suburbia and occurs in obese, diabetic, infertile women, who often have irregular menses resulting from failure in ovulation. Exfoliative cytology is a highly sensitive and inexpensive screening technique for cervical cancer and its precursors, and it has led to a significant fall in cancer incidence and death in areas where this was a common disease. Annual Pap smears are still advised for high-risk, sexually active women. However, for other women, after three negative annual Pap smears, the frequency may be reduced at the physician's discretion. For endometrial cancer detection, aspiration curettage taken from the endometrial cavity is advised for those at risk as a quick, relatively painless outpatient method not requiring anesthesia.

Breast Cancer. The value of self-examination and mammography has been established in patients who are at high risk for breast cancer: personal history (5× increased risk), family history (3×), multiparity or first birth after 35 years of age (3×), fibrocystic disease (1.5 to 3.8×). For women at high risk, baseline mammograms are advised between the ages of 35 and 40 years and then annually after 40. There is controversy regarding appropriate utilization of mammography in women with standard risk. Most of the data support a baseline study at 35 and annual studies after 50. Special screening procedures may be indicated in patients with known genetic lesions that predispose them to breast or ovarian cancer, or both (e.g., *BRCA1, BRCA2*).

Colorectal Cancer. Fecal occult blood testing with flexible sigmoidoscopy or a total colon examination is advised annually in those individuals who are 50 years of age and older.[125] Colonoscopy and barium enema are reserved for symptomatic patients or to clarify positive tests for occult blood in the stool. Individuals with a family history of colorectal cancers or with other risk factors (familial adenomatous polyposis, inflammatory bowel disease) are especially urged to comply with screening recommendations. Genetic testing is available for some known genes involved in familial colon carcinogenesis (e.g., *APC, HNPCC*).

Head and Neck Cancers. Too often, examinations for rectal and pelvic cancers are performed with alacrity, but careful inspection and palpation of the oral cavity, oropharynx, hypopharynx, and larynx are frequently ignored. Any sore or lump, hoarseness, or dysphagia should be carefully evaluated because secondary malignant tumors in the aerodigestive tract are common in patients with previously successfully treated tumors in this region.[126] The cumulative incidence can be as high as 25% to 35%. Learning how to visualize the larynx and pharynx is a simple, underused examination.

Molecular Pathology of Cancer

Once cancer is suspected, a careful work-up is essential and proper consultation is necessary. Questionable findings require periodic follow-up or surgical intervention to establish or exclude the diagnosis. Most importantly, clinical leads should be pursued and investigative studies should not be unduly procrastinated. *Surgical biopsy or excision is the single most important procedure in establishing a firm diagnosis*[127] because neoplasms can masquerade as benign or inflammatory conditions. Whenever possible, a histologic diagnosis is essential before undertaking radical treatment. Oncologic imaging can precede or follow the surgical biopsy, depending on clinical circumstances and is described further in Chapter 15, Principles of Oncologic Imaging and Tumor Imaging Strategies. Once the pathologic diagnosis is made, certain additional tests are advised to determine the anatomic extent or stage of the advancement.

Examination of cells and tissue specimens has been amplified and extended to establish the diagnosis of malignancy by the new molecular biology methodology available. Only a brief overview is provided here; this is more comprehensively presented in Chapter 3, The Pathology of Cancer.

Immunohistochemistry

The expanding role of immunohistochemistry in diagnostic pathology has been greatly abetted by the increasing number of commercially available antibodies directed against tumor antigenic determinants for differential diagnostic purposes. Correct interpretation can contribute to distinguishing benign from malignant disease, but in general has been applied more to the classification of malignancy than to primary diagnosis. Immunohistochemistry can aid in identifying metastatic cells at distant sites by dissecting multiple cell populations from nonhomogeneous tumoral tissues.

Diagnostic Molecular Markers: Chromosomal Rearrangements

A large and important class of molecular markers for cancer diagnosis are chromosomal rearrangements[128] re-

TABLE 1–10. **Characteristic Karyotypic Abnormalities in Solid Tumors**

Tumor Type	Type of Rearrangement
Epithelial Tumors	
Pleomorphic adenoma	Translocation of 12q13–15, t(3;8) (p21;q12)
Lung carcinoma	del(3) (p14–23)
Kidney carcinoma	del(3) (p14–23), t(3;5) (p13;q22)
Bladder carcinoma	i(5p), trisomy 7, monosomy 9
Wilms' tumor	del(11) (p13)
Ovarian carcinoma	add (19) (p13)
Prostate carcinoma	del(7) (q22), del(10) (q24)
Mesenchymal Tumors	
Lipoma	Translocations of 12q13–15, ring chromosomes
Leiomyoma	Structural changes of 12q13–15, del(7) (q21q31), trisomy 12
Liposarcoma (myxoid)	t(12;16) (q13.3;p11.2)
Synovial sarcoma	t(X;18) (p11;q11)
Rhabdomyosarcoma	t(2;13) (q35–37;q14)
Malignant fibrous histiocytoma	add (19) (p13)
Neurogenic, Neuroectodermal, and Germ Cell Tumors	
Meningioma	Monosomy 22, del(22) (q12–13)
Astrocytoma	del(9) (p13–24), dmin
Neuroblastoma	del(1) (32–26), hsr/dmin
Retinoblastoma	del(13) (q14), i(6) (p10)
Malignant melanoma	Deletions of 6q, i(6) (p10)
Ewing's sarcoma, Askin tumor, peripheral neuroepithelioma	t(11;22) (q24;q12)
Germ cell tumors	i(12) (p10)

From Le Beau MM: Molecular biology of cancer. In: DeVita VT Jr, Hellman S, Rosenberg SA (eds): Cancer: Principles & Practice of Oncology, 5th ed, p 103. Philadelphia, Lippincott-Raven Publishers, 1997, with permission. Modified from Rowley JD, Mitelman F: Principles of molecular cell biology of cancer: chromosome abnormalities in human cancer and leukemia. In: DeVita VT Jr, Hellman S, Rosenberg SA (eds): Cancer: Principles & Practice of Oncology, 4th ed. Philadelphia, J.B. Lippincott, 1993.

sulting in karyotypic abnormalities that are characteristic for specific tumors (Table 1–10).[129, 130] Using fluorescence *in situ* hybridization, analysis of chromosomal abnormalities and karyotypes can yield portraits of cytogenetic aberrations and provide specific *in loci* genomes. The following rearrangements correspond to chromosomal abnormalities detected by cytogenetic analysis:

- duplications: additions of chromosomes
- deletions: loss of whole or part of chromosomes
- segmental amplifications: segments randomly reiterated or extra fragments
- translocations: exchange between chromosomes
- inversions: orientations are reversed

Diagnostic Molecular Genetics

This form of molecular genetic testing involves the analysis of nucleotide sequences within nucleic acid to detect the presence of malignant cells in fluids and tissues. DNA is, in general, stable in tissues and cells after removal, in contrast to RNA, which is unstable and highly degradable by endogenous RNAses released by lysosomes or dead cells. Consequently, analysis is usually done on total cellular DNA using a Southern blot procedure or polymerase chain reactions in which regions of DNA in a complex genome are amplified and more easily identified. RNA from tumors can be measured by a number of techniques. These include Northern blots, reverse transcription–polymerase chain reactions, and *in situ* hybridization.

Some interesting applications of these techniques, beginning to be applied clinically, have been found in the identification of tumor margins to facilitate complete removal of cancers, and in labeling micrometastases in lymph nodes and bone marrow aspirates. Molecular assessment of resected primary tumor margins by Brennan and colleagues[131] has led to the restaging of squamous cell cancer of the head and neck. Detection of micrometastases, using reverse transcription–polymerase chain reaction amplification of carcinoembryonic antigen mRNA in lymph nodes from patients with stage II colorectal cancer, was associated with a significant reduction in 5-year survival rate, from 91% to 50% in the positive subset.[132] More controversial has been the finding of circulating cancer cells and analysis of their prognostic significance as a result of differences in antibodies and markers used for their determination.[133, 134]

Oncologic Imaging

An increasing array of medical imaging procedures exists. These include sophisticated radiography, selective arteriography, radioisotopic scanning studies, ultrasound studies, and, most importantly, computed tomography (CT) and magnetic resonance imaging (MRI).[135, 136] Tests must be ordered with discrimination to avoid reduplication and huge medical bills.[137, 138] In addition to identification of primary tumors, the search for metastatic disease in regional nodal and distant visceral sites is important. A diagnostic oncologic imaging algorithm shows the disease process as it relates to cancer management and treatment (Fig. 1–10).

Computed Tomography Scans. CT scanning has revolutionized tumor imaging in diagnostic radiology. The ability to visualize inaccessible structures, as in the mediastinum

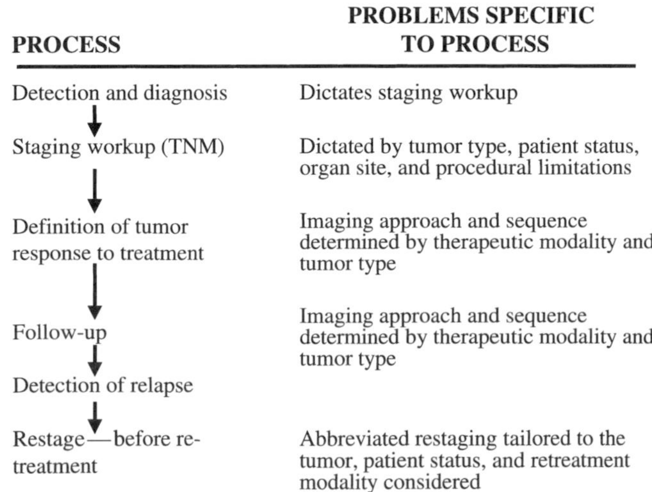

PROCESS
PROBLEMS SPECIFIC TO PROCESS
Detection and diagnosis
Dictates staging workup
Staging workup (TNM)
Dictated by tumor type, patient status, organ site, and procedural limitations
Definition of tumor response to treatment
Imaging approach and sequence determined by therapeutic modality and tumor type
Follow-up
Imaging approach and sequence determined by therapeutic modality and tumor type
Detection of relapse
Restage—before retreatment
Abbreviated restaging tailored to the tumor, patient status, and retreatment modality considered

Figure 1–10. Sequence of imaging process—staging and follow-up. (From Bragg DG, Rubin P, Youker JE [eds]: Oncologic Imaging. Elmsford, Pergamon Press, 1985, with permission.)

and retroperitoneal area, has completely changed work-up procedures. The impact and cost of this new technology, and recommendations formulated in decision trees as to sequencing diagnostic studies in a coordinated and non-competitive fashion, are outlined in *Oncologic Imaging* by Bragg and associates.[139] Spiral CT allows for finer definition and three-dimensional reconstruction in different planes. CT is superior in searching for pulmonary metastases and confirming lytic and blastic foci identified on scintibone scans.

There are newer imaging techniques on the horizon, such as holographic radiographic imaging, nuclear magnetic resonance spectroscopy, and three-dimensional anatomic and functional displays, which will further augment our understanding of tumor behavior and lead to more accurate diagnoses. The ultimate goal is specific labeling or targeting of tumor metabolic products, antigens, or antibodies. The threshold size for tumor detection is currently 2 to 5 mm, but with cellular and molecular imaging becomes less than 1 mm.

Magnetic Resonance Imaging and Magnetic Resonance Spectroscopy. The use of high-intensity magnetic fields to gain images of the anatomy and regional chemistry is one of the most advanced, but also one of the more costly, technologies. This technique has revolutionized the imaging of tumors by providing beautifully detailed, three-dimensional planar views in sagittal, coronal, and transverse cuts. Adjusting pulse sequences to emphasize different aspects of nuclear magnetic relaxation can optimize imaging. Images that emphasize blood flow, water density, tumor edema, and tumor chemistry are all possible. Specific paramagnetic contrast agents, such as gadolinium, can be used to enhance leaky tumor blood vessels.

In addition to MRI, there is the ability to use surface coils and obtain spectral analysis of specific chemical constituents in the region. As spatial resolution improves, research continues to discover unique characteristics or signatures to allow the detection of cancer, monitor its response to therapy, and determine if there is tumor viability at the end of treatment. Considerable research is directed to this area, with the recent creation of a biomedical imaging branch at the National Cancer Institute. MRI three-dimensional tumor reconstruction is likely to prove to be a powerful tool for delineation of central nervous system and spinal cord lesions and other masses in critical locations.

Nuclear Imaging. Nuclear imaging plays an important role in tumor imaging, particularly with regard to osseous or skeletal lesions, especially in the initial search or survey for metastatic foci detectable by total body ^{99m}Tc scanning. Although sensitive, the procedure lacks specificity. For most potential metastatic sites, such as liver and brain, CT and MRI are preferred to nuclear scans. Gallium-67 scintigraphy has been used in Hodgkin's disease and lung cancer to specifically identify occult deposits in extensions not appreciated on routine filming, and investigators have reported gallium-67 to have an accuracy of 76% to 100%.[140]

Ultrasound. Ultrasound remains a less expensive, and less hazardous, alternative to the above techniques. However, the hope for tissue or tumor signatures of the "echo" signal has not emerged. For children, ultrasound presents an alternative to CT for tumor imaging because exposures to ionizing irradiation are avoided. However, the images are definitely inferior and less preferable to most physicians. There has been interest in ultrasound for imaging of cancerous prostate glands and for aiding brachytherapy implantation to produce optimal three-dimensional distributions. Real-time image-guided brachytherapy, using ultrasound, is now a reality.[140a]

New Imaging Techniques. New techniques are on the horizon and relate to functional, metabolic, or molecular imaging:

- Magnetic resonance spectroscopy should allow for biochemical analysis of voxels and, when combined with MRI, can allow for spatial and chemical analysis of tumors noninvasively.[141–143]
- Monoclonal antibody imaging or specific labeling or targeting of antigens and antibodies with homing characteristics can be used to image microdeposits of cancer ranging from microns to millimeters.[143–145] Monoclonal antibodies are under investigation for both tumor detection and treatment. Some successes have already become clinically useful. There are 10^2 to 10^5 antigenic sites per tumor cell and 10^6 cells in 1 mm^3; thus, the potential exists for tagging subclinical metastatic foci of cancer with 10^8 to 10^{11} radiolabeled antibodies.
- Positron emission tomography scanning for tumor metabolism has been used to distinguish recurrent gliomas from brain necrosis.[146] In addition, uptake of (^{18}F)fluorodeoxyglucose has been used to predict early recurrence.[147]

Classification and Anatomic Staging

It is essential to develop a classification[148] of cancer based on both anatomic and histologic considerations. Such a dual classification is the keystone to cancer decision making as a multidisciplinary process. It is apparent in a review of the literature that differences in classification or language have made cross-comparisons of different cancers virtually impossible. Thus, a statement referring to early, moderate, and advanced cancers without further description leaves those who are unfamiliar, and even those with experience, uncertain as to where the line is being drawn. Because criteria change for each surgeon with time and the improvement of techniques, terms such as *operable, inoperable, resectable,* and *nonresectable* are not illuminating without qualifications.

Many national and international committees are attempting to standardize nomenclature. The main problem is keeping the descriptions from being so complex that they inhibit their clinical use. Simplicity is important; otherwise, even a large clinical series can be subdivided to the point that it is impossible to have sufficient numbers of patients in any category in the lifetime of an investigator. The two major agencies concerned with the classification of malignant disease are the American Joint Committee for Cancer (AJCC)[149] and the International Union Against Cancer (UICC).[150] The objectives of classification are as follows:

- Aid the clinician in the planning of primary and adjuvant treatment.
- Give some indication of prognosis.
- Assist in the evaluation of results of treatment.
- Facilitate the exchange of information.
- Contribute in the continuing investigation of cancer.

There have been five editions of the *AJCC Cancer Staging Manual*, starting in 1959, with the most recent published in 1997. Revisions in this edition have been made in gynecologic sites, prostate cancer, head and neck, lung, soft tissue sarcoma, testes, and brain. The UICC's manual has also had five editions, and its classification and staging now are identical to that of the AJCC.

Histopathologic Classification

The histopathologic classification is of equal importance to the anatomic stage in planning treatment and predicting outcome. The need for a standardized nomenclature is evident, and reference to the World Health Organization monographs, a 25-volume series,[151] and the *Atlas of Tumor Pathology* from the Armed Forces Institute of Pathology[2] provide a basis for uniformity in criteria by illustrative photomicrographs. The World Health Organization's *International Classification of Diseases for Oncology,*[152] second edition, is a numerical coding system for neoplasms by topography and morphology and is identical to the morphology field for neoplasms in the Systematized Nomenclature of Medicine. This should facilitate international collaboration in cancer research and multi-institutional clinical trials. The two essential features are the type of tumor and the grade for one dominant type.

Histologic Type. The need to appreciate the histopathologic type of cancer can be readily recognized when considering ovarian and testicular neoplasms. A testicular choriocarcinoma carries a much poorer prognosis and demands different therapy than a similar-stage seminoma. The appreciation of different types of testicular tumors, ovarian cancers, and brain neoplasms is essential to understanding management.

Tumor Grade. The value of *grading* carcinomas (e.g., Broders' classification of squamous cell carcinomas[153]) to express their degree of malignancy is well known. Similar grading systems have been evolved for cancers of the breast, prostate, sarcoma, and bladder. Grading is often more important than type in affecting prognosis, and this is well illustrated in soft tissue sarcomas.

Most tumors are graded on a scale of 3 or 4. *The highest grades generally indicate the most aggressive biology.* Grades (G) are typically defined as G1 = well differentiated; G2 = moderately well differentiated; G3 to G4 = poorly to very poorly differentiated. An accurate histologic diagnosis therefore is an essential element in evaluating tumor behavior, but in the future, certain types of cancer, biochemical, genetic, or immunologic measures, as described in previous sections, will become increasingly important elements in classifying tumor aggressiveness.

Cytogenetics. One may anticipate that special techniques such as immunohistochemical staining, tissue culture, cytogenetics, and molecular biomarkers will be used more routinely for typing and characterizing cancer behavior.[149]

Anatomic Staging and Classification

Since Pierre Denoix introduced the tumor, node, metastasis (TNM) system for classification of malignant cancers in 1944,[154] different users have introduced numerous variations. This is the antithesis of standardization, and to correct this deficiency, in 1982, national committees agreed to formulate a single set of TNM staging criteria to be used by the UICC and AJCC. Throughout this volume, these rules for classification will be used and have been published in the fifth editions of the UICC and the AJCC manuals. A common language is essential for assessing the results of treatment. The essence of a meaningful classification depends on quantifying the extent of disease. This is carried out in three compartments:

- T for primary tumor
- N for regional lymph nodes
- M for metastases

Most new classifications attempt to define the primary site with a TNM classification as follows: T1, T2, T3, or T4 with increasing extent, advancing nodal disease as N0, N1, N2, or N3, and the presence or absence of metastases, respectively, as M0 or M+ (Fig. 1–11). These categories may or may not be feasible for all sites and they tend to become unwieldy when attempting to maintain complete coverage of all clinical cases. This system allows for considering modes of malignant spread; that is, T for primary or direct extension, N for secondary lymphatic involvement, and M for vascular dissemination.

T Categories with Model for Unified Classification

The criterion for categorizing a primary tumor (T) is the apparent anatomic extent of the disease. Extent is commonly based on three features: depth of invasion, surface spread, and size. Following review of existing classifica-

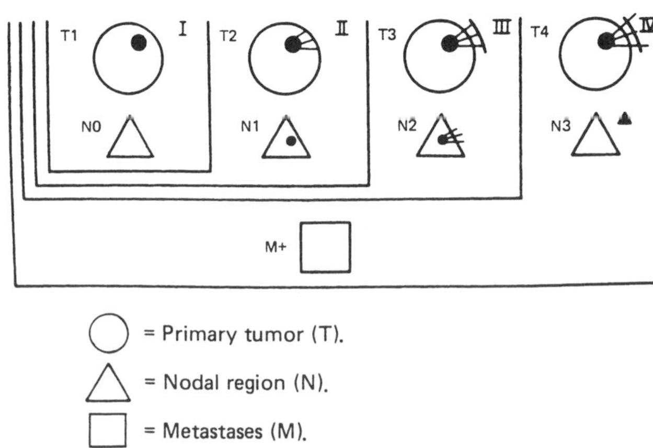

Figure 1–11. Stage grouping. The stage grouping is based on clustering TNM categories (see text).

TABLE 1–11. **Specific Criteria Related to T Categories**

	T1	T2	T3	T4
Depth of invasion				
Solid organs	Confined	Capsule muscle	Bone cartilage	Viscera
Hollow organs	Submucosa	Muscularis	Serosa	
Mobility	Mobile	Partial mobility	Fixed	Fixed and destructive
Neighboring structures	Not invaded	Adjacent (attached)	Surrounding (detached)	Viscera
Surface spread				
Regions (R)	1/2 or R_1	R_1	R_1+R_2	$R_1+R_2+R_3$
Circumference	<1/3	1/3 to 1/2	>1/2 to 2/3	>2/3
Size				
Diameter	<2 cm	2 to 4–5 cm	>4–5 cm	>10 cm

From Rubin P: A unified classification of tumors: an oncotaxonomy with symbols. Cancer 1973; 31:963.

tions, an attempt has been made to define the clinical basis for placement of a tumor in T1, T2, T3, or T4 category by the criteria in Table 1–11.[155]

As a model, the following approximation is valid for most TNM staging systems:

T0: No evidence of a primary lesion found grossly or microscopically. Evidence of malignant change without microinvasion and without a target lesion identifiable clinically.

T1: A lesion confined to the organ of origin. It is mobile, does not invade adjacent or surrounding structures or tissues, and is often superficial. T1 lesions are resectable.

T2: A localized but more infiltrative lesion characterized by deep extension into adjacent structures or tissues. Invasion is into capsules, ligaments, intrinsic muscle, and adjacent attached structures of similar tissue or function. There is some loss of tumor mobility, but it is not complete; therefore, fixation is not present.

T3: An advanced lesion that is confined to the region rather than to the organ of origin, whether solid or hollow. The critical criterion is fixation, which indicates invasion into a fixed structure or past a boundary. These structures are most often bone and cartilage, but invasion of the extrinsic muscle walls, serosa, and skin are also included. Surrounding detached structures of different anatomy or function are in this category; however, this inclusion can be debated because of the varieties of anatomic structures. T3 lesions are marginally resectable, or can only be debulked. In some malignancies, as in breast cancer, size alone may be sufficient to qualify for T3 designation.

T4: A massive lesion extending into another hollow organ, causing a fistula, or into another solid organ, causing a sinus. Invasions into major nerves, arteries, and veins are placed in this category. Destruction of bone in addition to fixation is an advanced sign. At most anatomic locations, T4 tumors are difficult to approach by any treatment modality.

N Categories and Unified Model for Classification

The establishment of lymph node categories should be as critical in design as the T or primary categories; however, the criteria currently used are more varied. The criteria consist of size, firmness, encapsulation, number of nodes, and ipsilateral or contralateral location. These are further defined in Table 1–12.[155]

N0: No evidence of disease in lymph nodes.

N1: These nodes are usually palpable and movable and are limited to the first lymphatic drainage station. For small nodes, a distinction between an uninvolved and an involved node must be made. Clinical determination of tumor involvement depends on the firmness and roundness of a node and its size, which is generally greater than 1 cm, and usually up to 3 cm in size and solitary. Alternatively, positivity of small nodes

TABLE 1–12. **Specific Criteria Related to N Categories***

	N1	**N2**	**N3**	**N4**
Station	***First***	***First***	***First***	***Second***
Drainage				
Unilateral	Ipsilateral	Ipsilateral	Ipsilateral	Contralateral
Bilateral	Ipsilateral	Contralateral or bilateral	Ipsilateral or contralateral	Distant
Number	Solitary	Multiple		
Size	<2–3 cm	>3 cm–>5 cm	>10 cm	
Mobility	Mobile	Partial matted muscle invasion	Fixed to vessels, bone, skin	Fixed and destructive

*To distinguish N_a from N_1, the specific criteria include size between 1 and 2 cm; firmness—soft to hard; roundness—½ to 1 cm.

From Rubin P: A unified classification of tumors: an oncotaxonomy with symbols. Cancer 1973; 31:963.

can be made pathologically after needle biopsy or excision. N1 nodes are usually encapsulated.

N2: These nodes are usually larger than N1 nodes or are multiple. They usually involve regional nodes in addition to first station nodes. N2 nodes frequently have extracapsular extension, and though often tethered to surrounding tissues, are not fixed.

N3: These nodes are usually fixed to surrounding structures by tumor that extends beyond the capsule. N3 nodes can involve bone, large blood vessels, skin, or nerves. They are usually 6 cm or larger in size.

NX: Nodes inaccessible to clinical evaluation.

N− or N+: Nodes are evaluated by microscopic study and designated as negative or positive depending on findings.

M Categories and a Unified Model for Classification

The lack of a consistent and thorough attempt to categorize an anatomic extent of metastases is conspicuous in the current schema. The important feature is the presence or absence of metastasis, that is, M0 versus M1. The reason for this reflects the poor prognosis if metastases are present. Nevertheless, cure—though rare—is possible for some solitary metastases. As chemotherapy becomes more effective, and results are assessed, there will be a need to categorize and subclassify this group of patients.

M0: No evidence of metastases.
M1: Distant metastases.
MX: No metastatic work-up done.

The categories M1 can be clinical (cM1) or pathologic (pM1). Each organ can be designated with special notations such as pulmonary (PUL), osseous (OSS), hepatic (HEP), brain (BRA), bone marrow (MAR), adrenals (ADR), and skin (SKI).

Principles in Developing an Effective Staging System

It is important to distinguish cancer staging classification. Staging is an attempt to define the true extent of cancer in its three compartments (TNM) at a point in time, usually at the time of detection. A classification is a multidimensional and multitemporal framework to include all possibilities of cancer presentations and spread at an organ site. There are at least 40 combinations with five Ts (including T0) and four Ns (including N0) and two M categories, but *for each patient at diagnosis or presentation, there is only one stage!* Staging does not imply a regular and predictable progression. Although some cancers proceed in a typical course, advancing from a primary tumor into secondary nodal disease and eventually to remote metastases, many variations exist. Metastases, in fact, can be the first sign of cancer, with the primary lesion being smaller and even microscopic in size. The staging is arbitrary and its effectiveness is determined by whether a consensus exists to use it as standard terminology for treatment selection and end-stage reporting. However, the exact criteria depend on each organ site and these definitions are offered as general guides only. A typical type of stage grouping is illustrated in Figure 1–11 and usually is limited to four groupings or stages.

Stage I, T1,N0,M0: Clinical examination reveals a mass limited to organ of origin. The lesion is operable and resectable with only local involvement and there is no nodal or vascular spread. This stage affords the best chance of curability (70% to 90%).

Stage II, T1 or T2,N1,M0: Clinical examination shows evidence of local spread into surrounding tissue and first station lymph nodes. The lesion is operable and resectable, but because of greater local extent, there is uncertainty about completeness of removal. The specimen shows evidence of microinvasion into capsule and lymphatics. This stage affords a good chance of curability (about 50% ± 5%).

Stage III, any T3, or any N2,M0: Clinical examination reveals an extensive primary tumor with fixation to deeper structures, bone invasion, and lymph nodes of a similar nature. The lesion is operable but not resectable and gross disease is left behind. This stage affords some chance of survival (20% ± 5%).

Stage IV, T4,N3,M+: Evidence of distant metastases beyond the local site or organ. The primary lesion is inoperable. There is little to no chance of cure in most sites (<5%).

There are two approaches with regard to stage grouping. The UICC,[150] with few exceptions, does not favor stage grouping, but stresses the need for careful definition of each TNM category. The AJCC[149] favors stage grouping into four stages because it tends to standardize end-result reporting; if derived from a carefully executed protocol, this will yield excellent data that relate to prognosis. The exact criteria for clustering will vary with each site. A valid system is based on the knowledge of spread and the clinical evolution of the specific cancer and will differ at each anatomic site, depending on the equivalence of T and N categories in terms of prognosis. In the following chapters, for every major disease site, a diagram illustrates the TNM categories and stage grouping and AJCC/UICC criteria are presented in tabular form.

Staging Work-Up

Tumor Staging. A consistent classification of cancer requires a consistent staging work-up. There are usually two phases: first, a clinical-radiographic imaging that is noninvasive; the second is invasive, in which specimens verify presence of cancer locally and in nodes or distant sites. Imaging is becoming increasingly sophisticated. As a result, more small tumors are being detected at an earlier point in the disease course (Table 1–13).

Primary Tumor (T). Clinical examination of accessible lesions is recommended, preferably under anesthesia if the lesion is internal (e.g., cervix or bladder tumors). Radiographs of the site, including special contrast and tomographic techniques, and direct and indirect visualization by endoscopic means are essential studies.

TABLE 1–13. **Imaging Procedures: Limitations and Applications**

Imaging Procedure	Relative Cost	Relative Sensitivity	Relative Specificity	Comments
Plain film radiography	Low	Varied	High	Plain films have excellent sensitivity and specificity in soft tissues (mammography) and bones. In the chest, low-contrast tumor targets are a problem, and CT is preferred for staging primary and nodes.
Computed tomography				
Brain	Moderate	High	Moderate	Procedure of choice for screening suspected mass/lesion using contrast enhancement only.
Lung	Moderate	High	Moderate	Highest sensitivity of all studies in detection of lung nodules.
Abdomen	Moderate	High	Moderate	High false-positive.
Magnetic resonance	High	High	High	Resolution better than CT in CNS, soft tissue, and head and neck cancers. Elimination of bone artifacts makes CNS images better than CT. In the chest, tumor and hilar node imaging improved in the mediastinum over CT. Useful in the GI, genitourinary, and gynecologic tumors, but CT is adequate for staging.
Ultrasound, abdominal	Moderate	High	Moderate	Lack of radiation exposure, cost, and availability lend ultrasound to abdominal screening. Technique is operator-dependent. Initial procedure in pediatric tumors.
Radionuclide scan				
Bone	Moderate	High	Low	Procedure of choice in skeletal scanning. Abnormal sites must be verified by film radiography. MRI resolves problem diagnosis.
Brain	Moderate	Moderate	Low	MRI/CT has replaced radionuclide brain scanning.
Liver	Moderate	Moderate	Low	Displaced by CT/US as liver screening imaging modality of choice.
Contrast GI studies	Moderate	High	High	Cancer screening applications can be justified for high-risk groups (esophagus, stomach, colon). CT provides depth of invasion and involved nodes.
Angiography	High	High	Moderate	Cost, invasiveness, and time limit applications.
Lymphangiography	High	High	Moderate	Advanced to CT for pelvic and retroperitoneal nodes.

CNS = central nervous system; CT = computed tomography; GI = gastrointestinal; MRI = magnetic resonance imaging; US = ultrasound.

From Rubin P, Chen Y, Brasacchio RA: Staging and classification of the cancer and the host: a unified approach versus neotaxonomy. In: Perez CA, Brady LW (eds): Principles and Practice of Radiation Oncology, 3rd ed, p 213. Philadelphia, Lippincott-Raven Publishers, 1997, with permission. Modified from Bragg DG, Rubin P, Youker JE (eds): Oncologic Imaging. Elmsford, NY, Pergamon Press, 1985.

Lymph Nodes (N). Clinical examination is important when nodes are accessible. Lymphangiography by means of contrast agents is of value, but is rarely being done currently; CT and MRI are the preferred imaging procedures. Needle biopsy, more recently combined with CT, is being used for confirmation of positive nodes.

Metastases (M). The most common metastases are to the lung, liver, bone, bone marrow, and brain, and each site has a most favored methodology. For lung, CT scans are more accurate than chest films. For liver, CT scans are also favored over nuclear scans or ultrasound. For bone, ^{99m}Tc scans are best for initial survey, with bone radiographs for verification. For bone marrow and brain, MRI is the most sensitive, but is also more costly.

Clinical Versus Surgical Versus Pathologic Criteria for Staging. Two different types of evaluative evidence are used for classification of the true extent of disease at different anatomic sites. Checklists and the standard AJCC anatomic diagrams should be used for careful geographic mapping of cancer extent by clinical oncologists, surgeons, and pathologists.

Clinical-Diagnostic Staging (cTNM). This staging is noninvasive and relies on careful physical examination and generally available laboratory and radiographic studies. This can be applied to accessible sites, such as the head and neck region, especially where more than one modality can be used, and allows for reasonable accuracy in comparison of results.

Surgical-Pathologic Staging (pTNM). This staging is based on information obtained by surgical procedures and is generally useful at inaccessible sites, such as in cancers of the ovary, stomach, colon, and kidney. Biopsies and histopathologic analysis are an essential part of this staging category. Complete resection of organs, with drainage of regional lymph nodes, is designed for such clinically inaccessible sites as the ovaries and pancreas. Correlation of the pathologic findings is important for an evaluation of the accuracy of staging procedures.

It is important to distinguish each type of stage classification, whether clinical-diagnostic, surgical-evaluative, or postsurgical-pathologic, by the prefix c or p, before TNM categories. A new addition to the postsurgical classification is the concept of residual disease after surgery.

The major impact of the clinical versus surgical staging work-up can be seen in Hodgkin's disease, in which the surgical effort is directed at defining the true extent of the disease, which in turn influences the logical choice and aggressiveness of treatment modalities. This redirection of the surgical effort into staging procedures is the foundation of multidisciplinary conferences for cancer decision making. Uniform criteria and uniform categories are necessary to make reported series comparable between different specialties.

Geographic Mapping of Primary Tumor and Regional Nodes. For many malignancies, accurate mapping of the primary tumor and regional nodes is possible and completes the surgical-pathologic staging process. In some cases, where neoadjuvant approaches are used to shrink tumors progressively, surgeons may be asked to "mark" the initial site of lesion involvement. In addition to the operative note, a series of anatomic diagrams, preferably three-dimensional, should be widely adopted for identification of macroresidual and microresidual tumor. The AJCC[149] has checklists and anatomic site diagrams that can be correlated with surgical clips and should allow radiation oncologists to plan treatment more accurately. Pathologists should use these same diagrams to verify residual disease. The concept of accurate geographic mapping, so widely adopted in Hodgkin's disease and non-Hodgkin's lymphoma, is now being increasingly applied to gastrointestinal tumors, particularly rectal cancers, and is applicable to all sites. Multimodal treatment requires accurate imaging and mapping of disease, preferably on one set of anatomic forms before therapy.

C-Factor. The C-factor, or certainty factor, reflects the validity of classification according to the diagnostic methods used. Its use is optional. The C-factor definitions are:

- C1: Evidence from standard diagnostic means such as inspection, palpation, and standard radiography, intraluminal endoscopy for tumors of certain organs.
- C2: Evidence obtained by special diagnostic means such as radiographic imaging in special projections, tomography, CT, ultrasonography, lymphography, angiography, scintigraphy, MRI, endoscopy, biopsy, and cytology.
- C3: Evidence from surgical exploration, including biopsy and cytology.
- C4: Evidence of the extent of disease following definitive surgery and pathologic examination of the resected specimen.
- C5: Evidence from autopsy.

Stage Migration and Conversion Rate. Stage migration is a major factor in the literature of cancer results. An effect known as the *Will Rogers phenomenon* can result from the intermixing of clinical-diagnostic and surgical-pathologic staging, ultimately having an impact on the reporting of end results. As patients with more advanced (pathologically determined) disease progress to the higher stages, there is the apparent removal of more advanced or less favorable disease from the earlier stages, so that results are artificially improved. However, this results in patients with similar surgical-pathologic rather than clinical-diagnostic stage groupings being compared, although overall survival remains the same. Ulfelder[156] demonstrated this phenomenon in ovarian cancer staging; Figure 1–12 illustrates the importance of comparing patients using the same criteria. The current rules in clinical staging give the patient the benefit of the doubt and downstage their tumor classification. This allows questionable stage II patients to remain stage I, making results for the latter appear worse.

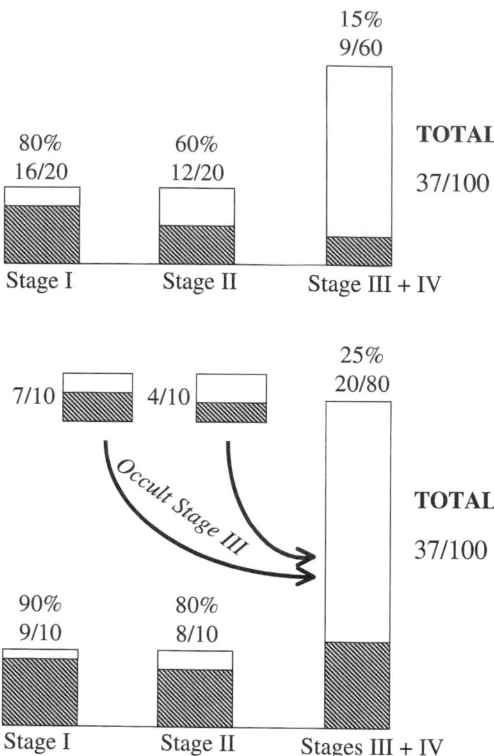

Figure 1–12. The Will Rogers phenomenon. Hypothetical graph of 5-year survival rate (hatched columns) by stage of 100 patients with ovarian carcinoma. The upper row indicates the original staging; the lower row shows reassignment of one half of each group into stages I and II due to the discovery of occult, biopsy-proven extension to either the diaphragmatic peritoneum or the retroperitoneal nodes. Although the overall cure rate is unchanged (37%), the rate in each stage is significantly increased. (From Ulfelder H: Current concepts in cancer: ovary. Classification systems. Int J Radiat Oncol Biol Phys 1981; 7:1083, with permission from Elsevier Science.)

Occasionally, a neoplastic disease undergoes a dynamic change and a new staging system emerges, as was seen for Kaposi's sarcoma appearing in patients with acquired immunodeficiency syndrome.[157] In addition, some of the more common cancer classifications have responded to new imaging approaches and required refinement, as with breast cancer,[158, 159] or there have been changes in diagnostic or pathologic approaches, as with colorectal cancer[160] or genitourinary cancers, such as prostate[161] and testicular tumors.[162] Gynecologic cancer classification and staging systems have been similarly affected by diagnostic operative procedures, such as laparotomy for staging of nodes to increase accuracy.[163]

Molecular genetic detection of micrometastases in lymph nodes and in bone marrow aspirates will lead to increased cure rates independent of treatment as a result of stage migration, as noted by Coleman and Harris.[164] That is, the unfavorable node-positive patients, who would be undetected by routine methods at present, will be uncovered, purifying localized stages and allowing for adjuvant treatment therapy for more advanced stages with micrometastases that are more likely to be cured by the addition of radiation or chemotherapy, or both.[132] Nonetheless, clinical

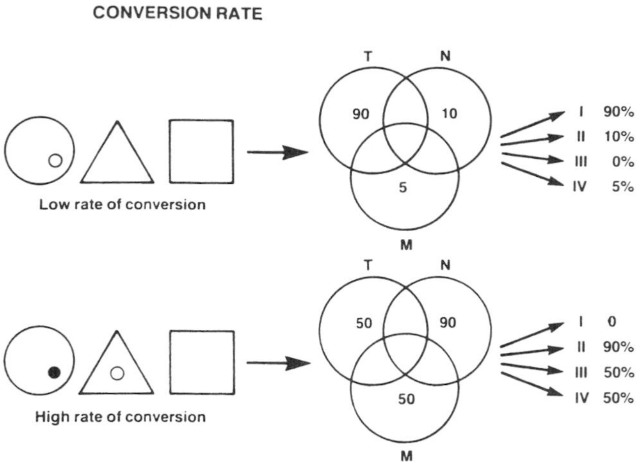

Figure 1–13. Conversion rate. The high and low conversion rate of a malignancy is illustrated. A low conversion rate cancer is suggested by a squamous cell cancer of the skin 2 cm in diameter. It is identified in the T compartment, and 90% of the time, it is confined within this compartment. If a nodular melanoma of the same size is found clinically, on a full work-up and follow-up, nodes would be positive 90% and metastases 50%. This is a high conversion rate. T = tumor; N = node; M = metastases.

staging is imperfect with today's technology since it is impossible to detect microscopic extensions or deposits in all potential foci. Despite improvements in diagnosis, a gap in knowledge exists between the apparent clinical stage and the true pathologic stage. This difference may be expressed as a *conversion rate* and is critical to cancer management. In low conversion rate cancers, such as skin cancers, i.e. squamous cell or basal cell carcinoma, precise local treatment can be prescribed. However, in high conversion rate cancers, such as melanoma or lung cancer, local therapy alone is often ineffective for cure. The concept of conversion rate is illustrated in Figure 1–13.

The conversion rate is the factor that determines how aggressive or radical a treatment the oncologist should choose. Most cancers are treated at least one stage beyond their clinically defined stage. Very aggressive cancers, such as small cell anaplastic cancer of the lung, Wilms' tumor, and choriocarcinoma, are treated as stage IV, or as if they have occult hematogenous metastases, even if they are defined as localized stage I malignancies. Information on conversion rates is sparse but can be collected in well-designed studies.

The conversion rate for metastatic disease to distant sites often can be determined for localized and regionalized disease by subtracting the 5-year survival rate from 100. For example, for localized bladder cancer, the conversion rate to metastases is 15% (100 − 85), whereas for regionalized bladder malignancy, it is as high as 80% (100 − 20).

Dual Classification. Where possible, dual anatomic-histologic classifications should be used because this is the essence of good reporting. The comparison of one series with another, that is, surgery versus radiation therapy, depends on the presence of similar groups of cancer patients in each category. True randomization in any series must pass this simple test both retrospectively and prospectively. This is always regulated in prospective studies by stratifying patients into prognostic categories prior to randomization. The only way in which confusion can be eliminated during the next decade is to accept the AJCC-UICC classification on a wider basis, and for journal editors to encourage authors to follow these ground rules when reporting end results.

Host Classification

Performance Classification. There has been widespread acceptance of the Karnofsky Performance Scale and many cooperative groups have adopted its use. The Karnofsky Performance Scale determines the ability of a patient to perform daily functions, and defines quality rather than quantity of life (Table 1–14).[148, 165] This modification pro-

TABLE 1–14. **Criteria for Performance Status on the Karnofsky Performance Scale and ECOG Performance Scale**

Karnofsky Performance Scale		ECOG Performance Scale	
100	Normal; no complaints; no evidence of disease	0	Normal activity; asymptomatic
90	Able to carry on normal activity; minor signs or symptoms of disease	1	Symptomatic; fully ambulatory
80	Normal activity with effort; some signs or symptoms of disease		
70	Cares for self; unable to carry on normal activity or to do active work	2	Symptomatic; in bed < 50% of time
60	Requires occasional assistance but is able to care for most needs		
50	Requires considerable assistance and frequent medical care	3	Symptomatic; in bed > 50% of time; bedridden
40	Disabled; requires special care and assistance		
30	Severely disabled; hospitalization is indicated although death not imminent		
20	Very sick; hospitalization necessary; active support treatment is necessary	4	100% bedridden
10	Moribund, fatal processes progressing rapidly		
0	Dead	5	Dead

ECOG = Eastern Cooperative Oncology Group.

From Rubin P, Chen Y, Brasacchio RA: Staging and classification of the cancer and the host: a unified approach versus neotaxonomy. In: Perez CA, Brady LW (eds): Principles and Practice of Radiation Oncology, 3rd ed, p 213. Philadelphia, Lippincott-Raven Publishers, 1997, with permission. Modified from Karnofsky DA, Abelmann WH, Craver LF, et al: The use of nitrogen mustards in the palliative treatment of carcinoma with particular reference to bronchogenic carcinoma. Cancer 1948; 1:634.

posal is determined at the time of clinical-diagnostic classification, and recorded at subsequent times of classification as well as at each follow-up examination to measure the quality of life.

Quality of Life. A major assessment of the quality of life (QOL) issue has been initiated by a National Cancer Institute workshop, and this has been moved into cooperative group research.[166] As patients are entered onto different protocols, both the acute and long-term toxicities are known to have an impact on lifestyle. Five broad categories are used to describe quality of life: normal life, happiness/satisfaction, achievement of personal goals, social utility, and natural capacity.[167] Normal life can be defined as the ability to function at a level similar to healthy persons of the same age; happiness suggests short-term positive feelings, whereas satisfaction implies a longer cognitive experience, according to Ferrans.[167] Other commonly used QOL scales are Functional Assessment of Cancer Therapy and Profile of Moods States.[168, 169] Both consist of multiple psychological and social questions rated on a scale of 1 to 5, rating symptoms such as pain, fatigue, and nausea on a scale of none to worst. The QOL evaluation differs from traditional outcome parameters in two ways: it incorporates a wider range of outcomes with a less tangible quality, such as well-being and satisfaction, and concerns the patient's perspective, not the physician's. In addition, sexual functional evaluation may be measured with the Sexual Adjustment Questionnaire developed by Waterhouse and Metcalfe.[170] The Sexual Adjustment Questionnaire has five subscales: desire, activity level, arousal, orgasm, and satisfaction. Data are being collected to quantify and analyze these effects. Analysis of QOL is particularly important when long-term survival may be adversely affected by toxicities or in cases where tumor responses may be less than dramatic.

Toxicity Scales. Late Effects of Normal Tissues–Subjective, Objective, Management Analytic (LENT-SOMA) criteria is a system currently being validated by Radiation Therapy Oncology Group/European Organization Treatment of Cancer investigators and used for scoring late effects in normal tissues.[171] Thirty-five organ sites have been assessed and for each clinical measure, there are four grades: mild, moderate, severe, and life threatening. This system allows for a comparison between the perception of morbidity by the patient (QOL scales) and the physician assessments, thereby providing a better database to establish the therapeutic benefit of different treatments.

Comorbidity factors have been assessed by Piccirillo and Feinstein, who emphasized a clinical biologic classification of cancer that illustrates the significance of symptoms and comorbidity.[172] They have gone on to show that comorbidity factors, such as severe heart disease and diabetes, can lead to significant differences in survival for similar stages of disease in different organs.[173–175]

Radiation Therapy Oncology Group statisticians have introduced recursive partitioning analysis into brain and lung cancer trial protocols. The results are then based on a number of elements stratified into prognostic classes. The value of this method can be seen in Figure 1–14,[176] illustrating survival curves formed through a decision tree based on various factors such as histopathologic grade, Karnofsky Performance Scale, age, type of resection, and neurologic findings.

Principles of Treatment

The finality of treatment in a patient with malignant disease demands that only those who are capable and properly trained undertake therapy. There are few situations in medicine where the stakes are as high and the therapeutic procedure as decisive for cure or death. The responsibility is great and the judgment is critical. This is reflected in the emergence of subspecialties in virtually all major disciplines, that is, radiation oncology, medical oncology, surgi-

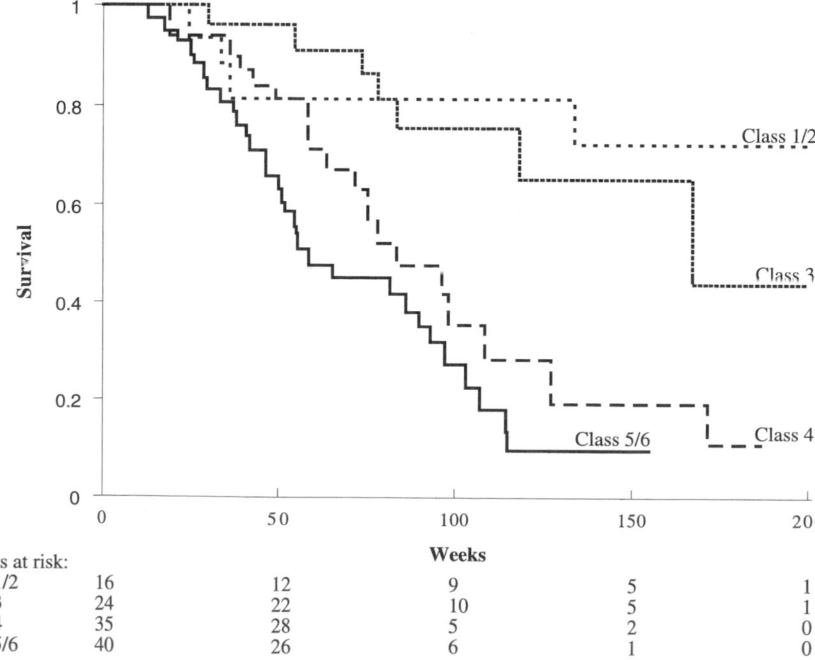

Figure 1–14. Survival in weeks for patients with anaplastic astrocytoma or glioblastoma multiforme, treated with stereotactic radiosurgery, stratified by prognostic class as defined by the RTOG recursive partitioning analysis ($p < 0.001$). The numbers below the horizontal axis correspond to the number of patients at risk in each prognostic group at each time point. (From Sarkaria JN, Mehta MP, Loeffler JS, et al: Radiosurgery in the initial management of malignant gliomas: survival comparison with the RTOG recursive partitioning analysis. Int J Radiat Oncol Biol Phys 1995; 32:931, with permission from Elsevier Science.)

cal oncology, gynecologic oncology, and pediatric oncology. *The first decision is the most important determinant of success in treatment and this should be a multimodal effort.*

The basic principle in therapy is to cure the patient with minimal functional and structural impairment. The decision as to how radical treatment should be is determined by a combination of factors:

- aggressiveness of the cancer
- predictability in regard to its spread—the conversion factor
- morbidity and mortality of the therapeutic procedure
- cure rate for the therapeutic procedure under consideration
- the therapeutic ratio or window

As the chance for cure decreases, the tendency for treatment to be more radical appears justified. In many circumstances, unfortunately, there may not be a decision that will allow for a successful result; indeed, a conservative approach may lead to an increased mortality. As in many problems in medicine, the choice is relative. What percentage of survival is acceptable for a debilitating therapeutic modality, be it surgery, radiation therapy, or chemotherapy? There is no formula or figure other than personal perspective. If cure is virtually impossible, one must be guided by palliation.

Although there is general agreement on many principles of management, controversy exists over the different procedures that offer limited success. Teamwork between a tumor pathologist, a diagnostic radiologist, and surgical, radiation and medical oncologists is required for the best effort. However, "togetherness" is not a substitute for individual responsibility and judgment on the part of every physician involved. The physician will gradually reconcile the differences and assimilate the areas of agreement by carefully monitoring each patient and reading the literature. Maturity of decision rests on clinical experience and is tempered by long-term follow-up experience.

Ideally, each cancer patient should be treated with a highly individual prescription. Optimal treatment is usually designed to treat the defined overt cancer and, where methods are available, suspected occult deposits. Lacking such precision, the selection of treatment should be multidisciplinary because the evidence in many cancers indicates that combinations of treatment are more effective than single modalities in the majority of instances.

Surgical Oncology

Surgical oncology (see Chapter 4, Principles of Surgical Oncology) is not a well-defined discipline as a result of the variety of surgical specialties that are based on disease site or organ, and therefore it differs from radiation oncology and medical oncology, which allow application of their respective modality to a wide anatomy. Generally, the role of surgical oncology can be defined as

- providing selection of definitive surgical treatment of localized malignancies based on a careful staging diagnostic procedure
- knowledge of and ability to consult with other modalities in choosing adjuvant therapy preoperatively and postoperatively
- reconstruction and rehabilitation for resected organs
- when the tumor is unresectable, providing debulking of residual cancer to improve effectiveness of other modes of treatment
- surgery for palliation and for some oncologic emergencies

Radiation Oncology

Radiation (see Chapter 6, Principles of Radiation Oncology and Cancer Radiotherapy) has proven to be the most effective single modality available for the treatment of cancer and is used with the anatomic goal of local tumor control, an approach shared with surgery. However, radiation may also be used in a locoregional approach, effectively sterilizing the tumor within a field, including first-station lymph nodes, an approach shared with surgery. In the case of certain lymphomas and leukemias, radiation also can be used as a systemic control.

Technical progress in this area has been greatly aided by advances in imaging technologies and computers, allowing for near conformal radiation treatments with three-dimensional attention to tumor location in relation to sensitive normal organs and structures. Pharmacologically, the focus has been on the use of drugs to improve the therapeutic ratio. Specifically, the drugs take advantage of biologic or physiologic differences between tumor and normal cells, sensitizing the tumor to radiation while leaving the normal tissue response unaffected. Alternatively, the approach has been to specifically protect normal tissues from the radiation, while maintaining tumor sensitivity.

Clinically, radiation therapy is divided into two categories: curative and palliative therapies. These categories do not always clearly differentiate one from the other, but are useful for devising therapies at the appropriate dose and potential toxicity.

- Curative therapy is administered to patients who have a high probability of achieving permanent and lasting tumor control. It is delivered to the tumor itself, the immediate regions at risk from tumor infiltration, the area where the tumor was located prior to surgery, or some combination of the above. Curative therapy is commonly associated with acute or chronic side effects of varying degrees. However, it is felt that the development of minor or moderate toxicity is justified by the possibility of cure.
- Palliative therapy is given to patients who have little potential for a prolonged survival. The goal is to relieve symptoms, and to do so with minimal impact on the quality of life. Treatments are therefore usually low to moderate doses with fewer associated side effects.

Medical Oncology

In the period following World War II, there was a rapid introduction of cancer chemotherapeutic agents, beginning with successes in leukemias, lymphomas, and Hodgkin's disease, followed by pediatric malignancies. This activity, fostered through a National Cancer Institute drug development program, screened thousands if not millions of potential pharmaceuticals over a 50-year span for adult solid tumors. Medical oncology (see Chapter 8, Basic Concepts of Cancer Chemotherapy and Principles of Medical Oncology) responded to the challenges of managing cancer patients and created this relatively new specialty to encompass a multidisciplinary approach of cancer care in the 1950s. Primary chemotherapy is distinct from adjuvant, neoadjuvant, and induction chemotherapy, where it is used in conjunction with other more curative treatment.

- Definitive primary chemotherapy is curative for leukemias, lymphomas, and Hodgkin's disease, as well as choriocarcinomas, some pediatric malignancies, and especially testicular cancers.
- Adjuvant chemotherapy is the use of systemic agents after surgery or irradiation, or both, has controlled the primary tumor, that is, postoperative chemotherapy regimens.
- Neoadjuvant chemotherapy refers to the use of chemotherapy as the initial therapy for localized cancers for which an alternative but less than completely effective local treatment is possible.
- Induction chemotherapy is used where no effective alternative treatment exists, such as for advanced cancers, and is prescribed when drugs are administered as the initial treatment for such cases.
- Concurrent chemotherapy, in the form of a radiosensitizer or radioprotector, and radiation is an expanding role for chemotherapy and is used in anal, esophageal, small cell lung cancer, and head and neck cancers to enhance the efficacy of radiation therapy.

Results and Prognosis

5-Year Versus 10-Year Survival Rate Increases

Survival rates have been used extensively to assess accomplishments of treatment. The most frequently used standard is 5-year survival, but as data have matured, later survival data have become available, particularly with the continuing maturation of the SEER program.[14] Survival rates, however, can be confounded by the earlier detection of cancer and improved by more definitive staging, both of which may add to or appear to lengthen survival, or do both. The Will Rogers phenomenon, aptly described by Ulfelder,[156] illustrates how improved staging appears to improve survival for each stage, but not overall survival. More recently, a better yardstick for measuring overall progress is decreasing the mortality rate. Mortality has the advantage of being a definitive end point, measurable by all investigators. Although overall cancer mortality is tending to fall, according to recent ACS data,[177] these figures are confounded by death from some cause, which at some time in each life is unavoidable.

The 5-year survival rate is most commonly chosen as a parameter to measure survival, and is indicative of the curability of the cancer (Fig. 1–15). It is a simple, convenient parameter but is based on a complex interplay of many factors. It depends on the accessibility of the cancer,

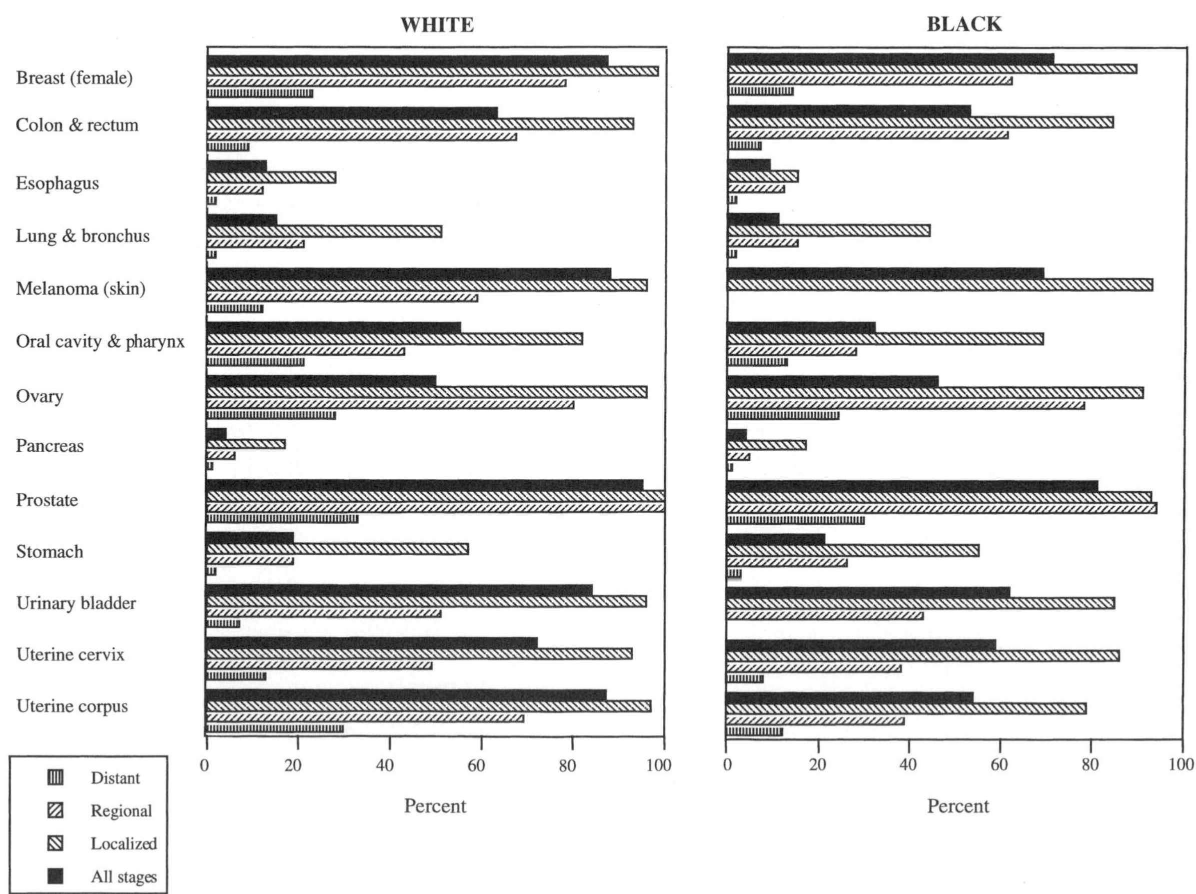

Figure 1–15. Five-year relative survival rates by race and stage at diagnosis, United States, 1986–1993. Staging is according to the SEER historical categories rather than AJCC staging system. The data source is the NCI Surveillance, Epidemiology and End Results Program, 1997. (From Landis SH, Murray T, Bolden S, et al: Cancer statistics, 1999. CA Cancer J Clin 1999; 49:8, with permission.)

TABLE 1–15. **Long-Term Relative Survival Rates for Patients Diagnosed, SEER Program, All Races, Men and Women**

	5-Year Relative Survival Rate (%)			10-Year Relative Survival Rate (%)	
Primary Site	***1973–75***	***1985***	***1989–94****	***1973–75***	***1985***
All sites	48	54	60†	41	48
Brain	18	26	30†	14	22
Breast	73	79	85†	60	69
Colon	48	60	63†	44	55
Esophagus	4	9	12†	3	6
Hodgkin's disease	66	80	82†	57	77
Kidney	49	57	61†	42	49
Larynx	64	69	66	51	56
Leukemias	33	42	43†	20	32
Liver	3	7	5†	2	7
Lung and bronchus	11	14	14†	8	10
Melanoma	76	86	88†	68	83
Multiple myeloma	23	28	29†	9	11
Non-Hodgkin's lymphomas	45	54	51†	33	44
Oral cavity and pharynx	51	54	53	41	45
Pancreas	3	3	4†	2	2
Prostate	67	78	93†	NA	68
Rectum	46	NA	61†	40	NA
Stomach	14	18	21†	11	15
Thyroid gland	91	93.2	95†	90	93
Urinary bladder	71	78.4	82†	63	75

SEER = Surveillance, Epidemiology and End Results; NCI = National Cancer Institute.
*Survival rates for 1989–1994 are adjusted for normal life expectancy and are based on follow-up of patients through 1995.
†The differences between 1973–1975 and 1989–1994 are statistically significant ($p < 0.05$).
Data sources are SEER statistics[13, 14] and NCI Surveillance, Epidemiology and End Results Program, 1998.

the stage in which the cancer is detected, the effectiveness of treatment, and the type of site harboring the cancer (Table 1–15). Some points of interest follow:

- Localized cancers are often highly curable, ranging from 50% to 80% in most sites.
- Regionalized lymph node involvement always portends more aggressive disease and is a poor prognostic factor, often reducing survival to 50% or less.
- Distant metastases are rarely curable, but still are compatible with 5-year survival ranging from 5% to 20%. This survival figure also reflects effective palliation by chemotherapeutic and hormonal agents.
- Survival is generally better in cancers located in accessible sites than in internal organs because they can be identified while in localized stages. This finding reflects the importance of early detection.

If one examines the trends in survival based upon End Results Group data and the SEER program over the past three decades using the 5-year results, there is evidence for a significant gain in survival for each decade for the majority of cancer sites (see Fig. 1–2 and Table 1–1). The most striking gains (>15%) have been made in colon, rectum, larynx, melanoma, breast (female), uterine (cervix and corpus), prostate, testis, bladder, kidney, thyroid, Hodgkin's, non-Hodgkin's lymphoma, multiple myeloma, and some of the leukemias. For long-term survival rates (all races, both sexes), the relative 5- and 10-year rates are 54% and 48%, respectively. The attrition rate is low and survival averages 57% (32% to 92%), indicating that most 5-year survivors live to 10 years, with a few exceptions such as in invasive cancers of the esophagus and pancreas. Table 1–15 provides the 5- and 10-year relative survival rates for 24 major primary sites; the relative rate is the ratio of observed survival rate to the general population survival rate and is an indirect adjustment for death due to causes other than cancer. The sites with the highest 10-year relative survival rates are thyroid (93%), melanoma (83%), bladder (75%), breast (69%), and Hodgkin's disease (77%).

Mortality (Premature or Cancer-Related Mortality) Rate Decreases

As noted, SEER data and ACS cancer statistics are now showing a decrease in mortality rates at virtually all sites, including lung, prostate, breast, and alimentary tract—the major sites. The decline has favored the white population over blacks, and men over women, −0.9% versus −0.1%, as a result of rising mortality from lung cancer for women.[177]

In a convincing analysis of years lost to cancer, Mettlin[178] illustrated the advances made through better diagnosis and treatment by age group as a function of decade. In the latest SEER data,[14] the largest percentage decrease in mortality rates was in the pediatric and young adult age group, from 0 to 14 years of age (48%). The mortality rates also have declined for the 15 to 34 years and 35 to 44 years age groups (28% and 26%, respectively), and even in the 45 to 54 years and 55 to 64 years groups, where rates have fallen 18% and 2%, respectively. A decline in mortality rate has occurred for most major cancer sites, even for lung cancer, although unfortunately the latter cancer continues to increase in incidence in the female population.[177]

In summary, standardized rates of years of life lost may be an excellent tool for measuring the success of cancer treatments. The evidence strongly suggests reductions in the cancer burden over the past three decades are real.

Lack of Uniformity in End-Stage Reporting

The lack of uniformity in end-stage reporting is a major source of confusion when comparing the results of different treatment modalities. As mentioned, this can be overcome by agreement on a dual anatomic-pathologic classification for each cancer site. Assuming that such a classification exists, the following common errors and points should be looked for:

1. The starting time for determination of survival recommended by the AJCC is the date of *treatment initiation* or the date tumor-directed treatment was decided on. This definition is used because it usually coincides with the date of clinical staging of the cancer.[149]
2. A probability of less than 5% ($p<0.05$) is generally considered to be of statistical significance in reference to 95% confidence limits.
3. The results should be in terms of *absolute survival*; that is, patients who are lost to follow-up are included. If they are excluded, the survival rate is inevitably better, and the survival figures are referred to as determinate or relative. Calculation by direct method is the simplest procedure for summarizing patient survival. This is done by calculating the percentage of patients alive at the end of the specified interval, such as 5 years, using only patients exposed to the risk of dying for the last 5 years.
4. The survival may be referred to as, for example, 3 months to 10 years with an "average" survival of 2.3 years. This is meaningless.
5. The 5-year survival rates should be designated *without recurrence* or, preferably, *disease-free*. For some carcinomas, such as breast cancer and thyroid neoplasm, this is not a long enough follow-up period.
6. Ideally, the presentation of data should be by "actuarial" or "life table" method, corrected for age and sex. This method is described by the AJCC[149]:
   a. Observed survival: "The actuarial or life table method uses all survival information accumulated to the closing date of the study and describes the manner in which patient depletion occurred during that period. It presents a survival pattern in which the patients who are lost to follow up are depleted in a mathematical calculation similar to the patent populations under continued follow-up; it is not a specified point in survival like the 5-year survival. Such data are often displayed graphically in journals as survival curves ranging from 1 year to 10 years."[179]
   b. Adjusted survival rate: This is usually higher than the observed survival and corrects for deaths from other causes for patients free of cancer at the time of death.
   c. Relative survival rate: The survival rate is adjusted for "normal mortality expectation" in a general population similar to the patient group in the study with respect to race, sex, age, and calendar period of observation.
   d. Disease-free survival rate: This is usually lower than the observed survival and corrects for patients living with cancer, either a local-regional recurrence or metastatic.

The pressure for investigators to publish and present early, and, therefore, to project survival rates, has led to false optimism regarding new forms of treatment. Premature survival curves plateau or are horizontal, reaching to infinity, or precipitously step vertically to zero, depending on the outcome of the first few patients treated. This was illustrated by a sobering analysis of a treatment of leukemia by Powles and co-workers,[180] who showed how the reported survival rate varied inversely with time from the completion of the study (Fig. 1–16).

Of additional note is that a statistical value of $p>0.05$ for median survival at the completion of a study, or shortly thereafter, does not predict improvement in later overall long-term survival. Only sufficient follow-up of a minimum of 5 years, or better 10 years, is the necessary test of time for true cancer cure. Also, it is a given rule that a significant number of patients must survive to project these 5-year and 10-year survival rates; otherwise, the numbers are misleading because of a large standard deviation.

Patterns of Failure and Corrective Strategies

In the analysis of treatment outcomes, patterns of failure—that is, the first evidence of relapse in recurrence of the cancer—are equally as important as survival rates. A corrective strategy will depend upon whether the primary tumor, the regional nodes, metastases, or combinations are formed at the time of the work-up of the first relapse. There are seven possible failure pathways, as noted in Figure 1–17.

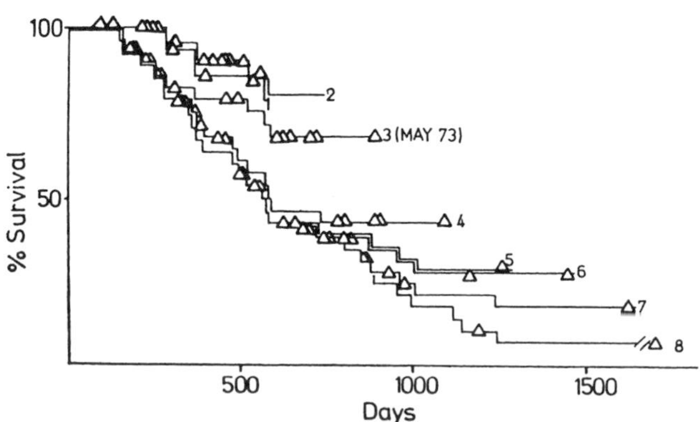

Figure 1–16. Sequential 6-month analysis of the duration of survival (from diagnosis) of 28 patients receiving chemo-immunotherapy. The first analysis (curve 1) was in May 1972; curve 3 (May 1973) corresponds to the entry of the last patient in the group; curves 4–8 are analyses at 6-month intervals thereafter. Triangles denote patients remaining alive and the curves drop each time a patient dies, by an amount proportional to the total number of patients in the study. (From Powles RL, Russell J, Lister TA, et al: Immunotherapy for acute myelogenous leukaemia: a controlled clinical study 2½ years after entry of the last patient. Br J Cancer 1977; 35:265, with permission.)

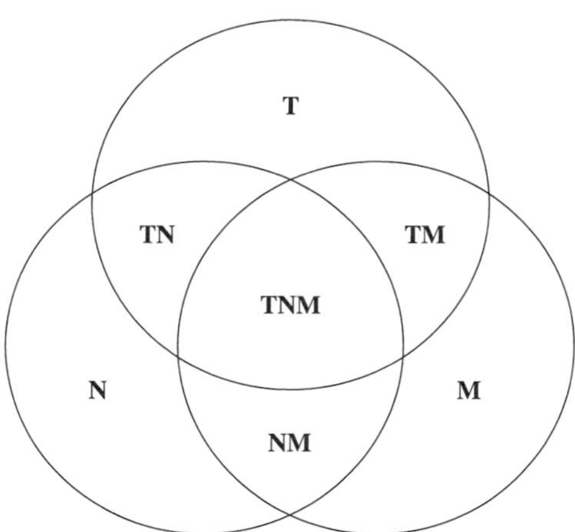

Figure 1–17. Venn diagram of seven failure pathways for tumor (T), node (N), metastases (M), and combinations.

Primary (T) Failures. Inability to control primary tumors, particularly in locally advanced stages when invasion of contiguous structures and viscera has occurred, remains a significant obstacle to cancer cure. As illustrated in Table 1–16, Suit[181] estimated the failure rate of advanced cancers at specific sites that are not easily eradicable: cancers of the oral cavity, oropharynx, and nasopharynx (T3, T4, N2, N3); gynecologic cancers of the cervix (stages III and IV), ovary (stage IIB), and vulva; and large advanced genitourinary cancers of the bladder (stages B and C) and prostate (stage C). Malignant brain tumors, such as glioblastoma multiforme, medulloblastoma, and mixed gliomas, which are locally invasive and rarely disseminate outside the central nervous system, illustrate the problem clearly.

Nodal (N) Failures. Nodal failures can occur at major node-bearing regions that drain the sites of invasive cancers. Metastatic lymph nodes, which can be difficult to control, include cervical nodes in head and neck cancer, axillary and supraclavicular nodes in breast cancer, mediastinal nodes in esophageal and lung cancers, para-aortic and pelvic nodes in gynecologic and genitourinary cancers, and mesenteric nodes in gastrointestinal cancers. As primary tumors are controlled, the N category is frequently seen as a major failure pathway; this failure has necessitated extended-field radiation treatment at many sites. The introduction of total nodal irradiation techniques for Hodgkin's and non-Hodgkin's lymphomas has focused on the control of nodal extensions, most often in contiguous or adjacent uninvolved nodes, by extending fields below the diaphragm for most presentations above the diaphragm.

TABLE 1–16. **Local/Regional Failure as Primary Cause of Death**

Tumor Site	Estimated No. of Deaths
Bone and connective tissue	1020
Breast	4774
Central nervous system	8277
Colorectal	20,760
Esophagus	3763
Head and neck	4700
Lung	8316
Lymphomas (excluding myeloma)	1872
Ovary	6480
Pancreas	12,000
Prostate	12,360
Skin	2240
Stomach	4380
Urinary bladder	4950
Uterine (cervix)	4366
Uterine (corpus)	1881
Total	102,139

From Suit HD: Statement of problem pertaining to the effect of dose fractionation and total treatment on the response to x-irradiation. In: Time and Dose Relationships in Radiation Biology as Applied to Radiotherapy. Upton, Brookhaven National Laboratory Report 50203 (C-57), 1969, with permission.

Metastatic (M) Failures. The majority of cancer patients fail as a result of disseminated disease. The most common cancers, breast and lung, are aggressive and metastasize in the early stages of growth, often before clinical detection. Undifferentiated and anaplastic cancers can metastasize aggressively; melanomas, sarcomas of the bone and soft tissue, choriocarcinomas, and ovarian cancers also may be widespread at the time of diagnosis. Although metastases affect more than one organ system, the documentation of the first metastatic site may suggest elective treatment to specific organs.

Combinations of TNM. Four additional failure pathways (TN, NM, TM, TNM) represent combinations of the TNM compartments (see Fig. 1–17). In many advanced cancers of the breast, lung, head and neck, and gynecologic sites (T3, T4, N2, N3 groupings in stages III and IV), both primary and nodal involvement are difficult to completely resect or eradicate by irradiation. For example, local control of the primary tumor may occur in testicular and ovarian tumors, but nodal and metastatic spread are the main failure pathways. Small cell cancer of the lung, other types of lung cancer, advanced gastric and rectal cancers, and pancreatic cancer can and often do fail in all three compartments. Although the T and N categories may be the overt areas of failure, better local control is certain to unmask occult metastases.

New therapeutic strategies for cancer control should be based on the failure patterns of a given cancer at each stage of presentation. Ideally, all modalities should be optimally combined to achieve the best control possible in the three compartments of TNM. Combined irradiation and chemotherapy will augment each other to control advanced disease in the primary (T) or nodal (N) compartments; in an additive and interactive manner, combined treatments can also be used to control overt or suspected occult metastases in the M compartment. Patients at high risk for recurrence are the optimal target group for clinical adjuvant trials and protocols investigating the elective addition of treatments.

Clinical Investigations

There is an increasing interest in the development of clinical trials[182, 183] to reconcile differences in therapeutic claims. This leads to combined-modality treatments in which various combinations of surgery, radiation therapy, and chemotherapy are used. A demonstration of significant gains from prospective trials and detailed protocols is essential for correct conclusions. The basis of the multidisciplinary approach to cancer management is for all responsible disciplines to be represented in the initial decision making. Unidisciplinary actions can determine a course of events that limits the application of other modalities. The clinical trial and the hospital tumor board offer a means of clinical interaction for patient care that is lacking in consultation following crisis and recurrence.

Cooperative controlled clinical studies are being developed to answer complex treatment questions. These are multidisciplinary undertakings, and they involve multiple universities and medical centers at both the national and, occasionally, the international levels. Although the hope for rapidly achieving good data lies in cooperative national protocols, this ideal will be difficult to achieve. It assumes that clinicians place all eligible patients on study, that pathologists at different institutions agree on classifications, and that treatment selection is unbiased. These criticisms notwithstanding, this seems to be the only practical solution to the dilemma presented by small patient series and long-term follow-up (5 to 10 years) for evaluation of results to become meaningful.[184]

The size and scope of clinical trials in cancer diagnosis and treatment are perhaps the largest such efforts undertaken in modern medicine. New procedures, new agents, and new combinations of agents and modalities are being evaluated in thousands of studies worldwide. These trials collectively cost hundreds of millions of dollars. Information on these trials is available from the National Institutes of Health, and includes phase I (toxicity), phase II (search for efficacy), and phase III (demonstrate if more effective than standard therapy). Computerized systems exist to provide on-line searching by key terminology of current trends and results.

Meta-Analysis

Meta-analysis is a quantitative summary of randomized clinical trials by combining results in one disease site, including all known studies that have been initiated, published and unpublished, and assessing therapeutic effectiveness or average results pooled across trials.[185] Meta-analysis is not an alternative to properly designed and sized randomized clinical trials.

Ethical Issues

Equipoise, as described by Fried, is a state of genuine uncertainty on the part of a clinical investigator or treating physicians regarding the comparative merit of different therapies for a specific disease process.[186] If equipoise exists, it is justifiable to conduct a randomized study. Nonetheless, when the medical community is faced by a sudden change in disease status, it has to be able to respond. This was seen in the response by the Food and Drug Administration to AIDS research. "Fast track" approval of promising cancer drugs, such as new AIDS agents, now allows for approval based on improvement of short-term "surrogate markers" rather than long-term survival and quality of life benefits.

Recommended Reading

There are many excellent general references on the subject of cancer and a large number of oncology journals exist entirely devoted to clinical and research reports. These include *Cancer*; *Seminars in Oncology*; *Journal of Clinical Oncology*; *American Journal of Clinical Oncology*; *International Journal of Radiation Oncology, Biology and Physics*; *Journal of Gynecologic Oncology*; and *Journal of Surgical Oncology*. Our favorite references for the student include the AFIP Tumor Fascicles in *Atlas of Tumor Pathology*[2] for detailed pathology at tumor sites, because these are beautifully illustrated. For general principles of cancer treatment, we recommend *Cancer: Principles & Practice of Oncology*, edited by DeVita and colleagues,[3] and also *Clinical Oncology*, edited by Abeloff and coworkers.[4] For the discipline of radiation oncology alone, the reader will be served well by *Principles and Practice of Radiation Oncology*, edited by Perez and Brady[5]; a relatively new addition to the literature is the highly informative *Textbook of Radiation Oncology*, in its first edition, edited by Leibel and Phillips.[6]

REFERENCES

General References

1. Ackerman LV, del Regato JA: Cancer: Diagnosis, Treatment and Prognosis. St. Louis, C.V. Mosby Co., 1977.
2. National Research Council Committee on Pathology: Atlas of Tumor Pathology. Washington, Armed Forces Institute of Pathology, 1950–present.
3. DeVita VT Jr, Hellman S, Rosenberg SA (eds): Cancer: Principles & Practice of Oncology, 5th ed. Philadelphia, Lippincott-Raven Publishers, 1997.
4. Abeloff MD, Armitage JO, Lichter AS, et al (eds): Clinical Oncology, 2nd ed. New York, Churchill Livingstone, 2000.
5. Perez CA, Brady LW (eds): Principles and Practice of Radiation Oncology, 3rd ed. Philadelphia, Lippincott-Raven Publishers, 1998.
6. Leibel SA, Phillips TL (eds): Textbook of Radiation Oncology. Philadelphia, W.B. Saunders Co., 1998.

Specific References

7. The Human Genome Project: Deciphering the Blueprint of Heredity. Mill Valley, University Science Books, 1994.
8. Culver KW: Gene Therapy. A Primer for Physicians, 2nd ed. Larchmont, Mary Ann Liebert Inc, 1996.
9. Greenlee RT, Murray T, Bolden S, et al: Cancer statistics, 2000. CA Cancer J Clin 2000; 50:7.
10. Landis SH, Murray T, Bolden S, et al: Cancer statistics, 1999. CA Cancer J Clin 1999; 49:8.
11. United States Bureau of the Census: Current Population Reports, P25–1127, National and State Population Estimates: 1990 to 1994. Washington, Government Printing Office, 1995.
12. United States Bureau of the Census: Current Population Reports, P25–1130, Population Projections of the United States, by Age, Sex, Race, and Hispanic Origin: 1995–2050. Washington, Government Printing Office, 1996.
13. SEER Cancer Statistics Review, 1973–1994: Tables and Graphs. NIH Publication No 97–2789. Bethesda, National Cancer Institute, 1997.
14. SEER Cancer Statistics Review, 1973–1995. NIH Publication No 98–2789. Bethesda, National Cancer Institute, 1998.
15. Simone JV, Lyons J: The evolution of cancer care for children and adults. J Clin Oncol 1998; 16:2904.
16. Rosenthal DS: Changing trends. CA Cancer J Clin 1998; 48:3.
17. Wingo PA, Landis S, Ries LAG: An adjustment to the 1997 estimate for new prostate cancer cases. CA Cancer J Clin 1997; 47:239.
18. Cole P, Rodu B: Declining cancer mortality in the United States. Cancer 1996; 78:2045.

19. Myers MH, Ries LAG: Cancer patient survival rates: SEER program results for 10 years of follow-up. CA Cancer J Clin 1989; 39:21.
20. National Center for Health Statistics: Vital Statistics of the United States, 1998. Washington, Public Health Service, 1998.
21. Miller BA, Kolonel LN, Bernstein L, et al: Racial/Ethnic Patterns of Cancer in the United States 1988–1992. NIH Publication No 96–4104. Bethesda, National Cancer Institute, 1996.
22. Parker SL, Johnston Davis K, Wingo PA, et al: Cancer statistics by race and ethnicity. CA Cancer J Clin 1998; 48:31.
23. Vijayakumar S, Winter K, Sause W, et al: Prostate-specific antigen levels are higher in African-Americans than in white patients in a multicenter registration study: Results of RTOG 94-12. Int J Radiat Oncol Biol Phys 1998; 40:17.
24. Chamberlain RM, Winter KA, Vijayakumar S, et al: Sociodemographic analysis of patients in radiation therapy oncology group clinical trials. Int J Radiat Oncol Biol Phys 1998; 40:9.
25. Renan MJ: Cancer genes: current status, future prospects, and applications in radiotherapy/oncology. Radiother Oncol 1990; 19:197.
26. Bishop JM: Molecular themes in oncogenesis. Cell 1991; 64:235.
27. Butz K, Hoppe-Seyler F: Viruses and cancer: molecular pathologic mechanisms of viral carcinogenesis. Immun Infekt 1995; 23:179.
28. Boice JD Jr, Lubin JH: Occupational and environmental radiation and cancer. Cancer Causes Control 1997; 8:309.
29. Weinstein IB, Carothers AM, Santella RM, et al: Molecular mechanisms of mutagenesis and multistage carcinogenesis. In: Mendelsohn J, Howley PM, Israel MA, et al (eds): The Molecular Basis of Cancer, p 59. Philadelphia, W.B. Saunders Co., 1995.
30. Stam K, Heisterkamp N, Grosveld G, et al: Evidence of a new chimeric bcr/c-abl mRNA in patients with chronic myelocytic leukemia and the Philadelphia chromosome. N Engl J Med 1985; 313:1429.
31. Wallace MR, Marchuk DA, Andersen LB, et al: Type 1 neurofibromatosis gene: identification of a large transcript disrupted in three NF1 patients. Science 1990; 249:181.
32. Miyoshi Y, Ando H, Nagase H, et al: Germ-line mutations of the APC gene in 53 familial adenomatous polyposis patients. Proc Natl Acad Sci U S A 1992; 89:4452.
33. Powell SM, Zilz N, Beazer-Barclay Y, et al: APC mutations occur early during colorectal tumorigenesis. Nature 1992; 359:235.
34. Wong AJ, Ruppert JM, Bigner SH, et al: Structural alterations of the epidermal growth factor receptor gene in human gliomas. Proc Natl Acad Sci U S A 1992; 89:2965.
35. Soussi T: p53 tumor suppressor gene. Bull Cancer 1993; 80:96.
36. Thibodeau SN, Bren G, Schaid D: Microsatellite instability in cancer of the proximal colon. Science 1993; 260:816.
37. Bronner CE, Morrison PT, Smith LG, et al: Mutation in the DNA mismatch repair gene homologue hMLH1 is associated with hereditary non-polyposis colon cancer. Nature 1994; 368:258.
38. Krontiris TG, Devlin B, Karp DD, et al: An association between the risk of cancer and mutations in the HRAS1 minisatellite locus. N Engl J Med 1993; 329:517.
39. Hastie ND, Dempster M, Dunlop MG, et al: Telomere reduction in human colorectal carcinoma and with aging. Nature 1990; 346:866.
40. Rainier S, Johnson LA, Dobry CJ, et al: Relaxation of imprinted genes in human cancer. Nature 1993; 362:747.
41. Makos M, Nelkin BD, Lerman MI, et al: Distinct hypermethylation patterns occur at altered chromosome loci in human lung and colon cancer. Proc Natl Acad Sci U S A 1992; 89:1929.
42. Harris CC: Chemical and physical carcinogenesis: advances and perspectives for the 1990s. Cancer Res 1991; 51(suppl 18):5023S.
43. Trosko JE: Role of low-level ionizing radiation in multi-step carcinogenic process. Health Physics 1996; 70:812.
44. Cho KR, Vogelstein B: Suppressor gene alterations in the colorectal adenoma-carcinoma sequence. J Cell Biochem Suppl 1992; 16G:137.
45. Moller H: Occurrence of carcinogens in the external environment: epidemiological investigations. Pharmacol Toxicol 1993; 72(suppl 1):39.
46. Stiller CA: International variations in the incidence of childhood carcinomas. Cancer Epidemiol Biomarkers Prev 1994; 3:305.
47. Hebert JR, Hurley TG, Olendzki BC, et al: Nutritional and socioeconomic factors in relation to prostate cancer mortality: a cross-national study. J Natl Cancer Inst 1998; 90:1637.
48. Trichopoulos D, Lipworth L, Petridou E, et al: Epidemiology of cancer. In: DeVita VT Jr, Hellman S, Rosenberg SA (eds): Cancer: Principles & Practice of Oncology, 5th ed, p 231. Philadelphia, Lippincott-Raven Publishers, 1997.
49. International Agency for Research on Cancer: IARC monographs 1 to 62. 1972–1995. Lyon, IARC Scientific Publications, 1972–1995.
50. Miller EC, Miller JA: Mechanisms of chemical carcinogenesis. Cancer 1981; 47:1055.
51. Robinson M, Bull RJ, Munch J, et al: Comparative carcinogenic and mutagenic activity of coal tar and petroleum asphalt paints used in potable water supply systems. J Appl Toxicol 1984; 4:49.
52. McKee RH, Plutnick RT: Carcinogenic potential of gasoline and diesel engine oils. Fundam Appl Toxicol 1989; 13:545.
53. Marczynski B, Marek W, Baur X: Ethylene oxide as a major factor in DNA and RNA evolution. Med Hypotheses 1995; 44:97.
54. Weiss W, Nash D: An epidemic of lung cancer due to chloromethyl ethers. 30 years of observation. J Occup Environ Med 1997; 39:1003.
55. Steenland K, Loomis D, Shy C, et al: Review of occupational lung carcinogens. Am J Ind Med 1996; 29:474.
56. Hayes RB: The carcinogenicity of metals in humans. Cancer Causes Control 1997; 8:371.
57. Vineis P, Pirastu R: Aromatic amines and cancer. Cancer Causes Control 1997; 8:346.
58. International Agency for Research on Cancer: IARC monographs evaluating carcinogenic risks to humans (suppl 7). Overall evaluations of carcinogenicity: An updating of IARC monographs 1–42. Lyon, IARC Scientific Publications, 1987.
59. International Agency for Research on Cancer: IARC monographs on the evaluation of the carcinogenic risk to humans, vol 50. Pharmaceutical Drugs. Lyon, IARC Scientific Publications, 1990.
60. Lipsett MB: Hormones, medications, and cancer. Cancer 1983; 51:2426.
61. Sagar SM: Oestrogen modulators and clear cell carcinoma of vagina. Lancet 1987; 1:913.
62. Sieber SM: The action of antitumor agents: a double-edged sword? Med Pediatr Oncol 1977; 3:123.
63. Urowitz MB, Lee P: The risks of antimalarial retinopathy, azathioprine lymphoma and methotrexate hepatotoxicity during the treatment of rheumatoid arthritis. Baillieres Clin Rheumatol 1991; 4:193.
64. Petru E, Schmahl D: Cytotoxic chemotherapy-induced second primary neoplasms: clinical aspects. Neoplasma 1991; 38:147.
65. Johansson SL, Cohen SM: Epidemiology and etiology of bladder cancer. Semin Surg Oncol 1997; 13:291.
66. Drake MJ, Nixon PM, Crew JP: Drug-induced bladder and urinary disorders. Incidence, prevention and management. Drug Safety 1998; 19:45.
67. Hirota Y, Matsumoto I, Aso T, et al: Hepatocellular carcinoma and bladder cancer as complications following five years of chemotherapy for acute myeloblastic leukemia. Jpn J Med 1990; 29:203.
68. Geissler K, Friedl J, Hauser I: Therapy of Hodgkin's disease. Wien Klin Wochenschr 1994; 106:309.
69. Hall EJ: Etiology of cancer: Physical factors. In: DeVita VT Jr, Hellman S, Rosenberg SA (eds): Cancer: Principles & Practice of Oncology, 5th ed, p 203. Philadelphia, Lippincott-Raven Publishers, 1997.
70. Modan B: Low-dose radiation carcinogenesis. Eur J Cancer 1992; 28A:1010.
71. Boice JD: Cancer following medical irradiation. Cancer 1981; 47:1081.
72. Howley PM, Ganem D, Kieff E: Etiology of cancer: Viruses. In: DeVita VT Jr, Hellman S, Rosenberg SA (eds): Cancer: Principles & Practice of Oncology, 5th ed, p 168. Philadelphia, Lippincott-Raven Publishers, 1997.
73. Hehlmann R, Schetters H, Kreeb G, et al: RNA-tumor viruses, oncogenes, and their possible role in human carcinogenesis. Klin Wochenschr 1983; 61:1217.
74. Hoppe-Seyler F, Butz K: Molecular mechanisms of virus-induced carcinogenesis: the interaction of viral factors with cellular tumor suppressor proteins. J Mol Med 1995; 73:529.
75. Fouchard N, Mahe A, Huerre M, et al: Cutaneous T cell lymphomas: Mycosis fungoides, Sézary syndrome and HTLV-I-associated adult T cell leukemia (ATL) in Mali, West Africa: a clinical, pathological and immunovirological study of 14 cases and a review of the African ATL cases. Leukemia 1998; 12:578.
76. Hisada M, Okayama A, Shioiri S, et al: Risk factors for adult T-cell leukemia among carriers of human T-lymphotropic virus type I. Blood 1998; 92:3557.

77. Wong SY, Sewell HF, MacGregor JE, et al: Epstein-Barr virus—a possible missing link in the initiation of cervical carcinogenesis? Med Hypotheses 1991; 35:219.
78. Chong JM, Fukayama M: Epstein-Barr virus associated gastric carcinoma: the genetic alteration and the expression of CD44 variant. Nippon Rinsho 1997; 55:381.
79. Brechot C: Molecular mechanisms of hepatitis B and C viruses related to liver carcinogenesis. Hepatogastroenterology 1998; 45(suppl 3):1189.
80. Buendia MA: Hepatitis B viruses and cancerogenesis. Biomed Pharmacother 1998; 52:34.
81. Burkitt DP: The discovery of Burkitt's lymphoma. Cancer 1983; 51:1777.
82. Lin CT, Dee AN, Chen W, et al: Association of Epstein-Barr virus, human papilloma virus, and cytomegalovirus with nine nasopharyngeal carcinoma cell lines. Lab Invest 1994; 71:731.
83. Rassekh CH, Rady PL, Arany I, et al: Combined Epstein-Barr virus and human papillomavirus infection in nasopharyngeal carcinoma. Laryngoscope 1998; 108:362.
84. Kingma DW, Weiss WB, Jaffe ES, et al: Epstein-Barr virus latent membrane protein-1 oncogene deletions: correlations with malignancy in Epstein-Barr virus-associated lymphoproliferative disorders and malignant lymphomas. Blood 1996; 88:242.
85. Lee DA, Hartman RP, Trenkner SW, et al: Lymphomas in solid organ transplantation. Abdom Imaging 1998; 23:553.
86. Koike K: Hepatitis B virus HBx gene and hepatocarcinogenesis. Intervirology 1995; 38:134.
87. Ren EC: Hepatitis B virus and hepatocellular carcinoma. Ann Acad Med Singapore 1996; 25:17.
88. Corboy JR, Garl PJ, Kleinschmidt-DeMasters BK: Human herpesvirus 8 DNA in CNS lymphomas from patients with and without AIDS. Neurology 1998; 50:335.
89. Fisher SG: Epidemiology: a tool for the study of human papillomavirus-related carcinogenesis. Intervirology 1994; 37:215.
90. Hoppe-Seyler F, Butz K: Cellular control of human papillomavirus oncogene transcription. Mol Carcinogen 1994; 10:134.
91. Villa LL: Human papillomaviruses and cervical cancer. Adv Cancer Res 1997; 71:321.
92. Mougin C, Bernard B, Lab M: Biology of papillomavirus II infections. Their role in the carcinogenesis of the cervix. Ann Biol Clin 1998; 56:21.
93. Huibregtse JM, Beaudenon SL: Mechanism of HPV E6 proteins in cellular transformation. Semin Cancer Biol 1996; 7:317.
94. De Luca A, Baldi A, Esposito V, et al: The retinoblastoma gene family pRb/p105, p107, pRb2/p130 and simian virus-40 large T-antigen in human mesotheliomas. Nat Med 1997; 3:913.
95. Mutti L, De Luca A, Claudio PP, et al: Simian virus 40-like DNA sequences and large-T antigen-retinoblastoma family protein pRb2/p130 interaction in human mesothelioma. Dev Biol Stand 1998; 94:47.
96. Ames BN, Gold LS: The causes and prevention of cancer: the role of environment. Biotherapy 1998; 11:205.
97. Bandera EV, Freudenheim JL, Graham S, et al: Alcohol consumption and lung cancer in white males. Cancer Causes Control 1992; 3:361.
98. Davidson BJ, Hsu TC, Schantz SP: The genetics of tobacco-induced malignancy. Arch Otolaryngol 1993; 119:1198.
99. Gupta PC, Murti PR, Bhonsle RB: Epidemiology of cancer by tobacco products and the significance of TSNA. Crit Rev Toxicol 1996; 26:183.
100. Berwick M, Schantz S: Chemoprevention of aerodigestive cancer. Cancer Metastasis Rev 1997; 16:329.
101. Palmer S: Diet, nutrition, and cancer. Prog Food Nutr Sci 1985; 9:283.
102. Eichholzer M: The significance of nutrition in primary prevention of cancer. Ther Umsch 1997; 54:457.
103. Willett WC: Nutrition and cancer. Salud Publica Mex 1997; 39:298.
104. Ferrone S, Chu T, Hellstrom KE: Tumor antigens recognized by monoclonal antibodies. In: DeVita VT Jr, Hellman S, Rosenberg SA (eds): Biologic Therapy of Cancer, 2nd ed, p 77. Philadelphia, Lippincott-Raven Publishers, 1995.
105. Ballesta AM, Molina R, Filella X, et al: Carcinoembryonic antigen in staging and follow-up of patients with solid tumors. Tumour Biol 1995; 16:32.
106. Olt G, Berchuck A, Bast RC Jr: The role of tumor markers in gynecologic oncology. Obstet Gynecol Surv 1990; 45:570.
107. Guadagni F, Roselli M, Cosimelli M, et al: TAG-72 expression and its role in the biological evaluation of human colorectal cancer. Anticancer Res 1996; 16:2141.
108. Posner MR, Mayer RJ: The use of serologic tumor markers in gastrointestinal malignancies. Hematol Oncol Clin North Am 1994; 8:533.
109. Grem J: The prognostic importance of tumor markers in adenocarcinomas of the gastrointestinal tract. Curr Opin Oncol 1997; 9:380.
110. Carrel S, Zografos L, Schreyer M, et al: Expression of CALLA/CD10 on human melanoma cells. Melanoma Res 1993; 3:319.
111. Anderson DR, Grillo-Lopez A, Varns C, et al: Targeted anti-cancer therapy using rituximab, a chimaeric anti-CD20 antibody (IDEC-C2B8) in the treatment of non-Hodgkin's B-cell lymphoma. Biochem Soc Trans 1997; 25:705.
112. Kemp JD, Smith KM, Mayer JM, et al: Effects of anti-transferrin receptor antibodies on the growth of neoplastic cells. Pathobiol 1992; 60:27.
113. Fan Z, Mendelsohn J: Therapeutic application of anti-growth factor receptor antibodies. Curr Opin Oncol 1998; 10:67.
114. Waldmann TA: Lymphokine receptors: a target for immunotherapy of lymphomas. Ann Oncol 1994; 5(suppl 1):13.
115. Witters LM, Kumar R, Chinchilli VM, et al: Enhanced anti-proliferative activity of the combination of tamoxifen plus HER-2-neu antibody. Breast Cancer Res Treat 1997; 42:1.
116. Torre EA, Salimbeni V, Fulco RA: The erbB 2 oncogene and chemotherapy: a mini-review. J Chemother 1997; 9:51.
117. Pegram MD, Lipton A, Hayes DF, et al: Phase II study of receptor-enhanced chemosensitivity using recombinant humanized anti-p185HER2/neu monoclonal antibody plus cisplatin in patients with HER2/neu-overexpressing metastatic breast cancer refractory to chemotherapy treatment. J Clin Oncol 1998; 16:2659.
118. Stevenson FK, George AJ, Glennie MJ: Anti-idiotypic therapy of leukemias and lymphomas. Chem Immunol 1990; 48:126.
119. Bhattacharya-Chatterjee M, Foon KA, Kohler H: Anti-idiotype monoclonal antibodies as vaccines for human cancer. Int Rev Immunol 1991; 7:289.
120. Tartour E, Fridman WH: Cytokines and cancer. Int Rev Immunol 1998; 16:683.
121. Kowalski LP, Medina JE: Nodal metastases: predictive factors. Otolaryngol Clin North Am 1998; 31:621.
122. Miller AB: Controversies in breast cancer screening. Cancer Prev Control 1997; 1:73.
123. Berry DA: Benefits and risks of screening mammography for women in their forties: a statistical appraisal. J Natl Cancer Inst 1998; 90:1431.
124. Taylor WR, Fontana RS, Uhlenhopp MA, et al: Some results of screening for early lung cancer. Cancer 1981; 47:1114.
125. Byers T, Levin B, Rothenberger D, et al: American Cancer Society guidelines for screening and surveillance for early detection of colorectal polyps and cancer: update 1997. CA Cancer J Clin 1997; 47:154.
126. Johnson BE, Linnoila RI, Williams JP, et al: Risk of second aerodigestive cancers increases in patients who survive free of small-cell lung cancer for more than 2 years. J Clin Oncol 1995; 13:101.
127. Underwood JCE: Introduction to Biopsy Interpretation and Surgical Pathology. New York, Springer-Verlag, 1987.
128. Sklar JL, Costa JC: Principles of cancer management: molecular pathology. In: DeVita VT Jr, Hellman S, Rosenberg SA (eds): Cancer: Principles & Practice of Oncology, 5th ed, p 259. Philadelphia, Lippincott-Raven Publishers, 1997.
129. Le Beau MM: Molecular biology of cancer. In: DeVita VT Jr, Hellman S, Rosenberg SA (eds): Cancer: Principles & Practice of Oncology, 5th ed, p 103. Philadelphia, Lippincott-Raven Publishers, 1997.
130. Rowley JD, Mitelman F: Principles of molecular cell biology of cancer: chromosome abnormalities in human cancer and leukemia. In: DeVita VT Jr, Hellman S, Rosenberg SA (eds): Cancer: Principles & Practice of Oncology, 4th ed. Philadelphia, J.B. Lippincott, 1993.
131. Brennan JA, Mao L, Hruban RH, et al: Molecular assessment of histopathological staging in squamous-cell carcinoma of the head and neck. N Engl J Med 1995; 332:429.
132. Liefers GJ, Cleton-Jansen AM, van de Velde CJ, et al: Micrometastases and survival in stage II colorectal cancer. N Engl J Med 1998; 339: 223.

133. Israeli RS, Miller WH Jr, Su SL, et al: Sensitive nested reverse transcription polymerase chain reaction detection of circulating prostatic tumor cells: comparison of prostate-specific membrane antigen and prostate-specific antigen-based assays. Cancer Res 1994; 54:6306.
134. Pelkey TJ, Frierson HF Jr, Bruns DE: Molecular and immunological detection of circulating tumor cells and micrometastases from solid tumors. Clin Chem 1996; 42:1369.
135. McLoud TC: CT and MR in pleural disease. Clin Chest Med 1998; 19:261.
136. Ott DJ, Wolfman NT, Scharling ES, et al: Overview of imaging in colorectal cancer. Dig Dis 1998; 16:175.
137. Kubal WS: The pathological globe: clinical and imaging analysis. Semin Ultrasound CT MR 1997; 18:423.
138. Brand RE, Matamoros A: Imaging techniques in the evaluation of adenocarcinoma of the pancreas. Dig Dis 1998; 16:242.
139. Bragg DG, Rubin P, Hricak H (eds): Oncologic Imaging, 2nd ed. Philadelphia, W.B. Saunders, 2001.
140. Front D, Bar-Shalom R, Israel O: The continuing clinical role of gallium 67 scintigraphy in the age of receptor imaging. Semin Nucl Med 1997; 27:68.
140a. Cheng G, Liu H, Yu Y: Image-guided brachytherapy. In: Bragg DG, Rubin P, Hricak H (eds): Oncologic Imaging, 2nd ed. Philadelphia, W.B. Saunders, 2001.
141. Del Maschio A, Panizza P: MR state of the art. Eur J Radiol 1998; 27(suppl 2):S250.
142. Castillo M, Kwock L, Scatliff J, et al: Proton MR spectroscopy in neoplastic and non-neoplastic brain disorders. Magn Reson Imaging Clin N Am 1998; 6:1.
143. Manyak MJ, Javitt MC: The role of computerized tomography, magnetic resonance imaging, bone scan, and monoclonal antibody nuclear scan for prognosis prediction in prostate cancer. Semin Urol Oncol 1998; 16:145.
144. Weynants P, Marchandise FX, Sibille Y: Pulmonary perspective: immunology in diagnosis and treatment of lung cancer. Eur Respir J 1997; 10:1703.
145. Goldenberg DM, Juweid M, Dunn RM, et al: Cancer imaging with radiolabeled antibodies: new advances with technetium-99m-labeled monoclonal antibody Fab fragments, especially CEA-scan and prospects for therapy. J Nucl Med Technol 1997; 25:18.
146. Sonoda Y, Kumabe T, Takahashi T, et al: Clinical usefulness of ^{11}C-MET PET and ^{201}T1 SPECT for differentiation of recurrent glioma from radiation necrosis. Neurol Med Chir 1998; 38:342.
147. Glantz MJ, Hoffman JM, Coleman RE, et al: Identification of early recurrence of primary central nervous system tumors by [^{18}F]fluorodeoxyglucose positron emission tomography. Ann Neurol 1991; 29:347.
148. Rubin P, Chen Y, Brasacchio RA: Staging and classification of the cancer and the host: a unified approach versus neotaxonomy. In: Perez CA, Brady LW (eds): Principles and Practice of Radiation Oncology, 3rd ed, p 213. Philadelphia, Lippincott-Raven Publishers, 1997.
149. AJCC Cancer Staging Manual, 5th ed. Philadelphia, Lippincott-Raven Publishers, 1997.
150. International Union Against Cancer: TNM Classification of Malignant Tumors, 5th ed. Berlin, Springer-Verlag, 1997.
151. World Health Organization: International Histological Classification of Tumors, Nos. 1–25. Geneva, World Health Organization, 1998.
152. World Health Organization: International Classification of Diseases for Oncology, 2nd ed. Geneva, World Health Organization, 1999.
153. Broders AC: The grading of carcinoma. Minn Med 1925; 8:726.
154. Denoix P: TNM classification. Bull Inst Nat Hyg (Paris) 1944; 1:1.
155. Rubin P: A unified classification of tumors: an oncotaxonomy with symbols. Cancer 1973; 31:963.
156. Ulfelder H: Current concepts in cancer: ovary. Classification systems. Int J Radiat Oncol Biol Phys 1981; 7:1083.
157. Krown SE, Testa MA, Huang J: AIDS-related Kaposi's sarcoma: prospective validation of the AIDS Clinical Trials Group staging classification. J Clin Oncol 1997; 15:3085.
158. Kessler M, Heywang-Kobrunner H, Westhaus R, et al: Imaging procedures in early cancer of the breast. Current status of screening and diagnosis. Chirurg 1991; 62:77.
159. Davis PL, McCarty KS Jr: Technologic considerations for breast tumor size assessment. Magn Reson Imag Clin North Am 1994; 2:623.
160. Mainprize KS, Mortensen NJ, Warren BF: Early colorectal cancer: recognition, classification and treatment. Br J Surg 1998; 85:469.
161. Okada K, Yamanaka Y, Hachiya T, et al: Clinical staging of prostate cancer. Nippon Rinsho 1998; 56:1963.
162. Nichols CR: Testicular cancer. Curr Probl Cancer 1998; 22:187.
163. Vinatier D, Dufour P, Cosson M, et al: Laparoscopy in gynaecological cancer. Surg Oncol 1996; 5:211.
164. Coleman CN, Harris JR: Current scientific issues related to clinical radiation oncology. Radiat Res 1998; 150:125.
165. Karnofsky DA, Abelmann WH, Craver LF, et al: The use of nitrogen mustards in the palliative treatment of carcinoma with particular reference to bronchogenic carcinoma. Cancer 1948; 1:634.
166. Cella DF, Bonomi AE: Measuring quality of life: 1995 update. Oncology 1995; 9:47.
167. Ferrans CE: Development of a conceptual model of quality of life. Sch Inq Nurs Pract 1996; 10:293.
168. Cella DF: Quality of life outcomes: measurement and validation. Oncology 1996; 10:233.
169. Bonomi AE, Cella DF, Hahn EA, et al: Multilingual translation of the Functional Assessment of Cancer Therapy (FACT) quality of life measurement system. Qual Life Res 1996; 5:309.
170. Waterhouse J, Metcalfe MC: Development of the sexual adjustment questionnaire. Oncol Nurs Forum 1986; 13:53.
171. Rubin P: Special issue: Late Effects of Normal Tissues (LENT) Consensus Conference, including RTOG/EORTC SOMA scales. San Francisco, California, August 26–28, 1992. Int J Radiat Oncol Biol Phys 1995; 31:1035.
172. Piccirillo JF, Feinstein AR: Clinical symptoms and comorbidity: significance for the prognostic classification of cancer. Cancer 1996; 77:834.
173. Piccirillo JF, Wells CK, Sasaki CT, et al: New clinical severity staging system for cancer of the larynx. Five-year survival rates. Ann Otol Rhinol Laryngol 1994; 103:83.
174. Piccirillo JF: Inclusion of comorbidity in a staging system for head and neck cancer. Oncology 1995; 9:831.
175. Pugliano FA, Piccirillo JF, Zequeira MR, et al: Clinical-severity staging system for oropharyngeal cancer: five-year survival rates. Arch Otolaryngol 1997; 123:1118.
176. Sarkaria JN, Mehta MP, Loeffler JS, et al: Radiosurgery in the initial management of malignant gliomas: survival comparison with the RTOG recursive partitioning analysis. Int J Radiat Oncol Biol Phys 1995; 32:931.
177. Wingo PA, Ries LA, Rosenberg HM, et al: Cancer incidence and mortality, 1973–1995: a report card for the U.S. Cancer 1998; 82:1197.
178. Mettlin C: Trends in years of life lost to cancer: 1970 to 1985. CA Cancer J Clin 1989; 39:33.
179. American Joint Committee on Cancer Staging and End-Results Reporting: Manual for Staging of Cancer, 3rd ed. Philadelphia, J.B. Lippincott, 1988.
180. Powles RL, Russell J, Lister TA, et al: Immunotherapy for acute myelogenous leukaemia: a controlled clinical study 2½ years after entry of the last patient. Br J Cancer 1977; 35:265.
181. Suit HD: Statement of problem pertaining to the effect of dose fractionation and total treatment on the response to X-irradiation. In: Time and Dose Relationships in Radiation Biology as Applied to Radiotherapy. Upton, Brookhaven National Laboratory Report 50203 (C-57), 1969.
182. Simon RM: Design and analysis of clinical trials. In: DeVita VT Jr, Hellman S, Rosenberg SA (eds): Cancer: Principles & Practice of Oncology, 5th ed, p 513. Philadelphia, Lippincott-Raven Publishers, 1997.
183. Pajak TF: Methodology of clinical trials. In: Perez CA, Brady LW (eds): Principles and Practice of Radiation Oncology, 3rd ed, p 231. Philadelphia, Lippincott-Raven Publishers, 1997.
184. Rubin P (ed): Current Concepts in Cancer: Cancer of the Urogenital Tracts, Parts I and II. Chicago, American Medical Association, 1969.
185. Collins R, Gray R, Godwin J, et al: Avoidance of large biases and large random errors in the assessment of moderate treatment effects: the need for systematic overviews. Stat Med 1987; 6:245.
186. Fried C: Medical Experimentation: Personal Integrity and Social Policy. Amsterdam, North-Holland Publishing, 1974.

2 *The Biology of Cancer*

RICHARD P. HILL, PHD, Experimental Therapeutics

The genetic code is the small dictionary which relates the four letter language of the nucleic acids to the twenty letter language of proteins.

FRANCIS CRICK
Life Itself: Its Origins and Nature

Perspective

It is often stated that cancer is many different diseases, and this is usually taken to mean that there are differences between cancers in different organs, such as breast or colon. However, it is also true that there is substantial variability between cancers of the same organ in different patients and that there is significant phenotypic heterogeneity among the cells of an individual cancer. It is this heterogeneity that makes cancer such a difficult disease to treat successfully and that provides the challenge to understanding the detailed causes of the disease. The unifying aspect of cancer is that it is a disease that involves the inappropriate and, ultimately, uncontrolled proliferation of cells. The loss of cellular growth control is the result of a series of genetic changes in the cells of the cancer, and it arises from a long process of variation and selection that is similar to the evolution of life itself. The variation arises because cancer cells tend to have an increased likelihood of undergoing genetic or epigenetic changes (i.e., they are genetically unstable), whereas the selection arises from the varied microenvironmental conditions to which the cells are exposed during tumor growth (and treatment). Tumor growth and development (progression) is thus both a cellular and a tissue phenomenon.

This chapter starts with a description of tumor progression, with an emphasis on genetic instability and on the basic concept that the development of cancer involves multiple genetic changes in cells. This is followed by a section on specific genetic changes associated with the development of individual cancers and on the role and known functions of oncogenes and tumor suppressor genes. The protein products of many of these genes are critical elements of the cellular pathways that control cell division and differentiation. This second section concludes with a brief discussion of how some viruses may be involved in the development of cancer in humans. The third section addresses the growth of tumors, with discussion of cell kinetics and current knowledge of the genes involved in control of the cell cycle. The death of cells by apoptosis is outlined, and the role of the extracellular matrix in the control of cellular growth and differentiation is described. Finally, there is a summary of current knowledge of the process of angiogenesis, which is critical for sustained tumor growth, and a discussion of metastasis formation.

Tumor Development

The Classic Model

The classic model of tumor development divides the process into three stages: initiation, promotion, and progression. *Initiation* is the process by which critical DNA damage becomes permanent in the cellular DNA as a result of cell division prior to repair or due to faulty repair. *Promotion* is defined as a process by which epigenetic events are thought to influence selectively the proliferation of the initiated cell(s), whereas *progression* involves further heritable changes that are acquired as the cell population divides and develops into a cancer. This classic model provides a convenient conceptual framework, but as discussed later, recent studies of the molecular basis of carcinogenesis have indicated that multiple changes in the genome are required for tumorigenesis, and these stages are better considered as part of a continuum of changes rather than as discrete steps.

Many of the important recent advances in our understanding of the malignancy process are dependent on information from earlier epidemiologic studies, which have identified familial predisposition to cancer. Such studies have assisted in the identification of genes in which mutations or deletions are associated with malignancy, such as the retinoblastoma *(RB1)* gene, the *TP53* gene in the Li-Fraumeni syndrome, the *BRCA1* and *BRCA2* genes involved in breast and ovarian cancer, and the *INK4A* gene in melanoma. Studies of cancer incidence in individuals who have inherited genetically based defects in DNA repair have also demonstrated the involvement of DNA repair genes in the prevention of malignancy, particularly the genes involved in mismatch repair (implicated in human nonpolyposis colon cancer) and in excision repair (implicated in skin cancers in xeroderma pigmentosum).

Epidemiologic studies have also identified various environmental factors as likely to be involved in cancer development. These include tobacco, alcohol, multiple components of diet, sun exposure, ionizing radiation, and various occupational exposures (e.g., asbestos). It is likely that chemicals in tobacco smoke, which may be converted to active carcinogens by metabolism in the body, result in

DNA damage and mutations in affected cells. Smokers have a 10- to 15-fold increased risk of lung cancer and lower, but significantly increased risks for other cancers, such as head and neck and bladder carcinomas. These risks may be partially affected by genetic susceptibilities associated with polymorphisms in the (cytochrome p450) enzymes that are responsible for metabolizing some of the chemicals to their active form.[1] Melanoma and skin cancers are also likely induced by DNA damage, in this case, caused by the ultraviolet component of sunlight. Cancer incidence is associated with increasing sun exposure, and up to 50% of skin cancers have been found to have mutations in the *TP53* gene, most of which are consistent with ultraviolet damage.[2]

Fat intake shows a strong association with the incidence of a number of cancers, including prostate, breast, and colorectal carcinoma, but detailed mechanisms explaining this association have not yet been established. Exposure to asbestos dust has been associated with mesothelioma, a rare cancer in the chest, but again the explanation for this effect is unknown. Extensive studies of the survivors of the A-bomb attack on Hiroshima and Nagasaki in 1945 have established that exposure to ionizing irradiation can cause an increased risk of cancers in many organs. Again, it is likely that this is due to DNA damage caused by the radiation exposure. The risk is directly related to the dose of radiation received and is different for different tissues. It appears to be highest for leukemia with people exposed to 1 sievert (Sv) having a four- to five-fold increased risk. For lung cancer, a similar dose increases risk by about two-fold. A comparison with the increased risk of lung cancer from smoking indicates that smoking about 10 cigarettes per day is equivalent to an exposure of about 3.5 Sv, which is over 1000 times the average yearly exposure level due to background radiation (2 to 3 mSv).[3]

Genetic Instability

Tumor progression was described originally by Foulds[4] as "the acquisition of permanent, irreversible, qualitative changes of one or more characteristics of a neoplasm." Nowell[5] hypothesized that progression occurs because acquired genetic changes in individual cancer cells result in a growth advantage for that cell and that this leads to the sequential selection of more aggressive subpopulations of cells as the cancer grows. Inherent in this idea is that one or more of these changes promotes genetic instability, which increases the probability that further genetic changes will occur. Recent studies of signal transduction pathways in cells have indicated that many aspects of normal cell growth, differentiation, and death are controlled by a balance of positive and negative signals arising from both inside and outside the cell. In cancers, this balance is disturbed as a result of alterations in the gene products involved. A change in its ability to respond to a specific signal can cause a cell to proliferate in the face of other signals that would normally prevent such proliferation. Many of these controlling signals are cell- and tissue-type specific, so the gene alterations that provide for a growth advantage may be different in different tissues. Thus, cancers of different organs are likely to contain cells with genetic alterations specific to that disease site, as well as those that are more general. There are also many redundancies in the genes involved in cellular growth control, so even in the same tissue, the development of a cancer can arise from different genetic changes.

The rapid evolution of techniques for characterization and cloning of genes has provided support for the Nowell hypothesis that multiple genetic changes are involved in the development of malignancy. Current estimates of the required number of genetic changes suggest as few as two to at least six changes for different malignancies. Also, individual tumor cells probably contain many other changes that are not essential for maintaining the malignant phenotype. These genetic changes may arise either directly or indirectly from such factors as inherited gene mutations, chemical- or radiation-induced DNA damage, incorporation of certain viruses into the cell, or random errors during DNA synthesis. A paradigm for tumor progression has been presented by Fearon and Vogelstein.[6] This model, which was developed for colon cancer (Fig. 2–1), proposes that a mutation in a gene called *APC* (adenomatous polyposis coli) results in an increased level of proliferation in a cell (or cells) in the normal mucosal tissue in the gut lining. Hypomethylation of DNA, activation of the *KRAS* proto-oncogene, and loss of the *DCC* (deleted in colon cancer) gene are involved in the progression to benign adenoma. Mutation of the *TP53* gene and other chromosomal losses are involved in the progression to malignant carcinoma and metastasis. Activating mutations of the *KRAS* gene have been found in 50% of colon cancers, and both copies of *DCC* appear to be inactivated in large adenomas and in carcinomas. Although many cancers may arise following this orderly sequence of events, all colon cancers are not likely to have the exact sequence, nor does the path to a colon cancer always involve all these genes.

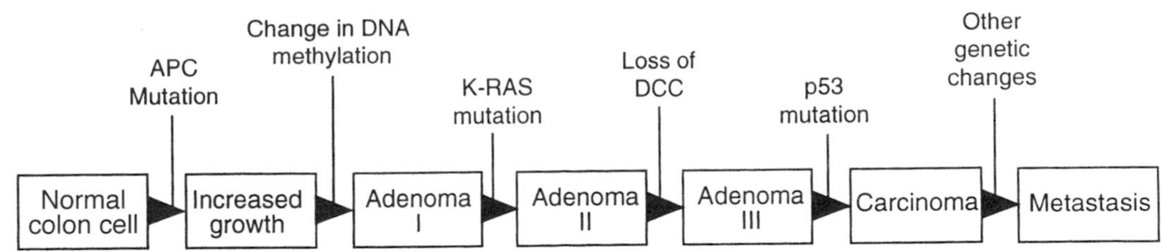

Figure 2–1. A model for genetic changes and progression in colon cancer. (Modified from Fearon ER, Vogelstein B: A genetic model for colorectal tumor genesis. Cell 1990; 61:759.)

Genetics of Cancer

Overview

Most mutations in cancer cells are somatic and therefore are found only in the tumor cells. However, about 1% of all cancers occur in individuals who carry an identified germline mutation in every cell in their body. The primary strategy for identifying inherited cancer genes has been *linkage analysis*. Large multigenerational families that have an unexpectedly high incidence of certain cancers, for example, that occur at unusually young ages, are studied to establish the gene or genes that cosegregate (i.e., that are found in the same family members) with the development of cancer. Using this approach, more than 20 cancer syndromes have been identified (Table 2–1). Most of the genes that have been identified are expressed in a wide range of tissues, but the individuals with those genes usually have a predisposition to only certain types of cancer. This factor emphasizes the importance of the interaction of the products of these genes with tissue-specific factors in the development of cancers.

The simplest classification of these genes is that those in which the function of both alleles is lost due to inactivating mutations or deletions are known as *tumor suppressor genes*, whereas those that have so-called gain-of-function or activating mutations are called *oncogenes*. Linkage analysis has limitations associated with variable penetrance and genetic heterogeneity. Studies of partially inbred populations, such as the Mormons in Utah, suggest that up to 10% to 15% of cancers may have inherited traits. Identification of the genes involved is difficult, however, and will require the application of one or more complex strategies, such as comparative genomic hybridization,[7] genomic mismatch scanning,[8] and analysis of differences in the DNA or mRNA in tumor and normal cells using gene-chip (DNA array) technologies.[9]

The cells of most cancers contain chromosomal abnormalities, and many of these aberrations influence the functioning of oncogenes and tumor suppressor genes. The best-known chromosomal abnormality is the Philadelphia chromosome that is present in about 90% of patients with chronic myelogenous leukemia (CML). This reciprocal translocation, which occurs between the long arms of chromosomes 9 and 22, results in the juxtaposition of the *ABL* oncogene from chromosome 9 with the *BCR* gene on chromosome 22. The fusion protein that results has ele-

TABLE 2–1. **Some Inherited Cancer Syndromes and (Tumor Suppressor) Genes Involved**

Syndrome	Tumor	Tumor Suppressor Gene	Chromosome Location	Proposed Function
Familial retinoblastoma	Retinoblastoma Osteosarcoma	*RB1*	13q14.3	Cell cycle and transcriptional regulator; E2F binding
Li-Fraumeni syndrome	Sarcoma, breast, brain, leukemia	*TP53*	17p12–13	Transcription factor, responds to DNA damage and stress, apoptosis
Familial adenomatous polyposis	Colorectal	*APC*	5q21	Regulation of β-catenin
Neurofibromatosis types 1 and 2	Neurofibroma	*NF1*	17q11.2	GTP-activating protein (GAP) for ras signalling
	Acoustic neuroma	*NF2*	22q12.2	Links membrane proteins to cytoskeleton
Multiple endocrine neoplasia types 1 and 2	Pancreatic (islet cell)	*MEN1*	11q13	Unknown
	Medullary thyroid	*RET*	10q11.2	Receptor tyrosine kinase
Familial breast cancer	Breast, ovarian	*BRCA1*	17q21	Involved in cellular growth control and DNA repair
	Breast	*BRCA2*	13q12	
Wilms' tumor	Wilms' tumor (kidney)	*WT1*	11p13	Transcriptional repressor
Nevoid basal cell cancer	Basal cell	*PTCH*	9q22.3	Transmembrane receptor
Von Hippel–Lindau syndrome	Renal (clear cell)	*VHL*	3p25	Regulates production of VEGF under oxic conditions
Hereditary papillary renal cancer	Renal (papillary type)	*MET*	7q31	Receptor for hepatocyte growth factor
Hereditary nonpolyposis colorectal cancer	Colorectal	*MSH2*	2p16	DNA mismatch repair
		MLH1	3p21	
		PMS1	2q32	
		PMS2	7p22	
Familial melanoma	Melanoma	*INK4A* (p16)	9p21	Cyclin-dependent kinase inhibitor
		CDK4	12q13	Cyclin-dependent kinase
Ataxia telangiectasia	Lymphoma	*ATM*	11q22	DNA repair; induction of p53
Bloom's syndrome	Solid tumors	*BLM*	15q26.1	DNA helicase
Xeroderma pigmentosum	Skin	*XPA*	9q34	DNA repair helicases
		XPB	2q21	Nucleotide excision repair
		XPC	3p25	
		XPD	19q13.2	
		XPE		
		XPF	16p13	
		XPG	13q32–33	
Fanconi's anemia	Acute myeloid leukemia	*FACC*	9q22.3	DNA repair
		FACA	16q24.3	

vated levels of tyrosine-specific protein kinase activity, and transfection of murine bone marrow cells with this fusion protein has resulted in induction of a condition similar to CML.

Tumor Suppressor Genes

Inactivation of tumor suppressor genes (see Table 2–1) can occur by mutation or deletion. Analysis of constitutively deleted regions on chromosome 13, associated with inherited retinoblastoma, led to the development of the "two-hit" model of carcinogenesis in which it was postulated that, for certain genes, both alleles needed to be inactivated for tumorigenesis to occur.[10] This inactivation of both alleles often occurs by a process known as *loss-of-heterozygosity (LOH)*. For many genetic loci, there is heterogeneity between the alleles of genes on the paternal and maternal chromosomes. One allele of a tumor suppressor gene may be inactivated in the germline, or it may be inactivated by a somatic mutation. Recombination may then occur prior to division, resulting in the mutated allele being carried on both copies of the chromosome in a cell. This loss of heterozygosity results in inactivation of the gene, since both copies in the cell are mutated or deleted. Thus, sites of LOH in tumor cells may give clues about the location of putative tumor suppressor genes.

The analyses of deleted regions of chromosome 13 eventually led to the identification of the first tumor suppressor gene, the retinoblastoma gene *RB1*, which, as discussed in this chapter (see "Genetic Control of the Cell Cycle"), codes for an important protein in the control of the cell cycle. In inherited cases of retinoblastoma, one allele is mutated in the germline. In both inherited and sporadic cases, both alleles are inactivated in the tumor cells, with about 70% of the cases showing LOH and the other 30% showing an independent mutation of the second allele. Inactivation of *RB1* predisposes to osteosarcoma, as well as retinoblastoma, and there may be some association with breast, bladder, and lung cancer. Since the *RB1* gene is expressed in all cells, it is not understood why the loss of RB protein predisposes to retinoblastoma and osteosarcoma in particular. Molecular analysis of regions showing loss of heterozygosity in tumors has allowed the identification of a number of other tumor suppressor genes, including *NF2*, the neurofibromatosis type 2 gene, and *MEN1*, the multiple endocrine neoplasia type 1 gene.

The best-known tumor suppressor gene is the *TP53* gene, since mutations in this gene are among the most common in human cancers. The gene is located on the short arm of chromosome 17 and codes for a 393-amino acid nuclear phosphoprotein that forms a tetramer, which has a number of different functions including that of a transcription factor. The protein is not required for normal development, since p53 knockout mice develop normally, but it appears to act as a critical component of the cellular machinery for response to DNA damage. Following DNA damage, levels of the p53 protein in the cell rise to initiate either a block in the cell cycle (in G_1 phase by upregulation of the p21 protein; see "Genetic Control of the Cell Cycle") or to induce apoptosis (see "Angiogenesis"). There is also evidence that the p53 protein may participate in protein complexes involved in DNA repair. Mutations in the *TP53* gene in cancers have been found to occur primarily in the specific DNA binding region and a number of hot spots have been identified.[5–7] Lack of function of *TP53* allows cells that have sustained genetic damage to survive and proliferate, and such cells have been found to have a higher incidence of genetic instability and gene amplification. It is likely that the failure to block proliferation or induce apoptosis in such cells is the reason that the inactivation of *TP53* contributes to malignancy. Mutant *TP53* may also have properties of an oncogene, because certain mutations lead to mutant protein products that can block the function of normal p53 protein, presumably because tetramers that contain one or more mutant subunits are inactive. Heterozygous mutations of the *TP53* gene are carried in the germline of about 70% of patients with the Li-Fraumeni syndrome, a rare condition that is characterized by the occurrence, at an early age, of diverse mesenchymal and epithelial tumors.

DNA repair proteins may also act as tumor suppressor genes. A number of syndromes that are known to involve defective DNA repair are associated with increased risk of malignancy. These include ataxia-telangiectasia syndrome (AT), xeroderma pigmentosum (XP), Fanconi's anemia, and Bloom's syndrome, as well as hereditary nonpolyposis colon cancer. The cells of patients with XP are defective in excision repair as a result of a mutation in one of the various genes involved in this pathway, and these patients have a high incidence of skin cancer associated with exposure to sunlight. Cells from patients with AT are extremely sensitive to ionizing radiation and have delayed upregulation of p53 protein levels following irradiation. Patients with AT have an increased incidence of lymphomas. The gene responsible for AT, *ATM*, codes for a large protein that is believed to act in a signal transduction pathway, which is activated in cells in the presence of DNA damage, probably upstream of p53. Cells from AT heterozygotes are often found to have a radiosensitivity intermediate between homozygotes and normals. Epidemiologic studies suggest that AT heterozygotes have an increased risk of breast cancer, but results from recent molecular studies are equivocal on this issue.[11]

Hereditary nonpolyposis colon cancer is a common inherited cancer syndrome that may account for about 5% of all colon cancers. It is associated with defective mismatch repair. Mismatch repair (also known as replication error repair) is a system capable of repairing DNA mispairs, which may arise in regions of repeating mono- or dinucleotides, where the DNA polymerase can apparently slip sideways leaving small 3 to 4 base deletions or insertions that result in single-stranded loops in the replicated DNA. Lack of a mismatch repair system leads to an increased frequency of mutations which, in turn, predisposes to the development of malignancy. Some of the genes involved in this repair process (see Table 2–1) were identified as a result of their homology with known mismatch repair genes in *Escherichia coli*.

The identified genes associated with familial breast and ovarian cancer, *BRCA1* and *BRCA2*, may also act as tumor suppressor genes through a role in DNA repair. Both gene products have been shown to interact either directly or indirectly with the yeast Rad 51 protein, which functions in the repair of DNA double-strand breaks. Unlike other inherited tumor suppressor genes, *BRCA1* or *BRCA2* mutations are rare in sporadic forms of breast and ovarian cancer. Between them, *BRCA1* and *BRCA2* mutations are believed to be involved in about 90% of familial breast cancers, which accounts for about 5% of all breast cancer patients.

Oncogenes

The initial identification of oncogenes (Table 2–2) arose from the finding that these genes (so-called v-oncs) were critical elements in cancer-causing, RNA-containing (retro) viruses, although it soon became apparent that these genes were closely related to normal cellular genes (known as proto-oncogenes or c-oncs). These proto-oncogenes had become incorporated into the viral genome and various alterations in their structure and regulation had occurred. Other oncogenes have been identified in tumors of nonviral origin by strategies such as transfection of DNA from tumor cells into immortal (see "Characteristics of Tumor Cells") rodent cells in culture and identification of the DNA segments responsible for the transformation that can occur in some of the cells. Such a strategy was used to identify the *HRAS* oncogene in human EJ bladder carcinoma cells. This oncogene was found to carry an activating point mutation in codon 12 that resulted in a change from a valine to a glycine in the corresponding p21-ras protein. Other forms of this proto-oncogene, which are often found to be mutated in human tumors, include the *KRAS* and *NRAS* genes. Activating mutations in the 13th and 61st codons have also been identified in activated forms of the *RAS* genes. In normal cells in culture (not immortal), it is often found that transfecting mutant *RAS* alone is insufficient to convert the cells to transformed cells and that the action of a second oncogene or tumor suppressor gene such as *MYC* or *TP53* is required for transformation. This necessity for interaction between oncogenes is consistent with the multihit concept of tumor development discussed above and may arise because the activity of a single oncogene can result in unbalanced growth stimulation leading to the induction of apoptosis (see "Cell Death and Apoptosis"). In this model, the second oncogene is thought to be required to block this effect.

The other main mechanisms by which oncogenes may be activated are translocation and gene amplification, which may result in an altered gene product or a change in the regulation of the level of expression of the gene product. The activation of the *ABL* oncogene as a result of translocation was discussed earlier in relation to the Philadelphia chromosome in CML. A similar situation arises in Burkitt's lymphoma, in which the *MYC* oncogene on chromosome 8 becomes translocated close to one of the immunoglobulin genes on either chromosomes 2 (κ-light chain), 14 (constant region heavy chain), or 22 (λ-light chain); this results in a change in the control of the expression of the *MYC* gene.

Gene amplification occurs as a result of regions of the genome undergoing several rounds of DNA synthesis during the same cell cycle. The amplified region is often several hundred kilobases in size, so that more than one gene may be involved and there may be multiple copies. Regions of amplification may be present in the chromosome at the original site of the genes involved, as small extrachromosomal fragments called double minutes (DMs), or as homologously staining regions (HSRs) in chromosomes that do not normally contain the gene. For example, cells from human neuroblastomas often contain HSRs that contain amplified copies of the *NMYC* gene, whereas amplified copies of the *LMYC* gene are often found in cell lines derived from human small cell lung cancer. The *HER2/NEU* oncogene (also known as *ERBB2*) is often found to be amplified in breast and ovarian cancers.

Oncogenes and Signal Transduction

A list of oncogenes that were identified primarily by their actions in rodent cells, together with their known functions and associated human cancers, if known, is given in Table 2–2. Most of these oncogenes encode proteins with a range of functions associated with the regulation of cellular response to external signals that induce cellular growth and

TABLE 2–2. **Some Oncogenes, Their Functions and Associated Human Cancers**

Oncogene	Function	Associated Human Cancer
SIS	Platelet-derived growth factor	
ERBB1	Epidermal growth factor receptor	
FMS	CSF-1 receptor	
KIT	Stem cell growth factor receptor	
MET	Hepatic growth factor receptor	Papillary renal cancer
HER2/NEU/ERBB2	Heregulin receptor	Breast cancer, ovarian cancer, bladder cancer, glioblastoma
RET	Neurotrophic factor receptor	Medullary thyroid cancer
TRKA	Nerve growth factor receptor	
ERBA	Thyroid hormone receptor (nuclear)	
RAS (H, K, N)	GTPase	Lung cancer, pancreatic cancer, bladder cancer, colorectal cancer
BCR-ABL	Cytoplasmic tyrosine kinase	Chronic myelogenous leukemia
RAF	Cytoplasmic tyrosine kinase	
SRC	Cytoplasmic tyrosine kinase	
FOS	Transcription factor	
JUN	Transcription factor	
MYC (c, L, N)	Transcription factor	Burkitt's lymphoma, neuroblastoma, lung cancer
BCL6	Transcription factor	Large-cell lymphoma
BCL2	Anti-apoptosis	Prostate cancer, lymphoma

differentiation. These proteins include growth factors, growth factor receptors, members of the MAP (mitogen-activated protein) kinase signal transduction pathways and transcription factors, which control the expression of other genes. The linkage of these various functions is illustrated in Figure 2–2,[12] which shows an extracellular growth factor interacting with its specific (growth factor) receptor, resulting in the formation of receptor dimer. The receptor is a transmembrane protein, and the intracellular portion contains a region that has tyrosine kinase activity. The formation of a dimer following binding to the growth factor facilitates autophosphorylation of tyrosine residues in the intracellular region of the receptor. These phosphorylated tyrosine residues can, in turn, bind to SH-2 (src homology-2) domains in linking molecules that are required for interaction with the RAS-GDP complex. This complex is associated with the inner surface of the plasma membrane and acts as a form of on-off switch. RAS-GDP is the *off* configuration; binding to the linker molecules catalyzes the exchange of GDP for GTP and its conversion to the *on* form, the RAS-GTP complex. This activated form of RAS-GTP can then phosphorylate the serine-threonine kinase RAF1, which initiates a signal cascade through the MAP (ERK)-kinase mitogenic signal transduction pathways. This culminates in the activation of transcription factors, such as *fos, jun*, and *myc*, which can initiate the production of the proteins necessary for cell proliferation.

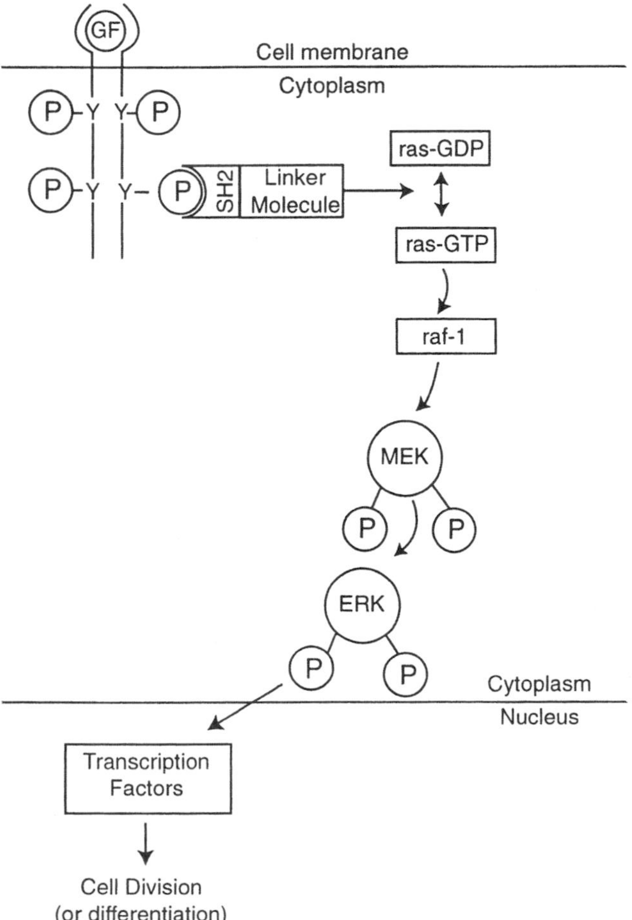

Figure 2–2. Cytoplasmic signaling cascade in the MAP (ERK)-kinase pathway. For description see text. (Modified from Tannock IF, Hill RP (eds): The Basic Science of Oncology, 3rd ed. New York, McGraw-Hill, 1998.)

The ERK-kinase (extracellular regulated kinase) pathway is one of three similar signal MAP-kinase pathways in cells and is primarily involved in stimulation of proliferation or differentiation. The other two MAP-kinase pathways, the SAPK (stress-activated protein kinase) and $p38^{HOG}$ pathways, are associated with the response of cells to stress and can initiate an apoptotic response leading to cell death or the production of inflammatory cytokines. Blocking the activation of the SAPK pathway can result in cells surviving stresses, such as heat-shock and some forms of chemotherapy, that would otherwise cause cell death, whereas blocking the $p38^{HOG}$ pathway has an anti-inflammatory effect. The stress response pathways have a parallel kinase cascade to that of the ERK-kinase pathway. All of these pathways are further regulated by specific kinases or phosphorylases that can reverse the action of the kinases or activate other kinases, which can initiate inactivating phosphorylation events at other sites on the proteins involved.

Aberrant levels of expression of growth factors produced by cancer cells can stimulate the ERK-kinase mitogenic pathway, although few growth factors have yet been definitively linked to the induction of human cancers. Several viral and cellular oncogenes encode mutated growth factor receptors that are not dependent on their (growth factor) ligand for activation, such as the ERBB receptors, which are analogues of the epidermal growth factor receptor (EGFR). One of these, *HER2/NEU*, can be activated by a single point mutation that results in constitutive dimerization. Amplification of these receptors, which leads to amplification of the signal, has been observed in a number of human cancers, including breast and bladder carcinoma and glioblastoma.

The normal RAS-GTP complex has GTPase activity, which results in the conversion of RAS-bound GTP to GDP and therefore to autoinactivation of the complex. Activating mutations in the *RAS* gene result in the loss of this GTPase activity and hence to the complex being more likely to be in the RAS-GTP *on* mode. Mutations in *KRAS* are commonly observed in lung, colorectal, and pancreatic carcinomas in humans, whereas *HRAS* is often mutated in oral and bladder cancers. Deregulation of the expression of transcription factors, such as *jun* or *myc*, through mutation or amplification as discussed above, can lead to abnormalities of the control of growth and cell differentiation.

Viruses and Cancer Development

Many different retroviruses have been found to be capable of inducing transformation of animal cells and of inducing cancer in animals. These viruses have a high efficiency for (random) integration into the host genome of cells, and they either carry an oncogene as part of their genome or act by inserting close to, and modifying the expression of, cellular proto-oncogenes. The only human cancer known to be associated with a retrovirus is adult T-cell leukemia (ATL), which is a rare form of leukemia endemic in certain parts of Japan, South America, Africa, and the southeastern United States. The virus involved is HTLV-1 (human T-cell leukemia virus 1), which is related to HIV, the human immunodeficiency virus implicated in AIDS. The HTLV-1 infects T-cells, but it does not carry an oncogene or act by insertional mutagenesis. The exact mechanism of transformation remains unclear, but one of the proteins encoded by the viral genome, *TAX,* has transcriptional activity for a number of cellular proteins, including interleukin-2 (IL-2), the IL-2 receptor and the proto-oncogenes, *SIS* and *FOS*. Recently, Kaposi's sarcoma (KS), which is frequently associated with HIV infection, has been associated with the TAT protein, which is encoded by HIV. This protein can be released by infected T-cells and has been found to act as a growth factor for KS cells. There is also evidence that a DNA-containing virus, human herpes virus 8 (HHV-8), may play a role in the development of Kaposi's sarcoma.

Several other DNA-containing viruses also have been associated with malignancy. The papovaviruses, SV40 and polyoma, and a few adenoviruses cause tumors in rodents and can transform their cells in culture, but they have not been associated directly with human cancers. In contrast, papillomaviruses are implicated in a number of human tumors, including benign warts and anogenital tumors. Viral DNA from certain high-risk papillomaviruses, including HPV 16 and 18, is found in the cells of about 90% of all cervical carcinomas. However, most women with clinically apparent infection with one of the high-risk types do not develop cervical cancers, probably because such infections are often transient, and it is likely that it is persistent infection that contributes to the development of these tumors. Furthermore, HPV infection alone is probably not sufficient for tumor development. In benign warts, the papillomavirus genome is maintained in an episomal form (i.e., a circular form that is not integrated into the host genome), but in cervical cancer, the viral genome is randomly integrated into the host cell DNA.

The products of two HPV genes, *E6* and *E7*, are consistently expressed in cervical cancers. The E6 protein binds to the p53 protein and targets it for degradation by the ubiquitin-mediated proteosomal pathway. E7 binds to RB (and related) proteins, resulting in the release of the transcription factor E2F, which is involved in the transition from G_1 to S phase in the cell cycle. However, transfection of the *E6* and *E7* genes into human epithelial cells in culture results only in an extension of their lifetime, and such cells do not cause tumor formation in immune-deprived mice. This is consistent with the epidemiologic data that HPV infection alone is insufficient to cause malignant transformation of these human cells and with the concept that multiple changes are required in cells for cancer development. Interestingly, the large T-antigen of SV40 virus and the *E1A* and *E1B* gene products of adenoviruses act in a similar way in rodent cells to inactivate the function of the RB and p53 proteins. Transfection of *E1A* alone into normal cells can cause them to undergo apoptosis, whereas concurrent transfection of *E1B* blocks this effect, allowing the cells to survive and proliferate.

Other DNA-containing viruses that have been associated with human malignancies include the Epstein-Barr virus (EBV) and the hepatitis B virus (HBV). The EBV is a herpes virus that was found to be released from cells of Burkitt's lymphoma in African children, and it also has been implicated in nasopharyngeal carcinoma and Hodgkin's disease. This virus infects B-cells in culture and immortalizes them with high efficiency. An increased number of divisions by these cells due to their chronic stimulation by malaria is thought to increase the likelihood of the occurrence of the tumorigenic *MYC/IG* translocation found in the endemic form of Burkitt's lymphoma seen in Africa (see "Oncogenes"). Chronic infection with the hepatitis B virus has been associated with hepatocellular carcinoma (HCC), one of the most common cancers worldwide. The viral genome is often integrated into the cells of hepatocellular carcinoma. Two genes, *HBX* and *PRES2/S*, are usually retained intact after viral DNA integration. Transfection of *HBX* into immortalized mouse hepatocytes in culture causes their transformation, and mice that have been modified to inherit the gene as a transgene develop liver cancer.

Tumor Growth

Characteristics of Tumor Cells

Tumor growth depends on the uncontrolled proliferation of the malignant cell population. However, most tumors show some differentiation consistent with their tissue of origin, which indicates that tumor cell growth is rarely completely without control. Such differentiation is an important aspect of the pathologic identification and grading of tumors. The appearance of tumor cells is also different from that of normal cells, and pathologists use certain criteria, such as increased nuclear size, increased nuclear-to-cytoplasmic ratio, irregular chromatin distribution, and prominent nucleoli, to make a diagnosis of malignancy. When growing in culture, tumor cells also display features that are different from those of normal cells: Notably they grow to higher cell density, they have a reduced dependence on serum concentration, and they will grow over the top of each other, forming irregular piles of cells called *foci*. In contrast, growth of normal cells is dependent on higher serum concentrations (believed to reflect a greater requirement for growth factors present in the serum) and usually ceases when the cells make contact with each other. Such cells are said to be contact inhibited in their growth. Normal cells, with the exception of hematopoietic cells, also must be attached to a surface to be able to grow; that is, they are anchorage dependent. Tumor cells can usually be grown in suspension in an agarose or methyl cellulose medium, which prevents them from adhering to a solid surface. This property of anchorage-independence and the ability to form foci when grown attached to a surface are often regarded as diagnostic of a transformed cell. The ability to form a tumor if injected back into a suitable host provides the final proof that such transformed cells are tumorigenic.

Normal cells have a limited life span in culture (for fibroblasts about 50 to 60 doublings), and at that limit, they remain viable but cease proliferation; that is, they undergo *senescence*. Some cells may attain spontaneously the ability to grow indefinitely in culture, in which case they are said to be *immortal*. Such cells do not necessarily demonstrate the features of transformed cells discussed earlier, but they may acquire these properties spontaneously during further growth, thereby undergoing *malignant transformation*. Rodent cells are relatively prone to immortalization and malignant transformation in culture, but human cells are much more resistant to these processes for reasons that are largely unknown. The senescence of normal cells is associated with the shortening of the ends of the chromosomes, the telomeres, which consist of multiple repeats of specific DNA sequences and proteins. The loss of some of these repeats occurs at each cell division, and it is hypothesized that once the telomeres reach a critical size, they can no longer stabilize the chromosomes effectively.[13] It is postulated that the cells recognize these shortened chromosomes as damaged DNA and turn on the cell cycle inhibitor p21 (see "Genetic Control of the Cell Cycle"), which arrests the cell in G_1 phase. The enzyme telomerase can act to extend the length of telomeres, but it is expressed in only a few normal cells (e.g., embryonic cells, germ cells, certain lymphocytes). The enzyme is usually active in immortal and malignant cells, which has stimulated research to develop therapeutic agents that would specifically inhibit the enzyme.

Cell Kinetics

Extensive studies, initially using radiolabeled precursors that were incorporated into DNA during the S phase of the cell cycle and visualized by autoradiography and, more recently, using fluorescent dyes and flow cytometry, have provided information about the growth kinetics of cells in tumors and normal tissues. These studies have indicated that only a fraction of cells in a tumor are in the proliferative cycle at any one time. This fraction, the growth fraction, can vary widely from one tumor to another (from a few percent to more than 30%), but it tends to be lower in slowly growing tumors. For the cells that are actively in the proliferative cycle, the cell cycle time can also be quite variable, but it is usually in the range of 2 to 3 days for human tumors other than hematologic malignancies, for which it can be shorter than 1 day. A major conclusion to emerge from studies of tumor growth kinetics is that tumor cells do not grow faster (i.e., have a shorter cell cycle time) than cells in normal proliferative tissues, such as the bone marrow or intestinal mucosa.

The rate of growth of a cell population depends on the relationship between the production of new cells and cell death (or loss). In the normal proliferative tissues of an adult, these two are in balance, except in cases of injury, in which cell production may exceed cell loss until the tissue is restored. In tumors, the balance is permanently disturbed, with cell loss occurring less frequently than new cell production, although the rate of cell loss may be as high as 90% of the rate of new cell production in slowly growing tumors. Thus, the growth of a tumor depends on three factors: the average cell cycle time for the proliferating cells, the growth fraction, and the rate of cell loss. The first two of these factors are often combined to define a parameter called the *potential doubling time* (T_{POT}), which is the theoretical doubling time of the tumor cell population in the absence of cell loss. Estimates of T_{POT} for human tumors range from a low of about 3 days to greater than 20, mainly owing to variation in the growth fraction. For many tumor types, the median value is in the range 4 to 6 days. The difference between this value and the actual volume doubling time of a tumor (median for human tumors is 60 to 90 days) is accounted for by cell loss. The T_{POT} value is an important parameter for tumor treatment, because it may reflect the rate of increase of viable cells during protracted treatment with radiation or chemotherapy.

The binary nature of cell division predicts that the unrestricted growth of a cell population would be exponential, meaning that it requires a constant time to double in size. Tumors are often observed to grow exponentially, despite the fact that not every cell is in the proliferative cycle, and the rate of growth can thus be defined by the volume doubling time. In rodent tumors, the volume doubling time often increases when the tumor becomes large, implying a reduction in the rate of growth; measurements made on human tumors have usually been consistent with exponential growth, but little is known about the growth rate prior to detection. Tumors are rarely detected before they reach a diameter of 1 cm. At this size (approximately half a gram), a tumor will likely contain 100 million (10^8) to 1 billion (10^9) tumor cells, depending on the amount of stroma. For a single cell to produce 10^9 cells requires 30 doublings; a further 10 to 13 doublings would result in a tumor that is over a kilogram in size and is likely to be lethal. Thus, an important consequence of exponential growth is that the majority of the life of a tumor occurs before it is detectable.

Not every tumor cell is necessarily capable of indefinite proliferation and of regrowing the tumor should it survive treatment (i.e., is a tumor stem cell). When cells are taken directly from a primary human tumor and plated in culture, the fraction of those that can grow to form colonies is usually very low (less than 1%). Furthermore, analysis of the expected level of cell killing associated with curative doses of radiation therapy suggests that only a small fraction of the cells in a tumor must be killed to achieve a cure. These observations imply that the proportion of cells in a tumor that are tumor stem cells may be quite low. This is not surprising in well-differentiated tumors, in which many tumor cells have undergone differentiation, but it is also likely true for tumors that show little differentiation. Moreover, although tumor stem cells are defined as cells having high proliferative capacity, they are not necessarily all proliferating in a growing tumor (c.f., the situation in bone marrow, where the pluripotent stem cells are largely quiescent). This has implications for the response of tumors (and normal tissues) to treatment, because most anticancer drugs are selectively toxic to proliferating cells. Another implication is that studies of the phenotype of the bulk of cells in a tumor (partial or complete response) may not necessarily provide information about the (tumor stem) cells that are critical to long-term success or failure of treatment.

Genetic Control of the Cell Cycle

The cell cycle is regulated by a series of proteins known as cyclins, cyclin-dependent kinases (CDKs), and cyclin-dependent kinase inhibitors (CDKIs) that participate in activating and inactivating phosphorylation events on specific protein targets. These events regulate biochemical pathways or checkpoints that control mitogenic and growth inhibitory signals, and coordinate the orderly sequence of cell cycle transitions. Important checkpoints occur in late G_1, when cells must commit to and then complete DNA synthesis, and in G_2, when cells must commit to and complete mitosis. The cyclins act as positive regulators of the activity of the cyclin-dependent kinases, because the activity of CDKs is dependent on their binding to the appropriate cyclin. The CDKIs act as negative regulators of this activity.

The CDKs are small serine-threonine kinases (32 to 40 kDa), which are expressed throughout the cell cycle. However, cyclin levels fluctuate through the cell cycle (Fig. 2–3), and production peaks at the time of maximum kinase activity. Tight control of the degradation of cyclins in various parts of the cell cycle also contributes to the regulation of cyclin-dependent kinase activity. As indicated in Figure 2–3, passage from G_1 to S phase is controlled by the activities of CDKs associated with cyclins D, E, and A. Cyclin D and its associated CDKs (2, 4, 5, and 6) are responsible for the phosphorylation of the retinoblastoma protein pRB, which is required for transition of cells from G_1 to S phase. In its hypophosphorylated form, pRB binds to the transcription factor E2F and inhibits the transcription of proteins essential for entry into S phase. Phosphorylation of pRB releases E2F and transcription is activated. Both cyclin E– and cyclin A–associated CDKs play a role in modulating this transcriptional activity and are important for progression through S phase. Cyclin D/CDK complexes also appear to be involved in the re-entry of quiescent (G_0) cells into the cycle. Cyclin-dependent kinase-1 (also known as CDC-2) is associated with cyclin B and plays a major role in controlling entry of cells into mitosis. The rapid degradation of cyclin B is important for the exit of cells from mitosis.

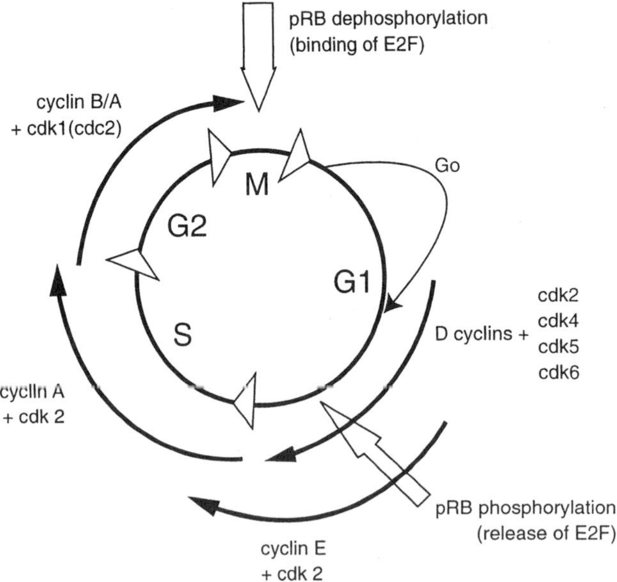

Figure 2–3. The cell cycle and associated cyclins and cyclin-dependent kinases (CDKs). The inner circle represents the cell cycle with the heavy arrows indicating when the various cyclins and their associated CDKs are active. The open arrows indicate the change in the phosphorylation of the retinoblastoma protein (pRB). (Modified from Tannock IF, Hill RP (eds): The Basic Science of Oncology, 3rd ed. New York, McGraw-Hill, 1998.)

There are two different families of CDK inhibitors (CDKIs): the KIP (kinase inhibitory protein) and INK4 (inhibitor of CDK4) families. The KIP family includes CIP1/WAF1, also known as p21, SDI1, KIP1, and KIP2. These proteins bind to the cyclin-CDK complex and inhibit its activity. Small variations in the KIP/CDK concentration in the cells control cyclin-dependent kinase activity at critical points in the cell cycle. Increased levels of KIPs in cells usually result in G_1 arrest, and these proteins play important roles in differentiation, senescence, and cellular responses to growth regulatory cytokines and DNA damage. In particular, p21 is upregulated in cells undergoing senescence and following DNA damage, when it acts to arrest cells in G_1 or to cause cessation of DNA synthesis. There is also evidence that upregulation of p21WAF1/CIP1 and KIP1 are among the effects caused by the growth inhibitory cytokine, transforming growth factor-β (TGFβ). The INK4 family of CDKIs includes p15INK4b, p16INK4a, p18INK4c, and p19INK4d. These proteins destabilize the cyclin D-CDK4 or -CDK6 complexes and may impair the ability of cells to leave G_1 phase.

The genes that regulate cell cycle control are frequently disrupted in cancer cells. Genetic changes in cyclin D are common in human cancer and overexpression of cyclin D1 is reported to occur in up to 45% of breast cancers.[14] The INK4a gene is one of the most commonly mutated (deleted) genes in human cancers and is implicated in familial melanoma.[15] Disruption of pathways regulating pRB activity is also common in human tumors. Mutations of the CIP or KIP genes, *WAF1/CIP1, KIP1,* and *KIP2*, appear to be infrequent in human cancers, but their function may be affected at the level of regulation or protein stability. For example, mutation and inactivation of the *TP53* gene influences the *WAF1* response to DNA damage, possibly allowing the proliferation of genetically altered cells.

Cell Death and Apoptosis

Cell death occurs by two main mechanisms; necrosis and apoptosis. *Necrosis* is a passive response to cellular injury in which cells swell and lyse, releasing their contents into the interstitial space, which may elicit an inflammatory response. In contrast, *apoptosis*, or programmed cell death, is an active process by which cells are eliminated from the organism. Activation of the apoptotic pathway in cells that have sustained DNA damage minimizes the risk of the growth of mutated or transformed cells. Apoptotic cells have a characteristic appearance that involves chromosomal condensation and nuclear fragmentation, shrinkage of the cell, and loss of contact with neighboring cells. Subsequently, there is blebbing of the cell membrane and the formation of apoptotic bodies that contain parts of the chromatin surrounded by cellular membranes. These bodies are phagocytosed by neighboring cells, and there is minimal inflammation. Inside the cell there is an influx of calcium from the endoplasmic reticulum into the cytoplasm, loss of mitochondrial membrane potential, and activation of endonucleases. The endonucleases cleave DNA at specific sites between the nucleosomes, leading to DNA fragments of sizes that are multiples of about 180 base pairs. When the DNA from such cells is subjected to gel electrophoresis, it forms a ladder pattern that is characteristic of apoptotic cells. It is these cut ends of the DNA that are labeled in the well-known TUNEL assay for detecting apoptotic cells.

Apoptosis can be triggered in cells by a variety of different stimuli, including unbalanced growth signals and damage to the cell membrane or DNA. These trigger several incompletely understood signal transduction pathways, some of which involve regulation by *TP53*. Following DNA damage as a result of oxidative stress or treatment with certain drugs or radiation, induction of apoptosis involves increased expression of the p53 protein. Cells that have a mutated *TP53* gene may not be triggered into apoptosis by such damage. The molecular mechanisms controlling the apoptotic process in cells are not completely understood, but the main effectors of apoptosis are a series of cysteine proteases, called *caspases*, which are activated by cleavage of precursor molecules and act to cleave specific substrates that are targets of the apoptotic pathway. The protein product of the *BCL2* oncogene has been found to be a major negative regulator of apoptosis. Various analogues of this protein, such as MCL2 and $BCLX_L$, also inhibit apoptosis, whereas other analogues, such as BAX, BAD, and $BCLX_S$, stimulate apoptosis. These proteins interact to form homodimers and heterodimers and the ratio of inhibitor/activator determines whether induction or inhibition of apoptosis occurs. BAX/BAX dimers induce apoptosis, whereas BCL2/BAX dimers do not. Overexpression of BCL2 does not inhibit apoptosis in all cell types, nor does it inhibit apoptosis induced by all stimuli in one cell type. These proteins are bound to the mitochrondrial membrane, and in some cell types, this binding appears to be essential for *BCL2* function, which includes inhibition of calcium efflux from the endoplasmic reticulum and enhancement of the mitochrondrial membrane potential.

Many cancer cells have a decreased ability to undergo apoptosis in response to various stimuli, including DNA damage, and this may be reflective of their ability to tolerate increased levels of genetic instability. Overexpression of BCL2 is found in many cancers and has been associated with poor prognosis in prostate carcinoma.[16] It has been suggested that it may also confer resistance to certain chemotherapeutic drugs that induce apoptosis as one mechanism of cell killing.

The Extracellular Matrix

In the earlier sections of this chapter, the discussion focused primarily on the dysregulation of the growth control of individual cells. However, in a multicellular organism, cells interact with each other and with the extracellular matrix (ECM). Disruption of these interactions also plays an important role in the development and growth of a cancer. The ECM has a structure and composition that varies for different tissue types and locations. Most epithelial cells are in contact with a basement membrane, which contains mainly laminin, type IV collagen, entactin, and heparan sulfate proteoglycans. These components interact with each other and with the smaller amounts of other proteins, such as fibronectin, vitronectin, tenascin, fibrinogen, and thrombospondin, to form a highly organized three-dimensional (noncellular) matrix, which provides support for and interacts with the cells. Interaction occurs through specific domains on the proteins, which bind to cell adhesion molecules attached to the surface of the cells, particularly integrins. The best-known domain is the RGD (arginine, glycine, aspartic acid) motif that binds to integrins and has been found in many ECM proteins. Interaction between the ECM and normal cells is essential for their survival and growth; depriving them of such interactions will cause apoptosis in epithelial cells and cell-cycle arrest in fibroblasts. A common property of malignant cells is that they may continue to survive and proliferate in the absence of these interactions with the ECM.

An important aspect of the ECM is that its components (particularly proteoglycans) can interact with and bind growth factors, such as basic fibroblast growth factor (b-FGF) or TGFβ, thus providing control of the availability of these growth factors to the cells. The growth factors can be released by the action of proteolytic enzymes, such as plasmin. This may be important in the growth of tumors, because cancer cells often produce plasminogen activator, which catalyses the breakdown of plasminogen to plasmin. During invasion and metastasis, interactions of cells with the ECM may induce the production of proteolytic enzymes, which degrade ECM components, allowing for invasion of the cells through the matrix (see "Metastasis"). The degraded matrix components (e.g., fibronectin fragments) may then induce further protease production, accelerating the process. Release of growth factors by these proteases may also assist in the growth of the metastatic cells.

Cells express a wide range of different cell adhesion molecules (CAMs) on their surface, including integrins, which are primarily involved in cell-ECM interactions, cadherins, which are involved in cell-cell interactions, and members of the immunoglobulin (Ig) superfamily, which are also involved in cell-cell interactions. Integrins are dimers formed as a pair of one α and one β subunit, each of which spans the plasma membrane. Various combinations of the 16α and 9β subunits provide for diversity, and the different combinations bind preferentially to different ECM proteins, although there is considerable overlap and redundancy. The cytoplasmic domain of the β subunit is believed to interact directly with talin and α-actinin, which are components of the actin cytoskeleton of cells, in localized regions called focal adhesion plaques. These plaques provide a structural bridge linking the ECM to the cellular cytoskeleton. Focal adhesion plaques also contain a number of protein tyrosine kinases, such as the focal adhesion kinase, $p125^{FAK}$. These kinases play an important role in the regulation of integrin function. Another protein kinase associated with the cytoplasmic domain of the β subunit is $p59^{ILK}$ (integrin-linked kinase), and it is now well accepted that integrin-induced kinase activity can activate the mitogenic MAP (ERK)-kinase signal transduction pathway through interaction with the RAS protein. The expression of integrins is altered on malignant cells relative to their normal counterparts, but the loss or gain of specific integrins has not been linked directly to malignant transformation.

Cadherins are components of the specialized intercellular attachment sites known as adherent junctions and desmosomes, and they mediate calcium-dependent adhesion between similar cells. Distinct members of the cadherin family are found in different tissues and in different intercellular junctions. Cadherins are also transmembrane proteins and their intracellular domains have been found to interact with three proteins known as α-, β-, and λ-catenin, which mediate binding to the actin cytoskeleton and link cadherins to components of signal transduction pathways in the cell. The APC tumor-suppressor protein, which is mutated in about 70% of colon cancers (see "Genetic Instability"), also binds to β-catenin. Mutations in the protein prevent this binding, which results in increased levels of free β-catenin that are believed to cause deregulated growth through interaction with the T-cell factor-4 (Tcf-4) transcription factors. The major epithelial cadherin, E-cadherin, has been found to be downregulated in many carcinomas and low levels of E-cadherin have been associated with poorly differentiated invasive carcinomas of bladder, breast, colon, and lung.[17]

Some members of the Ig superfamily of proteins can act as cellular adhesion molecules (e.g., I-CAM, V-CAM, N-CAM) and are involved in interactions between cells of the same or different types. Both I-CAM and V-CAM are involved in interactions of lymphocytes with activated endothelial cells. One member of this family is DCC, which is often deleted in colon cancers. It is believed that this molecule may act as a receptor for specific intercellular or cell-matrix interactions.

Angiogenesis

Progressive growth of a solid tumor beyond a size of about 0.5 to 1.0 mm in diameter requires angiogenesis (i.e., the formation of new blood vessels) to supply nutrients to the growing mass. Angiogenesis is a normal part of embryonic development and wound healing, but tumor blood vessels show many differences from those in most normal tissues. Tumor capillaries are often longer than those in normal tissues and tend to be dilated and tortuous. They are often quite leaky, and blood flow can be erratic and prone to stasis and can even reverse within individual vessels. The leakiness of the vessels, combined with the lack of functional lymphatic vessels in tumors, leads to an increased interstitial fluid pressure (IFP) within the tumor that may itself affect blood flow. The arrangement of tumor blood vessels is often chaotic, which results in regional variations in nutrient supply and removal of catabolites. Cells distant from functional blood vessels can become hypoxic, and the tumor interstitium may become acidic owing to impaired clearance of lactic acid and carbonic acid. These factors may influence the efficacy of treatment, because hypoxic cells are more resistant to radiation and some drugs. Furthermore, increased IFP and diffusion distances can adversely affect drug delivery to the tumor cells. There is evidence that hypoxia may also be associated with an increased probability of metastasis formation.[18]

Angiogenesis is stimulated by several different growth factors (e.g., platelet-derived growth factor and basic fibroblast growth factor), but the most important appears to be vascular endothelial growth factor (VEGF). These growth factors are usually produced by the tumor cells themselves, and their production can be affected by the microenvironmental conditions in the tumor. For example, the level of VEGF in cells is upregulated by hypoxia and can be influenced by the expression of certain oncogenes, such as mutant *RAS* and *SRC*. The VEGF protein was identified initially as a factor that caused increased vascular permeability (VPF), but it is also a highly selective mitogen for endothelial cells and acts as a differentiation and survival factor for endothelial cells in newly formed vessels. Receptors for VEGF are expressed primarily on activated endothelial cells that are capable of proliferation. Nearly all types of human tumors express VEGF, and VEGF receptors are expressed on endothelial cells of blood vessels in and surrounding tumors. The importance of VEGF for angiogenesis is shown by the fact that VEGF knockout mice develop severe vascular abnormalities and do not survive as embryos. Furthermore, even the loss of one VEGF allele can cause vascular defects and lethality in embryos. It has been found that many types of human primary tumors, such as breast, prostate, lung, and cervical carcinomas, may contain localized regions of high vascular density (vascular hot spots), and counts of vessels in these regions indicate that high vascular density correlates strongly with poor survival, suggesting a relationship between angiogenesis, VEGF expression, and metastasis.[19]

It has been proposed that agents that inhibit angiogenesis might inhibit tumor growth with minimal toxicity. A large number of such agents has been identified, including thalidomide and α- and β-interferon, but these have limited activity. Recently two naturally occurring agents with high activity have been identified: angiostatin, which is a degradation product of plasminogen produced by the action of elastase, and endostatin, which is a proteolytic fragment of collagen XVIII. Both of these agents were isolated originally from tumor-bearing mice and have been found to induce regression of certain rapidly growing rodent tumors.[20] Clinical trials of these agents are just starting.

Metastasis

The ability of tumor cells to spread and form metastases at sites distinct from the primary tumor can be regarded as one of the last stages of tumor progression, although it is likely that genetic changes will continue to occur within both the primary tumor and its metastases as they continue to grow. The primary routes of metastatic spread are via the lymphatic vessels to local lymph nodes and via the blood vessels to more distant sites. Different types of tumors tend to have different patterns of spread. For example, tumors of the head and neck usually spread initially to regional lymph nodes, and only to distant sites when the tumors are more advanced. In contrast, tumors of the breast can spread early to distant sites as well as to local axillary nodes; about 25% of breast cancer patients with no evidence of lymph node involvement at the time of primary treatment are later found to have distant metastases. The lungs, liver, and bone are common sites of distant spread, but metastases from specific types of tumors also tend to occur in specific target organs. For example, prostate tumors almost invariably metastasize to bone, as do breast cancers, whereas small cell carcinoma of the lung often forms metastases in the brain. This organ preference of metastasis led to the development by Paget in 1889 of the *"soil and seed" hypothesis*,[21] which postulated that tumor cell and host-organ interactions can occur that are more or less favorable for metastatic cell growth. This concept can be understood in terms of the requirement that tumor cells be in an environment in which growth factors stimulate growth and negative growth signals fail to inhibit growth. Thus, how a particular tumor cell responds to the balance of positive and negative growth signals to which it is exposed in a specific organ environment will dictate whether or not a micrometastasis forms. The detailed mechanisms of organ preference for specific tumor types remain to be elucidated.

The process of metastasis can be broken down into a number of steps (Fig. 2–4) that include:

- escape from the primary tumor into the circulation (intravasation)
- survival in the circulation
- arrest at a new site
- escape from the circulation (extravasation)
- migration into the interstitial space at the new site and initiation of growth

This is followed by the initiation of new vessel formation (angiogenesis) to provide nutrients to the growing tumor mass. There is strong evidence that many more tumor cells escape into the circulation than ever form metastatic growths. This has led to the concept that metastasis is a very inefficient process and that specific genetic changes may be required in the cells for successful formation and growth of metastases.

The early stages of the metastatic process are believed to require changes in the adhesive properties of the cells and in the expression of proteolytic enzymes required for the breakdown of basement membranes and other extracellular matrix components (see "The Extracellular Matrix"). In experimental systems, changes in the expression of cell adhesion molecules, such as integrins and cadherins, have been found to affect the metastatic ability of tumor cells; biochemical and immunohistochemical analyses of human tumors have suggested an association between the expression of these molecules and biologic aggressiveness of the disease. For example, the expression of E-cadherin is often low in poorly differentiated and invasive carcinomas. The levels of expression of proteolytic enzymes, such as plasminogen activators, cathepsins, and particularly metalloproteinases and their inhibitors, have also been found to influence the metastatic ability of tumor cells in experimental systems, and have been reported to correlate with the aggressiveness of disease in clinical studies. High levels of expression of cathepsin D have been associated with more aggressive disease in breast cancer. Paradoxically, high expression of the plasminogen activator inhibitor PAI-1 has also been associated with more aggressive disease in a variety of cancers including breast cancer.[22] This seems counterintuitive, but there is evidence that PAI-1 may play a role in blocking cell adhesion mediated by interaction of the plasminogen activator receptor and vitronectin, a cell matrix protein. Thus, proteins can have multiple roles in tissue that may appear to be conflicting under certain circumstances.

These two factors—expression of cellular adhesion molecules and proteolytic activity—plus the ability to initiate growth at the new site are the three primary controlling elements of metastasis formation. However, studies of the properties of metastatic cells have found them to be extremely heterogeneous, and beyond these three broad classes it has been difficult to identify specific changes that are important in all or even a majority of different metastatic cell populations. Changes in the expression of gene products associated with these three classes may be the result of changes in the expression of oncogenes and tumor suppressor genes. The overexpression of an activated *RAS* gene can, for example, cause changes in expression of multiple genes, including both proteolytic enzymes and adhesion molecules.

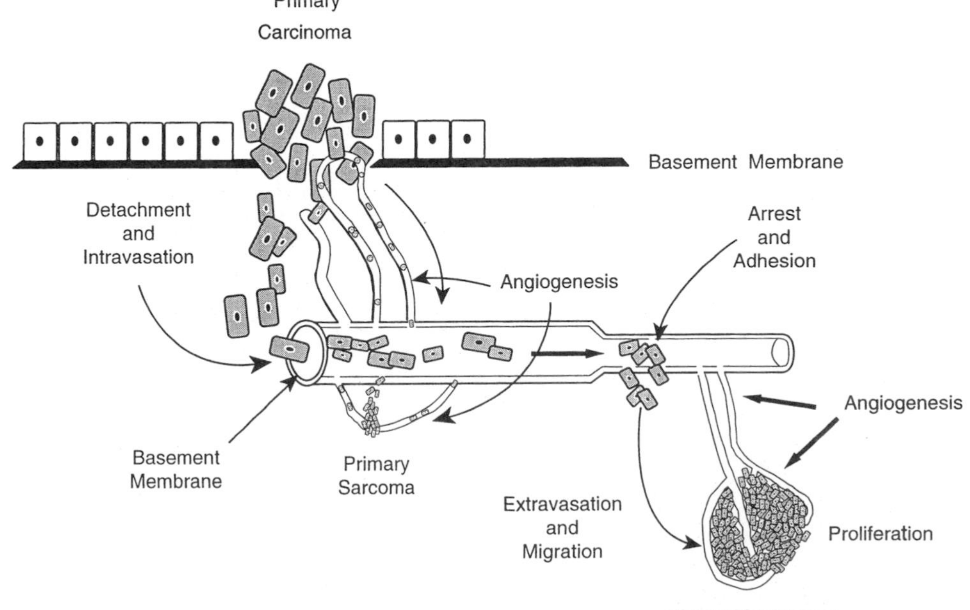

Figure 2–4. The major steps in metastasis formation. Primary tumors (carcinoma or sarcoma) develop a blood supply by inducing angiogenesis. Some tumor cells may detach and intravasate into blood vessels where they will enter the circulation and be transported to another site. They can arrest (usually in the capillary bed of another organ) and extravasate out of the vessel into the tissue. If suitable growth conditions exist at this new location, they may grow into a metastasis that eventually needs to stimulate angiogenesis to supply nutrients for further growth. (Modified from Tannock IF, Hill RP (eds): The Basic Science of Oncology, 3rd ed. New York, McGraw-Hill, 1998.)

A number of genes have been identified as metastasis-associated genes by strategies such as screening of c-DNA libraries obtained from populations of metastatic and nonmetastatic cells or by individual chromosome transfer into metastatic cells. The protein products of most of these genes fall into the three broad categories described earlier and are specifically associated with metastasis in one or a few cell lines. The most extensively studied of these genes is the *NM23* gene, which codes for a protein with nucleoside diphosphate (NDP) kinase activity and appears to be involved in cellular development and differentiation. Low levels of expression of this gene have been associated with more aggressive disease in various cancers, including breast cancer and melanoma, but in other cancers, such as colon or prostate carcinoma, no relationship was found with aggressiveness of the disease.

Metastases represent a major barrier to effective therapy of human cancers. Most treatment strategies use the same drugs to treat both the primary tumor and its metastases. Drugs that target specific steps of the metastatic process, such as inhibitors of metalloproteinase activity, are becoming available, and some drugs are being tested for their efficacy in inhibiting metastasis formation. Even if they are successful, however, their clinical utility may be limited, because in many patients metastases will have been seeded before the detection of the primary tumor.

Summary

The development of cancer involves mutations or genetic alterations that arise predominantly in somatic cells, but they may, in a small percentage of tumors, be inherited. Cells in advanced malignancies contain multiple genetic changes. These genetic alterations may arise directly or indirectly in cells from such factors as chemical- or radiation-induced DNA damage, incorporation of certain viruses into the cell, or random errors during DNA synthesis or repair of DNA damage. The changes that are critical for carcinogenesis affect oncogenes or tumor suppressor genes. Most oncogenes encode proteins that are involved in the mitogenic signal transduction pathways that control cell growth and differentiation. Some tumor suppressor genes encode proteins that also act in these pathways, but there is a wider range of functions for the products of such genes. For example, they may be cyclin-dependent kinase inhibitors, cellular adhesion molecules, or DNA repair enzymes. There has been considerable progress in understanding the mechanisms by which individual genes may contribute to tumor development over the last 10 years. Challenges for the future include developing an understanding of how different mutations act together to cause cancer growth, determining why the same molecular defect has a different influence on tumor development in different tissues in the body, and translating our increased molecular knowledge of the causes of cancer into improved strategies for treatment and prevention.

Recommended Reading

An excellent review article is "From Molecular Genetics to Clinical Medicine" by Blackwood and Weber.[23] Fearon's 1997 article,[24] "Human Cancer Syndromes: Clues to the Origin and Nature of Cancer" in *Science* is another outstanding oncologic background resource. Also in this category are articles by Heppner and Miller,[25] "The Cellular Basis of Tumor Progression," one by Ligget and Sidransky,[26] "Role of the p16 Tumor Suppressor Gene in Cancer," and "Cancer Cells Exhibit a Mutator Phenotype" by Loeb.[27] The textbook, *The Basic Science of Oncology,* 3rd edition, by Tannock and Hill is a comprehensive reference.[12] Recent articles provide important additional insights.[28–32]

REFERENCES

1. Nakachi K, Imai K, Hayashi S, et al: Polymorphisms of the CYP1A1 and glutathione-S-transferase genes associated with susceptibility to lung cancer in relation to cigarette dose in a Japanese population. Cancer Res 1993; 53:2994–2999.
2. Daya-Grosjean L, Dumaz N, Sarasin A: The specificity of p53 mutation spectra in sunlight-induced human cancers. J Photochem Photobiol B 1995; 28:115–124.
3. Boice JD, Lubin JH: Lung cancer risks: comparing radiation with tobacco. Radiat Res 1996; 146:356–357.
4. Foulds L: Neoplastic Development. London, Academic Press, 1975.
5. Nowell P: Mechanisms of tumor progression. Cancer Res 1986; 46:2203–2207.
6. Fearon ER, Vogelstein B: A genetic model for colorectal tumorigenesis. Cell 1990; 61:759–767.
7. Bryndorf T, Kirchhoff M, Rose H, et al: Comparative genomic hybridization in clinical cytogenetics. Am J Hum Genet 1995; 57:1211–1220.
8. Cheung VG, Gregg JP, Gogolin-Ewens KJ, et al: Linkage-disequilibrium mapping without genotype. Nature Genet 1998; 18:225–230.
9. DeRisi J, Penland L, Brown PO, et al: Use of cDNA microarray to analyse gene expression patterns in human cancer. Nature Genet 1996; 14:457–460.
10. Moolgavkar SH, Knudsen AG, Jr: Mutation and cancer: a model for human carcinogenesis. J Natl Cancer Inst 1981; 66:1037–1052.
11. Chen J, Birkholtz GG, Lindblom P, et al: The role of ataxia-telangiectasia heterozygotes in familial breast cancer. Cancer Res 1998; 58:1376–1379.
12. Tannock IF, Hill RP (eds): The Basic Science of Oncology, 3rd ed. New York, McGraw-Hill, 1998.
13. Bacchetti S, Counter CM: Telomeres and telomerase in human cancer. Int J Oncol 1995; 7:423–432.
14. Hunter T, Pines P: Cyclins and cancer II: cyclin D and cdk inhibitors come of age. Cell 1994; 79:573–582.
15. Ranade K, Hussussian CJ, Sikorski RS, et al: Mutations associated with familial melanoma impair p16INK4A function. Nature Genet 1995; 10:114–116.
16. Johnson MI, Hamdy FC: Apoptosis regulating genes in prostate cancer. Oncol Rep 1998; 5(3):553–557.
17. Birchmeyer W, Behrens J: Cadherin expression in carcinomas: role in the formation of cell junctions and the prevention of invasiveness. Biochim Biophys Acta 1994; 1198:11–26.
18. Brown JM, Giaccia AJ: The unique physiology of solid tumors: opportunities (and problems) for cancer therapy. Cancer Res 1998; 58:1408–1416.
19. Weidner N, Semple JP, Welch WR, et al: Tumor angiogenesis and metastasis: correlation in invasive breast carcinoma. N Engl J Med 1991; 324:1–8.
20. Boehm T, Folkman J, Browder T, et al: Antiangiogenic therapy of experimental cancer does not induce acquired drug resistance. Nature 1997; 390:404–407.
21. Paget S: The distribution of secondary growths in cancer of the breast. Lancet 1889; 1:371–573.
22. Kute TE, Grondahl-Hansen J, Shao SM, et al: Low cathepsin D and low plasminogen activator type 1 inhibitor in tumor cytosols defines a group of node negative breast cancer patients with low risk of recurrence. Breast Cancer Res Treat 1998; 47:9–16.
23. Blackwood MA, Weber BL: *BRCA1* and *BRCA2*: from molecular genetics to clinical medicine. J Clin Oncol 1998; 16:1969–1977.

24. Fearon EC: Human cancer syndromes: clues to the origin and nature of cancer. Science 1997; 278:1043–1058.
25. Heppner GH, Miller FR: The cellular basis of tumor progression. Int Rev Cytol 1998; 177:1–56.
26. Liggett WH, Sidransky D: Role of the p16 tumor suppressor gene in cancer. J Clin Oncol 1998; 16:1197–1206.
27. Loeb LA: Cancer cells exhibit a mutator phenotype. Adv Cancer Res 1998; 72:25–56.
28. Aumailley M, Gayraud B: Structure and biological activity of the extracellular matrix. J Mol Med 1998; 76:253.
29. Talks KL, Harris AL: Current status of antiangiogenic factors. Br J Haematol 2000; 109:477.
30. Deng CX, Brodie SG: Roles of BRCA1 and its interacting proteins. Bioessays 2000; 22:728.
31. DeClerck YA: Interactions between tumour cells and stromal cells and proteolytic modification of the extracellular matrix by metalloproteinases in cancer. Eur J Cancer 2000; 36:1258.
32. Johnson DE: Programmed cell death regulation: basic mechanisms and therapeutic opportunities. Leukemia 2000; 14:1340.

3 *The Pathology of Cancer*

PATRICE F. SPITALNIK, MD, Pathology and Laboratory Medicine
P. ANTHONY DI SANT'AGNESE, MD, Pathology and Laboratory Medicine

Acquired genetic lability permits stepwise selection of variant sublines and underlies tumor progression.

PETER NOWELL[7]

Perspective

Pathology is the study of the basic mechanisms and processes of disease, including the etiology, pathogenesis, and morphologic manifestations. The pathologist, in concert with the clinician, correlates this information with clinical signs and symptoms to arrive at a diagnosis and to help determine a therapeutic approach. The diagnostic material provided to the anatomic pathologist includes needle biopsies and aspirates, incisional and excisional biopsies, and cells in fluids, brushings, and scrapings. The so-called tools of the trade include light microscopy, electron microscopy, immunohistochemistry, cytogenetics, flow cytometry, and molecular diagnosis.

Definitions

- *Neoplasia* means "new growth." Neoplastic cells in a group or mass compose a tumor (swelling) or neoplasm.
- *Neoplasms* are now known to be a group of cells, derived from a single progenitor cell, in which at least one mutation causes its progeny to have a growth advantage over the normal surrounding cells. This results in a proliferation of cells within the tissue. The initial mutation is followed by other mutations, which allow the growing clone to become a clinically significant neoplasm.
- A neoplasm is *benign* if the mutations allow the tumor only a growth advantage over the adjacent normal tissue. A benign neoplasm remains confined to its original site.
- A tumor is *malignant* if sequential mutations take place that allow the neoplasm to invade surrounding structures destructively and metastasize to distant sites in the body. Cancer is a malignant neoplasm.
- The process of successive multiple mutations, leading ultimately to a heterogeneous malignant neoplasm, is known as the *clonal evolution model of tumor development*. This model is explained further in the section on carcinogenesis. The cellular genetic alterations in this process result in the acquisition of abnormal growth stimuli or the loss of inhibitory signals.

Clinical Aspects of Cancer

Diagnosis

To make a complete and correct diagnosis of a neoplasm, the pathologist and the clinician must work together closely. Efficient transmission of information from the clinician to the pathologist regarding the patient's history and other relevant clinical information is crucial. For example, a history of prior irradiation to an organ might indicate that identified atypical cells are probably benign, whereas without this information the cells might be considered malignant. In another example, a nodule of adenocarcinoma of the lung could be primary or metastatic; a history of previous malignancy and its tissue type might influence the final pathologic diagnosis. Of note, specimens submitted to determine whether a neoplasm has been entirely removed in surgery must have clearly demarcated borders with spatial orientation provided by the surgeon.

The diagnosis of cancer is made by a pathologist based on tissue and cells submitted for examination. In most cases, for an experienced pathologist, the diagnosis is straightforward. In some cases, however, difficulties arise when clear histologic and cytologic distinctions are not present. Severely inflamed and markedly hyperplastic lesions can mimic cancer, whereas some very well-differentiated carcinomas can resemble benign tissue. As described in the previous chapter and earlier, it has become evident that numerous sequential genetic alterations are the basis for neoplastic transformation in cells. These genetic alterations result in diagnostic morphologic changes in the cell and tissue patterns, as well as in the proliferative and invasive behavior of the neoplastic cells. In the past, pathology relied on tumor morphology or phenotype alone to make most diagnoses and predict future behavior of the neoplasm. The pathologist now uses this new genetic information to characterize tumors at the molecular level, hoping that the more specific information will allow for better diagnosis, disease prognosis, and treatment (Table 3–1).

TABLE 3–1. **Summary of Cancer Diagnosis**

Definitive diagnosis requires histologic or cytologic examination with specific cellular characteristics elucidated:	
Surgical biopsy	Tissue examination
Cytopathology	Examination of exfoliated cells
	Examination of tissue/cells obtained by fine-needle aspiration
Molecular cytogenetics	Specific chromosomal/genetic rearrangements identified
Flow cytometry	Immunophenotyping of cells
Molecular diagnosis	Polymerase chain reaction (PCR)
	Reverse transcriptase–polymerase chain reaction (RT-PCR)
	Fluorescence *in situ* hybridization (FISH)
Validity of the interpretation depends on both the pathologist and the clinician:	
	Representative sample must be obtained
	All material must be properly processed
	All pertinent patient data and history must be available to the pathologist
	The clinician and pathologist must work together in order to make a proper diagnosis

Methods of Diagnosis

SURGICAL BIOPSY

Histologic examination of tissue removed by excisional or incisional biopsy is the traditional and most widely used method of diagnostic verification of a suspected malignancy. Incisional biopsy removes only a portion of a suspected lesion for diagnostic purposes, whereas an excisional biopsy removes the entire tumor with a rim of normal surrounding tissue and can be used for therapeutic as well as diagnostic purposes. The reason for performing either an incisional or excisional biopsy is usually related to the size of the lesion. The larger the tumor, the more likely that an incisional biopsy will be taken. Once a diagnosis is made on the incisional biopsy, then proper excision of the tumor can be carried out and appropriate staging of the tumor can take place. Care must be taken during the biopsy to remove a representative piece of tissue.

FROZEN SECTION

The frozen section is a valuable tool for intraoperative diagnosis. It is used to establish the existence and type of tumor present, to verify that enough tissue is available for accurate diagnosis, and to determine that adequate surgical resection margins are taken. It should be used only when the information gained by the frozen section will influence the course of the surgical procedure.

CYTOPATHOLOGY

Cytopathology, as its name implies, involves the microscopic examination of individual cells or groups of cells that are not in the context of a tissue or organ. Cytopathology is most often used as a screening method to detect malignancy in the uterine cervix. Characteristic cellular morphology allows the pathologist to diagnose early dysplasia, as well as invasive malignancy (Fig. 3–1). Widespread use of the Papanicolaou (Pap) smear of the uterine cervix as a screening test for women in the general population has significantly lowered the mortality rate for those with cervical carcinoma over the last 30 years.

Exfoliative cytology is a reliable method of diagnosis. It involves the microscopic study of cells exfoliated from surfaces or floating in fluid; typically, these include the respiratory epithelium, pleural space, peritoneal space, urinary tract, skin, uterus, or most commonly, the uterine cervix. The Pap stain is used to examine the cells' morphologic characteristics.

Fine-needle aspiration of tumors is a widely used, mini-

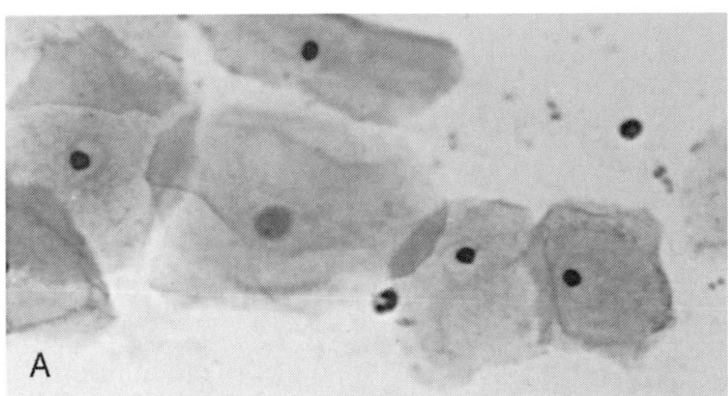

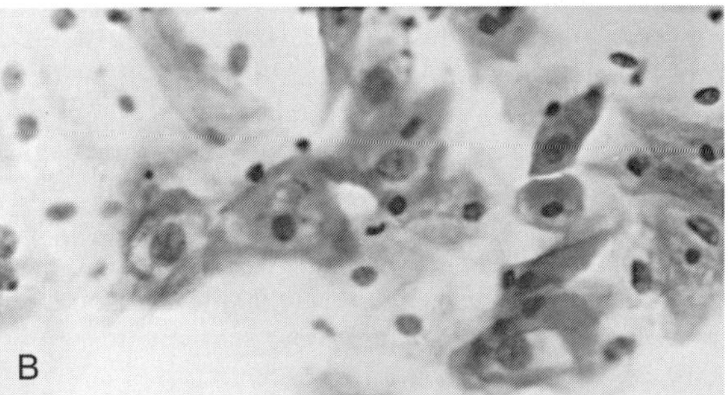

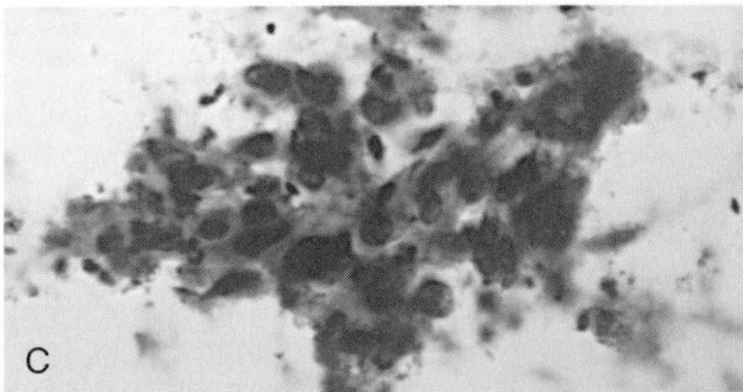

Figure 3–1. (A) Normal superficial and intermediate squamous cells are large, polygonal cells with abundant, translucent cytoplasm and low nuclear-to-cytoplasmic (N:C) ratios. Nuclei in superficial cells are round and pyknotic, whereas those in intermediate cells are round with smooth, delicate nuclear membranes and evenly distributed vesicular chromatin. (B) In contrast to normal superficial and intermediate cells, these dysplastic squamous cells are smaller with more opaque cytoplasm, larger nuclei, and higher N:C ratios. The hyperchromatic nuclei have slightly irregular contours and smudged chromatin. The sharply demarcated, perinuclear halo, together with the other nuclear features, is characteristic of human papillomavirus infection. (C) This irregular aggregate from an invasive squamous cell carcinoma is composed of crowded cells with opaque cytoplasm and high N:C ratios. Nuclei are pleomorphic and markedly hyperchromatic. Granular, necrotic debris is in the background. (A–C: Papanicolaou stain, original magnification 400×.) (Contributed by Lisa Teot, MD, University of Rochester Medical Center.)

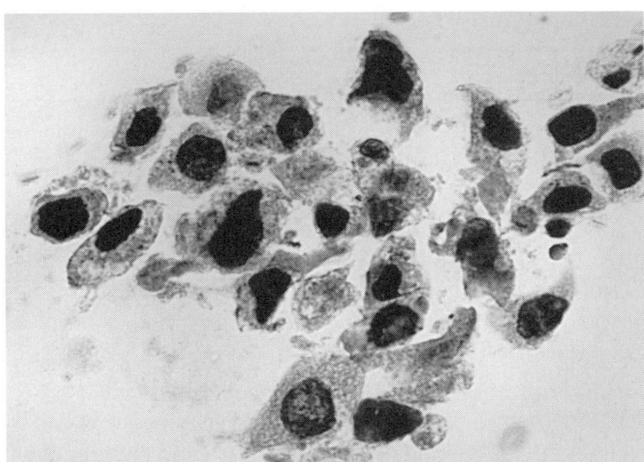

Figure 3–2. Needle aspiration specimen with malignant tumor cells derived from a well-differentiated squamous cell carcinoma of lung. Note cellular pleomorphism and hyperchromatic nuclei. (800×, Pap stain).

mally invasive method that produces samples of small tissue fragments and individual cells. Cells and tissue can be sampled from nearly all solid organs in the body using this approach (Fig. 3–2).

IMMUNOHISTOCHEMISTRY

Immunohistochemistry aids the pathologist by using functional characteristics of the cells in the neoplasm to make a specific diagnosis. It is used in conjunction with the hematoxylin and eosin (H&E) stain on the biopsy specimen. This technique is particularly helpful when diagnosing undifferentiated tumors or metastases that lack histologic criteria to allow the determination of the tissue type or site of origin. Polyclonal or monoclonal antibodies to cellular components and cell-surface markers, as well as *in situ* hybridization of cellular RNA, give the pathologist the necessary information to diagnose and distinguish general categories of malignancy from each other.

Some useful immunohistochemical reagents include desmin; vimentin; prostate-specific antigen; chromogranin; alpha-fetoprotein; S-100; estrogen and progesterone receptors; CD15, CD31, CD34, CD43, CD45RO, and CD68; and several specific cytokeratins; these can distinguish cells of lymphoid, muscle, nerve, neuroendocrine, mesenchymal, or epithelial origin (Table 3–2). Of note, it is frequently necessary to use a panel of different antibodies to classify a malignancy because some antibodies are positive for a broader range of cells than is usually expected. For example, epithelial membrane antigen can be expressed by some lymphomas and vimentin can stain some carcinomas, even though vimentin is used most often to define sarcomas. An example of a simple scheme used to classify some undifferentiated tumors using immunohistochemistry is illustrated in Table 3–3. Once the general category of tumor is determined, subphenotyping, using many of the available tumor markers, is possible. For example, lymphomas can be separated into B- and T-cell neoplasms. In addition, sarcomas can be classified using muscle and neural tumor markers.[8] To characterize some poorly differentiated carcinomas, patterns of expression of cytokeratins 7 and 20 can prove useful[9] (Table 3–4).

Immunocytochemistry may also be used to characterize cytopathology specimens. Particular attention must be paid to ensure that proper cytology controls are used when evaluating immunocytochemistry results. The reagents are generally the same as those used in biopsy immunohistochemistry and are found in Table 3–2.

CYTOGENETICS

Many neoplasms involve translocation or deletion of genes. Cytogenetics uses karyotypic visualization of chromosomes to detect these alterations. The Philadelphia chromosome was the first consistent genetic alteration to be demonstrated in a neoplasm, chronic myelogenous leukemia (CML). It involves the reciprocal translocation of a portion of the *ABL* proto-oncogene, a growth regulatory gene on

TABLE 3–2. **Diagnostically Useful Immunohistochemical Tumor/Tissue Markers**

Marker	Target of Marker
Alpha-fetoprotein	Germ cell tumors, hepatocellular carcinoma
Beta–human chorionic gonadotropin	Trophoblastic tissue and germ cell tumors
CD15 (Leu M-1)	Reed-Sternberg cells, Hodgkin's disease, granulocytes
CD20	B-lymphocytes
CD31	Endothelial cells
CD34	Endothelial cells and hematopoietic stem cells
CD43	T-lymphocytes, small proportion of B-lymphocytes
CD45 (leukocyte common antigen)	Leukocytes
CD45RO	T-lymphocytes
CD68	Macrophages
CD79a	B-lymphocytes
Calcitonin	Medullary carcinoma of the thyroid
Chromogranin	Neuroendocrine secretory granules
Cytokeratins (AE 1,3)	Epithelial cells or mesothelium
Cytokeratins (7,20)	Epithelial cells
Desmin	Smooth, cardiac, or skeletal muscle
EBV (*in situ* hybridization)	Post-transplant lymphoproliferative disorder
Epithelial membrane antigen	Epithelial cells
Factor VIII	Endothelial cells
Glial fibrillary acidic protein (GFAP)	Neural and glial cells
HMB-45, melanin (monoclonal antibody)	Melanoma
Ham-56	Macrophages
Kappa and lambda light chains (*in situ* hybridization)	Immunoglobulin light chains in evaluation of lymphoid and plasmacytic proliferations
Ki-67	Cell proliferation marker
Prostate-specific antigen	Prostatic epithelium
S-100	Neural tissue, melanoma Some macrophages (Histiocytosis X) Dendritic cells
Vimentin	Most mesenchymal tissues (sarcomas) Some carcinomas Melanoma

TABLE 3–3. **Immunohistochemical Panel for an Undifferentiated Neoplasm**

Type of Malignancy	Antibodies				
	S-100	*Cytokeratins*	*HMB-45*	*Vimentin*	*CD45 (LCA)*
Carcinoma	–	+	–	–	–
Sarcoma	+/–	–	–	+	–
Lymphoma	–	–	–	+	+
Melanoma	+	–	+	+	–

chromosome 9 with the breakpoint cluster region (BCR) on chromosome 22.[10] This rearrangement creates the fusion protein BCR-ABL with tyrosine kinase activity, and therefore has a positive proliferative effect on cell growth (Fig. 3–3).

Translocation of the *MYC* proto-oncogene (a gene that encodes a transcription factor) on chromosome 8 to the immunoglobulin heavy chain gene on chromosome 14 is found in Burkitt's lymphoma.[11] This translocation results in constitutive expression of the normal *MYC* gene in its new position and contributes to neoplastic transformation in affected cells. Cytogenetics, along with the molecular diagnostic methods of reverse transcriptase–polymerase chain reaction (RT-PCR) and Southern blotting (see "Molecular Diagnosis") are used clinically to diagnose patients with CML, lymphomas, and many hematologic malignancies. Cytogenetics is also used to follow patients during treatment to detect evidence of minimal residual disease and monitor response to treatment.

FLOW CYTOMETRY

Immunophenotyping by flow cytometry is usually performed to evaluate cell-surface antigen receptors on lymphocytes and hematopoietic cells. A few intracellular proteins can also be evaluated by flow cytometry using special cell permeabilization techniques. A monoclonal population of lymphocytes with identical kappa or lambda light chains can be diagnostic for a neoplastic process (Fig. 3–4). Flow cytometry is also used to assess DNA ploidy in clinical samples and can have prognostic value. For example, hyperdiploidy in acute lymphocytic leukemia is associated with a good prognosis.[12]

MOLECULAR DIAGNOSIS

Molecular methods are used to aid in diagnosis, as well as to predict behavior and response to treatment of some neoplasms. These methods include the polymerase chain reaction (PCR), RT-PCR (Fig. 3–5), and fluorescence *in situ* hybridization (FISH). These techniques are used for detecting translocations or gene rearrangements in leukemias, lymphomas, and some sarcomas; gene amplifications in neuroblastoma; minimal residual disease in leukemias or lymphomas; and inherited germline mutations in family members of affected patients. Amplification of the *MYCN* gene (an oncogene that encodes a transcription factor) in neuroblastoma is an indicator of a poor prognosis. In conjunction with histology and immunohistochemistry, it is used to monitor disease progression and severity.[13] These methods are being used to a greater extent as more oncogenes are identified and the molecular patterns of neoplastic transformation are elucidated.

General Histologic and Cytologic Features of Cancer

In most cases, benign neoplasia differs considerably from malignant neoplasia. At times, malignant tumors may appear benign, and features between the two can overlap; however, certain features are characteristic for malignancy. Cellular phenotype and overall tissue structure are all-important in the diagnosis of neoplasia. It must be stressed that all diagnoses are predictions of future biologic behavior, and pathologists rely on morphology and molecular characteristics to make these as accurate as possible. The principal histologic and cytologic features of cancer are discussed in the following sections.

Invasiveness

- A benign neoplasm is limited to its original site and usually has a well-defined connective tissue capsule (Fig. 3–6). Where this fibrous capsule is present, it compresses surrounding normal tissue and makes the mass freely movable and easily resected surgically.

TABLE 3–4. **C7/C20 Immunophenotypic Grouping**

CK7+ CK20+	CK7+ CK20–	CK7– CK20+	CK7– CK20–
Transitional cell carcinoma	Breast carcinoma (ductal and lobular)	Colorectal adenocarcinoma	Hepatocellular carcinoma
Ovarian carcinoma (mucinous)	Lung adenocarcinoma (non–small cell)		Renal cell carcinoma
Pancreatic carcinoma	Ovarian carcinoma (serous)		Prostatic adenocarcinoma
	Endometrial adenocarcinoma		Squamous cell carcinoma
	Epithelial mesothelioma		Small cell (neuroendocrine) carcinoma
	Thymoma		

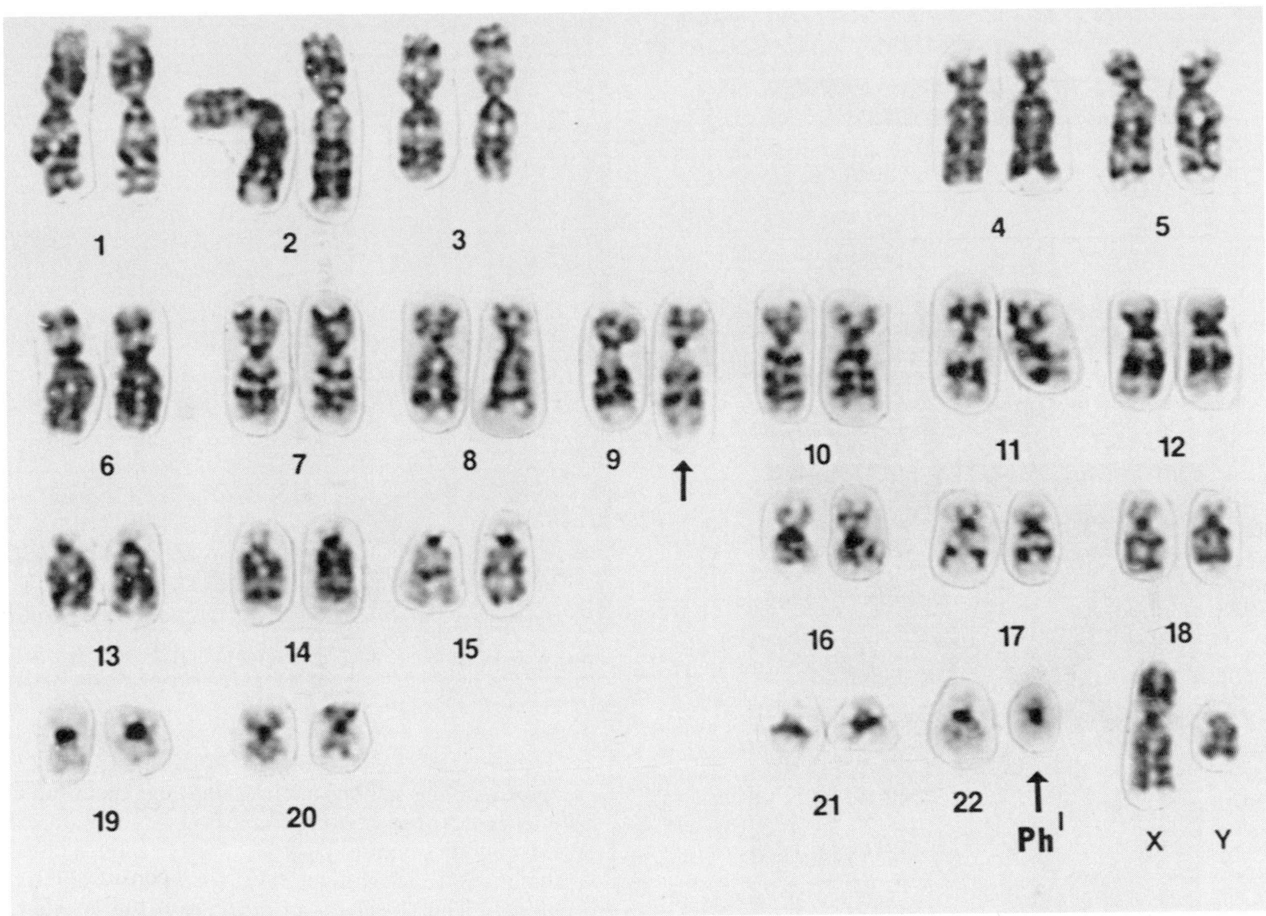

Figure 3–3. Karyotype of a leukemic cell from a patient with chronic myelogenous leukemia, showing the typical t(9;22) translocation producing the Philadelphia chromosome (Ph). (Contributed by Peter Nowell, MD, University of Pennsylvania School of Medicine.)

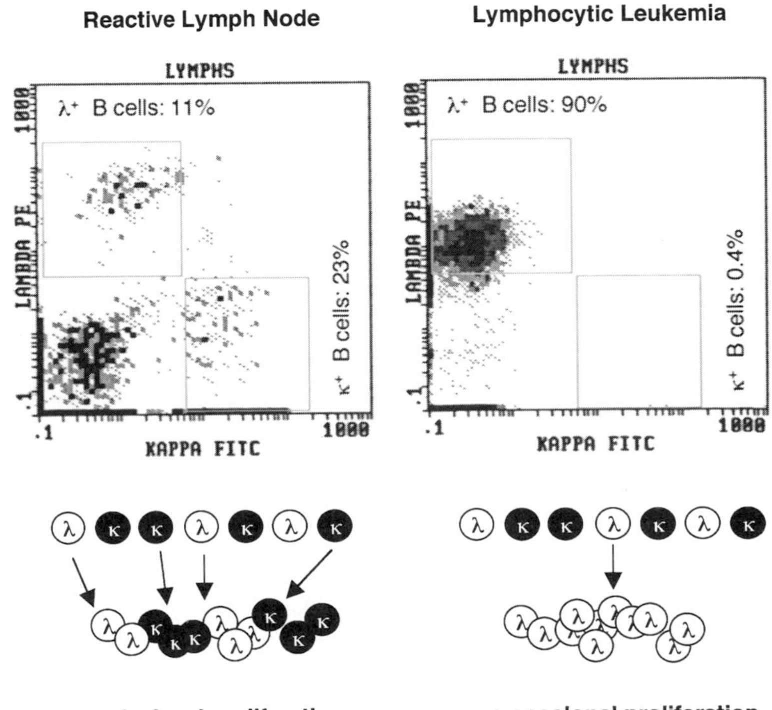

Figure 3–4. Detection of monoclonality by flow cytometry. Fluorescence histograms of anti-kappa versus anti-lambda in a reactive lymph node *(left)* or a lymph node replaced by B-cell chronic lymphocytic lymphoma *(right)*. Note the separate kappa+/lambda− (23%) and kappa−/lambda+ (11%) populations in the benign reactive node. In contrast, the B-cell lymphoma contains a large kappa−/lambda+ (90%) population without a corresponding kappa+/lambda− (0.4%) population, consistent with a monoclonal proliferation. The population of cells in the left lower quadrant is T-lymphocytes and is kappa−/lambda−. Below the flow cytometry histograms is an illustration of the polyclonal nature of the proliferation resulting in distinct kappa+ and lambda+ populations as contrasted to a monoclonal expansion of a transformed malignant lambda-expressing B-cell. (Contributed by Daniel Ryan, MD, University of Rochester Medical Center.)

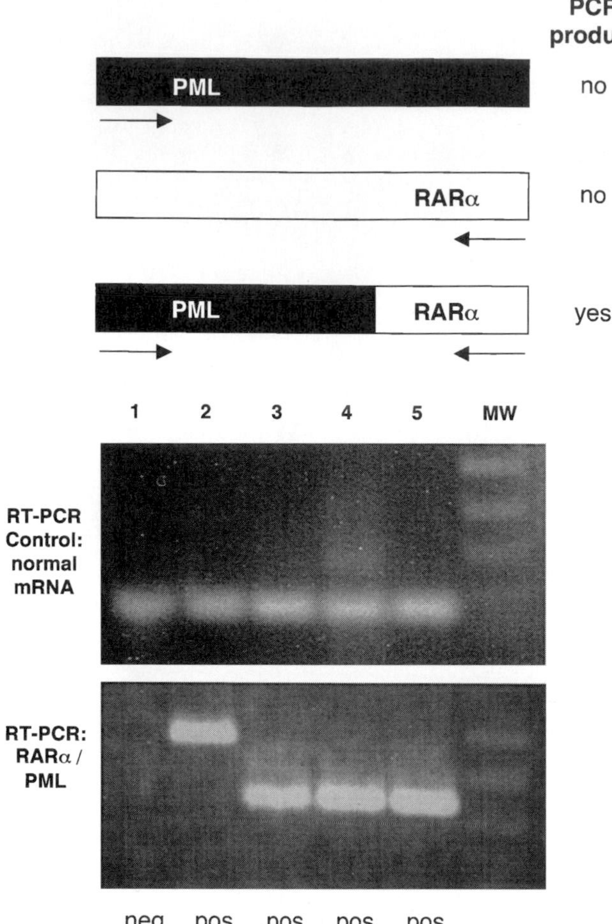

Figure 3–5. Detection of gene rearrangement by reverse transcriptase–PCR (RT-PCR). Acute promyelocytic leukemia (APL) is characterized by a gene translocation resulting in a chimeric PML/RARα gene product, which aberrantly affects transcription of multiple genes in myeloid progenitors. This product can be identified by PCR using one primer specific for each involved gene—only sequences in which the two genes are joined and transcribed as mRNA will place the two PCR primers in proximity and thus result in generation of a PCR product. Gels below show RT-PCR of a patient with APL in remission (1) and APL at diagnosis (2–5). Upper gel shows that each sample contains amplifiable cDNA derived from mRNA of a normal cellular gene. Lower gel shows that the four patients with diagnosed APL express the abnormal chimeric transcript (one is a different size due to different breakpoint of the translocation), whereas the patient in remission has no detectable abnormal PML/RARα transcript. This assay is sensitive to about one malignant cell in 1000–10,000 normal cells. (Contributed by Daniel Ryan, MD, University of Rochester Medical Center.)

- Malignant tumors are not limited by the confines of normal tissue. Their borders are indistinct, and the malignant cells and structures merge with the surrounding tissue. A few malignant tumors may appear to have a defined border and close scrutiny must be applied to inspect for invasion of adjacent tissue.
- Malignant cells aggressively invade tissue locally, and they can also metastasize by invading blood vessels and lymphatic channels within the tumor and travel to distant organs.
- Perineural invasion and peritoneal seeding of tumor cells are also known mechanisms of local and distant spread of the neoplasm. Invasion and metastasis are the most dependable diagnostic criteria for malignancy. Destruction of normal tissue is seen in some aggressive tumors and ensues as a result of invasive infiltrative growth. Thus, necrosis of adjacent tissue is often observed (Fig. 3–7).

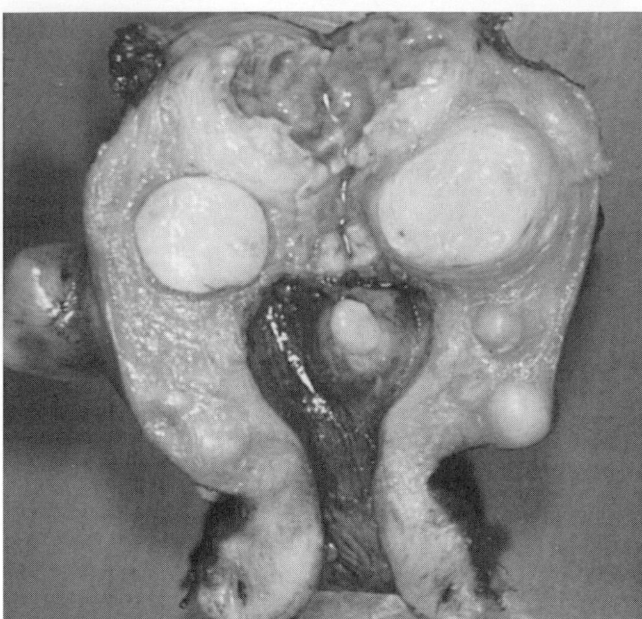

Figure 3–6. Leiomyomas of the uterus. Note the well-defined nature of these benign tumor nodules. There is cystic degeneration of the nodule at the top.

Differentiation and Atypical Tissue Structure (Anaplasia)

- Well-differentiated tumors consist of cells and structures that most closely resemble the tissue of origin of the neoplasm (Figs. 3–8 and 3–9).
- Poorly differentiated and undifferentiated tumors have more aggressive behavior and typically do not resem-

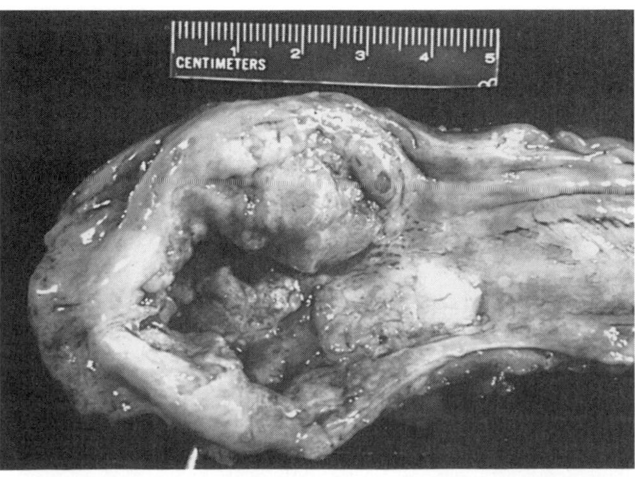

Figure 3–7. Squamous cell carcinoma of the esophagus. A large, destructive, ulcerative tumor has replaced the esophageal mucosa and wall.

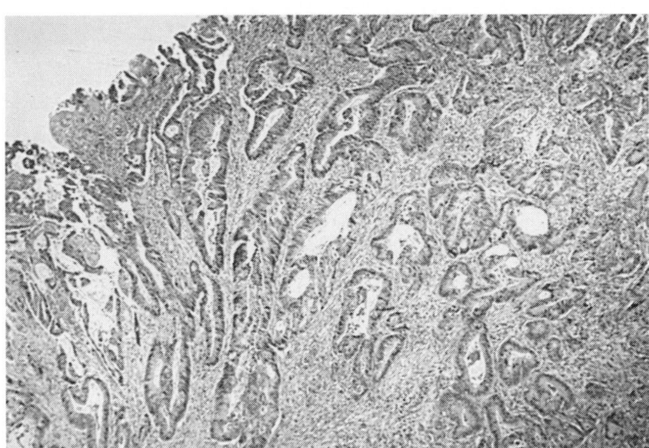

Figure 3–8. Well-differentiated adenocarcinoma of the colon. Note well-formed glandular structures and resemblance to normal colonic glands. (160×, H&E.)

ble the tissue of origin in structure or function (Fig. 3–10). The growth patterns and resulting tissue architecture are disorderly, with cellular arrangements that often deviate considerably from normal.

Often, immunohistochemistry is needed to discern the cellular functional phenotype: benign tumors are usually well differentiated; malignant tumors can be well or poorly differentiated, or undifferentiated; anaplastic tumor cells lack differentiation. Neoplasia, thus, results from a lack of maturation from an original cell type and not loss of differentiation

Pleomorphism

Because of the multistep progression of neoplastic tumor growth, there is considerable genetic heterogeneity within a single mass and from the original mass to its metastases. Thus, tissue patterns can vary within the same tumor, and individual tumor cells also often vary considerably in their morphologic characteristics.

Growth Rate

Malignant tumor cells usually proliferate at a higher rate than their normal counterparts. This is often manifested by increased numbers of mitotic figures in tissue sections. In addition, accelerated growth and inadequate angiogenesis result in areas of necrosis within certain aggressive tumors. It should be noted that in some slow-growing lymphoid tumors, expansion is due mainly to a lack of apoptosis from overexpression of the *BCL2* gene, rather than from an increase in cell growth factors and proliferation. Mitoses in these types of tumors are infrequent.

Aneuploidy

The DNA content of malignant cells is typically abnormal. Whereas normal or hyperplastic cells have diploid or some multiple of the normal diploid content, cancer cells often have irregular and variable numbers of chromosomes. This is reflected histologically by the presence of hyperchromasia and chromatin irregularities within cell nuclei, as well as abnormal mitotic figures.

Classification of Neoplasia

Standardization in the classification of tumors is important. The gold standards for the classification of tumors are the World Health Organization's (WHO) *International Histologic Classification of Tumours* manuals,[5] which are available for most tumor sites and are a collaborative effort of a variety of national experts in the field. The classification of neoplasms is illustrated in pictures with accompanying narrative descriptions. A complementary series is the Armed Forces Institute of Pathology's *Atlas of Tumor Pathology*,[6] which is a compendium of gross and microscopic characteristics that is more detailed and all-inclusive, describing gray and controversial areas; this series also deals with the behavior of neoplasms. The WHO's *International Histologic Classification of Tumours* and the *Atlas of Tumor Pathology* should serve as primary and complementary references, respectively. The tumor classification system used throughout this volume is the one advocated by the WHO.

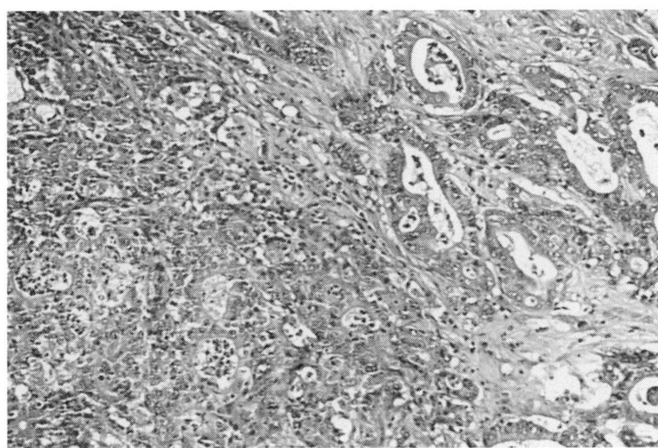

Figure 3–9. Moderately differentiated adenocarcinoma. The glandular structures are less well-formed, particularly on the left. (200×, H&E.)

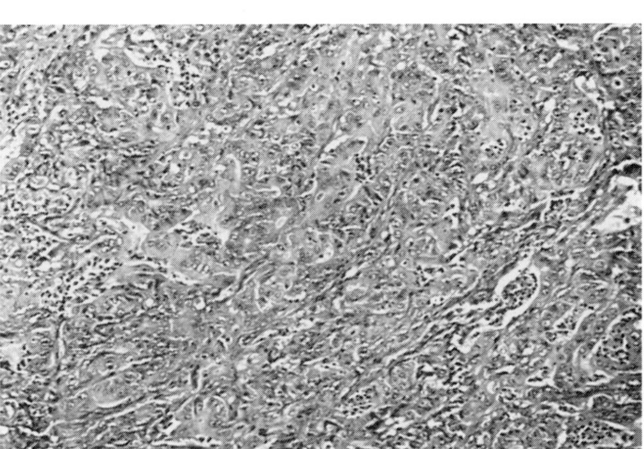

Figure 3–10. Poorly differentiated adenocarcinoma. There is little resemblance to normal glandular structures, with the tumor growing mainly in ill-defined sheets. (200×, H&E.)

TABLE 3–5. **Classification of Neoplasms**

Tissue Origin	Benign	Malignant	Examples
Epithelial/Glandular	Adenoma	Adenocarcinoma	Thyroid follicular adenoma; adenocarcinoma of the lung
Squamous	Squamous papilloma	Squamous cell carcinoma	Squamous papilloma of skin; squamous cell carcinoma of cervix
Connective tissue	Tissue type + (-oma)	Tissue type + (-sarcoma)	Osteoma; osteosarcoma
Hematopoietic and lymphoreticular	Lymphoma	Leukemia	Follicular lymphoma, small, cleaved cell-type; acute myelocytic leukemia
Neural tissue	Neuroma	Blastoma	Acoustic neuroma; neuroblastoma
Germ cell	Teratoma	Teratocarcinoma	Benign cystic teratoma of ovary; immature teratoma of testis

Neoplasms are classified based on the tissue or cell, the type of differentiation, and the anatomic site. In addition, neoplasms are divided into benign and malignant groups, based on their potential biologic behavior. Benign neoplasms are generally innocuous masses that do not metastasize and do little harm to the host, whereas malignant tumors are aggressive neoplasms, which, if untreated, generally result in metastases and death. Some benign neoplasms may undergo malignant transformation. Benign tumors are usually named by adding the suffix *-oma* to the name of a type of cell or tissue, as in *neuroma* or *osteoma*. Malignant tumors are divided into two groups: sarcomas (those of mesenchymal origin) and carcinomas (those of epithelial origin). These terms are then used with the tissue of origin, as in *fibrosarcoma* or *squamous cell carcinoma*.

Like most classifications, there are numerous exceptions. Malignancies of hematopoietic and lymphocytic origin are classified separately. In many instances, eponyms are used in the practice of pathology, particularly when the cell of origin is not clearly established, as with Ewing's sarcoma or Hodgkin's disease. An example of the classification and nomenclature of tumors is shown in Table 3–5. It is beyond the scope of this chapter to provide a comprehensive listing of all of the classified neoplasms, but numerous comprehensive works have been devoted to this topic.

Another category in the early development of malignant neoplasms is the so-called preinvasive or *in situ* dysplasia or malignancy. These terms are generally applicable to malignant epithelial neoplasms, which arise in compartments confined by a basement membrane. Changes in these neoplasms can usually be observed sequentially, such as in carcinoma of the cervix. The preinvasive changes of dysplasia and carcinoma *in situ* can be observed via serial Pap smears and biopsies. In contrast, sarcomas generally arise over rather diffuse areas, but, although conceptually there may be an *in situ* phase, in practice this is not generally observable. Carcinomas *in situ* have most of the morphologic features of malignancy, but they lack one cardinal feature—invasiveness. These generally represent a stage in developing cancer in which the tumor is confined to the epithelium (Fig. 3–11).

Grading and Staging of Cancer

Malignant neoplasms are further classified by grade and stage. Grading and staging are important to assess prognosis and to help determine the type of therapeutic intervention. Grading is an assessment of the potential biologic aggressiveness of the tumor and staging is an assessment of the extent of spread (i.e., size of primary, local spread, and metastases).

Grading

Grading is usually based on cytologic characteristics (e.g., nuclear pleomorphism, hyperchromasia, increased nucleus-to-cytoplasm ratio, number of mitoses, and abnormal mitotic figures) or histologic features that indicate the degree of differentiation (e.g., gland formation, keratin production), or both.

Over the years, there has been a proliferation of grading systems for various organ system cancers. In general, the American Joint Committee on Cancer (AJCC)[14] and the International Union Against Cancer (UICC)[15] recommends a generic grading system for most malignancies: well differentiated, moderately differentiated, poorly differentiated, or grade cannot be assessed. However, there are specific grading systems that have become widely recognized and accepted in association with certain malignancies, including the modified Scarf-Bloom-Richardson grading system for breast cancer[16] and the Gleason grading system for prostate cancer.[17] The Scarf-Bloom-Richardson grading system combines architectural and cytologic features whereas the Gleason grading system is based on architectural features alone.

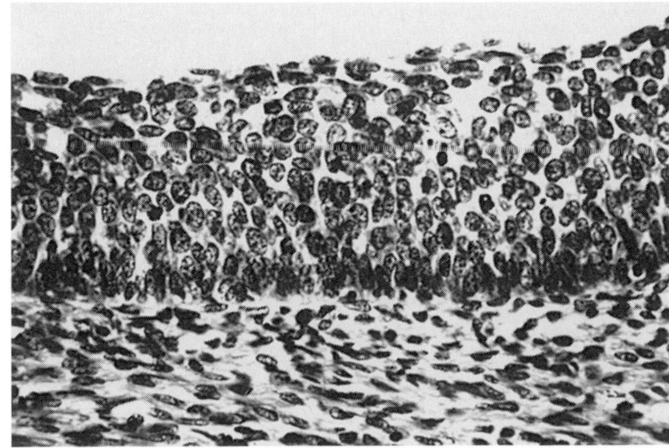

Figure 3–11. Carcinoma *in situ* of the uterine cervix. The epithelium is replaced by small, poorly differentiated cells with many of the cytologic features of malignancy. (160×, H&E.)

Staging

Standardization is important so that a common language exists to facilitate communication between clinicians and researchers. This is especially important for patients enrolled in multi-institutional, cooperative study-group protocols on the cutting edge of developing new therapeutic approaches. The TNM (tumor, node, metastasis) staging system was developed through the joint efforts of the AJCC and the UICC. These organizations have also worked closely together with the International Federation of Gynecology and Obstetrics (FIGO) to classify gynecologic malignancies. Over the years, the AJCC[14] and the UICC[15] have gradually brought their classification systems together and are now identical. Under the TNM staging system, T refers to tumor size and local spread within or outside the organ of origin; N refers to presence or absence of lymph node metastases, and their size and distribution; M refers to metastases. These may be broken down further to indicate, for example, localized metastatic spread versus widespread metastatic disease.

The histologic grade and the stage are useful in determining the prognosis of the tumor. In general, the higher the grade and stage, the poorer the prognosis. Grading of tumors is basically subjective but still prognostically valuable. The tumor grade correlates with patient outcome. Population studies show that stage for stage, patients with low-grade tumors have better survival rates than patients with high-grade neoplasms (Fig. 3–12).

Basic Science of Cancer

Carcinogenesis

In order to understand the basis of the molecular and cellular diagnostic techniques described in this chapter, it is necessary to highlight the principles of abnormal growth regulation in neoplasia:

- Tumor initiation followed by clonal expansion is based on changes in the function of growth regulatory genes.
- These altered genes, *oncogenes*, encode for abnormal growth stimulatory proteins and allow the transformed cell to grow without dependence on normal growth factors and extracellular stimuli.
- These proteins can be growth factors, growth factor receptors, signal-transducing proteins, nonreceptor tyrosine kinases, nuclear transcription factors, or proteins in cellular apoptotic pathways.
- Inhibition of cell growth at the genetic level is controlled by *tumor suppressor genes*. Mutations in these genes result in abnormal growth through loss of function.
- In the multistep process of neoplasia, mutations of genes that regulate apoptosis, such as *BCL2* and *TP53*, are also components that facilitate neoplastic progression. Identification of these oncogenes (altered tumor suppressor and apoptotic genes) in neoplasms has led to a better understanding of their functions.

Based on the finding that chromosomal, cytogenetic alterations were present in malignant cells, Nowell proposed the clonal evolution model of tumor progression.[18] It stated that certain mutations in a single cell lead to further mutations of cells and, eventually, subclones with progressively more aggressive behavior. This model had been postulated since the 1960s and 1970s,[7] although definitive confirmatory experimental methods were not yet available. At that time, Loeb and colleagues also postulated that the mutator phenotype "causing infidelity of DNA replication may be responsible for tumor oncogenesis and progression."[19] Thus, genetic instability increased with tumor progression.

During the 1970s, chromosomal banding techniques made identification of individual chromosomes possible. This was then followed by the characterization of gene rearrangements and translocations that helped to confirm the hypothesis that somatic genetic changes were responsible for the development of cancer. Cytogenetic identification of some childhood acute leukemias, the 9,22 translocation of chronic myelogenous leukemia, the 8,14 translocation of Burkitt's lymphoma, as well as some adult solid tumors became available. Knudson and associates' investigations of pediatric tumors revealed the genetic basis of tumor suppression.[20] They elucidated the relationship between inherited mutations in growth inhibitory genes

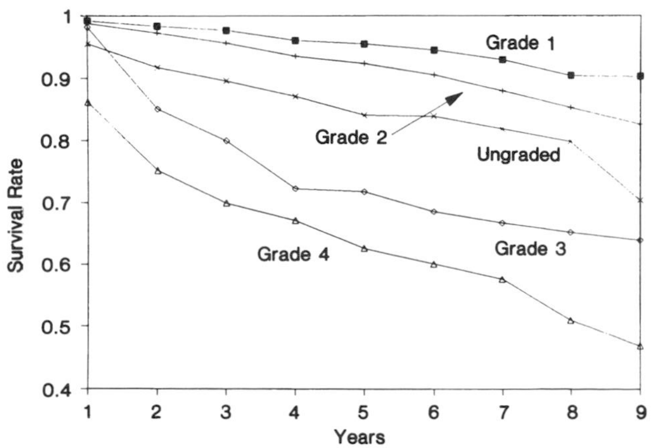

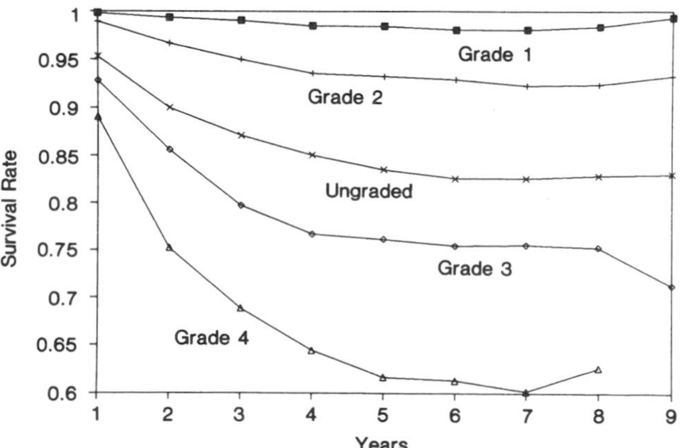

Figure 3–12. Survival rates as related to neoplastic grade in patients with transitional cell carcinoma of the urinary bladder *(left)* and adenocarcinoma of the endometrium *(right)*. From Henson DE: The histologic grading of neoplasms. Arch Pathol Lab Med 1988; 112:1091–1096, with permission.)

and the subsequent somatic mutation that results in loss of growth inhibition and thus tumor development. This process is known as the *two-hit model* of carcinogenesis and was first identified in inherited retinoblastoma (RB). The retinoblastoma tumor suppressor gene was found to be deleted or mutated in sporadic and inherited osteosarcoma and has been implicated, in part, in many common adult malignancies, such as lung, breast, prostate, and bladder carcinomas.[21–24]

Molecular genetics and cytogenetics in the 1980s further confirmed the model of the genetic basis of cancer by cloning individual oncogenes and characterizing their expressed proteins in many different neoplasms. Polymerase chain reactions are now widely used in molecular diagnosis to detect translocations in leukemias, such as chronic myelogenous leukemia, in particular when cytogenetics is unable to visualize the translocation.

Agents of Carcinogenesis

Several viruses, ultraviolet rays, ionizing radiation, and some chemicals have been shown to be mutagenic, and thus participate, in part, in the multistage process of carcinogenesis.

VIRUSES

Viruses, either RNA or DNA, generally exert their effects in cells by causing damage and inducing polyclonal hyperplastic cell growth.

- Hepatitis B virus, a DNA virus, usually leads to chronic inflammation of the liver. Chronic hepatitis B virus infection is epidemiologically associated with hepatocellular carcinoma and follows chronic inflammation and regeneration of hepatocytes. A *TP53* mutation is found in all hepatocellular neoplasms studied.
- Infection with Epstein-Barr virus (EBV), a DNA virus, is associated with B-cell lymphomas. The virus is known to cause a polyclonal expansion of B-lymphocytes and, therefore, a mutation in the actively dividing cells is more likely to occur. In particular, the specific translocation (8,14) causes constitutive expression of the transcription factor *MYC,* when it is translocated to the region of the immunoglobulin heavy chain and leads eventually to a clonal neoplasm of B-lymphocytes. EBV infection therefore appears to be a component in the multistep process of tumor progression. Most individuals are able to suppress this effect before significant polyclonal expansion takes place, but in patients experiencing immunosuppression there is a greater likelihood of neoplastic transformation.
- In contrast to the first two examples, human papilloma virus (HPV), a DNA virus, appears to cause tumors by integrating viral DNA (*E6* and *E7* genes) directly into the genome of the infected cells. This integration can result in downregulation of the cellular tumor suppressor gene products. The viral E7 protein binds to the RB protein and prevents its normal functioning. It also activates *TP53* and causes cellular apoptosis in infected cells. As a result of this *TP53* activation, the E6 oncogene protein product binds to *TP53* and causes its ubiquitin-dependent degradation. The frequency of HPV infection in the uterine cervix and the abovementioned evidence points to its role in the neoplastic transformation in the uterine cervix from dysplasia to invasive carcinoma. Because cancer is a multistep process, these mutations, along with other factors, including smoking, early pregnancy, and immunologic and hormonal status, contribute to mechanisms leading to the ultimate development of a significant neoplasm.[25, 26]

CHEMICALS

Chemicals exert their effect as initiators of carcinogenesis either by direct action, as highly reactive electrophiles forming a covalent adduct with the DNA, or indirect action, requiring metabolic enzymatic conversion to produce a carcinogen.

- Alkylating agents used as cancer chemotherapeutic drugs have been found to cause hematologic malignancies, as well as some solid tumors, after a latent period.
- Aromatic amines and azo dyes are metabolized by the cytochrome P-450 enzyme system in the liver and can induce hepatocellular carcinoma.
- Polycyclic aromatic hydrocarbons are metabolized by the cytochrome P-450 enzyme system and have a high degree of carcinogenic potency. In particular, benzo-[a]pyrene, formed by incomplete combustion of tobacco, has been found to produce lung tumors in laboratory animals.[27]
- Aflatoxin B1, a potent carcinogen and indirect-acting initiator, is a large health problem in the Third World, where it is produced by the fungus *Aspergillus flavus* in moist peanuts and grains. It has been shown to induce neoplasms that are epidemiologically related to hepatocellular carcinoma, all of which have a characteristic mutation of the *TP53* gene.
- Environmental exposure to asbestos, an indirect-acting agent associated with the shipping and mining industries, has been associated with an increased incidence of bronchogenic carcinoma and malignant mesothelioma. Smoking increases the already high risk of lung cancer in this population, but it does not seem to have an effect on the development of malignant mesothelioma.

ULTRAVIOLET RADIATION

Ultraviolet (UV) radiation, particularly ultraviolet B (UVB; 280 320 nm), induces malignant transformation through the formation of pyrimidine dimers in the DNA of the cells in the skin. This induced DNA damage must be repaired by the nucleotide excision repair (NER) pathway, which involves recognition of the DNA damage followed by extensive repair processes. The pathway uses a large number of gene products, and subsequent mutations in these genes can lead to the development of cancer of the skin, in particular, squamous cell carcinoma and basal cell carcinoma. Excessive exposure to sunlight is believed to exceed the capabilities of the NER pathway, and DNA damage is not repaired fully.

An extreme example of the importance of a functioning DNA repair pathway is seen in patients with xeroderma pigmentosum. This is an autosomal recessive disease that predisposes a sensitivity to sunlight in those born with a mutation in one of several genes in the NER pathway. Affected individuals have a high incidence of skin cancers in areas of sun exposure.

IONIZING RADIATION

Ionizing radiation in the form of electromagnetic (x-rays and γ-rays) and particulate (α- and β-particles, protons and neutrons) irradiation is most often associated with thyroid neoplasms and some leukemias. Other cancers include those of the breast, lung, and salivary gland.

Multistep Progression of Neoplasia

Neoplastic transformation is a multistep process of mutations, resulting from a genetic alteration of a single cell, giving rise to a clonal proliferation. Ultimately, the original clone becomes a heterogeneous mass of cells with abnormally regulated growth, local invasiveness, and the ability to penetrate vessels and metastasize. In some neoplasms (e.g., the uterine cervical neoplasm), the progression occurs sequentially from dysplasia to carcinoma *in situ*, to carcinoma with local invasion, and finally to carcinoma with distant metastasis; the pathologist and cytopathologist can observe these steps by light microscopy (see Fig. 3–1).

As a neoplasm grows and progresses within a patient, subpopulations or subclones of cells predominate within the tumor. Individual clones within the tumor create genetic heterogeneity. Some subclones have a genetic advantage and thus grow better than neighboring cells and represent those with the more aggressive growth characteristics. Sampling of neoplastic cells from either the primary or metastatic tumor masses will usually reflect this genetic heterogeneity between neighboring cells. More aggressive tumor growth behavior is manifested histologically by poor differentiation of the cells, cellular crowding, cellular pleomorphism, and atypical mitotic figures reflecting aneuploidy an (abnormal chromosome number). Aneuploidy is correlated with persistent genetic instability throughout tumor progression and may be critical in all colorectal cancers.[28] Some subpopulations are also more able to evade immunologic attack from the patient's immune system and thus have an additional growth advantage. This phenomenon has been named *tumor escape* and may reflect poor presentation of tumor antigens, as well as several other mechanisms.[29]

Experimental work by Vogelstein and colleagues[30, 31] has elucidated the individual steps of the clonal evolution model in colon cancer. An initial mutation in the adenomatous polyposis coli (*APC*) tumor suppressor gene leads to excessive proliferation of colonic epithelial cells within the mucosa. Loss of DNA methylation and further mutations of growth regulatory genes (e.g., *RAS*) lead to increased cell proliferation and a benign adenoma. Additional other mutations in DNA repair genes (e.g., in hereditary nonpolyposis colorectal cancer) and loss of control of cell apoptosis genes (e.g., *TP53*) result in more genetic instability without subsequent cell death within the developing neoplasm.

In more advanced carcinomas, mutations or deletions of the tumor suppressor genes *TP53* and *DCC* (deleted in colon cancer) may also be found. The *DCC* gene has been shown to encode a cell-surface, transmembrane protein that participates in cell-extracellular matrix or cell-cell interactions. Mutations in *TP53* and *DCC* have been shown to account for the more aggressive tendency of malignant neoplasms to leave the confines of the original tumor and invade locally through basement membrane, which leads to invasion of connective tissue collagen and blood vessels or lymphatics and travel to distant organs. This temporal sequence of mutations has been shown to be essential for tumor development and malignant behavior.

Gatekeeper and Caretaker Genes

The *APC* gene controls the early stages of colon carcinogenesis and is known as a *gatekeeper gene*. Gatekeeper genes control cell growth and are important in the initiation phase of neoplasia. Other examples of gatekeeper genes are *RB* and *NF1*. *NF1* is a gene that is mutated in neurofibromatosis type I and some sarcomas, and it functions normally by inhibiting signal transduction in the cell. Cells also have *caretaker genes* that control genomic stability by repairing damaged or mismatched DNA. Caretaker genes include *MSH2*, which is associated with hereditary nonpolyposis coli, and *BRCA1* and *BRCA2*, breast cancer susceptibility genes. *BRCA1* and *BRCA2* have been implicated in the generation of familial breast and ovarian cancers. Mutations of caretaker genes lead to greater genetic instability of all genes within a developing neoplasm.[31] Identification of these mutations in tumors will lead not only to a more definitive diagnosis but also to an understanding of which tumors will respond to certain types of treatment.

TP53 has been called the *cellular gatekeeper for growth and division*. This is a transcription factor that activates a number of genes that are responsible for proteins that cause cell cycle arrest, apoptosis, and DNA repair. Stress on the cell, such as DNA damage and hypoxia, activates *TP53*, and in this way, *TP53* functions to protect the cell as a gatekeeper against the formation of cancers. Large tumors with insufficient angiogenesis undergo apoptosis because of *TP53*-mediated cell death due to hypoxia. It has been shown that over 50% of human tumors have mutations of *TP53*, and chemotherapy and radiotherapy with DNA-damaging effects may be more therapeutically successful in those tumors with wild-type *TP53*.[32] Knowledge of the presence of a *TP53* mutation in specific tumors may prove to be useful in the development of specific therapeutic decisions in the future.[25]

Inherited Predisposition to Cancer

Prevention of cancer is one of the best methods of dealing with malignancy. The tools of molecular biology are now available to detect known, inherited genetic mutations in familial syndromes such as retinoblastoma, Li-Fraumeni, familial ADC, hereditary nonpolyposis colorectal cancer (HNPCC), neurofibromatosis, Wilms' tumor, familial breast cancer, von Hippel–Lindau, multiple endocrine neoplasia type 1 or 2, as well as many others. However, in total, only about 1% of cancer patients has one of these syndromes. Thus, inherited cancer represents only a very small fraction of the patients with malignancy.

The acquisition of a mutant allele and the subsequent risk of cancer depends on other genes present in the cell, as well as diet, environment, and personal lifestyle. Examination of these syndromes and identification of their mutant alleles and oncoproteins will lead to a much better understanding of carcinogenesis in sporadic and common cancers. It will also lead to better identification of affected individuals. Prenatal testing is important in families with these syndromes and can lead to informed family planning. Screening of family members is also essential for identification of those carrying mutations to prevent malignancy or to diagnose affected individuals early. For example, patients with inherited mutations of the DNA mismatch repair gene in HNPCC can benefit from close monitoring of polyps by regular colonoscopy. Prophylactic mastectomy or oophorectomy in those with the *BRCA1* mutation could prevent malignancy and death with this screening.[33, 34]

Growth, Invasion, and Metastatic Spread of Malignancy

A neoplasm develops from a single cell and therefore represents a clonal proliferation. Benign lesions do not yet possess the ability to invade or metastasize and are confined to their original site of growth. In a solid tumor, once the neoplastic mass of cells is large enough to be clinically detectable, a large proportion of its life cycle has passed (Fig. 3–13), it has undergone clonal progression and is quite heterogeneous. In addition, in malignant tumors, areas of cell disassociation or dedifferentiation are found within the mass and at the invading borders. As tumor progression proceeds, some subclones will be more aggressive than neighboring ones and will possess greater ability to grow, invade, and metastasize.

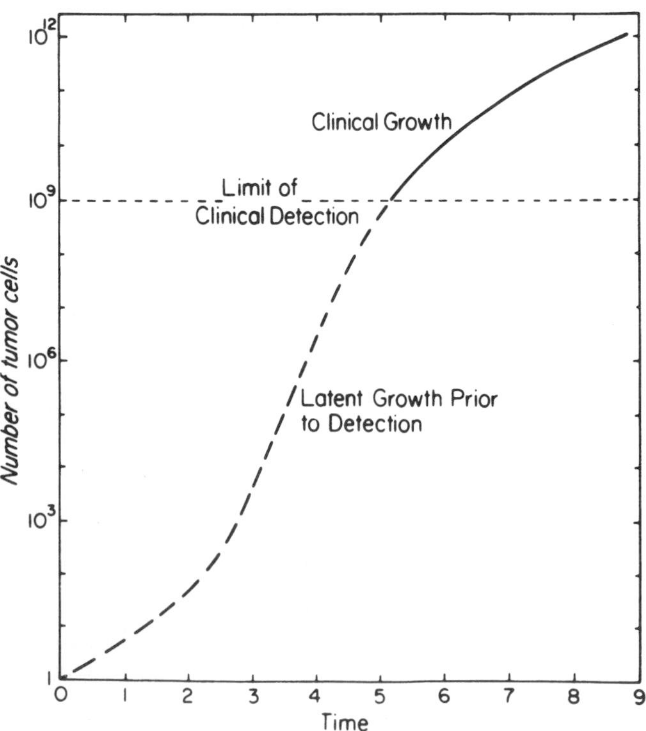

Figure 3–13. Hypothetical growth curve for a human tumor, showing the long latent period prior to detection. Tumors may show an early lag phase and progressive slowing of growth at large size. (From Tannock IF, Hill RP: The Basic Science of Oncology. Elmsford, NY, Pergamon Press PLC, 1988, with permission.)

In order to separate from an expanding tumor mass, malignant cells must acquire specific genetic alterations that allow them to decrease cell-cell adhesiveness. Genetic downregulation and inactivation of the (epithelial) E-cadherin cell adhesion system plays a significant role in the loss of cell-cell adhesiveness and the initial phase of clonal progression in some epithelial malignancies. E-cadherin expression is strong in well-differentiated tumors, but it is reduced in undifferentiated or highly invasive tumors. Expression of E-cadherin is well correlated with a positive clinical outcome in patients.[35]

Malignant epithelial cells must cross the basement membrane and invade surrounding connective tissue, as well as small vessels and lymphatics (Fig. 3–14). Invasion is facilitated by increased expression of cell-surface laminin receptors for basement membrane on cancer cells. Integrins interact with components of connective tissue, and certain integrins have been implicated in carcinogenesis and invasion.[36, 37] Tumor cells also generate a number of proteolytic enzymes to penetrate the extracellular matrix. These include collagenases and cathepsin D. Host macrophages are stimulated to produce proteases that include matrix metalloproteinases (MMP). Levels of type IV collagenase (MMP-2) found in tumors correlate directly with tumor invasiveness.[37]

Once in the circulation, malignant cells usually travel as tumor emboli. In order to metastasize, they must adhere to the endothelium at a distant site and invade through the vessel wall into the tissue. Anatomic drainage patterns of the tissue of origin, as well as cellular and tissue factors related to the tumor cells and sites of metastasis, are important in determining the ultimate location of metastasis (Figs. 3–15 and 3–16). Local growth factors are associated both with tumor cells and target organ capillaries. The synthesis of these factors may play a role in homing or attracting certain tumor emboli to specific distant locations. Metastasis is considered a late stage of carcinogenesis and requires a number of mutations in order to occur. Downregulation of E-cadherin and elaboration of proteases are cellular genetic alterations that promote malignancy.

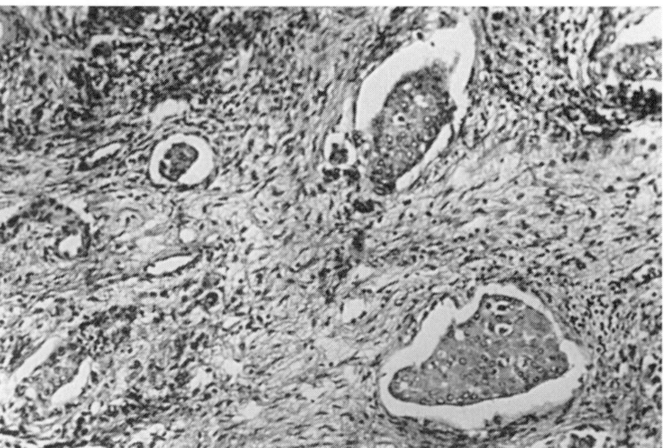

Figure 3–14. Carcinoma of the breast with tumor cells within lymphatic channels. (400×, H&E.)

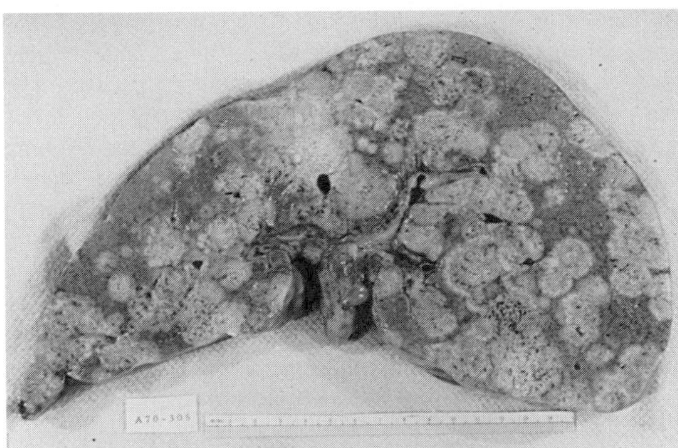

Figure 3–15. Carcinoma of breast metastatic to liver.

Tumor Angiogenesis

Because of oxygen and nutrient requirements, a neoplasm cannot grow beyond 1 to 2 mm unless there is neovascularization. Therefore, tumor growth, expansion, and metastasis are dependent on the ability of the neoplasm to stimulate angiogenesis. Poorly differentiated, large tumors often have blood vessels that are not well formed, and they are disorganized and inadequately spaced; these tumors are more likely to have tissue hypoxia and large areas of tumor necrosis, and new vessel growth allows the neoplasm to avoid these conditions. Without angiogenesis, only those cells at the periphery of the expanding mass will remain viable; therefore, many large tumors, which grow rapidly and aggressively, require constant angiogenesis to survive. In addition, angiogenesis provides tumor cells with access to the vasculature for metastatic spread. It has been shown that in breast and prostate cancer, microvessel density correlates with metastasis and prognosis.[38–40]

Tumor cells and activated macrophages produce a number of angiogenic factors that stimulate angiogenesis. These include vascular endothelial growth factor (VEGF), basic and acidic fibroblast growth factor (FGFA, FGFB), and epidermal growth factor (EGF). Malignant tumors also generate antiangiogenic factors. Antiangiogenic factors include angiostatin and endostatin. It has recently become clear that angiogenesis and therefore neoplastic proliferation result from a net imbalance favoring the production of angiogenic factors over those that are antiangiogenic. Drugs aimed at inhibiting neovascularization are being investigated. Experimental trials using purified inhibitors of angiogenesis in animals have been promising.[41–43]

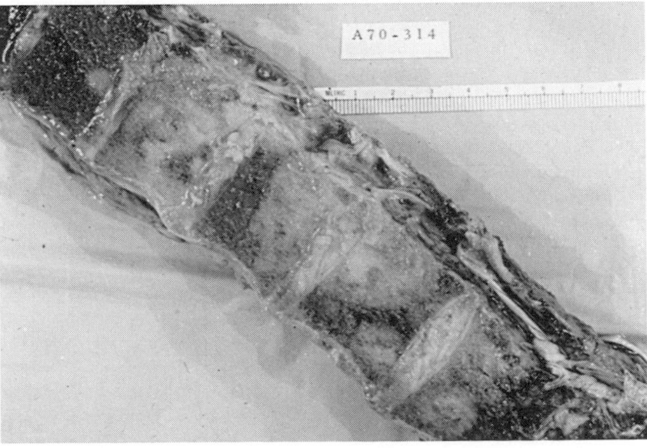

Figure 3–16. Carcinoma of breast metastatic to vertebral bodies.

Molecular Pathology and Oncogene-Specific Therapeutics

It has long been the goal of oncology to tailor specific therapies directly for tumor cells and spare the host cells from the toxicity of conventional chemotherapy and radiotherapy. Monoclonal antibodies are now being developed and used in some cases of lymphoma and breast cancer. Other therapies are also available, that take advantage of newly discovered mutations in the genome of the neoplastic cells. Table 3–6 lists some important tumor markers with prognostic and therapeutic relevance.

It appears that for a subset of lymphomas and a small number other malignancies, monoclonal antibody therapy is becoming a reality. A genetically engineered, chimeric, murine and human monoclonal antibody directed against CD20, a B-cell specific antigen expressed on non-Hodgkin's lymphomas, has been synthesized recently,[44] and a clinical response without dose-limiting toxicity in relapsed low-grade non-Hodgkin's lymphoma has been demonstrated. In order to determine which patients are likely to respond to monoclonal antibody therapy, immunohistochemistry on biopsied tumor material must be positive for CD20 in those undergoing therapy. Because this assay is part of a standard panel in the classification of lymphomas, the success of this therapy reinforces the necessity for the collaboration of the pathologist and clinician to ensure the proper diagnosis and provide the best therapy for the patient.

TABLE 3–6. **Prognostically/Therapeutically Important Tumor Markers**

Marker (Oncogene/Receptor)	Implication
ERBB2	Oncogene is amplified and the protein is overexpressed in some breast cancers. *ERBB2* is associated with a poorer clinical outcome. Successful therapy with a monoclonal antibody to the overexpressed antigen
Estrogen and progesterone receptors	Positive in most breast cancers; a positive result indicates a better prognosis and response with tamoxifen therapy
CD20	Receptor is expressed on some B-cell lymphomas. When the result is positive, the condition is amenable to therapy with monoclonal antibody to this receptor
MYCN	Amplification of oncogene in neuroblastoma is associated with a poorer clinical outcome

Another monoclonal antibody therapy is showing clinical response in some breast cancers. *HER2/NEU (ERBB2)*, an amplified oncogene encoding an overexpressed growth factor receptor, has been found in a subset of breast cancers with a poor prognosis. This subset of breast cancers represents an example of a neoplasm that has become the target of an oncogene-specific therapy. The monoclonal antibody Herceptin (trastuzumab) has been developed against this overexpressed cell surface receptor and has shown promise in the treatment of these breast neoplasms.[45] Pathologists are now able to use immunohistochemistry to detect the presence of the product of the amplified oncogene in biopsies of breast tumors. This detection method has led to more specific and successful therapy for this neoplasm.[46, 47]

Many breast tumors are also evaluated by immunohistochemistry for the presence of estrogen and progesterone receptors. If these receptors are positive in the tumor, this is a good predictor of clinical outcome. Tamoxifen, a nonsteroidal antiestrogen, has been shown to be an effective therapy in combination with other drugs, when estrogen and progesterone receptors are positive in this tumor.[48]

Oncogene-specific therapy is also part of the chemotherapeutic regimen of acute promyelocytic leukemia (APL). The t(15,17) translocation found in APL results in the chimeric *PML/RAR*α gene product that causes aberrant transcription of a number of genes in myeloid progenitor cells. This gene product is detected using RT-PCR and is diagnostic for APL (see Fig. 3–5).[49] Molecular diagnosis is essential to confirm the morphologic histologic diagnosis because malignant immature promyelocytic leukemic cells can be induced to differentiate terminally by treatment with retinoic acid in 90% of cases.

Chemotherapy with retinoic acid in combination with other agents has been very successful in patients with APL. If retinoic acid is used alone, these patients will relapse and new tumors will be insensitive to retinoic acid treatment. Recent experimental work has shown that further mutations in the chimeric *PML/RAR*α oncogene are responsible for subsequent resistance to treatment with retinoic acid.[50] This finding is consistent with the clonal evolution model of neoplasia. Accurate, specific diagnosis is particularly important in APL because treatment with retinoic acid can have significant adverse side effects and should only be used when the diagnosis is confirmed. In addition, rapid, definitive diagnosis is essential, because many patients with APL can have a consumptive coagulopathy and require prompt treatment to prevent this life-threatening sequela. Treatment of APL with retinoic acid was discovered empirically before the oncogene was elucidated, but this chemotherapy represents the first example of specific targeting of a drug to an oncogene. It seems clear that further research will continue to uncover more genotype-specific therapy of neoplasia.

Recommended Reading

The literature on the pathology of cancer is quite extensive and ranges from basic and descriptive texts to detailed and very specific ones. Numerous journals and textbooks are available relating to basic pathology, histologic and cytologic diagnosis, and research aspects of neoplasia. The chapter on neoplasia in *Robbins' Pathologic Basis of Disease*, edited by Cotran, Kumar, and Collins, is an excellent introduction to the principles of neoplastic disease.[1] For more detailed information about specific types of cancer, *Ackerman's Surgical Pathology*, written and edited by Juan Rosai, is an excellent source.[2] For basic science references, *The Genetic Basis of Human Cancer*, edited by Vogelstein and Kinzler,[3] and *The Basic Science of Oncology*, edited by Tannock and Hill,[4] are both useful sources on this subject. The gold standards for the classification of tumors are the WHO's *International Histological Classification of Tumours*[5] and the complementary series, *Atlas of Tumor Pathology*, by the Armed Forces Institute of Pathology.[6]

ACKNOWLEDGMENTS

The authors wish to thank Dr. Thomas Bonfiglio and Dr. Mark Stoler, coauthors of this chapter in previous editions, for permission to retain figures and information from those editions.

REFERENCES

General References

1. Cotran RS, Kumar V, Collins T (eds): Robbins' Pathologic Basis of Disease, 6th ed. Philadelphia, W.B. Saunders, 1999.
2. Rosai J: Ackerman's Surgical Pathology, 8th ed. St. Louis, Mosby, 1996.
3. Vogelstein B, Kinzler K (eds): The Genetic Basis of Human Cancer. New York, McGraw-Hill, 1998.
4. Tannock IF, Hill RP (eds): The Basic Science of Oncology, 3rd ed. New York, McGraw-Hill, 1998.
5. World Health Organization: International Histological Classification of Tumours, 2nd ed. New York, Springer-Verlag, 1989.
6. Rosai J (ed): Atlas of Tumor Pathology, 3rd ser. Washington, Armed Forces Institute of Pathology, 1997–98.

Specific References

7. Nowell PC: The clonal evolution of tumor progression. Science 1976; 194:23–28.
8. Enzinger FM, Weiss SW (eds): Soft Tissue Tumors, 3rd ed, pp 139–163. St. Louis, Mosby, 1995.
9. Wang NP, Zee S, Zarbo RJ, et al: Coordinate expression of cytokeratins 7 and 20 defines unique subsets of carcinomas. Applied Immunohistochemistry 1995; 3:99–107.
10. Pasternak G, Hochhaus A, Schultheis B, et al: Chronic myelogenous leukemia: molecular and cellular aspects. J Cancer Res Clin Oncol 1998; 124:643–660.
11. Croce CM: Molecular biology of lymphomas. Semin Oncol 1993; 20:31–46.
12. Secker-Walker LM, Prentice HG, Durrant J, et al: Cytogenetics adds independent prognostic information in adults with acute lymphoblastic leukaemia on MRC trial UKALL XA. MRC Leukaemia Working Party. Br J Haematol 1997; 96:601–610.
13. Thorner PS, Squire JA: Molecular genetics in the diagnosis and prognosis of solid pediatric tumors. Pediatric and Developmental Pathology 1998; 1:337–365.
14. Fleming ID, Cooper JS, Henson DE, et al (eds), for the American Joint Committee on Cancer: AJCC Cancer Staging Manual, 5th ed. Philadelphia, Lippincott-Raven, 1998.
15. Sobin LH, Wittekind C (eds), for the International Union Against Cancer: TNM Classification of Malignant Tumours, 5th ed. New York, Wiley-Liss, 1997.
16. Elston CW, Ellis IO: Pathological prognostic factors in breast cancer. I. The value of histological grade in breast cancer: experience from a large study with long-term follow-up. Histopathology 1991; 19:403–410.
17. Gleason DF. The Veterans Administration Cooperative Urological Research Group: histological grading and clinical staging of prostatic carcinoma. In: Tannenbaum M (ed): Urologic Pathology: the Prostate, pp 171–197. Philadelphia, Lea & Febiger, 1977.

18. Nowell PC: Chromosomes and cancer: evolution of an idea. Adv Cancer Res 1993; 6:1–17.
19. Loeb LA, Springgate CF, Battula N: Errors in DNA replication as a basis of malignant disease. Cancer Res 1974; 34:2311–2321.
20. Knudson AG, Meadows AT, Nichols WW, et al: Chromosomal deletions and retinoblastoma N Engl J Med 1976; 295:1120–1123.
21. Reissmann PT, Koga H, Takahashi R, et al, and the Lung Cancer Study Group: Inactivation of the retinoblastoma susceptibility gene in non–small-cell lung cancer. Oncogene 1993; 8:1913–1919.
22. Bookstein R, Rio P, Madreperla SA, et al: Promoter deletion and loss of retinoblastoma gene expression in human prostate carcinoma. Proc Natl Acad Sci U S A 1990; 87:7762–7766.
23. Ishikawa J, Xu H-J, Hu S-X, et al: Inactivation of the retinoblastoma gene in human bladder and renal cell carcinomas. Cancer Res 1991; 51:5736–5743.
24. Wadayama B, Toguchida J, Shimizu T, et al: Mutation spectrum of the retinoblastoma gene in osteosarcomas Cancer Res 1994; 54:3042–3048.
25. Levine AJ: p53, the cellular gatekeeper for growth and division. Cell 1997; 88:323–331.
26. Stoler M: The biology of human papillomaviruses. Pathology Case Reviews 1997; 2:8–20.
27. Hecht SS: Tobacco and cancer: approaches using carcinogen biomarkers and chemoprevention. Ann N Y Acad Sci 1997; 833:91–111.
28. Lengauer C, Kinzler KW, Vogelstein B: Genetic instability in colorectal cancers. Nature 1997; 386:623–627.
29. Shu S, Plautz GE, Krauss JC, Chang AE: Tumor immunology. JAMA 1997; 278:1972–1980.
30. Kinzler KW, Vogelstein B: Lessons from hereditary colorectal cancer. Cell 1996; 87:159–170.
31. Kinzler KW, Vogelstein B: Cancer-susceptibility genes. Gatekeepers and caretakers. Nature 1997; 386:761, 763.
32. Blank KR, Rudoltz MS, Kao GD, et al: The molecular regulation of apoptosis and implications for radiation oncology. Int J Radiat Biol 1997; 71:455–466.
33. Fearon ER: Human cancer syndromes: clues to the origin and nature of cancer. Science 1997; 278:1043–1058.
34. Blackwood MA, Weber BL: BRCA1 and BRCA2: from molecular genetics to clinical medicine. J Oncol 1998; 16:1969–1977.
35. Hirohashi S: Inactivation of the E-cadherin–mediated cell adhesion system in human cancer. Am J Pathol 1998; 153:333–338.
36. Strunck E, Vollmer G: Variants of integrin beta 4 subunit in human endometrial adenocarcinoma cells: mediators of ECM-induced differentiation? Biochem Cell Biol 1996; 74:867–873.
37. Crowe DL, Shuler CF: Regulation of tumor cell invasion by extracellular matrix. Histol Histopathol 1999; 14:665–671.
38. Weidner N, Semple JP, Welch WR, Folkman J: Tumor angiogenesis and metastasis—correlation in invasive breast carcinoma. N Engl J Med 1991; 324:1–8.
39. Weidner N: Intratumor microvessel density as a prognostic factor in cancer. Am J Pathol 1995; 147:9–18.
40. Folkman J: Tumor angiogenesis. In: Holland JF, et al (eds): Cancer Medicine, 4th ed, p 181. Baltimore, Williams and Wilkins, 1997.
41. O'Reilly MS, Holmgren L, Chen C, Folkman J: Angiostatin induces and sustains dormancy of human primary tumors in mice. Nature Med 1996; 2:689–692.
42. O'Reilly MS, Boehm T, Shing Y, et al: Endostatin: an endogenous inhibitor of angiogenesis and tumor growth. Cell 1997; 88:277–285.
43. Vogler WR, Liu J, Volpert O, et al: The anticancer drug edelfosine is a potent inhibitor of neovascularization in vivo. Cancer Invest 1998; 16:549–553.
44. Maloney DG, Grillo-Lopez AJ, White CA, et al: IDEC-C2B8 (Rituximab) anti-CD20 monoclonal antibody therapy in patients with relapsed low grade non-Hodgkin's lymphoma. Blood 1997; 90:2188–2195.
45. Goldhirsch A, Coates AS, Castiglione-Gertsch M, Gelber RD: New treatments for breast cancer: breakthroughs for patient care or just steps in the right direction? Ann Oncol 1998; 9:973–976.
46. Press MF, Hung G, Godolphin W, Slamon DJ: Sensitivity of HER-2/neu antibodies in archival tissue samples: potential source of error in immunohistochemical studies of oncogene expression. Cancer Res 1994; 54;2771–2777.
47. Ross JS, Fletcher JA: HER-2/neu (c-erb-B2) gene and protein in breast cancer. Am J Clin Pathol 1999; 112:S53–S67.
48. Locker GY: Hormonal therapy of breast cancer. Cancer Treat Rev 1998; 24:221–240.
49. Miller WH, Kakizuka A, Frankel SR, et al: Reverse transcriptase polymerase chain reaction for the rearranged retinoic acid receptor alpha clarifies diagnosis and detects minimal residual disease in acute promyelocytic leukemia. Proc Natl Acad Sci U S A 1992; 89:2694–2698.
50. Imaizumi M, Suzuki H, Yoshimari M, et al: Mutations in the E-domain of RAR portion of the PML/RAR chimeric gene may confer clinical resistance to all-trans retinoic acid in acute promyelocytic leukemia. Blood 1998; 92:374–382.

4 *Principles of Surgical Oncology*

ELIN R. SIGURDSON, MD, PHD, Surgical Oncology
JOHN A. RIDGE, MD, PHD, FACS, Head and Neck Surgery
ROBERT J. GINSBERG, MD, Thoracic Surgery

No good physician quavers incantations when the malady he's treating needs the knife.

SOPHOCLES, *Ajax*

Perspective

Complete surgical excision represents the most effective therapy for most solid tumors. Despite tremendous efforts and legitimate advances in cancer treatment with drugs, radiation, and biologic response modifiers, the majority of patients with solid tumors will have benefited from surgery alone.[8] However, the modern practice of cancer surgery demands an understanding of tumor biology and multidisciplinary cancer care that transcends the technical issues involved in the so-called radical resection of organs.

A thorough understanding of the principles of surgical oncology is essential to the appropriate therapy for patients with solid tumors. Surgeons from any specialty who care for cancer patients should understand and be prepared to pursue the following:

- diagnosis by appropriate biopsy of lesions
- adequate staging
- radical resection
- organ-sparing procedures
- multimodality therapy
- current reconstructive options
- palliative resections
- surgery for metastatic cancers

In addition, the surgeon should be fully familiar with oncologic emergencies, as well as the surgical complications that may be induced by treatment with other modalities. Finding a surgeon whose education, temperament, and technical ability will best serve the patient with a newly diagnosed solid tumor is perhaps the most important task confronting the primary care physician.

The distinct characteristics of cancer and the potential benefits of resection have been recognized for hundreds of years,[9] but surgical approaches to tumors were largely limited until anesthesia and infection control methods gained wide acceptance.[10] Effective surgery for cancers of the gastrointestinal tract, head and neck, breast, genitourinary system, and other sites was developed over the ensuing decades, and current methods of anesthesia and perioperative care have rendered most operations safe when performed by experienced surgeons.[11] Reviews suggest that even formidable undertakings, such as liver resection, pancreatectomy (Whipple procedure), and esophageal resection, may be performed safely today on all populations, including both young and elderly patients.[12–15] The latter represents an important issue in planning cancer care, because solid tumors primarily affect older patients who have an increasingly longer life expectancy in developed nations today.[16] There is little reason these days to withhold potentially lifesaving treatment from an individual based on age alone. Indeed, waiting until an emergency ensues, rather than addressing a cancer promptly when it is discovered, should be discouraged because older patients are less tolerant of the complications caused by emergency surgery.

Although the potential impact of a cancer removal is usually obvious, the surgeon should be prepared to discuss all aspects of treatment, including adjuvant or preoperative chemotherapy, radiation therapy, organ preservation, and reconstruction. The surgeon has an important role to play in educating patients and guiding them through the decision making and treatment planning. This is especially important when counseling patients with regard to radical resection or organ preservation (such as for tumors of the breast, prostate, bladder, or larynx).

Surgery for the Diagnosis of Cancer

Surgeons and their colleagues in radiology and internal medicine have important roles in the diagnosis of cancer. Many tumors are detected through imaging studies, or with endoscopic procedures; however, a biopsy is frequently necessary to establish the diagnosis. The diagnosis is rarely assigned following a therapeutic procedure, such as when a colon resection is performed for an obstructing or bleeding lesion, because in the majority of cases, a diagnostic biopsy has been performed before surgery. The technique chosen to obtain a tissue diagnosis is obvious for some tumors; however, in some situations, an incorrectly performed biopsy will compromise the patient's cancer care.

Needle Biopsy

Fine-needle aspiration biopsies and core-needle biopsies have become the most widely used techniques to diagnose tumors for which biopsies cannot be performed during endoscopic procedures. Fine-needle aspiration should be the first diagnostic procedure performed for palpable abnormalities. In the hands of experienced cytopathologists, the fine-needle aspiration provides a rapid and accurate diagnosis in a cost-effective manner.[17–19] The procedure is safe, effective, and does not produce a scar that may complicate later resection. This is particularly important for head and neck cancers and sarcomas, in which an inappropriately placed scar or violation of the tumor complicates the subsequent cancer treatment.

If the lesion is not palpable but can be imaged, a fine-needle aspiration or small caliber core-needle biopsy can be performed. This is true for many mammographic abnormalities, in which a diagnosis of breast cancer can be assigned with stereotactic or ultrasound-guided needle biopsics. Needle biopsies have largely replaced open diagnostic procedures for abnormalities within the chest, liver, head and neck, and retroperitoneum. However, for certain pulmonary and gastrointestinal cancers, biopsy could represent a significant risk of tumor spread from technical complications, such as bleeding. In these instances, if the lesion appears resectable, a biopsy should not be done.

Excisional and Incisional Open Biopsy

An excisional biopsy is generally preferred if a surgical biopsy is needed. This will remove the entire lesion if it proves benign, and it usually assures adequate tissue for the pathologist. However, in some instances, excising the entire lesion is inappropriate and an incisional biopsy should be performed. For example, a pigmented lesion on the face that may be benign should not be removed in its entirety if disfigurement would result; only the most suspicious area should be removed.

In planning a biopsy, the surgeon should consider several important issues:

- With the exception of small skin lesions, no worrisome abnormality should be removed in its entirety unless the doctor extirpating the lesion is prepared to render definitive surgical care.
- The incision must be placed in a manner that will not compromise resection and reconstruction (Fig. 4–1).[20] This is particularly important when organ or limb preservation is possible.
- Any biopsy should be performed with minimum disruption of normal tissues. Meticulous hemostasis is important in order to prevent hematomas, which may disrupt tissue planes and implant tumor cells far from the biopsy site.
- The specimen should be oriented and the clinical situation accurately described to the pathologist. The surgeon must communicate with the pathologist to confirm that adequate tissue has been removed for diagnosis.
- When an open biopsy of a neck node is performed, the surgeon and patient should both be prepared for a neck dissection at that time, rather than delaying definitive treatment.

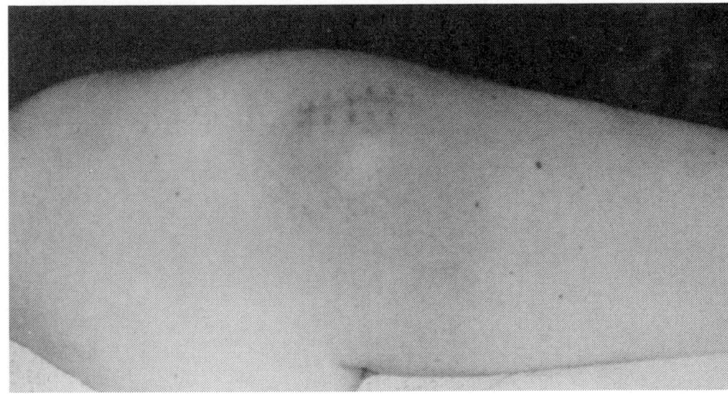

Figure 4–1. Incisional biopsies should be performed with consideration of the incision needed to remove the mass should it prove to be cancer. In this picture of a thigh mass, the incision is oriented longitudinally to allow for removal of the scar *en bloc* with the tumor if the biopsy is malignant. (From Shiu MH, Brennan M [eds]: Surgical Management of Soft Tissue Sarcoma, p 83. Philadelphia, Lea & Febiger, 1989, with permission.)

Open breast biopsy for a palpable lesion or needle localization for mammographically detected lesions is a commonly performed procedure (Fig. 4–2).[21] The appropriate incisions and techniques used to produce the best combination of cosmetic and sound oncologic results have been described in a number of reviews.[22, 23] In an axillary node dissection, the primary tumor excision should rarely be extended into the axilla; complications have led to this procedure no longer being standard practice.[24] In most other instances, surgery involves an incision directly over the lesion; tunneling to the tumor from a periareolar incision or through the breast from the site where the localiza-

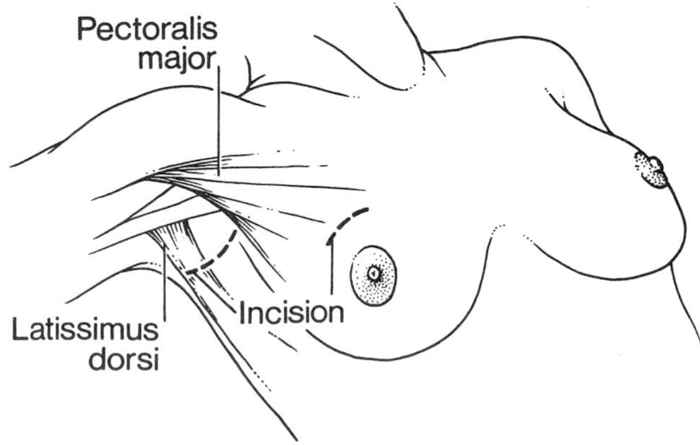

Figure 4–2. The placement of the incision for both the lumpectomy and the axillary dissection has an impact on the cosmetic result. The illustration depicts the ideal placement of the incisions. The lumpectomy incision should be curvilinear, placed directly over the tumor, with a separate axillary incision placed posterior to the pectoralis major muscle and at the lower hair line. (From Harris JR, Hellman S, Henderson IC, et al [eds]: Breast Diseases, p 270. Philadelphia, J.B. Lippincott, 1987, with permission.)

tion wire enters the skin should be avoided. Such approaches may result in excessive tissue loss and can spread the tumor through a large area of the breast; this becomes a problem for the radiation therapist if a cancer is discovered and breast preservation is advised. The major determinant for excellent postirradiation cosmesis is attention to surgical excision of the primary tumor.[24, 25]

Surgery for Staging of Cancer

Staging systems have been developed to correlate extent of disease with patient survival. Although all patients are individuals with their own relationship to their cancer, staging systems are designed to predict the anticipated survival of a large group of patients with a given tumor burden. Most solid tumors are staged according to the size of the primary cancer (T), whether lymph node metastases are present (N), and whether there are metastases beyond the lymph node basin draining the primary cancer (M).

Depending on the site of disease, primary tumor extent may vary from T1 to T4, nodes from N0 to N3, and metastases from M0 to M1. The extent of tumor, nodal, and metastatic disease is combined to predict survival rates in stages I to IV. The tumor, node, metastasis (TNM) staging system is designed primarily so that the disease-free 5-year survival rates for stages I, II, III, and IV are approximately 75%, 60%, 30%, and 5%, respectively. The staging system is reviewed regularly and adjusted to account for improvements in the understanding of the behavior of tumors and treatment changes. Cancers are staged only at clinical presentation (TNM) and, occasionally, after pathologic examination (pTNM). *Once a stage has been assigned to the cancer, it does not change*; that is, should a tumor recur after treatment, the stage will not be increased. For example, a patient who presents with bone metastases from a lung cancer has stage IV disease; if a stage I lung cancer has been appreciated and treated before the development of bone metastases, the cancer is a recurrent stage I lesion, and *not* a stage IV cancer.

The American Joint Committee on Cancer and the Union Internationale Contre le Cancer (International Union Against Cancer) have agreed upon a single staging system for solid tumors, which is based on the TNM and pTNM staging system.[26] Since 1991, the Joint Committee for the Accreditation of Healthcare Organizations has required that all cancer patients are staged according to the TNM system upon presentation, this information becoming part of the medical record. In many cases, the doctor who is best able to determine the stage of the patient's cancer is the surgeon. It is therefore imperative that all surgeons be familiar with this staging system. Only the surgeon operating on a patient is in a position to evaluate small-volume disease in a body cavity, in pleural or peritoneal fluid, and other sites of disease that cannot be assessed outside of the operating room. This requires a knowledge of the modes of spread of each cancer, so that an appropriate staging evaluation is performed in a timely and cost-effective manner, without a barrage of unnecessary tests. An excellent example of surgical-pathologic staging is found in the classification of regional lymph node stations in lung cancer, adopted by the American Joint Committee on Cancer.[27]

There are four classifications of staging:

- *Clinical classification*, designated cTNM, is based on all clinical evidence, including radiographic work-up and operative findings and includes all information available before the first definitive treatment.
- *Pathologic classification*, designated pTNM, includes the T and N staging provided by the pathologic evaluation of the resected tumor, as well as the preoperative staging for metastatic disease.
- *Retreatment classification*, designated rTNM, is used after a disease-free interval when further treatment is planned; the primary staging of the patient does not change.
- *Autopsy classification*, designated aTNM, is performed after the death of a patient.

If multiple tumors occur in the same organ, the suffix "m" is added, such as T(m)NM. This may be found in patients with two breast cancers in one breast, or with more than one colon cancer. In patients who have received neoadjuvant therapy before surgical staging, the prefix "y" is added to the clinical and pathologic staging, denoting the possibility of downstaging from the preoperative treatment. The staging is then recorded as yTNM for clinical, or ypTNM for pathologic staging.

All doctors treating patients with cancer should review in detail the American Joint Committee on Cancer's staging book. Most important in initial staging is the fact that evaluation of the clinical stage can involve any invasive modality including surgical exploration, but excluding the therapeutic excision. Therefore, invasive procedures such as laparotomy and laparoscopy, thoracotomy and thoracoscopy, biopsies at endoscopy, and the like, can be employed in the initial clinical staging. However, once the tumor is excised, pTNM is the appropriate staging.

Surgery for the Treatment of the Primary Cancer

Radical Cancer Treatment

In the majority of cases, the surgical resection of a primary solid tumor encompasses removal of the tumor *en bloc* together with the draining lymph nodes. This principle was first described during the eighteenth century; however, it was not until the advent of ether anesthesia that such resection became reasonable. Halsted, in the latter part of the nineteenth century, developed the radical mastectomy for the removal of large cancers of the breast and, in 1894, he presented the results of this operation on 50 women.[28] He performed radical excision of the breast and pectoralis major muscles, with *en bloc* excision of the fascia of the rectus abdominus, serratus, subscapularis, latissimus dorsi and teres major muscles, as well as the skin of the breast (Fig. 4–3). This procedure reduced local recurrences from approximately 60% (most of his patients had massive cancers or bulky axillary lymphadenopathy) to 6% and revolutionized the treatment of breast cancer. In later reports, Halsted described 5-year survival rates of 75% for patients with tumors confined to the breast and 31% for patients with axillary lymph node involvement. However, only 10%

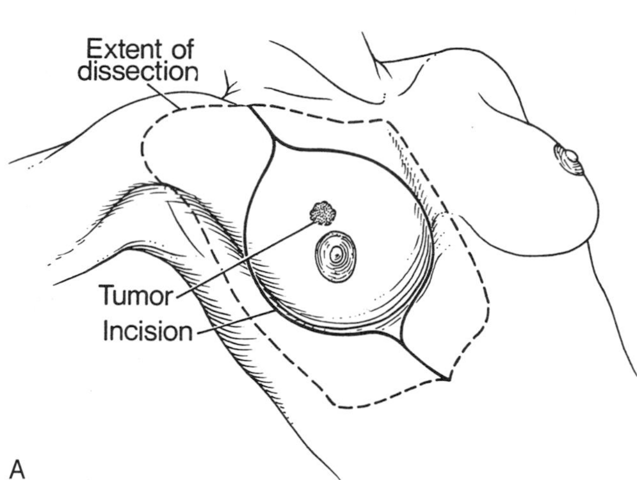

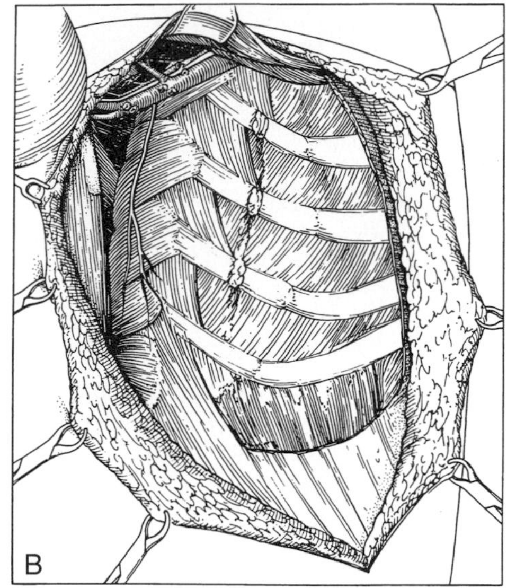

Figure 4–3. (A) The Halsted radical mastectomy was performed through a vertical incision, with removal of the skin overlying the breast as denoted by the solid line. The operation was completed with a skin graft to cover the defect. (B) The resection included the skin, breast, the sternal head of the pectoralis major muscle, the pectoralis minor muscle, and the axillary lymph nodes in levels 1, 2, and 3. (From Harris JR, Hellman S, Henderson IC, et al [eds]: Breast Diseases, p 268. Philadelphia, J.B. Lippincott, 1987, with permission.)

of the patients were alive at 5 years if supraclavicular node dissection was performed to remove involved nodes above the clavicle.[29] From this work, Halsted proposed that breast cancer spread in an orderly fashion: from the breast, to the regional lymph nodes, and then beyond. This has become known as the Halstedian model of cancer progression.

During the first half of the twentieth century, while anesthesia improved and the mortality of operations diminished, most patients presented with locally advanced disease. There was no chemotherapy and only primitive radiation therapy, and surgical resection represented the only chance to cure a patient. The early successes of Halsted and others led to aggressive operations that attempted to encompass all disease that was not yet metastatic. Crile described the radical neck dissection in 1906,[30] and Martin brought Halstedian principles to head and neck surgery. He advocated standard surgical procedures for the management of the neck lymph nodes synchronously with resection of the primary tumor.[31, 32]

For most of the twentieth century, the Halstedian model remained unchallenged. In the early 1980s, Fisher and colleagues described an alternative hypothesis.[33] They suggested that breast cancer becomes a systemic disease at a preclinical stage in its progression and that aggressive local and regional treatment would not improve survival. They and others brought breast-sparing approaches to the forefront of modern cancer surgery, placing an emphasis on the multidisciplinary management of the tumor:

- Extensive surgery was replaced with radiation therapy to control local and regional disease.
- Full axillary dissections in breast cancer have been replaced by sentinel node biopsies to identify the node-negative patient who does not need a node dissection (Fig. 4–4).
- Chemotherapy has been added to the treatment regimen in an effort to cure undetected metastases.

It is likely that neither Halsted's nor Fisher's models for tumor spread adequately explain the natural history of cancer,[34–36] and that the best approach for the management of patients with cancer will involve a synthesis of the two approaches. However, even after decades, these important principles continue to guide the surgical management of cancer.

Benign Lesion Management

Surgical therapy of benign problems removes the *smallest* amount of tissue possible that will cure the condition and leave the patient with near normal function. In contrast, surgical treatment of cancer removes the *largest* amount of involved, or potentially involved, tissue that may be sacrificed while maintaining near normal function. For example, operations for diverticulitis remove the involved bowel but not the mesentery of the colon, whereas both the colon and mesentery are removed during the resection of a colon cancer. Generally, so-called cancer operations are distinguished from those undertaken to treat benign disease by the removal of appropriate lymph node groups along with the primary tumor (Fig. 4–5).[37] Advances in surgical technique, such as sentinel node mapping,[38–41] are designed to identify patients who do not benefit from full node dissections.

Multimodal Therapy

For most solid tumors, failure to remove regional lymph nodes or to completely encompass the primary cancer during the resection represents the most important preventable

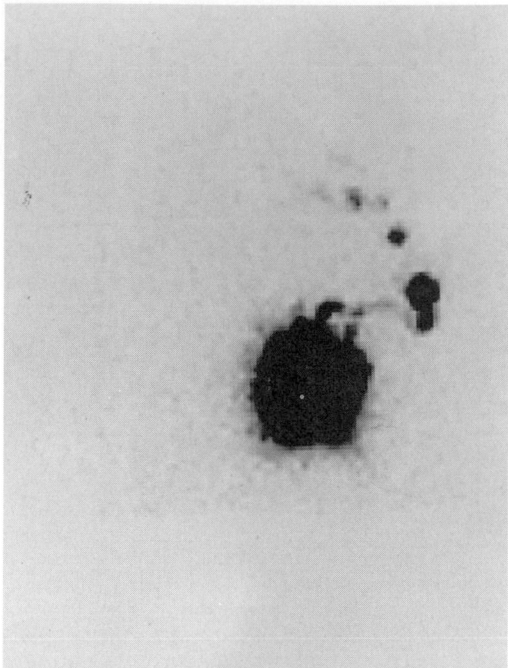

Figure 4–4. Lymphoscintigraphy in breast cancer identifies the sentinel node that represents the first lymph node draining that region of the breast. Technetium sulfur colloid is injected around the breast cancer, and the lymphoscintigram reveals two draining lymphatics that converge and drain to the lower axilla. Studies have confirmed that if this node does not contain cancer, the remainder of the axillary nodes will be cancer free.

cause of tumor recurrence. Radiation and chemotherapy represent powerful weapons against cancer; however, in general, the use of adjuvant radiotherapy or chemotherapy cannot overcome the damaging effects of insufficient surgery.[42–46] These modes of treatment should be used to extend the benefits of cancer operations rather than to compensate for having performed an inadequate operation.

Multimodality therapy has become the accepted approach for many solid tumors. Many clinical trials are currently under way to investigate the best way to employ surgery, radiotherapy, and chemotherapy. However, when devising new research protocols and planning treatments, it is important to remember the relative contribution of each form of therapy to cancer cure. One area that should be considered for each patient is the relative risk of local recurrence and distant metastases. For example, a patient with breast cancer with 10 involved nodes is likely to succumb to distant disease; therefore, systemic therapy should begin early in the course of treatment. Conversely, a patient with a very early breast cancer has a low risk of distant disease, and priorities should be placed on local and regional cancer control. Rectal cancer treatment involves all specialties, with most patients receiving adjuvant therapy following surgery. However, it should be remembered that total mesorectal resection (with nerve sparing) is an excellent procedure for organ, sphincter, and potentia coeundi preservation, and it is associated with low morbidity and low local recurrence (Fig. 4–6).[47]

If staging reveals no evidence of metastatic disease, surgical resection alone will cure about 80% of stage I tumors and 60% of stage II tumors. Apart from its role in organ-sparing procedures, radiation therapy can decrease local and regional recurrence of resected cancers. For instance, for patients with node-positive rectal cancer, local recurrences can be reduced from 30% to 10% with radiation therapy, although it increases overall survival by less than 5%.[48–50] Similarly, adjuvant chemotherapy increases overall survival for node-positive patients with colorectal and breast cancer by 5% to 7%.

Organ-Preserving Surgery

In most instances in which organ-preserving surgery is proposed, the reduction in volume of tissue removed still produces equivalent tumor control and survival to that achieved by surgical resection. Nonetheless, decreased local control or survival are occasionally accepted in order to achieve organ preservation or for cosmetic purposes. For example, in over 95% of women, ductal carcinoma *in situ* of the breast is cured with a simple mastectomy. However, with lumpectomy and breast irradiation, the local recurrence rate is 1% to 2% per year and one third of the recurrences are invasive cancers.[51] Thus, some women will die of breast cancer, but not for many years, and many women accept this risk in order to preserve the breast. Similar considerations may apply to cancers of the tongue base and rectum.

Reconstructive Surgery

In some instances, ablative (curative) surgery is associated with a significant cosmetic defect; this is sometimes true of head and neck and breast cancers. In other cases, a functional deficit may be caused following tumor resection. Under both circumstances, reconstruction provides improved quality of life. This procedure is common when sections of the mandible are resected and can be reconstructed with a free flap (Fig. 4–7).[52–54] It also is useful in exenterative pelvic surgery, where the vagina or bladder may need to be reconstructed.[55, 56] Improvements in reconstructive methods following resection of extremity sarcomas have significantly increased the chance of limb preservation with modern bone and joint reconstruction.[57]

Surgery for Advanced, Recurrent, or Metastatic Cancer

Surgery is important in treating patients with recurrent or metastatic cancer. When primary tumors present with metastatic disease, it is often still advisable to remove the primary tumor. If the primary cancer has been removed and the patient develops a local recurrence, surgery may be indicated to prevent adverse complications of local progression.

Palliative Tumor Resection

There is frequently a role for removing a primary tumor even in the presence of metastatic disease. This is true for many gastrointestinal malignancies, in which a tumor may cause bowel obstruction or bleeding before the patient dies of distant disease. In this situation, prior to beginning

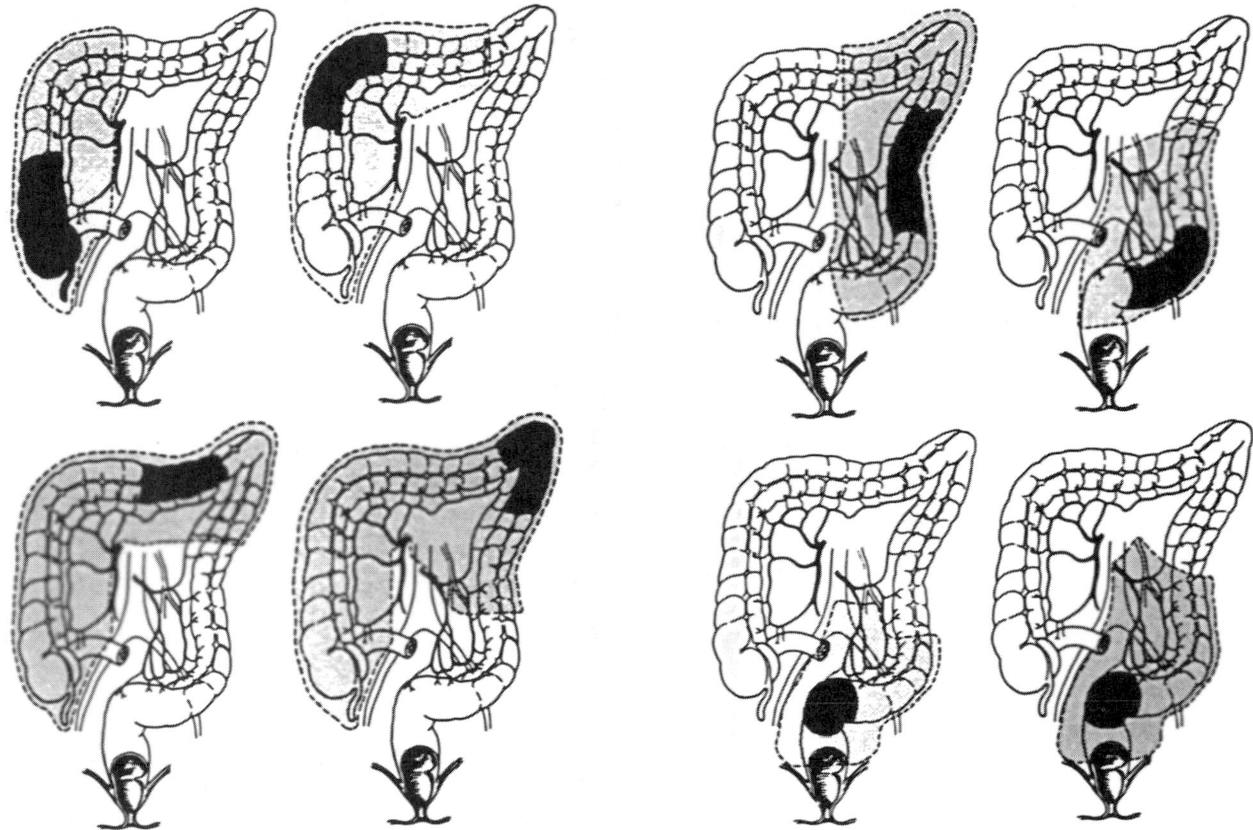

Figure 4–5. For most solid tumors, the lymphatic drainage is predictable, and curative operations entail the removal of the primary tumor with the draining lymphatic bed. These drawings illustrate the operations appropriate for colon cancer, depending on the site of the primary tumor, denoted by the solid shading. (From Cohen AM, Winawer SJ, Friedman MA, et al [eds]: Cancer of the Colon, Rectum, and Anus, p 433. New York, McGraw-Hill, 1995, with permission.)

chemotherapy, it is advisable to remove the tumor while the patient is still well and able to tolerate an operation, rather than waiting until the tumor causes complications in a weakened patient. This is particularly true with rectal cancer, even if a permanent colostomy will be needed, because control of disease in the pelvis is only achieved by surgical resection. If the patient has a life expectancy of months to 1 year, the tumor should be removed, because neither chemotherapy nor radiation can be expected to control the primary tumor and the patient will die with chronic discharge, bleeding, and uncontrolled pain. An important exception is the patient with clinical ascites from carcinomatosis. Such patients will not develop a bowel obstruction before succumbing to cancer; the life expectancy of patients with ascites from gastrointestinal cancers is measured in weeks.[58]

There are other tumors that, along with regional lymph nodes, should be removed even in the presence of distant disease. This is particularly true for cancers in which other therapies are ineffective. Uncontrolled, subcutaneous, local or regional tumors will often break through the skin, ulcerate, and develop a foul odor that may alienate patients from others. Melanoma and breast cancer represent common examples of such tumors. Removal of involved nodes before they create local problems and become unresectable is desired.

Potentially Curative Resections

There are some cases in which surgical resection of metastases not only provides palliation but also improves survival and, at times, cures. These include colon cancer metastatic to the liver[59, 60] or lung,[61] sarcoma metastatic to the lung,[62, 63] and lung cancer metastatic to the brain.[64] If a patient develops a solitary resectable metastasis from a resected primary tumor, a 5-year survival rate of 25% can be expected (Fig. 4–8) and, following resection of multiple pulmonary metastases, a 5-year survival rate of up to 20% of patients has been achieved. The term *oligometastases* has been used to identify those patients with more than one metastatic focus who may benefit from surgical resection or other curative therapy (e.g., stereotactic radiosurgery).

Pulmonary Metastases

At present, complete resection of pulmonary metastases via median sternotomy, allowing both lungs to be fully assessed, is the best or only mode of curative treatment for a number of cancers.[65–67] In addition, in conjunction with chemotherapy, some nonseminomatous testicular cancers have responded well to resection of pulmonary metastases in which complete resection of the metastases appears to be the most significant factor affecting prognosis.[68]

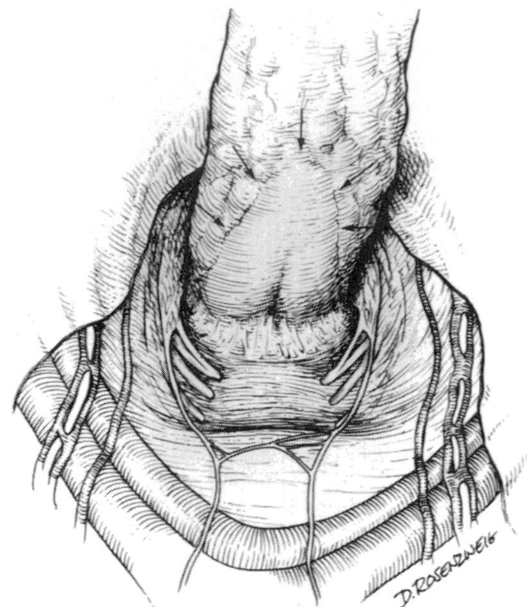

Figure 4–6. The principles of oncologic surgery are well demonstrated by the total mesorectal resection. The operation is performed with sharp dissection along the fascial planes to remove the entire mesorectum. Nerve preservation maximizes postoperative bladder and sexual function. Removal of the mesorectum significantly decreases local-regional failure. (From Enker WE: Total mesorectal excision with sphincter and autonomic-nerve preservation in the treatment of rectal cancer. Current Techniques in General Surgery 1996; 5:1, with permission.)

Hepatic Metastases

Patients with endocrine tumors, for example, carcinoids, will respond symptomatically if over 90% of the disease in the liver can be removed. Five-year survival rates of 24% to 39% have been reported by several groups after resection of liver metastases from colorectal cancer in selected patients (Table 4–1).[69–74] Prognostic factors are unilobular versus bilobular metastases, extent of liver resection, and negative versus positive resection margins. Liver metastases from other primary lesions, such as gastric, pancreatic, sarcoma, renal cell, Wilms', breast, melanoma, lung, and thyroid cancers, have been reported with variable results.[75–80]

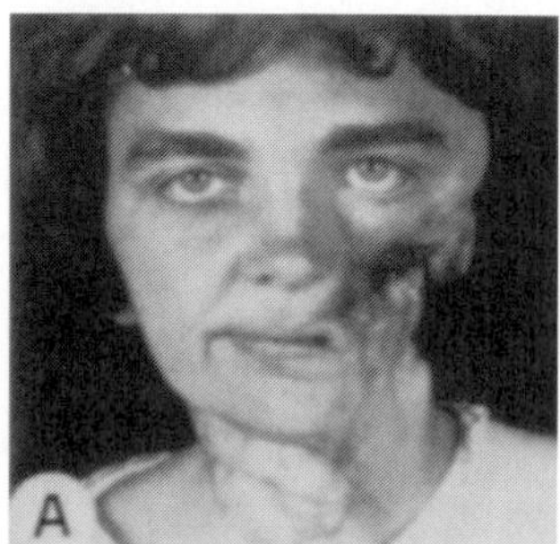

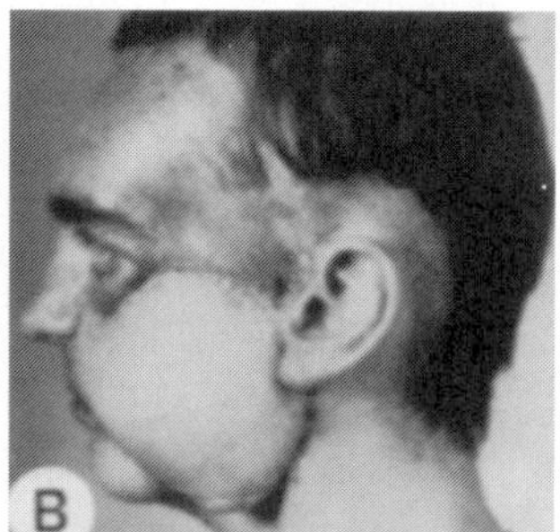

Figure 4–7. Palliative reconstruction of the face in a patient with recurrent sarcoma of the face. Photograph A is preoperative appearance. Photograph B shows final postoperative appearance. (From Bakamjian VY, Calamel PM: Oropharyngeal-esophageal reconstructive surgery. In Converse JM [ed]: Reconstructive Plastic Surgery, 2nd ed, vol 5, p 2697. Philadelphia, W.B. Saunders, 1977, with permission.)

Brain Metastases

Most patients with brain metastases are best managed with radiotherapy, although there is a small subset of patients who can improve with surgical excision. These are patients with solitary lesions, minimal neurologic impairment, and a long disease-free interval. Metastases from primary tumors, including lung, kidney, thyroid, colon, melanoma, and soft tissue sarcoma are most likely to respond favorably.[81, 82] Total resection plus radiotherapy gives the best results.[83]

Debulking Surgery

Debulking or cytoreductive procedures are tumor resections performed when it is known that removal of all of the disease is impossible. In general, such efforts do not benefit the patient, and they may actually do harm. However, some patients with selected types of tumors may benefit from debulking surgery, particularly when combined with an additional modality. For example, current chemotherapy protocols for ovarian cancer may prove curative with cytoreductive surgery, even if all of the gross tumor cannot be removed.[84, 85]

Other examples of tumors in which cytoreductive surgery may become important include thyroid cancers, endocrine cancers that maintain function and produce life-threatening hormonally mediated side effects, pediatric rhabdomyosarcomas, and glioblastoma multiforme. However, for the overwhelming majority of solid tumors, there is, as yet, no benefit from debulking operations.[86] This may change in the future if new and more effective treatments become available.

Palliative Bypass and Stents

Bypass surgery has a significant role in managing both primary gastrointestinal cancers and metastatic disease. This is true for small and large bowel obstruction, gastric outlet obstruction, obstructing esophageal tumors, and biliary obstructions. If a bypass is not feasible, occasional rectal or esophageal obstructions may be destroyed with a laser or held patent with a stent. The laser has been most effective for selected esophageal,[87] tracheobronchial,[88] and low rectal obstructions.[89] Similarly, stenting can often provide relief of biliary obstruction[90, 91] and some esophageal lesions when surgical bypass is not feasible.[92]

Orthopedic treatment of bone metastases can improve the quality of life of patients who would otherwise be unable to walk or to bear weight; submitting to such a procedure is often preferable to spending the remainder of one's life bedridden.[93] Examples of such procedures include prophylactic treatment of an impending femoral neck fracture or, in cases of metastatic disease to the vertebrae, stabilization with metallic rods to avoid spinal cord compression.

Surgical Emergencies

The surgeon often is confronted with emergencies in cancer patients. Surgical emergencies that arise in patients with

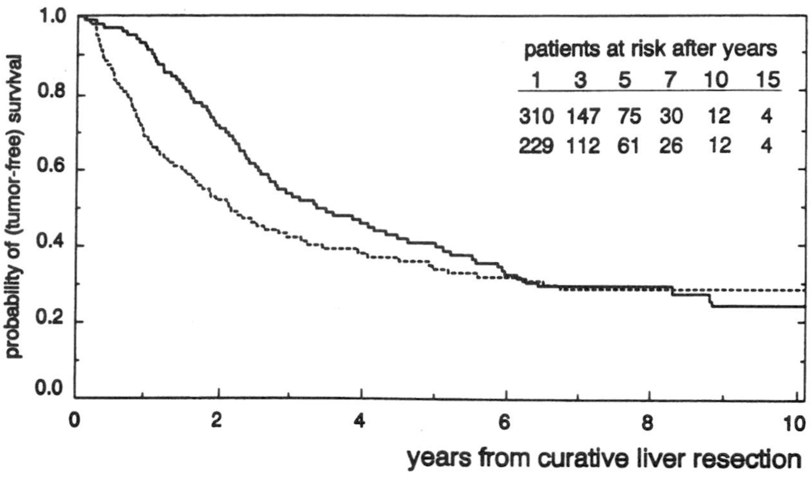

Figure 4–8. Surgical extirpation of metastatic disease results in a 25% to 30% 5-year survival in most patients with solid tumors. This shows the overall survival and disease-free survival of resection of liver metastases from colorectal cancer. Similar survival is found in pulmonary resection for metastatic sarcoma and for resection of intracranial metastases from lung cancer. (From Asbun HJ, Tsao JI, Hughes KS: Resection of hepatic metastases from colorectal carcinoma. The registry data. Cancer Treat Res 1994; 69:33, with permission.)

solid tumors are distinct from those that arise in patients with hematologic malignancies.

Oncologic Emergencies in Lymphomas and Leukemia Patients

Patients with lymphomas or leukemia frequently present with problems related to neutropenia:

- Prolonged neutropenia can place a patient at risk of sepsis from minor insults, such as anal fissures or skin infections. Anal fissures should be treated with sphincterotomy as soon as the patient's leukocyte counts recover, and the problem should be allowed to heal before the next course of chemotherapy.
- Perirectal inflammatory problems may not progress to frank abscesses when patients have few white blood cells, and they often resolve with the resolution of neutropenia.
- Typhlitis (inflammation of the cecum) also is associated with prolonged neutropenia. Patients have fever and right lower quadrant pain. A computed tomography scan is diagnostic, showing a phlegmon about the cecum. Typhlitis usually resolves with the return of white cells, and operations are seldom necessary unless full-thickness bowel necrosis ensues.[94]

Appendicitis, cholecystitis, and diverticulitis may occur in neutropenic patients. Although the inflammatory response in these patients often is blunted, a thorough history and physical examination usually will suggest the correct diagnosis. Unlike typhlitis, these acute conditions should be treated surgically, although surgical procedures have been associated with a high mortality rate in neutropenic patients.[95, 96]

TABLE 4–1. **5-Year Survival Rates after Resection of Liver Metastases from Colorectal Cancer**

Reference	No. of Patients	5-Year Survival
Lise et al[69]	64	30%
Nordlinger et al[70]	1568	28%
Scheele et al[71]	473	39±3%
Wanebo et al[72]	74	24%
Fong et al[73]	456	38%
Bakalakos et al[74]	301	29%

Complications in Patients with Solid Tumors

Oncologic emergencies can include bowel obstructions, acute urinary obstructions, complications related to increased intracranial pressure, impending paralysis from spinal cord tumors, and acute gastrointestinal bleeding that requires endoscopic or surgical intervention. This is just a short compendium of the various oncologic emergencies that require treatment.

Bowel Obstruction

Bowel obstructions are common problems for patients with solid tumors. Adhesions, rather than recurrent cancer, cause many of the small bowel obstructions. The erroneous assumption that a small bowel obstruction in a cancer patient is a manifestation of recurrence is common, and even in the presence of active intra-abdominal disease, small bowel obstructions should be managed as in other patients.[97, 98] However, it is advisable to obtain a preoperative barium enema to detect unheralded multiple points of narrowing from carcinomatosis.

Massive Hemoptysis

Massive hemoptysis frequently occurs in patients with primary lung cancers, but it is always wise to consider a differential diagnosis, because massive hemoptysis may also be seen with tuberculosis, fungal infections, and lung abscesses. Management is directed toward protecting the normal lung from aspiration of blood, as well as diagnosing the cause.

The first step in management of hemoptysis is bronchoscopy. Rigid bronchoscopy is helpful in removing as much blood clot as possible. The next step should be to protect the normal lung from aspiration by positioning the patient (with the normal lung up) and selective intubation of the so-called good lung. Controlling bleeding on the affected side is difficult, but in the upper airway, it may be possible to ablate tumor with a laser. Surgical resection of lung containing actively bleeding tumor is possible, but the mortality is high.[99] Massive hemoptysis in patients with esophageal cancer often results in death within 24 hours as a result of aortic perforation. There is little that can be done to avoid a fatal outcome.

Airway Obstruction

Patients presenting with stridor may have a tumor in the larynx or trachea. They may also have a paralyzed vocal cord, which limits the airway and requires immediate attention. Temporizing maneuvers include treatment with inhaled epinephrine, room-supplemented mixtures of helium and oxygen to reduce the viscosity of the air, and steroids to diminish inflammation. Endoscopy may be advisable in an effort to identify a cause for the stridor and to remove obstructing tumors.

A tracheotomy is frequently the first procedure performed for upper airway obstruction. However, a tracheotomy in patients with stridor is technically demanding, even for experienced surgeons, and deaths sometimes occur. Following establishment of control of the airway, diagnostic endoscopy with biopsy should be considered.

Arterial Rupture

Arteries are at risk from spontaneous rupture if chronically exposed to air in an open wound. The risk of this potentially disastrous complication is increased in a previously irradiated vessel or by contamination of the wound, such as with saliva or a fistula. The problem, therefore, is most commonly seen in patients with head and neck cancers, where an irradiated carotid artery may rupture or wound breakdown can occur as a result of saliva leakage into the neck. Extremity surgery combined with radiation or wound breakdown, or with both, also may lead to arterial rupture.

Massive hemorrhage may ensue, threatening life or limb. Most such episodes are preceded by loss of a small amount of bright red blood that appears in the wound; appreciation of this herald bleeding represents the best chance to control the problem. The vessel should be ligated or embolized in healthy tissue proximal and distal to the site of vessel injury. Once obvious arterial bleeding begins, the situation usually worsens rapidly; stroke and death occur frequently with major arterial rupture, and their incidence is heightened if frank bleeding ensues before the problem is resolved. Efforts at arterial reconstruction should be considered hazardous in this setting.

The majority of patients with exposed irradiated arteries do not experience this catastrophic complication, but those who do have severe morbidity and a high mortality rate. Therefore, patients with wound breakdown resulting in arterial exposure should be admitted to the hospital and local wound care measures should be instituted. Patients should be prepared for a reconstructive procedure; it is usually possible to prevent arterial rupture if well-vascularized healthy tissue can be used to cover the wound. The advent of modern reconstructive surgery has diminished dramatically the incidence of hemorrhage from arterial rupture because appropriate tissue flaps generally prevent the wound breakdown that precipitates the problem.

Vascular Access Procedures

The modern treatment of leukemia, lymphoma, and advanced solid tumors often involves intensive chemotherapy regimens. Patients frequently receive toxic drugs that damage their veins, and the use of cytotoxic agents is accompanied by side effects that often necessitate phlebotomy. Placement of vascular access devices in patients who have never undergone this procedure is usually straightforward; thrombocytopenia, which is common in patients with leukemia or recent chemotherapy, is only a minor impediment. Therefore, use of long-term central venous catheters has become more common in the care of patients with cancer, because they prevent superficial thrombophlebitis and increase patient tolerance of frequent blood tests.

Catheters are intravascular foreign bodies and, even with good nursing care, they can become infected, precipitating episodes of sepsis. In addition, thrombosis of the central veins is a recognized complication of long-term venous access catheters. Removing an infected catheter will usually simplify control of the infection, but it will not reverse the injury to a thrombosed vessel. Although these problems may necessitate removal of the device, it is often possible to save a vascular access catheter through appropriate use of antibiotics and anticoagulants,[100] particularly because placement of a second device is usually far more demanding than the original procedure.

Preoperative and Postoperative Care

Preoperative Care

The preoperative care of a cancer patient includes:

- assessment and assurance of patient fitness for surgery
- staging the tumor
- determining the goals of treatment (curative or palliative)
- determining the risk of treatment
- obtaining informed consent

Determinants of fitness for surgery include assessment of cardiac, pulmonary, renal, hepatic, and nutritional status. Uncontrolled angina, transient ischemic attacks, hypertension, and congestive heart failure should be addressed before any elective procedure begins. Optimizing pulmonary function in patients with reactive and chronic obstructive lung disease is important. Nicotine and smoke will increase morbidity and operative risk; therefore, cessation from smoking should be encouraged.

Assessment of nutritional status can frequently be accomplished from the medical history alone. If there has been significant weight loss, a possible nutritional deficit may be assessed by measuring serum markers and testing for cutaneous anergy. Preoperative nutritional support will not reverse the effects of cancer cachexia, but prolonged nutritional support will overcome the results of obstructive nutritional losses. In such instances, nutritional support will decrease the morbidity and mortality of patients undergoing major surgical procedures, although it has not been shown to improve survival rates in patients undergoing chemotherapy or radiation therapy. In cases in which nutritional support is indicated, use of the alimentary tract is preferred (enteral feeding); however, if this cannot be tolerated, total parenteral nutrition may be used. If preoperative total parenteral nutrition is used, typically 2 weeks of nutritional supplementation are required in order to derive a benefit.

Age is rarely a contraindication to surgery. With appropriate preoperative assessment and optimization of underlying physiology, most patients will tolerate the surgical procedure well. With most solid tumors, surgery most often provides the only chance of cure as well as the best palliation, and even extensive operations, such as pelvic exenterations, liver resection, and pancreaticoduodenectomy, can be performed in elderly patients with a very small risk of perioperative mortality. Patients who are otherwise well should not be denied the opportunity of a curative procedure based solely on age.

Informed consent is an important part of the preoperative care of the patient. It is important that the patient understands not only the risk of the operation but also the potential for the operation to cure or palliate the disease. Patients may have many reasonable treatment options, and making these choices can be difficult for some patients. This is especially true with respect to issues that are related to changes in body image and function that may have an impact on quality of life or cure of cancer. It is important that the relative prospects of cure for each procedure be explained to the patient and family. If one treatment choice entails a heightened risk of tumor recurrence, patients should also understand the subsequent chance for cure. The surgeon should not be persuaded to provide inappropriate procedures for patients who demand inappropriate care for their cancer. These patients are better served by allowing them to pursue other opinions, with the expectation that the patient will accept appropriate care when better informed.

Postoperative Care

Postoperative care of the cancer patient goes beyond hospital discharge; the surgeon also is responsible for planning adjuvant therapy and maintaining long-term follow-up. Follow-up for a cancer patient is performed not only to assure full rehabilitation but also to identify recurrence at a treatable stage and detect second primary cancers:

- Second cancers are common in patients cured of cancers of the breast, colon, head and neck, and lung.
- The frequency of follow-up should be proportional to the risk of recurrence and should focus on sites that are amenable to treatment. If no effective therapy exists, nothing can be gained by identifying recurrence before the patient is symptomatic.
- However, many recurrences are treatable and may even be cured, including nodal metastases from head and neck cancer, liver metastases from colon cancer, and recurrences in the treated breast. For example, in many solid tumors, the greatest risk of recurrence is in the first 2 to 3 years. The patient should be seen and assessed frequently during that period and then less often as the risk of recurrence decreases.

Summary

Caring for a patient with cancer is recognized as central to board certification in general surgery and most surgical specialties, and there are recognized subspecialty surgical fellowships in the disciplines of surgical oncology, as well as gynecologic, head and neck, thoracic, and urologic oncology. Surgical oncologists have extensive training and expertise, allowing them to perform the complex procedures necessary to cure patients with advanced disease. Surgical oncologists also understand and employ multidisciplinary approaches to cancer treatment and, therefore, are able to advise patients with respect to the overall management of their malignancy.

Recommended Reading

The National Comprehensive Cancer Network has developed guidelines that cover most cancers and that suggest management paradigms. These guidelines are updated regularly and are published according to disease site in the journal *Oncology.*

Several texts designed for specialists provide an overview of the multidisciplinary approach to the cancer patient and address the surgeon's role in managing cancer.[1] Additional texts are designed for subspecialists in gynecologic oncology,[2] head and neck oncology,[3] genitourinary oncology,[4] and pediatric oncology.[5] Excellent atlases demonstrate techniques of both common and less frequently performed procedures for cancer operations.[6, 7]

REFERENCES

General

1. DeVita VT Jr, Hellman S, Rosenberg SA (eds): Cancer: Principles & Practice of Oncology, 5th ed. Philadelphia, Lippincott-Raven, 1997.
2. Hoskins WJ, Perez CA, Young RC (eds): Principles and Practice of Gynecologic Oncology, 2nd ed. Philadelphia, Lippincott-Raven, 1997.
3. Thawley SE, Panje WR, Batsakis JG, et al (eds): Comprehensive Management of Head and Neck Tumors, 2nd ed. Philadelphia, W.B. Saunders, 1999.
4. Raghaven D, Scher HI, Leibel SA, et al (eds): Principles and Practice of Genitourinary Oncology. Philadelphia, Lippincott-Raven, 1997.
5. Pizzo PA, Poplack DG (eds): Principles and Practice of Pediatric Oncology, 3rd ed. Philadelphia, Lippincott-Raven, 1997.
6. Daly JM, Cady B, Low DW: Atlas of Surgical Oncology. St. Louis, Mosby, 1993.
7. Shah JP, McMinn RMH: Color Atlas of Head and Neck Anatomy. London, Mosby, 1997.

Specific

8. Gagandeep SP, Poston GJ, Kinsella AR: Gene therapy in surgical oncology. Ann Surg Oncol 1995; 2:179–188.
9. Brested JH: The Edwin Smith surgical papyrus. Chicago, University of Chicago Press, 1930.
10. Hill GJ: Historical milestones in cancer surgery. Semin Oncol 1979; 6:409–427.
11. Rosenberg SA: Principles of cancer management: surgical oncology. In: DeVita VT Jr, Hellman S, Rosenberg SA (eds): Cancer: Principles & Practice of Oncology, 5th ed, pp 295–306. Philadelphia, Lippincott-Raven, 1997.
12. Spencer MP, Sarr MG, Nagorney DM: Radical pancreatectomy for pancreatic cancer in the elderly. Is it safe and justified? Ann Surg 1990; 212:140–143.
13. Lubin MF: Is age a risk factor for surgery? Med Clin North Am 1993; 77:327–333.
14. Fong Y, Blumgart LH, Fortner JG, et al: Pancreatic or liver resection for malignancy is safe and effective for the elderly. Ann Surg 1995; 222:426–434.

15. Poon RT, Law SY, Chu KM, et al: Esophagectomy for carcinoma of the esophagus in the elderly: results of current surgical management. Ann Surg 1998; 227:357–364.
16. Manton KC, Vaupel JW: Survival after the age of 80 in the United States, Sweden, France, England, and Japan. N Engl J Med 1995; 333:1232–1235.
17. Peterson IM, Brink WJ: Fine-needle aspiration biopsy. When is it most beneficial? Postgrad Med 1990; 88:119–122.
18. Zakowski MF: Fine-needle aspiration cytology of tumors: diagnostic accuracy and potential pitfalls. Cancer Invest 1994; 12:505–515.
19. Rimm DL, Stastny JF, Rimm EB, et al: Comparison of the costs of fine-needle aspiration and open surgical biopsy as methods for obtaining a pathologic diagnosis. Cancer 1997; 81:51–56.
20. Shiu MH, Brennan M (eds): Surgical Management of Soft Tissue Sarcoma. Philadelphia, Lea & Febiger, 1989.
21. Harris JR, Hellman S, Henderson IC, et al (eds): Breast Diseases. Philadelphia, JB Lippincott, 1987.
22. Hansen N, Morrow M: Breast disease. Med Clin North Am 1998; 82: 203–333.
23. Dooley WC: Surgery for breast cancer. Curr Opin Oncol 1998; 10:504–512.
24. Mills JM, Schultz DJ, Solin LJ: Preservation of cosmesis with low complication risk after conservative surgery and radiotherapy for ductal carcinoma in situ of the breast. Int J Radiat Oncol Biol Phys 1997; 39:637–641.
25. Heimann R, Powers C, Halpem HJ, et al: Breast preservation in stage I and II carcinoma of the breast. The University of Chicago experience. Cancer 1996; 78:1722–1730.
26. American Joint Committee on Cancer: AJCC Cancer Staging Manual, 5th ed. Philadelphia, Lippincott-Raven, 1997.
27. Mountain CF, Dresler CM: Regional lymph node classification for lung cancer staging. Chest 1997; 111:1718–1723.
28. Halsted WS: The results of operations for the cure of cancer of the breast performed at the Johns Hopkins Hospital. Ann Surg 1894; 20:497–555.
29. Halsted WS: The results of radical operations for the cure of carcinoma of the breast. Ann Surg 1907; 46:1–19.
30. Crile GW: Excision of cancer of the head and neck with special reference to the plan of dissection based on one hundred and thirty-two operations. JAMA 1096; 47:1780–1785.
31. Martin HE: Cancer of the head and neck. JAMA 1948; 137:1306–1315.
32. Martin HE: Cancer of the head and neck. JAMA 1948; 137:1366–1376.
33. Fisher B, Redmond C, Fisher ER: The contribution of recent NSABP clinical trials of primary breast cancer therapy to an understanding of tumor biology—an overview of findings. Cancer 1980; 46(suppl):1009–1029.
34. Ridge JA: Regional lymph node dissection is both therapeutic and diagnostic. In: Harken AH (ed): Surgical Debates, pp 65–71. Philadelphia, Hanley & Belfus, 1988.
35. Hellman S: Karnofsky Memorial Lecture. Natural history of small breast cancers. J Clin Oncol 1994; 12:2229–2234.
36. Gardner B: William Stewart Halsted is alive and well. J Surg Oncol 1998; 68:1.
37. Cohen AM, Winawer SJ, Friedman MA, et al (eds): Cancer of the Colon, Rectum, and Anus. New York, McGraw-Hill, 1995.
38. Morton DL, Wen DR, Wong JH, et al: Technical details of intraoperative lymphatic mapping for early stage melanoma. Arch Surg 1992; 127:392–399.
39. Giuliano AE, Dale PS, Turner RR, et al: Improved axillary staging of breast cancer with sentinel lymphadenectomy. Ann Surg 1995; 222:394–399.
40. Krag D, Harlow S, Weaver D, et al: Technique of sentinel node resection in melanoma and breast cancer: probe-guided surgery and lymphatic mapping. Eur J Surg Oncol 1998; 24:89–93.
41. Cox CE, Pendas S, Cox JM, et al: Guidelines for sentinel node biopsy and lymphatic mapping of patients with breast cancer. Ann Surg 1998; 227:645–651.
42. Kim RY, Salter MM, Wepplemann B, et al: Analysis of treatment modalities and their failures in stage IB cancer of the cervix. Int J Radiat Oncol Biol Phys 1988; 15:831–835.
43. Adam IJ, Mohamdee MO, Martin IG, et al: Role of circumferential margin involvement in the local recurrence of rectal cancer. Lancet 1994; 344:707–711.
44. Arbman G, Nilsson E, Hallbook O, et al: Local recurrence following total mesorectal excision for rectal cancer. Br J Surg 1996; 83:375–379.
45. Gage I, Schnitt SJ, Nixon AJ, et al: Pathologic margin involvement and the risk of recurrence in patients treated with breast-conserving therapy. Cancer 1996; 78:1921–1928.
46. DiBase SJ, Komarnicky LT, Schwartz GF, et al: The number of positive margins influences the outcome of women treated with breast preservation for early stage breast carcinoma. Cancer 1998; 82:2212–2220.
47. Enker WE: Total mesorectal excision with sphincter and autonomic-nerve preservation in the treatment of rectal cancer. Current Techniques in General Surgery 1996; 5:1–8.
48. Gastrointestinal Tumor Study Group. Prolongation of the disease-free interval in surgically treated rectal carcinoma. Gastrointestinal Tumor Study Group. N Engl J Med 1985; 312:1465–1472.
49. Fisher B, Wolmark N, Rockette H, et al: Postoperative adjuvant chemotherapy or radiation therapy for rectal cancer: results from NSABP protocol R-01. J Natl Cancer Inst 1988; 80:21–29.
50. Krook JE, Moertal CG, Gunderson LL, et al: Effective surgical adjuvant therapy for high-risk rectal carcinoma. N Engl J Med 1991; 324:709–715.
51. Fisher B, Dignam J, Wolmark N, et al: Lumpectomy and radiation therapy for the treatment of intraductal breast cancer: findings from National Surgical Adjuvant Breast and Bowl Project B-17. J Clin Oncol 1998; 16:441–452.
52. Bakamjian VY, Calamel PM: Oropharyngeal-esophageal reconstructive surgery. In: Bakamjian VY, Calamel PM (eds): Reconstructive Plastic Surgery, 2nd ed, vol 5, pp 2697–2756. Philadelphia, W.B. Saunders, 1977.
53. Larson DL, Sanger JR: Management of the mandible in oral cancer. Semin Surg Oncol 1995; 11:190–199.
54. Burkey BB, Coleman JR Jr: Current concepts in oromandibular reconstruction. Otolaryngol Clin N Am 1997; 30:607–630.
55. Jain AK, DeFranzo AJ, Marks MW, et al: Reconstruction of pelvic exenterative wounds with transpelvic rectus abdominis flaps: a case series. Ann Plast Surg 1997; 38:115–122.
56. Miller SM, Schnurch HG, Ebert T, et al: Reconstructive surgery of the efferent urinary tract in pelvic exenteration of gynecological tumors. Urologe A 1999; 38:237–241.
57. Yasko AW, Reece GP, Gillis TA, et al: Limb-salvage strategies to optimize quality of life: the M.D. Anderson Cancer Center experience. CA Cancer J Clin 1997; 47:226–238.
58. Parsons SL, Lang MW, Steele RJ: Malignant ascites: a 2-year review from a teaching hospital. Eur J Surg Oncol 1996: 22:237–239.
59. Asbun HJ, Tsao JI, Hughes KS: Resection of hepatic metastases from colorectal carcinoma. The registry data. Cancer Treat Res 1994; 69:33–41.
60. Scheele J, Stang R, Altendorf-Hofmann A, et al: Resection of colorectal liver metastases. World J Surg 1995; 19:59–71.
61. McCormack PM, Burt ME, Bains MS, et al: Lung resection for colorectal metastases. 10-year results. Arch Surg 1992; 127:1403–1406.
62. The International Registry of Lung Metastases: Long-term results of lung metastasectomy: prognostic analyses based on 5206 cases. J Thorac Cardiovasc Surg 1997; 113:37–49.
63. Putnam JB Jr: Soft part sarcomas—metastases. Chest Surg Clin N Am 1998; 8:97–118.
64. Patchell RA, Tibbs PA, Walsh JW, et al: A randomized trial of surgery in the treatment of single metastases to the brain. N Engl J Med 1990; 322:494–500.
65. Vigneswaran WT: Management of pulmonary metastases from colorectal cancer. Semin Surg Oncol 1996; 12:264–266.
66. van der Veen AH, van Geel AN, Hop WC, et al: Median sternotomy: the preferred incision for resection of lung metastases. Eur J Surg 1998; 164:507–512.
67. de Oliviera-Filho AG, Neto LS, Epelamn S: Median sternotomy for the resection of bilateral pulmonary metastases in children. Pediatr Surg Int 1998; 13:560–563.
68. Anyanwu E, Krysa S, Buelzebruck H, et al: Pulmonary metastasectomy as secondary treatment for testicular tumors. Ann Thorac Surg 1994; 57:1222–1228.
69. Lise M, Da Pian PP, Nitti D, et al: Colorectal metastases to the liver: present results and future strategies. J Surg Oncol 1991; 2(suppl):69–73.

70. Nordlinger B, Guiguet M, Vaillant JC, et al: Surgical resection of colorectal carcinoma metastases to the liver. A prognostic scoring system to improve case selection, based on 1568 patients. Association Française de Chirurgie. Cancer 1996; 77:1254–1262.
71. Scheele J, Altendorf-Hofmann A, Stangl R, et al: Surgical resection of colorectal liver metastases: Gold standard for solitary and radically resectable lesions. Swiss Surg 1996; 4(suppl):4–17.
72. Wanebo HJ, Chu QD, Vezeridis MP, et al: Patient selection for hepatic resection of colorectal metastases. Arch Surg 1996; 131:322–329.
73. Fong Y, Cohen AM, Fortner JG, et al: Liver resection for colorectal metastases. J Clin Oncol 1997; 15:938–946.
74. Bakalakos EA, Kim JA, Young DC, et al: Determinants of survival following hepatic resection for metastatic colorectal cancer. World J Surg 1998; 22:399–404.
75. Takao S, Shinchi H, Uchikura K, et al: Liver metastases after curative resection in patients with distal bile cancer. Br J Surg 1999; 86:327–331.
76. Falconi M, Bassi C, Bonora A, et al: Role of chemoembolization in synchronous liver metastases from pancreatic endocrine tumours. Dig Surg 1999; 16:32–38.
77. Stief CG, Jahne J, Hagemann JH, et al: Surgery for metachronous solitary liver metastases of renal cell carcinoma. J Urol 1997; 158:375–377.
78. Schneebaum S, Walker MJ, Young D, et al: The regional treatment of liver metastases from breast cancer. J Surg Oncol 1994; 55:26–31.
79. Salmon RJ, Levy C, Plancher C, et al: Treatment of liver metastases from uveal melanoma by combined surgery-chemotherapy. Eur J Surg Oncol 1998; 24:127–130.
80. Berney T, Mentha G, Roth AD, et al: Results of surgical resection of liver metastases from non-colorectal primaries. Br J Surg 1998; 85:1423–1427.
81. Saitoh Y, Fujisawa T, Shiba M, et al: Prognostic factors in surgical treatment of solitary brain metastases after resection of non-small-cell lung cancer. Lung Cancer 1999; 24:99–106.
82. Wronski M, Arbit E: Resection of brain metastases from colorectal carcinoma in 73 patients. Cancer 1999; 85:1677–1685.
83. Agboola O, Benoit B, Cross P, et al: Prognostic factors derived from recursive partitiion analysis (RPA) of Radiation Therapy Oncology Group (RTOG) brain metastases trials applied to surgically resected and irradiated brain metastatic cases. Int J Radiat Oncol Biol Phys 1999; 42:155–159.
84. Boente MP, Chi DS, Hoskins WJ: The role of surgery in the management of ovarian cancer: primary and interval cytoreductive surgery. Semin Oncol 1998; 25:326–334.
85. Tarraza HM, Ellerkmann RM: Pelvic radical surgery. Surg Oncol Clin N Am 1998; 7:399–416.
86. Ridge JA: Debulking (cytoreductive) surgery. In: Harken AH, Moore EE (eds): Surgical Secrets, pp 204–206. Philadelphia, Hanley & Belfus, 1996.
87. Boyce GA: Palliation of malignant esophageal obstruction. Dysphagia 1990; 5:220–226.
88. Edell ES, Cortese DA, McDougall JC: Ancillary therapies in the management of lung cancer: photodynamic therapy, laser therapy, and endobronchial prosthetic devices. Mayo Clin Proc 1993; 68:685–690.
89. Dohmoto M, Hunerbein M, Schlag PM: Palliative endoscopic therapy of rectal carcinoma. Eur J Cancer 1996; 322A:25–29.
90. O'Brien S, Hatfield AR, Craig PI, et al: A three year follow up of self expanding metal stents in the endoscopic palliation of longterm survivors with malignant biliary obstruction. Gut 1995; 36:618–621.
91. Vitale GC, Larson GM, George M, et al: Management of malignant biliary stricture with self-expanding metallic stent. Surg Endosc 1996; 10:970–973.
92. Reed CE: Pitfalls and complications of esophageal prosthesis, laser therapy, and dilation. Chest Surg Clin N Am 1997; 7:623–636.
93. Schmidt RG: Management of extremity metastatic bone cancer. Curr Prob Cancer 1995; 19:166–181.
94. Wade DS, Nava HR, Douglass HO Jr: Neutropenic enterocolitis. Clinical diagnosis and treatment. Cancer 1992; 69:17–23.
95. Glenn J, Funkhouser WK, Schneider PS: Acute illnesses necessitating urgent abdominal surgery in neutropenic cancer patients: description of 14 cases and review of the literature. Surgery 1989; 105:778–789.
96. Wade DS, Douglass H Jr, Nava HR, et al: Abdominal pain in neutropenic patients. Arch Surg 1990; 125:1119–1127.
97. Tang E, Davis J, Silberman H: Bowel obstruction in cancer patients. Arch Surg 1995; 130:832–836.
98. Costa I, Conclaves F: Intestinal obstruction in cancer patients. Palliative treatment. Acta Med Port 1997; 10:381–385.
99. Yeh KA, Goldberg M: Palliative surgery for thoracic malignancies. Curr Prob Cancer 1995; 19:130–152.
100. Schwarz RE, Groeger JS, Coit DG: Subcutaneously implanted central venous access devices in cancer patients; a prospective analysis. Cancer 1997; 79:1635–1640.

5 *Basic Principles of Radiobiology*

JACQUELINE P. WILLIAMS, PHD, Radiation Oncology
PETER KENG, PHD, Radiation Oncology and Radiation Biology
ROBERT M. SUTHERLAND, PHD, Cellular Biology

You may call it coalition, you may call it the accidental and fortuitous concurrence of atoms.

LORD PALMERSTON, 1857

Perspective

The deposition of ionizing radiation within biologic material induces a series of interactions that can result in a wide variety of biologic end effects. Our understanding of these events, in terms of their molecular biology, has increased exponentially over the past few decades; however, the basic principles have remained the same. This chapter outlines those principles and their effects, and it attempts, when possible, to relate these responses to different stages of the radiation interaction. A convenient outline of these interactions follows.

Stages of Radiation Action

Physical Stage—Energy Absorption

Radiation produces activated (excited or ionized) molecules.

- approximate duration = 10^{-16} seconds

Physicochemical Stage—Ion Radical Formation

Unstable primary products undergo secondary reactions to produce stable molecules plus chemically reactive free atoms and free radicals (molecules with unpaired electrons).

- approximate duration = 10^{-12} seconds

Chemical Stage—Target Radicals

Chemically reactive species react with each other and with the milieu.

- approximate duration = 10^{-8} seconds

Biologic Stage

The organism responds sequentially to chemical products of irradiation.

- approximate duration = 10^{-2} seconds, up to many years.

A specific scheme has been proposed for inactivation of mammalian cells through these different stages (Fig. 5–1).

Physical Stage

Interaction with Matter

The absorption of radiation into matter results in an interaction between the radiation and the substance molecules.[8-10] This occurs through two mechanisms: excitation or ionization of the constituent atoms. Through excitation, electrons are shifted to higher orbits within the atom, enabling the atom to become more reactive chemically. During ionization, orbiting electrons are completely ejected from the atom, resulting in free radicals or broken chemical bonds, or both. Ionizing radiations of interest include high-energy (short-wavelength) electromagnetic radiation and high-speed subatomic particles. Charged particles, such as electrons or protons, are directly ionizing; that is, with sufficient kinetic energy, they can directly break chemical bonds. Electromagnetic radiations (x- and γ-rays), as well as neutrons, are indirectly ionizing; that is, they do not themselves disrupt chemical bonds, but through their energy dissipation, they produce charged particles with high kinetic energy that do. Neutrons interact with the nuclei of atoms of the absorbing material and impart kinetic energy to fast-recoil protons and other nuclear fragments.

Linear Energy Transfer

Linear energy transfer (LET) refers to the energy transferred per unit length of the radiation beam track in the absorbing material.[11] The unit commonly used for this quantity is the kiloelectron volt (keV) per micron of unit density material. Typical LET values for commonly used

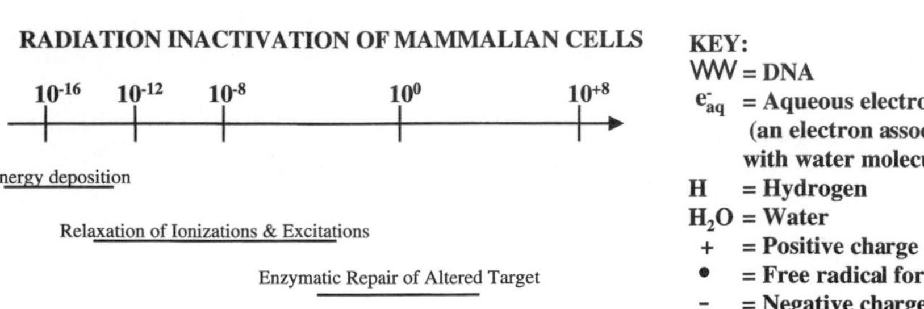

KEY:
WW = DNA
e^-_{aq} = Aqueous electron (an electron associated with water molecules)
H = Hydrogen
H_2O = Water
\+ = Positive charge
• = Free radical formation
\- = Negative charge
* = Excited state

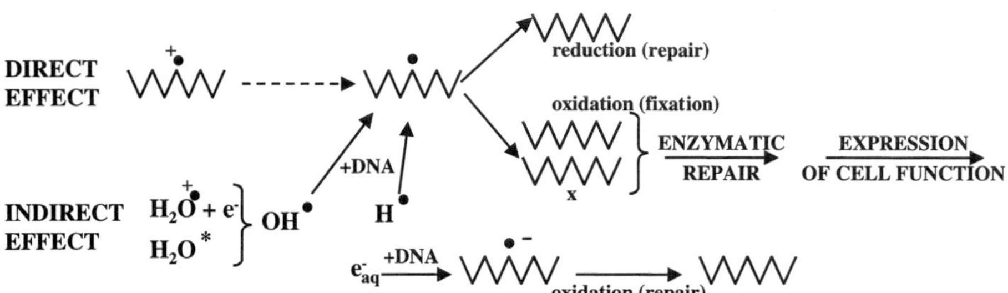

Figure 5–1. Schematic representation of stages of radiation action involved in inactivation of mammalian cells. The top line drawing represents the time scale in seconds. The lower panel shows direct and indirect effects of radiation on cellular DNA. (From Chapman JD, Dugle DL, Reuvers AP, et al: Studies on the radiosensitizing effect of oxygen in Chinese hamster cells. Int J Radiat Biol Rel Stud Phys Chem Med 1974; 26:383–389, with permission.)

radiations are cobalt-60 x-rays = 0.2 keV/μ; 250 kV x-rays = 2.0 keV/μ; 10 MeV protons = 4.7 keV/μ. Figure 5–2 provides a theoretical illustration of differences between ionization pathways created by particles with varying ionizing capabilities. LET can be measured either as a track average (dividing the track length into equal units and measuring the energy) or as an energy average (dividing the track into energy increments and measuring track length). For some forms of radiation, these two methods of calculation result in varying LET values (e.g., 14 MeV neutrons have a track average of 12 keV/μ, but their energy average is 100 keV/μ). For both x-rays and monoenergetic charged particles, the two methods yield approximately the same results.

Although different radiations usually produce qualitatively similar effects initially (ionizations), there can be marked quantitative differences between them, as well as different biologic end effects, owing to differences in LET. These differences result from dissimilarities in the spatial proximity of ionizations leading to *ionization clustering* and the influence of secondary processes, such as back reactions and chain reactions in the initial physical and chemical events. Biologic modification, as a result of structural organization and coupled systems, also plays a significant part in the final damage.

Relative Biologic Effectiveness

As suggested earlier, equal doses of different types of ionizing radiation do not produce equal biologic effects because of differences in LET. It is customary to express the biologic effectiveness of the test radiation as compared with 250 kV x-rays; that is, the relative biologic effectiveness (RBE) is the ratio of the doses of 250 kV x-rays to the test radiation required for equal biologic effect. Note that the RBE varies with the biologic system used and with

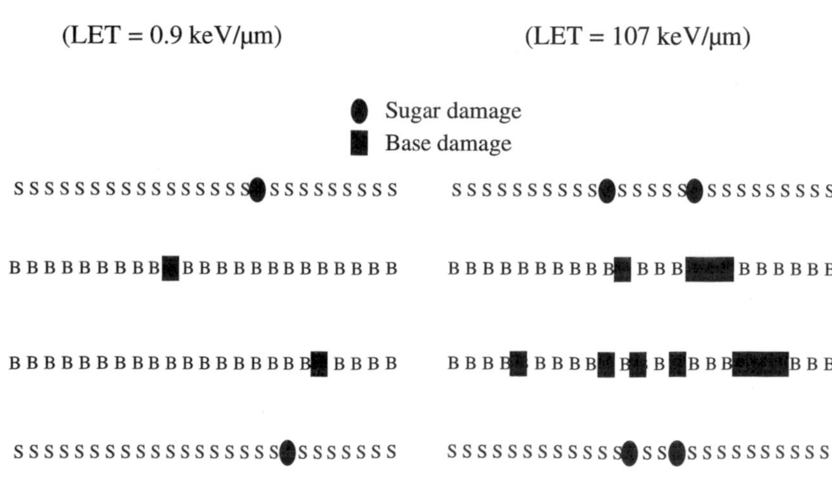

Figure 5–2. Representative single particle interactions with B-DNA: Interaction of a sparsely ionizing 1000 MeV/nucleon helium ion, average LET = 0.9 keV/μm *(left).* Interaction of a densely ionizing 1 MeV/nucleon helium ion, average LET = 107 keV/μm *(right).* Note the substantial clustering of DSBs and base and sugar damage in a local area at the higher LET value. The 1 MeV/nucleon helium ion will deposit approximately 120 times more dose in a typical cell than the 1000 MeV/nucleon helium ion. (From Blakely EA, Kronenberg A: Heavy-ion radiobiology: new approaches to delineate mechanisms underlying enhanced biological effectiveness. Radiat Res 1998; 150 (suppl):S126–S145, with permission. Courtesy of W. R. Holley and A. Chatterjee.)

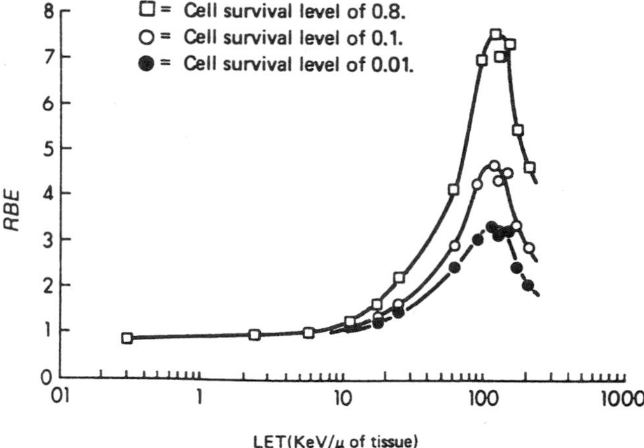

Figure 5–3. Variation of relative biologic effectiveness (RBE) with linear energy transfer (LET) for survival of mammalian cells of human origin. The RBE rises to a maximum at an LET of about 100 keV/μ, and subsequently falls for higher values of LET. The curves refer to various cell survival levels, illustrating that the absolute value of the RBE is not unique but depends on the level of biologic damage, and therefore on the dose level. (From Barendsen GW: Variation of RBE with LET for survival of mammalian cells of human origin. Curr Topics Radiat Res Q 1968; 4:293–356, with permission.)

the level of damage, which is related to the dose delivered, in that given system. The RBE for many cellular systems has been shown to increase with increasing LET, peaking at about 100 keV/μ, then decreasing (Fig. 5–3).[13] Thus, there appears to be an optimal LET (density of ionizations), after which there is a decline because of overkill.

Physicochemical Stage

To attempt to understand radiobiologic phenomena in living cells, we must know something about how radiation interacts with molecules and the relative radiosensitivity of these molecules. Methodology has been developed that allows us to sort out—from all of the numerous and complex radiation-induced interactions—those that are most likely to occur under conditions in which the quality of radiation, biologic material, radiation dose, and other factors are specified. The past decade has seen a remarkable advance in our appreciation of molecular biology as it relates to radiation events, chiefly owing to the development and application of powerful new techniques and methods to elucidate fundamental mechanisms that lead to cell survival, cell death, mutations, or genomic instability.[14] Nonetheless, interpretation of radiobiologic phenomena still depends on an understanding of how molecules exist in living cells and change over time.

Direct and Indirect Effects

Because ionizations produced by radiation are random processes, some molecules will escape ionization, but they may undergo radiation-related changes brought about by energy transfer from an ionized molecule (or its products) to undamaged molecules. Therefore, there are two types of chemical changes in irradiated molecules:

1. *Direct effect:* the release of energy in the structure of the molecule under discussion. This is the dominant process for radiation with high LET (neutrons or α-particles).
2. *Indirect effect:* the initial energy absorbed by one molecule transferred to another molecule being measured.

Metastable states exist in molecules after the direct action of irradiation and have been demonstrated—along with energy transfer processes—through electron spin resonance and thermoluminescence techniques. Energy is transferred, both within and between molecules, via special structures, such as tryptophan and benzene rings, and migration of dissociated small molecular fragments.

Important Physicochemical Reactions

Because cells consist of at least 80% water, most of the indirect effects seen in tissues involve reactive species derived from water molecules. Early radiation chemistry studies showed that water dissociates into free radicals H· and OH·, arising from primary ions H_2O^+ and H_2O^-.[15, 16] A further conceptual leap by Fricke[17] demonstrated that the resultant solutes and free radicals will, in all probability, undergo secondary interactions with other solute molecules or free radicals (radical-radical interactions), or both (Fig. 5–4). If all factors remain constant, then the resultant permanent damage will be linear with dose. Some biochemical and biologic consequences of free radical damage in DNA are enumerated in Table 5–1.

The advent and refinement of pulse radiolysis, together with the increasing power of simulation, have contributed greatly to our understanding of radiation absorption into matter through direct and simulated observation of the above-mentioned and other transient species in both water and other liquids.[19] In addition, the recognition that a large fraction of radiation damage results from the activity of free radicals or reactive oxygen species, or both, has led to a search for response modifiers to these specific agents. Radiation chemists and biologists continue to play a major role in the research into this field.[20]

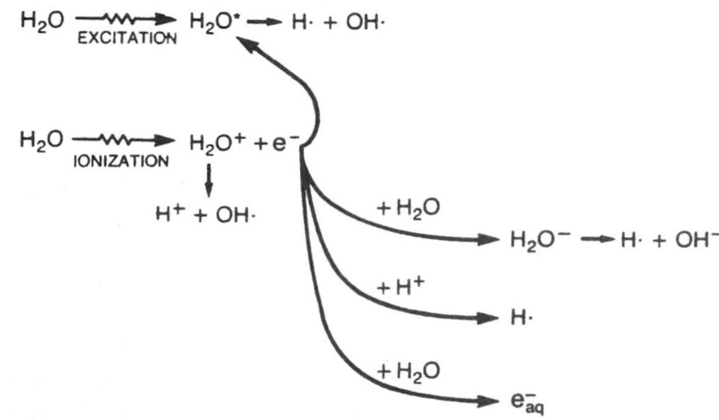

Figure 5–4. Direct action of ionizing radiation on water molecules, demonstrating the generation of reactive species. (From Chapman JD, Dugle DL, Reuvers AP, et al: Studies on the radiosensitizing effect of oxygen in Chinese hamster cells. International Journal of Radiation Biology and Related Studies in Physics, Chemistry and Medicine 1974; 26:383–389, with permission.)

TABLE 5–1. **Biochemical and Biological Consequences of Some Free Radical–Induced DNA Lesions**

Lesion	Block to DNA Polymerases	Lethal	Base Inserted Opposite *in vitro*	Mutagenic
Abasic sites	Yes	Yes	A>G>T	Yes
Thymine glycol	Yes	Yes	A>>>G	Poor
Dihydrothymine	No	No	A	No
5-Hydroxymethyluracil	No	n.d.*	A	n.d.
5-Formyluracil	No	n.d.	A>C	n.d.
Urea	Yes	Yes	A>G	Yes
β-Ureidoisobutyric acid	Yes	Yes	A>G>T	Yes
5-Hydroxycytosine	No	No	G>A	Yes
5-Hydroxyuracil	No	n.d.	A	n.d.
Uracil glycol	No	n.d.	A	n.d.
Dihydrouracil	No	n.d.	A	n.d.
Formamidopyrimidine	Yes	Yes	n.d.	n.d.
8-Oxoadenine	No	No	T>>G	Poor
2-Oxoadenine	No	No	T>A	Yes
8-Oxoguanine	No	No	C>A	Yes
α-Adenine	Yes	Yes	deletion	Yes

*Not determined.
From Wallace SS: Enzymatic processing of radiation-induced free radical damage in DNA. Radiat Res 1998; 150 (suppl):S60–S79, with permission.

Radiation-Sensitive Sites in Cells

The interaction between ionizing radiation and biologic matter can occur in any (and every) organelle and subcompartment of a cell.[5] The predominant changes that result from irradiation of different sites within cells and different classes of macromolecules, in solution or dry state, can be summarized as follows:

Nucleus: A variety of experiments over the years have shown that the target site responsible for cell killing is probably within the nucleus; the dose to the cytoplasm required to kill the cell is much higher than doses required in the nucleus.[21, 22] In general, these studies have involved localization of radiation damage to the nucleus versus the cytoplasm of cells through the use of microbeams, low-energy electrons, microdissection, nuclear transplantation, and the selective incorporation of lethal levels of radioisotopes into macromolecules such as DNA.

Proteins: Damage to side chain groups and changes in secondary and tertiary structures can occur following irradiation (conformation). These conformational changes are principally via the OH· radical from water hydrolysis.

Lipids: Damage to lipids may result in the formation of peroxides of unsaturated fatty acids.

DNA: DNA damage can be seen as a change in or loss of a base, hydrogen bond breakage between strands, single- and double-strand breakage, formation of cross-links between the double helix to other DNA molecules and to chromosomal proteins, or conformational changes.[23] DNA is generally recognized as the primary target for cell inactivation by ionizing radiation,[24] and the probability of direct and indirect action in DNA has been modeled in Monte Carlo–type calculations.[25]

Many studies have indicated positive correlations between DNA content and radiosensitivity in different cellular organisms. At biologically relevant doses, irradiation leads to a variety of sugar and base lesions in mammalian cell DNA, in addition to covalent cross-links within the DNA or nuclear proteins.[26, 27] For instance, 4 Gy of ionizing radiation will produce 4000 tracks per cell nucleus, which will result in approximately 4 times 10^{-5} to 10^{-6} mutations per loci per cell (Table 5–2). As a reference, background radiation, which is considered to be 2 mSv per year, results in approximately 2 tracks per cell per year. Damage to the deoxyribose backbone of the DNA disrupts phosphodiester bonds, frequently producing single-strand breaks (SSBs). In fact, ionizing radiation is thought to produce approximately 1000 SSBs and 25 to 40 double-strand breaks (DSBs) per gray per diploid cell[24] (Fig. 5–5).

In 1981, Ward introduced the concept of multiply damaged sites[28]; although not restricted to radiation damage, these sites are a hallmark of radiation injury. The inherent complexity of the lesions naturally leads to difficulties in repair, so there has been some recognition that cell death is most likely induced through repair (or misrepair) of these complex lesions. In addition, genetic changes, such as mutations and chromosomal aberrations, can arise at the site of the damaged DNA, leading to mutagenesis and possibly carcinogenesis.[29] Nonetheless, more recent concepts suggest that exposure of cell populations may produce nontargeted effects; that is, there are important genetic consequences occurring in cells that do not themselves receive direct radiation exposure.[29, 30] Signaling pathways are induced in cells not immediately affected by radiation or suffering from DNA damage, and this process has been described as a form of *bystander effect*.[31]

TABLE 5–2. **Genomic Damage Per Cell Following 4 Gy (Equivalent of 4000 Tracks Per Nucleus)**

4000	SSB (<4)*
4000	Bases (<4)*
100	DSB (<8)*
1	Chromosome deletion
1	Chromosome translocation 1:1 symmetric:asymmetric

*After repair.

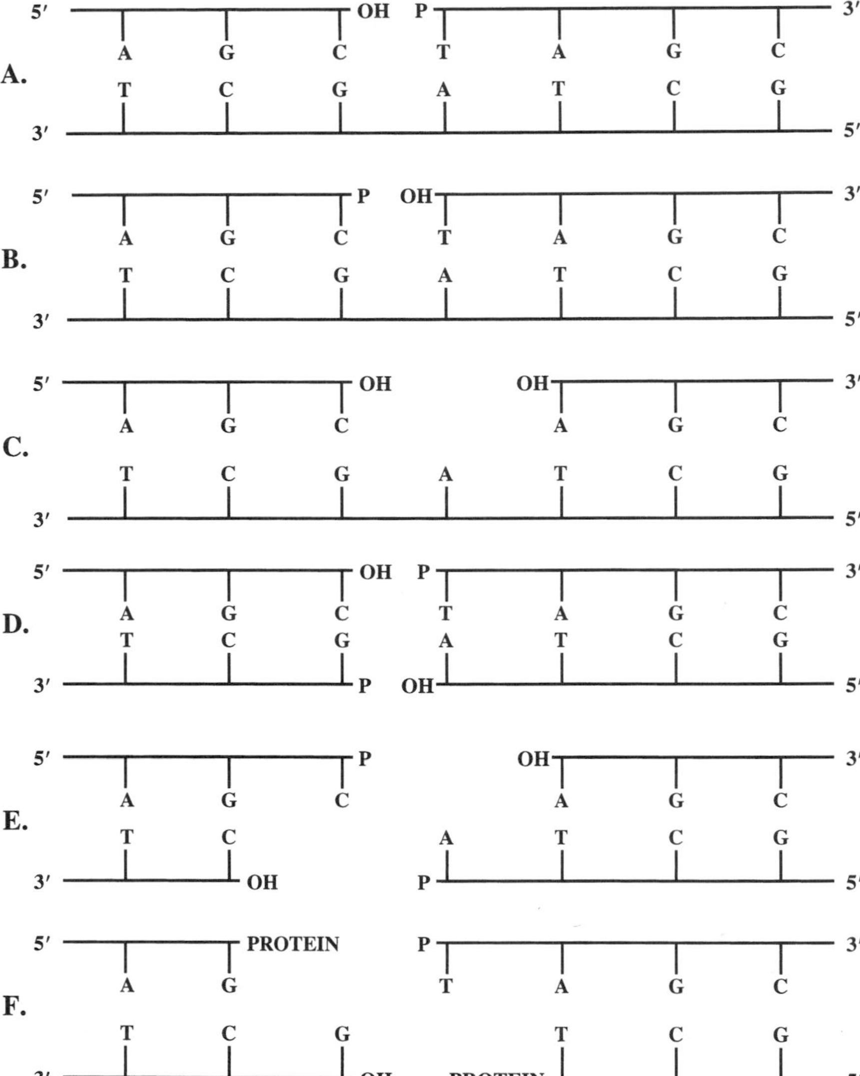

Figure 5–5. Examples of radiation-induced DNA single- and double-strand breaks. (A) Single-strand breaks containing a 3′-phosphate. (B) Single-strand breaks containing a 5′-phosphate. (C) A gap in the damaged deoxyribose with a thymine base loss and a modified 3′-terminus leading to 3′- and 5′-hydroxyl ends. (D) DNA double-strand breaks created by two adjacent single-strand breaks. (E) DNA double-strand breaks created by two adjacent gaps. (F) DNA double-strand breaks created by two adjacent gaps with termini modified by cross-linking to protein. (From Fuks Z, Weichselbaum RR: Radiation therapy. In Mendelsohn J, Howley PM, Israel MA, et al [eds]: The Molecular Basis of Cancer, pp 401–431. Philadelphia, W.B. Saunders Co., 1995, with permission.)

- Techniques have been developed to assess DNA damage in irradiated mammalian cells (Table 5–3).[32–45] Following the work of McGrath and Williams and their development of alkaline sucrose gradient sedimentation,[46] the initial focus of attention was on *single-strand breaks*. SSBs are common and increase in proportion to radiation dose. However, SSBs alone are not considered to be very lethal to mammalian cells and are highly reparable; their early postirradiation repair proceeds exponentially, according to first-order kinetics ($t_{1/2}$ of 2 to 10 minutes).[47]
- *DNA base damage* is frequently observed following irradiation and, although it has not been looked on as particularly lethal, is considered to be an important process in the genesis of mutations.[5] X-ray base damage is repaired in mammalian cells by excision through relatively poorly understood enzymatic pathways; nonetheless, these pathways appear to be highly efficient because 80% of base damage is removed from DNA within 15 minutes of irradiation.[48]
- Techniques have been gradually improving for the study of the most important lesions in DNA damage following ionizing irradiation, the *double-strand break* (see Table 5–1 and Fig. 5–5). DSBs may arise as intermediates during repair of other DNA damage, such as interstrand cross-links, or endogenously during certain processes that require rearrangement of DNA sequences, such as V(D)J recombination or meiosis. DSBs can arise from either a single event, which severs both DNA strands simultaneously, or two closely associated SSBs on the deoxyribose backbone. Because unrepaired DSBs are likely to prove lethal and, alternatively, DSB misrepair can give rise to rearrangements and deletions, DSBs represent a significant lesion in cell lethality, mutagenesis, and carcinogenesis.[49]

Radiation Damage Repair

The ability of normal cells to recover from radiation damage was demonstrated in experiments during the 1930s and 1940s,[50, 51] in which responses decreased as the dose rate decreased, and fractionation or split-dose techniques were

TABLE 5–3. **Methods Used to Detect DNA Breaks in Mammalian Cells**

Assay	Primary Lesion Detected	Influence of Chromatin Structure or Lesion Placement*	Approximate Range of Detection† (SSBs or DSBs per Diploid Cell)	Approximate Rejoining Half-time‡
ASGs (zonal rotor)[32]	SSB	No	1000–5000	3.5 min/2 hr (5%)
Alkaline elution[33]	SSB	No	100–5000	4 min/1.2 hr (8%)
Alkaline comet assay[34]	SSB	No	50–15,000	4 min/2 hr (5%)
Alkaline DNA precipitation[35]	SSB	No	500–25,000	5 min/1.1 hr (20%)
Alkaline unwinding[36]	SSB	Yes	50–50,000	2 min/2.7 hr (5%)
Nucleoid sedimentation[37]	SSB	Yes	100–20,000	5 min
Halo assay[38]	SSB	Yes	200–15,000	3.5 min
Neutral sucrose gradient sedimentation[39]	DSB	No	125–50,000	2 hr
Neutral DNA precipitation[40]	DSB	No	1000–10,000	45 min
Neutral gel electrophoresis[41]	DSB	No	125–2500	11 min/1 hr (25%)
Neutral gel electrophoresis[42]	DSB	No	125–2500	25 min/3 hr (30%)
Neutral comet assay[43]	DSB	No	125–7500	10 min/2 hr (35%)
NFE (pH 7.0)[33]	DSB	Yes	250–4000	45 min
NFE (pH 9.6)[33]	DSB	Yes	125–2500	15 min/1.5 hr (32%)
NFE (pH 11.1)[44]	DSB	Yes	25–1500	8 min/1 hr (30%)
Nonionic detergent NFE_{tx}[45]	Multiple DSBs	Yes	600–7500	30 min

*The possible influence of chromatin structure is based largely on the observation of differences in damage induction for different cell lines exposed to the same dose.

†Estimates of range of sensitivity are based on response to ionizing radiation, with 1 Gy producing 1000 SSBs and 25 DSBs per diploid mammalian cell.

‡Rejoining half-times show the fastest and slowest components, with the percentage rejoined by the slowest component given in parentheses. In cases in which only one value is given, there is either a single component of rejoining, or the half-time of only one (fast) component was reported. When repair is dependent on cell type or dose, results reported are approximations.

From Olive PL: The role of DNA single- and double-strand breaks in cell killing by ionizing radiation. Radiat Res 1998; 150 (suppl):S42–S51, with permission.

used to examine end points such as skin erythema and chromosome breaks. Major emphasis in this area developed after 1960, when it was shown that mammalian cells exhibited split-dose repair or sublethal damage (SLD) recovery. Elkind and colleagues, in a study on the so-called shoulder of cell survival curves (see "Cell Survival") demonstrated that if a radiation dose was divided (or split) and a temporal break of a few hours was allowed between the two doses, then the shoulder on the curve reappeared.[52] This phenomenon was explained by the ability of cells to repair a great proportion of damage that occurs after low doses of radiation, and it suggested that multiple small doses of radiation can preserve normal, healthy tissue, which is the basic principle underlying the use of fractionation.

Another form of recovery—repair of potentially lethal damage (PLD)—has been studied in both plateau phase cultures and solid tumors. This repair process, measured by varying the postirradiation incubation conditions of *in vitro* cell lines allowing for cell salvage, has now been shown to have some relevance to the clinical condition.[6] Weichselbaum and associates have demonstrated that a number of clinically radiation-resistant tumors have a greater capacity for PLD repair than other, more radiation-sensitive tumors,[53] although this is only one of a number of radiation parameters that accounts for therapy response.

DNA Repair Processes

All cell types have evolved multiple mechanisms for the repair and signaling of DNA damage. The considerable progress made in characterizing DNA repair processes is the result of work initially performed with bacterial strains exposed to germicidal ultraviolet (UV) irradiation. The repair processes now recognized include excision repair (base, nucleotide, and mismatch) and single-step repair[54]; mismatch repair is the one pathway that may enhance cytotoxicity.[55, 56] The repair of DSBs is principally performed through homologous recombination or by nonhomologous DNA end-joining. Postreplication repair (or replicative bypass), a potentially important repair-associated process, is not fully understood at present in terms of its molecular mechanisms.[57]

Single-Step Repair

Single-step repair is performed by alkyltransferase through the direct removal of an alkyl residue, or through the direct reversion of UV-induced cyclobutane pyrimidine dimers by photolyases in the presence of photoreactivating blue light.[58–60]

Excision Repair

Base Excision Repair (BER). A significant fraction (60% to 70%) of cellular DNA damage is caused by free radicals generated from water, notably the hydroxyl radical (OH·).[18] These free radicals can produce a wide spectrum of damage (e.g., damage to purine and pyrimidine rings, SSBs, and sites of base loss[61–63]), but all damage induced by hydroxyl radicals is removed by base excision repair.[64] In addition to free radical damage, BER is also involved in repairing other endogenous DNA damage, such as spontaneous depurinations, deaminations, and alkylations.[65]

Base excision repair of free radical–induced damage goes through a series of biochemical steps that involve the sequential operation of an endonuclease, a polymerase, and a ligase. This pathway is ubiquitous from bacteria to man and is illustrated in Figure 5–6. Although free radical damage (and, by association, BER) was thought to be unimportant in the late consequences of radiation injury, it

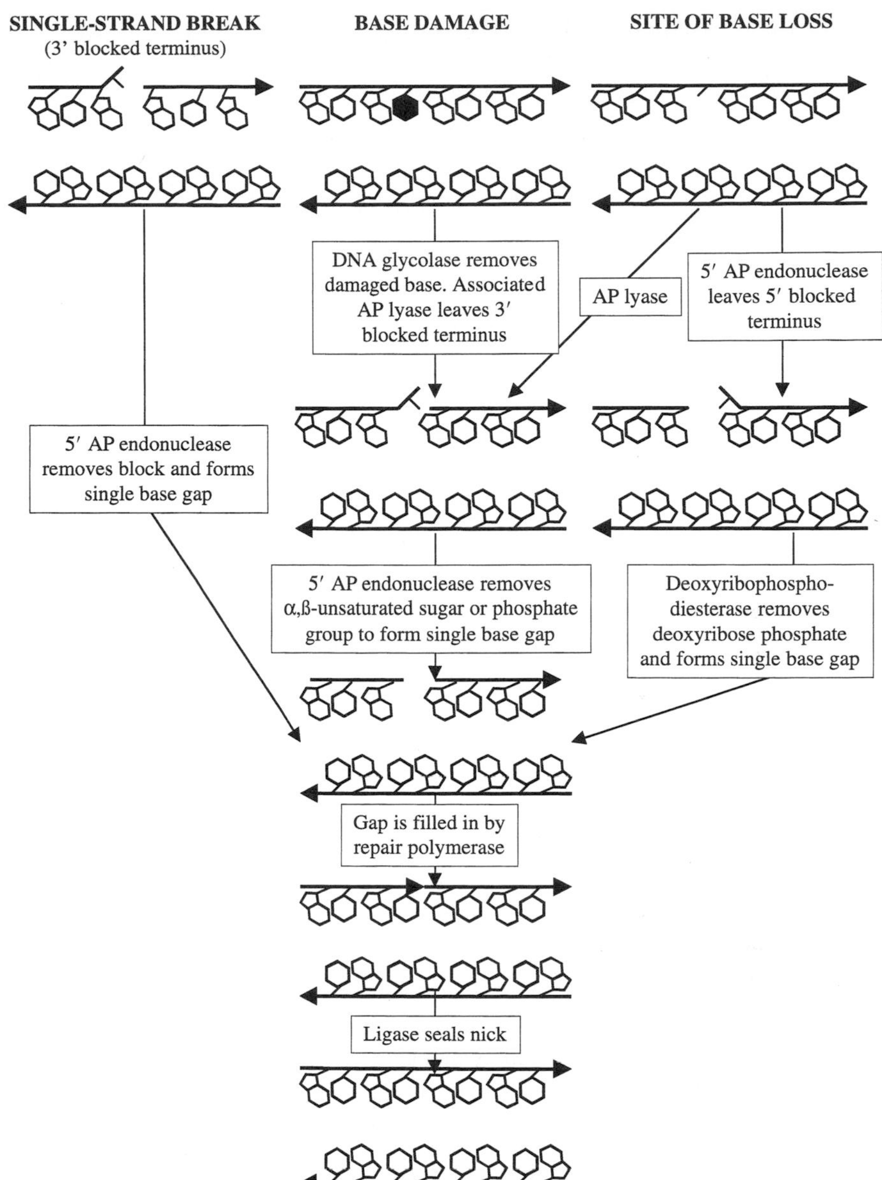
SINGLE-STRAND BREAK
(3' blocked terminus)
BASE DAMAGE
SITE OF BASE LOSS
DNA glycolase removes damaged base. Associated AP lyase leaves 3′ blocked terminus
AP lyase
5′ AP endonuclease leaves 5′ blocked terminus
5′ AP endonuclease removes block and forms single base gap
5′ AP endonuclease removes α,ß-unsaturated sugar or phosphate group to form single base gap
Deoxyribophospho-diesterase removes deoxyribose phosphate and forms single base gap
Gap is filled in by repair polymerase
Ligase seals nick

Figure 5–6. Base excision repair of free radical–induced damage. (From Wallace SS: Enzymatic processing of radiation-induced free radical damage in DNA. Radiat Res 1998; 150 [Suppl]:S60–S79, with permission.)

has become apparent that the yield of DSBs cannot fully account for their lethal effect.[66, 67] It has therefore been suggested, with some experimental support,[68–70] that during the process of repair, additional DSBs may be produced in closely opposed, but otherwise nonlethal, damaged sites, particularly in complex lesions. BER is therefore implicated in cell death, mutagenesis, and carcinogenesis, and upregulation or downregulation of this process may also affect cytotoxicity and mutagenicity.

Nucleotide Excision Repair (NER). A great deal of research has gone into the area of nucleotide excision repair, which is important in the removal of DNA adducts induced by UV light and various chemicals. This work has made use of repair-deficient mutant cell lines as well as patients sensitive to UV (e.g., those with Cockayne's syndrome or xeroderma pigmentosum). Of note, two pathways exist for nucleotide excision repair. One deals with the rapid removal of lesions that block transcription and, therefore, need to be removed with some speed and precision; this is known as transcription-coupled repair. The other, a slower, transcription-independent (and less efficient) pathway, performs more global genomic repair.[71] NER is a highly versatile pathway, acting upon a broad spectrum of structurally diverse DNA alterations (bulky DNA lesions) that cause substantial local distortions of the DNA helix.[72] Nonetheless, there is little redundancy in this pathway.

Double-Strand Break Repair

Homologous Recombination. Homologous recombination repair (HRR) has been studied assiduously in the yeast *Saccharomyces cerevisiae*, and it has been shown that during the HRR process, the damaged chromosome retrieves genetic information from an undamaged homologue under the control of the *RAD51* (formerly RecA) family of genes.[73, 74] However, in mammalian cells, although it has been known that HRR occurs, its relative importance in DNA repair has been unknown, and few of the gene products have been identified. However, *RAD51*-like genes have now been identified in mammals,[75] and though their role and functions are speculative, the combination of sequence conservation and gene expression patterns suggests that they function in the HRR pathway.[76]

Nonhomologous End-Joining. The majority of DSBs in mammalian cells are rejoined by nonhomologous end-joining (NHEJ), which does not depend on extensive regions of homology. Studies in DNA repair suggest that a DNA-dependent protein kinase (DNA-PK) may function in NHEJ pathways for DNA DSB repair and V(D)J recombination.[77–79] DNA-PK is a nuclear serine-threonine protein kinase composed of a catalytic subunit p350 and a DNA binding component termed Ku.[49, 80, 81] Ku consists of two tightly associated polypeptides of approximately 70 kDa and 80 kDa in length (Ku70/80). An intriguing feature of DNA-PK is that it binds to both DNA ends and other discontinuities in DNA, and it requires these structures for its activation. Deficiency in either the DNA–end-binding activity (Ku70/80) or the catalytic activity (p350) can reduce DNA DSB repair capacity and increase radiation sensitivity. For example, Ku DNA binding activity is absent in extracts of radiosensitive hamster *xrs6* cells, which are defective in DNA DSB repair[78]; introduction of the human gene encoding Ku80 complements the mutant DNA DSB repair defects. Another example is the radiosensitive human malignant glioma M059J cell line, which has been found to lack the p350 subunit and is therefore defective in DNA DSB repair.[82]

Targeting DNA Repair

The relationship between DNA damage and repair to cell death has not been easy to evaluate, but it has been supported by the fact that cells from patients with specific diseases associated with repair deficiencies are particularly sensitive to the cytotoxic action of ionizing radiation. For example, fibroblasts cultured from patients with ataxia telangiectasia (AT) are more sensitive to radiation compared with fibroblasts from normal individuals[83, 84] (Fig. 5–7). Furthermore, radiation sensitivity has been correlated with DSB induction and repair in several human tumor lines.[86–88] These features have been studied intensively in order to gain an insight into the underlying molecular and genetic mechanisms of DNA repair. In addition, mutant mouse models (e.g., SCID [severe combined immune deficiency] mice) demonstrate a genetic defect that affects both V(D)J recombination and DSB repair,[89, 90] and they lack the ability to undergo repair of sublethal damage.[91]

The signaling pathways that lead from DNA damage to either repair and survival or cell death are being continuously dissected, and revelations into underlying mechanisms are increasing with our understanding of events at both the molecular and genetic level. The studies mentioned previously, for instance, led Lohrer to conclude that "the signal chain from DNA damage to the cell cycle is the most important parameter in cell survival."[92] The components of this chain or pathway consist of, but are not limited to, recognition of injury, response in the form of direct or indirect initiation of a signaling cascade (an alarm signal), gene activation leading to either repair or

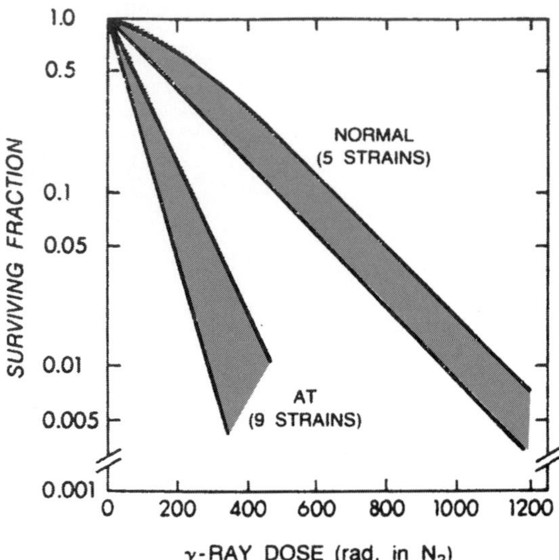

Figure 5–7. Range of surviving fractions of cultured diploid fibroblasts from nine ataxia telangectasia (AT) patients and five clinically normal subjects as a function of cobalt-60 γ-irradiation delivered under hypoxic conditions. (From Paterson MC, Smith PJ, Bech-Hansen NT, et al: Gamma ray hypersensitivity and faulty DNA repair in cultured cells from humans exhibiting familial cancer proneness. In Okada S, Imamura M, Terashima T, et al [eds]: Proceedings of the Sixth International Congress of Radiation Research, Japan, pp 484–495. Tokyo, Toppan Printing Co., 1979, with permission.)

cell death, and repair maintenance or fidelity of repair. Szumiel has published a fine review of some of the early components of this pathway, that is, the monitoring, signaling, and transduction following DNA damage.[93]

Several genes have now been identified that are intimately involved in DNA repair. For example, *XRCC5* encodes for the 80-kDa subunit of Ku, and *XRCC7*, the gene that is defective in SCID mice, encodes for p350, a DNA-dependent protein kinase.[81, 94] These genes and their downstream products are being actively researched for their potential use as therapeutic targets.[95, 96]

Biological Stage

Cell Cycle Effects

The concept of the cell cycle is essential to our understanding of cellular radiobiologic phenomena. A cell population in the exponential growth phase is made up of cells in various stages of the cell cycle with a constant ratio. The cell cycle is divided into two fundamental parts: interphase, which occupies the majority of the cell cycle, and mitosis, which lasts about 30 to 60 minutes, ending with the division of the cell. Interphase is divided into three discrete compartments: S phase (for DNA synthesis), G_1 phase (a gap before S phase), and G_2 phase (a gap after S phase). Rapidly dividing mammalian cells have a cell cycle that lasts about 24 hours, and in a typical cell cycle, G_1 lasts 12 to 14 hours, S phase lasts 6 hours, G_2 lasts 2 to 3 hours, and mitosis lasts about 1 hour.

Identification of the positions of individual cells in the different phases of the cell cycle can be determined by several methods. Cells in mitosis are easily recognized under the microscope; however, microscopy does not reveal whether an interphase cell is in G_1, S, or G_2 phase of the cell cycle. Cells in S phase can be detected by their ability to incorporate labeled DNA precursors, whose presence can be detected after killing the cells. This method can be modified to determine the fraction of cells in different parts of the cell cycle, but the experiments are time consuming and indirect. Most researchers use the technique of flow cytometry to study cell cycle effects.[97] This method measures the amount of DNA in each cell of a population that is treated with a fluorescent DNA-binding dye and passed, one at a time, through a sensitive optical device. A typical profile of DNA content in a rapidly dividing cell population is shown in Figure 5–8. For a given population, the DNA content of G_2/M cells is twice that of G_1 cells, whereas cells in S phase have an intermediate DNA content that increases with the extent of replication. Effects of radiation at different stages of the cell cycle have also been studied with synchronized cell populations obtained from both *in vitro* and *in vivo* conditions.[98, 99] There are several available methods to synchronize cells, such as mitotic selection, addition of drugs that stop cells at a certain cycle stage (e.g., hydroxyurea, colcemid, excess thymidine), temperature shock, centrifugal elutriation, and cell sorting by flow cytometry.

Variations in sensitivity to radiation at different stages of the cell cycle have been observed in mammalian cells.[100, 101] Radiation-induced cell cycle effects include changes in cell survival (age response), chromosome aberration, DNA synthesis and repair, and division delay. Survival curves obtained from *in vitro* studies indicate that, in general, whenever there is a long G_1 period, there appears to be a resistant state in early G_1, followed by a decline in survival toward S. Resistance begins to rise as soon as cells enter S, reaching a maximum in late S phase. Survival then falls sharply in G_2 to the value found in mitosis (Fig. 5–9). However, age-response functions depend strongly on the dose level applied; therefore, discussion of cell cycle–

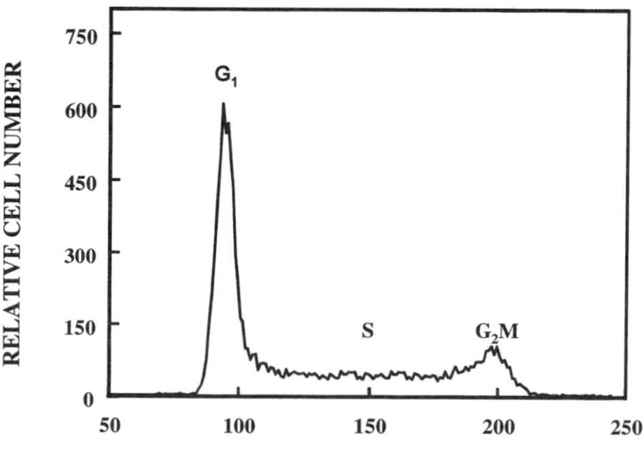

Figure 5–8. A typical profile of DNA content in an asynchronous, cycling population of mammalian cells measured by flow cytometry. DNA content varies during the cell cycle: Cells in G_2/M have twice as much DNA as do cells in G_1, whereas cells in S phase have an intermediate amount.

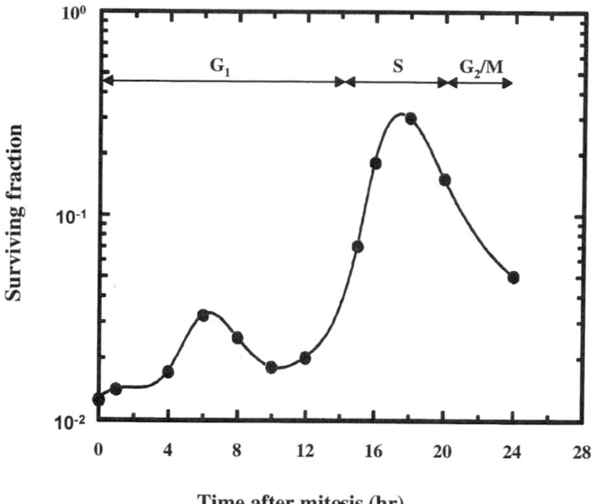

Figure 5–9. Age-response curve of Chinese hamster ovary cells after irradiation with 6 Gy Cs-137 γ rays at different times in the cell cycle. Cell survival is plotted versus time after mitotic detachment.

dependent response always requires specification of the radiation dose used. Variation in radiosensitivity over the cell cycle is often similar for hypoxic and well-oxygenated cells, although cell cycle–dependent variations in oxygen enhancement effect have occasionally been demonstrated.[102] High LET radiation, such as neutron and α-particles, reduces the variations in sensitivity to radiation at different stages of the cell cycle.[103] The main features of the cell cycle–dependent sensitivity measured from irradiated animal tumors are similar to those found in cultured cells.

When a rapidly dividing, asynchronous cell population is exposed to ionizing radiation, the earliest observable effect is a decline in the mitotic index, followed by its rise to, or above, the pre-exposure level. The delay in mitosis produced by ionizing radiation shows a cell cycle–dependent manner that is roughly the inverse of that for cell survival. After a moderate dose of ionizing radiation (4 to 8 Gy), S phase cells exhibit the longest mitotic delay, followed by cells in G_1, G_2, and M. The length of the G_2/M delay is also dependent on the dose and the quality of radiation used. An increased radiation dose causes a longer delay, although the exact shape of the curve relating them may vary between different cell types. The relative efficiencies of neutrons, γ-rays, and α-particles at producing division delay are approximately in the proportion of 4:2:1; this ratio reflects the relative extent of ionization produced by the different types of radiation. The cells eventually recover from the block and continue their cell cycle progression until the completion of mitosis. Studies show that the main cause of the mitotic delay is a temporary hold in cell cycle progression in the later part of the G_2 stage; this hold is termed *G_2/M block*.[104] Once the cells pass the G_2/M block checkpoint, radiation treatment produces little effect on cell cycle progression and the completion of mitosis.

Radiation-induced mitotic delay is mediated by a group of cell cycle regulatory proteins.[105] One of the key components is a kinase (a 34 kDa protein) encoded by the cdc2 genes and their homologs.[106] As a kinase, $p34^{cdc2}$ has been shown to phosphorylate multiple substrates and has been implicated in the activation of several cellular processes, including chromosome condensation, nuclear envelope breakdown, mitotic spindle formation, and the activation of DNA replication.[107] In a rapidly growing cell population, the level of $p34^{cdc2}$ protein is relatively constant throughout the cell cycle. The temporal regulation of $p34^{cdc2}$ kinase activity, however, involves its periodic association with regulatory subunits, cyclins, and its phosphorylation and dephosphorylation state.[108]

Type B cyclins are proteins whose abundance oscillates during the cell cycle, gradually accumulating in interphase and disappearing abruptly at the end of mitosis. During the late interphase, $p34^{cdc2}$ is complexed with cyclin B and is kept inactive as a kinase by phosphorylation at its inhibitory sites: threonine14, tyrosine15, and serine161 residues. At the G_2/M transition, this complex is dephosphorylated and becomes the active mitosis-promoting factor (MPF). MPF activity is required for the successful induction of mitosis in mammalian cells. A model of the G_2/M regulation is shown in Figure 5–10.

The involvement of $p34^{cdc2}$ and cyclin B in radiation-induced mitotic delay has been studied in cultured mammalian cells.[109–111] The $p34^{cdc2}$ kinase activity of asynchronous Chinese hamster ovary (CHO) cells is reduced after irradiation and then gradually returns to normal.[109] The inhibition and recovery of kinase activity takes place during the same time, when cells are blocked in the G_2/M phase of the cell cycle. This simultaneous activity suggests that G_2/M delay is the result of a radiation-induced inhibition of $p34^{cdc2}$ kinase activity. Other studies, using partially synchronized HeLa cells, indicate that delay in the accumulation of cyclin B mRNA and protein is responsible for the inhibition of kinase activity.[110, 111] These experiments provide a likely molecular pathway through which ionizing radiation induces mitotic delay.

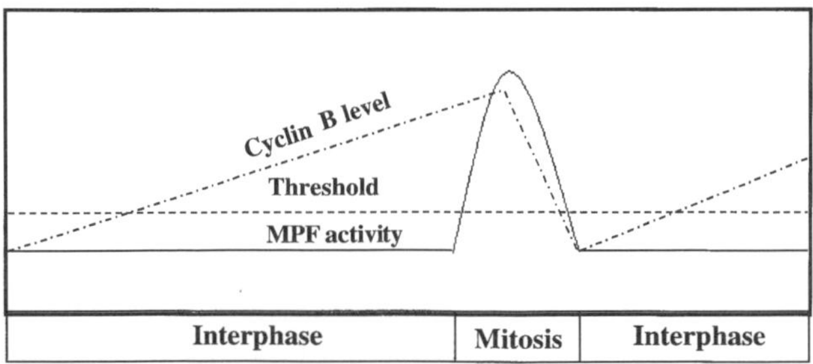

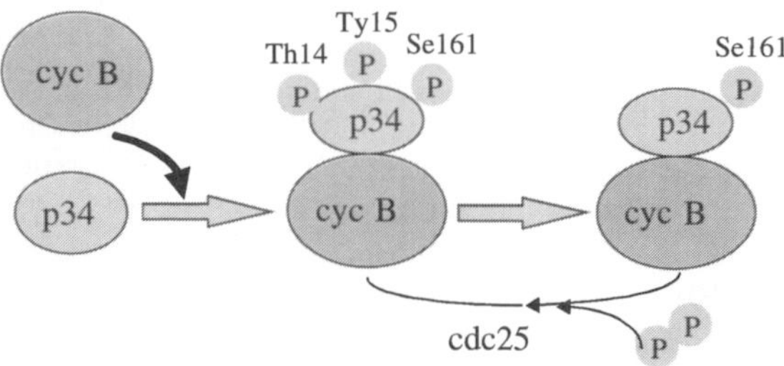

Figure 5–10. Biochemical model of G_2/M regulation. The upper section shows the fluctuation of cyclin B and MPF levels as predicted for normal cycling cells. The lower section shows the association of cyclin B with cdc25 during phosphorylation and dephosphorylation to activate and inactivate MPF.

It has been suggested that mitotic delay is a mechanism by which cells are given sufficient time to repair radiation-induced damage. Cells irradiated during the time between G_2/M block checkpoint and mitosis usually have a lower survival rate than those irradiated in G_2 phase before the checkpoint. Caffeine, an agent that is known to reduce or eliminate the radiation-induced mitotic delay, has been shown to increase the radiation sensitivity of mammalian cells. A similar G_1/S checkpoint regulation operates in mammalian cells through the function of the *TP53* gene. *TP53* is a tumor suppressor gene that encodes a nuclear phosphoprotein that normally activates G_1 cell cycle arrest in response to radiation injury. *TP53* activity can extend the time available for DNA repair before S phase entry and, perhaps, increase the cell's capacity to survive radiation damage.[112]

Cell Survival

The term *survival* must be defined, because lack of immediate cell death does not necessarily signify true survival.[1] An appropriate definition in differentiated cells is loss of a specific function. However, it must be noted that in proliferating cells, it is not sufficient to describe loss of reproductive integrity, because some cells may continue to divide through a number of divisions before eventually stopping. Surviving cells must demonstrate sustained proliferation, that is, *clonogenic survival.*

A cell survival curve describes the relationship between radiation dose received and the number of clonogenic cells that survive[1] and will be described in more detail in Chapter 6, Principles of Radiation Oncology and Cancer Radiotherapy. The dose-effect relationship is determined by *in vitro* colony formation assay techniques that give a survival function based on clonogenic reproductive capacity. In these techniques, a known number of cells are plated, that is, they are seeded into culture dishes, and the colonies forming from surviving cells are scored postradiation. Using this method, survival curves, which characterize the cell population, can be obtained. Survival curves for mammalian cells are commonly sigmoidal in shape, and a frequently used model is the single-hit, multitarget model of cell inactivation[52]:

$$SF = 1 - (1 - e^{-qD})^n$$

SF represents the surviving fraction, *D* is the radiation dose, and $-q$ is the final slope of the survival curve. When plotted on a semilogarithmic scale (Fig. 5–11), the curve is biphasic, and its parameters define the cell population under study. Survival curves permit us to express radiosensitivity using two parameters, D_0 and n. The shoulder on survival curves for mammalian cells after low LET radiation indicates that damage must be accumulated before lethal damage results. This is characterized by the extrapolation number *n* or the quasi-threshold dose D_q ($D_q = D_0 \ln n$), or both. The slope of the curve is equal to $-1/D_0$ with D_0 as the mean lethal dose, that is, the dose required to reduce survivors to 1/e (0.37) of the initial number.

Over the years, a number of *in vivo* assays for tumor

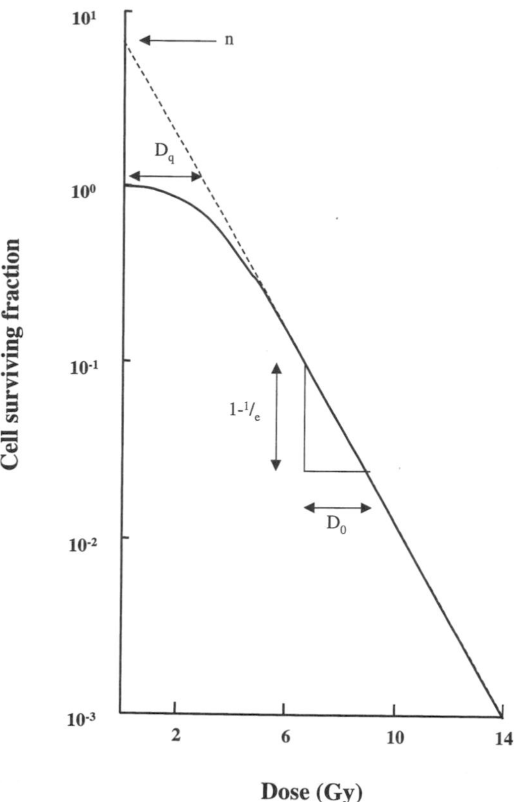

Figure 5–11. Typical mammalian cell survival curve for lower LET radiation such as x-rays. D_q = the "quasi-threshold" dose; D_0 = mean lethal dose; and n = the extrapolation number where D_q = D_0 ln n.

and normal tissue have also added significantly to our ability to quantitatively determine dose-effect relationships. These include the spleen colony assay for bone marrow cells, lung colony assays, skin and intestinal crypt cell assays, and transplantation assays for mammary, thyroid, and liver cells. The use of these and other assays for mammalian cells has revealed the following:

- the general presence of a shoulder on survival curves
- a comparatively narrow range of D_0 or slopes (0.5 to 2.5 Gy)
- modifications of slope and shoulders by radiations of different linear energy transfer
- a marked change in sensitivities produced by oxygen and certain chemicals

The emphasis in dose-effect relationship studies has been to assess the low-dose region, not only because of interest in fundamental mechanisms of accumulation of DNA damage but also because of applications to estimates of radiation hazards and to radiation therapy, in which smaller doses of radiation are more pertinent. Many curves applied to single, acute doses of radiation appear to fit a linear-quadratic equation,[8] in which the response is directly related to both the dose and the square of the dose:

$$SF = e^{-(\alpha D + \beta D^2)}$$

In terms of physical events, it is suggested that αD corresponds to single-event inactivation, or a linear component of cell kill, representing the $\log_e$ of the cells killed per gray, whereas βD^2 represents lethality, resulting from an interaction of two individual events and representing the $\log_e$ of the cells killed per Gy^2. The biologic implications are that the α or linear component represents nonreparable damage and that the β or quadratic component represents damage that must be accumulated before becoming lethal, and is therefore reparable under appropriate conditions. For many years, the linear α component was largely ignored, despite the fact that it assumes major significance at low doses (in the order of 2 Gy). This concept was reversed in the early 1970s when Dutreix and colleagues demonstrated that reducing the dose per fraction below 3 Gy did not result in additional tissue sparing.[113]

The relative contributions of the α and β components of cellular inactivation differ between tumors and various normal tissues. The dose at which the linear (α) and quadratic (β) components are equal is termed the α/β ratio, and this term is used to differentiate between tissues, particularly in terms of their radiation response. For example, early effects tend to be seen in rapidly proliferating tissues and, importantly, in tumors, whereas late effects occur in slow renewal tissues that proliferate more slowly. Survival curves for tumors and early responding tissues have relatively steep initial slopes (large component) and are characterized by a large ratio of the α and β coefficients (that is, a large α/β ratio). In contrast, the dose-response curves for late tissues are more curved and are typified by a reduced α/β ratio.

In relation to the LET and the RBE, as the LET increases, there is a decrease in the shoulder (D_q) and an increase in the slope (D_0) of survival curves (Fig. 5–12). Thus, the RBE increases with increasing LET. It should be noted that the RBE for a given type of radiation varies with the biologic test system and with the level of damage and consequently the dose of radiation. This is duc to the comparison of different shapes of the survival curves. At low LET, oxygen and other modifiers can alter the response

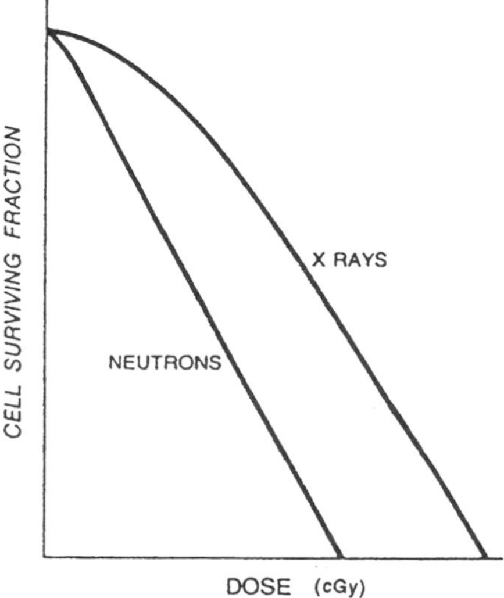

Figure 5–12. Typical survival curves of mammalian cells exposed to single doses of x-rays and fast neutrons. In the case of x-rays, the survival curve has a large initial shoulder; for fast neutrons, the initial shoulder is smaller and the final slope is steeper.

to irradiation; these are described later and in Chapter 6, Principles of Radiation Oncology and Cancer Radiotherapy.

Cell Death

There are two patterns of morphological changes that are associated with cell death in mammalian cells.[5] The most recognizable is *necrosis*, which is degenerative in nature and results from the more severe forms of cell injury. Necrosis is a result of the collapse of cellular metabolism and the depletion of its ATP stores,[114, 115] leading to a breakdown in the homeostatic mechanisms of the cell membrane.[116] When necrosis is seen *in vivo*, it is usually accompanied by exudative inflammation and, if covering a large enough volume of tissue, is followed by the development of scar tissue.

The second recognized element of radiation-induced cell death is *apoptosis*, often referred to as programmed cell death. This is a natural process and is essential during normal development and tissue homeostasis, being involved in organogenesis and T-lymphocyte elimination.[117–120] Because this process is inherent in cells and can be induced by specific stimuli, apoptosis has garnered special interest over the last decade as a potential means of inducing tumor cell death.

Apoptosis

Apoptosis has a number of morphologic features that distinguish the process from necrosis.[121, 122] These features include chromatin condensation (rather than chromatin degradation); cell shrinkage (compared with the cell swelling seen in necrosis), leading to a loss of cellular contact with neighboring cells; and degradation of the DNA in a nucleosomal pattern, resulting in a characteristic ladder seen on agarose gel electrophoresis.[123] Unlike necrosis, apoptosis is not accompanied by inflammation. Finally, apoptosis results from the activation of a specific program of genes, whereas the genetic control mechanism for necrosis, if present, is unknown.

Apoptosis occurs spontaneously in some types of solid tumors,[124, 125] but it is also inducible, because components are constitutively expressed in an inactive form in some cell populations and can be activated in others.[126] For instance, the process can be induced by ionizing radiation in the crypts of the small intestine, the parotid gland, thymocytes, lymphocytes, and hematopoietic cells, and in stem and undifferentiated progenitors of testicular, intestinal, renal, neuronal, and oligodendrocytic cell lineages.[127–130] Following a stimulating trigger, there is activation of a set of cysteine proteases (caspases) that serve as the effector mechanism for an orderly disintegration of defined subcellular structures.[93] The consequent biochemical sequence leads to the activation of unidentified calcium- and magnesium-dependent endonucleases that cleave the nuclear chromatin at selective internucleosomal linker sites, resulting in discrete nuclear fragments.[5] A concomitant elevation of cell-surface transglutaminase activity leads to the generation of surface signal molecules that are recognized by adjacent phagocytes.[131, 132] These phagocytes engulf the apoptotic cells without leakage of toxic intracellular components, which can damage surrounding tissue, and without inducing an inflammatory response.

Research into the genetic control of apoptotic pathways has revealed potential roles for tumor suppressor genes, for example, *TP53* and *RB*, the retinoblastoma gene product, and oncogenes such as *MYC* and *BCL2*.[96] For instance, expression of wild-type *TP53* has been shown to induce apoptosis in some tumor cell lines,[133, 134] leading to the suggestion that tumors that demonstrate wild-type *TP53* expression would be radiation sensitive. However, this has proved to be too simplistic an approach.

One outcome of the recent surge of interest in apoptosis was the recognition of at least two possible signaling mechanisms, one being based in the plasma membrane and the other being secondary to DNA damage (Fig. 5–13).[135] Work by Haimovitz-Friedman and associates at Sloan-Kettering[136] demonstrated that, in endothelial cell membrane preparations, radiation (as well as other stress factors) triggers activation of a sphingomyelin pathway, which is shown to be important in both tumor necrosis factor–α (TNFα)[137, 138] and *FAS*-mediated apoptosis.[139] This so-called early phase apoptotic pathway does not require signals from damaged DNA, and it appears to be regulated through a protein kinase C (PKC) pathway.[135, 140] Sphingomyelin hydrolysis, via acidic sphingomyelinase activity, leads to the generation of ceramide, a requirement for radiation-induced apoptosis, because it serves as a second messenger, stimulating a cascade of kinases and transcription factors that are involved in a variety of cellular responses.[141, 142] One of the responses includes employment of a stress-activated protein kinase (SAPK/JNK) pathway,[143] a functional component of apoptosis. This pathway is parallel to but distinct from the mitogen-activated protein kinase (MAPK/ERK) pathway,[144, 145] although in some cell types, these two pathways are thought to form a regulatory mechanism by acting in opposition.[146, 147]

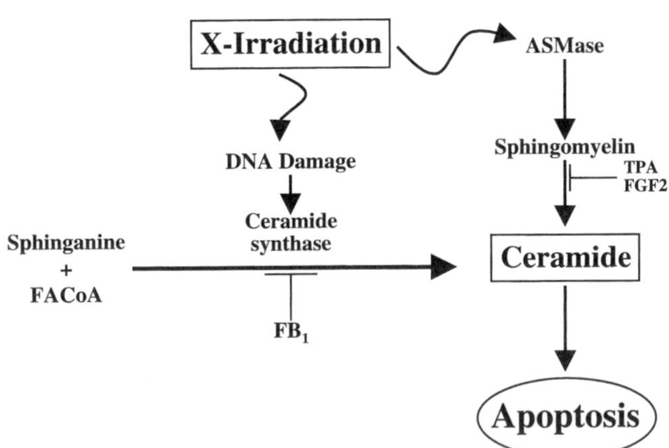

Figure 5–13. Radiation appears to target both the plasma membrane and the nucleus to induce two different signaling systems for apoptosis through the same second messenger, ceramide. Generation of ceramide mediated through the activation of ASMase induces so-called early-phase apoptosis and is regulated by the PKC pathway, whereas "late-phase" apoptosis is mediated by activation of CS. (From Haimovitz-Friedman A: Radiation-induced signal transduction and stress response. Radiat Res 1998; 150:S102–S108, with permission.)

Ceramide has also been shown to be involved in an apoptotic response to DNA damage, which does not involve generation of sphingomyelinase but activation of ceramide synthase (CS).[148] The suggested pathway for this so-called late phase apoptosis is via *de novo* synthesis of ceramide in the endoplasmic reticulum and mitochondria, through condensation of the sphingoid base sphinganine and fatty acyl-CoA. It is still to be determined whether this pathway is *TP53* dependent and to what degree it is involved in cell cycle checkpoint–associated apoptosis.[149]

Targeting Apoptosis

One aim of research in the late 1990s has been to find a means of activating apoptosis selectively in tumor cells but not in normal tissue, thereby inducing maximal tumor cell kill while minimizing normal tissue complications.[96] The importance of *TP53* in apoptosis regulation, particularly after its function had been found to be mutated in so many tumors, led to research into approaches for restoring or boosting its wild-type expression, thereby restoring or increasing apoptosis. These approaches have not yet come to fruition.

A reverse approach is to prevent apoptosis in normal tissue, thereby reducing complications and possible side effects of therapy. Prevention of apoptosis could be achieved by inhibiting or antagonizing normal apoptotic pathways or by increasing regulation. For instance, phorbol esters have been shown to antagonize ceramide-mediated apoptosis induced by TNF.[150] Similarly, basic fibroblast growth factor (FGF2) has been found to protect endothelial cells against radiation-induced apoptosis. Both of these agents appear to work through activation of PKC, which can inhibit ceramide-induced apoptosis at numerous sites in the sphingomyelin pathway.[151, 152]

As briefly described earlier, the SAPK and MAPK pathways are thought to act in opposition. Factors that enhance MAPK expression have been found to inhibit apoptosis and reduce SAPK activity. For example, both FGF2 and 12-0-tetradecanoyl-phorbol-13-acetate (TPA) have been found to activate MAPK secondary to activation of PKC.[153–155]

Radiation Response and Its Modification

The ability to modify radiation responses has continued to intrigue investigators, both from a mechanistic point of view and because of its obvious applications in radiation therapy and other fields. In order to modify the response, we must first understand the process under investigation. With that understanding, we can devise a better means of treatment.

Tissue Effects

Just as detectable cellular injury reflects the cumulative effects of ionizing radiation on cellular molecules, the effects of ionizing radiation on tissues represent the summation of damage to cells within that tissue. Because the functional integrity of many tissues is dependent on the organization of the parenchymal and stromal cells within it, cellular damage in critical tissue components can lead to death of the entire tissue and even the organism itself. Similarly, many organs and organ systems within animals are linked very closely to other organs; normal functioning of these related organs is required in order for each to function properly. It is therefore possible to produce functional, as well as structural, alterations in tissues that are not even included in the exposed area. Any assessment of tissue damage following radiation exposure should also include consideration of these *abscopal* (ab = away from; scopal = target) effects.

Of considerable import when assessing radiation tissue effects is the differentiation into acute- and late-responding tissues.

Acute-Responding Tissue. Acute or early responses are generally seen in those tissues with a high proliferative capacity and a rapid turnover of cells (rapid renewal systems), as exemplified by gastrointestinal mucosa, bone marrow, skin, and oropharyngeal and esophageal mucosa.[4] The classic organization of these tissues is hierarchical, with a small base population of stem cells that produces a highly proliferative compartment of progenitor cells. These progenitor cells will ultimately differentiate into a mature, nonproliferative, functional cell population. Irradiation chiefly affects the stem and progenitor cell populations; therefore, the acute tissue effects become evident as differentiated cells are lost through normal cell depreciation, and the depleted stem and progenitor cells fail to restore their numbers. The severity of the response is dose dependent; however, the rate of development of the effect is relatively dose independent. The dose-independent rate of development is determined by the rate of release into, and loss of cells from, the differentiated cell compartment.

Following the work of Dutreix and colleagues,[113] Withers introduced the concept of a *flexure dose* (D_f),[156] which is considered to be the point at which the dose-response curve begins to bend significantly. It is measured at approximately 0.1 α/β, that is, the curve bends at 0.1 of the dose when the linear and quadratic components are equal. The dose reflects the maximal single dose-sparing of late-responding tissues, and its value is used in hyperfractionation, discussed later. Examples of α/β and flexure dose values for typical acute-responding tissues can be seen in Table 5–4. Of note, the α/β ratio for these tissues is about 10 Gy.

Late- or Chronic-Responding Tissue. Late radiation effects classically are considered to be the response of slowly proliferating tissues, for example, central (oligodendrocytes) or peripheral (Schwann cells) nervous tissue, kidney (renal epithelium), dermis (fibroblasts), and bones (osteoclasts and chondroblasts). Typical examples are given in Table 5–4; of relevance to radiation therapy, the α/β ratio for late-responding tissues is about 2 Gy. In these tissues, compared with the above-mentioned early responding tissues, cells may be both functional and proliferative, and the tissues are therefore considered to be flexible rather than hierarchical.[157, 158] The tissues appear to be more dose dependent because the greater the radiation dose, the shorter the apparent latency. The dose-dependency of tissue is a consequence of not only the turnover time of the

TABLE 5–4. **Estimates of the α/β Ratio and Flexure Doses for Normal Tissues**

	α/β ratio	Flexure Dose
Acute-Responding Tissues		
Melanocytes	6.5	0.65
Hair follicles (depletion)	7	0.7
Lip mucosa desquamation	8	0.8
Colon epithelium*	8	0.8
Bone marrow	9	0.9
Skin epithelium	10	1.0
Jejunal epithelium*	13	1.3
Spermatogenic cells	13	1.3
Seminiferous epithelium*	14	1.4
Tumors:		
Mouse fibrosarcoma metastases	10	1.0
Human tumors	6–25	0.6–0.25
Experimental tumors	10–35	0.1–0.35
Late-Responding Tissues		
Kidney	0.5–5	0.05–0.5
Cartilage and submucosa	1.0–4.9	0.1–0.49
Liver	1.4–3.5	0.14–0.35
Lung	1.6–4.5	0.16–0.45
Human skin	1.6–4.5	0.16–0.45
Spinal cord	1.6–5	0.16–0.5
Bone	1.8–2.5	0.18–0.25
Dermis	2.5±1.0	0.25
Bladder	5.0–10.0	0.5–1.0

*Clonal assay results in which repopulation may affect results.

Adapted from Withers HR, McBride WH: Biologic basis of radiation therapy. In: Perez CA, Brady LW (eds): Principles and Practice of Radiation Oncology, 3rd ed, pp 79–118. Philadelphia, Lippincott-Raven, 1998.

resident cells but also the recruitment of other lethally irradiated cells into proliferation, leading to a cascade or avalanche of cell death. This response can be affected by additional insult, for example, chemotherapy or surgery, among other things.

Physical Modification

Fractionation

As described in Hall's book *Radiobiology for the Radiologist*, the concept of multifraction regimens for use in radiotherapy is a consequence of early studies performed in France during the 1920s and 1930s.[1] In these studies, it was shown that during the administration of a sterilizing radiation dose to the testes, unacceptable skin damage could be avoided if the treatment was spread out over several weeks using daily doses (or fractions) while still achieving full sterilization. It was postulated that this same scenario could be applied to the treatment of a tumor; that is, the tumor could be sterilized while sparing the surrounding normal tissue.

As discussed previously, the relative importance of the linear (α) component of the survival curve becomes of greater significance at lower doses, and the extent of the range over which the α component dominates depends on the relative values of α versus β. It becomes apparent that the higher the relative value of α, the more linear is the response at low doses, and the less sensitive it is to dose fractionation[4]; this can be seen in the acute curve in Figure 5–14.[159] As the α component is reduced relative to β, the survival curve becomes curvier and dose fractionation has more of an effect (see late curve, Fig. 5–14).

The difference between the dose-response curves for early and late-responding tissues (see Fig. 5–14) led to the following axiom: "Fraction size is the dominant factor in determining late effects, while overall treatment time has little influence. By contrast, fraction size and overall treatment time both determine the response of acutely responding tissues."[1] Supported by both research and clinical evidence, increasing dose fraction size and lengthening treatment tissue are disadvantageous. For instance, increasing the fraction size leads to dissociation between early and late-responding tissue, with an increase in the severity of late effects. Because tumors generally are early responders, the severity of late effects becomes a therapeutic disadvantage.

Hyperfractionation

The aim of hyperfractionation is to further separate early and late-responding tissue through the use of smaller-than-standard doses that are delivered as two or more fractions per day, with the overall treatment time remaining the same. This rationale exploits the differences in α/β ratios

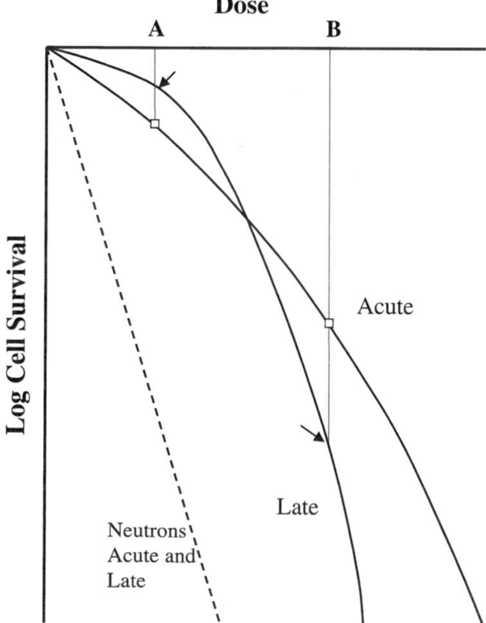

Figure 5–14. Hypothetical survival curves for the target cells for acute and late effects in normal tissues exposed to x-rays or neutrons. The α/β ratio is lower for late effects than acute effects in x-irradiated tissues, resulting in a greater alteration in effect in late-responding tissues with a change in dose. At dose A, survival of target cells is higher in late-responding tissues than in acute-responding tissues; at dose B, the reverse is true. Increasing the dose per fraction from A to B results in a relatively greater increase in late rather than acute injury. For neutrons, the α/β ratio is high, with no detectable influence of the quadratic function (βd^2) over the first two decades of reduction in cell survival, implying that accumulation of injury plays a negligible role in cell killing. (From Withers HR, Thames HD Jr, Peters LJ: Biological bases for high RBE values for late effects of neutron irradiation. Int J Radiat Oncol Biol Phys 1982; 8:2071–2076, with permission from Elsevier Science.)

for different tissues by reducing late effects in normal tissue while achieving the same or better tumor cell kill. By using doses at or below the flexure dose, there is a sparing of late-responding tissues; this will not be true for early responding tissues, for example, tumors, because of the differences in the flexure values (see Table 5–4). However, hyperfractionation is contraindicated in slowly proliferating tumors because their α/β ratio is low.[160]

It must be noted that a regimen of 2 fractions per day is not the limit for hyperfractionation. Further sparing would occur through the use of smaller doses, although this would necessitate 3 or 4 fractions per day. Hyperfractionation has already proven beneficial clinically, particularly in the treatment of head and neck cancer.[161]

Accelerated Treatment

An alternative strategy to hyperfractionation is to shorten treatment time while maintaining the conventional fraction number and dose. The aim is to reduce repopulation in a rapidly proliferating tumor, although this has the disadvantage of increasing toxicity in early responding tissues; that is, early effects may prove to be a limiting factor. Reducing treatment time can be achieved through a number of means, some of which are listed below:

1. *Multiple daily standard fractions* demonstrate good local control but a high frequency of severe complications.[162–164]
2. *Concomitant boosting* describes the so-called boost dose given to a coned-down field concomitantly with the initial treatment volume, instead of sequentially, with an interval of at least 6 hours between treatments.[165]
3. *Continuous hyperfractionated accelerated radiation (CHART)*, with fractions of 1.4 to 1.5 Gy, is given three times daily at 6-hour intervals for 12 consecutive days. This protocol has had some limited success in both head and neck and lung cancers,[166–169] although there has been a concomitant increase in early effects such as mucositis.[170]

When multiple daily fractions are used, sufficient time must be allowed between fractions to allow for sublethal damage (SLD) repair. Results from Sweden[171, 172] and from multicenter (Radiation Therapy Oncology Group) clinical trials[173, 174] have indicated that an interval of less than 4 hours *increases* the incidence of late effects, suggesting that SLD repair may be relatively slow in late-responding tissues. This belief has led to the current practice of using a minimum interval of 4 to 8 hours between fractions.

Dose Rate

In radiation biology, dose rates of ionizing radiation, which extend from a few centigray per day up to hundreds of Gy delivered in a fraction of a second, have been used in a variety of organisms. For mammalian cells, the largest effect of changing dose rate is observed between 0.01 to 1 Gy per minute. As the dose rate is lowered, the slope of the survival curve flattens out, that is, the D_0 increases. It increases because the lower dose rates allow more time for repair of sublethal radiation damage during irradiation. At dose rates below 0.01 Gy per minute there is little effect, because at this level essentially all sublethal damage is repaired during exposure and the residual cell-killing effect results from nonreparable injury.

Use of different dose rates of radiation confers some of the same advantages and disadvantages as fractionation. As the dose rate is lowered and the exposure time is extended, the resultant biologic effect is reduced, so that continuous very low dose rate irradiation can be considered a form of hyperfractionation.[1, 4]

Chemical Modification

The spectrum of agents that can be considered to fall within the field of radiation modifiers, either sensitizers or protectors, has grown markedly with the progress toward a deeper understanding of molecular and cellular mechanisms underlying oncogenesis and radiation effects.[175] The relatively simple, early concepts of radiation sensitization (overcoming chronic hypoxia and incorporating halogenated pyrimidines into DNA) and radiation protection (increasing the thiol content) have been replaced by complex fields of study: cellular microenvironment, angiogenesis, signal transduction processes, DNA damage and repair, gene pathways, and other areas. An arbitrary classification of sensitizers and protectors is listed in Table 5–5; a few of the classes are discussed here.

TABLE 5–5. **Radiation Sensitizers and Protectors**

Oxygen delivery:	Oxygen Nicotinamide Blood flow modifiers
Hypoxic radiation modifiers:	Hypoxic cell sensitizers Bioreductive agents–enhancers
Nonhypoxic radiation modifiers:	Halopyrimidines Boron neutron capture therapy Poly(ADP-ribose) polymerase inhibitors (?repair) Signal transduction modifiers
Biologics ("normal" biological molecules or processes):	Antibodies $\pm$ radioactivity Hormones Anti-inflammatory agents Inflammatory molecules Cytokines and growth factors Nitric oxide Apoptosis Differentiation
Chemotherapy (cytotoxic drugs):	Cisplatin Topoisomerase inhibitors Taxanes Thymidylate synthase inhibitors
Protectors (and antiprotectors):	Thiols and aminothiols Nitroxides Hematopoietic growth factors Thiol depletion (antiprotector) Pentoxifylline Superoxide dismutase
Angiogenesis modifiers	
Gene therapy:	Radiation inducible Hypoxia inducible Enzyme-prodrug
Other:	Novel delivery systems—biodegradable polymers Chelates

From Coleman CN: Chemical sensitizers and protectors. Int J Radiat Oncol Biol Phys 1998; 42:781–783, with permission from Elsevier Science.

Oxygen

Oxygen is considered to be the most potent, and possibly most important, of the chemical modifiers of radiation. Under scientific investigation throughout this century, and following the work of Read and Gray and associates,[176–178] the idea was finally realized that cells demonstrate profound differences in their response to radiation when under hypoxic versus oxic conditions. That is, hypoxic cells require greater doses of radiation to induce an equivalent cell kill than oxygenated cells. This sensitization has been termed the *oxygen enhancement ratio* (OER). It is the ratio of the radiation doses required to reduce survival to a specific level in hypoxic (N_2) compared with oxygenated (O_2) conditions. The OER for mammalian cells generally approaches 3.0 at high doses (Fig. 5–15[1, 179]). However, there is some evidence that the value may be lower at x-ray doses of less than 2 Gy, that is, the normal therapeutic dose. Thomlinson and Gray postulated that viable hypoxic cells may be one cause of radiotherapeutic failure,[180] because it is likely that many tumors contain hypoxic cells owing to their inherent rapid rate of growth, outgrowing their blood supply. Their postulation led to the scientific evaluation of hypoxia as a major target for tumor therapy.

Since the time of these initial findings, there has been an interest in characterizing hypoxic cells within tumors, driven principally by their resistance to radiation treatment.

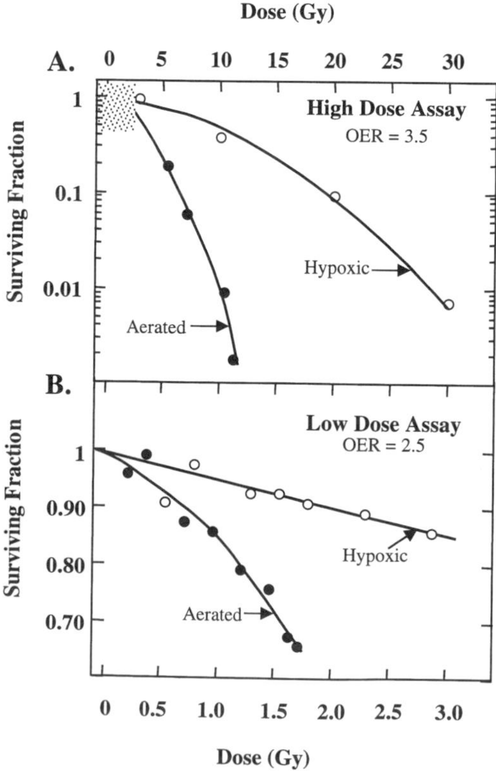

Figure 5–15. Cells are much more sensitive to x-rays under oxic versus hypoxic conditions. The OER has a value close to 3 at high doses, but may have a lower value of about 2 at x-ray doses below 2 Gy. (From Hall EJ: Radiobiology for the Radiologist, 4th ed. Philadelphia, J.B. Lippincott Co., 1994, with permission. Redrawn from Palcic B, Skarsgard LD: Reduced oxygen enhancement ratio at low doses of ionizing radiation. Radiat Res 1984; 100:328–339.)

In 1979, Brown suggested a further distinction that was later confirmed: some cell regions are transiently hypoxic because of a temporary cessation of blood flow.[181, 182] In general, hypoxia (both chronic and transient) affects a wide range of therapies in addition to radiation. The underlying cause of hypoxia, that is, abnormal blood networks, can adversely affect drug penetration and also create a microenvironment of reduced oxygenation and high pH levels.[183] Such conditions lead to cells persisting in states of quiescence or at least reduced proliferation, minimizing their susceptibility to many anticancer agents.[184] Hypoxia may also contribute to tumor progression through its direct effect on tumor suppressor proteins such as p53.[185–187]

Hypoxic Radiation Modifiers: Bioreductive Agents

Interest in modification of radiation damage led to research into the development of radiation-sensitizing chemicals, such as DNA-base analogues and electron affinic agents. High concentrations of one class of sensitizing agents, the nitroimidazoles, proved effective *in vitro* at producing enhancement ratios approaching those of oxygen.[188, 189] One nitroimidazole compound, misonidazole, entered phase I–II and phase III clinical trials, although it ultimately proved to have little or no therapeutic benefit.[190] Many of the agents tested in this endeavor were found, subsequently, to be either insufficiently potent or to have dose-limiting toxicities.

Studies on the mode of action of misonidazole and later, tirapazamine, showed that this group of drugs worked through the unmetabolized drug reacting with radiation-induced radicals in DNA.[191] Further study showed that, following extended exposure, reductive drug metabolism occurred, leading to selective cell killing even in the absence of radiation.[192, 193] Subsequently, three major classes of agents were shown to demonstrate significant bioreductive activation in hypoxic cells: quinones, nitroaromatics, and N-oxides.[194] Use of these agents leads to an alternative mode of therapeutic attack, that is, to *increase* tumor cell hypoxia, thereby increasing the potential for hypoxic cell kill.[195] Through modification of oxygen transport or manipulation of tumor blood flow, there is a possibility that the cytotoxicity of bioreductive agents can be potentiated, and clinical initiatives are now under way with encouraging results.[184]

Biologics: Cytokines

Cytokines and growth factors have been shown to be part of the cascade of events following radiation injury leading to late effects.[196] Nonetheless, due to their pleuripotential nature, many of the cytokine components can demonstrate both sensitizing or protective roles, depending on their position geographically and temporally, their threshold level of activation, synergism with other cytokines, and other factors.

Indirect evidence for the role of cytokines as modifiers of radiation was evidenced in early work by Ainsworth and Chase,[197] who demonstrated a radioprotective effect achieved through the preadministration of lipopolysaccharide (LPS) on the development of a lethal hematopoietic syndrome in mice. LPS has been shown to induce macrophages to produce several cytokines, including interleukin-1 (IL-1) and IL-6, tumor necrosis factor–α (TNFα) and –β (TNFβ), interferon-α (αIFN) and -β (βIFN), and transforming growth factor–β (TGFβ).[198–200] Studies have shown that both IL-1 and TNFα can substitute for LPS and protect bone marrow progenitor cells both *in vitro* and *in vivo*.[201] Neta and coworkers[202, 203] reported that low, otherwise ineffective doses of IL-1α could synergize the protective effects of granulocyte colony-stimulating factor (G-CSF) and granulocyte-macrophage colony-stimulating factor (GM-CSF) in mice receiving total body irradiation (TBI), suggesting that cytokine interactions may be necessary for radioprotection of hematopoietic progenitor cells. This idea has been supported by the successful use of other combinations of cytokines.[204]

Similar to IL-1, TNFα mediates the radioprotective effects of LPS.[201, 203] Administration of exogenous TNF has been shown to induce hematopoietic progenitor cell protection, and this could be reversed through administration of an anti-TNF antibody.[204] Although the mechanism of radiation protection is unknown, *in vitro* TNF has been shown to enhance tumor cell kill in some lines, provided that it is administered 4 to 12 hours before irradiation.[205, 206] This effect may be associated with a TNF-induction of apoptosis.[207] The complexity of the interactions of these cytokines and growth factors is underscored by work showing that TGFβ can sensitize mice to TBI by either down-regulating IL-1 receptor expression, or by reducing IL-1 and TNFα expression.[201] In addition, in patients receiving TBI, increased serum levels of TNF have been found during the preconditioning regimen before bone marrow transplant; these levels were associated with a higher risk of later radiation-related complications.[208, 209] The same has been found for TGFβ.[210, 211] How much these levels are a consequence of tumor burden relative to normal tissue reactions is still to be determined.

It is increasingly apparent that cellular and molecular events, mediated by autocrine, paracrine, and endocrine factors, play a major role in the response to radiation injury.[5, 196] Not limited to the brief, above-mentioned description, hundreds of cytokines, chemokines, and other factors are being investigated for their roles in tissue response to irradiation. Elucidation of the roles played by cytokines, growth factors, hormones, and their receptors in the biochemical pathways controlling radiation damage repair or leading to radiation-induced cell death could have immediate clinical application in the future through intervention in specific mechanisms.

Interactions: Radiation Therapy and Chemotherapy

Experimental studies have indicated that the radiation response of cultured cells *in vitro*, as well as tumor and normal tissue cells *in vivo*, can be greatly enhanced when radiation therapy is administered in conjunction with specific chemotherapeutic agents. The magnitude of response enhancement achieved is dependent on the chemotherapeutic agent chosen, the dose used, the sequence and timing of radiation treatment relative to drug administration and the tissue, as well as the biologic end point examined. However, there has also been an accumulation of data on potentiated late effects owing to the interactions of these modalities or an enhancement from their separate effects on different cell populations within the same organ.[212–216] This potentiation of effects is particularly true in the area of bone marrow transplantation, in which combined-modality therapy is frequently used in preconditioning regimens.[217–219] Although an increasing amount of experimental data has been accumulated over the past few years, space limitations restrict the discussion of this combined approach to therapy. The reader is therefore directed to an upcoming edition of *Seminars in Radiation Oncology*, edited by B. Movsas. This interaction is also discussed in Chapter 34, Late Effects of Cancer Treatment.

Radiation Carcinogenesis

The ability of radiation to induce cancer and leukemia was appreciated shortly after the discovery of radiation and its application to medicine, when pioneer radiologists, ignorant of the hazards, developed skin cancers and leukemias following exposure to radiation sources. Since that time, a great deal of effort has been expended in attempts to elucidate the mechanisms of radiation carcinogenesis because there are now substantial epidemiological data that implicate ionizing radiation as a causative agent for a broad range of human cancers.[220] In addition, good data relative to tumor induction in humans are available for relatively high dose exposures. This information comes from long-term studies of survivors of the atomic bomb blasts at Hiroshima and Nagasaki, populations accidentally exposed to radiation during weapons testing, workers exposed to radiation during clean-up of nuclear accidents (e.g., Chernobyl), and patients exposed to large amounts of radiation for diagnostic purposes or for the treatment of relatively benign diseases. Appropriate epidemiologic assessment and discussion of all the available data are not possible in this format. However, several generalizations about tumor induction resulting from exposure to ionizing radiation can be made:

- Nearly all tissues in the body are susceptible to tumor induction, but they vary considerably with respect to their sensitivity to cancer induction.
- Major sites of solid tumors induced by total-body exposure to radiation are the breast, thyroid, lung, and digestive organs.
- Latency period (the time from exposure to tumor detection) is frequently long, that is, years to decades. The shortest latency is for leukemia (5 to 7 years); for solid tumors, latency may be greater than 45 years.
- Interaction between host and environmental factors (e.g., hormonal influences, exposure to other carcinogenic agents) may play a significant role in tumor induction.
- Dose-response relationships for many animal model systems are qualitatively similar to those for human tumor induction. However, direct quantitative risk extrapolation from animals to humans would be inappropriate.

Over the past 25 years, our understanding of the mechanisms underlying carcinogenesis has improved considerably. The classic view of the radiation induction of carcinogenesis was that mutations occurred at sites of DNA damage, as described earlier. The damage is converted into a mutation during subsequent DNA replication or as a consequence of enzymatic repair.[221] However, some investigators now have proposed a process of genetic instability, transmissible over many generations of cell replication, as the earliest cellular event in the sequence,[222] which can occur at either the nucleotide or chromosomal levels.[223] This instability puts all cells at risk for mutation, but its major impact occurs when critical genes, such as *TP53*, are mutated as a secondary consequence of radiation exposure.[224] In all, tumorigenicity has been found to result from changes in control points governing cell cycle and cell differentiation, and molecular analysis of the multistep nature of carcinogenesis has classified two general classes of genetic changes: activation of a proto-oncogene, loss of a suppressor gene (e.g., *TP53*), or a combination of both.[225, 226] However, no causal relationship has yet been established that relates changes in specific genes to the development of radiation-induced cancers.

Proto-Oncogenes and Oncogenes

Proto-oncogenes have been found to be present in all mammalian cells and many are known to be involved in cell growth regulation.[227, 228] However, radiation (and other stress factors) can cause changes in the proto-oncogenes, activating them to oncogenes. These oncogenes will then act in a dominant fashion, even in the presence of normal copies, and their activation leads to transformation and immortalization of the normal cell phenotype.[229, 230] A large number of oncogenes have now been identified, with members of the *RAS* family being the most numerous.[229, 231, 232]

Suppressor Genes

Following experiments in the 1970s, looking at the hybridization of normal cells with tumor cells leading to a loss of tumorigenicity,[223] it was proposed that normal cells contained one or more genes that could suppress neoplastic potential. With the development of more sophisticated methodologies, microcell fusion became possible and single human chromosomes could now be shown to potentially carry tumor suppressor genes.

Most of the available dose-response information for radiation-induced carcinogenesis is for relatively high doses of radiation. Although many animal studies using lower doses of radiation have been reported, tumor induction information for extremely low doses (those of interest with respect to environmental exposures of large populations) has been difficult to obtain because of the large number of animals that would have to be included to detect statistically significant increases in the rate of tumor induction. To assess risk at low doses and establish protection standards, the shape of the dose-response curve in the low-dose region must be extrapolated from the higher dose regions. However, the dose-response model most appropriate for extrapolation to the low-dose region is a subject of great debate. For a more detailed discussion of this important issue, the reader is advised to read *Health Effects of Exposure to Low Levels of Ionizing Radiation: BEIR V*[234] and the recommendations of *ICRP Publication 60*.[235]

Total Body Irradiation

The total organism, when considered as a whole, is as sensitive as its most vulnerable vital tissues; the most sensitive of the vital tissues in the human body is considered to be the hematopoietic system. This sensitivity has led to patient deaths from acute, overwhelming infections following total body irradiation (TBI) as part of treatment therapies. The associated late effects of such therapy are discussed in detail in Chapter 34, Late Effects of Cancer Treatment. However, if part of the hematopoietic system is shielded, the tolerance of the individual for radiation is greatly increased, and the next most sensitive vital tissue, the GI tract, determines tolerance.

The tolerance of the organism, or its component collection of normal tissues, varies with the application of radiation depending on four characteristics: dose, time, volume, and quality. Too often, radiation effects are described and pharmacopathologic changes are presented without reference to these pertinent radiation factors.

$$\text{Biologic Effect} \sim \frac{\text{Dose} \times \text{Volume}}{\text{Time}}$$

Essentially, the biologic effect of radiation is directly proportional to the dose and volume, and inversely related to the time of administration. Some of the situations that occur are described below.

1. *Large dose, large volume of tissue exposed, and high dose rate (radiation accidents or explosions):*
   - dose: 4.5 to 100 Gy
   - time: seconds to hours or days
   - volume: total body

   This situation can occur during an atomic bomb explosion or, possibly, a nuclear reactor accident. The LD_{50} for humans, that is, the dose at which 50% of the exposed population would die, is 4.5 to 5.5 Gy. Levels of whole-body irradiation at 10 to 20 Gy are lethal for the entire population (LD_{100}); the syndromes that lead to lethality are dose dependent:

   Bone marrow syndrome: If the patient survives intestinal manifestations with levels of 4.5 to 10 Gy, then aplastic anemia and thrombocytopenia will occur within 1 to 3 weeks.

   GI syndrome: Death occurs within days, as a result of electrolyte imbalance and infection, with levels of 10 to 20 Gy.

   CNS syndrome: Death can occur instantly or within hours, with levels of 60 Gy or more.
2. *Small dose, large volume of tissue exposed, and low dose rate (background and occupational exposure)*:
   - dose: small, but variable
   - time: lifetime
   - volume: entire population; whole body, but organs of particular concern—gonads, bone marrow, and other tissues especially susceptible to radiation carcinogenesis (breast, thyroid, alimentary tract)
3. *Small dose, small volume of tissue exposed, and high dose rate (diagnostic radiography)*:

- dose: small (average individual exposure ~ 39 mrem/year)
- time: intermittent
- volume: variable; organs of particular concern—gonads, bone marrow, and other tissues especially susceptible to radiation carcinogenesis, and the fetus

4. *Large dose, small volume and high dose rate (radiation therapy)*:
   - dose: 40 to 100 Gy
   - time: 4 to 8 weeks
   - volume: usually limited to segments of the body or separate organs; attempts are made to include as little of normal structures as possible in the treatment beams so that segmental damage can be tolerated by the patient

For general reference, the average annual total body exposures for residents of the United States have been estimated as follows[236]:

natural background:	terrestrial	28 mrem/yr
	cosmic (extraterrestrial)	27 mrem/yr
	inhaled (e.g., radon)	200 mrem/yr
	biologic (radionuclides, e.g., ^{40}K)	40 mrem/yr
medical procedures:	x-ray	39 mrem/yr
	nuclear medicine	14 mrem/yr
consumer (fallout, nuclear power):		~10 mrem/yr
Other:		2 mrem/yr
Total		**~ 360 mrem/yr**

For the two types of exposure, medical and consumer, the genetically significant dose (GSD) is considerably lower than these estimates. For example, the total GSD is estimated to be approximately 110 mrem per year and approximately 23 mrem per year for medically related exposures. This difference reflects the fact that the gonads receive only a fraction of the doses listed earlier. Furthermore, only exposure to individuals with child-bearing potential are included in GSD estimates.

The major health-related concerns associated with medical and occupational exposure are radiation-induced cancer, genetic damage, and effects on the developing fetus. Genetic risk is considered to be extremely low at these doses, as is the risk of fetal injury. Carcinogenesis is, without a doubt, the major somatic effect of exposure of populations to low doses of ionizing radiation. However, the risk is considered to be relatively low at these exposure levels.

In the case of medical exposures to radiation, the important question to ask is whether the medical gain outweighs the risks associated with the procedures. If x-rays are ordered properly, then there is no question that the immediate and later gains outweigh any theoretical gonadal or carcinogenic hazard. The dose of 0.001 cGy to the gonads during a routine chest film is of no concern in terms of offspring and need not arouse fear in terms of radiation injury. The hazard of not finding an early tuberculous or neoplastic lesion presents a greater risk of morbidity and mortality. Nonetheless, we should minimize unnecessary exposure to radiation and use it only when it may benefit health.

Recommended Reading

The radiation biology literature is extensive; therefore, for the convenience of the interested reader, we suggest the following textbook material as excellent references to the various areas of radiation biology discussed in this chapter. *Radiobiology for the Radiologist* by Hall[1] is an excellent general reference text, being particularly valuable to medical practitioners. A similar book with equal reference to the medical community is the *Handbook of Radiobiology* by Prasad.[2] A detailed look at the molecular basis for many of the processes and mechanisms briefly discussed earlier may be found in Mendelsohn and colleagues' *The Molecular Basis of Cancer.*[3] For those readers who want a quick revision in general aspects (in addition to Chapter 6, Principles of Radiation Oncology and Cancer Radiotherapy), there are a number of informative chapters by leaders in this field. See Withers and McBride,[4] Fuks and Weichselbaum,[5] and Hellman's chapters[6] as part of highly recommended texts.

In addition to these references, we have included current references within many of the chapter subsections. These references provide the detailed discussions that we have frequently been unable to provide because of space limitations. The reader is strongly encouraged to pursue areas of interest by referring to the textbooks and the original material.

REFERENCES

General References

1. Hall EJ: Radiobiology for the Radiologist, 4th ed. Philadelphia, J.B. Lippincott Co., 1994.
2. Prasad KN: Handbook of Radiobiology, 2nd ed. Boca Raton, CRC Press, 1995.
3. Mendelsohn J, Howley PM, Israel MA, et al: The Molecular Basis of Cancer. Philadelphia, W.B. Saunders Co., 1995.
4. Withers HR, McBride WH: Biologic basis of radiation therapy. In: Perez CA, Brady LW (eds): Principles and Practice of Radiation Oncology, 3rd ed. pp 79–118. Philadelphia, Lippincott-Raven, 1998.
5. Fuks Z, Weichselbaum RR: Radiation therapy. In: Mendelsohn J, Howley PM, Israel MA, et al (eds): The Molecular Basis of Cancer, pp 401–431. Philadelphia, W.B. Saunders Co., 1995.
6. Hellman S: Principles of cancer management: radiation therapy. In: DeVita VT, Jr, Hellman S, Rosenberg SA (eds): Cancer, Principles & Practice of Oncology, 5th ed. pp 307–332. Philadelphia, Lippincott-Raven, 1997.

Specific References

7. Chapman JD, Dugle DL, Reuvers AP, et al: Studies on the radiosensitizing effect of oxygen in Chinese hamster cells. Int J Radiat Biol Rel Stud Phys Chem Med 1974; 26:383–389.
8. Kellerer AM, Rossi HH: The theory of dual radiation action. Curr Topics Radiat Res Q 1972; 8:85–158.
9. Tubiana M, Dutreix J, Wambersie A: Introduction to Radiobiology. London, Taylor & Francis, 1990.
10. Paretzke HG, Turner JE, Hamm RN, et al: Spatial distributions of inelastic events produced by electrons in gaseous and liquid water. Radiat Res 1991; 127:121–129.
11. Goodhead DT, Nikjoo H: Track structure analysis of ultrasoft x-rays compared to high- and low-LET radiations. Int J Radiat Biol 1989; 55:513–529.
12. Blakely EA, Kronenberg A: Heavy-ion radiobiology: new ap-

proaches to delineate mechanisms underlying enhanced biological effectiveness. Radiat Res 1998; 150 (suppl):S126–S145.
13. Barendsen GW: Variation of RBE with LET for survival of mammalian cells of human origin. Current Topics in Radiation Research Quarterly 1968; 4:293–356.
14. Stone HB, Dewey WC, Wallace SS, et al: Molecular biology to radiation oncology: a model for translational research? Opportunities in basic and translational research. Radiat Res 1998; 150:134–147.
15. Debierne MA: Recherches sur les gaz produits par les substances radioactives. Decomposition de l'eau. Annales de Physique 1914; 2:97–127.
16. Wourtzel E: Les actions chimiques du rayonnement α. Le Radium 1919; 11:19–22.
17. Fricke H: The reduction of oxygen to hydrogen peroxide by the irradiation of its aqueous solution with x-rays. Journal of Chemical Physics 1934; 2:556–559.
18. Wallace SS: Enzymatic processing of radiation-induced free radical damage in DNA. Radiat Res 1998; 150 (suppl):S60–S79.
19. Belloni J: Contribution of radiation chemistry to the study of metal clusters. Radiat Res 1998; 150 (suppl):S9–S20.
20. Whitmore GF: One hundred years of x-rays in biological research. Radiat Res 1995; 144:148–159.
21. Munro TR: The relative radiosensitivity of the nucleus and the cytoplasm of the Chinese hamster fibroblast. Radiat Res 1970; 42:451–470.
22. Coleman CN: Beneficial liaisons: radiobiology meets cellular and molecular biology. Radiother Oncol 1993; 28:1–15.
23. Fuciarelli AF, Zimbrick JD: Radiation Damage in DNA. Structure/Function Relationships at Early Times. Columbus, Battelle Press, 1995.
24. Olive PL: The role of DNA single- and double-strand breaks in cell killing by ionizing radiation. Radiat Res 1998; 150 (suppl):S42–S51.
25. Nikjoo H, Uehara S, Wilson WE, et al: Track structure in radiation biology: theory and applications. Int J Radiat Biol 1998; 73:355–364.
26. Oleinick NL, Chiu S, Ramakrishan N, et al: The formation, identification, and significance of DNA-protein cross-links in mammalian cells. Br J Cancer 1987; 55 (suppl):135–140.
27. Dizdaroglu M: Chemical determination of free radical–induced damage to DNA. Free Radic Biol Med 1991; 10:225–242.
28. Ward JF: Some biochemical consequences of the spatial distribution of ionizing radiation-produced free radicals. Radiat Res 1981; 86:185–195.
29. Little JB: Challenging the standard paradigms for radiation carcinogenesis. Proceedings of the Eleventh International Congress of Radiation Research, Dublin, Ireland, July 18–23, 1999 (Abstract); 4.
30. Ward JF: Non-targeted effects and DNA models. Proceedings of the Eleventh International Congress of Radiation Research; Dublin, Ireland, July 18–23, 1999 (Abstract); 7.
31. Azzam EI, de Toledo SM, Gooding T, et al: Intercellular communication is involved in the bystander regulation of gene expression in human cells exposed to very low fluences of alpha particles. Radiat Res 1998; 150:497–504.
32. Wheeler KT, Wierowski JV: DNA repair kinetics in irradiated undifferentiated and terminally differentiated cells. Radiat Environ Biophys 1983; 22:3–19.
33. vanAnkeren SC, Murray D, Meyn RE: Induction and rejoining of gamma-ray–induced DNA single- and double-strand breaks in Chinese hamster AA8 cells and in two radiosensitive clones. Radiat Res 1988; 116:511–525.
34. Olive PL, Banath JP: Induction and rejoining of radiation-induced DNA single-strand breaks: "tail moment" as a function of position in the cell cycle. Mutat Res 1993; 294:275–283.
35. Olive PL: DNA precipitation assay: a rapid and simple method for detecting DNA damage in mammalian cells. Environ Mol Mutagen 1988; 11:487–495.
36. Dikomey E, Franzke J: Three classes of DNA strand breaks induced by X-irradiation and internal beta-rays. Int J Radiat Biol Rel Stud Phys Chem Med 1986; 50:893–908.
37. Bryant PE, Warring R, Ahnstrom G: DNA repair kinetics after low doses of x-rays. A comparison of results obtained by the unwinding and nucleoid sedimentation methods. Mutat Res 1984; 131:19–26.
38. Taylor YC, Duncan PG, Zhang X, et al: Differences in the DNA supercoiling response of irradiated cell lines from ataxia-telangiectasia versus unaffected individuals. Int J Radiat Biol 1991; 59:359–371.
39. Blöcher D, Pohlit W: DNA double strand breaks in Ehrlich ascites tumour cells at low doses of x-rays. II. Can cell death be attributed to double strand breaks? Int J Radiat Biol Rel Stud Phys Chem Med 1982; 42:329–338.
40. Wlodek D, Olive PL: Chromatin structure influence on DNA damage measurements by four assays: Pulsed- and constant-field gel electrophoresis, DNA precipitation and non-denaturing filter elutriation. Nukleonika 1996; 41:23–34.
41. Stamato T, Guerriero S, Denko N: Two methods for assaying DNA double-strand break repair in mammalian cells by asymmetric field inversion gel electrophoresis. Radiat Res 1993; 133:60–66.
42. Nunez MI, Villalobos M, Olea N, et al: Radiation-induced DNA double-strand break rejoining in human tumour cells. Br J Cancer 1995; 71:311–316.
43. Olive PL, MacPhail SH, Banath JP: Lack of correlation between DNA double-strand break induction/rejoining and radiosensitivity in six human tumor cell lines. Cancer Res 1994; 54:3939–3946.
44. Kaur BS, Blazek ER: Subdenaturing (pH 11.1) filter elution: more sensitive quantification of DNA double-strand breaks. Radiat Res 1997; 147:569–578.
45. Johnston PJ, MacPhail SH, Banath JP, et al: Higher-order chromatin structure-dependent repair of DNA double-strand breaks: factors affecting elution of DNA from nucleoids. Radiat Res 1998; 149:533–542.
46. McGrath RA, Williams RW: Reconstruction *in vivo* of irradiated *Escherichia coli* deoxyribonucleic acid: the rejoining of broken pieces. Nature 1966; 212:534–535.
47. Dikomey E, Franzke J: DNA repair kinetics after exposure to X-irradiation and to internal beta-rays in CHO cells. Radiat Environ Biophys 1986; 25:189–194.
48. Mattern MR, Hariharan PV, Cerutti PA: Selective excision of gamma-ray damaged thymidine from the DNA of cultured mammalian cells. Biochim Biophys Acta 1975; 395:48–55.
49. Jeggo PA: Identification of genes involved in repair of DNA double-strand breaks in mammalian cells. Radiat Res 1998; 150 (suppl):S80–S91.
50. Elkind MM, Whitmore G: The Radiobiology of Cultured Mammalian Cells. New York, Gordon & Breach Publishers, 1967.
51. Metler FA, Moseley RD: Medical Effects of Ionizing Radiation. Orlando, Grune & Stratton, 1985.
52. Elkind MM, Sutton H: Radiation response of mammalian cells grown in culture. Part 1. Repair of x-ray damage in surviving Chinese hamster cells. Radiat Res 1960; 13:556–593.
53. Weichselbaum RR, Beckett M: The maximum recovery potential of human tumor cells may predict clinical outcome in radiotherapy. Int J Radiat Oncol Biol Phys 1987; 13:709–713.
54. Rajewsky MF, Engelbergs J, Thomale J, et al: Relevance of DNA repair to carcinogenesis and cancer therapy. Recent Results Cancer Res 1998; 154:127–146.
55. Mu D, Tursun M, Duckett DR, et al: Recognition and repair of compound DNA lesions (base damage and mismatch) by human mismatch repair and excision repair systems. Mol Cell Biol 1997; 17:760–769.
56. Nehme A, Baskaran R, Nebel S, et al: Induction of JNK and c-Abl signalling by cisplatin and oxaliplatin in mismatch repair-proficient and -deficient cells. Br J Cancer 1999; 79:1104–1110.
57. Naegeli H: Roadblocks and detours during DNA replication: mechanisms of mutagenesis in mammalian cells. Bioessays 1994; 16:557–564.
58. Singer B, Hang B: What structural features determine repair enzyme specificity and mechanism in chemically modified DNA? Chem Res Toxicol 1997; 10:713–732.
59. Zhao X, Mu D: (6-4) photolyase: light-dependent repair of DNA damage. Histol Histopathol 1998; 13:1179–1182.
60. Yasui A, McCready SJ: Alternative repair pathways for UV-induced DNA damage. Bioessays 1998; 20:291–297.
61. Von Sonntag V: The Chemical Basis of Radiation Biology. London, Taylor & Francis, 1987.
62. Kuwabara M: Chemical processes induced by OH attack on nucleic acids. Radiation Physics and Chemistry 1991; 37:690–704.
63. Breen AP, Murphy JA: Reactions of oxyl radicals with DNA. Free Radical Biol Med 1995; 18:1033–1077.
64. Wallace SS: Oxidative damage to DNA and its repair. In: Scandalios JG (ed): Oxidative Stress and the Molecular Biology of Antioxidant Defenses, pp 49–90. Cold Spring Harbor, Cold Spring Harbor Laboratory Press, 1997.

65. Wilson DM, III, Engelward BP, Samson L: Prokaryotic base excision repair. In: Nickoloff JA, Hoekstra MF (eds): DNA Damage and Repair, vol 1. DNA Repair in Prokaryotes and Lower Eukaryotes, pp 29–64. Totowa, Humana Press, 1998.
66. Ward JF: Biochemistry of DNA lesions. Radiat Res 1985; 104 (suppl):S103–S111.
67. Ward JF: DNA damage produced by ionizing radiation in mammalian cells: identities, mechanisms of formation and reparability. Prog Nucleic Acid Res Mol Biol 1988; 35:95–125.
68. Ahnstrom G, Bryant PE: DNA double-strand breaks generated by repair of x-ray damage in Chinese hamster cells. Int J Radiat Biol Rel Stud Phys Chem Med 1982; 41:671–676.
69. Ventur Y, Schulte-Frohlinde D: Does the enzymatic conversion of DNA single-strand damage into double-strand breaks contribute to biological inactivation of γ-irradiated plasmid DNA? Int J Radiat Biol 1993; 63:167–171.
70. Goodhead DT: Initial events in the cellular effects of ionizing radiations: clustered damage in DNA. Int J Radiat Biol 1994; 65:7–17.
71. Weeda G, de Boer J, Donker I, et al. Molecular basis of DNA repair mechanisms and syndromes. Recent Results Cancer Res 1998; 154:147–155.
72. Gunz D, Hess MT, Naegeli H: Recognition of DNA adducts by human nucleotide excision repair. Evidence for a thermodynamic probing mechanism. J Biol Chem 1996; 271:25089–25098.
73. Shinohara A, Ogawa T: Homologous recombination and the roles of double-strand breaks. Trends Biochem Sci 1995; 20:387–391.
74. Shinohara A, Shinohara M, Ohta T, et al: Rad52 forms ring structures and co-operates with RPA in single-strand DNA annealing. Genes Cells 1998; 3:145–156.
75. Ogawa T, Shinohara A, Ikeya T: A species-specific interaction of rad51 and rad52 proteins in eukaryotes. Adv Biophys 1995; 31:93–100.
76. Thacker J: The role of homologous recombination processes in the repair of severe forms of DNA damage in mammalian cells. Biochimie 1999; 81:77–85.
77. Rathmell WK, Chu G: Involvement of the Ku autoantigen in the cellular response to DNA double-strand breaks. Proc Natl Acad Sci USA 1994; 91:7623–7627.
78. Getts RC, Stamato TD: Absence of a Ku-like DNA end binding activity in the xrs double-strand DNA repair-deficient mutant. J Biol Chem 1994; 269:15981–15984.
79. Rathmell WK, Chu G: A DNA end-binding factor involved in double-strand break repair and V(D)J recombination. Mol Cell Biol 1994; 14:4741–4748.
80. Peterson SR, Kurimasa A, Oshimura M, et al: Loss of the catalytic subunit of the DNA-dependent protein kinase in DNA double-strand-break-repair mutant mammalian cells. Proc Natl Acad Sci USA 1995; 92:3171–3174.
81. Kirchgessner CU, Patil CK, Evans JW, et al: DNA-dependent kinase (p350) as a candidate gene for the murine SCID defect. Science 1995; 267:1178–1183.
82. Lees-Miller SP, Godbout R, Chan DW, et al: Absence of p350 subunit of DNA-activated protein kinase from a radiosensitive human cell line. Science 1995; 267:1183–1185.
83. Pandita TK, Hittelman WN: The contribution of DNA and chromosome repair deficiencies to the radiosensitivity of ataxia-telangiectasia. Radiat Res 1992; 131:214–223.
84. Hallahan DE, Dunphy E, Kuchibhotla J, et al: Prolonged c-jun expression in irradiated ataxia telangiectasia fibroblasts. Int J Radiat Oncol Biol Phys 1996; 36:355–360.
85. Paterson MC, Smith PJ, Bech-Hansen NT, et al: Gamma ray hypersensitivity and faulty DNA repair in cultured cells from humans exhibiting familial cancer proneness. In: Okada S, Imamura M, Terashima T, et al. (eds): Proceedings of the Sixth International Congress of Radiation Research, Japan, May 1979, pp 484–495. Tokyo, Toppan Printing Co., 1979.
86. Kelland LR, Edwards SM, Steel GG: Induction and rejoining of DNA double-strand breaks in human cervix carcinoma cell lines of differing radiosensitivity. Radiat Res 1988; 116:526–538.
87. Schwartz JL, Rotmensch J, Giovanazzi S, et al: Faster repair of DNA double-strand breaks in radioresistant human tumor cells. Int J Radiat Oncol Biol Phys 1988; 15:907–912.
88. Wlodek D, Hittelman WN: The relationship of DNA and chromosome damage to survival of synchronized X-irradiated L5178Y cells. II. Repair. Radiat Res 1988; 115:566–575.
89. Biedermann KA, Sun JR, Giaccia AJ, et al: scid mutation in mice confers hypersensitivity to ionizing radiation and a deficiency in DNA double-strand break repair. Proc Natl Acad Sci USA 1991; 88:1394–1397.
90. Hendrickson EA, Qin XQ, Bump EA, et al: A link between double-strand break related repair and V(D)J recombination: the scid mutation. Proc Natl Acad Sci USA 1991; 88:4061–4065.
91. Nevaldine B, Longo JA, Hahn PJ: The scid defect results in much slower repair of DNA double-strand breaks but not high levels of residual breaks. Radiat Res 1997; 147:535–540.
92. Lohrer HD: Regulation of the cell cycle following DNA damage in normal and ataxia telangiectasia cells. Experientia 1996; 52:316–328.
93. Szumiel I: Monitoring and signaling of radiation-induced damage in mammalian cells. Radiat Res 1998; 150:S92–S101.
94. Jeggo PA, Taccioli GE, Jackson SP: Ménagè trois: Double strand break repair, V(D)J recombination and DNA-PK. Bioessays 1995; 17:949–957.
95. Kiehntopf M, Esquivel EL, Brach MA, et al: Clinical applications of ribozymes. Lancet 1995; 345:1027–1031.
96. Maity A, Kao GD, Muschel RJ, et al: Potential molecular targets for manipulating the radiation response. Int J Radiat Oncol Biol Phys 1997; 37:639–653.
97. Keng PC: Use of flow cytometry in the measurement of cell mitotic cycle. International Journal of Cell Cloning 1986; 4:295–311.
98. Keng PC, Siemann DW, Wheeler KT: Comparison of tumour age response to radiation for cells derived from tissue culture or solid tumours. Br J Cancer 1984; 50:519–526.
99. Masunaga S, Keng PC: Effect of caffeine on gamma-ray induced G_2 arrest in well-synchronized Chinese hamster ovary cells in vitro. Radiat Med 1996; 14:309–313.
100. Terasima T, Tolmach LJ: Changes in the x-ray sensitivity of HeLa cells during the division cycle. Nature 1961; 190:1210–1211.
101. Keng PC, Wheeler KT: Radiation response of synchronized 9L rat brain tumor cells separated by centrifugal elutriation. Radiat Res 1980; 83:633–643.
102. Freyer JP, Jarrett K, Carpenter S, et al: Oxygen enhancement ratio as a function of dose and cell cycle phase for radiation-resistant and sensitive CHO cells. Radiat Res 1991; 127:297–307.
103. Elkind MM: Cell-cycle sensitivity, recovery from radiation damage and a new paradigm for risk assessment. Int J Radiat Biol 1997; 71:657–665.
104. Norbury C, Nurse P: Animal cell cycles and their control. Annual Review of Biochemistry 1992; 61:441–470.
105. Elledge SJ: Cell cycle checkpoints: preventing an identity crisis. Science 1996; 274:1664–1672.
106. Morgan DO: Principles of CDK regulation. Nature 1995; 374:131–134.
107. Sherr CJ: Cancer cell cycles. Science 1996; 274:1672–1677.
108. Pines J, Hunter T: p34cdc2: the S and M kinase? New Biologist 1990; 2:389–401.
109. Lock RB, Ross WE: Inhibition of p34cdc2 kinase activity by etoposide or irradiation as a mechanism of G2 arrest in Chinese hamster ovary cells. Cancer Res 1990; 50:3761–3766.
110. Muschel RJ, Zhang HB, Iliakis G, et al: Cyclin B expression in HeLa cells during the G2 block induced by ionizing radiation. Cancer Res 1991; 51:5113–5117.
111. Muschel RJ, Zhang HB, McKenna WG: Differential effect of ionizing radiation on the expression of cyclin A and cyclin B in HeLa cells. Cancer Res 1993; 53:1128–1135.
112. Kastan MB, Onyekwere O, Sidransky D, et al: Participation of p53 protein in the cellular response to DNA damage. Cancer Res 1991; 51:6304–6311.
113. Dutreix J, Wambersie A, Bounik C: Cellular recovery in human skin reactions: application to dose fraction number overall time relationship in radiotherapy. Eur J Cancer 1973; 9:159–167.
114. Nicotera P, Leist M, Ferrando-May E: Intracellular ATP, a switch in the decision between apoptosis and necrosis. Toxicol Lett 1998; 102–103:139–142.
115. McConkey DJ: Biochemical determinants of apoptosis and necrosis. Toxicol Lett 1998; 99:157–168.
116. Farber JL: Biology of disease: membrane injury and calcium homeostasis in the pathogenesis of coagulative necrosis. Lab Invest 1982; 47:114–123.
117. Zucker RM, Hunter S, Rogers JM: Confocal laser scanning micros-

copy of apoptosis in organogenesis-stage mouse embryos. Cytometry 1998; 33:348–354.
118. Araki T, Saruta T, Okano H, et al: Caspase activity is required for nephrogenesis in the developing mouse metanephros. Exp Cell Res 1999; 248:423–429.
119. Pender MP: Activation-induced apoptosis of autoreactive and alloreactive T lymphocytes in the target organ as a major mechanism of tolerance. Immunol Cell Biol 1999; 77:216–223.
120. Genestier L, Bonnefoy-Berard N, Revillard JP: Apoptosis of activated peripheral T cells. Transplant Proc 1999; 31:33S–38S.
121. Fawthrop DJ, Boobis AR, Davies DS: Mechanisms of cell death. Arch Toxicol 1991; 65:437–444.
122. Renvoize C, Biola A, Pallardy M, et al: Apoptosis: identification of dying cells. Cell Biol Toxicol 1998; 14:111–120.
123. Walker PR, Leblanc J, Smith B, et al: Detection of DNA fragmentation and endonucleases in apoptosis. Methods 1999; 17:329–338.
124. Whiteside TL: Immune cells in the tumor microenvironment. Mechanisms responsible for functional and signaling defects. Adv Exp Med Biol 1998; 451:167–171.
125. Gorczyca W, Bedner E, Burfeind P, et al: Analysis of apoptosis in solid tumors by laser-scanning cytometry. Mod Pathol 1998; 11:1052–1058.
126. Weil M, Jacobson MD, Coles HS, et al: Constitutive expression of the machinery for programmed cell death. J Cell Biol 1996; 133:1053–1059.
127. Allan DJ: Radiation-induced apoptosis: its role in a MADCaT (mitosis-apoptosis-differentiation-calcium toxicity) scheme of cytotoxicity mechanisms. Int J Radiat Biol 1992; 62:145–152.
128. Harmon BV, Allan DJ: Apoptosis. Adv Genet 1997; 35:35–56.
129. Billis W, Fuks Z, Kolesnick R: Signaling in and regulation of ionizing radiation-induced apoptosis in endothelial cells. Recent Prog Horm Res 1998; 53:85–92.
130. Wright EG: Radiation-induced genomic instability in haemopoietic cells. Int J Radiat Biol 1998; 74:681–687.
131. Hart SP, Haslett C, Dransfield I: Recognition of apoptotic cells by phagocytes. Experientia 1996; 52:950–956.
132. Ren Y, Savill J: Apoptosis: the importance of being eaten. Cell Death & Differentiation 1998; 5:563–568.
133. Wang TH, Wang HS: p53, apoptosis and human cancers. J Formos Med Assoc 1996; 95:509–522.
134. Wiman KG: New p53-based anti-cancer therapeutic strategies. Med Oncol 1998; 15:222–228.
135. Haimovitz-Friedman A: Radiation-induced signal transduction and stress response. Radiat Res 1998; 150:S102–S108.
136. Haimovitz-Friedman A, Kan CC, Ehleiter D, et al: Ionizing radiation acts on cellular membranes to generate ceramide and initiate apoptosis. J Exp Med 1994; 180:525–535.
137. Kolesnick RN, Haimovitz-Friedman A, Fuks Z: The sphingomyelin signal transduction pathway mediates apoptosis for tumor necrosis factor, Fas, and ionizing radiation. Biochem Cell Biol 1994; 72:471–474.
138. Bettaieb A, Record M, Come MG, et al: Opposite effects of tumor necrosis factor alpha on the sphingomyelin-ceramide pathway in two myeloid leukemia cell lines: role of transverse sphingomyelin distribution in the plasma membrane. Blood 1996; 88:1465–1472.
139. Foghi A, Ravandi A, Teerds KJ, et al: Fas-induced apoptosis in rat thecal/interstitial cells signals through sphingomyelin-ceramide pathway. Endocrinology 1998; 139:2041–2047.
140. Chmura SJ, Nodzenski E, Crane MA, et al: Cross-talk between ceramide and PKC activity in the control of apoptosis in WEHI-231. Adv Exp Med Biol 1996; 406:39–55.
141. Gomez-Munoz A: Modulation of cell signalling by ceramides. Biochim Biophys Acta 1998; 1391:92–109.
142. Sharma K, Shi Y: The yins and yangs of ceramide. Cell Res 1999; 9:1–10.
143. Verheij M, Bose R, Lin XH, et al: Requirement for ceramide-initiated SAPK/JNK signalling in stress-induced apoptosis. Nature 1996; 380:75–79.
144. Cano E, Mahadevan LC: Parallel signal processing among mammalian MAPKs. Trends Biochem Sci 1995; 20:117–122.
145. Schlesinger TK, Fanger GR, Yujiri T, et al: The TAO of MEKK. Front Biosci 1998; 3:Dl181–Dl186.
146. Yujiri T, Sather S, Fanger GR, et al: Role of MEKK1 in cell survival and activation of JNK and ERK pathways defined by targeted gene disruption. Science 1998; 282:1911–1914.
147. Gupta K, Kshirsagar S, Li W, et al: VEGF prevents apoptosis of human microvascular endothelial cells via opposing effects on MAPK/ERK and SAPK/JNK signaling. Exp Cell Res 1999; 247:495–504.
148. Liao W-C, Fuks Z, Persaud R, et al: Radiation-induced DNA damage initiates late-phase apoptosis via activation of ceramide synthase. Proceedings of the 89th Annual Meeting of the American Association of Cancer Research, New Orleans, Louisiana, March 28–April 1, 1998 (Abstract); 30:531.
149. Radford IR: Initiation of ionizing radiation-induced apoptosis: DNA damage-mediated or does ceramide have a role? Int J Radiat Biol 1999; 75:521–528.
150. Hannun YA, Obeid LM: Mechanisms of ceramide-mediated apoptosis. Adv Exp Med Biol 1997; 407:145–149.
151. Fuks Z, Haimovitz-Friedman A, Kolesnick RN: The role of the sphingomyelin pathway and protein kinase C in radiation-induced cell kill. Important Adv Oncol 1995; 19–31.
152. Chmura SJ, Nodzenski E, Weichselbaum RR, et al: Protein kinase C inhibition induces apoptosis and ceramide production through activation of a neutral sphingomyelinase. Cancer Res 1996; 56:2711–2714.
153. Gardner AM, Johnson GL: Fibroblast growth factor-2 suppression of tumor necrosis factor alpha-mediated apoptosis requires Ras and the activation of mitogen-activated protein kinase. J Biol Chem 1996; 271:14560–14566.
154. Stadheim TA, Kucera GL: Extracellular signal-regulated kinase (ERK) activity is required for TPA-mediated inhibition of drug-induced apoptosis. Biochem Biophys Res Commun 1998; 245:266–271.
155. Skaletz-Rorowski A, Waltenberger J, Muller JG, et al: Protein kinase C mediates basic fibroblast growth factor-induced proliferation through mitogen-activated protein kinase in coronary smooth muscle cells. Arterioscler Thromb Vasc Biol 1999; 19:1608–1614.
156. Withers HR: Response of tissues to multiple small dose fractions. Radiat Res 1977; 71:24–33.
157. Wheldon TE, Michalowski AS, Kirk J: The effect of irradiation on function in self-renewing normal tissues with differing proliferative organisation. Br J Radiol 1982; 55:759–766.
158. Michalowski AS: Post-irradiation modification of normal-tissue injury: lessons from the clinic. Br J Radiol 1992; 24 (Suppl):183–186.
159. Withers HR, Thames HD Jr, Peters LJ: Biological bases for high RBE values for late effects of neutron irradiation. Int J Radiat Oncol Biol Phys 1982; 8:2071–2076.
160. Ang KK, Thames HD, Peters LJ: Altered fractionation schedules. In: Perez CA, Brady LW (eds): Principles and Practice of Radiation Oncology, 3rd ed. pp 119–142. Philadelphia, Lippincott-Raven, 1997.
161. Stuschke M, Thames HD: Hyperfractionated radiotherapy of human tumors: overview of the randomized clinical trials. Int J Radiat Oncol Biol Phys 1997; 37:259–267.
162. Nguyen TD, Panis X, Froissart D, et al: Analysis of late complications after rapid hyperfractionated radiotherapy in advanced head and neck cancers. Int J Radiat Oncol Biol Phys 1988; 14:23–25.
163. Ball D, Bishop J, Smith J, et al: A phase III study of accelerated radiotherapy with and without carboplatin in nonsmall cell lung cancer: an interim toxicity analysis of the first 100 patients. Int J Radiat Oncol Biol Phys 1995; 31:267–272.
164. Nguyen LN, Komaki R, Allen P, et al: Effectiveness of accelerated radiotherapy for patients with inoperable non–small cell lung cancer (NSCLC) and borderline prognostic factors without distant metastasis: a retrospective review. Int J Radiat Oncol Biol Phys 1999; 44:1053–1056.
165. King SC, Acker JC, Kussin PS, et al: High-dose, hyperfractionated, accelerated radiotherapy using a concurrent boost for the treatment of nonsmall cell lung cancer: unusual toxicity and promising early results. Int J Radiat Oncol Biol Phys 1996; 36:593–599.
166. Saunders MI: Fractionation and dose in thoracic radiotherapy. Lung Cancer 1994; 10 (Suppl 1):S245–S252.
167. Saunders MI, Dische S, Barrett A, et al: Randomised multicentre trials of CHART vs conventional radiotherapy in head and neck and non-small-cell lung cancer: an interim report. CHART Steering Committee. Br J Cancer 1996; 73:1455–1462.
168. Powell ME, Hoskin PJ, Saunders MI, et al: Continuous hyperfractionated accelerated radiotherapy (CHART) in localized cancer of the esophagus. Int J Radiat Oncol Biol Phys 1997; 38:133–136.

169. Goodchild K, Hoskin P, Dische S, et al: A feasibility study of continuous hyperfractionated accelerated radiotherapy (CHART) and brachytherapy in patients with early oral or oropharyngeal carcinomas. Radiother Oncol 1999; 50:29–31.
170. Symonds RP: Treatment-induced mucositis: an old problem with new remedies. Br J Cancer 1998; 77:1689–1695.
171. Turesson I, Notter G: Accelerated versus conventional fractionation. The degree of incomplete repair in human skin with a four-hour-fraction interval studied after postmastectomy irradiation. Acta Oncol 1988; 27:169–179.
172. Nyman J, Turesson I: Does the interval between fractions matter in the range of 4–8 h in radiotherapy? A study of acute and late human skin reactions. Radiother Oncol 1995; 34:171–178.
173. Sause WT, Scott C, Krisch R, et al: Phase I/II trial of accelerated fractionation in brain metastases RTOG 85-28. Int J Radiat Oncol Biol Phys 1993; 26:653–657.
174. Fu KK, Clery M, Ang KK, et al: Randomized phase I/II trial of two variants of accelerated fractionated radiotherapy regimens for advanced head and neck cancer: results of RTOG 88-09. Int J Radiat Oncol Biol Phys 1995; 32:589–597.
175. Coleman CN: Chemical sensitizers and protectors. Int J Radiat Oncol Biol Phys 1998; 42:781–783.
176. Read J: The effect of ionizing radiations on the broad bean root: I. The dependence of the alpha ray sensitivity on dissolved oxygen. Br J Radiol 1952; 25:651–661.
177. Read J: The effect of ionizing irradiations on the broad bean root: X. The dependence on the x-ray sensitivity of dissolved oxygen. Br J Radiol 1952; 26:89–99.
178. Gray LH, Conger AD, Ebert M, et al: The concentration of oxygen dissolved in tissues at the time of irradiation as a factor in radiotherapy. Br J Radiol 1953; 26:628–654.
179. Palcic B, Skarsgard LD: Reduced oxygen enhancement ratio at low doses of ionizing radiation. Radiat Res 1984; 100:328–339.
180. Thomlinson RH, Gray LH: The histological structure of some human lung cancers and the possible implications for radiotherapy. Br J Cancer 1955; 9:539–549.
181. Brown JM: Evidence for acutely hypoxic cells in mouse tumours, and a possible mechanism of reoxygenation. Br J Radiol 1979; 52:650–656.
182. Chaplin DJ, Olive PL, Durand RE: Intermittent blood flow in a murine tumor: radiobiological effects. Cancer Res 1987; 47:597–601.
183. Tannock IF: The relation between cell proliferation and the vascular system in a transplanted mouse mammary tumour. Br J Cancer 1968; 22:258–273.
184. Siemann DW: The tumor microenvironment: a double-edged sword. Int J Radiat Oncol Biol Phys 1998; 42:697–699.
185. Graeber TG, Osmanian C, Jacks T, et al: Hypoxia-mediated selection of cells with diminished apoptotic potential in solid tumours. Nature 1996; 379:88–91.
186. Green SL, Giaccia AJ: Tumor hypoxia and the cell cycle: implications for malignant progression and response to therapy. Cancer J Sci Am 1998; 4:218–223.
187. Sutherland RM: Tumor hypoxia and gene expression—implications for malignant progression and therapy. Acta Oncol 1998; 37:567–574.
188. Taylor YC, Brown JM: Radiosensitization in multifraction schedules. II. Greater sensitization by 2-nitroimidazoles than by oxygen. Radiat Res 1987; 112:134–145.
189. Stratford IJ, Hickson ID, Robson CN, et al: Radiosensitizing and cytotoxic effects of nitroimidazoles in CHO cells expressing elevated levels of glutathione-S-transferase. Int J Radiat Oncol Biol Phys 1989; 16:1307–1310.
190. Lee DJ, Pajak TF, Stetz J, et al: A phase I/II study of the hypoxic cell sensitizer misonidazole as an adjunct to high fractional dose radiotherapy in patients with unresectable squamous cell carcinoma of the head and neck: a RTOG randomized study (79-04). Int J Radiat Oncol Biol Phys 1989; 16:465–470.
191. Rauth AM, Melo T, Misra V: Bioreductive therapies: an overview of drugs and their mechanisms of action. Int J Radiat Oncol Biol Phys 1998; 42:755–762.
192. Sutherland RM: Selective chemotherapy of noncycling cells in an *in vitro* tumor model. Cancer Res 1974; 34:3501–3503.
193. Hall EJ, Roizin-Towle L: Hypoxic sensitizers: radiobiological studies at the cellular level. Radiology 1975; 117:453–457.
194. Brown JM: The potential benefit of hypoxic cytotoxins in radio-oncology. In: Molls M, Vaupel P (eds): Medical Radiology: Blood Perfusion and Microenvironment of Human Tumors, pp 219–229. Heidelberg, Springer-Verlag, 1998.
195. Brown JM, Giaccia AJ: Tumour hypoxia: the picture has changed in the 1990s. Int J Radiat Biol 1994; 65:95–102.
196. Rubin P, Johnston CJ, Williams JP, et al: A perpetual cascade of cytokines postirradiation leads to pulmonary fibrosis. Int J Radiat Oncol Biol Phys 1995; 33:99–109.
197. Ainsworth EJ, Chase HB: Effect of microbial antigens on irradiation mortality in mice. Proc Soc Exp Biol Med 1959; 102:483–490.
198. Cavaillon JM, Haeffner-Cavaillon N: Signals involved in interleukin 1 synthesis and release by lipopolysaccharide-stimulated monocytes/macrophages. Cytokine 1990; 2:313–329.
199. Trinchieri G: Regulation of tumor necrosis factor production by monocyte-macrophages and lymphocytes. Immunol Res 1991; 10:89–103.
200. DeFranco AL, Hambleton J, McMahon M, et al: Examination of the role of MAP kinase in the response of macrophages to lipopolysaccharide. Prog Clin Biol Res 1995; 392:407–420.
201. Neta R, Oppenheim JJ, Schreiber RD, et al: Role of cytokines (interleukin 1, tumor necrosis factor, and transforming growth factor beta) in natural and lipopolysaccharide-enhanced radioresistance. J Exp Med 1991; 173:1177–1182.
202. Neta R, Oppenheim JJ, Douches SD: Interdependence of the radioprotective effects of human recombinant interleukin 1 alpha, tumor necrosis factor alpha, granulocyte colony-stimulating factor, and murine recombinant granulocyte-macrophage colony-stimulating factor. J Immunol 1988; 140:108–111.
203. Neta R: Modulation of radiation damage by cytokines. Stem Cells 1997; 15 (Suppl 2):87–94.
204. Neta R, Oppenheim JJ: Radioprotection with cytokines—learning from nature to cope with radiation damage. Cancer Cells 1991; 3:391–396.
205. Hallahan DE, Spriggs DR, Beckett MA, et al: Increased tumor necrosis factor alpha mRNA after cellular exposure to ionizing radiation. Proc Natl Acad Sci USA 1989; 86:10104–10107.
206. Hallahan DE, Virudachalam S, Sherman ML, et al: Tumor necrosis factor gene expression is mediated by protein kinase C following activation by ionizing radiation. Cancer Res 1991; 51:4565–4569.
207. Jeremias I, Debatin KM: TRAIL induces apoptosis and activation of NFkappaB. Eur Cytokine Netw 1998; 9:687–688.
208. Abe Y, Watanabe Y, Kimura S: The role of tumor necrosis factor receptors in cell signaling and the significance of soluble form levels in the serum. Surg Today 1994; 24:197–202.
209. Holler E, Ertl B, Hintermeier-Knabe R, et al: Inflammatory reactions induced by pretransplant conditioning—an alternative target for modulation of acute GvHD and complications following allogeneic bone marrow transplantation? Leuk Lymph 1997; 25:217–224.
210. Anscher MS, Peters WP, Reisenbichler H, et al: Transforming growth factor-β as a predictor of liver and lung fibrosis after autologous bone marrow transplantation for advanced breast cancer. N Engl J Med 1993; 328:1592–1598.
211. Anscher MS, Kong FM, Jirtle RL: The relevance of transforming growth factor beta 1 in pulmonary injury after radiation therapy. Lung Cancer 1998; 19:109–120.
212. Cassady JR, Carabell SC, Jaffe N: Chemotherapy-irradiation related hepatic dysfunction in patients with Wilms' tumor. In: Vaeth JM (ed): Combined Effects of Chemotherapy and Radiotherapy on Normal Tissue Tolerance, pp 147–160. Basel, Karger, 1979.
213. Johnson FL, Balis FM: Hepatopathy following irradiation and chemotherapy for Wilms' tumor. American Journal of Pediatric Hematology-Oncology 1982; 4:217–221.
214. Hancock SL, Donaldson SS, Hoppe RT: Cardiac disease following treatment of Hodgkin's disease in children and adolescents. J Clin Oncol 1993; 11:1208–1215.
215. Moni J, Nori D: The pitfalls and complications of radiation therapy for esophageal carcinoma. Chest Surg Clin N Am 1997; 7:565–584.
216. de Graaf H, Dolsma WV, Willemse PH, et al: Cardiotoxicity from intensive chemotherapy combined with radiotherapy in breast cancer. Br J Cancer 1997; 76:943–945.
217. Mieli-Vergani G: Hepatic complications after bone marrow transplantation. Bone Marrow Transplant 1993; 12 (Suppl 1):96–97.
218. Cohen EP, Lawton CA, Moulder JE: Bone marrow transplant nephropathy: radiation nephritis revisited. Nephron 1995; 70:217–222.

219. Tabbara IA: Allogeneic bone marrow transplantation: acute and late complications. Anticancer Res 1996; 16:1019–1026.
220. United Nations Scientific Committee on the Effects of Atomic Radiation: UNSCEAR 1994: Report to the General Assembly, Annex E. Epidemiological Studies of Radiation Carcinogenesis. New York, United Nations, 1994.
221. Little JB: Radiation-induced genomic instability. Int J Radiat Biol 1998; 74:663–671.
222. Selvanayagam CS, Davis CM, Cornforth MN, et al: Latent expression of p53 mutations and radiation-induced mammary cancer. Cancer Res 1995; 55:3310–3317.
223. Lengauer C, Kinzler KW, Vogelstein B: Genetic instabilities in human cancers. Nature 1998; 396:643–649.
224. Ullrich RL, Ponnaiya B: Radiation-induced instability and its relation to radiation carcinogenesis. Int J Radiat Biol 1998; 74:747–754.
225. Kinzler KW, Vogelstein B: Life (and death) in a malignant tumour. Nature 1996; 379:19–20.
226. Mendonca MS, Temples TM, Farrington DL, et al: Evidence for a role of delayed death and genomic instability in radiation-induced neoplastic transformation of human hybrid cells. Int J Radiat Biol 1998; 74:755–764.
227. Matsukage A, Hirose F, Yamaguchi M: Transcriptional regulation of DNA replication-related genes in cell growth, differentiation and oncogenesis. Jpn J Cancer Res 1994; 85:1–8.
228. Hoffman B, Liebermann DA: Molecular controls of apoptosis: differentiation/growth arrest primary response genes, proto-oncogenes, and tumor suppressor genes as positive and negative modulators. Oncogene 1994; 9:1807–1812.
229. Rosen N: Oncogenes. In: Mendelsohn J, Howley PM, Israel MA, et al (eds): The Molecular Basis of Cancer, pp 105–116. Philadelphia, W.B. Saunders Co., 1995.
230. Namba M, Mihara K, Fushimi K: Immortalization of human cells and its mechanisms. Crit Rev Oncog 1996; 7:19–31.
231. Buzard GS: Studies of oncogene activation and tumor suppressor gene inactivation in normal and neoplastic rodent tissue. Mutat Res 1996; 365:43–58.
232. Arbelaez AM, Bernal C, Patarca R: Acute retroviruses and oncogenesis. Crit Rev Oncog 1999; 10:17–81.
233. Harris H, Miller OJ, Klein G, et al: Suppression of malignancy by cell fusion. Nature 1969; 223:363–368.
234. Committee on the Biological Effects of Ionizing Radiation: Health Effects of Exposure to Low Levels of Ionizing Radiation: BEIR V. Washington, National Academy Press, 1990.
235. International Commission on Radiological Protection: Recommendations. Annals of the ICRP Publication 60. Oxford, Pergamon Press, 1990.
236. National Council on Radiation Protection and Measurements: Exposure of the Population in the United States and Canada from Natural Background Radiation. NCRP No 94. Bethesda, National Council on Radiation Protection and Measurements, 1987.

6 Principles of Radiation Oncology and Cancer Radiotherapy

PHILIP RUBIN, MD, Radiation Oncology
JACQUELINE P. WILLIAMS, PhD, Radiation Oncology

The most efficient route to improvement in the response of cancer patients to radiotherapy is through understanding basic biological, radiological and physiological principles and then designing new therapies based on that knowledge.

STONE AND COLLEAGUES[10]

Perspective

The most exciting and challenging change in the radiation oncology discipline has been the introduction of molecular biology concepts that may be applicable to developing innovations in oncologic practice. These can be expressed by the cellular and molecular model proposed by Coleman and Harris (Fig. 6–1),[9] illustrating the many factors and pathways that are genetically controlled or affected by radiation, offering new potential targets for therapeutic intervention. Early and late-responding genes, growth factors, cytokines and their receptors, signal transduction, apoptosis, and stress response genes may all be exploited to improve therapeutic outcomes and reduce late-effect toxicity in normal tissues. In addition, molecular measurements of DNA damage and repair, single- and double-strand breaks, chromosomal aberrations, and alterations in cell cycle checkpoint regulation following radiation that lead to changes in cellular radiation resistance may also be useful both in terms of predictive assays and developing new radiation modifiers. Translational radiation research is needed to develop new clinical trials based on biologic models, using molecular biologic approaches to understand clinical observations; this approach should be viewed as a translational research bridge with a bidirectional flow of information: from the laboratory to the clinic and from the clinic back to the laboratory.

The ideal outcome for using radiation therapy in the treatment of malignant disease is achieved when a tumor is completely eradicated and the surrounding normal tissues show minimal evidence of structural or functional injury. This ideal has been described as the *selective effect* of irradiation. Although the ideal selective effect is being obtained more frequently in the majority of instances in clinical practice, one accepts a certain degree of permanent residual damage as a sequela to the destruction of a lethal tumor. The acceptable extent of an alteration in normal structures varies in different settings, but the integrity of vital tissues always must be maintained. The ability to eradicate a tumor without undue complication or destruction of normal tissues is the essential factor in tumor radiocurability and is referred to as the therapeutic ratio. Therefore, it is necessary to either (1) destroy the tumor cells more readily than vital normal tissues in the treatment field for the same dose absorbed or (2) focus the radiation beam so that a differential dose between the tumor volume and the normal surrounding tissue is achieved. Such improvements in therapy will result from research advances in molecular and cell biology in the former circumstance and radiation physics in the latter. It is our immediate purpose to elaborate on this concept and to develop its clinical implications, because one of the major frontiers of radiation research is to make radiation more selective and thus approach the ideal situation.[9, 10]

The cure of cancer, with preservation of structure, function, and esthetics, has become more evident with advances in modern radiation oncology, based on technologic gains in radiation physics and insights into radiation biology and pathophysiology. According to Wilson,[11] more than 37% of all U.S. cancer patients may be treated for cure with organ preservation using irradiation. Using present American Cancer Society statistics,[12] this translates to a favorable outcome for more than 502,000 U.S. cancer patients and pertains to more than 2 million people when applied globally (Table 6–1).[11]

Pediatric tumors[13] were among the first to be ablated without sacrifice of limbs and soft tissues, followed by patients with Hodgkin's disease,[14] which among the lymphomas, yielded to extended–radiation-field techniques, eliminating the use of radical neck node dissections. Improvements in effective screening and an increased awareness of the need for routine self-examination for breast cancer have allowed for improved long-term survival and

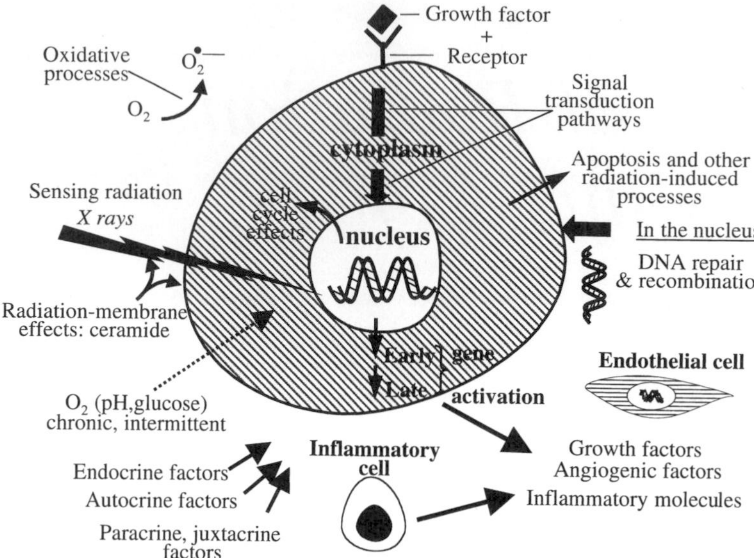

Figure 6–1. Potential radiation biologic targets for translational research. For each of the pathways, detailed molecular and cellular knowledge is continuously becoming available that explains cellular phenotype and provides novel therapeutic targets. (Modified from Coleman CN, Harris JR: Current scientific issues related to clinical radiation oncology. Radiat Res 1998; 150:125.)

conservation of structure and cosmesis in the majority of cases. Potency is maintained in both early and relatively advanced prostate cancer through radiation treatment, unlike in radical prostatectomy. With early detection techniques, gynecologic malignancies, such as cancer of the cervix[15, 16] and uterus,[17, 18] are highly curable, whereas head and neck cancers involving the larynx and other upper aerodigestive sites treated by radiation therapy allow for preservation of voice and swallowing.[19–21] With the continued improvements in imaging using computed tomography and magnetic resonance imaging, and the increasing accuracy of three-dimensional conformal treatment, tumors of the eye and selected brain tumors can be eliminated with preservation of vision and minimal neurologic impairment. Anal preservation also has been achieved in anal cancer patients by supplanting abdominoperineal surgery with combination chemoradiotherapy. Preoperative irradiation in rectal cancer allows lower-lying lesions to be removed, again with anal sphincter preservation.

TABLE 6–1. **Cancer Sites Amenable to Conservation Surgery and Radiation Therapy**

Site (Type)	No. of Patients
Major	
Breast	108,720
Eye—choroid (melanoma)	1,700
Prostate	39,600
Vocal cord	9,760
Other	
Head and neck	
Esophagus	
Bladder	
Cervix	
Uterus	
Central nervous system	
Soft-tissue (sarcomas)	
Retina (retinoblastoma)	
Anus	
Other	223,320
Total	383,100

From Wilson JF: Syllabus: A categorical course in radiation therapy: cure with preservation of function and aesthetics, p 5. Oak Brook, IL, Radiological Society of North America, 1998, with permission.

Molecular and Cellular Biology Aspects of Radiation Oncology

With the introduction of a large variety of new molecular experimental techniques, molecular radiation oncology is being actively explored in the laboratory, accompanied by the introduction of novel clinical approaches and new therapeutic strategies (Table 6–2).[22] These new techniques include DNA excision and splicing using restriction endonucleases; performing Southern, Northern, and Western blotting for DNA, RNA, and protein identification respectively; the creation of vectors for inserting foreign passenger DNA; the increasing use of genomic libraries of expressed genes; DNA amplification by polymerase chain reactions; fluorescence *in situ* hybridization for chromosomal location of genes and analysis of promoter regions; and RNA protection assays for identifying cytokine ladders. Some of the genes and pathways that are currently targets for therapeutic modification are listed below:

- *Early response genes*, such as *FOS*, *JUN*, and *MYC*, have mRNA levels that are dramatically induced following irradiation, mitogenic stimuli, and stress.[23–25]
- *Apoptosis* is a genetically controlled response by which eukaryotic cells undergo programmed cell death. The process can be identified by double-strand breaks that occur between nucleosomal sites, producing fragments in multiples of approximately 185 base pairs.[26, 27] These fragments will form so-called ladders in gels, thus differentiating this process from necrosis, which produces a diffuse smear of DNA. Cell proliferation and cell loss through apoptosis and extracellular matrix production are mediated by growth factors via regulation of cell cycle checkpoints[28]; however, cytocidal doses of radiation, as well as a large number of antineoplastic agents, have been shown to induce apoptosis.[29] Coordination of the cell cycle process is through the activity of a family of intracellular en-

TABLE 6–2. **Application of Molecular Biologic Concepts to Radiation Therapy**

Process	Potential Manipulation	Examples of Therapy*
DNA damage	Increase damage in tumor cells	Hypoxic-cell sensitizers, thymidine analogues
DNA repair	Decrease repair in tumor cells	Fluoropyrimidines, hydroxyurea, cisplatin
Signal transduction	Inhibit protective signaling cascades in tumor cells	Protein kinase C inhibitors (?), phosphotyrosine kinase inhibitors (?)
Radiation-induced gene expression	Use gene therapy	Tumor necrosis factor linked to radiation-responsive promotor (?)
Growth factor expression	Administer or increase expression of protective factors	Interleukin-1, granulocyte colony-stimulating factor, granulocyte-macrophage colony-stimulating factor, basic fibroblast growth factor (?)
	Block expression of factors producing long-term toxicity	Antibodies or antisense RNA against epidermal growth factor, transforming growth factor β (?)
Apoptosis	Force tumor cells to undergo apoptosis	Transfection of wild-type *TP53* (?)
Cell cycle	Synchronize tumor cells in sensitive phase of cycle (early S or M phase)	Antimetabolites (early S phase), paclitaxel phase (M), cyclin inhibitors (G_1 to S phase)
	Prevent G_2 arrest in tumor cells	Cyclin inhibitors (G_2 to M phase) (?)

*A question mark indicates potential therapy.

From Lichter AS, Lawrence TS: Recent advances in radiation oncology. N Engl J Med 1995; 332:371, with permission.

zymes, the cyclin-dependent kinases; these act through cyclins as specialized regulators of the cell cycle. In addition, the proto-oncogene *BCL* family plays a central role in both inhibiting and promoting apoptosis; the proto-oncogenes *BAK*, *BAD*, and *BAX* are all inducers and promoters.[30–33] Apoptosis is now being widely studied in the hopes that its modulation will improve the efficacy of anticancer treatment.[27, 34, 35]

- *Oncogenes* have been identified as genes capable of causing cancer that act in a dominant fashion, that is, a single copy can produce a malignant transformation. About 50 to 100 oncogenes have been identified; for example, activated *RAS*, which is present in 10% to 15% of human cancers, tends to be higher in leukemias and lower in solid tumors. Transfection of oncogenes into cells may confer radioresistance. Current evidence also suggests that molecular pathways that are involved in carcinogenesis also determine intrinsic cellular radiosensitivity,[36] and that oncogene expression could serve as a marker for predicting tumor response to therapy. Oncogenes also may serve as potential targets for improving radiation therapy.[37]
- *Suppressor genes* are recessive, and loss of both copies leads to a malignant phenotype. Retinoblastoma was the first human tumor associated with loss of a suppressor gene. The most common suppressor gene mutation is in *TP53*; the expression of wild-type p53 in a *TP53*-mutated tumor cell *in vitro* leads to cell cycle arrest, slower cell proliferation, and occasionally to apoptosis.[38, 39] *In vivo* introduction of wild-type *TP53* into human tumors has been achieved through viral vectors, and such gene therapy insertions into xenograft mouse models have demonstrated significant increases in tumor radiation sensitivity.[40, 41] However, loss of *TP53* function has been shown in only 50% of human cancer cases, and p53 loss has been associated with both enhanced and decreased chemosensitivity.[42, 43] Nonetheless, as a result of its involvement in apoptosis and cell cycle arrest, the *TP53* mutation is being pursued by a number of groups.[44–47] Although numerous human studies have been reported, the results are inconsistent and unconvincing.[48, 49] Although extrapolation of animal data to humans should be viewed with caution, clinical trials with *TP53* gene therapy are ongoing and appear to be well tolerated.
- *Progression through cell cycle* occurs through checkpoints, regulated by protein kinases in association with cyclins (Fig. 6–2). *TP53* is considered the guardian of the genome and mediates responses to DNA damaging agents, such as ionizing radiation at the G_1 checkpoint. For instance, radiation-induced G_1/S arrest is mediated by *TP53* through p21 transcriptional activation, which inhibits cyclin-dependent kinase activity; Dulic and associates[50] have shown that *TP53* tumor suppressor gene products increase after γ-irradiation and may be critical for G_1 checkpoint arrest. In addition, *TP53* has been implicated in having a secondary role in controlling G_2M checkpoint arrest.[10, 51, 52]
- *Growth factors or cytokines* are nonhormonal polypeptides that act through autocrine and paracrine (and possibly endocrine) mechanisms related to growth, differentiation, development, and maintenance of normal tissues. Irradiation leads to a perpetual, dysregulated cytokine cascade; this results in acute and late effects through the concurrent release of proinflammatory and profibrotic cytokines and chemokines.[53]
- Gene therapy[54] is increasingly possible through, for example, the use of radiation-induced genes paired with cytotoxic or protective agents, tumor suppressor genes,[38, 55] or the use of suicide genes, which involve infection with a viral vector containing thymidine kinase gene, followed by treatment with an antiviral agent such as ganciclovir.[56–58]

Radiocurability of Tumors

Therapeutic Ratio

There is a sigmoidal relationship between radiation dose and the probability of control of a homogeneous group of tumors; that is, with increasing radiation doses, more and

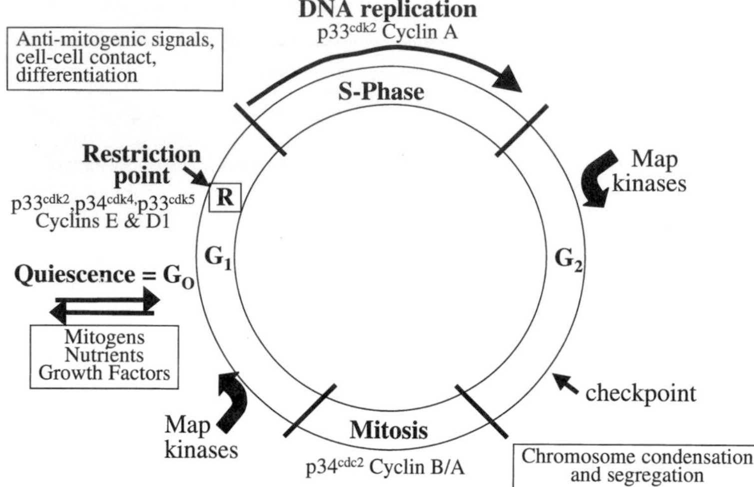

Figure 6–2. Cell cycle progression, with the major regulatory kinases indicated. Once a cell passes the restriction point (R), it is committed to progress through S-phase, even in the absence of mitogenic signals. Checkpoints (indicated in G_2) have also been identified in G_1, S, and mitosis.

more neoplastic cells are killed, until ultimately all clonogenic cells are destroyed and a cure is achieved. The same principle of radiation killing, however, also applies to normal cells and tissues, and so the probability of normal tissue complications and tumor cure are similar.[7, 59, 60] Because there are approximately 300 varieties of human tumors and 50 different normal organs and tissues, each with different cell types, the overlap in the tolerance dose of normal tissues and the tumor dose for ablation is inevitable. It is this relationship between normal tissue tolerance and the tumor lethal dose that determines the therapeutic ratio (Fig. 6–3).[11]

The therapeutic ratio is favorable (i.e., the tumor can be destroyed without excessive normal tissue complication) when the tumor cure curve is to the left of the normal tissue dose-effect curve (Fig. 6–4A). When the two curves are identical (Fig. 6–4B), the therapeutic ratio is less favorable, but may be improved by precise radiation physics treatment planning. This is increasingly true with the advent of three-dimensional conformal treatment planning and modern megavoltage or brachytherapy techniques, so that greater dose is delivered to the tumor than to the normal surrounding tissue. Finally, if the tumor ablation curve is to the right of the vital normal tissue (Fig. 6–4C), the circumstance is most unfavorable. To reverse this situation, innovations and combined-modality approaches are essential to a good outcome.

Tumor Control Dose in Clinical Setting

A dose may be chosen for each type of tumor that will cause destruction of a high proportion of cells and lead, in turn, to local cure. The prescribed dose for different human tumors is not a fixed dose but varies with tumor size and extent, tumor type, pathologic grade and differentiation, and its response to irradiation. The tumor lethal dose may be defined as the dose that has a 95% probability of achieving tumor control (cure)—the TCD_{95}. Practical guides for tumor radiocurability have been developed. Table 6–3 illustrates the TCD_{95} for different tumor types, and Table 6–4 shows tumor control probability correlated with radiation dose and volume of cancer.[61]

According to the cell survival theory, tumor size is a critical factor in tumor cure by radiation therapy. Using the tumor, node, metastases (TNM) designation, T0 and N0 refer to occult stage or microscopic foci (millimeters), which are pathologically positive but clinically negative. Localized lesions are T1 and T2, usually less than 4 cm in diameter, and T3 and T4 are extensive tumors, usually greater than 4 cm.

1. *Highly radiocurable tumors (TCD_{95} range 35 to 60 Gy)*, such as seminomas, lymphosarcomas, Hodgkin's disease, neuroblastomas, Wilms' tumors, histiocytic cell sarcomas, medulloblastomas, retinoblastomas, dysgerminomas, and Ewing's sarcomas are treated in this dose range, as are occult cancers—either squamous cell or adenocarcinomas—suspected or residuum after surgery. T1 cancers of the larynx and skin are readily controlled completely. Metastatic lymph nodes with microdeposits are also treated within these dose levels. These doses are well tolerated by normal tissues and complications are minimal.
2. *Radiocurable tumors (TCD_{95} range 60 to 75 Gy)* are those requiring the risk of exceeding normal tissue tolerance to assure a high degree of curability. These are moderate to large tumors (T2 and T3) of the oral cavity, pharynx, bladder, cervix, uterus, ovary, and lung.

   Some of the best data available have resulted from thousands of well-documented and well-followed squamous cell cancers in the head and neck region at M.D. Anderson Hospital. Fletcher and colleagues[61] made careful analyses and built an excellent series of dose-response relationships relating to cancers at different sites in the nasopharynx, oral cavity, oropharynx, hypopharynx, superglottis, and larynx (see Table 6–4). Complications are usually modest.
3. *The least radiocurable tumors (TCD_{95} range 80 Gy and above)* are those large-to-massive squamous cell and adenocarcinomas (T3 and T4) that are less consistently cured by irradiation alone and in which the 95% tumor cure level is not reached. The lack of tumor control by irradiation may result from a number of factors, such as shifts in cell cycle kinetics, poor oxygenation, shifts from proliferative to nonproliferative compartments, or inherent radioresistance. Normal tissue tolerance is often exceeded and compli-

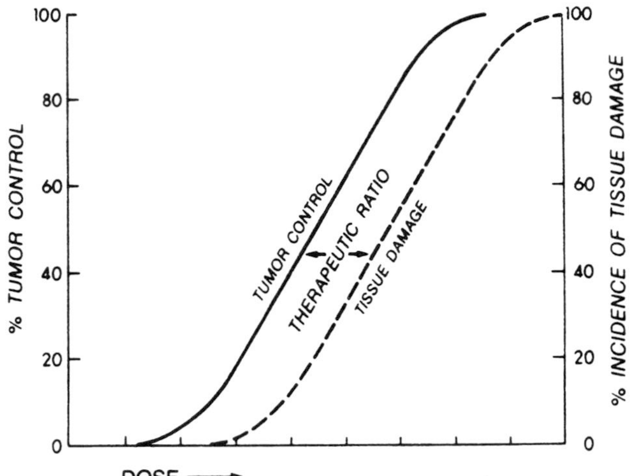

Figure 6–3. Therapeutic ratio. The response curves of both tumor cure and normal tissue complication are sigmoidal. The differential in dose to achieve these effects is the therapeutic ratio.

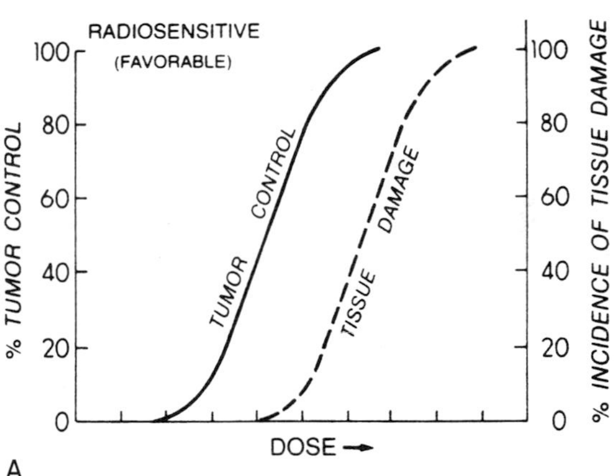

Figure 6–4. Different therapeutic ratios exist in different clinical circumstances depending on the relative radiosensitivities (dose-response curves) of tumor versus the critical normal tissue in the treatment field. These figures show (A) a favorable ratio, (B) a less favorable ratio, and (C) an unfavorable ratio.

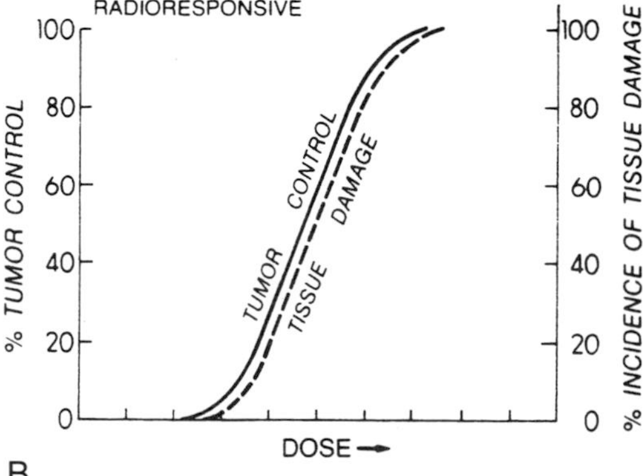

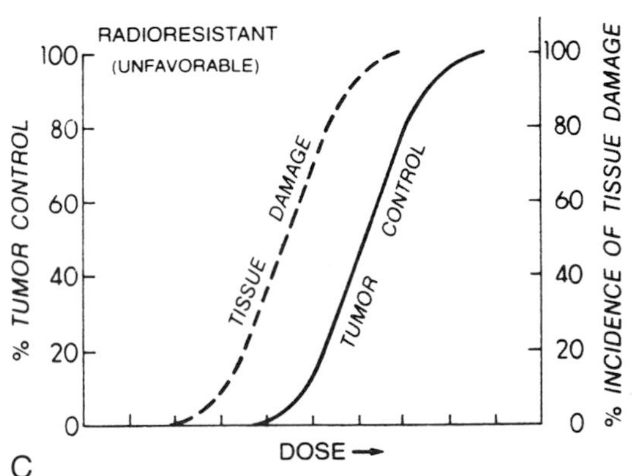

TABLE 6–3. **Curative Doses of Radiation for Different Tumor Types**

20–30 Gy
Seminoma
Acute lymphocytic leukemia (CNS)

30–40 Gy
Seminoma
Wilms' tumor
Neuroblastoma

40–50 Gy
Hodgkin's disease
Lymphosarcoma
Histiocytic cell sarcoma
Skin cancer (basal and squamous)

50–60 Gy
Lymph nodes, microscopic foci
Squamous cell carcinoma, cervix cancer, and head and neck cancer
Embryonal cancer
Breast cancer, ovarian cancer
Medulloblastoma
Retinoblastoma
Ewing's tumor
Dysgerminoma

60–65 Gy
Larynx (<1 cm)
Breast cancer, lumpectomy

70–75 Gy
Oral cavity (<2 cm, 2–4 cm)
Oro-nasal-laryngo-pharyngeal cancer
Bladder cancer
Cervix cancer
Uterine fundal cancer
Ovarian cancer
Lymph nodes, metastatic (1–3 cm)
Lung cancer (<3 cm)
Prostate cancer

80 Gy or above*
Head and neck cancer (>4 cm)
Breast cancer (>5 cm)
Glioblastoma (glioma)
Osteogenic sarcoma (bone sarcoma)
Melanoma
Soft tissue sarcoma (>5 cm)
Thyroid cancer
Lymph nodes, metastatic (>6 cm)
Prostate cancer

*External radiation often combined with brachytherapy to attain dose level.

cations are part of the cost of cure. If interstitial and intracavitary irradiation is applicable in addition to external irradiation, these doses are achievable in some sites within tolerance levels. Tumors arising from mature tissues, such as neural, renal, and osseous tissues, frequently give rise to radioresistant neoplasms such as glioblastoma multiforme, hypernephroma, and osteogenic sarcomas, respectively.[62] However, this can now be considered a simplistic viewpoint with the increase in understanding of the molecular mechanisms underlying inherent or acquired resistance to therapy modes.[63–65]

Various Aims of Radiation Oncology

Curative. The patient must be in good physical condition, and general supportive measures of hygiene, nutrition, and blood profiles need to be maintained. Radical irradiation is as effective as radical surgery in many of the cancers that have been mentioned; however, it should be recognized that both modalities can be debilitating and can carry a certain morbidity.[66] Overall, the patient will tolerate the course of radiation therapy, and most of the untoward acute reactions will clear up within a few weeks after treatment cessation. Some late effects, such as fibrosis and cellular depletion, may become evident years after treatment, but severe morbid or lethal complications are usually minimal.

Palliative. Palliation often requires curative levels of radiation therapy, although lower doses are also used. Palliative doses must be applied judiciously and may cause some untoward reaction. The aims of palliation are to

- allow for a symptom-free period appreciably longer than the debilitation caused by the irradiation treatment period
- prolong useful or comfortable survival, increase quality and quantity of life
- relieve distressing symptoms (e.g., hemorrhage, pain, and obstruction), though survival may not be prolonged
- avert impending symptoms such as hemorrhage, obstruction, and perforation
- ensure that therapy is not debilitating in itself and does not lead to worse complications than those caused by the neoplastic process itself

TABLE 6–4. **Tumor Control Probability* Correlated to Radiation Dose and Volume of Cancer**

	Squamous Cell Carcinoma of the Upper Respiratory and Digestive Tracts	Adenocarcinoma of the Breast
50 Gy†	>90% subclinical 60% T1 lesions of nasopharynx 50% 1–3 cm neck nodes	>90% subclinical
60 Gy†	90% T1 lesions of pharynx and larynx 50% T3+T4 lesions of tonsillar fossa	
70 Gy†	90% 1–3 cm neck nodes 70% 3–5 cm neck nodes 90% T2 lesions of tonsillar fossa and supraglottic larynx 80% T3+T4 lesions of tonsillar fossa	90% clinically positive Axillary nodes
70–80 Gy primary	⟶	65% 2–3 cm
(8–9 weeks) primary		30% >5 cm
80–90 Gy primary **(8–10 weeks)**	⟶	56% >5 cm
80–100 Gy primary **(10–12 weeks)**	⟶	75% 5–15 cm

*The control rate is corrected for the percentage of nodes that would be positive histologically had a dissection of the axilla been performed.
†10 Gy in five fractions per week.
Adapted from Fletcher GH: Textbook of Radiotherapy. Philadelphia, Lea & Febiger, 1980.

Tumor Radiosensitivity and Radioresistance: Concepts and Criteria

In describing the radiobiologic basis for radiation oncology, two basic concepts are used in most of the scientific data presented in this chapter.[63, 67] They are the dose-response or dose-effect curve and the clonogenic cell survival fraction.

1. The dose-response or dose-effect curve characterizes the relationship between the radiation dose and the tumor response or tissue effect, such as tumor control or normal tissue damage, and is plotted on a linear scale. This type of graph refers to the radiation response of *in vivo* systems (Fig. 6–5).
2. The clonogenic cell survival fraction represents the proportion of cells surviving irradiation based on measurements made on cells in tissue culture (*in vitro*). The data are displayed on a semilog plot (Fig. 6–6).[5] However, it must be noted that *in vitro* radiosensitivity of cells derived from tumors does not necessarily predict for local control[68] and that radiocurability is complex as a result of the interactions of inherent radiobiologic parameters.

The R's of Radiobiology

The ability of radiation therapy to cure tumors is well established.[5, 59, 69, 70] As the radiation dose increases, more cells are destroyed and, depending on the radiosensitivity of the tumor cells, a cumulative dose can be achieved to completely eradicate the tumor. The resultant dose-response or dose-effect curves in most biologic systems irradiated are sigmoidal. The sigmoidal quality indicates that the dose-response curves are steep and that a small difference in dose (10% to 20%) can determine whether few to all clonogenic cells will be ablated. A family of hypothetical dose-response curves, indicating a range of radiation sensitivities, is illustrated in Figure 6–5.

Different normal tissues and organs in the body have different tolerance doses, depending on whether an early or late effect is studied. From this, it follows that many tumors arising from radiosensitive tissues are themselves radiosensitive, and those arising from radioresistant tissues are often radioresistant (Table 6–5).[7] Again, this is a highly generalized statement because the radiosensitivity of tumors can vary widely between individuals and is dependent on a large number of parameters, including cell cycle time, growth fraction, and tumor volume. Nonetheless, the testes and ovaries are exquisitely sensitive, as are the lymphoid and bone marrow systems. Tissues with predominantly proliferating cells are more sensitive than mature tissues that have slow or nondividing cells. Thus, in the adult, neurons, mature bone and cartilage, muscle, and endocrine cells—where they are no longer growing—are more radioresistant. By contrast, in infancy, when neural tissue is rapidly proliferating, it is highly vulnerable to irradiation, particularly *in utero* and the first years of life. The same is true of rapidly growing cartilage and bone, muscle, and endocrine glands in the infant and child.

Cellular radiosensitivity can be owed to a variety of factors, both intrinsic and extrinsic, and their interaction. In addition to the inherent radiation sensitivity, the overall tumor response to radiation therapy will also depend on variations in the capacity of tissues and cells to reoxygenate, reassort in the cell cycle, repair, repopulate, and be recruited from resting to proliferating compartments. These mechanisms and their effect on cellular radioresponsiveness are often referred to as the R's of radiobiology and each are briefly reviewed, beginning with intrinsic radiosensitivity.

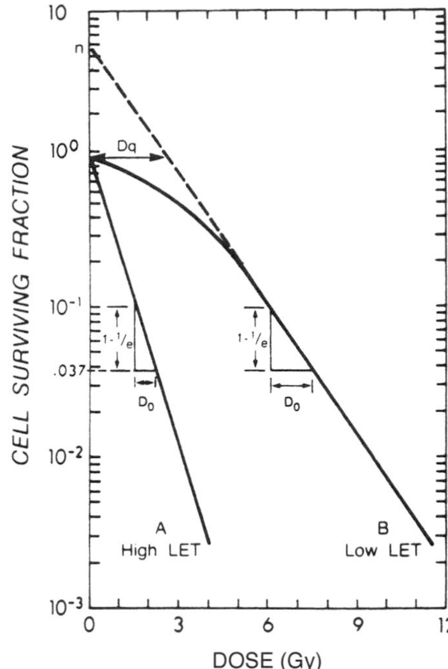

Figure 6–6. A clonogenic cell survival curve represents the fraction or proportion of cells surviving irradiation. On a semilog plot, after an initial shoulder, the curve bends sharply downward and radiation killing becomes more effective with each additional Gy absorbed. Cell survival curves are described by their shoulder (Dq) and slope (D_0) parameters. These cell survival parameters ultimately contribute to the width of the therapeutic ratio. LET = linear energy transfer. (From Hall EJ: Radiobiology for the Radiologist, 4th ed. Philadelphia, J.B. Lippincott Co., 1994, with permission.)

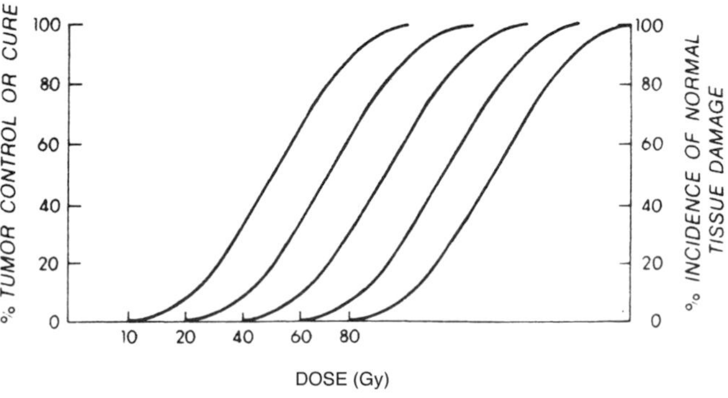

Figure 6–5. A sigmoidal dose-response curve characterizes the relationship between tumor control and normal tissue damage versus dose. As the radiation dose increases, a threshold is reached beyond which both tumor control and normal tissue injury increase. Several such curves are illustrated, reflecting the variation in radiation sensitivity of the hundreds of varieties of tumors and more than 50 different normal tissues and organs in the human.

TABLE 6–5. **Various Tumors and Tissues in Decreasing Order of Radiosensitivity**

Tumors	Relative Radiosensitivity	Tissues of Origin
Lymphoma, leukemia, seminoma, dysgerminoma	High	Lymphoid, hematopoietic (marrow), spermatogenic epithelium, and ovarian follicular epithelium
Squamous cell cancer of the oropharyngeal, glottis, bladder, skin, and cervical epithelia; adenocarcinoma of alimentary tract; breast	Fairly high	Oropharyngeal stratified epithelium, sebaceous gland epithelium, urinary bladder epithelium, optic lens epithelium, gastric gland epithelium, colon epithelium, and breast epithelium
Salivary gland tumor, hepatoma, renal cancer, pancreatic cancer, chondrosarcoma, and osteogenic sarcoma	Fairly low	Mature cartilage or bone tissue, salivary gland epithelium, renal epithelium, hepatic epithelium, chondrocytes, and osteocytes
Rhabdomyosarcoma, leiomyosarcoma, and ganglioneurofibrosarcoma	Low	Muscle tissue and neuronal tissue

Adapted from Rubin P, Casarett GW: Clinical Radiation Pathology. Philadelphia, W.B. Saunders, 1968.

Intrinsic Radiosensitivity and Cell Survival Theory

Figure 6–6[5] illustrates the characteristics of radiation survival curves of mammalian cells following treatment with low linear energy transfer (LET) (x-rays and γ-rays) and with high LET (neutrons) radiation. The survival curve, plotted on a semilog scale, displays the surviving fraction of cells as a function of dose.[71–73] Following an initial shoulder region, the radiation killing is essentially logarithmic or exponential. These survival curves can be described by their shoulder (D_q or n) and their slope (D_0). The radiosensitivity is referred to by the D_0, or the dose required to reduce the survival rate to 37% along the exponential portion of the curves. Irradiating cells with high LET radiation alters both the slope and shoulder of the survival curve.[74] For clinical purposes, the dose required to reduce the surviving fraction to 10% on the exponential portion of the curve, or to provide a log kill, is often a more convenient quantity and is referred to as the $D_{10} = 2.3\ D_0$.[59]

With the possibility of using an *in vitro* clonogenic assay for measuring cellular radiosensitivity of animal and human cell lines, various attempts at expressing radiosensitivity have been made.[75, 76] The range of D_0 values typically observed does not explain the variation in response of different human tumors, and it was realized that the shoulder region of the survival curve should be considered to have greater influence than the slope. Fertil and Malaise[77] suggested cell survival at a dose of 2 Gy to be a good measure of inherent radiosensitivity. They correlated the data from *in vitro* survival measurements at 2 Gy with the clinically estimated TCD_{90} values for different histologic types and found a correlation between the 2 Gy dose and the perceived clinical radioresponsiveness. Later, however, this and other groups proposed a discrepancy between results following doses higher than 1 Gy, suggesting a differential in repair response.[78, 79]

Reoxygenation: Oxygen Effect

The level of cell killing by low LET radiation is dependent on the degree of oxygenation at the time of irradiation.[5, 80, 81] This effect is directly related to the cellular oxygen tension, so that with increasing oxygen concentration, radiation sensitivity usually reaches a plateau at a partial pressure of oxygen of 20 to 30 mm Hg (Fig. 6–7A).[5] Further increases in oxygen concentration have little additional effect. Cell survival curves obtained under both oxic and completely hypoxic (absence of oxygen) conditions indicate that the dose required to produce the same biologic effect under hypoxic conditions is approximately 2.5 to 3 times greater than the dose required under fully oxygenated circumstances. Consequently, larger radiation doses would be necessary to eradicate a tumor containing hypoxic cells than one that did not.

Most animal tumors have a hypoxic cell component of 10% to 20%,[82, 83] and evidence has shown that hypoxic cells in at least some tumors constitute a major limiting factor in cure by conventional radiation therapy.[84–86] A diagram illustrating how the percentage of hypoxic cells in a tumor affects a single dose-survival curve for the tumor as a whole is shown in Figure 6–7B.[87, 88] The data show the survival of fully oxygenated cells as well as the survival of the same cells in the absence of oxygen. When oxygen-deficient cells are present in a tumor, the final slope of the cell survival curve is seen ultimately to parallel the slope of the fully hypoxic curve. Consequently, even if only 1.0% or 0.1% of the tumor cells are hypoxic, the relative radiation resistance of these cells will limit the curability of the tumor by single-dose radiation therapy.

Fortunately, tumors may reoxygenate during fractionated radiation treatments through a variety of mechanisms.[81, 89] For example, as a tumor shrinks, its parenchymal cells are lost and the vascular density increases, decreasing intercapillary distances, producing a supervascular state, and increasing oxygen diffusion. Reoxygenation can also occur when alternately oxygenated cells die and do not use oxygen, allowing the oxygen to diffuse further to persistent hypoxic cells in tumor cords. The additional complications of transient hypoxia[90] and varying levels of hypoxia[91] must also be considered when developing new therapeutic strategies.[92]

Reassortment: Cell Cycle Kinetics and Age Response Function

The patterns of radiosensitivity change through the cell cycle (Fig. 6–8).[5, 28, 93–95] This change is an age-response function and varies widely among different cell types. Cells in mitosis are almost always sensitive, followed by cells at

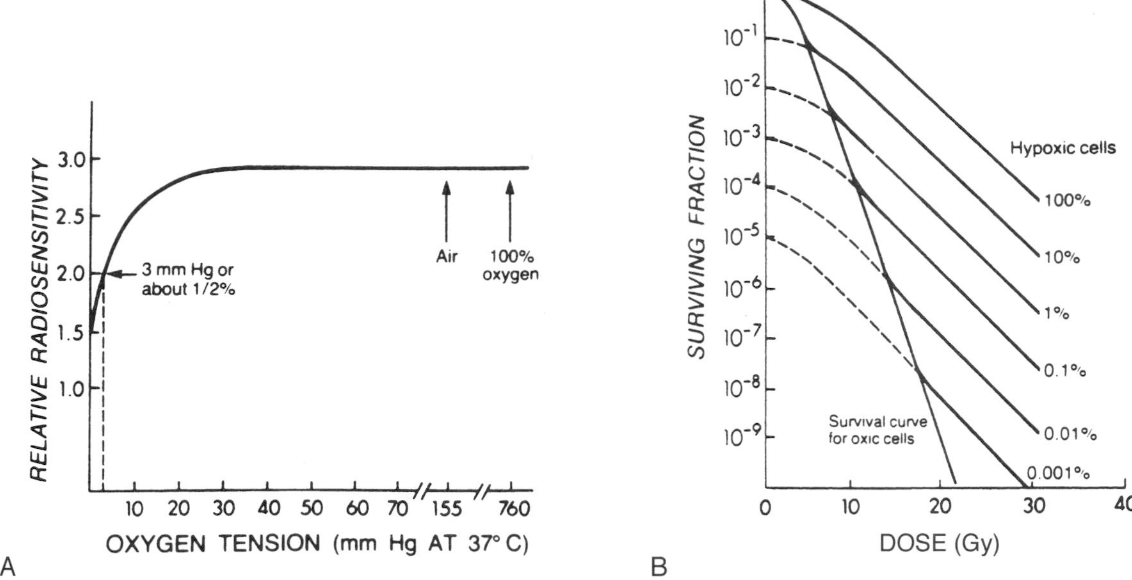

Figure 6–7. (A) Oxygen effect. The oxygen effect is illustrated as the curve relating relative radiation sensitivity to oxygen tension in tissues. As the oxygen increases, the relative radiosensitivity of cells increases by a factor of approximately 3 for the same dose. (From Hall EJ: Radiobiology for the Radiologist, 4th ed. Philadelphia, J.B. Lippincott Co., 1994, with permission.) (B) Survival curves illustrate the effect of various proportions of oxygen deficient or hypoxic cells on the resultant shape of the survival curve of mixed cell populations. Because of the resistant tail (shallow slope), even a small percentage of hypoxic cells (<1%) may determine whether irradiation can successfully eradicate a tumor. (Based on a model proposed by van Putten LM, Kallman RF: Oxygenation status of a transplantable tumor during fractionated radiation therapy. J Natl Cancer Inst 1968; 40:441. Modified from Hewitt HB, Wilson CW: The effect of tissue oxygen tension on the radiosensitivity of leukaemia cells irradiated *in situ* in the livers of leukaemic mice. Br J Cancer 1959; 13:675, with permission of Oxford University Press.)

the G_1/S boundary, whereas the period of greatest resistance usually is late S. However, in cells having a long G_1, a second resistant period in the early G_1 phase may also be seen. Reassortment occurs as cells in the sensitive cycle die and surviving radioresistant cells redistribute into more sensitive phases of cell cycle. Thus, it is conceivable that during fractionated radiation therapy, cells reassort and enter into radiosensitive phases. However, as a result of the long and varying cell cycle times, as well as small growth fractions, the impact of favorable cell reassortment on clinical radiation therapy is likely to be small.

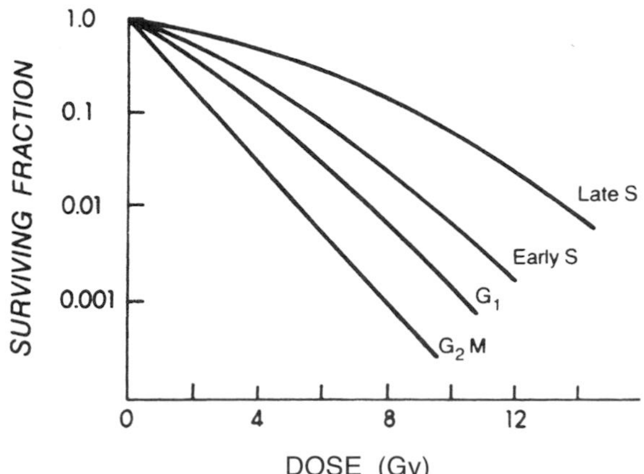

Figure 6–8. Patterns of radiosensitivity change through the cell cycle. This change is known as the "age function," and varies widely among different cell types. Cells in mitosis are almost always sensitive, followed by cells at the G_1/S boundary, whereas the period of greatest resistance is at late S. G = gaps; G_1 = first gap before DNA synthesis; G_2M = second gap before mitosis; S = DNA synthetic phase. (Adapted from Sinclair WK: Cyclic X-ray responses in mammalian cells in vitro. Radiat Res 1968; 33:620, with permission. Copyright © 1967 OPA (Overseas Publishers Association) N.V.)

Repair and the Fractionation Effect

The shoulder of the cell survival curve, the D_q (see Fig. 6–6),[5] represents the minimum number of targets in each cell that must be hit before the target is inactivated, thereby killing the cell. After irradiation, a cell may have received an ionizing event in some, but not all, of its critical sites, so that it has been damaged but not killed. Given time, the cell can repair the effects of this sublethal damage and completely recover from it. Consequently, if the time interval between successive doses is sufficiently long, each fractional dose will re-establish the shoulder on the survival curve, thus making divided daily doses less effective than a single dose. Figure 6–9 shows an idealized fractionation experiment from Elkind and Whitmore[96] using cultured cells *in vitro*. The survival curve for single acute exposures of x-rays is Curve A; whole Curve S is obtained if the total dose is given as a series of small fractions of the size D_1, with the time interval between fractions sufficient for repair of sublethal damage to take place. From this, it is evident that a much larger total dose of radiation is required to achieve the same degree of killing if it is given in a series of small fractions as compared with a single large exposure. To achieve a clinical advantage, it is important

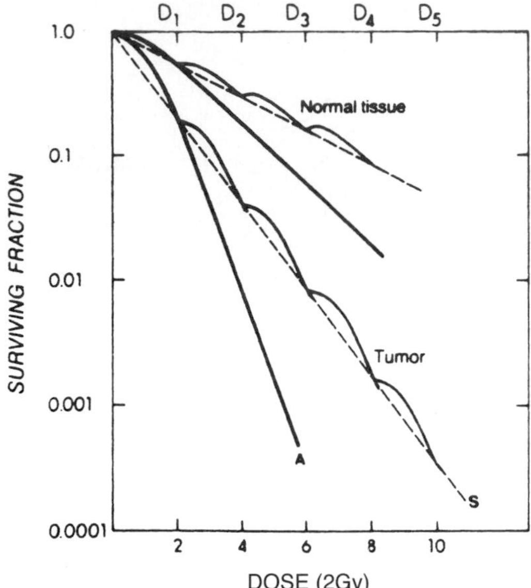

Figure 6–9. Cell repair and fractionation effect. Each repeated fractional dose allows for cell repair of sublethal damage and is expressed by the recapitulation of the shoulder of the survival curve. If 10 Gy is given as a divided fractional dose (D_1, D_2, D_3, D_4, D_5) of 2 Gy daily, it achieves a similar degree of cell kill (S on the dashed line) as 6 Gy given in one single exposure. The survival curve for single acute exposures of x-rays is curve A. This diagram also shows a differential effect on the therapeutic ratio between tumor cells and normal cells that increases with divided or fractional doses of radiation. This is displayed by the increasing differences in the slopes of the solid lines (single dose) versus the dashed lines (fractional dose). (Adapted from Elkind MM, Whitmore G: The Radiobiology of Cultured Mammalian Cells. New York, Gordon & Breach, 1967, with permission. Copyright © 1967 OPA [Overseas Publishers Association] N.V.)

that the D_0 and D_q of the tumor be smaller than that of the normal tissue in the treatment field.

In addition to sublethal repair,[97] another form of cell recovery, observed if cells are held under nonoptimal growth conditions, is referred to as potential lethal damage repair. The effect of potential lethal damage repair typically leads to a shallower slope on the cell survival curve. However, potential lethal damage repair has proved difficult to assess clinically and its role in radiotherapy remains to be determined.

Repopulation

Another possible means of obtaining a differential effect between normal tissues and tumors is seen if the cellular repopulation that occurs between fractionated doses is greater in the normal tissue at risk than in the tumor. This is illustrated schematically in Figure 6–10, in which there is regeneration or repopulation of the tissues between each fractional dose. If, as shown, the normal tissue could repopulate itself to a greater extent than the tumor, a differential effect is established between the tumor and the normal tissue with regard to cell kill per radiation dose. On the other hand, if the tumor repopulates more quickly, the reverse is true. The tumor repopulating more quickly occasionally occurs in highly anaplastic tumors with large growth fractions and short cell cycle times. Such a tumor

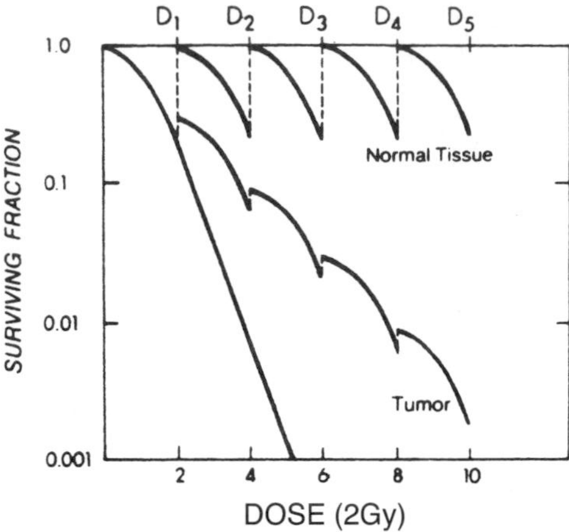

Figure 6–10. Repopulation. In a rapid renewal system, repopulation or regeneration of cells within the fractional interval occurs. This figure illustrates that even if the tumor and normal tissue have the same radiation response, the therapeutic ratio is improved through the more rapid regeneration of normal tissue versus tumor.

appears to be radioresistant because it appears to be unchanged, whereas in fact it is radioresponsive, but is repopulating between fractions. A hyperfractionation schedule is the therapeutic strategy developed to overcome this clinical happenstance.

Recruitment

Recruitment is a special circumstance and applies to the recruitment of nonproliferating G_0 cells into cell cycle (Fig. 6–11).[5] The assumption is that the majority of cells are more vulnerable to irradiation during mitosis or proliferation than if they are in the nonproliferating compartment. Generally speaking, proliferating cells tend to be more radiosensitive than G_0 cells, which in turn are more sensitive than mature cells. G_0 cells are often stem cells in tissues with a potential for proliferation, whereas mature cells usually, but not always, have lost the capacity to proliferate. As proliferating cells are ablated, cells are recruited from nonproliferating into proliferating compartments. If tumors behave thus, they become more radiosensitive and curable, producing a favorable therapeutic ratio.

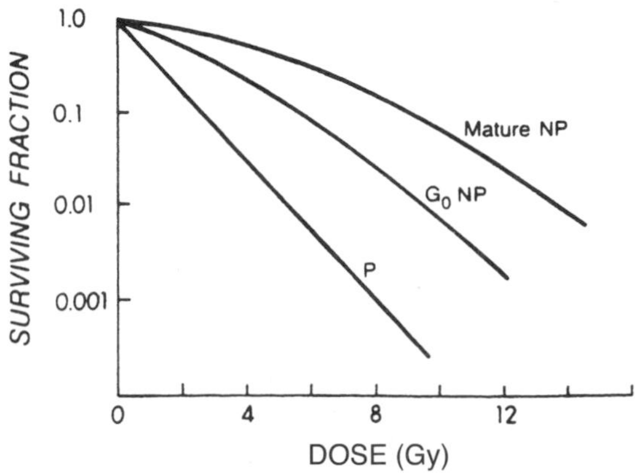

Figure 6–11. Recruitment. The gap (G_0) compartment has nonproliferating cells (NP) that can be recruited into the cycle, becoming proliferating cells (P).

The reverse is true for a critical normal tissue. This process has become more important with the growing use of combined-modality therapies.[98]

Normal Tissue Tolerance

Molecular Biology Aspects of Normal Tissue Radiation Biology

With the introduction of increasingly sophisticated molecular biologic techniques, we have extended our original paradigm of the clinical pathologic course of events induced by irradiation and chemotherapy from target cells per se to include the intercellular communication between targets—principally the cytokine conversation between cells—and this inclusion represents a series of paradigm shifts leading to a better understanding of the mechanisms underlying cytotoxic-induced late effects.[99–101] In our current paradigm, the emphasis has moved from the target cells themselves to the autocrine, paracrine, and, possibly, endocrine mRNA messages and proteins that are passed between cells. A target organ being irradiated, with its multiple cellular components, results in the development of persistent or "perpetual" cytokine cascades, and we believe it is the incremental sustenance of these messages that allows surviving cells to recover or express the late effects, or do both.[53, 100] In Figure 6–12,[100] the four basic cell components are shown—the parenchymal cell, the endothelial cell, the macrophage, and the fibroblast—along with some of the associated proinflammatory and profibrotic cytokines released following irradiation. A more detailed account of the mechanisms of dysregulated cytokine cascades and the resultant late effect syndromes can be found in Chapter 34, Late Effects of Cancer Treatment.

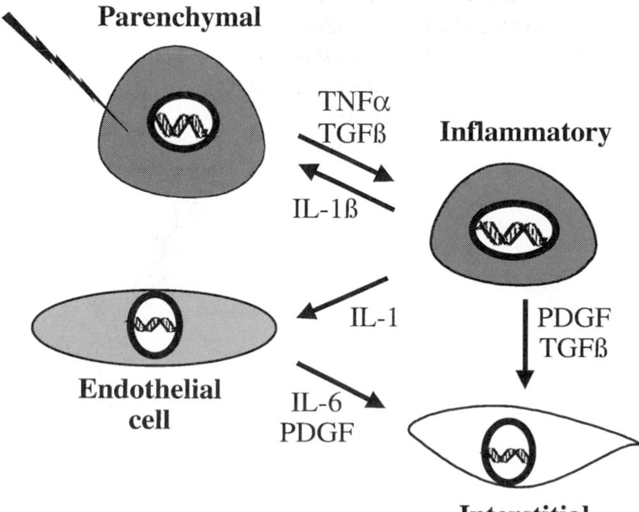

Figure 6–12. Hypothetical pathway indicating a chain of events beginning with initial injury to the primary target cell—the type II pneumocyte—and culminating in activation of the fibroblasts to lay down extracellular matrix proteins. (From Rubin P, Finkelstein JN, Williams JP: Paradigm shifts in the radiation pathophysiology of late effects in normal tissues: molecular vs classic concepts. In Tobias JS, Thomas PRM [eds]: Current Radiation Oncology, 3rd ed, p 1. London, Arnold, 1998, with permission.)

Relative Cell Radiosensitivity and Kinetics of Radiation Response

Radiation acts at a cellular level, and tissue effects represent a summation of cellular effects.[102, 103] Because the key target cells for the survival of a complex organ depend on the organization of all its tissues, cellular damage in one key cell population may result in death of the whole tissue. For example, small blood vessels are fairly sensitive to irradiation, so the effects on a tissue from disruption of its blood supply may be greater than those from the irradiation of the parenchymal cells themselves.

A relative cell radiosensitivity is illustrated in Figure 6–13,[7] which is based on the classification schema related to cellular division and differentiation by Cowdry.[104] The uncommitted stem cell is a vegetative intermitotic cell; the committed stem cell is a differentiating intermitotic cell. Reverting postmitotic cells have the ability to divide when conditioned or challenged, such as hepatocytes after liver resection. The organization of tissues and organs by these cell types determines their radiosensitivity, which is based on their most radiosensitive cells. Table 6–5 reviews cell and tissue radiosensitivity.

The histologic manifestations of radiation cellular death are pyknosis and karyolysis, swollen vacuolated cells with loss of staining capacity and altered permeability, with eventual degeneration and phagocytosis. The events following exposure to radiation doses are determined, in part, by the radiosensitivity of the cells in the parenchymal compartment as well as related to the radiosensitivity of vascular stroma and its turnover rate.[105, 106] A *rapid renewal system,* illustrated in Figure 6–14,[7] consists of vegetative intermitotic cells, differentiating intermitotic cells, and fixed postmitotic cells as found in skin or the mucous membrane of the alimentary tract or in the testes. The initial fractional doses of irradiation destroy the stem cell compartments (vegetative intermitotic cells and differentiating intermitotic cells) and reduce the production of cells that normally flow into the postmitotic compartment. The lining or mucous membrane thins and, as the dose increases, the connective tissue becomes edematous. With large doses, the parenchymal compartment may be lifted or sloughed as a result of the edema. The ability of the tissue to regenerate depends on the survival of stem cells (vegetative intermitotic cells), which gradually increase in

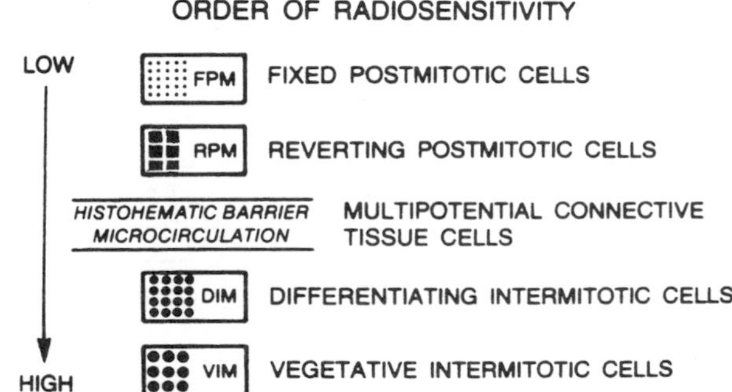

Figure 6–13. Relative cell radiosensitivity. (From Rubin P, Casarett GW: Clinical Radiation Pathology. Philadelphia, W.B. Saunders, 1968, with permission.)

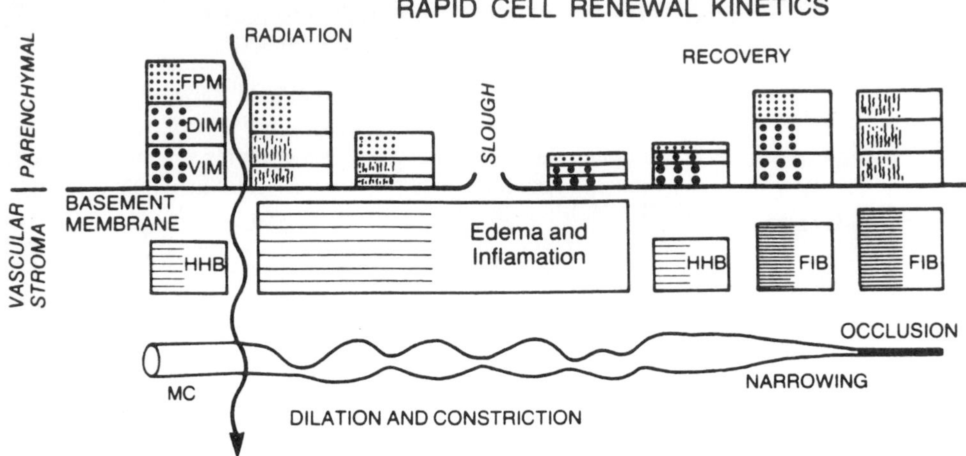

Figure 6–14. Rapid renewal system illustrating radiation effects on both parenchyma and microvasculature compartments. VIM = vegetative intermitotic cells; DIM = differentiating intermitotic cells; FPM = fixed postmitotic cells; HHB = histohematic barrier; FIB = increased fibrosis; MC = microcirculation. (From Rubin P, Casarett GW: Clinical Radiation Pathology. Philadelphia, W.B. Saunders, 1968, with permission.)

number, differentiate, and rebuild the postmitotic compartment. The compartments eventually stabilize, but they might be relatively reduced as a result of increased fibrosis and an increased histohematic barrier. If large doses have been given, the microcirculation might become occluded at a later time, leading to frank delayed necrosis. With lesser degrees of fibrosis, the parenchymal compartment might atrophy, and when stressed, as by infection, might show its limited stem cell reserve capacity or mitotic potential to respond.

The sequence of events differs in a *slow renewal system* or *nonrenewal system* (Fig. 6–15).[7] The parenchymal compartment consists of reverting postmitotic cells or fixed postmitotic cells. Little or no change occurs in the parenchymal compartment with the fractional dose schemes used clinically. The vascular stromal compartment more often determines the course of events, although there are effects that can be attributed to a direct effect on parenchymal cells.[107, 108] The late expression of injury of these cells is caused by their slow renewal, hence the slow expression of injury.

Clinical Pathologic Course

The sequence of clinical events after the initiation of radiation therapy will be considered in terms of four successive time periods of arbitrary length: acute clinical period (first 6 months), subacute clinical period (second 6 months), chronic clinical period (second through fifth year), and late clinical period (after 5 years) (Fig. 6–16).[7] Two curves are shown, illustrating two courses of a potentially infinite number of variations of early and late effect events.

Subclinical damage occurs when moderate doses are administered, below tissue tolerance, while clinically evident damage exceeds clinical threshold and results in both early and late effects. Events such as trauma (surgery), infection, or chemotherapy may shift subclinical residual injury to a clinical phase. This is illustrated by the addition of doxorubicin to mediastinal irradiation for Hodgkin's disease patients, who, years after the administration of so-called safe doses of both radiation therapy and chemotherapy, develop cardiac decompensation and cardiomyopathy.[109, 110]

Normal Tissue Tolerance Dose

The tolerance dose[101, 111] is an attempt to express the minimal and maximal injurious doses acceptable to the clinician and is also expressed as the normal tissue complication probability.[112, 113] These calculations require the assignment of an arbitrary—but useful—percentage for the risk of complications. The *minimal tolerance dose* is defined as the $TD_{5/5}$, that is, the dose to which a given population of patients is exposed under a standard set of treatment conditions, resulting in no more than a 5% severe complication rate within 5 years after treatment. The *maximal tolerance dose* is defined as the $TD_{50/5}$, that is, the dose that results in a 50% severe complication rate 5 years after

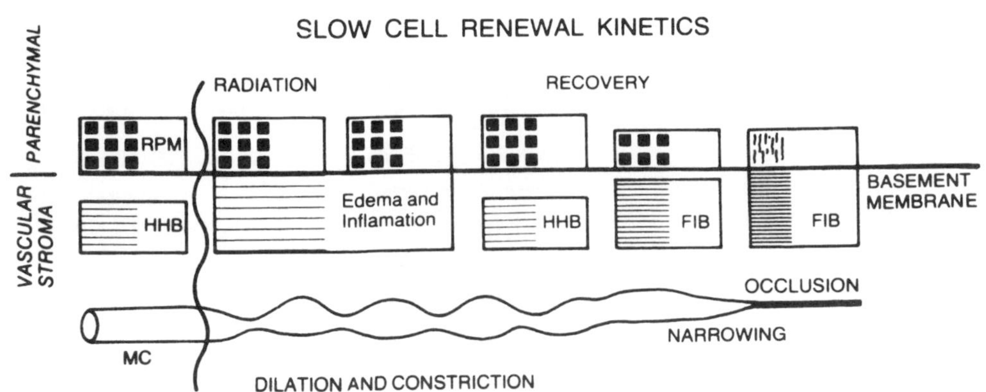

Figure 6–15. Slow renewal system illustrating effects on the vascular compartment, which leads to a late effect in the parenchymal cells as the capillary sclerosis and fibrosis increases. RPM = reverting postmitotic cells. (From Rubin P, Casarett GW: Clinical Radiation Pathology. Philadelphia, W.B. Saunders, 1968, with permission.)

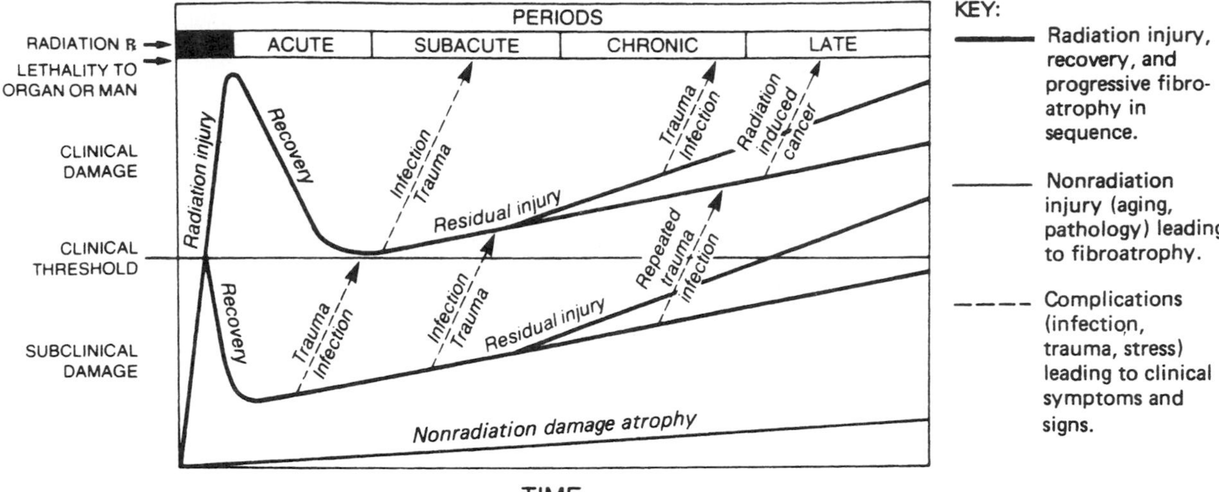

Figure 6–16. Sequence of clinical events after radiation. Note that the clinical course can be accelerated by trauma, infection, or chemotherapy. (From Rubin P, Casarett GW: Clinical Radiation Pathology. Philadelphia, W.B. Saunders, 1968, with permission.)

treatment. Because of the sigmoidal nature of the dose-response curve, this is a steep response; that is, a difference in 5% to 10% in dose can change an acceptable complication rate from 5% to 50%—unacceptably high.

The dose-limiting tissues or organs in radiation therapy are based on our inability to define an optimal tumor dose (many biologic factors are unknown clinically), so that the radiation oncologist is often required to treat to tolerance. These dose-limiting tissues or organs are defined according to dose. The dose limits specified are based on the best and most current dose-time data available. These dose limits assume a standard set of conditions:

- supervoltage irradiation (1 to 10 MeV)
- dose delivery of 2 ± 10% Gy per day, 5 fractions weekly, or 10 Gy, with 2-day rest intervals
- completion of treatment in 6 to 8 weeks
- doses conditioned by partial-volume organ irradiation

Our longest clinical experience is with limited-field irradiation to part of an organ, and this experience has provided insights into tissue and organ radiation sensitivity[110, 114]:

2 to 10 Gy. With fractionated doses of less than 10 Gy, the testes spermatogonia, ovarian oogonia, and lens epithelium are injured. The testes spermatogonia are very sensitive to smaller fractional doses and are destroyed more efficiently than ovarian tissue. Lymphocytes and lymphoid tissues also will be suppressed with trivial doses.

10 to 20 Gy. With fractionated doses of 10 to 20 Gy, the normal bone marrow hematopoietic stem cells will be depressed, but larger doses will be required to achieve suppression with limited volumes. In disease states, unlike in the normal state, smaller fractional doses (<10 Gy) may ablate the bone marrow. Growing cartilage and growing bone also will be arrested within this dose range.

20 to 30 Gy. Between 20 and 30 Gy, a number of vital organs reach their radiation threshold and decompensate, despite fractionation. This is most apparent when an entire organ is so treated. The kidneys and lungs are both vulnerable to this dose range and demonstrate a combination of injury to the microvasculature and epithelial cells.

30 to 40 Gy. The liver becomes vulnerable at this level. For many organs, there are limited data on whole-organ fractional therapy schedules, but skin and oropharyngeal mucosa can become acutely reactive. The liver displays a special veno-occlusive event secondary to platelet adhesion to central veins at or somewhat above this dose level.

40 to 50 Gy. At this dose level, the heart and gastrointestinal organs are likely to experience severe and life-threatening injury, particularly with large-volume or whole-organ irradiation.

50 to 60 Gy. The majority of organs are vulnerable to fractionated schedules in the 50 to 60 Gy range. Gastrointestinal injury is significant, and the colorectal tissues become vulnerable. The spinal cord and brain may become demyelinated. Vascular connective tissue stroma is affected at this dose range, which has a major effect even with partial-organ irradiation. Long-term fibrosis may occur in lung, liver, kidney, and bone marrow even when smaller volumes are irradiated.

60 to 70 Gy. At this range, the brain is more likely to react to irradiation by undergoing demyelination at the TD_{5-50} levels. The rectum and bladder become vulnerable to major injury at the TD_5 level. However, mature cartilage and bone are able to withstand these doses, as are pancreas, peripheral nerves, and muscle.

Dose Selection

The choice of dose depends on weighing the probability of cure versus the probability of complication (Fig. 6–17).[115] Models for decision making include cost-benefit analysis in clinical terms in which negative outcomes are evaluated. The Bayesian model and the ratio operating characteristic

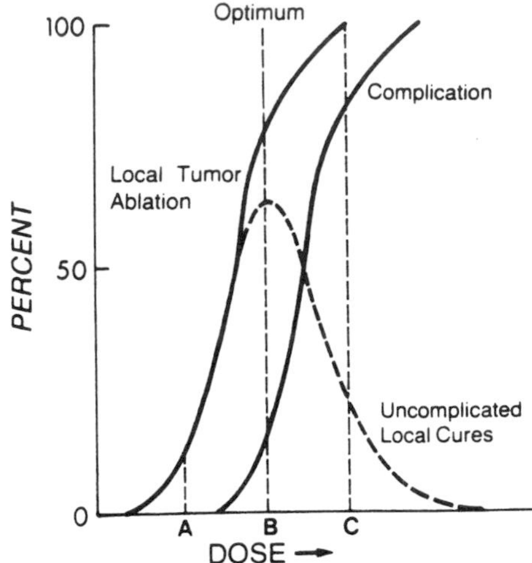

Figure 6–17. Treatment outcomes. Uncomplicated cures *(dashed lines)* are the desired result of treatment. This is illustrated as a function of the therapeutic ratio, i.e. the greater the separation between the tumor control (ablation) curve and the normal tissue complication curve, the greater the number of uncomplicated cures that will result. A, B, and C represent three different dose levels that if chosen, would lead to three different outcomes. *A* would result in few tumor cures but no complications. *C* would lead to complete cure in many cases, but virtually all patients would suffer complications. The optimal choice in this group of dose levels is *B*, which would result in the greatest number of cured patients without complications. (Adapted from Mendelsohn ML: The biology of dose-limiting tissues. In Time and Dose Relationships in Radiation Biology as Applied to Radiotherapy, Brookhaven National Laboratory [BNL] Report 5023 (C-57), p 154. Upton, Brookhaven National Laboratory, 1969, with permission.)

curves have been suggested for clinical decision making. (The term *ratio operating characteristic* is applied to decision making when there is a negative and a positive outcome.) In these systems, values are assigned to four potential outcomes:

- uncomplicated cure — preferred or positive outcome
- complicated cure
- uncomplicated recurrence
- complicated recurrence

} negative outcomes

When cure rates are similar for different modalities—that is, surgery versus radiation therapy—the negative outcomes, their frequency and severity, often are the basis of the final choice. When results are equivalent for different forms of therapy, the state of the host is also critical to treatment selection. Better survival results for one modality compared with another may be more related to the state of health of the host than the treatment effectiveness.

State of the Host. The associated medical problems of the host, rather than the malignancy itself, may determine the choice of treatment. For example, when a very elderly patient has bladder cancer, surgery is often contraindicated because of comorbidity problems, such as heart disease. Although radiation therapy places physical demands on a patient, it is more often better tolerated, with less risk of mortality. The role of natural immunologic factors in radiation therapy is being studied, and the means to affect their response, through cytokines or drugs, is now available. However, such factors may augment as well as inhibit radiation response, and such manipulation therefore requires more careful clinical investigations.

Tolerance Volume. The concept of a tolerance volume needs to be defined in the same fashion as tolerance dose. The volume frequently proves to be more critical to complications outcome and also serves as a clinical guide because it is possible to obliterate or lose a certain volume of a vital organ with large doses; exceeding the TD_{90-100} is akin to surgical resection. Loss of some volume generally does not affect organ survival because the organ can often compensate for volume loss, up to a threshold volume, through regeneration or hypertrophy and remain, although impaired, within functional tolerance for survival. Different organs demonstrate a range of tolerance volume (TV) parameters:

1. TV_{5-25}: 5% to 25% of the organ volume irradiated can result in a life-threatening or lethal complication.
2. TV_{50-90}: 50% to 90% of the organ volume irradiated can result in a life-threatening or lethal complication.

There are generally two levels of critical volume for dose-limiting or vital organs. Only the gastrointestinal tract and the central nervous system (CNS) can have disastrous outcomes after small volumes (TV 5% to 10%) are exposed to doses exceeding TD_{5-50}. However, it is important to note that necrotic bowel and, on occasion, CNS necrotic foci can be resected successfully. For the majority of organs considered dosc limiting, such as bone marrow, lung, kidney, and, in all probability, heart and liver, high doses can be tolerated to smaller volumes. Such organs may decompensate when more than 50% of the total volume (as applied to paired organs) is exceeded.

The time when organ decompensation begins clearly depends on the compensatory regenerative mechanisms that come into play when significant organ volume loss occurs. The dose-response curve is not an absolute or fixed effect but varies as a function of volume (Fig. 6–18A).[116] This is an important concept because it allows the radiation oncologist to give much larger doses to partial volumes. For TD_5 and TD_{50}, the dose increases as the volume decreases (Fig. 6–18B). Note that the slope changes as more than 50% of the whole organ is included. Small increments in dose, that is, 10% to 20% of the total dose, can be lethal. The dose-volume histogram is being adopted by numerous investigators to predict unfavorable outcomes as a result of volume loss in a critical structure.[116, 117]

Predictive Assays for Radiation Response: Tumors Versus Normal Tissues

- Clonogenic assays of human tumors in mammalian cell cultures have been commonly used to determine radioresponsiveness.[5] The intrinsic cellular radiosensitivity concept mentioned previously was proposed by Fertil and Malaise[77] and can be measured as the SF_2—the cell survival at 2 Gy using an *in vitro* clonogenic cell survival assay. Tumors have been divided into six histologic groups based on their SF_2, ranging from the most radiosensitive to the most radioresistant:

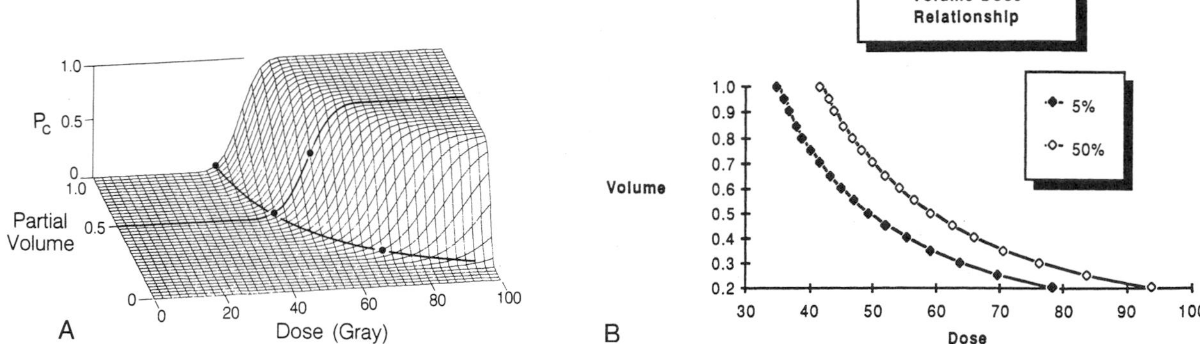

Figure 6–18. Volume effect: (A) The dose response curve is not an absolute or fixed effect but varies as a function of volume. This important concept allows the radiation oncologist to give much larger doses to partial volumes. (From Lyman JT, Wolbarst AB: Optimization of radiation therapy, III: a method of assessing complication probabilities from dose-volume histograms. Int J Radiat Oncol Biol Phys 1987; 13:103, with permission from Elsevier Science.) (B) For TD_5 and TD_{50}, the dose increases as the volume decreases. Note that the slope changes as more than 50% of the whole organ is included. Small increments in dose, that is, 10% to 20%, can prove to be lethal.

oat cell carcinomas, lymphomas, adenocarcinomas, squamous cell cancers, melanomas, and glioblastomas. However, SF_2 values are based on *in vitro* assays and have proved contradictory in patients, with West and coworkers finding a lower local control in cancer of the cervix with SF_2 greater than 0.55,[79] whereas others have found little or no correlation between SF_2 and clinical tumors.[118–120]

- A technique that involves counting chromosomal aberrations after a single 2 Gy exposure and biopsy uses premature chromosomes under condensation or fluorescent *in situ* hybridization techniques; this assay is being evaluated.
- Nonclonogenic assays have been developed based on cell growth in multiwell dishes; growth is measured by stain density and has the advantage of being rapid and automated. Colorimetric assays, such as the 3-(4,5-dimethylthiazol-2-yl)-2,5-diphenyl tetrazolium bromide (MTT) cytotoxicity assay or its derivatives, are based on the ability of viable cells to metabolize or reduce a visually appropriate compound or by evaluating DNA or RNA content of a cell colony after irradiation. However, such assays have been found to be better applied to drug sensitivity. Cell adhesive index is based on cell growth, not clonogenicity, and utilizes a specially prepared surface so that cells from a biopsy will attach and grow. However, none of these assays have proved to be predictive to date.
- The oxygen status of tumors can be determined using polarographic oxygen probes (e.g., the Eppendorf probe) or, conversely, by measuring the levels of hypoxia using deposited ^{123}I-labeled nitroimidazoles, visualized by single photon emission computed tomography. A clinical trial performed in advanced cervical cancer patients by a team from Germany[121] demonstrated improved survival if pO_2 values were 5 mm Hg or lower using Eppendorf probes. Positron emission tomography imaging of hypoxia, with ^{18}F fluoromisonidazole or ^{18}F fluorodeoxyglucose to measure metabolic activity, has been used to predict tumor response to bioreductive drugs, such as tirapazamine, and radiation.[122]
- Potential doubling time (Tpot) is based on a tumor's proliferative potential, using cell cycle time and growth fraction, and can be measured using flow cytometry on a single tumor cell biopsy specimen taken a few hours after 5-bromo-2′-deoxyuridine injection. One European Organization for Research and Treatment of Cancer trial, in preliminary analysis, showed improved local control of fast-growing tumors (Tpot < 4 days) following twice-a-day accelerated fractionation versus conventional once-a-day therapy (Fig. 6–19).[123, 124]
- The radiation or chemotherapy response of both normal tissues and tumors, as measured by a combination of cytogenetic assays, may be predictive of later outcomes to cytotoxic therapy. According to Streffer and colleagues,[125] such assays include micronuclei assay, DNA repair kinetics by comet assay, and cell proliferation by flow cytometry. The comet assay is useful for recognizing radiosensitive patients in whom severe damage will occur, whereas cell proliferation plus micronuclei counts predict for tumor response. Telomerase activity has been used to predict mitotic potential of tumors, and a number of investigators have found it a useful correlate with outcome following irradiation and chemotherapy in cancers of the oral cavity and oropharynx[126, 127]; that is, a decline indicated response to therapy.
- Tumor angiogenesis as measured by the mean vascular density has been used to predict metastases[128] and tumor cell radiosensitivity.[129]
- Plasma cytokine assays have been used by investigators to predict normal tissue toxicity both before therapy and after treatment. For instance, Anscher and associates[130, 131] have used serum levels of transforming growth factor–β, to predict for both pneumonitis and hepatitis in bone marrow transplantation patients. A Radiation Therapy Oncology Group study has preliminary data indicating that the level of tumor necrosis

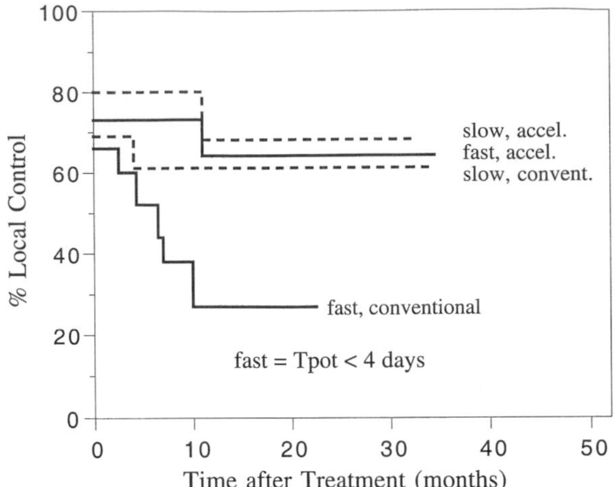

Figure 6–19. Illustrating the results of an EORTC cooperative trial to compare conventional fractionation (2 Gy once per day to 70 Gy in 7 weeks) with accelerated treatment (1.6 Gy three times daily to 72 Gy in 5 weeks). Fast-growing tumors were those with a Tpot less than 4 days. Slow-growing tumors had a measured Tpot greater than 4 days. (From Hall EJ: Radiobiology for the Radiologist, 4th ed. Philadelphia, J.B. Lippincott Co., 1994, with permission. Redrawn from Begg AC, Hofland I, Van Glabbeke M, et al: Predictive value of potential doubling time for radiotherapy of head and neck tumor patients: Results from the EORTC cooperative trial 22851. Semin Radiat Oncol 1992; 1:22.)

factor–α was elevated in patients with pulmonary toxicity of fibrosis and pneumonitis (W. Hartsell, unpublished data). In addition, in our hands, interleukin-6 has proved to be predictive of pneumonitis in both clinical and experimental studies.[132]

In summary, many predictive assays are being explored in clinical trials and show promise in selecting patients for modifiers of radiation response: time, dose, fractionation (hyperfractionated versus conventional versus accelerated), hypoxic cell radiosensitizers, chemotherapy and biologic response modifiers, radioprotectors of normal tissues, and physical modifiers (three-dimensional conformal therapy, neutrons, protons, and x-rays).

Modifiers of Radiation Response

Response and recovery are as basic to the laws of radiobiologic and radiopathologic mechanisms as are action and reaction to the laws of physical motion.[59, 133–138] Following the initial interaction of ionizing radiation and biologic matter, a sequence of events begins that may result in a lethal alteration in a living cellular system, be it host tissue or malignant tumor. From the physical event of energy transfer, a chemical reaction occurs with the release of free radicals and the decomposition of water into hydrogen and hydroxyl ionic forms. The biochemical targets affected are believed to be nucleic acids, such as DNA and RNA, and vital enzymes and proteins. This results in recognizable biologic injury in the form of mitotic-linked deaths, in which chromosomal aberrations are evident microscopically. In radiotherapeutic terms, this cell death results in tumor destruction. Biochemical recovery and biologic repair also can occur; consequently, host tissues may maintain their integrity, allowing successful organ function, thereby preserving the organism or patient. The radiopathologic end effect is the summation of these events, which it is hoped will result in long-term survival of the patient, free from recurrence of the neoplasm.

Mathematical Modeling

A number of mathematic models have been developed to consider the different treatment fractions of dose-time fractionation based on clinical and experimental data.[5] A variety of valuable clinically applicable formulae exist (normal standard dose [NSD], time-dose fraction [TDF], cumulative radiation effect [CRE], and new computer-based formulations), but all have limitations. In addition, the α/β ratio and linear quadratic equation are applicable to cellular populations, but do not always provide guides to safe doses for *in vivo* organ tolerances.

Strandqvist Lines. The dose-time isoeffect line introduced by Strandqvist[139] is based on the concept that the total dose in the total period of time determines the effects, independent of fractionation (Fig. 6–20).[5] As a result of the phenomena of cell and tissue repair, it is apparent that a greater total dose needs to be given if fractional doses are used that extend the period of time in which the dose is delivered. Using his observations in treating skin cancer and oropharyngeal cancers and comparing them with skin erythema reactions, Strandqvist was able to construct a family of curves in which an optimal zone could be found favoring tumor cure with minimal complications.

Normal Standard Dose. The NSD[140, 141] is a single reference dose developed by Ellis[140] for the biologic effect of a fractionated radiation therapy regimen. This index facilitates the comparison of treatment plans that have widely

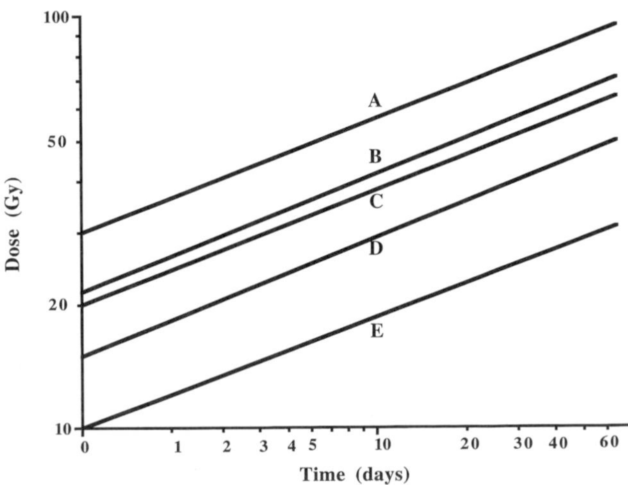

Figure 6–20. Strandqvist lines: The dose-time isoeffect line relates total dose delivered and total time independent of fractionation for different tissue end points: A = skin necrosis; B = cure of skin carcinoma; C = moist desquamation of the skin; D = dry desquamation of the skin; and E = skin erythema. (From Hall EJ: Radiobiology for the Radiologist, 4th ed. Philadelphia, J.B. Lippincott Co., 1994, with permission. Redrawn from Strandqvist M: Studien uber die Kumulative Wirkung der Rontgenstrahlen bei Fraktionierung. Acta Radiol 1944; 55(Suppl Stockh):1.)

different fractionation patterns and overall treatment times. The unit for NSD is the rad equivalent therapy (ret) and is determined by a formula that converts the Gy dose. The NSD corresponds to the tolerance of the normal tissue at the tumor site and represents the normal connective tissue tolerance, which is given as 1800 ret. The NSD tolerance level varies with different organs and tissues.

The difference between the NSD concept and the Strandqvist line is that the NSD formulation allows for the separation of fraction number and time variables. In general, it is the size of the dose per fraction that most influences the shape of the isoeffect curves. However, it should be recognized as unlikely that any one isoeffect formulation will hold for all tissues because of the extreme complexities and variations in the responses of different tissues to radiation therapy.[142]

Time-Dose Fraction and Cumulative Radiation Effect. The modification of the NSD concept proposed by Orton[143, 144] introduced the concept of partial tolerance and defined a TDF so that one could have guidelines for combining two split courses or continuous irradiation, as in brachytherapy. A standard radium therapy regimen was used in comparison with equivalent techniques (60 Gy/168 h). Data derived from different dose-rate effects of different radioisotopes were plotted as isoeffect curves. Ellis's equivalent dose for fractionated external irradiation is 1800 ret, and in a thorough review by Ellis, the NSD-TDF concept was related to radiation therapy.[142]

The CRE concept of Kirk and coworkers[145] was based on the need to assess the biologic effect of various fractionated schemas on the basis of the accumulated subtolerance radiation injury. The application by Turresen and Notter[146–148] of CRE in predicting late effects in normal tissue gave validity to the concept. However, whatever formulation or computer-generated guidelines are employed, caution must be used in selecting safe doses that are unorthodox. Indeed, few of the aforementioned indices are in wide use, and they have been supplanted by the linear quadratic survival relationship.

The Linear Quadratic Survival Relationship (α/β Ratio).[5, 59] Experiments with isoeffect curves for a variety of acute- and late-responding normal tissues in animals have shown that the isoeffect lines for late responses are steeper than those for early responses (Fig. 6–21).[149] Thames and associates[150, 151] consequently suggested a greater capacity for repair of damage that is expressed late than for damage that is expressed early. The observed differences in the slopes of the isoeffect lines between acute- and late-responding normal tissues can be related to differences in the shapes of cell survival curves. The linear quadratic survival curve model is represented by the equation:

$$\text{Log}_e\, S = \alpha D + \beta D^2$$

A small α/β ratio (Fig. 6–22)[152] would be characteristic of a late-responding normal tissue. Consequently, decreasing the fraction size would preferentially spare late-effects tissues. Thus, in hyperfractionation protocols, greater total doses are delivered by giving smaller fractional doses more than once a day. The increased total doses should cause late effects similar to those with standard fractionation but should give increased tumor responses because it is thought

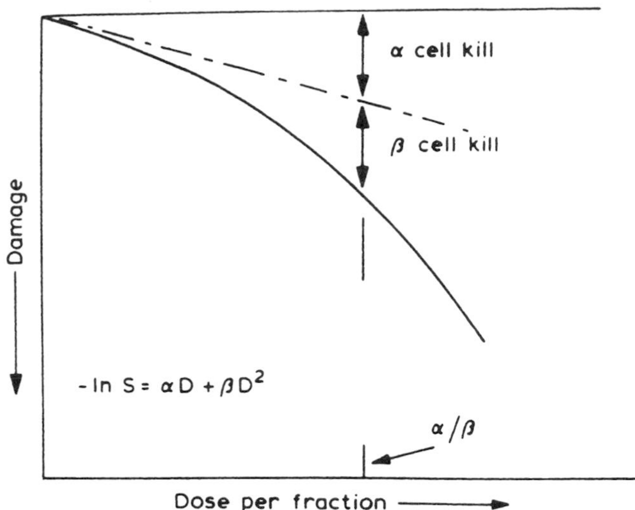

Figure 6–21. At the dose equivalent of the α/β ratio, the log cell kill due to the α-process (nonreparable) is equal to that due to the β-process (reparable injury). In general, acutely reacting tissues have a high α/β ratio (8 to 15 Gy), whereas tissues involved in late effects have a low α/β ratio (1 to 5 Gy). (From Fowler JR: Fractionation and therapeutic gain. In Steel GG, Adams GED, Peckham MJ [eds]: Biological Basis of Radiotherapy, p 181. Amsterdam, Elsevier Science, 1983.)

that tumors respond to fractionated treatments like early responding normal tissues. Thus, with such an approach, a therapeutic benefit is expected.

Dose-Time Relationship Modifiers of Fractionation

The magnitude of the radiation dose is not the only important variable; of equal importance is the distribution of the dose with respect to time—the fractionation factor.[40, 153–156] It has been observed that as the interval of time between treatments is extended, the total dose must be

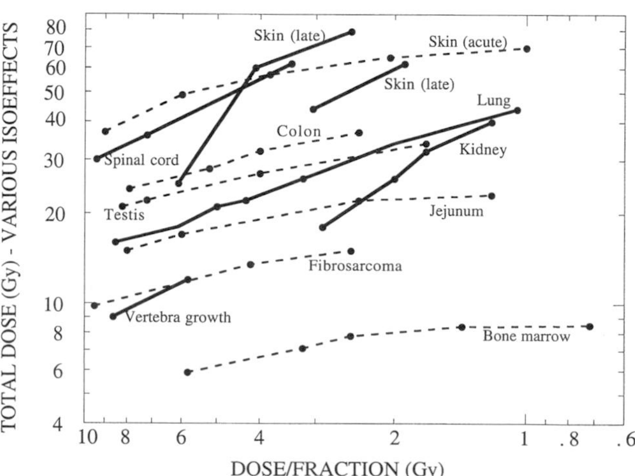

Figure 6–22. Total dose for isoeffect as a function of dose per fraction. Late effects = solid lines; acute effects = broken lines. (From Withers HR: Biologic basis for altered fractionation schemes. Cancer 1985; 55:2086. Copyright © 1985 American Cancer Society. Reprinted with permission of Wiley-Liss, Inc., a subsidiary of John Wiley & Sons, Inc.)

raised to produce the same effect.[157] This can be explained only on the basis that a certain amount of tissue recovery takes place during the interval. However, clinical experience has also shown that, in general, normal tissues recover more rapidly than neoplastic tissues. Therefore, by increasing the total dose delivered over a longer period of time, the differential between the tumor lethal dose and tissue tolerance dose can be accentuated in three ways: (1) *fractionation*—high-intensity dosage in short intervals, that is, external irradiation; (2) *protraction*—low-intensity dosage over a long period of time, that is, interstitial radioisotopes; and (3) combinations of low- and high-dose ratio (see Tables 6–3 and 6–4).

The required tumor lethal dose for different human tumors ranges from 20 Gy in 2 weeks to 80 Gy in 8 weeks, with the vast majority of tumors receiving doses between 45 and 75 Gy. A daily fractionation schema of 2 ± 10% Gy is used, delivering 60 to 70 Gy at 10 Gy per week, depending on the primary tumor size in current conventional or standard regimen. The number of daily fractions varies from 2 to 5. Using a standard dose of 60 Gy (6 weeks times five daily doses), the following three major treatment tactics, often using combinations of high-and-low dose rates, have been selected by radiation therapists:

Higher-Than-Standard Dose, Shorter Time. When the tumor dose needs to be high, combined internal and external irradiation is preferred over either technique alone. Doses from 60 to 100 Gy are most often given during combined doses of external and internal radiation. Because of different dose rates or protraction, better total dose-time levels can be achieved. The contrast between the dose rates of external and internal irradiation should be noted as intensity of radiation delivery, that is, low- versus high-dose rate in Gy/h. When interstitial or intracavitary irradiation is protracted, doses can be given at 10 Gy/d and 60 to 70 Gy/wk using radium or iridium sources.

Higher-Than-Standard Dose, Longer Time. Longer protracted doses leading to higher levels of radiation are usually used in tumors occupying large volumes. For these large volumes, a 60-Gy level may be delivered in 8 to 10 weeks. Doses between 60 and 80 Gy are often given with booster techniques, using small, coned-down fields of external irradiation or electrons to add another 10 to 20 Gy. This is referred to as the *shrinking field technique*. Interstitial implants or intracavitary sources can also add 10 to 20 Gy to an externally delivered dose of 50 to 60 Gy. This tactic is often used in split-course techniques, in which larger doses are given by interrupting treatment to allow for tumor regression and a reduced volume to be treated. The second course can then be carried to a higher dose level of 70 to 80 Gy in 8 to 10 weeks to a more limited target. Maximum doses used are most often at the 80-Gy level in spite of the time factor; some exceptions with levels as high as 90 or 100 Gy are noted for combined external and interstitial techniques in the cervix, metastatic neck nodes, inoperable breast cancer, and soft tissue sarcomas on limbs.

Lower-Than-Standard Dose, Longer Time. This tactic is a compromise, often resulting in less than the required tumor dose, and is generally ineffective with two exceptions: (1) radiosensitive tumors occupying large volumes or (2) microdeposits or millimeter-size foci in large volumes. Advanced ovarian cancer, with seedings through the abdomen, is treated by this technique.

Low-Dose Rate Versus High-Dose Rate Effects. The principal dose rate effect is cell killing, which occurs between 1 Gy/min and 0.01 Gy/min. This effect is due to repair of sublethal damage that occurs during the actual radiation exposure. At lower dose rates, cell division or repopulation occurs, whereas at higher dose rates, the 1 to 10 Gy/min used with external irradiation, little difference in kill occurs.[158] Steel introduced the concept of the Regaud dose rate, that is, a relatively low dose rate of 1 Gy/hr (0.01–0.02 Gy/min), which is approximately isoeffective with fractionated therapy using 2 Gy fractions.[156] At this dose rate, human tumor cell lines show a wide range of radiosensitivity, differing by a factor of 7, and may well be the most clinically relevant in the way of describing the radiosensitivity of tumor cells.

With intracavitary and interstitial brachytherapy, the commonly used dose rate is 10 Gy/24 h or 0.42 Gy/h or 0.69 cGy/min, which, in reference to variations of total dose and total treatment time to produce an equivalent to 60 Gy in 7 days (Fig. 6–23),[159] is a dose rate of 0.36 Gy/h. The general shape of the Patterson and Parker curves is similar to Ellis and is the basis for dose curves used clinically with some modification. High-dose–rate irradiation is comparable to low-dose irradiation[160, 161] and is in wide use clinically.[162] The major advantages are the physical placement, the control of dwell-time of single sources, and the use of highly computerized systems rather than the dose rate of the irradiation per se.[163] For instance, very high brachytherapy doses are being given to prostate cancer patients with permanent seed implants, using ^{125}I or ^{103}Pd. Ultrasound- or computed tomography–guided implants, using templates for accuracy, offer a rapid reconstruction, in real time, of isodose distribution curves in the prostate and anterior rectal wall. Doses for ^{125}I range between 150 and

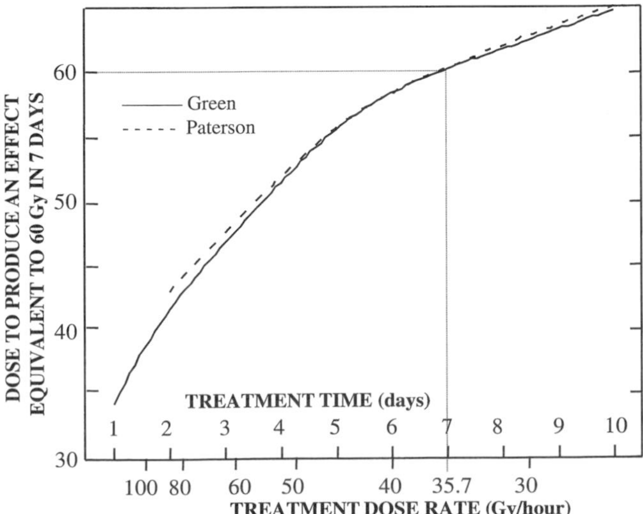

Figure 6–23. Variation of total dose with treatment time to produce an effect equivalent to 60 Gy in 7 days with a radium implant. (Redrawn from Orton CG: Time-dose factors [TDFs] in brachytherapy. Br J Radiol 1974; 47:603, with permission.)

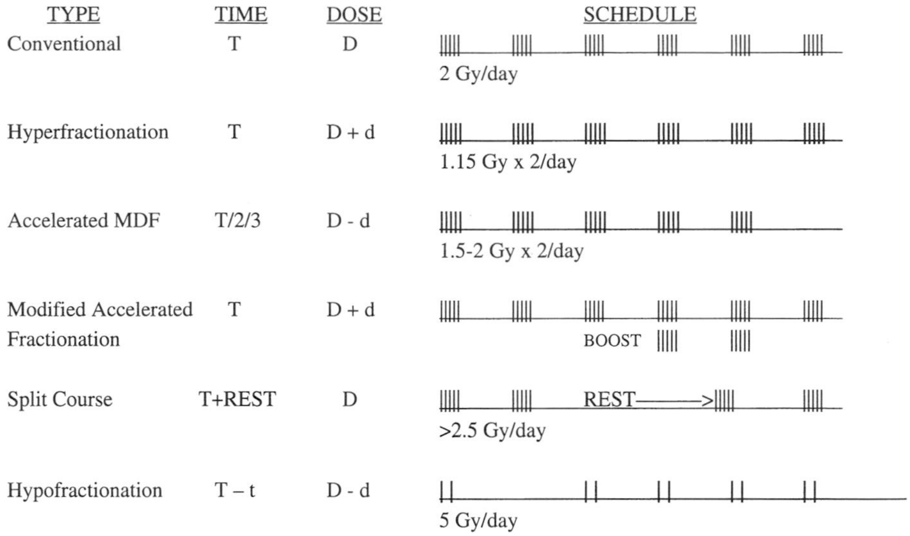

TYPE	TIME	DOSE	SCHEDULE
Conventional	T	D	2 Gy/day
Hyperfractionation	T	D + d	1.15 Gy x 2/day
Accelerated MDF	T/2/3	D - d	1.5-2 Gy x 2/day
Modified Accelerated Fractionation	T	D + d	BOOST
Split Course	T+REST	D	REST——> >2.5 Gy/day
Hypofractionation	T – t	D - d	5 Gy/day

Figure 6–24. Various types of fractionation schedules used in radiation therapy. (From Perez CA, Brady LW, Roti Roti JL: Overview. In Perez CA, Brady LW [eds]: Principles and Practice of Radiation Oncology, 3rd ed, p 1. Philadelphia, Lippincott-Raven, 1997, with permission.)

250 Gy ($T_{1/2}$ = 58 days); for ^{103}Pd ($T_{1/2}$ = 20 days), they range between 100 to 150 Gy over short periods of time. The majority of the dose is delivered over the first 3 half-lives; as the radioisotope decays, the dose rate falls dramatically, and this may be a factor in improved dose tolerance. Simply utilizing dose itself will require redefining tolerance for the rectal wall[164] because the doses used are double the levels currently prescribed for external irradiation. Further support can be found in a recent correlation by Jereczek-Fossa and coworkers of normalized total dose with the combined total doses of external and brachytherapy using a linear quadratic model[165]: brachytherapy dose rate, fractional dose, and normalized total dose were independent risk factors for late complications.

Altered Fractionation

One of the most actively investigated areas in radiation oncology has been altered fractionation schedules relative to the number of fractions used daily, fraction size, total dose, and total time of schedule. A concise review of the terminology as well as the advantages and disadvantages can be found in Figure 6–24[166] and Table 6–6.[166] These show the different fractionation schemes relative to fraction size, time interval, total dose, and total time; Table 6–7 lists the complication end points for major cells and organs. Based on the linear quadratic model, a separation of early and late effects can be demonstrated as a function of fraction size. Four strategies have emerged:

1. *Split-course irradiation* has been widely used and tested in clinical trials as being more or less effective than conventional irradiation. Larger fractions are used daily, causing an increased reaction that requires that the course be split with a few weeks' rest, rather than treating with continuous radiation on a daily basis as occurs with conventional small fraction doses of 1.5 to 2.0 Gy daily. Generally speaking, the split-course schedules have not proven to be any more effective than conventional irradiation fractionation schedules and therefore have been relegated to largely palliative use.[167]
2. *Hyperfractionation*: The basic aim of hyperfractionation is to deliver smaller, rather than standard frac-

TABLE 6–6. **Comparison of Various Fractionation Schedules**

	Conventional	Split-Course	Accelerated Fractionation	Hyperfractionation
Indication, in tumors, of growth rate	Average	Average or slow	Rapid	Slow (with large cell loss factors)
Normal tissue effects, acute	Standard	Standard or greater	Greater	Standard or greater
Normal tissue effects, late	Standard	Greater	Standard (if complete repair of sublethal damage occurs) or greater	Lower
Advantages		Shorter actual treatment time (fewer fractions)	Destroys more tumor cells; prevents tumor cell repopulation; less overall treatment time	(?) Lower OER with small doses; spares late damage; allows reoxygenation; allows stem cell repopulation
Disadvantages		May permit tumor repopulation		More fractions

OER = oxygen enhancement ratio.

From Perez CA, Brady LW, Roti Roti JL: Overview. In: Perez CA, Brady LW (eds): Principles and Practice of Radiation Oncology, 3rd ed, p 1. Philadelphia, Lippincott-Raven, 1997, with permission.

TABLE 6–7. **Tolerance Doses for Fractionated Doses to Whole or Partial Organs**

Target Cells	Complication End Point	$TD_{5/50}$–$TD_{50/5}$ (Gy)
2–10 Gy		
Lymphocytes and lymphoid	Lymphopenia	2–10
Testes, spermatogonia	Sterility	1–2
Ovarian oocytes	Sterility	6–10
Diseased bone marrow	Severe leukopenia and thrombocytopenia	3–5
10–20 Gy		
Lens	Cataract	6–12
Bone marrow stem cells	Acute aplasia	15–20
20–30 Gy		
Kidney: renal glomeruli	Arterionephrosclerosis	23–28
Lung: Type II cells, vascular connective tissue stroma	Pneumonitis or fibrosis	20–30
30–40 Gy		
Liver: central veins	Hepatopathy	35–40
Bone marrow	Hypoplasia	25–35
40–50 Gy		
Heart (whole organ)	Pericarditis or pancarditis	43–50
Bone marrow microenvironments	Permanent aplasia	45–50
50–60 Gy		
Gastrointestinal	Infarction necrosis	50–55
Heart (partial organ)	Cardiomyopathy	55–65
Spinal cord	Myelopathy	50–60
60–70 Gy		
Brain	Encephalopathy	60–70
Mucosa	Ulcer	65–75
Rectum	Ulcer	65–75
Bladder	Ulcer	65–75
Mature bones	Fracture	65–70
Pancreas	Pancreatitis	>70

tional doses (i.e., 1 to 1.2 Gy), 2 or 3 times daily (at 4- to 6-hour intervals) in order to separate early and late normal tissue reactions. The overall treatment time remains 6 to 8 weeks, but the total dose is increased to 75 to 80 Gy. The goal is to keep the late normal tissue reactions the same as those occurring following standard fractionation, although accepting somewhat increased acute reactions. This schedule is intended to reduce any tumor proliferation during the course of radiation treatment. Because most tumors appear to behave more like acutely responding normal tissues, it is hoped that the larger total dose will obtain greater regressions without increasing late complications. Usually the total dose is increased by 10% to 20%.

Clinical trials have demonstrated a gain in locoregional cancer control using this approach. A European Organization for Research and Treatment of Cancer phase IV trial by Horiot and associates used 80 Gy with twice-daily 1.15 Gy fractions with 6- to 8-hour interfraction intervals versus 70 Gy with single daily fraction of 2 Gy—both given in 7 weeks for T2, T3, N0, and N1 advanced head and neck cancer; in the final analysis at 5 years, locoregional control was increased from 40% to 59% by hyperfractionation.[168] Survival was also improved. In other sites, such as CNS gliomas[169, 170] and lung cancer,[171, 172] hyperfractionation has yielded modest survival benefits in clinical trials.

3. *Accelerated fractionation* involves delivering fractional doses (1.5 to 2 Gy) multiple times daily with intervals of 4 to 6 hours between fractions. The resulting higher total doses will increase both acute and late normal tissue effects, and consequently split-course regimens, requiring two courses of treatment, are needed. Wang and colleagues[173] presented large survival and local control gains in head and neck cancer patients when comparing accelerated fractionation schedules with conventional daily irradiation in retrospective, nonrandomized studies. The intent of this strategy was to reduce repopulation in rapidly growing tumors. Through the split-course technique, there is the anticipation of keeping the late reactions the same. Short intensive schedules known as CHART, for continuous hyperfractionated accelerated radiation treatment, devised by British investigators, consist of 1.5 Gy three times a day at 6-hour intervals for 12 consecutive days including weekends. Saunders and coworkers have reported improvements in survival rate in a multicenter trial in non–small cell lung cancer patients and a small, though nonsignificant, improvement in the disease-free interval in head and neck patients.[174]
4. *Hypofractionation* has usually been associated with large fractions and has led to increased late effects, unless tumor and target volumes are reduced as the total dose increases. When hypofractionation is combined with chemotherapy and other agents, it may prove more effective and efficient. Large, daily fractional doses (3 to 4 Gy) are very effective in relieving obstruction and compression, particularly in radiosensitive and radioresponsive tumors such as in spinal cord compression, superior vena cava obstruction, urethral obstruction, and bronchial or tracheal obstruction. A small field within a large field can also be effective in rapidly growing tumors with large growth fractions requiring large daily doses to be delivered in short time intervals. A once-a-week schedule, or a less-than-daily fractionation (hypofractionation) regimen can be effective for slower growing resistant tumors, tumors with large shoulder (D_q) cell populations, and palliative settings.[172]

Chemical Modifiers: Radiosensitizers and Radioprotectors

The potential effect of radiation modifiers in radiotherapy is illustrated schematically in Figure 6–25.[175, 176] This diagram shows that by protecting the normal tissue or enhancing the radiation damage to the tumor, it is possible to separate further the tumor control and normal tissue complication curves. Such an increased separation will consequently result in an improved therapeutic ratio. As a greater understanding of the underlying mechanisms of oncogene-

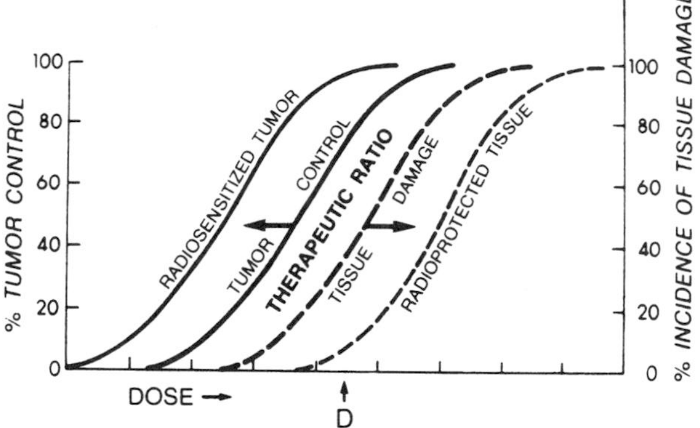

Figure 6–25. The concept of radiosensitization and radioprotection is based on the use of agents that can displace either the tumor dose-response curve to the left or the normal tissue damage curve to the right, thereby increasing the therapeutic ratio.

sis is achieved, a larger spectrum of chemical radiation sensitizers and protectors is now becoming available.[176]

Significant efforts have been expended to overcome the problem of tumor hypoxia,[177] in consideration of the following observations:

- The available oxygen tension in and around a cell determines its radiation response. Well-oxygenated cells can be eradicated more efficiently and effectively (factor of 2.5 to 3.0) by the same dose of x-irradiation.[5]
- Because normal tissues are believed to be fully oxygenated, attempts have been made to increase tumor oxygen tension. Means used have included atmospheric oxygen breathing with 5% CO_2[178]; the more direct means of vascular targeting is now in vogue.[179, 180]

Radiosensitizers. More than 80 randomized studies have been performed worldwide pursuing the goal of hypoxic cell radiosensitization with more than 10,000 patients entered in clinical trials. Horsman and Overgaard, in their analysis, found a 4.6% improvement in local tumor control with only a 2% gain in survival and an increase of 0.6% for the radiosensitizers.[181] The nitroimidazoles, used in approximately half of the patients (5304 in 36 randomized trials), yielded a similar benefit of 3.9% in local control with survival improving in 2.8%. Use of misonidazole was quickly replaced by metronidazole, and more recent drug generations—etanidazole (SR 2508) and pimonidazole—promised a fivefold increase in radiosensitivity; however, randomized clinical trials on both sides of the Atlantic with SR 2508, by the European Organization of Research and Treatment of Cancer[182] and Radiation Therapy Oncology Group,[183] proved to be of no benefit. Only nimorazole has yielded positive results in Denmark.[184] In addition, one compound—namely paclitaxel (taxol)—is currently receiving a great deal of attention. A cytotoxic agent in its own right, it has also proved to be a radiation potentiator and may well prove to be useful in settings with refractory tumors.[185]

Radioprotectors. Sulfhydryl-containing compounds, such as cystine and cysteamine, have long been known to be radioprotective.[175, 186] One of the thiophosphate derivatives of cysteamine, WR-2721, was reported to selectively protect normal tissues, including bone marrow, salivary glands, and intestinal mucosa.[187] It is believed that these sulfhydryl compounds act as radical scavengers that protect from radiation damage by reducing the yield of damaging radiochemical species. Some normal tissue protection has been seen against both radiation-induced and chemotherapy-induced toxicity using WR-2721 in clinical investigations of head and neck, lung, and rectal cancers.[188–190]

Bioreductive Drugs. Interest has turned to this new class of compounds that are drawn to hypoxic cells and preferentially kill them rather than simply causing radiosensitization alone.[191–193] Radiation is still required to eradicate the aerated cells, with bioreductive drugs killing the hypoxic cells. A promising compound is SR 4233 (tirapazamine), with the ability to log kill hypoxic cells efficiently in rodent tumor cells by a factor of 300, referred to as the *hypoxic cytotoxicity ratio*.[194] Tirapazamine is being used in both phase II radiotherapy and phase III chemotherapy trials, exploring this approach based on promising findings in the laboratory.[194]

Cytotoxic Agents

This remains one of the major therapeutic strategies in modern oncology—optimally combining or sequencing chemotherapy and radiation.[133, 195–197] A variety of mechanisms have been defined by Steel and Peckham,[198] including additivity, synergism, and supra-additivity, as well as radiosensitization and spatial cooperation, describing desirable chemotherapy radiation interactions. The isobologram provides a quantitative means to assess the potential effectiveness of combined regimens.[199] However, the modest gains have been somewhat disappointing, despite extensive randomized head and neck cancer clinical trials using simultaneous radiochemotherapy, particularly containing 5-fluorouracil (5-FU) or cisplatin, or both. Bourhis and associates in a large meta-analysis study of 76 trials (11,659 patients) found an absolute benefit of only 4% from chemotherapy[200]; the improvement in 5-year survival rates increased from 32% to 36% in advanced squamous cell cancers of aerodigestive passages.

Because of their spectrum of activities against human neoplasms, cytotoxic chemotherapeutic agents, such as doxorubicin and cyclophosphamide, have been evaluated in combination with radiation therapy as well as a number of other agents, both in the laboratory and in the clinic. However, to date, the optimal employment of cytotoxic agents plus radiation therapy to maximize tumor cell kill while minimizing normal tissue toxicity has not been fully realized. Simultaneous infusion of agents such as 5-fluorouracil, mitomycin C, and cisplatin—singly or in combination—allows for smaller quantities of chemotherapy to be used but increases the effect caused by concurrent administration. This has been successfully used in cancers such as anal cancer, esophageal cancer, and bladder cancer. Pilot phase I and II studies have indicated a tolerable level of toxicity and improved tumor control, requiring phase III clinical trials for confirmation.

Biologic Response Modifiers (Cytokines)

The use of cytokines and growth factors in oncologic treatment is increasing as molecular studies are elaborated, as discussed earlier in this chapter.[201–203] The use of the interferons, both alone and in combination with radiation or chemotherapy, or with both, is a major therapeutic strategy under investigation.

- Interferon-α acts as a differentiation modulator and antiproliferative cytokine, and also has been ascribed to affecting the radiosensitivity of tumors by interfering with cellular DNA repair processes, resulting in an accumulation of sublethal radiation damage. In combination with retinoic acid, it has been shown to be effective in therapy for squamous cell cancer of the skin, head and neck and cervical cancer.[204, 205]
- Interferon-β and radiation produce enhanced killing as a result of an induction of a G_2M block, accumulating cells in a radiosensitive cell cycle phase. The results from preliminary phase I and II trials in treatment of non–small cell lung cancer by McDonald and associates[206] were not confirmed in a larger Radiation Therapy Oncology Group randomized phase III study recently closed.
- Cytokines, such as granulocyte-macrophage colony-stimulating factors, have been used to reduce acute and late normal tissue toxicity to minimize mucositis and promote healing.[207, 208]

Physical Modifiers

Classic radiotherapeutic techniques, using x-irradiation and radium, have been designed to allow for a favorable distribution of dosage between the tumors and the normal tissues in the treatment beam; that is, one attempts to deliver a maximum dose to the tumor and a minimum dose to the normal tissues. Major advances are the use of telecobalt units and linear accelerators that produce megavoltage irradiation and high-energy electrons in the range of 1 to 25 million MeV. The advantages over orthovoltage are as follows:

- better depth doses—more efficient tumor treatment
- less side scatter—less radiation sickness
- no differential absorption by bone—more uniform dosage
- skin sparing effect—only slight radiation dermatitis

X-irradiation and electron irradiation, even in the range of 1 to 6 MeV, are considered low LET irradiations and are less effective in treating hypoxic compared with oxic cells. However, densely ionizing radiations, such as neutrons, negative pi mesons, and accelerated heavy ions, can reduce the importance of tumor hypoxia. The ionizations occur at such close ranges that most hydrogen and hydroxyl radicals tend to combine to form water instead of interacting with organic bases to form organic radicals. Therefore, the absence of oxygen is less influential in determining the quantity of biologic damage. Damage to the important compounds occurs by direct ionization.

One of the most important potential major advances has been the introduction of three-dimensional conformal treatment using computerized three-dimensional treatment planning systems and multileaf collimation to change the portal dynamically to contour, in a beam's eye view, the different tumor shapes from various angles.[209, 210] In Figure 6–26,[211] the probability of complications is seen to be reduced and tumor control improved with intensity modulation techniques in which protocols of dose escalation and normal organ volume reduction or exclusion are attempted. Examples of this new approach demonstrate sparing of the rectal wall in the treatment of prostate cancer, and in head and neck cancer, there is sparing of salivary glands.[212, 213] Proton beams with Bragg peaks are another modality testing tight precise tumor dose configurations.[214, 215] Stereotactic techniques are widely used for solitary CNS metastases and small malignant gliomas (<4 cm), with increasing success based on three-dimensional conformal treatment principles.[216, 217] More detail is provided in Chapter 7, Radiation Physics as Applied to Clinical Radiation Oncology.

Recommended Reading

There is a rich and wide-ranging literature on radiation oncology based on the sciences and advances of radiation

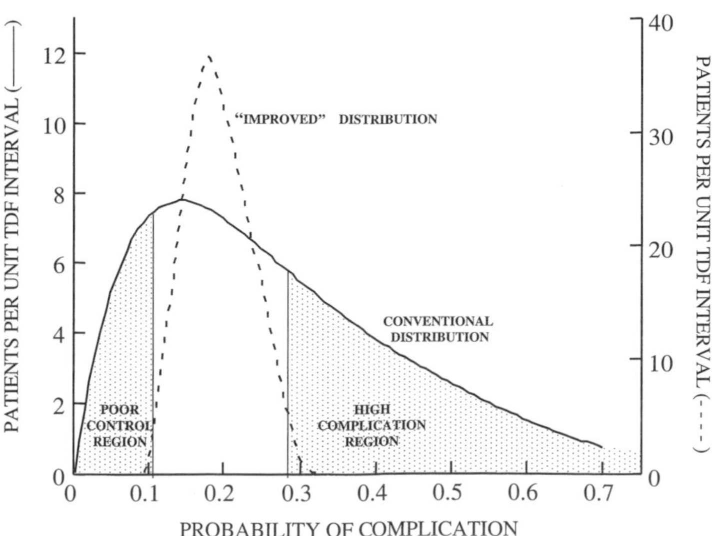

Figure 6–26. Frequency distribution of patients with different probabilities of complication. (From Orton CG: Other considerations in three-dimensional treatment planning. In Bagne F [ed]: Computerized Treatment Planning Systems, p 136. HHS Publications FDA 84-8223, 1984, with permission.)

biology and radiation physics. *Principles and Practice of Radiation Oncology* by Perez and Brady, in its recent third edition,[1] is an excellent starting place for an integrated approach to these elements, with an emphasis on the clinical and medical aspects of cancer at each disease site. Another major textbook in radiation oncology, published in 1998 and in its first, very comprehensive edition, is *Textbook of Radiation Oncology* edited by Leibel and Phillips.[2] New editions of major oncology textbooks have excellent chapters devoted to principles of radiation oncology—*Cancer: Principles & Practice of Oncology*, 5th edition,[3] edited by DeVita and associates, and *Clinical Oncology*, 2nd edition,[4] edited by Abeloff and colleagues. The radiobiologic basis of radiation oncology is addressed concisely and succinctly in Hall's *Radiobiology for the Radiologist*, 4th edition,[5] and Andrews offers a historical perspective on the development of radiation and its integration with other modes of therapy in *The Radiobiology of Human Cancer Radiotherapy*.[6] The study of radiation late effects is described fully in the now-classic *Clinical Radiation Pathology* by Rubin and Casarett.[7] *Progress in Radio-Oncology VI*, edited by Kogelnik and Sedlmayer, is devoted to innovations and advances and provides an excellent window on European, American, and Asian investigations.[8]

REFERENCES

General References

1. Perez CA, Brady LW (eds): Principles and Practice of Radiation Oncology, 3rd ed. Philadelphia, Lippincott-Raven, 1998.
2. Leibel SA, Phillips TL (eds): Textbook of Radiation Oncology. Philadelphia, WB Saunders, 1998.
3. DeVita VT Jr, Hellman S, Rosenberg SA (eds): Cancer: Principles & Practice of Oncology, 5th ed. Philadelphia, Lippincott-Raven, 1997.
4. Abeloff MD, Armitage JO, Lichter AS, Niederhuber JE (eds): Clinical Oncology, 2nd ed. New York, Churchill Livingstone, 2000.
5. Hall EJ: Radiobiology for the Radiologist, 4th ed. Philadelphia, JB Lippincott Co., 1994.
6. Andrews JR (ed): The Radiobiology of Human Cancer Radiotherapy, 2nd ed. Baltimore, University Park Press, 1978.
7. Rubin P, Casarett GW: Clinical Radiation Pathology. Philadelphia, W.B. Saunders, 1968.
8. Kogelnik HD, Sedlmayer F (eds): Progress in Radio-Oncology VI. Bologna, Monduzzi Editore, 1998.

Specific References

9. Coleman CN, Harris JR: Current scientific issues related to clinical radiation oncology. Radiat Res 1998; 150:125.
10. Stone HB, Dewey WC, Wallace SS, et al: Molecular biology to radiation oncology: a model for translational research? Opportunities in basic and translational research. Radiat Res 1998; 150:134.
11. Wilson JF: Syllabus: A Categorical Course in Radiation Therapy: Cure with Preservation of Function and Aesthetics, p 5. Oak Brook, IL, Radiological Society of North America, 1998.
12. Cancer Facts and Figures—1996. Atlanta, American Cancer Society, 1996.
13. Constine LS: Tumors in children. In: Wilson JF (ed): Syllabus: A Categorical Course in Radiation Therapy: Cure with Preservation of Function and Aesthetics, p 75. Oak Brook, IL, Radiological Society of North America, 1988.
14. Kaplan HS: Hodgkin's Disease, 2nd ed. Cambridge, Harvard University Press, 1980.
15. Morrow CP, Cozen W: Perspective on cervical cancer: Why prevent? J Cell Biochem 1995; 23(suppl):61.
16. Singer A: Cervical cancer screening: state of the art. Baillieres Clin Obstet Gynaecol 1995; 9:39.
17. Orth G, Croissant O: Human papillomaviruses and carcinogenesis of the uterine cervix: future prospects in the domain of detection and prevention. Bull Acad Natl Med 1997; 181:1365.
18. Mencaglia L, Valle RF, Perino A, et al: Endometrial carcinoma and its precursors: early detection and treatment. Int J Gynaecol Obstet 1990; 31:107.
19. Hazuka MB, Martel MK, Marsh L, et al: Preservation of parotid function after external beam irradiation in head and neck cancer patients: a feasibility study using 3-dimensional treatment planning. Int J Radiat Oncol Biol Phys 1993; 27:731.
20. Mittal BB: Advanced techniques in radiation therapy for head and neck cancers. Otolaryngol Clin North Am 1991; 24:1569.
21. Moller T: Head and neck cancer. Acta Oncol 1996; 35(suppl 7):22.
22. Lichter AS, Lawrence TS: Recent advances in radiation oncology. N Engl J Med 1995; 332:371.
23. Wilson RE, Taylor SL, Atherton GT, et al: Early response gene signalling cascades activated by ionizing radiation in primary human B cells. Oncogene 1993; 8:3229.
24. Usenius T, Tenhunen M, Koistinaho J: Ionizing radiation induces expression of immediate early genes in the rat brain. Neuroreport 1996; 7:2559.
25. Ferrer I, Olive M, Blanco R, et al: Selective c-Jun overexpression is associated with ionizing radiation-induced apoptosis in the developing cerebellum of the rat. Brain Res Mol Brain Res 1996; 38:91.
26. Bosman FT, Visser BC, van Oeveren J: Apoptosis: pathophysiology of programmed cell death. Pathol Res Prac 1996; 192:676.
27. Guchelaar HJ, Vermes A, Vermes I, et al: Apoptosis: molecular mechanisms and implications for cancer chemotherapy. Pharm World Sci 1997; 19:119.
28. O'Connor PM, Fan S: DNA damage checkpoints: implications for cancer therapy. Prog Cell Cycle Res 1996; 2:165.
29. Nishio K, Arioka H, Saijo N: Apoptosis and chemosensitivity. Gan To Kagaku Ryoho 1997; 24:216.
30. Dietrich JB: Apoptosis and anti-apoptosis genes in the Bcl-2 family. Arch Physiol Biochem 1997; 105:125.
31. Hawkins CJ, Vaux DL: The role of the Bcl-2 family of apoptosis regulatory proteins in the immune system. Semin Immunol 1997; 9:25.
32. McDonnell TJ, Beham A, Sarkiss M, et al: Importance of the Bcl-2 family in cell death regulation. Experientia 1996; 52:1008.
33. Asoh S: Mechanism of apoptosis induced by the Bax protein. Nippon Ika Daigaku Zasshi 1997; 64:463.
34. Lotem J, Sachs L: Control of apoptosis in hematopoiesis and leukemia by cytokines, tumor suppressor and oncogenes. Leukemia 1996; 10:925.
35. Larsen CJ: The Bcl2 gene, prototype of a gene family that controls programmed cell death (apoptosis). Ann Genet 1994; 37:121.
36. McBride WH, Dougherty GJ, Syljuasen R, et al: New molecular and genetic approaches aimed at improving radiation therapy. In: Kogelnik HD, Sedlmayer F (eds): Progress in Radio-Oncology VI, p 27. Bologna, Monduzzi Editore, 1998.
37. Kondo H, Nobuoka A: Clinical application of oncogene and antioncogene as a tumor marker. Nippon Rinsho 1996; 54:1494.
38. Spitz FR, Nguyen D, Skibber JM, et al: In vivo adenovirus-mediated p53 tumor suppressor gene therapy for colorectal cancer. Anticancer Res 1996; 16:3415.
39. Grasso L, Mercer WE: Pathways of p53-dependent apoptosis. Vitam Horm 1997; 53:139.
40. Pekkola-Heino K, Servomaa K, Kiuru A, et al: Increased radiosensitivity is associated with p53 mutations in cell lines derived from oral cavity carcinoma. Acta Otolaryngol (Stockh) 1996; 116:341.
41. Naida JD, Davis MA, Lawrence TS: The effect of activation of wild-type p53 function on fluoropyrimidine-mediated radiosensitization. Int J Radiat Oncol Biol Phys 1998; 41:675.
42. Weller M: Predicting response to cancer chemotherapy: the role of p53. Cell Tiss Res 1998; 292:435.
43. Mueller H, Eppenberger U: The dual role of mutant p53 protein in chemosensitivity of human cancers. Anticancer Res 1996; 16:3845.
44. Yount GL, Haas-Kogan DA, Vidair CA, et al: Cell cycle synchrony unmasks the influence of p53 function on radiosensitivity of human glioblastoma cells. Cancer Res 1996; 56:500.
45. Gjerset RA, Turla ST, Sobol RE, et al: Use of wild-type p53 to achieve complete treatment sensitization of tumor cells expressing endogenous mutant p53. Mol Carcinog 1995; 14:275.
46. Miyakoshi J, Yamagishi N, Ohtsu S, et al: Changes in radiation sensitivity of human osteosarcoma cells after p53 introduction. Jpn J Cancer Res 1995; 86:711.

47. Wang TH, Wang HS: p53, apoptosis and human cancers. J Formos Med Assoc 1996; 95:509.
48. Huang A, Gandour-Edwards R, Rosenthal SA, et al: p53 and bcl-2 immunohistochemical alterations in prostate cancer treated with radiation therapy. Urology 1998; 51:346.
49. Zellars RC, Naida JD, Davis MA, et al: Effect of p53 overexpression on radiation sensitivity of human colon cancer cells. Radiat Oncol Invest 1997; 5:43.
50. Dulic V, Kaufmann WK, Wilson SJ, et al: p53-dependent inhibition of cyclin-dependent kinase activities in human fibroblasts during radiation-induced G1 arrest. Cell 1994; 76:1013.
51. Hochhauser D: Modulation of chemosensitivity through altered expression of cell cycle regulatory genes in cancer. Anticancer Drugs 1997; 8:903.
52. Li YX, Weber-Johnson K, Sun LQ, et al: Effect of pentoxifylline on radiation-induced G2-phase delay and radiosensitivity of human colon and cervical cancer cells. Radiat Res 1998; 149:338.
53. Rubin P, Johnston CJ, Williams JP, et al: A perpetual cascade of cytokines postirradiation leads to pulmonary fibrosis. Int J Radiat Oncol Biol Phys 1995; 33:99.
54. Dachs GU, Dougherty GJ, Stratford IJ, et al: Targeting gene therapy to cancer: a review. Oncol Res 1997; 9:313.
55. Bertelsen AH, Beaudry GA, Stoller TJ, et al: Tumor suppressor genes: prospects for cancer therapies. Biotechnology 1995; 13:127.
56. Sokol DL, Gewirtz AM: Gene therapy: basic concepts and recent advances. Crit Rev Eukaryot Gene Expr 1996; 6:29.
57. Uckert W, Kammertons T, Haack K, et al: Double suicide gene (cytosine deaminase and herpes simplex virus thymidine kinase) but not single gene transfer allows reliable elimination of tumor cells in vivo. Hum Gene Ther 1998; 9:855.
58. Denning C, Pitts JD: Bystander effects of different enzyme-prodrug systems for cancer gene therapy depend on different pathways for intercellular transfer of toxic metabolites, a factor that will govern clinical choice of appropriate regimes. Hum Gene Ther 1997; 8:1825.
59. Withers HR, McBride WH: Biologic basis of radiation therapy. In: Perez CA, Brady LW (eds): Principles and Practice of Radiation Oncology, 3rd ed, p 79. Philadelphia, Lippincott-Raven, 1998.
60. Cosset JM, Peters LJ, Girinsky T, et al: Predictive tests of radiocurability: towards a custom-made radiotherapy? Bull Cancer (Paris) 1990; 77:83.
61. Fletcher GH: Textbook of Radiotherapy. Philadelphia, Lea & Febiger, 1980.
62. Weichselbaum RR, Beckett MA, Vokes EE, et al: Cellular and molecular mechanisms of radioresistance. Cancer Treat Res 1995; 74:131.
63. Bergman PJ, Harris D: Radioresistance, chemoresistance, and apoptosis resistance. The past, present, and future. Vet Clin North Am 1997; 27:47.
64. Meyn RE, Stephens LC, Milas L: Programmed cell death and radioresistance. Cancer Metastasis Rev 1996; 15:119.
65. Weichselbaum RR, Beckett MA, Hallahan DE, et al: Molecular targets to overcome radioresistance. Semin Oncol 1992; 19:14.
66. Hellman S: Principles of cancer management: radiation therapy. In: DeVita VT Jr, Hellman S, Rosenberg SA (eds): Cancer. Principles & Practice of Oncology, 5th edition, vol 1, p 307. Philadelphia, Lippincott-Raven, 1997.
67. Burnet NG, Wurm R, Nyman J, et al: Radiation sensitivity—from laboratory to clinic. In: Tobias JS, Thomas PRM (eds): Current Radiation Oncology, vol 3, p 27. London, Arnold, 1998.
68. Weichselbaum RR, Beckett MA, Vijayakumar S, et al: Radiobiological characterization of head and neck and sarcoma cells derived from patients prior to radiotherapy. Int J Radiat Oncol Biol Phys 1990; 19:313.
69. Sephton RG: Current concepts in radiobiology applied to radiotherapy. Australas Phys Eng Sci Med 1991; 14:130.
70. Bentzen SM: Quantitative clinical radiobiology. Acta Oncol 1993; 32:259.
71. West CM: Intrinsic radiosensitivity as a predictor of patient response to radiotherapy. Br J Radiol 1995; 68:827.
72. Malaise EP, Fertil B, Chavaudra N, et al: Distribution of radiation sensitivities for human tumor cells of specific histological types: comparison of in vitro to in vivo data. Int J Radiat Oncol Biol Phys 1986; 12:617.
73. West CM, Davidson SE, Elyan SA, et al: The intrinsic radiosensitivity of normal and tumour cells. Int J Radiat Biol 1998; 73:409.
74. Peters LJ, Brock WA, Chapman JD, et al: Predictive assays of tumor radiocurability. Am J Clin Oncol 1988; 11:275.
75. Sasai K, Evans JW, Kovacs MS, et al: Prediction of human cell radiosensitivity: comparison of clonogenic assay with chromosome aberrations scored using premature chromosome condensation with fluorescence in situ hybridization. Int J Radiat Oncol Biol Phys 1994; 30:1127.
76. Gerweck LE, Zaidi ST, Zietman A: Multivariate determinants of radiocurability. I: Prediction of single fraction tumor control doses. Int J Radiat Oncol Biol Phys 1994; 29:57.
77. Fertil B, Malaise EP: Intrinsic radiosensitivity of human cell lines is correlated with radioresponsiveness of human tumors: analysis of 101 published survival curves. Int J Radiat Oncol Biol Phys 1985; 11:1699.
78. Lambin P, Fertil B, Malaise EP, et al: Multiphasic survival curves for cells of human tumor cell lines: induced repair or hypersensitive subpopulation? Radiat Res 1994; 138:S32.
79. West CM, Davidson SE, Burt PA, et al: The intrinsic radiosensitivity of cervical carcinoma: correlations with clinical data. Int J Radiat Oncol Biol Phys 1995; 31:841.
80. Denekamp J, Fowler JF: ARCON—current status: summary of a workshop on preclinical and clinical studies. Acta Oncol 1997; 36:517.
81. Kallman RF: Reoxygenation and repopulation in irradiated tumors. Front Radiat Ther Oncol 1988; 22:30.
82. Brown JM: Evidence for acutely hypoxic cells in mouse tumours and a possible mechanism of reoxygenation. Br J Radiol 1979; 52:650.
83. Moulder JE, Rockwell S: Hypoxic fractions of solid tumors. Int J Radiat Oncol Biol Phys 1984; 10:695.
84. Stone HB, Brown JM, Phillips TL, et al: Oxygen in human tumors: Correlations between methods of measurement and response to therapy. Radiat Res 1993; 136:422.
85. Milas L, Hunter N, Peters LJ: Tumor bed effect-induced reduction of tumor radiocurability through the increase in hypoxic cell fraction. Int J Radiat Oncol Biol Phys 1989; 16:139.
86. Hockel M, Schlenger K, Arad D, et al: Association between tumor hypoxia and malignant progression in advanced cancer of the uterine cervix. Cancer Res 1996; 56:4509.
87. van Putten LM, Kallman RF: Oxygenation status of a transplantable tumor during fractionated radiation therapy. J Natl Cancer Inst 1968; 40:441.
88. Hewitt HB, Wilson CW: The effect of tissue oxygen tension on the radiosensitivity of leukaemia cells irradiated in situ in the livers of leukaemic mice. Br J Cancer 1959; 13:675.
89. Withers HR, Thames HD: Dose fractionation and volume effects in normal tissues and tumors. Am J Clin Oncol 1988; 11:313.
90. Pigott KH, Hill SA, Chaplin DJ, et al: Microregional fluctuations in perfusion within human tumours detected using laser Doppler flowmetry. Radiother Oncol 1996; 40:45.
91. Wouters BG, Brown JM: Cells at intermediate oxygen levels can be more important than the "hypoxic fraction" in determining tumor response to fractionated radiotherapy. Radiat Res 1997; 147:541.
92. Chaplin DJ, Hill SA, Bell KM, et al: Modification of tumor blood flow: current status and future directions. Semin Radiat Oncol 1998; 8:151.
93. Denekamp J: Cell kinetics and radiation biology. Int J Radiat Biol Rel Stud Phys Chem Med 1986; 49:357.
94. Kastan MB: Molecular biology of cancer: the cell cycle. In: DeVita VT Jr, Hellman S, Rosenberg SA (eds): Cancer: Principles & Practice of Oncology, 5th ed, vol 1, p 121. Philadelphia, Lippincott-Raven, 1997.
95. Sinclair WK: Cyclic X-ray responses in mammalian cells in vitro. Radiat Res 1968; 33:620.
96. Elkind MM, Whitmore G: The Radiobiology of Cultured Mammalian Cells. New York, Gordon & Breach, 1967.
97. van der Schueren E, Landuyt W, Scalliet P: Repair of 'sublethal damage': key factor in normal tissue tolerance to fractionated and low dose rate irradiation. Front Radiat Ther Oncol 1989; 23:60.
98. Fu KK: Biological basis for the interaction of chemotherapeutic agents and radiation therapy. Cancer 1985; 55:2123.
99. Hopewell JW: The volume effect in radiotherapy—its biological significance. Br J Radiol 1997; 70(suppl):S32.
100. Rubin P, Finkelstein JN, Williams JP: Paradigm shifts in the radiation pathophysiology of late effects in normal tissues: molecular vs classic concepts. In: Tobias JS, Thomas PRM (eds): Current Radiation Oncology, 3rd ed, p 1. London, Arnold, 1998.

101. Emami B, Lyman J, Brown A, et al: Tolerance of normal tissue to therapeutic irradiation. Int J Radiat Oncol Biol Phys 1991; 21:109.
102. Burnet NG, Wurm R, Nyman J, et al: Normal tissue radiosensitivity—how important is it? Clin Oncol 1996; 8:25.
103. Suit HD, Baumann M, Skates S, et al: Clinical interest in determinations of cellular radiation sensitivity. Int J Radiat Biol 1989; 56:725.
104. Cowdry EV: Textbook of Histology, 4th ed. Philadelphia, Lea & Febiger, 1950.
105. Hopewell JW: The importance of vascular damage in the development of late radiation effects in normal tissues. In: Meyn RE, Withers HR (eds): Radiation Biology in Cancer Research, p 449. New York, Raven Press, 1979.
106. Armitage RJ, Tough TW, Macduff BM, et al: CD40 ligand is a T cell growth factor. Eur J Immunol 1993; 23:2326.
107. Duchting W, Ulmer W, Ginsberg T, et al: Radiogenic responses of normal cells induced by fractionated irradiation—a simulation study. Part II. Late responses. Strahlenther Onkol 1995; 171:525.
108. Wheldon TE, Michalowski AS, Kirk J: The effect of irradiation on function in self-renewing normal tissues with differing proliferative organisation. Br J Radiol 1982; 55:759.
109. Billingham ME, Bristow MR, Glatstein E, et al: Adriamycin cardiotoxicity: endomyocardial biopsy evidence of enhancement by irradiation. Am J Surg Pathol 1977; 1:17.
110. Putterman C, Polliack A: Late cardiovascular and pulmonary complications of therapy in Hodgkin's disease: report of three unusual cases, with a review of relevant literature. Leuk Lymphoma 1992; 7:109.
111. Peters LJ: Radiation therapy tolerance limits. For one or for all? Cancer 1996; 77:2379.
112. Begnozzi L, Gentile FP, Di Nallo AM, et al: A simple method to calculate the influence of dose inhomogeneity and fractionation in normal tissue complication probability evaluation. Strahlenther Onkol 1994; 170:590.
113. Zaider M, Amols HI: A little to a lot or a lot to a little: is NTCP always minimized in multiport therapy? Int J Radiat Oncol Biol Phys 1998; 41:945.
114. Lyman JT, Wolbarst AB: Optimization of radiation therapy, IV: A dose-volume histogram reduction algorithm. Int J Radiat Oncol Biol Phys 1989; 17:433.
115. Mendelsohn ML: The biology of dose-limiting tissues. In: Time and Dose Relationships in Radiation Biology as Applied to Radiotherapy, Brookhaven National Laboratory (BNL) Report 5023 (C-57), p 154. Upton, NY, Brookhaven National Laboratory, 1969.
116. Lyman JT, Wolbarst AB: Optimization of radiation therapy, III: A method of assessing complication probabilities from dose-volume histograms. Int J Radiat Oncol Biol Phys 1987; 13:103.
117. Lawrence TS, Kessler ML, Ten Haken RK: Clinical interpretation of dose-volume histograms: the basis for normal tissue preservation and tumor dose escalation. Front Radiat Ther Oncol 1996; 29:57.
118. Brock WA, Tucker SL, Geara FB, et al: Fibroblast radiosensitivity versus acute and late normal skin responses in patients treated for breast cancer. Int J Radiat Oncol Biol Phys 1995; 32:1371.
119. Johansen J, Bentzen SM, Overgaard J, et al: Relationship between the in vitro radiosensitivity of skin fibroblasts and the expression of subcutaneous fibrosis, telangiectasia, and skin erythema after radiotherapy. Radiother Oncol 1996; 40:101.
120. Russell NS, Grummels A, Hart AA, et al: Low predictive value of intrinsic fibroblast radiosensitivity for fibrosis development following radiotherapy for breast cancer. Int J Radiat Biol 1998; 73:661.
121. Hansgen G, Hintner I, Krause V, et al: Intratumor pO_2, S-phase fraction and p53 status in cervix carcinomas. Strahlenther Onkol 1997; 173:385.
122. Peters L, Hicks R, Binns D, et al: Prediction of tumour response: cause-specific vs empiric factors. In: Kogelnik HD, Sedlmayer F (eds): Progress in Radio-Oncology VI, p 463. Bologna, Monduzzi Editore, 1998.
123. Begg AC, Hofland I, Moonen L, et al: The predictive value of cell kinetic measurements in a European trial of accelerated fractionation in advanced head and neck tumors: an interim report. Int J Radiat Oncol Biol Phys 1990; 19:1449.
124. Begg AC, Hofland I, Van Glabbeke M, et al: Predictive value of potential doubling time for radiotherapy of head and neck tumor patients: results from the EORTC cooperative trial 22851. Semin Radiat Oncol 1992; 1:22.
125. Streffer C, Bauch Th, Stüben G, et al: Predictive assays for individualization of cancer therapy. In Kogelnik HD, Sedlmayer F (eds): Progress in Radio-Oncology VI, p 501. Bologna, Monduzzi Editore, 1998.
126. Curran AJ, St Denis K, Irish J, et al: Telomerase activity in oral squamous cell carcinoma. Arch Otolaryngol 1998; 124:784.
127. Sumida T, Sogawa K, Hamakawa H, et al: Detection of telomerase activity in oral lesions. J Oral Pathol Med 1998; 27:111.
128. West CM, Davidson SE, Roberts SA, et al: The independence of intrinsic radiosensitivity as a prognostic factor for patient response to radiotherapy of carcinoma of the cervix. Br J Cancer 1997; 76:1184.
129. West CML, Cooper R, Davidson SE, et al: Optimising measurements of tumour radiosensitivity. In: Kogelnik HD, Sedlmayer F (eds): Progress in Radio-Oncology VI, p 517. Bologna, Monduzzi Editore, 1998.
130. Anscher MS, Peters WP, Reisenbichler H, et al: Transforming growth factor-β as a predictor of liver and lung fibrosis after autologous bone marrow transplantation for advanced breast cancer. N Engl J Med 1993; 328:1592.
131. Perez CA, Korba A, Zivnuska F, et al: 60Co moving strip technique in the management of carcinoma of the ovary: analysis of tumor control and morbidity. Int J Radiat Oncol Biol Phys 1978; 4:379.
132. Chen Y, Rubin P, Smudzin T, et al: IL-6 and circulating lymphocytes in the modulation of radiation pulmonary injury [Abstract]. Int J Radiat Oncol Biol Phys 1998; 42(1S):167.
133. John MJ, Flam MS, Legha SS, et al: Chemoradiation: An Integrated Approach to Cancer Treatment. Malvern, Lea & Febiger, 1993.
134. Myerson RJ, Moros E, Roti Roti JL: Hyperthermia. In: Perez CA, Brady LW (eds): Principles and Practice of Radiation Oncology, 3rd ed, p 637. Philadelphia, Lippincott-Raven, 1998.
135. Hallahan DE, Weichselbaum R: Role of gene therapy in radiation oncology. Cancer Treat Res 1998; 93:153.
136. Rockwell S: Oxygen delivery: implications for the biology and therapy of solid tumors. Oncol Res 1997; 9:383.
137. Langmuir VK: The use of radioimmunotherapy in combination with bioreductive agents. Recent Results Cancer Res 1996; 141:137.
138. Horsman MR: Nicotinamide and other benzamide analogs as agents for overcoming hypoxic cell radiation resistance in tumours. A review. Acta Oncol 1995; 34:571.
139. Strandqvist M: Studien uber die Kumulative Wirkung der Rontgenstrahlen bei Fraktionierung. Acta Radiol 1944; 55(Suppl Stockh):1.
140. Ellis F: Dose, time and fractionation: a clinical hypothesis. Clin Radiol 1969; 20:1.
141. Orton CG, Ellis F: A simplification in the use of the NSD concept in practical radiotherapy. Br J Radiol 1973; 46:529.
142. Ellis F: Is NSD-TDF useful to radiotherapy? Int J Radiat Oncol Biol Phys 1985; 11:1685.
143. Orton CG, Cohen L: A unified approach to dose-effect relationships in radiotherapy. I: Modified TDF and linear quadratic equations. Int J Radiat Oncol Biol Phys 1988; 14:549.
144. Orton CG: A unified approach to dose-effect relationships in radiotherapy. II: Inhomogeneous dose distributions. Int J Radiat Oncol Biol Phys 1988; 14:557.
145. Kirk G, Gray WM, Watson ER: Cumulative radiation effect, Part I. Fractionation treatment regimens. Clin Radiol 1971; 122:145.
146. Turesson I, Notter G: The influence of the overall treatment time in radiotherapy on the acute reaction: comparison of the effects of daily and twice-a-week fractionation on human skin. Int J Radiat Oncol Biol Phys 1984; 10:607.
147. Turesson I, Notter G: The influence of fraction size in radiotherapy on the late normal tissue reaction—I: Comparison of the effects of daily and once-a-week fractionation on human skin. Int J Radiat Oncol Biol Phys 1984; 10:593.
148. Turesson I, Notter G: The influence of fraction size in radiotherapy on the late normal tissue reaction—II: Comparison of the effects of daily and twice-a-week fractionation on human skin. Int J Radiat Oncol Biol Phys 1984; 10:599.
149. Fowler JR: Fractionation and therapeutic gain. In: Steel GG, Adams GED, Peckham MJ (eds): Biological Basis of Radiotherapy, p 181. Amsterdam, Elsevier Science, 1983.
150. Thames HD Jr, Withers HR, Peters LJ, et al: Changes in early and late radiation responses with altered dose fractionation: implications for dose-survival relationships. Int J Radiat Oncol Biol Phys 1982; 8:219.
151. Thames HD, Bentzen SM, Turesson I, et al: Time-dose factors in radiotherapy: a review of the human data. Radiother Oncol 1990; 19:219.

152. Withers HR: Biologic basis for altered fractionation schemes. Cancer 1985; 55:2086.
153. Barton MB, Withers HR: The effect of radiotherapy treatment time on tumour control. In: Tobias JS, Thomas PRM (eds): Current Radiation Oncology, vol 3, p 58. London, Arnold, 1997.
154. Fischer DB, Fischer JJ: Dose-response relationships in radiotherapy: applications of logistic regression model. Int J Radiat Oncol Biol Phys 1977; 2:773.
155. Trott KR, Kummermehr J: The time factor and repopulation in tumours and normal tissues. Semin Radiat Oncol 1993; 3:115.
156. Steel GG: The ESTRO Breur lecture. Cellular sensitivity to low dose-rate irradiation focuses the problem of tumour radioresistance. Radiother Oncol 1991; 20:71.
157. Overgaard J, Hjelm-Hansen M, Johansen V, et al: Comparison of conventional and split-course radiotherapy as primary treatment in carcinoma of the larynx. Acta Oncol 1988; 27:147.
158. Hall EJ: Radiation dose-rate: a factor of importance in radiobiology and radiotherapy. Br J Radiol 1972; 45:81.
159. Orton CG: Time-dose factors (TDFs) in brachytherapy. Br J Radiol 1974; 47:603.
160. Hall EJ: Weiss lecture. The dose-rate factor in radiation biology. Int J Radiat Biol 1991; 59:595.
161. Brenner DJ: Radiation biology in brachytherapy. J Surg Oncol 1997; 65:66.
162. Orton CG: High and low dose-rate brachytherapy for cervical carcinoma. Acta Oncol 1998; 37:117.
163. Dale RG, Jones B: The clinical radiobiology of brachytherapy. Br J Radiol 1998; 71:465.
164. Wallner K, Roy J, Harrison L: Dosimetry guidelines to minimize urethral and rectal morbidity following transperineal I-125 prostate brachytherapy. Int J Radiat Oncol Biol Phys 1995; 32:465.
165. Jereczek-Fossa B, Jassem J, Nowak R, et al: Late complications after postoperative radiotherapy in endometrial cancer: analysis of 317 consecutive cases with application of linear-quadratic model. Int J Radiat Oncol Biol Phys 1998; 41:329.
166. Perez CA, Brady LW, Roti Roti JL: Overview. In: Perez CA, Brady LW (eds): Principles and Practice of Radiation Oncology, 3rd ed, p 1. Philadelphia, Lippincott-Raven, 1997.
167. Marcial VA, Pajak TF, Rotman M, et al: "Compensated" split-course versus continuous radiation therapy of carcinoma of the tonsillar fossa. Final results of a prospective randomized clinical trial of the Radiation Therapy Oncology Group. Am J Clin Oncol 1993; 16:389.
168. Horiot JC, Le Fur R, N'Guyen T, et al: Hyperfractionation versus conventional fractionation in oropharyngeal carcinoma: final analysis of a randomized trial of the EORTC cooperative group of radiotherapy. Radiother Oncol 1992; 25:231.
169. Stuschke M, Thames HD: Hyperfractionated radiotherapy of human tumors: overview of the randomized clinical trials. Int J Radiat Oncol Biol Phys 1997; 37:259.
170. Beck-Bornholdt HP, Dubben HH, Liertz-Petersen C, et al: Hyperfractionation: where do we stand? Radiother Oncol 1997; 43:1.
171. Jeremic B, Shibamoto Y, Acimovic L, et al: Hyperfractionated radiotherapy alone for clinical stage I nonsmall cell lung cancer. Int J Radiat Oncol Biol Phys 1997; 38:521.
172. Palazzi M, Cerrotta A, Villa S: Altered fractionation radiotherapy in lung cancer. Tumori 1998; 84:171.
173. Wang CC, Blitzer PH, Suit HD: Twice-a-day radiation therapy for cancer of the head and neck. Cancer 1985; 55:2100.
174. Saunders MI, Dische S, Barrett A, et al: Randomised multicentre trials of CHART vs conventional radiotherapy in head and neck and non-small-cell lung cancer: an interim report. CHART Steering Committee. Br J Cancer 1996; 73:1455.
175. Brown JM, Hall EJ, Hirst DG, et al: Chemical modification of radiation and chemotherapy. Am J Clin Oncol 1988; 11:288.
176. Coleman CN: Chemical sensitizers and protectors. Int J Radiat Oncol Biol Phys 1998; 42:781.
177. Siemann DW: The tumor microenvironment: a double-edged sword. Int J Radiat Oncol Biol Phys 1998; 42:697.
178. Griffin RJ, Okajima K, Song CW: The optimal combination of hyperthermia and carbogen breathing to increase tumor oxygenation and radiation response. Int J Radiat Oncol Biol Phys 1998; 42:865.
179. Horsman MR, Ehrnrooth E, Ladekarl M, et al: The effect of combrestatin A-4 disodium phosphate in a C3H mammary carcinoma and a variety of murine spontaneous tumors. Int J Radiat Oncol Biol Phys 1998; 42:895.
180. Wilson WR, Li AE, Cowan SM, et al: Enhancement of tumor radiation response by the antivascular agent 5,6-dimethylxanthenone-4-acetic acid. Int J Radiat Oncol Biol Phys 1998; 42:905.
181. Horsman MR, Overgaard J: The oxygen effect. In: Steel GG (ed): Basic Clinical Radiobiology, p 132. London, Arnold, 1997.
182. Eschwege F, Sancho-Garnier H, Chassagne D, et al: Results of a European randomized trial of Etanidazole combined with radiotherapy in head and neck carcinomas. Int J Radiat Oncol Biol Phys 1997; 39:275.
183. Riese NE, Buswell L, Noll L, et al: Pharmacokinetic monitoring and dose modification of etanidazole in the RTOG 85-27 phase III head and neck trial. Int J Radiat Oncol Biol Phys 1997; 39:855.
184. Overgaard J, Sand Hansen H, Overgaard M, et al: Randomised double-blind phase III study of nimorazole as a hypoxic radiosensitizer of primary radiotherapy in supraglottic larynx and pharynx carcinoma. Results of the Danish Head and Neck Cancer Study (DAHANCA) protocol 5-85. Radiother Oncol 1998; 46:135.
185. Choy H, Yee L, Cole BF: Combined-modality therapy for advanced non-small cell lung cancer: paclitaxel and thoracic irradiation. Semin Oncol 1995; 22:38.
186. Uma Devi P: Normal tissue protection in cancer therapy—progress and prospects. Acta Oncol 1998; 37:247.
187. Schein PS: WR-2721: a chemotherapy and radiation-protective agent. Cancer Invest 1990; 8:265.
188. Tannehill SP, Mehta MP, Larson M, et al: Effect of amifostine on toxicities associated with sequential chemotherapy and radiation therapy for unresectable non-small-cell lung cancer: results of a phase II trial. J Clin Oncol 1997; 15:2850.
189. Wagner W, Prott FJ, Schonekas KG: Amifostine: a radioprotector in locally advanced head and neck tumors. Oncol Rep 1998; 5:1255.
190. Poplin EA, LoRusso P, Lokich JJ, et al: Randomized clinical trial of mitomycin-C with or without pretreatment with WR-2721 in patients with advanced colorectal cancer. Cancer Chemother Pharmacol 1994; 33:415.
191. Rauth AM, Melo T, Misra V: Bioreductive therapies: an overview of drugs and their mechanisms of action. Int J Radiat Oncol Biol Phys 1998; 42:755.
192. Kelson AB, McNamara JP, Pandey A, et al: 1,2,4-Benzotriazine 1,4-dioxides. An important class of hypoxic cytotoxins with antitumor activity. Anticancer Drug Des 1998; 13:575.
193. Patterson AV, Saunders MP, Chinje EC, et al: Enzymology of tirapazamine metabolism: a review. Anticancer Drug Des 1998; 13:541.
194. Brown JM, Wang LH: Tirapazamine: laboratory data relevant to clinical activity. Anticancer Drug Des 1998; 13:529.
195. Robertson JM, Shewach DS, Lawrence TS: Preclinical studies of chemotherapy and radiation therapy for pancreatic carcinoma. Cancer 1996; 78:674.
196. Aisner J, Hiponia D, Conley B, et al: Combined modalities in the treatment of head and neck cancers. Semin Oncol 1995; 22:28.
197. Hennequin C, Favaudon V, Balosso J, et al: Radio-chemotherapy combinations: from biology to clinics. Bull Cancer (Paris) 1994; 81:1005.
198. Steel GG, Peckham MJ: Exploitable mechanisms in combined radiotherapy-chemotherapy: the concept of additivity. Int J Radiat Oncol Biol Phys 1979; 5:85.
199. Gessner PK: Isobolographic analysis of interactions: an update on applications and utility. Toxicology 1995; 105:161.
200. Bourhis J, Pignon JP, Domenge C, et al: Meta-analysis of chemotherapy in head and neck cancer (MACH-NC): locoregional treatment versus same treatment + chemotherapy. In: Kogelnik HD, Sedlmayer F (eds): Progress in Radio-Oncology VI, p 793. Bologna, Monduzzi Editore, 1998.
201. Vokes EE: The promise of biochemical modulation in combined modality therapy. Semin Oncol 1994; 21:29.
202. Bear HD, Hamad GG, Kostuchenko PJ: Biologic therapy of melanoma with cytokines and lymphocytes. Semin Surg Oncol 1996; 12:436.
203. Ben-Efraim S: Cancer immunotherapy: hopes and pitfalls: a review. Anticancer Res 1996; 16:3235.
204. Hamasaki VK, Vokes EE: Interferons and other cytokines in head and neck cancer. Med Oncol 1995; 12:23.
205. Pelicano L, Chelbi-Alix MK: Interferon and retinoic acid in the treatment of human cancer: mechanisms of action. Bull Cancer (Paris) 1998; 85:313.

206. McDonald S, Chang AY, Rubin P, et al: Combined Betaseron R (recombinant human interferon beta) and radiation for inoperable non-small cell lung cancer. Int J Radiat Oncol Biol Phys 1993; 27:613.
207. Symonds RP: Treatment-induced mucositis: an old problem with new remedies. Br J Cancer 1998; 77:1689.
208. Rosso M, Blasi G, Gherlone E, et al: Effect of granulocyte-macrophage colony-stimulating factor on prevention of mucositis in head and neck cancer patients treated with chemo-radiotherapy. J Chemother 1997; 9:382.
209. Leibel SA, Ling CC, Kutcher GJ, et al: The biological basis for conformal three-dimensional radiation therapy. Int J Radiat Oncol Biol Phys 1991; 21:805.
210. Fontenla GT, Pelizzari CA, Chen E: Implications of 3-dimensional target shape and motion in aperture design. Med Phys 1996; 23:1431.
211. Orton CG: Other considerations in three-dimensional treatment planning. In: Bagne F (ed): Computerized Treatment Planning Systems, p 136. HHS Publications FDA 84-8223, 1984.
212. Roach M, Pickett B, Akazawa PF, et al: Implementation of newer radiotherapeutic technology in the management of prostate cancer. Cancer Treat Res 1998; 93:247.
213. Marsh L, Eisbruch A, Watson B, et al: Treatment planning for parotid sparing in the patient requiring bilateral neck irradiation. Med Dosim 1996; 21:7.
214. Bortfeld T, Schlegel W: An analytical approximation of depth-dose distributions for therapeutic proton beams. Phys Med Biol 1996; 41:1331.
215. Raju MR: Proton radiobiology, radiosurgery and radiotherapy. Int J Radiat Biol 1995; 67:237.
216. Mehta MP: The physical, biologic, and clinical basis of radiosurgery. Curr Probl Cancer 1995; 19:265.
217. Flickinger JC, Kondziolka D: Radiosurgery instead of resection for solitary brain metastasis: the gold standard redefined. Int J Radiat Oncol Biol Phys 1996; 35:185.

7 Radiation Physics as Applied to Clinical Radiation Oncology

MICHAEL C. SCHELL, PhD, Radiation Oncology
CALVIN R. MAURER, JR, PhD, Neurosurgery
J. ANTHONY SEIBERT, PhD, Radiology
FANG-FANG YIN, PhD, Radiation Oncology

I saw flaring atom-streams and torrents of her myriad universe.

ALFRED, LORD TENNYSON

Perspective

Given the ability of radiation to annihilate cells, it is a rational move to focus large doses of radiation on a cancerous lesion while attempting to spare the normal tissue adjacent to the lesion. This has been demonstrated with modern three-dimensional (3-D) conformal techniques, such as intensity modulation radiotherapy techniques (IMRTs), which can accomplish sharply differentiated dose distributions (Fig. 7–1). Therefore, the underlying strategy is to incur more damage in the tumor than in the surrounding normal tissue, thereby producing a favorable therapeutic gain; this and similar techniques will be discussed in more detail later in this chapter. A typical tumor control curve versus a tissue damage (complication) probability curve is shown in Figure 7–2. As stated above, the treatment goal is to incur the maximum tumor control or damage with the widest separation between the tumor control curve and the tissue damage curve, resulting in the maximum possible therapeutic gain factor. This strategy existed until approximately the mid-1980s, when more aggressive efforts were initiated to institute conformal therapy.

Impact of Advances in Radiation Physics on Radiation Oncology

Advances in the science of radiation physics have brought about fundamental and revolutionary advances in the diagnosis and treatment of cancer. In 1946, Robert Wilson recognized that the optimal dose delivery to a tumor may be achieved with the use of proton therapy beams through the enhanced ionization of the Bragg peak to concentrate delivery of the dose to the tumor.[1] However, hard evidence of the efficacy of proton therapy did not arrive until 20 years later. At that time, Kaplan[2] provided data in the form of the improved survival for Hodgkin's disease as a function of beam energy.

Feinstein and coworkers[3] provided the evidence of a second significant impact from radiation physics on the treatment planning of cancer patients. Feinstein demonstrated that improvements in the resolution of diagnostic procedures allowed for a more accurate staging of lung cancer (tumor, nodes, and metastases). The consequence of an increased accuracy of tumor status showed that the staging in previous decades led oncologists to diagnose the advanced tumors in the lower or less advanced stages. The net result was that the improved resolution of diagnostic procedures resulted in a stage migration, that is, an apparent increase in patient survival in the early stages. As a consequence, the patients' databases accrued in earlier decades were significantly less accurate than the current patient accrual.

Finally, the third impact was through the ability to escalate the dose to the tumor while maintaining the current normal tissue complication rates. Zelefsky and associates[4, 5] demonstrated that actuarial survival was improved for patients treated with 3-D conformal radiotherapy as opposed to conventional external beam therapy. In addition, despite the simultaneous dose escalation and increased survival for 3-D radiation therapy, the morbidity of the treatment for 3-D therapy was maintained at conventional levels.

Irradiation Techniques

Two basic methods exist for irradiating a tumor:

1. external beam irradiation with x-rays, γ-rays, or protons[1, 6]
2. the insertion of radioactive sources interstitially or into the cavities of the body of the patient

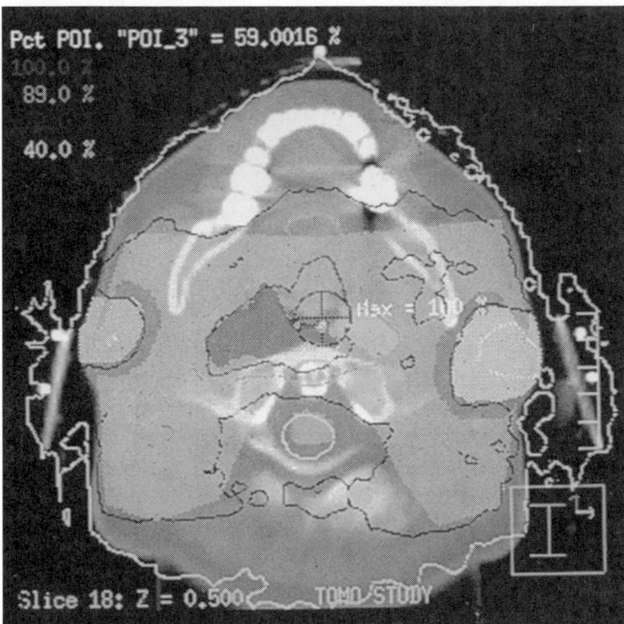

Figure 7–1. Dose distribution delivered by intensity modulation radiotherapy, used by the prototype tomography unit under development at the University of Wisconsin. Dose delivery to the tumor is 100%, whereas the lymph nodes receive 80% of the delivered dose. The parotid glands are spared, as well as the spinal cord. (Courtesy of Thomas R. Mackie, PhD, University of Wisconsin.)

The former approach involves the passage of radiation beams through normal tissue prior to focusing on the target whereas the latter approach relies on the rapid fall-off of the dose with short distances from the radioactive source. External beam irradiation is noninvasive; that is, there is no mechanical damage to the normal tissue between the beam entrance and the target within the patient. Brachytherapy (radioactive implants) frequently has the disadvantage of mechanically disturbing the normal tissue with the insertion of seeds or needles. However, brachytherapy has the dosimetric advantage of a rapid dose fall-off with minimal dose to normal tissue. Table 7–1 illustrates the range in energies of x-ray and γ-ray sources used in brachytherapy. Other radiations have been utilized in the attempt to achieve a therapeutic gain factor relative to x-irradiation of tumors.

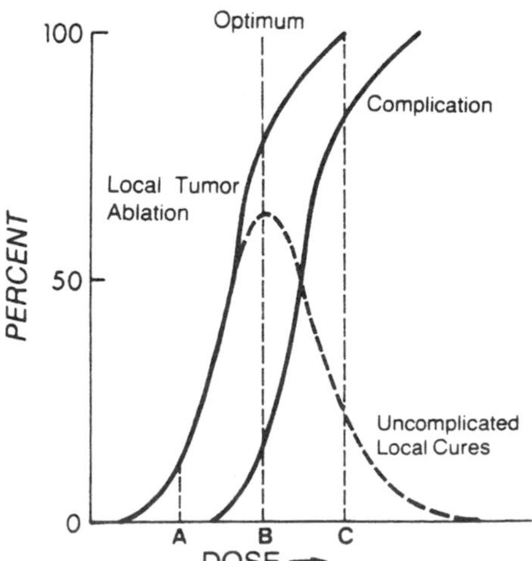

Figure 7–2. Tumor versus treatment outcomes. An uncomplicated curve (*dashed line*) is the desired result of treatment. A, B, and C represent three different dose levels, which, if chosen, would lead to three different outcomes: A would result in few tumor cures but no complications; C would lead to complete cure, but virtually all patients would suffer complications. The optimal choice is B. (Adapted from Mendelsohn ML: The biology of dose-limiting tissues. In: Time and Dose Relationships in Radiation Biology as Applied to Radiotherapy, Brookhaven National Laboratory [BNL] Report 5023 [C-57]. Upton, New York, BNL, 1969.)

TABLE 7–1. **Clinically Useful Radioactive Materials**

Radionuclide	Half-Life of Radiation	Useful Emission	Average Energy
Strontium-90	28.5 yrs	β	700 KeV
Radium-226	1622 yrs	photon & α	830 KeV
Cobalt-60	5.26 yrs	photon	6.25 MeV
Cesium-137	30.0 yrs	photon	662 KeV
Iridium-192	74.2 days	photon	370 KeV
Iodine-125	59.6 days	photon	28 KeV
Palladium-103	17 days	photon	21 KeV

Basic Physical Concepts

Basic radiation physics concepts are defined in Table 7–2[7]:

- Exposure is expressed in roentgens (R) and is defined as the number of ion pairs formed in air per unit mass by x-rays and γ-rays (Coulombs/kg).
- Absorbed dose is the energy absorbed locally by the medium from the incident radiation, and is expressed in the Système International (SI) unit Gray (Gy).
- Kerma is charged particle kinetic energy released in the medium per unit mass; it includes not only the locally absorbed dose but also the energy that is reirradiated away from the point of the photon interaction.
- The equivalent dose represents a rough approximate accounting of the relative biologic effectiveness of the ionizing radiation in question relative to 250-kVp orthovoltage x-rays. The equivalent dose is expressed in sievert (Sv) and is simply the absorbed dose multiplied by a biologic effectiveness factor. For example, the biologic factor for neutrons is a factor of 10.
- Activity is the expression of the decays or nuclear transformations per unit time with the initial unit of activity expressed in terms of curies (Ci). The SI unit of activity is the Bequerel (Bq). A Bequerel equals one disintegration per second.

Figure 7–3 illustrates the comparative depth dose curves along the beam axis for a variety of directly and indirectly ionizing radiation. The salient distinguishing factor between charged particle and indirectly ionizing radiation is the finite range for the charged particle beams as compared with the exponential attenuation of indirectly ionizing beams (photons and neutrons).

Birth of 3-D Megavoltage Radiation Therapy

The modern era of megavoltage therapy started on April 13, 1948, with the irradiation of a glioblastoma with a 22 MV x-ray beam produced by a betatron at the University of Illinois. A group led by Kerst[8] was investigating the

TABLE 7–2. **Radiologic Quantities—The Système International (SI) Units**

Radiation Quantity	Description	SI Units (abbreviation)	Symbol	Quantities
Exposure	Ionization per mass in air from x- and γ-rays	Coulombs/kg (C/kg)	X	1R = 2.58 × 10^{-4} C/kg
Absorbed dose	Energy imparted per mass by radiation	Gray (Gy)	D	1 rad = 1 cGy 1 joule/kg = 1 Gy
Kerma	Kinetic energy released per unit mass	—	K	K(mGy) = 3.39 × 10^2 × X(C/kg)
Equivalent dose	Relative biologic damage in man	Sievert (Sv)	H	H(Sv) = w_n × D(Gy) H(rem) = QF × D(rad) 1 rem = 10 mSv
Activity	Quantity of radioactive material expressed as the nuclear transformation rate	Bequerel (Bq)	A	1 Ci = 3.7 × 10^{10} Bq 1 Bq = 1 per sec^{-1} (dps)

Modified from Hendee WR, Ibbott GS: Radiation Therapy Physics, 2nd ed. St. Louis, Mosby–Year Book, 1996.

application of x-rays for industrial radiography and, at the same time, Quastler and his group[9] began radiobiology experiments at the betatron facility, in collaboration with the physics group. The motivation for the x-ray beam development stemmed from the unanticipated discovery of a brain lesion in a physics graduate student. Together, Kerst, Skaggs, Koch, Laughlin, and Lanzl focused their attention on the development of a radiotherapeutic x-ray beam.[10]

Within 2 weeks of the diagnosis, the physics research group had investigated and designed the primary and secondary collimation and electron contamination of the x-ray beam, the beam intensity flattener, the transmission ion chamber that monitored the delivered dose, and an anthropomorphic head phantom for the study of dose distribution. This effort yielded the first megavoltage radiotherapy beam, the 22 MV x-ray beam delivering 25 beams arranged in a noncoplanar geometry (3-D treatment geometry). Although the patient succumbed to his disease, the autopsy indicated that the tumor had completely regressed.

This event set the gold standard for decades to come in radiotherapy:

- The discussion had led, in a stepwise fashion, to the advantages of using 3-D beam geometries for the reduction of the normal tissue dose. In the case of the glioblastoma, 25 treatment fields had been used and distributed to yield a minimal normal tissue dose. Although the beam fields had overlapped at the surface of the scalp, the authors realized that the skin sparing of the high-energy x-ray beam eliminated the possibility of hot spots on the skin.
- The design of the 3-D plan had been discussed in detail, with extensive consideration given to beam geometry, in order to avoid entrance or exit of the beam through critical normal tissues such as the eye. Radio-opaque markers were used to locate the eyes in the portal films.
- Not only was a 3-D treatment executed but also the basic design for the head of the modern linear accelerator had been completed, with a quantum leap over the existing orthovoltage radiotherapy devices.
- The concept of isocentric treatment had also been introduced. In this case, the patient was rotated because of the unwieldy size of the betatron.
- The evaluation of the treatment plan was achieved through the use of two head phantoms, which were constructed out of pressed wood.

Radiation therapy with the betatron commenced on April 30, 1948. Subsets of five fields of the total of 25 were irradiated per day with a dose rate of approximately 30 R

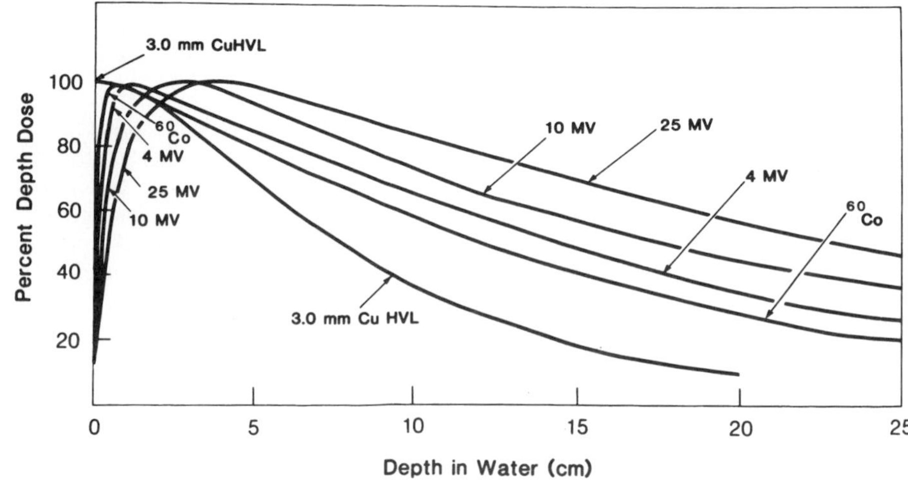

Figure 7–3. The central axis depth dose in water for orthovoltage x-rays; ^{60}Co; and 4, 10, and 25 MV x-ray beams. (From Khan FM [ed]: The Physics of Radiation Therapy, 2nd ed, p 181. Baltimore, Williams & Wilkins, 1994, with permission.)

per minute. The tumor was seen to regress, as evinced by the decompression. Treatment was discontinued on May 16, 1948 and the patient expired on June 3, 1948. Pulmonary congestion was the ultimate cause of death. Gail Adams, John Laughlin, and Larry Lanzl later cofounded and became presidents of the American Association of Physicists in Medicine.

The development of the betatron led to significant improvements in the beam energies and tissue penetration of units used in clinics around the world. This is illustrated in Figure 7–4 in the increased depth dose of a 10-MV x-ray beam relative to the older orthovoltage beam. This figure demonstrates the isodose distributions for beam energies ranging from 200 kVp through 10 MV, where the source-to-surface distance ranges from 50 cm to 100 cm. Observe that the dose distribution penetrates to a greater depth as the beam energy increases and also that the scatter dose outside of the collimator beam reduces with the increase in beam energy. Simple rectangular collimation is executed through the use of the four independent jaws of the accelerator, whereas the complex collimation is achieved with multileaf collimation (MLC). The typical multileaf collimator consists of forty pairs of leaves, with each leaf capable of independent static positioning for static beam collimation and dynamic movement for beam intensity modulation.[11–13]

Simple wedge shape dose distributions can be produced through the use of dynamic motion of the independent jaws. The jaw will sweep across the beam as the patient is irradiated. Variation of the jaw position thus produces an angle in the dose distribution with respect to the central beam access. The magnitude of the wedge angle is a

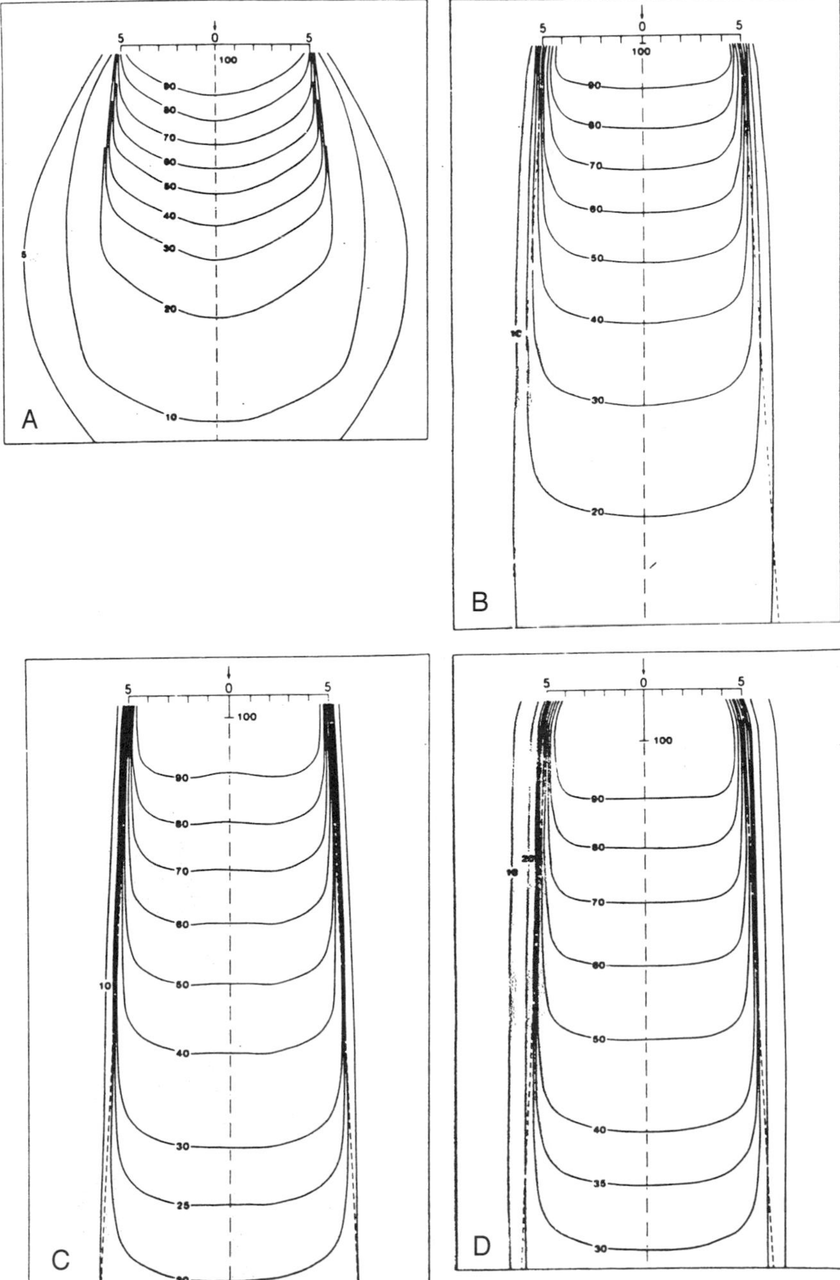

Figure 7–4. Two-dimensional depth dose curves for x-ray beams in order of increasing energy, beginning with orthovoltage x-rays. As the x-ray beam energy increases, the penetration of the beam increases and the penumbra width decreases. The beam profiles that are perpendicular to the central axis are relatively flat or uniform. (From Khan FM [ed]: The Physics of Radiation Therapy, 2nd ed, p 232. Baltimore, Williams & Wilkins, 1994, with permission.)

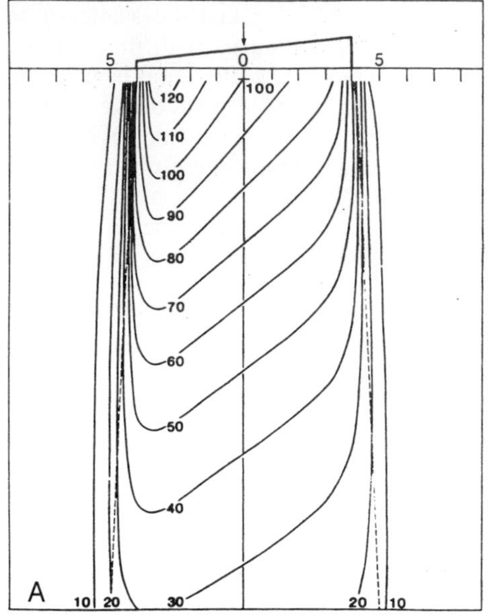

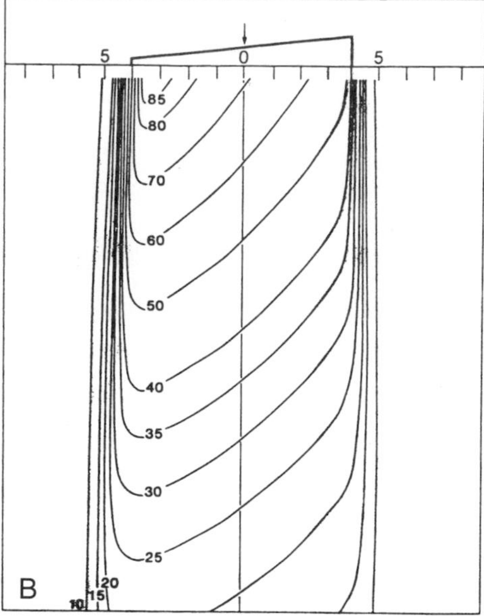

Figure 7–5. Wedge-shaped 2-D isodose curves for x-ray beams. The wedge is symbolized by the triangle at the surface of the phantom. The wedge is used to attenuate the x-ray beam to produce an angles beam profile perpendicular to the central axis. (From Khan FM [ed]: The Physics of Radiation Therapy, 2nd ed, p 234. Baltimore, Williams & Wilkins, 1994, with permission.)

function of the movement of the independent jaws across the beam profile (Fig. 7–5).

Tumor Dose Escalation and Conformal Therapy

In the early 1990s, Thames and associates[14] hypothesized that tumor control would increase if the tumor dose was increased by 20%. This was supported by studies with dose escalation conformal therapy and beam intensity modulation therapy of the prostate, which achieved significant local control while simultaneously decreasing the normal tissue complication rates.[15] At about the same time, Lichter[16] expanded on Thames' hypothesis to include cure rate, that is, a "3-D hypothesis," which simply stated that dose escalation would produce an increase in the cure rate. Increased tumor dose must be accompanied by increased protection to the normal tissue proximal to the target. Indeed, Hanks and others[17] have reported that conformal therapy of the prostate has reduced the acute grade II complication rates. Similarly, Sandler and associates, as well as Michalski and colleagues,[18, 19] have demonstrated a reduction in the complication rates in the bladder and rectum when treated conformally.

Perhaps the most persuasive article for the progression to beam intensity optimization techniques from conformal 3-D treatment planning was presented by De Gersem and coworkers.[20] This group investigated the use of figures of merit to evaluate treatment plans for both 3-D conformal techniques and IMRTs for 10 small cell lung cancer patients. The figures of merit were based on biophysical (dose histogram analysis of the plan)[21–25] and biologic models (the use of tumor control probability functions and normal tissue complication probability functions)[26–33] for the evaluation and intercomparison of the treatment plans for 3-D conformal techniques and IMRTs.

In their paper,[20] it was assumed that the parameters for tumor control probability (TCP) and normal tissue complication probability (NTCP) calculations are known; however, in reality, this is not the case. The uncertainty of these parameters is large and, therefore, the parameter values are not well known. In addition, for each planning technique, the dose gradient was allowed to vary, which is not the case for normal forward treatment planning. Nonetheless, the plans were compared for 3-D techniques and IMRTs with both biologic and biophysical figures of merit. NTCP values were calculated for the lung, heart, spinal cord, and esophagus. The conclusions were that higher TCP values were achievable with the IMRT approach for both figures of merit, as opposed to the 3-D conformal forward planning approach, while maintaining the NTCP values in approximately the same range for both plans. The main conclusion of the article was that, although the biologic parameters for calculation of the NTCPs and TCPs are not well known, the effort did give an estimate of the probable increase of tumor control rate. Specifically, the uncomplicated local control probability increased by 15% for 3-D and by 21% for IMRT. However, IMRT control rate was 63.5% as opposed to 42.5% with 3-D treatment planning.

In 1993, the International Commission on Radiation Units (ICRU) and Measurements published ICRU Report 50, which formalized conformal therapy volume descriptions.[34] The report gave a number of definitions (Fig. 7–6):

- *clinical target volume* (CTV): the volume that includes the macroscopic image of the tumor and the margin that accommodates the microscopic extent of the disease
- *planning target volume* (PTV): the treatment volume defined by the dose delivery affected by the treatment technique

The CTV is derived from 3-D images (data sets) from computed tomography (CT), magnetic resonance imaging (MRI), and occasionally, single-photon emission computed tomography (SPECT). The volumes are then inferred

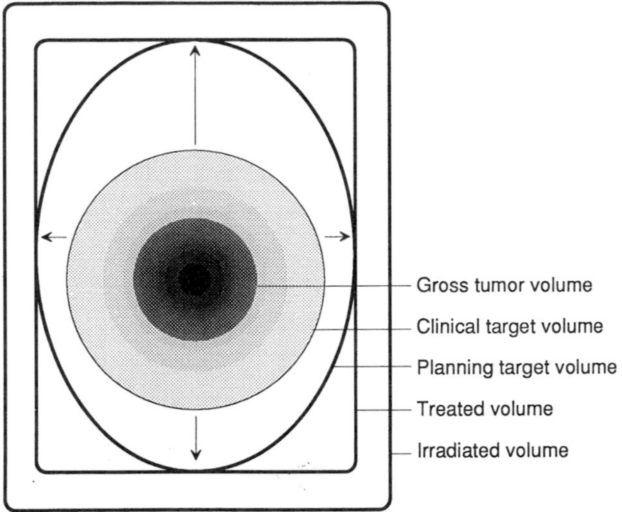

Figure 7–6. Gross tumor volume, clinical target volume, planning target volume, and treated volume are illustrated. ICRU Report 50 provides the foundation for three dimensional treatment planning parameters and dose reporting. (From International Commission on Radiation Units and Measurements: Prescribing, recording, and reporting photon beam therapy. ICRU Report 50. Bethesda, International Commission on Radiation Units and Measurements, 1993, with permission.)

through image correlation on planning systems using 3-D workstations.[35–38] This information forms the input for the 3-D treatment planning system and is provided by a collaboration of the diagnostic radiologist and the radiation oncologist.

The physics and dosimetry group then transfers the data set to the 3-D treatment planning system for the plan design. These data sets are large and incur a cost in terms of time as a result of the increased scan times and the need for physician input. Factors that may affect the identification of the planning target and clinical target volumes are:

- the volume definition, which can vary between observers; this issue was addressed in a study of the variability in target volume specification from 3-D image sets between physicians[39] (Fig. 7–7)
- the influence of organ movement during the scan procedure, which also has an impact on the definition of the CTV; the impact of respiration and, to lesser extent, the movement of the heart have been a concern in the determination of the volume error and set-up error for radiation therapy. Organ movement during the scan acquisition has led to gated image studies.[40] Roeske and associates[41] demonstrated that the prostate moves during therapy, in spite of use of external immobilization devices, and this movement can extend to as much as 1 cm in the anterior posterior direction. Balter and associates[42] determined that the optimal reproducibility, that is, minimization of internal organ motion due to respiration, could be achieved at the end of the exhale cycle

A change in patient position can produce a significant change in the target. For example, Breuer and Wynchank[43] investigated the position of the human brain within the skull and discovered that the set-up variability was between 1.5 and 4 millimeters.

Computer-Based Dose Calculation Algorithms

The evolution of computer-based dose calculation algorithms started in the mid-1960s with the Bentley-Milan calculation[44] and others[45]; the former technique was based on percent depth dose data. Shortly thereafter, a photon algorithm was expanded to include the effect of scatter from an irregularly shaped field, pioneered by Clarkson.[46] The calculation technique was extended by Cunningham[47] to use the tissue-air ratio table and the scatter-air ratio table, and it was used to calculate the effect of an irregularly shaped field around a central axis or any point within the phantom on a given plane. The caveat or restriction for this initial approach is that all beams are coplanar, that is, the axis of all beams converging on an isocenter is confined to one transverse plane in the patient.

Both calculation algorithms were developed prior to the evolution of computed or digital tomography. CT images the electron density of the medium in the transverse plane of the phantom (or patient). The determination of the electron density in a given volume then allows for the inference of the density and material type of the material contained within the phantom. An understanding of the structure of the "heterogeneities" that are observed within a patient then provides the data for the calculation of the effect of radiation on those heterogeneities within the patient because the depth dose along central axis will vary as it transits the region of heterogeneity. A phantom is comprised of water, with bone and lung located at given depth ranges along the central axis. There are two effects produced by the change in density on the dose distribution along the central axis[48–50]:

1. The transmission and absorption of the x-ray beam will be directly impacted by the density, with a de-

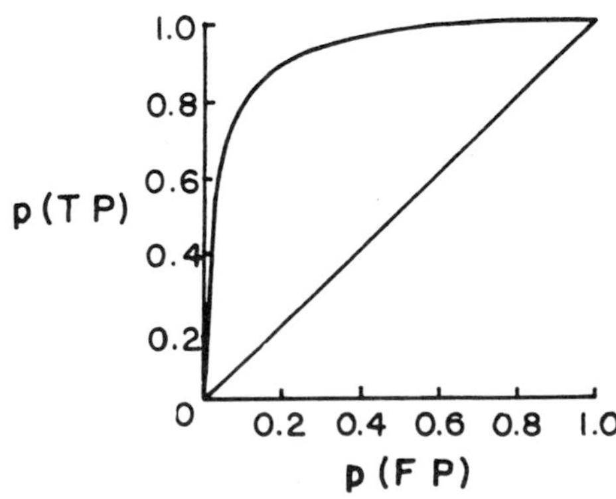

Figure 7–7. The receiver operator characteristics curve describes the characterization or the ability of a system or observer to correctly choose and diagnose objects in an image. A linear line indicates that there is an equal number of true and false choices made and reflects a random selection process. (From Hendee WR, Ibbott GS: Radiation Therapy Physics, 2nd ed. St. Louis, Mosby–Year Book Inc, 1996, with permission.)

crease by bone as well as an increase in transmission through lung.
2. There will exist a build-up or build-down of the dose as a result of the change in the electron fluence through the transition region.

Both effects have a significant impact on the treatment planning process and a treatment planning system. For example, the dose to a lung tumor is grossly underestimated by the assumption of a homogeneous patient. The omission of heterogeneity corrections for lung cancer can easily underestimate the dose by 15%.[51] Similarly, the transmission of high-energy x-ray beams through femoral heads can be reduced by several percent along the central axis.

The introduction of refinements in heterogeneity corrections led to variations in the basic photon dose algorithm, such as the equivalent tissue-air ratio method and the Batho Power Law.[52, 53] These algorithms were expanded as the capability of computers progressed to include the noncoplanar beam geometry and the calculation of doses and planes off the central axis plane. The general term describing this algorithm or planning approach was the *2.5-D treatment-planning algorithm.* The common feature of the photon dose calculation algorithms at this point in time is that they are based on a measurement of the depth dose and beam profiles for a particular x-ray beam in a water phantom. Consequently, these measurements contain the impact of the beam hardening of the particular x-ray spectrum only and the characteristics of charged particle scatter in the water phantom. The dose perturbations from heterogeneity within the patient are inferred and calculated by inference, based on the basic beam data in water.

The aforementioned dose calculation algorithms are model based and contain parameters that are inferred from the measured data set for the particular beam in question. Computer technology can accommodate radiation transport models in reasonable calculation times to execute clinical treatment plans. Two model-based calculations are available for clinical use: the convolution/superposition method and the Monte Carlo simulation technique. The convolution/superposition approach contains convolution kernels, which are usually derived from Monte Carlo simulation. The Monte Carlo simulation is, by definition, the reproduction of photon and recoil electron interactions with the materials in question. The calculation of these interactions is based on the probabilities (interaction cross sections) for the processes involved. Both approaches produce the dose per photon fluence and, consequently, the dose per monitor unit.

Convolution/Superposition Method

The convolution/superposition method delineates or partitions the primary interaction by the incident beam from the transport of the secondary recoil particles (charged particles and scattered photons), which are set in motion when the incident x-ray beam interacts with the medium.[54–58] The principal advantage of this approach is the ability to calculate the dose distributions, not only from the perturbations impacted on the incident primary beam but also from the effect of the perturbations on the scattered components of the beam. Consequently, the approach is capable of accounting for all of the complexities of the charge particle interactions with a complex medium, such as a patient. The convolution kernels represent the relative energy deposited in a voxel (volume element) as a function of position about the site of the primary interaction. The kernel for a polyenergetic x-ray beam is represented by the weighted summation of the kernel for each energy bin of the x-ray beam spectrum and is calculated as follows:

$$A(\vec{r}) = \sum_i w_i h\nu_i \left[\frac{\Delta E(\vec{r})}{N h\nu}\right]_i$$

where N is the number of photons with photon energy $h\nu$, $\Delta E(r)$ is the energy deposited at voxel position r, and w is the relative weight of the normalized incident photon fluence. The dose calculation in a homogeneous phantom becomes:

$$D(\vec{r}) = \iiint_{vol} \frac{\mu}{\rho} \psi(\vec{r'})\, A(\vec{r} - \vec{r'})\, dV$$

In this equation, μ/ρ is the mass attenuation coefficient and ψ is the photon fluence.

Direct Monte Carlo Treatment Planning

The Monte Carlo technique uses measured and analytic probability distributions governing the interactions of the directly ionizing and indirectly ionizing radiation to simulate particle transport through the phantom (or patient); patient heterogeneities are determined by inference from serial CT scans. The Monte Carlo approach tracks each particle until the energy of the particle is below a preset threshold. Each track is a score or history of the particle interactions. Large numbers of histories are generated in order to obtain a small statistical fluctuation in the average dose distribution within the medium. The Monte Carlo approach accounts for the effects of all materials on the incident x-ray and electron beams.[8, 59]

A prototype Monte Carlo–based treatment planning system has been developed by a group at the Lawrence Livermore National Laboratory[60]; this system is capable of calculating the dose distributions in patients. The treatment planning code commences the photon histories in the head of the clinical linear accelerator and transports the x-rays through the collimator and the intervening air and, finally, in the patient. This system has been successfully validated for external beam irradiation and brachytherapy implants.

Imaging

Accurate, patient-specific anatomic information is necessary to design an optimal treatment plan that delivers radiation to the entire extent of a lesion while minimizing exposure to normal tissue.[61–64] Because of this need, medical images play an important role in clinical radiation oncology. Images are used in many steps of the radiotherapy process, including diagnosis, staging, treatment planning, treatment delivery, and follow-up evaluation. Various kinds of images are used, including CT, magnetic resonance (MR), ultrasound, nuclear medicine (positron emission tomography [PET], SPECT), and projection images such as simulator and portal films.

Image Acquisition

Computed Tomography Imaging

The development of CT in the early 1970s revolutionized medical imaging. For the first time, physicians were able to obtain high-quality tomographic (cross-sectional) images of internal structures of the body. The first clinical scanner, introduced in the mid-1970s, was a "head-only" scanner that was able to produce two slices in 5 minutes. Technology has progressed significantly since that time, with state-of-the-art scanners able to acquire volume-based images in a single breath-hold by using continuous rotation (slip-ring scanners), simultaneous table translation (spiral, or helical, data acquisition), and multiple array detector geometry. However, despite the enhanced speed and patient throughput improvements, the information presented in the CT images essentially remains unchanged.

The major components of a modern CT scanner include an x-ray generator, x-ray tube, beam collimation, a linear array of detectors, data acquisition system, table and translation mechanics, gantry rotation motor, and a host of peripherals.

- X-rays are collimated in the direction perpendicular to the CT table, which defines the slice thickness; slice thicknesses are typically 1 to 10 mm, depending on the collimator adjustment.
- The slice sensitivity profile represents the actual distribution of x-rays in the object, is generally gaussian (bell-shaped), and is typically wider than the nominal (indicated) slice thickness.
- Perpendicular to this direction is the "fan beam" geometry, a fan-shaped divergent x-ray beam emanating from the focal spot.

Although several CT scanner geometries have been implemented, the most popular is the third-generation design, in which an array of discrete detectors (typically 900 to 1000) is found opposite the x-ray tube and is irradiated by the fan beam. Each detector has an aperture (active width), and the detector array sampling pitch is defined as the center-to-center distance between detectors and is nearly equal to the detector aperture. For most modern clinical scanners, the detector aperture is about 1 mm in width. Design criteria of most CT scanners ensure that resolution is not limited because of a focal spot dimension being too large. The detector aperture and the slice thickness thus define the voxel dimensions. The voxel dimensions are typically 0.5 mm × 0.5 mm × slice thickness.[65]

Tomographic slices are produced by the acquisition of x-ray projections measured at several angular positions about the object. A "sinogram" (a two-dimensional map of the x-ray projection values measured at each detector versus the detector array/tube angle around the patient) is produced and used in the subsequent filtered back-projection of the data during the image reconstruction process. The specific details of reconstruction are beyond the scope of this chapter, but the outcome is a map of linear attenuation coefficients of the anatomy within the beam, normalized to the linear attenuation coefficient of water at the effective energy of the x-ray beam. The attenuation values are represented as discrete digital numbers, known as CT numbers or Hounsfield units, by the following expression:

$$\text{CT number} = K\,(\mu_{\text{tissue}} - \mu_{\text{water}}) / \mu_{\text{water}}$$

where K is a constant (commonly 1000) and μ is the linear attenuation coefficient. Thus, it is the linear attenuation coefficient that is actually measured by a CT scan. The differences in attenuation coefficients are manifested in the CT image as differences in gray levels over a 12-bit ($2^{12} = 4096$) dynamic range. Because the linear attenuation coefficient is related to the electron density, the CT numbers can be used to estimate this quantity for treatment planning (Fig. 7–8).

CT images have been widely used in radiation treatment planning because they provide excellent contrast between bone, soft tissue, and air. There is no obvious geometric distortion in CT images, and the tissue density information is required for dose calculation. However, it should be noted that the anatomic structures may be degraded as a result of volume averaging (for example, the skull appears to be thicker around the curved region), organ motion, and tissue distortion from streak artifacts caused by metal in the imaging object. Occasionally, a tumor volume such as a low-grade brain tumor is difficult to diagnose with CT images as a result of poor soft-tissue discrimination. The use of MR images can alleviate this problem.

Magnetic Resonance Imaging

MR imaging is a clinically important medical imaging modality as a result of its exceptional soft tissue contrast. MR was invented in the early 1970s, and the first commercial scanners appeared about 10 years later. MR imaging exploits the existence of induced nuclear magnetism in the patient; materials with an odd number of protons or neutrons possess a weak, but observable, nuclear magnetic moment. Commonly, protons (^{1}H) are imaged, although carbon (^{13}C), phosphorus (^{31}P), sodium (^{23}Na), and fluorine (^{19}F) are also of significant interest. The nuclear moments are normally randomly oriented, but they align when placed in a strong magnetic field; typical field strengths for imaging range between 0.2 and 1.5 T, although spectroscopic and functional imaging work is often performed with higher field strengths. The nuclear magnetization is very weak; the ratio of the induced magnetization to the applied field is only 4×10^{-9}. The collection of nuclear moments often is referred to as magnetization or spins.

The basic technique underlying MRI is to measure the nuclear moment while it oscillates in a plane perpendicular to a static magnetic field. Firstly, one must tip the moment away from the static field. When perpendicular to the static field, the moment feels a torque proportional to the strength of the static magnetic field; the torque always points perpendicular to the magnetization and causes the spins to oscillate or precess in a plane perpendicular to the static field. The frequency of the rotation ω_0 is proportional to the field:

$$\omega_0 = -\gamma B_0$$

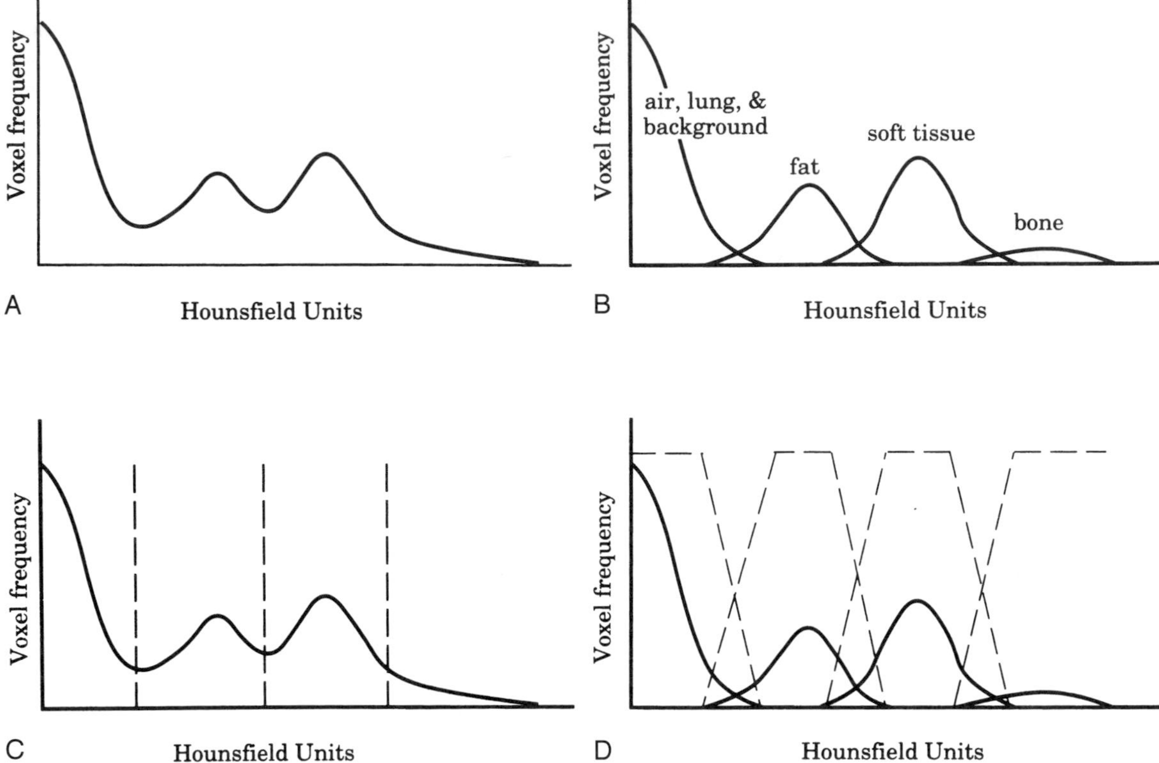

Figure 7–8. A histogram or frequency distribution is depicted for a CT scan of human anatomy, with the voxel frequency shown as a function of Hounsfield units. In B, the relative distribution for each tissue type is deconstructed, with the delineation of the density of the human tissues increasing as the Hounsfleld units increase. Symbolically, in C and D, the windows are placed on the frequency distribution at levels that are corresponding to the four basic tissues: lung, fat, soft tissue, and bone. This, in a simplistic manner, depicts how the window and leveling are used to discriminate preferentially for the tissue of interest. (From Kessler ML, Puff DT: Segmentation and visualization for treatment planning. In: Mackie TR, Palta JR [eds]: Teletherapy: Present and Future. Madison, Advanced Medical Publishing, 1996, with permission.)

where γ, the gyromagnetic ratio, is a constant specific to the nucleus, and B_0 is the magnetic field strength. The direction of B_0 defines the z axis. The precession frequency is called the Larmor frequency. The negative sign indicates the direction of the precession.

To observe this precession, we first need to tip the magnetization away from the static field. This is accomplished with a weak rotating radiofrequency field. Another useful radiofrequency pulse rotates spins by π radians (180°); this can be used to invert the spins and also to refocus transverse spins that have dephased. This is called spin echo and is widely used in imaging. The key innovation for MRI was to impose spatial variations on the magnetic field to distinguish spins by their location. Applying a magnetic field gradient causes each region of the volume to oscillate at a distinct frequency. The most effective nonuniform field is a linear gradient where the field and the resulting frequencies vary linearly with distance along the object being imaged. Fourier analysis of the signal obtains a map of the spatial distribution of spins.

The tremendous clinical utility of MR is due to the great variety of mechanisms that can be exploited to create image contrast. If MR images were restricted to water density alone, MR would be considerably less useful because most tissues would appear identical. Fortunately, many different MR contrast mechanisms can be employed to distinguish different tissues and disease processes. The primary contrast mechanisms exploit relaxation of the magnetization. The two types of relaxations are called spin-lattice (or longitudinal) relaxation, characterized by a relaxation time, T1, and spin-spin (or transverse) relaxation, characterized by a relaxation time, T2.

- *Spin-lattice relaxation* describes the rate of recovery of the z component of magnetization toward equilibrium after it has been disturbed by radiofrequency pulses. Differences in the T1 time constant can be used to produce image contrast by exciting the magnetization and then imaging before full recovery has been achieved. Tissue with a shorter T1 recovers faster and produces more signal relative to tissues with a longer T1 time constant.
- *Spin-spin relaxation* describes the rate at which the nuclear magnetic resonance signal decays after it has been created. Image contrast is produced by delaying the data acquisition. Tissue with a longer T2 produces more signal.

Figure 7–9 shows examples of these two basic types of contrast. The images are of identical axial sections through the brain of a patient. One image was acquired with an imaging method that produces T1 contrast. The very bright ring of subcutaneous fat results from its relatively short T1. In addition, white matter has a shorter T1 than gray matter, so it shows up brighter in this image. The other image was acquired with an imaging method that produces T2 contrast. Here the cerebrospinal fluid in the ventricles is bright as a result of its long T2. White matter has a shorter T2 than gray matter, so it is darker in this image.

In addition to the intrinsic tissue contrast, artificial MR contrast agents can be introduced. The most popular agents decrease both T1 and T2. One agent approved for clinical use is gadolinium diethylenetetraaminopentaacetic acid (DTPA). Gadolinium is toxic, but is rendered innocuous by chelation with DTPA. Decreasing T1 causes faster signal recovery and a higher signal on a T1-weighted image. The contrast-enhanced regions then show up brighter relative to the rest of the image.

MR images provide good soft tissue contrast. CT images have greater spatial resolution and image calcifications and bony detail far better, whereas with MR, bone cortex produces low signal and is therefore not visible; in MR, bones are identified by the presence of the marrow signal. Therefore, whereas MR provides more detail about soft tissues, CT provides more information about bones, and the two types of imaging can be considered complementary.

Nuclear Medicine Imaging

In CT, the regions under study are used in a transmission mode in the measurement of the attenuation coefficient; in nuclear medicine, the region under study becomes an active source. This is achieved through the administration of radioactive materials inasmuch as the body contains no natural radioactive sources. To be useful in imaging, either the radioactive material itself, or the chemical form it is bound in, must have properties that will cause it to be selectively taken up in specific regions of the anatomy. For example, glucose labeled with ^{11}C, or a glucose analogue labeled with ^{18}F, accumulates in the brain or tumors because glucose is used as a primary source of energy. Once taken up into the tissue of interest, the materials become "radiating" sources. Thus, the imaging problem in nuclear medicine is that of defining the radioactive source distribution rather than the distribution of attenuation coefficients. Not only the spatial but also the uptake distribution of radiopharmaceuticals depends on the biokinetic properties of the pharmaceuticals and the normal or abnormal state of the patient. Thus, sequences of nuclear medicine images can be used for tracer kinetic modeling for dynamic qualitative study and quantitative physiologic evaluation.

Radioactivity is detected by a rectilinear scanner, gamma camera, or tomographic imaging system (e.g., SPECT or PET scanner). The gamma camera is the most commonly used radionuclide detection system. A conventional gamma camera is a two-dimensional (2-D) planar imaging system and consists of a collimator for forming the radioactive distribution into a 2-D image, a detector for detecting the position of each γ-ray photon, and a recorder for producing an image from the detected photons. Typically the detectors are scintillating crystals that convert gamma energy into light, which is amplified by photomultiplier tubes. A variation of the gamma camera is the Anger camera, which overcomes the problem of having the resolution limited by the number of discrete detectors. The basic disadvantage of these cameras is that they produce a 2-D projection of 3-D source distribution.

SPECT and PET scanners obtain many projections with such cameras, and create a 3-D tomographic image using a mathematic reconstruction algorithm. One fundamental difference between SPECT and PET is the use of annihilation coincidence detection in PET.

- PET uses radionuclides such as ^{11}C, ^{13}N, ^{15}O, and ^{18}F that emit positrons. Each emitted positron immediately interacts with an electron to produce an annihilation event that generates two γ-rays, each having energies of 511 keV and at almost exactly opposite directions. The PET imaging system is designed to detect these two coincidence events. The PET radionuclides have very short half-lives, often requiring an on-site cyclotron for their production. Coincidence detection requires expensive instrumentation.

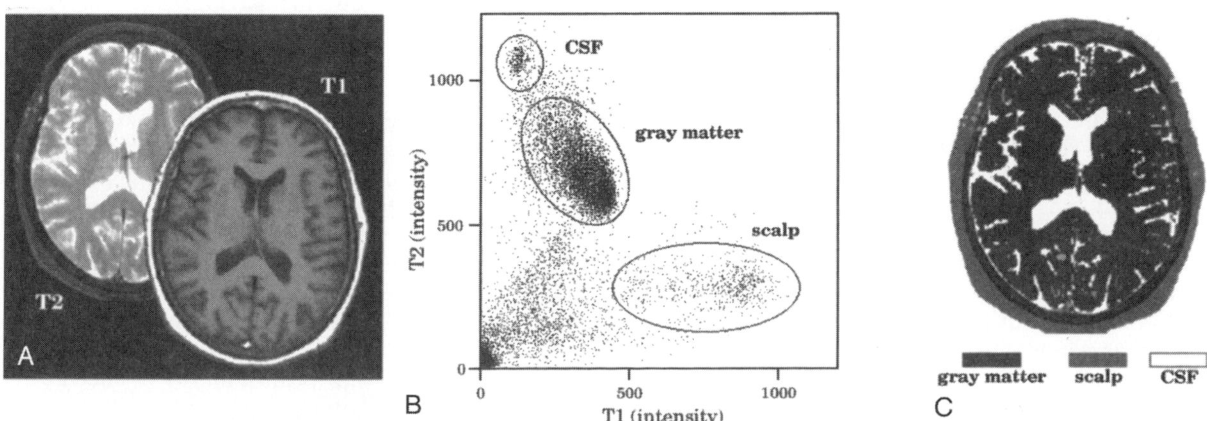

Figure 7–9. (A) Representative MR images in the axial plane of a human brain for T2- and T1-weighted pulse sequences. (B) Distribution of brain tissue as a function of T2 and T1 intensities. (C) Tissue discrimination as derived by the variation in pulse sequence. (From Kessler ML, Puff DT: Segmentation and visualization for treatment planning. In: Mackie TR, Palta JR [eds]: Teletherapy: Present and Future. Madison, Advanced Medical Publishing, 1996, with permission.)

- SPECT uses standard radionuclides normally found in nuclear medicine clinics and that emit individual γ-ray photons with energies that are much lower than 511 keV. Typical examples are the 140 keV photons from ^{99m}Tc and the 70 keV photons from ^{201}Tl.

Thus, the costs of SPECT instrumentation and of performing SPECT studies are substantially less than for PET. Resolution and signal-to-noise ratio of nuclear medicine images are relatively poorer than for anatomic images such as CT and MR. Nuclear medicine interpretation is generally aided by correlation to anatomic images using image registration software.

Projection Imaging (Simulator and Portal Imaging)

The key to success in radiation therapy is to accurately deliver the prescribed radiation to the target volume. Generally, each treatment field is simulated using a conventional fluoroscopic imaging system (called a simulator) to allow better understanding about treatment region and field design before delivery of MeV beams. Most diagnostic images are acquired using x-ray photons, with energies ranging from 20 kVp to 120 kVp to allow penetration of photons through imaging objects.[65–67] Phosphor screen/film combination is the typical detector used to acquire plane x-ray images. Fluoroscopic imaging uses a very low tube current (a few milliamperes) so that a relatively long exposure time is possible (several minutes) for real-time visualization of treatment regions. However, the signal-to-noise ratio of fluoroscopic images is relatively poor and conventional fluoroscopic imaging systems suffer geometric distortions called pincushion, although these can be corrected using a post–image-processing algorithm. The video signal of the fluoroscopic image is displayed on a dedicated monitor and can then be digitized as a digital image for effective storage, retrieval, and processing.

The delivery of radiation to the target is not always ideal as a result of potential systematic errors (such as wrong measurement data, wrong skin marks), random errors (day-to-day set-up errors, patient motion, and organ movement), and human mistakes during the setting of blocking and field. To ensure an accurate delivery, each treatment field should be verified by taking portal images in the treatment position. Conventionally, one portal film is taken before the beginning of the treatment, and once per week thereafter. A typical portal film imaging system is composed of a sheet of double-emulsion film and a cassette that has a metal sheet at the x-ray tube side and phosphor screens between film. The exposed film is developed with a regular film processor. This procedure takes 5 to 10 minutes before the film is available for review by a physician; therefore, the portal film imaging is not feasible for a real-time verification of treatment set-up.

The development of electronic portal imaging devices allows acquisition of portal images within a few seconds.[68] Electronic portal images and reference images are displayed on a video monitor for immediate comparison; therefore, it becomes possible to perform daily real-time set-up verification without substantially increasing cost and time. Differing from the conventional x-ray images that are acquired using keV energy ranges, portal images are acquired with MeV x-ray energies generated in the treatment machine. The photoelectric interaction is the dominant event for keV x-rays whereas the Compton scatter interaction is the dominant event for MeV x-rays. Unfortunately, this means that the image quality of portal images is relatively poor, particularly the contrast between bony structures and soft tissues. Nonetheless, another advantage to acquiring electronic portal images is that image-processing techniques can be applied to enhance the contrast of portal images and to perform computer-assisted verification for the improvement of verification efficiency.[69–72] Digital images also allow effective image storage and communication through a networking system.

Image Registration

Image registration is the determination of a one-to-one mapping or transformation between the coordinates in one image and those in another image or in the physical space occupied by the patient. Registration of multimodal images makes it possible to combine different types of structural information (e.g., CT and MR) or functional information (e.g., PET and SPECT), or both, for diagnosis and therapy planning. Registration of images acquired with the same modality at different times allows quantitative comparison of serial data for longitudinal monitoring of disease progression or regression and post-therapy follow-up. To make the registration beneficial in terms of medical diagnosis or treatment, the transformation or mapping that the registration produces must be applied in a clinically meaningful way by a system that will typically include registration as a subsystem. The larger system may combine the two registered images by producing a reoriented version of one image that can be "fused" with the other. This fusing of two images into one may be accomplished, for example, by simply summing intensity values in two images, by superimposing outlines from one image on the other image, or by encoding one image in hue and the other in brightness in a color image. Regardless of the method employed, image fusion should be distinguished from image registration, which is a necessary first step before fusion can be successful. Alternatively, the larger system may use the registration simply to provide a pair of movable cursors on two views linked via the registering transformation so that the cursors are displayed at corresponding points.

Image registration can be accomplished by matching corresponding pairs of points. The points can be anatomic landmarks, skin-affixed markers, or bone-implanted markers. Because markers used for point-based registration are taken as being reliable for the purpose of registration, they are often called *fiducial markers*, or simply *fiducials*. The determination of a precise point used for registration is called *fiducial localization*. Localization may involve interactive visual identification of anatomic landmarks or automatic identification and localization of a fiducial marker using a computer algorithm.

The three-dimensional boundary surface of an anatomic object or structure is an intuitive and easily characterized geometric feature that can be used for medical image registration. Surface-based registration methods involve determining corresponding surfaces in different images (or physical space) and computing the transformation that best aligns these surfaces. The skin boundary surface (air-skin interface) and the outer cranial surface are obvious choices that have frequently been used for both image-to-image and image-to-physical registration of head images. The surface representation can be simply a point set (i.e., a collection of points on the surface), a faceted surface (e.g., triangle set), an implicit surface, or a parametric surface (e.g., B-spline surface).

Extraction of a surface, such as the skin or bone, is relatively easy and fairly automatic for head CT and MR images; extraction of many soft tissue boundary surfaces is generally more difficult and less automatic. Image segmentation algorithms can generate 2-D contours in contiguous image slices that are linked together to form a 3-D surface, or they can generate 3-D surfaces directly from the image volume. In physical space, skin surface points can be easily determined using laser range finders; stereo video systems; and articulated mechanical, magnetic, active and passive optical, and ultrasonic 3-D localizers. Bone surface points can be found using track A-mode and B-mode ultrasound probes.

Alternatively, image intensity can be used for registration. Intensity-based registration involves calculating a transformation between two images using the pixel (picture element) or voxel values alone. In its purest form, the registration transformation is determined by optimizing some "similarity measure" that is calculated from all pixel or voxel values. Because of the predominance of 3-D images in medical imaging, we typically refer to these measures as *voxel similarity measures*. For example, if two images being registered are identical except for misalignment, an intuitively obvious similarity measure to use is the sum of squares of intensity differences. In this case, the similarity measure is zero when the images are correctly aligned, and will increase with misregistration. In the slightly more realistic scenario in which the two images differ by misalignment and gaussian noise, it has been shown that the sum of squares of intensity differences is the optimal measure. Certain image registration problems are reasonably close to this ideal case, such as serial registration of MR images. Registration of multimodal images, such as CT-MR registration, has been approached in many ways. The most successful voxel similarity algorithms use the joint probability distribution function of intensities in the two images and similarity measures calculated from the probability distribution function that are based on information theory.[73]

Research has demonstrated that the most effective and accurate algorithms for most types of image-to-image registration are those based on intensities. Point-based and surface-based methods can also be used for these applications, but they require a greater degree of user interaction and have typically exhibited lower accuracy than intensity-based methods. Techniques based on points and surfaces do, however, play an important role in the registration of image to physical space, which is important in image-guided surgery and radiosurgery because the internal information necessary for intensity-based registration is typically unavailable in physical space. In stereotactic radiosurgery, image-to-physical registration of the head is generally accomplished with a stereotactic frame. The frame provides rigid skull fixation using pins or screws and establishes a stereotactic coordinate system in physical space. Most frame systems relate image space to the physical coordinate space by attaching a localizing system consisting of N-shaped fiducials during image acquisition. These N-shaped objects appear as a set of dots in the image slices. The positions of the dots are used to obtain the image registration.

Image Characteristics and Limits of Planning

Several factors limit the accuracy of determining lesion boundaries in an image and of delivering radiation to a planned volume. It is important that the physician be aware of these uncertainties when making and interpreting a plan. The accuracy of lesion boundary identification is limited by partial volume averaging within the voxel, image display characteristics, and image perception. The accuracy is limited by set-up error and by assumptions and errors in the calculation of attenuation, scattering, and nonisotropic geometry of the unit voxel. In both CT and MR, the slice thickness is commonly 2 to 10 times larger than the in-plane pixel dimensions of the tomographic slices.

A digital image is a 2-D or 3-D array of elements called pixels (2-D) or voxels (3-D). Each pixel or voxel has an intensity value associated with it that represents the average value of some quantity. In CT, for example, the intensity represents the average x-ray attenuation coefficient over the region covered by the voxel. This causes a partial volume artifact and loss of accuracy in rendering attenuation changes. In the slice thickness direction, errors as large as the dimension of the slice thickness itself are possible, particularly when rendering multiplanar reconstruction from the stack of tomographic slices in a nonaxial direction. In the case of CT data acquired with 5-mm slice thickness, the voxel dimensions are typically 0.5 mm $\times$ 0.5 mm $\times$ 5 mm (Fig. 7–10). Up to a 5-mm error is possible when determining object boundaries (e.g., tumors for radiation treatment planning).

Spatial sampling of the underlying continuous image constitutes a loss of information by partial volume averaging (Fig. 7–11). Even if there were an infinitely small voxel, another source of inaccuracy is caused by the conversion of the continuous gray level distribution of analog image data into discrete integer values in the process of *quantization*—the process of digitization. In both instances (sampling and quantization), structural information on the scale of the voxel dimension and smaller is lost. The continuous intensity is also quantized, that is, mapped onto a limited number of discrete gray values. This process can cause perceptual limitations as a result of poor relative luminance resolution in dark parts of an image. It can also cause problems in images acquired with a low dynamic range (small number of gray values).

The geometric and intensity fidelity of an image is an important factor in the determination of lesion boundaries. Blurring, contrast, noise, distortion, and artifacts affect image fidelity. Blurring results from the imaging process and from the object. Geometric blurring is a product of the geometry of the imaging process and is influenced by the size of the radiation source and the distances between the

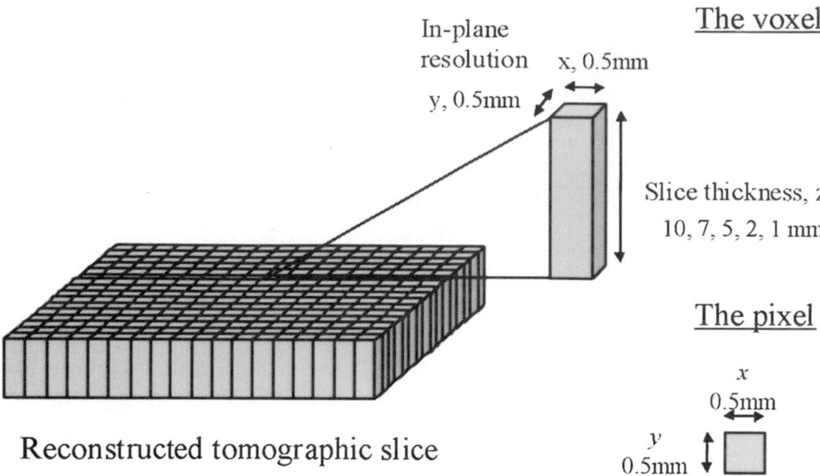

Figure 7–10. The parallelepiped is a simplistic representation of the pixel with dimensions of x and y. Pixel dimensions x and y and the slice thickness z depict the complete and basic representation of a voxel (volume element).

source and patient and between the patient and image receptor. In nuclear medicine, for example, blurring is relatively large and is influenced by the diameter and height of the holes in the collimator of the scintillation camera and the distance between the collimator and the patient. In conventional radiography, receptor blurring is determined by the characteristics of the intensifying screens used to convert impinging x-rays to light for absorption by the light-sensitive x-ray film. The spatial configuration of a structure of interest may prevent the reproduction of a sharp edge in the image. For example, the edge of a cross-sectional image through a cylinder will be sharper than one through a cone because the spatially varying edge of the cone is averaged over the thickness of the image slice.

All medical images are subject to blurring through motion of the radiation source, the anatomy of interest, or the image receptor. Patient motion (both voluntary and involuntary) is the major source of error in the final image. Motion artifacts are more pronounced when the moving object has a significantly different density than the surrounding objects in the region.[34, 35, 74–76] Respiration, the beating heart, an inability of the patient to remain still in a confined area, gas, and fluid flow can cause patient motion. Streak artifacts in CT images are caused by the presence of electron-dense materials with such high x-ray absorption that the attenuation is outside of the dynamic range of the scanner, for example, dental fillings and hip prostheses. Beam hardening artifacts in CT are a consequence of the fact that the x-ray beam is composed of a spectrum of photon energies. As the polychromatic x-ray beam transits through the patient and is increasingly attenuated, the lower energies are preferentially removed, causing an increase in the effective or average energy of the beam, thereby decreasing the calculated μ value.

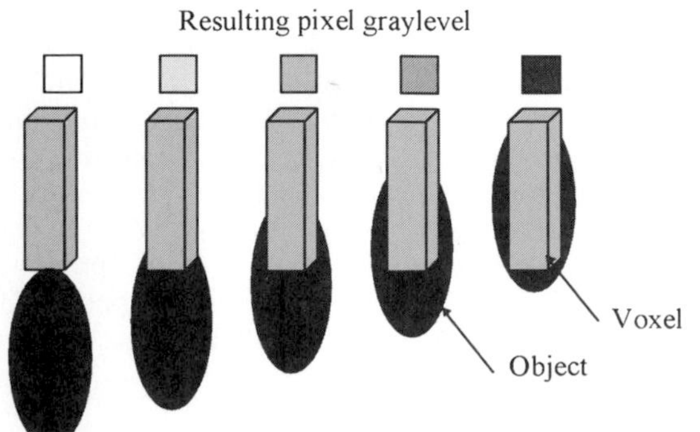

Figure 7–11. Partial volume averaging is caused by the mapping of only a portion of an object or a boundary within the voxel, having an attenuation coefficient significantly different from the surrounding tissues, which results in pixel values that can corrupt the true location of an object or boundary by as much as the slice thickness itself. The choice of a thinner slice thickness can minimize the errors produced by this artifact.

Image contrast is another critical characteristic of medical images. Contrast describes the ability of the image to reveal subtle differences in the composition of different structures in the anatomy of interest. In all imaging, the patient furnishes a certain level of intrinsic contrast. In CT, intrinsic contrast is determined by the difference in electron density between structures. In MR, intrinsic contrast is determined by differences in water proton density and relaxation times. In mammography, the differences are extremely subtle and the tissues are said to offer little intrinsic contrast. Most imaging techniques allow some adjustment of parameters to increase the contrast in the image. In mammography, using low-energy x-rays that undergo principally photoelectric reactions can help reveal subtle differences in tissues. In MR, many different types of pulse sequences and parameters can be used to improve image contrast.

When a video monitor is used to display digital medical images, there is great flexibility in image contrast. The user can display any desired intensity range in the image data as black-to-white on the screen by interactively adjusting the window and level. The level is the image intensity that is displayed as gray on the screen. The window is the range of image intensities displayed from black to white. Although this provides great flexibility, visually perceived boundaries often change as the window and level values are altered. As a rule of thumb, the level should be set halfway between the intensities of the two tissues that the user wishes to differentiate; the intensity of a voxel in CT is related to the electron density of the tissue (Fig. 7–12).

All medical images can have geometric distortions and

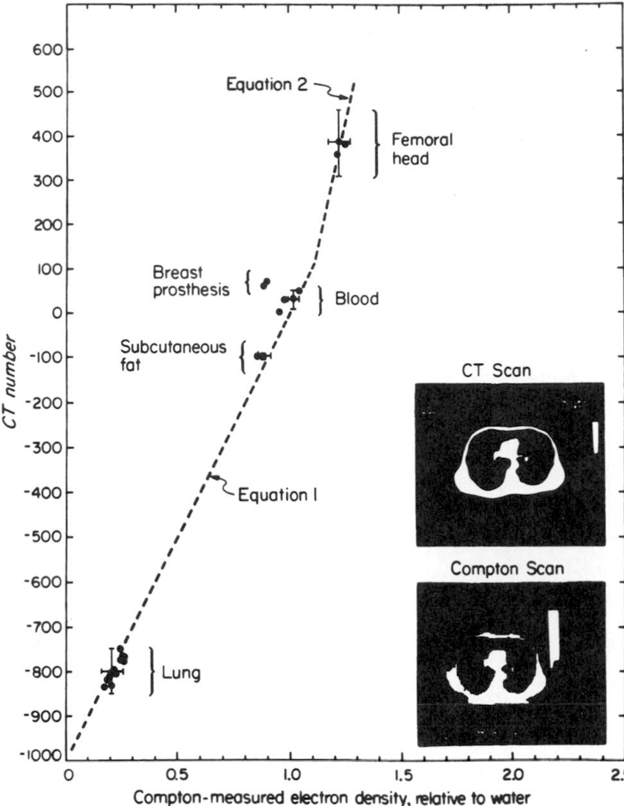

Figure 7–12. CT numbers plotted as a function of electron density relative to water. (From Battista JJ, Rider WD, Van Dyk J: Computed tomography for radiotherapy planning. Int J Radiat Oncol Biol Phys 1980; 6:99, with permission.)

artifacts. Geometric distortion is always present in projection images, for example, because structures that are nearer to the intensifying screen are magnified less than those farther away are. Linear or scale distortion results from uncertainty in the image voxel dimensions. Scale distortion of several percent, which is equivalent to geometric error of several millimeters at the edge of an image, is common in MR images. In CT images acquired with the gantry tilted, uncertainty in the tilt angle, which is not an infrequent problem, causes a shear distortion. A tilt angle error of 1 degree can cause geometric error on the order of 1 to 2 mm. Nonrigid distortion can occur in MR images because of inhomogeneity in the static magnetic field. Such inhomogeneity can arise from scanner imperfections, magnetic susceptibility differences between adjacent structures (e.g., air-tissue interfaces) in the object being imaged, and from magnetic resonance differences among tissues. The latter is the cause of the well-known fat shift in MR images. These factors can cause geometric errors of several millimeters in many typical diagnostic MR images. Most imaging modalities exhibit characteristic types of artifacts. In CT, streak artifacts are caused by thick bone, such as near the skull base and teeth, and by metal. In ultrasonography, multiple reflections within the patient give rise to reverberation artifacts that resemble multiple equally spaced interfaces. In MR, some pulse sequences produce images with substantial intensity drop-out near air-tissue interfaces.

Treatment Planning

The evolution of the technology has made possible the 3-D treatment protocols exemplified by Radiation Therapy Oncology Group protocol numbers 93-11 (dose escalation study for lung cancer), 94-06 (dose escalation study for prostate cancer), and 98-03 (dose escalation study for glioblastoma multiforme); more information on these protocols can be seen at www.rtog.org. These 3-D protocols were based on the volume definitions from ICRU 50 but did not anticipate the intricacies of an overall dose prescription for the final plan, which rigorously prescribed doses through each dose escalation. Furthermore, the protocols present challenges to each department or facility specific to the attributes of the dose escalation software algorithms and hardware:

- Axial and spiral tomotherapy are vulnerable to patient motion but also produce large dose gradients within both the target volume and immediately adjacent normal tissues; other IMRT approaches also produce large dose gradients.
- The dose escalation studies present or open unexplored domains in traditional treatment parameters, such as the dose per fraction to microscopic disease and tumor. IMRT techniques may allow for microscopic disease to receive 1.6 Gy per fraction, while the minimal tumor dose per fraction of the tumor is 1.8 Gy per fraction. Smaller volumes of the target can receive significantly higher doses per fraction.
- Dose escalation IMRT protocols also have encountered the problem of ever-increasing numbers of fractions per overall treatment. To remedy this peccadillo, a protocol has been designed to fix the number of fractions while increasing the dose per fraction.

Intrinsic in these variations is the nonlinear response to dose of the tumor[77] and the normal tissues. The protocols are, in effect, exploring virginal segments of the treatment parameter domain in radiation oncology. Furthermore, each protocol has a tendency to probe in a unique direction or subset of the unexplored territory. The complete recording of the 3-D treatment plan, including the dose-volume histograms and 3-D dose distributions through the pertinent tissues, alleviates this difficulty. The Radiation Therapy Oncology Group 3-D database will allow for the vigorous analysis of short- and long-term tissue response over the parameters of dose, dose rate, dose per fraction size, and total treatment time.

Image registration is predominantly performed for intracranial lesions. The rigidity of the skull and the confinement of the brain tissue by the skull facilitate the application of image fusion: correlation between CT and MRI studies or between preoperative and postoperative scans. Figure 7–13 contains the registration of the CT and MRI data sets for stereotactic radiosurgery. For this particular patient, the registration was performed via two methods:

1. surface matching of the skull between CT and MRI
2. intensity matching between CT and MRI

The accuracy of the fusion for both methods was significantly better than for the stereotactic frame localization method. In Figure 7–13, the alignment of the two scans

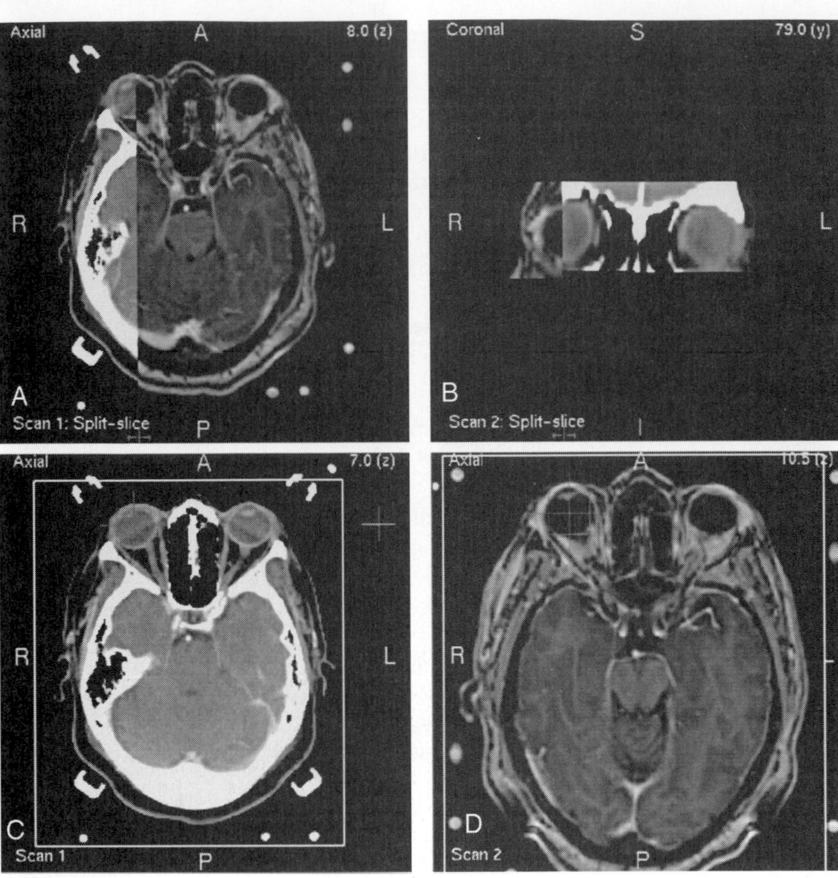

Figure 7–13. Image registration. (A) The comparison of CT with the reconstructed MR slice after correlation was performed using intensity matching. (B) Comparison in the coronal view. (C) The representative CT cut, complete with the corresponding MR reconstruction (D). (Courtesy of the Department of Radiation Oncology, University of Rochester, NY.)

is shown in the upper two panels. The MRI slices are reconstructed to the CT slice selected from the stereotactic frame study. The fidelity of the fusion or matching is well within 1 mm for this study. The fusion is initiated by the selection of identical anatomic sites within each data set, with a minimum of three sites required. The time required to fuse the two studies is on the order of 2 minutes. In this case, the maximum resolution of both CT and MRI scans was used. In summary, the image fusion is most applicable for sites where respiration and pulse have a minimal impact. Consequently, image fusion can be applied and satisfy the accuracy requirements for stereotactic radiosurgery.

Treatment Plan Examples

Computerized treatment planning in the 1960s and 1970s was typified by dose distributions overlaid on patient contours. The contours (body outlines) were derived mechanically and digitized into the computer system. All treatment beams were coplanar with heterogeneity regions estimated by the treatment planner. Figures 7–13A and 7–13B show the typical arrangement for a head-and-neck case with parallel-opposed cobalt-60 beams and an electron boost field for the neck nodes.

The transition to CT-based treatment planning and rigorous heterogeneity corrections is illustrated in Figure 7–14—a composite treatment plan for breast cancer. The chest wall is treated with a set of parallel-opposed beams and an *en face* electron beam with bolus. Heterogeneity corrections are derived from the CT data and the uncertainty in the dose delivery reduces from 7% to 5% overall. The composite plan evinces the impact of the heterogeneities as the beams pass through normal soft tissue and lung tissue. The lung tissue allows for greater transmission of the treatment beam.

A further example of the image manipulation in 3-D treatment planning is exemplified in Figure 7–15 for irradiation of mediastinal masses. The beam's eye view of

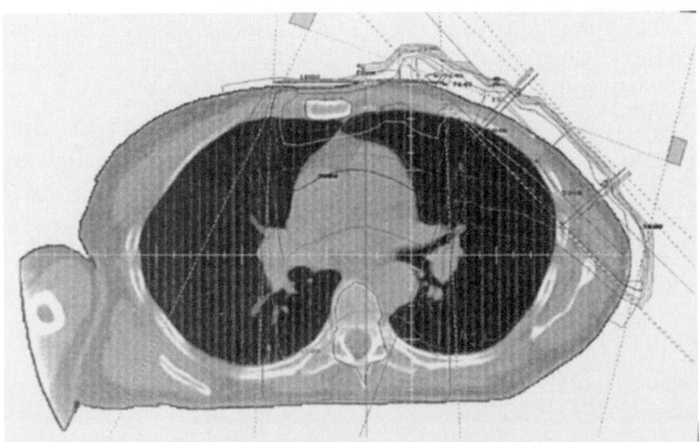

Figure 7–14. A composite plan for the treatment of breast cancer with parallel-opposed breast tangent x-ray beams and an electron beam. Bolus was deployed for the electron beam. Note the increased penetration of the lung in this 2-D composite plan. (Courtesy of the Department of Radiation Oncology, University of Rochester, NY.)

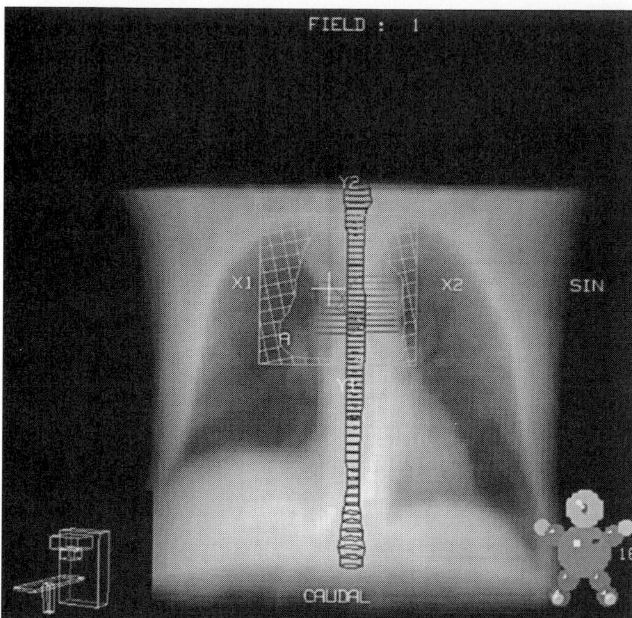

Figure 7–15. The digitally reconstructed radiograph for a patient with a mediastinal metastasis is shown with a beam's eye view for the posterior field. This posterior field is collimated with cerrobend blocking, easily visible in the DRR in the lungs, as well as the rib outlines, the heart, and the vertebral column. (Courtesy of the Department of Radiation Oncology, University of Rochester, NY.)

the blocked field illustrates the alignment targeting of the masses within the blocked field, as well as the outline of the spinal cord in the position of the field relative to the heart and the lungs. This treatment planning tool allows for the planner to spare critical normal tissues with the refinement of the block contour within the x-ray beam.[78, 79]

The second example of the digitally reconstructed radiograph[80] in the beam's eye view is depicted in Figure 7–16 for the irradiation of a large pituitary adenoma. In this view, the multileaf collimator is adjusted to target the adenoma and spare the patient's eyes and brain stem. In this example, a left lateral field is depicted with a wedge as part of a 3-D irradiation.

Tomotherapy[81] for irradiation of the nasal pharynx is depicted in Figure 7–1. A tumor is 1.5 cm anterior to the spinal cord and the tomotherapy dose delivery provides 100% coverage to the lesion; 89% of the tumor dose is delivered to the node. The spinal cord receives 40% of the tumor dose, allowing for a maximum tumor dose of 11.3 Gy if the spinal cord column is the only criterion. Seventy-two percent of the dose is delivered to areas of possible lymphatic involvement (microscopic), while sparing the parotid glands and the cord. The tomotherapy technique is comparable to the dose delivery in proton therapy. In this treatment plan, the dose gradient between the tumor and the spinal cord is 60% over 1.5 cm in the direction of the tumor and 32% fall-off in the last 6 mm anterior to the spinal cord. The ability of tomotherapy to conform the dose to the tumor and microscopic disease volumes, while sparing critical structure such as the spinal cord, is an accomplishment difficult to achieve in forward planning.

Three-dimensional treatment planning is founded on the image reconstruction of patient anatomy from images scanned through the anatomy of interest. Projection of the x-ray beam through the patient anatomy enables:

1. the production of a digitally reconstructed radiograph as shown in Figure 7–17
2. a 3-D representation of the anatomy (vertebral column and skull as shown in the center of Figure 7–17)
3. the 2-D photograph

Manipulation of the image reconstruction allows for the treatment planning team to optimize the treatment beam geometry in forward planning.

In the forward planning mode, the domain of optimal beam geometries is explored by the planning team and then further reviewed with direct dose calculation and dose-volume histogram analysis. The conformal 3-D irradiation of a liver metastasis is shown in Figure 7–18. This figure is an axial CT scan at the central axis level of this treatment plan. The lesion is irradiated with five fields, all conformally shaped to the projection of the lesion in the beam's eye view. The normal tissue sparing of this treatment plan allowed for an unusual dose fractionation schedule of 10 Gy per fraction for 5 fractions, delivering a total of 50 Gy to the lesion. The other critical structures, right and left kidneys and the spinal cord, received less than half the clinical tolerance that is typical of these structures.

Monte Carlo–generated plans for a mediastinal mass are compared with the equivalent path length calculations in Figure 7–19. The equivalent path length dose algorithm is capable of correcting for heterogeneities along the ray line projection. However, the equivalent path length dose algorithm fails to account for the increased penumbra width as the tissue density decreases. Note the enlarged dose

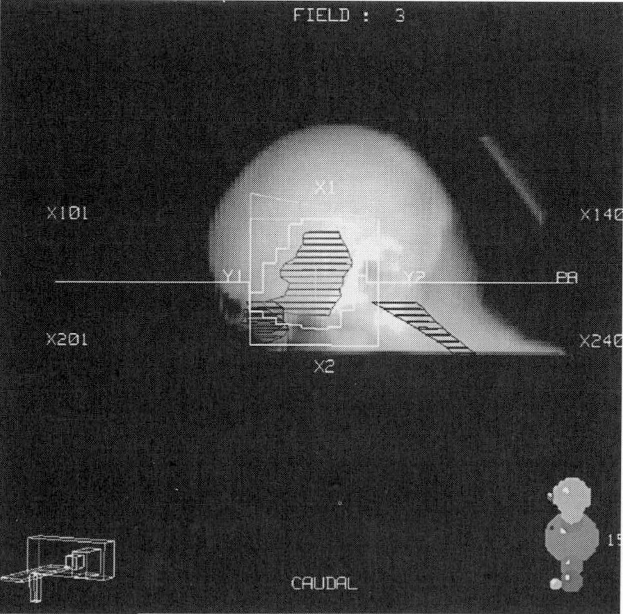

Figure 7–16. In this three-field pituitary plan, the beams are collimated with multileaf collimators. The margin about the tumor mass is varied to spare critical structures as they encroach upon the tumor mass. (Courtesy of the Department of Radiation Oncology, University of Rochester, NY.)

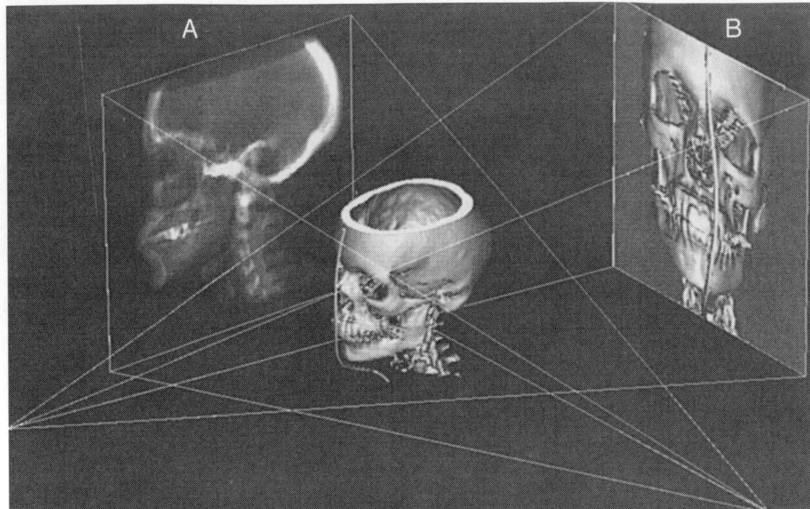

Figure 7–17. CT scans are used to reconstruct the surface of the human skull, as generated by the treatment planning system, PINNACLE (ADAC Corp.). A digitally reconstructed radiograph in the beam's eye view (A) and a 2-D photograph of the human skull (B) are shown. (From Kessler ML, Puff DT: Segmentation and visualization for treatment planning. In: Mackie TR, Palta JR [eds]: Teletherapy: Present and Future. Madison, Advanced Medical Publishing, 1996, with permission.)

distributions in the Monte Carlo plans as opposed to the equivalent path length curves. The effect is particularly pronounced in the sagittal views.

Future Directions in Treatment Plan Optimization

The principal goal of radiation oncology is to control local disease by delivering the maximum dose to the target volume while minimizing the dose to the adjacent normal tissues. A variety of approaches have emerged over the years and used the traditional approach to treatment planning known as forward treatment planning.[82–88] However, the difficulty with forward treatment planning or human optimization is the length of time required for the human operator to reach the global minimum or unique solution given the large domain of treatment plan options. Research developments in the late 1990s have focused on the automation of treatment plan optimization.[89–94] The search domain includes but is not limited to:

- the use of a larger number of treatment fields
- 3-D treatment geometry
- automated field shaping, with the use of multileaf collimators
- the introduction of IMRTs with the use of static MLC, dynamic motion of MLC leaves, or other more sophisticated IMRT approaches.[94, 95]

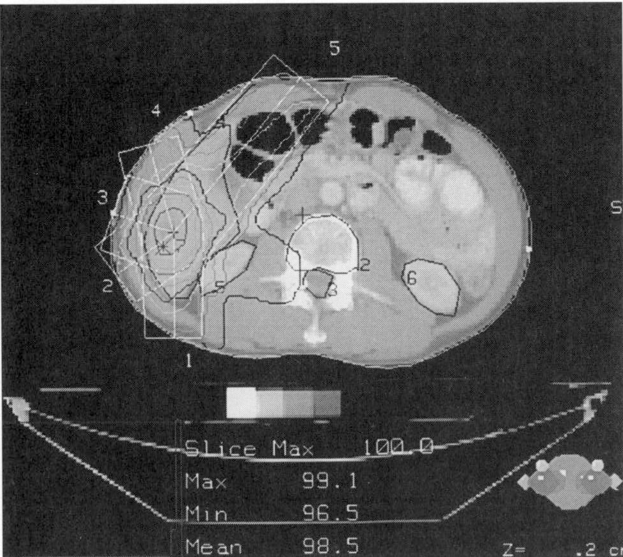

Figure 7–18. 3-D conformal irradiation of a liver lesion using CadPlan. The five beams focusing on one isocenter are collimated conformally with a multileaf collimator. The dose sparing of normal tissue was significant, and it allowed for the high dose of 5 Gy per fraction. (Courtesy of the Department of Radiation Oncology, University of Rochester, NY.)

All optimization techniques are, in a broad sense, inverse treatment planning approaches. The approach is to prescribe a dose distribution to the target volume and impose penalties on dose delivery to critical structures external to the target volume. The investigation of treatment optimization techniques has produced one commercial treatment planning and delivery system known as the Peacock system (NOMOS Corporation). Other approaches include the use of spiral tomotherapy,[81] dynamic MLC for IMRT,[92] and dynamic MLC during gantry rotation. As these treatment techniques progress, the use of circular collimators in linac-based stereotactic radiosurgery and the gamma knife will become increasingly obsolete. Stereotactic radiosurgery, with the μMLC, delivers a conformal dose distribution to irregularly shaped lesions and is significantly superior to the circular collimation technique in terms of dose uniformity, accuracy, and normal tissue dose-sparing. The exception is for lesion dimensions smaller than the μMLC leaf width.

In summary, 3-D dose escalation studies, IMRT, tomotherapy, and dynamic MLC techniques present unique opportunities and challenges. The initial 3-D dose escalation studies have explored the tumor and tissue dose response for variations in different independent treatment parameters. Concomitantly, each dose delivery technique may prove to be tumor-site dependent. The appropriate and necessary conditions for inverse treatment planning are, as yet, not well known.[96]

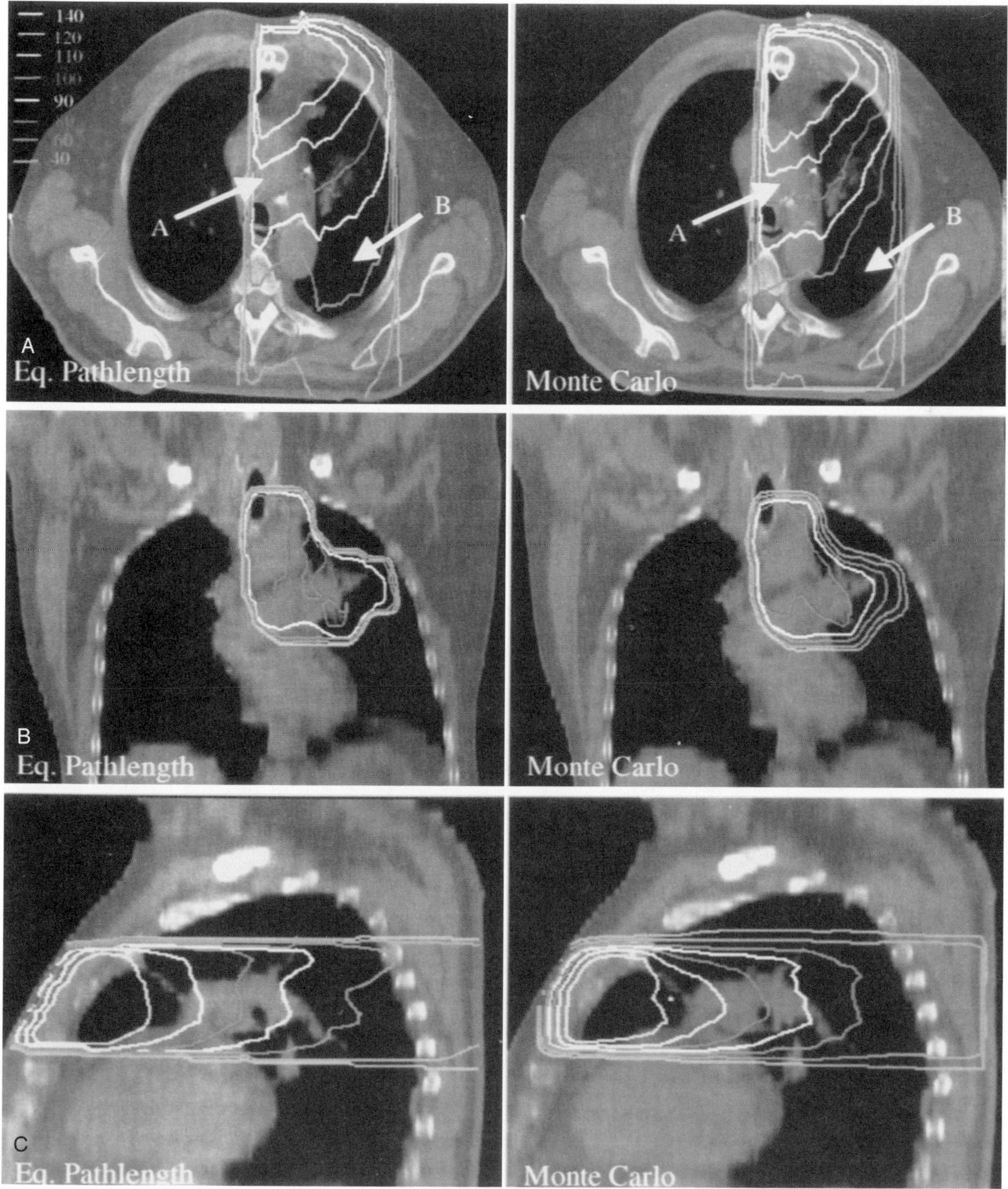

Figure 7–19. A comparison of dose distributions for opposed but oblique x-ray beams through the mediastinum and the left lung. Comparisons for both the equivalent path length and the Monte Carlo calculations are shown in the axial *(A)*, coronal *(B)*, and sagittal *(C)* views. Note that the Monte Carlo algorithm is capable of calculating the lateral disequilibrium as the penumbra spreads or broadens in the less dense lung tissue. (From Wang L, Chui CS, Lovelock M: A patient-specific Monte Carlo dose–calculation method for proton beams. Med Phys 1998; 25:867–878, with permission.)

REFERENCES

1. Wilson RR: Radiological use of fast protons. Radiology 1946; 47:487.
2. Kaplan HS: Hodgkin's Disease, 2nd ed. Cambridge, Harvard University Press, 1980.
3. Feinstein AR, Sosin DM, Wells CK: The Will Rogers phenomenon. Stage migration and new diagnostic techniques as a source of misleading statistics for survival in cancer. N Engl J Med 1985; 312:1604–1608.
4. Zelefsky MJ, Fuks Z, Wolfe T, et al: Locally advanced prostatic cancer: long-term toxicity outcome after three-dimensional conformal radiation therapy—a dose-escalation study. Radiology 1998; 209:169–174.
5. Zelefsky MJ, Wallner KE, Ling CC, et al: Comparison of the 5-year outcome and morbidity of three-dimensional conformal radiotherapy versus transperineal permanent iodine-125 implantation for early-stage prostatic cancer. J Clin Oncol 1999; 17:517–522.
6. Koehler AM, Preston WM: Protons in radiation therapy. Radiology 1972; 104:191–195.
7. Hendee WR, Ibbott GS: Radiation Therapy Physics, 2nd ed. St. Louis, Mosby-Year Book Inc, 1996.
8. Kerst DW: Betatron-Quastler era at the University of Illinois. Med Phys 1975; 2:297–300.
9. Quastler H, Adams GD, Almy GM, et al: Techniques for application of the betatron to medical therapy with report of one case. Am J Roentgenol Rad Ther 1949; 61:591–625.
10. Adams GD, Almy GM, Dancoff SM, et al: Techniques for application of the betatron to medical therapy. Am J Roentgenol Rad Ther 1948; 60:153–157.
11. Brucer M: An automatic controlled pattern cesium-137 teletherapy machine. AJR Am J Roentgenol 1956; 75:49–55.
12. Galvin JM, Smith AR, Lally B: Characterization of a multi-leaf collimator system. Int J Radiat Oncol Biol Phys 1993; 25:181–192.
13. Spirou SV, Chui CS: Generation of arbitrary intensity profiles by dynamic jaws or multileaf collimators. Med Phys 1994; 21:1031–1041.
14. Thames HD, Schultheiss TE, Hendry JH, et al: Can modest escalations of dose be detected as increased tumour control? Int J Radiat Oncol Biol Phys 1992; 22:241–246.
15. Leibel SA, Kutcher GJ, Mohan R: Three-dimensional conformal radiation therapy at the Memorial Sloan-Kettering Cancer Center. Semin Radiat Oncol 1992; 2:274–289.
16. Lichter AS: Three-dimensional conformal radiation therapy: a testable hypothesis. Int J Radiat Oncol Biol Phys 1991; 21:853–855.
17. Hanks GE, Hanlon AL, Pinover WH, et al: Survival advantage for prostate cancer patients treated with high-dose three-dimensional conformal radiotherapy. Cancer J Sci Am 1999; 5:152–158.
18. Sandler HM, Perez-Tamayo C, Ten Haken RK, et al: Dose escalation for stage C (T3) prostate cancer: minimal rectal toxicity observed using conformal therapy. Radiother Oncol 1992; 23:53–54.
19. Michalski JM, Purdy JA, Winter K, et al: Preliminary report of toxicity following 3D radiation therapy for prostate cancer on 3DOG/RTOG 9406. Int J Radiat Oncol Biol Phys 2000; 46:391–402.
20. De Gersem WRT, Derycke S, Colle CO, et al: Inhomogeneous target dose distributions: a dimension more for optimization? Int J Radiat Oncol Biol Phys 1999; 44:461–468.
21. Lawrence TS, Tesser RJ, Ten Haken RK: An application of dose volume histograms to the treatment of intrahepatic malignancies with radiation therapy. Int J Radiat Oncol Biol Phys 1990; 19:1041–1047.
22. Drzymala RE, Mohan R, Brewster L, et al: Dose-volume histograms. Int J Radiat Oncol Biol Phys 1991; 21:71–78.
23. Kutcher GJ, Burman C, Brewster L, et al: Histogram reduction method for calculating complication probabilities for three dimensional treatment planning evaluations. Int J Radiat Oncol Biol Phys 1991; 21:137–146.
24. Lawrence TS, Ten Haken RK, Kessler ML, et al: The use of 3D dose volume analysis to predict radiation hepatitis. Int J Radiat Oncol Biol Phys 1992; 23:781–788.
25. Levegrün S, Waschek T, van Kampen M, et al: Biological scoring of different target volume extensions in 3D radiotherapy treatment planning. Proceedings of the Symposium on Principles and Practice of 3-D Radiation Treatment Planning, Munich, 1996. Munich, Technische Universität, 1996.
26. Ling CC, Spiro IJ, Mitchell J, et al: The variation of OER with dose rate. Int J Radiat Oncol Biol Phys 1985; 11:1367–1373.
27. Kutcher GJ, Burman C: Calculation of complication probability factors for non uniform normal tissue irradiation: the effective volume method. Int J Radiat Oncol Biol Phys 1989; 16:1623–1630.
28. Niemierko A, Goitein M: Calculation of normal tissue complication probability and dose-volume histogram reduction schemes for tissues with a critical element architecture. Radiother Oncol 1991; 20:166–176.
29. Niemierko A, Goitein M: Implementation of a model for estimating tumor control probability for an inhomogeneously irradiated tumor. Radiother Oncol 1993; 29:140–147.
30. Niemierko A, Goitein M: Modeling of normal tissue response to radiation: the critical volume model. Int J Radiat Oncol Biol Phys 1993; 25:135–145.
31. Ten Haken RK, Martel MK, Kessler ML, et al: Use of veff and iso-NTCP in the implementation of dose escalation protocols. Int J Radiat Oncol Biol Phys 1993; 27:689–695.
32. Webb S, Nahum A: A model for calculating tumor control probability in radiotherapy including the effects of inhomogeneous distributions of dose and clonogenic cell density. Phys Med Biol 1993; 38:653–666.
33. Jackson A, Ten Haken RK, Robertson JM, et al: Analysis of clinical complication data for radiation hepatitis using a parallel architecture model. Int J Radiat Oncol Biol Phys 1995; 31:883–891.
34. International Commission on Radiation Units and Measurements: Prescribing, recording, and reporting photon beam therapy. ICRU Report 50. Bethesda, International Commission on Radiation Units and Measurements, 1993.
35. Sailer SL, Bourland JD, Rosenman JG, et al: 3D beams need 3D names. Int J Radiat Oncol Biol Phys 1990; 19:797–798.
36. Dickof P, Ladyke C: Naming 3D beams. Int J Radiat Oncol Biol Phys 1991; 21:1106–1107.
37. Van Dyk J, Barnett RB, Cygler JE, et al: Commissioning and quality assurance of treatment planning computers. Int J Radiat Oncol Biol Phys 1993; 26:261–273.
38. Kutcher GJ, Coia L, Gillin M, et al: Comprehensive QA for radiation oncology: report of AAPM Radiation Therapy Committee Task Group 40. Med Phys 1994; 21:581–618.
39. Ketting CH, Austin-Seymour M, Kalet I, et al: Automated planning target volume generation: an evaluation pitting a computer-based tool against human experts. Int J Radiat Oncol Biol Phys 1997; 37:697–704.
40. Kutcher GJ, Mageras GS, Leibel SA: Control, correction and modeling of setup errors and organ motion. Semin Radiat Oncol 1995; 5:134–145.
41. Roeske JC, Forman JD, Mesina CF, et al: Evaluation of changes in the size and location of the prostate, seminal vesicles, bladder, and rectum during a course of external beam radiotherapy. Int J Radiat Oncol Biol Phys 1995; 33:1321–1329.
42. Balter JM, Ten Haken RK, Lawrence TS, et al: Uncertainties in CT-based radiation therapy planning associated with patient breathing. Int J Radiat Oncol Biol Phys 1996; 36:167–174.
43. Breuer H, Wynchank S: Quantitation of brain movement within the skull associated with head position: its relevance to proton therapy planning. 23rd Proton Therapy Cooperative Groups (PTCOG) Meeting, Cape Town, 1995. Boston, PTCOG, 1996.
44. Milan J, Bentley RE: The storage and manipulation of radiation dose data in a small digital computer. Br J Radiol 1974; 47:115–121.
45. Van de Geijn J: The computation of two and three dimensional dose distributions in cobalt-60 teletherapy. Br J Radiol 1965; 38:369–367.
46. Clarkson JR: A note on depth doses in fields of irregular shape. Br J Radiol 1941; 14:265.
47. Cunningham JR: Scatter-air ratios. Phys Med Biol 1972; 17:42–51.
48. Shiu AS, Hogstrom KR: Dose in bone and tissue near bone-tissue interface from electron beam. Int J Radiat Oncol Biol Phys 1991; 21:695–702.
49. Shiu AS, Tung S, Hogstrom DR, et al: Verification data for electron beam dose algorithms. Med Phys 1992; 19:623–636.
50. Shiu AS, Tung SS, Nyerick CE, et al: Comprehensive analysis of electron-beam central-axis dose for a radiotherapy linear accelerator. Med Phys 1994; 21:559–566.
51. Orton CG, Mondalek PM, Spicka JT, et al: Lung corrections in photon beam treatment planning: are we ready? Int J Radiat Oncol Biol Phys 1984; 10:2191–2199.
52. Wong JW, Purdy JA: On methods of inhomogeneity corrections for photon transport. Med Phys 1990; 17:807–881.
53. Khan FM, Potish RA: Treatment Planning in Radiation Oncology. Baltimore, Williams & Wilkins, 1998.

54. Mohan R, Chui C, Lidofsky L: Differential pencil beam dose computation model for photons. Med Phys 1986; 13:64–73.
55. Van de Geijn J, Fraass BA: The net fractional depth dose; a basis for a unified analytical description of FDD, TAR, TMR, and TPR. Med Phys 1984; 11:784–793.
56. Mohan R, Wang X, Jackson A, et al: The potential and limitations of the inverse radiotherapy technique. Radiother Oncol 1994; 32:232–248.
57. Mohan R: Field shaping for three-dimensional conformal radiation therapy and multi-leaf collimation. Semin Radiat Oncol 1995; 5:86–99.
58. Mohan R: Intensity modulation in radiotherapy. In: Palta J, Mackie TR (eds): Teletherapy: Past and Future, pp 761–792. Madison, Advanced Medical Publishing, 1996.
59. Eyges L: Multiple scattering with energy loss. Phys Rev 1948; 74:1534.
60. Schach von Wittenau AE, Cox LJ, Bergstrom PM Jr, et al: Correlated histogram representation of Monte Carlo derived medical accelerator photon-output phase space. Med Phys 1999; 26:1196–1211.
61. Chaney EL, Pizer SM: Defining anatomical structures from medical images. Semin Radiat Oncol 1992; 2:215–225.
62. Wolbarst AB: Physics of Radiology. Norwalk, Appleton & Lange, 1993.
63. Robb RA: Three-Dimensional Biomedical Imaging: Principles and Practice. New York, VCH, 1995.
64. Pellizari CA, Grzeszczuk R, Chen GTY, et al: Volumetric visualization of anatomy for treatment planning. Med Phys 1996; 34:205–211.
65. Curry TS III, Dowdey JE, Murry RC Jr: Christensen's Physics of Diagnostic Radiology, 4th ed. Philadelphia, Williams & Wilkins, 1990.
66. Kessler ML, Pitluck S, Petti P, et al: Integration of multimodality imaging data for radiotherapy treatment planning. Int J Radiat Oncol Biol Phys 1991; 21:1653–1667.
67. Kuszyk BX, Ney DR, Fishman EK: The current state of the art in three dimensional oncologic imaging: an overview. Int J Radiat Oncol Biol Phys 1995; 33:1029–1039.
68. Munro P: Portal imaging technology: past, present, and future. Semin Radiat Oncol 1995; 5:115–133.
69. James M: Pattern Recognition. Oxford, BSP Professional Books, 1987.
70. Lorenson WE, Cline HE: Marching Cubes: a high resolution 3D surface construction algorithm. Computer Graphics 1987; 21:163–169.
71. Sherouse GW, Rosenman J, McMurry HL, et al: Automatic digital contrast enhancement of radiotherapy films. Int J Radiat Oncol Biol Phys 1987; 13:801–806.
72. Jain AK: Fundamentals of Digital Image Processing. Englewood Cliffs, Prentice Hall, 1989.
73. Fitzpatrick JM, Hill DLG, Maurer CR Jr: Image registration. In: Fitzpatrick JM, Sonka M (eds): Handbook of Medical Imaging, vol 2: Medical Image Processing and Analysis. Bellingham, SPIE Optical Engineering Press, 2000.
74. Korin H, Ehman R, Reiderer SJ, et al: Respiration kinematics of the upper abdominal organs: a quantitative study. Magn Reson Med 1992; 23:172–178.
75. Poncelet BP, Wedeen VJ, Weisskoff RM, et al: Brain parenchyma motion: measurement with cine echo-planar MR imaging. Radiology 1992; 185:645–651.
76. Balter JM, Sandler HM, Lam K, et al: Measurement of prostate movement over the course of routine radiotherapy using implanted markers. Int J Radiat Oncol Biol Phys 1995; 31:113–118.
77. Okunieff P, Morgan D, Niemierko A, et al: Radiation dose-response of human tumors. Int J Radiat Oncol Biol Phys 1995; 32:1227–1237.
78. Emami B, Lyman J, Brown A, et al: Tolerance of normal tissue to therapeutic irradiation. Int J Radiat Oncol Biol Phys 1991; 21:109–122.
79. Marks LB: The pulmonary effects of thoracic irradiation. Oncology 1994; 8:89–100.
80. Sherouse GW, Novins K, Chaney EL: Computation of digitally reconstructed radiographs for use in radiotherapy treatment design. Int J Radiat Oncol Biol Phys 1990; 18:651–658.
81. Mackie TR, Holmes T, Swerdloff S, et al: Tomotherapy: a new concept for the delivery of dynamic conformal radiotherapy. Med Phys 1993; 20:1709–1719.
82. Rosenman J, Sailer SL, Sherouse GW, et al: Virtual simulation: initial clinical results. Int J Radiat Oncol Biol Phys 1991; 20:843–851.
83. Gehring, MA, Mackit TR, Kubsad SS, et al: A three-dimensional volume visualization package applied to stereotactic radiosurgery treatment planning. Int J Radiat Oncol Biol Phys 1991; 21:491–500.
84. Hogstrom KR, Starkschall G, Shiu AS: Dose calculation algorithms for electron beams. In: Purdy J (ed): Advances in Radiation Oncology Physics, pp 900–924. New York, American Institute of Physics, 1991.
85. Niemierko A, Urie M, Goitein M: Optimization of 3-D radiation therapy with both physical and biological end points and constraints. Int J Radiat Oncol Biol Phys 1992; 23:99–108.
86. Convery DJ, Rosenbloom ME: The generation of intensity-modulated fields for conformal radiotherapy by dynamic collimation. Phys Med Biol 1992; 37:1359–1374.
87. LoSasso TJ, Chui CS, Kutcher GJ, et al: The use of a multi-leaf collimator for conformal radiotherapy of carcinomas of the prostate and nasopharynx. Int J Radiat Oncol Biol Phys 1993; 25:161–170.
88. Fraass BA, McShan DL: Three dimensional photon beam treatment planning. In: Smith AR (ed): Radiation Therapy Physics, pp 43–93. Berlin, Springer, 1995.
89. Brahme A: Treatment optimization using physical and radiobiological objective functions. In: Smith AR (ed): Radiation Therapy Physics, pp 209–246. Berlin, Springer, 1995.
90. Rosen II, Lam KS, Lane RG, et al: Comparison of simulated annealing algorithms for conformal therapy treatment planning. Int J Radiat Oncol Biol Phys 1995; 33:1091–1099.
91. Deasy JO: Multiple local minima in radiotherapy optimization problems with dose-volume constraints. Med Phys 1997; 24:1157–1161.
92. Ling CC, Burman C, Chui CS, et al: Conformal radiation treatment of prostate cancer using inversely-planned intensity-modulated photon beams produced with dynamic multileaf collimation. Int J Radiat Oncol Biol Phys 1996; 35:721–730.
93. Yu Y, Schell MC: A genetic algorithm for the optimization of prostate implants. Med Phys 1996; 23:2085–2091.
94. Chang SX, Deschesne KM, Cullip TJ, et al: A comparison of different intensity modulation treatment techniques for tangential breast irradiation. Int J Radiat Oncol Biol Phys 1999; 45:1305–1314.
95. Ling CC, Burman C, Chui CS, et al: Conformal radiation treatment of prostate cancer using inversely-planned intensity-modulated photon beams produced with dynamic multileaf collimation. Int J Radiat Oncol Biol Phys 1996; 35:721–730.
96. Xing L, Li JG, Donaldson S, et al: Optimization of importance factors in inverse planning. Phys Med Biol 1999; 44:2525–2536.

8 Basic Concepts of Cancer Chemotherapy and Principles of Medical Oncology

RICHARD F. BAKEMEIER, MD, FACP, Medical Oncology
RAMAN QAZI, MD, FACP, Hematology/Oncology

Work on, my medicine, work!

WILLIAM SHAKESPEARE, *Othello*

Perspective

The evolution of the field of cancer chemotherapy during the 30-plus years' history of this textbook presents an impressive panorama of the application of laboratory and clinical science to the challenges of clinical oncology.

- During the 1950s and early 1960s, a variety of chemical agents were demonstrated to have antitumor effects in experimental animal systems and were then investigated in the treatment of human cancers.
- By the end of the 1960s, it was apparent that systemic chemotherapy could induce long-lasting, complete clinical remissions in a variety of disseminated malignancies, such as choriocarcinoma in women, as well as acute lymphoblastic leukemia, Wilms' tumor, Burkitt's lymphoma, and Hodgkin's disease in children and young adults.
- The previously prevalent view that chemotherapy was appropriate only for disseminated stages of cancer became obsolete as benefit was demonstrated in certain groups of women given systemic, so-called "adjuvant" chemotherapy, following primary surgical or radiation therapy for breast cancer, with the intent of eradicating occult micrometastases.
- The introduction of a series of new agents in the past three decades has led to cancer remissions of variable completeness and duration. The demonstration of effectiveness of the vinca alkaloids, anthracycline antibiotics, and platinum derivatives in the 1970s, the epipodophyllotoxins in the 1980s, and the taxanes in the 1990s has provided an abundance of chemotherapy combinations.
- Intensive combination chemotherapy has achieved long-term and complete clinical remissions, and apparent cures in disseminated large cell non-Hodgkin's lymphomas and testicular carcinomas. However, the common adult cancers—breast, colon, lung, and prostate cancers—continue to show disappointing responses, either in completeness or in duration.

Clearly, new approaches to the aforementioned common cancers are needed; the answers may soon be forthcoming from the molecular biologists and geneticists who are intensively studying mechanisms of cell division and differentiation. It is reasonable to hope that, within the coming decade, the approach to a variety of cancers will shift from the application of cytotoxins, which damage both neoplastic cells and normal cells, to exploitation of recently acquired knowledge. For example, following DNA damage, the p53 protein plays a role in arresting cell division and contributes to "programmed cell death" or apoptosis; therefore, there exists the possibility of taking advantage of the role of the *TP53* suppressor gene products and other cell cycle control mechanisms. The complex interactions of this *TP53* system with other genes controlling cyclin-dependent kinase, retinoblastoma gene activation, E2F transcription factors, and a series of enzymes involved in DNA synthesis are gradually being clarified.

Another area of increasing importance is the evolving role played by monoclonal antibodies. Examples that are already in clinical trials are antibodies being directed against *HER2/neu* (Herceptin) in the case of breast cancer, and against CD20 (rituximab) in the case of non-Hodgkin's lymphoma. These agents are being administered alone or in combination with chemotherapy, and are discussed in greater detail in the relevant chapters (e.g., Chapters 17 and 18).

Mechanisms of resistance to common chemotherapeutic agents and the role of genes such as *MDR1,* which mediates resistance, are being actively studied. The biology of oncogene function (e.g., *RAS*), development of tumor blood supply, and the process of tumor invasion all provide new opportunities for intervention. When these and other molecular mechanisms are better understood, the window of opportunity will expand for designing chemotherapeutic strategies based on new targets. Thereby, the development of cancer cell resistance to chemotherapy, which frustrates the therapeutic approaches to the common malignancies, may be circumvented. Details of the current knowledge of these exciting new horizons are further discussed, and can be found in detail in the general references.[1–12]

Medical Oncology

In the last three decades, medical oncology has become firmly established as a subspecialty of internal medicine. It encompasses many facets of internal medicine, including infectious diseases and immunology, pulmonary medicine, gastroenterology, hematology, neurology, nephrology, and endocrinology.[13] The major functions of a medical oncologist are:

- the interpretation of the natural history of malignant diseases
- the appropriate application of cancer chemotherapeutic techniques, both in the adjuvant setting combined with surgery or radiation therapy for primary tumors and for disseminated malignancies
- the diagnosis and management of complications of the diseases
- the coordination of emotional, nutritional, and social support

Because approximately two thirds of the 1 million or more cancer patients diagnosed annually in the United States develop recurrent or disseminated neoplastic disease, a clear need exists for the widespread availability of physicians with skills in the discipline.[14–16]

The medical oncologist should be well informed in the basic principles of the pharmacology of cancer chemotherapy and pain control; tumor pathobiology, including cell kinetics; patterns of metastasis; immunologic aspects of neoplasia; cancer epidemiology; and early detection methods. The development of more effective chemotherapeutic techniques depends on using currently available drugs in optimal ways as well as on the development of new agents. Participation in clinical trials, including cooperative group trials, is important for progress to be maintained in this area (see Chapter 9, Basic Concepts in Drug Development and Clinical Trials). These clinical trials also involve the study of a variety of biologic response modifiers, about which the medical oncologist should stay informed. These are discussed in Chapter 11, Basic Concepts of Tumor Immunology and Principles of Immunotherapy.

History of Cancer Chemotherapy

The history of human cancer chemotherapy is relatively brief. The first clinical studies involving nitrogen mustard were undertaken by Gilman, Goodman, Lindskog, and Dougherty in 1942 (although the myelosuppressive and lympholytic properties of mustards were recognized as early as 1919).[9] Another major milestone was the demonstration, in 1948, by Farber and associates of a beneficial effect of a folic acid analogue in acute lymphoblastic leukemia of childhood. Following these, a variety of chemical compounds shown to have antitumor activity in experimental animal systems eventually entered into human clinical trials. The purine antagonist, 6-mercaptopurine, was described by Elion and Hitchings in 1952, one of a series of contributions that led to the receipt of a Nobel prize. In the early 1950s, Heidelberger synthesized 5-fluorouracil (5-FU) after reasoning correctly that an antimetabolite resembling uracil should block the formation of thymine nucleotides, and thereby prevent DNA synthesis. This antipyrimidine is still a mainstay of cancer chemotherapy 40 years later. In the 1960s and 1970s, many new antineoplastic drugs came into clinical use and, in subsequent years, the emphasis has been on developing new combinations of available drugs, optimizing their timing and dosage, and modulating their toxicities.

Treatment Decisions

The proper application of new drugs or new combinations of standard agents requires knowledge of the mechanisms of action and metabolism of the drugs involved, as well as their effects on normal tissues. Understanding effects on bone marrow cell kinetics and morphology is particularly important, as is knowledge of drug-induced alterations in renal, gastrointestinal, and pulmonary functions. The number and variety of available chemotherapeutic agents, each most useful with a particular group of malignancies, have made true expertise in this field a challenging—even formidable—goal. However, virtually all physicians whose responsibilities involve cancer patient management should have a general appreciation of the principles of cancer chemotherapy. This includes the indications for palliative and adjuvant drug treatment for the common malignancies, and the recognition and management of the most frequently experienced side effects of standard chemotherapeutic agents.

It is of primary importance that realistic goals be set for programs of chemotherapy because these goals will influence the choice of agents and the intensity of treatment. But the first decision that the medical oncologist must grapple with, following confirmation of the histologic diagnosis and staging of the patient, is whether to recommend active cytotoxic therapy at all. This decision requires an objective appraisal of a broad range of information, including:

- the natural history of the particular patient's disease
- the type and severity of symptoms
- the current activity level (performance status) of the patient
- the patient's age
- the likely response rate of this malignancy to available therapy
- the measurability of response to therapy
- the psychosocial aspects of the patient, including motivation for treatment, availability of support systems, and financial consequences of therapy for the patient and family

Once the decision to treat has been made, the optimal application of antineoplastic drugs requires consideration of:

1. the biologic characteristics of the neoplastic disease
2. the pharmacology of the agents to be used
3. the spectrum of drug effectiveness as determined through clinical trials and through currently available *in vitro* predictive tests
4. the clinical condition of the patient, including nutrition, infections, hematologic status, emotional profile, and general level of activity

The following discussion will briefly consider these topics, and the reader is referred to more extensive references for additional details (see General References).

Tumor Biologic Aspects of Cancer Chemotherapy

Malignant Transformation

Effective chemotherapeutic control of neoplastic cell growth is based ideally on knowledge of specific quantitative and qualitative changes in cellular biology resulting from malignant transformation. Such transformation involves a heritable change or changes in the stem cell of virtually any tissue, resulting in the production of daughter cells with absent or imperfect functioning of normal homeostatic controls or alteration of normal differentiation. Current knowledge leaves unanswered many relevant questions concerning the genotypic and phenotypic changes involved in the abnormal proliferative, invasive, and metastatic characteristics of cancer cells (see Chapter 2, The Biology of Cancer).

Some human neoplastic cell genomes have been shown to contain DNA similar to the oncogenes associated with neoplastic transformation in animal tumor systems caused by certain viruses. Furthermore, homologous sequences of DNA have been identified in normal human cells. These cellular proto-oncogenes function in normal processes of growth and differentiation, and in viral or chemical carcinogenesis, they may be activated through mutation, translocation, or gene amplification. Although the mechanisms by which oncogenes contribute to the changes associated with malignancy are still not fully explained, the products of these genes have been identified. They include tyrosine-specific protein kinase activity, growth factors or growth factor receptors, proteins with guanosine triphosphate–binding activity, and nuclear proteins that may be involved in chromatin remodeling or transcription regulation, or in both.[3]

As these mechanisms are clarified, it seems likely that specific biochemical targets will be identified toward which new chemotherapeutic agents can be directed. The resulting information may permit specific manipulation of the differentiation and proliferation of malignant cells in a manner that spares major alterations in normal cell functions.

Kinetic Basis of Chemotherapy

Tumor Cell Burden

Figure 8–1 provides a graphic representation of several concepts important in cancer chemotherapy. One of these concepts is that of *tumor cell burden*. The simplified growth curve of the tumor in Figure 8–1 begins at a hypothetical time-zero. An event occurs from which the first surviving tumor stem cell or clonogenic cell results, deviating from its normal counterparts in a manner that permits inappropriate differentiation and proliferation. As tumor cell division occurs, at intervals varying from hours to weeks, cells accumulate in one or more sites, in numbers that usually must approximate at least 10^9 cells in one location (a mass approximately 1 cm in diameter) for their detection at the so-called clinical horizon. Actually, many tumors demonstrate a progressive exponential slowing of growth in relation to tumor burden, referred to as gompertzian growth after a nineteenth-century mathematician. This tumor growth process will involve many cell divisions and tumor size doublings; during this time, a number of changes can occur that are important in an eventual interaction of the tumor cells with chemotherapeutic agents. These include changes in:

1. vascular supply and oxygenation, which eventually may become inadequate, providing poor nutrition of the central zone of the tumor and poor exposure to chemotherapeutic agents

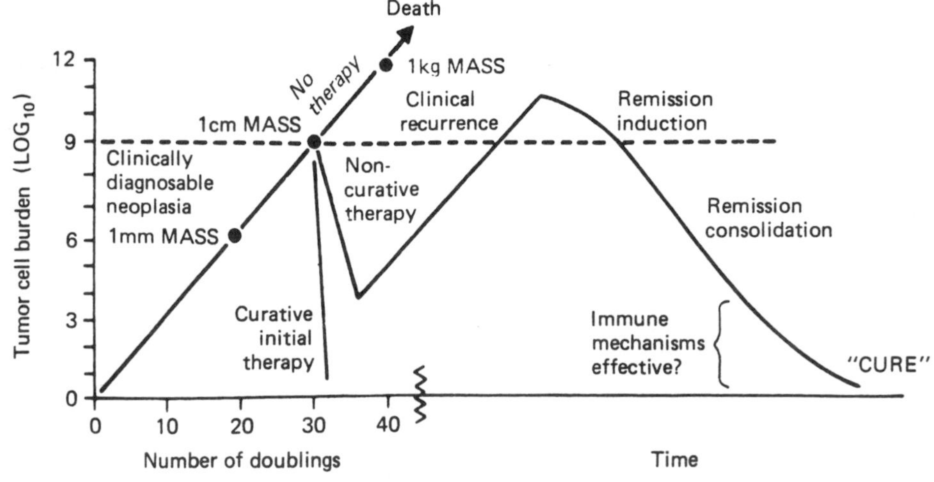

Figure 8–1. Concept of tumor cell burden and relation to phases of treatment.

2. the genetically determined resistance to chemotherapy, which may result from selective killing of cells in the tumor initially sensitive to the agent, overgrowth of residual chemoresistant cells (see discussion later in this chpater), and further development of heterogeneous populations of resistant cells by sequential mutations.

Figure 8–1 also indicates the various outcomes of tumor therapy. Initial therapy, whether it be surgery, radiation therapy, or cytotoxic chemotherapy, may be curative. However, if it is noncurative, the tumor cell burden may be reduced to 10^4 or 10^5 cells; cytotoxic agents characteristically kill tumor cells according to first-order kinetics, meaning that a constant percentage rather than a constant number of tumor cells is killed by a given exposure to the drug. Thus the killing of 99.999% of the cells when the tumor burden is 10^9 will leave 10^4 cells. Such relatively low tumor cell burdens are usually not detectable without the aid of a biochemical marker, such as the β-subunit of human chorionic gonadotropin in gestational trophoblastic malignancies and nonseminomatous testicular carcinomas. However, despite the appearance of a complete remission, the survival of this number of tumor cells may eventually lead to a clinical recurrence following additional tumor doublings, the rate of which depends on the summation of tumor cell divisions and cell death. One of the major roles of chemotherapy is the management of disseminated recurrences with regimens designed for remission induction and consolidation.

Cell Cycle and Growth Fraction

The growth and division of cells, both normal and neoplastic, can be diagrammed as in Figure 8–2. The phases of the cell cycle are termed G_1 (G = gap), S (synthesis of DNA), G_2 (premitotic interval), and M (mitosis). A prolonged G_1 phase, or resting phase, is commonly termed G_0. Consideration of the phase or phases in which a given cytotoxic agent has an effect and the time intervals involved is a potentially important factor in the choice of agents and the timing of their administration. Because the mechanism of action of most cytotoxic agents involves processes associated with cell division, the response of tumor cells to chemotherapeutic agents is generally enhanced by a large *growth fraction*, that is, a large percentage of the tumor cells proceeding through the mitotic cycle (i.e., dividing) at any given time. By choosing agents acting in different phases of the cell cycle, combinations of phase-specific drugs, such as those indicated in Figure 8–2, can be administered with increased tumor cell killing potential. It should also be noted, however, that actively growing *normal tissues*, such as bone marrow, gastrointestinal epithelium, and hair follicles, are also highly susceptible to the effects of most cytotoxic antineoplastic agents. Toxicity of these normal tissues affects the dose and frequency with which cytotoxic agents may be given safely.

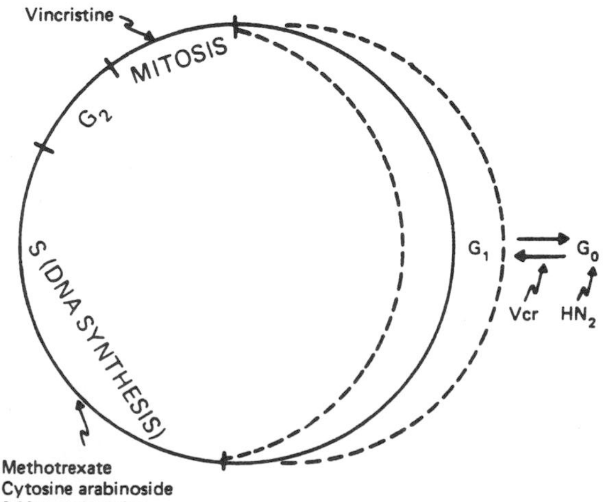

Figure 8–2. The mitotic cycle with sites of action of certain phase-specific antitumor agents. G_1 = (Gap 1) resting phase; G_2 = (Gap 2) premitotic interval; G_0 = prolonged G_1 or resting phase; Vcr = vincristine; HN_2 = nitrogen mustard.

Apoptosis, a form of cell death occurring in normal tissues as well as in malignant tumors, may be increased in tumors responding to chemotherapeutic agents as well as to irradiation. This process involves condensation and budding of the cell and characteristic cleavage of cellular DNA into fragments; unlike necrotic cell death, there is no associated inflammation. Apoptosis has received increased attention in relation to the influence of the suppressor gene *TP53*, which is required for its efficient activation.[17] *TP53* appears to provide a cell cycle checkpoint control following DNA damage, resulting either in slowing of cell division to permit DNA repair, or in initiation of apoptotic cell death. Acquired mutations in *TP53* are frequently observed in common human cancers, including colon, bladder, lung, prostate, and cervix cancers and melanoma, all of which demonstrate relative resistance to cytotoxic chemotherapeutic agents. Certain proto-oncogenes, such as *MYC,* also may initiate apoptosis,[18] whereas the proto-oncogene *BCL2* inhibits apoptosis in the presence of vincristine, vinblastine, methotrexate, 5-FU, cisplatin, and etoposide,[19] all widely used chemotherapeutic agents. The molecular consequences involving these genetic mechanisms are undergoing intense study, and their elucidation should facilitate the development of new approaches to minimizing tumor cell resistance.

Tumor Cell Resistance to Chemotherapy

Malignant tumors consist of heterogeneous populations of cells varying in their phase of the cell cycle, their distance from the vascular supply of nutrients and drugs, and their genetically determined resistance to cytotoxic drugs. The latter heterogeneity is illustrated by an initial tumor response to chemotherapy (representing the killing of chemosensitive cells), followed by progressive regrowth in spite of continued administration of the agent (representing the proliferation of initially chemoresistant cells that attain a selective advantage). Biochemical mechanisms of resistance (in addition to those involving *TP53* mutations described earlier) that have been demonstrated in animal or human tumor cells are:

- decreased drug uptake or increased export
- decreased drug-activating enzymes
- increased drug-inactivating enzymes

- increased levels of the inhibited target enzyme
- altered affinity of the target enzyme for the drug
- increased DNA repair
- increase in an alternative metabolic pathway bypassing the drug inhibition

Increased rates of drug removal from cells have been associated with multidrug (pleiotropic) resistance, in which tumor cells become resistant to several structurally unrelated agents.[20] Such cells have been found to be able to pump out these drugs, apparently as a result of high levels of a membrane glycoprotein (P-glycoprotein). Identification of increased levels of P-glycoprotein has the potential of identifying nonresponsive tumors. By identifying pleiotropic resistance, it may be possible to reverse this resistance with other drugs, such as verapamil or quinidine, which increase the intracellular accumulation of the cytotoxic drugs.

Other approaches to prevent the emergence of drug-resistant tumor cell populations include the use of combinations of drugs with independent mechanisms of action (Fig. 8–3). This approach can be extended to the use of two or more sequential or alternating non–cross-resistant combinations of several drugs each[10] and using maximal drug doses.[23] Much of the rationale for this approach to the problem is founded on the Goldie-Coldman hypothesis.[24] This assumed that drug-resistant cells arise spontaneously at a measurable mutation rate, and that the earlier and more intensively a tumor can be treated, the lower the likelihood that drug-resistant cells will emerge.

Much attention was devoted in the 1970s and 1980s to the development of predictive assays involving cultured human tumor cells exposed *in vitro* to cytotoxic drugs. An ideal predictive assay would indicate the likelihood of tumor cell chemosensitivity or resistance and would reduce the need to expose patients to sequential trials of toxic, but possibly ineffective, drugs. Unfortunately, all tumor specimens cannot be successfully cultured *in vitro*, and when they are, the prediction of clinically significant drug resistance results more commonly than prediction of sensitivity. Despite their cost and lack of widespread accessibility, such tests are potentially important and their investigation continues.

Pharmacologic Aspects of Cancer Chemotherapy

Optimal application of antineoplastic drugs also requires consideration of general principles of pharmacology, including drug absorption, distribution, biotransformation, bioavailability, and excretion.

Absorption

Absorption of drugs determines the route of administration appropriate for a given agent, such as oral (PO), intramuscular (IM), intravenous (IV), or intrathecal (IT). The rate of absorption affects the concentration achieved and thus

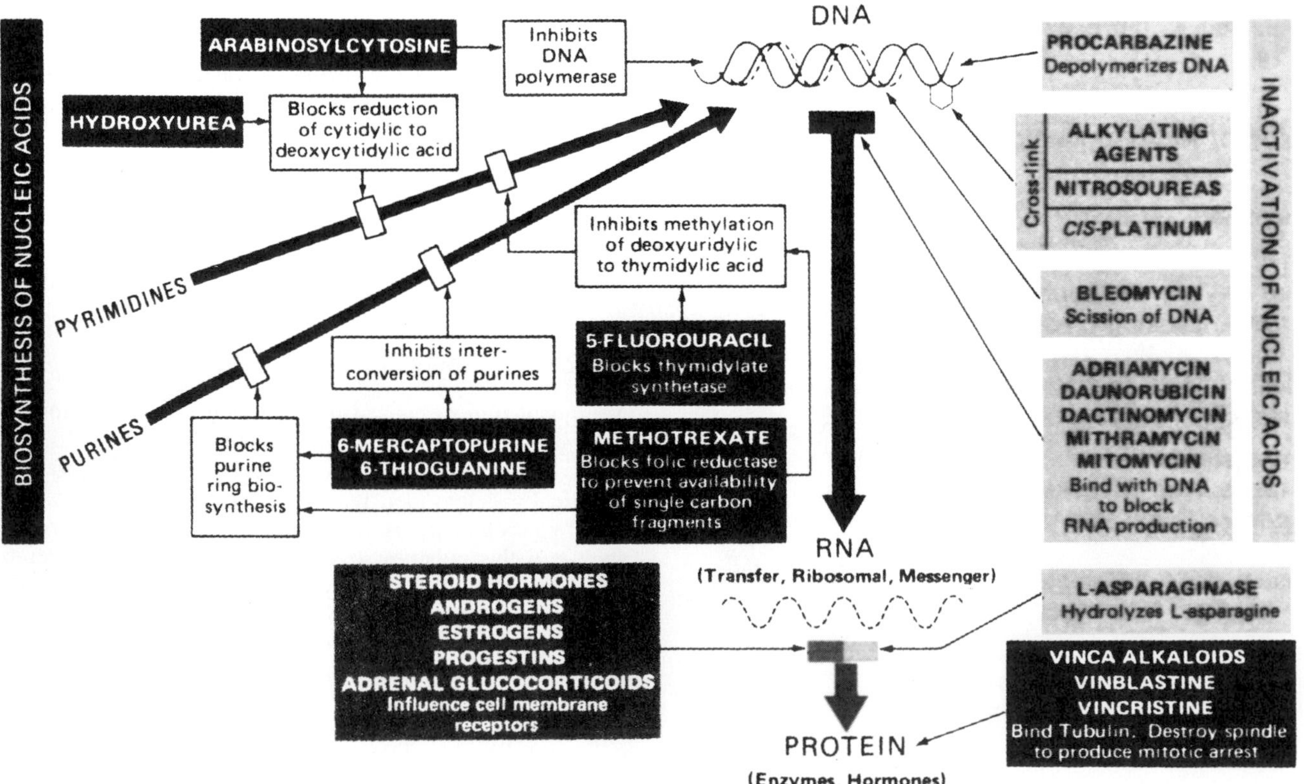

Figure 8–3. Sites of action of antineoplastic drugs. (From Krakoff IH: Systemic treatment of cancer. CA Cancer J Clin 1996; 46:137, with permission; as adapted from Karnofsky DA: Mechanism of action of anticancer drugs at a cellular level. CA Cancer J Clin 1968; 18:232–234.)

the bioavailability, which determines the duration and intensity of the exposure of cancer cells to the drug.

The pharmacokinetics, or alterations with time of drug concentration following administration, are important in determining the appropriate dose and intervals between doses. Optimal administration of a given drug may prove to be via the delivery of large, intermittent pulse doses, which will result in periodic high drug gradients across cell membranes with a large area under the plasma disappearance curve; constant infusion for several days; or, less commonly, daily oral dosage on a long-term basis.

Distribution

The concentration and effectiveness of antineoplastic drugs can sometimes be enhanced by local or regional administration, including instillation into a body cavity such as the pleural, peritoneal, or intrathecal space, or into an artery, with localization of the drug through infusion. These maneuvers may overcome barriers to the distribution of a drug into sanctuary sites, such as the central nervous system (CNS). The choice of the agent according to its tissue distribution characteristics also may be as important as its route of delivery. For example, the nitrosoureas have greater lipid solubility than most other agents, increasing their ability to enter the CNS.

Biotransformation

An example of biotransformation of a cancer chemotherapeutic agent is the activation of the alkylating agent, cyclophosphamide, by the mixed-function oxidase system of the liver, without which the agent is ineffective. Likewise, 5-FU must be phosphorylated before it is active. The *inactivation* of an antineoplastic agent must also be kept in mind when considering its use. For example, the purine analogue 6-mercaptopurine is catabolized by the enzyme xanthine oxidase. Its toxicity is increased when it is used concurrently with allopurinol, an inhibitor of the same enzyme. Because allopurinol is commonly used to prevent hyperuricemia in malignant diseases, the interaction of these two drugs is not a rare occurrence, and 6-mercaptopurine doses must be reduced in this situation.

Excretion

Excretion patterns of antineoplastic agents are important determinants of toxicity and of the need for alterations in drug dosage, especially when there is impairment of excretory organ function. Because methotrexate, a dihydrofolate reductase inhibitor, is largely excreted by the kidney, doses must be reduced if there is renal impairment. To compound the problem, high doses of methotrexate also may cause increased renal impairment by precipitating in renal tubules, particularly under acid conditions. In the presence of impaired liver function or biliary obstruction, vincristine and doxorubicin doses should be reduced because their excretion in bile is decreased under those circumstances. For a more extensive discussion of these subjects, the reader is referred to other sources.[2, 10, 11]

Mechanisms of Drug Action

Selection of Agents

Understanding the pharmacodynamics of antineoplastic agents is fundamental to their appropriate use. This includes knowledge of the mechanisms of action and physiologic effects of these agents (see Fig. 8–3). The majority of current cytotoxic agents act primarily on macromolecular synthesis, repair, or function, that is, on the production or function of DNA, RNA, or protein. Thus, although there are more than 35 available antineoplastic drugs from which to choose, there is considerable overlap in their mechanisms of action. These agents can be grouped into several classes (see Table 8–1 for more details):

- alkylating agents
- antimetabolites
- natural or semisynthetic products (antibiotics, plant alkaloids, enzymes, monoclonal antibodies, epipodophyllotoxins)
- miscellaneous agents
- hormones and hormone inhibitors

The choice of a chemotherapeutic agent for a given tumor type is generally not a consequence of *a priori* prediction of antitumor activity by the drug but is, instead, the result of empiric clinical trials (see Chapter 9).

Design of Combinations

Because single agents are, with few exceptions, unable to effect cures or even significant remissions, multiple agents are usually administered concurrently or sequentially. This process affords the advantages of maximizing the likelihood of tumor cell death by damaging several different biochemical sites, of minimizing the proliferation of resistant tumor cells, and of minimizing the toxicity to normal tissues by choosing agents with non-overlapping toxicities. Fundamentals to be noted in designing drug combinations are:

- Use only drugs that show some activity against the tumor type.
- Select drugs that differ in their mechanisms of action.
- Select drugs that differ in the site of their major toxicities (although bone marrow suppression is common to many and is difficult to avoid).
- Use optimal doses and timing for each drug (allowing adequate recovery from toxic changes in the most sensitive normal tissues between doses).

An example of the application of these principles is the four-drug CHOP combination for lymphoma (*c*yclophosphamide, *h*ydroxydaunomycin, *O*ncovin, and *p*rednisone). CHOP consists of intermittent doses of:

- cyclophosphamide, an alkylating agent whose major toxicities are marrow suppression and bladder irritation
- doxorubicin (also termed hydroxydaunorubicin), an antibiotic with topoisomerase (DNA repair)-inhibiting and DNA-intercalating properties whose major toxicities are marrow suppression and cardiac toxicity at higher doses

TABLE 8–1. **Antineoplastic Agents and Their Common Abbreviations**

Agent	Trade Name	Abbreviation
Alkylating Agents		
Nitrogen Mustards		
Mechlorethamine	Mustargen, nitrogen mustard	HN_2
Cyclophosphamide	Cytoxan, Endoxan	CTX
Ifosfamide	Ifex	IFS
Phenylalanine mustard	Melphalan (Alkeran)	L-PAM
Chlorambucil	Leukeran	CLR
Ethylenimine Derivatives		
Triethylenethiophosphor-amide	Thiotepa (Thioplex)	T-TEPA
Alkyl Sulfonates		
Busulfan	Myleran	MYL
Nitrosoureas		
Cyclohexylchloroethyl nitrosourea	Lomustine (CeeNU)	CCNU
1,3 bis-(2-chloroethyl)-1-nitrosourea	Carmustine (BiCNU)	BCNU
Streptozotocin	Zanosar	STZC
Triazenes		
Dimethyl triazenoimidazole carboxamide	Dacarbazine	DTIC
Antimetabolites		
Folic Acid Analogues		
Methotrexate	Amethopterin	MTX
Pyrimidine Analogues		
5-Fluorouracil	Fluorouracil	5-FU
Cytosine arabinoside	Cytarabine (Cytosar)	ARA-C
Gemcitabine	Gemzar	
Purine Analogues		
6-Mercaptopurine	Purinethol	6-MP
6-Thioguanine	Thioguanine	6-TG
Deoxycoformycin	Pentostatin	DCF
Natural or Semisynthetic Products		
Vinca Alkaloids		
Vinblastine	Velban	VLB
Vincristine	Oncovin	VCR
Vinorelbine	Navelbine	VNR
Antibiotics		
Doxorubicin	Adriamycin	ADR
Idarubicin	Idamycin, Zavedos	IDA/ZVD
Mitoxantrone	Novantrone	NOV
Daunorubicin	Daunomycin	DNR
Bleomycin	Blenoxane	BLEO
Dactinomycin, actinomycin D	Cosmegen	AMD
Mithramycin, plicamycin	Mithracin	MTM
Mitomycin C	Mutamycin	MITO-C
Enzymes		
L-asparaginase	Elspar	L-ASP
Monoclonal Antibodies		
Trastuzumab	Herceptin	
Rituximab	Rituxan	
Epipodophyllotoxins		
Etoposide	VePesid	VP-16
Teniposide	Vumon	VM-26
Miscellaneous		
Platinum Coordination Complexes		
cis-diammine-dichloroplatinum II	Cisplatin (Platinol)	DDP
Carboplatin	Paraplatin	CBP
Miscellaneous *Continued*		
Taxanes		
Paclitaxel	Taxol	
Docetaxel	Taxotere	
Camptothecins		
Irinotecan	Camptosar	CPT-11
Topotecan	Hycamtin	TPT
Adenosine Analogues		
Fludarabine	Fludara	FLU
Cladribine	Leustatin	2-CDA
Substituted Urea		
Hydroxyurea	Hydrea	HXU
Methylhydrazine Derivative		
Procarbazine	Matulane	PRO
Antimicrotubule Agent		
Estramustine	Emcyt	EM
Acridine Derivative		
Amsacrine	Amsidyl	m-AMSA
Liposomal Chemotherapy		
Doxorubicin liposome	Doxil, DaunoXome	
Interferons		
Interferon alfa-2a	Roferon-A	$IFN\alpha_{2a}$
Interferon alfa-2b	Intron A	$INF\alpha_{2b}$
Cardioprotective Agent		
Dexrazoxane	Zinecard, Cardioxane	DEX
Hormones and Hormone Inhibitors		
Estrogens		
Diethylstilbestrol		DES
Conjugated estrogens	Premarin	
Ethinyl estradiol	Estinyl	
Androgens		
Testosterone propionate		TES/TP
Fluoxymesterone	Halotestin	
Progestins		
Medroxyprogesterone acetate	Provera	MPA
Megestrol acetate	Megace	MA
Luteinizing Hormone-Releasing Hormone (LHRH) Analogues		
Leuprolide	Lupron	
Goserelin	Zoladex	
Adrenocorticosteroids		
Dexamethasone		
Antiestrogens		
Tamoxifen	Nolvadex	TAM
Toremifene	Fareston	TOR
Hormone Synthesis Inhibitors		
Aminoglutethimide	Cytadren	AG
Anastrozole	Arimidex	
Letrozole	Femara	
Antiandrogens		
Flutamide	Eulexin	
Bicalutamide	Casodex	
Nilutamide	Anandron, Nilandron	
Vitamin Derivative		
All-trans retinoic acid		ATRA
Photoporphyrin		
Porfimer sodium	Photofrin	

- vincristine, a vinca alkaloid with peripheral nerve toxicity, but very little bone marrow suppression
- prednisone, a synthetic corticosteroid hormone with effects on glucose metabolism and bone matrix

Other non–marrow-suppressive drugs, such as bleomycin or methotrexate with leucovorin (folinic acid) rescue, may be used with this CHOP combination in the intervals when blood cell counts are low from cyclophosphamide and doxorubicin. The first letters of the drug names are often combined to provide a useful abbreviation, for example:

MOPP:(*m*echlorethamine/vincristine (*O*ncovin)/*p*rocarbazine/*p*rednisone),
CMF:(*c*yclophosphamide/*m*ethotrexate/5-*F*U), and
CAF:(*c*yclophosphamide/doxorubicin (*A*driamycin)/5-*F*U).

Dose Intensity

One of the potential pitfalls of applying combination chemotherapy to clinical oncologic problems is the temptation to decrease doses of one or more of the drugs in the combination to reduce toxicity. There is evidence that such dose reduction may significantly limit therapeutic effectiveness in terms of cure or long-term relapse-free survival, even though complete remission rates appear unchanged. The studies of Hyrniuk[23] and others over the past decade have indicated the importance of *dose intensity*, which is defined as the amount of drug delivered per unit of time, expressed as milligrams per square meter per week. This calculation, performed for each drug in a given combination, can be converted into *relative dose intensity* by calculating the ratio of the average dose intensity of all drugs of the test combination to that of a standard regimen. Differences in response rates and durations of response can then be related to this dose intensity, which has been demonstrated to have a positive relation to response rates for advanced breast, colon, lung, and ovarian cancers, and for lymphomas.[10]

Synergy and Antagonism of Drugs

A phenomenon that deserves increased attention in its ability to improve the results of combination chemotherapy is that of *biochemical modulation*, by which two or more drugs interact to enhance their effects (*synergy*) or decrease them (*antagonism*). Knowledge of mechanisms of action of drugs, and of intermediary cell metabolism, allows the oncologic pharmacologist to predict possible interactions. Examples of such interactions are leucovorin (folinic acid) rescue from 5-FU action, and diethyldithiocarbamate and thiourea rescue from cisplatin toxicity.

Clinical Aspects of Cancer Chemotherapy

Although every potential chemotherapy patient should be approached as an individual, with consideration of a broad range of physiologic and psychologic factors, certain generalizations are useful. Table 8–2 describes criteria for categorizing the performance status of a patient, as described by Karnofsky and colleagues.[25] These categories, based on easily assessed daily activities, permit a functional classification of patients to accompany data from physical examinations and laboratory determinations. A performance status below 40% often predicts an unsatisfactory tumor response and poor tolerance of side effects of drugs.

The Eastern Cooperative Oncology Group (ECOG), a multi-institutional cooperative group for cancer studies, uses a slightly simpler performance status scale (Table 8–3). It is uncommon for a patient with a performance status below 3 to be given chemotherapy unless a response of the particular tumor is highly likely and the patient is highly motivated to be treated. At the other end of the clinical spectrum, it may be difficult to justify side effects from chemotherapy in a patient whose tumor-related symptoms are not very severe. However, when major symptoms develop and palliative chemotherapy is elected in the presence of a markedly decreased performance status, the patient's ability to tolerate effective doses of drugs may be

TABLE 8–2. **Karnofsky Performance Status Scale**

	Percent	
Able to carry on normal activity; no special care is required	100	Normal; no complaints; no evidence of disease
	90	Able to carry on normal activity; minor signs or symptoms of disease
	80	Normal activity with effort; some signs or symptoms of disease
Unable to work; able to live at home; cares for most personal needs; a varying amount of assistance is needed	70	Cares for self; unable to carry on normal activity or do active work
	60	Requires occasional assistance, but is able to care for most needs
	50	Requires considerable assistance and frequent medical care
Unable to care for self; requires equivalent of institutional or hospital care; disease may be progressing rapidly	40	Disabled, requires special care and assistance
	30	Severely disabled; hospitalization is indicated though death is not imminent
	20	Very sick; hospitalization is necessary
	10	Moribund; fatal processes progressing rapidly
	0	Dead

From Karnofsky DA, Abelman WH, Kraver LF, et al: The use of nitrogen mustards in the palliative treatment of carcinoma with particular reference to bronchogenic carcinoma. Cancer 1948; 1:634–669.

TABLE 8–3. **ECOG Performance Status Scale**

Status	Definition
0	Normal activity
1	Symptoms, but ambulatory
2	In bed <50% of time
3	In bed >50% of time
4	100% bedridden

ECOG = Eastern Cooperative Oncology Group.

significantly limited. The art of chemotherapy involves recognizing the transition between these two phases of the natural history of the malignancy. The use of chemotherapy is reviewed in each of the disease-oriented chapters. Table 8–4 lists cancers in which chemotherapy has been incorporated into clinical practice.

Nutritional Status

Related to but not specifically included in the performance status criteria is the patient's nutrition. In general, a cachectic, anorectic patient is less likely to tolerate a meaningful course of chemotherapy, and is therefore less likely to attain a good clinical response. Corrective nutritional supplementation may be necessary before beginning cytotoxic chemotherapy, including use of a nasogastric feeding tube, gastrostomy, jejunostomy, central venous hyperalimentation, or simply discussing the patient's diet in detail with the patient and family in an attempt to find appetizing and nutritious foods.[26, 27] Similarly, nutritional support may improve outcomes when unusually harsh chemotherapeutic regimens are used, such as those in bone marrow transplantation or leukemic induction, or both, or when chemotherapy is combined with radiation therapy.

TABLE 8–4. **Indications for Use of Chemotherapy**

Neoplasms in Which Chemotherapy is the Primary Therapeutic Modality for Localized Tumors

Large cell lymphomas
Burkitt's lymphoma
Childhood and some adult stages of Hodgkin's disease
Wilms' tumor
Embryonal rhabdomyosarcoma
Small cell lung cancer
Central nervous system lymphomas

Neoplasms in Which Primary Chemotherapy Can Allow for Less Mutilating Surgery

Anal carcinoma
Bladder carcinoma
Breast cancer
Laryngeal cancer
Osteogenic sarcoma
Soft tissue sarcomas

Neoplasms in Which Clinical Trials Indicate an Expanding Role for Primary Chemotherapy in the Future

Non–small cell lung cancer
Breast cancer
Esophageal cancer
Nasopharyngeal cancer
Other cancers of the head and neck region
Pancreatic cancer
Gastric cancer
Prostate cancer (hormones)
Cervical carcinoma

Neoplasms in Which Chemotherapy May Be Used for Metastases and/or Widespread Disease

Embryonal carcinoma
Choriocarcinoma
Non-Hodgkin's lymphoma
Leukemias (acute lymphoblastic leukemia, acute myeloid leukemia)

Adapted from DeVita VT Jr: Principles of cancer management: chemotherapy. In: DeVita VT Jr, Hellman S, Rosenberg SA (eds): Cancer. Principles and Practice of Oncology, 5th ed, pp 333–347. Philadelphia, Lippincott-Raven, 1997, with permission.

Infections, Anemia, and Bleeding Tendencies

Because many of the antitumor drugs cause bone marrow suppression and immunosuppression (of humoral and cellular immune functions), any pre-existing infections should be controlled before lowering polymorphonuclear leukocyte counts and inhibiting immune mechanisms. Appropriate use of antibiotics and hematopoietic growth factors is important. Bleeding tendencies should be evaluated and corrected, if possible prior to chemotherapy, with platelet transfusions, vitamin K, or other appropriate therapy. The widespread availability of granulocyte colony-stimulating factor may permit more intensive, myelosuppressive chemotherapy in patients whose bone marrow otherwise would not be able to tolerate such therapy.[28–30] The autotransplantation of a large number of undamaged autologous bone marrow or peripheral blood stem cells, which have been preserved *in vitro* during exposure of the patient to cytotoxic chemotherapy, is another technique used to protect the patient from cytopenic complications. (See the discussion relating to high-dose chemotherapy later in this chapter.)

Pain

Uncontrolled pain can markedly lower a patient's performance status and contribute to making tolerance of chemotherapy less satisfactory. Proper use of analgesic agents is an art that all physicians who manage cancer patients should strive to master.[31] The cancer chemotherapy itself may be aimed at pain relief and result in a gradual lessening of narcotic or other analgesic requirements. However, before such a response, adequate pain control may allow a patient to become a candidate for an effective chemotherapy program and to have less difficulty with side effects. This subject is discussed in detail later in this book.

Psychosocial Status

The final host factors to be considered, important in assessing a patient's suitability for chemotherapy, can be summarized under the term *psychosocial status*.[32] In general, patients referred for chemotherapy are aware, to varying degrees, that they have a malignancy, and often that it has spread beyond the possibility of its removal by surgery or local treatment by radiation therapy. Cautious and sympathetic openness on the part of the medical oncologist is advisable so that the patient is made aware that the physician is willing to discuss the disease frankly and that there are treatments available for such a disease. Such communication will permit the oncologist to assess how highly motivated to undertake therapy are the patient, the patient's family, and other support systems. Patient motivation will influence the oncologist's decision to undertake a prolonged, intensive, and possibly expensive course of chemotherapy with resultant side effects. Concomitantly, the patient is reassured that the physician understands the doubts and anxiety one feels as a result of a diagnosis of cancer.

A satisfactory explanation of possible toxic side effects by the oncologist when seeking the patient's informed consent for any investigational chemotherapeutic approach is very important at both a psychological and a medicolegal level. Although insufficient explanation puts the patient at a disadvantage in making important decisions, the oncologist can err in the other direction. Hope and optimism that help a patient continue to be active, to maintain nutrition, and to interact with family and friends may be devastated by an overzealous cataloging of major, minor, and rare toxicities and by survival statistics that the patient cannot handle objectively. Therefore, maintaining a supportive, trusting rapport between physician and patient and patient's family will contribute to better patient compliance during chemotherapy. Additional aspects of this subject are discussed in Chapter 14, Principles of Psychosocial Oncology.

Drug Toxicity

Physicians administering antineoplastic drugs have an obligation to understand and anticipate the potential toxic side effects that patients may experience while receiving chemotherapy. Although the toxicities of most of these agents for normal tissues are significant, they often assume exaggerated emphasis in the minds of patients and the lay public because of anecdotes from acquaintances and from the press and television describing primarily the most severe reactions. The therapeutic index, or relationship between the therapeutic benefit and toxicity, is relatively small for many anticancer drugs. Nevertheless, with astute surveillance for signs of toxicity, and with adequate appreciation of techniques for controlling side effects and for modifying doses when necessary, life-threatening toxicity is generally avoidable.

In general, as noted above in the section on the kinetic basis of chemotherapy, actively dividing cells are more susceptible than are nondividing cells to the effects of many antineoplastic drugs. Therefore, toxicity is generally a reflection of varying degrees of damage to actively dividing normal cells in the bone marrow, gastrointestinal tract, hair follicles, and gonads. Less common toxic reactions, such as pulmonary fibrosis (bleomycin, busulfan, and mitomycin C) and cardiotoxicity (doxorubicin, daunomycin, mitoxantrone, and idarubicin), should also be looked for and limited in their severity by restricting total doses to recommended limits and by discontinuing the drug and starting appropriate supportive therapy if toxicity appears. The toxicity of specific agents has been described in the section on classification of antineoplastic chemotherapeutic agents. General comments are included there, and the reader is referred to other sources for more extensive descriptions.[1–12, 33]

The screening and development programs for new drugs described in Chapter 9 are designed not only to detect antitumor activity but also to eliminate drugs whose toxicity would be intolerable. Those drugs that enter clinical use usually cause moderate side effects that can be controlled by proper dosage and judicious use of antiemetic agents. Brief comments on bone marrow suppression, immunosuppression, nausea and vomiting, alopecia, sterility, miscellaneous organ toxicities, and second malignancies are presented in the following discussions.

Bone Marrow Suppression

Bone marrow suppression can be minimized by using intermittent schedules of cell cycle–specific agents that damage dividing hematopoietic stem cells. Most bone marrow stem cells are resting at any given time, and are recruited into the mitotic pool following damage to more mature cells by chemotherapeutic agents. Figure 8–4[34] indicates the course of the peripheral granulocyte count following a pulse dose of various agents. With most myelosuppressive agents, the lowest peripheral granulocyte counts (the nadir) are reached in about 8 to 10 days. At that point, bone marrow stem cell proliferation is at a maximum. Cycle-specific agents should be avoided at this point to reduce hematopoietic damage, if response of the tumor will permit such a drug-free interval. Granulocyte counts less than 500/dL lasting for more than 5 to 7 days are associated with significant increases in infectious complications. If the interval between treatments can be extended to 17 to 21 days, then most of the stem cells will have returned to the resting state, and exposure to the antitumor agents at this time will have minimal effect on the stem cells.[34]

Certain exceptions to these generalizations, however, are important in designing drug regimens employing nitrosoureas or melphalan. These agents produce a biphasic suppression of peripheral granulocytes, the first at 8 to 10 days after a pulse dose, and the second at approximately 27 to 32 days (see Fig. 8–4). Retreatment should be delayed until 6 to 8 weeks have elapsed to permit return of the hematopoietic stem cells to the resting state. Large intermittent doses can be tolerated over many months by observing these intervals. By using dose adjustments, excessive myelosuppression can be prevented in the presence of decreased blood cell counts, although therapeutic results may be compromised. Such dose adjustments may be especially necessary in treating older patients, the marrow tolerance of whom is often decreased.

Nausea

Nausea is widely associated with cancer chemotherapy, especially with cisplatin-based regimens, and may lead to the patient's refusal to continue therapy. Some nausea in chemotherapy patients is clearly psychogenic, because it may occur before a patient is treated, suggesting a conditioned response. Attempts are being made to distract such patients with music or psychotherapy. Nausea and vomiting following the chemotherapy treatment by the usual 3 to 6 hours are more likely the result of physiologic effects on

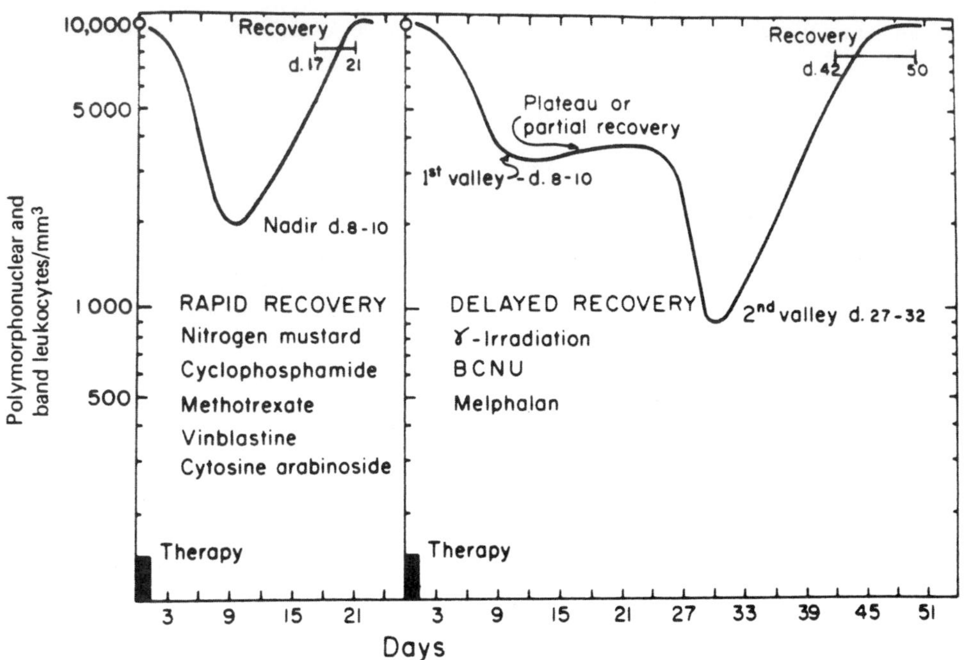

Figure 8–4. Times to recovery of peripheral granulocyte counts following administration of pulse doses of antineoplastic drugs. (From Bergsagel DE: An assessment of massive doses of chemotherapy of malignant disease. Can Med Assoc J 1971; 104:31–36, with permission.)

the CNS. Granisetron, ondansetron, dexamethasone, and metoclopramide have gained wide usage.[35, 36] Marijuana and tetrahydrocannabinol have been used with limited success for control of nausea and vomiting.

Alopecia

Alopecia is especially notable with cyclophosphamide, vincristine, doxorubicin, and bleomycin. Patients should be forewarned of this side effect and advised to have a photograph before treatment so a realistic wig can be made. Patients should be reassured that their hair usually will return even with continuing therapy, and that regrown hair may be even more attractive than its predecessor. Attempts to reduce hair loss with scalp cooling and tourniquet constriction have met with mixed success.[37]

Specific Organ Toxicity

Specific organ toxicity may involve the kidney, liver, heart, lung, central nervous system, and gonads.

RENAL TUBULAR NECROSIS

Renal tubular necrosis can result from the use of cisplatin without adequate hydration and diuretics to assure a large urine flow. Likewise, high doses of methotrexate can lead to precipitation in the renal tubules, particularly in association with an acidic or concentrated urine. Hydration, alkalinization of the urine with sodium bicarbonate, and diuretics can prevent the renal damage. Creatinine clearance should be checked periodically when these agents are used.

LIVER TOXICITY

Liver toxicity may occasionally result from L-asparaginase therapy or from prolonged treatment with methotrexate or 6-mercaptopurine. Mithramycin in antitumor doses may cause liver damage, although rarely, if ever, with the smaller doses used for controlling hypercalcemia.

CARDIOTOXICITY

Cardiotoxicity has been associated primarily with the anthracycline antibiotics doxorubicin and daunorubicin, but it may also be seen with high-dose cyclophosphamide therapy. It may be sudden in onset, irreversible, and associated with a high mortality rate. There may be transient electrocardiographic changes or a delayed cardiomyopathy, with congestive heart failure, particularly with cumulative doses of doxorubicin over 550 mg/m^2 or over 450 mg/m^2 with associated radiation therapy. Histologic examinations of patients dying with this complication have shown degeneration of myocardial cells and interstitial edema. Doxorubicin, daunorubicin, mitoxantrone, and idarubicin should be used with extra caution in patients with pre-existing cardiac disease, particularly if they have also received irradiation to an area of the heart or cyclophosphamide therapy, both of which appear to augment cardiomyopathy. Periodic monitoring of left ventricular ejection fractions should be conducted to detect the cardiotoxicity early enough to avoid serious and irreversible consequences.[8, 38]

PULMONARY TOXICITY

Pulmonary toxicity has been most closely associated with bleomycin, which selectively localizes in the lung. Decrease in diffusion capacity and in total lung capacity may occur in one third to one half of patients who receive bleomycin, with clinically apparent pulmonary fibrosis in approximately 5% of patients. Such fibrosis is usually associated with doses of over 400 units total cumulative dose or over 30 units in a single dose, although it may occur with doses of 100 units or less. The toxicity may be reversible on cessation of drug administration and institution of supportive care, including corticosteroids. Pulmonary fibrosis is an uncommon complication of busulfan, bis-chloroethyl-nitrosourea, and mitomycin C therapy.[39]

NEUROTOXICITY

Neurotoxicity has been most commonly associated with vincristine, which causes peripheral neuropathy characterized by loss of deep tendon reflexes, paresthesias, motor weakness, and occasionally jaw or other pain. Such changes are usually reversible over several months. Cisplatin and taxane neurotoxicity is also characterized by peripheral neuropathy. Ototoxicity, observed in 31% of patients treated with cisplatin, is usually characterized by tinnitus or hearing loss in the high frequency range, or both. Procarbazine and L-asparaginase may cause CNS symptoms, including somnolence, hallucinations, and depression. When given after cranial radiation therapy, methotrexate can lead to increased brain tissue drug concentrations and produce leukoencephalopathy as a result of white matter necrosis, particularly in children.

GONADAL DAMAGE

Gonadal damage and consequent sterility have been associated with a number of drugs, including a variety of alkylating agents, vinblastine, procarbazine, cytosine arabinoside, and cisplatin. Combination chemotherapy, such as MOPP chemotherapy for Hodgkin's disease, is particularly damaging, with more than 80% of male patients developing azoospermia, testicular atrophy, and elevated gonadotrophin levels. Ovarian failure may occur; women older than 40 years of age are particularly likely to have permanent amenorrhea after adjuvant combination chemotherapy for breast cancer.

SECOND MALIGNANCIES

Second malignancies attributable to genetic damage from chemotherapy have become a major concern as more and more patients have achieved long-term remissions and cures. Because many of the agents used have demonstrable mutagenic properties, this association seems understandable. Studies of patients in complete remission following combination chemotherapy for Hodgkin's disease have indicated the following[40, 41]:

- Chemotherapy alone or chemotherapy plus radiation therapy seems more likely to predispose to secondary acute leukemia than radiation therapy alone.
- Peak incidence of the onset of secondary acute leukemia is between 3 and 9 years following previous chemotherapy, with a declining frequency thereafter.
- Certain drugs, including alkylating agents, procarbazine, and nitrosoureas, appear to have more leukemogenic potential than other drugs. This observation increases expectations that appropriate modifications of current combination chemotherapy may decrease the likelihood of this complication.
- The risk of secondary leukemia rises with increasing patient age at the time of treatment, especially in those older than 40 years of age.

Combined-Modality Treatment

To improve therapeutic index as measured by local tumor control and improved survival, *both* radiation and chemotherapy are being used increasingly in the management of many types of cancer. Benefit from such combined-modality treatment might occur from synergistic drug-radiation interaction and eradication of occult metastases that were seeded before or during radiation treatment. Combined-modality treatment may also lead to increased acute and late toxicity, which may limit its benefits.[42, 43]

- Several studies of cancer of the anal canal have shown that concurrent therapy with radiation and 5-FU plus mitomycin C or cisplatin can lead to 75% to 90% long-term disease-free survival, in contrast to the frequent relapses observed after radical surgery alone.[44] This approach avoids abdominoperineal resection and colostomy and has become the preferred treatment, with surgery reserved for local failure.
- A National Institutes of Health Consensus Conference has recommended combined radiation and chemotherapy as standard postoperative treatment for patients with rectal cancer.[45]
- The prognosis for patients with esophageal cancer with surgery or radiation therapy, or with both, is poor, even in the absence of demonstrable metastases. A multi-institutional trial comparing combined chemotherapy and radiation therapy with radiation therapy alone showed marked improvement in survival (38% vs. 10% at 2 years; $p < 0.001$). These results have been supported by other trials, albeit with increased toxicity.[46, 47] Results achieved with chemoradiation may be comparable to those achieved by the addition of surgery.
- Significant improvement in disease-free and overall survival has also been demonstrated in locally advanced prostate cancer with radiation therapy and luteinizing hormone-releasing hormone agonists as compared with radiation therapy alone.[48]
- Several randomized trials in patients with locally advanced non–small cell lung cancer with good performance status have evaluated the use of chemotherapy either before or concurrent with radiation therapy. Most have shown small, but definite, improvement in survival of patients receiving both cisplatin-based chemotherapy and radiation therapy compared with those receiving radiation therapy alone.[49]
- Combined-modality treatment with cisplatin and 5-FU followed by radiation may be beneficial in avoiding laryngectomy in laryngeal carcinoma with no compromise in survival and 60% of patients retaining their larynx in the combined-modality arm.[50]
- Addition of consolidation involved-field radiation to an abbreviated course of CHOP appears to obviate the need for six cycles of chemotherapy in patients with low-stage, high-risk non-Hodgkin's lymphoma without compromising survival and improving toxicity profile.[51, 52]

High-Dose Chemotherapy with Peripheral Stem Cell Transplantation

The use of peripheral stem cell transplantation following high-dose chemotherapy for a variety of malignancies has expanded exponentially over the last decade. The rationale for dose intensification in cancer treatment resulting in marrow ablation, followed by marrow rescue with allogeneic, autologous, or peripheral stem cell transplant, follows Thomas's attempts in 1950 to cure leukemia using total body irradiation and marrow from identical twins. Introduction of various colony-stimulating factors to reduce duration of marrow aplasia has spurred clinical investigation in this field, and also has helped optimize collection of peripheral stem cells when used in conjunction with mobilization chemotherapy. The major advantages of peripheral stem cell transplantation over autologous marrow transplantation include rapid neutrophil and platelet recovery, reduced tumor cell contamination, and reduced cost.[53]

High-dose chemotherapy with peripheral stem cell transplantation and colony-stimulating factors allows higher dose escalation. It has demonstrated that drug resistance can be overcome, and previously refractory patients with lymphoma, acute leukemia, myeloma, and testicular carcinoma can be cured or have long disease-free periods.[54–56] Despite high response rates, evidence for improvement in survival of patients with breast or ovarian cancer with high-dose chemotherapy is still lacking. These are areas of intense ongoing research.

Summary

Increasingly, cancer chemotherapy is being used early in the clinical history of malignant diseases, as in the adjuvant or neoadjuvant therapy for primary breast, colorectal, and head and neck cancers, and as in definitive, potentially curative therapy for certain disseminated malignancies, including Hodgkin's disease, intermediate-grade non-Hodgkin's lymphomas, testicular carcinoma, choriocarcinoma in women, and rhabdomyosarcoma and acute lymphoblastic leukemia of childhood. It should be clear from the foregoing description of concepts of cancer chemotherapy that the medical oncologist must also be very conversant with broad areas of clinical pharmacology and increasingly familiar with molecular biology and molecular genetics in order to use cancer treatment modalities optimally. A major challenge of medical oncology is to use available agents with an understanding of their mechanisms of action and interaction, thus rising above the level of using chemotherapeutic regimens in a "cookbook" fashion.

Medical oncologists often find themselves in the primary care role of supporting and palliating terminal cancer patients. The doctor-patient relationship engendered during a prolonged chemotherapy program often leads patients to turn primarily to the medical oncologist for help with their problems, even after active chemotherapeutic approaches have been exhausted. This supportive role of the medical oncologist is very challenging. It mandates adequate knowledge not only of chemotherapy but also of nutrition, pain control, gastrointestinal function, treatment of infectious complications, and psychosocial aspects of cancer. Familiarity with community resources for home and institutional care, financial help, nursing support, rehabilitation services, and transportation is also important. A team approach is often highly effective, with oncologists, primary care physicians, nurses, pharmacists, social workers, physical therapists, psychiatrists, and nutritionists complementing each other's functions. The training and personal characteristics of many medical oncologists make them well suited to coordinate such a group in the total care of cancer patients.

Recommended Reading

The following references will assist the reader in pursuing this subject in more depth. The text by Pratt and colleagues, *The Anticancer Drugs*,[2] is excellent as a well-written, lucid introduction to cancer chemotherapeutic agents. Complementing that book, and explaining the biologic basis of cancer and cancer therapy, is Ruddon's revised book *Cancer Biology.*[3] DeVita's chapter "Principles of Cancer Management: Chemotherapy" in the classic textbook of oncology by DeVita, Hellman, and Rosenberg[10] is an excellent summary of the topic, followed by detailed chapters on the pharmacology, toxicity, and application of each major group of chemotherapeutic agents. The chapter "Chemotherapy" in the textbook edited by Gross and Roath[8] incorporates much of the most relevant principles into a readable narrative centered on an actual non-Hodgkin's lymphoma case. *The Chemotherapy Sourcebook*[11] is a recently revised reference book. The pocket-sized paperbacks edited by Rosenthal and coworkers[1] and by Skeel and Lachant[4] provide a broad view of malignant diseases and their treatment, and are books suitable to be carried on ward rounds. Deeper exploration of individual topics can be achieved through the Specific References.

REFERENCES

General References

1. Rosenthal S, Carignan JR, Smith BD (eds): Medical Care of the Cancer Patient, 2nd ed. Philadelphia, W.B. Saunders Co., 1993.
2. Pratt WB, Ruddon RW, Ensminger WD, Maybaum J: The Anticancer Drugs, 2nd ed. New York, Oxford University Press, 1994.
3. Ruddon RW: Cancer Biology, 3rd ed. New York, Oxford University Press, 1995.
4. Skeel RT, Lachant NA (eds): Handbook of Cancer Chemotherapy, 4th ed. Boston, Little, Brown & Co., 1995.
5. Haskell CM: Principles of cancer chemotherapy. In: Haskell CM (ed): Cancer Treatment, 4th ed, pp 31–57. Philadelphia, W.B. Saunders Co, 1995. See also Antineoplastic Agents, pp 78–165.
6. Salmon SE, Bertino JR: Principles of cancer therapy. In: Bennett JC, Plum F (eds): Cecil. Textbook of Medicine, 20th ed, pp 1036–1049. Philadelphia, W.B. Saunders Co., 1996.
7. Kirkwood JM, Lotze MT, Yasko JM (eds): Current Cancer Therapeutics, 2nd ed. Philadelphia, Churchill Livingstone, 1996.
8. Bakemeier RF: Chemotherapy. In: Gross S, Roath S (eds): Hematology. A Problem-Oriented Approach, pp 661–670. Baltimore, Williams & Wilkins, 1996.
9. Chabner BA, Allegra CJ, Curt GA, Calabresi P: Antineoplastic agents. In: Hardman JG, Limbird LE, Molinoff PB, et al (eds): Goodman & Gilman's The Pharmacological Basis of Therapeutics, 9th ed, pp 1233–1287. New York, McGraw-Hill, 1996.
10. DeVita VT Jr: Principles of cancer management: chemotherapy. In: DeVita VT Jr, Hellman S, Rosenberg SA (eds): Cancer. Principles and Practice of Oncology, 5th ed, pp 333–347. Philadelphia, Lippincott-Raven, 1997. See also Pharmacology of Cancer Chemotherapy, pp 375–508.
11. Perry MC (ed): The Chemotherapy Sourcebook, 2nd ed. Baltimore, Williams & Wilkins, 1997.
12. Foley JF, Vose JM, Armitage JO: Current Therapy in Cancer, 2nd ed. Philadelphia, W.B. Saunders Co., 1998.

Specific References

13. Edwards MH, Myers WPL, Kennedy BJ, et al: Graduate education in medical oncology. Bethesda, National Cancer Institute Monograph, 1978.

14. Mayer RJ: Manpower needs in medical oncology. J Cancer Educ 1989; 4:225–226.
15. Ginder GD, Kennedy BJ: Impact of technology change and managed care on medical oncology. J Cancer Educ 1997; 12:73–76.
16. Seligman PA, Ross DD: Palliative care education—can we respond to the challenge? J Cancer Educ 1999; 14:127–128.
17. Peller S: Clinical implications of p53: effect of prognosis, tumor progression and chemotherapy response. Semin Cancer Biol 1998; 8:379–387.
18. Prendergast GC: Mechanisms of apoptosis by c-Myc. Oncogene 1999; 18:2967–2987.
19. Simonian PL, Grillot DAM, Nunez G: Bcl-2 and Bcl-XL can differentially block chemotherapy-induced cell death. Blood 1997; 90:1208–1216.
20. Beck WT, Dalton WS: Mechanisms of drug resistance. In: DeVita VT Jr, Hellman S, Rosenberg SA (eds): Cancer. Principles and Practice of Oncology, 5th ed, pp 498–512. Philadelphia, Lippincott-Raven, 1997.
21. Krakoff IH: Systemic treatment of cancer. CA Cancer J Clin 1996; 46:137.
22. Karnofsky DA: Mechanism of action of anticancer drugs at a cellular level. CA Cancer J Clin 1968; 18:232–234.
23. Hyrniuk WM: Average relative dose intensity and the impact on design of clinical trials. Semin Oncol 1987; 14:65–74.
24. Coldman AJ, Goldie JH: Impact of dose-intense chemotherapy on the development of permanent drug resistance. Semin Oncol 1987; 14(suppl):29–33.
25. Karnofsky DA, Abelman WH, Kraver LF, et al: The use of nitrogen mustards in the palliative treatment of carcinoma with particular reference to bronchogenic carcinoma. Cancer 1948; 1:634–669.
26. Brennan MF, Piser PWT, Posner M, et al: A prospective randomized trial of total parenteral nutrition after major pancreatic resection for malignancy. Ann Surg 1994; 304:220–236.
27. Souba WW: Nutritional support. In: DeVita VT Jr, Hellman S, Rosenberg SA (eds): Cancer. Principles and Practice of Oncology, 5th ed, pp 2841–2857. Philadelphia, Lippincott-Raven, 1997.
28. Bodey GP, Anaissie E, Gutterman J, et al: Role of granulocyte-macrophage colony stimulating factor as adjuvant treatment in neutropenic patients with bacterial and fungal infections. Eur J Clin Microbiol Infect Dis 1994; 13:518–523.
29. Glaspy J: The impact of epoetin alfa on quality of life during cancer chemotherapy: a fresh look at an old problem. Semin Hematol 1997; 34(suppl 2):20–26.
30. Haus U, Farber L, Ullrich S, Burger KJ: The effect of recombinant human granulocyte macrophage colony stimulating factor after chemotherapy of various tumors. Anticancer Drugs 1997; 8:597–602.
31. Foley KM: Management of cancer pain. In: DeVita VT Jr, Hellman S, Rosenberg SA (eds): Cancer. Principles and Practice of Oncology, 5th ed, pp 2807–2841. Philadelphia, Lippincott-Raven, 1997.
32. Indeck BA, Bunney MA: Community resources. In: DeVita VT Jr, Hellman S, Rosenberg SA (eds): Cancer. Principles and Practice of Oncology, 5th ed, pp 2891–2904. Philadelphia, Lippincott-Raven, 1997.
33. Foley JF: Complications and side effects of chemotherapy agents. In: Foley JF, Vose JM, Armitage JO (eds): Current Therapy in Cancer, 2nd ed, pp 385–388. Philadelphia, W.B. Saunders Co., 1998.
34. Bergsagel DE: An assessment of massive doses of chemotherapy of malignant disease. Can Med Assoc J 1971; 104:31–36.
35. Navari R, Gandara D, Hesketh P, et al: Comparative clinical trial of granisetron and ondansetron in the prophylaxis of cisplatin induced emesis. J Clin Oncol 1995; 13:1242–1248.
36. Perez EA, Tiemeier T, Solberg LA: Antiemetic therapy for high-dose chemotherapy with transplantation: report of a retrospective analysis of a 5-HT(3) regimen and literature review. Support Care Cancer 1999; 7:413–424.
37. Seipp CA: Adverse effects of treatment. Hair loss. In: DeVita VT Jr, Hellman S, Rosenberg SA (eds): Cancer. Principles and Practice of Oncology, 5th ed, pp 2757–2758. Philadelphia, Lippincott-Raven, 1997.
38. Speyer JL, Green MD, Sanger J, et al: A prospective randomized trial of ICRF-187 for prevention of cumulative doxorubicin induced cardiac toxicity in women with breast cancer. Cancer Treat Rev 1990; 17:161–163.
39. Stover DE, Kaner RJ: Pulmonary toxicity. In: DeVita VT Jr, Hellman S, Rosenberg SA (eds): Principles and Practice of Oncology, 5th ed, pp 2729–2737. Philadelphia, Lippincott-Raven, 1997.
40. Blayney DW, Longo DL, Young RL, et al: Decreasing risk of leukemia with prolonged follow-up after chemotherapy and radiation therapy for Hodgkin's Disease. N Engl J Med 1987; 316:710–714.
41. Grunwald H, Rosner F: Chemicals and leukemia. In: Henderson ES, Lister TA, Greaves MF (eds): Leukemia, 6th ed, pp 179–194. Philadelphia, W.B. Saunders Co., 1996.
42. Tannock IF: Treatment of cancer with radiation and drugs. J Clin Oncol 1996; 14:3156–3174.
43. Vokes E: Combined modality therapy of solid tumors. Lancet 1997; 397(suppl):4–6.
44. Flam MS, John M, Pajak TF, et al: Role of mitomycin in combination with fluorouracil and radiotherapy and of salvage chemoradiation in the definitive non-surgical treatment of epidermoid carcinoma of the anal canal: results of phase III randomized intergroup study. J Clin Oncol 1996; 14:2527–2539.
45. NIH Consensus Conference: Adjuvant therapy for patients with colon and rectal cancer. JAMA 1990; 264:1444–1450.
46. Herskovic A, Martz K, Al Sarraf M, et al: Combined chemotherapy and radiotherapy compared with radiotherapy alone in patients with cancer of the esophagus. N Engl J Med 1992; 326:1593–1598.
47. Bosset JF, Gignoux M, Tribould JP, et al: Chemoradiotherapy followed by surgery compared with surgery alone in squamous cell cancer of the esophagus. N Engl J Med 1997; 337:161–167.
48. Bolla M, Gonzalez D, Warde P, et al: Improved survival in patients with locally advanced prostate cancer treated with radiotherapy and goserelin. N Engl J Med 1997; 337:295–300.
49. Non-Small Cell Lung Cancer Collaborative Group: Chemotherapy in non-small cell lung cancer: a meta-analysis using updated data on individual patients from 52 randomized trials. BMJ 1995; 311: 899–909.
50. The Department of Veterans Affairs Laryngeal Cancer Study Group: Induction chemotherapy plus radiation compared with surgery plus radiation in patients with advanced laryngeal cancer. N Engl J Med 1991; 324:1685–1690.
51. Miller TP, Dahlberg S, Cassidy JR, et al: Three cycles of CHOP (3) plus radiotherapy (RT) is superior to eight cycles of CHOP (8) alone for localized intermediate and high grade non-Hodgkin's lymphoma (NHL). A Southwest Oncology Group Study. J Clin Oncol 1996; 15:1257.
52. Canellos GP, Lister TA, Sklar JL (eds): The Lymphomas, 1st ed. Philadelphia, W.B. Saunders Co., 1998.
53. Mangan K. Peripheral blood stem cell transplantation: from laboratory to clinical practice. Semin Oncol 1995; 22:202–209.
54. Attal M, Harousseau JI, Stoppa AM, et al: A prospective randomized trial of autologous bone marrow transplantation and chemotherapy in multiple myeloma. N Engl J Med 1996; 335:91–97.
55. Margolin K, Doroshen JH, Ahn C, et al: Treatment of germ cell cancer with two cycles of high dose ifosfamide, carboplatin and etoposide with autologous stem cell support. J Clin Oncol 1996; 14:2631–2637.
56. Gianni A: High dose chemotherapy and autologous bone marrow transplantation compared with MACOP-B in aggressive B cell lymphoma. N Engl J Med 1997; 336:1290–1297.

9 *Basic Concepts in Drug Development and Clinical Trials*

FRANCES COLLICHIO, MD, Hematology and Oncology
JENNIFER GRIGGS, MD, MPH, Medical Oncology
JOSEPH D. ROSENBLATT, MD, Medical Oncology

That which purifies us is trial, and trial is by what is contrary.

JOHN MILTON

Perspective

The process of drug development, from the ideas to commercial use, takes years and is complex. This chapter describes how drugs are developed and includes an overview of the preclinical testing as well as the later phases of clinical trials that drugs must go through. We examine new drugs under development and how unique mechanisms of action may require new methods of clinical trial design. We also examine some important statistical tools, such as meta-analysis, interim analysis, and randomization. Two important facets of clinical trial research—quality of life and health services research—are discussed.

Drug Exploration and Development

One method of drug development is to screen natural products in preclinical systems for their effectiveness against cancer. Of 46 nonhormonal antitumor drugs marketed in the United States, 24 (52%) were originated from a natural source.[1] From 1960 to 1982, the National Cancer Institute (NCI) screened thousands of potential marine, microbial, and plant extracts in the P388 mouse leukemia model. Several that became available through this technique are active against rapidly proliferating tumors, such as leukemia and lymphoma, but show little effect on more slowly growing tumors, such as breast, colon cancer, and other solid tumors. In the early 1980s, this program was discontinued because it was determined that few novel agents were being isolated from natural sources.[2]

From 1985 to 1990, a new *in vitro* screen based on a diverse panel of human tumor cell lines was developed.[3] The NCI screen comprises 60 cell lines derived from nine cancer types and is organized into subpanels, representing leukemia, lung, colon, central nervous system, melanoma, ovarian, renal, prostrate, and breast cancers. The NCI turned back to nature with these new screening tools in 1986.[2] Agents showing significant activity in the primary *in vitro* screens are selected for secondary testing in several *in vivo* systems. Those agents exhibiting significant *in vivo* activity are advanced into preclinical and clinical development. In addition, contacts with the NCI and countries all over the world exist to facilitate the exploration of land and sea. Twenty-three anticancer agents are in active preclinical and clinical development as a result of this program.[2] Paclitaxel, which is used to treat breast, ovarian, and lung cancer, is one of the agents developed through this program.

Another system that is used to develop new drugs is to synthesize analogues of active drugs that may be safer or have a wider range of action than the parent drug. In this case, known structures of chemical agents are subtly modified in an attempt to enhance therapeutic effectiveness and minimize toxicity. Examples of such drugs include carboplatin, which exhibits similar efficacy to cisplatin with no renal, oto-, or neurotoxicity; gemcitabine, which exhibits increased activity against solid tumors compared with cytosine arabinoside, from which it was derived; and doxorubicin, which, compared with daunorubicin, exhibits a broader range of activity.[1] However, except for these rare examples, drug analogues have not been as helpful to the field of oncology as one would have liked.

Since the beginning of the 1990s, the molecular biology of cancer cell growth has been explored in greater depth than ever before. The discovery of molecular mechanisms of growth, metastatic behavior, growth modulation, gene rearrangement, and gene mutations has led to new classes of drugs that target these mechanisms:

- The protein kinase C modulators interfere with cellular signal transduction.
- The antisense oligonucleotides may alter the expression of oncogenes.

- Antiangiogenesis agents impede the angiogenic process crucial for tumor growth.[1]
- Newer matrix metalloproteinase inhibitors may interfere with tumor implantation and metastasis.
- Farnesyl transferase inhibitors may directly inhibit the action of certain mutated oncogenes such as *RAS* by interfering with crucial modification of *RAS* structure.

Several dozen new agents that specifically target newly identified biologic pathways are under active preclinical or clinical investigation. Our belief is that this kind of rational drug development may be especially productive in coming years. Malignant cells express antigens that can be recognized by antibodies or lymphocytes, or both. A wide variety of genetic abnormalities has been identified in cancer cells, many of which may provide suitable immunologic targets. These include translocations that generate fusion proteins (e.g., BCR-ABL, EWS-fl1), mutated oncogenes (e.g., *RAS*), tumor suppressor genes (e.g., retinoblastoma, *TP53*), or aberrantly expressed normal proteins such as oncofetal antigens (e.g., CEA), mucins, or tyrosine kinases (e.g., HER2/neu). Some tumor antigens are unique to the malignant cells; other antigens are overexposed or abnormally exposed on the malignant cell compared with the normal cell. These differences between tumor and normal tissues can be explored to develop vaccines, antitumor antibodies, and antibodies that are modified to carry toxin molecules.

Cancer vaccines have been studied for at least 20 years, but their therapeutic effect is thus far limited[4]; newer approaches are being tested that combine vaccines with cytokines or insert genes that augment immunogenicity. Likewise, early work on antibody therapy was largely unsuccessful for several reasons, including poor antibody delivery to tumors and the development of human antimouse antibodies. With the development of mouse-human chimeric antibodies or fully humanized antibodies, some of the difficulties in mouse-derived monoclonal antibodies are overcome. The use of C2B8 (rituximab) against CD20 on B-cell lymphoma[5] and the 4D5 anti-HER2/neu antibody (trastuzumab) in breast and ovarian cancer[6] are examples of successful applications of antibody-based therapies.

Newer technology for synthesizing compounds that might have antitumor activity has also been developed, allowing testing of so-called designer drugs. Protein structure–based drug design incorporates the use of atomic-level structural information about a macromolecule (an enzyme, receptor, or nucleic acid), typically obtained by x-ray crystallography, computational chemistry, molecular graphics, and magnetic resonance spectrometry.[7] Several human immunodeficiency virus protease inhibitors were developed by structure-based drug design. The high-resolution crystal structures of several matrix metalloproteinases have made possible the design of several inhibitors such as marimastat that are being tested in clinical trials. The matrix metalloproteinases are involved in cancer cell invasion and dispersion through the extracellular matrix, and are also linked with the metastatic and angiogenic properties of tumors.[1] We expect to see increasing numbers of so-called designer drugs as the technology matures and the number of oncogenic targets increases.

Clinical Trials in Cancer

In the sections that follow, we first describe the traditional methods of bringing compounds from the preclinical arena into clinical trials. We start by describing clinical protocols. Next, we cover phase I, II, III, and IV trials. We conclude with the problems encountered in analyzing the effectiveness of some of the newer classes of drugs and cancer prevention strategies.

Design of Clinical Trials

A successful clinical trial requires careful planning. Key questions should be asked:

1. What are the major and minor objectives of the trial?
2. How many patients will be necessary? Do we have the patients in our area to achieve this goal in a reasonable length of time (approximately 2 years)?
3. How long will it take to complete the accrual of patients onto the trial? How much time will be needed for adequate follow-up to reach preliminary conclusions?
4. How will the study be funded?

Funding can come from university budgets for clinical research, grants from government and private groups, fellowships, and the pharmaceutical industry. A grant proposal is necessary in many instances. Pharmaceutical companies frequently require a *letter of intent*. An example of the contents of a letter of intent is shown in Table 9–1.

After this planning stage, a protocol is written. The protocol starts with an introduction, justifying the study based on the state-of-the-art treatment of the disease in question and how the study may improve care. After the introduction, the protocol proceeds systematically to define eligibility requirements, registration procedures, the treatment protocol, required tests for follow-up, measurement of response, and provisions for reporting adverse events and for trial termination. The primary end point and secondary end points should be stated clearly in the protocol. An outline is shown in Table 9–2.

Phase I Studies

A phase I clinical trial is the first attempt at evaluating a novel drug or new combinations in human beings. The primary objective is to determine the maximum tolerated dose (MTD), as defined by acceptable toxicity. The secondary objectives are to study clinical pharmacology and to describe any tumor responses noted in the study.

There are several different designs for phase I trials. One

TABLE 9–1. **Elements of a Letter of Intent**

A. Objectives of the study
B. Background
   1. Rationale for implementing the study
   2. Prior experience in this treatment area
   3. Appropriate references of published and unpublished data
C. Number of patients to be treated
D. Dose, schedule, and duration of all drugs used in the study
E. Evaluation criteria
   1. How response will be evaluated
   2. Biologic end points
F. Characteristics of the patient population to be included/excluded

TABLE 9–2. **Subheadings in a Typical Clinical Research Protocol**

A. Introduction
B. Objectives
C. Selection of patients
  1. Eligibility criteria
  2. Exclusion criteria
D. Registration
E. Treatment plan
F. Measurement of effect
G. Study parameters
  1. Tests
  2. Exam requirements
H. Drug formulation
I. Statistical considerations
J. Records to be kept/case report forms
K. Patient consent
L. References

such design is the modified Fibonacci series.[8] The initial dose is 1⁄10 the acceptable dose in animal toxicology studies. The dose is then increased in large increments (100%, 67%, 50%, 40%), followed by more conservative dose increments (30% to 35%) in the later phases of the study. Dose escalation for subsequent patients occurs only after sufficient time (e.g., 2–3 months) has passed to document any acute toxic effects in patients treated at lower doses. The definitions of toxicity vary from study to study; however, MTD is usually defined as the dose at which dose-limiting toxicity is seen in at least two of six patients enrolled at that dose level. The dose used for further testing is usually one level below the MTD.

There are several arguments in place to change the design of phase I trials:

- The modified Fibonacci series results in exploring many dose levels before the MTD is reached.
- The MTD may be imprecise.
- Most responses on phase I studies occur close to MTD or at 80% to 120% of the dose below the MTD.[9]

Newer designs expose fewer patients to the lower doses. Accelerated titration designs have been shown to decrease the number of patients treated at subtherapeutic dose levels and to reduce the duration of the study. Doses are evaluated within patients until toxicity is seen.[10] The continuous reassessment method observes each subject (or group of subjects) for a response and then calculates the dose to be administered to the next individual or group.[11] Variants of the continuous reassessment method exist.[12–14] The Bayesian decision method is similar, with a dose-based or fixed number of patients treated at one time, with the clinical dose requiring knowledge of the responses of all previous patients.[15] In a study of quantitative assessment design, the dose was adjusted to a small cohort of patients based on toxicity before proceeding. The number of patients required to complete the study was smaller than the traditional phase I approach.[16] Finally, in random walk rules, patients are treated with the next higher, same, or next lower dose according to a probability distribution and the patient's response.[17]

There is also a push to better define the starting dose. In compound-oriented testing, each compound is tested in a fashion identical to its proposed use in humans in terms of dose, route, and schedule of administration.[18] Second, consideration given to the mechanisms of action of the drugs may enable researchers to choose the most appropriate animal model before the phase I trial is done. For example, the dog model is more appropriate for studying thymidylate synthase inhibitors than are the mouse and rat models because extracellular thymidine concentrations are similar in dogs and humans.[19]

Some phase I trials are very complicated in that they involve the simultaneous escalation of two or more drugs. The design of these trials has been discussed by Korn and Simon.[20] So-called phase Ib trials attempt to assess the relationship between the dosing of a biologic agent to toxicity and the anticipated immunologic effects. However, because the relevance of many immunologic end points to desired clinical results is still poorly understood, the validity of Ib studies has been questioned.[21]

Phase II Trials

There are two types of phase II studies: trials of single agents and trials of combinations of agents. Both are called phase II trials because eligibility is limited to patients with a specific diagnosis and there is no internal control group. The objective of most phase II trials is to determine if the drug has antitumor activity against the tumor type in question. For this objective, response rate is an appropriate end point. Tumor response rate is recorded as follows:

1. *Complete response:* disappearance of all measurable tumor.
2. *Partial response:* greater or equal to 50% regression of one or more evaluable lesions, with no progression of any lesion.
3. *Stable disease:* less than 50% reduction in tumor volume or the lack of progression.
4. *Progressive disease:* the occurrence of any new lesion during treatment or an increase in size by 25% of one or more lesion. A decline in functional performance status is occasionally classified as progressive disease.

Patients occasionally have nonmeasurable but evaluable disease; such disease presents in the skin, as pleural effusions, or interstitial lung disease. In these cases, the protocol should specify whether nonmeasurable disease can be evaluated on the study. Such evaluation is usually achieved by taking photographs or radiographs prior to, during, and after therapy. Many trials employ an independent response evaluation committee to avoid investigator bias.

In phase II studies of combinations of agents, the activity of the drugs as single agents is usually known. It is speculated that the combination will be more active than the single agents. For example, the response rate to doxorubicin (Adriamycin) in metastatic breast cancer is approximately 36% to 38%[22, 23]; the response rate to paclitaxel (Taxol) is approximately 40%.[24] In the late 1990s, when these two agents were combined, the response rate was 70% to 80%.[25, 26] In phase II studies of drug combinations, the rationale for using the combination, including speculation regarding potential additive or synergistic toxicities, must be developed in great detail.

Phase III Studies

Phase III studies are designed to establish the value of new treatment in comparison with standard therapy. The trials should have relevant and objective end points, such as symptom control, disease-free interval, and survival. In general, response rates should not be the sole measure of benefit because they may not correlate with patient survival. When paclitaxel and doxorubicin as single agents were compared with the combination in a phase III trial, the response rate of the combination was higher than that of the single agents, but the survival was the same,[27] illustrating inadequacy of either survival or response as sole outcome measures. Phase III trials are often done in the adjuvant (after surgery) or neoadjuvant (before planned surgery) setting. The end points for efficacy in an adjuvant setting are disease-free, as well as overall, survival.

Figure 9–1 shows a schema of a typical phase III trial. Choosing a sample size and patient eligibility takes place before the schema is followed. Schemas are used in phase I and II studies as well, but they are more complex in phase III studies. Sometimes, designs may involve second and third randomizations, adding to the complexity of the phase III schema.

Sample Size

The protocol for a phase III trial should specify the number of patients to be accrued, the duration of follow-up after enrollment closes, and when the final analysis will be performed. Methods to plan sample size are based on the assumption that at the end of the follow-up period, a statistical test is to be performed comparing the experimental treatment with the control treatment with regard to a single primary end point. Usually a statistical significance of 0.05 is chosen in the analysis. This means that if there is no true difference between the treatments, the probability of obtaining the difference that was seen is only 5%. When a trial has few patients, differences in observed outcomes must be extreme in order to obtain statistical significance. As sample size and extent of follow-up increase, the power of a study increases, and statistical significance can be achieved with small differences in outcome. Therefore, in order to determine sample size, the investigator must decide ahead of time what difference between the groups will be clinically significant.

The sample size for phase III trials can be very large, sometimes requiring thousands of patients. Pharmaceutical companies, private industry, and the NCI have set up consortia in order to increase accrual onto trials. The NCI cooperative groups are called Eastern Cooperative Oncology Group, Cancer and Leukemia Group B, Gynecologic Oncology Group, Pediatric Oncology Group, National Surgical Adjuvant Breast Project, and the Community Clinical Oncology Program. Comparative groups may involve hundreds of sites, with variable technical and treatment philosophies and capabilities, and may facilitate careful evaluation of treatment feasibility and efficacy in community as well as academic settings. As an example, the study comparing doxorubicin alone, paclitaxel alone, or the combination of both was done by the Eastern Cooperative Oncology Group and involved more than 700 patients.[27]

Eligibility Criteria

In the past, eligibility criteria were often excessively stringent, requiring patients to be in excellent physical condition with little prior treatment, leading to expensive work-ups and, in the end, results that were not applicable to the community of cancer patients at large. For these and other reasons, there is an evolving trend to broaden eligibility

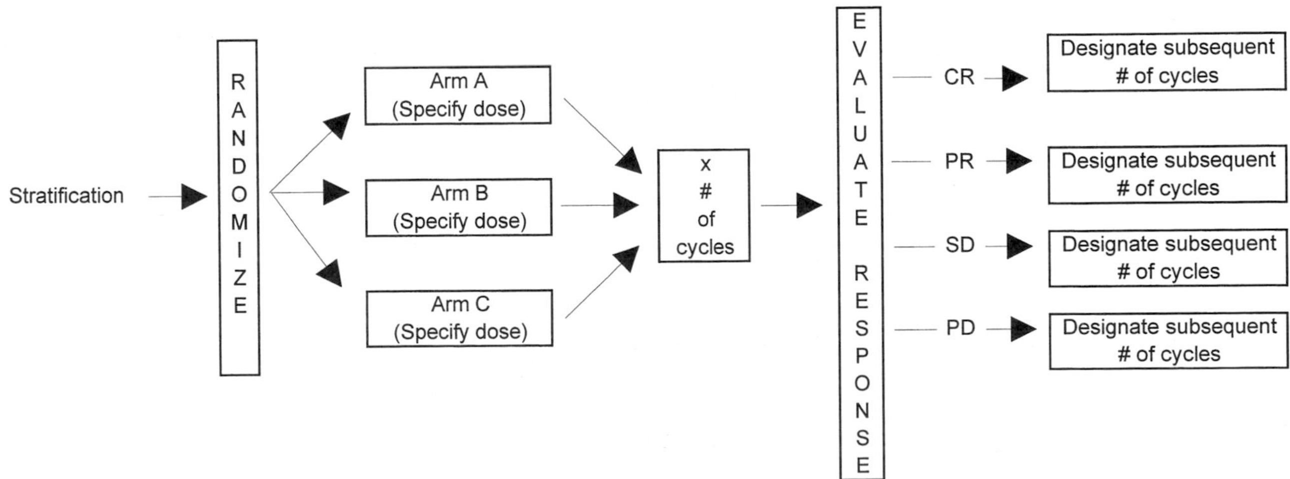

Figure 9–1. A typical phase III trial, with the major points emphasized: stratification, randomization, and evaluation. CR = complete response; PR = partial response; SD = stable disease; PD = progressive disease.

requirements. For example, a study could compare two antiestrogens in the treatment of breast cancer: tamoxifen and toremifene. The study should enroll premenopausal women who have received any form of adjuvant chemotherapy (including none) before starting the antiestrogen. In the past, the type of preceding adjuvant chemotherapy might have been specified, limiting patient accrual and preventing generalization of the results. Because the study would be comparing tamoxifen and toremifene, the type of adjuvant chemotherapy patients received should not, in theory, affect the result in a large study of this type.

Stratification

Stratification, that is, the selection of patients into groups based on entry characteristics, may be done for several reasons. First, it may be important to be certain that groups of patients are evenly matched at the start of the trial. For example, in a treatment comparing two different hormonal agents in the adjuvant treatment of breast cancer, it may be important to stratify based on the number of positive axillary lymph nodes, menopausal status, and presence or absence of the estrogen receptor. Second, the end points of a trial may be stratified. In the previous example, survival may be the major end point of the trial. A secondary end point may be survival based on menopausal status. When patient characteristics and study end points are stratified, the number of patients required to demonstrate treatment differences increases.

Randomization

Randomization is critically important for producing reliable results. With randomization, patients are assigned to the different treatment choices of the study, known as treatment arms, by selection of a random number at a central registration office. In nonrandomized studies, controls and treatment groups may differ by disease and patient characteristics (clinical and nonclinical) and may receive different diagnostic procedures, supportive care, secondary treatments, methods of evaluation, and follow-up.[21] These differences can lead to a bias in noticing and reporting the side effects of one treatment over another. Furthermore, younger patients or those felt to have a better or worse prognosis may be subtly shunted to a more aggressive treatment arm.

Phase IV Studies

Once a new program is shown to be an improvement over previous treatment for a given disease site and stage of disease, it becomes the standard of care. Further investigation of feasibility and efficacy in new and different settings has been referred to as phase IV testing. In some instances, community oncologists may be asked to evaluate a new program to ensure that it can be given safely to large numbers of patients and that it demonstrates efficacy. For example, a study could be done of gemcitabine in metastatic pancreatic cancer in the community setting. Because gemcitabine is already approved for metastatic pancreatic cancer, it is a phase IV study.

Analysis of Clinical Trials

Phase I trials are analyzed primarily by toxicity data (see earlier discussion) and phase II studies primarily by response rates (see earlier discussion). The concepts discussed in the following sections apply primarily to phase III and IV studies.

Intention-to-Treat Analysis

The intention-to-treat principle means that all randomized patients should be included in the primary analysis of the trial. For cancer, this often means all eligible patients. Excluding patients arbitrarily because of early death, poor compliance, excessive toxicity, and other reasons makes it difficult to interpret the results and apply the treatment later to other patients. For example, the side effects of a chemotherapy treatment may make a patient too exhausted to come for follow-up. If this patient and others are excluded from the analysis, then the treatment will appear to be less toxic than it really is.

Interim Analysis

If statistical tests are performed repeatedly, then the probability that the difference in outcome will be found statistically significant (at the 0.05 level) at some point may be considerably higher than 5%; this is called a type I error. It has been shown that type I error can be as high as 26% if the significance test is performed every 3 months of a 3-year trial.[28] Interim analyses can be very misleading. The random trends seen in interim analyses can destroy accrual to a clinical trial and interfere with a physician being able to state honestly that there is no reliable evidence indicating that one treatment option or the other is preferable. It is standard practice for a multicenter trial to have a data monitoring committee review interim results, rather than the treating physicians or the physician authors of the trial, so that no bias is introduced into the study. The data monitoring committee determines when the results are mature and can be released.

Calculation of Survival Curves

Most cancer clinical trials display results by showing survival curves or disease-free survival curves. An example of a typical survival curve is given in Figure 9–2. Time is shown on the horizontal axis, and the percentage of patients surviving is shown on the vertical axis. Other time-to-event distributions can be similarly represented. There are basically two methods to follow: the life table (or actuarial method),[21] and the Kaplan-Meier method.[29] The Kaplan-Meier method is very useful in studies with few patients or variable follow-up. In the Kaplan-Meier method, follow-up information is obtained on all patients and the curve takes into account usable length of follow-up. Tick marks are placed on the curve to represent the follow-up times of living patients. Censoring leads to misrepresentation of the data. For example, if a patient is too sick to come to clinic to make the follow-up appointment as a result of toxicity of the treatment and his data are censored, then important information about the treatment is left out. Similarly, if

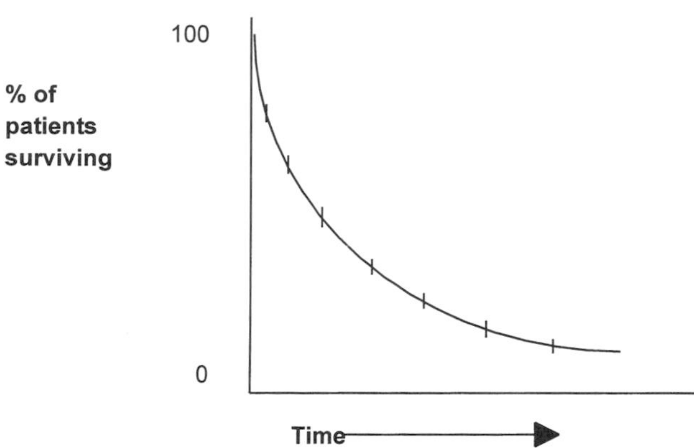

Figure 9–2. Demonstrates a survival curve generated from data obtained during a clinical trial.

follow-up times are short, then examination of the curve would indicate that data for larger follow-up periods are not yet mature.

Meta-Analysis

Meta-analysis has become a popular statistical tool in the last few years. This is a quantitative summary of different research protocols in a particular area, distinguished from the traditional literature by its emphasis on quantifying results of individual studies and on combining results across studies. The approach uses only randomized clinical trials that have been studied, regardless of whether they have been published, excludes nonrandomized studies from the analysis, and assesses therapeutic effectiveness based on the average results pooled from the trials.[21] In calculating average treatment effects, a measure of difference in outcome between treatments is calculated separately for each trial. For example, a comparison of mortalities can be computed for each trial. A weighted average of these differences is then computed and the statistical significance of this average is evaluated. This approach requires access to all patient data and cooperation from leaders of the trials included in the analysis.[21]

Meta-analysis is not a substitute for properly designed large, randomized trials. The individual trials may have subtle differences in treatment that make comparisons difficult. Likewise, patient populations may be slightly different in the analyzed studies, making pooling of the results somewhat inaccurate and obscuring real differences that may be applicable to subjects within the larger groups.

Reporting Results of Clinical Trials

Simon gives guidelines for effective reporting of clinical results as follows[21]:

1. The methods should be discussed, including response criteria.
2. The methods of statistical analysis should be described.
3. The patients studied should be adequately described.
4. The sample size should be sufficient to establish the effect of the conclusions. For a negative study, confidence limits for treatment differences should be presented.
5. All patients registered on the study should be properly accounted for and study drop-out rate reported.
6. The target sample size, number of interim analyses, and decision process for stopping accrual and reporting results should be presented.
7. In randomized trials, comparisons should be made for eligible patients, with exclusions only for ineligible patients.
8. Claims of superior efficacy should not be made on the basis of nonrandomized phase II trials unless the disease is so rare or the prognosis so poor that properly controlled randomized trials are not possible.

Health Services Research

A newer field called health services research is emerging, and it is receiving greater emphasis than ever before. A global assessment of health care, health services research is being advocated as a means for providing information needed to support decision making in health care.[30] This field covers five broad areas: technology assessment, practice variations, medical decision making, cost-effectiveness analysis, and clinical practice guidelines. Several other areas are also considered, such as gender inequity, race inequity, quality of life, and methods to measure quality of services. Health systems research is being incorporated into many clinical trials, and it is especially applicable when costly resources (bone marrow transplantation or stem cell harvest) or extreme toxicity (high-dose interferon for metastatic melanoma) is being used.

Regulatory and financial authorities—both in the health sector and government—are interested in quality-of-life measures to assist in resource allocation and policy decisions.[31] For example, when meager increases in the length of survival are afforded by the use of chemotherapy for poorly treatable solid tumors, an analysis of quality-of-life on versus off treatment may help determine whether a treatment is worthwhile or cost-effective.

Quality of Life

The term *quality of life* has emerged to summarize the assessment of the combined impact of disease and treatment and the trade-off between the two.[32] Quality of life is increasingly assessed as part of phase II, III, and IV trials. Cancer is frequently incurable, and treatments are given to relieve symptoms, to prevent serious complications of the disease, and to prolong life. These goals often include the maximum relief of symptoms with minimal treatment-related toxicity.

Several tools have been developed to measure quality of life.[33] One popular tool is the Functional Assessment of Cancer Therapy scale (FACT) developed by David Cella, Ph.D., and coworkers.[34] The scale was developed and extensively validated before widespread use. It is a simple, brief questionnaire that can be completed easily in 5 minutes, usually without assistance. It is scored so that results may be quantified. Modified FACT scales for different malignancies and other chronic illnesses (e.g., FACT-B, for breast cancer) have been developed.[35]

New Methods of Clinical Trial Design and Analysis

With the development of many new compounds with new mechanisms of action, there is an emerging need to modify clinical trials and develop newer methods for analyzing the effect of treatment. Tests of antitumor vaccines represent a case in point. Animal data and results in earlier clinical trials suggested that trials to test the antitumor efficacy of vaccines should be done in the adjuvant setting.[4] However, trials of this type are large and expensive, and frequently phase II data demonstrating efficacy of treatment are lacking. Single-arm studies comparing outcome with historic controls have been done, but these can be criticized for the potentially biased patient selection (treated patients were healthier or went through more rigorous staging tests than the historic controls). Attempts have been made to correlate immune response with clinical response. These are, however, hampered by being unable to determine if the immune response correlates with the baseline clinical status of the patients or with the treatment.[21] As an alternative, adjuvant trials can be postponed until more potent immunotherapies are developed that cause sufficient antitumor activity in advanced disease. Until these limitations have been clarified, analysis of vaccine trials should continue to require large phase III randomized trials.

Antiangiogenic agents are being tested by the usual paradigm of phase I to phase III trials, but it may be more appropriate to develop new strategies. Antiangiogenic agents are cytostatic in nature, preventing tumor growth rather than inducing reduction in tumor size. The therapy may be administered in several different settings: as adjuvant therapy; as a maintenance therapy after tumor reduction, given to those with advanced, metastatic, or recurrent disease; in conjunction with radiation therapy or surgery; in combination with chemotherapy; and, perhaps, as a chemopreventive agent.[36] To be suitable for long-term use, these agents should possess little toxicity and preferably have oral bioavailability. Phase I studies should not search for the MTD, but they should demonstrate a biologically active dose with little toxicity, suitable for disease administration. These studies may require extensive laboratory and biologic evaluation. Phase II studies may need to be modified or to use other biologic end points such as tumor markers for efficacy. For example, marimastat, a matrix metalloproteinase inhibitor, has been shown to cause a decrease in the tumor markers CA 19-9, PSA, and CA125 in 50% of patients.[36] With cytostatic approaches, randomized studies are needed to demonstrate efficacy.

Cancer prevention has been increasingly studied. As with other forms of cancer therapy, chemopreventive agents go though an *in vitro* and animal model screening process before being tested in phase I clinical safety studies. But unlike the other agents we have discussed, the usual end points of response rate (in phase II trials) and survival (in phase III trials) are impractical. The U.S. Food and Drug Administration and the NCI have developed guidelines for phase II and III testing.[37] They recommend that phase II trials should be small randomized studies to assess chronic drug toxicity, measure biomarker modulation (such as reversal of intraepithelial neoplasia, changes in differentiation signals, changes in genetic and regulatory signals, changes in proliferation), and standardize assays and quality control procedures. Among other end points, phase III studies should demonstrate a significant reduction in incidence or delay in occurrence of cancer. Several such agents are in phase II and III chemoprevention trials, including retinoids, tamoxifen, nonsteroidal anti-inflammatory drugs (including aspirin), vitamins D and E, and others.[38]

Research Data Management

Research data management is the discipline devoted to the collection, storage, retrieval, and quality control of the data required for evaluating the scientific objective of the study.[39] It plays a crucial role in determining the success or failure of the study. There are four main components—protocol development, data collection, computing, and quality control. Data managers should have a sufficient knowledge of tumor biology, medical terminology, and the medical record to allow adequate data collection for subsequent interpretation.

The process of data collection is facilitated by data collection forms (case report forms) and checklists. The forms should contain the key objectives of the study, such as the important side effects of the treatment, the response of the tumor to treatment at specified end points, survival, and quality of life. Unexpected toxicity and death within 30 days are called into the central office. The forms should contain number codes so that they can be easily decoded into a computer for analysis and retrieval at any time.

The conduct of multi-institutional studies presents a special challenge. The coordinating center must ensure compliance with the protocol, data collection, and timing of data collection from a large geographic area. The coordinating center is responsible for registration and randomization of patients, creation of a computer database, and statistical analysis.

Inclusion of Minorities and Women in Clinical Trials

The National Institutes of Health Revitalization Act of 1993 was passed in response to the gaps in medical knowledge that had resulted from the historic exclusion of women and minorities from clinical research.[40] Such exclusions had previously been justified on the grounds of creating a homogenous study population. The policy of the National Institutes of Health is that all federally funded research studies include women and minorities unless there is "clear and compelling rationale" for the exclusion. In addition, all studies must include enough members of the groups to allow sufficient power to conduct analyses of differences in effects of health care interventions. This may require oversampling of some groups. Costs associated with conducting such studies are not allowed as an acceptable excuse for the exclusion of women and minorities. Outreach efforts for recruitment of minorities and women into clinical studies are also required.

Summary

To make progress in the therapy of a variety of different cancers, clinical trials require the study of large numbers of patients. In adjuvant trials, such as in breast and colon cases, histologic variables, the various strata for the number of nodes involved, extent of disease, and other factors demand hundreds of patients to establish potential significance of an intervention. Although only a modest improvement may be documented, this may have a considerable impact if applied to the general population.

It has been disappointing that only 1% to 3% of the potentially eligible patients enter such clinical trials. Even within the cooperative groups, the percentage of eligible patients who enter trials is low. Easier trials with less stringent eligibility requirements, logical end points, assessments of quality of life, and health systems resources should increase accrual onto studies. Greater attention by the media and acceptance by insurance companies should also help. Clinical practice guidelines should incorporate clinical research into case pathways. This has been done by the National Comprehensive Cancer Network.[41] Advances in oncology are slow and usually occur in small steps. Well-performed clinical trials are the only means of realizing these advances. A substantial commitment on the part of the country and treatment establishment to carry out clinical research would ultimately lower the cost and drastically improve efficacy of future cancer therapies.

REFERENCES

1. Weiss RB: Introduction: New sources and new antitumor drugs in development. Semin Oncol 1997; 24:153–155.
2. Gordon MC, Newman DJ, Weiss RB: Coral reefs, forests, and thermal vents: The worldwide exploration of nature for novel antitumor agents. Semin Oncol 1997; 24:156–163.
3. Boyd MR, Paul KD: Some practical considerations and applications of the National Cancer Institute in vitro anticancer drug discovery screen. Drug Development Research 1995; 34:91–109.
4. Sznol M, Holmlund J: Antigen-specific agents in development. Semin Oncol 1997; 24:173–186.
5. Piro LD, White CA, Grillo-Lopez AJ, et al: Extended rituximab (anti-CD20 monoclonal antibody) therapy for relapsed or refractory low-grade or follicular non-Hodgkin's lymphoma. Ann Oncol 1999; 10:655–661.
6. Baselga J, Tripathy D, Mendelsohn J, et al: Phase II study of weekly intravenous trastuzumab (Herceptin) in patients with HER2/neu-overexpressing metastatic breast cancer. Semin Oncol 1999; 26:78–83.
7. Jackson RC: Contributions of protein structure-based drug design to cancer chemotherapy. Semin Oncol 1997; 24:164–172.
8. Carter SK, Selawry O, Slavik M: Phase I clinical trials. Monogr Natl Cancer Inst 1977; 45:75–80.
9. Van Hoff DD, Turner J: Response rates, duration of response, and dose response effects in phase I studies of antineoplastics. Invest New Drugs 1991; 9:115–122.
10. Simon R, Freidlin B, Rubinstein L, et al: Accelerated titration designs for phase I clinical trials in oncology. J Natl Cancer Inst 1997; 89:1138–1147.
11. Mani S, Ratain M: New phase I methodology. Semin Oncol 1997; 24:253–261.
12. Faries D: Practical modifications of the continual reassessment method for phase I cancer clinical trials. J Biopharm Stat 1994; 4:147–164.
13. Moler S: An extension of the continual reassessment methods using a preliminary up-and-down design in a dose finding study in cancer patients, in order to investigate a greater range of doses. Stat Med 1995; 14:911–922.
14. Piantadosi S, Fisher JD, Grossman S: Practical implementation of a modified continual reassessment method for dose-finding trials. Cancer Chemother Pharmacol 1998; 41:429–436.
15. Whitehead J, Brunier H: Bayesian decision procedures for dose determining experiments. Stat Med 1995; 149:885–893.
16. Mick R, Ratain MJ: Model guided determination of maximum tolerated dose in phase I clinical trials: evidence for increased precision. J Natl Cancer Inst 1993; 85:217–223.
17. Durham SD, Flournoy N, Rosenberger WF: A random walk rule for phase I clinical trials. Biometrics 1997; 53:745–760.
18. Collins JM, Grieshaber CK, Chabner BA: Pharmacologically guided phase I clinical trials based upon preclinical drug development. J Natl Cancer Inst 1990; 82:1321–1326.
19. Jackman AL, Taylor GA, Calvert H, et al: Modulation of antimetabolite effects. Effects of thymidine on the efficacy of the quinazoline-based thymidylate synthetase inhibitor CB3717. Biochem Pharmacol 1984; 33:3269–3275.
20. Korn EL, Simon R: Using the tolerable-dose diagram in the design of phase I combination chemotherapy trials. J Clin Oncol 1993; 11:794.
21. Simon R: Clinical trials in cancer. In: DeVita VT, Hellman S, Rosenberg SA (eds): Cancer: Principles and Practice of Oncology, 5th ed, pp 513–528. Philadelphia, Lippincott, 1997.
22. Bontenbal M, Andersson M, Wildiers J, et al: Doxorubicin vs epirubicin, report of a second-line randomized phase II/III study in advanced breast cancer. EORTC Breast Cancer Cooperative Group. Br J Cancer 1998; 77:2257–2263.
23. Amadori D, Frassineti GL, De Matteis A, et al: Modulating effect of lonamide in response to doxorubicin in metastatic breast cancer patients: results from a multicenter prospective randomized trial. Breast Cancer Res Treat 1998; 49:209–217.
24. Geyer CE Jr, Green SJ, Moinpour CM, et al: Expanded phase II trial of paclitaxel in metastatic breast cancer: a Southwest Oncology Group study. Breast Cancer Res Treat 1998; 51:169–181.
25. Schwartsmann G, Mans DR, Menke CH, et al: A phase II study of doxorubicin/paclitaxel plus G-CSF for metastatic breast cancer. Oncology 1997; 11:24–29.
26. Martin M, Lluch A, Ojeda B, et al: Paclitaxel plus doxorubicin in metastatic breast cancer: preliminary analysis of cardiotoxicity. Semin Oncol 1997; 24:S26–S30.
27. Sledge GW, Neuberg D, Ingle S, et al: Phase III trial of doxorubicin (A) vs. paclitaxel (T) vs doxorubin + paclitaxel (A+T) as first-line therapy for metastatic breast cancer (MBC): an intergroup trial [Abstract]. Proc Am Soc Clin Oncol 1997; 15:1a.
28. Fleming TR, Green SJ, Harrington DP: Considerations of monitoring and evaluating treatment effects in clinical trials. Control Clin Trials 1984; 5:55.
29. Kaplan EI, Meier P: Nonparametric estimation from incomplete observations. Journal of the American Statistical Association 1958; 53:457.
30. Jones J, Hunter D: Consensus methods for medical and health services research. BMJ 1995; 311:376–380.
31. Rogerson RJ: Environmental and health related quality of life: conceptual and methodological similarities. Social Science and Medicine 1995; 41:1373–1382.
32. O'Boyle CA, Waldron D: Quality of life issues in palliative medicine. J Neurol 1997; 244(Suppl):S18–S25.
33. Scott CB: Issues in quality of life assessment during cancer therapy. Semin Radiat Oncol 1998; 8(Suppl):5–9.
34. Cella DF, Tulsky DS, Gray G, et al: The functional assessment of cancer therapy scale: development and validation of the general measure. J Clin Oncol 1993; 11:570–579.
35. Brady MJ, Cella DF, Mo F, et al: Reliability and validity of the Functional Assessment of Cancer Therapy-Breast quality-of-life instrument. J Clin Oncol 1997; 15:974–986.
36. Pluda JM: Tumor-associated angiogenesis: mechanisms, clinical implications, and therapeutic strategies. Semin Oncol 1997; 24:203–218.
37. Kelloff GJ, Johnson JR, Crowell JA, et al: Approaches to the development and marketing approval of drugs that prevent cancer. Cancer Epidemiol Biomarkers Prev 1995; 4:1–10.
38. Kelloff GJ, Hawk T, Karp JE, et al: Progress in clinical chemoprevention. Semin Oncol 1997; 24:1–13.
39. Begg CB: Research data management. In: DeVita VT, Hellman S, Rosenberg SA (eds): Cancer: Principles and Practice of Oncology, 5th ed, pp 513–528. Philadelphia, Lippincott, 1997.
40. NIH Guideline on the Inclusions of Women and Minorities as Subjects in Clinical Research. NIH Guide, vol 23, no 11, March 18, 1994.
41. Carlson RW, Goldstein LJ, Gradishar WJ, et al: NCCN breast cancer practice guidelines. Oncology 1996; 11(Suppl):47–75.

10 *Gene Therapy for Cancer*

KHALED A. TOLBA, MD, Hematology and Oncology
HOWARD J. FEDEROFF, MD, Neurology
JOSEPH D. ROSENBLATT, MD, Medical Oncology

And all our knowledge is, ourselves to know.
ALEXANDER POPE

Perspective

The remarkable progress made toward understanding the genetic basis of disease in general and cancer in particular, coupled with expanding knowledge in virology, molecular genetics, recombinant DNA technology, and immunology, transformed the discipline of gene therapy from a theoretic concept to a reality.[1–5] The first truly effective gene transfer vectors based on murine retroviruses were developed in 1981 and 1982.[6, 7] Limitations of retroviruses led to efforts to develop different vectors, both viral and nonviral. Expectations generated in the early days of gene therapy led to clinical trials before the technology matured.[8, 9, 10] In the few years since the National Institutes of Health launched its first protocol for gene therapy by Anderson, Blaese, and Rosenberg,[11] involving *ex vivo* retroviral gene transfer of a neomycin resistance gene into tumor infiltrating lymphocytes from patients with melanoma, the field witnessed such rapid growth that, by 1996, the number of studies reviewed and approved by the Recombinant DNA Advisory Committee of the National Institutes of Health had already surpassed 100[12] and involved a large variety of vectors and approaches. More than 200 trials have been activated as of the time of this writing.[13]

In this chapter, gene therapy is discussed, focusing on its use in cancer. Discussed also are the available delivery systems, both viral and nonviral, as well as genetic and immunologic anticancer strategies. The first sections cover viral vectors, including a discussion of replication-competent oncolytic viruses for gene transfer, followed by nonviral vectors for gene transfer. We also cover specific strategies for cancer gene therapy, such as use the of antisense nucleic acid and ribozymes targeting mutated oncogenes, delivery of tumor suppressor genes, and immunotherapy.

Gene Transfer Methodology

Viral Vectors

Retroviral Vectors

Retroviruses were the first vectors to enter clinical trials and, arguably, are the most intensively studied of all the now-available vectors. The retrovirus genome is composed of two identical copies of a single-stranded RNA molecule. The virus genome is approximately 10 kb and it has an insert capacity of 9 to 12 kb. Retroviruses have only one promoter located in the viral long terminal repeat. All retroviruses contain three essential genes: *gag*, *pol*, and *env*. *Gag* codes for a polyprotein precursor, which is cleaved by the viral protease into three or four structural proteins; *pol* encodes the viral reverse transcriptase, protease, and integrase, whereas *env* encodes the envelope glycoprotein. Replication-defective retroviral vectors are generated by replacing most or all of the viral genome with the transgene of interest; thus the virus is incapable of making proteins necessary for its replication (Fig. 10–1). Viral proteins needed for the initial round of packaging are provided by a packaging cell line engineered to produce these proteins.[14] The resulting viruses are replication defective. Retroviruses are divided into three main classes: oncoviruses, lentiviruses, and spumaviruses.

ONCOVIRUSES

Oncoviruses are the simplest retroviruses and contain three open reading frames (*gag*, *pol*, *env*). The viral genome is made up of two copies of a single-stranded RNA. Fusion of the viral envelope with the host cell membrane is followed by viral entry and reverse transcription of the viral RNA into a DNA copy that can gain access to the host DNA during mitosis. The viral cDNA is integrated into the host cell DNA, and the integrated copy is designated the provirus.[15] Viral RNA and proteins are then expressed. New virions are assembled in the cytoplasm, and, as long as a packaging sequence is present, they are released by budding.

Most of the early work on retroviral vectors focused on murine leukemia virus (MLV) 11.[16] These vectors have a number of advantages,[17, 18] including:

- the ability to integrate into the host genome
- an insert size of 6 to 7 kb that can accommodate most cDNAs
- a safe packaging system that essentially eliminated helper virus contamination

On the other hand, this virus system still has significant disadvantages that preclude universal application for gene therapy, including low transduction efficiency, and requirement for host cell proliferation for provirus integration.[19] The latter disadvantage, particularly, hampers its use for

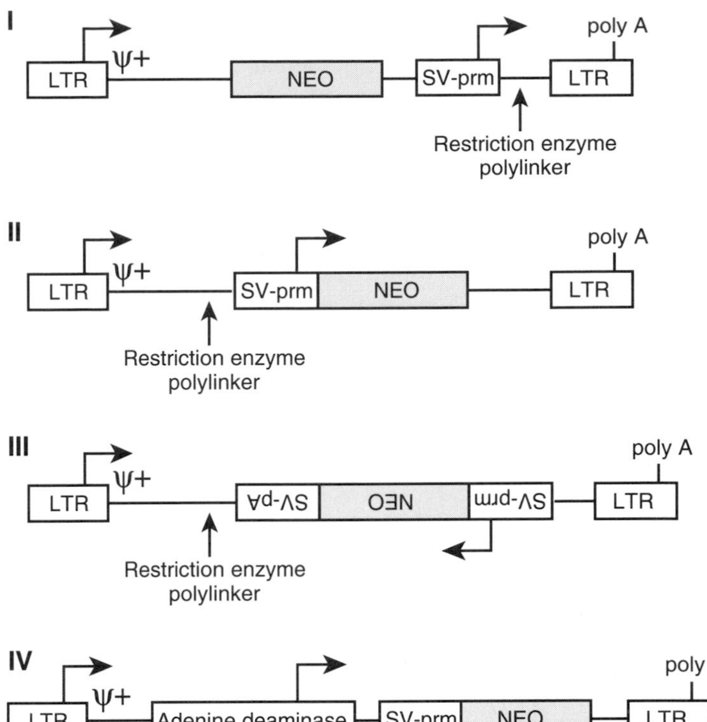

Figure 10–1. Recombinant retroviral vectors: four different retroviral vectors each encoding a selection marker, a neomycin resistance gene (NEO), and a restriction enzyme polylinker site for cloning the transgene of interest. Both genes (NEO and the transgene) can be driven by either the LTR promoter or an SV40 promoter.

both hematopoietic stem cell and tumor cell transduction, in which the majority of cells are in the resting phase. There is also a potential for carcinogenesis as a result of insertional mutagenesis secondary to random integration of the provirus and the lack of target cell specificity.[20]

The initial step in a cell transduction by a retrovirus, and a primary determinant of retrovirus infectivity, is the interaction between the env glycoprotein and specific receptors on the host cell.[21] A great deal of work has been expended on manipulating this process for efficient and target tissue–specific gene delivery[22]; however, few naturally occurring retroviral infections are strictly limited to one cell type. MLVs are either ecotropic (can infect all rodent cells) or amphotropic (can infect all mammalian cells). Ecotropic Moloney MLV confers a restricted host range because it attaches selectively to a peptide loop in the murine cationic amino acid transporter, found only on cells of mouse and rat origin,[23, 24] whereas amphotropic MLV envelopes attach to an epitope on the ubiquitous RAM-1 phosphate transporter, which is conserved throughout mammalian species, and hence confers a widened host range, including human cells.[25, 26] Env proteins can be genetically exchanged among retroviruses allowing viruses to acquire the host range of the env protein, a process known as pseudotyping. Pseudotypes usually retain the native *gag* and *pol* genes while using a new env protein. In some cases, retroviral pseudotypes can incorporate nonretroviral env proteins, such as the envelope of the rhabdovirus vesicular stomatitis virus (VSV).[27, 28] Pseudotyping can potentially improve viral gene transfer through two mechanisms:

- It allows viral entry into a cell line that originally expresses very low levels of the viral receptor, such as mammalian hematopoietic stem cells. Because stem cells express low levels of the amphotropic receptor, pseudotyping with vesicular stomatitis virus envelope can confer enhanced tropism for human cells.
- Pseudotyping can bypass virus interference by using *env* genes from different interference groups. Virus interference is a phenomenon in which cells infected by a retrovirus cannot be superinfected by other retroviruses of the same interference group as a result of blocking of the receptor by endogenous env protein synthesized in the infected cell. So far, eight interference groups have been identified for retroviruses that can infect human cells where each group is presumed to interact with a different receptor.

LENTIVIRUSES

Lentiviruses include human immunodeficiency virus (HIV)-1, HIV-2, simian immunodeficiency virus, and Visna virus, among others. These viruses contain a nuclear localization signal that enables the viral RNA genome to be trafficked to the nucleus without a requirement for breakdown of the nuclear membrane, as is the case for oncoviruses.[29–31] This process, in turn, leads to the potential transduction of nondividing cells. HIV vectors pseudotyped with MLV amphotropic, ecotropic, and vesicular stomatitis virus-G *env* have been constructed.[32, 33] Studies have shown that HIV vectors are more efficient than MLV vectors in transducing nondividing cells, though transduction rates are still higher in dividing cells.[34, 35] Although HIV appears to be a promising vector for gene therapy, numerous safety concerns such as the potential for generation of a replication-competent helper virus will need to be thoroughly addressed before lentiviral vectors are considered for clinical use.

SPUMAVIRUSES

Spumaviruses, or foamy viruses, represent the third class of retroviruses. They have been isolated from many vertebrates, including primates, but are not convincingly associated with any known disease, even in accidentally infected research personnel.[36] Human foamy virus (HFV) was originally isolated from a human nasopharyngeal cell line, but it may be a chimpanzee virus variant.[37] HFV constructs have been used for gene delivery, and, compared with those of MLV, HFV holds certain advantages over MLV, including capacity to transduce nondividing cells, larger packaging capacity, and a wide host range. Similar to HIV, HFV provirus appears to survive in nondividing cells and efficiently express its transgene when the cell divides later. Vectors based on spumaviruses are under development.

Adenovirus

Adenoviruses are double-stranded DNA viruses. The genome is 36 kb in length, surrounded by an icosahedral protein capsid with a diameter of approximately 140 nm. The capsid is composed of two major proteins: the hexon and penton complex, with the penton comprised of two units, the base and the fiber. Viral entry into cells is a two-step process. First, the fiber protein attaches to an unidentified receptor on the cell surface,[38] and this is followed by internalization, which is mediated by the RGD-containing domain of the penton base that binds to α_v-type integrins (the cellular receptors for the extracellular protein vitronectin).[39] This two-step entry mechanism has been the focus of intense efforts to target the adenovirus to certain cell types.

Adenoviruses were first discovered by Rowe and associates in 1953 while trying to cultivate epithelial cells from the adenoids.[40] More than 100 different serotypes of adenovirus (Ad) have been identified, about half of which are derived from humans.[41] The 47 different human serotypes are grouped A to F according to their ability to cause tumors in newborn hamsters. Certain Ad serotypes are oncogenic in newborn rodents (the first such observation for a human virus).[42]

The adenovirus genome has been divided into two major regions: early and late (with regard to the onset of DNA synthesis). The switch from early to late usually takes place approximately 7 hours after infection. There are six distinct early regions numbered in the order of their synthesis: E1A, E1B, E2A, E2B, E3, and E4. E1A encodes transcriptional regulators of viral DNA, which are required for replication. E1B proteins counteract the E1A-induced apoptosis, which is explained in detail in the section entitled "Oncolytic Adenovirus." They also code for a DNA polymerase and a 72 kDa DNA-binding protein. The E3 region is not necessary for viral replication in culture, but it modulates the host immune response to virally infected cells.[43] The E4 region facilitates DNA replication, enhances late viral gene expression, and decreases host protein synthesis. At least seven open reading frames map to this region, the most functionally significant of which is the ORF6 protein.[44] This 34 kDa protein complexes with the 55 kDa protein from the E1B region, and the complex might have a role in host protein synthesis shutoff.[45]

ADENOVIRUS GENE VECTORS

First-generation Ad vectors were constructed using serotypes 2 and 5 because they were the best characterized of all serotypes,[46] and they can be produced in higher titers than most other serotypes. They also belong to subgroup C, which is nononcogenic in rodents. Deletion of the E1A region, an integral process in the preparation of most vectors, would render the most oncogenic serotypes nononcogenic. Without any viral genome deletion, it is possible to accommodate a DNA insert size up to 1.8 to 2 kb. An additional 3.2 kb can be added, through the deletion of the E1 region, without affecting the growth of the virus by using the 293 helper cell line, which is a human embryonic kidney line transformed by the E1 region of Ad5.[47] Deletion of the E3 region alone—up to 3.1 kb can be deleted—produces a replication-competent virus that can accommodate up to 5 kb in insert.[48] When both the E1 and E3 regions are deleted, the resulting replication-deficient vector can accommodate up to 7.5 kb of exogenous DNA. Most Ad vectors now used are deleted in both the E1 and E3 region.

Adenovirus vectors offer a number of advantages: They can be produced to very high titers, they can efficiently transfer genetic information to replicating as well as nonreplicating cells, and they do not integrate into the host genome, thus avoiding the potential for insertional mutagenesis. The viral genome remains epichromosomal; therefore, the risks of insertional mutagenesis are eliminated. However, adenovirus vectors have certain disadvantages. Most significantly, a persistent basal level of viral gene expression, noted both *in vitro*[49] and *in vivo*,[50] eventually generates an immune response against the Ad and limits the therapeutic utility of the vector, particularly in which prolonged expression of the transgene or repeated vector administration is desired. Another problem is inadvertent generation of replication-competent adenovirus. The presence of replication-competent adenovirus will boost the level of late gene expression in target cells, resulting in a heightened immune response against the vector and the infected cell. Second, replication-competent adenovirus can act as a helper virus for replication of the recombinant vector, potentially moving the transgene into unintended tissues within the patient, and, in theory, from one individual to another.

An adenovirus mutant that preferentially replicates in and kills *TP53*-mutated tumor cells has raised considerable interest as a cancer cell–specific therapy. This virus is discussed in the section entitled "Oncolytic Adenovirus."

The discipline of gene therapy has been the subject of intense scrutiny both from supervising federal agencies and the media. This scrutiny was prompted by the unfortunate death of an 18-year-old patient, who was enrolled in a gene therapy clinical trial at the University of Pennsylvania to correct a hereditary enzyme deficiency (ornithine transcarbamoylase [OTC]). In its severe form, OTC deficiency is fatal in infancy. Because this was a phase I safety study with no expected clear and immediate benefit to the participants, only consenting adults were enrolled. Restriction of entry to healthy consenting adults was mandated by the existing laws that protect infants and children from participating in clinical studies to which they cannot consent, except when a clear benefit is realistically achievable.

The death of a healthy adult as a direct consequence of an experimental treatment that was not expected to provide much benefit has pointed to the need for better scrutiny of gene therapy trials. The direct cause of the patient's death was believed to be adult respiratory distress syndrome and multiorgan failure as a result of an inflammatory response elicited by the viral proteins. Adenoviral vectors are known to trigger a host immune response, which is initiated in the first few hours by the delivered viral proteins. Immune response against these proteins is associated with a cytokine storm and mobilization of immune effector cells; this was most likely at the center of events that led to the death of the patient.

Long before the events at the University of Pennsylvania, efforts had been under way to develop a helper-dependent or so-called gutless adenovector that lacks all of the native viral genes. These genes have been replaced by an expression cassette encoding the therapeutic gene and a packaging signal similar to the herpes simplex virus (HSV) amplicon. It is hoped that these efforts will produce a virus with far less toxicity than the currently available adenoviral vectors. However, this tragic death illustrates the potential for unexpected adverse events and toxicity, and emphasizes the need to develop useful models for preclinical testing and safer vectors.

HERPES SIMPLEX

HSV-1 is a human neurotropic virus that primarily infects epithelial cells of the skin and mucous membranes, where it undergoes a productive (lytic) cycle in the nucleus of infected cells.[51] From there it is carried by retrograde axonal transport to neuronal cells, primarily sensory ganglia, where it establishes a latent state with the genome existing as an intranuclear extrachromosomal episome for the life of the host. During this latency phase, gene expression is limited to several intranuclear RNA species, known as latency associated transcripts (LATs).[52, 53] LATs do not appear to perturb nerve cell function. HSV-1 can be reactivated from latency, resulting in viral replication and clinical signs of infection. Virus mutants, engineered to be defective for both growth and reactivation, can still establish latency with repression of lytic genes and expression of LATs.

Interest in HSV-1 as a gene therapy vector is derived from this natural tendency to remain dormant in the host cell for several years, while still being able to express certain genes. Because of its natural tropism for neurons and remarkably large coding capacity, most of the work on HSV so far has been on delivery and expression of genes to the central nervous system (CNS), or for the purpose of selective destruction of cancer cells, particularly CNS tumors.

HSV is a double-stranded DNA virus with an icosahedral protein capsid surrounded by a glycoprotein-containing lipid envelope.[54] A layer of proteins known as the tegument separates the two. The genome is 152 kb long and consists of a unique long and unique short segment, each flanked by inverted repeat sequences that contain several genes involved in latency, transcriptional control of viral promoters, and prevention of apoptosis in infected cells.[55]

There are at least 83 different genes identified so far in the viral genome; of these, 5 *orf* are present in two copies. These viral genes are classified as immediate-early (IE or α), early (E or β) or late (L or γ). These groups of genes are expressed in an orderly fashion with the α-genes expressed first, then β-genes, and both are required for the expression of γ-genes. α-proteins perform regulatory functions or prevent a host response to infection. β-proteins are necessary for nucleic acid metabolism or viral DNA synthesis as well as post-translational modification of proteins. The γ-proteins are mostly structural components of the virions.

Of the known 81 genes on the HSV genome, at least 43 are dispensable for viral replication, encoding accessory functions that contribute to the virus life cycle in the host but that can be deleted without preventing virus replication in at least some cell cultures. The remaining 38 genes cannot be deleted without ablating viral replication.

During lytic infection, the first genes to be expressed are the IE genes, which include infected cell proteins (ICP) 0, 4, 22, 27, and 47. With the exception of ICP47, all the other proteins regulate the expression of other viral genes at both the transcriptional and post-transcriptional level.

When the virus enters the latent state, lytic gene expression is rapidly repressed, and a single region of the genome, the inverted repeats flanking the unique long, remains active, producing a family of LATs. These sequences have been the focus of intense research because of their implications for gene therapy. Two promoters have been linked to this site, latency-associated promoter (LAP) 1 and 2.[56] Both LAP1 and LAP2 are independently capable of expressing LAT during latency, though LAP2 is considerably weaker. The LATs that accumulate during latency are unusually stable introns measuring 2 and 1.5 kb in length, both believed to be spliced out from an unstable and difficult-to-detect 8.3 kb precursor. These introns are antisense to the IE gene ICP0 and may serve to control its level of expression by destabilizing the ICP0 mRNA. Successful expression of therapeutic genes has been achieved by placing the transgene downstream of LAP1, near the start of LAT mRNA.

HSV vectors employed in cancer gene therapy generally fall into two categories, amplicons and replicating HSV vectors engineered to selectively kill tumor cells.

AMPLICONS

HSV amplicons are plasmids engineered to contain an HSV origin of replication (oriS), an HSV packaging signal ('a'), and a bacterial origin of replication[57, 58] (Fig. 10–2). Amplicons usually represent ~1% of the 150 kb HSV genome. They do not encode viral proteins and must, therefore, be supplied with both viral structural proteins and proteins required for viral DNA synthesis and exocytosis. Amplicons are propagated as plasmids in bacteria and then transfected into complementing cells infected with a defective HSV helper virus to create a mixed population of HSV particles containing either the defective HSV helper genome or concatemers of the amplicon plasmid (containing the gene of interest), and packaged in an HSV capsid.[59, 60] Amplicon vectors retain the wide tropism of HSV-1, but the viral stocks tend to have lower titers (HSV can be prepared at titers up to 109 versus ~108 seen in

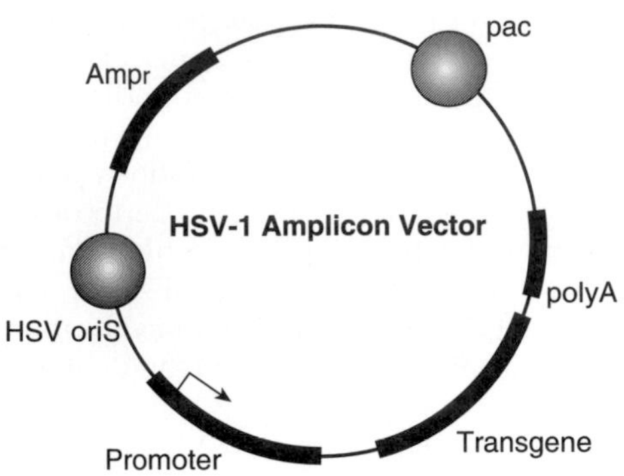

Figure 10–2. HSV amplicon plasmid containing the HSV DNA origin of replication (HSV oriS), the IE 3/4 promoter, transgene, amplicon packaging signal (pac), and ampicillin resistance gene (Ampr).

amplicon preparations). Production of amplicons used to require repeated passaging of the amplicon-helper preparation to increase amplicon vector titer. The end product is a mixture of amplicons and defective helper viruses. Amplicon-helper preparations are still quite toxic to most cells because of the helper virus, and this has inspired efforts to produce helper-free amplicon systems. True helper virus–free amplicon preparations have been produced by some groups, but virus yield produced by this method is relatively low.[61] This involves deletion of the cleavage and packaging signal from a set of cosmids that represent the HSV genome. Contransfection of cells with this modified cosmid set and vector DNA (plasmid) results in the production of vector stocks free of detectable helper virus.[62, 63] More efficient helper-free amplicon methods using bacterial artificial chromosomes are under development (Fig. 10–3).[64, 65] In theory, amplicons could accommodate as much as 150 kb of copies of the transgene in concatemers. Although prolonged expression of a gene is possible in postmitotic cells, nonreplicating amplicon genomes are segregated in dividing cells and result in progressive dilution. One attempt to address this issue led to the inclusion of Epstein-Barr virus (EBV) sequences required to maintain the plasmid, as an episome, in the nucleus of transfected cells.[66] EBV has been shown to contain a unique latent replication origin (oriP) that directs viral self-replication and maintenance in cells without entering the lytic cycle: EBV nuclear antigen 1 (EBNA-1) is a DNA-binding transactivator for oriP. However, amplicon vectors carrying the combination of EBNA-1 and EBV oriP are only marginally more effective for eukaryotic expression.[67] Amplicons have been used to transfer genes to neurons both *in vitro*,[68, 69, 70] and *in vivo*.[71, 72] Amplicons have been used to shuttle an immune-stimulating gene (e.g., B 7-1 or interleukin [IL]-12) or a drug-susceptibility gene (e.g., HSV-tk).

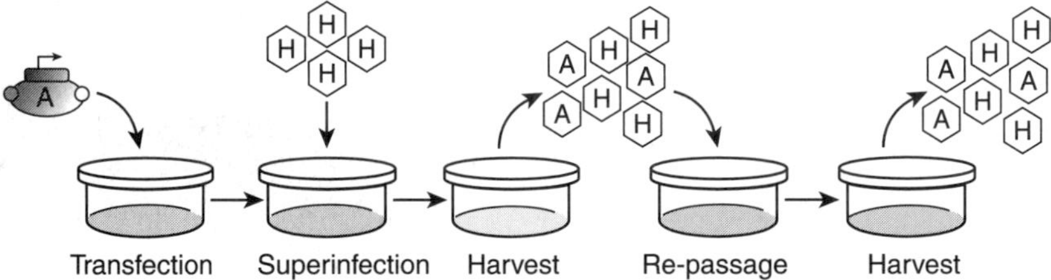

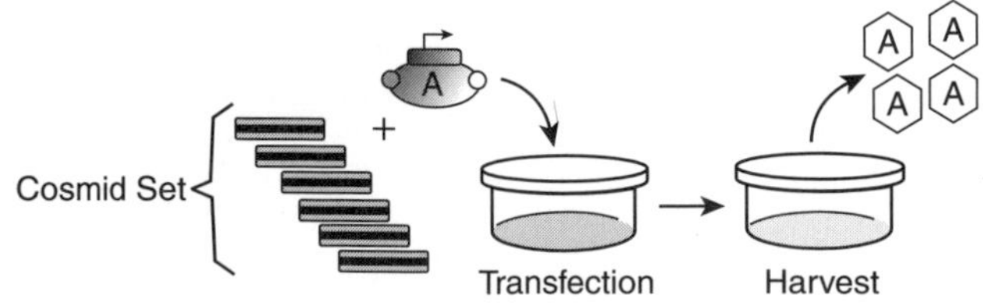

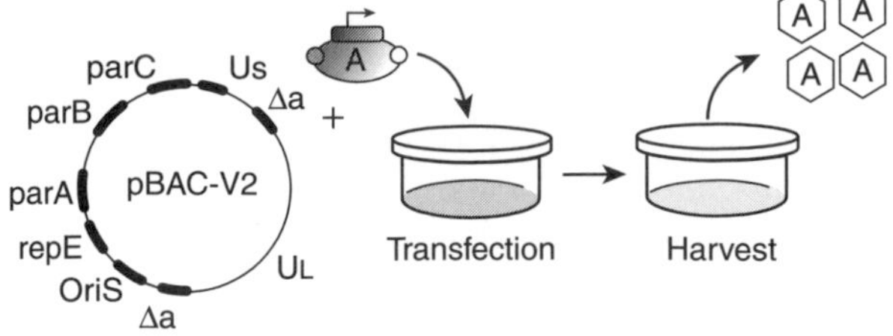

Figure 10–3. First-generation amplicon packaging: using a mixture of amplicon plasmid and helper virus. Second-generation amplicon packaging: using a set of cosmids encoding the HSV genome minus the packaging signal. Third-generation amplicon packaging: using a bacterial artificial chromosome (BAC) to encode the HSV genome minus the packaging signal.

REPLICATING HSV VECTORS ENGINEERED TO SELECTIVELY KILL TUMOR CELLS

These vectors, although sparing the normal host tissues, are similar in concept to adenoviral vectors designed to selectively replicate in tumor cells. They are discussed in more detail in the "Replication-Competent Oncolytic Viruses" section.

ADENO-ASSOCIATED VIRUS

Adeno-associated virus (AAV) is a 4.7 kb single-stranded DNA, nonpathogenic human parvovirus.[73] It commonly inhabits the respiratory and gastrointestinal tract but is not associated with any known disease. It is a dependent virus that requires adenovirus or herpesvirus as a helper virus for replication. Without a helper virus, AAV establishes a latent infection, integrating as a tandem array of several genomic equivalents oriented as head-to-tail or tail-to-tail.[74, 75] Two thirds of integrated wild-type AAV provirus are found at a specific chromosome 19 site, 19q13-qter[76, 77] (AAV vectors do not integrate site specifically).[78, 79] This is believed to be mediated by the viral *rep* gene because viruses with deletions in this gene integrate randomly.[80, 81] The preintegration site has been narrowed to an 8 kb fragment, the first 4 kb of which had been sequenced.[82] The preintegration site contains the AAV *rep* binding sequence (GCTC)3.[83]

AAV vectors are produced by deleting most of the viral coding sequence and cotransfection of adenovirus infected cells.[84] Vectors greater than 115% of the wild-type genome size are not packaged efficiently.[85] AAV vectors generally fall into two types: the first replaces the capsid gene with the transgene (about 2 kb), while the *rep* gene is maintained, allowing for site-specific integration. A second type has been constructed by placing the AAV terminal repeats on either side of the foreign gene, allowing for 4 to 4.5 kb insert size. This vector type can integrate with greater than 50%, but the incidence of chromosome 19 site-specific integration is significantly reduced.[86]

A number of questions remain unanswered regarding the mechanisms by which AAV transfects its target tissues, such as the surface receptor, mechanism of viral integration, and whether transcription of target genes takes place before or after integration. Research in the late 1990s shed some light on these topics. A 150 kDa glycoprotein has been identified as a candidate receptor for AAV serotype 2, the most commonly used serotype.[87] It appears that human CD34 cells lack this receptor molecule, raising questions about the utility of AAV for long-term stem cell transduction. Heparan sulfate proteoglycan has been identified as an AAV receptor,[88] with the human fibroblast growth factor receptor 1[89] and αVβ5 integrin[90] acting as coreceptors for successful viral entry.

AAV vector integration is another poorly understood area of that virus life cycle. AAV vectors do not contain their integration proteins and as a result have to rely on cellular factors for the recombination process. Evidence suggests that viral integration occurs through nonhomologous recombination after variable degradation at vector termini, which results in proviruses with variable deletions. It is not known whether the substrate for integration is the single-stranded vector genome that originally enters the cell or a double-stranded DNA molecule produced after second strand synthesis. Transient gene expression from the episomal AAV can take place prior to integration.

AAV has a number of favorable characteristics as a gene therapy vector including the ability to integrate and establish a stable latent provirus in 19% to 70% of exposed cells, the ability to infect and transform nondividing cells, and a lack of association with any known disease. AAV vectors can be constructed without any viral genes expressed on the infected cell surface, thus avoiding antiviral immune response. AAV has aroused considerable interest as a vector for stable long-term gene transfer for genetic defects such as cystic fibrosis.[91, 92]

VACCINIA

Vaccinia virus has been used for 200 years as a safe vaccine against smallpox, a disease that had been officially eradicated in 1971. It was originally isolated from a horse, and it replaced cowpox as a vaccine for humans against smallpox. Though routine vaccination with vaccinia virus is no longer conducted, experience gained over the years by using the virus makes it one of the best studied and safest vectors for gene transfer. In addition to a remarkably safe track record, vaccinia virus has a number of advantages suited for gene transfer, including:

- ability to transduce both dividing and nondividing cells
- large coding capacity, up to 25 kb
- relatively high levels of transgene expression
- ability to produce recombinant virus in high titers

Vaccinia is an orthopox virus with a linear double-stranded DNA genome, 186 kb in size.[93] A large portion of this, up to 25 kb, is dispensable and can be replaced with a therapeutic gene. The viral DNA does not integrate into the host genome and has no carcinogenic potential. Viral transcription and replication occur in the cytoplasm, with gene expression occurring in a temporal manner governed by different early, intermediate, and late promoters.[94] A curious and potentially advantageous feature of the recombinant vaccinia vectors is their propensity to localize to tumor tissue when injected systemically. Viral titer levels of 106 plaque-forming units (pfu)/g of tumor tissue were noted, compared with undetectable levels (<20 pfu/g) in liver and spleen tissue at day 9 in a murine tumor model.[95] The combination of a high efficiency of gene transduction, preferential localization to tumor cells, and cytopathic effects seen in infected cells makes vaccinia virus an attractive vector for cancer gene therapy and for purposes of immunization.

Vaccinia vectors were first used for gene expression in mammalian cells in 1982; since then, they have been the subject of intense studies. Clinical trials with recombinant vaccinia virus coding for an HIV envelope protein were among the first such studies.[96] The virus has also been explored for vaccination against tumor-associated antigens such as prostate specific antigen, and carcinoembryonic antigen.[97] Several cytokines and immune modulatory molecules have been expressed from vaccinia virus such as IL-1β,[98] IL-12,[99] and B-7100.

REPLICATION-COMPETENT ONCOLYTIC VIRUSES

Viruses that selectively replicate in and lyse tumor cells as opposed to normal host tissue represent an attractive new class of anticancer agent. Among these, a mutant adenovirus (ONYX-015) and an HSV-1 with a deletion of the γ-34 gene have been studied most intensively and are in Phase I clinical trials.

ONCOLYTIC ADENOVIRUS

Wild-type adenovirus is a transforming virus for murine cells. In an attempt to elucidate this function of the virus, an adenovirus with deletion of the 55 kDa protein (and subsequently designated ONYX-015) was generated in 1987 and subsequently found to be lytic for tumor cells lacking wild-type p53 protein. Adenovirus' E1A gene codes for a protein capable of initiating cell cycle and transforming the cell. This is accomplished through interaction with two regulators of the cell cycle, the retinoblastoma protein[101] and cyclin A.[102] However, E1A also usually triggers apoptosis mediated by p53 that will eliminate the cell and abort the virus's replicative cycle. In an attempt to thwart this, adenovirus' E1B region codes for two proteins that inactivate *TP53*, namely 19 kDa and 55 kDa. The 19 kDa protein was originally discovered as an inhibitor of apoptosis in cells productively infected with Ad.[103, 104] Adenovirus mutants that fail to express a functional 19 kDa protein induce apoptosis that severely compromises virus yield. The ability of 19 kDa to inhibit apoptosis is not limited to cells infected by an adenovirus; 19 kDa can also inhibit apoptosis induced by such diverse factors as TNFα and Fas ligand.

In 1987, Barker and Berk engineered a group C adenovirus (dl 1520) with an 827-base deletion in the E1B region of the *TP55* gene, and a point mutation at codon 2022 that generates a stop codon, preventing expression of a truncated protein from the deleted gene.[105] The E1B 19 kDa gene is not affected by this deletion. In 1996, Bischoff and colleagues described the potential of dl 1520 as an anticancer agent that selectively replicates in and kills tumor cells lacking *TP53*, and the virus was renamed ONYX-015, after the biotech company that introduced it into clinical work.[106] Activity of ONYX-015 against *TP53* mutant tumors was demonstrated both in tumor cell lines, and in tumor xenografts in athymic mice.[107] Although the wild-type virus can proliferate in and lyse *TP53*-positive and -negative tumor lines equally well, dl 1520 grew poorly in *TP53*-positive tumors, producing about 100 times less infectious virus particles than did the wild-type virus. Animal studies showed efficacy of ONYX-015 when administered both intratumorally and intravenously. Combining ONYX-015 with chemotherapy (cisplatin and 5-fluorouracil) was more efficient than use of either agent alone. Based on this set of data, the FDA approved ONYX-015 for clinical trials. *TP53* is mutated in 60% of head and neck cancers. This, coupled with close proximity of most lesions to the surface, makes head and neck tumors suitable targets for direct intratumoral inoculation by the virus. Two phase I–II trials in patients with head and neck cancer and with ovarian carcinoma were launched in late 1996, the results of which are awaited. Subsequent trials will likely target tumors with distant metastases because animal data showed some activity of the virus delivered intravenously.

Despite some very promising *in vitro* and *in vivo* data, a number of questions still remain. The ability of ONYX-015 to discriminate between malignant and normal cells is still a concern. Because adenovirus does not infect mouse cells, mouse studies are insufficient to predict whether the virus will be discriminating enough to restrict killing to tumor cells alone when used in humans. The interaction between the virus and the immune system is another area of speculation. Most persons have been infected with an adenovirus at some point and may have immune memory for viral antigens. Whereas this could not be examined in athymic mice, it remains to be seen whether such an immune response will limit viral spread in an immunocompetent individual. This has been a limiting factor when using adenovirus for gene delivery in patients with cystic fibrosis.

ONCOLYTIC HERPES SIMPLEX VIRUS

A variety of HSV mutants selectively grow in tumor cells. The genes deleted include those coding for enzymes involved in nucleic acid metabolism (e.g., thymidine kinase, DNA polymerase, ribonucleotide reductase) that would not be available in postmitotic neurons or other differentiated cells but are available in dividing tumor cells. Such mutants may have other limitations, including[108]:

- lack of efficacy (DNA polymerase mutants)
- resistance to the two main HSV therapeutics in clinical use, acyclovir and ganciclovir (thymidine kinase–negative mutants)
- retained capacity to induce encephalitis (thymidine kinase and DNA polymerase mutants)
- lack of an animal model as a result of significant differences in human and mouse or rat susceptibility to genetically engineered HSV (ribonucleotide reductase mutants)
- potential loss of susceptibility of tumor cells previously treated with alkylating agents (ribonucleotide reductase mutants)

HSV mutants lacking the γ34.5 gene (G207) have been tested for experimental treatment of brain tumors.[109] γ34.5 is present in two copies and encodes a 263–amino acid protein. The 70–amino acid carboxyl terminus is highly homologous to the mammalian growth arrest and DNA damage gene *GADD34*, and the carboxyl terminus of *GADD34* effectively replaces γ34.5 in the viral genome.[110, 111] Viral infection normally triggers a host stress response that shuts off protein synthesis and causes apoptosis aborting viral replication. γ34.5 effectively prevents this protein shutoff and allows viral replication to proceed. Specifically, HSV-1 infection activates the host cell PKR kinase, and, in the absence of a functional γ34.5, this leads to phosphorylation of the α-subunit of the translation initiation factor e1F-α, and total shutoff of protein synthesis.[112] A second function of γ34.5 is to enable the virus to multiply efficiently in the CNS. Viruses constructed with mutations in this gene are highly attenuated in experimental animals.[113, 114] This function of γ34.5 appears to be independent of its ability to preclude the protein shutoff. Evidence in support of this is based on the observation that viruses carrying *GADD34* in place of γ34.5 show no evidence of protein shutoff but still are attenuated (i.e., replicate poorly in neural tissue[108]).

A number of HSV-1 mutants for γ34.5 have been tested as a treatment for CNS tumors in experimental animals with a high degree of success and no incidence of encephalitis in any of these animals.[109] In addition, these mutants are still sensitive to acyclovir, thus adding a safety feature to eliminate the virus, should an unforeseen complication arise.

The success of these mutants prompted others to try them in other solid tumors of non-CNS origin. Kucharczuck and coworkers[115] showed the effectiveness of an HSV mutant for γ34.5 in an animal model for mesothelioma. Sensitive polymerase chain reaction assays showed no evidence of the viral genome in the brain of infected animals. A clinical trial with G207 for glioblastoma has already been initiated, the outcome of which is awaited.

NEW CASTLE DISEASE VIRUSES

New Castle disease viruses (NDVs) are the paramyxovirus of chickens that can cause mild conjunctivitis and laryngitis in humans. Tumor lysis by NDV was first reported in 1955 in numerous tumor cell lines, including both carcinoma (cervical and bladder) and sarcoma (neuroblastoma and fibrosarcoma).[116, 117] On the other hand, nine human fibroblast cell lines were resistant to NDV *in vitro*. The mechanism by which NDV causes tumor cell lysis has not been elucidated yet. Clinical experience with NDV includes both administration of suspensions of tumor cells and virus as well as the virus alone in patients with melanoma, but no conclusions about efficacy have been reported.[118]

AUTONOMOUS PARVOVIRUSES

Parvoviruses are single-stranded DNA viruses with a small genome (5 kb).[119] They are subdivided into three groups[120, 121]:

- Densoviruses, which are exclusive to arthropods
- Dependoviruses (AAVs), which require helper viruses for replication (e.g., adenovirus)
- Autonomous parvoviruses, such as B-19 and H-1, which replicate in target cells causing cell lysis

Replication is limited to cells that enter the S phase and, unlike AAV, do not integrate or cause latent infection. Toolan was the first to describe the antineoplastic activity of autonomous parvoviruses,[122, 123] and subsequent studies showed that both the minute virus of mice and the rodent parvovirus H-1 have an antitumor activity selectively replicating in and lysing tumor cells,[124] both *in vitro* and *in vivo*.[125] Recombinant vectors based on the minute virus of mice and LuIII, another autonomous parvovirus, have been described.[126, 127] Whether recombinant parvovirus–based vectors will be useful remains to be seen.

Nonviral Gene Transfer Strategies

This category includes liposomes, molecular conjugates, and naked DNA. They have several advantages over viral vectors, namely an almost unrestricted size of DNA construct, safety, and ease of preparation.

MODIFIED DNA CONJUGATES

DNA can be chemically modified to preferentially target certain cell types or intracellular compartments. Complexes of DNA plus a protein, such as poly(L-)lysine, can be modified to target specific cell types through the use of different ligands, such as asialo-orosomucoid covalently linked to the poly(L-)lysine to target the liver through the asialoglycoprotein receptor. The system still suffered from transient and ineffective gene expression because of DNA trapping in the endosomes. As an attempt to bypass this hurdle, defective Ad particles or peptides derived from the N-terminal influenza hemagglutinin HA-2 protein have been added to enable the DNA to exit the endosomes into the cytoplasm and eventually enter the nucleus where it is transcribed.

LIPOSOMES

Polycationic lipids can be complexed with plasmid DNA of any size to form complexes capable of fusing with cell membranes and delivering foreign DNA.[128] Several lipid formulations are available, such as mixtures of dioleoyl phosphatidylethanolamine with N-[1-(2,3-dioleoyloxy)propyl]-N,N,N-trimethylammonium chloride (lipofectin), 2,3-dioleyloxy-N-[2(sperminecarboxamido)ethyl]-N,N-dimethyl-1-propanaminium trifluoroacetate (Lipofectamine), dimethyl dioctadecylammonium bromide (Lipofectace), and dioctadecylamidoglycyl spermine (Transfectam).[129] This approach is highly efficient for gene transfer *in vitro* and is being investigated for use *in vivo*.

NAKED DNA

This is probably the most simple means of delivering foreign DNA into tissues. A variation of this technique involves the use of a high-velocity gene gun to inject complexes of DNA-coated gold particles.[130] The technique is readily suited for DNA delivery into subcutaneous tissues because of their close proximity to the surface. An operative procedure will be required for gene delivery to visceral tissues because the particles are unlikely to travel into such a depth on their own. The technique may be suitable for vaccination against infectious agents[131] and cancer immune therapy because the translated proteins are efficiently processed by host antigen presenting cells. Levels and duration of gene expression are limited because of lysosomal degradation of the internalized particles.

Ribozymes and Antisense Nucleic Acid

The goal of gene therapy has been to introduce new genetic material into a cell in order to replace a defective gene or confer new functional attributes to a certain cell. However, as our understanding of the biology of cancer expands, it has become clear that silencing of a mutated oncogene or tumor suppressor gene may also be a more appropriate therapeutic goal. Gene silencing is a more complicated task than introducing new sequences partly because it needs to occur in the majority of tumor cells. However, significant progress has been made over the past decade to make this a potential clinical strategy for cancer therapy. In the mid-1990s a clinical trial with *BCR-ABL* antisense oligodeoxynucleotides (ODNs) in chronic myeloid leukemia (CML) was reported,[132] and clinical trials for *ex vivo* purging of CD34+ with antisense DNA targeting *MYB* gene mRNA have been initiated. Tools used for gene silencing are reverse complementary antisense ODNs and ribozymes. The sites of action are either at the level of gene transcription or translation. We will briefly review some salient features of these two therapeutic modalities; however, a thorough review of the topic is beyond the scope of this chapter, and the reader is referred to a number of excellent reviews on the subject.[133–136]

ANTISENSE NUCLEIC ACID

Antisense ODNs are the most commonly used tools to perturb mRNA transcription. These are short nucleotide sequences synthesized as exact reverse complements of the target mRNA. Antisense ODNs will hybridize with a complementary mRNA target. The resulting duplex will interfere with ribosomal translation and target the mRNA for destruction as explained later in this chapter. Paterson was the first to inhibit gene expression through an exogenous nucleic acid when he used single-stranded DNA complementary to RNA in a cell-free system in 1977.[137] Zamecnik and Stephenson are generally credited as the first to identify the therapeutic potential of antisense nucleic acids by using a 13-nucleotide antisense DNA sequence to the Rous sarcoma virus that was capable of inhibiting viral replication in culture.[138]

Inhibition of gene expression can be accomplished either at the transcriptional or the translational level. Inhibition of gene expression at the translational level usually involves interference with the mRNA and has traditionally been referred to as the *antisense* approach. The antisense message can be either DNA or RNA, and it can be either introduced into the target cell or expressed *in situ* from a transfected viral or plasmid vector. Through reverse complementation, the antisense message will hybridize with the target mRNA and the resulting duplex will render the mRNA message unreadable by the ribosomal complex. This concept is not foolproof, and the RNA-RNA or RNA-DNA duplex is subject to a variety of enzymes such as helicases, unwindases, as well as the ribosomal complex's own unwindase activity that permits a read-through of the mRNA. This is particularly true for antisense sequences hybridizing downstream of the translation initiation site. A number of mechanisms enable the antisense ODN to destroy its cognate mRNA; most significant among these is the activation of RNase H. A ubiquitous nuclear enzyme required for DNA synthesis, human RNase H requires only one DNA-RNA base pair for binding, followed by efficient destruction of the mRNA, leaving the DNA half of the duplex free to engage several other mRNA molecules. Antisense RNA molecules exert their disruptive activity through a different mechanism. A double-stranded RNA duplex may serve as a substrate for the double-stranded RNA adenosine deaminase that deaminates adenosine to inosine. Conversion to inosine may tag the mRNA molecule for degradation or render the message unreadable.

Inhibition of gene expression at the transcriptional level may be achieved through homologous recombination using a plasmid containing a selectable gene marker (e.g., an antibiotic resistance gene) flanked by sequences complementary to the gene of interest in the genomic DNA. Crossover events during cell division will insert the targeting sequences into the genomic DNA and effectively destroy the targeted gene. This method is restricted for cell lines and animal models. Another option to disrupt gene transcription is synthetic ODN capable of hybridizing with double-stranded DNA, thereby creating a triple-stranded molecule unable to bind transcription factors. The triple helix also interferes with duplex unwinding and mRNA synthesis. A third approach to inhibit DNA transcription is to use specific DNA sequences that act as decoys, competing with native DNA for transcription factors *in vivo*. A major drawback of this approach is the lack of specificity and the requirement for high levels of the DNA decoy.

RIBOZYMES

Ribozymes are catalytic RNA molecules with enzymatic activity capable of cleaving RNA. They catalyze endoribonucleolytic cleavage of RNA in a sequence-specific manner and hence hold a therapeutic potential as cancer gene therapy agents. Ribozymes were first isolated from the *Tetrahymena thermophilia* pre-rRNA that was found to catalyze its own excision.[139] Ribozymes are usually designed to incorporate a site-specific cleaving motif into a single-stranded RNA molecule, with the 5′ and 3′ ends capable of hybridizing with complementary sequences flanking an available catalytic cleavage site on the target mRNA. Once the ribozyme hybridizes with its target mRNA, a specific mRNA cleaving molecule results. This molecule can then destroy multiple mRNA molecules in a successive fashion.

Examples of RNAs that can be targeted in this manner include those coding for mutated oncogenes, tumor suppressor genes, and drug resistance genes. The mutated *RAS* oncogene has been studied for that purpose, and anti-*RAS* ribozymes have been studied in several tumor models. A specific anti-*HRAS* ribozyme has been developed that can target the frequently mutated GUC of codon 12 in the *HRAS* oncogene.[140] This has been tested in a human bladder cancer model transfected with anti-*HRAS* ribozyme in athymic mice. The ribozyme was found to be more effective in suppressing tumorigenicity than a mutant ribozyme that did not possess catalytic activity.[141]

KRAS point mutations are found in 90% of pancreatic cancers, and 95% of these are located in codon 12. This codon can serve as the target for a ribozyme specific for this mutation, suggesting that it can be used as a pancreatic cancer–specific treatment.[142] Other potential targets for ribozymes include other oncogenes such as *MYCN* in neuroblastoma and viral mRNA such as HIV-1 mRNA. A particularly clever strategy is ribozyme-mediated repair of the β-globin gene mRNA in cells from patients with sickle cell disease, through ribozyme-mediated cleavage and trans-splicing. Therapeutic trials of ribozyme introduction into tumor stem cells, or T-cells designed to inhibit HIV-1, have been initiated in both the United States and Australia.

Gene Therapy

Chronic Myeloid Leukemia as a Model for Nucleic Acid Therapeutics

CML has served as a paradigm for developing antisense therapeutics in the field of cancer. This stems largely from the presence of an obvious mRNA target that lends itself for this therapy in the form of the *BCR-ABL* translocation with its undisputed contribution to the development and pathogenesis of CML.[143] The majority of clinical trials using antisense therapeutics for CML have focused on *ex vivo* marrow purging that requires relatively small doses of the ODN mostly out of cost considerations. Szczylik and associates[144] were among the first to point out the therapeutic potential of oligonucleotides in CML when they showed that an 18 nt ODN complementary to the *BCR-ABL* junction was able to inhibit the leukemic cell colony formation *in vitro*. Ribozymes have been applied against the *BCR-ABL* fusion sequence as well with partial success.[145–146] Part of the difficulty of targeting the *BCR-ABL* fusion junction stems from its relative inaccessibility for hybridization with complementary sequences,[147] and more accessible portions of the mRNA have been suggested as better targets for hybridization. Despite partial success both *in vitro* and *in vivo* for anti–*BCR-ABL* ODN, *BCR-ABL* itself has been largely discarded as a target for CML gene therapy and superseded by less obvious targets. The rationale behind this includes the relative absence of *BCR-ABL* mRNA in the CML stem cells (though they have the translocation)[148] restricting the treatment effect to the level of the progenitor cells, and the lack of evidence that transient downregulation of the message will eventually kill the CML cell.[149, 150] Because of this, other targets for nucleic acid therapeutics were sought and *myb*,[151] a transcription factor essential for both normal and leukemic hematopoiesis, was identified as an appropriate target. *Myc*, a transcription factor located downstream from the *BCR-ABL*, has been suggested as another target for oligonucleotide therapy of CML, and simultaneous targeting of both messages was more effective than each separately in a severe combined immunodeficient mouse model.[152] Early data from a clinical trial with ODN for patients with CML have been published.[153] Phosphorothioate-modified ODN antisense to the *MYB* gene was used as a marrow purging agent. Early data were promising, with seven of eight patients engrafting, and four of six having essentially normal metaphases 3 months after engraftment, which suggests a significant purge. Five patients showed normal blood counts, with follow-ups ranging from 6 months to 2 years.

Potential cancer-related targets for antisense therapy include *BCL2, TP53, fos, jun, abl, RB1, HOX,* PKC, NFkB, and TGFβ.[154]

Suicide Gene Therapy

Suicide genes are negative selectable marker genes whose protein product will kill transduced cells under certain conditions.[155] Herpes simplex virus thymidine kinase (HSV-tk) is a classic example of genes in that category, rendering transduced cells susceptible to killing by ganciclovir. Ganciclovir is a prodrug that needs to be phosphorylated in order to exert its therapeutic potential. HSV-tk phosphorylates ganciclovir to its monophosphate form approximately 1000-fold more efficiently than the mammalian form.[156] The mammalian counterpart will then dephosphorylate and triphosphorylate the monophosphate form, and the end product is a drug that will eventually inhibit DNA polymerase.[157] Ganciclovir, at the therapeutic concentration (1 to 10 μmol/L) is essentially nontoxic in the absence of HSV-tk because of the relative inefficiency of the cellular enzyme to activate the drug into its active form. The intracellular half-life of the phosphorylated ganciclovir is six times longer (18 to 24 hours) than that of the parent drug because of the difficulty of the phosphorylated form to cross cell membranes, which, in turn, limits toxicity.

Moolten was the first to exploit this concept as a cancer therapy when he reported that mice injected with tumor cells transduced with HSV-tk could be cured by systemic ganciclovir treatment.[158] However, because of the relative inefficiency of then-available gene transfer technology, the suicide gene concept would have remained a mere curiosity, if it were not for the bystander effect associated with its use. The bystander effect is the killing of neighboring cells that have not been transduced by the suicide gene in the presence of transduced cells. A number of mechanisms have been proposed to explain this effect, including the transfer of the phosphorylated ganciclovir through gap junctions between neighboring cells, an antitumor host immune response mediated against antigens released from dead tumor cells, and transduction of vascular endothelium with impaired blood flow to the tumor bed.[159, 160] It has been estimated that transduction of at least 10% of the tumor cells is required to see a response based on bystander effect.

The first clinical trial of HSV-tk in cancer was approved to treat ovarian cancer[161] using allogeneic ovarian cancer cells transduced by HSV-tk, followed by ganciclovir. This was administered intraperitoneally to patients with stage III disease. No significant toxicity was observed in the first nine patients treated. One patient achieved complete clinical remission with disappearance of ascites and normalization of CA-125 for almost 1 year.

Another trial enrolled patients with brain tumors.[162] Producer cells generating retrovirus particles containing HSV-tk were infused into the tumor beds. Antitumor response was reported in five out of eight patients treated, with complete remission seen in one patient for more than a year. The HSV-tk gene has also been used to modulate graft-versus-host disease in bone marrow transplant recipients. By transducing donor leukocytes with HSV-tk, one can allow the graft-versus-leukemia process, mediated by donor leukocytes, to proceed until onset of toxicity from graft-versus-host disease, then administer systemic ganciclovir to suppress the donor leukocytes. This approach has been used in patients who have received bone marrow transplantation for CML and post-transplant non-Hodgkin's lymphoma.

Other suicide genes under study include cytosine deaminase (CD), which can convert the prodrug 5-fluorocytosine (5-FC) to 5-fluorouracil (5-FU).[163, 164] 5-FU is phosphorylated into the monophosphate and triphosphate forms, which block thymidylate synthetase and mRNA transcription, respectively. The HSV-tk system has been compared with CD/5-FC in a colorectal cell line transfected *in vitro*. CD induced 963-fold chemosensitivity to 5-FC, whereas HSV-tk induced 139-fold chemosensitivity to ganciclovir.[165] This discrepancy might be due in part to the fact that the toxic metabolite of the CD/5-FC system is not phosphorylated. Thus, 5-FU might cross cell membranes more readily than the phosphorylated ganciclovir, allowing for a more pronounced bystander effect. Ganciclovir must enter the cell by nucleoside transport systems, which is postulated to be the rate-limiting factor in that system.[166]

This theory remains speculative and further work on the bystander mechanisms of CD/5-FC is needed before it is confirmed.

Tumor Suppressor Genes

Tumor suppressor genes maintain tissue homeostasis by controlling cell proliferation, differentiation, and apoptosis.[167, 168] The crucial role they play in the pathogenesis of cancer, and the high rate of tumor suppressor gene mutations and inactivation in human cancers makes them a natural target for gene therapy.

TP53

TP53 is arguably the most significant tumor suppressor gene studied so far. Our understanding of *TP53*'s role in cell biology and its relevance to human cancer has undergone several modifications before it was recognized as, perhaps, the most relevant tumor suppressor gene. *TP53* was first recognized as a tumor antigen in SV40-transformed cells[169, 170] and, subsequently, as an oncogene when the mutated form of the gene, cloned in the early 1980s,[171, 172] cooperated with the *RAS* oncogene in transforming rat cells.[173, 174] The role of *TP53* as a tumor suppressor gene was recognized in the late 1980s.[175] Subsequent work led to the recognition that the gene was mutated in more than 50% of human cancers.[176]

Acting as a checkpoint in the cell cycle, *TP53* functions mainly as a guardian of the genome in DNA repair and induction of apoptosis. DNA damage upregulates *TP53* and leads to either cell cycle arrest at the G_1/S boundary to allow for DNA repair, or apoptosis. *TP53* transcriptionally upregulates p21 (CIP1), which binds to and inhibits cyclin and cyclin-dependent kinase complexes that propel the cell beyond the G_1 restriction point. p21 also binds to proliferating cell nuclear antigen,[177, 178] and *TP53* upregulates *GADD45*, which stimulates DNA excision repair.[179]

The high frequency of *TP53* mutations among different human cancers, as well as its central role in control of the cell cycle, made it an obvious target for cancer gene therapy. Adenovirus-mediated *TP53* gene transfer into *TP53*-deficient human prostate cancer mice led to apoptosis.[180] Expression of wild-type *TP53* in cervical cancer cells led to apoptosis and cell growth suppression both *in vitro* and *in vivo*.[181] Similar data have been obtained in squamous cell carcinoma of the head and neck,[182] small cell lung cancer,[183] human melanoma cell lines,[184] and an ovarian cancer cell line.[185] Wild-type *TP53* has also been used to experimentally purge metastatic breast cancer cells from bone marrow. Wild-type *TP53* was transferred into breast cancer cells, but not into bone marrow progenitors, resulting in loss of tumor cell clonogenicity.[186]

Systemic therapy with *TP53* has been explored using a liposome-*TP53* DNA complex injected systemically into nude mice harboring breast carcinoma cells and resulted in a marked tumor reduction with no relapse for up to 1 month after cessation of treatment.[187]

The first clinical trial with *TP53* in human cancer was initiated by Roth and coworkers using recombinant retrovirus expressing wild-type *TP53* to replace defective *TP53*. Nine patients with unresectable non–small cell lung cancer (NSCLC) or isolated metastases were enrolled.[188, 189] Six out of seven patients showed evidence of enhanced apoptosis by terminal deoxynucleotidyl transferase-mediated deoxyuridine 5′ triphosphate nick end-labeling (TUNEL) staining of post-treatment versus pretreatment tumor biopsy specimens. Three out of seven patients evaluable for response showed evidence of local tumor regression in the treated lesions. Of the remaining four patients, three had stable disease at the injection site for 8 to 9 weeks (with progressive lesions at the untreated sites), and the remaining patient had progressive disease. In all seven evaluable patients, no toxic effect directly attributable to the vector was reported. None of these patients had retroviral sequences at any tissue other than the injected tumor site.

Swisher and associates initiated another protocol to evaluate wild-type *TP53* gene transfer using adenovirus for patients with NSCLC.[190] It included 53 patients with advanced NSCLC and *TP53* mutations whose conventional treatments had failed. Patients received monthly injections of escalating doses of Ad-*TP53* (106 to 1011 pfu) with or without cisplatinum at 80 mg/m^2 IV for 3 days prior to Ad-*TP53* injections. Clinical responses with greater than 50% regression of the injected tumor were observed for 4 to 11+ months. Long-term follow-ups are needed.

p21

p21 is a cyclin-dependent kinase inhibitor that interferes with cell cycle progression from the G_1 to the S phase. p21 also binds to proliferating cell nuclear antigen,[191] a subunit of the DNA polymerase σ-holoenzyme complex that is involved in DNA replication and repair. p21 has been explored for gene therapy in prostate cancer cells, where it suppressed tumor cell growth *in vitro* and was associated with a reduction in tumor size and improved survival.[192] The study compared the effectiveness of p21 with p53 and found p21 more effective than p53.

Retinoblastoma

Retinoblastoma gene (*RB*) was the first tumor suppressor gene to be identified. *RB* was also one of the first genes to be positionally cloned (i.e., the gene was isolated based on its location and without prior knowledge of its sequence).[193] The gene, which extends over more than 100 kb of genomic DNA, codes for a nuclear phosphoprotein (pRB^{110}) with a molecular weight of 110 kDa. It is constitutively expressed in a large number of cell types at all phases of the cell cycle. pRB^{110} activity is modulated through its level of phosphorylation. pRB is dephosphorylated during the G_1 phase and phosphorylated during the remainder of the cell cycle. Progression of the cell through G_1-S phase boundary is dependent on phosphorylation, which is carried out by cyclin-dependent G_1 kinases. pRB^{110} acts through sequestering several transcription factors, which are released on phosphorylation of the protein.

Replacement of the wild-type retinoblastoma into *RB*-deficient tumor cells including retinoblastoma, osteosarcoma, and carcinomas of the bladder, breast, lung, and prostate suppresses their tumorigenic activity in nude mice.[194, 195] Studies in the mid-1990s suggested a number of mechanisms for antitumor activity including enhancement of tumor immunogenicity,[196] an antiangiogenesis effect,[197] and suppression of tumor invasiveness.[198] A truncated form of RB protein of about 94 kDa (pRB^{94}) lacking the N-terminal 112 amino acids was reported to have more potent tumor cell suppression, as compared with the full-length RB protein (pRB^{110}).[199] It had a slower turnover and a tendency to remain unphosphorylated or hypophosphorylated in host tumor cells. pRB^{94} inhibited the growth of not only the RB-deficient tumor cells but also those with normal RB alleles. Gene therapy of established human *RB+* and *RB−* bladder xenografts in nude mice by recombinant adenovirus vectors encoding either pRB^{94} variant or full-length pRB^{110} showed both were capable of suppressing tumor growth, but the pRB^{94} was more potent than the full-length protein.[200]

BCL-x$_S$

BCL-x is a genetic homologue of *BCL2* that undergoes alternative splicing of its mRNA message into long (*BCL-x*$_L$) and short (*BCL-x*$_S$) forms.[201] The long form, similar to *BCL2*, is an inhibitor of apoptosis, whereas the short form functions as a dominant negative inhibitor of *BCL2* and *BCL-x*$_L$, and can thereby promote apoptosis. Overexpression of *BCL-x*$_S$ in MCF-7 breast cancer cells, which express *BCL2* and overexpress *BCL-x*$_L$, sensitized these cells to apoptosis induced by etoposide and paclitaxel.[202] Adenovirus-mediated transfer of *BCL-x*$_S$ into MCF-7 solid tumors in nude mice resulted in a 50% reduction in tumor size.[203] Direct mediators of apoptosis may represent attractive targets for gene therapy.

Immune Therapy–Based Gene Therapy

Most tumors manage to evade the host immune surveillance as a result of a number of mechanisms. Nevertheless, most tumors possess a variety of antigens such as mutated oncogenes *(RAS)*, tumor suppressor genes (*TP53*, retinoblastoma protein), fusion proteins arising from chromosomal translocations (BCR-ABL, PML-RAR) and aberrantly expressed embryonic proteins (CEA and AFP) that could, in theory, allow targeting of tumor cells for elimination by the immune system. Gene therapy–based immune strategies have been used to restore or enhance tumor immunogenicity and recruit immune effector cells. A variety of immune-based gene therapy strategies have targeted the tumor cell either *ex vivo* or *in vivo*. Such an approach takes advantage of the tumor's native antigens generated through mutations of oncogenes, tumor suppressor genes, and fusion proteins arising out of chromosomal translocations. This approach does not necessarily require manipulations of the whole tumor cell population, and treatment of a small fraction of the tumor mass is usually sufficient. This is often accomplished *ex vivo*, with the tumor cells reinfused back as a vaccine. A large number of immunostimulatory cytokines have been explored such as IL-2,[204, 205] IL-4,[206] IL-12,[207–209] IL-13,[210] granulocyte-macrophage colony-stimulating factor (GM-CSF),[211, 212] tumor necrosis factor (TNF)–α,[213] as well as the costimulatory molecule B7.1.[214–217] Animal models have repeatedly demonstrated the feasibility of generating systemic immunity against parental tumors using a variety of vectors and immune strategies. An example of this type of approach using chemokines and costimulatory ligand transduction using HSV amplicon vectors was published in 1999 (Fig. 10–4).[218] Clinical trials testing this concept (i.e., reinfusing tumor cells transduced with an immune-modulating cytokine, IL-2, and GM-CSF) have been conducted in patients with melanoma[219] and renal cell carcinoma,[220] and both studies documented partial tumor regression in some patients. *In vivo* manipulation of the tumor cells has been accomplished using a cationic liposomal DNA preparation.

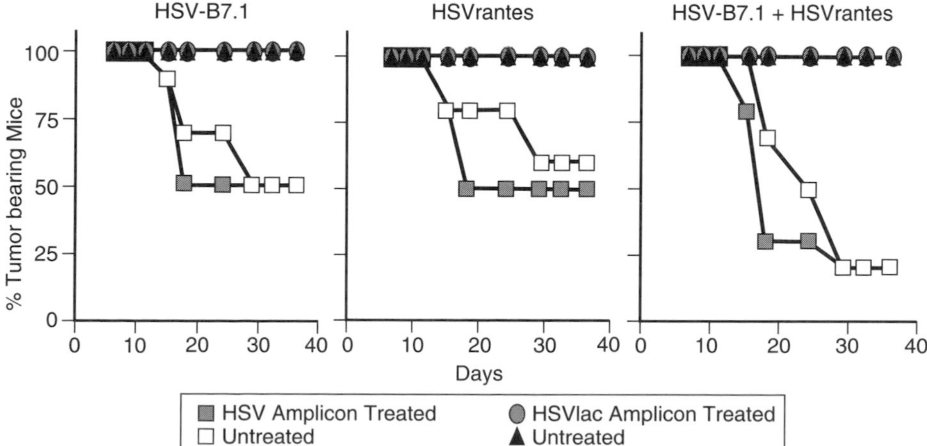

Figure 10–4. Tumor incidence in mice inoculated with HSV amplicon into pre-established EL4 tumor and parental ELA cells injected contralaterally. Viable EL4 cells were implanted subcutaneously on both hind limbs of 106 8-week-old C57BL/6 mice. Tumors were allowed to develop to a size of 5 to 6 mm in diameter. HSV amplicon virus (2×10^6 amplicon containing virus particles) was injected into the right tumor on days 7 and 14, and tumor growth on HSV amplicon treated and untreated side was monitored every 3 days. The HSVlac treated tumor or the contralateral untreated tumor is also shown. The graph represents the percentage of tumor bearing mice over time. (Modified from Kutubuddin M, Federoff HJ, Challita-Eid PM, et al: Eradication of pre-established lymphoma using herpes simplex virus amplicon vectors. Blood 1999; 93:643.)

This approach was explored in patients with melanoma who received intratumoral injections of plasmids encoding allogeneic major histocompatibility complex molecules. Local immunologic reactions, as well as responses at distant uninjected sites, were seen in some patients.[221] However, the remarkable success in animal systems has yet to translate into proven clinical strategies.

A novel approach to tumor immunotherapy is the use of dendritic cells (DCs), an antigen presenting cell (APC), to express tumor-specific antigens. DCs are potent APCs, and they can be generated in sufficient numbers for therapeutic purposes using peripheral blood mononuclear cells cultured in IL-4 and GM-CSF with or without TNFα, as well as other cytokines (SCF, FLT3 ligand). Using DCs to present tumor antigens to the immune system bypasses a major hurdle toward successful tumor immunotherapy, namely, the tumor cell's own inefficiency as an APC as a result of lack of MHC-I or II, costimulatory molecules (B7.1), or adequate peptide processing molecules such as TAP-1. Use of DCs transduced by known tumor antigens delivered either through a viral vector such as adenovirus,[222] DNA plasmid, or through introduction of tumor-cell derived mRNA into DCs[223] are all undergoing active study. DCs pulsed with melanoma cell lysates, or a cocktail of peptides recognizable by cytotoxic T-cells, have been used to immunize melanoma patients with advanced disease, and objective responses have been seen.[224] Newer immune strategies using more potent vectors such as HSV, modified adenovirus, and other vectors are an area of very active investigation.

The past decade has seen an explosion in the use of gene transfer strategies to treat cancer. Improved vector systems, both viral and nonviral, should allow more efficient and specific targeting of tumor cells. Newer systems may allow targeting of micrometastatic tumor as well as large tumor deposits. Improved immunologic strategies may result in more vigorous antitumor immune responses. Gene therapy has made great strides since its conception. The rapid progress made over the past two decades suggests that this modality will continue to grow as a highly efficient and potent tool against cancer.

REFERENCES

1. Friedmann T, Roblin R. Gene therapy for human genetic disease. Science 1972; 175:949–955.
2. Mulligan RC: The basic science of gene therapy. Science 1993; 260:926–932.
3. Brenner MK. Human somatic gene therapy: progress and problems. J Intern Med 1995; 237:229–239.
4. Miller AD. Human gene therapy comes of age. Nature 1992; 357:455–460.
5. Anderson WF: Human gene therapy. Science 1992; 256:808–813.
6. Tabin CJ, Hoffmann JW, Goff SP, et al: Adaptation of a retrovirus as a eukaryotic vector transmitting the herpes simplex thymidine kinase gene. Mol Cell Biol 1982; 2:426–436.
7. Wei C, Gibson M, Spear PG, et al: Construction and isolation of a transmissible retrovirus containing the src gene from Harvey Murine Sarcoma Virus and the thymidine kinase gene from herpes simplex virus type 1. J Virol 1981; 39:935–944.
8. Varmus H. NIH review of gene therapy protocols. Science 1995; 267:1889.
9. Marshall E. Varmus orders up a review of the science of gene therapy. Science 1995; 267:1588.
10. Friedmann T. Gene therapy, an immature genie but certainly out of the bottle. Nat Med 1996; 2:144–147.
11. Rosenberg SA, Aebersold P, Cornetta A, et al: Gene transfer into humans: immunotherapy of patients with with advanced melanoma using tumor infiltrating lymphocytes modified by retroviral gene transduction. N Engl J Med 1990; 323:570–578.
12. Crystal RG: Transfer of genes to humans: early lessons and obstacles to success. Science 1995; 270:404–410.
13. Verma IM, Somia N: Gene therapy—promises, problems and prospects. Nature 1997; 389:239.
14. Miller AD: Retroviral vectors. Curr Top Microbiol Immunol 1992; 158:1–24.
15. Varmus HE: Form and function of retroviral proviruses. Science 1982; 216:812–820.
16. McLachlin JR, Cornetta K, Eglitis MA, et al: Retroviral-mediated gene transfer. Prog Nucleic Acid Res Mol Biol 1990; 38:91–135.
17. Cone Rd, Mulligan RC: High-efficiency gene transfer into mammalian cells: generation of helper free recombinant retrovirus with broad mammalian host range. Proc Natl Acad Sci U S A 1984; 81:6349–6353.
18. Danos O, Mulligan RC: Safe and efficient generation of recombinant retroviruses with amphotropic and ecotropic host ranges. Proc Natl Acad Sci U S A 1988; 85:6460–6464.
19. Miller DG, Adam MA, Miller AD: Gene transfer by retrovirus vectors occurs only in cells that are actively replicating at the time of infection. Mol Cell Biol 1990; 10:4239–4242.
20. Miller AD. Retroviral vectors. Curr Top Microbiol Immunol 1992; 158:1–24.
21. Weiss RA, Tailor CS: Retrovirus receptors. Cell 1995; 82:531–533.
22. Miller AD: Cell-surface receptors for retroviruses and implications for gene transfer. Proc Natl Acad Sci U S A 1996; 93:11407–11413.
23. Kim JW, Closs EI, Albritton LM, et al: Transport of cationic amino acids by the mouse ecotropic retrovirus receptor. Nature 1991; 352:725–728.
24. Wang H, Kavanaugh MP, North RA, et al: Cell-surface receptor for ecotropic murine retroviruses is a basic amino-acid transporter. Nature 1991; 352:729–731.
25. van Zeijl M, Johann SV, Closs E, et al: A human amphotropic retrovirus receptor is a second member of the gibbon ape leukemia virus receptor family. Proc Natl Acad Sci U S A 1994; 91:1168–1172.
26. Miller DG, Edwards RH, Miller AD: Cloning of the cellular receptor for amphotropic murine retroviruses reveals homology to that for gibbon ape leukemia virus. Proc Natl Acad Sci U S A 1994; 91:78–82.
27. Yang Y, Vanin EF, Whitt MA, et al: Inducible, high-level production of infectious murine leukemia retroviral vector particles pseudotyped with vesicular stomatitis virus G envelope protein. Hum Gene Ther 1995; 6:1203–1213.
28. Ory DS, Neugeboren BA, Mulligan RC: A stable human-derived packaging cell line for production of high titer retrovirus/vesicular stomatitis virus G pseudotypes. Proc Natl Acad Sci U S A 1996; 93:11400–11406.
29. Trowbridge RS, Lehmann J, Torchio C, et al: Visna virus synthesized in absence of host-cell division and DNA synthesis. Microbios 1980; 29:71–80.
30. Weinberg JB, Matthews TJ, Cullen BR, et al: Productive human immunodeficiency virus type 1 (HIV-1) infection of nonproliferating human monocytes. J Exp Med 1991; 174:1477–1482.
31. Lewis P, Hensel M, Emerman M: Human immunodeficiency virus infection of cells arrested in the cell cycle. EMBO J 1992; 11:3053–3058.
32. Poeschla E, Corbeau P, Wong-Staal F: Development of HIV vectors for anti-HIV gene therapy. Proc Natl Acad Sci U S A 1996; 93:11395–11399.
33. Akkina RK, Walton RM, Chen ML, et al: High-efficiency gene transfer into CD34+ cells with a human immunodeficiency virus type 1-based retroviral vector pseudotyped with vesicular stomatitis virus envelope glycoprotein G. J Virol 1996; 70:2581–2585.
34. Naldini L, Blomer U, Gallay P, et al: In vivo gene delivery and stable transduction of non-dividing cells by a lentiviral vector. Science 1996; 272:263–267.
35. Reiser J, Harmison G, Kluepfel-Stahl S, et al: Transduction of non-dividing cells using pseudotyped defective high-titer HIV type 1 particles. Proc Natl Acad Sci U S A 1996; 93:15266–15271.
36. Scheizer M, Turek R, Hahn H, et al: Markers of foamy virus infections in monkeys, apes, and accidentally infected humans: ap-

propriate testing fails to confirm suspected foamy virus prevalence in humans. AIDS Res Hum Retroviruses 1995; 11:161–170.

37. Brown P, Nemo G, Gajdusek DC. Human foamy virus: further characterization, seroepidemiology and relationship to chimpanzee foamy viruses. J Infect Dis 1978; 137:421–427.
38. Defer C, Belin MT, Caillet-Boudin, et al: Human adenovirus–host cell interactions: comparative study with members of subgroups B and C. J Virol 1990; 64:3661–3673.
39. Wickham TJ, Mathias P, Cheresh DA, et al: Integrins α v β 3 and α v β 5 promote adenovirus internalization but not virus attachment. Cell 1993; 73:309–319.
40. Rowe WP, Huebner RJ, Gilmore LK, et al: Isolation of a cytopathogenic agent from human adenoids undergoing spontaneous degeneration in tissue culture. Proc Soc Exp Biol Med 1953; 84:570–573.
41. Hierholzer JC, Wigand R, Anderson LJ, et al: Adenoviruses from patients with AIDS: a plethora of serotypes and a description of five new serotypes of of subgenus D (types 43–47) J Infect Dis 1988; 158:804–813.
42. Branton PE, Bayley ST, Graham FL: Transformation by human adenoviruses. Biochim Biophys Acta 1985; 780:67–94.
43. Wold WS, Gooding LR: Adenovirus region E3 proteins that prevent cytolysis by cytotoxic T-cells and tumor necrosis factor. Molecular Biology and Medicine 1989; 6:433–452.
44. Cutt JR, Shenk T, Hearing P, et al: Analysis of adenovirus early region 4-encoded polypeptides synthesized in productively infected cells. J Virol 1987; 61:543–552.
45. Pilder S, Moore M, Logan J, et al: The adenovirus E1B-55k transforming polypeptide modulates transport or cytoplasmic stabilization of viral and host cell mRNA. Mol Cell Biol 1986; 6:470–476.
46. Chroboczek J, Bieber F, Jacrot B: The sequence of the genome of adenovirus type 5 and its comparison with the genome of adenovirus type 2. Virology 1992; 186:280–285.
47. Graham FL, Smiley J, Russell WC, et al: Characteristics of a human cell line transformed by DNA from human adenovirus 5. J Gen Virol 1977; 36:59–72.
48. Bett AJ, Haddara W, Prevec L, et al: An efficient and flexible system for construction of adenovirus vectors with inserts or deletions in early region 1 and 3. Proc Natl Acad Sci U S A 1994; 91:8802–8806.
49. Rich DP, Couture LA, Cardoza LM, et al: Development and analysis of recombinant adenoviruses for gene therapy of cystic fibrosis. Hum Gene Ther 1993; 4:461–476.
50. Yang Y, Nunes FA, Berencsi K, et al: Cellular immunity to viral antigens limits E1-deleted adenoviruses for gene therapy. Proc Natl Acad Sci U S A 1994; 91:4407–4411.
51. Roizman B, Sears AE: Herpes simplex virus and their replication. In: Roizman B, Whitley RJ, Lopez C (eds): The Human Herpesviruses, pp 11–68. New York, Raven, 1993.
52. Croen KD, Ostrove JM, Dragovic LJ, et al: Latent herpes simplex virus in human trigeminal ganglia. Detection of an immediate early gene "anti-sense" transcript by in situ hybridization. N Engl J Med 1987; 317:1427–1432.
53. Deatly AM, Spivack JG, Lavi E, et al: Latent herpes simplex virus type 1 transcripts in peripheral and central nervous system tissues of mice map to similar regions of the viral genome. J Virol 1988; 62:749–756.
54. Roizman B, Sears AE: Herpes simplex viruses and their replication. In: Fields BN, Knipe DM, Howley P, et al (eds): Fields Virology, 3rd ed, pp 2231–2295. Philadelphia, Lippincott-Raven, 1996.
55. Roizman B: The function of herpes simplex virus genes: a primer for genetic engineering of novel vectors. Proc Natl Acad Sci U S A 1996; 93:11319–11320.
56. Marconi P, Krisky D, Oligino T, et al: Replication-defective herpes simplex virus vectors for gene transfer in vivo. Proc Natl Acad Sci U S A 1996; 93:11307–11312.
57. Spaete R, Frenkel N:The herpes simplex virus amplicon: a new eucaryotic defective–virus cloning amplifying vector. Cell 1982; 30:295–304.
58. Frenkel N, Singer O, Kwong AD: The herpes simplex virus amplicon: a versatile defective virus vector. Gene Therapy 1994; 1(Suppl 1):S40–S46.
59. Geller A, Breakfield X: A defective HSV-1 vector expresses Escherichia coli β-galactosidase in cultured peripheral neurons. Science 1988; 241:1667–1669.
60. Geller A, During M, Haycock J, et al: Long term increase in neurotransmitter release from neuronal cells expressing a constitutively active adenylate cyclase from a herpes simplex virus type 1 vector. Proc Natl Acad Sci U S A 1993; 90:7603–7607.
61. Fraefel C, Song S, Lim F, et al: An efficient helper virus-free packaging system for herpes simplex type 1 plasmid vectors. Paper presented at 20th International Herpes Virus workshop, p 32. Groningen, The Netherlands, 1996.
62. Fraefel C, Song S, Lim F, et al: Helper virus-free transfer of herpes simplex virus type 1 plasmid vectors into neural cells. J Virol 1996; 70:7190–7197.
63. Geller AI, Yu L, Wang Y, Fraefel C: Helper virus-free herpes simplex virus-1 plasmid vectors for gene therapy of Parkinson's disease and other neurological disorders. Exp Neurol 1997; 144:98–102.
64. Stavropoulos TA, Strathdee CA: An enhanced packaging system for helper-dependent herpessimplex virus vectors. J Virol 1998; 72:7137–43.
65. Saeki Y, Ichikawa T, Saeki A, et al: Herpes simplex virus type 1 DNA amplified as bacterial artificial chromosome in Escherichia coli: rescue of replication-competent virus progeny and packaging of amplicon vectors. Hum Gene Ther 1998; 9:2787–2794.
66. Wang S, Di S, Young W-B, et al: A novel herpes amplicon system for in vivo gene delivery. Gene Ther 1997; 4:1132–1141.
67. Yates JL, Warren N, Sugden B: Stable replication of plasmids derived from Epstein-Barr virus in various mammalian cells. Nature 1985; 313:812–815.
68. Battleman,D, Geller A, Chao M: HSV-1 vector-mediated gene transfer of the human nerve growth factor receptor p75hNGFR defines high-affinity NGF binding. J Neurosci 1993; 13:941–951.
69. Geller A, During M, Haycock J, et al: Long-term increases in neurotransmitter release from neuronal cells expressing a constitutively active adenylate cyclase from a herpes simplex virus type 1 vector. Proc Natl Acad Sci U S A 1993; 90:7603-7607.
70. Geschwind M, Kessler J, Geller A, et al: Transfer of the nerve growth factor gene into cell lines and cultured neurons using a defective herpes simplex virus vector. Transfer of the NGF gene into cells by a HSV-1 vector. Brain Res 1994; 24:327–335.
71. During M, Naegele J, O'Malley K, et al: Long-term behavioral recovery in parkinsonian rats by an HSV vector expressing tyrosine hydroxylase. Science 1994; 266:1399–1403.
72. Kaplitt M, Kwong A, Kleopoulos S, et al: Preproenkephalin promoter yields region-specific and long-term expression in adult brain after direct in vivo gene transfer via a defective herpes simplex viral vector. Proc Natl Acad Sci U S A 1994; 91:8979–8983.
73. Berns KI: Parvovirus replication. Microbiol Rev 1990; 54(3):316–329.
74. Berns KI, Cheung AKM, Ostrove JM, et al: Adeno-associated virus latent infection. In: Mahy BWJ, Minson AC, Darby GK (eds): Virus Persistence, p 249. Cambridge, Cambridge University Press, 1982.
75. Kotin RM, Berns KI: Organization of adeno-associated virus DNA in latently infected Detroit 6 cells. Virology 1989; 170:460.
76. Kotin RM, Siniscalco M, Samulski RJ, et al: Site-specific integration by adeno-associated virus. Proc Natl Acad Sci U S A 1990; 87:2211–2215.
77. Samulski RJ, Zhu X, Xiao X, et al: Targeted integration of adeno-associated virus (AAV) into human chromosome 19. EMBO J 1991; 10:3941–3950.
78. Kearns WG, Afione SA, Fulmer SB, et al: Recombinant adeno-associated virus (AAV-CFTR) vectors do not integrate in a site-specific fashion in an immortalized epithelial cell line. Gene Ther 1996; 3:748–755.
79. Ponnazhagen S, et al: Lack of site specific integration of the recombinant adeno-associated virus 2 genomes in human cells. Hum Gene Ther 1997; 8:275–284.
80. Walsh CE, Liu JM, Xio X, et al: Regulated high level expression of a human gamma-globin gene introduced into erythroid cells by an adeno-associated virus vector. Proc Natl Acad Sci U S A 1992; 89:7257–7261.
81. Russell DW, Miller AD, Alexander IE: Adeno-associated virus vectors preferentially transduce cells in S phase. Proc Natl Acad Sci U S A 1994; 91:8915–8919.
82. Kotin RM, Linden RM, Berns KI: Characterization of a preferred site on human chromosome 19q for integration of adeno-associated virus DNA by non-homologous recombination. EMBO J 1992; 11:5071.
83. Weitzman MD, Kyostio SRM, Kotin RM, et al: Adeno-associated

virus (AAV) rep proteins mediate complete formation between AAV DNA and the human integration site. Proc Natl Acad Sci U S A 1994; 91:5808.

84. Muzyczka N: Use of adeno-associated virus as a general transduction vector for mammalian cells. Curr Top Microbiol Immunol 1992; 158:97–129.
85. Muzyczka N: Use of AAV as a general transduction vector for mammalian cells. Curr Top Micro Immunol 1992; 158:97–129.
86. Zhu X: Characterization of adeno-associated virus proviral structure in latently infected human cells [PhD thesis]. Pittsburgh, PA: University of Pittsburgh, 1993.
87. Mizukami H, Young NS, Brown KE: Adeno-associated virus type 2 binds to a 150-kilodalton cell membrane glycoprotein. Virology 1996; 217:124–130.
88. Summerford C, Samulski RJ, et al: Membrane associated heparansulfate proteoglycan is a receptor for adeno-associated virus type 2 virions. J Virol 1998; 72:1438–1445.
89. Qing K, Mah C, Hansen J, et al: Human fibroblast growth factor receptor 1 is a co-receptor for infection by adeno-associated virus 2. Nat Med 1999; 5:71–77.
90. Summerford C, Bartlett JS, Samulski RJ. $\alpha V\beta 5$ integrin: a coreceptor for adeno-associated virus type 2 infection. Nat Med 1999; 5:78–82.
91. Flotte TR, Afione SA, Solow R, et al: Expression of the cystic fibrosis transmembrane conductance regulator from a novel adeno-associated virus promoter. J Biol Chem 1993; 268:3781.
92. Flotte TR, Solow R, Owens RA, et al: Gene expression from adeno-associated virus vectors in airway epithelial cells. Am J Respir Cell Mol Biol 1992; 7:349.
93. Moss B: Poxviridae and their replication. In: Fields BN, Knipe DM (eds): Virology, 2nd ed, p 207. New York, Raven, 1990.
94. Moss B: Vaccinia virus: a tool for research and vaccine development. Science 1991; 252:1662–1667.
95. Peplinski GR, Tsung K, Casey MJ, et al: In vivo murine tumor gene delivery and expression by systemic recombinant vaccinia virus encoding interleukin-1. Cancer Journal Scientific America 1996; 2:21–27.
96. Cooney EL, McElrath MJ, Corey L, et al: Enhanced immunity to human immunodeficiency virus (HIV) envelope elicited by a combined vaccine regimen consisting of priming with a vaccinia recombinant expressing HIV envelope and boosting with gp160 protein. Proc Natl Acad Sci U S A 1993; 90:1882–1886.
97. Kantor J, Irvine K, Abrams S, et al: Antitumor activity and immune responses induced by a recombinant carcinoembryonic antigen-vaccinia virus vaccine. J Natl Cancer Inst 1992; 84:1084–1091.
98. Peplinski GR, Tsung K, Whitman ED, et al: Construction and expression in tumor cells of a recombinant vaccinia virus encoding human interleukin-1 beta. Ann Surg Oncol 1995; 2:151.
99. Meko JB, Yim JH, Tsung K, et al: High cytokine production and effective anti-tumor activity of recombinant vaccinia virus encoding murine IL-12. Cancer Res 1995; 55:4765–4770.
100. Hodge JW, Abrams S, Schlom J, et al: Induction of antitumor immunity by recombinant vaccinia viruses expressing B-7.1 or B-7.2 costimulatory molecules. Cancer Res 1994; 54:5552.
101. Whyte P, Buchkovich K, Horowitz JM, et al: Association between an oncogene and an antioncogene: the adenovirus E1A proteins bind to the retinoblastoma gene product. Nature 1988; 334:124–129.
102. Pines J, Hunter T: Human cyclin A is adenovirus E1A associated protein p60 and behaves differently from cyclin B. Nature 1990; 346:760–763.
103. Pilder S, Logan J, Shenk T: Deletion of the gene encoding the adenovirus 5 early region 1B-21,000-molecular weight polypeptide leads to degradation of viral and cellular DNA. J Virol 1984; 52:664–671.
104. White E, Grodzicker T, Stillman BW, et al: Mutations in the gene encoding the adenovirus E1B 19 K tumor antigen causes degradation of chromosomal DNA. J Virol 1984; 52:410–419.
105. Barker D, Berk AJ: Adenovirus proteins from both E1B reading frames are required for transformation of rodent cells by viral infection and DNA transfection. Virology 1987; 156:107–121.
106. Bischoff JR, Kirn DH, Williams A, et al: An adenovirus mutant that replicates selectively in p53-deficient human tumor cells. Science 1996; 274:373–376.
107. Heise C, Sampson-Johannes A, Williams A, et al: ONYX-015, an E1B gene attenuated adeno-virus, causes tumor-specific cytolysis and anti-tumoral efficacy that can be augmented by standard chemotherapeutic agents. Nat Med 1997; 3:639–645.
108. Andreansky S, He B, Gillespie Y, et al: The application of genetically engineered Herpes simplex viruses to the treatment of experimental brain tumors. Proc Natl Acad Sci U S A 1996; 11:313–318.
109. Andreansky S, Soroceanu L, Flotte E, et al: Evaluation of genetically engineered Herpes Simplex viruses as oncolytic agents for human malignant brain tumors. Cancer Res 1997; 57:1502–1509.
110. Chou J, Roizman B: Herpes Simplex virus 1 $\gamma(1)34.5$ gene function which blocks the host response to infection maps in the homologous domain of the genes expressed during growth arrest and DNA damage. Proc Natl Acad Sci U S A 1994; 91:5427–5251.
111. Chou J, Poon AP, Johnson J, et al: Differential response of human cells to deletions and stop codons in the $\gamma 34.5$ gene of herpes simplex virus. J Virol 1994; 68:8304–8311.
112. Chou J, Chen JJ, Gross M, et al: Association of a novel M 90,000 phosphoprotein with PKR kinase in cells exhibiting enhanced phosphorylation of EIF-2α and premature shutoff of protein synthesis after infection with $\gamma 134.5$-mutants of herpes simplex virus 1. Proc Natl Acad Sci U S A 1995; 92:10516–10520.
113. Chou J, Kern ER, Whitley RJ, et al: Mapping of herpes simplex virus-1 neurovirulence to $\gamma 134.5$, a gene nonessential for growth in culture. Science 1990; 250:1262–1266.
114. Bolovan CA, Sawtell NM, Thompson RL: ICP34.5 mutants of herpes simplex virus type 1 strain 17syn+ are attenuated for neurovirulence in mice and for replication in confluent primary mouse embryo cell cultures. J Virol 1994; 68:48–55.
115. Kucharczuk JC, Randazzo B, Chang MY, et al: Use of replication-restricted Herpes virus to treat experimental human malignant mesothelioma. Cancer Res 1997; 57:466–471.
116. Reichard KW, Lorence RM, Cascino CJ, et al: Newcastle disease virus selectively kills human tumor cells. J Surg Res 1992; 52:448–453.
117. Lorence RM, Reichard KW, Katubig BB, et al: Complete regression of human neuroblastoma xenografts in athymic mice after local Newcastle disease virus therapy. J Natl Cancer Inst 1994; 86:1228–1233.
118. Cassel WA, Murray DR, Phillips HS: A phase II study on the postsurgical management of Stage II malignant melanoma with a Newcastle disease virus oncolysate. Cancer 1983; 52:856–860.
119. Shaughnessy E, Lu D, Chatterjee S, et al: Parvoviral vectors for the gene therapy of cancer. Semin Oncol 1996; 23:159–171.
120. Op De Beeck A, Anouja F, Mousset S, et al: The nonstructural proteins of the autonomous parvoviruses minute virus of mice interfere with the cell cycle, inducing accumulation in G2. Cell Growth Differ 1995; 6:781–787.
121. Rommelaere J, Cornelis JJ: Antineoplastic activity of parvoviruses. J Virol Methods 1991; 33:233–251.
122. Toolan HW, Saunders EL, Southam CM, et al: H-1 virus viremia in the human. Proc Soc Exp Biol Med 1965; 119:711–715.
123. Toolan HW, Ledinko N: Inhibition by H-1 virus on the incidence of tumors produced by adenovirus 12 in hamsters. Virology 1968; 35:475–478.
124. Van Pachterbeke C, Tuynder M, Cosyn JP, et al: Parvovirus H-1 inhibits growth of short-term tumor-derived but not normal mammary tissue cultures. Int J Cancer 1993; 55:672–677.
125. Dupressoir T, Vanacker JM, Cornelis J, et al: Inhibition by parvovirus H-1 of the formation of tumors in nude mice and colonies in vitro by transformed human mammary epithelial cells. Cancer Res 1989; 49:3203–3208.
126. Russell SJ, Brandenburger A, Flemming CL, et al: Transformation-dependent expression of interleukin genes delivered by a recombinant parvovirus. J Virol 1992; 66:2821–2828.
127. Maxwell IH, Maxwell F, Rhode SL III, et al: Recombinant LuIII autonomous parvovirus as a transient transducing vector for human cells. Hum Gene Ther 1993; 4:441–450.
128. Felgner PL, Ringold GM: Cationic liposome mediated transfection. Nature 1989; 337:387–388.
129. Felgner PL, Zaugg RH, Norman JA: Synthetic recombinant DNA delivery for cancer therapeutics. Cancer Gene Ther 1995; 2:61–65.
130. Yang NS, Burkholder J, Roberts B, et al: In vivo and in vitro gene transfer to mammalian somatic cells by particle bombardment. Proc Natl Acad Sci U S A 1990; 87:9568–9572.
131. Wang B, Ugen KE, Srikantan V, et al: Gene inoculation generates immune responses against human immunodeficiency virus type 1. Proc Natl Acad Sci U S A 1993; 90:4156–4160.

132. de Fabritis P, Amadori S, Petti MC, et al: In vitro purging with BCR-ABL antisense oligodeoxynucleotides does not prevent haematologic reconstitution after autologous bone marrow transplantation. Leukemia 1995; 9:662.
133. Kmiec EB: Genomic targeting and genetic conversion in cancer therapy. Semin Oncol 1996; 23:188–193.
134. Maher L Jr: Prospects for the therapeutic use of antigene oligonucleotides. Cancer Invest 1996; 14:66.
135. Gewirtz AM, Sokol DL, Ratajczak MZ: Nucleic acid therapeutics: state of the art and future prospects. Blood 1998; 92:712–736.
136. Crooke ST: Advances in understanding the pharmacological properties of antisense oligonucleotides. Adv Pharmacol 1997; 40:1–41.
137. Paterson BM, Roberts BE, Kuff EL: Structural gene identification and mapping by DNA-mRNA hybrid-arrested cell-free translation. Proc Natl Acad Sci U S A 1977; 74:4370.
138. Zamecnik PC, Stephenson ML: Inhibition of Rous sarcoma virus replication and cell transformation by a specific oligodeoxynucleotide. Proc Natl Acad Sci U S A 1978; 75:280.
139. Irie A, Kijima H, Ohkawa T, et al: Anti-oncogene ribozymes for cancer therapy. Adv Pharmacol 1997; 40:207–257.
140. Koizumi M, Kamiya H, Ohtsuka E: Ribosymes designed to inhibit transformation of of NIH 3T3 cells by the activated c–Ha-ras gene. Gene 1992; 117:179–184.
141. Tone T, Kashani-Sabet M, Funato T, et al: Suppression of EJ cells tumorigenecity. In Vivo 1993; 7:471–476.
142. Kijima H, Bouffard DY, Scanlon KJ: Ribozyme-mediated reversal of human pancreatic carcinoma phenotype. In: Ikehara S (ed): Proceedings of International Symposium of Bone Marrow Transplantation, pp 153–163. Berlin, Springer, 1997.
143. Melo JV: The diversity of BCR-ABL fusion proteins and their relationship to leukemia phenotype. Blood 1996; 88:2375.
144. Szczylik C, Skoeski T, Nicolaides NC, et al: Selective inhibition of leukemia cell proliferation by BCR-ABL antisense oligonucleotides. Science 1991; 253:562.
145. Leopold LH, Shore SK, Reddy EP: Multi-unit anti BCR-ABL ribozyme therapy therapy in chronic myelogenous leukemia. Leuk Lymphoma 1996; 22:365.
146. Pachuk CJ, Yoon K, Moelling K, et al: Selective cleavage of BCR-ABL chimeric RNAs by a ribozyme targeted to non-contiguous sequences. Nucleic Acids Res 1994; 22:301.
147. Kronenwett R, Haas R, Sczakiel G: Kinetic selectivity of complementary nucleic acids: bcr-abl directed antisense RNA and ribozymes. J Mol Biol 1996; 259:632.
148. Bedi A, Zehnbauer BA, Collector MI, et al: BCR-ABL gene rearrangement and expression of primitive hematopoietic progenitors in chronic myeloid leukemia. Blood 1993; 81:2898.
149. Bedi A, Zehnbauer BA, Barber JP, et al: Inhibition of apoptosis by BCR-ABL in chronic myeloid leukemia. Blood 1994; 83:2038.
150. McGahon A, Bissonnette R, Schmitt M, et al: BCR-ABL maintains resistance of chronic myelogenous leukemia cells to apoptotic cell death. Blood 1994; 83:1179.
151. Kanei-Ishii C, Nomura T, Ogata K, et al: Structure and function of the proteins encoded by the myb gene family. Curr Top Microbiol Immunol 1996; 211:89.
152. Skorski T, Perrotti D, Nieborowska-Skorska M, et al: Antileukemia effect of c-myc N3–p5 phosphoramidate antisense oligonucleotides in vivo. Proc Natl Acad Sci U S A 1997; 94:3966.
153. Gewirtz AM, Luger S, Sokol D, et al: Oligodeoxynucleotides therapeutics for human myelogenous leukemia: interim results [Abstract]. Blood 1996; 88(Suppl 1):270a.
154. Adams SW, Emerson SG: Gene therapy for leukemia and lymphoma. Hematol Oncol Clin North Am 1998; 12:631–648.
155. Freeman SM, Whartenby KA, Freeman JL, et al: In situ use of suicide genes for cancer therapy. Semin Oncol 1996; 23:31–45.
156. Elion GB, Furman PA, Fyfe JA, et al: Selectivity of action of an antiherpetic agent, 9-(2-hydroxyethoxymethyl) guanine. Proc Natl Acad Sci U S A 1977; 74:5716–5720.
157. Davidson RL, Kaufman ER, Crumpacker CS, et al: Inhibition of herpes simplex virus transformed and nontransformed cells by acycloguanosine: mechanisms of uptake and toxicity. Virology 1981; 113:9–19.
158. Moolten FL: Tumor chemosensitivity conferred by inserted herpes thymidine kinase genes: paradigm for a prospective cancer control strategy. Cancer Res 1986; 46:5276–5281.
159. Bi WL, Parysek LM, Warnick R, et al: In vitro evidence that metabolic cooperation is responsible for the bystander effect observed with HSV-tk retroviral gene therapy. Hum Gene Ther 1993; 4:725–731.
160. Freeman SM, Ramesh R, Marrogi AJ: In vivo studies on the mechanism of the "bystander effect." Cancer Gene Ther 1994; 4:326–332.
161. Freeman SM, McCune C, Angel C, et al: Treatment of ovarian cancer using HSV-TK gene-modified vaccine regulatory issues. Hum Gene Ther 1992; 3:342–49.
162. Oldfield EH, Ram Z, Culver KW, et al: Clinical protocol: gene therapy for the treatment of brain tumors using intratumoral transduction with thymidine kinase gene and intravenous ganciclovir. Hum Gene Ther 1993; 4:39–69.
163. Mullen CA, Kilstrup M, Blease RM: Transfer of the bacterial gene for cytosine deaminase to mammalian cells confers lethal sensitivity to 5-fluorocytosine: a negative selection system. Proc Natl Acad Sci U S A 1992; 89:33–37.
164. Mullen CA, Coale MM, Lowe R, et al: Tumors expressing cytosine deaminase suicide gene can be eliminated in vivo with 5-fluorocytosine and induce protective immunity to wild type tumor. Cancer Res 1994; 54:1503–1506.
165. Trinh QT, Austin EA, Murray DM, et al: Enzyme/prodrug gene therapy: comparison of cytosine deaminase/5-fluorocytosine versus thymidine kinase/ganciclovir enzyme/prodrug systems in a human colorectal carcinoma cell line. Cancer Res 1995; 55:4808–4812.
166. Haberkorn U, Altmann A, Morr I, et al: Monitoring gene therapy with herpes simplex virus thymidine kinase in hepatoma cells: uptake of specific substrates. J Nucl Med 1997; 38:287–294.
167. Weinberg RA: Tumor-suppressor genes. Science 1991; 254:1138–1146.
168. Levine AJ: The tumor suppressor genes. Annu Rev Biochem 1993; 62:623–651.
169. Lane DP, Crawford LV: T antigen is bound to a host protein in SV40-transformed cells. Nature 1979; 278:261–263.
170. Linzer DI, Levine AJ: Characterization of a 54 K dalton cellular SV40 tumor antigen present in SV40 transformed cells and uninfected embryonal carcinoma cells. Cell 1979; 17:43–52.
171. Oren M, Levine AJ: Molecular cloning of a cDNA specific for the murine p53 cellular tumor antigen. Proc Natl Acad Sci U S A 1983; 80:56–59.
172. Matlashewski G, Lamb P, Pim D, et al: Isolation and characterization of a human p53 cDNA clone: expression of the human p53 gene. EMBO J 1984; 3:3257–3262.
173. Eliyahu D, Raz A, Gruss P, et al: Participation of p53 cellular tumor antigen in transformation of normal embryonic cells. Nature 1984; 312:646–649.
174. Parada LF, Land H, Weinberg RA, et al: Cooperation between gene encoding p53 tumor antigen and ras in cellular transformation. Nature 1984; 312:649–651.
175. Finlay CA, Hinds PW, Levine AJ: The p53 proto-ocogene can act as a suppressor of transformation. Cell 1989; 57:1083–1093.
176. Harris CC, Hollstein M: Clinical implications of the p53 tumor-suppressor gene. N Engl J Med 1993; 329:1318–1327.
177. Waga S, Hannon GJ, Beach D, et al: The p21 inhibitor of cyclin-dependent kinases controls DNA replication by interaction with PCNA. Nature 1994; 369:574–578.
178. Li R, Waga S, Hannon GJ, et al: Differential effects by the p21 CDK inhibitor on PCNA-dependent DNA replication and repair. Nature 1994; 371:534–537.
179. Smith ML, Chen I-T, Zhan Q, et al: Interaction of the p53 regulated protein GADD45 with proliferating cell nuclear antigen. Science 1994; 266:1376–1380.
180. Yang C, Cirielli C, Capogrossi MC, et al: Adenovirus-mediated wild-type p53 expression induces apoptosis and suppresses tumorigenesis of prostatic cancer cells. Cancer Res 1995; 55:4210–4213.
181. Hamade K, Alemny R, Zhang WW, et al: Adenovirus-mediated transfer of a wild-type p53 gene and induction of apoptosis in cervical cancer. Cancer Res 1996; 56:3047–3054.
182. Clayman GL, el-Naggar AK, Roth JA, et al: In vivo molecular therapy with p53 adenovirus for microscopic residual head and neck squamous carcinoma. Cancer Res 1995; 55:1–6.
183. Gjerset PA, Turla ST, Sobol RE, et al: Use of wild-type p53 to achieve complete treatment sensitization of tumor cells expressing endogenous mutant p53. Mol Carcinog 1995; 14:275–285.
184. Cirielli C, Riccioni T, Yang C, et al: Adenovirus-mediated gene transfer of wild-type p53 results in melanoma cell apoptosis in vitro and in vivo. Int J Cancer 1995; 63:673–679.

185. Santoso JT, Tang DC, Lane SB, et al: Adenovirus-based p53 gene therapy in ovarian cancer. Gynecol Oncol 1995; 59:171–178.
186. Seth P, Brinkmann U, Schwartz GN, et al: Adenovirus-mediated gene transfer to human breast tumor cells: an approach for cancer gene therapy and bone marrow purging. Cancer Res 1996; 56:1346–1351.
187. Lesoon-Wood LA, Kim WH, Kleinman HK, et al: Systemic gene therapy with p53 reduces growth and metastases of a malignant human breast cancer in nude mice. Hum Gene Ther 1995; 6:395–405.
188. Roth JA: Modification of tumor suppressor gene expression and induction of apoptosis in non-small cell lung cancer (NSCLC) with an adenovirus vector expressing wildtype p53 and cisplatin. Hum Gene Ther 1996; 7(8):1013–1030.
189. Roth JA, Nguyen D, Lawrence DD, et al: Retrovirus-mediated wild-type p53 gene transfer to tumors of patients with lung cancer. Nat Med 1996; 2:985–991.
190. Swisher SG, Roth JA, Lawrence D, et al: Persistent transgene expression following repeated injections of a recombinant adenovirus containing the p53 wild type gene in patients with non-small cell lung cancer [Abstract]. Proceedings of the American Association for Cancer Research 1997; 38:342.
191. Flores-Rozas H, Kelman Z, Dean FB, et al: Cdk-interacting protein 1 directly binds with proliferating cell nuclear antigen and inhibits DNA replication catalyzed by the DNA polymerase δ holoenzyme. Proc Natl Acad Sci U S A 1995; 91:8655–8659.
192. Eastham JA, Hall SJ, Sehgal I, et al: In vivo gene therapy with p53 or p21 adenovirus for prostate cancer. Cancer Res 1995; 55:5151–5155.
193. Friend SH, Bernards R, Rogel S, et al: A human DNA segment with properties of the gene that predisposes to retinoblastoma and osteosarcoma. Nature 1986; 323:643–646.
194. Goodrich DW, Lee WH: Molecular characterization of the retinoblastoma susceptibility gene. Biochem Biophys Acta 1993; 1155:43–61.
195. Zhou Y, Li J, Xu K, et al: Further characterization of retinoblastoma gene-mediated cell growth and tumor suppression in human cancer cells. Proc Natl Acad Sci U S A 1994; 91:4165–4169.
196. Lu Y, Ussery GD, Muncaster MM, et al: Evidence for retinoblastoma protein (RB) dependent and independent INF-gamma responses: RB coordinately rescues INF-gamma induction of MHC class II gene trascription in non-inducible breast carcinoma cells. Oncogene 1994; 9:1015–1019.
197. Dawson DW, Tolsma SS, Volpert OV, et al: Retinoblastoma gene expression alters angiogenic phenotype. Proceedings of the American Association for Cancer Research 1995; 36:88a.
198. Li J, Hu S-X, Xu K, et al: Effects of expression of the retinoblastoma (RB) and p53 tumor suppressor genes on tumor cell invasion in vitro. Proc AACR 1995; 36:78a.
199. Xu HJ, Xu K, Zhou Y et al: Enhanced tumor cell growth suppression by an N-terminal truncated retinoblastoma protein. Proc Natl Acad Sci U S A 1994; 91:9837–9841.
200. Xu HJ, Zhou Y, Seigne J, et al: Enhanced tumor suppressor gene therapy via replication-deficient adenovirus vectors expressing an N-terminal truncated retinoblastoma protein. Cancer Res 1996; 56:2245–2249.
201. Boise LH, Gonzalez-Garcia M, Postema CE, et al: bcl-x, a bcl-2–related gene that functions as a dominant regulator of apoptotic cell death. Cell 1993; 74:597–608.
202. Sumantran VN, Ealovega MW, Nunez G, et al: Overexpression of bcl-xs sensitizes MCF-7 cells to chemotherapy-induced apoptosis. Cancer Res 1995; 55:2507–2510.
203. Ealovega MW, McGinnis PK, Sumantran VN, et al: bcl-xs gene therapy induces apoptosis of human mammary tumors in nude mice. Cancer Res 1996; 56:1965–1969.
204. Fearon ER, Pardoll DM, Itaya T, et al: Interleukin-2 production by tumor cells bypasses T helper function in the generation of an antitumor response. Cell 1990; 60:397–403.
205. Gansbacher B, Zier K, Daniels B, et al: Interleukin 2 gene transfer into tumor cells abrogates tumorigenicity and induces protective immunity. J Exp Med 1990; 172:1217–1224.
206. Golumbek PT, Lazenby AJ, Levitsky HI, et al: Treatment of established renal cancer by tumor cells engineered to secrete interleukin 4. Science 1991; 254:713–716.
207. Bramson JL, Hitt M, Addison CL, et al: Direct intratumoral injection of an adenovirus expressing interleukin-12 induces regression and long-lasting immunity that is associated with highly localized expression of interleukin-12. Hum Gene Ther 1996; 7:1995–2002.
208. Tahara H, Zitvogel L, Storkus WJ, et al: Effective eradication of established murine tumors with IL-12 gene therapy using a polycistronic retroviral vector. J Immunol 1995; 154:6466–6474.
209. Meko JB, Yim JH, Tsung K, et al: High cytokine production and effective antitumor activity of a recombinant vaccinia virus encoding murine interleukin 12. Cancer Res 1995; 55:4765–4770.
210. Lebel-Biay S, Laguerre B, Quintin-Colonna F, et al: Experimental gene therapy of cancer using tumor cells engineered to secrete interleukin 13. Eur J Immunol 1995; 25:2340–2348.
211. Colombo MP, Ferrari G, Stoppacciaro A, et al: Granulocyte monocyte colony stimulating factor gene trasnfer suppresses tumorigenicity of a murine adenocarcinoma in vivo. J Exp Med 1991; 173:889–897.
212. Dranoff G, Jaffee E, Lazenby A, et al: Vaccination with irradiated tumor cells engineered to secrete murine granulocyte-macrophage colony-stimulating factor stimulate potent specific and long lasting anti-tumor immunity. Proc Natl Acad Sci U S A 1993; 90:3539–3543.
213. Tos AG, Cignetti A, Rovera G, et al: Retroviral vector mediated transfer of the tumor necrosis factor alpha gene into human cancer cells restores an apoptotic cell death program and induces a bystander-killing effect. Blood 1996; 87:2486–2495.
214. Chen L, Ashe S, Brady WA, et al: Costimulation of anti-tumor immunity by the B7 counterreceptor for the T lymphocyte molecules CD28 and CTLA-4. Cell 1992; 71:1093–1102.
215. Townsend SE, Allison JP. Tumor rejection after direct costimulation of CD8+ T cells by B7-transfected melanoma cells. Science 1993; 259:368–370.
216. Hirano N, Takahashi T, Takahashi T, et al: Protective and therapeutic immunity against leukemia induced by irradiated B7-1 (CD80)-transduced leukemic cells. Hum Gene Ther 1997; 8:1375–1384.
217. Yang G, Hellstrom KE, Hellstrom I, et al: Anti-tumor immunity elicited by tumor cells transfected with B7-2, a second ligand for CD28/CTLA-4 costimulatory molecules. J Immunol 1995; 154:2794–2800.
218. Kutubuddin M, Federoff HJ, Challita-Eid PM, et al: Eradication of pre-established lymphoma using herpes simplex virus amplicon vectors. Blood 1999; 93:643–654.
219. Belli F, Arienti F, Sule-Suso J, et al: Active immunization of metastatic melanoma patients with interleukin-2 transduced allogenic melanoma cells: evaluation of efficacy and tolerability. Cancer Immunol Immunother 1997; 44:197–203.
220. Simons JW, Jaffee EM, Weber CE, et al: Bioactivity of autologous irradiated renal cell carcinoma vaccines generated by ex vivo granulocyte-macrophage colony-stimulating factor gene transfer. Cancer Res 1997; 57:1537–1546.
221. Nabel G, Gordon D, Bishop D, et al: Immune response in human melanoma after transfer of an allogenic class I major histocompatibility complex gene with DNA liposome complexes. Proc Natl Acad Sci U S A 1996; 93:15388–15393.
222. Kaplan J, Pennington S, Nicolette C, et al: Induction of tumor-specific immunity by dendritic cells transduced with recombinant adenovirus. American Society of Gene Therapy 1st annual meeting, Abstract 720, p 180a, 1998.
223. Boczkowski D, Nair SK, Snyder D, et al: Dendritic cells pulsed with RNA are potent antigen presenting cells in vitro and in vivo. J Exp Med 1996; 184:465–472.
224. Nestle FO, Alijagic S, Gilliet M, et al: Vaccination of melanoma patients with peptide- or tumor lysate-pulsed dendritic cells. Nat Med 1998; 4:328–332.

11 Basic Concepts of Tumor Immunology and Principles of Immunotherapy

JACQUELINE P. WILLIAMS, PHD, Radiation Oncology
EDITH LORD, PHD, Immunology
STANLEY E. ORDER, MD, FACR, Molecular Oncology

And nothing, not God, is greater to one than one's self is.
WALT WHITMAN (1819–1892)

Perspective

The foundation of the immune system is its ability to develop a concept of *self,* which, when combined with an ability to distinguish *self* from *nonself,* has provided the body with the means to recognize and remove foreign materials, cells, and organisms. In order to carry out this role, the immune system has evolved an elaborate, interactive system of checks and balances.[3, 8] In addition, the process of immune recognition is specific and has memory.

If a material is recognized by the immune system as foreign, it is said to be *antigenic*. In the event that the immune system subsequently can mount an active response against it, the material or antigen is said to be *immunogenic*. This feature has led decades of researchers to investigate whether the immune system per se could be used as a means of therapy, and cancer is one of the obvious disease targets for the evolving use of immunotherapy. The theory of *immune surveillance* presumes that tumor cells are antigenic in nature and that the immune system can be used to eliminate such cells before they can grow and spread. Thus, progressive tumor growth may be attributed to an ineffective immune system. Most approaches to tumor immunotherapy have tried to make the tumor appear more foreign compared with normal tissues, or they have attempted to amplify host immune reactions to growing tumors.

In order to review the potential role of the immune system in affecting tumor development and progression, it is useful to discuss briefly the basic biology of the immune system and its responses.

Basic Principles of the Immune System

In humans, a variety of lymphoreticular cells arise from the bone marrow and, with their products, mediate the immune response. These cells move freely throughout the circulatory and lymphatic systems of the body. It is only through the concerted interaction of these cells, which include lymphocytes, monocytes, macrophages, dendritic cells (DCs), endothelial cells, basophils, and eosinophils, that immune responses can occur. In addition, specialized epithelial and stromal cells interact with the cells of the immune system, frequently by secreting factors that regulate and control the immune cells and by providing the environment within which the immune response takes place.[8]

There is a defined time course to an immune response (Fig. 11–1). Following exposure to an antigen, there is a latent period or *lag phase*, during which there is accumulation of the antigen load until it reaches a specific immunogenic threshold level. There then follows an *activation phase*; this phase involves the activation and maturation of specific lymphocytes, which leads to the clearance of the antigen (the *response*). As the antigen levels subsequently decline, the lymphocytes undergo programmed cell death, although a few remain as specific memory cells that can activate should antigen presentation recur.

Select populations of immune cells, notably the B-lymphocytes, are capable of producing soluble effector molecules, and the first immune molecule to be recognized was the *antibody.* Antibodies can be defined as a ubiquitous group of secreted proteins that are part of the immunoglobulin (Ig) family, which forms the crux of the humoral immune response.[9] The antibody molecule is constructed of one or more units that are called *monomers,* and each monomer is composed of four polypeptide chains: two identical large chains of approximately 55 kD, designated

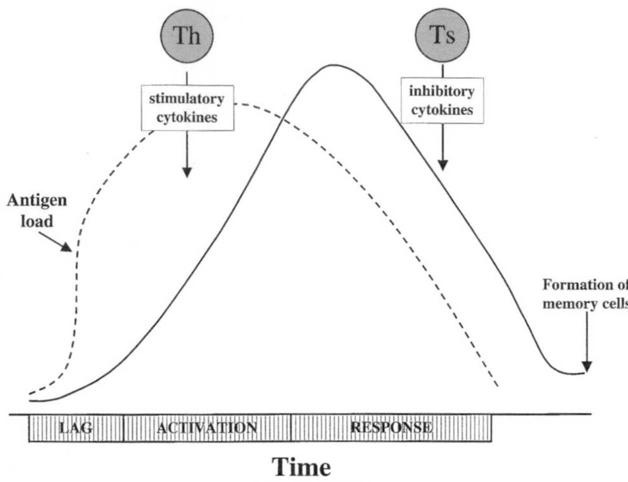

Figure 11–1. The time course of an immune response. The activation and maturation of the lymphocytes occur under the stimulation of cytokines released by helper T-cells (Th). The decline in the immune response is mediated by inhibitory cytokines released by suppressor T-cells (Ts). (Modified from Spaner D, Radvanyi L, Miller RG: Immunology related to cancer. In: Tannock IF, Hill RP [eds]: The Basic Science of Oncology, 3rd ed, p 240. New York, McGraw-Hill, 1998, with permission of The McGraw-Hill Companies.)

heavy chains, and two identical small chains of 25 kD, termed *light chains.*[9] Each heavy and light chain pair is stabilized by disulfide bonds and contains a single antigen-binding site. Therefore, each complete antibody molecule is divalent, that is, has two sites that are capable of specifically joining with an immunizing antigen. The unique bond between antigen and antibody forms the basis for the exquisite sensitivity that is the hallmark of immunologic reactions.

Major Histocompatibility Antigens—Recognition of Self

The ability of the immune system to differentiate self from nonself is determined largely through products of the genetic region known as the major histocompatibility complex (MHC), whose genes are coded on chromosome 6 in the human and chromosome 17 in the mouse. The antigens of self-recognition that are encoded in this region are expressed as integral membrane proteins, and they are divided into two main classes: class I (HLA-A, -B, and -C) and class II (HLA-DR, -DP, and -DQ).[10]

- Class I MHC molecules are composed of a polymorphic α-polypeptide chain, which is noncovalently linked to a β_2-microglobulin molecule, and they are cell-surface glycoproteins found on most normal cells. The function of these molecules is to bind and display the cell's own peptides to specific immune cells, notably T-cells; this process is known as *antigen presentation*. Although these peptides or antigens should represent the person (self), at least in the case of MHC I, MHC I molecules are crucial for recognition of nonself; once the presented antigen is recognized as foreign, it is with their help that tumor cells become susceptible to T-cell–mediated killing.[11]
- Unlike class I molecules, class II MHC molecules have a more limited distribution, and they are found on B-cells, macrophages, DCs, epidermal Langerhans' cells, thymic epithelial cells, and in the human, in activated T-cells. These are heterodimeric membrane glycoproteins, and their constituent chains are designated α and β.

The molecular structure of both classes of MHC proteins contains the formation of specialized grooves. Following proteolysis, a peptide of the presenting antigen becomes bound within one of these grooves, forming a peptide-MHC complex; the peptide-MHC complex is the *ligand* that is recognized by T-cells.

Antigen Processing and Presentation

Antigen-presenting cells accomplish the mechanism by which the foreign material or antigen is processed and bound with MHC; this process has to occur before it can be presented to the T-cells. Antigen-presenting cells include DCs, B-cells, monocytes, macrophages, and Langerhans' cells. However, in order for this process to be accomplished, the antigen must be unfolded, degraded, and broken into peptide fragments. In *exogenous processing*, the antigen first undergoes endocytosis, followed by degradation within lysosomes, and it is then associated with class II MHC products and transported to the cell surface. During *endogenous processing*, the antigen is formed intracellularly, it undergoes degradation outside the lysosomes, and it becomes associated with class I MHC products before transport to the cell surface. In addition, exogenous elements can be presented through an endogenous pathway, termed *cross priming*, activating CD8+ T-cells.[12, 13] It is this pathway that provides the underlying basis for tumor vaccines.[14]

Cells of the Immune System

LYMPHOCYTES

Lymphocytes are critical cells of the adaptive immune system, comprising one fifth of blood leukocytes. Detailed studies of the molecules displayed on the cell surface of these cells have revealed a considerable heterogeneity among the different types of human lymphocytes; however, further molecular analysis has delineated these lymphocytes into groups, defined by their selective response to structurally similar antigens. The receptors present on each lymphocyte's surface membrane have been shown to be specific to an antigen's determinants (*epitopes*). In addition, *clusters of differentiation* are now used to describe the cell-surface components on leukocytes and also have been used to define lymphoreticular tumors. Thus, lymphocytes are divided into three main classes on the basis of their lineage and function: T-cells, B-cells, and null or double-negative cells.

T-Cells. The name *T-cells* was derived from the role of the thymus in the differentiation of these lymphocytes. T-cells complete their early differentiation within the thymus, migrate through the peripheral circulation, and return through the lymphatic circulation to seed secondary lymphoid tissues.[8] They interact with cell-surface antigens through a diversity of surface receptors,[15,16] but they are only able to "see" antigens on the surface of another cell when they are appropriately displayed as a peptide-MHC ligand. Thus, T-cell activation is dependent on the interaction between the ligand and the T-cell receptors for the antigen,[17] which are themselves associated with glycoprotein complexes, the CD3 polypeptides.[18,19] These complexes are present on all human, mature T-cells and are critical for intracellular signaling. Following contact with appropriately presented antigens, in the presence of stimulatory secondary signals, a series of complex signaling pathways are activated that ultimately result in division to form functional T-cell clones.[20] After encountering a foreign antigen, a population of long-lived *memory T-cells* persists, capable of re-expanding when they are challenged by that same antigen.

T-cells have been subdivided based on cell-surface molecule displays, as well as their functional roles:

- In general, T-cells help B-cells to produce Ig, activate monocytes and increase their microbicidal action, inhibit certain types of immune responses, direct killing of target cells, and mobilize the inflammatory response. However, different subtypes of T-cells have been defined based on their display of the coreceptor surface markers, CD4 and CD8. These T-cell subtypes perform different tasks; for example, CD4+ cells are capable of recognizing class II MHC, whereas CD8+ cells recognize class I MHC.
- In general, *suppressor T-cells* are thought to express the CD8+ phenotype and are capable of modulating both B-cell and T-cell populations, as well as hematopoietic precursors. However, the acknowledged suppressive roles of some T-cells may reflect the activities of different subsets that have contradictory cytokine-producing phenotypes.
- A major activity of T-cells is the lysis of cells expressing specific antigens. These cytolytic T-lymphocytes (CTLs) usually express the CD8+ phenotype,[21,22] although some CD4+ T-cells also express CTL activity.[23] However, CD4+ T-cells tend to play more of a helper cell role in cytolytic activities.[21]

Helper T-cells themselves can be divided into three subpopulations (Th0, Th1, Th2), based on their capacity to produce specific cytokines:

1. *Th0 cells* elaborate a mixture of cytokines and may reflect a helper T-cell precursor population.
2. *Th1 cells* produce a number of cytokines, including interleukin (IL)-2, interferon-gamma (γIFN), and tumor necrosis factor-beta (TNFβ), and they induce delayed hypersensitivity reactions.[24]
3. *Th2 cells* produce certain interleukins (e.g., IL-4, IL-5, IL-10, IL-13) that assist in humoral immune responses.[24]

In general, the immune response is activated by the presence of a foreign antigen, but it is modulated by the ability of an individual's MHC to present the antigenic peptides. Other factors affecting the response include the presence of appropriate cytokines and the prevailing balance between the activities of the helper and suppressor T-cells.

B-Cells. The term *B-cells* originated from early studies in birds, in which similar lymphoid cells developed within a special organ called the *bursa of Fabricius*; no anatomic counterpart of this bursa exists in humans. Human B-cells originate in the bone marrow and acquire surface Ig molecules, where they act as antigen receptors, *B-cell receptors*. There is a transition of B-cells from immature to mature, which centers about the expression and maturation of the surface Ig gene arrangements, as well as a migration from the bone marrow to the periphery. This entire process is beyond the scope of this chapter, but it is presented in detail in a number of excellent textbooks.[3,4,25]

Unlike T-cells, mature B-cells may be activated by soluble antigens, either directly, through a cross-linkage of the membrane Ig molecules with the antigen, or indirectly, which often occurs through an intimate interaction with a helper T-cell, referred to as *cognate help*. Following direct cross-linkage–dependent B-cell activation, B-cell responses may be increased through the binding of complement components.[26,27] In contrast, cognate help is dependent on a series of pathways that ultimately lead to the expression of a class II MHC-peptide complex on the cell surface.[28] This complex then acts as the ligand for the antigen-specific CD4+ T-cells. Following interaction with T-cell–derived cytokines, individual B-cell clones differentiate into plasma cells that produce multiple copies of a specific antibody for that antigen.[29] Antibody production may be enhanced through the actions of helper T-cells or downregulated by macrophage-mediated suppression or the activity of CD8+ suppressor T-cells.

Null or Double-Negative Cells. The third class of lymphocytes, *null cells*, express neither T-cell– nor B-cell–surface markers. Null cells appear to be a distinct lineage of lymphoid cells that display certain T-cell markers early in their development, then later acquire markers also found on macrophages and neutrophils. Although the primary role of null cells is not known, natural killer (NK) cells and lymphokine-activated killer (LAK) cells originate from within this subpopulation:

- The *NK cell* population presents with large intracytoplasmic granules that contain perforin (a pore-forming protein), serine proteases, such as the granzymes, as well as other enzymes. Both in the presence and absence of previous sensitizing stimuli, NK cells can lyse certain cultured target cells. Their activity can be increased in the presence of a number of cytokines (IL-2, αIFN, γIFN, and IL-12).[30]
- Peripheral blood mononuclear cells, which are removed from patients and cultured *in vitro* with IL-2 or alloantigens, produce a subset of cells that are capable of killing a broad spectrum of tumor cells. Although these cells appear to be derived primarily from NK cells, LAK cells are able to lyse some fresh tumor cell isolates that resist killing by NK cells.[31] LAK cells require the continued presence of IL-2 for optimal cytotoxicity, and they must establish direct contact with the tumor target for killing to occur. LAK cell activity is not dependent on specific antigen recognition and is not MHC restricted, yet LAK cells are selectively cytotoxic for tumor, not normal cells.

- The cells participating in antibody-dependent cellular cytotoxicity (ADCC) are found within the null cell population.

Monocytes and Macrophages. Monocytes and macrophages are also capable of presenting antigen to lymphocytes. Monocytes are long-lived, circulating cells that are recruited into the tissue from the bone marrow and circulating populations, where they differentiate into tissue macrophages. Macrophages are highly phagocytic cells that possess a variety of physiologic protective functions.[32, 33] They are also capable of presenting antigen to lymphocytes and may play a role in carrying antigen from the periphery to other immune sites. In addition, monocytes are capable of producing cytokines, such as the interferons, prostaglandins, IL-1, IL-6, TNFα, and other factors that can modulate the function of the T-lymphocytes and B-lymphocytes.[34]

Dendritic Cells. Originating from bone marrow precursors, DCs are scattered throughout the tissues of the body, including the lymphatic system, and when they are pulsed with antigens, DCs are capable of presenting immunogens for several days.[35] DCs are typically 30 to 100 times more efficient at their pivotal role in stimulating T-cells than are macrophages or B-cells,[36] and their abundant surface area enables them to sample antigens from large regions of their environment, enabling extensive cell-cell interaction.

Cytokines

Although intimate cell contact is essential for peak immune cell responses, T-cells, monocytes, and macrophages also can elaborate cytokines that affect target cells within and beyond the immune system. Cytokines are soluble polypeptides secreted by activated lymphocytes or mononuclear cells. They can exert regulatory activity on other cells of the immune system or target cells involved in immune reactions, and they may influence the magnitude of inflammatory or immune responses. As noted earlier, the nonspecificity of cytokine activity can lead to either a limiting or increasing effect on target cells.

Cytokines produced by lymphocytes are sometimes referred to as *lymphokines*, and cytokines produced by monocytes are termed *monokines*. Because they act on target cells at a distance from the secreting cells, cytokines may be considered to be true hormones.

Tumor Immunology

Tumor immunity arises when effector cells recognize small differences between normal and tumor cells and, through a cascade of cellular and humoral interactions, direct cytotoxic cells and antibodies to the tumor targets. [37]

Tumor-Associated Antigens

Normal cells display a variety of molecules that are recognized by the immune system as self and, therefore, do not provoke an immune response. However, during the transition from a normal to a malignant cell, alterations may occur in the nature and display of these cell-surface molecules and, once these molecules become sufficiently altered, they can allow the host to recognize a tumor as nonself, initiating immune rejection. Unfortunately, it appears that only a limited spectrum of tumor antigens differs from those on normal cells, and the majority of tumor-associated antigens (TAAs) can usually be found on at least one, if not more, types of normal cells. Nonetheless, increasing numbers of human TAAs now have been recognized.[38–41]

Evidence for the existence of TAAs that could mediate the immunologic rejection of tumor cells was first obtained from animal studies.[37] Following the development of inbred strains of mice, oncogenic viruses, radiation, and chemical carcinogens were used to induce animal tumors that could then be transplanted between members of the same strain. From these studies it was shown that excision of a tumor before metastasis, followed by transplant of the same tumor back into the same mouse, resulted in rejection, that is, *immunity*.[42–44] However, not all induced animal tumors evoke an immune response, that is, are *immunogenic*; resistance is most often seen with tumors that have been induced using large doses of chemical carcinogens, DNA viruses, or ultraviolet light.[45, 46]

In order to evoke immunity, B-cells, macrophages, or DCs must be able to detect TAAs on human tumors and then initiate antigen processing. In addition, the distribution of the TAAs must be limited to either no normal cells or a relatively small population of normal cells that are not essential for survival, thereby limiting the potential side effects of the immunotherapy. For example, although the oncogene *HER2-neu (ERBB2)* and its proteins are present on a number of normal tissues, they are dramatically overexpressed in a large percentage of breast and ovarian cancers.[47, 48]

Antibodies that recognize TAAs have been detected in sera from cancer patients, but in the majority of cases, they are found in both normal and tumor sera.[37] In a large percentage of patients, antibodies can be detected that bind to cells from other donors that have the same histologic tumor type. In far fewer patients, antibodies have been isolated that are specific to the patient's own tumor cells. To date, production of human monoclonal antibodies that are capable of recognizing specific TAAs has proved to be technically difficult, although owing to refinements, this technology is improving steadily.[49, 50] A number of monoclonal antibody-defined TAAs that are used as markers in clinical trials are shown in Table 11–1.

Superantigens

In contrast to conventional TAAs, superantigens (SAgs) are potent immunostimulatory molecules that are capable of activating T-cells without internalization and processing by antigen-presenting cells.[51] Like conventional antigens, SAgs must first bind to a class II MHC–expressing target cell before being presented to the effector T-cell. However, SAgs are capable of initiating tumor cell killing by direct activation of CTLs, cytokine-induced activation of NK cells, and SAg-dependent cell-mediated cytotoxicity.[52–54]

Cells Involved in Tumor Cell Killing

A number of cell populations within the conglomeration of immune cells are capable of cytotoxic activity against tumor cells.

TABLE 11–1. **Monoclonal Antibody-Defined TAAs Used as Targets in Clinical Trials**

Tumor Type	TAA	Clinical Application
Breast	*HER2/neu*	
	Carcinoembryonic antigen	Immunoscintigraphy
Ovary	CA125	Immunodiagnosis
Pancarcinoma	TAG-72	Immunoscintigraphy
	Leγ	Passive immunotherapy
Lung	Carcinoembryonic antigen	Immunoscintigraphy
	Epidermal growth factor receptor	Immunoscintigraphy
Gastrointestinal	Carcinoembryonic antigen	Immunoscintigraphy
	gp72	Active specific immunotherapy
Prostate	PSA	Immunodiagnosis
	Ganglioside	Passive immunotherapy
Melanoma	Ganglioside	Passive immunotherapy
	gp100	Immunodiagnosis
	MAGE	
	Mart-1	

TAG = tumor-associated glycoprotein; Leγ = Lewis gamma; gp = glycoprotein; PSA = prostate-specific antigen; MAGE = human melanoma associated gene; Mart = melanoma antigen recognized by T-cells.

Cytotoxic T-Lymphocytes and Tumor-Infiltrating Lymphocytes

Using animal models, investigators were able to show that a T-cell subpopulation, CTLs, was able to recognize and eliminate tumors bearing specific antigens. It was seen that, in order to initiate tumor cell killing, CTLs had to be in contact with the tumor surface. Although the underlying pathways leading to CTL-mediated tumor cell destruction remain an enigma, direct membrane interactions, lymphotoxins, perforins, phospholipases, cytokine secretion by helper T-cells, and the induction of apoptosis have been implicated in CTL-mediated tumor cell killing (Fig. 11–2).[55, 56] In view of these animal models, clinical investigators looked for T-cells in humans that similarly recognized specific TAAs and, indeed, tumor-infiltrating lymphocytes (TILs)[57] were isolated from patients by culturing solid tumor explants. These cells appear to be predominantly T-lymphocytes, and they have been isolated from patients with melanoma, sarcoma, renal cell, breast, ovarian, colon, pancreatic, and head and neck carcinomas and should be considered to be activated CTLs.[58–60]

Natural Killer Cells

Like CTLs, NK cells[61] contain cytotoxic granules, which consist of components such as perforin (a complement-related molecule) and granzymes. Both CTLs and NK cells participate in tumor cell killing by first establishing direct cell contact with their targets. Following adherence to the tumor cell surface, the NK cell granules are released and the contents are transferred to the tumor cell, where they mediate apoptosis. Although the mechanism by which NK cells recognize tumor targets is unclear, NK cells do possess a number of specific cellular receptors, one of which is CD16, which is associated with the high affinity Fc portion of IgG.[62, 63] Activation of this receptor triggers ADCC against targets coated with IgG.[61]

Lymphokine-Activated Killer Cells

During a search for cytotoxic lymphocytes, it was shown that a subpopulation of peripheral blood lymphocytes could be activated *in vitro* using high doses of IL-2, generating cells that were cytotoxic to tumor cells that were otherwise resistant to NK activity.[64] Indeed, a major difference between the LAK cells and CTLs is that LAK cells demonstrate MHC-unrestricted cytolysis against a wide spectrum of both fresh and cultured tumor cells.[65] LAK precursor

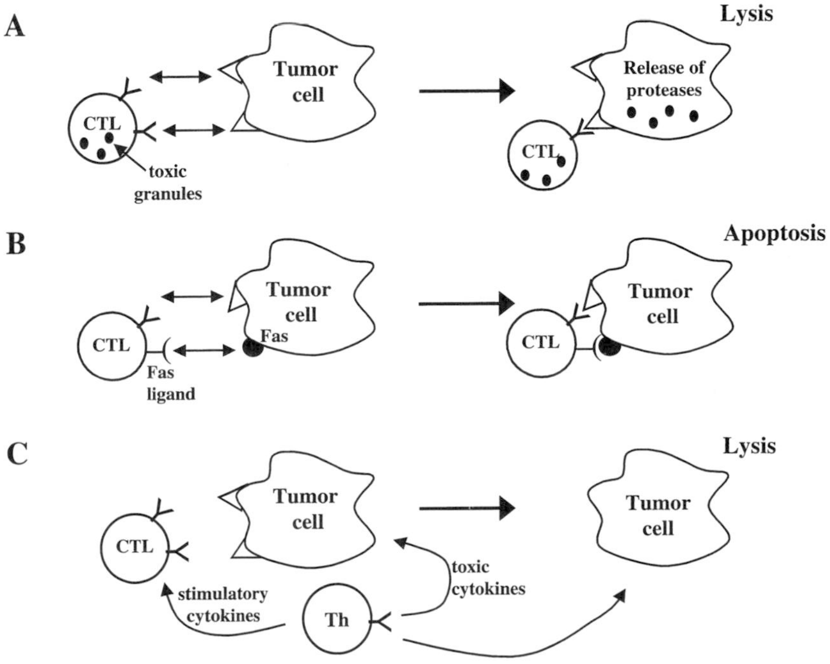

Figure 11–2. Mechanisms by which cytotoxic T-lymphocytes (CTLs) may kill tumor cells. (A) The recognition of tumor cells by the CTLs induces the secretion of cytotoxic granules that can penetrate the tumor cells, leading to lysis. (B) CTLs that express the Fas (TNFRSF6) ligand may induce apoptosis in tumor cells that express the Fas (TNFRSF6) antigen. (C) Activation of helper T-cells leads to the release of cytokines that stimulate CTLs and, also, may be directly toxic to tumor cells. (Modified from Spaner D, Radvanyi L, Miller RG: Immunology related to cancer. In: Tannock IF, Hill RP [eds]: The Basic Science of Oncology, 3rd ed, p 240. New York, McGraw-Hill, 1998, with permission of The McGraw-Hill Companies.)

and effector cells can be identified within the lymphocyte population as being CD3-/CD56+, the same as NK cells.[66]

Tumor Immunotherapy

As our understanding of the cellular and molecular mechanisms that are operable in the human immune system has advanced, efforts have been directed at using the patient's own immune system for cancer surveillance and even cancer destruction. One of the avenues for such manipulation is through *active immunotherapy*, which refers to the administration of agents that mimic or enhance a patient's immune response to recognize tumor-specific antigens (TSAs) and eliminate tumor cells, and such therapy includes both specific and nonspecific stimulators. *Passive immunotherapy* refers to the administration of active immunologic agents that can, directly or indirectly, bring about tumor regression. The possibility of enhancing antitumor immunity through tumor vaccines, adoptive transfer of cytotoxic cells, monoclonal antibodies, and cytokines, or genetic manipulation is now being studied and is discussed here.

Passive Immunotherapy

Serotherapy

The concept of using antibodies as so-called magic bullets was first proposed early in the twentieth century, with the idea of directing specific effector molecules toward antigens on the cell surface. Initial attempts at using polyclonal antibodies for cancer treatment (i.e., serotherapy) were hampered by the nonspecific diversity in antibody recognition and a perceived lack of commercial value. In addition, there were limitations because large volumes of high-titer, monoclonal, specific moieties for TAAs could be achieved only with murine-derived monoclonal antibodies. However, with the rise in the availability of monoclonal antibodies of defined specificity and high purity, together with the increase in successful manipulations by molecular and genetic biologists, the clinical assessment of serotherapy, using both unconjugated and conjugated moieties, has greatly advanced.[37]

In general, the binding of an antibody to tumor cell–surface antigens is a necessary stage in the therapy process; however, it is not always sufficient to inhibit tumor growth, although some limited success has been seen.[67] However, human tumors express high levels of many growth factors and their receptors, so that, in addition to antibody research, receptor-directed therapies have been examined. Monoclonal antibodies have been raised against a number of receptors, including epidermal growth factor, HER2, and IL-1, IL-2, and IL-6, and many have been studied in clinical trial.[68–71] For example, in a series of studies from 1999, an anti-HER2 receptor antibody (trastuzumab) produced a 14% response rate among patients with breast cancer whose tumors overexpressed the receptor.[72]

In addition to the sheer heterogeneity of antigen expression, several factors may impede the efficient use of monoclonal antibodies[37]: the formation of antibody complexes with shed antigen[73]; a failure to penetrate the target tissue[74]; induction of antibody-induced antigenic modulation[75]; and the development of human antimouse, antitoxin, or antichimeric antibodies (HAMA, HARA, HACA).[76] With respect to the development of HAMA, HARA, and HACA, the majority of monoclonal antibodies now are humanized, by inserting their antigen-recognizing (Fab) regions into the framework of human Ig or by glycolylating the fragments in order to minimize the development of the reactions.[77]

Radioimmunotherapy

The function of many of the antibodies used in serotherapy is to trigger complement-dependent cytotoxicity or to participate in ADCC. However, any number of extraneous factors can combine to impair these processes, for example, resistance by the tumor cells, poor recruitment into the tumor, and the presence of antibody-antigen complexes. In order to overcome some of these deficiencies, antibodies have been combined with conjugates, such as radioisotopes, and in this way, *radioimmunotherapy* (RIT) becomes a form of systemically targeted radiation therapy. The tumoricidal activity of RIT is primarily because of the radioisotope, localized through the antigen-antibody interaction, although in some situations the antibody itself may contribute to tumor cell killing. Because the radioisotope emits continuous, exponentially decreasing, low-dose-rate irradiation to the targeted tissue, the radionuclide conjugates also may have the ability to kill adjacent antigen-negative tumor cells as bystanders.

In the late 1970s, Order and colleagues pioneered the experimental and clinical use of ^{131}I-antiferritin,* a radiolabeled antibody, for the imaging and therapy of hepatocellular carcinoma.[78, 79] Since that time, a number of radiolabeled antibodies have been used for various cancers, including antibodies directed against carcinoembryonic antigen (CEA), human hepatoma, and malignant lymphocytes.[80–83] For example, in patients with ovarian cancer without clinically apparent disease, infusions of ^{90}Y-labeled HMFG1† (an antimucin) antibody have induced a significant survival advantage.[84] Similar antitumor effects against microscopic disease were seen after intraperitoneal administration of ^{177}Lu-labeled CC49‡, a monoclonal antibody, in patients with chemotherapy-resistant ovarian cancer.[85] The greatest successes for radioimmunoconjugates and radionuclides have been seen in the induction of regression in lymphomas after intravenous injection.[86–88] Some of the reported phase I and II trials and their results are listed in Table 11–2.[86, 88, 89–95] New approaches for increasing the therapeutic index of RIT include novel targets, such as CDs, and its use in combination therapies.[96–98]

The effectiveness of RIT may be affected by several factors,[99] including the following:

- the antibody itself (specificity, affinity, avidity, and immunoreactivity)
- the radioisotope (chemical stability of the radioisotope-antibody conjugate, emission characteristics, and half-life)

*Iodine-131–anti-human ferritin.
†Yttrium-90–labeled human milk fat globule antigen 1.
‡Lutetium-177–labeled CC49.

TABLE 11–2. **Results of Radioimmunotherapy Clinical Trials**

Investigator	Disease	Trial Phase	Radiopharmaceutical	Antigen	CR	PR
Knox et al[89]	Lymphoma	I/II	^{90}Y-2B8	CD20	13/51	21/51
Kaminski et al[90]	Lymphoma	I/II	^{131}I-Anti-B1	CD20	20/53	22/53
Kaminski et al[91]	Lymphoma	II	^{131}I-Anti-B1	CD20	14/45	13/45
Kaminski et al[92]	Lymphoma	II	^{131}I-Anti-B1	CD20	17/32	7/32
Kaminski et al[93]	Lymphoma	III	^{131}I-Anti-B1	CD20	10/60	29/60
Press et al[86]	Lymphoma	I/II	^{131}I-Anti-B1/BMT	CD20	16/19	2/19
Press et al[88]	Lymphoma	II	^{131}I-Anti-B1/BMT	CD20	16/21	2/21
DeNardo et al[94]	Lymphoma	I/II	^{131}I-Lym-1	CD20	3/30	14/30
DeNardo et al[95]	Lymphoma	I/II	^{131}I-Lym-1	CD20	7/21	4/21

CR = complete response; PR = partial response, a decrease in the sum of all products of tumor dimension of ≥50% or all tumor volumes by ≥70%; ^{90}Y-2B8 = yttrium-90–labeled anti-CD20 antibody; ^{131}I-Anti-B1 = iodine-131–labeled anti-B1 antibody; BMT = bone marrow transplantation; ^{131}I-Lym-1 = iodine-131–labeled anti-lymphoma antibody.

Modified from DeNardo SJ, Kroger LA, DeNardo GL: A new era for radiolabeled antibodies in cancer? Curr Opin Immunol 1999; 11:563, with permission from Elsevier Science.

- the tumor antigenic target (density, location, heterogeneity of display, stability, and modulation)
- the characteristics of the targeted tumor, including the volume, proliferative rate, and intrinsic radiosensitivity

Despite advances in the field of RIT, several problems remain:

- a relatively low uptake of radiolabeled antibody by the tumor
- nonspecific uptake of radiolabeled antibody
- chemical instability of radioimmunoconjugates
- development of human reactivity to the infused monoclonal antibodies

Immunotoxins

Another approach of serotherapy is to conjugate antibodies to protein toxin chains (immunotoxins), using antibodies, antibody fragments (Fv, Fab, and others), or growth factors to target the cancer cells. Fusion of the toxin to one of the target cell's surface antigens occurs, followed by internalization of the conjugated molecules, ultimately leading to the death of the cell[100]; many of the toxins used are based on gelonin, diphtheria, ricin, or *Pseudomonas*.[101–104]

Early phase I and II clinical studies were reported for metastatic melanoma,[105, 106] although more recent efforts have concentrated on lymphomas and primary brain tumors[74, 107–109]; some limited successes have been recorded. Some additional clinical studies are listed in Table 11–3.[109–116] There has been some concern that the administration of immunotoxins has been associated with side effects, such as unexpected neurotoxicity and vascular leak syndrome.[117] However, these side effects appear to be related to the antibody used rather than to a direct effect of the toxins themselves.[118, 119]

Adoptive Immunotherapy

Adoptive immunotherapy involves extracting tumor reactive cells from a host, for example, a cancer patient, manipulating these cells, then returning them to the patient or donating them to another target subject. In early preclinical models, however, this form of therapy was found to work well only when large numbers of cells were extracted from intensely immune donors, and then returned to subjects with only small tumor burdens. Nonetheless, because of the specificity of the therapy, adoptive immunotherapy lends itself to use in metastatic disease, and it has been heavily investigated in the treatment of immunogenic metastatic cancers, for example, melanoma and renal cell carcinoma.[120]

The cells most investigated in this field have been TILs,

TABLE 11–3. **Results of Immunotoxin Trials**

Investigator	Disease	Trial Phase	Chimeric Toxin	Antigen	CR	PR	Toxicity
Martin et al[110]	Acute GVHD	III	H65-RTA	CD5	51/12		Allergy, VLS
LeMaistre et al[111]	CTCL, NHL	I	DAB_{389}IL-2	IL-2R	6/52	10/52	Mild VLS
Grossbard et al[112]	rel B-NHL	I	Anti-B4-bR	CD19	2/34	3/34	↑ AST, ↑ ALT
Multani et al[109]	rel B-NHL	II	Anti-B4-bR	CD19	0/16		PLTs
Grossbard et al[113]	rel B-NHL*	II	Anti-B4-bR	CD19	26/49		
Lynch et al[114]	rel SCLC	I	N901-bR	CD56	0/21	1/21	VLS
Frankel et al[115]	TCL	I	Anti-CD7-dgA	CD7	0/11	2/11	VLS
Schnell et al[116]	rel HD	I/II	RFT5-SMPT-dgA	CD25	0/17	2/17	VLS

CR = complete response; PR = partial response; GVHD = graft-versus-host disease; CTCL = cutaneous T-cell lymphoma; NHL = non-Hodgkin's lymphoma; rel = relapsed; rel B = relapsed B-cell; SCLC = small cell lung cancer; TCL = T-cell lymphoma; HD = Hodgkin's disease; H65-RTA = H65-RTA; DAB_{389}IL-2 = diphtheria toxin fused to IL-2; Anti-B4-bR = anti-B4-blocked ricin; N901-bR = N901-blocked ricin; Anti-CD7-dgA = anti-human CD7 antibody coupled with deglycosylated ricin A chain; RFT5-SMPT-dgA = anti-CD25 immunotoxin–RFT5 monoclonal antibody coupled with a deglycosylated ricin A chain via a sterically hindered disulfide link; VLS = vascular leak syndrome; AST = hepatic transaminases or aspartate aminotransferase; ALT = alanine aminotransferase; PLT = thrombocytopenia.

*Patients in complete remission following allogeneic bone marrow transplant.

Modified from Kreitman RJ: Immunotoxins in cancer therapy. Curr Opin Immunol 1999; 11:570.

LAKs, and autolymphocyte therapy, with present research becoming more focused on DCs.[120]

Tumor-Infiltrating Lymphocytes

T-cell–mediated immunity has been detected against the E6 and E7 proteins of human papillomavirus–16,[121] which is associated with the development of cervical cancer. In addition, studies have demonstrated that human T-cell–mediated cytotoxicity against oncogenic peptides derived from mutant and wild-type *TP53*,[122] mutant *RAS*,[123, 124] and p210$^{bcr\text{-}abl}$.[124] Because of these and similar activities, TILs have been used in adoptive immunotherapy protocols.

TIL populations are expanded in culture *in vitro* using relatively low concentrations of IL-2, then they are returned to cancer patients.[58, 125] In one trial performed at UCLA,[126] patients with metastatic renal cell carcinoma received TILs isolated from primary tumors, administered with infusions of IL-2. An objective response rate of 34.6% was seen, including a 9% complete response. The actuarial survival rate was 65% at 1 year and 43% at 2 years, which compared well with predicted survival rates without immunotherapy.[127] This result led to a phase III randomized trial; however, the study failed to show a benefit for the addition of the TILs to the IL-2 therapy.[128]

Dendritic Cells

Preclinical studies have shown that a strong antitumor immunity may be rapidly induced when animals are vaccinated with DCs pulsed with tumor proteins.[129] Clinical application of DCs became feasible when it was discovered that growth factors, such as granulocyte-macrophage colony-stimulating factor (GM-CSF), can be used to promote peripheral blood DC growth *in vitro*.[130] A sample of a patient's peripheral blood cells is cultured *in vitro* under conditions that amplify the number and proportion of DCs. These cells are then pulsed with tumor-specific antigens in the form of peptides, proteins, cDNAs, or even mRNAs encoding the antigens, with the aim of loading peptides from a TAA onto the DCs' MHC molecules. Introduced back into the patient by infusion, these cells then stimulate a primary CTL response against the tumor antigen and can promote tumor regression.

One human vaccine trial using autologous DCs has been reported in detail. In this study, all patients vaccinated with DCs pulsed *ex vivo* with tumor-specific protein developed antitumor immune responses, and cytolytic effects of the DCs on tumor targets were demonstrated.[35] Studies incorporating DCs into active vaccine and passive cellular immunotherapeutic strategies are expanding quickly, with a number of clinical trials being reported on a variety of tumors.[131–135]

Active Immunotherapy

Because our understanding of the immune system has expanded, we now recognize the existence of CTLs, TSAs, and antibodies. Therefore, it has become apparent that if uncontrolled malignant growth occurs, it is not owing to an inability of the immune system to recognize tumor cells but, rather, that the tumor cells are not providing the necessary signals needed to trigger an effective immune response. Active immunotherapy represents an attempt to present tumor antigens in a more immunogenic form in order to fix this deficiency in tumor surveillance.

Bacterial Immunostimulants

Following observations over the past three centuries, there have been indications that the toxins released during wound infection can lead to tumor regression in some types of cancers.[136] Subsequent research has indicated that the mechanism for this process is due, in all probability, to the toxins' ability to induce the release of TNF. However, the precise mechanisms by which immunostimulants affect tumor growth are yet to be defined.

Of the potential bacterial immunostimulants, bacille Calmette-Guérin (BCG), an attenuated strain of *Mycobacterium bovis* that is used as a tuberculosis vaccine, has gained the most attention. Although there were some early reports of beneficial results using BCG in advanced melanoma patients,[137, 138] most attempts to use BCG for this disease have failed to show any benefit.[139] In contrast, intravesicular delivery of BCG has proved to be useful in the treatment of carcinoma *in situ* of bladder cancer, for delaying tumor recurrence, and for inhibiting the development of new neoplasms in superficial bladder cancer, and it now constitutes standard treatment.[140, 141]

Chemically Defined Immunomodulators

Some investigators have attempted to increase the tumoricidal activities of immune cells, notably the macrophages, through the use of chemically defined agents.[142] Examples of such agents are muramyl dipeptide and trehalose dimycolate, both of which have demonstrated beneficial biologic effects in preclinical and early clinical trials, but they have yet to reliably result in tumor regression.[143–145]

Cytokines

Many specific and nonspecific cellular interactions result in the release of a large number of cytokines. Therefore, some cytokines have been investigated for their antitumor effects.

Interleukin-2. IL-2 is classed as a type I cytokine, and it was the first of this superfamily of cytokines to be cloned. It is produced solely by activated T-lymphocytes, and it is a growth and differentiation factor that is critical for clonal T-lymphocyte expansion and function.[146] When applied *in vitro*, high-dose IL-2 can expand T-lymphocyte numbers in the absence of any known antigen.[147] However, if the T-cells were previously activated, their ability to respond to IL-2 is dramatically enhanced through a rapid upregulation of the high affinity IL-2 receptor.[148] Of interest, because the high affinity IL-2 receptor is not expressed on normal cells but is seen on abnormal lymphocytes associated with certain lymphoid malignancies and in individuals during allograft rejection, the IL-2 receptor increasingly is being seen as a potential target for therapy.[149, 150]

As described previously, IL-2 has been used extensively in adoptive immunotherapy. In addition, it has been shown to have direct antitumor activity. In Europe, in small phase I and II trials, infusion of recombinant IL-2 in patients with metastatic disease has proved to be a feasible therapy, producing durable responses.[151–153] Nonetheless, in general, it appears that IL-2's direct antitumor activity is modest, so investigators are now examining its usefulness in combination therapies.[154] However, in at least one randomized trial performed in Italy, no clinical difference was seen when IL-2 was added to a combination treatment of cisplatin and 5-fluorouracil for head and neck cancers.[155]

Interferons. Classified as type II cytokines because of their binding through type II receptors, the interferons are a conserved family that should be considered to be a separate group of cytokines from the remainder.[156] The interferon family itself is subdivided into types I and II; type I interferons include αIFN, βIFN, ωIFN, and δIFN, whereas the only recognized type II interferon is γIFN. Interferons have been shown to inhibit growth in a number of different malignancies; however, their mechanism of action is unclear at present. One hypothesized mode of action is through interferon's inhibitory effect on key cell cycle regulatory genes.[157, 158] Intriguingly, certain interferons (notably γIFN) are able to upregulate the yield of peptides that are available for MHC binding and presentation,[159] as well as enhancing the expression of some TSAs,[160] which may, in turn, make tumor cells more immunogenic.

Of the interferon family, αIFN (or interferon-alfa, the synthetic form) has been the most intensively studied and, especially at present, is the most used as part of combination therapies.[161–163] Major or complete cytogenetic response rates have been observed with αIFN alone in chronic myelogenous leukemia (20% to 25%),[164, 165] multiple myeloma (20%),[161] malignant melanoma (15% to 25%),[166, 167] and renal cell carcinoma (15%).[163, 167] In addition, there is good evidence that the addition of interferon to chemotherapeutic regimens improves the response rates and prolongs survival. For example, there is strong evidence that αIFN enhances the activity of 5-fluorouracil in the treatment of renal cell carcinomas and colorectal cancer.[168–170] Some of the mechanisms for this activity have been identified.[170]

Of interest, because of studies that have shown that IL-2 and αIFN work synergistically in the generation of LAK cells *in vitro*, the European Organization for the Research and Treatment of Cancer (EORTC) has looked at combining the two agents with chemotherapeutic regimens to improve treatment response rates for advanced stage melanoma. However, to date, although improved response rates have been demonstrated, no survival benefits have been observed.[171]

Tumor Vaccines

Since the first vaccines were developed against infectious diseases, physicians have dreamed of using vaccines against cancer. For tumors with a viral carcinogenesis, it is logical to assume that preventive vaccines can be used to reduce the risk of tumor development, but until the late 1990s, therapeutic vaccination had proved to be elusive. However, with the identification of TAAs and TSAs and an understanding of their role in immunogenicity together with the rapid evolution of recombinant DNA technology, several vaccines, composed of either TAAs, tumor cells, or anti-idiotypic antibodies, are beginning to enter clinical trials[172–174]:

- Several TAAs have been incorporated into vaccinia virus and other potentially immunogenic viruses. For example, rV-CEA, a recombinant CEA-vaccinia vaccine against CEA, has been entered in a number of phase I trials in breast, lung, and colorectal cancer patients.[175, 176] CTL responses specifically against CEA were demonstrated, although most patients still showed tumor progression. Similar results now have been seen using a prostate-specific antigen vaccine.[177]
- Whole (tumor) cell vaccines also have been investigated, using either autologous tumor cells exposed to radiation, frequently engineered to secrete GM-CSF,[178, 179] or by using allogeneic tumor cells coadministered with immunostimulants (BCG, Detox) or other agents.[180] Early phase I trials have proved to be encouraging.
- Examples of consistently immunogenic molecules that have come under intense research scrutiny at Memorial Sloan-Kettering are the gangliosides. These are glycosphingolipids found in the cell membrane that are overexpressed in a number of different tumors and induce cytotoxic IgM antibodies in most patients.[181] Using these molecules as targets, ganglioside antibodies have been conjugated to moieties, such as keyhole-limpet hemocyanin,[182] and together with the immunologic adjuvant QS-21, they have been used in patients with melanoma or prostate cancer with promising results.[183–185]

Escape Mechanisms for Tumor Cells

In order for a successful immunization to take place, we must understand the evasive maneuvers that tumor cells may undergo to escape. Several events may contribute to failure in mounting an effective antitumor response in the cancer patient.

Heterogeneity in Antigen Expression

The cellular heterogeneity of many human tumors has been known for some time, both in terms of their phenotype and genotype.[186] This fact becomes relevant to some modes of immunotherapy when TAAs are not globally expressed by all cells within a tumor; indeed, some subpopulations of cells may lack immunogenic antigens altogether.[187] It has been suggested that this observed heterogeneity in antigen expression occasionally may relate to different phases of the cell cycle, although this has been demonstrated only *in vitro*.[188, 189] Nonetheless, researchers must be aware that even if potentially immunogenic antigens are produced by a tumor cell, they may not be displayed because of inadequate processing or failure to be presented along with the appropriate MHC determinants.[190]

Circulating Antigen

Certain antibodies are able to induce antigenic modulation at the cell surface, which may result in the shedding of substantial amounts of antigen into the circulation and, in some cases, circulating TAAs have been found to suppress effector cell function. There are two suggested pathways for this activity: circulating TAA induction of regulatory suppressor T-cells has been demonstrated, although their mechanism of action is unknown,[191] and the antigens may form direct complexes with the potential effector cells, reducing their cytolytic activities.[192]

Suppressor Cells and Factors

Several studies have shown that the tumor-bearing host is immunosuppressed by the growing tumor, thus producing an intrinsic disadvantage for attempts at active immunotherapy. Suppressor cells have been identified among subpopulations of NK cells, T-cells, and mononuclear phagocytes.[193, 194] In addition, the release of humoral suppressor factors has also been demonstrated.[195]

Patient Immunocompetence

- The ability of a patient's immune system to recognize and kill a tumor varies directly with his or her nutritional status and inversely with the tumor burden. Cell-mediated immunity appears to be most affected by protein-calorie malnutrition, although humoral immunity and phagocytic function are also impaired.
- Cellular immune defects have been observed in a variety of human cancers, for example, Hodgkin's disease, disseminated carcinomas, chronic lymphocytic leukemia, and ovarian carcinoma.
- Cancer therapy can also reduce a patient's immunocompetence. There is a transient depression of T-cell and B-cell levels following both surgery and radiation therapy, and certain chemotherapeutic drugs may be immunosuppressive.

Summary

In general, by the time human tumors become clinically detectable, they have been established for a long time; a 1-cm^3 tumor can contain more than a billion malignant cells at diagnosis. Therefore, once established, such a tumor burden may simply overwhelm the cytotoxic capacity of even an enhanced immune response. Thus, the most significant effects of immunotherapy might be seen only in patients with microscopic disease in an adjuvant setting, following elimination of all clinically evident tumor with more conventional forms of treatment, such as surgery, radiation, or chemotherapy.

Recommended Reading

Basic concepts of immunology can be reviewed in a variety of texts, including the fourth edition of *Fundamental Immunology* by W.E. Paul[1] and the third edition of Rosenberg's *Principles and Practice of the Biological Therapy of Cancer.*[2] An overview of tumor immunology and immunotherapy also can be found in *Biologic Therapy of Cancer,*[3] *Cancer Chemotherapy and Biotherapy: Principles and Practice,*[4] and *Cancer Medicine.*[5] An article by Meredith and associates provides the reader with a concise overview of RIT,[6] and a 1999 issue of *Current Opinion in Immunology* was devoted to cancer-oriented immunologic therapy.[7]

REFERENCES

General

1. Paul WE (ed): Fundamental Immunology, 4th ed. Philadelphia, Lippincott-Raven, 1999.
2. Rosenberg SA (ed): Principles and Practice of the Biological Therapy of Cancer, 3rd ed. Philadelphia, Lippincott Williams & Wilkins, 2000.
3. DeVita VT, Hellman S, Rosenberg SA (eds): Biologic Therapy of Cancer, 2nd ed. Philadelphia, Lippincott, 1995.
4. Chabner BA, Longo DL (eds): Cancer Chemotherapy and Biotherapy: Principles and Practice, 2nd ed. Philadelphia, Lippincott-Raven, 1996.
5. Holland JF, Bast RC Jr, Morton DL, et al (eds): Cancer Medicine, 4th ed. Baltimore, Williams & Wilkins, 1997.
6. Meredith RF, LoBuglio AF, Spenser EB: Recent progress in radioimmunotherapy for cancer. Oncology 1997; 11:979.
7. Vitetta E: Cancer. Editorial overview. Curr Opin Immunol 1999; 11:539.

Specific

8. Paul WE: The immune system: an introduction. In: Paul WE (ed): Fundamental Immunology, 4th ed, p 1. Philadelphia, Lippincott-Raven, 1999.
9. Frazer JK, Capra JD: Immunoglobulins: structure and function. In: Paul WE (ed): Fundamental Immunology, 4th ed, p 37. Philadelphia, Lippincott-Raven, 1999.
10. Margulies DH: The major histocompatibility complex. In: Paul WE (ed): Fundamental Immunology, 4th ed, p 263. Philadelphia, Lippincott-Raven, 1999.
11. Tait BD: HLA class I expression on human cancer cells. Implications for effective immunotherapy. Human Immunol 2000; 61:158.
12. Rock KL: A new foreign policy: MHC class I molecules monitor the outside world. Immunol Today 1996; 17:131.
13. Bennett SR, Carbone FR, Karamalis F, et al: Induction of a CD8+ cytotoxic T lymphocyte response by cross-priming requires cognate CD4+ T cell help. J Exp Med 1997; 186:65.
14. Armstrong TD, Pulaski BA, Ostrand-Rosenberg S: Tumor antigen presentation: changing the rules. Cancer Immunol Immunother 1998; 46:70.
15. Weiss A, Kadlecek T, Iwashima M, et al: Molecular and genetic insights into T-cell antigen receptor signalling. Ann NY Acad Sci 1995; 766:149.
16. Davis MM, Chin Y-H: T-cell antigen receptors. In: Paul WE (ed): Fundamental Immunology, 4th ed, p 341. Philadelphia, Lippincott-Raven, 1999.
17. Fremont DH, Rees WA, Kozono H: Biophysical studies of T-cell receptors and their ligands. Curr Opin Immunol 1996; 8:93.
18. Van Boehmer H, Fehling HJ: Structure and function of the pre-T cell receptor. Annu Rev Immunol 1997; 15:433.
19. Malissen B, Ardouin L, Lin SY, et al: Function of the CD3 subunits of the pre-TCR and TCR complexes during T cell development. Adv Immunol 1999; 72:103.
20. Guse AH: Ca^{2+} signaling in T-lymphocytes. Crit Rev Immunol 1998; 18:419.
21. Doherty PC, Topham DJ, Tripp RA, et al: Effector $CD4^+$ and $CD8^+$ T-cell mechanisms in the control of respiratory virus infections. Immunol Rev 1997; 159:105.
22. De Panfilis G: $CD8^+$ cytolytic T lymphocytes and the skin. Exp Dermatol 1998; 7:121.
23. Mauri D, Pichler WJ: Involvement of CD80 in the generation of $CD4^+$ cytotoxic T cells. Immunol Res 1996; 15:126.
24. Chaturvedi P, Yu Q, Southwood S, et al: Peptide analogs with different affinities for MHC alter the cytokine profile of T helper cells. Int Immunol 1996; 8:745.
25. Melchers F, Rolink A: B-lymphocyte development and biology. In: Paul WE (ed): Fundamental Immunology, 4th ed, p 183. Philadelphia, Lippincott-Raven, 1999.

26. Fearon DT: The complement system and adaptive immunity. Semin Immunol 1998; 10:355.
27. Carroll MC: The role of complement and complement receptors in induction and regulation of immunity. Annu Rev Immunol 1998; 16:545.
28. Takatsu K: Cytokines involved in B-cell differentiation and their sties of action. Proc Soc Exp Biol Med 1997; 215:121.
29. Gray D, Bergthorsdottir S, van Essen D, et al: Observations on memory B-cell development. Semin Immunol 1997; 9:249.
30. Rashleigh SP, Kusher DI, Endicott JN, et al: Interleukins 2 and 12 activate natural killer cytolytic responses of peripheral blood mononuclear cells from patients with head and neck squamous cell carcinoma. Arch Otolaryngol Head Neck Surg 1996; 122:541.
31. Bradley M, Zeytun A, Rafi-Janajreh A, et al: Role of spontaneous and interleukin-2-induced natural killer cell activity in the cytotoxicity and rejection of Fas+ and Fas− tumor cells. Blood 1998; 92:4248.
32. Aderem A, Underhill DM: Mechanisms of phagocytosis in macrophages. Annu Rev Immunol 1999; 17:593.
33. Gordon S: Macrophages and the immune response. In: Paul WE (ed): Fundamental Immunology, 4th ed, p 533. Philadelphia, Lippincott-Raven, 1999.
34. Belardelli F: Role of interferons and other cytokines in the regulation of the immune response. APMIS 1995; 103:161.
35. Hsu FJ, Benike C, Fagnoni F, et al: Vaccination of patients with B-cell lymphoma using autologous antigen-pulsed dendritic cells. Nat Med 1996; 2:52.
36. Rosenberg SA, Yannelli JR, Yang JC, et al: Treatment of patients with metastatic melanoma with autologous tumor-infiltrating lymphocytes and interleukin 2. J Natl Cancer Inst 1994; 86:1159.
37. Bast RC Jr, Mills GB, Gibson S, et al: Tumor immunology. In: Holland JF, Bast RC Jr, Morton DL, et al (eds): Cancer Medicine, 4th ed, p 207. Baltimore, Williams & Wilkins, 1997.
38. Roselli M, Guadagni F, Buonomo O, et al: Tumor markers as targets for selective diagnostic and therapeutic procedures. Anticancer Res 1996; 16:2187.
39. Colcher D, Pavlinkova G, Beresford G, et al: Single-chain antibodies in pancreatic cancer. Ann NY Acad Sci 1999; 880:263.
40. Balzar M, Winter MJ, de Boer CJ, et al: The biology of the 17-1A antigen (Ep-CAM). J Mol Med 1999; 77:699.
41. Hadden JW: The immunology and immunotherapy of breast cancer: an update. Int J Immunopharmacol 1999; 21:79.
42. Foley EJ: Antigenic properties of methylcholanthrene-induced tumors in mice of the strain of origin. Cancer Res 1953; 13:835.
43. Klein G, Sögren HO, Klein E, et al: Demonstration of resistance against methylcholanthrene-induced sarcoma in the primary autochthonous host. Cancer Res 1960; 20:1561.
44. Herberman RB: Immunogenicity of tumor antigens. Biochim Biophys Acta 1977; 473:93.
45. Chieco-Bianchi L, Collavo D, Biasi G: Immunologic unresponsiveness to murine leukemia virus antigens: mechanisms and role in tumor development. Adv Cancer Res 1988; 51:277.
46. Ullrich SE: Modulation of immunity by ultraviolet radiation: key effects on antigen presentation. J Invest Dermatol 1995; 105 (suppl):30S.
47. Bast RC Jr, Pusztai L, Kerns BJ, et al: Coexpression of the HER-2 gene product, p185HER-2, and epidermal growth factor receptor, p170EGF-R, on epithelial ovarian cancers and normal tissues. Hybridoma 1998; 17:313.
48. Ross JS, Fletcher JA: HER-2/neu (c-erb-B2) gene and protein in breast cancer. Am J Clin Pathol 1999; 112 (suppl):S53.
49. Saleh MN, Tilden AB, Meredith RF, et al: Chimeric antibodies with specificity for tumor antigens: demonstration of in situ localization to tumors after antibody therapy. Biotech Histochem 1998; 73:186.
50. Molema G, Kroesen BJ, Helfrich W, et al: The use of bispecific antibodies in tumor cell and tumor vasculature directed immunotherapy. Journal of Controlled Release 2000; 64:229.
51. Kotb M: Superantigens of gram-positive bacteria: structure-function analyses and their implications for biological activity. Curr Opin Microbiol 1998; 1:56.
52. Riesbeck K, Billstrom A, Tordsson J, et al: Endothelial cells expressing an inflammatory phenotype are lysed by superantigen-targeted cytotoxic T cells. Clin Diagn Lab Immunol 1998; 5:675.
53. Dobashi H, Seki S, Habu Y, et al: Activation of mouse liver natural killer cells and NK1.1(+) T cells by bacterial superantigen-primed Kupffer cells. Hepatology 1999; 30:430.
54. Mason KM, Dryden TD, Bigley NJ, et al: Staphylococcal enterotoxin B primes cytokine secretion and lytic activity in response to native bacterial antigens. Infect Immun 1998; 66:5082.
55. Tschopp J, Nabholz M: Perforin-mediated target cell lysis by cytolytic T lymphocytes. Annu Rev Immunol 1990; 8:279.
56. Lui C-C, Young LHY, Young JD-E: Lymphocyte-mediated cytolysis and disease. N Engl J Med 1996; 335:1651.
57. Halapi E: Oligoclonal T cells in human cancer. Med Oncol 1998; 15:203.
58. Lewko WM, Good RW, Bowman D, et al: Growth of tumor derived activated T-cells for the treatment of cancer. Cancer Biother 1994; 9:211.
59. Cross DS, Platt JL, Juhn SK, et al: Tumor infiltrating lymphocytes in squamous cell carcinoma of the head and neck: mechanisms of enhancement using prostaglandin synthetase inhibitors. Adv Exp Med Biol 1997; 400B:1013.
60. Peoples GE, Anderson BW, Fisk B, et al: Ovarian cancer-associated lymphocyte recognition of folate binding protein peptides. Ann Surg Oncol 1998; 5:743.
61. Yokoyama WM: Natural killer cells. In: Paul WE (ed): Fundamental Immunology, 4th ed, p 575. Philadelphia, Lippincott-Raven, 1999.
62. Trinchieri G, Valiante N: Receptors for the Fc fragment of IgG on natural killer cells. Nat Immun 1993; 12:218.
63. Morel PA, Ernst LK, Metes D: Functional CD32 molecules on human NK cells. Leuk Lymphoma 1999; 35:47.
64. Rosenstein M, Yron I, Kaufmann Y, et al: Lymphokine-activated killer cells: lysis of fresh syngeneic natural killer-resistant murine tumor cells by lymphocytes cultured in interleukin 2. Cancer Res 1984; 44:1946.
65. Bean P, Agah R, Mazumder A: Differential lysis of tumor target cells displayed by lymphokine activated killer (LAK) cell clones. Int J Cell Cloning 1992; 10:190.
66. Podack ER, Penichet KO, Lin BY, et al: Increased cytotoxicity and CD16 (Leu 11) expression in long-term, IL-2-activated human peripheral blood mononuclear cells. Blood Cells 1987; 13:117.
67. Nasi ML, Meyers M, Livingston PO, et al: Anti-melanoma effects of R24, a monoclonal antibody against GD3 ganglioside. Melanoma Res 1997; 7 (suppl):S155.
68. Modjtahedi H, Hickish T, Nicolson M, et al: Phase I trial and tumour localization of the anti-EGFR monoclonal antibody ICR62 in head and neck or lung cancer. Br J Cancer 1996; 73:228.
69. Nichols J, Foss F, Kuzel TM, et al: Interleukin-2 fusion protein: an investigational therapy for interleukin-2 receptor expressing malignancies. Eur J Cancer 1997; 33 (suppl):S34.
70. Mackiewicz A, Kapcinska M, Wiznerowicz M, et al: Immunogene therapy of human melanoma. Phase I/II clinical trial. Adv Exp Med Biol 1998; 451:557.
71. Jiang Y, Genant HK, Watt I, et al: A multicenter, double-blind, dose-ranging, randomized, placebo-controlled study of recombinant human interleukin-1 receptor antagonist in patients with rheumatoid arthritis: radiologic progression and correlation of Genant and Larsen scores. Arthritis Rheum 2000; 43:1001.
72. Goldenberg MM: Trastuzumab, a recombinant DNA-derived humanized monoclonal antibody, a novel agent for the treatment of metastatic breast cancer. Clin Ther 1999; 21:309.
73. Gopalkrishna P, Begum Z, Khar A: Stress induced shedding of a tumor antigen by a rat histiocytic cell line AK-5: a possible mechanism of immune evasion. Cell Mol Biol (Noisy-le-grand) 1998; 44:563.
74. Multani PS, O'Day S, Nadler LM, et al: Phase II clinical trial of bolus infusion anti-B4 blocked ricin immunoconjugate in patients with relapsed B-cell non-Hodgkin's lymphoma. Clin Cancer Res 1998; 4:2599.
75. Pulczynski S: Antibody-induced modulation and intracellular transport of CD10 and CD19 antigens in human malignant B cells. Leuk Lymphoma 1994; 15:243.
76. Engert A, Sausville EA, Vitetta E: The emerging role of ricin A-chain immunotoxins in leukemia and lymphoma. Curr Top Microbiol Immunol 1998; 234:13.
77. Kricka LJ: Human anti-animal antibody interferences in immunological assays. Clin Chem 1999; 45:942.
78. Order SE, Klein JL, Ettinger D, et al: Phase I-II study of radiolabeled antibody integrated in the treatment of primary hepatic malignancies. Int J Radiat Oncol Biol Phys 1980; 6:703.
79. Order SE, Stillwagon GB, Klein JL, et al: Iodine-131 antiferritin, a

new treatment modality in hepatoma: a Radiation Therapy Oncology Group study. J Clin Oncol 1985; 3:1573.
80. Zeng ZC, Tang ZY, Liu KD, et al: Improved long-term survival for unresectable hepatocellular carcinoma (HCC) with a combination of surgery and intrahepatic arterial infusion of ^{131}I-anti-HCC mAb. Phase I/II clinical trials. J Cancer Res Clin Oncol 1998; 124:275.
81. Juweid ME, Hajjar G, Swayne LC, et al: Phase I/II trial of (131)I-MN-14F(ab)2 anti-carcinoembryonic antigen monoclonal antibody in the treatment of patients with metastatic medullary thyroid carcinoma. Cancer 1999; 85:1828.
82. Vriesendorp HM, Quadri SM, Wyllie CT, et al: Fractionated radiolabeled antiferritin therapy for patients with recurrent Hodgkin's disease. Clin Cancer Res 1999; 5 (suppl):3324s.
83. DeNardo GL, DeNardo SJ, Shen S, et al: Factors affecting ^{131}I-Lym-1 pharmacokinetics and radiation dosimetry in patients with non-Hodgkin's lymphoma and chronic lymphocytic leukemia. J Nucl Med 1999; 40:1317.
84. Hird V, Maraveyas A, Snook D, et al: Adjuvant therapy of ovarian cancer with radioactive monoclonal antibody. Br J Cancer 1993; 68:403.
85. Alvarez RD, Partridge EE, Khazaeli MB, et al: Intraperitoneal radioimmunotherapy of ovarian cancer with ^{177}Lu-CC49: a phase I/II study. Gynecol Oncol 1997; 65:94.
86. Press OW, Eary JF, Appelbaum FR, et al: Radiolabeled-antibody therapy of B-cell lymphoma with autologous bone marrow support. N Engl J Med 1993; 329:1219.
87. Lewis JP, DeNardo GL, DeNardo SJ: Radioimmunotherapy of lymphoma: a UC Davis experience. Hybridoma 1995; 14:115.
88. Press OW, Eary JF, Appelbaum FR, et al: Phase II trial of ^{131}I-B1 (anti-CD20) antibody therapy with autologous stem cell transplantation for relapsed B cell lymphomas. Lancet 1995; 346:336.
89. Knox SJ, Goris ML, Trisler K, et al: Yttrium-90-labeled anti-CD20 monoclonal antibody therapy of recurrent B-cell lymphoma. Clin Cancer Res 1996; 2:457.
90. Kaminski MS, Zasadny KR, Francis IR, et al: Iodine-131-anti-B1 radioimmunotherapy for B-cell lymphoma. J Clin Oncol 1996; 14:1974.
91. Kaminski MS, Vose J, Saleh M, et al: A multicenter phase II study of iodine-131 anti-B1 antibody in patients with chemotherapy-relapsed/refractory low-grade or transformed low-grade B-cell non-Hodgkin's lymphoma (NHL). Blood 1997; 90:509.
92. Kaminski MS, Gribbin T, Estes J, et al: I-131 anti-B1 antibody for previously untreated follicular lymphoma (FL): clinical and molecular remissions [Abstract]. Proceedings of the American Society of Clinical Oncology 1998; 17:2a.
93. Kaminski MS, Zelenetz AD, Press OW, et al: Multicenter, phase III study of iodine-131 tositumomab (anti-B1 antibody) for chemotherapy-refractory low-grade or transformed low-grade non-Hodgkin's lymphoma (NHL). Blood 1998; 92:316.
94. DeNardo GL, DeNardo SJ, Lamborn KR, et al: Low-dose fractionated immunotherapy for B-cell malignancies using ^{131}I-Lym-1 antibody. Cancer Biother Radiopharm 1998; 13:239.
95. DeNardo GL, DeNardo SJ, Goldstein DS, et al: Maximum tolerated dose, toxicity, and efficacy of ^{131}I-Lym-1 antibody for fractionated radioimmunotherapy of non-Hodgkin's lymphoma. J Clin Oncol 1998; 16:3246.
96. Matthews DC, Appelbaum FR, Eary JF, et al: Phase I study of (131)I-anti-CD45 antibody plus cyclophosphamide and total body irradiation for advanced acute leukemia and myelodysplastic syndrome. Blood 1999; 94:1237.
97. Zelenetz AD: Radioimmunotherapy for lymphoma. Curr Opin Oncol 1999; 11:375.
98. DeNardo GL, O'Donnell RT, Kroger LA, et al: Strategies for developing effective radioimmunotherapy for solid tumors. Clin Cancer Res 1999; 5 (suppl):3219s.
99. Knox S: Overview of studies on experimental radioimmunotherapy. Cancer Res 1995; 55:5832s.
100. Kreitman RJ: Immunotoxins in cancer therapy. Curr Opin Immunol 1999; 11:570.
101. Chandler JC, Frankel AE, Tagge EP: Genetic engineering of immunotoxins. Semin Pediatr Surg 1996; 5:206.
102. Perentesis JP, Gunther R, Waurzyniak B, et al: In vivo biotherapy of HL-60 myeloid leukemia with a genetically engineered recombinant fusion toxin directed against the human granulocyte macrophage colony-stimulating factor receptor. Clin Cancer Res 1997; 3:2217.
103. Rosenblum MG, Marks JW, Cheung LH: Comparative cytotoxicity and pharmacokinetics of antimelanoma immunotoxins containing either natural or recombinant gelonin. Cancer Chemother Pharmacol 1999; 44:343.
104. Klimka A, Barth S, Matthey B, et al: An anti-CD30 single-chain Fv selected by phage display and fused to Pseudomonas exotoxin A (Ki-4(scFv)-ETA′) is a potent immunotoxin against a Hodgkin-derived cell line. Br J Cancer 1999; 80:1214.
105. Gonzalez R, Salem P, Bunn PA Jr, et al: Single-dose murine monoclonal antibody ricin A chain immunotoxin in the treatment of metastatic melanoma: a phase I trial. Mol Biol 1991; 3:192.
106. Selvaggi K, Saria R, Schwartz R, et al: Phase I/II study of murine monoclonal antibody-ricin A chain (XOMAZYME-Mel) immunoconjugate plus cyclosporine A in patients with metastatic melanoma. J Immunother 1993; 13:201.
107. Stone MJ, Sausville EA, Fay JW, et al: A phase I study of bolus versus continuous infusion of the anti-CD19 immunotoxin, IgG-HD37-dgA, in patients with B-cell lymphoma. Blood 1996; 88:1188.
108. Laske DW, Muraszko KM, Oldfield EH, et al: Intraventricular therapy for leptomeningeal neoplasia. Neurosurgery 1997; 41:1039.
109. Multani PS, O'Day S, Nadler LM, et al: Phase II clinical trial of bolus infusion anti-B4 blocked ricin immunoconjugate in patients with relapsed B-cell non-Hodgkin's lymphoma. Clin Cancer Res 1998; 4:2599.
110. Martin PJ, Nelson BJ, Appelbaum FR, et al: Evaluation of a CD5-specific immunotoxin for treatment of acute graft-versus-host-disease after allogeneic bone marrow transplantation. Blood 1996; 88:824.
111. LeMaistre CF, Saleh MN, Kuzel TM, et al: Phase I trial of a ligand fusion-protein (DAB389IL-2) in lymphomas expressing the receptor for interleukin-2. Blood 1998; 91:399.
112. Grossbard ML, Lambert JM, Goldmacher VS, et al: Anti-B4-blocked ricin: a phase I trial of 7-day continuous infusion in patients with B-cell neoplasms. J Clin Oncol 1993; 11:726.
113. Grossbard ML, Multani PS, Freedman AS, et al: A phase II study of adjuvant therapy with anti-B4-blocked ricin after autologous bone marrow transplantation for patients with relapsed B-cell non-Hodgkin's lymphoma. Clin Cancer Res 1999; 5:2392.
114. Lynch TJ Jr, Lambert JM, Coral F, et al: Immunotoxin therapy of small-cell lung cancer: a phase I study of N9010-blocked ricin. J Clin Oncol 1997; 15:723.
115. Frankel AE, Laver JH, Willingham MC, et al: Therapy of patients with T-cell lymphomas and leukemias using an anti-CD7 monoclonal antibody-ricin A chain immunotoxin. Leuk Lymphoma 1997; 26:287.
116. Schnell R, Vitetta E, Schindler J, et al: Treatment of refractory Hodgkin's lymphoma patients with anti-CD25 ricin A-chain immunotoxin. Leukemia 2000; 14:129.
117. Frankel AE, Tagge EP, Willingham MC: Clinical trials of targeted toxins. Semin Cancer Biol 1995; 6:307.
118. Kuan CT, Pai LH, Pastan I: Immunotoxins containing Pseudomonas exotoxin that targets LeY damage to human endothelial cells in an antibody-specific mode: relevance to vascular leak syndrome. Clin Cancer Res 1995; 1:1589.
119. Baluna R, Sausville EA, Stone MJ, et al: Decreases in levels of serum fibronectin predict the severity of vascular leak syndrome in patients treated with ricin A chain-containing immunotoxin. Clin Cancer Res 1996; 2:1705.
120. Hoffman DMJ, Gitlitz BJ, Belldegrun A, et al: Adoptive cellular therapy. Semin Oncol 2000; 27:221.
121. Schoell WM, Mirhashemi R, Liu B, et al: Generation of tumor-specific cytotoxic T lymphocytes by stimulation with HPV type 16 E7 peptide-pulsed dendritic cells: an approach to immunotherapy of cervical cancer. Gynecol Oncol 1999; 74:448.
122. Houbiers JGA, Nijman HW, van der Burg SH, et al: In vitro induction of human cytotoxic T lymphocyte responses against peptides of mutant and wild-type p53. Eur J Immunol 1993; 23:2072.
123. Jung S, Schluesener HJ: Human T lymphocytes recognize a peptide of single point-mutated, oncogenic ras protein. J Exp Med 1991; 173:273.
124. Cheever MA, Chen W, Disis ML, et al: T-cell immunity to oncogenic proteins including mutated ras and chimeric bcr-abl. Ann NY Acad Sci 1993; 690:101.
125. Economou JS, Belldegrun AS, Glaspy J, et al: In vivo trafficking of adoptively transferred interleukin-2 expanded tumor-infiltrating

lymphocytes and peripheral blood lymphocytes. Results of a double gene marking trial. J Clin Invest 1996; 97:515.
126. Figlin RA, Pierce WC, Kaboo R, et al: Treatment of metastatic renal cell carcinoma with nephrectomy, interleukin-2 and cytokine-primed or CD8(+) selected tumor infiltrating lymphocytes from primary tumor. J Urol 1997; 158:740.
127. Elson PJ, Witte RS, Trump DL: Prognostic factors for survival in patients with recurrent or metastatic renal cell carcinoma. Cancer Res 1988; 48:7310.
128. Figlin RA, Thompson C, Roudet P, et al: Multi-center randomized placebo-controlled phase II/III trial of CD8(+) tumor infiltrating lymphocyte therapy (CD8(+)TIL/recombinant interleukin-2 (IL-2) in metastatic renal cell carcinoma (MRCC) [Abstract]. Proceedings of the American Society of Clinical Oncology 1998; 17:318a.
129. Mayordomo JI, Zorina T, Storkus WJ, et al: Bone marrow-derived dendritic cells serve as potent adjuvants for peptide-based antitumor vaccines. Stem Cells 1997; 15:94.
130. Sallusto F, Lanzavecchia A: Efficient presentation of soluble antigen by cultured human dendritic cells is maintained by granulocyte/macrophage colony-stimulating factor plus interleukin 4 and down regulated by tumor necrosis factor alpha. J Exp Med 1994; 179:1109.
131. Salgaller ML, Thurnher M, Bartsch G, et al: Report from the International Union Against Cancer (UICC) Tumor Biology Committee: UICC workshop on the use of dendritic cells in cancer clinical trials. Cancer 1999; 86:2674.
132. Nair SK, Hull S, Coleman D, et al: Induction of carcinoembryonic antigen (CEA)-specific cytotoxic T-lymphocyte responses in vitro using autologous dendritic cells loaded with CEA peptide or CEA RNA in patients with metastatic malignancies expressing CEA. Int J Cancer 1999; 82:121.
133. Thomas R, Chambers M, Boytar R, et al: Immature human monocyte-derived dendritic cells migrate rapidly to draining lymph nodes after intradermal injection for melanoma immunotherapy. Melanoma Res 1999; 9:474.
134. Tjoa BA, Simmons SJ, Elgamal A, et al: Follow-up evaluation of a phase II prostate cancer vaccine trial. Prostate 1999; 40:125.
135. Lodge PA, Jones LA, Bader RA, et al: Dendritic cell-based immunotherapy of prostate cancer: immune monitoring of a phase II clinical trial. Cancer Res 2000; 60:829.
136. Wiemann B, Starnes CO: Coley's toxins, tumor necrosis factor and cancer research: a historical perspective. Pharmacol Ther 1994; 64:529.
137. Morton DL, Eilber FR, Holmes EC, et al: Preliminary results of a randomized trial of adjuvant immunotherapy in patients with malignant melanoma who have lymph node metastases. Austral NZ J Surg 1978; 48:49.
138. Bast RC Jr, Zbar B, Borsos T, et al: BCG and cancer. N Engl J Med 1974; 290:1458.
139. Agarwala SS, Kirkwood JM: Adjuvant therapy of melanoma. Semin Surg Oncol 1998; 14:302.
140. Crawford ED: Diagnosis and treatment of superficial bladder cancer: an update. Semin Urol Oncol 1996; 14 (suppl):1.
141. Schmitz-Drager BJ, Muller M: Intravesical treatment of bladder cancer: current problems and needs. Urol Int 1998; 61:199.
142. Killion JJ, Fidler IJ: Therapy of cancer metastasis by tumoricidal activation of tissue macrophages using liposome-encapsulated immunomodulators. Pharmacol Ther 1998; 78:141.
143. Murray JL, Kleinerman ES, Cunningham JE, et al: Phase I trial of liposomal muramyl tripeptide phosphatidylethanolamine in cancer patients. J Clin Oncol 1989; 7:1915.
144. Kleinerman ES: Biologic therapy for osteosarcoma using liposome-encapsulated muramyl tripeptide. Hematol Oncol Clin North Am 1995; 9:927.
145. Watanabe R, Yoo YC, Hata K, et al: Inhibitory effect of trehalose dimycolate (TDM) and its stereoisometric derivatives, trehalose dicorynomycolates (TDCMs), with low toxicity on lung metastasis of tumour cells in mice. Vaccine 1999; 17:1484.
146. Hollander GA: On the stochastic regulation of interleukin-2 transcription. Semin Immunol 1999; 11:357.
147. Mookerjee BK, Pauly JL: Mitogenic effect of interleukin-2 on unstimulated human T cells: an editorial review. J Clin Lab Anal 1990; 4:138.
148. Overwijk WW, Theoret MR, Restifo NP: The future of interleukin-2: enhancing therapeutic anticancer vaccines. Cancer J Sci Am 2000; 6 (suppl):S76.
149. Nichols J, Foss F, Kuzel TM, et al: Interleukin-2 fusion protein: an investigational therapy for interleukin-2 receptor expressing malignancies. Eur J Cancer 1997; 33 (suppl):S34.
150. Waldmann TA: T-cell receptors for cytokines: targets for immunotherapy of leukemia/lymphoma. Ann Oncol 2000; 11 (suppl):101.
151. Dummer R, Gore ME, Hancock BW, et al: A multicenter phase II clinical trial using dacarbazine and continuous infusion interleukin-2 for metastatic melanoma. Clinical data and immunomonitoring. Cancer 1995; 75:1038.
152. Peest D, Leo R, Deicher H: Tumor-directed cytotoxicity in multiple myeloma—the basis for an experimental treatment approach with interleukin-2. Stem Cells 1995; 13 (suppl):72.
153. Tagliaferri P, Barile C, Caraglia M, et al: Daily low-dose subcutaneous recombinant interleukin-2 by alternate weekly administration: antitumor activity and immunomodulatory effects. Am J Clin Oncol 1998; 21:48.
154. Bear HD, Hamad GG, Kostuchenko PJ: Biologic therapy of melanoma with cytokines and lymphocytes. Semin Surg Oncol 1996; 12:436.
155. Mantovani G, Gebbia V, Airoldi M, et al: Neo-adjuvant chemo-(immuno-)therapy of advanced squamous-cell head and neck carcinoma: a multicenter, phase III, randomized study comparing cisplatin + 5-fluorouracil (5-FU) with cisplatin + 5-FU + recombinant interleukin 2. Cancer Immunol Immunother 1998; 47:149.
156. Sen GC, Lengyel P: The interferon system. A bird's eye view of its biochemistry. J Biol Chem 1992; 267:5017.
157. Saunders N, Dahler A, Jones S, et al: Interferon-gamma as a regulator of squamous differentiation. J Dermatol Sci 1996; 13:98.
158. Grander D, Sangfelt O, Erickson S: How does interferon exert its cell growth inhibitory effect? Eur J Haematol 1997; 59:129.
159. York IA, Goldberg AL, Mo XY, et al: Proteolysis and class I major histocompatability complex antigen presentation. Immunol Rev 1999; 172:49.
160. Guadagni F, Roselli M, Schlom J, et al: In vitro and in vivo regulation of human tumor antigen expression by human recombinant interferons: a review. Int J Biol Markers 1994; 9:53.
161. Gisslinger H: Interferon alpha in the therapy of multiple myeloma. Leukemia 1997; 11 (suppl):S52.
162. Fiorani C, Tonelli S, Casolari B, et al: The role of interferon-alpha in the treatment of myeloproliferative disorders. Curr Pharm Des 1999; 5:987.
163. Fossa SD: Interferon in metastatic renal cell carcinoma. Semin Oncol 2000; 27:187.
164. Shepherd PC, Richards SM, Allan NC: Progress with interferon in CML—results of the MRC UK CML III study. Bone Marrow Transplant 1996; 17 (suppl):S15.
165. Cortes J, Fayad L, Kantarjian H, et al: Association of HLA phenotype and response to interferon-alpha in patients with chronic myelogenous leukemia. Leukemia 1998; 12:455.
166. Legha SS: The role of interferon alfa in the treatment of metastatic melanoma. Semin Oncol 1997; 24 (suppl):S24.
167. Hernberg M, Pyrhonen S, Muhonen T: Regimens with or without interferon-alpha as treatment for metastatic melanoma and renal cell carcinoma: an overview of randomized trials. J Immunother 1999; 22:145.
168. Meadows LM, Lindley C, Ozer H: Treatment of gastrointestinal and renal adenocarcinomas with interferon-alpha. Biotherapy 1992; 4:179.
169. Igarashi T, Marumo K, Onishi T, et al: Interferon-alpha and 5-fluorouracil therapy in patients with metastatic renal cell cancer: an open multicenter trial. The Japanese Study Group Against Renal Cancer. Urology 1999; 53:53.
170. Makower D, Wadler S: Interferons as biomodulators of fluoropyrimidines in the treatment of colorectal cancer. Semin Oncol 1999; 26:663.
171. Keilholz U, Eggermont AM: The role of interleukin-2 in the management of stage IV melanoma: the EORTC Melanoma Cooperative Group program. Cancer J Sci Am 2000; 6 (suppl):S99.
172. Herlyn D, Birebent B: Advances in cancer vaccine development. Ann Med 1999; 31:66.
173. Del Vecchio M, Parmiani G: Cancer vaccination. Forum 1999; 9:239.
174. Brinckerhoff LH, Thompson LW, Slingluff CL Jr: Melanoma vaccines. Curr Opin Oncol 2000; 12:163.
175. Schlom J, Kantor J, Abrams, S, et al: Strategies for the development

of recombinant vaccines for the immunotherapy of breast cancer. Breast Cancer Res Treat 1996; 38:27.
176. McAneny D, Ryan CA, Beazley RM, et al: Results of a phase I trial of a recombinant vaccinia virus that expresses carcinoembryonic antigen in patients with advanced colorectal cancer. Ann Surg Oncol 1996; 3:495.
177. Meidenbauer N, Harris DT, Spitler LE, et al: Generation of PSA-reactive effector cells after vaccination with a PSA-based vaccine in patients with prostate cancer. Prostate 2000; 43:88.
178. Soiffer R, Lynch T, Mihm M, et al: Vaccination with irradiated autologous melanoma cells engineered to secrete human granulocyte-macrophage colony-stimulating factor generates potent antitumor immunity in patients with metastatic melanoma. Proc Natl Acad Sci USA 1998; 95:13141.
179. Simons JW, Mikhak B, Chang JF, et al: Induction of immunity to prostate cancer antigens: results of a clinical trial of vaccination with irradiated autologous prostate tumor cells engineered to secrete human granulocyte-macrophage colony-stimulating factor using ex vivo gene transfer. Cancer Res 1999; 59:5160.
180. Trefzer U, Weingart G, Chen Y, et al: Hybrid cell vaccination for cancer immune therapy: first clinical trial with metastatic melanoma. Int J Cancer 2000; 85:618.
181. Livingstone PO: Approaches to augmenting the immunogenicity of melanoma gangliosides: from whole melanoma cells to ganglioside-KLH conjugate vaccines. Immunol Rev 1995; 145:147.
182. Harris JR, Markl J: Keyhole limpet hemocyanin (KLH): a biomedical review. Micron 1999; 30:597.
183. Livingstone P: Ganglioside vaccines with emphasis on GM2. Semin Oncol 1998; 25:636.
184. Slovin SE, Scher HI: Peptide and carbohydrate vaccines in relapsed prostate cancer: immunogenicity of synthetic vaccines in man—clinical trials at Memorial Sloan-Kettering Cancer Center. Semin Oncol 1999; 26:448.
185. Yao TJ, Meyers M, Livingstone PO, et al: Immunization of melanoma patients with BEC2-keyhole limpet hemocyanin plus BCG intradermally followed by intravenous booster immunization with BEC2 to induce anti-GD3 ganglioside antibodies. Clin Cancer Res 1999; 5:77.
186. Shackney SE, Shankey TV: Genetic and phenotypic heterogeneity of human malignancies: finding order in chaos. Cytometry 1995; 21:2.
187. Arvan D: Tumor cell heterogeneity: an overview. Clin Chim Acta 1992; 206:3.
188. Colombatti M, Dipasquale B, Del-l'Arciprete L, et al: Heterogeneity and modulation of tumor-associated antigens in human glioblastoma cell lines. J Neurosurg 1989; 71:388.
189. Song S, Statsny JJ, Chen H, et al: Expression of sarcoma-associated antigens p102 and p200 in human sarcoma cell lines. Anticancer Res 1996; 16:1171.
190. Restifo NP, Kawakami Y, Marincola F, et al: Molecular mechanisms used by tumors to escape immune recognition: immunogenetherapy and the cell biology of major histocompatability complex class I. J Immunother 1993; 14:182.
191. Jiang S, Tugulea S, Pennesi G, et al: Induction of MHC-class I restricted human suppressor T cells by peptide priming in vitro. Human Immunol 1998; 59:690.
192. Koyama S: Immunosuppressive effect of shedding intercellular adhesion molecules 1 antigen on cell-mediated cytotoxicity against tumor cells. Jpn J Cancer Res 1994; 85:131.
193. Jaffe ML, Arai H, Nabel GJ: Mechanisms of tumor-induced immunosuppression: evidence for contact-dependent T cell suppression by monocytes. Mol Med 1996; 2:6925.
194. Mathe G: Suppressor T-cells. Biomed Pharmacother 1999; 53:213.
195. Chen W, Jin W, Wahl SM: Engagement of cytotoxic T lymphocyte-associated antigen 4 (CTLA-4) induces transforming growth factor beta (TGF-beta) production by murine CD4(+) T cells. J Exp Med 1998; 188:1849.

12 *HIV-Associated Malignancies*

BERNADINE R. DONAHUE, MD, Radiation Oncology
JAMES C. WERNZ, MD, Medical Oncology
JAY S. COOPER, MD, Radiation Oncology

The same medicine does not cure every patient.
AURELIUS CORNELIUS CELSUS, *1st century physician*

Perspective

Approximately 16,000 people throughout the world are infected each day with human immunodeficiency virus (HIV).[1] It is estimated that in 1996 alone, over 1 million people died of acquired immunodeficiency syndrome (AIDS)–related diseases. Although the most common source of morbidity and mortality has been opportunistic infections, AIDS-related malignancies are a well-recognized and potentially lethal manifestation of the disease.

In some HIV-infected individuals, the development of a malignancy becomes an AIDS-defining event. During the 1980s and 1990s, the incidence rates of three specific malignancies, in conjunction with HIV, increased sufficiently to be considered AIDS-defining conditions: Kaposi's sarcoma (KS), non-Hodgkin's lymphoma (NHL), and carcinoma of the uterine cervix.

In 1997, the National Cancer Institute sponsored the first National AIDS Malignancy Conference. This chapter represents the state of the art in the year 2000. AIDS is not a static disease. Both its associated morbidities and treatments evolve over time; however, many of the basic principles of its management should remain steadfast.

AIDS-Defining Malignancies in the Highly Active Antiretroviral Therapy (HAART) Era

Assessing the risk of cancer in the AIDS population before and after widespread use of HAART, rate ratios of AIDS-defining cancers were calculated for the period 1992 to 1996 and compared with the rate ratios in 1997 to 1999, when HAART was widely available in resource-rich areas of the world. Overall, the rate of KS fell from 15.2 to 4.9 per 1000 patient years in these two periods, with a rate ratio of 0.32, indicating a highly significant decrease in this tumor, coinciding with the use of HAART. For NHL, the rate fell from 6.2 to 3.6 per 1000 patient years, indicating a significant decline, although not as great as that seen in KS. The rate ratio for NHL between the two time periods was 0.58. Of interest, a greater reduction was observed in the rate ratio of primary central nervous system NHL; furthermore, no decline in certain specific types of NHL, such as Burkitt's lymphoma, was seen. No significant decline in cervical cancer was found.[1a]

Kaposi's sarcoma, occurring in young homosexual men, heralded the onset of the AIDS epidemic in 1981.[2] Intermediate- or high-grade B-cell lymphomas in HIV-infected individuals became AIDS-defining conditions in 1985,[3] and cervical carcinoma was recognized in 1993 as an AIDS-defining illness for HIV-infected women.[4] In 1997 it was reported that HIV-infected individuals had a risk of developing KS and NHL that was 1000 and 150 times higher, respectively, than the general population.[5]

The second decade of the AIDS pandemic was characterized both by better strategies to prevent the transmission of HIV and improved treatment for infection. The development of progressively more effective multiple-drug antiretroviral therapy (HAART), including protease inhibitors, has altered the clinical behavior of AIDS by slowing the progression of AIDS and reducing mortality.[6] HIV can be suppressed to undetectable levels in a substantial percentage of HIV-infected individuals who are compliant with the drug regimens, which leads to a marked decrease in AIDS-related infectious complications and other illnesses. Our impression is that with suppression of HIV and consequent reconstitution of the immune system, there has been a decrease in AIDS-related malignancies.

Many factors contribute to the development of neoplasms in the setting of HIV infection. These factors include chronic defects in cellular and humoral immunity, dysregulated B-cell and monocyte stimulation, and, in some instances, possible infection with HIV-associated viruses such as the Kaposi's sarcoma herpes virus and the Epstein-Barr virus.[7–9] The decision to provide definitive or palliative care in the setting of HIV-associated malignancies must take into consideration not only the specific nature of the malignancy to be treated but also the host's status, viral load, and the timeline of the patient's disease. The benefit-risk ratio for any treatment, including surgery, chemotherapy, and radiation therapy, must be weighed for each patient. Little information exists about the possible immunosuppressive effects of chemotherapy or radiation therapy on HIV replication. However, until these issues are clarified, it seems prudent to remember that if curative treatment of an existing malignancy is possible, it should not be compromised by fear of possible immunosuppression.

Kaposi's Sarcoma

Epidemiology

Kaposi's sarcoma (KS) is the most common neoplasm occurring in persons who have AIDS. Approximately 15% to 20% of AIDS patients develop this neoplasm, which rarely occurs in immunocompetent individuals and virtually never before age 50.[10] Early on in the epidemic, people infected with HIV had at least a 20,000 times greater risk of developing KS than uninfected individuals.[9] The KS associated with HIV became known as "epidemic" KS to distinguish it from the classic form of KS. The discovery that HIV-infected gay or bisexual men were more likely than HIV-infected heterosexual men to develop KS was one of the first clues that KS, or its etiologic agent, might somehow be sexually transmitted. The theory was later reinforced by the finding that women who acquired HIV infection from bisexual men had an approximately fourfold greater risk of developing KS than women who contracted the virus from either exclusively heterosexual men or by intravenous drug use.[10]

At the start of the epidemic in the early 1980s, approximately 50% of HIV-infected patients were considered to have AIDS on the basis of having Kaposi's sarcoma.[11] By the early 1990s, the incidence of KS as an AIDS-defining illness had fallen to 14%.[12, 13] The explanations given for this decline include the recognition of other risk groups (e.g., intravenous drug users), changes in the definition of AIDS, and changes in sexual transmission of HIV since the gay community became active in advocating safe-sex practices.

In December 1994, a herpes virus that appeared to be associated with the etiology of Kaposi's sarcoma was identified.[14] This virus has now been termed *human herpes virus 8* (HHV8), and it has been detected in both AIDS-associated forms of Kaposi's sarcoma, as well as classic KS. Whether HHV8 is the sole etiologic agent is yet unclear; if HHV8 is the cause of KS, then infection with the virus should precede the clinical development of Kaposi's sarcoma lesions in all cases. In a 1996 report from the Multicenter AIDS Cohort Study, antibodies to HHV8 were detected in 80% of HIV-infected men who subsequently went on to develop Kaposi's sarcoma.[15] The antibodies to HHV8 were identified at a median of 2½ years before any clinical sign of disease. The virus was identified in only 18% of the men who never developed Kaposi's sarcoma. Outcomes of the study suggest that Kaposi's sarcoma results from or is at least facilitated by infection with HHV8.

HHV8 has now been isolated, and it has been cultured with and shown to be cytotoxic to human epithelial cells.[16] Additionally, HHV8 DNA has now been sequenced. It is now thought that the HIV *tat* gene, which may somehow be influenced by HHV8, may be the initiating factor that transforms a normal mesenchymal cell into a proliferating KS lesion.[17] In addition to its transactivating potential, HIV-1 tat protein also enhances angiogenesis in KS.[18] *In vivo* experiments with nude mice have demonstrated that extracellular tat protein upregulates the inflammatory cytokines that are increased in KS lesions (e.g., γIFN, TNFα, IL-1β), activate endothelial cells, and induce the expression of the angiogenic factors, bFGF and vascular endothelial growth factor (VEGF).[17] Additionally, HIV-induced inflammatory cytokines may induce KS cells to grow by autocrine stimulation.

Diagnosis

Kaposi's sarcoma is characterized by purplish lesions on the skin or mucosal surfaces. It is a vascular tumor, and a number of angiogenic growth factors are produced by KS tumor cells or the surrounding supportive network of stromal cells and extracellular matrix, or both. The lesions can be macular, plaquelike, or nodular, with or without associated lymphadenopathy or lymphedema. At presentation, skin lesions can be either single or multiple. Visceral Kaposi's sarcoma typically involves the bronchi and the gastrointestinal tract. KS lesions may cause pain, bleeding, or disfigurement. As involvement of lymph nodes and lymphatic spaces occurs, progressive edema can result. This occurrence is seen most commonly in lesions involving the lower extremity, the groin, the genitalia, and the face. Oropharyngeal lesions can result in life-threatening airway obstruction. Pulmonary involvement can result in life-threatening respiratory failure. Although we generally advocate biopsy confirmation, before the initiation of therapy, it is most feasible with skin lesions. Biopsy of bronchial lesions may be contraindicated because of the risk of hemorrhage, and in these settings characteristic endoscopic and radiographic findings should be used to establish the diagnosis.

Treatment

Local

Kaposi's sarcoma typically exhibits multifocal distribution at the time of presentation; therefore, it frequently requires a systemic approach. In some settings, however, patients require localized therapy. Some lesions can be excised surgically, but this is rarely the case. Cryotherapy with liquid nitrogen and intralesional therapy with vinblastine have become the most popular forms of local control of Kaposi's sarcoma.[19] Caution must be used when using cryotherapy with deeply pigmented lesions, because the healed area may be hypopigmented. Intralesional interferon alfa[20] or, more recently, human chorionic gonadotropin (β-HCG)[21] has also been used with some success, and Panretin gel was recently made available. Radiation therapy often represents the optimal choice for palliation of pain, bleeding, or edema. One of the more commonly used dose-fractionation schemes is 30 Gy in 10 fractions delivered over 2 weeks, which has resulted in substantial benefit without substantial toxicity.[22] However, in treatment of extensive lesions in patients who have far advanced AIDS, when a briefer duration of palliation will suffice, a dose of 8 Gy in one fraction may be used.[23] Treatment of symptomatic oropharyngeal lesions with radiation has been problematic because of the high degree of radiation-induced mucositis that these patients develop even following low-dose radiation therapy.[24] Symptomatic visceral involvement nearly always requires a systemic approach. However, there are instances in which patients' lesions have failed to respond to systemic chemotherapy or in which patients are unable to tolerate systemic chemotherapy. These patients may require local radiation to palliate bleeding or obstructive lesions. In one report of 25 patients who had pulmonary lesions treated with radiation therapy, subjective improvement was observed in nearly 90% of patients, although only one third of patients survived for 3 months.[25]

Systemic

Systemic therapy has been used in the treatment of epidemic KS since the beginning of the AIDS epidemic. However, owing to the recent advent of more potent antiretroviral agents (e.g., protease inhibitors), there has been a marked change. Very few patients are now requiring ongoing chronic chemotherapy to control their disease. Interferons have been used for many years to treat epidemic KS.[26] In early trials, the interferons were found to be antiviral and antiproliferative, as well as immunomodulating, which made them candidates for study in KS.[27, 28] Interferon alfa has been found to inhibit HIV *in vitro*[29] and also to be antiangiogenic.[30] Response to interferon alfa as a single agent is very much determined by the immune status of the patient. Patients with CD4 counts greater than or equal to 400 are much more likely to respond than those with CD4 counts less than 150.[26]

Interferon alfa was initially approved by the FDA for treatment of epidemic KS at high doses, (e.g., 30 million units [MU], three injections weekly), which were rarely tolerated; such high doses are no longer thought to be appropriate. In the early years of the epidemic, interferon alfa was given at these high doses as an oncologic antiproliferative agent.[31] Trials performed by the AIDS Clinical Trial Group showed activity of lower doses of interferon alfa (9 MU subcutaneously [subQ] daily) in combination with zidovudine (AZT; 3′-azido-3′-deoxythymidine).[32, 33] It was subsequently observed that doses as low as 1 MU subQ daily when administered with a single nucleoside analogue, for example, didanosine, resulted in substantial activity.[29] Now with our expanded knowledge of the pathogenesis of KS, the mechanism of this action is better understood.

Systemic chemotherapy has been reserved for patients with symptomatic disease for whom treatment with systemic interferon alfa would be inappropriate. The concern has always been whether it would further compromise the immune system. Very early on in the AIDS epidemic, there was a major concern over the toxicity of chemotherapy in treating KS.[34, 35] The standard doses of chemotherapy used for solid tumors resulted in unacceptable morbidity for these AIDS patients. Consequently, treatment protocols were developed with low-dose chemotherapy to which epidemic KS was responsive.[36, 37] There are a number of drug regimens that are active in KS; however, the regimen of Adriamycin, bleomycin, and vincristine (ABV) had become the standard of care as the years of clinical trials progressed.[34] In randomized trials reported in 1998, the response rate to ABV was in the range of 31% with a median duration of response of 6 months.[38]

Liposomal daunorubicin and doxorubicin are now approved by the FDA for the treatment of epidemic KS. Randomized studies comparing these drugs with the standard ABV have shown at least comparable activity with a more favorable toxicity profile.[38–40] Since these drugs have become available, they are frequently used as first-line therapy. Paclitaxel is also now approved for treatment. It is active when given at doses of 100 mg/m^2 every 14 days. Toxicity is infrequent except for myelosuppression, which can be dealt with by growth factors when necessary.[41] Even though there are other active drugs available, such as VP-16, paclitaxel has become a favorite second- or third-line drug following the liposomal agents, owing to its activity and acceptable toxicity. Its activity may be mediated by its known antiangiogenic effects; it is possible that as new antiangiogenic agents become available for clinical trials, a role for their use in the treatment of KS will be defined.

Results and Prognosis

All of the above-mentioned treatments are aimed at decreasing the burden of disease and effectively palliating symptoms for the duration of a patient's lifetime. Effective improvement of symptoms can be achieved in the vast majority of patients, using one or a combination of therapeutic interventions. Of interest is the observation that the introduction of protease inhibitors in some patients who have KS can result not only in the stabilization of existing lesions and the slowing of the progression of the disease but in bringing about measurable regression of existing lesions.[42] Before effective combination drug therapy (HAART) was able to suppress HIV over long periods of time, patients required ongoing therapy to control their symptomatic KS. It has now been shown that when effective combination antiretroviral therapy is instituted, resulting in a drop of HIV RNA, as measured by polymerase chain reaction, to undetectable levels, chronic chemotherapy for epidemic KS frequently can be discontinued.[43]

Systemic Non-Hodgkin's Lymphoma (NHL)

Epidemiology

The incidence of lymphoma in association with AIDS has been approximately 60 to 100 times greater than expected in the general population.[44, 45] Whereas primary central nervous system lymphoma (PCNSL) was one of the initial criteria approved by the Centers for Disease Control and Prevention for a diagnosis of AIDS,[46] the inclusion of systemic high-grade B-cell lymphoma did not occur until 1985;[3] PCNSL is discussed separately later in this chapter. For purposes of clarity, all manifestations of NHL other than PCNSL are referred to here as systemic NHL. Systemic, AIDS-related, non-Hodgkin's lymphoma (AIDS-NHL) has been considered a late manifestation of infection by HIV, and more than one step appears to be involved in its pathogenesis. Epstein-Barr virus has been implicated in its etiology by the finding of anti-EBV immunoglobulins and circulating of EBV-infected B-cells in the setting of HIV.[9, 47] However, additional factors probably need to be present to cause malignant transformation of B-cells, such as *MYC* gene rearrangements.[48]

Diagnosis

Rapidly developing adenopathy or constitutional B symptoms (fevers, unexplained weight loss, night sweats), or both, are the most common presentations of AIDS-NHL. Nearly 75% of all patients present with advanced stage disease (stage III or stage IV) and most manifest B symptomatology.[49] In general, diagnosis by histologic analysis is most readily accomplished by biopsy of a clinically suspicious peripheral lymph node. The most common histologic subtypes are high-grade B-cell lymphoma or Burkitt's lymphoma; however, intermediate-grade (diffuse large cell–type) lymphomas are not uncommon. Because patients who have AIDS-NHL frequently have extranodal involvement, staging evaluation should include chest, abdomen, and pelvic CT scans; bone marrow biopsy; and CSF analysis.

Treatment

Early on in the AIDS epidemic, treatment for AIDS-NHL lymphoma was based on high-dose chemotherapy regimens that had been developed for non–AIDS-related lymphomas.[50, 51] These treatments were not well tolerated, and they resulted in substantial toxicity, as well as high rates of infectious complications, both opportunistic and bacterial. Later, therapy relied on attenuated doses of cytotoxic chemotherapy or standard-dose chemotherapy plus cytokine support.[52–55] Most studies have shown complete remission rates of approximately 50%, with approximately 25% of all patients treated sustaining long-term remissions.[50–52, 56] In 1994, Sparano and coworkers defined a regimen with high efficacy and acceptable toxicity using infusional cyclophosphamide, doxorubicin, and etoposide.[57]

The role of consolidative radiation therapy following systemic treatment in AIDS patients who have non-Hodgkin's lymphomas has not been consistently addressed. It has been suggested that radiation should be used as a consolidative boost in patients with bulky disease who have demonstrated slow or partial response to chemotherapy.[39] Radiation, however, is also indicated for palliation of bulky lesions, and it is frequently used to provide palliative therapy for patients who develop lymphomatous meningitis. The majority of these patients have far-advanced AIDS, and because of concerns about further bone marrow suppression in these already very compromised patients, treatment usually is limited to cranial radiation (not cranio*spinal*), and intrathecal chemotherapy is administered in an attempt to clear the cerebral spinal fluid of malignant cells. Patients who have grossly evident spinal meningeal disease have generally been treated only to a limited volume, encompassing the gross disease and a small margin. Unfortunately, it is not uncommon for previously undetectable spinal meningeal involvement outside the irradiated volume to become evident and symptomatic before the patient's death.[57a]

Results and Prognosis

Despite our best therapies, patients who have AIDS-NHL generally survive only 6 months after diagnosis. However, prognostic factors have been identified that correlate with the length of survival.[58–60] Patients who have bone marrow involvement, low performance status at diagnosis (Karnofsky Performance Status [KPS] < 70), low CD4 count, and a prior diagnosis of AIDS have a median survival of 4 months. Those without these adverse features have a median survival of 11 months.

A newly described form of lymphoma called *primary effusion* or *body cavity lymphoma* has been identified in some HIV-infected patients.[61] There appears to be an association between infection with HHV8 and this particular type of lymphoma.[62] Typically, such patients present with an effusion in a body cavity, in the absence of widespread lymphadenopathy. Survival of patients who have primary effusion lymphoma is very short, 2 to 5 months, even with aggressive therapy.

Primary Central Nervous System Non-Hodgkin's Lymphoma

Epidemiology

The incidence of primary central nervous system lymphoma (PCNSL) has increased steadily since the onset of the AIDS epidemic. Ten percent to twenty percent of all AIDS-related non-Hodgkin's lymphomas originated in the brain without evidence of systemic involvement.[63] In general, PCNSL is seen later in the course of HIV infection than are systemic non-Hodgkin's lymphomas. Patients usually have CD4 counts less than 50 cells/mm^3 before PCNSL becomes evident.[64] The majority of these lymphomas are B-cell, large immunoblastic types, and Epstein-Barr virus DNA is identifiable in nearly all cases.[8, 65]

Diagnosis

In most patients who have HIV-associated PCNSL, the diagnosis is suggested by the onset of headaches or a change in mental status.[66] Unfortunately, PCNSL often is clinically and radiographically indistinguishable from some other pathologic neurologic processes (most notably toxoplasmosis) in HIV-infected patients. A so-called negative toxoplasmosis titer does not eliminate the diagnosis of toxoplasmosis, and, similarly, a so-called positive toxoplasmosis titer does not preclude the presence of PCNSL.[67, 68] Because of the high incidence of toxoplasmosis in the HIV-infected population, the standard first-line treatment for an HIV-infected patient who develops a neurologic abnormality and has a radiographically visible brain lesion consistent with either toxoplasmosis or central nervous system lymphoma is the institution of anti-toxoplasmosis antibiotics. Previously, it had been common to administer empiric cranial radiation therapy in patients who did not manifest clinical or radiographic improvement by the second or third week of anti-toxoplasmosis treatment. However, as our knowledge of the myriad HIV-related opportunistic infections expanded and the poor outcome with this empiric approach was recognized, the emphasis shifted to recommending biopsy for definitive diagnosis. This can frequently be performed safely using stereotactic guidance. It may be possible in the future, with further refinement of noninvasive radiographic imaging (such as evolving nuclear studies using tagged antibodies), that the diagnosis can be made in a noninvasive fashion.[69]

Treatment

Radiation therapy of the brain and meninges has been the mainstay of treatment for HIV-associated PCNSL. Various regimens of radiotherapy have been employed, and there is unquestionable clinical and radiographic evidence of tumor response. However, regardless of the nature of the course of radiation therapy delivered (a short palliative-intent course of 30 Gy in 10 fractions over 2 weeks versus a more definitive-intent 50 Gy course delivered in 1.8 to 2 Gy per fraction over 5 to 6 weeks), the mean overall survival time has been in the range of 2 to 5 months.[62, 70–72] Although methotrexate-based chemotherapy has been shown to prolong the median survival in immunocompetent patients who have PCNSL, many HIV-infected patients have been unable to tolerate this systemic approach. Therefore, a palliative regimen of 30 Gy in 10 fractions, or its equivalent, continues to be widely used.[38, 62] This dosage, however, may change in the era of HAART. Some HIV-infected patients may be able to tolerate chemotherapy for PCNSL, and they may be better served by conventionally fractionated radiation.

Results and Prognosis

Although the overall median survival of patients with PCNSL is poor, patients no older than 35 years who have Karnofsky performance scores of at least 80 tend to survive 5 to 6 months, rather than 2 months.[67] Such patients should be considered for enrollment in ongoing trials seeking to evaluate the efficacy of novel radiation schemes or chemoradiation.

Cervical Carcinoma

Epidemiology

Cervical carcinoma in the presence of HIV infection has been accepted by the CDC as an AIDS-defining illness.[4] In a retrospective study of women registered from 1987 through 1995 by the New York City Department of Health and institutional tumor registries, cervical cancer was the sixth most common initial AIDS-defining illness in women.[73] For women, cervical cancer was the most common AIDS-related malignancy, representing 55% of the cases, followed by lymphoma (29%) and Kaposi's sarcoma (16%). As is true in HIV-uninfected populations, cervical dysplasia appears to be a precursor to cervical malignancies, and cervical dysplasia occurs in 40% of HIV-infected women.[74] Etiologically, there appears to be an association between human papillomavirus infection and risk for cervical epithelial abnormalities in HIV-infected women.[75] Specifically, compared with HIV-seronegative women, HIV-infected women have a higher rate of persistent infection with human papillomavirus (HPV)-16 or HPV-18, the viral types that are most strongly associated with cervical carcinoma.[76] Moreover, the frequency and severity of dysplasia appear to correlate inversely with CD4 counts, thus implying a role for immunosuppression.[77]

Diagnosis

Routine gynecologic evaluation, including Pap smears (and colposcopy, when warranted), is the most successful means of detecting the dysplastic and *in situ* lesions that give rise to invasive lesions. Unfortunately, HIV-infected women have presented with more advanced-stage disease than is seen in the noninfected population. As many as 50% of HIV-infected women have stage III or IV disease at the time of diagnosis, as compared with approximately 20% of noninfected women diagnosed as having cervical carcinoma.[78]

Treatment

Treatment of cervical carcinoma in HIV-infected women should be dictated by the extent of disease, taking into account the patient's history of opportunistic infections and overall medical status. The small proportion of patients who have early-stage, nonbulky disease can be approached surgically, with a radical hysterectomy and pelvic node dissection. The more typical patients, who have more advanced local-regional disease, should receive external beam radiotherapy accompanied by an intracavitary boost. There is now evidence from randomized trials that the use of platinum-based chemotherapy with external beam radiation therapy improves outcome in women with locally advanced cervical cancer, stages IB to IVA, as well as in women with stage I to IIA disease with involved pelvic lymph nodes, parametrial disease, or positive surgical margins.[78a] This approach should be considered in HIV-infected individuals with similar stages of cervical carcinoma if it is felt that chemotherapy will be tolerated. Patients who have hematogenously borne metastatic disease may benefit from palliative chemotherapy or radiation therapy in an effort to reduce symptoms such as pain and bleeding.

Results and Prognosis

Although there initially was concern over the ability to deliver so-called standard treatment to HIV-infected patients with cervical carcinoma, available data suggest treatment can be delivered, albeit with a higher risk of complications.[79, 80] HIV-infected women treated with laser (cone) therapy or cryotherapy for cervical intraepithelial neoplasia (CIN) have an increased risk of excessive bleeding or infection compared with uninfected patients.[75] In one series of patients treated with standard radiation for advanced disease, 50% of patients had no or minimal response to treatment, and at a median follow-up of 3 months, all patients had progression of disease.[76] Unfortunately, as is true of other malignancies, cervical carcinoma appears to be more aggressive in the HIV-infected population than in the immunocompetent population. This may reflect the more aggressive biology of the disease in these patients, the more advanced stage with which they present, or both. In one study of 16 HIV-infected women who had cervical carcinoma, more than 50% of the patients (9 of 16) died of cervical cancer, at a mean interval of only 9.2 months from diagnosis.[74]

Early diagnosis of cervical abnormalities, before the development of invasive cancer, appears to be critical if we are to hope for increased cure rates. Because there appears to be a 10% to 20% progression rate from CIN1 to CIN2 or -3 over 1 to 2 years in the HIV population,[73] it is imperative that close surveillance with gynecological evaluations, including Pap smears and colposcopy, be offered to all HIV-infected women.

Other Malignancies

Anal Carcinoma

The incidence of anal carcinoma in the general population has increased in the past several years.[81] Although there appears to be a relationship between the presence of condylomata and male homosexual contact, it is controversial as to whether the increase in anal cancer is due to HIV. Although HIV infection has been implicated as an independent risk factor for anal cancer,[82] recent studies of homosexual men in New York City and San Francisco show a greater increase in the incidence of anal cancer in HIV-seronegative men than in HIV-seropositive men.[83]

Anal neoplasia, like cervical carcinoma, also appears to be related to sexually transmitted human papillomavirus (primarily HPV-16), with anal intercourse being a risk factor.[84] HIV-infected homosexual men have increased serum HPV DNA as compared with HIV-seronegative homosexual men.[85] Sixty percent of HIV-infected men have been identified at baseline examination as having an anogenital abnormality, and progression from low- to high-grade disease is approximately 60% over a 2-year period.[80] As with cervical carcinoma, the key to diagnosis is rigorous surveillance for anal intraepithelial neoplasia in the population at risk, with anal cytology and anoscopy.[86]

Carcinoma *in situ* can frequently be approached with measures employed for the treatment of genital warts, that is, topical podophyllin, topical 5-fluorouracil (5-FU) and laser therapy. In patients with low-grade, early-stage lesions (T1 and possibly some T2) without any evidence of nodal involvement, local excision with wide margins may be acceptable if the sphincter function is preserved. However, the majority of patients with HIV anal carcinoma present with more advanced primary anal tumors, nodal involvement, or both, and if treatment is to be administered in a definitive fashion, then chemoradiation is the treatment of choice. Both the EORTC phase III randomized trial showing the benefit of the addition of chemotherapy to radiation, and the RTOG phase III randomized trial showing the benefit of adding mitomycin to 5-FU and radiation have led to the general acceptance of 5-FU, mitomycin-C and radiation therapy as the standard of care.[87, 88] This treatment should be offered to HIV-infected patients with appropriately staged anal carcinoma, if possible. However, consideration should be given to withholding mitomycin in patients with advanced HIV because of the potential for severe myelosuppression and hemolytic uremic syndrome. Although the RTOG data has shown a higher incidence of recurrence and need for colostomy in patients with breaks greater than 10 days during the course of radiation, radiation administered in conjunction with chemotherapy in the treatment of anal cancer frequently results in marked moist desquamation, necessitating temporary cessation of therapy. Data from University of California at San Francisco (UCSF) have shown that patients with HIV infection require longer breaks from therapy because of severe skin reactions, and they uniformly require chemotherapy dose reductions because of neutropenia.[89] Again, as in the treatment of all HIV-infected patients, the patient's overall condition and comorbid existing diseases must influence the choice of therapy, including the extent of the radiation portal and the specific drugs and drug dosages that are prescribed.

As compared with the non–HIV-infected population, there is a suggestion that HIV-infected patients with anal carcinoma appear to have a shorter survival and a higher incidence of local failure. In the UCSF series, four of the seven HIV-positive patients died at mean of 8 months following therapy, and three of these four patients experienced local recurrence prior to their death.[85] However, eight HIV-infected patients treated with chemotherapy and reduced dose radiation (30 Gy in 15 fractions) at Kaiser Permanente achieved complete response.[90] At a median follow-up of 38 months, four patients were alive and free of disease. The remaining four were dead of AIDS-related causes, but they remained free of anal cancer until death. The variable outcome is probably due to multiple factors, including the heterogeneity of patients and the extent of their immunosuppression.

Hodgkin's Disease

The relationship between Hodgkin's disease and HIV infection is not clearly understood.[91] Although there may be an increased risk of Hodgkin's disease in patients who are infected with HIV, this increase is difficult to measure because both diseases typically occur in the same age population. Consequently, only a very large increase would be detected early. It is clear, however, that the Hodgkin's disease that occurs in patients who are HIV infected tends to be of advanced extent, tends to be associated with B symptoms, and is not likely to be cured.[92] Although immunologic function appears better preserved in HIV-associated Hodgkin's disease than in HIV-associated non-Hodgkin's lymphoma, the outcome of treatment of HIV-associated Hodgkin's disease is worse than that observed in the uninfected population. Only 50% of patients have complete resolution of this disease following combination chemotherapy, and only 40% will be free of disease after 1 year.[93, 94]

Pediatric Malignancies

Despite a decline in perinatally acquired HIV infection (most likely attributable to zidovudine therapy of pregnant

HIV-infected women), a substantial number of children develop AIDS.[95] These children appear to be at increased risk of developing tumors of smooth muscle origin and lymphomas.[96, 97] Several groups, including the Pediatric Oncology Group and the Children's Cancer Group, are now attempting to quantify the scope of the problem in the pediatric population.

Special Considerations

Treatment of malignancies in the AIDS population is particularly challenging. Not only do the majority of HIV-infected patients who present with malignancies do so with advanced stage disease but treatment is frequently made difficult by the complicating factors of their immunosuppressed state and coexisting opportunistic infections. It is crucial to individualize care to each patient's needs and abilities. The decision to provide definitive versus palliative care must take into consideration not only the specific nature of the malignancy being treated but also the host's status, viral load, and the timeline of the patient's disease. The benefit-risk ratio of treatment must be weighed. Concern may be warranted over the potential immunosuppressive effects of high-dose chemotherapy or large-field radiation. Intensive chemotherapy and radiation therapy can compromise a so-called normal immune system, and the effect on an immune status already compromised by HIV infection may be even more burdensome. At present, HAART should be instituted in patients who will undergo intensive chemotherapeutic and radiotherapeutic regimens to reduce the viral load.[98, 99] Consideration should be given to the potential drug-drug interactions that could result. Prophylaxis should be instituted against *Pneumocystis carinii,* and it should be considered for *Mycobacterium avium-intracellulare* and cytomegalovirus.[100] Yet, it is unclear whether potential immunosuppressive effects of radiation therapy clinically influence outcome or the likelihood of HIV replication. In fact, the pathogenesis of HIV infection is so complex that there are tantalizing, seemingly paradoxical, suggestions that whole-body radiation therapy may be beneficial in the setting of HIV.[101, 102] In terms of toxicity, HIV-infected patients who have CD4 counts above 200 cells/mm^3 have been reported to tolerate, at least acutely, the short-term effects of radiation therapy as well as HIV-uninfected patients.[38]

Conclusion

Malignancies have been associated with HIV infection since the beginning of the epidemic. The unifying characteristics of the various AIDS-related malignancies include their nearly always advanced stage at presentation and the less salutary outcome following conventional treatment as compared with histologically similar tumors in HIV-uninfected populations. The advent of more effective combination antiretroviral therapy has changed the face of AIDS. It is hoped that if HAART antiretrovirals are instituted in a timely fashion and tolerated by HIV-infected patients, the incidence of HIV-related malignancies will decrease. We must remain attuned to these changes, and as the spectrum of AIDS continues to change in the future, so too must our therapeutic approaches. We must continue to individualize patient care with careful consideration of benefits and risks. The challenge of identifying and treating AIDS-related malignancies remains great. A heightened awareness of the incidence of clinical presentation of these neoplasms will lead to earlier diagnoses and, in association with continued research efforts, improve outcome.

Recommended Reading

A general overview of malignancies associated with the HIV epidemic can be found in the review article by Safai, Diaz, and Schwartz.[49] A more extensive review of various aspects of these diseases is provided in *Hematologic and Oncologic Aspects of HIV Infection*. Specific discussion of the role of radiation in the treatment of HIV-associated malignancies can be found in the excellent article by Swift.[42]

REFERENCES

1. Pear R: New estimate doubles rate of H.I.V. spread. New York Times, November 26, 1997:A6.

1a. Medscape HIV Journal 2000: Conference Report, vol 6, no 3/mha0627, 4th International AIDS Malignancy Conference.

2. Centers for Disease Control: Kaposi's sarcoma and pneumocystis pneumonia among homosexual men—New York City and California. MMWR Morb Mortal Wkly Rep 1981; 30:305–308.

3. Centers for Disease Control: Revision of the case definition of acquired immunodeficiency syndrome for national reporting—United States. Ann Intern Med 1985; 103:402–403.

4. Centers for Disease Control and Prevention: 1993 revised classification system for HIV infection and expanded surveillance case definition for AIDS among adolescents and adults. JAMA 1993; 269:729–730.

5. Serraino D, Pezzotti P, Dorrucci M, et al: Cancer incidence in a cohort of human immunodeficiency virus seroconverters. Cancer 1997; 79:1004–1008.

6. Carpenter CC, Fischl MA, Hammer SM, et al: Antiretroviral therapy for HIV infection in 1996: recommendations of an international panel. International AIDS Society—USA. JAMA 1996; 276:146–154.

7. Bowen DL, Lane HC, Fauci AS: Immunopathogenesis of the acquired immunodeficiency syndrome. Ann Intern Med 1985; 103:704–709.

8. Herndier BG, Kaplan LD, McGrath MS: Pathogenesis of AIDS lymphomas. AIDS 1994; 8:1025–1049.

9. Birx DL, Redfield RR, Tosato G: Defective regulation of Epstein-Barr virus infection in patients with acquired immunodeficiency syndrome (AIDS) or AIDS-related disorders. N Engl J Med 1986; 314:874–879.

10. Beral V, Peterman TA, Berkelman RL, et al: Kaposi's sarcoma among persons with AIDS: a sexually transmitted infection? Lancet 1990; 335:123–128.

11. De Jarlais DC, Marmor M, Thomas P, et al: Kaposi's sarcoma among four different AIDS risk groups. N Engl J Med 1984; 310:1119.

12. Armenian HK, Hoover DR, Rubb S, et al: Composite risk score for Kaposi's sarcoma based on a case-control and longitudinal study in the Multicenter AIDS Cohort Study (MACS) population. Am J Epidemiol 1993; 138:256–265.

13. Gallant JE, Moore RD, Richman DD, et al: Risk factors for Kaposi's sarcoma in patients with advanced human immunodeficiency virus disease treated with zidovudine: Zidovudine Epidemiology Study Group. Arch Intern Med 1994; 154:566–572.

14. Chang Y, Cesarman E, Pessin MS, et al: Identification of herpesvirus-like DNA sequences in AIDS-associated Kaposi's sarcoma. Science 1994; 266:1865–1869.

15. Gao SJ, Kingsley L, Hoover DR, et al: Seroconversion to antibodies

against Kaposi's sarcoma–associated herpesvirus-related latent nuclear antigens before the development of Kaposi's sarcoma. N Engl J Med 1996; 335:233–241.
16. Foreman KE, Friberg J, Kong WP, et al: Propagation of a human herpesvirus from AIDS-associated Kaposi's sarcoma. N Engl J Med 1997; 336:163–171.
17. Ensoli B, Barillari G, Salahuddin SZ, et al: Tat protein of HIV-1 stimulates growth of cells derived from Kaposi's sarcoma lesions of AIDS patients. Nature 1990; 345:84–86.
18. Barillari G, Fiorelli V, Gendelman R, et al: HIV-1 tat protein enhances angiogenesis and Kaposi's sarcoma (KS) development triggered by inflammatory cytokines (IC) of bFGF by engaging the avB integrin [Abstract]. 1st National AIDS Malignancy Conference, Bethesda, Maryland. J Acquir Immune Defic Syndr Hum Retrovirol 1997; 14:A33.
19. Boudreaux AA, Smith LL, Cosby CD, et al: Intralesional vinblastine for cutaneous Kaposi's sarcoma associated with acquired immunodeficiency syndrome: a clinical trial to evaluate efficacy and discomfort associated with injection. J Am Acad Dermatol 1993; 28:61–65.
20. Dupuy J, Price M, Lynch G, et al: Intralesional interferon-alpha and zidovudine in epidemic Kaposi's sarcoma. J Am Acad Dermatol 1993; 28:966–972.
21. Gill PS, Lunardi-Ishkandar Y, Louie S, et al: The effects of preparations of human chorionic gonadotropin on AIDS-related Kaposi's sarcoma. N Engl J Med 1996; 335:1261–1269.
22. Cooper JS, Steinfeld AS, Lerch IA: The prognostic significance of residual pigmentation following radiotherapy of epidemic Kaposi's sarcoma. J Clin Oncol 1989; 7:619–621.
23. Berson AM, Quivey JM, Aarris JW, et al: Radiation therapy for AIDS-related Kaposi's sarcoma. Int J Radiat Oncol Biol Phys 1990; 19:569–575.
24. Cooper JS, Fried PR: Toxicity of oral radiotherapy in patients having AIDS. Arch Otolaryngol Head Neck Surg 1987; 113:327–328.
25. Meyer JL: Whole lung irradiation for Kaposi's sarcoma. Am J Clin Oncol 1993; 16:372–376.
26. Krown SE, Real FX, Cunningham-Rundles S, et al: Preliminary observations on the effect of recombinant leukocyte A interferon in homosexual men with Kaposi's sarcoma. N Engl J Med 1983; 308:1071–1076.
27. Borden EC, Hogan TF, Voelkel JG: Comparative antiproliferative activity in vitro of natural interferons alpha and beta for diploid and human cells. Cancer Res 1982; 42:4948–4953.
28. Lane HC, Kovacs JA, Feinberg J, et al: Anti-retroviral effects of interferon-alpha in AIDS-associated Kaposi's sarcoma. Lancet 1988; 2:1218–1222.
29. Poli G, Oronstein JM, Kinter A, et al: Interferon-alpha but not AZT suppresses HIV expression in chronically infected cell lines. Science 1989; 244:575–577.
30. Sidky YA, Borden EC: Inhibition of angiogenesis by interferons: effects on tumor- and lymphocyte-induced vascular response. Cancer Res 1987; 47:5155–5156.
31. Krown SE: Biology and therapy of HIV-associated Kaposi's sarcoma. The PRN Notebook 1997; 2:2–6.
32. Krown SE, Gold JM, Niedzwiecki D, et al: Interferon-alpha with zidovudine: safety, tolerance and clinical and virologic effects in patients with Kaposi's sarcoma associated with the acquired immunodeficiency syndrome (AIDS). Ann Intern Med 1990; 112:812–821.
33. Fischl MA, Uttamchandani RB, Resnick L, et al: A phase I study of recombinant human interferon-alpha or human lymphoblastoid interferon-alpha and concomitant zidovudine in patients with AIDS-related Kaposi's sarcoma. J Acquir Immune Defic Syndr Hum Retroviral 1991; 4:1–10.
34. Laubenstein LJ, Krigel RL, Odajnky CM, et al: Treatment of epidemic Kaposi's sarcoma with etoposide or a combination of doxorubicin, bleomycin, and vincristine. J Clin Oncol 1984; 2:1115–1120.
35. Gelmann E, Longo D, Lane H, et al: Combination chemotherapy of disseminated Kaposi's sarcoma in patients with the acquired immune deficiency syndrome. Am J Med 1987; 82:456–461.
36. Gill PS, Rarick MU, McCutchan JA, et al: Systemic treatment of AIDS-related Kaposi's sarcoma: results of a randomized trial. Am J Med 1991; 90:427–433.
37. Aversa SM, Cattelan AM, Salvagno L, et al: Chemo-immunotherapy of advanced AIDS-related Kaposi's sarcoma. Tumori 1999; 85:54–59.
38. Stewart S, Jablonowski H, Goebel FD, et al: Randomized comparative trial of pegylated liposomal doxorubicin versus bleomycin and vincristine in the treatment of AIDS-related Kaposi's sarcoma. J Clin Oncol 1998; 16:683–691.
39. Gill PS, Wernz J, Scadden D, et al: Randomized phase III trial of liposomal daunorubicin versus doxorubicin, bleomycin, and vincristine in AIDS-related Kaposi's sarcoma. J Clin Oncol 1996; 14:2353–2364.
40. Northfelt D, Stewart S: DOXIL (Pegylated liposomal doxorubicin) as first-line therapy of AIDS-related Kaposi's sarcoma (KS): integrated efficacy and safety results from two comparative trials [Abstract]. Abstracts of the 4th Conference on Retroviruses and Opportunistic Infections 1997; 736:200.
41. Gill PS, Tulpule A, Reynolds T, et al: Paclitaxel (Taxol) in the treatment of relapsed or refractory advanced AIDS-related Kaposi's sarcoma [Abstract]. Proceedings of the American Society of Clinical Oncology 1996; 15:A854.
42. Swift PS: Radiation therapy for malignancies in the setting of HIV disease. Oncology 1997; 11:683–694.
43. Volm M, Wernz J: Patients with advanced AIDS-related Kaposi's sarcoma (EKS) no longer require systemic chemotherapy after introduction of effective antiretroviral therapy [Abstract]. Proceedings of the American Society of Clinical Oncology 1997; 16:A46.
44. Beral V, Peterman T, Berkleman R, et al: AIDS-associated non-Hodgkin's lymphoma. Lancet 1991; 337:805–809.
45. Biggan RJ, Rabkin CS: The epidemiology of acquired immunodeficiency syndrome-related lymphomas. Curr Opin Oncol 1992; 4:883–893.
46. Centers for Disease Control: Update on acquired immune deficiency syndrome (AIDS)—United States. MMWR Morb Mortal Wkly Rep 1981; 31:507–514.
47. Lane HC, Fauci AS: Immunologic abnormalities in the acquired immunodeficiency syndrome. Annual Review of Immunology 1985; 3:477–500.
48. Laurence J, Astrin SM: Human immunodeficiency virus induction of malignant transformation in human B lymphocytes. Proc Natl Acad Sci USA 1991; 88:7635–7639.
49. Safai B, Diaz B, Schwartz J: Malignant neoplasms associated with human immunodeficiency virus infection. CA Cancer J Clin 1996; 42:74–90.
50. Gill PS, Levine AM, Krailo M, et al: AIDS-related malignant lymphoma: Results of prospective treatment trials. J Clin Oncol 1987; 5:1322–1328.
51. Kaplan LD, Abrams DI, Feigel E, et al: AIDS-associated non-Hodgkin's lymphomas in San Francisco. JAMA 1989; 261:719–724.
52. Levine AM, Sullivan-Halley J, Pike MC, et al: Human immunodeficiency virus–related lymphoma. Prognostic factors predictive of survival. Cancer 1991; 68:2466–2472.
53. Levine AM, Wernz JC, Kaplan L, et al: Low dose chemotherapy with central nervous system prophylaxis and zidovudine maintenance in AIDS-related lymphoma. JAMA 1991; 226:84–88.
54. Bermudez AM, Grant K, Rodvien R, et al: Non-Hodgkin's lymphoma in a population with or at risk for acquired immunodeficiency syndrome: indications for intensive chemotherapy. Am J Med 1989; 86:71–76.
55. Levine AM, Espina BE, Tulpule A, et al: Low dose mBACOD with concomitant dideoxycytidine (ddC): an effective regimen in AIDS-related lymphoma [Abstract]. Blood 1993; 82(suppl):A1531.
56. Gisselbracht C, Oskenhendler E, Tirelli U, et al: Human immunodeficiency virus–related lymphoma treatment with intensive combination chemotherapy. Am J Med 1993; 95:188–196.
57. Sparano JA, Wiernik PH, Strack M, et al: Infusional cyclophosphamide, doxorubicin and etoposide in HIV-related non-Hodgkin's lymphoma: a follow-up report of a highly active regimen. Leuk Lymphoma 1994; 14:263–271.
57a. Donahue B: Lymphomatous meningitis in HIV-associated non-Hodgkin's lymphoma: An unexpected pattern of relapse. Pages presented at: Ninth Inernational Congress on Anti-Cancer Treatment; January 1999; Paris.
58. Levine AM, Goll PS, Meyer PR, et al: Retrovirus and malignant lymphoma in homosexual men. JAMA 1985; 254:1921–1925.
59. Lowenthal DA, Strauss DJ, Campbell SW, et al: AIDS-related lymphoid neoplasia: the Memorial Hospital experience. Cancer 1988; 61:2325–2337.
60. Knowles DM, Chemulak GA, Subar M, et al: Lymphoid neoplasia

associated with the acquired immunodeficiency syndrome (AIDS). Ann Intern Med 1988; 108:744–753.
61. Ansari MQ, Dawson DB, Nadon R, et al: Primary body cavity–based AIDS-related lymphomas. Am J Clin Pathol 1996; 105:221–229.
62. Jaffe ES: Primary body cavity–based AIDS-related lymphomas: evolution of a new disease entity. Am J Clin Pathol 1996; 105:141–143.
63. Formenti SC, Gill PS, Lean E, et al: Primary central nervous system lymphoma in AIDS—results of radiation therapy. Cancer 1989; 63:1101–1107.
64. Levine AM: AIDS-associated malignant lymphoma. Med Clin North Am 1992; 76:253–268.
65. Tachikawa N, Goto M, Hoshino Y, et al: Detection of Toxoplasma gondii, Epstein-Barr virus, and JC virus DNAs in the cerebrospinal fluid in acquired immunodeficiency patients with focal central nervous system complications. Intern Med 1999; 38:556–562.
66. Donahue BR, Sullivan JW, Cooper JS: Additional experience with empiric radiotherapy for HIV-associated primary CNS lymphoma. Cancer 1995; 76:328–332.
67. Loureiro C, Gill PS, Meyer PR, et al: Autopsy findings in AIDS-related lymphoma. Cancer 1988; 62:735–739.
68. Porter SB, Sarde MA: Toxoplasmosis of the central nervous system in the acquired immunodeficiency syndrome. N Engl J Med 1992; 327:1640–1643.
69. Kramer EL, Wasserheit C, Sanger J, et al: Identification of AIDS-related lymphoma using Tc-99m FAB fragment of Immu-LL2 antibody (Lymphoscan TM). Journal of the International Society of Tumor Targeting 1996; 2:18.
70. Baumgartner JE, Rachlin JR, Beckstead JH, et al: Primary central nervous system lymphomas: natural history: response to radiation therapy in 55 patients with acquired immunodeficiency syndrome. J Neurosurg 1990; 73:206–211.
71. Remick SC, Diamond C, Migliozzi JA, et al: Primary central nervous system lymphoma in patients with and without the acquired immunodeficiency syndrome—a retrospective analysis and review of the literature. Medicine 1990; 69:345–360.
72. Corn B, Donahue B, Rosenstock J, et al: Performance status and age as independent predictors of survival among AIDS patients with primary CNS lymphoma: a multivariate analysis of a multi-institutional experience. Cancer J Sci Am 1997; 3:52–56.
73. Maiman M, Fruchter RG, Clark M, et al: Cervical cancer as an AIDS-defining illness. Obstet Gynecol 1997; 89:76–80.
74. Schafer A, Friedman W, Mielke M, et al: The increased frequency of cervical dysplasia-neoplasia in women infected with the human immunodeficiency virus is related to the degree of immunosuppression. Am J Obstet Gynecol 1991; 164:593–599.
75. Williams AB, Darragh TM, Vranizar K, et al: Analysis of cervical human papilloma virus infection and risk of anal and cervical epithelial abnormalities in human immunodeficiency virus-infected women. Obstet Gynecol 1994; 83:205–211.
76. Sun XW, Kuhn L, Ellenbrock TV, et al: Human papillomavirus infection in women infected with the human immunodeficiency virus. N Engl J Med 1997; 337:1343–1349.
77. Varmuad SH, Kelley KF, Klein RS, et al: High risk of human papillomavirus infection and cervical squamous intraepithelial lesions among women with symptomatic human immunodeficiency virus infection. Am J Obstet Gynecol 1991; 165:392–400.
78. Maiman M, Fruchter RG, Guy L, et al: Human immunodeficiency virus infection and invasive cervical carcinoma. Cancer 1993; 71:402–406.
78a. National Cancer Institute Clinical Announcement: Concurrent chemoradiation for cervical carcinoma. U.S. Department of Health and Human Services, Public Health Service, National Institutes of Health. February 1999.
79. Cuthill S, Maiman M, Fruchter RG: Complications after treatment of cervical intraepithelial neoplasia in women infected with the human immunodeficiency virus. J Reprod Med 1995; 40:823–828.
80. Chadha M, Sood B, Stanson R: Patients with human immunodeficiency virus (HIV): infections and cervical neoplasia [Abstract]. Int J Radiat Oncol Biol Phys 1984; 30 (Suppl 1):284.
81. Melbye M, Rabkin CS, Frisch M, et al: Changing patterns of anal cancer incidence in the United States, 1946–1989. Am J Epidemiol 1994; 139:772–780.
82. Melbye M, Coté TR, Kessler L: High incidence of anal cancer among AIDS patients. Lancet 1994; 343:636–639.
83. Carlson RH: Increase in anal cancer rates not due to AIDS. Oncology Times: October 1996:52.
84. Northfelt DW, Swift PS, Palefsky JM: Anal dysplasia: pathogenesis, diagnosis and management. In: Krown SE, von Roenn JH (eds): Hematologic and Oncologic Aspects of HIV Infection, pp 1177–1188. Hematology Oncology Clinics of North America. Philadelphia, W.B. Saunders, 1996.
85. Frisch M, Glimelius B, Van Der Brule AJC, et al: Sexually transmitted infection as a cause of anal cancer. N Engl J Med 1997; 337:1350–1358.
86. Palefsky JM, Holly EA, Hogeboom CJ: Anal cytology as a screening tool for anal squamous intraepithelial lesions. J Acquir Immune Defic Syndr Hum Retrovirol 1997; 14:415–422.
87. Bartelink H, Roelofsen F, Eschwege F, et al: Concomitant radiotherapy and chemotherapy is superior to radiotherapy alone in the treatment of locally advanced anal cancer: results of a phase III randomized trial of the European Organization for Research and Treatment of Cancer Radiotherapy and Gastrointestinal Cooperative Groups. J Clin Oncol 1997; 15:2040–2049.
88. Flam M, John M, Pajak TF, et al: Role of mitomycin in combination with fluorouracil and radiotherapy, and of salvage chemoradiation in the definitive nonsurgical treatment of epidermoid carcinoma of the anal canal: results of a phase III randomized intergroup study. J Clin Oncol 1996; 14:2527–2539.
89. Hollan JM, Swift PS: Tolerance of patients with human immunodeficiency virus and anal carcinoma to treatment with combined chemotherapy and radiation therapy. Radiology 1994; 193:251–254.
90. Peddada AV, Smith PE, Rao AR: Chemotherapy and low-dose radiotherapy in the treatment of HIV-infected patients with carcinoma of the anal canal. Int J Radiat Oncol Biol Phys 1997; 37:1101–1105.
91. Hessol NA, Katz MH, Liu JY, et al: Increased incidence of Hodgkin's disease in homosexual men with HIV infection. Ann Intern Med 1992; 117:309–311.
92. Errante D, Zaganel V, Vaccher E, et al: Hodgkin's disease in patients with HIV infection and in the general population: comparison of clinicopathologic features and survival. Ann Oncol 1994; 2:37–40.
93. Pelstring RJ, Zellmer RB, Sulak LE, et al: Hodgkin's disease in association with human immunodeficiency virus infection: pathologic and immunologic features. Cancer 1991; 67:1865–1873.
94. Ames ED, Conjalka MS, Goldberg AF, et al: Hodgkin's disease and AIDS: twenty-three new cases and a review of the literature. Hematol Oncol Clin North Am 1991; 5:343–356.
95. Centers for Disease Control and Prevention: AIDS among children—United States, 1996. MMWR Morb Mortal Wkly Rep 1996; 45:1005–1010.
96. Chadwick EG, Connor EJ, Hanson IC, et al: Tumors of smooth-muscle origin in HIV-infected children. JAMA 1990; 263:3182–3184.
97. Epstein LG, DiCarlo FJ, Joshi VV, et al: Primary lymphomas of the central nervous system in two children with acquired immunodeficiency syndrome. Ann J Clin Pathol 1990; 94:722–728.
98. Hammer SM, Katzenstein DA, Hughes MD, et al: A trial comparing nucleoside monotherapy with combination therapy in HIV-infected adults with CD4 counts from 200 to 500 per cubic millimeter. N Engl J Med 1996; 335:1081–1090.
99. Delta Coordinating Committee: A randomized double-blind controlled trial comparing combinations of Zidovudine plus didanosine and Zalcitabine with Zidovudine alone in HIV-infected individuals. Lancet 1996; 348:283–291.
100. USPHS/ISDA: Guidelines for the prevention of opportunistic infections in persons infected with human immunodeficiency virus: a summary. Ann Intern Med 1997; 124:349–368.
101. del Regato JA: Trial of fractionated total-body irradiation in the treatment of patients with acquired immunodeficiency syndrome: a preliminary report. Am J Clin Oncol 1989; 12:365.
102. Fricker J: Baboon xenotransplant fails but patient improves. Lancet 1996; 347:457.

13 *Oncologic Emergencies*

JAMES W. KELLER, MD, Radiation Oncology
JAMES B. BENTON, MD, Radiation Oncology

Ignorance more frequently begets confidence than does knowledge: it is those who know little, and not those who know much, who so positively assert that this or that problem will never be solved by science.

CHARLES DARWIN
Introduction, *THE DESCENT OF MAN* (1871)

Perspective

Oncologic emergencies in this chapter have been arbitrarily divided into three categories: Anatomical/Mechanical, Metabolic, and Hematologic. Most present themselves in a setting of known cancer; however, this is not always the case. It is usually mandatory to establish a diagnosis of malignancy before embarking on therapies with potentially serious side effects, such as radiation or chemotherapy. The oncologist with the prepared mind will recognize the potential for an emergency earlier, which will lead to earlier diagnosis and treatment that should be associated with a better outcome and less morbidity.[5] The emergency may herald a poor prognosis and need for palliative care; on the other hand, in some situations, the condition may lead to an early diagnosis, effective treatment, and cure. It is a truism that the development of new problems in the cancer setting are always ascribed to the cancer, but a more benign process may be responsible. These clinical conditions are not always true emergencies requiring urgent care; clinical judgment is no less important in these instances. With the recognition of the need for hospice, comfort care during the natural history of advanced cancers, the emergent situation may be the patient's so-called friend.

Anatomical/Mechanical

Increased Intracranial Pressure

Increased intracranial pressure (ICP) may accompany primary or metastatic neoplasms of the central nervous system (CNS). The causative tumors are usually located in the brain parenchyma; leptomeningeal metastatic disease also produces increased ICP. As mass lesions within the brain expand, pressure in the semirigid cranial compartment rises. Eventually the autoregulatory mechanisms that preserve cerebral blood flow are defeated and CNS hypoxia develops. More importantly, brain shifts occur, leading to central and uncal tentorial herniation and to life-threatening brain stem injury. Leptomeningeal metastases interfere with cerebrospinal fluid (CSF) absorption and raise ICP by an indirect mechanism.

Brain metastases occur in 20% to 30% of all cancer patients.[6] In adults, brain lesions are usually metastases from melanoma or lung, breast, kidney, or GI carcinomas, and they are characteristically multiple. Primary brain tumors in adults are most commonly gliomas (astrocytomas, ependymomas, or oligodendrogliomas) and are usually solitary lesions. Leptomeningeal metastases are most often associated with acute leukemias and lymphomas, but they are also seen with solid tumors, especially lung and breast carcinomas.[7, 8]

Diagnosis

1. Symptoms of ICP include headache, nausea and vomiting, blurred vision, diplopia, unsteadiness, and altered mentation. Headache is classically worse in the morning, clears then recurs later in the day, is exacerbated by coughing or straining, and is relieved with vomiting.
2. Signs of ICP include bilateral papilledema (present in only 50% of cases) and nuchal rigidity (in patients with meningeal disease). New onset of seizures may herald CNS metastases. Focal neurologic deficits referable to the tumor location also are observed, for example, hemiparesis, ataxia, and difficulty with calculations, speech, or writing. Herniation is usually associated with severe headache, vomiting, third nerve palsy with unilateral pupillary dilatation, systemic hypertension, bradycardia, hemiparesis, and decerebrate rigidity or coma.[9]
3. Contrast computed tomography (CT) or magnetic resonance imaging (MRI) scan of the brain is urgently needed. MRI is more specific, but it may not be as immediately available and may be more expensive. Frequent findings include hydrocephalus, vasogenic edema, mass effect, and contrast-enhanced lesions. Lumbar puncture is contraindicated in patients with intracranial masses because removal of CSF may precipitate brain shift and herniation.
4. MRI with gadolinium contrast of the spine or cytologic evaluation of the CSF is required to confirm leptomeningeal metastases. Repeated sampling may be needed to detect abnormal cells.

5. In most clinical situations, the development of neurologic symptoms or signs and a positive brain CT or MRI scan are enough to diagnose metastatic disease. If not, then a stereotactic biopsy may be necessary.

Therapy

1. Corticosteroids are the mainstay of the initial therapy to reduce edema. Ten to 50 mg IV (intravenously) of dexamethasone is given as a loading dose, followed by 4 to 6 mg PO (orally) every 6 hours. Anticonvulsants are given if seizures are present.
2. Patients with rapidly evolving herniation require intubation and mechanical hyperventilation to maintain the pulmonary arterial pressure of CO_2 around 30 mm Hg. The osmotic diuretic mannitol is administered 1.5 to 2.0 g/kg IV, repeated every 4 to 6 hours. Monitoring of ICP by ventriculostomy or other indwelling cerebral monitoring devices may be required.[10]
3. Radiation therapy is usually used for patients with brain metastases. Treatment consists of 30 Gy in 10 fractions delivered to the whole brain. Data suggest that patients with a good performance status and a single brain metastasis do much better with surgery, followed by radiation.[6, 11, 12] Radiosurgery appears to be a promising alternative to craniotomy, and it is being used to treat suitable solitary metastases in some situations. Median survival is 4 to 6 months with whole brain radiation and 10 months with surgery and radiation, or radiosurgery.[6, 13–15]
4. Surgical exploration is indicated for patients with suspected primary brain tumors. Radiation therapy is administered after resection because residual disease is invariably present.
5. Chemotherapy does not have a role in the emergency treatment of intraparenchymal brain lesions; however, intrathecal or intraventricular (via an Ommaya reservoir) chemotherapy (methotrexate, cytarabine) is the treatment of choice for leptomeningeal metastases. It is sometimes combined with radiation therapy to the whole brain or areas of bulk meningeal disease.

Spinal Cord Compression

Advanced spinal cord compression by tumor has devastating sequelae, including paraplegia, incontinence, and quadriplegia, with all of the emotional and nursing consequences of such conditions. Recognition of incipient cord compression is important, because expeditious treatment at this stage prevents irreversible neurologic injury. Neoplastic cord compression is almost always secondary to extramedullary, extradural metastases (most often from breast, lung, prostate, lymphoma, or kidney); primary spinal cord tumors are unusual. Compression of the cord develops by posterior expansion of vertebral metastatic disease or by extension of paraspinal metastases through the intervertebral foramina. In 70% of cases, the thoracic spinal cord is involved. The lumbar and cervical spine are involved in 20% and 10% of cases, respectively.[16, 17]

Diagnosis

1. Almost all patients present initially with neck or back pain, which may be central or radicular. Leg weakness, numbness, and paresthesias follow; loss of sphincter control is a late event. Spine tenderness is common, and neck flexion or straight leg raising may provoke radicular pain. The specific neurologic findings depend on the level of the cord lesion (Table 13–1).
2. Plain films of the spine frequently demonstrate associated vertebral blastic or lytic lesions. MRI of the spine is the procedure of choice for detection and localization of cord compression. If MRI is not available, then myelography may be employed and combined with CT. At the time of myelography, the CSF should be sent for cytology.

Therapy

1. Dexamethasone should be administered immediately to reduce edema. Frequently prescribed doses are 4 mg every 6 hours, but loading doses as high as 100 mg have been used.
2. Decompression laminectomy is indicated initially if a tissue diagnosis is required, if the cord compression is in a previously irradiated area, or if neurologic deterioration occurs during radiation treatment. Laminectomy may also be considered for patients with radioresistant tumors or in those patients with rapid evolution of paraplegia. Now, with the increasing skill of interventional radiologists and pathologists, diagnoses are increasingly being made by needle aspirates. Spine surgeons also are more aware that surgery in these situations may demand stabilization of the spine rather than a simple laminectomy.[18, 19, 20]

TABLE 13–1. **Clinical Findings in Spinal Cord Compression**

Sign/Deficit	Spinal Cord	Conus Medullaris	Cauda Equina
Weakness	Symmetric, profound	Symmetrical, variable	Asymmetric, may be mild
Deep tendon reflexes	Increased or absent	Increased knee, decreased ankle	Decreased
Plantar reflex	Extensor	Extensor	Plantar
Sensory	Symmetric sensory level	Symmetric saddle	Asymmetric, radicular
Sphincters	Late onset	Early onset	Spared possibly
Progression	Rapid	Variable	Variable

3. Radiation therapy alone is used for patients with radiosensitive cancer, lesions below the conus medullaris, slow onset of compression, medical contraindications to surgery, or surgically unapproachable disease. Patients treated initially with decompression should also receive postoperative radiotherapy. Initially, high doses of radiation should be administered (4 Gy × 3). Subsequently, the daily fraction size can be reduced to conventional dose size and the total dose adjusted appropriately to biologic cord tolerance.
4. If effective chemotherapeutic agents are available for patients who can no longer benefit from surgical intervention or radiation therapy, they obviously should be employed.
5. The results of treatment are best in patients who present with minimal or no neurologic impairment and poorest in those with established paraplegia. About 60% to 70% of patients with minimal or no neurologic impairment are able to walk after treatment, compared with 55% of patients with established paraplegia. There is very little that is more satisfying to an oncologist than to see the patient walking into the office several months after treatment for spinal cord compression.[16, 21]

Superior Vena Cava Syndrome

Obstruction of the superior vena cava produces a unique clinical syndrome of facial, neck, and, occasionally, arm or truncal edema, with facial erythema and frequently the presence of chest venous collaterals. It is produced by the tumor compressing the cava (or a blood clot within), which, in turn, is associated with the development of collaterals. Collaterals allow blood to circumvent the obstruction and return to the right side of the heart[22]; the rate of caval obstruction and degree of compensatory venous collateralization determine the severity. It is infrequently a true emergency, unless there is accompanying cerebral edema with impending herniation, stridor with laryngeal edema or tracheal compression, or accompanying pericardial effusion or significant pleural effusion. The cause for the external compression now is almost always (>80%) neoplastic, with lung cancer accounting for approximately 70% of cases, lymphomas 15%, and a smaller number related to sarcomas, testicular cancers, or metastases. Thrombosis related to central venous catheters may be another cause, and thrombosis superimposed upon the obstruction may occur as well.[23–25]

Diagnosis

1. Dyspnea, facial swelling with erythema, upper extremity and truncal edema, chest pains, and cough are frequent. Headaches, nausea and vomiting, visual disturbances, and syncope usually suggest more serious aspects of the syndrome or concomitant central nervous system metastases. Hoarseness, stridor, dysphagia, and back pain suggest involvement of laryngeal nerves, trachea or larynx, esophagus, or vertebral bodies. Upper body venous distention is a common physical finding. Facial cyanosis is not common.
2. A chest film usually reveals a right-sided paratracheal or mediastinal mass; rarely, this mass may be very subtle and delay the diagnosis. A chest CT scan with contrast is diagnostic and also helps define the extent of the disease. Venography is rarely indicated unless there is a question of thrombosis and need for thrombolytic therapy.
3. A tissue diagnosis is mandatory and is usually obtained via bronchoscopy, fine-needle aspiration, excisional biopsy of a supraclavicular node, or CT-directed biopsy of a mass or lymph node in the chest. The tissue diagnosis could be pursued during the treatment if the patient is severely symptomatic and urgent therapy is indicated.

Therapy

1. Initial treatment is dependent upon the diagnosis. The mainstay of treatment is usually radiation therapy because most of the causes are related to lung cancer. Symptomatic relief occurs in 70% to 90% of cases, with only approximately 10% to 15% being nonresponders.[23]
2. The fractionation of radiation is important, and usually several high-dose fractions (3 to 4 Gy) are given initially to achieve rapid tumor reduction and relief of symptoms. Accelerated hyperfractionation (twice-daily treatments separated by at least 6 hours with fraction size greater than 1.5 Gy) also would be reasonable.
3. Small cell lung cancer, non-Hodgkin's lymphomas, and non-seminoma testicular cancers can be treated initially with chemotherapy, with or without radiation, depending upon the severity of the condition.
4. Although many patients are treated with corticosteroids, their role in this disease is questionable. Most oncologists do not use corticosteroids or administer them for a short course and continue only if response is noted or there is evidence of cerebral edema. It is theoretically possible that use of corticosteroids might confuse a diagnosis of a lymphoma.
5. The role of thrombolytic therapy in this condition remains unresolved. Because most patients respond to treatment, it has not been routine but reserved for those patients who are not responding or progressing. Intraluminal stenting, as used in other vascular situations, has also been used as an adjunct in this situation.
6. The survival of patients with non–small cell lung cancer presenting with this syndrome varies from 15% to 20% at 1 year and is related to the initial extent of disease; an occasional patient may survive over 5 years. The role of concomitant chemotherapy or subsequent chemotherapy in this setting has not been clearly established.

Pleural Effusion

Malignant pleural effusions are exudates (rather than transudates) and are related to tumor cell implants on the visceral or parietal pleura. Less commonly, the effusion may develop because of impairment of pleural lymphatic drainage by a mediastinal tumor. Metastatic breast and lung cancer and lymphoma account for more than 75% of malignant pleural effusions. A large pleural effusion can severely restrict ventilation and contributes to respiratory insufficiency in the cancer patient.

Diagnosis

1. Patients complain of dyspnea, unproductive cough, and dull chest discomfort. Physical findings include decreased breath sounds and dullness to percussion in the area of effusion.
2. Significant pleural effusions are visible on chest x-ray films. Lateral decubitus films will demonstrate layering of the fluid if it is not loculated.
3. Diagnostic thoracentesis is required to confirm a malignant etiology. Cytologic examination confirms the diagnosis in most cases, although, occasionally, a pleural biopsy or laparoscopic thoracoscopy is necessary.[26] Pleural fluid chemistries (L-lactate dehydrogenase [LDH], protein, glucose, pH), cultures, and blood cell count should also be obtained. Exudates are generally defined by a pleural fluid protein/serum protein level higher than 0.5 or a pleural fluid LDH/serum LDH level higher than 0.6 or an LDH level higher than ⅔ of the upper limit in serum.[27]

Therapy

1. Removal of the fluid provides immediate relief of the dyspnea. However, this is rarely longlasting without more definitive therapy, such as sclerosis or treatment of the underlying condition.
2. Nowadays, recurrent symptomatic effusion is treated with chest tube drainage and a sclerosing agent, such as doxycycline, bleomycin, or talc.[28] This strategy is effective in 70% to 85% cases. Investigational drainage systems into the peritoneal cavity are also being evaluated.[29]
3. Effusions related to lymphomas, breast cancer, and lung cancer frequently respond to chemotherapy and radiation. A course of radiation to the mediastinum is the mainstay of treatment for a chylous effusion because of malignant invasion or obstruction of the thoracic duct.[30]

Hemoptysis

Hemoptysis can be a life-threatening condition. Massive hemoptysis is defined as the expectoration of at least 600 cm^3 of blood in a 24-hour period.[31] The most common cause for hemoptysis is infection followed by bronchogenic cancer. In the lung cancer patient, the most frequent site is from erosion of the cancer into a blood vessel or from friable neovascular tissue. Other causes of hemoptysis could include tracheal and laryngeal cancers, and nonmalignant diseases, such as tuberculosis, bronchiectasis, bronchitis, pulmonary thromboembolism, or congestive heart failure; metastatic disease to the lung is rarely associated with hemoptysis.[25, 32, 33]

Diagnosis

1. It is essential to determine that the blood is coming from the respiratory tract.
2. Patients should be closely monitored, given supplemental oxygen (and possibly a mixture of helium and oxygen), and suctioned judiciously.
3. A complete blood count, coagulation studies, sputum examination, and a chest x-ray film should be obtained immediately.
4. A thorough examination of the upper aerodigestive tract is warranted. This usually requires bronchoscopy using a ventilation scope.
5. Subsequent exams should include a CT scan of the chest. Angiography should be considered for those patients without an identifiable source.

Therapy

1. The mainstays of therapy are bed rest and cough suppression.
2. Patients who are unstable should be admitted to the intensive care unit for close monitoring and given blood or blood products, as warranted.
3. A skilled pulmonologist or thoracic surgeon may contain the bleeding endoscopically with laser therapy, catheter tamponade, iced saline, or selective bronchial intubation.
4. If the patient is not a surgical candidate and has a malignancy, he or she should be considered for external beam radiation therapy, or high dose rate brachytherapy.[34]
5. Some patients may require embolization of a vessel with the assistance of interventional radiology.

Airway Obstruction

Neoplasms of the head and neck, thyroid, parathyroids, esophagus, trachea, lung, and lymphomas may cause airway obstruction by compressing the airway or invading it anywhere from the base of tongue to the carina. An 80% reduction in the luminal cross sectional area is generally required before the patient's symptoms become acute.[25]

Diagnosis

1. Symptoms include wheezing, dyspnea, orthopnea, and stridor, but these problems are often accompanied and preceded by pain, hoarseness, dysphagia, odynophagia, and speech difficulties.
2. Physical findings may be minimal, except for the obvious shortness of breath and retraction of the suprasternal and intercostal spaces, but they may include a neck mass. A high index of suspicion is often necessary to make a diagnosis.
3. A chest x-ray film may reveal a superior mediastinal mass or widening and deviation or compression of the trachea. Obviously, a thorough indirect or flexible laryngoscopy ear, nose, and throat examination is paramount to identifying more proximal upper airway lesions. However, it is important to perform endoscopy gingerly because repeated attempts may precipitate complete respiratory decompression. Nowadays, a CT scan of the neck and chest is performed, if time and symptoms permit, to help localize the problem. Pulmonary function tests with flow-loop studies can

help identify the anatomical site and physiologic implications of these tumors.

4. Pathologic diagnosis can be made on the basis of sputum cytology, needle aspiration, biopsy of suspicious peripheral nodes, or via ventilated bronchoscopy with brushings, washings, or biopsy.

Therapy

1. The patient should be monitored closely and given supplemental humidified oxygen; equipment for a tracheotomy or intubation should be immediately available.
2. Corticosteroids can be given and may produce some decrease in surrounding edema, allowing more time for investigation.
3. If the situation is critical and the obstruction is not subglottic, then the first approach is insertion of a large bore needle into the cricothyroid membrane. Oral endotracheal tubes are fraught with problems and require an experienced individual to insert one without worsening the situation. When bleeding is a problem related to a bleeding diathesis, thrombocytopenia, or a clotting abnormality, endotracheal tube insertion may be preferable to surgery if this problem cannot be quickly corrected with replacement therapy.
4. A tracheotomy is generally preferable to a cricothyroidotomy because there are more potential complications related to the cricothyroidotomy. Nonetheless, the cricothyroid membrane approach is attractive because it is superficial and lacks blood vessels; however, infections, necrosis, glottic edema, subglottic stenosis, and the need for a tracheotomy are drawbacks.
5. Therapy should follow based on a thorough evaluation of the condition. Radiation therapy has been the mainstay of treatment for obstruction. Initially, high dose fractions (3 to 4 Gy) are given, followed by more conventional fraction sizes. The total dose will depend on the final goals of treatment and the clinical situation.
6. Bronchoscopic laser or photodynamic therapy may alleviate intraluminal tracheal obstruction. The success rate for these approaches in selected patients exceeds 90%.[35, 36] In addition, intraluminal radioisotope therapy using high dose rate brachytherapy within bronchial catheters has been used to deliver rapid, short, intense courses of radiation and has produced very successful palliation.[34, 37]

Pericardial Effusion and Cardiac Tamponade

Malignant pericardial effusion can be a complication of malignancy and, if left untreated, may occasionally lead to tamponade. Cardiac tamponade is a life-threatening emergency resulting from fluid accumulating in the pericardium under pressure with impaired filling of the cardiac chambers and decreased cardiac output. The most common etiologies are malignancy and postradiation pericarditis, but cardiac tamponade may also be related to previous pericarditis, cardiac trauma, or myocardial perforation from a catheter placement. Pericardial effusion and tamponade are most often associated with the following malignancies: lung, breast, gastrointestinal, lymphoma, leukemia, melanoma, sarcoma, or mesotheliomas.[13, 23, 25]

Diagnosis

1. Symptoms of tamponade include dyspnea, cough, altered mental state, retrosternal chest pain exacerbated by leaning forward or lying down, and, less commonly, hoarseness, hiccups, epigastric pain, or nausea and vomiting. Symptoms may resemble congestive heart failure, and the wide spectrum of presentation is related to the degree of compression, the rapidity of onset, and the ability of the patient's cardiorespiratory system to compensate.[13, 25] Physical findings include tachypnea, tachycardia, cyanosis, hypotension, increased central venous pressure, distended neck veins, pulsus paradoxus (which is an exaggeration of the normal inspiratory fall in systolic blood pressure of more than 10 mm Hg), narrowed pulse pressure, Kussmaul's sign (paradoxical filling of neck veins during inspiration), and a quiet heart with diminished heart sounds and diminished point of maximal impulse.[13, 25] If the effusion occurs in a more chronic manner, then hepatomegaly, peripheral edema, and ascites may be present.
2. The chest x-ray film may reveal a normal size heart if the fluid has accumulated rapidly; however, more often there is an enlarged cardiac silhouette or the classic so-called water bottle, if the effusion is large. A pleural effusion often accompanies these changes. The electrocardiogram demonstrates nonspecific changes, such as tachycardia, low voltage, ST elevation, and T-wave changes, and sometimes the pathognomonic changes of electrical alternans, which is the sinusoidal variation in the P waves and QRS complexes related to the heart swinging in the pericardial fluid.[25]
3. Echocardiography is the diagnostic procedure of choice, and it is likely to reveal fluid surrounding the heart within the pericardial sac and the swinging motion of the heart within the fluid. The right-sided chambers collapse during diastole.[38]
4. Cardiac catheterization is rarely required to make the diagnosis, but it would demonstrate equalization of pressures in all four chambers.[38]

Therapy

1. Immediate pericardiocentesis and volume expansion are required for relief of cardiac tamponade. The fluid should be sent for cytology, culture, and chemistry profile. Cytology is diagnostic of malignancy in 85% of cases.[39]
2. Long-term control of malignant pericardial effusion is obtained by surgical creation of a pericardial window or, less often, a pericardiectomy.[40] An alternative approach involves sclerosis of the pericardial space by doxycycline or bleomycin, using a pericardial catheter.[41]
3. Systemic chemotherapy or radiation therapy may be effective in controlling malignant effusions in stable

patients who have sensitive tumors such as lymphomas or small cell lung carcinomas.[42]

Bowel Obstruction

Gastrointestinal tract obstruction is a common complication for patients with a history of colon, gynecologic, or any pelvic cancer. However, one should not immediately conclude that it is related to the underlying malignancy, because it could be related to previous surgery and adhesions or hernia, among other things, especially if the primary is not in an advanced stage at diagnosis. The obstruction may be unifocal or multifocal. Unifocal obstruction is typically produced by a localized but constrictive carcinoma of the colon. Ovarian, gastrointestinal (GI), or breast cancer can give rise to carcinomatosis, which is associated with multifocal small and large bowel obstructions.[43, 44]

Diagnosis

1. Patients frequently present with nausea and vomiting, abdominal bloating, cramping, abdominal pain, and inability to have a bowel movement or pass flatus.
2. Physical examination reveals abdominal distention, high-pitched, hyperactive bowel sounds, and tenderness.
3. Flat and upright abdominal films show multiple air-fluid levels or dilated bowel loops. An upper GI series is considered contraindicated; a barium enema or colonoscopy can be performed safely, if clinically indicated.[45]
4. Patients with a competent ileocecal valve and distal occlusion are at risk for cecal perforation, because of the closed loop obstruction. Progressive pain and distention with a palpable mass and acute cecal dilatation of more than 12 to 14 cm seen on an abdominal film is associated with a high possibility of rupture.[9]

Therapy

1. Electrolyte disturbances and dehydration should be corrected.
2. Decompression nasogastric suction should be initiated.
3. Surgery is generally indicated, especially if there are signs of peritonitis or ischemia (fever, elevated white blood cell [WBC] count, and localized tenderness). It is often employed to relieve the obstruction, to determine the extent of the problem, and to establish whether the obstruction is related to the cancer or some other cause. Partial bowel obstruction may resolve with conservative therapy, but frequently even patients with partial bowel obstruction eventually require surgical exploration.
4. Patients with carcinomatosis should be managed in a palliative manner with antiemetic, narcotics, or a celiac nerve block when feasible.[46] If all of these measures fail, then one can consider subcutaneous injections of octreotide, a somatostatin analogue that reduces the volume of gastrointestinal secretions.[47] The efficacy of this therapy continues to be examined.

Gastrointestinal Bleeding

Gastrointestinal bleeding may occur in patients with malignancies of the GI tract, such as large exophytic tumors of the esophagus, stomach, or intestine. However, most causes are not necessarily related to the malignancy. In the upper portion of the GI tract, causes may include esophageal varices, Mallory-Weiss tears, *Candida* esophagitis, reflux esophagitis, and gastritis related to medication, thrombocytopenia, and peptic ulcer disease. Metastatic cancers associated with upper GI bleeding include lymphomas, leiomyosarcomas, carcinoid, and metastatic melanoma; cancers of the small intestine are rare. Bleeding from the large intestines can occur and can be exacerbated by coagulation defects or thrombocytopenia, or can be related to diverticulitis, polyps, angiodysplasia, as well as from various forms of colitis.[48]

Diagnosis

1. Hematemesis suggests a lesion proximal to the ligament of Treitz, while bright red blood in the rectum usually indicates a lesion in the large bowel.
2. Upper endoscopy is highly reliable for identifying sources of esophageal and gastroduodenal bleeding. Gastroscopy may be hampered by blood clots and saline lavage or prokinetic drugs may be needed to evacuate the bleeding and obtain better visualization. Urgent colonoscopy is useful in the evaluation of lower GI bleeding, but it also may be difficult in massively bleeding or unstable patients.
3. Nuclear bleeding scans (radiolabeled red-cell or sulfur colloid studies) may be helpful in localizing lower tract bleeding.
4. Angiography is the gold standard for individuals with ongoing massive GI bleeding, particularly in the hemodynamically unstable patient.

Therapy

1. Patients should be carefully monitored, given intravenous fluids, and transfused when clinically indicated. Coagulopathy and thrombocytopenia should be corrected.
2. Bleeding gastroduodenal ulcers or gastritis requires therapy with H2-receptor antagonist and antacids. Endoscopic electrocautery or laser photocoagulation is an option for patients with a high risk of rebleeding or with stigmata of active hemorrhage.
3. Threatened variceal exsanguination has traditionally been treated with balloon tamponade (Sengstaken-Blakemore tube) and infusion of a splanchnic vasoconstrictor, such as vasopressin. Endoscopic sclerotherapy of the varices is subsequently performed; this may be used as initial therapy when bleeding is less massive.
4. Selective arteriographic infusion of vasopressin may provide temporary control of persistent colonic hemorrhage; it is usually followed by segmental resection of the bleeding site.[46]

Carotid Artery Hemorrhage

Hemorrhage from the carotid artery can be a catastrophe. The usual settings include wound disruption, external or internal carotid exposure, history of previous radiation, or in the presence of a salivary fistula. It can usually be anticipated if the artery is bathed in saliva from a fistula, if a small harbinger leak is found, or if the wall becomes avascular and dark. Airway control and maintenance of blood pressure are critical. Direct finger pressure may be helpful initially, and bilateral carotid artery ligation is usually performed below and above the point of rupture. Obviously, this needs to be performed by an experienced surgeon.

Metabolic

Hypercalcemia

Hypercalcemia is an important complication of cancer that can seriously affect a patient's quality of life, as well as being life threatening. The most common histologic types of cancer associated with hypercalcemia are breast, lung, and multiple myeloma, with head and neck, esophagus, lymphomas, hypernephromas, leukemia, cervical, and colon being less common. Approximately 10% to 20% of patients with cancer will experience this complication sometime during their illness; this can be as high as 20% to 40% of patients with myeloma or breast or lung cancer,[9, 49] but almost any kind of cancer may be associated with the condition.

The mechanism of production is usually mediated by increased osteoclastic activity, and most but not all patients will have bone metastases. Other conditions that are associated with elevation of calcium and need to be excluded include hyperparathyroidism (which is rarely associated with acute hypercalcemia), hypophosphatemia, sarcoidosis, and vitamin A and D intoxication.

The pathogenesis of hypercalcemia includes increased bone resorption, local bone destruction, decreased renal excretion, and enhanced intestinal absorption, which is uncommon in the malignant setting. Factors leading to increased bone resorption are numerous and include a parathormone (PTH)–like substance produced by the tumor (considered quite rare nowadays), prostaglandins, and PTH-related protein (which usually serves a paracrine function, but more is produced in malignancy and it becomes a circulating hormone). Cytokines that stimulate bone resorption and are produced by white cells also have been shown to be associated with hypercalcemia; these cytokines include lymphotoxin and tumor necrosis factor. Another mechanism is increased amounts of 1,25 dihydroxyvitamin D_3, as found in patients with non-Hodgkin's lymphomas and Hodgkin's disease.[50] Factors known to aggravate hypercalcemia include patient immobilization and decreased oral intake of fluids producing dehydration.

Diagnosis

1. Symptoms of hypercalcemia include fatigue, anorexia, bone pain, constipation, nausea and vomiting, polyuria, and polydipsia. Neurologic symptoms may range from lethargy, confusion, psychosis, seizures, obtundation, coma, even to death.[13, 49]
2. Physical findings are nonspecific and include signs of dehydration related to the obligate fluid loss of the hypercalcinuria and diminished reflexes. Changes in the electrocardiogram may occur, but they are rarely diagnostic unless the serum calcium is greater than 16; these include a lengthening of the PR interval, shortening of the QT interval and a wide, coved T wave.[9]
3. The diagnosis is established by an elevated serum calcium, the height of which will determine the need for immediate therapy. One should also measure blood urea nitrogen (BUN), creatinine, serum phosphate, alkaline phosphatase, albumin, magnesium, and electrolytes. The serum calcium should be adjusted upward or downward for every gram of albumin above or below 4.0 g/dL by 0.8 mg/dL. Depending upon the available laboratory facilities, one can also measure ionized calcium directly; it is the ionized or unbound calcium that mediates the calcium effects.

Therapy

The four principles of treatment include hydration, increasing renal excretion, inhibiting bone resorption, and treatment of the cancer.

1. Forced normal saline diuresis (200 to 300 mL per hour) should be initiated promptly to reverse volume contraction and promote calciuresis. Fluid balance and cardiopulmonary status must be monitored closely to avoid volume overload and congestive heart failure in elderly patients. Furosemide may be required to maintain volume equilibrium. Saline hydration significantly reduces the serum calcium level in 1 to 2 days. This may be the only strategy necessary for calcium values less than 14 mg/dL. For values greater than 14 mg/dL, treatment will depend upon hepatic, renal, and hematologic parameters; the symptoms; need for rapid reduction; and the availability of effective antineoplastic therapy.
2. Salmon calcitonin has been used for many years in the treatment of hypercalcemia. It inhibits osteoclastic bone resorption and increases renal excretion of calcium. Calcitonin has a rapid onset of action, and serum concentrations begin to decline within a few hours; the nadir may be reached within 24 hours. Tachyphylaxis is well known to occur with calcitonin, which limits its repeated use. The usual starting dose is 1 to 4 IU/kg administered by subcutaneous or intramuscular injection every 6 hours for a maximum of eight consecutive doses.[49]
3. Bisphosphate can induce osteoclast cytotoxicity and inhibit osteoclast precursors. The two drugs available in the United States are etidronate disodium (Didronel) and pamidronate disodium (Aredia). The onset of action is usually 2 days and the nadir is reached in 7 days. The recommended dose of etidronate is 7.5 mg/kg IV over 2 to 4 hours, once daily for 3 to 7 days. The dose for pamidronate is 60 to 90 mg IV

over 4 to 24 hours and is repeated in 7 days as needed. The 90-mg dose is recommended for patients with severe hypercalcemia. Both the single dose of pamidronate and its effectiveness make it more attractive.[49, 51]

4. Corticosteroids promote urinary calcium excretion and decrease intestinal absorption. They are most useful for treatment of hypercalcemia in lymphoma, myeloma, or breast cancer. Their therapeutic benefits are observed after 5 to 10 days of administration. Doses vary considerably and include prednisone 60 to 100 mg per day given in divided doses or IV equivalent drugs.
5. Gallium nitrate inhibits PTH-induced calcium resorption from bone. Its onset of action is 24 to 48 hours and the nadir of effect is 6 to 10 days. The recommended dose is 200 mg/m^2 per day IV as a continuous infusion for 5 consecutive days. The drug is associated with renal toxicity, but its duration of response is quite long.[49]
6. Plicamycin (mithramycin) is an effective inhibitor of RNA synthesis in osteoclasts. The onset of action is 12 hours and the nadir of effect is 2 to 3 days. The recommended dose is 25 μg/kg IV over 4 to 6 hours. The dose can be repeated every 24 to 48 hours, remembering that adverse hepatic, renal, myelotoxicity, and clotting events occur more often with increasing dosage. Because of the potential side effects, this drug is often reserved for patients refractory to other strategies.[49]

Hyponatremia

The serum concentration of sodium is in part regulated by vasopressin (antidiuretic hormone [ADH]), which is produced in the hypothalamus and stored in the posterior pituitary gland. The maintenance of body osmolality in a narrow range between 286 to 292 mOsmol/L is achieved through a balance of ADH and thirst.[52] In certain clinical situations, there may be an inappropriate amount of ADH, either secondary to pituitary secretion or due to secretion by a tumor of a protein immunologically similar to ADH; this leads to the syndrome of inappropriate ADH (SIADH). This syndrome can be associated with many conditions, but about two thirds of cases are associated with cancer, and mostly with small cell lung cancer. Other associated cancers include pancreas, neuroendocrine, non–small cell lung cancers, and lymphomas.[9] SIADH may also occur secondarily in the setting of brain metastasis or after treatment with drugs such as cyclophosphamide or vincristine[53]; in these cases, the hypothalamus-pituitary axis is the culprit. This scenario should be considered at any time if the serum sodium is less than or equal to 130 mEq/L in a patient without edema and with no evidence of hypovolemia, hypotension, or renal, adrenal, or thyroid disease. It is important to understand that the development of the syndrome is dependent upon inappropriate water intake in addition to inappropriate ADH secretion.[50] Hyponatremia due to ectopic hormone production can, occasionally, antedate the diagnosis of malignancy by months, but the tumor is usually clinically overt when hyponatremia is manifest.

Diagnosis

1. Symptoms are nonspecific, but they may include weakness, anorexia, nausea, headaches, muscle cramps, lethargy, and confusion.
2. Physical signs may not be present. If they are, then they will include altered mental status (memory loss, apathy, impaired abstract thinking), pathologic reflexes, extrapyramidal signs, pseudobulbar palsy, coma, seizures, and, rarely, death, which is usually associated with serum sodium of less than 115 mEq/L. The clinical signs and symptoms depend on the rapidity with which the syndrome has occurred. It is important to note that, clinically, these patients do not have edema, hypotension, or signs of hypovolemia.
3. In most cases, a serum sodium concentration less than 130 mEq/L is the first clue to the diagnosis. The three most important tests to make the diagnosis are:
   - low serum sodium
   - an elevated urine osmolality (>20 mOsmol/L)
   - a low plasma osmolality (<270 mOsmol/L)

   The urine specific gravity is greater than 1.0002 and the urine sodium is usually greater than 20 mEq/L. The BUN and creatinine test are normal or low due to dilution. It is wise to exclude adrenal insufficiency with a cortisol determination and thyroid deficiency.[52]

Therapy

1. If effective chemotherapy is available (e.g., in cases related to small cell lung cancer), it will eliminate the ectopic hormone production and correct hyponatremia in a few weeks.[54]
2. Mild to moderate hyponatremia, secondary to SIADH, is treated with a restriction of free water intake to 500 mL per day. However, this is often difficult for the patient to endure.
3. Demeclocycline, an antibiotic that causes nephrogenic diabetes insipidus, may be administered. The usual dose is 200 mg three times per day. Side effects include reversible elevation in BUN and photosensitivity.
4. Severe hyponatremia may require careful slow infusion of 3% hypertonic saline. If the serum sodium rises more than 1 mEq per hour, then there may be a risk of central pontine myelinolysis manifested by quadriparesis, dysphagia, and dysarthria.[23, 52] Resolution of the hyponatremia and avoidance of circulatory overload are facilitated by administering furosemide.[53]
5. Administration of oral salt or urea, with or without furosemide, has also been used.[9, 23, 52]

Tumor Lysis

The tumor lysis syndrome encompasses a group of metabolic disorders that complicate the treatment of bulky and highly proliferative neoplasms. This disorder rarely occurs spontaneously, but it typically occurs in patients when treated with chemotherapy. The most frequently associated neoplasms include Burkitt's lymphoma, lymphoblastic lymphoma, acute lymphoblastic leukemia with hyperleukocytosis, and lymphoma; it is rare in solid tumors, but it has been reported in some cases of small cell lung and breast cancer.[23, 55] These neoplasms are exquisitely chemosensitive; therefore, marked cytoreduction occurs with treatment. The resultant lysis of tumor cells liberates large quantities of intracellular urate, phosphate, and potassium into the circulation. The volume of these waste products overwhelms the excretory capacity of the kidneys and, as a result, hyperkalemia, hyperuricemia, hyperphosphatemia, and secondary hypocalcemia (related to the excess phosphate and sequestration of calcium phosphate) develop. Precipitation of urate or calcium phosphate in the renal tubules causes acute renal failure and worsening metabolic dysfunction.[56, 57]

Diagnosis

1. Patients may complain of weakness, irritability, and muscle cramps.
2. On examination, the patient may have tetany or be confused, and seizures or serious ventricular cardiac arrhythmias may occur. Death has been reported, related to acute renal failure and cardiac arrhythmias. Serial blood chemistry measurements reveal the metabolic disarray of hyperuricemia, hyperkalemia, hyperphosphatemia, hypocalcemia, and increase in creatinine and LDH. Phosphate crystals may be grossly visible in the urine sediment.

Therapy

This is a situation in which an ounce of prevention is worth a pound of gold. The following measures should be initiated 24 to 48 hours before the administration of any chemotherapy, then continued for 3 to 5 days.

1. IV hydration (3 L/m^2 per day) is given to promote the excretion of urates and phosphates. Allopurinol, at a dose of 500 mg/m^2 per day PO, will suppress uric acid formation.
2. If urine uric acid level exceeds 7 mg/dL, then urine alkalinization with IV sodium bicarbonate is recommended. Urinary pH should be maintained above 7 until hyperuricemia has resolved.[57, 58]
3. Hemodialysis is indicated in severe cases of tumor lysis syndrome.

Hematologic

Thrombocytopenia

Thrombocytopenia is an important clinical problem in the management of patients with cancer, and low levels of platelets, generally less than 20,000/μL, can be associated with spontaneous and life-threatening bleeding in the GI tract and brain. Thrombocytopenia occurs because there is a decreased or ineffective production of platelets or an increase in destruction or sequestration. The most common causes in the former include:

- chemotherapy drugs
- extensive radiation that includes a sizable portion of the bones that contain marrow
- hematologic diseases that originate in the bone marrow (leukemias, myeloma, lymphomas)
- less frequently, solid tumors that invade the marrow cavities

Causes of increased destruction would include disseminated intravascular coagulation (DIC), sepsis, hemorrhage, and conditions not necessarily associated with the malignancy, such as idiopathic thrombocytopenic purpura, microangiopathic hemolytic anemia, or drugs such as heparin or quinidine. There may also be qualitative defects in platelets leading to bleeding, and drugs (e.g., aspirin and nonsteroidal anti-inflammatory drugs [NSAIDs]), may accentuate this. Obviously, spontaneous bleeding can occur at higher platelet levels in this situation.[59]

Diagnosis

1. Purpura, ecchymoses, epistaxis, menometrorrhagia, hematuria, or gastrointestinal bleeding may occur.
2. Complete blood counts, including a platelet count, and a smear and differential should be obtained. If the cause of the thrombocytopenia is not immediately clinically apparent, then a bone marrow aspirate should be performed to look for hematologic disease, as well as to assess megakaryocyte production.

Therapy

1. Platelet transfusions are indicated when bleeding occurs with thrombocytopenia. Prophylactic transfusions are given when the platelet count is less than 20,000/μL. In the absence of fever or hemorrhage in patients with solid tumors, a platelet count of 10,000/μL may be an acceptable cutoff point for prophylactic transfusion.[60]
2. Platelet transfusions are usually not effective in immune-mediated thrombocytopenia or DIC unless other coagulation factors are replaced as well. Situations in which there is increased destruction may require other measures, such as corticosteroids, intravenous gamma globulin, or splenectomy.
3. Treatment of the underlying neoplastic disease obviously should be initiated.
4. The most exciting development in the treatment of thrombocytopenia is the development of recombinant thrombopoietin. It is being used in some chemotherapy regimens to obviate prolonged thrombocytopenia. It is anticipated that its role will be greatly expanded in the future.[61, 62]
5. Any agents that impair platelet function (such as NSAIDs) should be avoided until the thrombocytopenia resolves.

Neutropenia/Infection

Neutrophils or granulocytes are produced by marrow stem cells, divide and mature within the bone marrow for 9 to 10 days, then move to the blood stream where their half-life is relatively short (4 to 5 hours). Finally, the cells enter the tissues, where they function and die. The absolute neutrophil count (WBC × [percent segs + bands]) varies between 1600 to 8000/μL.[59] Neutropenia, in the oncologic setting, can be related to chemotherapy drugs, marrow replacement by hematologic or metastatic tumor, or, less frequently, radiation. The relationship between neutropenia and the incidence of infection has long been recognized[63]; an absolute neutrophil count below 1000/μL indicates an increased risk of infection, and the risk is most pronounced at neutrophil counts under 500/μL. The susceptibility of the neutropenic patient to infection may be increased due to a concomitant immunoglobulin deficiency, T-cell immunodeficiency, asplenia, or monocytopenia.[64]

All episodes of fever in these patients are considered to be infectious until proven otherwise. Bacteria and viruses are the usual types of infection early in the neutropenia, whereas resistant bacteria, fungi, protozoa, and viruses occur later. Initial infections historically were most often gram-negative, including *Escherichia coli* and *Pseudomonas.* They are now being replaced by gram-positive organisms, especially coagulase-positive staphylococci, and we are beginning to see cases of vancomycin-resistant enterococci. Indwelling central venous catheters have been increasingly identified with infections, predominantly of the gram-positive variety. However, in 30% to 40% of patients, a source of infection may not be found,[64] and despite appropriate interventions, 5% to 10% of cancer patients will succumb to infectious complication associated with neutropenia.[65]

Diagnosis

1. A temperature above 38°C in a setting of neutropenia requires prompt evaluation with a thorough examination. Symptoms may include rigors, myalgias, tachycardia, tachypnea, irritability, and lethargy, and they can range to more serious conditions such as shock, lactic acidosis, adult respiratory distress syndrome, respiratory failure requiring ventilator assistance, gastrointestinal hemorrhage, DIC, and death. Particular attention should paid to the gingiva, pharynx, perirectal region, lungs, skin, and vascular access sites.
2. Laboratory evaluation includes multiple blood cultures, as well as cultures of the urine, sputum, pharynx, and other sites as clinically indicated. If a central venous catheter is in place, then comparative quantitative blood cultures obtained from each lumen of the catheter and peripheral site should be used. A chest x-ray film should be obtained.

Therapy

1. It is standard practice to start broad spectrum antibiotic coverage immediately in the febrile neutropenic patients, even in the absence of signs of infection on physical examination after appropriate cultures are taken. A combination of an aminoglycoside and an antipseudomonal β-lactam was traditionally the initial choice. Monotherapy with ceftazidime or imipenem is now being used. There has been much written about the appropriate antibiotic combination to start in this setting, and the optimal combination may vary depending on the antimicrobial susceptibility pattern at a given institution.[63, 65]
2. Initial use of vancomycin, an antistaphylococcal agent, is warranted if gram-positive bacterial or catheter-related infection is suspected. However, caution should be used with the recent reported cases of vancomycin-resistant organisms.[63, 65]
3. Outpatient antibiotic therapy (ciprofloxacin and clindamycin) has been recommended in low-risk, neutropenic patients.[66]
4. Persistent, unexplained fever in the neutropenic patient on antibiotics after 5 to 7 days is an indication for empirical antifungal treatment with amphotericin B, with or without fluconazole or itraconazole.[65]
5. Colony-stimulating factors G-CSF and GM-CSF are one way of avoiding prolonged neutropenia by accelerating recovery. Use of these drugs has been shown to decrease the duration and severity of the neutropenia, as well as the incidence of infections.[67]
6. The role of neutrophil transfusion in this setting has been controversial. Where available, it has been used in select patients with profound neutropenia unresponsive to the above measures, and now there has been the additional modification of giving G-CSF to the donor to improve the yield.[68]

Disseminated Intravascular Coagulation

Disseminated intravascular coagulation (DIC) is a pathologic process mediated by activation of thrombin in the circulation, leading to the production of fibrin, consumption of certain clotting factors, aggregation and diminution of platelets, and activation of the fibrinolytic system. The clinical spectrum produced is related to hemorrhage, thrombus formation, or both. The process is believed to be an intermediary in many diseases and may be acute and self-limited, subacute, or chronic. The simplest way to understand the consequences of DIC on coagulation is to picture it as a conversion of plasma to serum. When this occurs certain factors are consumed (I, II, V, VIII, and XIII) plus platelets, and the fibrinolytic system is activated to produce fibrin degradation products (FDP), which act as circulating anticoagulants.

One of the causes of this process is cancer. The malignant disease most notably associated with DIC is acute promyelocytic leukemia; approximately 80% of cases have evidence of DIC at diagnosis, which is worsened by chemotherapy. Other causes of this disorder may result from metastatic carcinoma, major surgery or trauma, shock, infections (especially bacterial), hepatic disease, extensive burns, and massive transfusion reactions.[59, 69]

Diagnosis

1. Bleeding and thrombosis are the hallmarks of DIC. Hemorrhage in the form of petechiae, purpura, hematomas, hemorrhagic bullae, cyanosis, and gangrene of the digits, nose and ear lobes may be seen. Bleeding at sites of surgery, trauma, or venipunctures may be a clue. Migratory thrombophlebitis (Trousseau's syndrome, a paraneoplastic syndrome of thrombosis

associated with malignancy) or recurrent thrombotic events can be other manifestations of DIC.

2. Laboratory studies in most cases will demonstrate the following:
   - platelet count below 100,000/μL
   - fibrinogen less than 125 mg/dL
   - prothrombin time greater than 15 seconds

The activated partial thromboplastin time is abnormal in most patients, and FDPs are generally greater than 40 mg/mL in over half of the cases. Examination of the blood smear may demonstrate schistocytes to suggest microangiopathic hemolysis.[70]

Therapy

1. Controlling the underlying disease is the goal, but this is infrequently accomplished. If an infection is present, then antibiotic therapy should be initiated. Treatment of the cancer is usually indicated in situations of prostate, breast cancer, or a hematologic malignancy.[70]
2. The treatment of acute promyelocytic leukemia (French, American, and British classification M3) has undergone some revision, because initiation of treatment with chemotherapy was often associated with worsening DIC. It was then discovered that all-*trans* retinoic acid (ATRA) could promote terminal differentiation of the promyelocytes without the exacerbation of the DIC. Now chemotherapy is administered after a complete remission is obtained with ATRA.[69]
3. The treatment of DIC in other situations is far from satisfactory. Certainly, if there are no clinical manifestations but only laboratory ones, close observation is most prudent. If, on the other hand, bleeding is the predominant picture, then treatment usually includes replacement of platelets and the coagulation factors with cryoprecipitates or fresh frozen plasma. If thrombosis is predominant, then heparin is tried. The role of heparin in the face of bleeding is controversial but has been used. It is extremely important to follow the patient clinically, with coagulation tests and platelets counts to assess response.[70]

REFERENCES

General References

1. DeVita VT, Hellman S, Rosenberg SA (eds): Cancer: Principles and Practice of Oncology, 5th ed. Philadelphia, Lippincott-Raven, 1997.
2. Perez CA, Brady LW (eds): Principles and Practice of Radiation Oncology, 3rd ed. Philadelphia, Lippincott-Raven, 1997.
3. Hurst JW, Bourke E (eds): Medicine for the Practicing Physician, 4th ed. Stanford, Connecticut, Appleton and Lange, 1996.
4. Isselbacher KJ, Braunwald E, Wilson J, et al (eds): Harrison's Principles of Internal Medicine, 13th ed. New York, McGraw-Hill, Inc, 1994.

Specific References

5. Mayer DK: Prevention, early detection, and management of oncologic emergencies. Recent Results Cancer Res 1991; 121:360–365.
6. Patchell RA, Tibbs PA, Walsh JW, et al: A randomized trial of surgery in the treatment of single metastases to the brain. N Engl J Med 1990; 322:494–505.
7. Bleyer WA, Byrne TN: Leptomeningeal cancer in leukemia and solid tumors. Curr Probl Cancer 1988; 12:181–238.
8. Chamberlain MC, Kormanik PR: Carcinomatous meningitis secondary to breast cancer: predictors of response to combined modality therapy. J Neurol Oncol 1997; 35:55–64.
9. Kalia S, Tintinalli JE: Emergency evaluation of the cancer patient. Ann Emerg Med 1984; 13:723–30.
10. Guyot LL, Dowling C, Diaz FG, et al: Cerebral monitoring devices: analysis of complications. Acta Neurochir Suppl (Wein) 1998:47–49.
11. DeAngelis L, Mandell L, Thaler H, et al: The role of postoperative radiotherapy after resection of single brain metastases. Neurosurg 1989; 24:798–805.
12. Vecht CJ, Haaxma-Reiche H, Noordiijk EM, et al: Treatment of single brain metastases: radiotherapy alone or in combination with neurosurgery? Ann Neurol 1993; 33:583–590.
13. Neilan BA: Oncologic emergencies, treating acute problems resulting from cancer and chemotherapy. Postgrad Med J 1994; 95:125–128, 131–32.
14. Ciezki J, Macklis M: The palliative role of radiotherapy in the management of the cancer patient. Semin Oncol 1995; 22(suppl):82–90.
15. Auchter RM, Lamond JP, Alexander E, et al: A multi-institutional outcome and prognostic factor analysis of radiosurgery for resectable single brain metastasis. Int J Radiat Oncol Biol Phys 1996; 35:27–35.
16. Bruckmann JE, Bloomer WD: Management of spinal cord compression. Semin Oncol 1978; 5:135–140.
17. Byrne TN: Spinal cord compression from epidural metastases. N Engl J Med 1992; 327:614–618.
18. Siegal T, Siegal T: Current considerations in the management of neoplastic spinal compression. Spine 1989; 14:223–238.
19. Hosono N, Yonenobu K, Fuji T, et al: Orthopaedic management of spinal metastases. Clin Orthop 1995; 312:148–159.
20. Sundaresan N, Sachdev VP, Holland JF, et al: Surgical treatment of spinal cord compression for epidural metastasis. J Clin Oncol 1995; 13:2330–2335.
21. Glover DJ, Glick JH: Managing oncologic emergencies involving structural dysfunction. CA Cancer J Clin 1985; 35:238–251.
22. Kim HJ, Kim HS, Chung SH: CT diagnosis of superior vena cava syndrome: importance of collateral vessels. American Journal of Roentgenology 1993; 161:539–542.
23. Markman M: Common complications and emergencies associated with cancer and its therapy. Cleve Clin J Med 1994; 61:105–114.
24. Bell DR, Woods RL, Levi JA: Superior vena caval obstruction: a 10-year experience. Med J Aust 1986; 145:566–568.
25. Maguire WM: Mechanical complications of cancer. Emerg Med Clin North Am 1993; 11:421–430.
26. Menzies R, Charbonneau M: Thoracoscopy for diagnosis of pleural disease. Ann Intern Med 1991; 114:271–276.
27. Light RN, MacGregor MI, Luchsinger PC, et al: Pleural effusions: the diagnostic separation of transudates and exudates. Ann Intern Med 1972; 77:507–513.
28. Ruckdeschel JC: Management of malignant pleural effusion. Semin Oncol 1995; 22(suppl):58–63.
29. Reich H, Beattie EJ, Harvey JD: Pleuroperitoneal shunt for malignant pleural effusions: a one year experience. Semin Surg Oncol 1993; 9:160–162.
30. Yeam I, Sassoon C: Hemothorax and chylothorax. Curr Opin Pulm Med 1997; 3:310–314.
31. Crocco JA, Rooney JJ, Frakushen DS, et al: Massive hemoptysis. Arch Intern Med 1968; 121:495–498.
32. Santiago S, Tobias J, Williams AJ: A reappraisal of the causes of hemoptysis. Arch Intern Med 1991; 151:2249–2251.
33. DiLeo MD, Amedee RG, Butcher RB: Hemoptysis and pseudohemoptysis: the patient expectorating blood. Ear Nose Throat J 1995; 74:822–824.
34. Speiser BL, Spratling L: Remote afterloading brachytherapy for the local control of endobronchial carcinoma. Int J Radiat Oncol Biol Phys 1993; 25:579–587.
35. Turner JF Jr, Wang KP: Endobronchial laser therapy. Clin Chest Med 1999; 20:107–122.
36. Lam S: Photodynamic therapy of lung cancer. Semin Oncol 1994; 21(suppl):15–19.
37. Macha HN, Wahlers B, Reichle C, et al: Endobronchial radiation therapy for obstructing malignancies: ten years' experience with iridium-192 high-dose radiation brachytherapy afterloading technique in 365 patients. Lung 1995; 173:271–280.
38. Braunwald E: Pericardial disease. In: Isselbacher KJ, Braunwald E,

Wilson J, et al (eds): Harrison's Principles of Internal Medicine, 13th ed, pp 1094–1101. New York, McGraw-Hill Inc, 1994.

39. Posner MR, Cohen GI, Sharin AT: Pericardial disease in patients with cancer: the differentiation of malignant from idiopathic and radiation-induced pericarditis. Am J Med 1986; 71:407–413.
40. Fiocco M, Krasna MJ: The management of malignant pleural and pericardial effusions. Hematol Oncol Clin North Am 1997; 11:253–265.
41. Liu G, Crump M, Goss PE, et al: Prospective comparison of the sclerosing agents doxycycline and bleomycin for the primary management of malignant pericardial effusion and cardiac tamponade. J Clin Oncol 1996; 14:3141–3147.
42. Vaitkus PT, Hermann HC, LeWinter MM: Treatment of malignant pericardial effusion. JAMA 1994; 272:59–64.
43. Ripamonti C: Management of bowel obstruction in advanced cancer. Curr Opin Oncol 1994; 6:351–357.
44. Perez JA, Cardemil B, del Pozo M, et al: Intestinal obstruction caused by peritoneal carcinomatosis due to signet ring cell carcinoma of the breast. Rev Med Chil 1995; 123:617–623.
45. Thomas DR, Carter IK, Leslie WT, et al: Common emergencies in cancer medicine: hematologic and gastrointestinal syndromes. J Natl Med Assoc 1992; 84:165–176.
46. Frank C: Medical management of intestinal obstruction in the terminal care. Can Fam Physician 1997; 43:259–265.
47. Mercadante S, Spoldi E, Caraceni A, et al: Octreotide in relieving gastrointestinal symptoms due to bowel obstruction. Palliat Med 1993; 7:295–299.
48. Potter GD, Sellin JA: Lower gastrointestinal bleeding. Gastroenterol Clin North Am 1988; 17:341–356.
49. Chisholm MA, Mulloy AL, Taylor AT: Acute management of cancer-related hypercalcemia. Ann Pharmacother 1996; 30:507–513.
50. Odell WD: Endocrine/metabolic syndromes of cancer. Semin Oncol 1997; 24:299–317.
51. Bilezikian JP: Management of acute hypercalcemia. N Engl J Med 1992; 326:1196–1203.
52. Vokes T, Robertson GL: Syndrome of inappropriate antidiuretic hormone secretion. In: Hurst JW, Ambrose SS (eds): Medicine for the Practicing Physician, 2nd ed, pp 562–565. Boston, Butterworths, 1988.
53. Ayus JC, Krothpall RK, Ariett AJ: Treatment of symptomatic hyponatremia and its relationship to brain damage: a prospective study. N Engl J Med 1987; 317:1190–94.
54. Thomas CR, Dodhia N: Common emergencies in cancer medicine: metabolic syndromes. J Natl Med Assoc 1991; 83:809–818.
55. Kalemkerian GP, Darwish B, Vatrerasian ML: Tumor lysis syndrome in small cell carcinoma and other solid tumors. Am J Med 1997; 103:363–367.
56. Arrambide K, Toto RD: Tumour lysis syndrome. Br J Hosp Med 1993; 49:273–280.
57. Veenstra J, Krediet RT, Somers R, et al: Tumour lysis syndrome and acute renal failure in Burkitt's lymphoma. Description of 2 cases and a review of the literature on prevention and management. Neth J Med 1994; 45:211–216.
58. Jones DP, Mahmoud H, Chesney RW: Tumor lysis syndrome: pathogenesis and management. Pediatr Nephrol 1995; 9:206–212.
59. Keller JW: Surgery in the patient with hematopoietic disease. In: Lubin MF, Walker HK, Smith RB (eds): Medical Management of the Surgical Patient, pp 371–410. Boston, Butterworths, 1982.
60. Kempin SJ: Hemostatic defects in cancer patients. Cancer Invest 1997; 15:23–36.
61. Fanucchi M, Glaspy J, Crawford J, et al: Effects of polyethylene glycol-conjugated recombinant human megakaryocyte growth and development factor on platelet count after chemotherapy for lung cancer. N Engl J Med 1997; 336:404–409.
62. Miyazaki H: Update on thrombopoietin in preclinical and clinical trials. Curr Opin Hematol 1998; 5:197–202.
63. Chanock SJ, Pizzo PA: Fever in the neutropenic host. Infect Dis Clin North Am 1996; 10:777–790.
64. Thomas CR, Wood LV, Douglas JG, et al: Common emergencies in cancer medicine: infectious and treatment-related syndromes. Part I. J Natl Med Assoc 1994; 86:765–774.
65. Chanock SJ, Pizzo PA: Infectious complications of patients undergoing therapy for acute leukemia: current status and future prospects. Semin Oncol 1997; 24:132–140.
66. Rolston KV, Rubenstein EB, Freifeld A: Early empiric antibiotic therapy for febrile neutropenia patients at low risk. Infect Dis Clin North Am 1996; 10:223–236.
67. American Society of Clinical Oncology: Recommendations for the use of hematopoietic colony-stimulating factors: evidence-based clinical practice guidelines. J Clin Oncol 1994; 12:2471–2508.
68. Grigg A, Vecchi L, Bardy P, et al: G-CSF stimulated donor granulocyte collections for prophylaxis and therapy of neutropenic sepsis. Aust N Z J Med 1996; 26:813–818.
69. Fenaux P, Chomienne C, Degos L: Acute promyelocytic leukemia: biology and treatment. Semin Oncol 1997; 24:92–102.
70. Coleman RW, Rubin RN: Disseminated intravascular coagulation due to malignancy. Semin Oncol 1990; 17:172–186.

14 *Principles of Psychosocial Oncology*

ANDREW J. ROTH, MD, Psychiatry and Behavioral Sciences
WILLIAM BREITBART, MD, Psychiatry and Behavioral Sciences

At the rider's back sits dark Anxiety.

HORACE

Perspective

The patient with cancer faces many stressors during the course of illness, including fears of a painful death, disability, disfigurement, and dependency. Although such concerns are universal, the level of psychological distress is quite variable depending on personality, coping ability, social support, and medical factors. This chapter discusses the prevalence, assessment, and treatment methods of the major psychiatric syndromes seen in cancer patients. As people with cancer are living longer today because of improved cancer treatment, quality-of-life issues that include psychological well-being, both during and after treatment, take on even greater importance.

Psychiatric Disorders in Cancer Patients

In 1983, the Psychosocial Collaborative Oncology Group determined the prevalence of psychiatric disorders seen in three cancer centers in 215 cancer patients (ambulatory or hospitalized, with a wide range of cancer diagnoses and stages of disease) utilizing the criteria from the Diagnostic and Statistical Manual (DSM) III classification of disorders.[1] About half (53%) of the patients evaluated were adjusting normally to the stresses of cancer with no diagnosable psychiatric disorder; however, 47% had clinically apparent psychiatric disorders. Of the 47% who had psychiatric disorders, 68% had reactive anxiety and depression (adjustment disorders with depressed or anxious mood), 13% had major depression, and 8% had an organic mental disorder (delirium).

The incidences of pain, depression, and delirium all increase with higher levels of physical debilitation and advanced illness.[2–5] Approximately 25% of all cancer patients experience severe depressive symptoms, with the prevalence increasing in those with advanced illness. The prevalence of organic mental disorders (delirium) among cancer patients requiring psychiatric consultation has been found to range from 25% to 40%, and as high as 85% during the terminal stages of illness.[2] Narcotic analgesics, such as meperidine, levorphanol, and morphine sulfate, commonly cause confusional states, particularly in the elderly and terminally ill.[6, 7] Cancer patients with pain are twice as likely to develop a psychiatric complication of cancer than patients without pain. Of the patients who received a psychiatric diagnosis, 39% reported significant pain. In contrast, only 19% of patients without a psychiatric diagnosis had significant pain.[1] The psychiatric diagnoses of these patients with pain were predominantly adjustment disorder with depressed or mixed mood (69%) and major depression (15%).

Anxiety in the Cancer Patient

Assessment and Diagnosis

The recognition of anxious symptoms requiring treatment can be challenging. It is important that the physician inquire about anxiety symptoms when distress is suspected because patients may be embarrassed by their present concerns or by a history of phobias or panic. Table 14–1[8] provides some questions that are useful to ask.

Patients with anxiety complain of tension or restlessness, or they exhibit jitteriness, autonomic hyperactivity, insomnia, shortness of breath, numbness, or worry. Often the physical or somatic manifestations of anxiety overshadow the psychological or cognitive ones, and are the symptoms that the patient most often presents.[9] The consultant must use these symptoms as a cue to inquire about the patient's psychological state, which is commonly one of fear, worry, or apprehension. The assumption that a high level of anxiety is inevitably encountered during the terminal phase of illness is neither helpful nor accurate for diagnostic and treatment purposes. In deciding whether to treat anxiety during the terminal phase of illness, the patient's subjective level of distress is the primary impetus for the initiation of treatment. Other considerations include problematic patient behavior such as noncompliance as a result of anxiety, family and staff reactions to the patient's distress, and the balancing of the risks and benefits of treatment.[10]

Anxiety, like fever, is a symptom in this population that can have many causes. Additionally, in the cancer patient, symptoms of anxiety often arise from some medical complication of the illness or treatment such as organic anxiety disorder, delirium, or other organic mental disorders.[9, 10] Hypoxia, sepsis, poorly controlled pain, and adverse drug

TABLE 14–1. **Questions to Assess Anxiety Symptoms in Cancer Patients**

Have you experienced any of the following symptoms since your cancer diagnosis or treatment?
If yes, when do they occur (i.e., days prior to treatment, during procedures, at night, no specific time), and how long do they last?

- Do you feel nervous, shaky, or jittery?
- Have you felt fearful, apprehensive, tense?
- Have you had to avoid certain places or activities because of fear?
- Have you experienced your heart pounding or racing?
- Have you had trouble catching your breath when nervous?
- Have you had any unjustified sweating or trembling?
- Have you felt a knot in the pit in your stomach?
- Have you felt a lump in your throat when getting upset?
- Do you find yourself pacing back and forth?
- Are you afraid to close your eyes at night for fear that you will die in your sleep?
- Do you find yourself worrying about the next diagnostic test, or the results of it weeks in advance?
- Have you had the sudden onset of a fear of losing control or going crazy?
- Have you had the sudden onset of a fear of dying?
- Do you often worry about when your pain will return and how bad it will get?
- Do you worry about whether you'll be able to get your next dose of pain medication on schedule?
- Do you spend more time in bed than you should because you fear intensification of pain if you stand up or move about?

Modified from Roth AJ, Massie MJ, Redd WH: Consultation to the cancer patient. In: Jacobson AM, Jacobson JL (eds): Psychiatric Secrets. Philadelphia, Hanley & Belfus, 1995.

reactions, such as akathisia or withdrawal states, are specific entities that often present as anxiety.

It is important to consider the need to slowly taper benzodiazepines and opioid analgesics, used in the control of anxiety or pain, in order to prevent acute withdrawal states. Withdrawal states in cancer patients often present first as agitation or anxiety and become clinically evident days later than might be expected in younger, healthier patients as a result of impaired metabolism. Benzodiazepine withdrawal, for example, can present first as agitation or anxiety, though the diagnosis is often missed in terminally ill patients and, especially, the elderly, where physiologic dependence on these medications is often unrecognized.[11] In the dying patient, anxiety can represent impending cardiac or respiratory arrest, pulmonary embolism, electrolyte imbalance, or dehydration.[12]

Despite the fact that anxiety in terminal illness commonly results from medical complications, it is important not to forget that psychological factors related to death and dying or existential issues play a role in anxiety, particularly in patients who are alert and not confused.[9] Patients frequently fear the isolation and separation of death. Claustrophobic patients may be afraid of the idea of being confined and buried in a coffin. These issues can be disconcerting to consultants, who may find themselves at a loss for words that are consoling to the patient. Nonetheless, one should not avoid eliciting these concerns, listening empathetically to them, and enlisting pastoral involvement where appropriate.

Post-traumatic stress disorder (PTSD) is a specific type of anxiety disorder resulting from the effects of traumatic experiences. Recall of prior painful or frightening treatment is a common cause of PTSD in cancer patients, especially children. Illness can exacerbate feelings about earlier traumas, noted particularly in cancer patients who are Holocaust survivors. Symptoms can develop at various stages of illness, but are frequent at the time of diagnosis. In general, pediatric and geriatric populations have more difficulty coping with stressful events and are at greater risk for PTSD. The underdeveloped emotional state of children prevents them from using various adaptive strategies, and the elderly are likely to have fixed coping mechanisms that minimize their flexibility in dealing with trauma. In adults, the typical presenting symptoms include periods of intrusive repetition of the stressful event, along with denial, emotional numbness, and depression. PTSD has been described in children treated for cancer.[13] In both adults and children, use of denial is prominent and minimizes the painful event. The nonspecific emotional symptoms can make the diagnosis difficult to distinguish from a generalized anxiety disorder, depression, or panic disorder. Questions about intrusive phenomena help to determine the specific diagnosis. Many patients are relieved to understand their symptoms are an expected response to severe stress.

The specific treatment of anxiety in the terminally ill often depends on etiology, presentation, and setting. For instance, anxiety associated with hypoxia and dyspnea in a patient with diffuse lung metastases is most responsive to treatment with oxygen and opioid analgesics. If the same patient's presentation includes hallucinations and agitation, a neuroleptic would be added to the regimen. An arterial blood gas provides confirmatory information but is not essential to considering and treating hypoxia and so may be unnecessary when attempting to maximize the patient's comfort.

Pharmacologic Treatment

The pharmacotherapy of anxiety in cancer patients (Table 14–2) involves the judicious use of the following classes of medications: benzodiazepines, neuroleptics, antihistamines, antidepressants, and opioid analgesics.[9, 10, 14]

Benzodiazepines

Benzodiazepines are the mainstay of the pharmacologic treatment of anxiety in cancer patients. The shorter-acting benzodiazepines, such as lorazepam, alprazolam, and oxazepam, are safest in this population. The selection of these drugs avoids toxic accumulation due to impaired metabolism in debilitated individuals.[15] Lorazepam, oxazepam, and temazepam are metabolized by conjugation in the liver and are therefore safest in patients with hepatic disease. This is in contrast to alprazolam and other benzodiazepines, which are metabolized through oxidative pathways in the liver that are more vulnerable to interference through hepatic damage. However, the disadvantage of using short-acting benzodiazepines is that patients often experience breakthrough anxiety or end-of-dose failure. Such patients benefit from switching to longer acting benzodiazepines, such as diazepam or clonazepam. In addition, patients with advanced disease often benefit from parenteral administration of these drugs. Rectal diazepam[16] has been used widely

TABLE 14–2. **Anxiolytic Medications Used in Cancer Patients**

Generic Name	Approximate Daily Dosage Range (mg)	Route
Benzodiazepines		
Very Short-Acting		
Midazolam	10–60 per 24 hr	IV, SC
Short-Acting		
Alprazolam	0.25–2.0 tid–qid	PO, SL
Oxazepam	10–15 tid–qid	PO
Lorazepam	0.5–2 tid–qid	PO, SL, IV, IM
Intermediate-Acting		
Chlordiazepoxide	10–50 tid–qid	PO, IM
Long-Acting		
Diazepam	5–10 bid–tid	PO, IM, IV, PR
Clorazepate	7.5–15 bid–tid	PO
Clonazepam	0.5–2 bid–tid	PO
Nonbenzodiazepines		
Buspirone	5–20 tid	PO
Neuroleptics		
Haloperidol	0.5–5 q2–12 hr	PO, IV, SC, IM
Methotrimeprazine	10–20 q4–8 hr	PO, IV, SC
Thioridazine	10–75 tid–qid	PO
Chlorpromazine	12.5–50 q4–12 hr	PO, IM, IV
Antihistamines		
Hydroxyzine	25–50 q4–6 hr	PO, IV, SC
Tricyclic Antidepressants		
Imipramine	12.5–150	PO, IM
Clomipramine	10–150	PO

IM = intramuscular; IV = intravenous; PO = by mouth; PR = through the rectum; SC = subcutaneous; SL = sublingual.

in the palliative care field to control anxiety, restlessness, and agitation associated with the final days of life.

- *Midazolam*, a very short-acting, water-soluble benzodiazepine, is usually administered as an intravenous infusion in critical care settings where sedation is the goal in an agitated or anxious patient on a respirator. Midazolam may also prove useful in controlling anxiety and agitation in terminal phases of illness.[17] Unlike diazepam, midazolam has a short duration of action and seems to be less irritating to subcutaneous tissues when given by subcutaneous infusion.
- *Clonazepam*, a longer-acting benzodiazepine, has been found to be extremely useful in the palliative care setting for the treatment of anxiety, depersonalization, or derealization in patients with seizure disorders, brain tumors, and mild organic mental disorders. Patients who experience end-of-dose failure with recurrence of anxiety on shorter-acting drugs also find clonazepam helpful. Clonazepam is also useful in patients with organic mood disorders who have symptoms of mania, and as an adjuvant analgesic in patients with neuropathic pain.[18, 19]

Fears of causing respiratory depression should not prevent the clinician from using adequate dosages of benzodiazepines to control anxiety. The likelihood of respiratory depression is minimized when one utilizes shorter-acting drugs, increases the dosages in small increments, and ultimately switches to longer-acting drugs.

Nonbenzodiazepine Anxiolytics

- *Buspirone* is a nonbenzodiazepine anxiolytic that is useful in patients with chronic anxiety or anxiety related to adjustment disorders.[20] The onset of anxiolytic action is delayed in comparison to the benzodiazepines, taking 5 to 10 days for relief of anxiety to begin. Because of its delayed onset of action and indication for use in chronic anxiety states, buspirone may be of limited usefulness to the clinician treating anxiety and agitation in the terminally ill.
- Neuroleptics, such as *thioridazine*, *haloperidol*, and *alanzapine*, are useful in the treatment of anxiety when benzodiazepines are not sufficient for symptom control.[9] They are also indicated when an organic etiology is suspected or when psychotic symptoms, such as delusions or hallucinations, accompany the anxiety. Typically, haloperidol is sufficient to control anxious symptoms and avoid excessive sedation. Low-potency neuroleptics, such as thioridazine, are also effective anxiolytics and can help with insomnia and agitation. Neuroleptics are perhaps the safest class of anxiolytics in patients where there is legitimate concern regarding respiratory depression or compromise.
- *Chlorpromazine* has similar side effects that limit its application in this setting. However, it can be useful in patients where sedation is desirable. With this class of drugs in general, one must be aware of extrapyramidal side effects (particularly when patients are taking additional neuroleptics for antiemetic purposes) and the remote possibility of neuroleptic malignant syndrome.
- *Antidepressants* are the standard treatment for anxiety accompanying depression and are helpful in treating panic disorder.[21–24] Guidelines for their use are discussed in the section on depression later in the chapter. Their usefulness is often limited in the dying patient as a result of anticholinergic and sedative side effects. Because the consultant very often is faced with the task of relieving symptoms in a short period of time, drugs that require a period of weeks to achieve therapeutic effect are unsatisfactory.
- Opioid drugs such as the narcotic analgesics are primarily indicated for the control of pain. However, these drugs are also effective in the relief of dyspnea resulting from cardiopulmonary processes and the anxiety associated with them.[25] Opioid drugs are particularly useful in the treatment of dying patients who are in respiratory distress. Continuous intravenous infusions of morphine or other narcotic analgesics allow for careful titration and control of respiratory distress, anxiety, pain, and agitation.[26] When respiratory distress is not a major problem, it is preferable to use the opioid drugs solely for analgesic purposes and to add more specific anxiolytics (such as the benzodiazepines) to control concomitant anxiety.

Nonpharmacologic Treatment

Nonpharmacologic interventions for anxiety and distress include supportive psychotherapy and behavioral interventions, which are used alone or in combination. Brief supportive psychotherapy is often useful in dealing with both crisis-related issues and existential issues confronted by cancer patients.[27] Psychotherapeutic interventions should include both the patient and family, particularly as the patient with advanced illness becomes increasingly debilitated and less able to interact.

Relaxation, guided imagery, and hypnosis may help reduce anxiety and thereby increase the patient's sense of control. Even patients with advanced illness are still appropriate candidates for useful application of behavioral techniques despite physical debilitation. In assessing the utility of such interventions, the clinician should, however, take into account the mental clarity of the patient. Confusional states interfere dramatically with a patient's ability to focus attention and thus limit the usefulness of these techniques.[28] Occasionally these techniques can be modified so as to include even mildly cognitively impaired patients. This often involves the therapist taking a more active role by orienting the patient, creating a safe and secure environment, and evoking a conditioned response to the therapist's voice or presence.

A typical behavioral intervention for anxiety in a cancer patient would include a relaxation exercise, combined with some distraction or imagery technique. Typically, the patient is first taught to relax with passive breathing accompanied by either passive or active muscle relaxation. Once in such a relaxed state, the patient is taught a pleasant, distracting imagery exercise. In a randomized study comparing a relaxation technique to alprazolam in the treatment of anxiety and distress in nonterminally ill cancer patients, both treatments were demonstrated to be quite effective for mild to moderate degrees of anxiety or distress.[29] The drug intervention (alprazolam) was more effective for greater levels of distress or anxiety and had more rapid onset of beneficial effect. Relaxation techniques can be prescribed concurrently with anxiolytic medications in highly anxious cancer patients.

Terminal Care

Mental health professionals can assist in seeing that the emotional needs of patients and families are met during the terminal phase of illness. Such needs include continuous, updated information regarding the disease status and treatment options available. This information must be delivered repeatedly and with sensitivity as to what they are currently prepared and able to hear and absorb. Families, especially, require a great deal of reassurance that they and the medical staff have done everything possible for the patient. The goals of psychotherapy with the patient are as follows:

- to establish a bond that decreases the sense of isolation experienced with terminal illness
- to help the patient face death with a sense of self-worth
- to correct misconceptions about the past and present
- to integrate the present illness into a continuum of life experiences
- to explore issues of separation, loss, and the unknown that lies ahead

The therapist should emphasize past strengths and support previously successful ways of coping. This helps the patient mobilize inner resources, modify plans for the future, and perhaps even accept the inevitability of death.

It is during the terminal phase of illness that we have the greatest opportunity to affect the process of adaptation to loss. Mental health professionals must extend their supportive stance to include both the patient and family. Anticipatory bereavement is a common experience that allows patients, loved ones, and health care providers the opportunity to mentally prepare for the impending death. Patients and family members should be encouraged to use this period to reconcile differences, extend important final communications, and reaffirm feelings and wishes. It is a time of vital importance that can often set the tone for the subsequent bereavement course.[30]

Depression in the Cancer Patient

Prevalence

The incidence of depression in cancer patients ranges from 10% to 25% and increases with higher levels of disability, advanced illness, and pain.[31] Certain types of cancer are associated with an increased incidence of depression. Patients with pancreatic cancer, for example, are more likely to develop depression than patients with other types of intra-abdominal malignancies.[32] The somatic symptoms of depression, such as anorexia, insomnia, fatigue, and weight loss, can be unreliable and lack specificity in the cancer patient.[33] Thus, the psychological symptoms of depression take on greater diagnostic value and include the following: dysphoric mood, hopelessness, worthlessness, guilt, and suicidal ideation.[29, 31, 32]

Chochinov and associates[34] studied the prevalence of depression in a cohort of 130 terminally ill patients in a palliative care facility. They reported that 9.2% of patients met Research Diagnostic Criteria (RDC) for major depression when using high-severity thresholds for RDC criteria A symptoms (equivalent to the symptom threshold judgments specified in DSM-IV). This approach yielded the identical prevalence of major depression, whether or not one included somatic symptoms in the diagnostic criteria or used Endicott revised criteria[33] (involving replacement of somatic symptoms with nonsomatic alternatives). Although concern has been raised about the nonspecificity of somatic symptoms in the medically ill, these results—along with those of other investigations[35, 36]—indicate that their inclusion may not overinfluence the diagnostic classification of major depression. Not only have investigators found a relatively high prevalence of depression in patients with advanced cancer, but reports also suggest that depression is associated with increased morbidity in cancer patients.[4, 37, 38]

A family history of depression and a history of previous depressive episodes further suggest the reliability of a diagnosis. Evaluation of cancer-related organic factors, such as corticosteroids,[39] chemotherapeutic agents (e.g., vincristine, interferon, interleukin),[40–42] amphotericin,[43] brain radiation,[44] central nervous system metabolic-endocrine complications,[45] and paraneoplastic syndromes[46, 47] that can present as depression, must precede initiation of treatment.

Assessment and Diagnosis

Depressed mood and sadness can be appropriate responses in a cancer patient, and one must first distinguish between symptoms and syndromes; the symptom of sadness or depressed mood is not equivalent to the syndrome of major depression. Several of the studies cited earlier on prevalence of depression examine levels of severity of depressive symptoms (often as reported by patients on self-report measures such as the Beck Depression Inventory) and do not reflect rates of diagnosis of the specific clinical syndrome of major depression (although they may be highly correlative). Distinguishing between normal sadness and the syndrome of major depression in cancer patients has important treatment implications.

Table 14–3 lists the DSM-IV criteria for a diagnosis of major depressive syndrome; this classification system for psychiatric disorders is the most widely used diagnostic system in North America. These emotions can be manifestations of anticipatory grief over the potential loss of one's health, life, loved ones, and autonomy. Table 14–4[48] lists questions that a physician can ask in order to do a rapid assessment of mood.

The diagnosis of a major depressive syndrome in a cancer patient often relies more on the psychological or cognitive symptoms of major depression (worthlessness, hopelessness, excessive guilt, and suicidal ideation), rather than the neurovegetative or somatic signs and symptoms of major depression.[31, 32] The presence of neurovegetative signs and symptoms of depression, such as fatigue, loss of energy and other somatic symptoms, is often not helpful in establishing a diagnosis of depression in those who are more physically ill. Cancer and its treatment can produce many of the physical symptoms characteristic of major depression in the physically healthy. The strategy of relying on the psychological or cognitive signs and symptoms of depression for diagnostic specificity is itself not without problems. Nonetheless, feelings of hopelessness, worthlessness, or suicidal ideation must be explored in detail. Hopelessness that is pervasive and accompanied by a sense of despair or despondency is more likely to represent a symptom of a depressive disorder. Similarly, patients often state that they feel they are burdening their families unfairly, causing them great pain and inconvenience. Suicidal ideation, even rather mild and passive forms, is very likely associated with significant degrees of depression in cancer patients.[49]

TABLE 14–3. **DSM-IV Criteria for Major Depressive Syndromes**

At least five of the following symptoms have been persistent for 2 weeks or more:

- depressed mood, dysphoria, loss of interest or pleasure, or anhedonia (at least one symptom must be from this group)
- physical/somatic symptoms: sleep disorder, appetite or weight change, or fatigue or loss of energy
- psychological/cognitive symptoms: worthlessness/guilt, indecisiveness/poor concentration, or thoughts of death/suicidal ideation

DSM-IV = Diagnostic and Statistical Manual of Mental Disorders IV.

TABLE 14–4. **Questions to Assess Depressive Symptoms in Patients with Cancer**

Question	Symptom
Mood	
1. How well are you coping with your cancer? Well? Poorly?	(Well-being)
2. How are your spirits since diagnosis? Down? Blue? During treatment?	(Mood)
3. Do you cry sometimes? How often? Only alone?	
4. Are there things you still enjoy doing, or have you lost pleasure in things you used to do before you had cancer?	(Anhedonia)
5. How does the future look to you? Bright? Black?	(Hopelessness)
6. Do you feel you can influence your care or is your care totally under others' control?	
7. Do you worry about being a burden to family/friends during treatment for cancer?	(Worthlessness)
8. Feel others might be better off without you?	(Guilt)
Physical Symptoms (evaluate in the context of cancer-related symptoms)	
1. Do you have pain that is not controlled?	(Pain)
2. How much time do you spend in bed? Weak? Fatigue easily? Rested after sleep?	(Fatigue)
3. Any relationship to change in treatment or how you feel otherwise physically?	
4. How is your sleeping? Trouble going to sleep? Awake early? Often?	(Insomnia)
5. How is your appetite? Food tastes good? Weight loss or gain?	(Appetite)
6. How is your interest in sex? Extent of sexual activity?	(Libido)
7. Do you think or move more slowly?	(Psychomotor slowing)

Modified from Roth AJ, Holland JH: Psychiatric complications in cancer patients. In: Brain MC, Carbone PP (eds): Current Therapy in Hematology-Oncology, 5th ed. St. Louis, Mosby, 1995.

Four different approaches to the diagnosis of major depression in the cancer patient have been described:

- an inclusive approach—including all symptoms whether or not they may be secondary to cancer illness or treatment
- an exclusive approach—disregarding all physical symptoms from consideration, not allowing them to contribute to a diagnosis of major depressive syndrome
- an etiologic approach—determining if the physical symptom is due to cancer illness or treatment, or due to a depressive disorder
- a substitutive approach—where physical symptoms of uncertain etiology are replaced by other nonsomatic symptoms

The last approach is best exemplified by the Endicott substitution criteria[33] and utilized in studies by Chochinov and associates[34] and Kathol and coworkers.[35] Chochinov and associates studied the prevalence of depression in a terminally ill cancer population, and compared low versus high diagnostic thresholds, as well as Endicott substitution criteria. Interestingly, identical prevalence rates of 9.2% for major depression and 3.8% for minor depression (total = 13%) were found using both Endicott and RDC high threshold criteria.

Research assessment methods for depressive disorders in cancer patients have become more sophisticated, valid, and reliable. Table 14–5 lists a number of available assessment methods for depression, including diagnostic classification systems, structured diagnostic interviews, and screening instruments. Unfortunately, few studies of depression in terminally ill or advanced cancer patients have used such research assessment methods to date. Additionally, in their application to populations with advanced cancer, further work is still required in order to compensate for the limitations of such methods.

Treatment of Depression

Depression in cancer patients with advanced disease is optimally managed utilizing a combination of supportive psychotherapy, cognitive-behavioral techniques, and antidepressant medications. Psychotherapeutic interventions, either in the form of individual or group counseling, have been shown to effectively reduce psychological distress and depressive symptoms in cancer patients.[50, 51] Cognitive-behavioral interventions, such as relaxation and distraction with pleasant imagery, have also been shown to decrease depressive symptoms in patients with mild to moderate levels of depression.[28] Psychopharmacologic interventions (i.e., antidepressant medications) however, are the mainstay of management in the treatment of cancer patients with severe depressive symptoms who meet criteria for a major depressive episode.[29] The efficacy of antidepressants in the treatment of depression in cancer patients has been well established.[29, 52, 53]

Pharmacologic Treatment

Any treatment for major depression in cancer patients will be less effective if given in a context devoid of psychotherapeutic support. Although both psychotherapy and cognitive behavioral therapy have proven effective in reducing psychological distressive and mild to moderate depressive symptomatology in the cancer setting, pharmacotherapy is the mainstay for treating terminally ill patients meeting diagnosis criteria for major depression.[29] Table 14–6[48] outlines the common antidepressants used in these patients.

Factors such as prognosis and the time frame for treatment may play an important role in determining the type of pharmacotherapy for depression. A depressed patient with several months or years of life expectancy can afford to wait the 2 to 4 weeks it may take to respond to a tricyclic antidepressant. The depressed dying patient with less than 3 weeks to live may do best with a rapid-acting psychostimulant. Patients who are within hours to days of death and in distress are likely to benefit most from the use of sedatives or narcotic analgesic infusions.

Tricyclic Antidepressants

Tricyclic antidepressants (TCAs) have been the cornerstone for treating depression in the general cancer setting since the early 1960s. Their application, however, requires a careful risk-benefit ratio analysis. Although nearly 70% of patients treated with a tricyclic for nonpsychotic depression can anticipate a positive response, these medications are associated with a side effect profile that can be particularly troublesome for many patients.[54] The tertiary amines (amitriptyline, doxepin, imipramine) have a greater propensity to cause side effects than do secondary amines (nortriptyline, desipramine)[55]; thus, the secondary amines are more often a preferable choice for medically sicker patients.

The anticholinergic side effects can include constipation, dry mouth, and urinary retention. To avoid exacerbating symptoms associated with genitourinary outlet obstruction, decreased gastric motility, or stomatitis, a relatively nonanticholinergic tricyclic such as desipramine or nortriptyline is a reasonable choice. Those patients who are receiving medication with anticholinergic properties (such as pethidine, atropine, diphenhydramine, phenothiazines) are at risk for developing an anticholinergic delirium, and thus antidepressants that are potently anticholinergic should be avoided.[56] The anticholinergic actions of TCAs can also cause serious tachycardia, which may be problematic for terminally ill patients with cardiac insufficiency. The quinidine-like effects of TCAs can also lead to arrhythmias by virtue of their ability to delay conduction via the His-Purkinje system (associated with nonspecific ST-T changes and T waves on the electrocardiograph). These effects are particularly concerning for those terminally ill patients with pre-existing conduction defects, especially second- or third-degree heart block.

Tricyclic antidepressants should be started at low doses and increased in 10- to 25-mg increments every 2 to 4 days until a therapeutic dose is attained or side effects become a dose-limiting factor. Depressed cancer patients often achieve a therapeutic response at significantly lower doses of TCAs than are necessary in the physically well.[30] There is also evidence to suggest that patients with advanced cancer achieve higher serum tricyclic levels at modest doses.[57] In order to minimize drug toxicity and more carefully guide the process of drug titration, prescribing tricyclics (desipramine, nortriptyline, amitriptyline, imipramine) with well-established therapeutic plasma levels may be advantageous.[58] Desipramine and nortriptyline

TABLE 14–5. **Research Assessment Methods for Depression in Cancer Patients**

Diagnostic Classification Systems
Diagnostic and Statistical Manual (DSM-IV)
Endicott Substitution Criteria
Research Diagnostic Criteria (RDC)
Structured Diagnostic Interviews
Schedule for Affective Disorders and Schizophrenia (SADS)*
Diagnostic Interview Schedule (DIS)†
Structured Clinical Interview for DSM-III-R (SCID)
Screening Instruments—Self-Report
General Health Questionnaire (GHQ)
Hospital Anxiety and Depression Scale (HADS)
Beck Depression Inventory 0 (BDI)

*Designed for use with RDC criteria.
†Designed for use with DSM-III criteria.

TABLE 14–6. **Antidepressant Use in Cancer Patients**

Medication	Start/Daily Dose (mg)	Primary Side Effects/Comments
Tricyclics (TCAs)		All TCAs can cause cardiac arrhythmias; blood levels are available for all but doxepin; get baseline EKG
Amitriptyline (Elavil)	10–25/50–100	Sedation; anticholinergic; orthostasis
Imipramine (Tofranil)	10–25/50–150	Intermediate sedation; anticholinergic; orthostasis
Desipramine (Norpramin)	25/75–150	Little sedation or orthostasis; moderate anticholinergic
Nortriptyline (Pamelor)	10–25/75–150	Little anticholinergic or orthostasis; intermediate sedation; blood level provides useful therapeutic window
Doxepin (Sinequan)	25/75–150	Very sedating; orthostatic hypotension; intermediate anticholinergic effects; potent antihistamine
Second Generation		
Bupropion (Wellbutrin)	75/200–450	May cause seizures in those with low seizure threshold/brain tumors; initially activating; sexual dysfunction
Trazodone (Desyrel)	50/150–200	Sedating; not anticholinergic; risk of priapism
Selective Serotonin Reuptake Inhibitors (SSRIs)		SSRIs have few anticholinergic or cardiovascular side effects. Sexual dysfunction including anorgasmia.
Fluoxetine (Prozac)	10/20–40	Headache; nausea; anxiety; insomnia; has very long half-life; may be even longer in debilitated patient
Sertraline (Zoloft)	25/50–150	Nausea; insomnia
Paroxetine (Paxil)	10/20–50	Nausea; somnolence; asthenia; no active metabolites
Citalopram	20/20–40	Reportedly fewer GI and sexual side effects; fewer problematic interactions with other medications
Psychostimulants		All psychostimulants may cause:
Dextroamphetamine (Dexedrine)	2.5/5–30	Nightmares, insomnia, psychosis anorexia, agitation, and restlessness; possible cardiac complications; they should be given in two divided doses at 8 A.M. and noon; can be used as analgesic adjuvant and to counter sedation of opiates
Methylphenidate (Ritalin)	2.5/5–30	
Pemoline (Cylert)	18.75/37.5–150	Monitor liver tests
Others		
Venlafaxine (Effexor)	75/225–375	Inhibits reuptake of both serotonin and norepinephrine; achieves steady state in 3 days; may increase blood pressure
Nefazodone (Serzone)	100/200–500	Affects serotonin, $5HT_2$, and norepinephrine; sedating; decreased cardiotoxicity; less reported sexual dysfunction than SSRIs
Mirtazapine (Remeron)	15/15–45	Sedating at lower doses, useful for agitated depression; less reported nausea, GI problems, sexual dysfunction; may cause weight gain

EKG = electrocardiogram; GI = gastrointestinal; $5HT_2$ = 5-hydroxytryptamine-2 receptor.
Modified from Roth AJ, Holland JH: Psychiatric complications in cancer patients. In: Brain MC, Carbone PP (eds): Current Therapy in Hematology-Oncology, 5th ed. St. Louis, Mosby, 1995.

are generally better tolerated in this population than amitriptyline or imipramine.

For the depressed cancer patient, the choice of TCA can be made on the basis of a side effect profile that will be the least incompatible with the patient's overall medical condition. Most tricyclics are available as rectal suppositories for patients who are no longer able to take medication orally. Although not very practical, amitriptyline, imipramine, and doxepin can also be given intramuscularly. However, it must be borne in mind that a therapeutic response to TCAs (as with all antidepressants) has a latency time of 3 to 6 weeks. For the terminally ill, depressed patient whose life expectancy is anticipated to be less than this, psychostimulants may offer a more viable, rapid response alternative.

Second Generation Antidepressants

SELECTIVE SEROTONIN REUPTAKE INHIBITORS

The selective serotonin reuptake inhibitors (SSRIs) are an important addition to the available antidepressant medications. They have been found to be as effective in the treatment of depression as the tricyclics[59, 60] and have a number of features that may be particularly advantageous for the cancer patient. The SSRIs have a very low affinity for adrenergic, cholinergic, and histamine receptors, thus accounting for negligible orthostatic hypotension, urinary retention, memory impairment, sedation, or reduced awareness.[61] Most of them have not been found to cause clinically significant alterations in cardiac conduction, and are generally well tolerated along with a wider margin of safety than the TCAs in the event of an overdose. They do not therefore require therapeutic drug level monitoring.

Most of the side effects of SSRIs result from their selective central and peripheral serotonin reuptake. These include increased intestinal motility (loose stools), nausea, vomiting, insomnia, headaches, and sexual dysfunction. Some patients may experience anxiety, tremor, and restlessness.[62] These side effects tend to be dose related and may be problematic for patients with advanced disease.

There are six SSRIs currently being marketed: *sertraline, fluoxetine, paroxetine, nefazodone, fluvoxamine*, and *citalopram*. With the exception of fluoxetine, whose elimination half-life is 2 to 4 days, the SSRIs have an elimination half-life of about 24 hours. Fluoxetine is the only SSRI with a potent active metabolite—norfluoxetine—whose elimination half-life is 7 to 14 days. Fluoxetine can cause mild nausea and a brief period of increased anxiety, as well as appetite suppression that usually lasts for a period of several weeks. The anorectic properties of fluoxetine have not been limiting factors in the use of this drug in cancer patients. Fluoxetine and norfluoxetine do not reach a steady state for 5 to 6 weeks, compared with 4 to 14 days for paroxetine, fluvoxamine, and sertraline. These differences are important in situations where a switch from an SSRI to another anti-depressant is being considered. Following a switch to a monoamine oxidase inhibitor (MAOI), the washout period for fluoxetine is at least 5 weeks; since fluoxetine has entered the market, there have been several reports of significant drug-drug interactions.[63, 64] Paroxetine, fluvoxamine, and sertraline, on the other hand, require considerably shorter washout periods (10–14 days) under similar circumstances.

All the SSRIs have the ability to inhibit the hepatic isoenzyme P450 2D6, with sertraline being least potent in this regard. This is important with respect to ratios of dose to plasma level, and with drug interactions, because the SSRIs are dependent upon hepatic metabolism. In the case of paroxetine (the most potent inhibitor), small dosage increases can result in dramatic elevations in plasma levels. Paroxetine and, to a somewhat lesser extent, fluoxetine appear to inhibit the hepatic enzymes responsible for their own clearance.[55] The coadministration of these medications with other drugs that are dependent on this enzyme system for their catabolism (e.g., tricyclics, phenothiazines, type IC antiarrhythmics, and quinidine) should be approached cautiously. Fluvoxamine has been shown in some instances to elevate the blood levels of propranolol and warfarin by as much as twofold and should thus not be prescribed together with these agents. SSRIs should be avoided with the chemotherapeutic agent procarbazine, which has MAOI-like properties.

SSRIs can generally be started at their minimally effective doses. For cancer patients, this usually means initiating therapy at approximately half the usual starting dose used in an otherwise healthy patient. If patients experience activating effects on SSRIs, they should not be given at bedtime but rather administered earlier in the day. Gastrointestinal upset can be reduced by ensuring the patient does not take medication on an empty stomach. Citalopram, the newest antidepressant to date, is reported to have fewer gastrointestinal and sexual side effects, as well as fewer problematic interactions with other medications than other SSRIs; however, it has not been studied in cancer patients.

SEROTONIN-NOREPINEPHRINE REUPTAKE INHIBITORS

Venlafaxine (Effexor) and mirtazapine (Remeron) are new antidepressants in the class of serotonin-norepinephrine reuptake inhibitors (SNRIs). Venlafaxine is a potent inhibitor of neuronal serotonin and norepinephrine reuptake; some patients may experience a modest sustained increase in blood pressure, especially at doses above the recommended initiating dose. Like other antidepressants, venlafaxine should not be used in patients receiving MAOIs. Although there are currently no data addressing its use in the depressed cancer patient, its pharmacokinetic properties and generally well-tolerated side effect profile suggest it may have a role to play. Mirtazapine is a sedating antidepressant, useful in depressed patients with associated anxiety and insomnia. It has few gastrointestinal and sexual side effects, and may induce weight gain.

TRAZODONE

If given in sufficient doses, trazodone can be an effective antidepressant. Trazodone is very sedating and, at low doses, is helpful in the treatment of the depressed cancer patient with insomnia. Although its anticholinergic profile is almost negligible, it has considerable affinity for α_1-adrenoceptors and therefore may predispose patients to orthostatic hypotension and its problematic sequelae (i.e., falls, fractures, and head injuries). In addition, it is highly serotonergic and its use should be considered when the patient requires adjunct analgesic effect in addition to antidepressant effects. Trazodone has little effect on cardiac conduction but can cause arrhythmias in patients with premorbid cardiac disease.[65] Trazodone has also been associated with priapism, and should thus be used with caution in male patients.[66]

BUPROPION

Bupropion (Wellbutrin), at present, is not the first drug of choice for depressed patients with cancer. However, one might consider prescribing bupropion if patients have a poor response to a reasonable trial of other antidepressants. Bupropion may have a role in the treatment of the psychomotor-retarded, depressed, terminally ill patient because it has energizing effects similar to the stimulant drugs.[67] However, because of a slightly increased incidence of seizures, it should be avoided in patients with central nervous system (CNS) disorders.[68] Bupropion is now marketed in a slow-release formula (Zyban), useful for smoking cessation.

Heterocyclic Antidepressants

The heterocyclic antidepressants have side effect profiles that are similar to the TCAs.

- *Maprotiline* should be avoided in patients with brain tumors and in those who are at risk for seizures, because the incidence of seizures is increased with this medication.[69]
- *Amoxapine* has mild dopamine-blocking activity. Hence, patients who are taking other dopamine blockers (e.g., antiemetics) have an increased risk of developing extrapyramidal symptoms and dyskinesias.[70]
- *Mianserin* (not available in the United States) is a serotonergic antidepressant with adjuvant analgesic properties that is used widely in Europe and Latin America. Van Heeringen and Zivkov[71] showed mianserin to be a safe and effective drug for the treatment of depression in cancer.

Psychostimulants

The psychostimulants (*dextroamphetamine, methylphenidate*, and *pemoline*) offer an alternative and effective pharmacologic approach to the treatment of depression in cancer patients.[72–74] These drugs have a more rapid onset of action than the tricyclics and are often energizing. They are most helpful in the treatment of depression in cancer patients with advanced disease and those where dysphoric mood is associated with severe psychomotor slowing and even mild cognitive impairment. Psychostimulants have been shown to improve attention, concentration, and overall performance on neuropsychological testing in the medically ill.[75] In relatively low doses, psychostimulants stimulate appetite, promote a sense of well-being, and improve feelings of weakness and fatigue in cancer patients.

Treatment with dextroamphetamine or methylphenidate is slowly increased over several days until a desired effect is achieved or side effects (overstimulation, anxiety, insomnia, paranoia, confusion) intervene. In general, patients are maintained on methylphenidate for 1 to 2 months, and approximately two thirds will be able to be withdrawn from methylphenidate without a recurrence of depressive symptoms. Those whose symptoms do recur can be maintained on a psychostimulant for up to 1 year without significant abuse problems. Tolerance will develop and adjustment of dose may be necessary. An additional benefit of these drugs is that they have been shown to reduce sedation secondary to opioid analgesics and provide adjuvant analgesia in cancer patients.[5] Common side effects of stimulants include nervousness, overstimulation, mild increase in blood pressure and pulse rate, and tremor. More rare side effects include dyskinesias or motor tics, as well as a paranoid psychosis or exacerbation of an underlying and unrecognized confusional state.

Pemoline is a unique psychostimulant chemically unrelated to amphetamine, and it is a less potent stimulant with little abuse potential. Advantages of pemoline as a psychostimulant in cancer patients include the lack of abuse potential, the lack of federal regulation through special triplicate prescriptions, the mild sympathomimetic effects, and the fact that it comes in a chewable tablet form that can be absorbed through the buccal mucosa and be used by cancer patients who have difficulty swallowing or have intestinal obstruction. Pemoline appears to be as effective as methylphenidate or dextroamphetamine in the treatment of depressive symptoms in cancer patients.[76] Pemoline should be used with caution in patients with liver impairment, and liver function tests should be monitored periodically with longer term treatment.[77]

Monoamine Oxidase Inhibitors

In general, MAOIs have been considered a less desirable alternative for treating depression in cancer patients. Because of their mode of action, patients who receive MAOIs must avoid foods rich in tyramine, sympathomimetic drugs (amphetamines, methylphenidate), and medications containing phenylpropranolamine and pseudoephedrine; the combination of these agents with MAOIs may cause hypertensive crisis, leading to strokes and fatalities. MAOIs in combination with opioid analgesics have also been reported to be associated with myoclonus and delirium and must therefore be used together cautiously.[6] The use of meperidine while taking MAOIs is **absolutely contraindicated** and can lead to hyperpyrexia, cardiovascular collapse, and death.[78] MAOIs can also cause considerable orthostatic hypotension.

The new reversible inhibitors of monoamine oxidase-A (RIMAs) may reduce some of the problems associated with the older MAOIs. There are no studies on the role of RIMAs in the depressed cancer patient, but there are interesting theoretical reasons to suggest they may eventually have a larger role to play than the nonselective MAOIs. RIMAs selectively inhibit MAO-A enzyme, thereby leaving MAO-B enzyme available to deal with any tyramine challenge.

MOCLOBEMIDE

Moclobemide, a RIMA first introduced onto the Canadian market, appears to be loosely bound to the MAO-A receptor and is thus relatively easily displaced by tyramine from its binding site. It has a very short half-life that further reduces the possibility of any prolonged adverse effects such as hypertensive crisis. Dietary restrictions avoiding tyramine-containing foods are thus not required. The side effect profile of moclobemide is far more favorable than that of nonselective MAOIs, and it tends to be well tolerated. Although the risk of hypertensive crisis is significantly reduced, it is not however entirely eliminated. Agents such as meperidine, procarbazine, dextromethorphan, or other ephedrine-containing agents are still best avoided. Coadministration with cimetidine will increase its plasma concentration, thus requiring appropriate dosage adjustments. Although RIMAs may offer some advantages in the terminally ill, depressed patient over tranylcypromine and isocarboxazid, they will likely remain a second-line choice to other available non-MAOI antidepressants.

Mood Stabilizers

Patients who have been receiving lithium carbonate for bipolar affective disorder prior to cancer should be maintained on it throughout cancer treatment, although close monitoring is necessary when the intake of fluids and electrolytes is restricted, such as during the preoperative and postoperative periods. The maintenance dose of lithium may need reduction in seriously ill patients. Lithium should be prescribed with caution in patients receiving cisplatin or other potentially nephrotoxic drugs. Use of carbamazepine as a mood stabilizer can be problematic in cancer patients because of its marrow suppressing properties. Valproic acid, on the other hand, though also not specifically studied in this population, is better tolerated than carbamazepine and is efficacious.

Choosing an Antidepressant

The choice of antidepressants depends on the nature of the depressive symptoms, medical problems present, and the side effects of the specific drug that one may want to exploit or avoid. The depressed patient who is agitated and has insomnia will benefit from the use of an antidepressant that has sedating effects, such as amitriptyline, doxepine, or mirtazapine. Patients with psychomotor slowing will benefit from the use of compounds with the least sedating effects, such as fluoxetine or bupropion. The patient who has stomatitis secondary to chemotherapy or radiotherapy, or who has slowed intestinal motility or urinary retention, should receive an antidepressant with the least anticholinergic effects, such as desipramine, nortriptyline, or one of the newer serotonin-based drugs. Low doses of TCAs can be especially useful as adjuvant pain medications in those patients with neuropathic pain syndromes.

Patients who are unable to swallow pills may be able to take an antidepressant in an elixir, intramuscular, or rectal suppository form, although absorption by this latter route has not been studied in cancer patients. Although three TCAs (amitriptyline, imipramine, and clomipramine) are available in injectable form, the U.S. Food and Drug Administration has approved imipramine and amitriptyline for oral and muscular administration and clomipramine for oral use only. Cardiac monitoring is suggested for the parenteral route of administration. The psychostimulant pemoline may be absorbed through the buccal mucosa and obviate the need for swallowing.

Nonpharmacologic Treatment

Supportive psychotherapy is a useful treatment approach to depression in cancer patients. Psychotherapy with these patients consists of active listening with supportive verbal interventions and the occasional interpretation.[51] Despite the seriousness of the patient's plight, it is not necessary for the psychiatrist or psychologist to appear overly solemn or emotionally restrained. Often it is only the psychotherapist, of all the patient's caregivers, who is comfortable enough to converse lightheartedly and allow patients to talk about their life and experiences rather than focus solely on impending death. The patient who wishes to talk or ask questions about death should be allowed to do so freely, with the therapist maintaining an interested, interactive stance. It is not uncommon for the patient to benefit from pastoral counseling. If a chaplaincy service is available, it should be offered to the patient and family.

Electroconvulsive Therapy

Occasionally, it is necessary to consider electroconvulsive therapy (ECT) for depressed cancer patients who have depression with psychotic features, in whom treatment with antidepressants has been ineffective or poses unacceptable side effects. Others have reviewed the safe effective use of ECT in the medically ill.

Suicide in the Cancer Patient

Cancer patients are at increased risk of suicide relative to the general population, particularly in the terminal stage of illness. Factors associated with increased risk of suicide in patients with advanced disease[48, 49] are listed in Table 14–7. Patients with advanced illness are at highest risk, perhaps because they are most likely to have such complications as pain, depression, delirium, and deficit symptoms. Psychiatric disorders are frequently present in hospitalized cancer patients who are suicidal. A review of the psychiatric consultation data from Memorial Sloan-Kettering Cancer Center showed that one third of suicidal cancer patients had a major depression, about 20% suffered from a delirium, and 50% were diagnosed with an adjustment disorder with both anxious and depressed features at the time of evaluation.[48, 49]

Thoughts of suicide probably occur quite frequently, particularly in the setting of advanced cancer, and seem to act as a steam valve for feelings often expressed by patients as, "if it gets too bad, I always have a way out." Once they develop a trusting and safe relationship, patients almost universally reveal occasional thoughts of suicide as a means of escaping the threat of being overwhelmed by cancer. Published reports, however, suggest that persistent suicidal ideation is relatively infrequent in cancer and is limited to those who are significantly depressed. Chochinov and coworkers found that of 200 terminally ill patients in a palliative care facility, 44.5% acknowledged at least a fleeting desire to die, but these episodes were brief and did not reflect a sustained or committed desire to die.[79] However, 17 patients (8.5%) reported an unequivocal desire for death to come soon and indicated that they had held this desire consistently over time. Among this group, 10 (58.8%) received a diagnosis of depression, compared with a prevalence of 7.7% in patients who did not endorse a genuine, consistent desire for death. Patients with a desire for death were also found to have significantly more pain and less social support than those patients without. At Memorial Hospital, suicide risk evaluation accounted for 8.6% of psychiatric consultations and was usually requested by staff in response to a patient verbalizing suicidal wishes.[49] Among 185 cancer patients with pain studied at Memorial Hospital, suicidal ideation was found in 17% of the study population.[48] The actual prevalence of suicidal ideation may be considerably higher in that patients often disclose these thoughts only after a stable, ongoing physician-patient relationship has been established.

Cancer patients commit suicide most frequently in the advanced stages of disease.[80, 81] Poor prognosis and advanced illness usually go hand-in-hand. With advancing disease, the incidence of significant cancer pain increases. Uncontrolled pain in cancer patients is a dramatically important risk factor for suicide.[82]

Depression is a factor in 50% of all suicides; those suffering from depression are at a much greater risk of suicide than the general population.[83] The role that depression plays in cancer suicide is equally significant. Approximately 25% of all cancer patients experience severe depressive symptoms, with about 6% fulfilling DSM-III criteria for the diagnosis of major depression.[1, 31] Among those with advanced illness and progressively impaired

TABLE 14–7. **Suicide Vulnerability Factors in Patients with Cancer**

Factor	Effect/Consequence
Pain	Suffering
Advanced illness	Poor prognosis
Depression	Hopelessness
Delirium	Disinhibition
Loss of control	Helplessness
Pre-existing psychopathology	
Substance/alcohol abuse	
Suicide history	Family history
Fatigue	Exhaustion
Lack of social support	Social isolation

Modified from Breitbart W: Cancer pain and suicide. In: Foley KM, Bonica JJ, Ventafridda V (eds): Advances in Pain Research and Therapy, vol 16, p 399. New York, Raven Press, 1990.

physical function, symptoms of severe depression rise to 77%. Depression also appears to be important in terms of patient preferences for life-sustaining medical therapy. Ganzini and associates reported that, among elderly depressed patients, an increase in desire for life-sustaining medical therapies followed treatment of depression, particularly in those subjects who had been initially more severely depressed and were therefore more likely to overestimate the risks and to underestimate the benefits of treatment.[84] They concluded that although patients with mild to moderate depression are unlikely to alter their decisions regarding life-sustaining medical treatment in spite of treatment for their depression, severely depressed patients should be encouraged to defer advance treatment directives. In these patients, decisions should be discouraged until after treatment of their depression.

Hopelessness is the key variable that links depression and suicide in the general population. Further, hopelessness is a significantly better predictor of completed suicide than is depression alone. With the typical cancer suicide being characterized by advanced illness and poor prognosis, hopelessness is commonly experienced.[85] Being left to face illness alone creates a sense of isolation and abandonment that is critical to the development of hopelessness. The prevalence of organic mental disorders among cancer patients requiring psychiatric consultation ranges from 25% to 40% and can be as high as 85% during the terminal stages of illness.[4, 5] Although earlier work suggested that delirium was a protective factor in regard to cancer suicide, clinical experience has found these confusional states to be a major contributing factor in impulsive suicide attempts, especially in the hospital setting.

Fatigue, in the form of emotional, spiritual, financial, familial, communal, and other resource exhaustion, increases risk of suicide in the cancer patient.[49] Nowadays, cancer is often a chronic illness, and increased survival is accompanied by an increased number of hospitalizations, complications, and expenses. Thus, symptom control becomes a prolonged process with frequent advances and setbacks. The dying process also can become extremely long and arduous for all concerned. It is not uncommon for both family members and health care providers to withdraw prematurely from the cancer patient under these circumstances. A suicidal patient can thus feel even more isolated and abandoned. The presence of a strong support system for the patient that may act as an external control of suicidal behavior reduces risk of cancer suicide significantly.

TABLE 14–8. **Evaluation of the Suicidal, Terminally Ill Cancer Patient**

Establish rapport with an empathic approach.
Obtain patient's understanding of illness and present symptoms.
Assess mental status (internal control).
Assess vulnerability variables; pain control.
Assess support system (external control).
Obtain history of prior emotional/psychiatric problems.
Obtain family history.
Record prior suicide threats, attempts.
Assess suicidal thinking, intent, plans.
Evaluate need for one-to-one nurse/companion in hospital/home.
Formulate treatment plan, immediate and long-term.

Modified from Breitbart W: Cancer pain and suicide. In: Foley KM, Bonica JJ, Ventafridda V (eds): Advances in Pain Research and Therapy, vol 16, p 399. New York, Raven Press, 1990.

TABLE 14–9. **Questions to Assess Suicidal Risk in Cancer Patients**

(Open with statement; asking does not enhance risk.)
Most patients with cancer have passing thoughts about suicide, such as "I might do something if it gets bad enough."

• Have you ever had thoughts like that?	(Acknowledge normality)
• Any thoughts of not wanting to live or that it would be easier if you were to die?	
• Do you have thoughts of suicide? Plan?	(Seriousness)
• Have you thought about how you would do it?	
• Have you ever been depressed or made a suicide attempt?	(Prior history)
• Have you ever been treated for other psychiatric problems, or have you been psychiatrically hospitalized before getting diagnosed with cancer?	
• Have you had a problem with alcohol or drugs?	(Substance use)
• Have you lost anyone close to you recently (family, friends, copatients)?	(Bereavement)

Modified from Roth AJ, Holland JH: Psychiatric complications in cancer patients. In: Brain MC, Carbone PP (eds): Current Therapy in Hematology-Oncology, 5th ed. St. Louis, Mosby, 1995.

The frequency of suicide attempts in cancer patients has not been well studied. Although the frequency of suicidal thinking in the cancer setting may be in question, its relationship to suicide attempts or completions is clearer. Reports have shown that many cancer suicides have previously conveyed suicidal thoughts or intentions to relatives, and many of the completed cancer suicides had been preceded by an attempted suicide. This is consistent with the statistics of suicide in general, which show that a previous suicide attempt greatly increases the risk of completed suicide.[86] A family history of suicide is of increasing relevance in assessing suicide risk.

Assessment

Assessment of suicide risk and appropriate intervention are critical. Early and comprehensive psychiatric involvement with high-risk individuals can often avert suicide in the cancer setting. A careful evaluation includes a search for the meaning of suicidal thoughts, as well as an exploration of the seriousness of the risk. Tables 14–8 and 14–9[48, 49] describe an approach to the assessment of suicidal ideation in cancer patients.

The clinician's ability to establish rapport and elicit a patient's thoughts is essential as he or she assesses history, degree of intent, and quality of internal and external controls. One must listen sympathetically; allowing the patient to discuss suicidal thoughts often decreases the risk of suicide. The myth that asking about suicidal thoughts "puts the idea in their head" is one that should be dispelled, especially in cancer.[87] Patients often reconsider and reject the idea of suicide when the physician acknowledges the legitimacy of their option and the need to retain a sense of control over aspects of their death.

The suicide vulnerability factors (see Table 14–7) should

be utilized as a guide to evaluation and management. Once the setting has been made secure, assessment of the relevant mental status and adequacy of pain control can begin. Analgesics, neuroleptics, or antidepressant drugs should be utilized when appropriate. Underlying causes of delirium or pain should be addressed specifically when possible. Initiation of a crisis intervention–oriented psychotherapeutic approach, mobilizing as much of the patient's support system as possible, is important. A close family member or friend should be involved in order to support the patient, provide information, and assist in treatment planning. Psychiatric hospitalization can sometimes be helpful, but it is usually not desirable in the terminally ill patient. Thus, the medical hospital or home is the setting in which management most often takes place. Although it is appropriate to intervene when medical or psychiatric factors are clearly the driving force in a cancer suicide, there are circumstances when usurping control from the patient and family with overly aggressive intervention may be less helpful. This is most evident in those with advanced illness where comfort and symptom control are the primary concerns.

The goal of the intervention should not be to prevent suicide at all cost, but to prevent suicide that is driven by desperation. Prolonged suffering resulting from poorly controlled symptoms leads to such desperation, and it is the consultant's role to provide effective management of such problems as an alternative to suicide in the cancer patient.

Euthanasia and Physician-Assisted Suicide

In a 1988 survey of California physicians, 57% of those responding reported that they had been asked by terminally ill patients to hasten death.[88] Persistent pain and terminal illness were the primary reasons for requesting for physician-assisted euthanasia. What is the appropriate response to such a request?

The clinician in the oncology setting faces a dilemma when confronting the issue of assisted suicide or euthanasia in the cancer patient. From the medical perspective, professional training reinforces the view of suicide as a manifestation of psychiatric disturbance to be prevented at all costs. However, from the philosophical perspective, many in our society view suicide as rational in those who face the distress of an often fatal and painful disease such as cancer, and a means to regain control and maintain a dignified death. Thus, an internal debate often takes place within the cancer care professional environment that is not dissimilar to the public debate that surrounds celebrated cases, in which the rights of patients to terminate life-sustaining measures or receive active euthanasia are at issue.

Those who provide clinical care for cancer patients with pain and advanced illness are sympathetic to the goals of symptom control and relief of suffering, but they are also obviously influenced by those who view suicide or active voluntary euthanasia as rational alternatives for those already dying and in distress. Danger lies in the premature assumption that suicidal ideation or a request to hasten death by the cancer patient represents a rational act that is unencumbered by psychiatric disturbance. Proposed criteria for rational suicide have included the following:

- The person must have clear mental processes that are unimpaired by psychological illness or severe emotional distress, such as depression.
- The person must have a realistic assessment of the situation.
- The motives for the decision of suicide are understandable to most uninvolved observers.

Clearly there are suicides that occur in the cancer setting that meet these criteria for rationality; however, the majority do not, by virtue of the fact that significant psychiatric comorbidity exists. The current research data on cancer suicide and the role of such factors as pain, depression, and delirium provide a factual framework on which to base guidelines for managing this vulnerable group of patients.

Delirium and Dementia in the Cancer Patient

Assessment and Diagnosis

In spite of very little being known about the neuropathogenesis of delirium, its symptoms suggest that it is a dysfunction of multiple regions of the brain.[89] Delirium has been characterized as an etiologically nonspecific, global, cerebral dysfunction with concurrent disturbances of level of consciousness, attention, thinking, perception, memory, psychomotor behavior, emotion, and the sleep-wake cycle. Disorientation, fluctuation, or waxing and waning of these symptoms, as well as acute or abrupt onset of such disturbances, are other critical features of delirium.

Despite changes in the classification of organic mental disorders or cognitive impairment disorders made in the evolution from DSM-III to DSM-III-R to DSM-IV, the essential nature of delirium as a syndrome has been maintained. Table 14–10[90] lists the DSM-IV criteria for delirium. The essential features of acute onset of disordered attention and cognition are retained. Associated phenomena such as psychomotor behavioral changes, perceptual disturbances, hallucinations, or delusions are no longer viewed as essential to the diagnosis of delirium. Research assessment methods for delirium in advanced cancer patients have been reviewed extensively elsewhere.[91–96] Only a limited

TABLE 14–10. **DSM-IV Criteria for Delirium**

Delirium due to a general medical condition:

1. Disturbance of consciousness (that is, reduced clarity of awareness of the environment) with reduced ability to focus, sustain, or shift attention.
2. Change in cognition (such as memory deficit, disorientation, language disturbance, or perceptual disturbance) that is not better accounted for by a pre-existing, established, or evolving dementia.
3. The disturbance develops over a short period of time (usually hours to days) and tends to fluctuate during the course of the day.
4. There is evidence from the history, physical examination, or laboratory findings of a general medical condition judged to be etiologically related to the disturbance.

Modified from Smith MJ, Breitbart WS, Platt MM: A critique of instruments and methods to detect, diagnose, and rate delirium. J Pain Symptom Manage 1995; 10:35–77.

number of studies of cognitive impairment disorders in palliative care settings have used such research assessment methods.

Delirium, in contrast with dementia, is conceptualized as a reversible process. Reversibility of the process of delirium is often possible even in the patient with advanced illness; however, it may not be reversible in the last 24 to 48 hours of life. This is most likely due to the fact that irreversible processes, such as multiple organ failure, are occurring in the final hours of life. Delirium occurring in these last days of life is often referred to as terminal restlessness or terminal agitation in the palliative care literature.

At times, it is difficult to differentiate delirium from dementia because they frequently share such common clinical features as impaired memory, thinking, and judgment, as well as disorientation. Dementia appears in relatively alert individuals, with little or no clouding of consciousness. The temporal onset of symptoms in dementia is more subacute or chronically progressive, and the sleep-wake cycle seems less impaired. Most prominent in dementia are difficulties in short- and long-term memory, impaired judgment and abstract thinking, as well as disturbed higher cortical functions (such as aphasia and apraxia). Occasionally, one will encounter delirium superimposed on an underlying dementia such as in the case of an elderly patient, an acquired immunodeficiency syndrome (AIDS) patient, or a patient with a paraneoplastic syndrome. Clinically, we often utilize a number of scales or instruments that aid us in the diagnosis of delirium, dementia, or cognitive failure.

The Delirium Rating Scale, developed by Trzepacz and associates[91] is a 10-item clinician-rated symptom rating scale for delirium (Table 14–11). The scale is based on DSM-III-R diagnostic criteria for delirium and is designed to be used by the clinician to identify delirium and distinguish it reliably from dementia or other neuropsychiatric disorders. Each item is scored by choosing one best rating and carries a numeric weight chosen to distinguish the phenomenologic characteristic of delirium. A score of 12 or greater is diagnostic of delirium.

The Mini-Mental State Examination[97] also is useful in screening for cognitive failure, but it does not distinguish between delirium and dementia. The Mini-Mental State Examination provides a quantitative assessment of the cognitive performance and capacity of a patient, and is a measure of severity of cognitive impairment. It is most sensitive to cortical dementias, such as Alzheimer's disease, but less sensitive in detecting subcortical deficits, such as those found in AIDS dementia.

TABLE 14–11. **Items from the Delirium Rating Scale**

1. Temporal onset of symptoms
2. Perceptual disturbances
3. Hallucination type
4. Delusions
5. Psychomotor behavior
6. Cognitive status during formal testing
7. Physical disorder
8. Sleep-wake cycle disturbance
9. Liability of mood
10. Variability of symptoms

Modified from Trzepacz PT, Baker RW, Greenhouse J: A symptom rating scale for delirium. Psychiatry Res 1988; 23:89–97.

TABLE 14–12. **Causes of Delirium in Patients with Advanced Cancer**

Direct Causes

Central nervous system (CNS) causes
- Primary brain tumor
- Metastatic spread to CNS
- Seizures

Indirect Causes

Metabolic encephalopathy due to organ failure
Electrolyte imbalance
Treatment side effects from:
- Chemotherapeutic agents
- Steroids
- Radiation
- Narcotics
- Anticholinergics
- Antiemetics
- Antivirals

Infection
Hematologic abnormalities
Nutritional deficiencies
Paraneoplastic syndromes

Modified from Fleishman SB, Lesko LM: Delirium and dementia. In: Holland J, Rowland J (eds): Handbook of Psychooncology: Psychological Care of the Patient with Cancer, p 342. New York, Oxford University Press, 1989.

Delirium is common in patients with far advanced cancer; between 15% and 20% of hospitalized cancer patients have organic mental disorders.[98] Massie and colleagues[2] found delirium in more than 75% of terminally ill cancer patients they studied. Delirium can be due either to the direct effects of cancer on the CNS or to indirect CNS effects of the disease or treatments (Table 14–12). Early symptoms of delirium can be misdiagnosed; however, in any patient showing acute onset of agitation, impaired cognitive function, altered attention span, or a fluctuating level of consciousness, a diagnosis of delirium should be considered.[99] A common error among medical and nursing staff is to conclude that a new psychological symptom is functional without completely ruling out all possible organic etiologies. Given the large numbers of drugs cancer patients require, and the fragile state of their physiologic functioning, even routinely ordered hypnotics are enough to tip patients over into a delirium.

Chemotherapeutic agents known to cause delirium include methotrexate, fluorouracil, vincristine, vinblastine, bleomycin, bis-chloroethyl-nitrosourea, cisplatinum, asparaginase, procarbazine, and the glucocorticosteroids.[38–42] However, except for steroids, the majority of patients receiving these agents will not develop prominent CNS effects. In addition, immunotherapeutic agents such as interleukin-2 can cause delirious symptoms, including hallucinations, disorientation, and confusion.[100]

The spectrum of mental disturbances related to steroids includes minor mood lability, affective disorders (mania or depression), cognitive impairment (reversible dementia), and delirium (steroid psychosis). The incidence of these disorders ranges from 3% to 57% in noncancer populations, and they occur most commonly on higher doses. Symptoms usually develop within the first 2 weeks on steroids but in fact can occur at any time, on any dose, even during the tapering phase. Prior psychiatric illness, or prior disturbance on steroids is not a good predictor of susceptibility to, or the nature of, mental disturbance with steroids. These disorders are often rapidly reversible upon dose reduction or discontinuation.

Amphotericin B, used regularly for the treatment of fungal infections in immunologically compromised cancer patients, can cause delirium, particularly with intrathecal administration. It may be difficult to distinguish CNS effects of antifungal medication from those of fever, CNS infection, or metabolic abnormalities. Acyclovir, an antiviral drug that has proved efficacious for the prophylaxis and treatment of herpes simplex and varicella zoster virus, also can cause neurotoxicity, including lethargy, agitation, tremor, and disorientation. Cyclosporine, which is a potent immunosuppressive agent used in transplantation, can have neurotoxicity, though this is generally mild in bone marrow transplant patients.[101]

Paraneoplastic syndromes (limbic and bulbar encephalitis, subacute cerebellar degeneration) are remote effects of primary tumors, most commonly small cell lung cancer or breast cancer, but may include stomach, uterine, renal, testicular, thyroid, and colon cancers. These syndromes are thought to be caused by the cancer inducing an antibody that cross-reacts with antigens in normal tissue. Symptoms may include a mental status change, hallucinations, cognitive deficits, depression, and anxiety.[102]

Treatment of Delirium

A standard approach for managing delirium in the cancer patient includes a search for underlying causes, correction of those factors, and management of the symptoms of delirium. The treatment of delirium in the dying cancer patient is unique, however, for the following reasons:

- Most often, the etiology of terminal delirium is multifactorial or may not be found.
- When a distinct cause is found, it is often irreversible (such as hepatic failure or brain metastases).
- Work-up may be limited by the setting (home, hospice).
- The consultant's focus is usually on the patient's comfort; ordinarily helpful diagnostic procedures that are unpleasant or painful (i.e., computed tomography scan, lumbar puncture) may be avoided.

When confronted with a delirium in the terminally ill or dying cancer patient, the consultant should always formulate a differential diagnosis. However, studies should be pursued only when a suspected factor can be identified easily and treated effectively. Interestingly, Bruera and associates[103] reported that an etiology was discovered in less than 50% of terminally ill patients with cognitive failure.

In addition to seeking out and correcting the underlying cause for delirium, symptomatic and supportive therapies are important.[99] Fluid and electrolyte balance, nutrition, and vitamins may be helpful. Measures to help reduce anxiety and disorientation (i.e., structure and familiarity) may include a quiet, well-lit room with familiar objects, a visible clock or calendar, and the presence of family. Often, these supportive techniques alone are not effective and symptomatic treatment with neuroleptic or sedative medications is necessary (Table 14–13). Sedation may be necessary to relieve severe agitation or insomnia.[99] Judicious use of physical restraints, along with one-to-one nursing observation, may also be necessary and useful.

Pharmacologic Treatment

- *Haloperidol*, a neuroleptic agent that is a potent dopamine blocker, is the drug of choice in the treatment of delirium in the medically ill.[87, 99, 104, 105] Haloperidol in low doses is usually effective in targeting agitation, paranoia, and fear.[2, 30] Parenteral doses are approximately twice as potent as oral doses, although the majority of delirious patients can be managed with oral haloperidol. Many palliative care practitioners utilize delivery of haloperidol by the subcutaneous route.
- A common strategy in the management of symptoms related to delirium is to add parenteral *lorazepam* to a regimen of haloperidol,[87, 106] which may be more effective in rapidly sedating the agitated delirious patient. In a double-blind, randomized comparison trial of haloperidol versus chlorpromazine versus lorazepam, Breitbart and coworkers demonstrated that lorazepam alone was ineffective in the treatment of delirium and, in fact, contributed to worsening delirium and cognitive impairment.[107] However, in low doses, both neuroleptic drugs were highly effective in controlling the symptoms of delirium (dramatic improvement in Delirium Rating Scale scores) and improving cognitive function (dramatic improvement in Mini-Mental Status Examination scores).
- Newer atypical agents such as *risperidone* and *olanzapine* have not been studied in cancer patients. They show promise because of improved side effect profiles, in particular fewer extrapyramidal symptoms.[108] However, their use in delirious patients is limited by lack of parenteral administration.

TABLE 14–13. **Medications Useful in Managing Delirium**

Generic Name	Approximate Daily Dosage Range (mg)	Route
Neuroleptics		
Haloperidol	0.5–5 q2–12 hr	IV, SC, IM, PO
Thioridazine	10–75 q4–8 hr	PO
Chlorpromazine	12.5–50 q4–12 hr	IV, IM, PO
Molindone	10–50 q8–12 hr	PO
Droperidol	0.5–5 q12 hr	IV, IM
Methotrimeprazine	12.5–50 q4–8 hr	IV, SC, PO
Novel Antipsychotics		
Risperidone	1–3 q12 hr	PO
Olanzapine	2.5–5 q12 hr	PO
Benzodiazepines		
Lorazepam	0.5–2.0 q1–4 hr	IV, SC
Midazolam	30–100 per 24 hr	IV, SC
Anesthetics		
Propofol	10–50 q1 hr	IV

IM = intramuscular; IV = intravenous; PO = by mouth; SC = subcutaneous.

- *Methotrimeprazine* (intravenous or subcutaneous) is often utilized to control confusion and agitation in terminal delirium. Hypotension and excessive sedation are problematic limitations of this drug.
- *Midazolam* is also used to control agitation related to delirium in the terminal stages.[16] The goal of treatment with midazolam, and to some extent with methotrimeprazine, is quiet sedation only. As opposed to neuroleptic drugs such as haloperidol, a midazolam infusion does not clear a delirious patient's sensorium or improve cognition. These clinical differences may be due to the underlying pathophysiology of delirium. One hypothesis postulates that an imbalance of central cholinergic and adrenergic mechanisms underlies delirium, and so a dopamine-blocking drug may initiate a rebalancing of these systems.

Although neuroleptic drugs such as haloperidol are most effective in diminishing agitation, clearing the sensorium, and improving cognition in the delirious patient, this is not always possible in the last days of life. Processes causing delirium may be ongoing and irreversible during the active dying phase. Ventafridda and colleagues[109] and Fainsinger and associates[110] have reported that a significant group (10% to 20%) of terminally ill patients experience delirium that can only be controlled by sedation to the point of a significantly decreased level of consciousness.

The use of neuroleptics in the management of delirium in the dying patient remains controversial in some circles. Some have argued pharmacologic interventions with neuroleptics or benzodiazepines are inappropriate in the dying patient because they view delirium as a natural part of the dying process that should not be altered. Another rationale often raised is that these patients are so close to death that aggressive treatment is unnecessary. Parenteral neuroleptics or sedatives may be mistakenly avoided because of exaggerated fears that they might hasten death through hypotension or respiratory depression. Many practitioners are unnecessarily pessimistic about the possible results of neuroleptic treatment for delirium. They argue that because the underlying pathophysiologic process often continues unabated (such as hepatic or renal failure), no improvement can be expected in the patient's mental status. There is concern that neuroleptics or sedatives may worsen a delirium by making the patient more confused or sedated. However, clinical experience in managing delirium in dying cancer patients suggests that the use of neuroleptics in the management of agitation, paranoia, hallucinations, and altered sensorium is safe, effective, and quite appropriate.

Management of delirium on a case by case basis seems wisest. The agitated, delirious dying patient should probably be given neuroleptics to help restore calm. A "wait and see" approach, before using neuroleptics, may be most appropriate with patients who have a lethargic or somnolent presentation of delirium. The consultant must educate staff and patients and weigh each of these issues in making the decision of whether to use pharmacologic interventions for the dying patient who presents with delirium.

Physical Effects of Cancer

Pain

Pain management in patients with advanced cancer or AIDS requires a multidisciplinary approach, enlisting expertise from a wide variety of clinical specialties including neurology, neurosurgery, anesthesiology, and rehabilitation medicine.[111] Psychiatric involvement in the treatment of both cancer and AIDS patients with pain has now also become an integral part of a comprehensive approach.[7, 28, 112] This topic is discussed in detail in Chapter 32, Cancer Pain Management: An Essential Component of Comprehensive Cancer Care.

Pain is a common problem for cancer patients, with approximately 70% of patients experiencing severe pain at some time in the course of their illness. Yet, despite its prevalence, studies have shown that pain is frequently underdiagnosed and inadequately treated.[113] Guidelines have recently been published by the Agency for Health Care Policy and Research that advocates the World Health Organization stepladder approach to treating pain in cancer patients.[114]

Pharmacologic Treatment

ADJUVANT ANALGESICS

In addition to opioids and nonsteroidal analgesics, adjuvant analgesics are a class of medications frequently prescribed for the treatment of chronic pain and have important applications in the management of pain in cancer (Table 14–14). Adjuvant analgesic drugs are used to enhance the analgesic efficacy of opioids, treat concurrent symptoms that exacerbate pain, and provide independent analgesia. They may be used in all stages of the analgesic ladder. Commonly used adjuvant drugs include antidepressants, neuroleptics, psychostimulants, anticonvulsants, corticosteroids, and oral anesthetics.[114–116] This subject is covered extensively in Chapter 32.

Nonpharmacologic Treatment

Behavioral interventions are effective in the management of acute procedure-related cancer pain and as an adjunct in the management of chronic cancer pain. Hypnosis, biofeedback, and multicomponent cognitive behavioral interventions have been used to provide comfort and minimize pain in adults, children, and adolescents undergoing bone marrow aspirations, spinal taps, and other painful procedures.[117, 118] Typically, behavioral interventions used in the

TABLE 14–14. **Adjuvant Analgesic Drugs for Cancer Pain Patients**

Generic Name	Approximate Daily Dosage Range (mg)	Route
Anticonvulsants		
Carbamazepine	200 tid–400 tid	PO
Valproate	500 tid–1000 tid	PO
Gabapentin	300 tid–1000 tid	PO
Oral Local Anesthetics		
Corticosteroids	600–900	PO
Dexamethasone	4–16	PO, IV

IV = intravenous; PO = by mouth.

management of acute procedure-related pain employ the basic elements of relaxation and distraction or diversion of attention.

In chronic cancer pain, cognitive behavioral techniques are most effective when they are employed as part of a multimodal, multidisciplinary approach.[27] Adequate medical assessment and management of cancer pain is essential. Mild to moderate levels of residual pain can be effectively managed with behavioral techniques that are quite similar to those used for anxiety, phobias, and anticipatory nausea and vomiting. Relaxation techniques are used to help the patient achieve a relaxed state. Once in a relaxed state, the cancer patient with pain can use a variety of imagery techniques including pleasant distracting imagery, transformational imagery, and dissociative imagery[27]:

- Transformational imagery involves the imaginative transformation of either the painful sensation itself or the context of pain, or both. Patients can imaginatively transform a sensation of pain in their arm, for instance, into a sensation of warmth or cold. They can use such imagery as "dipping their arm into a bucket of cold spring water," or "into a vat of warm honey." Such techniques can also be used to alter the context of the pain.
- Dissociative imagery or dissociated somatization refers to the use of one's imagination to disconnect or dissociate from the pain experience. Specifically, patients can sometimes imagine that they leave their pain-racked body in bed and walk about for 5 or 10 minutes pain free. Patients can also imagine that a particularly painful part of their body becomes disconnected or dissociated from the rest of them, resulting in a period of freedom from pain.

These techniques can provide much needed respite from pain. Even short periods of relief from pain can break the vicious pain cycle that entraps many cancer patients.

Anorexia and Weight Loss

Cancer patients and their families find weight loss demoralizing, perplexing, and distressing. Weight loss and anorexia in the cancer patient are complex problems that can arise from a number of sources. Although most often a variety of medical factors account for the anorexia and cachexia associated with terminal illness, psychological and psychiatric factors may also play a role in the etiology of anorexia and weight loss. Among the most frequent of such causes are anxiety, depression, and conditioned food aversions.[119]

The treatment of anorexia and weight loss begins with the identification and correction of its reversible causes. For example, when uncontrolled opioid-induced nausea is identified as a key factor in a patient's inability to eat, adding an antiemetic may completely control the subsequent anorexia. Once specific causes have been ruled out or corrected, subsequent treatment relies upon environmental manipulations. Frequent administration of favorite foods, nutritional supplements, and fluids can reverse weight loss.

When poor appetite is a symptom of underlying major depression or significant anxiety, psychopharmacologic interventions with antidepressants and anxiolytics are indicated. Conditioned nausea and vomiting is often quite responsive to relaxation training and other behavioral techniques. These interventions can be employed even by patients with advanced disease if their sensorium is clear and they are capable of concentrating.

Asthenia

Asthenia is defined as generalized weakness and physical or mental fatigue. Studies suggest that as many as two thirds of advanced cancer patients complain of weakness. Unfortunately, a treatable cause of asthenia will be identified and corrected in only a minority of cases. The role of psychiatric factors in the presentation of asthenia in the cancer patient is small in comparison to that of physical factors. However, psychiatric factors are probably enlisted too often by frustrated house staff who have seen a number of treatments fail and then view the patient's continuing malaise as a sign of depression. More likely, asthenia arises from some of the following causes: malnutrition, infection, profound anemia, metabolic abnormalities, and reactions to medication. Chemotherapeutic agents and radiotherapy, frequently employed as palliative therapies in patients with cancer, can both cause significant weakness that may resolve after treatment is completed.

The psychological and psychiatric treatment of asthenic patients includes patient and family education (especially to address the nonpsychological nature of the problem in many cases). An ongoing supportive relationship that permits the patient to express fears and concerns about the meaning of continued weakness and to address distorted ideas that they may have about its prognostic significance is critically important.[120] Some patients who suffer with temporary asthenia from chemotherapy or radiotherapy feel that their weakness is a sign of imminent death.

The literature in support of the pharmacotherapy of asthenia in cancer patients is largely anecdotal. Some patients respond to steroids (e.g., methylprednisolone) with improvement in mood, appetite, and physical well-being; unfortunately, this response tends to be fleeting. Also problematic is the fact that prolonged use of steroids can exacerbate weakness by causing proximal myopathy. Steroids have several other potentially distressing adverse effects, including severe psychiatric syndromes such as organic mood syndromes and delirium. Psychostimulants have been used in the treatment of asthenia with mixed results. However, certain patients do respond well to amphetamine, methylphenidate, or pemoline, and it is thus appropriate to use stimulants, not only for depressive syndromes, but for the asthenia-weakness syndrome as well. Despite the appetite-suppressing effects of amphetamine-like drugs, stimulants often improve energy and appetite in asthenic medically ill patients.

Nausea and Vomiting

Approximately 50% of patients with advanced cancer experience nausea and vomiting during the course of their illness.[93, 121] Common causes of nausea and vomiting in cancer patients include radiation, medications, toxins, metabolic derangements, obstruction of the gastrointestinal tract, and chemotherapy. During the course of chemotherapy, many patients become sensitized to the treatment, develop phobic-like reactions, and even develop conditioned responses to stimuli in the hospital setting. As a result of being conditioned by the experience of profound nausea and vomiting secondary to highly emetic chemotherapy agents, patients report being nauseated in anticipation of treatment. A conservative estimate of the prevalence of anticipatory nausea and vomiting (ANV) is at least 33%. The factors that increase the likelihood of developing ANV are as follows:

- severity of post-treatment nausea and vomiting (high density, duration, and frequency)
- a pattern of increasing nausea and vomiting
- receiving highly emetic drugs (cisplatinum) or combinations of chemotherapies

Given the relationship between the intensity of postchemotherapy nausea and vomiting and the development of ANV, the efficacy of antiemetic regimens in the management of these symptoms becomes increasingly important. Antiemetic drugs are the mainstay of managing chemotherapy-induced nausea and vomiting in patients with advanced disease. Several antiemetic drugs have dopamine-blocking properties and so can cause a variety of extrapyramidal side effects. Akathisia is a common extrapyramidal symptom experienced by the patient as an intense inner sense of restlessness, often accompanied by outward manifestations of agitation. Physicians and nurses often confuse this with anxiety related to illness. Patients can often differentiate feelings of anxiety and nervousness from a sense of motor restlessness. Additionally, akathisia is often accompanied by other extrapyramidal symptoms such as mild tremor or cogwheel rigidity. Treatment of akathisia secondary to antiemetics may involve lowering the dose of the antiemetic, switching to a non–dopamine-blocking agent, such as ondansetron, or adding a benzodiazepine or an anticholinergic agent. Newer atypical neuroleptics (e.g., olanzapine) have not been studied for this use in cancer patients but may prove to have fewer extrapyramidal symptoms.

Rapid-onset, short-acting benzodiazepines are helpful in controlling ANV once it has developed. Alprazolam has been shown to be clinically effective in reducing ANV.[122] Behavioral control of ANV also has proven to be highly effective. The techniques that have been studied include relaxation training with guided imagery, video game distraction (in children), and systematic desensitization. It is unclear whether muscular relaxation or cognitive-attentional distraction is the key element in the efficacy of some of these techniques. Chemotherapy nurses trained in these techniques can improve markedly the quality of life in chemotherapy patients.

Insomnia

Behavioral interventions have been successfully applied to the treatment of insomnia in cancer patients; behavioral and relaxation approaches have shown an improvement in sleep onset and sleep duration.[123] Such techniques are useful nonpharmacologic interventions that help keep medication use to a minimum. Occasionally, sleep disturbance in cancer patients may be due to a concomitant psychiatric disorder such as depression or delirium. Obviously, in these cases, specific treatment for the underlying disorder is a preferred approach. Pharmacotherapy utilizing benzodiazepines, neuroleptics, or sedating antidepressants may also be indicated when sleep disturbance is due to medication side effects or to some other organic etiology.

Survivor Issues

Advances in the treatment of cancer in the last 30 years have led to the improvement not only in quantity of survival but also in the quality of living as well. Consequently, professional attention has turned from death, dying, and biologic survival issues to the emotional, physical, and behavioral consequences of rigorous treatment regimens on quality of life. The reported prevalence of PTSD in cancer survivors ranges from 4% to 25%.[124, 125] Newer research, utilizing more stringent diagnostic criteria, is providing the clinician with a more accurate understanding of the magnitude of the problem in patients, survivors, and parents of children.

In coping with a variety of physical, social, sexual, employment, and insurance problems, survivors often report psychological distress at subsyndromal levels. They may vary by site of cancer and treatment (e.g., bone marrow transplant)[126] and usually do not interfere with re-entry into family, social, or employment networks. Cured cancer patients have special medical and psychiatric concerns: fears of ending treatment; worry about disease recurrence and minor physical problems; a sense of greater vulnerability to illness and second malignancies; increased awareness of mortality and difficulty with re-entering into normal life; diminished self-esteem or confidence; perceived loss of job mobility, and fear of insurance discrimination. Concerns about infertility may reappear when patients consider marrying. There may also be persistent body image concerns, somatic preoccupation, disruptions in intimate relationships, and deficits in social competence.

Individual characteristics of survivors, such as their knowledge and view of cancer and related health beliefs, personality traits, premorbid adjustment, and sociodemographic factors, as well as their cancer experience, will affect the survivor's ability to adapt after cancer.[126]

Summary

As cancer treatments have become more aggressive and successful, there has been an increasing recognition of the psychological and psychiatric sequelae of cancer diagnosis, relapse, and survivorship. This chapter highlights the diagnosis and treatment of the psychiatric syndromes related to cancer treatment and the physical manifestations of this disease, such as pain, nausea and vomiting, asthenia, and insomnia. It is hoped that earlier recognition of these symptoms by oncology physicians and nurses will lead to less distress and an overall improvement in the quality of life of people with cancer.

REFERENCES

1. Derogatis LR, Morrow GR, Fetting J, et al: The prevalence of psychiatric disorders among cancer patients. JAMA 1983; 249:751–757.

2. Massie MJ, Holland JC, Glass E: Delirium in terminally ill cancer patients. Am J Psychiatry 1983; 140:1048–1050.
3. Massie MJ, Holland JC: The cancer patient with pain: psychiatric complications and their management. Med Clin North Am 1987; 71:243–258.
4. Spiegel D: Cancer and depression. Br J Psychiatry 1996; 30:109–116.
5. Stiefel F: Delirium is the confusion slowly clearing up. Support Care Cancer 1996; 4:325–326.
6. Bruera E, MacMillan K, Hanson J, et al: The cognitive effects of the administration of narcotic analgesics in patients with cancer pain. Pain 1989; 39:13–16.
7. Breitbart W: Psychotropic adjuvant analgesics for pain in cancer and AIDS. Psychooncology 1998; 7:333–345.
8. Roth AJ, Massie MJ, Redd WH: Consultation to the cancer patient. In: Jacobson AM, Jacobson JL (eds): Psychiatric Secrets. Philadelphia, Hanley & Belfus, 1995.
9. Holland JC: Anxiety and cancer: the patient and family. J Clin Psychiatry 1989; 50(suppl):20–25.
10. Massie MJ: Anxiety, panic and phobias. In: Holland JC, Rowland J (eds): Handbook of Psychooncology: Psychological Care of the Patient with Cancer, p 300. New York, Oxford University Press, 1989.
11. Ozdemir V, Fourie J, Busto U, et al: Pharmacokinetic changes in the elderly. Do they contribute to drug abuse and dependence? Clin Pharmacokinet 1996; 31:372–385.
12. Stoudemire A: Epidemiology and psychopharmacology of anxiety in medical patients. J Clin Psychiatry 1996; 57(suppl):64–72.
13. Hill JM, Stuber ML: The child with cancer: long term adaptation, psychiatric sequelae, and PTSD. In: Holland JC (ed): Psychooncology, p 923. New York, Oxford University Press, 1998.
14. Wald TG, Kathol RG, Noyes R Jr, et al: Rapid relief of anxiety in cancer patients with both alprazolam and placebo. Psychosomatics 1993; 34:324–332.
15. Chouinard G, Lefko-Singh K, Teboul E: Metabolism of anxiolytics and hypnotics: benzodiazepines, buspirone, zoplicone, and zolpidem. Cell Mol Neurobiol 1999; 19:533–552.
16. Burke AL: Palliative care: an update on "terminal restlessness." Med J Austral 1997; 166:39–42.
17. Bottomley DM, Hanks GW: Subcutaneous midazolam infusion in palliative care. J Pain Symptom Manage 1990; 5:259–261.
18. Walsh TD: Adjunct analgesic therapy in cancer pain. In: Foley KM, Bonica JJ, Ventafridda V (eds): Advances in Pain Research and Therapy, vol 16, p 155. New York, Raven Press, 1990.
19. Keck PE Jr, McElroy SL, Nemeroff CB: Anticonvulsants in the treatment of bipolar disorder. J Neuropsychiatry Clin Neurosci 1992; 4:395–405.
20. Sramek JJ, Hong WW, Hamid S, et al: Meta-analysis of the safety and tolerability of two dose regimens of buspirone in patients with persistent anxiety. Depression and Anxiety 1999; 9:131–134.
21. Popkin MK, Callies AL, Mackenzie TB: The outcome of antidepressant use in the medically ill. Arch Gen Psychiatry 1985; 42:1160–1163.
22. Chaturvedi SK, Hopwood P, Maguire P: Non-organic somatic symptoms in cancer. Eur J Cancer 1993; 29A:1006–1008.
23. Rubey RN, Lydiard RB: Pharmacological treatment of anxiety in the medically ill patient. Semin Clin Neuropsychiatry 1999; 4:133–147.
24. Cvjetkovic-Bosnjak M, Knezevic A, Soldatovic-Stajic B: Comparison of the efficacy of traditional antidepressive agents and the new generation of antidepressives in the treatment of depressive disorders. Med Pregl 1999; 52:108–111.
25. Bruera E, Macmillan K, Pither J, et al: Effects of morphine on the dyspnea of terminal cancer patients. J Pain Symptom Manage 1990; 5:341–344.
26. Radbruch L, Loick G, Schulzeck S, et al: Intravenous titration with morphine for severe cancer pain: report of 28 cases. Clin J Pain 1999; 15:173–178.
27. Massie MJ, Holland JC, Straker N: Psychotherapeutic interventions. In: Holland JC, Rowland JH (eds): Handbook of Psychooncology: Psychological Care of the Patient with Cancer, p 455. New York, Oxford University Press, 1989.
28. Breitbart W: Psychiatric management of cancer pain. Cancer 1989; 63(suppl):2336–2342.
29. Holland JC, Morrow GR, Schmale A, et al: A randomized clinical trial of alprazolam versus progressive muscle relaxation in cancer patients with anxiety and depressive symptoms. J Clin Oncol 1991; 9:1004–1011.
30. Chochinov HM, Holland JC: Bereavement. In: Holland JC, Rowland JH (eds): Handbook of Psychooncology: Psychological Care of the Patient with Cancer, p 612. New York, Oxford University Press, 1989.
31. Massie MJ, Holland JC: Depression and the cancer patient. J Clin Psychiatry 1990; 51(suppl):12–17.
32. Green AI, Austin CP: Psychopathology of pancreatic cancer. A psychobiologic probe. Psychosomatics 1993; 34:208–221.
33. Endicott J: Measurement of depression in patients with cancer. Cancer 1984; 53(suppl):2243–2249.
34. Chochinov HMC, Wilson KG, Enns M, et al: Prevalence of depression in the terminally ill: effects of diagnostic criteria and symptom threshold judgments. Am J Psychiatry 1994; 151:537–540.
35. Kathol RG, Mutgi A, Williams J, et al: Diagnosis of major depression in cancer patients according to four sets of criteria. Am J Psychiatry 1990; 147:1021–1024.
36. Zimmerman M, Coryell WH, Black DW: Variability in the application of contemporary diagnostic criteria; endogenous depression as an example. Am J Psychiatry 1990; 147:1173–1179.
37. Clarke DM: Psychological factors in illness and recovery. N Z Med J 1998; 111:410–412.
38. Hammerlid E, Ahlner-Elmqvist M, Bjordal K, et al: A prospective multicentre study in Sweden and Norway of mental distress and psychiatric morbidity in head and neck cancer patients. Br J Cancer 1999; 80:766–774.
39. Stiefel FC, Breitbart WS, Holland JC: Corticosteroids in cancer: neuropsychiatric complications. Cancer Invest 1989; 7:479–491.
40. Denicoff KD, Rubinow DR, Papa MZ, et al: The neuropsychiatric effects of treatment with interleukin-2 and lymphokine-activated killer cells. Ann Intern Med 1987; 107:293–300.
41. Patten SB, Love EJ: Drug-induced depression. Psychother Psychosom 1997; 66:63–73.
42. Lerner DM, Stoudemire A, Rosenstein DL: Neuropsychiatric toxicity associated with cytokine therapies. Psychosomatics 1999; 40:428–435.
43. Weddington WW: Delirium and depression associated with amphotericin B. Psychosomatics 1982; 23:1076–1078.
44. Vigliani MC, Duyckaerts C, Hauw JJ, et al: Dementia following treatment of brain tumors with radiotherapy administered alone or in combination with nitrosourea-based chemotherapy: a clinical and pathological study. J Neurooncol 1999; 41:137–149.
45. Geffken GR, Ward HE, Staab JP, et al: Psychiatric morbidity in endocrine disorders. Psychiatr Clin North Am 1998; 21:473–489.
46. Posner JB: Nonmetastatic effects of cancer on the nervous system. In: Wyngaarden JB, Smith LH (eds): Cecil's Textbook of Medicine, p 1104. Philadelphia, W.B. Saunders, 1988.
47. Patchell RA, Posner JB: Cancer and the nervous system. In: Holland J, Rowland J (eds): The Handbook of Psychooncology: The Psychological Care of the Cancer Patient, p 327. New York, Oxford Press, 1989.
48. Roth AJ, Holland JH: Psychiatric complications in cancer patients. In: Brain MC, Carbone PP (eds): Current Therapy in Hematology-Oncology, 5th ed. St. Louis, Mosby, 1995.
49. Breitbart W: Cancer pain and suicide. In: Foley KM, Bonica JJ, Ventafridda V (eds): Advances in Pain Research and Therapy, vol 16, p 399. New York, Raven Press, 1990.
50. Edelman S, Bell DR, Kidman AD: A group cognitive behaviour therapy programme with metastatic breast cancer patients. Psychooncology 1999; 8:295–300.
51. Sellick SM, Crooks DL: Depression and cancer: an appraisal of the literature for prevalence, detection, and practice guideline development for psychological interventions. Psychooncology 1999; 8:315–333.
52. Kugaya A, Akechi T, Nakano T, et al: Successful antidepressant treatment for five terminally ill cancer patients with major depression, suicidal ideation and a desire for death. Support Care Cancer 1999; 7:432–436.
53. Pirl WF, Roth AJ: Diagnosis and treatment of depression in cancer patients: Oncology (Huntingt) 1999; 13:1293–1301.
54. David JM, Glassman AH: Anti-depressant drugs. In: Kaplan HI, Sadock BJ (eds): Comprehensive Textbook of Psychiatry, 5th ed, p 1627. Baltimore, Williams & Wilkins, 1989.
55. Preskorn SH: Recent pharmacologic advances in anti-depressant therapy for the elderly. Am J Med 1993; 94:2S–12S.

56. Breitbart W, Passik SD: Psychiatric aspects of palliative care. In: Doyle D, Hanks GW, MacDonald N (eds): Oxford Textbook of Palliative Medicine, p 607. New York, Oxford University Press, 1993.
57. Stoudemire A, Fogel BS: Psychopharmacology in the medically ill. In: Stoudemire A, Fogel BS (eds): Principles of Medical Psychiatry, p 79. Orlando, Grune & Stratton, 1987.
58. Preskorn SH, Jerkovich GS: Central nervous system toxicity of tricyclic antidepressants: phenomenology, course, risk factors, and role of therapeutic drug monitoring. J Clin Psychopharmacol 1990; 10:88–95.
59. Montgomery SA, Kasper S: Comparison of compliance between serotonin reuptake inhibitors and tricyclic antidepressants: a meta-analysis. Int Clin Psychopharmacol 1995; 9(suppl):33–40.
60. Nurnberg HG, Thompson PM, Hensley PL: Antidepressant medication change in a clinical treatment setting: a comparison of the effectiveness of selective serotonin reuptake inhibitors. J Clin Psychiatry 1999; 60:574–579.
61. Pacher P, Ungvari Z, Nanasi PP, et al: Speculations on difference between tricyclic and selective serotonin reuptake inhibitor antidepressants on their cardiac effects. Is there any? Curr Med Chem 1999; 6:469–480.
62. Preskorn SH, Burke M: Somatic therapy for major depressive disorder: selection of an antidepressant. J Clin Psychiatry 1992; 53 (suppl):5–18.
63. Ciraulo DA, Shader RI: Fluoxetine drug-drug interactions: I. Antidepressants and antipsychotics. J Clin Psychopharmacol 1990; 10:48–50.
64. Cookson J, Duffett R: Fluoxetine: therapeutic and undesirable effects. Hosp Med 1998; 59:622–626.
65. Rudorfer MV, Manji HK, Potter WZ: Comparative tolerability profiles of the newer versus older antidepressants. Drug Safety 1994; 10:18–46.
66. Costabile RA, Spevak M: Oral trazodone is not effective therapy for erectile dysfunction: a double-blind, placebo controlled trial. J Urol 1999; 161:1819–1822.
67. Rush CR, Kollins SH, Pazzaglia PJ: Discriminative-stimulus and participant-rated effects of methylphenidate, bupropion, and triazolam in d-amphetamine-trained humans. Exp Clin Psychopharmacol 1998; 6:32–44.
68. Harris CR, Gualtieri J, Stark G: Fatal bupropion overdose. J Toxicol Clin Toxicol 1997; 35:321–324.
69. Bernard PG, Levine MS: Maprotiline-induced seizures. South Med J 1986; 79:1179–1180.
70. Madakasira S: Amoxapine-induced neuroleptic malignant syndrome. DICP 1989; 23:50–51.
71. van Heeringen K, Zivkov M: Pharmacological treatment of depression in cancer patients. A placebo-controlled study of mianserin. Br J Psychiatry 1996; 169:440–443.
72. Olin J, Masand P: Psychostimulants for depression in hospitalized cancer patients. Psychosomatics 1996; 37:57–62.
73. Masand PS, Tesar GE: Use of stimulants in the medically ill. Psychiatr Clin North Am 1996; 19:515–547.
74. Burns MM, Eisendrath SJ: Dextroamphetamine treatment for depression in terminally ill patients. Psychosomatics 1994; 35:80–83.
75. Weitzner MA, Meyers CA, Valentine AD: Methylphenidate in the treatment of neurobehavioral slowing associated with cancer and cancer treatment. J Neuropsychiatry Clin Neurosci 1995; 7:347–350.
76. Breitbart W, Mermelstein H: Pemoline. An alternative psychostimulant for the management of depressive disorders in cancer patients. Psychosomatics 1992; 33:352–356.
77. Nehra A, Mullick F, Ishak KG, et al: Pemoline-associated hepatic injury. Gastroenterology 1990; 99:1517–1519.
78. Smith MS, Muir H, Hall R: Perioperative management of drug therapy, clinical considerations. Drugs 1996; 51:238–259.
79. Chochinov HMC, Wilson KG, Enns M, et al: Desire for death in the terminally ill. Am J Psychiatry 1995; 152: 1185–1191.
80. Stiefel F, Volkenandt M, Breitbart W: Suicide and cancer. J Schweiz Med Wochenschr 1989; 119:891–895.
81. Breitbart W: Identifying patients at risk for, and treatment of major psychiatric complications of cancer. Support Care Cancer 1995; 3:45–60.
82. Foley KM: The relationship of pain and symptom management to patient requests for physician-assisted suicide. J Pain Symptom Manage 1991; 6:289–297.
83. Goldman LS, Nielsen NH, Champion HC: Awareness, diagnosis, and treatment of depression. J Gen Intern Med 1999; 14:569–580.
84. Ganzini L, Lec MA, Heintz RT, et al: The effect of depression treatment on elderly patients' preferences for life-sustaining medical therapy. Am J Psychiatry 1994; 151:1631–1636.
85. Chochinov HM, Wilson KG, Enns M, et al: Depression, hopelessness, and suicidal ideation in the terminally ill. Psychosomatics 1998; 39:366–370.
86. Zweig RA, Hinrichsen GA: Factors associated with suicide attempts by depressed older adults: a prospective study. Am J Psychiatry 1993; 150:1687–1692.
87. Murray GB: Confusion, delirium, and dementia. In: Hackett TP, Cassem NH (eds): Massachusetts General Hospital Handbook of General Hospital Psychiatry, 2nd ed, p 84. Littleton, MA, PSG Publishing, 1987.
88. Helig S: The San Francisco Medical Society euthanasia survey. Results and analysis. San Francisco Med J 1988; 61:24.
89. Trzepacz PT: The neuropathogenesis of delirium. A need to focus our research. Psychosomatics 1994; 35:374–391.
90. Tucker GJ: DSM-IV: proposals for revision of diagnostic criteria for delirium. APA Work Group on Organic Disorders of the DSM-IV Task Force and Major Contributors. Int Psychogeriatr 1991; 3:197–208.
91. Trzepacz PT, Baker RW, Greenhouse J: A symptom rating scale for delirium. Psychiatr Res 1988; 23:89–97.
92. Inouye SK, van Dyck CH, Alessi CA, et al: Clarifying confusion: the confusion assessment method. A new method for detection of delirium. Ann Intern Med 1990; 113:941–948.
93. Albert MS, Levkoff SE, Reilly C, et al: The delirium symptom interview: an interview for the detection of delirium symptoms in hospitalized patients. J Geriatr Psychiatry Neurol 1992; 5:14–21.
94. Williams MA: Delirium/acute confusional states: evaluation devices in nursing. Int Psychogeriatr 1991; 3:301–308.
95. Levkoff S, Liptzin B, Cleary P, et al: Review of research instruments and techniques used to detect delirium. Int Psychogeriatr 1991; 3:253–271.
96. Smith MJ, Breitbart WS, Platt MM: A critique of instruments and methods to detect, diagnose, and rate delirium. J Pain Symptom Manage 1995; 10:35–77.
97. Folstein MF, Folstein SE, McHugh PR: "Mini-mental state." A practical method for grading the cognitive state of patients for the clinician. J Psychiatr Res 1975; 12:189–198.
98. Fleishman SB, Lesko LM: Delirium and dementia. In: Holland J, Rowland J (eds): Handbook of Psychooncology: Psychological Care of the Patient with Cancer, p 342. New York, Oxford University Press, 1989.
99. Stiefel F, Razavi D: Common psychiatric disorders in cancer patients. II. Anxiety and acute confusional states. Support Care Cancer 1994; 2:233–237.
100. Walker LG, Walker MB, Heys SD, et al: The psychological and psychiatric effects of rIL-2 therapy: a controlled clinical trial. Psychooncology 1997; 6:290–301.
101. Palmer BF, Toto RD: Severe neurologic toxicity induced by cyclosporine A in three renal transplant patients. Am J Kidney Dis 1991; 18:116–121.
102. Breitbart W, Wein SE: Metabolic disorders and neuropsychiatric symptoms. Psychooncology 1998; 56: 639.
103. Bruera E, Miller L, McCallion J, et al: Cognitive failure in patients with terminal cancer: a prospective study. J Pain Symptom Manage 1992; 7:192–195.
104. Stiefel F, Holland J: Delirium in cancer patients. Int Psychogeriatr 1991; 3:333–336.
105. Akechi T, Uchitomi Y, Okamura H, et al: Usage of haloperidol for delirium in cancer patients. Support Care Cancer 1996; 4:390–392.
106. Fernandez F, Levy JK, Mansell PWA: Management of delirium in terminally ill AIDS patients. Int J Psychiatr Med 1989; 19:165–172.
107. Breitbart W, Platt M, Marotta R, et al: Low-dose neuroleptic treatment for AIDS delirium [Abstract]. 144th Annual Meeting of the American Psychiatric Association, May 11–16, 1991.
108. Green B: Focus on olanzapine. Curr Med Res Opin 1999; 15:79–85.
109. Ventafridda V, Ripamonti C, DeConno F, et al: Symptom prevalence and control during cancer patients' last days of life. J Palliat Care 1990; 6:7–11.
110. Fainsinger R, Miller MJ, Bruera E, et al: Symptom control during the last week of life in a palliative care unit. J Palliat Care 1991; 7:5–11.

111. Breitbart W, Holland J: Psychiatric aspects of cancer pain. In: Foley KM, Bonica JJ, Ventafridda V (eds): Advances in Pain Research and Therapy, vol 16, p 73. New York, Raven Press, 1990.
112. Hewitt DJ, McDonald M, Portenoy RK, et al: Pain syndromes and etiologies in ambulatory AIDS patients. Pain 1997; 70:117–123.
113. Breitbart W, Rosenfeld B, Passik SD: The Network Project: a multidisciplinary cancer education and training program in pain management, rehabilitation, and psychosocial issues. J Pain Symptom Manage 1998; 15:18–26.
114. Jacox A, Carr D, Payne R, et al: Clinical Practice Guideline Number 9: Management of Cancer Pain. AHCPR Publication No. 94-0592. Washington, U.S. Department of Health and Human Services, 1994.
115. Breitbart W: Psychotropic adjuvant analgesics for cancer pain. J Pain Symptom Manage 1989; 4(suppl):2–4.
116. Portenoy RK: Adjuvant analgesics in pain management. In: Doyle D, Hanks GWC, McDonald N (eds): Oxford Textbook of Palliative Medicine, 2nd ed, p 361. New York, Oxford University Press, 1998.
117. Sellick SM, Zaza C: Critical review of 5 nonpharmacologic strategies for managing cancer pain. Cancer Prevent Control 1998; 2:7–14.
118. Liossi C, Hatira P: Clinical hypnosis versus cognitive behavioral training for pain management with pediatric cancer patients undergoing bone marrow aspirations. Int J Clin Exp Hypnosis 1999; 47:104–116.
119. Lesko L: Anorexia. In: Holland JC, Rowland J (eds): Handbook of Psychooncology: Psychological Care of the Patient with Cancer, p 434. New York, Oxford University Press, 1989.
120. MacDonald N, Alexander HR, Bruera E: Cachexia-anorexia-asthenia. J Pain Symptom Manage 1995; 10:151–155.
121. Fessele KS: Managing the multiple causes of nausea and vomiting in the patient with cancer. Oncol Nurs Forum 1996; 23:1409–1415.
122. Razavi D, Delvaux N, Farvacques C, et al: Prevention of adjustment disorders and anticipatory nausea secondary to adjuvant chemotherapy: a double-blind, placebo-controlled study assessing the usefulness of alprazolam. J Clin Oncol 1993; 11:1384–1390.
123. NIH Technology Assessment Panel on Integration of Behavioral and Relaxation Approaches into the Treatment of Chronic Pain and Insomnia: Integration of behavioral and relaxation approaches into the treatment of chronic pain and insomnia. JAMA 1996; 276:313–318.
124. Green BL, Rowland JH, Krupnick JL, et al: Prevalence of posttraumatic stress disorder in women with breast cancer. Psychosomatics 1998; 39:102–111.
125. Jacobsen PB, Widows MR, Hann DM, et al: Posttraumatic stress disorder symptoms after bone marrow transplantation for breast cancer. Psychosom Med 1998; 60:366–371.
126. Kornblith AB: Psychological adaptation to cancer: Cancer survivor's adaptation. In: Holland JC (ed): Psychooncology, p 223. New York, Oxford University Press, 1998.

15 Principles of Oncologic Imaging and Tumor Imaging Strategies

PHILIP RUBIN, MD, Radiation Oncology
DAVID G. BRAGG, MD, FACR, Diagnostic Radiology

And all that lamentation of the leaves,
Could but compose man's image and his cry.

W. B. YEATS

Perspective

The technical advances of tumor imaging in radiologic diagnosis have been as dramatic as the multimodal advances in cancer treatment. In fact, they may be more so when we consider the innovations of the past few decades, such as computerized tomography (CT), ultrasound (US), magnetic resonance imaging (MRI), positron emission tomography (PET), and the potential of molecular imaging. These newer modalities, particularly when coupled with computer-controlled electronic video displays and digitally captured images that enable quantification of images in both static and dynamic modes, are revolutionary when compared with the old diagnostic roentgenographic procedures.

In medical imaging techniques over the past three decades, advances have been more dramatic than in the majority of other medical sciences. As a result, the boundaries of anatomic imaging have been pushed virtually to their limits, and this advancement has placed us at the realistic threshold of being able to harvest functional imaging, metabolic signals, and even molecular or microscopic imaging events. It is hoped that the next wave of advances in the medical imaging field will be the translation of *in vitro* into *in vivo* images, with amplification techniques allowing microscopic, metabolic, and even genetic changes to be translated into visual images. To this end, the overall trend for future progress in the field of imaging appears to be a shift from the refinement of anatomic end points toward functional and molecular imaging. This shift would allow for improved definition of the tumor's microenvironment, including cell density at its infiltrating edges, and its metastatic potential to regional lymph nodes and distant sites.

Even the most standard of radiologic procedures has improved. The accuracy in tumor visualization available today is due to:

- better films with finer grains and higher resolution qualities, as seen in mammography
- better contrast media
- selective catheterization for the imaging of tumor vascularity
- specialized procedure rooms
- improved dynamic imaging guidance
- precise biopsies, via skinny needles, for pathologic confirmation of suspected malignant disease at primary sites, regional lymph nodes, and remote visceral metastases, usually through CT or US guidance

The entire field of digital image capture promises new horizons for oncologic imaging, including postprocessing, archiving, transmission, and digital consultation, and tumors can be diagnosed earlier and more precisely because of these advances.

Those of us engaged in oncologic care and management have realized that tumors are now better defined because of three-dimensional volumetrics and are more accurately staged. However, one issue that is more debatable is what impact improved tumor imaging has had upon treatment and cancer curability, and the caveat to this issue is the rising cost of medical care, particularly the high cost of tumor imaging using the newer techniques. To justify this type of investment in equipment, resources, and time, it would be highly desirable to show both a correlation and a distinct contribution by improved tumor imaging on treatment and cancer curability at numerous disease sites. Such controlled studies are difficult to conduct, but at some sites they are under way and they provide both suggestive and definite evidence of contributing to increasing survival rates and decreasing death rates.[4, 5]

Parameters of an Imaging System

For any radiologic imaging system, the quality of the images and their value in cancer detection can be character-

TABLE 15–1. **Imaging Characteristics of Selected Diagnostic Systems**

Modality	Spatial Resolution	Contrast Discrimination	Temporal Resolution	Signal-to-Noise Ratio	Distortion and Artifacts	Widespread Application	Cost
Radiography	F	P	E	E	E	E	L
CT	E	E	F	E	F	F	M
MRI	E	E	P	E	F	F	M
US	F	F	E	F	F	F	L
PET	F	F	P	F	F	P	H
MRS	E	E	P	F	F	P	H

MRS = magnetic resonance spectroscopy; E = excellent; F = fair; P = poor; L = low cost; M = moderate cost; H = high cost.

ized, according to Hendee, in terms of four fundamental properties[6]: spatial resolution, contrast discrimination, image noise, and the presence of distortion and artifacts. These and other properties are presented in Table 15–1 for a select number of imaging systems. It is clear that no single procedure is best in all categories; contrast discrimination probably requires the greatest improvement. The emerging technologies, which are important to oncologic diagnosis, are dependent on the availability of computers and their sophisticated software packages for data handling, image capture, and display.

The concept of tumor threshold size is difficult to define. From an imaging standpoint, we can generally characterize the limits of resolution of the various imaging systems in use today. There are both objective and subjective limitations to these detection parameters, of which we all must be aware. In part, they are related to equipment (spatial and contrast resolution), patient considerations, target organ considerations, and interobserver variations. Equipment design advances and new techniques and systems have reduced these limitations somewhat, but we have now reached some practical end points in lesion size resolution. Table 15–2 summarizes several common imaging techniques, broadly defines the advantages and limitations of each, and assigns an estimate of the tumor detection threshold by organ site for each system. A number of assumptions have been made for the purposes of estimating rough approximations of tumor size thresholds visible by each technique to serve the purposes of comparison.

Decision Theory

Most oncologists understand the definitions of the terms *sensitivity, specificity, true* and *false, positive* and *negative*; however, the simple illustration provided in Table 15–3 serves as a review.[6] Any imaging procedure or laboratory test will have an accuracy or predictive value based on whether the result or time (positive or negative) correlates to the presence of disease.

- The *sensitivity* of a certain test or study is a function of the true positive rate compared with the sum of the true positives and false negatives.

$$\text{Sensitivity} = \frac{\text{true positives}}{\text{true positives} + \text{false negatives}}$$

- The *specificity* of a test relates to the relationship of the true negative yield compared with the sum of the true negative plus false positive rate for the study.

$$\text{Specificity} = \frac{\text{true negatives}}{\text{true negatives} + \text{false positives}}$$

TABLE 15–2. **Imaging Technology Status: Minimal Threshold Size**

Technique	Resolution (mm)	Functional Potential	Threshold Reached?	Sensitivity / Specificity	Metabolic Imaging Potential	Comments
Radiographs	5–10	4	Yes	2/3	4	Size threshold reached; digital imaging potential
CT	5	3	Yes	2/3	3	Virtual endoscopy potential
MRI / MRS	5	1	Probably	2/2	2	Potential for improved functional data
US	5–10	3	Probably	3/3	4	
Mammography	5	4	Yes	2/2	4	Digital mammography should improve specificity
PET	10–15	1	Probably	2/1	1	Increasing use for tumor staging and response; high potential for metabolic measures
SPECT	10–15	3	Probably	3/2	2–3	Improvement with better radionuclides
Angiography	5–10	3	Yes	2/2	4	Potential for interventional angiography
Conventional nuclear medicine	10–15	3	Yes	3/2	3	Improvement with better radionuclides

SPECT = single photon emission computed tomography; Scores: 1 = very high; 2 = high; 3 = low; 4 = very low.

TABLE 15–3.

	Disease Present	Disease Absent
Exam Positive	True positive	False positive
Exam Negative	False negative	True negative
Parameter	Sensitivity	Specificity

- The *predictive value* of a study is a more important parameter of the potential usefulness of an examination in a certain disease state. The predictive value of a positive exam is determined by the true positive and false positive rate.

$$\text{Predictive value of a positive test} = \frac{\text{true positives}}{\text{true positives} + \text{false positives}}$$

$$\text{Predictive value of a negative test} = \frac{\text{true negatives}}{\text{true negatives} + \text{false negatives}}$$

- The *accuracy rate* of a procedure is the product of the sensitivity and specificity.

$$\text{Accuracy} = \text{sensitivity} \times \text{specificity}$$

This brief review of some of the more common and useful terms involved in the decision process can be supplemented by consulting other bibliographic references.[7–9] In addition, Table 15–4 places the imaging sensitivity and specificity potentials for individual organ sites relative to detection accuracy, staging, and the ability to gauge tumor response. When reviewing the arbitrary numbers used to compare imaging accuracy in these organ sites, it becomes apparent that future efforts must be devoted to improving lymph node staging, evaluating metastatic sites, and developing more specific indicators of tumor response. In certain anatomic sites, the impact of the basic tumor biology represents the major obstacle.

The Oncologic Decision Process and Tumor Imaging Strategies

The first decision in cancer management most often determines whether the outcome will be successful. The most important factors in this decision are definition of the true anatomic extent or stage of the cancer and a multidisciplinary approach to treatment after the histopathologic diagnosis of cancer is made. The oncologic decision process and imaging strategies need to be consistent and logical, and there are several steps in the process (Table 15–5).

Accurate Diagnosis and Early Detection

To begin the oncologic decision process, the cancer needs to be detected and the diagnosis firmly established. In general, this occurs in two populations—symptomatic or asymptomatic patients. The ability to detect a cancer depends on the accuracy of the method, which is discussed later. The *gold standard* of diagnosis is the histopathologic verification of the cancer in the tissue in question, and the

TABLE 15–4. **Imaging Status per Cancer Site**

	Detection Accuracy	Specificity	Sensitivity	N Staging	M Staging	Follow-Up Ability	
Cancer Site	*1 = high / 4 = poor*			*1 = good / 4 = poor*			**Comments**
Brain	1	1	1	N/A	N/A	2	Major issue: tumor biology; functional yield should increase
Head / Neck	2	2	2	1–2	1–2	1–2	Anatomic end points reached; improvement unlikely
Breast	1	2	1–2	2–3	2–3	1–2	Digital imaging may improve specificity; N-M imaging needed
Lung	1–2	2	1–2	2	2–3	1–2	Improved specificity with PET; better detection needed
GI tract	1–2	2	1–2	2–3	2–3	1–2	Potential with virtual endoscopy; staging potential limited
Liver	1–2	1–2	1–2	N/A	1–2	1–2	Anatomic end points reached
Pancreas	2–3	3	3	4	3	2–3	Major issue: tumor biology; improved detection and staging needed
Kidney	1–2	1–2	1–2	2	2	1–2	Size end points reached
Bladder	2–3	2	3	3	2	2	Potential with virtual endoscopy
Prostate	2–3	3	2	3	2	2	Issues: tumor biology and behavior; T-N problems with multifocal tumors
Ovary	3	3	3	N/A	3–4	2–3	Major issue: tumor biology; challenges: detection and staging
Cervix	1–2	2–3	3	N/A	2	2	CT and MR underutilized
Testis	N/A	2–3	2	2	2	2	Imaging used in staging and follow-up
Soft tissue	N/A	N/A	N/A	2–3	1–2	2	Improved N-M imaging needed
Bone	1	1–2	1	N/A	1–2	2	Imaging end points reached
Lymphoma	N/A	2–3	2	2	2	2	PET/radionuclide roles need testing
Thyroid	2	2	2	2	1–2	1–2	Imaging good if thyroid functional

GI = gastrointestinal.

TABLE 15–5. **Sequence of Image-Guided Treatment**

Process	Problems Specific to Process
Screening and detection ↓	Detection of tumor at noninvasive or early stage
Detection and diagnosis ↓	Dictates staging work-up
Staging work-up (TNM) ↓	Dictated by tumor type, patient status, organ site, and procedural limitations
Definition of tumor response to treatment ↓	Imaging approach and sequence determined by therapeutic modality and tumor type
Post-treatment follow-up ↓	Imaging approach and sequence determined by therapeutic modality and tumor type
Detection of relapse ↓	Differential diagnosis—recurrent tumor vs. tissue necrosis
Restage—before retreatment	Abbreviated restaging tailored to the tumor, patient status, and retreatment modalities considered

essential element in establishing the accuracy of an imaging procedure is to demonstrate high sensitivity and specificity. The use of an imaging technique for screening purposes is also contingent on the population, cost of the procedure, and potential curability of a cancer at the time of detection. Clearly, early detection of incurable cancers is of little value.

Precise Staging

At each major anatomic site, it is essential to have a classification of cancer that is meaningful in terms of both treatment and prognosis. A consistent cancer language and categorization allows the oncologist to develop treatment strategies in a multidisciplinary fashion. The tumor, node, metastases (TNM) system is used by the American Joint Committee on Cancer (AJCC) and the International Union Against Cancer (UICC) for cancer staging and end results reporting,[10] or when appropriate, other specific classifications are advocated.

The role of oncologic imaging is complex and varies with each organ site and, often, tumor type. In addition, the imaging process frequently has to be tailored to suit the individual needs of the patient, the unique features of the tumor, and the presenting characteristics of the disease. To clarify the concept of tumor staging, decision flow diagrams may be used (Fig. 15–1). Staging work-up is necessary at the time of diagnosis to define the true extent of the cancer in its three compartments (TNM) before the best treatment can be chosen. In general, CT and MRI are the critical noninvasive procedures for accurate clinical staging in most anatomic sites. However, it must be noted that a distinction between clinical-radiographic versus surgical-pathologic staging is essential when reporting end results.

Table 15–5 outlines the sequence of imaging procedures that needs to be performed to achieve the TNM end points of staging, treatment, and follow-up. However, each compartment offers its own challenge to the diagnostic oncologist:

- With the T compartment, specific definitions of the tumor at a few anatomic sites are yet to be defined, for example, central nervous system brain tumors. In addition, there are no universally accepted means to achieve these definitions.
- Attempts to accurately assess the N compartment have been frustrated in both the past and present, in spite of the availability of numerous procedures to image lymph node sites. In order to improve our specificity and sensitivity in defining the N compartment, there is a need to develop tumor-seeking agents with the capability of identifying involved lymph nodes with only small burdens of tumor cells. Such advances would allow minimally invasive diagnostic and therapeutic techniques to be used.
- Because there is no clear answer to whether or not the outcome of this study will modify the therapeutic approach to the patient, assessment of the M compartment has been one of the most controversial elements in the imaging approach to the cancer patient. Some oncologists feel that this question should precede the application of any imaging procedure, but frequently this philosophy is lacking in this setting.

The most common organs targeted by the metastatic process are the brain, lung, liver, and skeletal system; however, imaging sensitivity and specificity vary with each of the organ sites—the lowest being in the liver and most accurate with the brain. Nonetheless, we are faced with the identification of sizable tumor

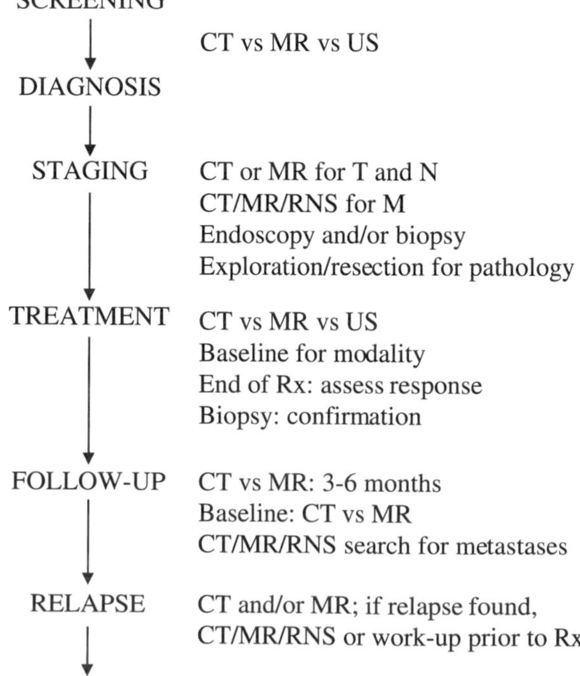

Figure 15–1. Decision flow diagram. (CT = computer tomography; MR = magnetic resonance imaging; US = ultrasound; RNS = radionuclide scan.)

burdens in each site and are unable to image micrometastases (or oligometastases), although attempts in this field are being made.[11] Micrometastases are defined as solitary or limited numbers of metastases at one organ site, in contrast to polyorgan, diffuse metastases. The realization of an ability to image micrometastases will transform the cancer imaging and management process; with certain tumors, micrometastatic surveillance will thrust imaging of the M compartment to the initial priority event. The treatment decision will therefore hinge on the outcome of the discovery of micrometastases because, potentially, such micrometastases may be cured using combinations of radiation, chemotherapy, and immunotherapy.

One major problem that requires emphasis is the need for consistent and universal definitions. For the radiation oncologist, tumor volume is characterized by the term *gross tumor volume* (GTV). Additional descriptors, *clinical target volume* (CTV) and *planning target volume* (PTV), are variable margins added to the GTV for treatment planning purposes. CTV reflects the immediate microscopic pathways of tumor extension that must be covered, and PTV reflects the setup variables and organ motion (Fig. 15–2). However, there is a critical need for both a universally accepted definition *and* a defined sequence of acquisition (imaging approach) for the GTV at each anatomic site. These definitions would give the oncology community the interinstitutional consistency and comparisons that we so desperately need, because such concepts are equally applicable to oncologic surgeons in order to define resection margins and to quantitate tumor volume response for the medical oncologists.

Future approaches to the definitions of GTV and CTV should incorporate tumor phenotype,[12] and they should include such elements as assessment of cell density, features of the tumor's microenvironment (e.g., metabolism), angiogenesis, aggressiveness, and metastatic potential.[13] In order to achieve these end points, there needs to be fundamental adaptations in our imaging approaches, for instance, incorporating amplification techniques that will allow microscopic-level events to become macroscopically integrated into the imaging system. Amplification of this magnitude requires the development of newer classes of contrast agents and radiopharmaceutical agents because our existing contrast agents suffer from the common faults of leaking from vessels, breakdown, and excretion. In addition, there is a need for *compartmental* contrast agents, that is, agents that remain localized in order to monitor many of the events in question. Fundamental to these changes in our past imaging research paradigm is an improved scientific communication among industry, the federal sector, scientists in disciplines outside radiology departments, as well as our research personnel, in an effort to set imaging research priorities that encompass critical clinical and biologic needs.

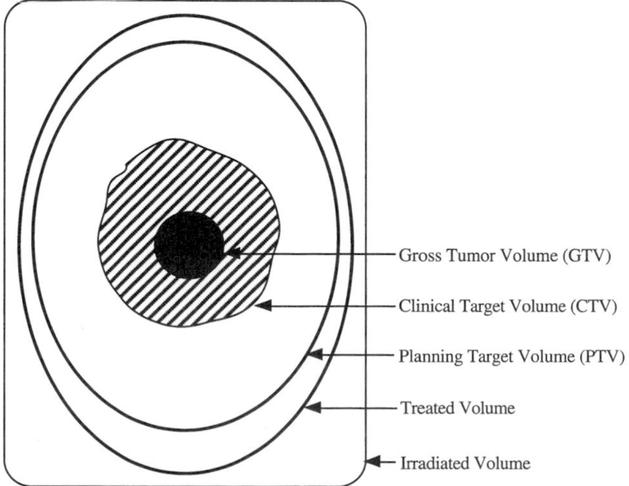

Figure 15–2. Volume definitions used in radiation oncology. (Modified from International Commission on Radiation Units and Measurements: Prescribing, recording, and reporting photon beam therapy. ICRU Report 50. Bethesda, International Commission on Radiation Units and Measurements, 1993.)

Optimum Treatment—Clinical Trials

The treatment of choice is a function of those clinicians who make that choice, and it is not based solely on the cancer and its presentation. Optimal treatment today is based on multidisciplinary decision making in which all involved specialists participate and plan treatments, frequently using combined modalities rather than a single mode of therapy. The multimodal treatment selection is based on staging as a first step, and it is most evident in clinical trial design.

Selecting a carefully defined and similarly targeted group of patients is the first step in protocol development. Such protocols are usually part of a cooperative group effort and are designed to assess therapeutic options; however, they are equally effective in testing diagnostic procedures. Optimal protocols should allow complementary imaging techniques to evolve, as well as identify methods of triaging patients through a maze of alternate imaging modalities. Of note, there is a newly formed national cooperative group—American College of Radiology Imaging Network (ACRIN)[14]—assigned to design and assess competitive imaging procedures in the context of national cooperative groups.

Better Follow-Up

Clinical trials are based on careful diagnostic criteria and staging to determine target groups for study and road maps for follow-up studies. Therefore, it is important to determine cancer persistence or early relapse as soon as possible so that salvage therapy or an alternate can be applied. At the time of first recurrence, a careful restaging work-up should document the precise failure pattern. This process is important, because patterns of failure allow us to determine whether the lack of success resulted from a local (T), nodal (N), or metastatic (M) failure; from complications of the treatment; or from unrelated disease. Once the reasons for failure are known, corrective measures can be taken or new therapeutic strategies can be developed for investigation.

Relapse and Restaging

Whenever possible, a strategy for post-treatment follow-up is recommended, with similar assumptions and guidelines that were developed for the initial staging work-up before treatment. Because the selection and outcome of the imaging study will depend on the therapeutic approach, it is more important for the radiologist to understand the treatment program during the follow-up interval than at any other time. If tumor persistence or tumor progression is noted in the face of treatment, then crossover to a new mode of therapy or new combination of agents is usually advised. Once a locoregional tumor relapse has been recognized, the staging process begins again, usually in a similar but modified form to be sure that there is no metastatic disease. Restaging and biopsy proof are essential at the time of relapse or recurrence, before retreatment, with very few exceptions.

In summary, the diagnostic radiologist and oncologist need to anneal the process of diagnostic imaging to therapeutic imaging, that is, image-guided therapeutic oncologic treatment. The basis of the multidisciplinary decision-making process rests on serial imaging procedures and begins with imaging strategies for staging and definition of tumor volumes in the TNM categories. Imaging guidance of the treatment, which is targeted to a well-defined, three-dimensional tumor volume for both surgeons and radiation oncologists, follows this direction. Imaging also defines the response to therapy—complete or partial regression—and is used in follow-up to detect persistence or recurrence, allowing for salvage therapy.

Impact of Tumor Imaging Strategies on Cancer Curability: Five Hypotheses

A number of hypotheses have been advanced suggesting that improvements in tumor imaging may lead to the selection of optimal multimodal therapy and, thereby, improve outcome and survival:

1. *Early diagnosis in symptomatic patients implies that smaller, more localized tumors, without metastatic spread to nodes or viscera, will be found, increasing the potential for cure.* Prostate cancer is now being diagnosed earlier through a combination of PSA, US, and MRI,[15, 16] which supports this hyphothesis.
2. Similarly, *improved screening procedures for occult tumors in asymptomatic patient cohorts will allow for the detection of smaller or minimal noninvasive cancers with a greater potential for cure,* although many authors have questioned the value of such widespread cancer screening.[17–19] Nonetheless, similar to use of the Pap smear for cervix cancer, with widespread mammographic screening, breast cancer increasingly is being diagnosed in the noninvasive and early stage of disease (<2 cm).[19]
3. *Precise staging and better tumor definition of extensions of the primary, lymph node involvement, and visceral metastases will lead to more accurate staging and, in turn, more optimal treatment.* With the wider use of imaging, particularly spiral CT and MRI, Hodgkin's disease is becoming so well defined that use of laparotomy for staging is now seldom required.[20, 21]
4. *More precise, three-dimensional outlining of the tumor volume leads to better local-regional treatment.* Improved survival rates in patients with head and neck cancers exemplify the use of CT or MRI for better staging and definition of gross tumor volumes for both primary tumors and nodes.[22–24]
5. *Evaluation of responses or detection of early relapses allows for the determination and application of another modality for salvage, hopefully leading to a better cure rate.* Simple postorchidectomy surveillance in testicular tumors, especially nonseminomas such as embryonal cell carcinoma and teratocarcinomas, has been shown to be a reasonable strategy to follow.[25] When the first signs of nodal or pulmonary metastases appear, salvage chemotherapy is virtually 100% effective; its prophylactic use is, therefore, not required in all patients. This spares a significant percentage of patients (>50%) from receiving unnecessary toxic multidrug therapy.

Comparative Survey of Major Organ Systems: The Gold Standard in Oncoimaging

The gold standard in tumor imaging must accurately reflect the true pathologic state of the cancer being diagnosed or staged in the primary (T), nodal (N), or metastatic (M) compartment. At the present time, CT and MRI are the most powerful tools available for noninvasive assessments of cancer invasion and dissemination, with US often directing interventional biopsy procedures. A brief overview of the comparison between CT, MRI, and US can be found in Table 15–6, with gold standard designations favoring the imaging procedure with the highest predictive value. As shown in the table, both CT and MRI contribute to staging, but when both are equal, CT is often used first, owing to availability and lower cost. Nevertheless, MRI, with its sharp multiplanar imaging, is increasingly gaining the edge in many organ sites.

TABLE 15–6. **Gold Standard in Oncologic Imaging Applied to Diagnosis and Staging**

Site	CT (CE)	MRI (CE)	US
Central Nervous System	++	+++	0
Head and Neck	+++	+++	+
Lung	+++	++	0
Breast	+	+++	++
Gastrointestinal			
Esophagus	+++	++	++
Gastric	+	+	++
Colon	+	+	0
Rectal	+	++	++
Pancreatic	+++	++	++
Liver	+++	+++	++
Genitourinary			
Kidney	+++	+++	++
Bladder	++	+++	++
Prostate	++	+++	+++
Musculoskeletal			
Osseous	+++	+++	0
Soft tissue sarcoma	++	+++	+
Lymphoid	+++	++	+

CE = contrast-enhanced; + = low; ++ = high; +++ = highest.

In most areas of the body imaged, CT has become the standard against which other tumor imaging systems are measured. CT plays a dominant role in the staging of most anatomic areas,[26–30] with particular advantages in lesion detection and definition in a number of specific organ sites. However, MRI is playing an increasingly important role in the staging process and at numerous anatomic sites, challenging the superiority of CT.

MRI provides an advantage because of its ability to provide multiplanar views with great clarity and, through its T1- and T2-weighted images, to spin echoes producing different signal intensities that can often discriminate between normal tissue and tumors. Nonetheless, the cost of using MRI is greater than that of a CT exam, and one needs to be certain of its value over a CT exam. Its role in central nervous system imaging is more easily understood and accepted than when used for other body sites.[26, 31, 32]

Imaging Surveillance Strategies for Metastases

Lung

Certain key questions should be addressed in the patient at risk for, or who is suspected of having, metastases, in particular, pulmonary metastases:

- How might the detection of pulmonary metastases modify therapy, including both primary treatment and salvage approaches?
- How should the initial and follow-up thoracic surveillance be structured?
- How does the detected pulmonary abnormality fit with the behavior of the primary tumor?

With respect to the last question, although exceptions do occur, metastatic disease patterns from primary extrathoracic neoplasms tend to have predictable radiologic patterns, which should be placed in the perspective of the patient's status when detected. Therefore, clinicians and radiologists should review presumed lung metastases within the context of the patient's primary tumor.

For imaging of pulmonary metastases, routine chest x-ray films have been used to detect lung metastases in low-risk patients; however, spiral (helical) CT is the modality of choice.[33, 34] This technology allows for minimal motion artifact and optimizes contrast enhancement of normal vascular structures, thereby improving the detection of pulmonary parenchymal nodules and nodal metastatic disease. CT does have its limitations—high sensitivity but poorer specificity, requiring additional procedures to evaluate discovered nodules. However, MRI has not proved to be as effective as CT for the detection of pulmonary metastases.

Brain

The design of an imaging surveillance system for metastatic brain disease should be based on the likelihood of the known primary tumor's ability to spread to the central nervous system. Although patients' symptoms generally indicate the presence of metastatic brain disease and signal the need for an imaging study, occasionally asymptomatic patient surveillance is indicated, such as for the patient with an adenocarcinoma of the lung. In such patients, occult brain metastases may be present within the first 3 to 6 months of detection of the primary in a significant percentage of the patients.

The most cost-effective surveillance technique for identification of metastatic brain lesions remains contrast-enhanced CT.[35] Nonetheless, contrast-enhanced MRI is increasingly used as it has become more available and competitive in terms of cost.[36, 37] Indeed, MRI is the most effective procedure for central nervous system malignancies.

Liver

The challenge of identifying metastatic liver disease[38] has been the subject of debate for years. The surgical proof of the effectiveness of imaging procedures is dependent on operative proof; frequently, surgeons simply use surgical palpation of surface lesions at the time of exploratory laparotomy. Therefore, the gold standard is lacking in many of the reported competitive series.

The so-called art of contrast-enhanced CT and MR imaging is an essential ingredient in tailoring studies to maximize the potential harvest of mass lesions in the liver, and most centers favor the application of timed, high contrast–enhanced CT for the evaluation of space occupying lesions in the liver.[39] US has less sensitivity in diagnosis and, in practice, is used less often. However, angiography offers an avenue to palliate metastatic and primary tumors of the liver.

Osseous

The identification and characterization of metastatic bone disease remain in the province of radionuclide bone scanning. The yield of these sensitive studies is high but nonspecific, and the results require identification and verification with film-screen radiographs and, occasionally, additional histologic verification. One exception to this is with myeloma, because in this patient setting, the radionuclide bone scan may be normal, with osseous involvement apparent only on the radiographic film scan. As in the lung, the use of bone scans should be dependent on the likelihood of the primary tumor to metastasize to the osseous system. For example, the primary tumors found to spread most frequently to bone are those from the breast, prostate, and lung.

New Advances and Horizons in Tumor Imaging

A well-designed imaging strategy is an implicit component of the therapeutic approach to a cancer patient. Although the goal of oncologic imaging in the past was focused on detailed anatomic tumor end points, now, in order to improve survival, oncologists require information on the phenotypic characteristics of the tumor in addition to the simple margins of the neoplasm. These details include the need to define such elements as the cellular density of the tumor, the percentage and location of hypoxic areas, vascular characteristics (e.g., perfusion and microvascular density), and the metastatic potential of the tumor. The ability of current technologies to look at these metabolic end points is summarized in Table 15–2. Of note, with reference to Table 15–2, which tabulates the present status of a number of common imaging technologies, under the column "Threshold Reached?," the authors have made an arbitrary judgment as to whether the end point has been achieved for each. In addition, in the "Comments" section of the table, a few points need clarification:

- For MRI technologies, there is a significant opportunity to achieve functional data through the efforts of spectroscopy and functional MRI.
- Several promising trials are under way comparing the diagnostic use of virtual CT endoscopy with actual endoscopy.[40] This technique is appropriate for any hollow organ imaging and may eventually replace diagnostic endoscopy.
- For both single photon emission computed tomography (SPECT) and PET, improvement is possible through increasing the specificity of the radionuclides. In addition, there is increasing evidence of the ability to gauge tumor response to treatment, particularly using PET. PET imaging with 2-[^{18}F]fluoro-2-deoxy-D-glucose (FDG) also has been used to define the nature of solitary pulmonary nodules in lung cancer[41] and in mediastinal staging for involved lymph nodes.[42]

Over the past decade, with the introduction and refinement of film or screen mammography, breast cancer imaging has changed dramatically. Further refinement with digital mammography should extend the specificity of breast cancer detection, although this methodology adds to the cost of diagnosis because of the threefold increase in capital equipment expenditures. However, the ultimate gain is not known as yet, because initial clinical trials comparing film or screen and digital techniques are still under way.[43]

Minimally invasive diagnosis and treatment techniques have been made possible with improved imaging systems, with the greatest acceptance being in the brain and abdomen. This field will advance significantly as more sophisticated techniques and trained physicians enter it. Dedicated MRI, CT, and biplane imaging systems have been developed to extend the diagnostic and therapeutic reach of these minimally invasive techniques.

Improving Imaging Technologies

Magnetic Resonance Spectroscopy

Magnetic resonance spectroscopy (MRS),[44–46] coupled with MRI, is a powerful investigational tool to study tumor biology and has enormous potential for use in tumor diagnosis and management. Just as MRI can generate high-resolution anatomic images based on proton density maps and intensity signals based on the water proton content, MRS can provide information on regional metabolism by tracking specific nuclei, including ^{31}P, ^{1}H, ^{13}C, and ^{23}Na.

- *Plasma ^{1}H-MRS:* An exciting discovery, which proved ultimately to be disappointing, was the report by Fossel and associates[47] on the ability of MRS to detect the presence of a malignant tumor from the analysis of blood plasma. However, further clinical studies have shown little or no differences between cancer, benign tumor, and normal patients.[48, 49]
- *Tumor characteristics (pathochemistry):* The search for a specific tumor signature has been thoroughly explored, endlessly and elusively, with T2-weighted MRIs and US signals. However, if a suspicious lesion is found by MRI and is suspected of being cancerous, then MRS may eventually prove of value for further analysis, particularly using ^{31}P. Various studies have demonstrated high concentrations of phosphomonoesters, as well as alterations in inorganic phosphate (P_I), phosphodiester, and nucleoside triphosphate levels that, in comparison to normal tissue, have correlations with malignancy.[50, 51]
- *Tumor pathophysiology:* Tumor bioenergetics may be characterized using ^{31}P MRS: levels decrease with increasing tumor size and perfusion and are consistent with biochemical evidence that adenosine triphosphate levels are low in larger human cancers, such as breast cancer.[52] Metastatic potential also has been associated with features of MRS proton spectra of cancer cells,[53] and tumor metabolism, through various catabolic and anabolic pathways, may be used to study growth potential. That is, rapidly growing tumors have a high metabolic rate that correlates with enzyme kinetics, such as the turnover of P_I, which tend to decline as tumors grow larger and slow down in proliferation.[54] In addition, the observation that MRS is sensitive to tumor hypoxia *in vivo* is now accepted and can be used to determine sensitizing therapeutic strategies.[55]
- *Drug sensitivity and resistance:* MRS has the potential to offer a noninvasive means of monitoring tumor response to treatment using ^{31}P determinators in human tumor xenografts and some patient tumors.[56, 57] Studies of different cell sublines (e.g., insensitive and resistant to drugs such as mitomycin or Adriamycin) show differences in ^{31}P MRS, although this may reflect tumor killing mechanisms and growth delay.[58, 59] *In vivo* pharmacokinetic studies also may be possible using fluoridated compounds.[58, 60]

Positron Emission Tomography

The basis of PET is that positrons decay by emitting two γ-rays at 180-degree angles, so that their point of origin can be identified using twin detectors. Particular use has been made of 2-[^{18}F]fluoro-2-deoxy-D-glucose (^{18}FDG-PET). Through the appropriate labeling of similar such key compounds, which can enter tumors through metabolic pathways, unique perfusion patterns can identify areas of metabolic activity, as well as hypoxia, in tumors, assisting in tumor diagnosis, monitoring, and staging. However, PET has been slow in its introduction to medicine and oncology as a result of its expense and complexity. A facility requires a cyclotron, a so-called hot laboratory for producing short-lived positron-emitting radioisotopes, and special multiheaded PET scanners with detector rings.

Applications of PET in oncology include use with brain tumors in differentiating between benign and malignant tissue.[61] The results obtained thus far have provided important data that indicate the usefulness of PET as a relatively noninvasive method for studying a variety of fundamental properties of tumors that could be very important for clinical management.[62] Some of the areas that can be studied with PET include oxygen consumption and extraction efficiency, regional blood flow and volume, glucose consumption, pH, amino acid uptake or protein synthesis, metabolic effects of antitumor therapy, drug pharmacokinetics, and binding of agents to receptors.

- *Hypoxia in tumors:* Tumors that contain hypoxic cells are resistant to radiation therapy and to many drugs.[63] There is also reason to believe that hypoxia and the associated pathophysiologic microenvironments that occur as tumors progress may be causally related to the development of therapeutically resistant phenotypes. A major research effort has been directed at the use of PET to predict which tumors may be hypoxic and to overcome hypoxia-associated resistance.[64, 65]
- *Tumor metabolism versus prognosis:* There are indications that certain metabolic parameters measurable with PET may be related to tumor grade and patient survival.[66] For example, glucose consumption is often high in brain tumors and has been correlated to grade.[67]
- *Monitoring effects of therapy:* There are now significant data for human tumors that suggest that PET may be used to monitor the effectiveness of therapy.[68, 69] In addition, glucose consumption has been shown to remain decreased in tumors that are controlled and to increase again in recurrent tumors.[70] Of note, radiation necrosis can be distinguished from tumor recurrence using ^{18}FDG-PET.[31, 62]
- *Tumor pharmacokinetics:* The ability to take up drugs throughout the tumor is a critical determinant of therapeutic response. Drug uptake may be very heterogeneous within a large tumor or among different tumors of apparently similar pathology. For example, in brain tumors, variability in the integrity of the blood-brain barrier may cause a correlated and significant variability in drug uptake. Published results with variously labeled drugs indicate the potential of PET for such studies.[71, 72]
- *Assistance in staging tumors:* Some reports suggest that PET sometimes defines tumor margins that extend beyond what is observed by other diagnostic methods, such as CT scan.[73] This may occur when the tumor cell population is metabolically heterogeneous and irregularly distributed, morphologically, within the tumor. Therefore, comparison of results with PET versus CT and MRI may provide important information for the therapist.
- *Binding to receptors:* PET may be useful to monitor binding kinetics and to optimize development of reagents and their use in conjunction with other therapy modalities. Therefore, antibodies, with or without attached cytotoxins to tumor-associated antigens or to appropriate growth factor receptors, may be useful in both diagnosis and therapy of malignancy.

Radioautoimmunodetection (RAID)

Perhaps the most challenging and potentially wide-ranging technique is that of using radiolabeled monoclonal antibodies (mAbs) to malignant tumor antigens for diagnostic and therapeutic purposes.[74, 75] Considerable advances have been made in immunochemistry (improving antibody preparation and labeling), coupled with improvements in instrumentation, especially SPECT.

- *Radiolabeled monoclonal antibodies:* In general, these are cell surface antigens, commonly glycoproteins, and may be labeled with a diverse group of radioisotopes: ^{131}I, ^{111}In, ^{123}I, and ^{99m}Tc. They are usually produced by murine hybridomas (fusion of an immunized donor lymphocyte with a mouse myeloma cell) that will elaborate the antibody. Two limiting factors are that less than 1% of radiolabeled mAbs usually enters the tumor (signal-to-noise background obscures detection) and toxicity. Toxicity is a result of, in part, the use of murine factors, which have led to the development of human antibodies to murine proteins.
- *SPECT:* The most commonly used methods of *in vivo* detection of radiolabeled mAbs have utilized planar gamma camera imaging with background subtraction techniques. However, SPECT allows for the detection of small lesions at depth (>2.5 cm). Using radiolabeled antibodies, SPECT has yielded high sensitivities in some studies, approaching 90%.[76]

Interventional Ultrasonography

Although US per se is an established and effective medical technique, with the design of smaller probes that have allowed for its physical introduction into body cavities, the technique is being used more frequently.[77, 78] For example, transrectal US is used for prostate cancer and for determining rectal wall invasion and, coupled with guided needle biopsy, has increased the accuracy of diagnosis and staging.[16] Other examples of endocavitary US applications are for staging gastrointestinal neoplasms,[79] aiding in intravascular assessments,[80] and sampling nodes via transtracheobronchial US.[81]

Clinical Investigations: Future of Imaging in Oncology

As we enter the second century of our field of radiology, we may anticipate that advances in our imaging sciences will be equally as dramatic as we have experienced during the first century. Clearly, the imaging paradigm will shift from anatomic and spatial two-dimensional or three-dimensional images to ones focused on molecular, functional, biologic, and genetic imaging. In both diagnosis and therapy, minimally invasive techniques will continue to evolve, tapping the unique abilities of imaging to explore the environment of the body.

- Molecular and genetic imaging will provide quantitative data for developing intermediate surrogate indices for normal and tumor tissue response.[82]
- Fusion of anatomic (CT and MRI) with functional (MRS and PET) modalities will allow so-called dose painting or sculpting in the simulations for three-dimensional conformal treatment and intensity modulated radiation therapy.[83]

- Incorporating applied transformation matrices and multiple data sets into three-dimensional treatment planning will allow for the peeling away of normal tissues and organs that obscure the tumor.[13]

Recommended Reading

A number of excellent textbooks devoted to cancer imaging have appeared. *Oncologic Imaging,* a second edition edited by David Bragg, Philip Rubin, and Hedvig Hricak, is based on imaging strategies for different organ cancer sites and is multiauthored primarily by American investigators.[1] *Imaging in Oncology,* two volumes edited by Janet Husband and Rodney Reznek, approaches cancer imaging by staging and site.[2] This European, multiauthored textbook is beautifully illustrated by ISIS Medical and contains text highlights that present concepts concisely. A very readable and clinical version of *Oncologic Imaging: A Clinical Perspective,* a first edition, is offered by Berman, Brodsky, and Clark and is well illustrated with standard CT and MRI views.[3]

REFERENCES

General References

1. Bragg D, Rubin P, Hricak H (eds): Oncologic Imaging, 2nd ed. Philadelphia, W.B. Saunders, 2001.
2. Husband JES, Reznek RH (eds): Imaging in Oncology. Oxford, Isis Medical Media, 1998.
3. Berman CG, Brodsky NJ, Clark RA (eds): Oncologic Imaging: A Clinical Perspective. Philadelphia, McGraw-Hill, 1998.

Specific References

4. Pelley RJ, Bukowski RM: Recent advances in diagnosis and therapy of neuroendocrine tumors of the gastrointestinal tract. Curr Opin Oncol 1997; 9:68–74.
5. Blackmore CC, Black WC, Jarvik JG, et al: A critical synopsis of the diagnostic and screening radiology outcomes literature. Acad Radiol 1999; 6(suppl):S8–S18.
6. Hendee WR: The impact of future technology on oncologic diagnosis. In: Bragg DG, Rubin P, Youker JE (eds): Oncologic Imaging, 1st ed, pp 629–644. New York, Pergamon Press, 1985.
7. Dixon AK: The impact of medical imaging on the physician's diagnostic and therapeutic thinking. Eur Radiol 1998; 8:488–490.
8. Goldstein JH, Phillips CD: Current indications and techniques in evaluating inflammatory disease and neoplasia in the sinonasal cavities. Curr Prob Diag Radiol 1998; 27:41–71.
9. Fajardo LL: Measuring and incorporating patient preferences and utilities in the assessment of diagnostic technology. Acad Radiol 1999; 6(suppl):S113–S114.
10. American Joint Committee on Cancer: AJCC Cancer Staging Manual, 5th ed. Philadelphia, Lippincott-Raven, 1997.
11. Yang M, Baranov E, Jiang P, et al: Whole-body optical imaging of green fluorescent protein-expressing tumors and micrometastases. Proc Natl Acad Sci (USA) 2000; 97:1206–1211.
12. Hellman S: Preface. In: Bragg D, Rubin P, Hricak H (eds): Oncologic Imaging, 2nd ed. Philadelphia, W.B. Saunders, 2001.
13. Chen G: Image processing in oncologic imaging. In: Bragg D, Rubin P, Hricak H (eds): Oncologic Imaging, 2nd ed. Philadelphia, W.B. Saunders, 2001.
14. Hillman BJ, Gatsonis C, Sullivan DC: American College of Radiology Imaging Network: new national cooperative group for conducting clinical trials of medical imaging technologies. Radiology 1999; 213:641–645.
15. Barentsz JO, Engelbrecht MR, Witjes JA, et al: MR imaging of the male pelvis. Eur Radiol 1999; 9:1722–1736.
16. Yu KK, Hricak H: Imaging prostate cancer. Radiol Clin N Am 2000; 38:59–85.
17. Black WC, Welch HG: Screening for disease. American Journal of Roentgenology 1997; 168:3–11.
18. Whitty CJ, Sudlow CL, Warlow CP: Investigating individual subjects and screening populations for asymptomatic carotid stenosis can be harmful. J Neurol Neurosurg Psychiatry 1998; 64:619–623.
19. Feig SA: Role and evaluation of mammography and other imaging methods for breast cancer detection, diagnosis, and staging. Semin Nucl Med 1999; 29:3–15.
20. Bonomo L, Ciccotosto C, Guidotti A, et al: Staging of thoracic lymphoma by radiologic imaging. Eur Radiol 1997; 7:1179–1189.
21. Goldschmidt H, Wallmeier M, Hegenbart U, et al: Malignant lymphoma. Pathology, diagnosis, therapy. Radiologe 1997; 37:1–9.
22. Adams S, Baum RP, Stuckensen T, et al: Prospective comparison of ^{18}F-FDG PET with conventional imaging modalities (CT, MRI, US) in lymph node staging of head and neck cancer. Eur J Nucl Med 1998; 25:1255–1260.
23. Weissman JL, Akindele R: Current imaging techniques for head and neck tumors. Oncology (Huntingt) 1999; 13:697–709.
24. Fischbein N, Anzai Y, Mukherji SK: Application of new imaging techniques for the evaluation of squamous cell carcinoma of the head and neck. Semin Ultrasound CT MR 1999; 20:187–212.
25. Kagan AR, Steckel RJ: Surveillance of patients with prostate cancer after treatment: the roles of serologic and imaging studies. Med Pediatr Oncol 1993; 21:327–332.
26. Ricci PE: Imaging of adult brain tumors. Neuroimaging Clin N Am 1999; 9:651–669.
27. Foster RS, Nichols CR: Testicular cancer: what's new in staging, prognosis, and therapy. Oncology (Huntingt) 1999; 13:1689–1694.
28. Freeny PC: Computed tomography in the diagnosis and staging of cholangiocarcinoma and pancreatic carcinoma. Ann Oncol 1999; 10(suppl):12–17.
29. Urban BA, Fishman EK: Renal lymphoma: CT patterns with emphasis on helical CT. Radiographics 2000; 20:197–212.
30. Lau CL, Harpole DH Jr: Noninvasive clinical staging modalities for lung cancer. Semin Surg Oncol 2000; 18:116–123.
31. Nelson SJ: Imaging of brain tumors after therapy. Neuroimag Clin N Am 1999; 9:801–819.
32. Nelson SJ, Vigneron DB, Dillon WP: Serial evaluation of patients with brain tumors using volume MRI and 3D ^{1}H MRSI. NMR Biomed 1999; 12:123–138.
33. Hirakata K, Nakata H, Nakagawa T: CT of pulmonary metastases with pathological correlation. Semin Ultrasound CT MR 1995; 16:379–394.
34. Hatanaka K: CT evaluation of pulmonary metastases: usefulness in comparison with chest radiography. Nippon Igaku Hoshasen Gakkai Zasshi 1999; 59:663–669.
35. Sighvatsson V, Ericson K, Tomasson H: Optimising contrast-enhanced cranial CT for detection of brain metastases. Acta Radiol 1998; 39:718–722.
36. Wen PY, Loeffler JS: Management of brain metastases. Oncology (Huntingt) 1999; 13:941–954.
37. Yokoi K, Kamiya N, Matsuguma H, et al: Detection of brain metastases in potentially operable non–small cell lung cancer: a comparison of CT and MRI. Chest 1999; 115:714–719.
38. Helmberger T, Rau H, Linke R, et al: Diagnosis and staging of liver metastases with imaging methods. Chirurg 1999; 70:114–122.
39. Schmidt J, Strotzer M, Fraunhofer S, et al: Intraoperative ultrasonography versus helical computed tomography and computed tomography with arterioportography in diagnosing colorectal liver metastases: lesion-by-lesion analysis. World J Surg 2000; 24:43–47.
40. Ogata I, Komohara Y, Yamashita Y, et al: CT evaluation of gastric lesions with three-dimensional display and interactive virtual endoscopy: comparison with conventional barium study and endoscopy. American Journal of Roentgenology 1999; 172:1263–1270.
41. Gould MK, Lillington GA: Strategy and cost in investigating solitary pulmonary nodules. Thorax 1998; 53(suppl):S32–S37.
42. Stokkel MP, Bakker PF, Heine R, et al: Staging of lymph nodes with FDG dual-headed PET in patients with non–small-cell lung cancer. Nucl Med Comm 1999; 20:1001–1007.
43. Anonymous: Digital mammography. Why hasn't it been approved for U.S. hospitals? Health Devices 2000; 29:14–21.
44. Foxall PJ, Nicholson JK: Nuclear magnetic resonance spectroscopy: a non-invasive probe of kidney metabolism and function. Exp Nephrol 1998; 6:409–414.
45. McCully K, Mancini D, Levine S: Nuclear magnetic resonance spec-

troscopy: its role in providing valuable insight into diverse clinical problems. Chest 1999; 116:1434–1441.
46. Rudkin TM, Arnold DL: Proton magnetic resonance spectroscopy for the diagnosis and management of cerebral disorders. Arch Neurol 1999; 56:919–926.
47. Fossel ET, Carr JM, McDonagh J: Detection of malignant tumors: water-suppressed proton nuclear magnetic resonance spectroscopy of plasma. New Engl J Med 1986; 315:1369–1376.
48. Engan T, Bjerve KS, Hoe AL, Krane J: Characterization of plasma lipids in patients with malignant disease by ^{13}C nuclear magnetic resonance spectroscopy and gas liquid chromatography. Blood 1995; 85:1323–1330.
49. Fluge O, Gilje KS, Sletten E, et al: Proton nuclear magnetic resonance spectroscopy of serum from patients with colorectal neoplasia. Eur J Surg Oncol 1996; 22:78–83.
50. Dagnelie PC, Sijens PE, Kraus DJ, et al: Abnormal liver metabolism in cancer patients detected by (31)P MR spectroscopy. NMR Biomed 1999; 12:535–544.
51. Leij-Halfwerk S, van den Berg JW, Sijens PE, et al: Altered hepatic gluconeogenesis during L-alanine infusion in weight-losing lung cancer patients as observed by phosphorus magnetic resonance spectroscopy and turnover measurements. Cancer Res 2000; 60:618–623.
52. Singer S, Souza K, Thilly WG: Pyruvate utilization, phosphocholine and adenosine triphosphate (ATP) are markers of human breast tumor progression: a ^{31}P- and ^{13}C-nuclear magnetic resonance (NMR) spectroscopy study. Cancer Res 1995; 55:5140–5145.
53. Singer S, Sivaraja M, Souza K, et al: ^{1}H-NMR detectable fatty acyl chain unsaturation in excised leiomyosarcoma correlate with grade and mitotic activity. J Clin Invest 1996; 98:244–250.
54. Westin T, Soussi B, Idstrom JP, et al: Energetics of nutrition and polyamine-related tumor growth alterations in experimental cancer. Br J Cancer 1993; 68:662–667.
55. Aboagye EO, Kelson AB, Tracy M, Workman P: Preclinical development and current status of the fluorinated 2-nitroimidazole hypoxia probe N-(2-hydroxy-3,3,3-trifluoropropyl)-2-(2-nitro-1-imidazolyl) acetamide (SR 4554, CRC 94/17): a non-invasive diagnostic probe for the measurement of tumor hypoxia by magnetic spectroscopy and imaging, and by positron emission tomography. Anticancer Drug Des 1998; 13:703–730.
56. Kuliszkiewicz-Janus M, Baczynski S: Chemotherapy-associated changes in ^{31}P MRS spectra of sera from patients with multiple myeloma. NMR Biomed 1995; 8:127–132.
57. Moller HE, Vermathen P, Rummeny E, et al: In vivo ^{31}P NMR spectroscopy of human musculoskeletal tumors as a measure of response to chemotherapy. NMR Biomed 1996; 9:347–358.
58. Kaplan O, Kushnir T, Askenazy N, et al: Role of nuclear magnetic resonance spectroscopy (MRS) in cancer diagnosis and treatment: ^{31}P, ^{23}Na, and ^{1}H MRS studies of three models of pancreatic cancer. Cancer Res 1997; 57:1452–1459.
59. Venkatesan PV, Saravanan K, Nagarajan B: Characterization of multidrug resistance and monitoring of tumor response by combined ^{31}P and ^{1}H nuclear magnetic resonance spectroscopic analysis. Anticancer Drugs 1998; 9:449–456.
60. Baldwin NJ, Wang Y, Ng TC: *In situ* ^{19}F MRS measurement of RIF-1 tumor blood volume: corroboration by radioisotope-labeled [^{125}I]-albumin and correlation to tumor size. Magn Reson Imaging 1996; 14:275–280.
61. Gupta NC, Nicholson P, Bloomfield SM: FDG-PET in the staging work-up of patients with suspected intracranial metastatic tumors. Ann Surg 1999; 230:202–206.
62. Deshmukh A, Scott JA, Palmer EL, et al: Impact of fluorodeoxyglucose positron emission tomography on the clinical management of patients with glioma. Clin Nucl Med 1996; 21:720–725.
63. Chapman JD, Engelhardt EL, Stobbe CC, et al: Measuring hypoxia and predicting tumor radioresistance with nuclear medicine assays. Radiother Oncol 1998; 46:229–237.
64. Koh WJ, Bergman KS, Rasey J, et al: Evaluation of oxygenation status during fractionated radiotherapy in human nonsmall cell lung cancers using [F-18]fluoromisonidazole positron emission tomography. Int J Radiat Oncol Biol Phys 1995; 33:391–398.
65. Cook GJ, Houston S, Barrington SF, et al: Technetium-99m-labeled HL91 to identify tumor hypoxia: correlation with fluorine-18-FDG. J Nucl Med 1998; 39:99–103.
66. Benard F, Sterman D, Smith RJ, et al: Prognostic value of FDG PET imaging in malignant pleural mesothelioma. J Nucl Med 1999; 40:1241–1245.
67. Woesler B, Kuwert T, Morgenroth C, et al: Non-invasive grading of primary brain tumours: results of a comparative study between SPET with ^{123}I-alpha-methyl tyrosine and PET with ^{18}F-deoxyglucose. Eur J Nucl Med 1997; 24:428–434.
68. MacVicar D, Husband JE: Assessment of response following treatment for malignant disease. Br J Radiol 1997; 70:S41–S49.
69. Shields AF, Ho PT, Grierson JR: The role of imaging in the development of oncologic agents. J Clin Pharmacol 1999; (suppl):40S–44S.
70. Bader JB, Samnick S, Moringlane JR, et al: Evaluation of 1–3-[^{123}I]iodo-alpha-methyltyrosine SPET and [^{18}F]fluorodeoxyglucose PET in the detection and grading of recurrences in patients pretreated for gliomas at follow-up: a comparative study with stereotactic biopsy. Eur J Nucl Med 1999; 26:144–151.
71. Carnochan P, Trivedi M, Young H, et al: Biodistribution and kinetics of radiolabelled pyrrolidino-4-iodo-tamoxifen: prospects for pharmacokinetic studies using PET. J Nucl Biol Med 1994; 38(suppl):96–98.
72. Imahori Y, Ueda S, Ohmori Y, et al: Positron emission tomography-based boron neutron capture therapy using borophenylalanine for high-grade gliomas: part I. Clin Cancer Res 1998; 4:1825–1832.
73. Wong WL, Hussain K, Chevretton E, et al: Validation and clinical application of computer-combined computed tomography and positron emission tomography with 2-[^{18}F]fluoro-2-deoxyglucose head and neck images. Am J Surg 1996; 172:628–632.
74. Divgi CR: Status of radiolabeled monoclonal antibodies for diagnosis and therapy of cancer. Oncology (Huntingt) 1996; 10:939–953.
75. Manyak MJ, Javitt MC: The role of computerized tomography, magnetic resonance imaging, bone scan, and monoclonal antibody nuclear scan for prognosis prediction in prostate cancer. Semin Urol Oncol 1998; 16:145–152.
76. Volpe CM, Abdel-Nabi HH, Kulaylat MN, et al: Results of immunoscintigraphy using a cocktail of radiolabeled monoclonal antibodies in the detection of colorectal cancer. Ann Surg Oncol 1998; 5:489–494.
77. Mallery S, Van Dam J: Interventional endoscopic ultrasonography: current status and future directions. J Clin Gastroenterol 1999; 29:297–305.
78. Bhutani MS: Interventional endoscopic ultrasonography: state of the art at the new millenium. Endoscopy 2000; 32:62–71.
79. Hawes RH: Endoscopic ultrasound. Gastrointest Clin North Am 2000; 10:161–174.
80. Nishanian G, Kopchok GE, Donayre CE, et al: The impact of intravascular ultrasound (IVUS) on endovascular interventions. Semin Vasc Surg 1999; 12:285–299.
81. Lewis JD, Faigel DO, Dowdy Y, et al: Hodgkin's disease diagnosed by endoscopic ultrasound-guided fine needle aspiration of a periduodenal lymph node. Am J Gastroenterol 1998; 93:834–836.
82. Sullivan DC, Tatum JL: Imaging at the cellular and molecular level. In: Bragg D, Rubin P, Hricak H (eds): Oncologic Imaging, 2nd ed. Philadelphia, W.B. Saunders, 2001.
83. Burman CM, Hunt MA, Chui C-S, et al: Three-dimensional and conformal treatment planning. In: Bragg D, Rubin P, Hricak H (eds): Oncologic Imaging, 2nd ed. Philadelphia, W.B. Saunders, 2001.

16 *Skin Cancer*

MERRILL J. SOLAN, MD, Radiation Oncology
LUTHER W. BRADY, MD, Radiation Oncology

Nonmelanoma Skin Cancer

It was the fatal flaw of humanity which Nature, in one shape or another, stamps ineffaceably on all her productions . . . to imply that they are temporary and finite.

NATHANIEL HAWTHORNE

Perspective

Skin cancers are the most common of all malignancies and the most preventable. In general, nonmelanoma skin cancers are readily treatable, rarely metastasize, and only infrequently cause death. In spite of these characteristics, the overall incidence of nonmelanoma skin cancer has increased dramatically over the past 20 years.[6, 7] With predictions of 900,000 to 1,200,000 new cases per year in the United States, nonmelanoma skin cancer approaches the overall incidence of all noncutaneous malignancies.[8] Fortunately, the mortality from nonmelanoma skin cancer has decreased by 20% to 30%, with about 1200 deaths per year in the United States.[9] Skin cancers are usually caused by excessive sun exposure and occur most often on the exposed areas of the head and neck. This chapter will cover nonmelanoma skin cancer in the first section, and then malignant melanoma is discussed in the second section.

Epidemiology and Etiology

Epidemiology

Most skin cancers arise from pre-existing lesions or in damaged skin. Premalignant skin lesions include actinic (solar) keratoses, epithelial hyperplasia, leukoplakia, nevi, and burn scars. Of the malignant skin cancers, basal cell carcinoma (BCC) is the most common skin cancer, followed in incidence by squamous cell carcinoma (SCC) (Fig. 16–1). Malignant skin lesions include:

- basal cell carcinoma
- intraepithelial carcinoma (Bowen's disease)
- squamous cell carcinoma
- keratoacanthoma (acute epithelial cancer)
- melanoma
- Merkel cell carcinoma
- adnexal and connective tissue tumors
- mycosis fungoides
- malignant lymphomas
- Kaposi's sarcoma
- secondary metastases

Skin cancers occur most frequently in people with fair complexions who have a history of excessive sun exposure, and are found most often on exposed hair-bearing areas of the head and neck; involvement of the palm of the hand and sole of the foot is rare. The male:female ratio of nonmelanoma skin cancer is approximately 2:1.[10] The incidence of sun-related skin cancer is extremely low in blacks, but it occurs with equal frequency in both blacks and whites when it arises from an atrophic skin lesion or burn scar (Marjolin's ulcer). Mortality rates from skin cancer are disproportionately high in blacks; this may be a result of the lower incidence of favorable-prognosis sun-induced skin cancer in this population, presentation with more advanced disease,[11] or higher incidence of more aggressive squamous cell carcinoma than basal cell carcinoma.[10]

Etiology

Sun Damage

Chronic exposure to ultraviolet (UV) B light (290–320 nm) is, by far, the most recognized cause of skin cancer. The mechanism of cancer induction appears to be both damage to DNA within the epidermis and induction of immunologic changes that inhibit an immune response against the tumor.[10, 12, 13] The increasing incidence of sun-induced nonmelanoma skin cancer is at least in part attributed to depletion of the ozone layer that absorbs UVB radiation.[14, 15] In addition, the increasing incidence of sun-induced cancer with advancing age suggests that cumulative exposure is an important factor; however, it is believed that, in spite of appearance of these tumors in older individuals, it is childhood exposure that determines ultimate risk.[14–18]

Genetics

Several inherited syndromes are associated with an increased risk of nonmelanoma skin cancer[10, 15, 18]:

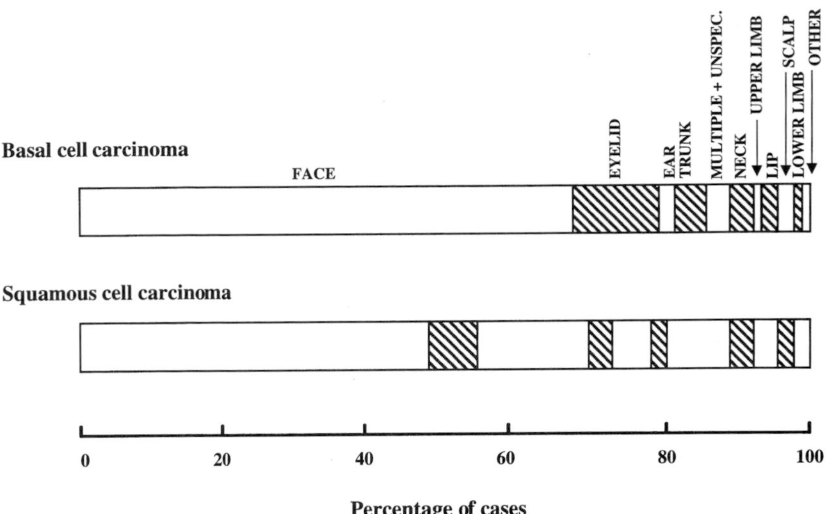

Figure 16–1. Incidence rate line graph for basal cell carcinoma (BCC) and squamous cell carcinoma (SCC).

- xeroderma pigmentosum—an autosomal recessive defect in DNA repair
- basal cell nevus syndrome—autosomal dominant or mosaic, associated with multiple BCCs
- albinism—an autosomal recessive failure to produce melanin, resulting in increased susceptibility to sun damage
- epidermodysplasia verruciformis—an autosomal recessive disorder associated with widespread human papilloma virus, leading to the development of warts that degenerate to SCCs[10]

Chemical Exposure

Both occupational and environmental exposure to some chemicals has resulted in an increased risk of skin cancers. For example, long-term exposure to arsenic has been shown to induce keratoses that increase the risk of SCC.[14] Exposure of chimney sweeps to coal tar has been described in the development of scrotal skin cancer,[19] and cigarette smoking is associated with an increased risk of SCC of the lip and mouth.[10, 18] Treatment of psoriasis with oral psoralens and UVA photochemotherapy has resulted in a dose-dependent risk of SCC.[10, 14]

Immunosuppression

The risk of nonmelanoma skin cancer, especially SCC, is increased in immunosuppressed patients, such as transplant patients on immunosuppressive drugs to prevent rejection and in patients with acquired immunodeficiency syndrome. Papillomavirus and oncoviruses have been implicated as etiologic agents, particularly in cases of keratoacanthoma.[10, 18, 20–22]

Chronic Irritation or Inflammation

Squamous cell skin cancers have been noted in old burn scars as well as in areas associated with skin diseases that have a chronic inflammatory or irritant course, such as syphilis, lupus, granulomas, and chronic ulcers. In general, SCCs rarely metastasize; however, SCCs that arise in a burn scar or other areas of chronic inflammation may be more aggressive, with regional nodal or distant metastases in as many as 20% of patients.[16]

Detection and Diagnosis

Clinical Detection

Medical history should include information about age, race, occupation, family history, and geographic background. Careful attention should be paid to a history of chronic sun exposure, blistering sunburn during childhood, prior radiation exposure, or chemical exposure. Any skin lesion should be examined thoroughly, with documentation of size, color, location, date of onset, symptoms (such as pain, pruritus, or bleeding), prior treatment, extension into other adjacent areas, and depth of penetration. Photographs of the lesion before and after treatment should be taken. Examination of all skin-bearing areas for the presence of other lesions requires that the patient be fully undressed for the examination.[23] Palpation of regional lymph nodes is essential, with biopsy of any suspicious adenopathy. Of note, the scalp is an area where a skin lesion can go undetected for some time without adequate palpation and visualization. Tools for the assessment of skin cancers include magnifying loops, Wood's light, potassium hydroxide (KOH) preparations, and biopsies.[23] Computed tomography scans and x-rays will help detect the degree of extension, depth, and the presence of bone or cartilage invasion.

Diagnostic Procedures

Biopsies should be performed on *all* suspicious skin lesions for histologic diagnosis.

Excisional Biopsy. This procedure is both diagnostic and therapeutic. The entire lesion is removed along with a 0.5- to 2-cm margin of surrounding normal tissue. This procedure is best suited for small lesions in areas where cosmesis will not be compromised. Additional treatment might be required for inadequate surgical margins, deep tumor infiltration, or extension into adjacent critical structures.

Incisional Biopsy. This procedure is performed for diagnostic purposes on a lesion that is too large or too deeply infiltrating for a cosmetically acceptable complete excision. Once the diagnosis is established, the definitive treatment modality is determined by tumor location and cosmetic considerations.

Classification and Staging

Histopathology

Premalignant and Benign Skin Lesions

Actinic (Solar) Keratoses. Actinic keratoses are rough, scaly, erythematous patches. These lesions tend to be multiple and occur most often on sun-exposed areas such as the face, neck, and hands; frequency increases with age. The incidence of malignant transformation is about 1%, with lesions forming a thick "cutaneous horn" or with induration at the base or ulceration at highest risk.[24]

Seborrheic Keratoses. These benign skin lesions are brown and flat, with sharply demarcated borders. They do not undergo malignant transformation.

Radiation Dermatitis. Any area of the body that has been exposed to ionizing radiation may develop changes as a result of radiation dermatitis. The skin becomes atrophic and thinned, with a reduction of subcutaneous tissue and the appearance of telangiectatic vessels and keratoses, and the skin is susceptible to ulceration and trauma. Most of the reported radiogenic skin cancers have occurred in patients receiving irradiation for benign dermatoses despite the fact that, in general, these patients received lower total radiation doses over more protracted periods of time than patients receiving radiation for malignant tumors. A latent period of at least 10 years is reported in the development of radiogenic cutaneous tumors, and the frequency of these tumors is related to the dose of radiation received and the patient's age at the time of radiation exposure, with younger patients being affected most frequently.[25]

Malignant Skin Lesions

Basal Cell Carcinoma. BCC is the most common skin cancer and arises from the basal layer of the epidermis, where the involved basal cells fail to mature into keratinocytes. The tumor steadily grows in bulk and, in most cases, retains its dependency on the skin for viability. Untreated, these lesions can burrow deeply, infiltrate vital areas, and may cause marked deformity (rodent ulcers). Most BCCs occur on the head and neck, nearly always on hair-bearing skin, with a predilection for the head above the line joining the earlobe to the angle of the mouth. BCCs tend to infiltrate more deeply at embryologic junctions.

There are four major subtypes of BCC[10, 17]:

- The nodular ulcerative type constitutes 45% to 60% of all BCCs. Lesions are smooth, small, translucent or pearly pink papules, with a characteristic central depression (secondary to necrosis) and prominent telangiectatic vessels in or around the lesion. There is a tendency to bleed with minor trauma and to ulcerate or crust with growth. These bleeding lesions with central depressions have been described as *rodent ulcers*.
- Superficial BCCs appear as red, scaly macules, frequently on the extremities or trunk, which enlarge into patches with crusting. They may invade along superficial nerve roots and embryonal fusion planes.
- *Morphea* are sclerosing BCCs that appear as flat, fibrotic, white-yellow macules or plaques that become firm and depressed as they enlarge. Lesions have indistinct borders and spread laterally within the dermis.
- Pigmented BCCs may be confused with malignant melanoma. Clinical behavior is the same as with the nonpigmented form.

BCCs rarely metastasize to lymph nodes (0.04%) or other organs (<1 in 4000 cases).[10]

Squamous Cell Carcinoma. Squamous cell carcinomas involve epidermal keratinizing cells that invade the dermal-epidermal junction. Typical SCCs are irregular exophytic lesions with a warty, keratotic scale. They may become crusted and ulcerated with growth, may bleed with minor trauma, and may develop conical mounds of keratin called *cutaneous horns*. Squamous cell carcinomas that develop in pre-existing actinic keratoses rarely metastasize; overall, 1% to 2% of patients with SCC develop nodal metastases.[18] The incidence of lymph node metastases in SCC increases with recurrent lesions and in SCCs developing in Marjolin's ulcer. Survival also is decreased in extremity lesions.

Bowen's Disease (Squamous Cell Carcinoma *in situ*). This skin lesion appears as a superficial, velvety, red-brown nodule or plaque that may be seen on any area of the body. Lesions may be mildly pruritic and tend to be indolent, growing slowly over several years before degenerating into an invasive SCC. The incidence of invasion is estimated at 5%; once invasion occurs, as many as one third will metastasize.[22]

Keratoacanthoma. These hyperkeratotic lesions are often classified as benign and self-healing, and are domed papules with a central keratotic plug. Keratoacanthomas are capable of rapid growth with considerable soft tissue destruction and may be associated with SCCs.

Melanoma. For a complete discussion of malignant melanoma, see the second section of this chapter.

Merkel Cell Carcinoma. This cutaneous tumor is characterized by an appearance in the seventh and eighth decades, a high rate of local recurrence, and frequent nodal and distant metastases. The cell of origin is felt to lie in the basal layer of the epidermis, and ultrastructural and immunohistochemical analysis suggests a neuroectodermal derivation; solid, trabecular, and diffuse variants exist. The lesions appear as firm, pink-red nodules with an intact epidermis that can involve the reticular dermis and subcutaneous tissue. Merkel cell tumors occur with greatest fre-

TABLE 16–1. **Staging of Nonmelanoma Skin Cancer**

Stage	Grouping	Descriptors*
Stage 0	Tis, N0, M0	Tis: Carcinoma *in situ* N0: No regional metastasis M0: No distant metastasis
Stage I	T1, N0, M0	T1: Tumor ≤2 cm in greatest dimension
Stage II	T2, N0, M0	T2: Tumor >2 cm, but not more than 5 cm in greatest dimension
	T3, N0, M0	T3: Tumor >5 cm in greatest dimension
Stage III	T4, N0, M0	T4: Tumor invades deep extradermal structures (i.e., cartilage, skeletal muscle, or bone)
	Any T, N1, M0	N1: Regional lymph node metastasis
Stage IV	Any T, Any N, M1	M1: Distant metastasis

*TX would indicate that primary tumor cannot be assessed; T0, that there is no evidence of primary tumor.

Used with the permission of the American Joint Committee on Cancer (AJCC®), Chicago, Illinois. The original source for this material is the AJCC® Cancer Staging Manual, 5th edition, 1997, published by Lippincott-Raven Publishers, Philadelphia, Pennsylvania.

quency on the head and neck region (50%) or extremities, but rarely on the trunk.[26]

Mycosis Fungoides. This cutaneous T-cell lymphoma is referred to as Sézary syndrome when it is associated with circulating malignant cells. There are three recognized clinical stages of mycosis fungoides: premycotic or eczematous, infiltrative plaque, and tumoral.

Kaposi's Sarcoma. Kaposi's sarcoma is a cutaneous malignancy, characterized by endothelial and fibroblastic proliferation and formation of new blood vessels. Lesions appear as violet-red to brown nodules and plaques, and the classic form is most common in elderly males of Mediterranean extraction. A more fulminant epidemic form is seen in patients with acquired immunodeficiency syndrome, and is associated with deep infiltration and adenopathy.

Cutaneous Metastases. Primary cancers originating in other organs may metastasize to the skin. They can be multiple, and may occur on any area of the body. Carcinomatous metastases usually are firm nodules with an intact epidermis; as they grow, epidermal invasion may lead to ulceration and bleeding. Cutaneous nodules from lymphoma tend to be softer and more rubbery in texture.

Staging

Anatomic staging for nonmelanoma skin cancer (excluding eyelid, vulva, and penis) is illustrated in Table 16–1[27] and Figure 16–2. The American Joint Committee on Cancer and the International Union Against Cancer staging classification is based on the Tumor (T), Node (N), Metastasis (M) system. Separate staging is employed for carcinoma of the eyelid, vulva, and penis.

Principles of Treatment

There are multiple, potentially curative treatment options for cutaneous BCC and SCC that should result in eradication of disease in more than 90% of patients. The decision regarding the best treatment for any given patient is determined by consideration of multiple factors[10, 16]:

- size of lesion
- anatomic location
- depth of invasion
- involvement of cartilage or bone
- prior treatment
- general medical condition of patient
- patient preference or convenience

The treatment modality selected should give the greatest likelihood of cure with acceptable cosmesis in a manner that is both practical and convenient for the patient (Table 16–2).

Surgery

Surgical excision is often the treatment of choice for lesions smaller than 3 cm that can be removed with little cosmetic deformity or functional impairment. Surgery is especially suited to scalp lesions because it avoids hair loss in the treated field inherent in radiation therapy. Advantages of surgical excision include short treatment time and pathologic assessment of the adequacy of resection margins.

Once a skin cancer is excised, the resultant tissue defect must be repaired. This can be accomplished by primary closure for most small lesions but may require skin grafts or other cosmetic reconstruction for large defects or in cases of deep infiltration or exposed bone or cartilage. Surgical techniques for the eradication of skin cancer include the methods listed in the following paragraphs.

Curettage with Electrodesiccation for Hemostasis. A curette is used to excise the tumor by an experienced

TABLE 16–2. **Multidisciplinary Treatment Decisions for Nonmelanoma Cancer**

Stage	Surgery	Radiation Therapy	Chemotherapy
Stage I	Excision or Mohs' technique	CRT 3 Gy × 15 = 45 Gy/3 wk	NR
Stage II	Mohs' technique	CRT 2.5 Gy × 20 = 50 Gy/4 wk CRT 2 Gy × 30 = 60 Gy/6 wk	NR
Stage III	Mohs' technique	CRT 2 Gy × 30–35 = 60–70 Gy/6–7 wk	NR
Stage IV	Excision if possible	PRT if feasible	IC II

CRT = curative radiation therapy; PRT = palliative radiation therapy; IC II = investigational chemotherapy, phase I/II clinical trials; NR = not recommended.
Adapted from National Cancer Institute. Information from PDQ—for Health Professionals: Skin Cancer. July 1999. CancerNet. Electronic database.

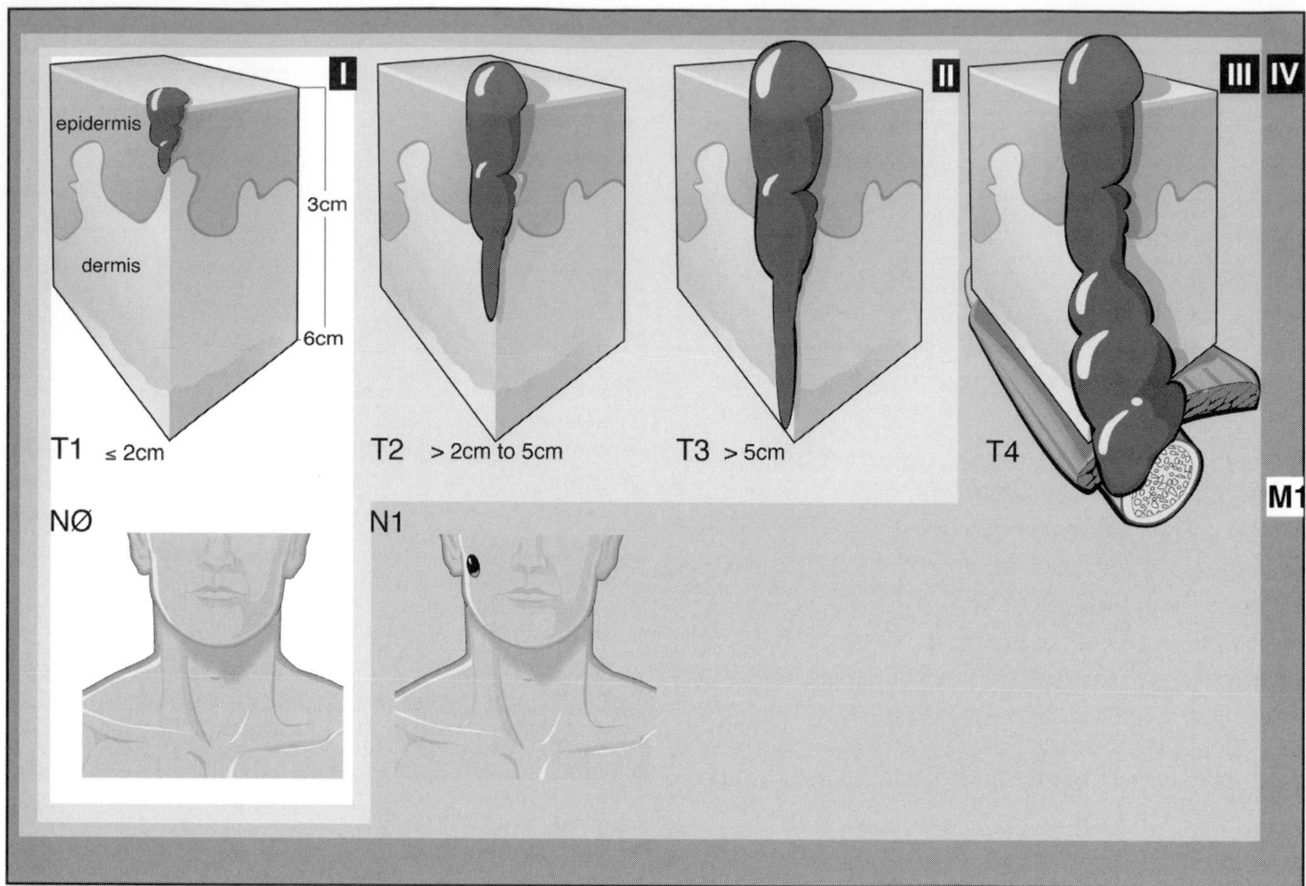

Figure 16–2. Anatomic staging for skin cancer.

clinician via a scraping technique. Healing is by secondary intention, and the patient usually is left with a scar. No assessment of surgical margins is possible.

Mohs' Surgery (Microscopically Controlled Surgery). Mohs' microscopically controlled surgery is named after general surgeon Fredrick Mohs, who developed this technique more than 50 years ago.[28, 29] The tumor is accurately mapped and meticulously excised, with multiple microscopic sections examined under light microscopy until resection margins are pathologically clear. The technique requires considerable skill and is very time consuming, but it results in the removal of minimal amounts of tissue. The defect can be sutured by an appropriate technique or can heal by secondary intention. The Mohs' technique is especially recommended in cases of morphea-type BCCs with indistinct margins and in multifocal recurrent BCCs and SCCs.[16] It offers the advantage of decreased functional and cosmetic morbidity.[29, 30]

Cryotherapy and Lasers. Cryotherapy is performed after gross tumor curettage and employs liquid nitrogen for controlled freezing of the tumor. Cryotherapy is rarely used in the treatment of SCC or BCC but frequently is employed to treat benign lesions such as actinic keratoses and warts.

Carbon dioxide lasers may be used to excise skin tumors and offer the advantage of minimal blood loss.[31] The lasers emit invisible infrared light (wavelength 10,600 nm), which is absorbed by water in the tissue and is converted from light energy to heat that vaporizes tissue.[32]

Radiation Therapy

Large skin cancers and those with deep infiltration or invasion of adjacent structures, or with both, may be best suited for treatment with radiation. When surgical excision would likely result in inadequate resection margins or a defect requiring extensive plastic surgical reconstruction, radiation can usually offer a better cosmetic and functional result. Radiation has an advantage over surgery, even for small lesions on the lip, eyelid, ear, or nose, or in situations in which the tumor overlies or invades bone or cartilage. Radiation is preferable over surgery in cases of multiple lesions and lymph node metastasis with respect to coverage.

Modern radiation therapy equipment makes possible the use of a variety of treatment techniques depending on the location and extent of the tumor. Orthovoltage, supervoltage, or electron beam energies can be chosen for controlled treatment depth. Lead cutouts and masks may be employed to collimate and shape the treatment fields to conform to the contour of the tumor and to protect the critical adjacent structures such as the eye, cartilage, or bone. The end cosmetic result is, in large part, determined by treatment fractionation and the total dose delivered.

The definitive irradiation doses vary with the histologic type, size and depth of the lesion, size of the treatment field, fraction size, and overall time of delivery.[26] Most skin cancers are readily treated to a dose of about 48 Gy, using 16 daily 3-Gy treatment fractions. Large lesions with deep extension or lesions involving the lip, eyelid, ear, or nose are often treated in a more protracted regimen of 2 Gy per fraction to a total of 60 Gy, with a resultant improvement in cosmesis. Shorter courses of treatment with higher daily fraction sizes offer the advantage of decreased cost and patient convenience but must be weighed against potential compromised cosmesis.

Very large, deeply infiltrating lesions, especially where bone and cartilage are involved, may be best treated in a combined-modality approach. Preoperative irradiation can be employed to shrink bulk disease and sterilize tumor margins, allowing more limited surgical resection with less morbidity. Postoperative irradiation is indicated where surgical margins are close or frankly positive and where multiple metastatic lymph nodes are involved.

Late radionecrosis rarely should be seen with the use of modern radiation techniques and attention to fractionation regimen.[25] The incidence of secondary radiogenic skin tumors within an area previously irradiated for skin cancer has been reported at about 3.5% (2% SCC and 1.5% BCC). It is notable that all of these tumors developed in sun-exposed skin and tended to occur after an average latent period of over 13 years. Irradiation, therefore, poses little practical risk in the elderly but should be used with caution in very young patients.[25] Irradiation-induced ulcers are seen more often than tumors and increase in incidence with increasing dose.

Chemotherapy and Other Pharmaceuticals

- Topical 5-fluorouracil (5-FU) is used most often in the treatment of actinic keratoses and, much less frequently, for superficial BCCs and Bowen's disease.[10] Treatment depth is only superficial, making its use contraindicated for deeper tumors. Recurrence rates may be higher than with other treatment modalities.
- Systemic retinoids have been used orally as chemopreventive agents in patients at high risk for developing cutaneous BCC and SCC. Their application is limited because of toxicity even at low doses.[33] Systemic retinoids have been shown to induce a regression of skin cancers but not cures.[17]
- Intralesional interferon-α (αIFN) has been employed to treat nodular and superficial BCCs and SCCs. Recurrence rates of up to 19% have been reported at 1 year, and application is mostly investigational.[10]
- Photodynamic therapy[10] employs the systemic photosensitizer intravenous porfimer sodium (Photofrin II) and nonionizing radiation (630-nm light wavelength), but is still investigational. Topical aminolevulinic acid also may be used as a photosensitizer.[34]

Results and Prognosis

Local Control and Survival

The cure rates for BCC and SCC of the skin are excellent at 90% to 100% with either surgery or radiation therapy for tumors smaller than 1 cm. With increasing size of lesion and depth of penetration, local control falls to 75% to 90%. BCC has an overall higher cure rate than SCC. The risk of metastatic spread to regional lymph nodes is higher for SCC; SCCs developing in non–sun-exposed areas or in sites of chronic ulceration or burn scars can be particularly aggressive, with a high risk of metastatic spread. Treatment-related complications with either surgery or radiation therapy increase with increasing size of the lesion, but are most often cosmetic in nature.

Recurrence

Recurrence rates for BCC are 5% to 10% and for SCC, 25% to 30%. Risk of recurrence is related to the following factors[35, 36]:

- size and depth of lesion
- development of lesion in non–sun-exposed site
- inadequate surgical excision with positive excision margins
- inadequate size of radiation field or treatment depth
- previous skin cancer

Recurrent skin cancers have a lower cure rate and the potential for increased treatment complications and poorer cosmesis than the initial lesions. Positive surgical margins can be treated with re-excision, radiation therapy, or Mohs' chemosurgery after the initial surgical procedure and before clinical recurrence is apparent to increase the likelihood of local control. For BCC, a positive, deep surgical margin is of greater concern than a positive lateral margin, with a 33% versus 17% recurrence rate respectively.[37] Retreatment of recurrent BCC results in 85% to 90% control. Squamous cell carcinomas excised with positive margins should always receive additional treatment because of the risk of metastasis. Radiation therapy failures are generally treated with surgery.

Prevention

Skin cancer prevention is possible only with increased public awareness.[15] Public education with regard to skin cancer must stress the following[17]:

- attention to changes in size or color, scaling, or bleeding of a pre-existing skin lesion or mole
- the importance of self-examination for early detection and treatment
- the advisement that UV radiation avoidance and protection is important for everyone, and should begin from early childhood
- the special attention that darkly pigmented individuals require because they are not immune to the development of skin cancers and the lesions may be more difficult to detect
- the significance of early diagnosis and treatment in the improvement of control and survival
- the fact that solar radiation is carcinogenic and should be avoided

Patients who have been treated for a skin cancer are at increased risk for developing another. For these patients, meticulous regular follow-up is necessary to search for recurrences or new lesions.[17] Exposure to solar radiation should be limited from childhood and sunscreens should be used regularly because, in addition to reducing the oncogenic effect of UV radiation in the epidermis, sunscreens have been shown to inhibit UVB-induced immunosuppression.[12, 35] Diets low in fat have been reported to decrease the risk of nonmelanoma skin cancer.[38]

Recommended Reading

Excellent comprehensive discussions of the diagnosis and treatment of skin cancers can be found in most standard texts of dermatology, medical oncology, and radiation oncology. The reader is referred to the chapters "Tumors of the Skin" by Koh and Bhawan in Moschella and Hurley's *Dermatology*[1]; "Dermal and Subcutaneous Tumors" and "Epidermal Nevi, Neoplasms, and Cysts" in *Andrews' Diseases of the Skin* edited by Arnold and colleagues[2]; "Premalignant and Malignant Nonmelanoma Skin Tumors" by Habif in *Clinical Dermatology*[3]; "Cutaneous Cancer and Malignant Melanoma" by Swetter and associates in *Clinical Oncology*[4]; and "Cancer of the Skin" by Brash in *Cancer: Principles & Practice of Oncology*.[5]

Malignant Melanoma

Malignant melanoma writes its message in the skin with its own ink and it is there for all of us to see. Some see but do not comprehend.[39]

Perspective

Melanomas are malignant cutaneous tumors that develop from melanocytes, ectodermal cells that migrate to the skin from the neural crest, and they are located in the basal layer of the epidermis. Although it is believed that most melanomas begin *de novo*, 30% to 50% may arise from pre-existing nevi. Melanocytes, and therefore malignant melanomas, may be seen in any area of the skin as well as in the eye, central nervous system, and respiratory, gastrointestinal, and genitourinary tracts.

The incidence of malignant melanoma has been increasing at the alarming rate of 6% per year since the early 1950s,[40, 41] and this tumor is now the fifth most common malignancy in the United States. The projected 2000 incidence of new melanoma cases in the United States was 47,700.[42] Because of the increased incidence of the tumor, melanoma mortality figures have increased at about 2% per year.

In the last decade, heightened physician and patient awareness of the problem of malignant melanoma and the implementation of large-scale skin cancer screening programs have resulted in earlier detection and improved survival. Malignant melanoma is curable in over 90% of early stage lesions and has an overall cure rate greater than 80%.[43] Nonetheless, the treatment of advanced melanoma remains a clinical and investigational challenge. There has been a constant evolution in the surgical and medical management of malignant melanoma, but continued efforts toward earlier detection and improved adjuvant treatment will be necessary to keep up with the rapidly increasing incidence of this disease.

Epidemiology and Etiology

Etiology

Malignant melanoma risk is related to the following factors[36, 44, 45]:

- excessive sun exposure
- race (pigmentation)
- change in an existing nevus
- presence of a large number of nevi
- history of previous melanoma
- family history of melanoma
- personal history of nonmelanoma skin cancer
- xeroderma pigmentosum

Sun Exposure

Studies of malignant melanoma support a solar etiology as the most important risk factor, based on the following observations[36, 44, 45]:

- The highest incidence is seen in lower latitudes, with the risk highest near the equator.
- A history of childhood sunburn produces increased risk.
- Early childhood sun exposure is important, with a decreased melanoma risk seen in persons whose excessive sun exposure occurred after the age of 15.
- The incidence of melanoma is markedly higher in white-skinned races with little protective melanin pigment, compared with blacks with similar sun exposure history.
- White-skinned individuals with very fair complexions, who sunburn easily and tan poorly, are at highest risk for developing melanoma.
- Habits of dress and patterns of sun exposure affect melanoma risk and determine the pattern of melanoma location and type of melanoma. These are briefly described later.

Race

Malignant melanoma is most common in fair-skinned individuals and rare in blacks, with a 13-fold difference in invasive melanoma and a 23-fold difference in *in situ* melanoma rates. Race also is a factor in determining anatomic site of melanoma, with lesions on the face most common in whites and lesions of the lower extremities, soles, and subungual skin prevalent in blacks.[43] Most of the increase in incidence of malignant melanoma has been seen in whites.

Nevi

Dysplastic and congenital nevi are believed to be precursor lesions to the development of malignant melanoma; dysplastic (simple) nevi are strong markers for melanoma risk. Persons with multiple dysplastic nevi and a family history of melanoma are at highest risk; an inherited familial dysplastic nevus syndrome and other inherited patterns may account for up to 10% of melanoma cases. Large congenital nevi may undergo malignant degeneration to melanoma in up to 20% of cases, prompting the recommendation for prophylactic excision of all congenital nevi greater than 2 cm.

Sex

The incidence of melanoma is 29% higher in white males than in white females, with an equal sex distribution seen in blacks.[43]

Anatomic Distribution

Melanomas of the face, ear, scalp, neck, and trunk predominate in white males, whereas tumors of the skin of the lower extremities predominate in white females.[43] Distribution in blacks, Asians, and Hispanics favors the lower extremities, soles, and subungual areas.

Age

Malignant melanoma affects a broad range of age groups and the distribution of ages resembles a bell curve. Rare in childhood, the incidence increases in the age group 20 to 30 years, has an average age of development of 57 years, and three quarters of all melanomas occur under the age of 70.[43]

Socioeconomic Status

Malignant melanoma risk in males has been reported as significantly higher in high-paying versus low-paying occupations.[46] No significant difference was seen between indoor and outdoor occupations, perhaps reflecting differences in recreational lifestyle.

Detection and Diagnosis

The successful management of malignant melanoma depends on early detection and treatment. With this in mind, education of the general public, as well as of physicians, about the risk factors and early warning signs of melanoma becomes increasingly important.[15] The New York University Melanoma Cooperative Group has devised the "A, B, C, D" rules for increasing awareness of the appearance of potential melanoma lesions[44]:

Asymmetry of the lesion
Border irregularity (or indistinctness)
Color variegation
Diameter greater than 6 mm

Additional important history and symptomatology include:

- change in appearance of a pre-existing melanocytic nevus (color, size, shape, elevation, surface texture, appearance of the surrounding skin)
- appearance of a new pigmented lesion, especially in persons older than 40 years of age

All cutaneous lesions that raise suspicion of melanoma should undergo excisional biopsy with a margin of normal-appearing surrounding skin.

Early Detection

Skin self-examination takes advantage of patient participation in early detection efforts.[44] Self-examination requires total examination of all skin surfaces in a stepwise fashion, and should be performed in good light, while completely disrobed, and with the aid of full-length and hand-held mirrors as well as a blow-dryer for examination of hair-bearing skin surfaces.

Physician examination requires total cutaneous inspection, under conditions of good lighting and with the patient completely disrobed.[23] A magnifying lens may be helpful as well as a blow-dryer for scalp examination. *Dermatoscopy* (epiluminescence microscopy) is a diagnostic technique that employs a dermatoscope to examine pigmented lesions under 10× oil magnification that renders the stratum corneum translucent for improved visualization of the lesion.[43] Baseline full-body photographs facilitate follow-up of patents with atypical nevi.

Skin cancer screening programs are becoming increasingly important, both in the early detection of melanoma and in public education. Organizations such as the American Academy of Dermatology and the American Cancer Society participate in nationwide skin cancer screening programs. Skin cancer lends itself to cost-effective screening because the lesions are readily visualized with inexpensive evaluation techniques and equipment.[47]

A major aspect of the National Melanoma/Skin Cancer Prevention Program is patient education. Guidelines are available for the development of workshops to train physicians and ancillary personnel in the most efficient and effective ways to set up and implement local skin cancer screening programs or clinics.[48]

Classification and Staging

Histopathology

Benign Pigmented Skin Lesions[44]

Simple Lentigo. Simple lentigo is a 1- to 5-mm macular pigmented lesion with well-demarcated, round borders, and brown to black pigmentation that may occur on any cutaneous area of the body, but most commonly on sun-exposed areas. The lesion tends to arise in childhood.

Junctional Nevus. Junctional nevus is a macular, well-defined lesion smaller than 6 mm with a smooth surface and uniform pigmentation. These lesions appear concentrated on sun-exposed areas, usually appear during childhood, and are rare in adults over age 40.

Compound Nevus. Compound nevus is a well-defined pigmented raised papule smaller than 6 mm. The distinction *compound* refers to the presence of the pigmented cells both at the dermal-epidermal junction and within the dermis. These lesions arise in childhood and early adulthood and may be hair bearing.

Intradermal Nevus. Intradermal nevus appears as a well-defined papule smaller than 6 mm with uniform pigmentation located within the dermis. Lesions may be hair bearing.

Solar Lentigo. Solar lentigo is a macule with uniform pigmentation that is found primarily on sun-exposed, sun-damaged skin.

Seborrheic Keratosis. Seborrheic keratosis is a verrucous, well-circumscribed papule or plaque with a "dull" or "warty" surface seen most often on the face, neck, or trunk. The cell of origin is the epidermal keratinocyte, not the melanocyte.

Malignant Melanoma

There are 4 major subtypes of malignant melanoma:

- lentigo maligna melanoma
- superficial spreading melanoma
- nodular melanoma
- acral lentiginous melanoma

Superficial spreading melanomas are associated with recreational sun exposure, occurring most frequently on sites of intermittent exposure such as the trunk and limbs, and are typically associated with precursor nevi. In contrast, lentigo maligna melanoma is associated with occupational sun exposure, seen predominantly on head and neck sites in older males, and not associated with pre-existing nevi. Acral lentiginous melanoma may be the form of melanoma more likely associated with causative factors other than sun exposure because it occurs on sun-protected palms and soles, is not associated with nevi, and has an equal incidence in all races.[43]

Lentigo maligna melanomas, superficial spreading melanoma, and acral lentiginous melanoma are characterized by initial indolent enlargement of a primarily flat lesion in a radial (horizontal) growth phase with low metastatic potential that may last for several years. The radial growth phase of these lesions is the most curable; the vertical growth phase follows and signals deeper penetration and increased metastatic potential, usually occurring rapidly over a period of weeks to months.

Lentigo Maligna Melanoma. Lentigo maligna melanoma comprises 4% to 15% of all malignant melanoma lesions and is the most benign in behavior. These lesions are seen most often on sun-exposed skin of the head and neck and dorsum of the hands. More common in women than in men, lentigo maligna melanoma has a median age of incidence of 70 years. In the radial growth phase, the lesions are flat and variegated with tan to brown coloration. There is very slow radial growth, and then the lesions become elevated with the onset of the vertical phase.

Superficial Spreading Melanoma. Superficial spreading melanoma comprises about 70% of malignant melanoma lesions in whites, and most develop in a precursor nevus. The radial growth phase is characterized by an inflammatory response, which results in epidermal hyperplasia and slight elevation, and color variegation with a rose-pink component to the tan to brown lesion. Radial growth may progress over 1 to 12 years and is characterized by a 5% metastatic potential. Vertical growth phase proceeds much more rapidly, with the formation of a nodule with red, white, and blue coloration and 35% to 85% metastatic potential depending upon depth. Superficial spreading melanomas occur most frequently on the back in males and the lower extremity in females.

Nodular Melanoma. Nodular melanoma constitutes about 12% to 30% of malignant melanomas and is the most malignant form. The male:female incidence ratio is 2:1, and the median age of occurrence is 50 years. This lesion has only a vertical growth phase and evolves relatively quickly over several months to a year. Nodular melanoma usually develops on trunk or head and neck sites and arises *de novo* without a precursor lesion. There is a characteristic blue-black coloration, and lesions often ulcerate or bleed.

Acral Lentiginous Melanoma. Acral lentiginous melanoma represents 2% to 8% of all malignant melanomas but 35% to 90% of all malignant melanomas occurring in blacks, Asians, and Hispanics; it occurs on the palms and soles and in subungual regions. Lesions are characterized by a flat radial phase that may last for several years, followed by a more rapid vertical phase. Acral lentiginous melanoma is most common in the sixth decade and metastases are common.

Staging

The staging system employed for malignant melanoma is based on the American Joint Committee on Cancer and International Union Against Cancer's Tumor (T), Nodal (N), and Metastasis (M) classification illustrated in Table 16–3.[27] This system requires pathologic evaluation of the primary lesion, and correlates T stage with depth and level of invasion as described by Breslow[49] and Clark,[50] respectively.

Principles of Treatment

Surgery

Surgery is the mainstay of treatment (Table 16–4) for malignant melanoma, both for the primary lesion and, often, for metastatic sites. However, the appropriate margin of excision has been the subject of considerable controversy. Based on a series of prospective randomized trials, it is now generally accepted that initial excision with conservative margins is indicated first for histopathologic diagnosis. Once diagnosis is confirmed, definitive re-excision is performed with clinical margins of 0.5 cm for *in situ* melanoma; 1.0 cm for invasive melanomas less than 1 mm

TABLE 16–3. **Staging of Malignant Melanoma**

Stage	Grouping	Descriptors*
Stage 0	pTis, N0, M0	pTis: Melanoma *in situ* (atypical melanocytic hyperplasia, severe melanocytic dysplasia), not an invasive malignant lesion (Clark's Level I). N0: No regional lymph node metastasis. M0: No distant metastasis.
Stage I	pT1, N0, M0	pT1: Tumor ≤0.75 mm in thickness and invades the papillary dermis (Clark's Level II).
	pT2, N0, M0	pT2: Tumor >0.75 mm but <1.5 mm in thickness and/or invades the reticular dermis (Clark's Level III).
Stage II	pT3, N0, M0	pT3: Tumor >1.5 mm, but <4 mm in thickness and/or invades the reticular dermis (Clark's Level IV).
Stage III	pT4, N0, M0	pT4: Tumor >4 mm in thickness and/or invades the subcutaneous tissue (Clark's Level V) and/or satellite(s) within 2 cm of the primary tumor.
	Any pT, N1, M0	N1: Metastasis 3 cm or less in greatest dimension in any regional lymph node(s).
	Any pT, N2, M0	N2: Metastasis >3 cm in greatest dimension in any regional lymph node(s) and/ or in-transit metastasis.
Stage IV	Any pT, Any N, M1	M1: Distant metastasis.

*pTX would indicate that primary tumor cannot be assessed; pT0, that there is no evidence of primary tumor.

Used with the permission of the American Joint Committee on Cancer (AJCC®), Chicago, Illinois. The original source for this material is the AJCC® Cancer Staging Manual, 5th edition, 1997, published by Lippincott-Raven Publishers, Philadelphia, Pennsylvania.

thick; 2.0 to 3.0 cm for lesions 1 to 4 mm in thickness, and more than 2.0 cm for lesions greater than 4 mm in thickness.[2, 51–53] Whenever possible, primary wound closure is preferable to grafting and reconstruction.[52]

Management of Lymph Nodes

Therapeutic lymph node dissection is indicated when nodes are pathologically involved because most patients with lymph node metastasis from malignant melanoma ultimately develop distant metastatic disease. Although therapeutic lymph node dissection may be beneficial for palliation of symptoms and improved local control, it may not have much impact on survival. Investigational use of melanoma-involved nodal tissue to produce melanoma vaccines is another potential indication for therapeutic dissection.

The management of clinically uninvolved regional lymph nodes in cutaneous melanoma has been a very controversial issue. *Elective lymph node dissection* (ELND) in patients with clinically negative nodes has been advocated by some as having prognostic relevance, and in some studies it showed a potential survival advantage in certain patient subgroups[54]; however, other studies failed to confirm this benefit.[52] It now appears that ELND is not indicated for patients whose primary melanoma is less than 1 mm thick because the potential for nodal metastasis in these patients is extremely low. ELND also is probably not indicated in patients whose melanoma primaries are located in areas of ambiguous nodal drainage (as in midline trunk lesions), in very elderly or debilitated patients, and in patients with known distant metastatic disease.[51, 55] Results from a prospective randomized multi-institutional trial involving 740 stage I and II malignant melanoma patients were reported by the Intergroup Melanoma Surgical Program; they showed a survival advantage to ELND over observation alone in intermediate-thickness (1–4 mm) melanoma patients. Benefit was seen especially in patients younger than 60 years of age with intermediate-thickness melanoma, especially in patients with nonulcerative lesions and lesions 1 to 2 mm thick.[53]

Sentinel lymph node mapping and biopsy has emerged as an alternative to ELND for malignant melanoma.[56–58] Morton and associates[59] introduced the concept that each area of skin drains preferentially to a specific "sentinel" lymph node within the nodal basin. Lymph node mapping techniques could identify the sentinel node for each malignant melanoma lesion, and biopsy of the sentinel node was predictive of involvement of other nodes within the nodal basin. A sentinel node biopsy with negative results spares

TABLE 16–4. **Multidisciplinary Treatment Decisions for Melanoma**

Stage	Surgery	Radiation Therapy	Chemotherapy
Stage I	Adequate resection with 2-cm margin No elective node dissection	NR	IC II or IM
Stage II	Radical resection with 2-cm margin Elective node dissection optional	NR	IC II or IM
Stage III	2–3-cm margin Therapeutic node dissection	NR	IC II or IM
Stage IV	As above if feasible and few metastases	If unresectable, PRT 30–60 Gy If unresectable, resect postop PRT 30–60 Gy	IC II
Recurrence	Re-excision if possible with 2–3-cm margin		IC II

PRT = palliative radiation therapy; ART = adjuvant radiation therapy; IC II = investigational chemotherapy, phase I/II clinical trials; IM = Immunotherapy; NR = not recommended.

Adapted from National Cancer Institute. Information from PDQ—for Health Professionals: Melanoma. January 2000. CancerNet. Electronic database.

the patient further aggressive node dissection, whereas positive results indicate the need for therapeutic dissection.

The technique of sentinel node mapping, employed by Morton and others, uses vital blue dye (Lymphazurin or Patent Blue-V), which has been shown to localize the sentinel node 80% to 85% of the time, with a false-negative rate of less than 10%. Occult nodal metastases are identified in 15% of stage I to stage II malignant melanoma lesions and are directly related to tumor thickness. Improved sentinel node mapping techniques employ an intradermal injection of a technetium-labeled sulfur colloid in addition to the blue dye, as well as use of an intraoperative hand-held gamma probe to localize the sentinel node at the time of surgery by both intensity of radioactive signal and amount of dye uptake.[58] Staging patients with sentinel node mapping and biopsy rather than formal ELND offers the advantage of decreased patient morbidity and cost.

Adjuvant Treatment of Malignant Melanoma

Interferon-α is the first adjuvant treatment for malignant melanoma identified as showing a survival benefit in high-risk patients, defined as patients with lesions greater than 4-mm thick or with involved lymph nodes, or with both.[60] In a prospective randomized trial of 280 patients, the Eastern Cooperative Oncology Group (ECOG) demonstrated improved disease-free and overall survival in node-positive patients who received dose-intensive interferon-α-2b.[61] The regimen, reported by Kirkwood and colleagues,[61] involves administration of high-dose interferon-α intravenously for 5 to 7 days weekly for 1 month, followed by 48 additional weeks of subcutaneous interferon given thrice weekly. Quality-of-life analysis for patients treated on the ECOG trial indicated that treatment benefit may outweigh toxicity problems in patients with nodal involvement.[62] Dose reduction studies are under way because of the significant toxicity of the dose-intensive ECOG regimen.

Vaccine therapy against malignant melanoma is the subject of much interest and investigation. Various investigators have employed autologous or allogenic whole-cell vaccines or specific melanoma-associated antigen peptide vaccines. Many vaccine preparations also include immunologic adjuvants (BCG, DETOX, and QS-21) to enhance the immune response. ECOG is conducting a study comparing high-dose interferon-α with a melanoma ganglioside vaccine (GM2) using QS-21 as the immunologic enhancer.

Radiation Therapy

Radiation therapy is not an alternative to surgery in the management of primary malignant melanoma because melanoma cells are generally considered relatively radioresistant when compared with other malignancies. Some investigators believe large fraction sizes are required to treat melanoma; although data exist supporting large fractions, several studies have shown that large fraction sizes are not necessarily better than lower fraction sizes.[63–65]

Radiation therapy often is an important part of the palliative treatment of metastatic melanoma and has been advocated as a postoperative adjuvant for cutaneous melanoma of the head and neck region. Ang and coworkers[66] reported a series of 174 patients with melanoma of the head and neck who received nodal irradiation postoperatively, either electively for high-risk disease or after nodal resection in the presence of known nodal metastasis. They found an improved 5-year actuarial locoregional control rate of 88% versus 50% in the historic literature. The Radiation Therapy Oncology Group (RTOG) is now conducting a prospective randomized trial to better define the role of adjuvant irradiation in head and neck melanoma patients with regional nodal involvement.

Chemotherapy

Chemotherapy as an adjuvant to surgery in the treatment of malignant melanoma has been disappointing in that no effective single or combination drug regimens have been identified. Dacarbazine and carmustine are the only single agents with consistent responses in the range of 20%.[5, 67] Taxanes have shown variable activity, with some reports as high as 20%.[5, 68]

Combination chemotherapy has been tried with limited success and, in fact, several trials using combination chemotherapy have seen disappointing results.[69, 70] Attempts at increasing dose intensity of various chemotherapeutic agents without increasing toxicity have employed intra-arterial hyperthermic infusion of an affected limb. Although local tumor responses have been observed, no clear survival benefit is evident.[71]

Treatment of Metastatic (Stage IV) Malignant Melanoma

Patients with distant metastasis from malignant melanoma have an expected 5-year survival rate of less than 10%. The most frequent metastatic sites are skin, subcutaneous tissues, and lymph nodes, followed by lung, liver, brain, and bone. Treatment usually employs systemic chemotherapy, but response rates are low (20% to 40%) and durability of response is short[72]; median survival is only 4 to 6 months.[73] Surgery may be useful for palliation of bleeding, obstruction, or ulceration, and has been advocated for removing solitary brain metastasis. Resection of visceral metastasis has not been helpful, and the morbidity makes the procedure rarely warranted. Wong and associates have reported benefit from aggressive surgical intervention in a subset of patients, representing about 10% of all patients, with nonregional metastatic malignant melanoma using surgery for solitary lesions of the subcutaneous tissues, lymph nodes, or lung.[73]

Radiation therapy is helpful in the treatment of metastatic malignant melanoma lesions for relief of bleeding, pain, or obstruction and is commonly employed in the management of brain metastasis and skin lesions.[72] Hyperthermia may be employed in conjunction with radiation therapy to enhance treatment response.[74, 75]

As mentioned earlier, chemotherapy has not proved very effective. The response rate for single agent chemotherapy is generally less than 10%.[5] The most effective single chemotherapeutic agent, dacarbazine, has a response rate of 20%. Lower response rates are reported for single-agent nitrosoureas (10% to 20%), cisplatin (15% to 20%), and paclitaxel (Taxol) (15%). Response is best seen in skin, subcutaneous, and lymph node metastases, with essentially no response in brain metastasis.

Combination chemotherapy has resulted in response rates as high as 40% and may be effective even for visceral metastasis.[72] The addition of tamoxifen to cisplatin has resulted in decreased cisplatin resistance in malignant melanoma,[70, 76, 77] and use of the Dartmouth regimen is being investigated in phase II trials.[78] Intensive chemotherapy programs with autologous bone marrow support have resulted in response rates of 40% to 65%, but duration of response has been less than 6 months and toxicity has been high.[72]

Immunotherapy has shown some promise in the treatment of advanced melanoma; however, much improvement is still needed. Interferon-α is being used as an adjuvant therapy and is described above. Interleukin-2 (IL-2) has been used with similar results. Response rates alone are low, approaching 20%, but 5% to 6% of patients have durable complete remission. Eighty percent of patients who achieve complete remission do not have a recurrence and represent a cure of metastatic disease.

Although not yet definitively proven, it is likely that combinations of multiagent chemotherapy and biotherapy result in higher response rates with some longterm complete remission in patients with metastatic melanoma. A study published in 1999 comparing tamoxifen and dacarbazine with tamoxifen and dacarbazine followed by IL-2 and αIFN showed improved median survival from 10.7 to 15.8 months with the latter combination.[79] *Chemoimmunotherapy* also is showing promise in the treatment of advanced melanoma; however, both IL-2 and αIFN have substantial toxicities and careful patient selection must be conducted before these aggressive regimens can be started.[80]

New applications of cytokines, such as IL-12 and granulocyte-macrophage colony stimulating factor, may result in some additional benefit.[81] The combination of IL-2 with autologous immune cells (lymphokine-activated killer cells and tumor-infiltrating lymphocytes) improves the response rate in some series.[80]

Results and Prognosis

The following prognostic factors are recognized as the most important predictors of local recurrence or distant metastatic spread, or both, in malignant melanoma:

- thickness/depth of invasion of primary lesion
- ulceration of primary lesion
- histologic subtype
- anatomic location of primary lesion
- sex and age of patient
- extent of lymph node involvement

Depth of Invasion

Depth of tumor invasion,[51] or tumor thickness, is the single most important prognostic factor in malignant melanoma. It is generally felt that tumor thickness is a more accurate measurement than depth of invasion, with less observer-dependent variability. Patients with *in situ* melanoma have a greater than 99% longterm disease-free survival after adequate surgical excision, and even early invasive melanoma (<1 mm thick) has a greater than 90% longterm survival. Risk of locoregional recurrence and distant metastasis increases dramatically with intermediate-risk (1–4 mm thick) and high-risk (>4 mm thick) lesions.

Ulceration

Degree of tumor ulceration is the best predictor of metastatic regional node involvement and is an independent prognostic factor for nodal failure with worsening prognosis as ulceration widens and deepens. Degree of ulceration is related to tumor thickness, and 10-year survival rates of 20% are seen in thick (>4 mm) lesions with ulceration versus 35% without ulceration. Ulceration is more common in trunk lesions in males. Extremity lesions tend not to ulcerate and are observed most frequently in females.

Histologic Subtype

Prognosis in malignant melanoma is related to histologic subtype of the primary lesion. Survival for more than 10 years is 90% for patients with lentigo maligna melanoma, 65% for patients with superficial spreading melanoma or nodular melanoma, and 50% for patients with acral lentiginous melanoma.

Anatomic Site

The anatomic distribution of a malignant melanoma has an impact on long-term prognosis. Lesions of the head, neck, and trunk are associated with poorer prognosis than are lesions of the extremities. Thick lesions (>4 mm) have a 5-year survival of 8% on the trunk and 82% on the extremities, when lymph nodes are negative. Distribution of lentigo maligna melanoma is about 53% extremities, 31% trunk, and 16% head and neck sites, with 10-year survival rates of 85% to 90%, 70%, and 70%, respectively.[82]

Sex and Age

Female sex is associated with a better prognosis in malignant melanoma than is male sex. In part, this may be explained by female predominance of extremity lesions, which rarely ulcerate. In addition, although survival in females is not related to age, males with stage II malignant melanoma who are younger than 50 years of age have a better prognosis than older stage III males. In males, 60% to 70% of malignant melanomas are stage III at presentation and 48% stages I to II.

Extent of Nodal Involvement

For patients with stage III malignant melanoma, the number of metastatic regional lymph nodes predicts long-term survival at 40% with 1 involved node, 26% with 2 to 4 involved nodes, and 15% with more than 5 involved nodes.

Metastasis

Patients with stage IV malignant melanoma have a mean duration of survival of 6 to 18 months. Median survival decreases with increasing number of metastatic sites: 7 months for 1 site; 4 months for 2 sites; and 2 months for more than 3 sites. Patients with nonvisceral metastasis involving skin, subcutaneous tissue, or nonregional lymph nodes have an 8-month median duration of survival versus 3 months for patients with visceral metastasis involving lung, brain, or liver. Patients with nonvisceral metastasis have a 1-year survival of 46% versus 18% for patients with visceral metastasis.

Other Less Important Factors

- *Tumor regression:* Thin melanomas with extensive areas of tumor regression within the primary lesion (white areas) have an increased metastatic rate and poorer prognosis.
- *Mitotic rate:* Increasing mitotic rate is associated with decreased survival. At 8 years, survival of 95% is seen with 0 mitosis, 80% with less than 6 mitoses/mm^2, and 38% with more than 6 mitoses/mm^2.
- *Prognostic index:* Product of mitotic rate and tumor thickness.
- *Host inflammatory response:* The presence of a lymphoid infiltrate at the primary tumor site improves prognosis.
- *Microscopic satellite lesions:* The presence of microscopic dermal satellite lesions in the primary resected specimen decreases prognosis.

Summary

Overall survival for very thin (<0.76 mm) malignant melanomas is about 96%. For very thick (>4 mm) lesions, or in patients with involved regional lymph nodes or distant metastasis, or with both, the 10-year survival is less than 10%. A four-variable prognostic model that considers tumor thickness, site of primary lesion, patient age, and patient sex is useful to determine prognosis in intermediate lesions.[83] The most important prognostic factors based on stage of disease are:

Stage I-II: thickness of primary lesion; presence of ulceration; anatomic site

Stage III: number of involved lymph nodes; presence of ulceration; thickness of primary lesion; anatomic site

Stage IV: number of metastatic lesions; site(s) of metastasis

Follow-Up

An estimated 3% to 5% of malignant melanoma patients will develop a second primary malignant melanoma within 3 years of initial presentation and treatment.[41] This number increases to a 5-year risk of 33% in patients with numerous atypical moles from melanoma-prone families. Although most malignant melanomas that recur either locoregionally or distantly do so within the first 3 years after treatment, late failures are still seen. Lifetime physician follow-up is therefore necessary as surveillance for the development of new primary melanomas, for early detection of locoregional or distant metastatic failure, and for reinforcement of patient education. However, Shumate and coworkers[84] studied recurrence patterns in 1475 malignant melanoma patients and found that, in greater than 90% of those who experienced recurrence, the patients were symptomatic at the time of recurrence. Despite some delay in detection of recurrence in patients not under routine medical surveillance, there was no impact on survival. The authors recommended a combination of physician- and patient-directed surveillance, but they argued against routine radiographic and laboratory studies, pointing to a lack of survival benefit with early detection of asymptomatic distant metastasis. For patients treated for early melanoma with no atypical moles and a negative family history, follow-up at 6-month intervals for the first 2 to 3 years and yearly thereafter seems adequate. For patients with high recurrence risk based on stage of initial lesion, and personal and family risk factors, follow-up every 3 to 6 months is indicated during the first 3-year period and every 6 to 12 months thereafter. Between physician follow-up visits, monthly patient self-examination is essential.

Recommended Reading

Excellent general chapters on malignant melanoma can be found in a number of comprehensive texts in dermatology, medical oncology, and radiation oncology. The reader is referred to the chapters on malignant melanoma in the General References.

REFERENCES

General References

1. Moschella S, Hurley HJ: Dermatology. Philadelphia, Harcourt Brace Jovanovich, 1992.
2. Odom RB, James WD, Berger TG: Andrews' Diseases of the Skin: Clinical Dermatology. Philadelphia, W.B. Saunders, 2000.
3. Habif TP: Clinical dermatology: a color guide to diagnosis and therapy. St. Louis, Mosby–Year Book, 1996.
4. Abeloff MD, Armitage JO, Lichter AS, Niederhuber JE: Clinical Oncology. New York, Churchill Livingstone, 2000.
5. DeVita VT, Hellman S, Rosenberg SA: Cancer: Principles and Practice of Oncology. Philadelphia, Lippincott-Raven, 1997.

Specific References

Nonmelanoma Skin Cancer

6. Gray DT, Suman VJ, Su WP, et al: Trends in population-based incidence of squamous cell carcinoma of the skin first diagnosed between 1984 and 1992. Arch Dermatol 1997; 133:735–740.
7. Karagas MR, Greenberg ER, Spencer SK, et al: Increase in incidence rates of basal cell and squamous cell cancer in New Hampshire, USA. New Hampshire Skin Cancer Study Group. Int J Cancer 1999; 81: 555–559.
8. Miller DL, Weinstock MA: Nonmelanoma skin cancer in the United States: incidence. J Am Acad Dermatol 1994; 30:774–778.
9. Weinstock MA: Nonmelanoma skin cancer mortality in the United States, 1969 through 1988. Arch Dermatol 1993; 129:1286–1290.
10. Preston DS, Stern RS: Nonmelanoma cancers of the skin. N Engl J Med 1992; 327:1649–1662.
11. Halder RM, Bridgeman-Shah S: Skin cancer in African Americans. Cancer 1995; 75:667–673.
12. Granstein RD: Evidence that sunscreens prevent UV radiation-induced immunosuppression in humans. Arch Dermatol 1995; 131:1201–1204.
13. Whitmore SE, Morrison WL: Prevention of UVB-induced immunosuppression in humans by a high sun protection factor sunscreen. Arch Dermatol 1995; 131:1128–1133.
14. Marks R: An overview of skin cancers. Cancer 1994; 75:607–612.

15. Rhodes AR: Public education and cancer of the skin: what do people need to know about melanoma and nonmelanoma skin cancer? Cancer 1995; 75:613–636.
16. Fleming ID, Amonette R, Monaghan T, Fleming MD: Principles of management of basal and squamous cell carcinoma of the skin. Cancer 1995; 75:699–704.
17. Goldberg LH: Basal cell carcinoma. Lancet 1996; 347:663–667.
18. Marks R: Squamous cell carcinoma. Lancet 1996; 347:735–738.
19. Boffetta P, Jourenkova N, Gustavsson P: Cancer risk from occupational and environmental exposure to polycyclic aromatic hydrocarbons. Cancer Causes Control 1997; 8:444–472.
20. Barr BBB, Benton EC, McLaren D, et al: Human papilloma virus infection and skin cancer in renal allograft recipients. Lancet 1989; 1(8630):124–129.
21. Moy R, Eliezri YD: Significance of human papillomavirus-induced squamous cell carcinoma to dermatologists. Arch Dermatol 1994; 130:235–238.
22. Sober AJ, Burstein JM: Precursors to skin cancer. Cancer 1995; 75:645–650.
23. Kopf AW, Salopek TG, Slade J, et al: Techniques of cutaneous examination for the detection of skin cancer. Cancer 1995; 75:684–690.
24. Marks R, Rennie G, Selwood TS: Malignant transformation of solar keratoses to squamous cell carcinoma. Lancet 1988; 1(8589):795–797.
25. Landthaler M, Hagspiel HJ, Braun-Falco O: Late irradiation damage to the skin caused by soft x-ray radiation therapy of cutaneous tumors. Arch Dermatol 1995; 131:182–186.
26. Solan MJ, Brady LW, Binnick SA, Fitzpatrick PJ: Skin. In: Brady LW, Perez CA (eds): Principles and Practice of Radiation Oncology, 3rd ed, pp 723–762. Philadelphia, Lippincott-Raven, 1997.
27. American Joint Committee on Cancer: AJCC Cancer Staging Manual, 5th ed. Philadelphia, Lippincott-Raven, 1997.
28. Rosin MP, Miller SJ, Schwab D, et al: Molecular analysis of effectiveness of Mohs' surgical technique. Lancet 1996; 347:1692–1693.
29. Lawrence CM: Mohs' micrographic surgery for basal cell carcinoma. Clin Exp Dermatol 1999; 24:130–133.
30. Dzubow LM: Mohs surgery. Lancet 1994; 343:433–434.
31. Kopera D: Treatment of lentigo maligna with the carbon dioxide laser. Arch Dermatol 1995; 131:735–736.
32. Gordon KB, Robinson J: Carbon dioxide laser vaporization for Bowen's disease of the finger. Arch Dermatol 1994; 130:1250–1252.
33. Tangrea JA, Edwards BK, Taylot PR, et al: Long-term therapy with low-dose isotretinoin for prevention of basal cell carcinoma: a multicenter clinical trial. J Natl Cancer Inst 1992; 84:328–332.
34. Liu H: Photodynamic therapy of nonmelanoma skin cancer with topical aminolevulenic acid: a clinical and histologic study. Arch Dermatol 1995; 131:737–738.
35. Karagas MR, Stutkel TA, Greenberg ER, et al: Risk of subsequent basal cell carcinoma and squamous cell carcinoma of the skin among patients with prior skin cancer. JAMA 1992; 267:3305–3310.
36. Marghoob AA, Slade J, Salopek TG, et al: Basal cell and squamous cell carcinomas are important risk factors for cutaneous malignant melanoma: screening implications. Cancer 1995; 75:707–714.
37. Liu FF, Maki E, Warde P, et al: A management approach to incompletely excised basal cell carcinomas of the skin. Int J Radiat Oncol Biol Phys 1991; 20:423–428.
38. Black HS, Thornby JI, Wolf JE, et al: Evidence that a low-fat diet reduces the occurrence of non-melanoma skin cancer. Int J Cancer 1995; 62:165–169.

Malignant Melanoma

39. Davis N: Modern concepts of melanoma and its management. Ann Plast Surg 1978; 1(6):628–629.
40. Urist MM, Karnell LH: The National Cancer Data Base. Report on melanoma. Cancer 1994; 74:782–788.
41. Rigel DS: Malignant melanoma: incidence issues and their effect on diagnosis and treatment in the 1990s. Mayo Clin Proc 1997; 72:367–371.
42. Landis SH, Murray T, Bolden S, Wingo PA: Cancer statistics. CA Cancer J Clin 1999; 49:8–31.
43. Elder DE: Skin cancer. Melanoma and other specific nonmelanoma skin cancers. Cancer 1995; 75(suppl):245–256.
44. Friedman RJ, Rigel DS, Silverman MK, et al: Malignant melanoma in the 1990s: the continued importance of early detection and the role of physician examination and self-examination of the skin. CA Cancer J Clin 1991; 41:201–226.
45. Austoker J: Melanoma: prevention and early diagnosis. BMJ 1994; 308:1682–1686.
46. Pion IA, Rigel DS, Garfinkel L, et al: Occupation and the risk of malignant melanoma. Cancer 1995; 75(Suppl):637–644.
47. McDonald CJ: Status of screening for skin cancer. Cancer 1993; 72(suppl):1066–1070.
48. Dobes WL Jr: Melanoma skin cancer screenings. A how-to approach. Cancer 1995; 75(suppl):705–706.
49. Breslow A: Thickness, cross-sectional areas and depth of invasion in the prognosis of cutaneous melanoma. Ann Surg 1970; 172:902–908.
50. Clark WH Jr, From L, Bernardino EA, et al: The histogenesis and biologic behavior of primary human malignant melanomas of the skin. Cancer Res 1969; 29:705–727.
51. NIH Consensus conference. Diagnosis and treatment of early melanoma. JAMA 1992; 268:1314–1319.
52. Harris MN, Shapiro RL, Roses DF: Malignant melanoma. Primary surgical management (excision and node dissection) based on pathology and staging. Cancer 1995; 75(suppl):715–725.
53. Balch CM, Soong SJ, Bartolucci AA, et al: Efficacy of an elective regional lymph node dissection of 1 to 4 mm thick melanomas for patients 60 years of age and younger. Ann Surg 1996; 224:255–263.
54. Drepper H, Kohler CO, Bastian B, et al: Benefit of elective lymph node dissection in subgroups of melanoma patients. Results of a multicenter study of 3616 patients. Cancer 1993; 72:741–749.
55. Stone CA, Goodacre TE: Surgical management of regional lymph nodes in primary cutaneous malignant melanoma. Br J Surg 1995; 82:1015–1022.
56. Godellas CV, Berman CG, Lyman G, et al: The identification and mapping of melanoma regional nodal metastases: minimally invasive surgery for the diagnosis of nodal metastases. Am Surg 1995; 61:97–101.
57. Krag DN, Meijer SJ, Weaver DL, et al: Minimal-access surgery for staging of malignant melanoma. Arch Surg 1995; 130:654–658.
58. Albertini JJ, Cruse CW, Rapaport D, et al: Intraoperative radiolymphoscintigraphy improves sentinel lymph node identification for patients with melanoma. Ann Surg 1996; 223:217–224.
59. Morton DL, Wen DR, Wong JH, et al: Technical details of intraoperative lymphatic mapping for early stage melanoma. Arch Surg 1992; 127:392–399.
60. Nathanson L: Interferon adjuvant therapy of melanoma. Cancer 1996; 78:944–947.
61. Kirkwood JM, Strawderman MH, Ernstoff MS, et al: Interferon alfa-2b adjuvant therapy of high-risk resected cutaneous melanoma: the Eastern Cooperative Oncology Group Trial EST 1684. J Clin Oncol 1996; 14:7–17.
62. Cole BF, Gelber RD, Kirkwood JM, et al: Quality-of-life-adjusted survival analysis of interferon alfa-2b adjuvant treatment of high-risk resected cutaneous melanoma: an Eastern Cooperative Oncology Group study. J Clin Oncol 1996; 14:2666–2673.
63. Konefal JB, Emami B, Pilepich MV: Malignant melanoma: analysis of dose fractionation in radiation therapy. Radiology 1987; 164:607–610.
64. Sause WT, Cooper JS, Rush S, et al: Fraction size in external beam radiation therapy in the treatment of melanoma. Int J Radiat Oncol Biol Phys 1991; 20:429–432.
65. Geara FB, Ang KK: Radiation therapy for malignant melanoma. Surg Clin North Am 1996; 76:1383–1398.
66. Ang KK, Peters LJ, Weber RS, et al: Postoperative radiotherapy for cutaneous melanoma of the head and neck region. Int J Radiat Oncol Biol Phys 1994; 30:795–798.
67. Comis RL: DTIC (NSC-45388) in malignant melanoma: a perspective. Cancer Treat Rep 1976; 60:165–176.
68. Legha SS, Ring S, Papadopoulos N, et al: A phase II trial of taxol in metastatic melanoma. Cancer 1990; 65:2478–2481.
69. Fletcher WS, Daniels DS, Sondak VK, et al: Evaluation of cisplatin and DTIC in inoperable stage III and IV melanoma. A Southwest Oncology Group study. Am J Clin Oncol 1993; 16:359–362.
70. Flaherty LE, Liu PY, Unger J, Sondak VK: Comparison of patient characteristics and outcome between a single-institution phase II trial and a cooperative-group phase II trial with identical eligibility in metastatic melanoma. Am J Clin Oncol 1997; 20:600–604.
71. Barth A, Morton DL: The role of adjuvant therapy in melanoma management. Cancer 1995; 75(suppl):726–734.

72. Ho RC: Medical management of stage IV malignant melanoma. Medical issues. Cancer 1995; 75(suppl):735–741.
73. Wong JH, Skinner KA, Kim KA, et al: The role of surgery in the treatment of nonregionally recurrent melanoma. Surgery 1993; 113:389–394.
74. Engin K, Leeper DB, Tupchong L, et al: Thermoradiation therapy for superficial malignant tumors. Cancer 1993; 72:287–296.
75. Overgaard J, Gonzalez Gonzalez D, Hulshof MC, et al: Randomised trial of hyperthermia as adjuvant to radiotherapy for recurrent or metastatic malignant melanoma. European Society for Hyperthermic Oncology. Lancet 1995; 345:540–543.
76. McClay EF, McClay ME, Albright KD, et al: Tamoxifen modulation of cisplatin resistance in patients with metastatic melanoma. A biologically important observation. Cancer 1993; 72:1914–1918.
77. McClay EF, McClay ME, Jones JA, et al: A phase I and pharmacokinetic study of high dose tamoxifen and weekly cisplatin in patients with metastatic melanoma. Cancer 1997; 79:1037–1043.
78. McClay EF, Berd D, Mastrangelo MJ: The Dartmouth regimen: gone or going strong? Cancer Invest 1998; 16:374–380.
79. Rosenberg SA, Yang JC, Schwartzentruber DJ, et al: Prospective randomized trial of the treatment of patients with metastatic melanoma using chemotherapy with cisplatin, dacarbazine, and tamoxifen alone or in combination with interleukin-2 and interferon alfa-2b. J Clin Oncol 1999; 17:968–975.
80. Rosenberg SA, Yannelli JR, Yang JC, et al: Treatment of patients with metastatic melanoma with autologous tumor-infiltrating lymphocytes and interleukin 2. J Natl Cancer Inst 1994; 86:1159–1166.
81. Armitage JO: Emerging applications of recombinant human granulocyte-macrophage colony-stimulating factor. Blood 1998; 92:4491–4508.
82. Balch CM, Urist MM, Karakousis CP, et al: Efficacy of 2-cm surgical margins for intermediate-thickness melanomas (1 to 4 mm). Results of a multi-institutional randomized surgical trial. Ann Surg 1993; 218:262–267.
83. Schuchter L, Schultz DJ, Synnestvedt M, et al: A prognostic model for predicting 10-year survival in patients with primary melanoma. The Pigmented Lesion Group. Ann Intern Med 1996; 125:369–375.
84. Shumate CR, Urist MM, Maddox WA: Melanoma recurrence surveillance. Patient or physician based? Ann Surg 1995; 221:566–569.

17 *Breast Cancer*

LEONARD R. PROSNITZ, MD, FACR, Radiation Oncology
JAMES DIRK IGLEHART, MD, Surgery and Genetics
ERIC P. WINER, MD, Medical Oncology

And she forgot the stars, the moon, the sun,
And she forgot the blue above the trees

JOHN KEATS

Perspective

Breast cancer is the most common malignancy affecting women in North America and Europe. In 2000, approximately 184,200 new cases of invasive breast cancer were diagnosed in the United States.[1] The number of noninvasive breast cancers is harder to verify, but it probably accounts for an additional 20,000 to 30,000 new cases[2]; thus, the number of invasive and noninvasive breast cancers treated in 2000 approximates to 200,000. Rates of breast cancer increased by nearly 4% per year during the 1980s; the increase stabilized during the 1990s to an overall annual incidence of 110 cases per 100,000. The availability of effective mammography and its widespread use led to the discovery of prevalent cases in the population between 1975 and 1990; therefore, improved detection accounts for a proportion of the increase in disease rates. In addition, after remaining stable for many years, rates of death from breast cancer have declined among white Americans and perhaps in young black women.

Despite the modest gains made in overall mortality rates, modern treatment of breast cancer has allowed dramatic improvements in quantity and quality of life after the diagnosis of a breast malignancy. These advances are due to improvements in treatment after diagnosis. The most noteworthy improvements are the use of lesser surgical procedures for appropriate patients, improvements in hormonal therapies, and the more effective use of adjuvant cytotoxic therapies. In addition, survival after the diagnosis of metastatic breast cancer has also improved as a result of more effective palliative treatments. The 5-year survival rate for breast cancer at all stages was 63% in 1960, increased to 75% in 1977, and was reported as 82% in 1990.[3]

The following sections briefly review the epidemiology of breast cancer, highlight current screening and diagnostic methodologies, and review the pathology and staging of this disease. Sections on treatment detail the approach to the primary disease localized to the breast and briefly introduce concepts used to treat systemic breast cancer.

Epidemiology and Etiology

Epidemiology

Cancer of the breast is the most common solid-organ malignancy diagnosed in North American women. Behind bronchogenic carcinoma, breast cancer is the second leading cause of cancer-related death in American women.[1] Data collected by the Surveillance, Epidemiology and End Results (SEER) program of the National Cancer Institute (NCI) place the lifetime risk of breast cancer at about 12.2%, which translates to the 1 in 8 figure that is frequently quoted. The lifetime chance of dying from breast cancer is much lower. One in 28 women (3.6%) will die from this disease. Overall, approximately 60% of women who contract breast cancer will be counted as "cured" of the disease, whereas one third will die from the complications of metastatic breast cancer.[3, 4]

Cumulative lifetime risk figures overstate the actual risks that are experienced by individual women. Conditional risk estimates refer to the chance of getting breast cancer during a future interval of life for a woman who is currently breast cancer–free. Looking at risk this way is more realistic to most people. The common question asked by 40-year-old women who have not had breast cancer is what is the chance of getting breast cancer during the next 20 years of life? When examined in this way, baseline risk factors for individual patients are more realistic and less threatening.

Estimates of conditional risk are available from several sources. The estimates used in Table 17–1 were calculated

TABLE 17–1. **Probability of Breast Cancer for Women of Various Ages**

Age	Cumulative Probability (%)	Probability by Age 80 (%)	Probability Over Next 20 Years (%)
29	0.1	8.2	1.2
39	0.4	7.9	2.8
49	1.3	7.1	4.5
59	3.2	5.2	5.2
69	5.8	2.6	4.5
79	8.3	—	—

Adapted from Claus EB, Risch N, Thompson WD: Autosomal dominant inheritance of early-onset breast cancer. Implications for risk prediction. Cancer 1994; 73:643–651.

from tables provided by Claus and associates, who described a simple means to determine conditional risks based on different family histories.[5] Risk estimates were calculated for American women of various ages whose family histories are essentially negative for cases of breast cancer. Cumulative probabilities refer to the chances that a woman of specified age has or has had breast cancer; with increasing age, a history of breast cancer becomes more common. The second column presents the chances of getting breast cancer by age 80 for women who have achieved various ages unaffected by breast cancer. The final column presents the likelihood that a woman will get breast cancer over 20 years of future life after reaching various ages breast cancer–free.

Risk factors for breast cancer are those factors in a person's medical history that affect her chance of getting breast cancer. Table 17–2 divides risk factors into those that are important in general clinical practice and those that are important to epidemiologists and clinical biologists who study the trends of breast cancer in a population. Risk factors for breast cancer were summarized in an NCI monograph.[6] Gender is listed at the top because male breast cancer does occur, although it is very uncommon; there are about 1000 new cases in the American male population each year. Therefore, the vast majority of masses in the breasts of boys or men are benign, usually unilateral or bilateral gynecomastia. Age is a very important and practical risk factor. As shown in Table 17–1, the proportion of U.S. women with breast cancer diagnosed before age 40 is only 0.5%; however, a 59-year-old woman has a 5.2% chance of developing the disease during the next 20 years. A family history of breast cancer is important, but it may be overemphasized. A clinically significant history should include first-degree relatives (mothers, sisters, and daughters) with breast cancer at a young age (before age 50). Ovarian cancer in a family with multiple cases of breast cancer is highly informative and suggests a breast-ovarian cancer syndrome.

Table 17–3 uses the cumulative estimates from Claus and associates to calculate conditional risk estimates over 20 years of life for women of various ages and with first-degree relatives with breast cancer within specified decades of life.[5] As seen, age at the onset of cancer in first-degree relatives influences the magnitude of risk for unaffected women at all ages. Additional first- or second-degree relatives add proportionally to the risk estimates; pedigree structure (the relationship of affected family members) also modifies the risk when more than one relative is considered.

TABLE 17–2. **Risk Factors for Breast Cancer**

Clinically Important Risks	Other Risk Factors
1. Gender (female >> male)	1. Early menarche, late menopause
2. Increasing age	2. Nulliparity
3. Family history in primary relatives (mother, daughter, sister)	3. Increasing age at first birth
4. History of breast cancer (ipsilateral, conserved, or contralateral)	4. Oral contraceptives
5. LCIS or atypical hyperplasia	5. Postmenopausal hormone replacement therapy (estrogen)

LCIS = lobular carcinoma *in situ.*

TABLE 17–3. **The Probability of Breast Cancer in Women Who Have One Primary Relative with Breast Cancer***

Age of Woman	Age of First-Degree Relative			
	20–29	*30–39*	*40–49*	*50–59*
29	5.5%†	3.9%	2.9%	2.1%
39	9.3	7.0	5.3	4.1
49	11.6	9.0	7.1	6.0

*Probability of breast cancer over 20 subsequent years of life, calculated for women of three different ages.

†Probability of acquiring breast cancer, percent risk over 20 years of life from each age indicated.

Adapted from Claus EB, Risch N, Thompson WD: Autosomal dominant inheritance of early-onset breast cancer. Implications for risk prediction. Cancer 1994; 73:643–651.

Women who appear to be cured of their initial breast cancer are at increased risk of a second primary in the opposite breast or in the conserved breast if mastectomy was not part of the initial therapy. This risk is slightly less than 1% per year of subsequent life.[7] Certain pathologic conditions are markers of increased risk; these conditions are themselves not considered malignant. Atypical epithelial hyperplasia, with or without other features of fibrocystic breast disease, increases risk by a factor of four- to fivefold over baseline.[8] Lobular carcinoma *in situ* (LCIS), also termed lobular neoplasia, increases risk by a factor of seven- to ninefold over baseline.[9, 10] Risk associated with atypical hyperplasia or LCIS is not confined to the breast containing the diagnostic tissue but is bilateral.

Table 17–2 also tabulates risk factors that are important but play less of a practical, clinical role. In general, these factors increase baseline risk by a factor of threefold or less. Exogenous estrogen use is listed in Table 17–2 as a weak risk factor. Estrogens are used either in premenopausal oral contraceptive preparations (OCPs) or as postmenopausal hormone replacement therapy (HRT). A large body of literature has accumulated about OCP and HRT and the risk of breast cancer. For OCP use, there is no convincing evidence that the relative risk of breast cancer is affected, either positively or negatively. Relative risks of using OCPs are in the range of 1.0 to 1.4; use at a young age, use before first pregnancy, and use for 10 or more years are associated with slightly higher risk ratios for breast cancer.[11] HRT modestly increases the risk of breast cancer; duration of use appears to be the most important variable. Short-term use (<10 years) is associated with a negligible risk increase. Postmenopausal use for 10 years or more is associated with a relative risk of between 1.2 and 1.4 times baseline.[11]

Etiology

Based on the high risk for breast cancer seen in women with two or more first-degree relatives with the disease, genetic epidemiologists postulated the existence of autosomal dominant genetic factors. In 1990, *BRCA1* was identified by Dr. M. C. King as the first inherited susceptibility gene for early-onset breast cancer (breast cancer with a mean age of onset significantly younger than expected in the general population).[12] In 1994, *BRCA2,* a second dominant inherited gene, was identified.[13] These remarkable discoveries have made it possible to perform presymptomatic tests for breast cancer risk, at least in patients with a suggestive family history. On the basis of knowledge that is incomplete and evolving, it is possible to make a few conclusions about breast cancer in patients with *BRCA1* or *BRCA2* mutations:

1. Mutations in these two genes account for 2% or 3% of all breast cancers and somewhat less than one half of heritable breast cancer syndromes.
2. Inheritance of disease-associated mutations in one of these two genes results in a life long risk for breast cancer (penetrance) of between 50% and 80%.
3. Cancers in *BRCA1* and *BRCA2* carriers appear to have a similar prognosis to that of sporadic cancers. There are many more uncertainties about genetic breast cancer, and the benefits of testing are not clearly established, principally because strategies for prevention of cancer in susceptible individuals are not well defined.[14]

In addition, an increasing number of tumor markers have been identified that may have value in determining outcome (Table 17–4), and they form three general categories. The first group consists of plasma or serum proteins that are detected by immunoassays and are designated *tumor-associated antigens* (TAAs), for example, carcinoembryonic antigen (CEA), tissue polypeptide antigen (TPA), and gross cystic disease protein (GCDP). Use also is made of a family of mucin-like, high-molecular-weight glycoproteins that are related to or are products of the *MUC1* gene, for example, CA 15–3, CA 27–29, and mammary serum antigen (MSA).[15] The second group of markers includes identification of genetic mutations and gene deletions or substitutions as part of the tumor biology, as well as markers for angiogenesis and cell proliferation. The resultant markers and oncogenes include *HRAS, MYC, FOS,* and *ERBB2* (*HER2/neu*).[16] A final group of markers being investigated are antibody responses to particular tumor-associated antigens that also may be detected in patient plasma or serum, for example, tumor suppressor gene *TP53* (p53) on chromosome 17p.

Detection and Diagnosis

Clinical Detection

The most common abnormality reaching clinical attention is a mass within the breast. There are four basic breast masses: benign tumor, usually a fibroadenoma; breast cyst; functional or fibrocystic mass; and breast cancer.

1. Fibroadenomas are benign tumors containing both stromal and epithelial elements that may be tiny or may grow to very large sizes (giant fibroadenomas). Fibroadenoma is the most common benign tumor in the breast; these tumors are commonly found in young women in their teens and twenties.
2. Breast cysts contain fluid produced by the glandular cells that line the inside of their walls. Cysts cannot be distinguished from solid tumors, such as fibroadenomas, by physical examination alone. Age is an important discriminating factor; cysts are common in the fourth and fifth decades of life, whereas fibroadenomas occur predominately in younger women. Both

TABLE 17–4. **Tumor Markers Investigated in Breast Cancer**

Tumor Marker	Association/Use
Tumor-associated antigens (TAA)	
Carcinoembryonic antigen (CEA)	Stage / prognosis / metastasis*
Tissue polypeptide antigen (TPA)	Diagnosis / stage
Tissue polypeptide-specific antigen (TPS)	Stage† / progression / prognosis
Related to or products of *MUC1* gene:	
CA 15-3	Stage / progression / prognosis
CA 27-29	Stage / metastasis
Mammary serum antigen (MSA)	Stage / metastasis
Tumor biology markers	
Growth factors associated with angiogenesis:	
Vascular endothelial growth factor (VEGF)	↑ Levels = angiogenesis / ↑ recurrence
Basic fibroblast growth factor (bFGF)	↓ Levels = worse prognosis / ↑ recurrence
Hepatocyte growth factor (HGF)	↑ Levels = progression
Molecules of adhesion and invasion:	
E-selectin	Metastasis
Cathepsin D	Tumor growth / metastasis
Intracellular adhesion molecule-1 (ICAM-1)	Stage
ERBB2 (HER2/neu)	Prognosis
Oncogene/proto-oncogene coexpression‡:	
HRAS, FOS	Survival
Antibody response against TAAs	
Antibodies to p53	Stage

*If used in a panel with TPA and CA 15-3.
†When used with CA 15-3.
‡Coexpression correlates with recurrence.[16]
Modified from Stearns V, Yamauchi H, Hayes D: Circulating tumor markers in breast cancer: accepted utilities and novel aspects. Recent Cancer Res Treat 1998; 52:239–259.

cysts and fibroadenomas present as singular masses with smooth borders and are frequently freely mobile.

3. Functional masses are sometimes referred to as fibrocystic masses. However, they do not necessarily contain cystic elements or other hallmarks of fibrocystic disease. These tumors are typically found in women over the age of 30 who are still menstruating. They may be singular, tender, and are likely to regress during passage of a menstrual cycle. Presumably, they arise by local increased glandular activity and stromal tissue edema.
4. The most common presentation of invasive breast cancer is a mass in the breast; 80% of all invasive breast cancers are detected as an asymptomatic mass in the breast.[17] In contrast, noninvasive breast cancers, an increasing fraction of early breast cancer, are rarely detected as a mass in the breast. The vast majority of intraductal carcinomas (ductal carcinoma *in situ* [DCIS]) present as a mammographic finding, usually a cluster of microcalcifications, with or without an associated mass effect. The majority of LCIS neoplasms are discovered as an incidental finding, presenting as neither a mass nor a mammographic finding.

Most masses are discovered by patients on a casual self-examination, for instance, during bathing. Clinical breast exam performed by a health professional does contribute to the discovery of early breast cancer in screening trials.[18] Despite the controversies surrounding screening for breast cancer, the average size of breast cancer at the time of presentation for treatment has decreased steadily over the modern era of surgical treatment. In earlier decades, the average size of breast cancer presenting for treatment was approximately 2 cm; in the Breast Cancer Detection Demonstration Project (BCDDP), 42% of all breast cancers were nonpalpable and 32% were less than 1 cm in size or *in situ* cancers.[19]

Breast cancer presents as a single, dominant, and asymptomatic mass in the breast. Three criteria help the clinician to discriminate benign from malignant masses:

- The first criterion is the presence of symptoms; breast cancer usually is asymptomatic and painless. Functional masses in the breast are frequently associated with pain and tenderness, particularly during the menstrual cycle.
- The second criterion is age. Breast cancer is very uncommon below the age of 30; a painless mass in a young woman or teenage girl is usually a fibroadenoma; a new mass in a postmenopausal woman is usually a breast cancer.
- The third criterion is the relation of the mass to the surrounding breast tissue. A mobile mass that moves freely within the breast tissue is commonly a cyst or fibroadenoma. Cysts are common in women after age 30 and remain prevalent until the time of menopause. As noted earlier, fibroadenomas are common benign tumors in the breasts of adolescents and young women.

In summary, breast cancers are asymptomatic masses that become more common as women grow older. Breast cancers are characterized by infiltration of the surrounding breast tissue and are frequently partially fixed and not as mobile as cysts or fibroadenomas.

Several other important physical findings during the breast examination should be mentioned:

- *Skin dimpling* is a frequent sign that can be detected on direct visual inspection of the breast, often elicited by raising the ipsilateral arm and pulling up on the breast. Dimpling is a result of entrapment and shortening of Cooper's ligaments by an infiltrating lesion that tugs on the overlying skin. Around the areola, this process can cause inversion of the nipple.
- *Peau d'orange* (orange peel skin) is edema of the skin of the breast caused by infiltration of the dermal lymphatics by cancer cells. This finding at presentation usually signifies inflammatory breast cancer, a disease characterized by diffuse lymphatic permeation by cancer cells, but it may also be seen occasionally in patients with conserved breasts after axillary lymph node dissection and radiation.
- *Nipple discharge* is a common symptom that is usually benign. Watery, opaque, or greenish discharge that can be demonstrated to originate from more than one nipple duct orifice, or from both nipples, is a benign finding. Bloody nipple discharge from a single, unique duct orifice on one nipple is a surgically significant finding that demands biopsy. The usual finding is intraductal papilloma; however, intraductal carcinoma in subareolar ducts can cause bloody discharge.
- Finally, *Paget's disease* of the nipple is an eczematoid eruption that starts on the nipple and may spread outward to involve the areola. Paget's disease is caused by intraepithelial spread of intraductal carcinoma arising in the lactiferous sinuses and large ducts of the nipple. In its pure form, Paget's disease is a form of intraductal or noninvasive carcinoma. Full-thickness biopsy of the surface of the nipple is required to make the diagnosis, frequently accomplished by a punch biopsy in the clinic. A deeper biopsy usually shows intraductal carcinoma, which may or may not be associated with invasive cancer.

Diagnostic Procedures

Modern radiology of the breast uses molybdenum radiation sources and intensifying screens to produce a negative image viewed as a standard x-ray film (Table 17–5). Effective screening mammography is performed on a dedicated machine and consists of a medial lateral oblique and a craniocaudal view (two views) of each breast. These four films are reviewed at a later time by a radiologist and a report is issued. This system is suited to a high volume of tests and minimizes the cost of each screening study. If abnormalities are found, additional diagnostic views or procedures are requested. Diagnostic mammography is performed with a physician on site who can direct magnification, compression or spot views, and ultrasonography, and perform physical examination. As implied, the goal of diagnostic mammography is to provide a differential diagnosis and suggestions for further evaluation.

TABLE 17–5. **Diagnostic Capabilities of Current Imaging Modalities in Breast Cancer**

Method	Diagnosis and Staging Capability	Recommended for Use
Primary tumor and regional nodes		
Mammography	Visualizes approximately 90% of breast cancers	Film / screen and xeromammography have similar diagnostic accuracy.
Ultrasound (dedicated)	Limited to identification of cystic lesions and evaluation of dense breast	Dedicated units are expensive and not suitable for stand-alone screening.
CT	Limited to evaluation of chest wall and internal mammary node involvement	Use of dedicated CT breast imaging systems has been abandoned.
MRI	Good for discrete lesions; calcifications are difficult to distinguish	Dedicated units are expensive. Useful for follow-up and for women with implants.
Metastatic breast cancer (as required)		
Chest x-ray film	Adequate for diagnosis; CT usually not needed	Essential for all tumor types
Radionuclide bone scans	Essential for baseline verification and evaluation of symptomatic patients	Abnormal bone scans require film.
Liver and adrenal imaging	Indicated with abnormal chemistries or symptoms	Initial imaging study: radionuclide scan (requires validation of abnormal scan by ultrasound or CT).

CT = computed tomography; MRI = magnetic resonance imaging.
Modified from Bragg DG, Rubin P, Youker JE (eds): Oncologic Imaging. Elmsford, NY, Pergamon Press, 1985.

Abnormal mammogram findings can be divided into four categories: masses, microcalcifications, asymmetries, and architectural distortions, described as follows:

1. *Masses* are either well demarcated and have smooth borders (typical of cysts or fibroadenomas) or they may be irregular with spiculated borders (typical of breast cancer).
2. *Microcalcifications* may display a variety of different morphologies. The most worrisome are numerous fine linear or linear branching forms.
3. *Asymmetries* refer to differences in the density and quantity of fibroglandular tissue when one breast is compared with the same area on the opposite side.
4. *Architectural distortion* refers to an alteration in the lacy or honeycombed pattern of glandular tissue against the background fat of the breast; spiculation is a form of architectural distortion.

At this time, film screen mammography is the most sensitive and specific test for the detection of breast cancers. Overall, mammography detects 85% to 90% of all subsequently confirmed breast cancers; false-negative rates of 10% to 15% are widely quoted.[18] The positive predictive value of mammography (the chance that a woman with a positive mammogram actually has a cancer) depends on many variables. Mammography results are not reported as simply positive or negative. In order to standardize the highly qualitative nature of mammography reporting, the American College of Radiology BIRADS system was written to assist in results reporting. This system has been applied to reporting mammogram findings. The following five categories of interpretation have been suggested:

1. Negative mammograms: Standard follow-up is recommended.
2. Benign negative: A benign finding requiring no special follow-up.
3. Probably benign: A short interval of follow-up is requested.
4. Indeterminate: Risk of cancer is measurable and biopsy is recommended. The positive predictive value of mammography in this category may range from as low as 2% to 3% to as high as 50%.
5. Likely malignant: The risk of cancer in this category is greater than 50%. Biopsy is mandated.

The use of mammography as a screening test is based on its high sensitivity and acceptable specificity. The utility of screening mammography in asymptomatic populations at standard risk has been studied. Eight prospective randomized studies have been carried out to evaluate the ability of screening mammography to reduce mortality. The design and randomization methods have varied. Both meta-analyses and consensus reports are available to assist in the interpretation of these randomized studies.[18, 20] In addition, other nonrandomized studies have been done in the United States and Europe; the best-known (and largest) study is the U.S. BCDDP.[19]

Results of the randomized trials of screening mammography fail to show a benefit in reduction of mortality for women younger than 50 years of age (the risk ratio lies between 0.85 and 1.16, but confidence limits span 1.0). The area is quite controversial, however, and benefit has been shown in some nonrandomized trials. From these results, it has been suggested that annual screening of women aged 40 to 50 is appropriate. However, guidelines from national organizations (American Cancer Society, National Cancer Institute, and the American College of Radiology) are conflicting. For women 50 years and older, the data are conclusive, positive, and in favor of screening. Trial results are consistent for women between 50 and 70 years of age; there is an average reduction in breast cancer mortality of about 30% (risk ratio of 0.71) when the results of the randomized trials are combined (the confidence limit is between 0.5 and 0.90). The advantage of screening disappears in women over the age of 70, but the numbers of older women included in screening studies are small.

There is consensus that screening mammography in intervals of 1 to 2 years benefits women between ages 49 and 71.[21] The benefits of screening younger women are less certain; no nationally accepted standard exists. Screening after age 70 is of unproven benefit and is left up to women and their health professionals. A special group is women at an increased risk for breast cancer because of family or personal history; for these patients, no data exist. One clinic active in counseling women with hereditary risk recommends screening beginning 5 to 10 years before the earliest age of onset in the family.[22]

Management of the Abnormal Mammogram

An indeterminate or likely malignant finding on screening mammography, and confirmed further by diagnostic imaging studies, leads to more invasive testing. The goal of these tests is to arrive at a pathologic diagnosis of the nonpalpable lesion. The choice of strategies and technologies is varied.

Aspiration cytology, or large core needle biopsies, can be obtained using either mammographic or ultrasound guidance. Aspiration through a small gauge needle obtains a cytologic preparation and is quite accurate (positive predictive value >95%).[23] Aspiration of nonpalpable lesions is done for distinct mammographic masses but rarely for microcalcifications alone. Both masses and microcalcifications may be sampled by needle core biopsy under ultrasound or stereotactic guidance. Core biopsies range from 14 to 18 gauge in diameter and are from 1 to 3 cm in length; these samples are large enough for embedding and histologic sectioning and for magnified specimen radiographs. These specimen radiographs are performed when microcalcifications are targeted and are required to confirm adequate sampling of the underlying pathology. Correlation of the pathology with the mammographic differential diagnosis is required to avoid false-negative biopsies. For instance, finding only normal breast tissue when a distinct mass is targeted implies inadequate sampling. Aspiration cytology and core biopsies are relatively noninvasive ways to achieve a reliable diagnosis of nonpalpable mammographic abnormalities. The alternative to these procedures is open biopsy after needle localization.

Needle localization is done in a standard mammogram apparatus through a compression plate with an open port and a grid system for placing the needle. After placement of the needle adjacent or through the abnormality, a wire can be passed through the needle that is secured in the tissue by a barbed tip. Placement is confirmed in two views and the mammographic abnormality removed by an open procedure using a surgical incision. Specimen mammography is used to confirm adequate sampling or removal of the radiographic lesion. The specimen is oriented and submitted to pathology with the specimen radiograph. This procedure, although more invasive than needle biopsy, can be used to completely remove suspicious mammographic findings. Several authors[24–26] review other techniques for diagnosis of nonpalpable, mammographic abnormalities.

Management of the Patient with a Palpable Mass and Negative Mammogram

As previously stated, 10% to 15% of patients with breast cancer will have negative findings on a mammogram. This is more likely in younger women with radiographically dense breasts. Patients with clinically suspicious masses should have biopsy performed even if mammograms are negative.

Classification and Staging

Histopathology

Most cancer of the breast is a carcinoma of the epithelial cells that line breast ducts and lobules. Rarer forms of cancer occurring in the breast arise from the stromal cells that surround the epithelial glands. These include benign phyllode tumors, malignant cytosarcoma phyllodes, and angiosarcomas. Description of the pathology and natural history of these rare forms of breast cancer can be found in many sources, some of which are referenced here.[27, 28]

A widely used classification of epithelial breast carcinomas, or adenocarcinomas of the breast, is provided by the World Health Organization (WHO).[29] The major elements of this classification are presented in Table 17–6. In practice, the most important distinction is between invasive and noninvasive breast carcinoma. Further distinction is made between lobular and ductal carcinomas, which can both be invasive or noninvasive.

Noninvasive ductal carcinoma is also known as DCIS or intraductal carcinoma. The malignant cells in this disease are confined to the ductal basement membrane. Intraductal proliferations are further classified according to their growth pattern as presented in Table 17–6. The comedo form of DCIS is prone to develop the calcifications that can be seen on high quality mammograms and lead to an early diagnosis.[30] LCIS is composed of smaller lobular or acinar cells and fills the terminal breast lobule with a homogeneous proliferation. Most clinicians currently regard LCIS as a risk factor for the development of invasive breast cancer, both lobular and ductal, but not as a premalignant condition per se. Consequently, LCIS is usually not treated, but affected women are placed under frequent surveillance.[31, 32]

The most common form of invasive ductal cancer is referred to as infiltrating ductal carcinoma, NOS (not otherwise specified). Infiltrating lobular carcinoma refers to a

TABLE 17–6. **WHO Classification of Breast Cancer (Selected)**

Histological Subtypes	Incidence
Noninvasive Carcinomas	
Intraductal carcinoma (DCIS)	15%
Lobular carcinoma *in situ* (LCIS)	2%
Invasive Adenocarcinomas	
Infiltrating ductal carcinoma, NOS	60%
Infiltrating lobular carcinoma	5–10%
Mucinous (colloid) carcinoma	2–5%
Medullary carcinoma	1–5%
Tubular carcinoma	2–5%
Papillary carcinoma	2–5%
Other types	1–5%

NOS = not otherwise specified.

distinct classification of breast adenocarcinomas. These tumors are recognized by the presence of small round cells that infiltrate a reactive stroma in cords that are one cell across (Indian file infiltration). The malignant cells in lobular carcinoma also grow circumferentially around ducts and lobules (targetoid growth). It is common for lobular characteristics to coincide with features of invasive ductal carcinomas, a variant frequently referred to as tubulolobular carcinoma. With certain exceptions, pure lobular and tubulolobular carcinomas have a similar prognosis to the more common infiltrating ductal carcinoma, NOS.[28]

Other special types of breast cancer that do not represent distinct pathologic subtypes include inflammatory carcinoma and Paget's disease. Inflammatory carcinoma is an aggressive infiltrating ductal carcinoma, or an NOS that has a tendency to infiltrate breast lymphatics early during its growth. Infiltration of dermal lymphatics with tumor cells produces dermal edema, erythema and the classic peau d'orange appearance of the breast. Paget's disease is DCIS in subareolar breast ducts that invade above the basement membrane of the squamous epithelium on the surface of the nipple. This invasion produces a psoriasis-like dry scaling lesion that always originates on the surface of the nipple. Like DCIS elsewhere in the breast, Paget's intraductal disease may be associated with more diffuse intraductal carcinoma under the areola or with an invasive component.

Staging

Staging systems for cancer attempt to stratify the extent of disease in a way that predicts outcome. For a system with four stages, ideal staging would result in an even distribution of outcomes (usually survival) proceeding from lowest to highest stage. In practice, an even distribution is usually not possible because of the heterogeneity of cancer and the multiple combinations of factors that influence outcome. For this reason, staging systems are continually revised within subcommittees of the American Joint Committee on Cancer (AJCC). The scheme presented in Table 17–7 summarizes the 1997 AJCC definition.[33]

The AJCC tumor, node, metastasis (TNM) staging system is used to define a stage grouping to summarize the status of the primary tumor and lymph nodes and the presence of distant metastases. In general, these four stages divide patients with breast cancer into a continuum of outcomes (Fig. 17–1). Stage I breast cancer is "cured" (remains disease-free at an arbitrary follow-up interval) about 80% of the time. Stage II breast cancer is a heterogeneous group, but on average it is cured 50% to 60% of the time. Stage III breast cancer is also heterogeneous, but it has an average long-term relapse-free rate of 30% to 40%. Finally, nearly all patients with metastatic breast cancer will succumb to their disease; the majority of women with stage IV breast cancer have died by 2 years of follow-up (Fig. 17–2).[34, 35]

Principles of Treatment

The goal of any oncologic treatment is to maximize the cure and at the same time optimize the quality of life. This is especially important for carcinoma of the breast in which late relapses are common. *Cure generally is defined as that point in time when the survival curve of patients with the disease in question becomes parallel to that of an age-matched population.* In breast carcinoma, cure does not occur until approximately 20 years after initial therapy.[36]

An optimal therapeutic outcome for any malignancy, but especially for breast carcinoma, requires a multidisciplinary approach, that is, input from surgical, radiation, and medical oncologists, diagnostic radiologists, and pathologists, as well as other professionals to provide psychosocial support. How to accomplish this in a cost-effective, efficient manner in an era of diminishing resources with increasing cost constraints is a challenging and unsolved problem (Table 17–8).

TABLE 17–7. **TNM Classification and Stage Grouping for Breast Cancer**

Stage	Grouping	Descriptor
Stage 0	Tis N0 M0	Tis: carcinoma *in situ* (pure DCIS, LCIS, and Paget's disease) N0: no regional lymph node metastasis M0: no distant metastasis
Stage I	T1* N0 M0	T1: tumor ≤2 cm in diameter; category includes T1mic: microinvasion ≤0.1 cm
Stage IIA	T0 N1 M0	T0: no evidence of primary tumor
	T1 N1 M0	N1: metastasis to movable ipsilateral axillary lymph nodes
	T2 N0 M0	T2: tumor >2 cm in diameter but less than 5 cm
Stage IIB	T2 N1 M0	
	T3 N0 M0	T3: tumor >5 cm
Stage IIIA	T0 N2 M0	N2: metastasis to ipsilateral axillary lymph nodes fixed to one another or to other structures
	T1 N2 M0	
	T2 N2 M0	
	T3 N1 M0	
	T3 N2 M0	
Stage IIIB	T4 Any N M0	T4†: tumor extending into skin or chest wall
	Any T N3 M0	N3: metastasis to ipsilateral internal mammary lymph nodes
Stage IV	Any T Any N M1	M1: distant metastases are present, including metastasis to ipsilateral supraclavicular nodes

*T1 is further subdivided: T1mic (see above); T1a: tumor >0.1 cm but ≤0.5 cm; T1b: tumor >0.5 cm but ≤1 cm; T1c: tumor >1 cm but ≤2 cm.

†T4 is further subdivided: T4a: extension to chest wall; T4b: edema or ulceration of the breast or satellite skin nodules confined to one breast; T4c: both T4a and T4b; T4d: inflammatory carcinoma (see text).

Used with the permission of the American Joint Committee on Cancer (AJCC®), Chicago, Illinois. The original source for this material is the AJCC® Cancer Staging Manual, 5th edition, 1997, published by Lippincott-Raven Publishers, Philadelphia, Pennsylvania.

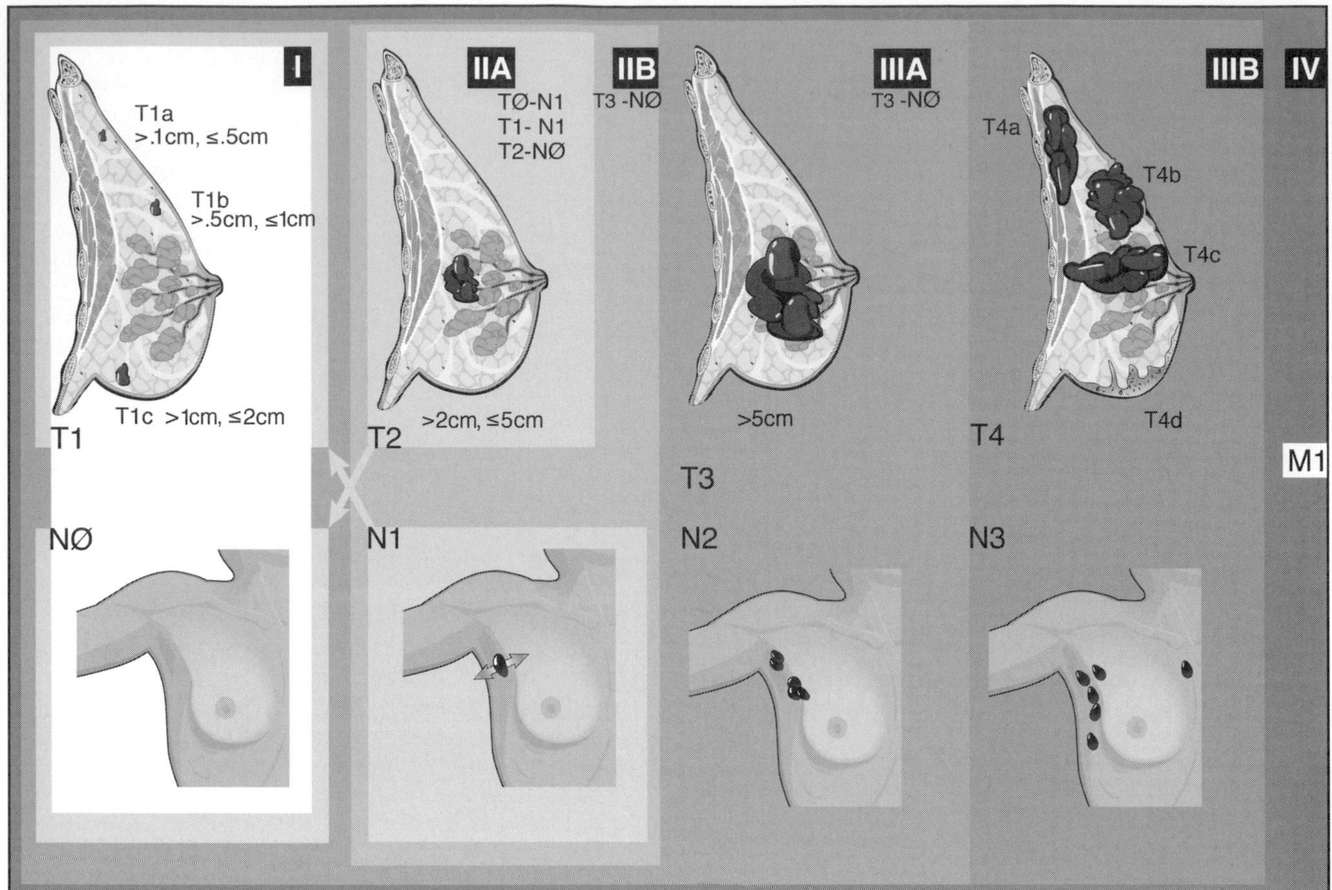

Figure 17–1. Anatomic staging for breast cancer.

TABLE 17–8. **Multidisciplinary Treatment Decisions in Breast Cancer**

Stage (Clinical)	Surgery	Radiation Therapy	Chemotherapy	Tamoxifen	Comments
Stage 0 (DCIS)	TM ± RC	0	0	±	Consider Tam as chemo prevention
	PM	+	0	±	Consider Tam as chemo prevention and to improve local control
Stage I	MRM ± RC	±	±	±	RT for node +ive patients
	PM ± ALND ± SLND	+	±	±	Chemo ± Tam depending on node status, tumor size, hormone receptor status, and patient age
Stage II	MRM ± RC	±	±	±	RT for node +ive or T3 patients
	PM ± ALND ± SLND	+	±	±	Chemo ± Tam depending on node status, tumor size, hormone receptor status, and patient age
Stage III					Tam for receptor +ive patients
Resectable	MRM + RC	+	+	±	
Unresectable:		+	+	+	
Chemo responders	MRM ± RC	+	+	±	
Nonresponders		Individualize Rx			
Stage IV		Individualize Rx			See text
Local recurrence					
Following BCT	0	0	±	±	
Following TM or MRM		Individualize Rx			

BCT = breast conservation therapy; TM = total mastectomy; MRM = modified radical mastectomy; RC = reconstruction; PM = partial mastectomy (lumpectomy); ALND = axillary lymph node dissection; SLND = sentinel lymph node dissection; Tam = tamoxifen.

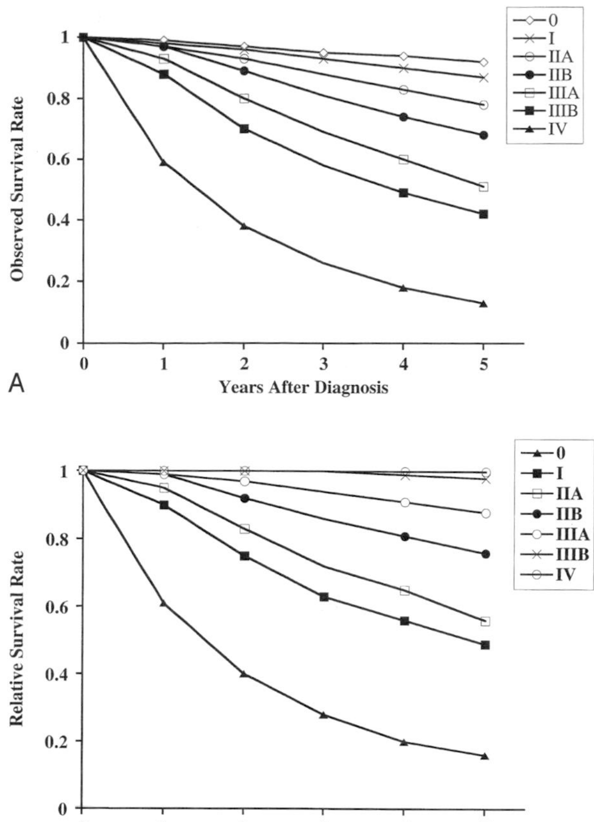

Figure 17–2. AJCC figures of (A) observed survival rate and (B) relative survival rate, up to 5 years after diagnosis. Used with the permission of the American Joint Committee on Cancer (AJCC®), Chicago, Illinois. The original source for this material is the AJCC® Cancer Staging Manual, 5th edition, 1997, published by Lippincott-Raven Publishers, Philadelphia, Pennsylvania.

In the following section, the principles of management of both clinically localized and generalized (i.e., metastatic) breast carcinoma are discussed, including indications for mastectomy, breast conserving therapy (BCT), adjuvant systemic therapy, postmastectomy radiation, axillary lymph node dissection, and breast reconstruction. Results of treatment are discussed in a later section, as well as the special categories of DCIS, a condition often referred to as breast cancer but really a premalignant lesion, and locally advanced breast carcinoma (LABC).

Clinically Localized Breast Carcinoma

Historically, breast cancer, as well as most other malignancies, was believed to originate in a single cell, growing and spreading in an orderly fashion from the primary site to regional lymph nodes and, subsequently, to distant sites. This concept was popularized by Halsted at the beginning of the twentieth century,[37] and a logical outgrowth of this idea was that a large operation that encompassed the entire breast, immediate surrounding tissues, and regional lymph nodes would generally result in a better cure rate. Thus, the Halsted radical mastectomy (RM) was developed, which removed not only the breast but also underlying muscle and the immediate regional lymph nodes in the axilla *en bloc*.[38] A further extension of RM was attempted in the 1950s and 1960s with the development of the supraradical (or extended radical) mastectomy, in which not only axillary but also internal mammary nodes were removed.[39] Despite some misgivings, the Halstedian hypothesis dominated surgical oncologic thinking until the 1970s. However, beginning in the 1940s and 1950s, there were attempts by investigators, such as McWhirter and Johansen and coworkers, to decrease the extent of surgery and replace it with radiation therapy by comparing procedures such as total mastectomy and radiation therapy with radical or extended radical mastectomy.[40, 41] However, these attempts remained essentially Halstedian in concept, with radiation simply substituting for a more extensive surgical procedure.

In the 1960s and 1970s, the concept of early dissemination and biologic predetermination was introduced by Fisher and his colleagues at the National Surgical Adjuvant Breast Project (NSABP).[42] This hypothesis, known as the alternate or Fisher hypothesis, suggested that breast carcinoma began as a small focus of malignant cells in the breast, but that inherent biologic characteristics of the tumor determined the outcome. By the time the tumor was clinically detectable in the breast, the carcinoma was believed to have been present for several years, during which time there had been ample opportunity for distant spread to occur. Lymph node involvement was an indicator of the propensity for distant spread but not a direct pathway for such. Therefore, more aggressive local-regional treatment might improve local-regional control, but it would not be expected to have an impact on survival; effective systemic therapy (adjuvant chemotherapy or hormonal therapy) would be necessary. The concept of micrometastases (or subclinical disease) was introduced; lymph node–positive patients were felt to be at high risk for harboring such clinically undetectable metastases in the majority of instances, with the risk directly related to the number of involved nodes.

Several NSABP studies supported this hypothesis. Fisher reported relapse rates of 50% and 60% at 5 and 10 years, respectively, for patients with operable breast carcinoma of any size and one to three involved axillary nodes. This increased to relapse rates of 80% at 5 years and 90% at 10 years, for patients with four or more axillary nodes involved with carcinoma.[34] NSABP protocol BO4 compared three different local forms of treatment (a total mastectomy [TM], a modified radical mastectomy [MRM], and a TM combined with radiation therapy) and found no difference in survival, despite improved local-regional control in the patients treated with MRM or TM plus radiation.[43] It was also in the 1970s that the first reports of the effectiveness of adjuvant systemic therapy appeared.[44, 45] All of these factors served to emphasize the importance of control of systemic micrometastases in patients with ostensibly clinically localized disease and also de-emphasized the importance of local therapy. The use of radiation therapy following mastectomy declined markedly, largely as a consequence of NSABP BO4 and the increased emphasis on adjuvant systemic therapy, despite the better local control that had been achieved in BO4.

Recent developments, however, presage a move of the pendulum back toward the center. Investigators in Europe and Canada have demonstrated that better local therapy in the presence of adjuvant systemic therapy can increase survival, with the magnitude of the benefit approaching that seen with adjuvant systemic therapy.[46, 47] This suggests that either there are some patients with nodal involvement without systemic micrometastases who are cured by better local-regional therapy or that, whereas node-positive patients may have systemic disease, the tumor burden is greater in the local-regional area and that radiation, as well as chemotherapy, is needed to control the local-regional disease.[48] It would appear, therefore, that the best outcome results from therapy that is optimal from both the local and systemic standpoint.

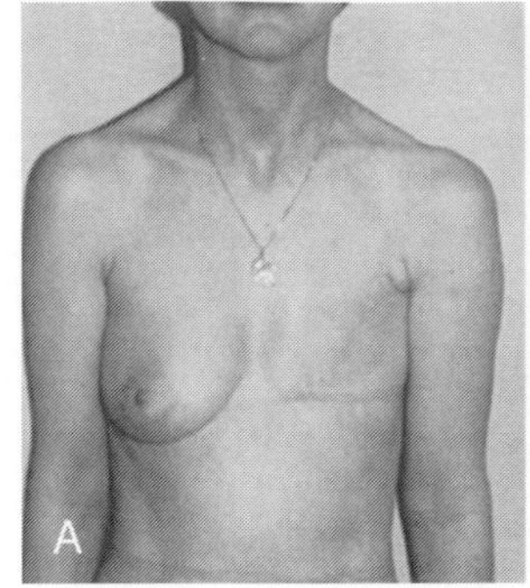

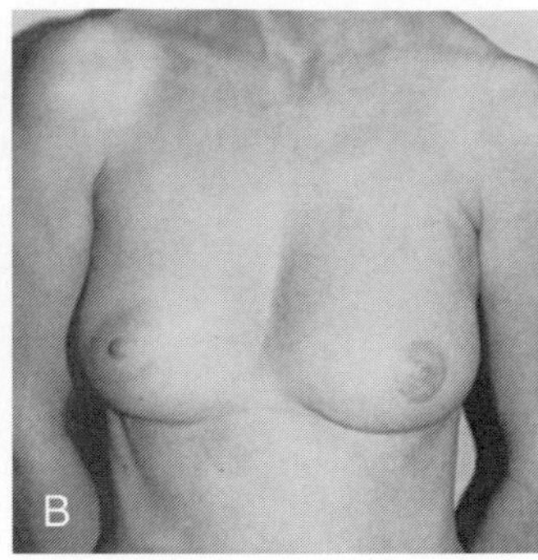

Figure 17–3. Surgical reconstruction: (A) Thirty-eight-year-old woman after modified radical mastectomy. (B) Two years after reconstruction with transverse abdominal island flap. No alloplastic material was used in either breast. (Courtesy of C. R. Hartrampf.)

Local Therapies

Mastectomy

Traditionally, RM was the treatment for localized small breast carcinomas, as outlined earlier. Removal of the entire breast was thought necessary because of the multicentric and multifocal nature of the disease in many patients. Because of the known morbidity of the operation, however, attempts at lesser surgical procedures, such as MRM or TM, were introduced, principally in Europe in the 1930s and 1940s.[40] Usually, radiation was added to the lesser operation. Studies comparing different surgical procedures, with or without postoperative radiation, have generally shown very similar outcomes, although almost all of the studies lacked sufficient power to detect small survival rate differences in the range of 5% to 10%.[49, 50]

These data, along with the increased emphasis on the systemic aspects of ostensibly localized disease, led to the MRM becoming the standard surgical procedure in the United States in the 1960s and 1970s, and the majority of patients today are still treated in this fashion. The MRM removes the entire breast, sometimes the pectoralis minor muscle (but not the pectoralis major) and level 1 and 2 axillary lymph nodes. Removal of nodes at these levels achieves excellent local control in the axilla as well as providing a highly accurate representation of axillary nodal status.[51] The Halstedian mastectomy removed much of the skin overlying the breast as well, with a skin graft often used, but this is believed to be no longer necessary. In the MRM, only the skin overlying the nipple areolar complex is removed by most surgeons, as well as any biopsy scar. Interestingly, MRM was adopted as the standard surgical procedure in the absence of any phase III trials demonstrating its equivalency to RM, with two relevant phase III trials being published much later.[52, 53]

Mastectomy produces some degree of psychological trauma in most patients. Breast reconstruction can alleviate this trauma considerably. In the past, reconstruction was only done 6 to 12 months after all therapy, including adjuvant chemotherapy, had been completed. There was concern that an early local recurrence might be masked, but as the prosthesis is usually placed under the pectoralis major muscle, a recurrence still should be detected easily. Therefore, there is no reason to delay breast reconstruction for long periods. In fact, immediate reconstruction at the time of mastectomy in selected patients is well tolerated, is welcomed by patients, and does not compromise or delay the use of adjuvant chemotherapy[54] (Fig. 17–3).

Most breast reconstructions use an implant filled with saline. When local tissues are inadequate, an expander that can gradually be filled with saline may be used, giving time for the tissues to stretch. When the local soft tissue is of poor quality because of previous radiation therapy, radical mastectomy, or skin grafting (and as a result of the moratorium on silicone gel implants), it may be necessary to perform a myocutaneous flap using the latissimus dorsi, TRAM (transverse rectus abdominis muscle), or free flap to cover the prosthesis. It is also possible to reconstruct the breast in some patients without an implant by using autologous tissue from the lower abdominal wall.[55]

Breast Conserving Therapy

The demonstration that a lesser surgical operation, such as TM, was as effective as RM, particularly when combined with radiation therapy, led to the use of breast conserving therapy (BCT). In this procedure, the gross tumor is surgically removed (variously termed lumpectomy, partial mastectomy, or excisional biopsy). Axillary lymph node dissection (ALND) may or may not be done through a separate incision, and radiation therapy is relied on to control subclinical disease elsewhere in the breast and sometimes in nodal areas, such as the internal mammary or supraclavicular nodes, particularly when the axillary nodes are demonstrably positive surgically. This procedure has been termed *breast conservation therapy* or *breast conserving therapy.* It is not conservative treatment; it is the radiation therapy equivalent of a radical or extended radical mastectomy when the nodes are treated.

BCT was first proposed in the 1930s by Sir Geoffrey Keynes,[56] although its widespread use did not occur until the 1990s. BCT has been facilitated by a number of developments over the last several decades:

1. The increased use of mammography, better mammographic techniques, and an increased awareness of breast carcinoma on the part of women have all led to earlier diagnosis and the finding of small carcinomas lending themselves more readily to lumpectomy.
2. Radiation therapy techniques and equipment, particularly the development of supervoltage radiation with consequent skin sparing in the 1960s and its dissemination by the 1970s, have made BCT much more practical and desirable.
3. Women have increasingly taken a more active role

TABLE 17–9. **Breast Conserving Therapy (BCT) Trials**

Trial	Yr of Entry	No of Pts	Follow-Up (yrs)	Survival (%)		RFS (%)		Local Recurrence (%)	
				Mast	*BCT*	*Mast*	*BCT*	*Mast*	*BCT*
EORTC[63]	1980–86	902	8	73	71			9	15
DBCG[64]	1983–89	905	6	82	79	66	70	4	3
NCI[65]	1979–87	247	10	75	77	69	72	10	18
Milan[66]	1973–80	701	16	68	71			3	7
NSABP[67]	1976–84	2105	12	62	62	51	50	8+	15
Gustave-Roussy[68]	1972–79	179	15	65	73	44	55	14	9

RFS = relapse-free survival; Mast = mastectomy.

in their medical management and forced a greater emphasis on quality-of-life issues. BCT has obvious advantages in this respect compared with mastectomy, given equal therapeutic efficacy. Without the influence of many female patients, however, it is doubtful that BCT would enjoy the position that it does today.

There is little doubt that BCT is as effective as more traditional procedures such as MRM; this is one of the most studied procedures in all of cancer therapy. Literally thousands of patients treated with BCT have been reported in retrospective analyses.[57–62] Thousands more have been reported in prospective phase III trials.[63–69] With only occasional exceptions, all trials show an equivalency for the two procedures in terms of survival, distant metastases rates, and local control (Table 17–9). A recent meta-analysis of these trials even suggests a small survival advantage for BCT, particularly in patients who are lymph node positive, a finding consistent with the survival benefits found in patients who are node positive and receiving postmastectomy radiation.[70] A National Institutes of Health Consensus Conference has recommended the adoption of BCT as the local therapy of choice for most women with carcinoma of the breast.[71]

SURGICAL ASPECTS OF BCT

BCT is a complex procedure that requires close cooperation between all relevant specialties if optimal results are to be obtained in terms of curing the patient, minimizing complications, and achieving good cosmesis (Fig. 17–4).

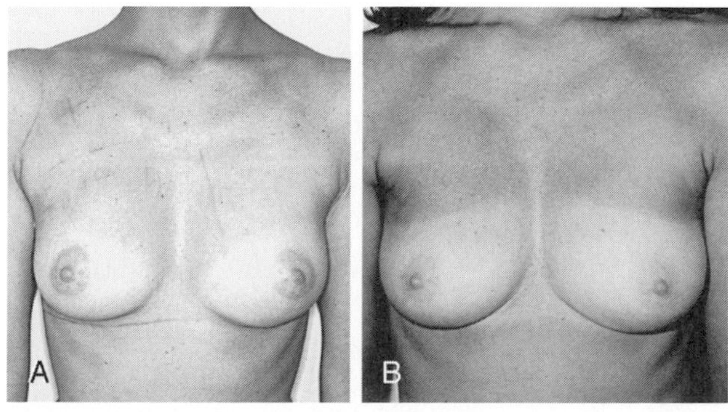

Figure 17–4. Radiation cosmesis: excellent cosmesis results from the selective effect of irradiation. If breast surgery does not distort or disfigure the fine surgical result, often lumpectomy is maintained by radiation therapy.

Mammograms are mandatory to outline the lump in question and to be sure there are no others elsewhere in the breast that are not clinically appreciated. The surgical incision should be placed directly over the tumor. The radiation oncologist will wish to give a concentrated dose of radiation to the tumor bed and biopsy scar (the boost field). Tunneling to biopsy a lump via a circumareolar incision makes the subsequent delivery of the radiation boost field more difficult and is to be avoided. Incisions in the superior half of the breast should be curvilinear and follow the natural creases of the skin[72]; wide margins of normal tissue appear to be unnecessary. The pathologic specimen should be inked for margin determination. A pathologically negative margin microscopically is all that is necessary. Local control rates appear to be equivalent if that margin is just a few cells away from the cancer or 1 to 2 cm away[73–75]; the greater the amount of normal tissue that is removed, the worse the cosmetic outcome. Surgical technique appears to be the most important factor in achieving good cosmesis.[76]

NODAL MANAGEMENT

Axillary lymph node dissection (ALND), as a part of BCT, remains as a standard procedure in most centers. Historically, ALND was performed to improve both local control and cure, according to Halstedian principles. With the advent of adjuvant systemic therapy and the recognition that the most important prognostic variable is lymph node status, ALND became a staging procedure, designed to guide decisions regarding systemic therapy. ALND is necessary as a staging procedure to determine pathologic axillary status because of the common occurrence of histologically positive lymph nodes in patients with clinically negative axillae. This status varies from 5% (in patients with microinvasive carcinoma only) to as high as 50% (in patients with T2 or T3 primary tumors).[77]

In the early days of adjuvant systemic therapy, it was common to treat patients with pathologically positive lymph nodes with systemic therapy but withhold it from those whose nodes were negative. With the recognition of the benefits for adjuvant systemic therapy in patients with negative nodes, however, it has come to be employed for the great majority of women with breast cancers over 1 cm in size, irrespective of nodal status, calling into question the performance of ALND.[78–81] Axillary radiation may be effectively used for the control of subclinical disease.[80, 82]

Sentinel node biopsies have recently been introduced.[83, 84] In experienced hands, the sentinel node biopsy has a high specificity and sensitivity. If sentinel nodes are negative, full axillary dissection yields positive nodes in about 1% of instances. If sentinel nodes are positive, then full axillary node dissection is usually carried out for optimization of local control. Thus, the entire area of management of the axilla is under very active investigation. It is likely that the frequency and extent of axillary surgery will decline in the future.

For palpable axillary disease, ALND is still mandatory, because doses of radiation therapy that are required for local control of clinically evident disease are associated with an unacceptable complication rate.[82] For patients without clinically apparent axillary disease who are undergoing BCT and will be irradiated anyway, axillary radiation instead of dissection can be considered; the patient should be involved in the decision-making process.

RADIATION

Careful radiation techniques are also of critical importance if good results are to be obtained with BCT. A detailed description of the technical aspects of radiation therapy for breast carcinoma is beyond the scope of this chapter but can be found in several excellent texts.[85, 86] Some points to emphasize are as follows:

1. Supervoltage equipment is mandatory, preferably a 6-MeV accelerator in the United States, where cobalt is seldom used. 4-MeV accelerators generally have less favorable dose distribution characteristics.
2. For day to day reproducibility, good patient immobilization is important, using a device such as an alpha cradle.
3. The entire breast is treated to a dose of 45 to 50 Gy, with 1.8 to 2 Gy per treatment over approximately 5 weeks.
4. A boost dose to the tumor bed, for an approximate additional 15 Gy, is appropriate and of demonstrable benefit in improving local control, shown in numerous retrospective studies as well as one phase III trial.[87]
5. Treatment planning, preferably CT based, with tissue compensators to maximize dose homogeneity and also limit the lung and heart dose, is important for optimal results. Generally, bolus should not be used in early stage disease.

Nodal radiation along with breast treatment is controversial; phase III trials on the issue are lacking and one must draw inferences, largely from postmastectomy data. If ALND has been performed and all nodes are negative, most authorities would agree to limit radiation to the breast, because the risk of supraclavicular (SC) or internal mammary (IM) nodal involvement is low. If ALND reveals positive lymph nodes, our policy is to treat the SC and IM nodes, because risk of IM nodal involvement is about 30% in these circumstances (regardless of site of primary tumor in the breast). The lateral axilla is not treated, because axillary failure is rare after adequate surgery alone and axillary radiation in combination with ALND results in an increased rate of complications, particularly arm edema.[88] There is broad consensus for this treatment philosophy in patients with four or more axillary nodes involved, but there is less agreement for patients with one to three positive nodes. If the IM nodes are to be treated, technical issues assume an even greater importance if excessive cardiac toxicity is to be avoided.[88, 89] Nodes should be localized by CT and appropriate planning used to determine if they can be included safely in tangent fields or if a separate internal mammary field is needed. If a separate internal mammary field is employed, it must be a mixed photon-electron beam to decrease the cardiac dose.

There is little doubt that radiation therapy can effectively sterilize subclinical disease in nodes in greater than 95% of instances. If an ALND is not performed, whether to irradiate nodes or not constitutes a clinical judgment based on the likelihood that they are involved. That probability is derived from the characteristics of primary tumor (e.g., size). Overall, the expected survival benefit from treating clinically uninvolved nodal sites is small.

SELECTION OF PATIENTS

According to NCI recommendations, the majority of patients with small breast carcinomas are suitable for BCT. However, most do not receive it for complex reasons, including physician bias, access to radiation oncology facilities, and economic issues.[90] Increasing patient and physician education will be necessary to improve this situation.

Ideally, the patient for BCT has a small, less-than-4-cm, well-circumscribed tumor, normal-sized breasts, is not overweight, and has a small tumor-to-breast ratio so that excision of the tumor leaves a minor defect in the breast. Contraindications may be either tumor- or patient-related and stem from expectations of either a high local failure rate, increased normal tissue complications, or both. Most contraindications should be considered relative rather than absolute. Some patients may desire breast preservation so strongly that they are willing to accept an increased risk of local failure, an increased risk of normal tissue damage, or both.

Relative contraindications are shown in Table 17–10.[91] Regarding tumor-related factors, two or more carcinomas in different areas of the breast could perhaps be excised and the remaining breast radiated, but the local failure rate under these circumstances appears unacceptably high.[92] Obviously, patients with diffuse microcalcifications throughout the breast cannot have these excised short of mastectomy. Radiation is possible, but again the local failure rate is high. Similarly, the inability to obtain negative pathologic margins worsens the local control rate, although a focally positive margin may not be significant.[73, 74] For patients in whom

TABLE 17–10. **Relative Contraindications to BCT**

Tumor-related
Two or more pathologically separate tumors
Diffuse microcalcifications
Inability to obtain microscopically negative margins
Large tumor-to-breast ratio
Patient-related
Obesity or large breast size
Collagen-vascular disease, particularly scleroderma
History of previous breast radiation
Pregnancy

Modified from American College of Radiology, American Cancer Society, Society of Surgical Oncology guidelines.

there is a large tumor-to-breast ratio, excision of the tumor may so compromise the cosmesis that breast preservation is no longer meaningful.

A subareolar tumor location used to be considered a contraindication for breast preservation because of the need to excise the nipple-areolar complex. However, such excision may leave the patient with a perfectly acceptable breast otherwise and, of course, subsequent plastic surgical reconstruction of a nipple-areolar complex is always possible.

In almost all of the BCT trials reported to date, an increased failure rate in the breast (e.g., in patients with positive margins) has not been associated with worsened survival. Nevertheless, it is logical that local failure of invasive carcinoma in the breast must carry with it some risk of dissemination, and it may simply take a long time for this to become apparent. Recent data suggest that this is true.[93]

Patient characteristics are important. Previous breast radiation therapy generally rules out BCT. That situation may arise, for example, in patients with Hodgkin's disease who develop a radiation-induced carcinoma. Pregnancy is another contraindication, although some pregnant patients, particularly those in their third trimester, may be treated with local excision and chemotherapy with radiation delayed until after delivery. Most patients with collagen-vascular diseases, such as lupus erythematosus, may be irradiated, but severe late fibrosis of the breast and associated soft tissues has been reported in patients with scleroderma.[94]

The most common patient characteristic influencing the decision for BCT is overall weight or breast size. A number of published reports demonstrate that larger patients tend to have worse long-term cosmetic results.[95, 96] This may be partly because of technical problems with treatment, such as difficulty with immobilization or greater dose inhomogeneity. Acute skin reactions are invariably worse due to skin folding, which reduces the skin sparing of supervoltage. There may also be a greater tendency for excess fatty tissue to scar and fibrose. Obese patients or those with a large breast size, unfortunately, also present a greater problem for breast reconstruction. Patient involvement in the decision-making process is critical, as well as multidisciplinary consultation, in order to select the best approach for any one individual. Certain patients may wish to select the therapy that their physician would regard as second choice, accepting an increased risk of either local failure or greater complications.

Postmastectomy Radiation Therapy

Despite the efficacy of BCT and the recommendations of the National Institutes of Health Consensus Conference, the majority of patients in the United States and throughout the world continues to be treated with mastectomy. Adjuvant systemic therapy (ASRx) has become increasingly used, with almost all patients in the United States with a primary tumor larger than 1 cm receiving some form of ASRx (see "Adjuvant Systemic Therapy" in this chapter). Historically, before the introduction of adjuvant systemic therapy, postmastectomy radiation therapy was commonly used for patients deemed to be high risk for local failure, as well as systemic recurrence following RM or MRM[97]; it was routinely employed for patients undergoing TM. Criteria varied somewhat, but generally patients considered to be high risk for local-regional recurrence (LRR) are the same ones most at risk for distant metastases, that is, those with positive axillary nodes, large primary tumors, or both.[77] The relationship between the extent of disease and the risk of local failure (and probably distant metastases) is roughly linear. Subdivisions into categories such as one to three positive nodes or greater than four positive nodes may be convenient analytically, but they should not be interpreted as having biologic significance.

The rationale, initially, for postmastectomy radiation therapy was to improve survival through better local-regional treatment. A secondary objective was to improve local control, even if survival benefits were not realized; LRR following mastectomy is often difficult to control with subsequent measures. The generally accepted outcome for treatment of a local recurrence is that approximately 50% of patients will achieve local control.[49, 50, 97] Failure results in significant morbidity and occasional mortality.

Over the years, a voluminous and controversial literature has been published regarding postmastectomy radiation therapy. Although many trials have been carried out, they have occurred over several decades and have been heterogeneous in nature. Problems include greatly varying radiation techniques and equipment, inconsistent use of adjuvant systemic therapy, inclusion of low-risk patients (i.e., those who are node negative), as well as those at much higher risk for failure and, not least, a number of statistical problems, such as inadequate numbers of patients in the trials to detect small differences, unequal patient distribution among the treatment arms, and lack of a consistent randomization process.[49, 50, 98] Despite these criticisms, some general conclusions arise:

- Postmastectomy radiation decreases the risk of local failure by approximately 66% to 75%. This has been a consistent finding in almost all the trials.
- To achieve maximum decrease in LRR requires irradiation of all the local-regional sites at risk, that is, the chest wall and regional lymph nodes, although the most common site of LRR is clearly the chest wall, followed by the supraclavicular area.
- Axillary failure, with or without radiation to the full axilla, is very uncommon (1%) following axillary lymph node dissection in which at least 10 lymph nodes are removed.[82]
- The inclusion of internal mammary lymph nodes in the radiation fields is particularly controversial, given a lesser failure rate in these nodes compared with the other sites, as well as an increased complication rate if good technique is not employed.[48, 89, 99, 100] Further discussion of the IM node controversy is beyond the scope of this chapter.

Although a decrease in LRR is a highly desirable objective in its own right, improved survival remains the ultimate goal of any cancer treatment. The evidence regarding postmastectomy radiation therapy in this respect is less clear-cut. Before adjuvant systemic therapy, the question was whether postmastectomy radiation therapy could improve survival compared with mastectomy alone. Some limitations of earlier studies have already been mentioned;

however, in general, these individual trials did not show any survival benefit for the radiated patients. Much new information, however, has been forthcoming. Data from eight phase III trials were subjected to meta-analysis by Cuzick and associates in 1987, then reanalyzed in 1994 by the same authors in a highly unusual publication, which essentially stated that the previous report was in error.[101, 102] The later analysis demonstrated a decrease in breast cancer–related deaths in patients receiving postmastectomy radiation therapy, with an approximate 5% to 10% absolute increase in breast cancer–related survival. Unfortunately, those results were offset by an increase in non–cancer-related deaths in the patients who were irradiated, principally owing to excessive cardiac mortality. In these patients, those with left-sided breast carcinoma fared worse than those with a right-sided lesion, patients treated with orthovoltage did worse than those treated with supervoltage, and patients in the earlier trials did worse than those in more modern trials. The authors concluded that better techniques would undoubtedly decrease the frequency of cardiac problems and would, in all probability, increase overall survival.

A second meta-analysis was carried out in 1995 by the Early Breast Cancer Trialists' Collaborative Group.[98] Thirty-six trials, initiated before 1985, some of which included adjuvant systemic therapy, were evaluated and analyzed. A two-thirds reduction in LRR was found in the patients who were irradiated and the effect was greater in patients with positive nodes. Again, there was some improvement in cancer-related deaths offset by an increased toxicity from the radiation, particularly in older women.

Given the proven benefit of ASRx, the appropriate question is the worth of postmastectomy radiation therapy in patients who are receiving ASRx. The rationale is twofold and encompasses both the Halsted and Fisher hypotheses. If breast carcinoma spreads in an orderly fashion, then some additional patients will be cured by better local-regional treatment. If the disease is disseminated shortly after onset, chemotherapy might control distant sites but fail locally because of an increased tumor burden locally. The addition of radiation therapy would prevent these local failures and hence increase the likelihood of cure of the patient.[48, 98]

Approximately 15 phase III trials have explored the worth of radiation in addition to adjuvant systemic therapy in both patients who were node positive and node negative.[50] These trials have consistently shown a decrease in local-regional recurrence, a general increase in disease-free survival, but a variable effect on overall survival. However, many of the trials have enrolled insufficient numbers of patients to demonstrate small survival advantages. Nonetheless, two of the larger trials, updated trials from Denmark and Canada, have both shown an approximate 10% absolute increase in survival, an improvement of the same order of magnitude as obtained with adjuvant systemic therapy. This lends further support to the use of radiation in addition to systemic therapy.[46, 47]

Therefore, what conclusions are reasonable at this time regarding postmastectomy radiation therapy, drawing not only on the breast cancer data but also on our knowledge of tumor biology and experience in other malignancies? Carcinomas that exhibit local-regional failure as a significant component of the pattern of failure generally benefit from combined treatment using both local and systemic therapies. The evidence is clear that local control is improved with the addition of radiation to both surgery and systemic therapy. Patients with positive nodes are the greatest beneficiaries, because they are at highest risk and exhibit an improved survival (as far as cancer deaths are concerned) when treated with radiation in addition to systemic therapy. This is the case for patients undergoing BCT as well as mastectomy. In older series, there has been a clear increase in cardiovascular deaths as a consequence of the radiation therapy; however, it is likely that modern radiation techniques will prevent future excessive cardiovascular mortality.

Systemic Therapy

Systemic therapy is the main element of treatment for patients with metastatic disease and is widely used for breast cancer, generally with the majority of patients with localized disease receiving some form of adjuvant therapy with either chemotherapy, hormonal agents, or both. The rationale for adjuvant systemic therapy is straightforward: many patients with ostensibly localized breast carcinoma will subsequently develop distant metastases, despite effective local therapy, and will eventually succumb to their disease. Because such patients are presumed to have subclinical metastases at the time of the diagnosis, effective systemic therapy is necessary, as well as optimal local-regional treatment. Systemic therapy is thought to be more effective when the tumor burden is small (i.e., there is no clinically detectable metastatic disease), hence early administration of systemic therapy at this time has a strong rationale.[35, 42]

An enormous research effort has been undertaken in this area in the last three decades, with literally thousands of published reports and greater than 120 prospective randomized trials of adjuvant systemic therapy. Those research efforts have resulted in the following:

1. *Identification of prognostic variables to determine which patients are most likely to be cured with local-regional treatment alone.* Despite examination of many prognostic variables (at least 30 in many published series), only two have gained widespread acceptance: primary tumor size and nodal status.[77, 103–105] For data analysis, patients are routinely grouped according to these two variables, as well as age and hormonal receptor status. Age and hormonal receptor status are important for their impact on the choice of, and response to, adjuvant systemic therapy.
2. *Identification of active agents against disseminated disease.* An underlying principle of adjuvant systemic therapy is that one should preferably use agents with demonstrated activity in the metastatic disease setting. However, the treatment of metastatic disease remains far from satisfactory, so that identification of agents active against metastases is a major research goal with the dual purpose of improving the therapy of both overt metastatic disease as well as adjuvant treatment.

TABLE 17–11. **Common Pharmacologic Agents for Breast Carcinoma**

	Agent	Comment
Hormonal:	Tamoxifen	Antiestrogen; generally first hormonal treatment of choice
	Anastrozole	Aromatase inhibitor; second-line treatment only for postmenopausal women
	Megestrol acetate	Progestin; second-line treatment
	Leuprolide acetate	LHRH agonist; produces medical oophorectomy; for premenopausal women
Chemotherapy:	Doxorubicin	Widely used, highly active anthracycline
	Paclitaxel	FDA-approved in 1990s; widely used, highly active
	Cyclophosphamide	Alkylating agent in use for decades; most often combined with doxorubicin or methotrexate and 5-fluorouracil (5-FU)
	Methotrexate	Antimetabolite; used for decades in combination with cyclophosphamide and 5-FU
	5-Fluorouracil (5-FU)	Antimetabolite; used for decades; generally in combination with cyclophosphamide and methotrexate; new oral formulations

3. *Randomized trials.* Multiple protocols in the adjuvant setting have the goal of improving both disease-free and, more importantly, overall survival. Toward this end, randomized trials have attempted to find the optimal combination of agents, duration of therapy, doses, and scheduling.

Table 17–11 lists some of the commonly used pharmacologic agents in the management of breast carcinoma. To organize and make sense of the vast amount of data that have been accrued, the Early Breast Cancer Trialists' Collaborative Group was formed about 20 years ago. That group has subsequently published a number of key overviews and meta-analyses of the data, which form the basis for much of the practice of adjuvant systemic therapy today.[106–108] Results of these analyses are presented in detail in a subsequent section (see "Results and Prognosis"), but a number of important principles have been demonstrated to date:

1. The impact of a systemic therapy, in terms of the *reduction in relative risk of relapse or death,* appears to be the same for groups of patients with different prognoses, although it is not the same in terms of absolute benefit. In other words, a patient with a good prognosis, for example, a woman with negative nodes who has a small primary tumor, would derive the same relative risk reduction from chemotherapy as would a high-risk patient with positive nodes. A patient with a higher risk of relapse and death, however, would derive a larger absolute benefit.
2. Chemotherapy is effective both in women younger than 50 and in those aged 50 to 69. The reduction in relative risk of relapse or death, however, is approximately twice as great in those younger than 50 than those 50 to 69. After adjustment for age, proportional reductions in risk are similar for women who are node negative and node positive and are also unrelated to menopausal status and whether or not hormonal manipulations, such as tamoxifen, have been employed.
3. Regarding the type and dosage of administration of chemotherapy, an overview analysis indicates that polychemotherapy (i.e., two or three drugs) is better than single-agent chemotherapy, although there was no indication of benefit for administration of more than three drugs. Three to six months of chemotherapy seems adequate, with no additional benefits from longer administration. As yet, there is no demonstrable benefit for high-dose chemotherapy in conjunction with stem cell support, and there is no definite indication that any one type of chemotherapy is superior to another. However, there is a small but not significant trend in favor of doxorubicin containing combinations, particularly for women over the age of 50.
4. For women younger than age 50, the reduction in recurrence rates with chemotherapy is the same, approximately, for women who are either receptor negative or positive. In contrast, for women 50 or older, the reduction in relative risk of relapse is twice as great for women who are receptor negative versus receptor positive.
5. Tamoxifen has been found to be highly effective in reducing risk of relapse or death as a result of breast cancer, although its effects are limited to patients who are receptor positive. The reduction in risk of relapse with 5 years of tamoxifen is double that for 1 year of therapy, and proportional mortality and risk reductions are similar for women with node-positive or node-negative disease. Benefits are unrelated to age, menopausal status, and whether or not chemotherapy has been given.

Principles of Management

Unfortunately, about 40% of all breast cancer patients will develop distant metastases and succumb to their disease. Most metastases are manifest within the first 5 years of diagnosis, but late relapses are frequent and may occur 10 or even 20 years after the diagnosis of the primary disease. The time to relapse is inversely related to the size of the primary lesion and the nodal status.[51]

At the time of writing, metastatic disease remains incurable with conventional chemotherapy or hormonal therapy, although long survival is possible. High-dose chemotherapy (HDC) with stem cell support has been reported to achieve a 20% long-term survival in phase II trials.[109] This has led to a marked growth in the use of high-dose chemotherapy in both the United States and worldwide, so that breast cancer is now the commonest indication for this procedure. Other studies have suggested, however, that patient selection is largely responsible for the promising results reported with high-dose chemotherapy[110, 111]; the final results of phase III trials exploring this question are still unavailable. Given the toxicity and expense of HDC, it is probably wise to restrict its use to clinical trials.

There is no evidence that early treatment of metastatic breast carcinoma prolongs survival; therefore, early diagnosis of metastatic disease in asymptomatic patients is of no clear benefit. Hence, follow-up of patients with treated localized breast carcinoma is limited and governed by the objective of detecting situations that are potentially curable. In practice, this means a focus on early detection of opposite breast primaries or local recurrence in the breast of a patient treated with BCT. It is necessary, however, to investigate any symptoms suggestive of metastatic disease. The symptoms should be of new onset, persistent usually for at least several weeks, and be progressive. Routine bone and CT scans of chest or abdomen in the absence of symptoms are of little value and are no longer obtained in most centers.

The goal of managing metastatic disease is to palliate symptoms and maximize both the duration and quality of life for the patient. Factors that will influence how such management is undertaken include patient age, hormone receptor status of the tumor, the interval between the initial diagnosis of the primary lesion and relapse, and the extent of disease and sites of involvement at the time of relapse. Once a diagnosis of metastases has been established, it is usually appropriate to perform a number of imaging studies to determine the extent of disease. This approach will guide subsequent therapy and provide prognostic information. Patients with metastases are usually subdivided according to whether the pattern of disease is predominantly soft tissue (e.g., local-regional recurrence on the chest wall or in regional nodes), bone, or visceral organ in descending prognostic order. Other important prognostic variables are

- time interval between the diagnosis of the primary carcinoma and the development of metastases (the longer, the better)
- the number of involved sites and extent of involvement (the fewer, the better)
- the hormone receptor status (the more positive, the better)
- central nervous system (CNS) involvement (a poor prognostic sign)

As is the case in managing primary breast carcinoma, the approach to metastatic disease needs to be multidisciplinary in nature, and systemic therapy is the mainstay of treatment. Specific situations, however, often call for local treatment, usually in the form of radiation. Examples are CNS metastases, limited-in-volume bone metastases, and local-regional recurrence. The choice of systemic therapy is governed by a number of the prognostic variables already mentioned. The most important variable is the hormone receptor status. For estrogen receptor (ER) and/or progesterone receptor (PR) positive tumors, hormonal therapy is generally the initial treatment, because it is less toxic than chemotherapy. Increasingly, many patients have taken tamoxifen in the adjuvant setting, but in those who are tamoxifen naive or who have been off of tamoxifen for more than one year, this agent is usually the first choice. In patients who have never received tamoxifen, the response rate is 30% to 60%, with a median duration of response of 1 to 2 years.[112]

Ultimately, however, resistance develops to tamoxifen. Whether a patient has received the drug in the metastatic setting and responded, or has had disease progression on adjuvant tamoxifen, additional hormonal therapy is worthy of consideration. In women who are premenopausal, either ovarian ablation (medical, surgical, or radiotherapeutic) or megestrol acetate is a reasonable second-line approach. In postmenopausal women, treatment with either an aromatase inhibitor (anastrozole or letrozole) or megestrol acetate is appropriate.[113–115] With second-line treatment, objective response rates tend to be in the 10% to 20% range, with another 30% of patients experiencing disease stabilization for 6 months or longer. In patients who respond to a second-line hormonal approach, third-line treatment can also be considered.

Systemic chemotherapy is used for patients with metastatic disease who present with extensive visceral involvement, are refractory to hormonal therapy, or whose tumor hormone receptors are negative. Many single agents have demonstrated activity in metastatic breast carcinoma. The most active ones include doxorubicin, epirubicin, paclitaxel, docetaxel, vinorelbine, cyclophosphamide, 5-FU, methotrexate, vinblastine, and vincristine. Common practice has been to use various combinations of agents, although it is not clear that this is superior to single agents used in sequence.[116, 117] At least two recent trials have demonstrated the overall equivalence of single agents compared with combination treatment.[118, 119] Major advantages of single-agent therapy include the ability to deliver full drug doses and the possibility of avoiding additional toxicities.

Special Considerations

Ductal Carcinoma *In Situ*

DCIS may be defined as a proliferation of malignant epithelial cells within the confines of the mammary ducts and lobules, without invasion through the basement membrane. DCIS was first described in the 1930s, although the original reports did not clearly distinguish between cases with and without microinvasion. It was believed to be a malignant condition, however, and RM was recommended as the therapy of choice. The distinction between DCIS and invasive carcinoma did not become clear for several decades, with the term *DCIS* being introduced in the 1960s. The history of DCIS is nicely reviewed by Frykberg and associates.[30]

Initially, in the premammography era, DCIS was thought to be a rare condition constituting approximately 2% of all breast carcinomas. Its natural history was unclear because very few cases went untreated. Two small series, each with approximately 30 patients, from Vanderbilt University and Memorial Sloan-Kettering Cancer Center respectively, identified patients with biopsies originally thought to be benign, but that, on retrospective review, turned out to harbor DCIS.[120, 121] In both of these studies, in which the tumor was excised with no particular effort to obtain negative margins, the subsequent risk of invasive carcinoma was 30% to 50% over 10 to 15 years.

With the introduction of mammography and its subsequent widespread adaptation, the situation with respect to DCIS changed drastically. The incidence of DCIS increased markedly, and it is now estimated to be approximately 30% to 40% of all mammographically discovered carcinomas and 15% to 20% of the 200,000 new cases of breast carcinoma (invasive or noninvasive) diagnosed in the United States.[2] Because most DCIS cases are now diagnosed by mammography, the size of the average DCIS has markedly decreased, with most lesions now less then 2 cm in size.[122]

With increasing attention to the pathologic and biologic features of DCIS, it is now recognized that DCIS is quite heterogeneous biologically, as well as pathologically, and that the different forms undoubtedly have different risks of progression to frank invasive carcinoma.[123–125] Pathologically, DCIS has been subdivided into comedo and noncomedo types, with noncomedo including cribriform, papillary, micropapillary, and solid. Comedo types are frequently associated with a high nuclear grade, aneuploidy, high proliferative rate, and an overexpression of a number of oncogenes, such as *ERBB2,* cyclin D1, and p53; there may be an added mixture of histologic types.[126, 127] Silverstein and coworkers suggest the importance of nuclear grade, independent of comedo or noncomedo type, as a prognostic variable[125, 128]; the comedo type of DCIS may have a greater tendency for malignant progression or local recurrence following BCT compared with noncomedo types.

Much confusion has arisen regarding the issues of multicentricity or multifocality of DCIS; these entities have not always been clearly defined in the past. Now, however, multicentricity describes disease outside the original quadrant of the breast where the index lesion was found, whereas multifocality refers to the presence of malignant cells elsewhere within the same quadrant of the breast as the primary tumor. The elegant studies of Holland and colleagues have done much to clarify this situation,[129] with multicentricity being very unusual and multifocality being common. The Holland data also appear to relate the extent of the margin at the time of local excision to the likelihood that additional cells will be found in a mastectomy specimen—the wider the clear margin, the lesser the chance of residual cells. Thus, margin status should be thought of as a surrogate for local tumor burden.

The treatment of DCIS is perhaps even more controversial than that for invasive carcinoma. Reasons for controversy include the long natural history of the disease, making judgment of the efficacy of treatment more difficult, as well as DCIS still being much less common than invasive carcinoma and, therefore, having fewer patients available for entry into the large phase III trials that have resolved many controversial issues in invasive breast cancer. Some key points, however, need to be kept in mind:

- DCIS, almost by definition, does not metastasize. The frequency of axillary nodal involvement is less than 1% in all large series, and that percentage is believed to represent cases in which the invasive component was missed in the original diagnosis.[130, 131] Thus, neither axillary lymph node dissection is indicated nor is axillary radiation.
- There would appear to be no role for adjuvant chemotherapy because of the excellent prognosis (discussed later) and the lack of distant metastases. Tamoxifen, however, has been shown to reduce recurrences when combined with lumpectomy and radiation.[132]
- One must clearly distinguish between local control of DCIS in the breast and survival. Death as a result of breast cancer in all reported series of DCIS patients is rare. In reviews by Fowble and associates,[130] as well as Frykberg and colleagues,[30] the mortality in both mastectomy patients and those treated with BCT was 1% to 2% at 10 years. Again, most authorities would agree that the breast cancer deaths were likely due to unrecognized invasive carcinoma at the time of diagnosis.

Historically, the treatment of DCIS was RM (TM in recent years). A number of factors contributed to a reluctance to use BCT, including that the disease was believed to be multicentric, multifocal, or both, and the notion that DCIS was somehow more radioresistant than invasive breast cancer. This notion was based on the increased local failure rate noted with patients with invasive breast carcinoma that had an extensive intraductal component.[133] The presence of an extensive intraductal component, however, appears in retrospect to be a surrogate for tumor burden and does not convey any intrinsic radioresistance.[134]

However, with the success of BCT in invasive breast carcinoma, a number of investigators have turned their attention to the use of BCT in DCIS. Almost all of the published trials to date are phase II studies, involving relatively small numbers of patients.[135, 136] A number of phase III trials have been initiated, principally in Europe, but only one has been published to date.[137] Interestingly, none of the published or ongoing trials directly compare mastectomy with local excision, either alone or when combined with radiation, but all are trials of local excision versus local excision plus radiation therapy, with or without tamoxifen.

The results of treatment of DCIS with mastectomy have been reviewed by Frykberg and colleagues.[30] Data were combined from fourteen published series in which 1061 women underwent mastectomy for DCIS. The overall local recurrence rate was approximately 1%, with an overall cancer mortality of 1.7%. Overall, breast cancer recurrence rates at 10 to 15 years range from 10% to 19% in patients treated with BCT[30, 130, 131, 136] and breast cancer mortality has ranged from 1% to 4%. Most of these series are comprised of patients treated over many years, without particular separation for prognostic variables or particular attention to obtaining negative margins at the time of local excision. A more homogeneous group of patients are the 818 women in the NSABP trial who were randomized to receive local excision alone or local excision plus whole breast radiation, with negative margins required for entry into the trial[137] (Figs. 17–5 and 17–6). The trial was unable to identify *any* subset of patients who did not benefit from the addition of radiation, although the trial has been criticized for the lack of accurate information as to size of the tumors.

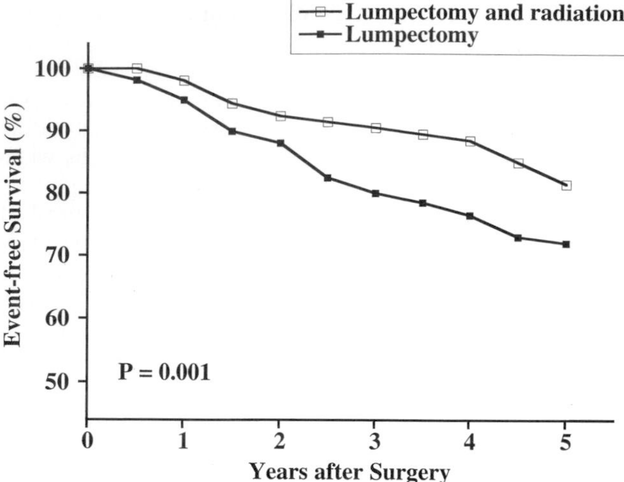

Figure 17–5. Event-free survival rate of women treated by lumpectomy or lumpectomy and radiation therapy. (Modified from Fisher B, Costantino J, Redmond C, et al: Lumpectomy compared with lumpectomy and radiation therapy for the treatment of intraductal breast cancer. N Engl J Med 1993; 328:1581–1586.)

In contrast to the NSABP trial, Silverstein, Lagios, and coworkers have suggested that prognostic variables may be important in determining outcome and treatment.[125, 128, 138] In a retrospective analysis, they determined that tumor size, width of the surgical margin, and pathologic classification (primarily nuclear grade and necrosis) could identify groups of patients with low, high, and intermediate risks of local failure. They suggested that the low-risk group did not need radiation at all, the high-risk group needed mastectomy, and the intermediate-risk group perhaps was the one that would most benefit from radiation plus excision. Additional prospective trials, involving large numbers of patients and controlling for prognostic variables, will be necessary to further resolve these issues. It does appear, however, that the risk of death as a result of breast cancer in patients diagnosed with DCIS is extraordinarily low, irrespective of the type of initial therapy.

Based on the previous discussion, our treatment recommendations are as follows:

- Patients with DCIS desirous of BCT should have the pathologic abnormality excised with negative margins.
- Patients with unfavorable histologic features (necrosis, high nuclear grade, comedo features) or tumor greater than 1 cm in size should receive postexcision radiation (46 to 50 Gy) to the entire breast, with a tumor bed boost of an additional 10 to 15 Gy.
- Axillary dissection is not necessary.
- Tamoxifen may be valuable for some patients.
- Patients with a favorable histologic picture and small primary lesions of less than 1 cm, whose tumor is widely excised, may be candidates for observation only.

Lobular Carcinoma *In Situ*

LCIS is a relatively uncommon incidental finding in breast tissue; the group at Columbia University introduced the term *lobular neoplasia* to emphasize, in their view, that this was not really a malignant or premalignant lesion but rather a marker for a subsequent risk of developing invasive carcinoma.[10] The microscopic appearance of LCIS is that of a solid proliferation of small cells, with generally uniform, round nuclei and scanty cytoplasm, and the basement membrane may or may not be disrupted. It may be difficult to distinguish this condition from invasive lobular carcinoma or even DCIS with lobular cancerization. Detailed pathologic descriptions may be found in literature from the late 1980s to the mid-1990s, as well as standard textbooks.[27, 28, 139, 140]

LCIS is almost always an incidental pathologic finding in breast tissue that was removed for some other reason. It does not result in tumors within the breast, nor is it usually visible mammographically, because it is usually not calcified. A recent report from NSABP does describe, however, calcification in 25% of LCIS lesions.[126] LCIS is an uncommon lesion with a reported incidence in biopsy specimens from 1% to 4%,[9, 31, 32, 141, 142] although it is more common in premenopausal women. Its frequency appears to be rising and the apparent increase in incidence may relate to the greater frequency with which breast biopsies are performed in recent years, owing to the heightened awareness of breast carcinoma.

The nature of LCIS is controversial. The appearance of the lesion under a microscope suggests malignancy in some respects, but the cells tend to have a low proliferative rate, and they are usually hormone receptor positive and negative for the expression of *HER2/neu*. There does not appear to be direct progression of the lesion of LCIS to invasive carcinoma; however, it represents a greatly increased risk of developing a subsequent breast cancer. The relative risk is estimated to be from 5 to 12 in a number of reports in the literature, with the 1996 update of the Columbia University series indicating a relative risk of 5.[10] NSABP data also suggest a lower frequency of subsequent invasive carcinoma (0.5% per year) than commonly supposed.[140] Invasive cancer may develop in either breast with equal frequency and there is no greater risk for the breast in which the LCIS was diagnosed. This finding in particular has led to the notion that LCIS is not a direct precursor of a subsequent cancer but rather a marker signifying a high risk of invasive cancer in either breast. In actuarial terms, the risk is approximately 1% per year, similar to the risk of a contralateral breast cancer in a woman who has had unilateral disease.

Treatment for LCIS has evolved in a conservative direction. The standard recommendation used to be mastectomy on the involved side. However, in view of the equal risk for the opposite breast, any therapy needs to be bilateral in nature. In the absence of established malignancy, radiation would appear to have no role; however, patients are candidates for chemoprevention with agents such as tamoxifen.[143–145] Most centers have adopted the policy of careful observation, although some patients, after careful discussion and assessment of the risks and benefits, may desire bilateral mastectomy. Observation must be a life long process, with mammograms performed at least annually. If a subsequent carcinoma develops, the histologic pattern is that most are usually seen in breast carcinoma; that is, the great majority of cases are infiltrating ductal and only a

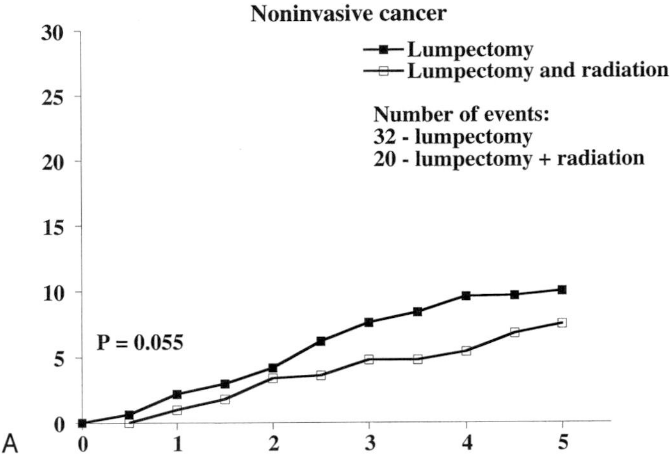

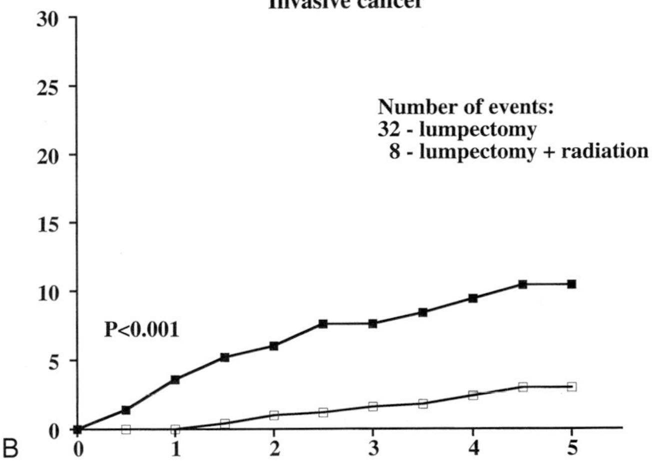

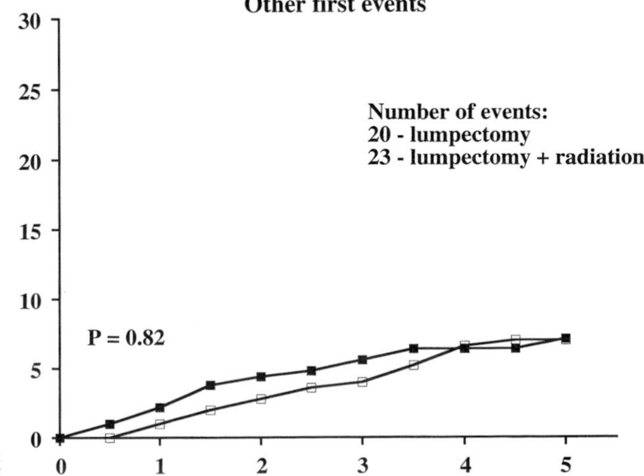

Figure 17–6. Cumulative incidence of noninvasive and invasive ipsilateral breast cancers and of all other first events in women treated by lumpectomy or lumpectomy and radiation therapy. (Modified from Fisher B, Costantino J, Redmond C, et al: Lumpectomy compared with lumpectomy and radiation therapy for the treatment of intraductal breast cancer. N Engl J Med 1993; 328:1581–1586.)

small minority infiltrating lobular, again suggesting that LCIS is not a direct precursor lesion.

Locally Advanced Breast Carcinoma

The category of locally advanced breast carcinoma (LABC) generally includes all patients with stage III disease, as defined by the AJCC classification system. The great majority of these patients have large primary tumors in the breast (T3 or T4), with or without axillary lymph node involvement. Technically, patients with small primary tumors with fixed nodes (N2 or N3) are stage III, but in practice such patients are rare. Inflammatory breast carcinoma (IBC) is a special type of LABC, characterized clinically by signs of inflammation in the breast and pathologically by tumor involvement of dermal lymphatics. Clinical signs of inflammation and pathologic involvement of skin lymphatics do not always accompany one another; the presence of either one alone is sufficient for the diagnosis of inflammatory cancer.

LABC patients are a heterogeneous group. Previous definitions included patients with T3N0 disease, who were primarily operable with an outlook not too different from stage II carcinoma, as well as those with rapidly progressive inflammatory carcinoma. Patients with T3N0 disease are now classified as having stage IIB disease, but they are included in many older literature reports as stage III. The vast majority of patients in stage III, however, have large, unresectable tumors with an unfavorable outlook. Fortunately, LABC is not common in developed countries and appears to be declining in frequency with the increasing use of mammography. It currently accounts for about 5% to 10% of cases in most major medical centers, with some correlation to the socioeconomic characteristics of the center's population, tending to be seen more often in those with less access to medical care. In developing countries, the frequency may be considerably higher.

The frequency of IBC is approximately 1% to 2% of all newly diagnosed breast cancer; however, its frequency is increasing rapidly.[146] The incidence of IBC among whites doubled from 0.3 to 0.7 cases per 100,000 person/years when comparing two periods of time (1975–1977 and 1990–1992). The frequency of IBC in black women is higher than that in whites: 5% to 10% of all breast cancers compared with 1% to 2% in the white population. The mean age of patients presenting with IBC appears to be similar to that of patients with noninflammatory cancer.[146]

Historically, most cases of LABC were considered to be not resectable. Indeed, surgery was believed to be contraindicated by authorities such as Haagensen, who declared that such patients were better treated by radiation therapy alone and that surgery would only hasten a poor outcome.[38] During the 1970s and 1980s, a number of reports were published of the results of therapy with radiation alone.[147, 148] Generally, these reports demonstrated 5-year survivals in the range of 30% to 50%, 10-year survivals at 20% to 30%, with 10-year disease-free survivals generally not exceeding 20%. Local control approximated 50% at 5 years, dropping to the range of 30% to 40% by 10 years.

These inadequate results, together with the well-known successes of adjuvant systemic therapy for earlier stage breast carcinoma, led rapidly to the introduction of systemic chemotherapy early in the treatment program for LABC. Additionally, a renewed interest in mastectomy developed, because local control achieved with radiation therapy alone, even with high doses in the range of 60 to 75 Gy, was disappointing, in the range of 30% to 40% long-term. Thus, therapy gradually evolved to employ all three modalities of systemic therapy (chemotherapy, hormone manipulations, or both), radiation, and mastectomy.

The trend is illustrated well in a report from Washington University in 1994.[149] The authors reported a series of 280 women treated from 1968 through 1989 with four different treatment methods (radiation alone, radiation plus mastectomy, radiation plus systemic therapy, and all modalities combined). Ten-year survival was 11% in the group treated with radiation alone with local control at only 31%. When all modalities were combined together, 10-year survival was 36% and local control was 91%. Combinations of radiation plus chemotherapy without surgery and radiation plus mastectomy without systemic therapy led to intermediate outcomes between the two levels already quoted.

During the last two decades, many phase II trials were reported in which various combinations of modalities were employed with results similar to those reported by Perez and coworkers,[149] suggestive of the value of combined-modality treatment for LABC.[150, 151] Phase III trials, however, were not initially encouraging, with three negative trials appearing in the literature.[152–154] Failure of these trials to show added benefits from systemic therapy may be attributed to relatively few patients enrolled in the trials, with insufficient power to demonstrate a small benefit. In addition, systemic therapy may be less effective in the setting of a presumed increased tumor burden present both systemically as well as locally in LABC. Nevertheless, a phase III 1997 EORTC trial with 410 enrolled patients did succeed in demonstrating a 35% reduction in the risk of death in patients receiving combined radiation, hormonal therapy, and chemotherapy when compared with those treated with radiation alone.[155] Local control was achieved in only 40% to 70% of patients; further benefits might be expected to accrue with the addition of mastectomy. Additionally, patients were not selected for hormonal therapy on the basis of estrogen receptor status, two thirds of the patients were postmenopausal, and the chemotherapy administered was CMF in conventional doses.

Current treatment strategies in the United States often employ induction chemotherapy with an anthracycline-containing combination followed by mastectomy, radiation, and additional chemotherapy[150, 151, 156]; hormonal therapy is generally added for patients who are receptor positive.[151] The optimal sequencing of these therapies remains uncertain, but there is little doubt that all are necessary for best results. Because the great majority of LABC patients still succumb to disseminated disease, further improvements in this area will need to come from advances in systemic therapy.

Inflammatory Breast Cancer

IBC is a special type of LABC. It is defined in the 1997 AJCC Cancer Staging Manual as "a clinicopathologic entity characterized by diffuse brawny induration of the skin of the breast with an erysipeloid edge, usually without an underlying palpable mass."[33] However, the clinical picture of IBC can be present without pathologic involvement of dermal lymphatics; whether such cases should be classified as IBC remains somewhat controversial. Authors describe a somewhat worse prognosis for patients with both clinical and pathologic features of IBC compared with those with either clinical or pathologic features alone.[157, 158] Even with the broadest definition, however, the prognosis for the patient with IBC is still considerably poorer than for patients with other varieties of breast cancer.

The frequency of IBC is dependent upon the precise definition. Most of the cases in the SEER program, reported by Chang and colleagues, were diagnosed clinically, and thus the frequency in the SEER data is about 5% of all cases of breast cancer.[146] With more restrictive definitions, such as requirement of both clinical and pathologic features, the frequency of IBC drops markedly to between 0.5% and 1% of all breast cancers. In black women, the incidence is about double that of whites, namely about 10% of all breast carcinomas. The mean age of presentation is about 52 years, similar to that of patients with other forms of breast carcinoma.

Clinically, patients with IBC typically present with a history of a fairly rapid development of increasing size of the breast, firmness, tenderness, and redness of the overlying skin. Although the AJCC definition of IBC suggests that most patients do not have a palpable mass, Haagensen found that about 60% of patients did indeed have an underlying mass that could be felt.[38] Mammographically, IBC patients may demonstrate an increase in the skin thickness of the breast, increased tissue density, and widening of subcutaneous lymphatic vessels, with or without a definite mass lesion. Axillary lymph node involvement is very common with reported rates from 50% to 100%.[158]

Before the advent of effective systemic therapy, treatment results for IBC were very disappointing. Five-year survival rates with local therapy alone, be it mastectomy, radiation therapy, or a combination of the two, ranged from 0% to 10%.[159, 160] Local control was reported as approximately 10% to 15% in patients treated with mastectomy alone and 30% to 40% in those treated with radiation alone.[157, 158, 160] The higher control rates were reported in those receiving large doses of radiation, but they still were optimistic estimates, considering many patients die of systemic disease before sufficient time elapses to manifest local failure. The extremely poor local control rates obtained with surgery alone led Haagensen to indicate that RM was contraindicated in such patients, indeed often making the situation worse.[38] Although radiation therapy alone was an improvement over surgery, local control remained far from satisfactory, even with the addition of chemotherapy, and only in recent years has tri-modality therapy become increasingly common for this disease.

With the advent of effective systemic chemotherapy, there has been a fairly dramatic improvement in survival, with 5-year rates ranging from 10% to 60% (more commonly toward the upper end of the range) and 10-year survival rates in the neighborhood of 20%.[157, 158] Optimal results appear to be achieved by the use of all three modalities—chemotherapy, radiation, and surgery—with local control achieved in approximately 75% of patients; although, as mentioned earlier, long-term disease-free survival is still uncommon (around 20% at 10 years). These data on IBC are derived almost entirely from retrospective analyses or prospective single-arm trials. Because of the extremely poor prognosis of the disease without systemic therapy, there has been a great reluctance to randomize patients into any trial that would withhold systemic therapy from one group of patients.

Treatment policies for IBC have thus evolved to include all three modalities of chemotherapy (with or without hormonal therapy), radiation, and surgery in a similar fashion to LABC in general. Generally, therapy is started with an anthracycline-containing drug combination, and depending on the response, one may proceed with mastectomy if the tumor becomes surgically resectable or with radiation if the tumor does not. Patients whose disease becomes resectable after chemotherapy usually have mastectomy performed, followed by additional chemotherapy and radiation. The addition of chemotherapy and radiation appears necessary for optimal local control and probably contributes to survival as well.

Occult Primary Breast Carcinoma with Axillary Nodal Metastases

Breast carcinoma that presents as axillary nodal metastases without any obvious primary in the breast itself is a very uncommon but most interesting problem. The three largest series in the literature are reported from the Memorial Sloan-Kettering Cancer Center, the University of Texas M. D. Anderson Cancer Center, and the Instituto Nazionale Tumori in Milan, and they consist of 35, 42, and 60 patients, respectively, for an estimated incidence in these institutions of about 0.5% of all breast carcinomas.[108, 161, 162] Despite the rarity of the condition, however, there are a number of common conclusions reached by the authors:

- In a woman presenting with axillary adenopathy in whom the histologic diagnosis is adenocarcinoma, the site of the primary tumor is almost certainly the breast. An extensive work-up for a primary tumor at a site other than the breast is generally unproductive and should not be done unless symptoms or histologic appearance of the tumor suggest otherwise.
- Diagnostic evaluation should be limited to mammography and a chest x-ray film. The positivity rate of the mammogram is quite variable, from approximately 10% to 50%. Indeed, when mastectomy is carried out, a primary lesion is found in the breast less than half the time, with the frequency of such a finding undoubtedly related to the extent of pathologic study of the breast.
- Tissue from lymph nodes should be analyzed for the presence of estrogen and progesterone receptors. If positive, this provides additional evidence for a primary lesion in the breast, as well as helpful information for appropriate choice of adjuvant systemic therapy. Negative receptor studies, however, should not be interpreted as evidence against a primary lesion in the breast.

Treatment recommendations cannot be made with great confidence, given the small number of patients reported in any one series. As a first step, axillary dissection should be carried out only if a biopsy has been obtained (at least level 1 and 2). In addition to providing staging information, optimal local control is obtained in this fashion. The ipsilateral breast should be treated either with mastectomy or radiation. Not treating the breast has resulted in a local failure rate of about 50% in both the M. D. Anderson and Milan series. Local control achieved with mastectomy appears to be excellent, in excess of 90%. There are theoretical reasons why radiation to the breast might be less effective than mastectomy: there is no obvious tumor on which to perform a lumpectomy or an area of the breast to select for a boost dose of radiation. Indeed, some patients in whom primary tumors have been discovered at mastectomy have been found to have multifocal tumors. Despite these theoretical problems, however, BCT has been successfully practiced in a number of patients in the above institutions with apparent local control ranging from 80% to 90%.

These patients appear to have a somewhat better prognosis than patients who present conventionally with a primary lesion in the breast and are found to have axillary nodal metastases. Five-year survival in the Memorial Sloan-Kettering series was approximately 75%, decreasing to approximately 60% at 10 years; M. D. Anderson and Milan data are very similar. The authors comment that this appears to be somewhat better than might be expected for patients who present with disease in the breast and then are discovered to have axillary nodes.

Adjuvant systemic therapy has often been given to these patients and indeed would appear to be standard practice in the United States if not much of the world. There are, of course, no phase III data in this rare subgroup of breast cancer patients to prove the value of adjuvant systemic therapy. There are actually no particularly suggestive data in the published retrospective series to support the use of adjuvant systemic therapy either, but given the usefulness of adjuvant systemic therapy for breast cancer generally, the approach certainly seems reasonable.

Results and Prognosis

This section addresses results of the treatment of breast carcinoma in the modern era, drawing largely on data from prospective randomized trials, supplemented by data from individual retrospective institutional studies when appropriate. The many prospective trials over the last decade provide a firm foundation for our knowledge of the outcomes of treatment for this disease.

Stages I and II

Considering first the local therapy of stages I and II breast carcinoma, it has been stated previously that BCT and MRM or RM have resulted in equivalent survival in many retrospective series. Six randomized trials have also addressed this issue, two U.S. and four European studies that commenced in the 1970s and were updated in the 1990s.[63–68] In addition, two overviews of these trials have been published.[70, 98] These landmark studies have contributed greatly to our knowledge of breast cancer therapy; there are probably more good data available regarding appropriate therapy of breast carcinoma and the outcome of treatment than for almost any other malignant disease.

The results of the six trials are considered in Table 17–9. Together they comprise just over 5000 patients, with the largest being the NSABP trial with 2105 patients.[67] Actuarial survival, relapse-free survival, and local recurrence are calculated at the follow-up year specified in the table. The data presented may be considered representative of expected outcomes for both mastectomy and BCT; all of these trials have demonstrated the equivalency of mastectomy and BCT, with no statistically significant differences in outcome.

Features of the trial designs are shown in Table 17–12. All of the studies required axillary dissection; the percentage of patients with positive lymph nodes ranged from 30% to 40%. In all trials except the Gustave-Roussy, patients with positive lymph nodes received adjuvant systemic therapy. In the four European trials, patients with positive lymph nodes in the mastectomy arm received postmastectomy radiation therapy. In all the trials except NSABP, patients with negative lymph nodes in the BCT arm received nodal as well as breast irradiation; radiation doses ranged from 45 to 50 Gy to the breast and lymph nodes if included. Five of the six trials specified a boost to the tumor site of 10 to 25 Gy.

Survivals in these trials ranged between 60% and 80%, with the lower numbers representing a reflection of a longer time of follow-up. Local recurrence in patients who received BCT was 3% to 15%, again largely a reflection of the length of follow-up. Local recurrence occurred, for the

TABLE 17–12. **Breast Conservation Trials: Study Features**

	Margin Status	Staging	Adjuvant Systemic Chemotherapy	Postmastectomy Radiation Therapy	Radiation Boost
EORTC[63]	51% (+)	20% T1; 80% T2 40% pN0, 60% pN1	+	±	+
DBCG[64]	7% (+)	?	+	+	+
NCI[65]	?	45% T1; 55% T2 60% pN0; 40% pN1	+	−	+
Milan[66]	(−)	all T1, 30% N(+)	+	−	+
NSABP[67]	(−)	30% T1; 50% T2 65% pN0; 35% pN1	+	−	−
Gustave-Roussy[68]	?	all T1, 33% N(+)	−	±	+

? = Not specified; + = Yes; − = No; ± = Sometimes.

most part, in the treated breast (as opposed to lymph nodes) with many of these patients subsequently salvaged with mastectomy. In general, failure in the ipsilateral breast appeared to occur with a frequency of 0.66% to 0.75% per year of follow-up. Most local recurrences, particularly in the first 5 years, tended to occur at the site of the original tumor and probably represented a failure to control the original disease. Beyond 5 years, more and more local failures occurred elsewhere in the breast and were felt to represent the development of a new primary cancer in the ipsilateral breast because patients with one breast cancer are more likely to develop a second primary in the opposite breast. Less well appreciated is that normal breast tissue in the ipsilateral breast is also at risk for a second primary cancer. This is the probable explanation for many of the so-called local failures seen in the ipsilateral breast beyond 5 years.

Local-regional recurrences in the mastectomy group were observed in 3% to 14% of patients. In most studies, local recurrences in the BCT arm exceeded those in the mastectomy arm, but the latter conveyed a much worse outlook than the former. The majority of patients experiencing local-regional recurrence following mastectomy will eventually develop distant disease and succumb to breast carcinoma.[163, 164] In contrast, over half of patients experiencing local failure in the breast after BCT will achieve long-term survival with subsequent mastectomy.[165, 166] Thus, the distant disease rates in all of these trials were equivalent.

A recent interesting meta-analysis of these trials has been carried out.[70] The authors obtained original data from some of the trials for analysis and derived data from the published reports for those trials in which original data were not available. This meta-analysis confirmed the equivalency of BCT and mastectomy, particularly for patients with negative nodes. A statistically significant improvement in survival was demonstrated, however, for patients who were node positive and receiving adjuvant nodal radiotherapy, compared with those who did not. Thus, mastectomy without adjuvant radiation therapy in a patient with positive nodes appears to be inferior to BCT (including lymph nodes) with respect to survival.

The pooled data from this meta-analysis also provide a useful benchmark for expected outcomes according to primary tumor size and nodal status. These data are shown in Table 17–13. The indication from this meta-analysis is that survival is improved in patients who are node positive and receive BCT compared with those undergoing mastectomy without adjuvant postmastectomy radiation therapy. This is consistent with recent published trials, demonstrating a benefit for postmastectomy radiation therapy compared with mastectomy alone, with both treatment arms receiving appropriate adjuvant systemic therapy.[46, 47]

TABLE 17–13. **Pooled Survival Rates from Breast Conservation Therapy Trials**

	BCT		Mastectomy*	
Subset	***5-yr (%)***	***10-yr (%)***	***5-yr (%)***	***10-yr (%)***
Node (−)	92	81	92	80
Node (+)	81	62	76	57
T1	93	78	89	76
T2	78	62	79	57

*Includes RM, TM, MRM.

In addition to the phase III trials cited earlier, there is a large body of literature consisting of retrospective analyses of patients treated at a number of institutions throughout the world. This literature has served to develop and refine the selection criteria for choosing patients appropriate for BCT, and it has examined a variety of potential prognostic factors for their impact on local control and survival. Among those prognostic factors are the following:

- Margin status is probably the most important variable impacting local control. A large series from the Joint Center for Radiotherapy at Harvard showed a 2% local failure rate at 5 years in all patients with negative margins, compared with 16% if margins were involved with either invasive carcinoma or DCIS but not LCIS.[74] Data from Duke and the University of North Carolina similarly demonstrated 5-year actuarial local control rates of 98% and 90% respectively for patients with negative versus positive margins.[73] Neither close margins (1 to 10 mm) nor focally positive margins have led to increased local failure rates compared with widely negative margins.

  Margin status appears to be a surrogate for tumor burden in the breast with a continuum of risk; a negative margin does not mean residual tumor is not present. Indeed, in the NSABP series, local failure rates at 8 to 10 years were 40% in patients with negative surgical margins who did not receive postexcision radiation therapy.[67] Conversely, positive margins do not constitute an absolute contraindication to BCT. Clearly, the local failure rate will be increased compared with patients with negative margins, although it has not been shown that survival is adversely affected. Certain patients may wish to accept an increased risk of local failure for a reasonable chance at breast preservation.

  In view of the importance of margin status, patients undergoing lumpectomy with a plan for breast preservation should have the operative specimen inked in order to facilitate margin determination. Patients with positive margins or those that are indeterminate because of specimen handling and who are desirous of BCT should undergo re-excision of the tumor area when feasible.
- Other factors thought to be important for risk of local failure include the presence of extensive intraductal carcinoma (EIC) in the pathologic specimen, young patient age, and the presence of vascular invasion.[133, 167] Much attention was formerly given to EIC, but it is probably a surrogate for margin status and tumor burden. Updated analyses of the JCRT series have shown that EIC does not adversely effect local control if negative margins are obtained surgically.[74, 134] Achieving negative margins is sometimes more difficult in the patient with EIC, however.
- Young age (less than 35 years) tends to be associated with EIC, positive margins, and a somewhat increased risk for distant metastases, as well as local failure following mastectomy or radiation therapy.[168, 169]

Young patients with negative lumpectomy margins may be offered BCT with the expectation of a slight increase in local failure but still an acceptable outcome. In a large series of 1026 patients from the Netherlands, vascular invasion was associated with an 8% risk of breast recurrence at 5 years compared with 1% for patients without adverse risk factors.[167]

- Initially, in the early days of BCT, there were concerns that patients with larger primary tumors (i.e., T2), positive axillary lymph nodes, or both were not good candidates for BCT because of a presumed increased tumor burden. Although such patients obviously have an increased risk of distant metastases and death compared with their node negative T1 counterparts, this has not been reflected in higher rates of local failure when treated with BCT. Indeed, one could argue for BCT in such patients in view of the desirability of postoperative radiation therapy should they undergo mastectomy.

Postmastectomy Radiation Therapy

The rationale for the use of postmastectomy radiation therapy (PMRT) in the era of adjuvant systemic therapy was presented earlier and some of the results cited. Focusing on phase III trials, however, we will quantify some of these data further.

All phase III trials comparing surgery alone (RM, MRM, or TM) with surgery plus radiation therapy, but without any adjuvant systemic therapy, and initiated before 1975 were updated and subjected to meta-analysis by Cuzick and associates.[101, 102] These trials used radiation therapy techniques and doses far from the optimal and included approximately 8000 women. Entry criteria varied, but most patients were node positive, had large primary tumors, or both. Overall, there were no survival differences between patients who received radiation therapy and those who did not, but this appeared to be a result of an excess of cardiac deaths in the patients who were irradiated, balanced by a reduction in breast cancer mortality in the same patients. In the Cuzick analysis, the later trials (1970s) tended to show a decrease in breast cancer mortality in patients who were irradiated, as well as no excess of cardiac deaths. However, the data were reported in terms of the effect on standard mortality ratios and thus are difficult to compare directly to survival benefits achieved by other modalities.

The findings were, however, similar to a second meta-analysis by the Early Breast Cancer Trialists' Collaborative Group.[98] This group examined 36 trials initiated before 1985, involving approximately 29,000 women. Surgery varied from lumpectomy to RM, but most patients had some variety of mastectomy. Both node negative and node positive women were included. A two-thirds reduction in local failure and a significant diminution in the odds of death as a result of breast carcinoma were seen, but this was again counterbalanced by an increased risk of cardiac deaths, particularly in women over age 60 who were irradiated. Overall, no survival differences between patients who were irradiated and those who did not receive radiation were observed.

Overall, 13 phase III trials have explored the use of PMRT in conjunction with adjuvant systemic therapy.[50] Most of these trials suffered from inadequate patient numbers and some from suboptimal radiation therapy techniques and doses. Two trials from Denmark and British Columbia, however, are noteworthy.[46, 47] Both of these trials included patients who were node positive or had T3 primary carcinomas; most patients had T1 or T2 primary lesions and one to three positive lymph nodes. The British Columbia trial demonstrated a 33% reduction in the risk of recurrent disease, a 29% reduction in the risk of breast cancer mortality, and a 26% reduction in overall mortality, corresponding to absolute gains in survival of 10% and 8%, respectively.[47] The Danish trial showed a 9% absolute improvement in survival between patients who received radiation therapy and those who did not, and a 54% 10-year survival rate in patients who received radiation therapy compared with 45% for those receiving surgery and systemic therapy without radiation.[46] On the other hand, a carefully controlled ECOG trial of PMRT for locally advanced breast carcinoma failed to show any benefit for the irradiated patients.[170]

A number of nonrandomized trials (reviewed by Fowble[50]) examined the risk of local-regional failure in patients treated with mastectomy and systemic adjuvant therapy. These studies showed that patients with primary tumors exceeding 5 cm or with four or more positive axillary nodes have an approximate 25% to 30% incidence of local-regional failure, despite adjuvant systemic therapy. In contrast, patients with primary tumors less than 2 cm or with negative axillary nodes have a low incidence of local-regional recurrence—5% to 10%. Patients with intermediate sized primaries and one to three positive nodes have a 10% to 20% risk of local-regional recurrence. These data have led to the recommendation by many U.S. authorities for PMRT in patients with four or more positive nodes and/or primary tumors greater than 5 cm. This is despite the fact that most patients who entered into the Danish and Canadian trials were intermediate in risk, that is, had primary tumors between 2 and 5 cm and one to three positive nodes.

Thus, the debate regarding the value of PMRT continues concerning the appropriate patients for treatment and whether or not it truly impacts survival. A large-scale, intergroup U.S. trial is planned to attempt resolution of some of these questions, but given the time required for patient entry and the necessity for long follow-up, answers from such a trial are at least 15 years away.

Adjuvant Systemic Therapy

The biologic rationale and principles of ASRx have already been discussed. Given the thousands of publications on this subject and the more than 120 phase III trials, the results to be expected for ASRx are best obtained from an examination of the overview data, updated in 1998.[106–108] These results are presented in Table 17–14.

Adjuvant chemotherapy appears to be more effective in women younger than age 50 compared with older women. The reduction in risk of relapse is approximately 35% for younger women; the reduction in risk of death for this group is 27%. The corresponding values for women older than age 50 are 20% and 11%, respectively. The relative

TABLE 17–14. **Effects of Adjuvant Polychemotherapy***

Patient Population	RRRR (%)	RRRM (%)	ASB (10-yr)	RRRC
<50 years	35	27		
N+	~35	~27	12	
N−	~35	~27	6	
ER+	33	~27		
ER−	40	~27		
>50 years	20	11		
N+	~20	~11	3	
N−	~20	~11	2	
ER+	18			
ER−	30			
All				20

RRRR = reduction in relative risk of relapse; RRRM = reduction in relative risk of mortality; ASB = absolute survival benefit; RRRC = reduction in relative risk of contralateral breast cancer; ER = estrogen receptor.

*The proportional risk reductions were the same for N+ and N− patients. The effect of chemotherapy is greater in ER− women >50 years compared with ER+, but is approximately equal in women <50 years.

benefit is similar for both women who are node positive and node negative. The absolute benefit will vary with the risk of relapse or death: the greater the risk, the higher the absolute benefit. The data are shown graphically in Figure 17–7. For women younger than age 50, the absolute benefits are greater in node positive compared with node negative women, because the overall risk of relapse or death is higher in those who are node positive.

The data are a benchmark for outcome in stages I and II breast cancer patients. Women under age 50 who are node negative and are treated with adjuvant chemotherapy have a 10-year survival rate of 77.6% and a relapse-free survival rate of 68.3%. Note how these numbers correspond to those in Table 17–13, in which the survival rates from breast conservation trials are presented. For patients who are node positive, are younger than 50, and receiving adjuvant chemotherapy, the 10-year, relapse-free survival rate is 47.6% and overall survival rate is 53.8%, compared with control values of 32.2% and 41.4%, respectively. For women older than age 50 who are node negative and receive adjuvant chemotherapy, the 10-year relapse-free survival rate is 65.6% and the overall survival rate is 71.2%, compared with control values of 59.8% and 64.8%, respectively. For women aged 50 to 69 who are node positive and receive adjuvant chemotherapy, the 10-year relapse-free survival rate is 43.4% and the overall survival rate is 48.6%, compared with untreated control values of 38.0% and 46.3%, respectively. These differences are all statistically significant. According to the overview authors, "the results are entirely compatible with there being little relevance of nodal status to the proportional mortality reductions in older as in younger women."[108]

Other findings from the overview analysis are as follows:

1. Polychemotherapy is more effective than single-agent treatment. Two or three drugs seem to provide optimum benefits without additional benefit from larger numbers of agents.
2. There is a trend for improved results from anthracycline-containing regimens in comparison with CMF (Fig. 17–8). This additional benefit from anthracyclines may be because of their greater efficacy in certain subgroups, such as *HER2/neu*-positive tumors.
3. The optimal duration of chemotherapy appears to be 3 to 6 months, with shorter duration regimens being less effective and no demonstrable benefit revealed as yet for regimens of longer duration.
4. The effects of tamoxifen and chemotherapy appear to be independent; that is, both agents would be expected to exert their effects on risk of relapse and survival independently of the other agent.

Finally, the role of high-dose chemotherapy with autologous stem cell support or autologous bone marrow transplantation should be mentioned. This procedure has been widely practiced in the United States, with an estimated 6000 procedures being performed, both adjuvant and for treatment of metastatic disease (in 1998). However, despite promising phase II data, the preliminary analysis of a long-awaited phase III trial shows no survival improvement for the use of high-dose chemotherapy in the adjuvant setting.[171]

Adjuvant Hormonal Treatment

Again, a highly significant reduction in relapse as well as mortality is achieved through the use of adjuvant tamoxifen in women with hormone receptor–positive breast carcinoma.[107] The data are shown in Table 17–15 and Figure 17–9. Five years of tamoxifen therapy appears to be superior to shorter intervals and results in an almost 50% reduction in the risk of relapse and a 26% reduction in the risk of dying. Figure 17–9 plots the relapse-free survival, as well as overall survival, for patients who are node negative and node positive. The data indicate that at a 10-year observation, 5-year adjuvant tamoxifen therapy leads

TABLE 17–15. **Effects of Adjuvant Tamoxifen***

	1-yr Tamoxifen			5-yr Tamoxifen			
Patient Population	*RRRR (%)*	*RRRM (%)*	*RRRC*	*RRRR*	*RRRM*	*ASB*	*RRRC*
All ER+	21	12	13	47	26		46
N+						11	
N−						5.6	

RRRR = reduction in relative risk of relapse; RRRM = reduction in relative risk of mortality; ASB = absolute survival benefit; RRRC = reduction in relative risk of contralateral breast cancer; ER = estrogen receptor.

*Tamoxifen was ineffective in ER− patients. Proportional risk reductions are the same for N+ and N− patients. Five years of tamoxifen is effective regardless of age.

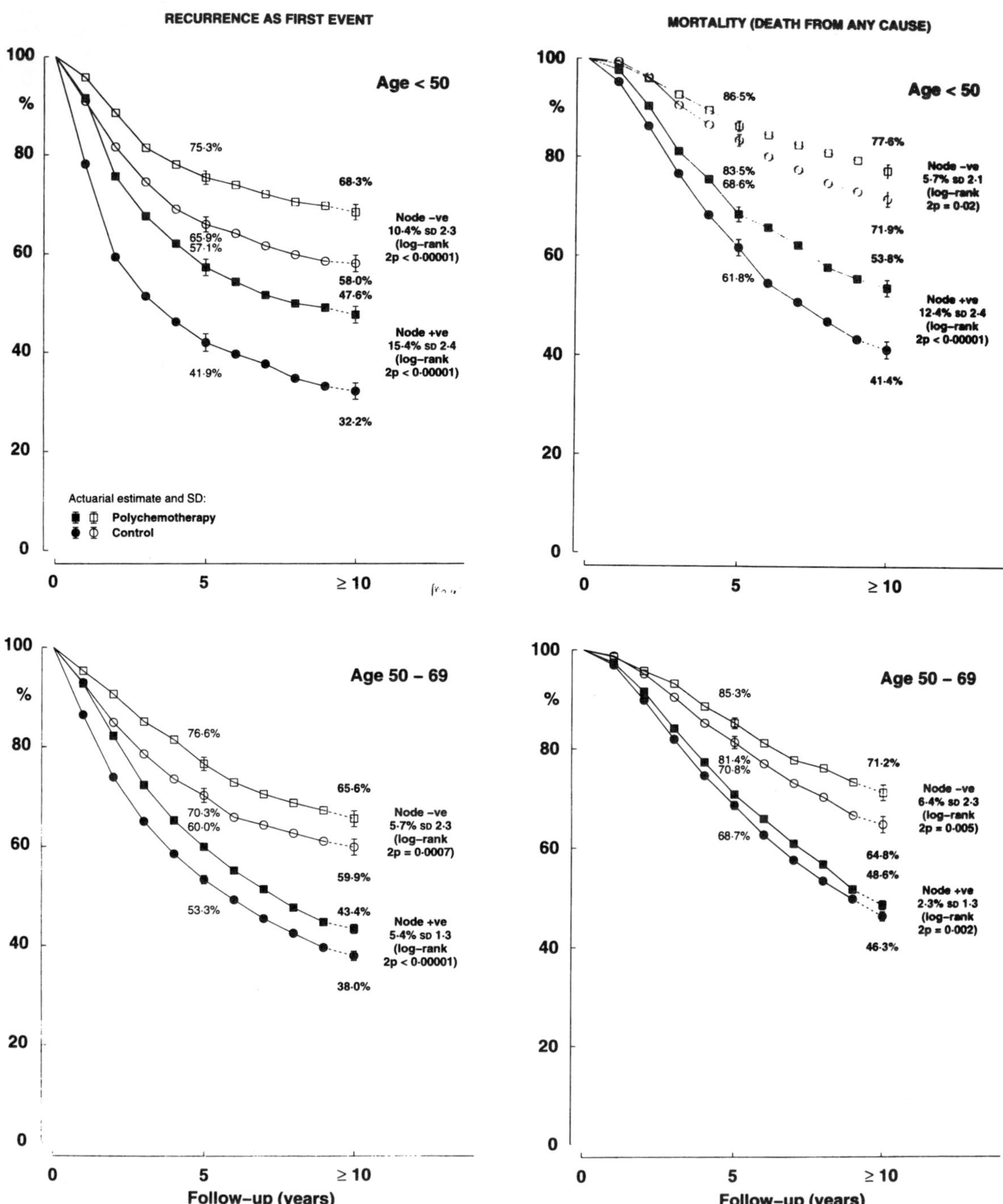

Figure 17–7. Overview estimates of relapse-free survival rates and survival rates for patients treated with chemotherapy versus untreated controls, with patients subdivided by age and nodal status. (From Early Breast Cancer Trialists' Collaborative Group: Polychemotherapy for early breast cancer: an overview of the randomised trials. Lancet 1998; 352:930–942, with permission. Copyright © 1998 The Lancet Ltd.)

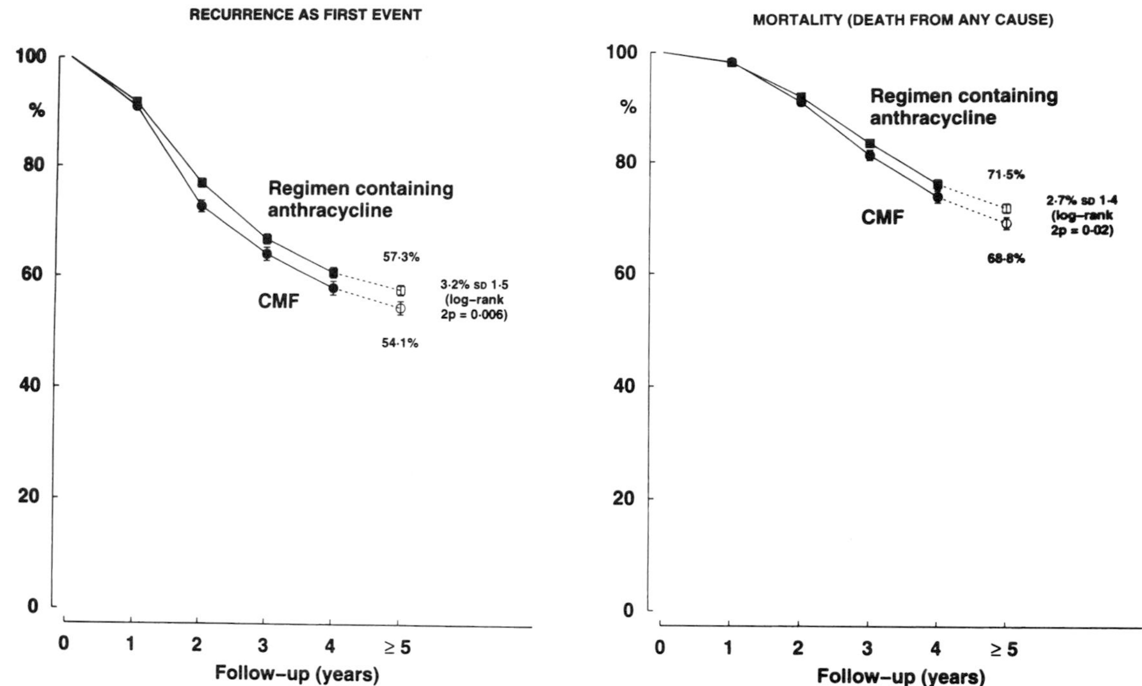

Figure 17–8. Overview estimates of relapse-free survival rates and survival rates for patients with regimens containing anthracycline versus CMF. (From Early Breast Cancer Trialists' Collaborative Group: Polychemotherapy for early breast cancer: an overview of the randomised trials. Lancet 1998; 352:930–942, with permission. Copyright © 1998 The Lancet Ltd.)

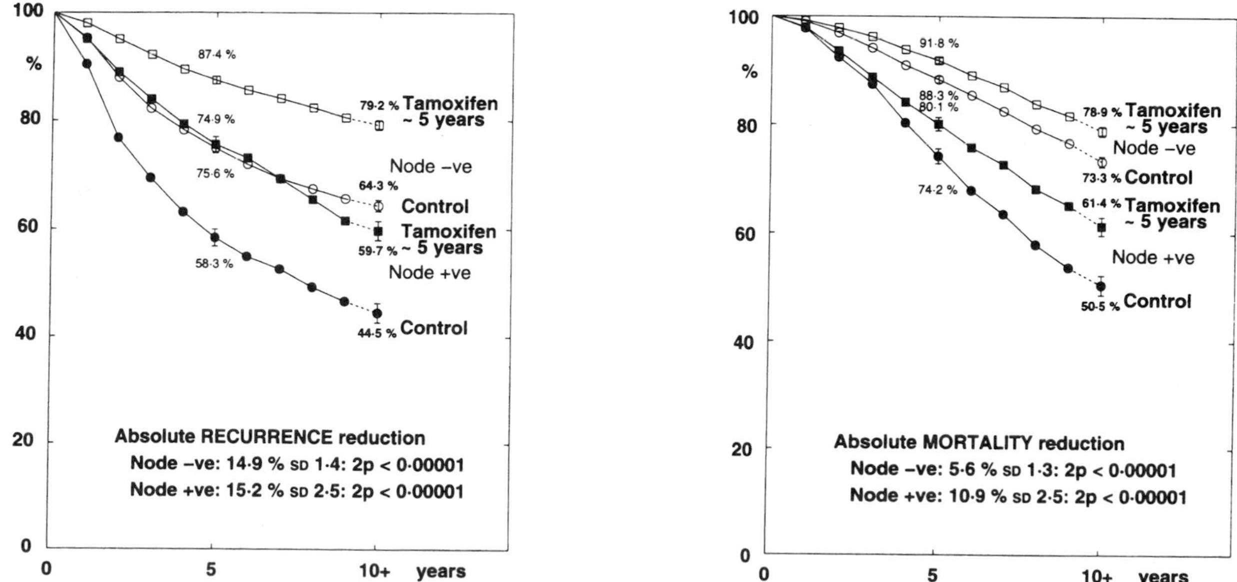

Figure 17–9. Overview estimates of relapse-free survival rates and survival rates for patients treated with tamoxifen for 5 years versus untreated controls, with patients subdivided by nodal status. (From Early Breast Cancer Trialists' Collaborative Group: Tamoxifen for early breast cancer: an overview of the randomised trials. Lancet 1998; 351:1451–1467, with permission. Copyright © 1998 The Lancet Ltd.)

to an absolute improvement of approximately 15% in relapse-free survival in both patients who are node negative and node positive. Overall survival has improved approximately 11% in those who are node positive and 5% in those who are node negative. The overall survival rate is approximately 80% at 10 years in patients who are node negative and treated with tamoxifen, and 60% in patients who are node positive, again a good correspondence with the pooled data from BCT. Unlike chemotherapy, there is no apparent influence of age on results. Efficacy does appear to directly correlate with the degree of ER positivity.

These overview data have led to the following set of recommendations regarding ASRx:

- Because ASRx produces the same relative benefit regardless of the actual risk of relapse, almost all patients, except those with the most favorable prognostic characteristics, are candidates for treatment. In practice, this has meant that almost all women with a tumor exceeding 1 cm in size, irrespective of nodal status, have been considered appropriate candidates for ASRx.
- Patients who are ER negative are not candidates for tamoxifen, irrespective of age.
- With chemotherapy, the relapse risk decreases by approximately one third in women younger than 50. Chemotherapy is recommended for almost all women who are ER negative and younger than 50, judged to be at significant risk for relapse. As the age of the patient increases, the benefits of adjuvant chemotherapy decrease, but they do not disappear. The decision to use chemotherapy in women older than 50 is still individualized and dependent on the extent of disease, receptor status, the patient's general medical condition, and individual patient preferences.
- For women older than age 50 with ER positive tumors, the efficacy of chemotherapy is considerably less than for younger women and, therefore, tamoxifen is the primary adjuvant systemic treatment. The greater the ER positivity, the more this is true. The decision to add chemotherapy to tamoxifen is individualized, dependent on patient preference, estimated risk of recurrence, general medical condition, and the age of the patient.

Metastatic Disease

Endocrine Therapy

As mentioned previously, hormonal therapy is the initial treatment of metastatic disease in patients with ER or PR positive tumors. Tamoxifen, a nonsteroidal antiestrogen first approved for the treatment of metastatic breast cancer over 20 years ago, is usually the first agent of choice because of its favorable toxicity profile.[112, 172] For patients who develop metastatic disease while taking tamoxifen or within a year of completing adjuvant tamoxifen, one of the other hormonal agents is usually considered. In patients with positive hormone receptors, first-line hormonal therapy can result in objective responses in up to 50% of patients; patients who respond to an initial hormonal treatment are thought to have an approximately 50% chance of responding to a second-line agent.[173, 174] Patients who do not respond to initial hormonal therapy are usually treated with chemotherapy. In some cases, however, particularly when the disease is indolent, a second-line hormonal treatment can be considered, even if there was no response to a first-line agent. The response duration to first-line tamoxifen therapy may range from 2 months to several years, with a median duration of 1 to 2 years. Occasionally, patients will have a prolonged response of many years' duration; response duration to second- and third-line hormonal therapy tends to be somewhat shorter.

In addition to tamoxifen, there are a variety of other hormonal therapies that are available. In premenopausal women who have responded to tamoxifen, ovarian oblation is a reasonable second-line consideration. Some unreported studies have attempted to determine if the combination of ovarian ablation plus tamoxifen would be more effective than tamoxifen alone in premenopausal patients with metastatic breast cancer. In postmenopausal women, the usual second-line therapy is treatment with an aromatase inhibitor.[113, 115, 173, 174] In the United States, the two modern aromatase inhibitors that are commercially available are anastrozole and letrozole. Both agents work by inhibiting the conversion of adrenally generated androstenedione to estrone; in premenopausal patients, aromatase inhibitors are not effective because of the high levels of ovarian-derived estrogen. In postmenopausal women, however, these agents can be highly effective and have been shown to be at least as effective (and less toxic) than megestrol acetate.[114, 115, 175] Options for third-line therapy, in both premenopausal and postmenopausal women, include megestrol acetate, androgens, and high-dose estrogen. The mechanism of action of megestrol acetate is unknown, but it has documented activity with objective response rates in the range of 10% to 20%. There are a number of new hormonal agents that are being evaluated in clinical trials, including more potent antiestrogens.

Do hormonal therapies improve survival for patients with metastatic breast cancer? There is no clinical trial that has addressed this issue in recent years, and the question may never be answered definitively. No oncologist would place a patient on a trial comparing placebo with a known hormonal therapy because of the established activity of these agents and their favorable side effect profile. There is no question that hormonal therapies can have a profound impact on quality of life, but they probably also prolong survival, at least in some patients.

Chemotherapy

For patients who have hormone receptor negative tumors, visceral crisis, or receptor positive tumors that have become refractory to hormonal therapy, chemotherapy is indicated. Many active agents are available; the most commonly used are listed in Table 17–11. Most active single agents produce responses in the range of 20% to 50% of previously untreated patients.[116–118] Three of the most common agents are doxorubicin, paclitaxel, and docetaxel.[117, 118, 176] Whereas combination regimens may, in some cases, yield higher response rates than single agents, they are slowly falling out of favor in the treatment of metastatic breast cancer.[119] Increasingly, oncologists are using sequential single agents in an effort to get as much as possible out of each drug and to spare patients added toxicity.

The duration of chemotherapy in the metastatic setting is flexible. Although stopping chemotherapy after only three cycles appears to compromise patient outcome, more than 6 months of treatment is probably not necessary.[177, 178] In practice, oncologists decide when to continue or discontinue a treatment that has been effective after considering a number of issues: patients' symptoms and relief of symptoms from chemotherapy, toxicity of the treatment regimen, and patient preference.

Greenberg and associates at M. D. Anderson Cancer Center have analyzed a large series of patients with metastatic breast cancer treated with chemotherapy between 1973 and 1982.[116] Of the 1581 patients in the database, the overall complete response rate was 16.6% and the partial response rate was 48.4%; the median duration of response was 19 months in responding patients. It must be recognized, however, that these patients were treated at a time when adjuvant therapy was less commonly used, suggesting that the patient population included a higher proportion of chemotherapy-naive patients than we could expect to see today. Those patients with prolonged complete responses tended to have a number of favorable parameters, including a prolonged disease-free interval and minimal tumor burden at relapse.

In the treatment of patients with metastatic breast cancer, the role of high-dose chemotherapy with peripheral stem cell support remains uncertain. This intensive treatment approach seems to increase the number of complete responses seen with treatment, and approximately 10% to 25% of patients with a complete response will remain free of disease progression for 2 to 3 years or longer. However, it is unknown if a fraction of these patients are truly cured or if the results with high-dose chemotherapy are truly superior to standard treatment.[179–182]

There have been more new drugs approved for breast cancer in the past several years than at any other time in recent history. The Food and Drug Administration has approved new chemotherapy agents and several new hormonal agents. These recent additions have broadened the treatment options for patients with advanced breast cancer. Among the recent advances is the drug Herceptin. This agent is the first monoclonal antibody to be effective in breast cancer and is a humanized monoclonal antibody directed against the *HER2/neu* receptor. In studies using Herceptin as a single agent, it appears to result in responses of 15% to 25% in patients with metastatic breast cancer.[183, 184] In addition, Herceptin has been shown to increase the response rates seen with doxorubicin-based chemotherapy and paclitaxel, although chemotherapy with doxorubicin led to unacceptable rates of cardiotoxicity. Herceptin is an important advance for the subgroup of patients with metastatic breast cancer whose tumors overexpress *HER2/neu,* but perhaps what is most exciting is the possibility that there will be other targeted therapies like Herceptin appearing in the years ahead.

Clinical Investigations

Many aspects of the clinical care of breast carcinoma remain under active investigation. A few of these are summarized briefly and questions likely to be addressed in the future are indicated:

1. *Prevention.* Measures to prevent breast cancer continue to be of great interest. Most prominent have been the tamoxifen trials both in the United States and Europe. The U.S. trial conducted by the NSABP is positive, but several European studies are still ongoing, which are negative to date.[143–145] Further follow-up to resolve these discrepancies will obviously be necessary. The use of antiestrogen compounds other than tamoxifen will undoubtedly be explored as well. Attention is also likely to focus on preventive measures for high-risk patients, such as those possessing the *BRCA1* or *BRCA2* genes, or patients at high risk for developing breast cancer because of previous radiation therapy (e.g., young women irradiated for Hodgkin's disease).
2. *Screening.* Screening mammography remains eminently successful, particularly for women over 50, but new screening and diagnostic tools to better detect or delineate breast cancer, particularly in younger women, are necessary. MRI is under active investigation in this regard, as well as other imaging modalities.
3. *Surgical therapy.* A trend toward less axillary surgery, in particular with increasing emphasis on sentinel node biopsy rather than full axillary dissection, or complete omission of axillary lymph node dissection based on decision analyses indicating minimal or no benefit is growing. Further studies are expected to better define the roles of these procedures. It is anticipated, however, that conventional full axillary dissection will continue to decline in frequency.
4. *Radiation therapy.* The role of radiation therapy in breast carcinoma will continue to be re-evaluated and better defined. Studies are under way, for example, to determine the need for radiation therapy in older women with small, ER positive tumors undergoing BCT. Additional investigations are anticipated to determine the role of radiation therapy in patients with DCIS. Despite the NSABP trial indicating benefit for radiation in all DCIS patients regardless of type, many clinicians feel it might be omitted in patients with widely excised, small DCIS lesions of favorable histologic characteristics.[135] Additional studies will undoubtedly be performed concerning the value of radiation therapy following mastectomy. Despite positive European and Canadian trials, there remains widespread concern in the United States regarding the exact role of radiation postmastectomy in patients with one to three positive lymph nodes and a general desire for confirmation of the European and Canadian results in U.S. studies.[100]
5. *Systemic therapy.* The search for better agents will continue, as well as for better combinations and appropriate doses. It is hoped that efforts will focus on identifying which patients benefit from current treatments; many thousands of patients are treated yearly in the adjuvant setting, and yet it is quite likely that only a small proportion actually derive benefit from the treatment. New biologic agents, including

angiogenesis inhibitors, differentiating agents, vaccines, and monoclonal antibody therapy, are all under active investigation and hold promise for the future, both in the adjuvant as well as the metastatic disease setting, and there is a need to increase participation of patients in clinical trials. Effective therapy of metastatic disease continues to be the most difficult therapeutic challenge facing breast oncologists.

Recommended Reading

The literature on breast cancer is voluminous to the point of being overwhelming. Fortunately, a number of excellent texts, as well as review articles, are available. The most useful text is perhaps *Diseases of the Breast* by Harris and associates.[185] For an in-depth discussion of ductal carcinoma *in situ,* consider the text edited by Silverstein.[186] We have attempted to cite a number of the pertinent review articles throughout this chapter; the interested reader is urged to consult the references list for the specific area in which one desires further information.

REFERENCES

1. Greenlee RT, Murray T, Bolden S, et al: Cancer Statistics, 2000. CA Cancer J Clin 2000; 50:7.
2. Ernster VL, Barclay J, Kerlikowske K, et al: Incidence of and treatment for ductal carcinoma in situ of the breast. JAMA 1996; 275:913–918.
3. Gloeckler Ries LA: Rates. In: Harris A, Edwards BK, Blot WJ, et al (eds): Cancer Rates and Risks, 4th ed, pp 42–43. Bethesda, National Institutes of Health Publication No 96–691, 1996.
4. Chu KC, Tarone RE, Kessler LG, et al: Recent trends in U.S. breast cancer incidence, survival and mortality rates. J Natl Cancer Inst 1996; 88:1571–1579.
5. Claus EB, Risch N, Thompson WD: Autosomal dominant inheritance of early-onset breast cancer. Implications for risk prediction. Cancer 1994; 73:643–651.
6. Byrne C: Risks for major cancers: breast. In: Harris A, Edwards BK, Blot WJ, et al (eds): Cancer Rates and Risks, 4th ed, pp 120–123. Bethesda, National Institutes of Health Publication No 96–691, 1996.
7. Rosen PP, Groshen S, Kinne DW, et al: Contralateral breast carcinoma: an assessment of risk and prognosis in stage I (T1N0M0) and stage II (T1N1M0) patients with 20-year follow-up. Surg 1989; 106:904–910.
8. Dupont WD, Page DL: Risk factors for breast cancer in women with proliferative breast disease. N Engl J Med 1985; 312:146–151.
9. Frykberg ER, Santiago F, Betsill WL Jr, et al: Lobular carcinoma in situ of the breast. Surgery, Gynecology and Obstetrics 1987; 164:285–301.
10. Bodian CA, Perzin KH, Lattes R: Lobular neoplasia. Long term risk of breast cancer and relation to other factors. Cancer 1996; 78:1024–1034.
11. Henderson BE, Bernstein L: Endogenous and exogenous hormonal factors. In: Harris JR, Lippman ME, Morrow M, et al (eds): Diseases of the Breast, pp 185–200. Philadelphia, Lippincott-Raven, 1996.
12. Friedman LS, Ostermeyer EA, Lynch ED, et al: The search for BRCA1. Cancer Res 1994; 54:6374–6382.
13. Wooster R, Neuhausen SL, Mangion J, et al: Localization of a breast cancer susceptibility gene, BRCA2, to chromosome 13q12–13. Science 1994; 265:2088–2090.
14. Warmuth MA, Sutton LM, Winer EP: A review of hereditary breast cancer: from screening to risk factor modification. Am J Med 1997; 102:407–415.
15. Stearns V, Yamauchi H, Hayes D: Circulating tumor markers in breast cancer: accepted utilities and novel aspects. Recent Cancer Res Treat 1998; 52:239–259.
16. Bland KI, Konstadoulakis MM, Vezeridis MP, et al: Oncogene protein co-expression. Value of Ha-ras, c-myc, c-fos, and p53 as prognostic discriminants for breast carcinoma. Ann Surg 1995; 221:706–718.
17. Donegan WL: Diagnosis. In: Donegan WL, Spratt JS (eds): Cancer of the Breast, 3rd ed, pp 126–166. Philadelphia, W.B. Saunders, 1988.
18. Rimer BK: Breast cancer screening. In: Harris JR, Lippman ME, Morrow M, et al (eds): Diseases of the Breast, pp 307–322. Philadelphia, Lippincott-Raven, 1996.
19. Smart CR, Byrne C, Smith RA, et al: Twenty-year follow-up of the breast cancers diagnosed during the Breast Cancer Detection Demonstration Project. CA Cancer J Clin 1997; 47:134–149.
20. Fletcher SW, Black W, Harris R, et al: Report of the International Workshop on Screening for Breast Cancer. J Natl Cancer Inst 1993; 85:1644–1656.
21. Kerlikowske K, Grady D, Rubin SM, et al: Efficacy of screening mammography. A meta-analysis. JAMA 1995; 273:149–154.
22. Lemon SJ, Tinley S, Fusaro R, et al: Cancer risk assessment in a hereditary cancer prevention clinic and its first year's experience. Cancer 1997; 80:606–613.
23. Pisano ED: Fine needle aspiration biopsy of breast lesions. In: Dershaw DD (ed): Interventional Breast Procedures. New York, Churchill Livingstone, 1996.
24. Dershaw DD (ed): Interventional Breast Procedures. New York, Churchill Livingstone, 1996.
25. Kopans D, Smith B: Preoperative imaging-guided needle localization and biopsy of nonpalpable breast lesions. In: Harris JR, Lippman ME, Morrow M, et al. (eds): Diseases of the Breast, pp 139–144. Philadelphia, Lippincott-Raven, 1996.
26. Friedrich M, Sickles E (eds): Radiological Diagnosis of Breast Diseases. Berlin, Springer-Verlag, 1997.
27. Page D, Anderson T: Diagnostic Histopathology of the Breast. Edinburgh, Churchill Livingstone, 1987.
28. Rosen PP: Breast Pathology. Philadelphia, Lippincott-Raven, 1997.
29. World Health Organization: Histological typing of breast tumors. In: International Histological Classification of Tumours, 2nd ed, p 19. Geneva, World Health Organization, 1981.
30. Frykberg ER, Masood S, Copeland EM, et al: Ductal carcinoma in situ of the breast. Surgery, Gynecology and Obstetrics 1993; 177:425–440.
31. Wood WC: Management of lobular carcinoma in situ and ductal carcinoma in situ of the breast. Semin Oncol 1996; 23:446–452.
32. Goldschmidt RA, Victor TA: Lobular carcinoma in situ of the breast. Semin Surg Oncol 1996; 12:314–320.
33. American Joint Committee on Cancer: AJCC Cancer Staging Manual, 5th ed. Philadelphia, Lippincott-Raven, 1997.
34. Fisher B, Bauer M, Wickerham DL, et al: Relation of number of positive axillary nodes to the prognosis of patients with primary breast cancer. An NSABP update. Cancer 1983; 52:1551–1557.
35. Harris JR, Lippman ME, Veronesi U, et al: Medical progress: breast cancer. N Engl J Med 1992; 327:319–328, 390–398, 473–480.
36. Hellman S: Natural history of small breast cancers. J Clin Oncol 1994; 12:2229–2234.
37. Halsted WC: The results of operations for the cure of cancer of the breast performed at the Johns Hopkins Hospitals. Ann Surg 1894; 20:497–555.
38. Haagensen CD: Diseases of the Breast, 2nd ed. Philadelphia, W.B. Saunders Co. 1971.
39. Urban JA, Baker HW: Radical mastectomy with en bloc excision of the internal mammary lymph node chain. Cancer 1952; 5:992–1008.
40. McWhirter R: Simple mastectomy and radiation therapy in the treatment of breast cancer. Br J Radiol 1955; 28:128–139.
41. Johansen H, Kaae S, Schiodt T: Simple mastectomy with postoperative irradiation versus extended radical mastectomy in breast cancer. A twenty-five-year follow-up of a randomized trial. Acta Oncol 1990; 29:709–715.
42. Fisher B: Biological and clinical considerations regarding the use of surgery and chemotherapy in the treatment of primary breast cancer. Cancer 1977; 40 (suppl):574–587.
43. Fisher B, Montague E, Redmond C, et al: Comparison of radical mastectomy with alternative treatments for primary breast cancer. A first report results from a prospective randomized clinical trial. Cancer 1977; 39(suppl):2827–2839.
44. Fisher B, Carbone P, Economou SG, et al: L-phenylalanine mustard (L-PAM) in the management of primary breast cancer. A report of early findings. N Engl J Med 1975; 292:117–122.

45. Bonadonna G, Brusamolino E, Valagussa P, et al: Combination chemotherapy as an adjuvant treatment in operable breast cancer. N Engl J Med 1976; 294:405–410.
46. Overgaard M, Hansen PS, Overgaard J, et al: Postoperative radiotherapy in high-risk premenopausal women with breast cancer who receive adjuvant chemotherapy. Danish Breast Cancer Cooperative Group 82b Trial. N Engl J Med. 1997; 337:949–955.
47. Ragaz J, Jackson SM, Le N, et al: Adjuvant radiation therapy and chemotherapy in node-positive premenopausal women with breast cancer. N Engl J Med. 1997; 337:956–962.
48. Hellman S: Stopping metastases at their source. N Engl J Med 1997; 337:996–997.
49. Pierce LJ, Glatstein E: Postmastectomy radiation therapy in the management of operable breast cancer. Cancer 1994; 74(suppl):477–485.
50. Fowble B: Postmastectomy radiation: then and now. Oncology 1997; 11:213–234.
51. Donegan WL: Surgical clinical trials. Cancer 1984; 53 (suppl):691–699.
52. Maddox WA, Carpenter JT, Laws HL, et al: A randomized prospective trial of radical (Halstead) mastectomy vs. modified radical mastectomy in 311 breast cancer patients. Ann Surg 1983; 198:207–212.
53. Martin JK, van Heerden JA, Taylor WF, et al: Is modified radical mastectomy really equivalent to radical mastectomy in treatment of carcinoma of the breast? Cancer 1986; 57:510–518.
54. Brewaeys P, Heymans O, Nizet J: Breast reconstruction. Rev Med Liege 1998; 53:483–489.
55. Evans GR, Kroll SS: Choice of technique for reconstruction. Clin Plastic Surg 1998; 25:311–316.
56. Keynes G: Conservative treatment of cancer of the breast. Br Med J 1937; 2:643–647.
57. Veronesi U, Salvadori B, Luini A, et al: Conservative treatment of early breast cancer. Long-term results of 1232 cases treated with quadrantectomy, axillary dissection and radiation therapy. Ann Surg 1990; 211:250–259.
58. Pierquin B, Huart J, Raynal M, et al: Conservative treatment for breast cancer: long-term results (15 years). Radiother Oncol 1991; 20:16–23.
59. Solin LJ, Schultz DJ, Fowble BL: Ten-year results of the treatment of early-stage breast carcinoma in elderly women using breast-conserving surgery and definitive breast irradiation. Int J Radiat Oncol Biol Phys 1995; 33:45–51.
60. Hurd TC, Sneige N, Allen PK, et al: Impact of extensive intraductal component on recurrence and survival in patients with stage I or II breast cancer treated with breast conservation therapy. Ann Surg Oncol 1997; 4:119–124.
61. Bouvet M, Ollila DW, Hunt KK, et al: Role of conservation therapy for invasive lobular carcinoma of the breast. Ann Surg Oncol 1997; 4:650–654.
62. Heaton KM, Peoples GE, Singletary SE, et al: Feasibility of breast conservation therapy in metachronous or synchronous bilateral breast cancer. Ann Surg Oncol 1999; 6:102–108.
63. van Dongen JA, Bartelink H, Fentiman IS, et al: Factors influencing local relapse and survival and results of salvage treatment after breast-conserving therapy in operable breast cancer: EORTC trial 10801, breast conservation compared with mastectomy in TNM stage I and II breast cancer. Eur J Cancer 1992; 28A:801–805.
64. Blichert-Toft M, Rose C, Andersen JA, et al: Danish randomized trial comparing breast conservation therapy with mastectomy: six years of life-table analysis. Danish Breast Cancer Cooperative Group. J Natl Cancer Inst Monogr 1992; 11:19–25.
65. Jacobson JA, Danforth DN, Cowan KH, et al: Ten-year results of a comparison of conservation with mastectomy in the treatment of stage I and II breast cancer. N Engl J Med 1995; 332:907–911.
66. Veronesi U, Salvadori B, Luini A, et al: Breast conservation is a safe method in patients with small cancer of the breast. Long-term results of three randomised trials on 1,973 patients. Eur J Cancer 1995; 31A:1574–1579.
67. Fisher B, Anderson S, Redmond CK, et al: Reanalysis and results after 12 years of follow-up in a randomized clinical trial comparing total mastectomy with lumpectomy with or without irradiation in the treatment of breast cancer. N Engl J Med 1995; 333:1456–1461.
68. Arriagada R, Le MG, Rochard F, et al: Conservative treatment versus mastectomy in early breast cancer: patterns of failure with 15 years of follow-up data. Institut Gustave-Roussy Breast Cancer Group. J Clin Oncol 1996; 14:1558–1564.
69. Forrest AP, Stewart HJ, Everington D, et al: Randomised controlled trial of conservation therapy for breast cancer: 6 year analysis of the Scottish trial. Lancet 1996; 348:708–713.
70. Morris AD, Morris RD, Wilson FJ, et al: Breast-conserving therapy vs. mastectomy in early-stage breast cancer: a meta-analysis of 10-year survival. Cancer J Sci Am 1997; 3:6–12.
71. Treatment of early stage breast cancer. NIH Consensus Statement. 1990; June 18–21; 8(6).
72. Margolese R, Poisson R, Shibata H, et al: The technique of segmental mastectomy (lumpectomy) and axillary dissection: a syllabus from the National Surgical Adjuvant Breast Project workshops. Surg 1987; 102:828–834.
73. Anscher MS, Jones P, Prosnitz LR, et al: Local failure and margin status in early-stage breast carcinoma treated with conservation surgery and radiation therapy. Ann Surg 1993; 218:22–28.
74. Gage I, Schnitt SJ, Nixon AJ, et al: Pathologic margin involvement and the risk of recurrence in patients treated with breast-conserving therapy. Cancer 1996; 78:1921–1928.
75. DiBiase SJ, Komarnicky LT, Schwartz GF, et al: The number of positive margins influences the outcome of women treated with breast preservation for early stage breast carcinoma. Cancer 1998; 82:2212–2220.
76. de la Rochefordiere A, Abner AL, Silver B, et al: Are cosmetic results following conservative surgery and radiation therapy for early breast cancer dependent on technique? Int J Radiat Oncol Biol Phys 1992; 23:925–931.
77. Carter CL, Allen C, Henson DE: Relation of tumor size, lymph node status, and survival in 24,740 breast cancer cases. Cancer 1989; 63:181–187.
78. Cady B: The need to reexamine axillary lymph node dissection in invasive breast cancer. Cancer 1994; 73:505–508.
79. Chadha M, Axelrod D: Is axillary dissection always indicated in invasive breast cancer? Oncology 1997; 11:1463–1468.
80. Haffty BG, Ward B, Pathare P, et al: Reappraisal of the role of axillary lymph node dissection in the conservative treatment of breast cancer. J Clin Oncol 1997; 15:691–700.
81. Parmigiani G, Berry DA, Winer EP, et al: Is axillary lymph node dissection indicated for early stage breast cancer? A decision analysis. J Clin Oncol 1999; 17:1465–1473.
82. Recht A, Houlihan MJ: Axillary lymph nodes and breast cancer: a review. Cancer 1995; 76:1491–1512.
83. Albertini JJ, Lyman GH, Cox C, et al: Lymphatic mapping and sentinel node biopsy in the patient with breast cancer. JAMA 1996; 276:1818–1822.
84. Cody HS III: Sentinel lymph node mapping in breast cancer. Oncology 1999; 13:25–34.
85. Bentel GC: Radiation Therapy Planning, 2nd ed. New York, McGraw-Hill, 1996.
86. Leibel SA, Phillips TL (eds): Textbook of Radiation Oncology. Philadelphia, W.B. Saunders Co. 1998.
87. Romestaing P, Lehingue Y, Carrie C, et al: Role of a 10-Gy boost in the conservative treatment of early breast cancer: results of a randomized clinical trial in Lyon, France. J Clin Oncol 1997; 15:963–968.
88. Larson D, Weinstein M, Goldberg I, et al: Edema of the arm as a function of the extent of axillary surgery in patients with stage I-II carcinoma of the breast treated with primary radiation therapy. Int J Radiat Oncol Biol Phys 1986; 12:1575–1582.
89. Hardenbergh P, Bentel G, Prosnitz L, et al: Postmastectomy radiotherapy: toxicities and techniques to reduce them. Semin Rad Oncol 1999; 9:1–11.
90. Nattinger AB, Gottleib MS, Veum J, et al: Geographic variation in the use of breast conserving treatment for breast cancer. N Engl J Med 1992; 326:1102–1107.
91. Recht A: Selection of patients with early stage invasive breast cancer for treatment with conservative surgery and radiation therapy. Semin Oncol 1996; 23(suppl):19–30.
92. Kurtz JM, Jacquemier J, Amalric R, et al: Breast-conserving therapy for macroscopically multiple cancers. Ann Surg 1990; 212:38–44.
93. Fortin A, Larochelle M, Laverdiere J, et al: Local failure is responsible for the decrease in survival for patients with breast cancer treated with conservative surgery and postoperative radiation therapy. J Clin Oncol 1999; 17:101–109.

94. Fleck R, McNeese MD, Ellerbroek NA, et al: Consequences of breast irradiation in patients with pre-existing collagen vascular diseases. Int J Radiat Oncol Biol Phys 1989; 17:829–833.
95. Gray JR, McCormick B, Cox L, et al: Primary breast irradiation in large breasted or heavy women: analysis of cosmetic outcome. Int J Radiat Oncol Biol Phys 1991; 21:347–354.
96. Moody AM, Mayles WPM, Bliss JM, et al: The influence of breast size on late radiation effects in association with radiation therapy dose inhomogeneity. Radiother Oncol 1994; 33:106–112.
97. Fletcher GH: History of irradiation in the primary management of apparently regionally confined breast cancer. Int J Radiat Oncol Biol Phys 1985; 11:2133–2142.
98. Early Breast Cancer Trialists' Collaborative Group. Effects of radiotherapy and surgery in early breast cancer: an overview of the randomized trials. N Engl J Med 1995; 333:1444–1455.
99. Arriagada R, Rutqvist LE, Mattsson A, et al: Adequate locoregional treatment for early breast cancer may prevent secondary dissemination. J Clin Oncol 1995; 13:2869–2878.
100. Recht A, Bartelink H, Fourquet A, et al: Postmastectomy radiotherapy: questions for the twenty-first century. J Clin Oncol 1998; 16:2886–2889.
101. Cuzick J, Stewart HJ, Peto R, et al: Overview of randomized trials comparing radical mastectomy without radiation therapy against simple mastectomy with radiation therapy in breast cancer. Cancer Treat Rep 1987; 71:7–14.
102. Cuzick J, Stewart H, Rutqvist L, et al: Cause-specific mortality in long-term survivors of breast cancer who participated in trials of radiation therapy. J Clin Oncol 1994; 12:447–453.
103. Clark GM, Wenger CR, Beardslee S, et al: How to integrate steroid hormone receptor, flow cytometric and other prognostic information in regard to primary breast cancer. Cancer 1993; 71:2157–2162.
104. Dorr FA: Prognostic factors observed in current clinical trials. Cancer 1993; 71:2163–2168.
105. Balslev I, Axelsson CK, Zedeler K, et al: The Nottingham prognostic index applied to 9,149 patients from the studies of the Danish Breast Cancer Cooperative Group (DBCG). Breast Cancer Res Treat 1994; 32:281–290.
106. Early Breast Cancer Trialists' Collaborative Group: Ovarian ablation in early breast cancer: overview of the randomised trials. Lancet 1996; 348:1189–1196.
107. Early Breast Cancer Trialists' Collaborative Group: Tamoxifen for early breast cancer: an overview of the randomised trials. Lancet 1998; 351:1451–1467.
108. Early Breast Cancer Trialists' Collaborative Group: Polychemotherapy for early breast cancer: an overview of the randomised trials. Lancet 1998; 352:930–942.
109. Ayash LJ, Wheeler C, Fairclough D, et al: Prognostic factors for prolonged progression-free survival with high-dose chemotherapy with autologous stem-cell support for advanced breast cancer. J Clin Oncol 1995; 13:2043–2049.
110. Rahman ZU, Frye DK, Buzdar AU, et al: Impact of selection process on response rate and long-term survival of potential high-dose chemotherapy candidates treated with standard-dose doxorubicin-containing chemotherapy in patients with metastatic breast cancer. J Clin Oncol 1997; 15:3171–3177.
111. Garcia-Carbonero R, Hidalgo M, Paz-Ares L, et al: Patient selection in high-dose chemotherapy trials: relevance in high-risk breast cancer. J Clin Oncol 1997; 15:3178–3184.
112. Powels TJ: Efficacy of tamoxifen as treatment of breast cancer. Semin Oncol 1997; 24(suppl):S1–48–S1–54.
113. Buzdar AU, Plourde PV, Hortobagyi GN: Aromatase inhibitors in metastastic breast cancer. Semin Oncol 1996; 23(suppl):28–32.
114. Buzdar A, Jonat W, Howell A, et al: Anastrozole, a potent and selective aromatase inhibitor, versus megestrol acetate in postmenopausal women with advanced breast cancer: results of overview analysis of two phase III trials. Arimidex Study Group. J Clin Oncol 1996; 14:2000–2011.
115. Dombernowsky P, Smith I, Falkson G, et al: Letrozole, a new oral aromatase inhibitor for advanced breast cancer: double-blind randomized trial showing a dose effect and improved efficacy and tolerability compared with megestrol acetate. J Clin Oncol 1998; 16:453–461.
116. Greenberg PA, Hortobagyi GN, Smith TL, et al: Long-term follow-up of patients with complete remission following combination chemotherapy for metastatic breast cancer. J Clin Oncol 1996; 14:2197–2205.
117. Fossati R, Confalonieri C, Torri V, et al: Cytotoxic and hormonal treatment for metastatic breast cancer: a systematic review of published randomized trials involving 31,510 women. J Clin Oncol 1998; 16:3439–3460.
118. Sledge GW, Neuberg D, Ingle J, et al: Phase III trial of doxorubicin (A) vs. Paclitaxel (T) vs. Doxorubicin + paclitaxel (A & T) as first-line therapy for metastatic breast cancer (MBC): an intergroup trial [Abstract]. Proceedings of the American Society of Clinical Oncology 1997; 16:1a.
119. Joensuu H, Holli K, Heikkinen M, et al: Combination chemotherapy versus single-agent therapy as first- and second-line treatment in metastatic breast cancer: a prospective randomized trial. J Clin Oncol 1998; 16:3720–3730.
120. Rosen PP, Braun DW, Kinne DW: The clinical significance of pre-invasive breast carcinoma. Cancer 1980; 46:919–925.
121. Page DL, Dupont WD, Rogers LW, et al: Intraductal carcinoma of the breast: follow-up after biopsy only. Cancer 1982; 49:751–758.
122. Schnitt SJ, Silen W, Sadowsky NL, et al: Ductal carcinoma in situ (intraductal carcinoma) of the breast. N Engl J Med 1988; 318:898–903.
123. Silverstein MJ: Noninvasive breast cancer: the dilemma of the 1990s. Obstet Gynecol Clin N Am 1994; 21:639–658.
124. Page DL, Jensen RA: Ductal carcinoma in situ of the breast: understanding the misunderstood stepchild. JAMA 1996; 275:948–949.
125. Silverstein MJ, Lagios MD: Use of predictors of recurrence to plan therapy for DCIS of the breast. Oncology 1997; 11:393–406.
126. Fisher ER, Costantino J, Fisher B, et al: Pathologic findings from the National Surgical Adjuvant Breast Project Protocol B-17. Cancer 1995; 75:1310–1319.
127. Lagios MD: Duct carcinoma in situ: biological implications for clinical practice. Semin Oncol 1996; 23(suppl):6–11.
128. Silverstein MJ, Lagios MD, Craig PH, et al: A prognostic index for ductal carcinoma in situ of the breast. Cancer 1996; 77:2267–2274.
129. Holland PA, Gandhi A, Knox WF, et al: The importance of complete excision in the prevention of local recurrence of ductal carcinoma in situ. Br J Cancer 1998; 77:110–114.
130. Fowble B: Intraductal noninvasive breast cancer: a comparison of three local treatments. Oncology 1989; 3:51–64.
131. Marks LB, Prosnitz LR: Lumpectomy with and without radiation for early-stage breast cancer and DCIS. Oncology 1997; 11:1361–1368.
132. Fisher B, Dignam J, Wolmark N, et al: Tamoxifen in treatment of intraductal breast cancer: National Surgical Adjuvant Breast and Bowel Project B-24 randomised controlled trial. Lancet 1999; 353:1993–2000.
133. Jacquemier J, Kurtz JM, Amalric R, et al: An assessment of extensive intraductal component as a risk factor for local recurrence after breast-conserving therapy. Br J Cancer 1990; 61:873–876.
134. Holland R, Connolly JL, Gelman R, et al: The presence of an extensive intraductal component following a limited excision correlates with prominent residual disease in the remainder of the breast. J Clin Oncol 1990; 8:113–118.
135. Silverstein MJ, Barth A, Pollar DN, et al: Ten year results comparing mastectomy to excision and radiation therapy for ductal carcinoma in situ of the breast. Eur J Cancer 1995; 31:1425–1427.
136. Solin LJ, Kurtz J, Fourquet A, et al: Fifteen-year results of breast-conserving surgery and definitive breast irradiation for the treatment of ductal carcinoma in situ of the breast. J Clin Oncol 1996; 14:754–763.
137. Fisher B, Costantino J, Redmond C, et al: Lumpectomy compared with lumpectomy and radiation therapy for the treatment of intraductal breast cancer. N Engl J Med 1993; 328:1581–1586.
138. Silverstein MJ, Poller DN, Waisman JR, et al: Prognostic classification of breast ductal carcinoma-in-situ. Lancet 1995; 345:1154–1157.
139. Cotran RS, Kumar V, Robbins SL (eds): Robbins Pathologic Basis of Disease, 5th ed. Philadelphia, W.B. Saunders Co., 1994.
140. Fisher ER, Costantino J, Fisher B, et al: Pathologic findings from the National Surgical Adjuvant Breast Project (NSABP) Protocol B-17. Five year observations concerning lobular carcinoma in situ. Cancer 1996; 78:1403–1416.
141. Levi F, Te VC, Randimbison L, et al: Trends of in situ carcinoma of the breast in Vaud, Switzerland. Eur J Cancer 1997; 33:903–906.
142. Winchester DJ, Menck HR, Winchester DP: National treatment trends for ductal carcinoma in situ of the breast. Arch Surg 1997; 132:660–665.
143. Fisher B, Costantino JP, Wickerham DL, et al: Tamoxifen for pre-

vention of breast cancer: report of the National Surgical Adjuvant Breast and Bowel Project P-1 Study. J Natl Cancer Inst 1998; 90:1371–1388.

144. Powles T, Eeles R, Ashley S, et al: Interim analysis of the incidence of breast cancer in the Royal Marsden Hospital tamoxifen randomised chemoprevention trial. Lancet 1998; 352:98–101.
145. Veronesi U, Maisonneuve P, Costa A, et al: Prevention of breast cancer with tamoxifen: preliminary findings from the Italian randomised trial among hysterectomised women. Lancet 1998; 352:93–97.
146. Chang S, Parker SL, Pham T, et al: Inflammatory breast carcinoma incidence and survival: the Surveillance, Epidemiology, and End Results Program of the National Cancer Institute, 1975–1992. Cancer 1998; 82:2366–2372.
147. Sheldon T, Hayes DF, Cady B, et al: Primary radiation therapy for locally advanced breast cancer. Cancer 1987; 60:1219–1225.
148. Dorr FA, Bader J, Friedman MA: Locally advanced breast cancer: current status and future directions. Int J Radiat Oncol Biol Phys 1989; 16:775–784.
149. Perez CA, Graham ML, Taylor ME, et al: Management of locally advanced carcinoma of the breast. Cancer 1994; 74:453–465.
150. Pierce LJ, Lippman M, Ben-Baruch N, et al: The effect of systemic therapy on local-regional control in locally advanced breast cancer. Int J Radiat Oncol Biol Phys 1992; 23:949–960.
151. Hortobagyi GN: Multidisciplinary management of advanced primary and metastatic breast cancer. Cancer 1994; 74:416–423.
152. Schaake-Koning C, van der Linden EH, Hart G, et al: Adjuvant chemo- and hormonal therapy in locally advanced breast cancer: a randomized clinical study. Int J Radiat Oncol Biol Phys 1985; 11:1759–1763.
153. Derman DP, Browde S, Kessel IL, et al: Adjuvant chemotherapy (CMF) for stage III breast cancer: a randomized trial. Int J Radiat Oncol Biol Phys 1989; 17:257–261.
154. Rodger A, Jack WJL, Hardman PDJ, et al: Locally advanced breast cancer: report of phase II study and subsequent phase III trial. Br J Cancer 1992; 65:761–765.
155. Bartelink H, Rubens RD, van der Schueren E, et al: Hormonal therapy prolongs survival in irradiated locally advanced breast cancer: a European Organization for Research and Treatment of Cancer randomized phase III trial. J Clin Oncol 1997; 15:207–215.
156. Kuerer HM, Newman LA, Smith TL, et al: Clinical course of breast cancer patients with complete pathologic primary tumor and axillary lymph node response to doxorubicin-based neoadjuvant chemotherapy. J Clin Oncol 1999; 17:460–469.
157. Fields JN, Perez CA, Kuske RR, et al: Inflammatory carcinoma of the breast: treatment results on 107 patients. Int J Radiat Oncol Biol Phys 1989; 17:249–255.
158. Jaiyesimi IA, Buzdar AU, Hortobagyi G: Inflammatory breast cancer: a review. J Clin Oncol 1992; 10:1014–1024.
159. Lamb CC, Eberlein TJ, Parker LM, et al: Results of radical radiotherapy for inflammatory breast cancer. Am J Surg 1991; 162:236–242.
160. Palangie T, Mosseri V, Mihura J, et al: Prognostic factors in inflammatory breast cancer and therapeutic implications. Eur J Cancer 1994; 80A:921–927.
161. Baron PL, Moore MP, Kinne DW, et al: Occult breast cancer presenting with axillary metastases. Arch Surg 1990; 125:210–215.
162. Ellerbroek N, Holmes F, Singletary E, et al: Treatment of patients with isolated axillary nodal metastases from an occult primary carcinoma consistent with breast origin. Cancer 1990; 66:1461–1467.
163. Merson M, Andreola S, Galimberti V, et al: Breast carcinoma presenting as axillary metastases without evidence of a primary tumor. Cancer 1992; 70:504–508.
164. Halverson KJ, Perez CA, Kuske RR, et al: Survival following regional recurrence of breast cancer. Int J Radiat Oncol Biol Phys 1992; 23:285–291.
165. Haffty BG, Fischer D, Beinfield M, et al: Prognosis following local recurrence in the conservatively treated breast cancer patient. Int J Radiat Oncol Biol Phys 1991; 21:293–298.
166. Abner AL, Recht A, Eberlein T, et al: Prognosis following salvage mastectomy for recurrence in the breast after conservative surgery and radiation therapy for early stage breast cancer. J Clin Oncol 1993; 11:44–48.
167. Borger J, Kemperman H, Hart A, et al: Risk factors in breast-conservation therapy. J Clin Oncol 1994; 12:653–660.
168. Solin LJ, Fowble B, Schultz DJ, et al: Age as a prognostic factor for patients treated with definitive irradiation for early stage breast cancer. Int J Radiat Oncol Biol Phys 1989; 16:373–381.
169. Kurtz JM, Jacquemier J, Amalric R, et al: Why are local recurrences after breast conserving therapy more frequent in younger patients? J Clin Oncol 1990; 8:591–59.
170. Olson JE, Neuberg D, Pandya KJ, et al: The role of radiation therapy in the management of operable locally advanced breast carcinoma: results of a randomized trial by the Eastern Cooperative Oncology Group. Cancer 1997; 79:1138–1149.
171. Peters W, Rosner G, Vredenburgh J, et al: A prospective randomized comparison of two doses of combination alkylating agents as consolidation after CAF in high risk primary breast cancer involving 10 or more axillary lymph nodes: preliminary results of CALGB 9082/SWOG 9114/NCICMA-13 [Abstract]. Proceedings of the American Society of Clinical Oncology 1999; 18:1a.
172. Sunderland MC, Osborne CK: Tamoxifen in premenopausal patients with metastatic breast cancer: a review. J Clin Oncol 1991; 9:1283–1297.
173. Howell A, Downey S, Anderson E: New endocrine therapies for breast cancer. Eur J Cancer 1996; 32A:576–588.
174. Brodie AMH, Njar VCO: Aromatase inhibitors and breast cancer. Semin Oncol 1996; 23(suppl):10–20.
175. Goss PE, Winer EP, Tannock IF, et al: Randomized phase III trial comparing the new potent and selective third generation aromatase inhibitor Vorozole with megestrol acetate in postmenopausal advanced breast cancer patients. J Clin Oncol 1999; 17:52–63.
176. Chevallier B, Fumoleau P, Kerbrat P, et al: Docetaxel is a major cytotoxic drug for the treatment of advanced breast cancer: a phase II trial of the clinical screening cooperative group of the European Organization for research and treatment of cancer. J Clin Oncol 1995; 13:314–322.
177. Muss HB, Case LD, Richards F, et al: Interrupted versus continuous chemotherapy in patients with metastatic breast cancer. The Piedmont Oncology Association. N Engl J Med 1991; 325:1342–1348.
178. Gregory RK, Powles TJ, Chang JC, et al: A randomised trial of six versus twelve courses of chemotherapy in metastatic carcinoma of the breast. Eur J Cancer 1997; 33:2194–2197.
179. Peters WP, Ross M, Vredenburgh JJ, et al: High-dose chemotherapy and autologous bone marrow support as consolidation after standard-dose adjuvant therapy for high-risk primary breast cancer. J Clin Oncol 1993; 11:1132–1143.
180. Bezwoda WR, Seymour L, Dansey RD: High-dose chemotherapy with hematopoietic rescue as primary treatment for metastatic breast cancer: a randomized trial. J Clin Oncol 1995; 13:2483–2489.
181. Gradishar WJ, Tallman MS, Abrams JS: High-dose chemotherapy for breast cancer. Ann Intern Med 1996; 125:599–604.
182. Stadmauer EA, O'Neill A, Goldstein LJ, et al: Phase III randomized trial of high dose chemotherapy and stem cell support shows no difference in overall survival or severe toxicity compared to maintenance chemotherapy with Cyclophosphamide, Methotrexate and 5FU for women with metastatic breast cancer who are responding to conventional induction chemotherapy [Abstract]. Proceedings of the American Society of Clinical Oncology 1999; 18:1a.
183. Cobleigh MA, Vogel CL, Tripathy D, et al: Efficacy and safety of herceptin (humanized anti-HER2 antibody) as a single agent in 222 women with HER2 overexpression who relapsed following chemotherapy for metastatic breast cancer [Abstract]. Proceedings of the American Society of Clinical Oncology, 1998; 17:97a.
184. Slamon D, Leyland-Jones B, Shak S, et al: Addition of herceptin (humanized anti-HER2 antibody) to first line chemotherapy for her2 overexpressing metastatic breast cancer (HER2+/MBC) markedly increases anticancer activity: a randomized multinational controlled phase III trial [Abstract]. Proceedings of the American Society of Clinical Oncology, 1998; 17:98a.
185. Harris JR, Lippman ME, Morrow M, et al. (eds): Diseases of the Breast. Philadelphia, Lippincott-Raven, 1996.
186. Silverstein MJ (ed): Ductal Carcinoma In Situ of the Breast. Baltimore, Williams and Wilkins, 1997.

18 *Hodgkin's Disease and the Lymphomas*

RICHARD T. HOPPE, MD, Radiation Oncology
LOUIS S. CONSTINE III, MD, Radiation Oncology
RAMAN QAZI, MD, FACP, Hematology/Oncology

This enlargement of the glands appeared to be a primitive affection of those bodies rather than the result of an irritation propagated to them from some ulcerated surface or other inflamed texture.

THOMAS HODGKIN, 1832

Perspective

Malignant lymphomas were first identified as a clinical entity in 1832, when Thomas Hodgkin described seven patients with enlarged lymph nodes that were not thought to result from inflammation, making this identification without the benefit of a microscope.[5] In 1845, Virchow distinguished lymphosarcoma from leukemia,[6] but it was not until later in the nineteenth century that histologic criteria for the diagnosis of both *Hodgkin's disease* and *malignant lymphoma* were developed.[7] Among the criteria for Hodgkin's disease was the recognition of pathognomonic giant cells, known as Reed-Sternberg (RS) cells.[8, 9] The twentieth century has seen continued effort to classify this heterogeneous group of diseases.

The lymphomas still present intriguing challenges to those seeking to clarify the etiology and pathogenesis of neoplasia. Progress in understanding the biology of the lymphomas has evolved with our greater understanding of the normal immune system.[1, 2] Moreover, investigations into the viral and immunologic aspects of Hodgkin's disease and Burkitt's lymphoma have stimulated analogous investigations of many other malignancies. The present management of these diseases is a clear example of the advantages of multidisciplinary collaboration in staging and treating malignancy.[3, 4] The increasing capacity for curing lymphomas has inspired oncologists to approach less responsive neoplasms with more determination and optimism.

Hodgkin's Disease

Epidemiology and Etiology

Epidemiology

Hodgkin's disease accounts for approximately 12% of all malignant lymphomas. The number of patients newly diagnosed each year in the United States has demonstrated a slight decrease over the last two decades,[10] with an annual incidence, at present, of about 7400 and a male-to-female ratio of 1.1:1.[11] More than 20 years ago, a striking pattern of age-related peaks was recognized in the incidence of Hodgkin's disease, with peaks appearing in children, young adults, and older adults.[12, 13] Curiously, the age range for the first peak varies according to the socioeconomic development of the country,[14] occurring before adolescence in underdeveloped countries but in the mid- to late twenties in industrialized countries. However, in general, the disease is regarded to be rare in those younger than the age of 5 years.

Patients with a congenital immunodeficiency disease, such as ataxia-telangiectasia, appear to have an increased risk for developing lymphomas, including Hodgkin's disease; non-Hodgkin's lymphomas are the most common.[15, 16] Similarly, Hodgkin's disease occurs more frequently in patients with iatrogenic or acquired immune system deficiency syndromes, including AIDS.[17, 18]

Although isolated clusters of Hodgkin's disease have been reported, leading to the possibility that there is an infectious nature to the malignancy, conclusive evidence of communicability is lacking.[19] One explanation for the possible infectious nature of Hodgkin's disease relates to its association with viruses. An increased incidence of

Hodgkin's disease is seen in patients with elevated titers of various antibodies to the Epstein-Barr virus (EBV), indicating an activated virus, and such elevations have been shown to predate the diagnosis of Hodgkin's disease.[20] Moreover, hybridization techniques have confirmed that a subset of patients with Hodgkin's disease have a clonal proliferation of EBV-infected cells and that EBV genomes are present in the RS cells, the pathognomonic cells of the disease.[21, 22] Reports of Hodgkin's disease in first-degree relatives of affected patients, especially of the same gender, and in parent-child concordant pairs support the hypothesis that EBV is a cofactor in the development of Hodgkin's disease.[23]

Etiology

The pathogenesis of Hodgkin's disease remains an enigma, although investigations have provided a greater understanding of its nature:

- Patients with untreated Hodgkin's disease have defective cellular immunity.[24, 25] The abnormality may be a consequence of the neoplasm itself producing inhibitory molecules[25, 26] or, alternatively, an inherent genetic defect that predisposes an individual to the development of Hodgkin's disease.
- Similar considerations relate to the association of Hodgkin's disease with EBV. Levels of expression of various antibodies (immunoglobulin [Ig]G or IgA against the EBV viral capsid antigen and early antigen D) are greater in the subset of individuals who develop Hodgkin's disease,[20, 27] which has led to the hypothesis that activation of EBV predisposes an individual to the induction of Hodgkin's disease by other unknown factors; that is, EBV acts as a cofactor. An alternative explanation is that the observed pattern of EBV activity is simply a marker of the effect of a more fundamental factor (viral, environmental, genetic, or a combination) that diminishes the immunologic control of latent infections in patients who develop Hodgkin's disease.
- The RS cell is the malignant cell in Hodgkin's disease. Sophisticated molecular biologic studies now support the concept that the RS cells are, in general, derived from germinal center B-cells that have lost their ability to express Ig.[28, 29] Demonstrations of clonal rearrangements of Ig heavy chain or light chain genes in tissue samples that contain large numbers of RS cells from patients with Hodgkin's disease, or even from individual RS cells, have been made.[30, 31] In addition, surface markers, such as the interleukin (IL)-2 and IL-4 receptors, can be demonstrated on RS cells that also are found on activated T-lymphocytes and B-lymphocytes.[32]

Detection and Diagnosis

Clinical Detection

The evolution of Hodgkin's disease has been well described.[1, 3] The process is likely to be unifocal in origin, and in 90% of patients, the disease presents in a pattern of involvement that suggests contiguous lymphatic spread, both at the time of presentation and the time of relapse, with contiguity between the supraclavicular and para-aortic regions assumed to be through the thoracic duct. Thus, clinical presentations fall into rather predictable patterns (Fig. 18–1).[33]

Patients with Hodgkin's disease usually present with painless lymph node enlargement. Constitutional symptoms occur in one third of patients, and they most prominently include unexplained fevers, drenching night sweats, or significant weight loss. Pruritus, malaise, or alcohol intolerance (intense pain in affected nodes after alcohol ingestion) may also occur. Most patients present with supradiaphragmatic nodal disease; the cervical and supraclavicular nodes are involved in 60% to 80% of patients. A primary mediastinal presentation is not very common despite the mediastinum being involved in the majority of patients, causing cough, dyspnea, and other respiratory symptoms.

A few patients (3% to 10%) present with isolated subdiaphragmatic involvement, usually with inguinal lymphadenopathy or, less commonly, an abdominal mass. The mesenteric nodes are rarely involved. In patients with generalized disease, the spleen is the most common site of subdiaphragmatic involvement. Although extralymphatic disease beyond the liver, lungs, and bone marrow is quite rare, if it occurs and is left unchecked, it progresses with involvement of multiple extralymphatic sites and potential organ failure.

Diagnostic Procedures

Recommended procedures for a complete evaluation and classification are as follows:

History and Physical Examination

- A *detailed history* records any systemic signs or symptoms (B symptoms) and evidence for cardiorespiratory

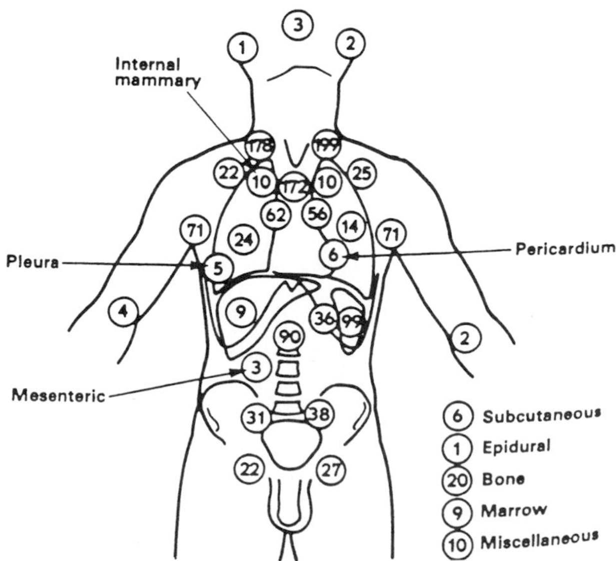

Figure 18–1. Anatomic distribution of sites of involvement. (From Kaplan HS, Dorfman RF, Nelson TS, et al: Staging laparotomy and splenectomy in Hodgkin's disease: analysis of indication and patterns of involvement in 285 consecutive cases, unselected patients. NCI Monograph 1973; 36:291.)

compromise and organ dysfunction. The *physical examination* includes a careful determination of the location and size of all palpable lymph nodes. An evaluation of Waldeyer's ring,[34] cardiorespiratory status, and organomegaly is vital.

- A *lymph node biopsy* is the usual method for diagnosis (see "Laboratory Procedure" for details).

Imaging

Imaging modalities for the detection and diagnosis of Hodgkin's disease are listed in Table 18–1 and detailed here:

- A *chest radiograph* (posteroanterior and lateral) should be taken, with measurement of the mass-to-thorax ratio. If the results of the chest x-ray study are positive, a *computed tomography (CT) scan* of the chest details the status of intrathoracic lymph node groups, lung parenchyma, pericardium, pleura, and the chest wall, and it is important for radiation therapy treatment planning.[35] A *magnetic resonance imaging (MRI)* scan of the chest may be used as an alternative to the CT scan of the chest when the interest is mainly in mediastinal adenopathy rather than pulmonary involvement.[36]
- An *abdominal CT scan* is effective for detecting enlarged abdominal and pelvic nodes. A node larger than 1 cm in the short axis diameter is considered to be abnormal. In addition, the CT scan can identify involvement of the spleen (focal nodules) or liver.
- A *bipedal lymphangiogram (LAG)* provides a detailed means for evaluating the size and architecture of the para-aortic, pericaval, and pelvic lymph nodes, and it also is helpful for planning radiation fields and assessing response to therapy. Unfortunately, the skill to perform lymphography is vanishing, and it is often impossible to obtain one, even in situations in which it would be especially helpful.
- In skilled hands, *gallium imaging* with single-photon emission CT is a helpful staging procedure.[37, 38] It also is useful in monitoring the response to therapy and evaluating patients with persistent mediastinal abnormalities on a CT scan of the chest.
- The value of *positron emission tomography* is unproved at this time, but it is being studied at several centers.[39, 40]

Laboratory Procedure

- A *complete blood cell count,* with differential white blood cell count, and the erythrocyte sedimentation rate (ESR) should be taken. Neutrophilic leukocytosis, mild normocytic, normochromic anemia and eosinophilia may occur. Patients with extensive disease sometimes have lymphocytopenia, another unfavorable prognostic indicator.[41]
- *Blood chemistries* should be taken, with particular attention to serum alkaline phosphatase, liver and renal function tests, and albumin. An elevated alkaline phosphatase level can reflect involvement of the liver, bone marrow, or bone. Hypergammaglobulinemia may be present, although hypogammaglobulinemia and hypoalbuminemia may be seen in patients with advanced disease and is associated with a worse prognosis.[41]
- *Bone marrow biopsy* should be taken in patients with

TABLE 18–1. **Imaging Modalities for Detection and Diagnosis of Hodgkin's Disease**

Method	Diagnosis and Staging Capability (Primary Tumor and Regional Nodes)	Recommended for Use
Chest x-ray study	Intrathoracic disease, if frequently assessed	Always
Chest CT scan	Provides additional evidence of intrathoracic disease; is the preferred study when the following situations are being addressed: • evaluation of a suspicious or equivocal mediastinum • evaluation of the "normal" mediastinum (may contain enlarged lymph nodes demonstrable by CT scan) • evaluation for chest wall involvement in the presence of bulky mediastinal disease • evaluation for pulmonary parenchymal lesions • evaluation for pleural or pericardial disease • anatomic extent of disease for treatment planning	Yes
Abdominal and pelvic CT scan	Delineates extent of bulky lymph node disease; normal-sized lymph nodes that contain tumor deposits, at times readily demonstrable by lymphography, however, will not be detected by CT scan; mesenteric lymphadenopathy is relatively reliable when shown by CT scan in the non-Hodgkin's lymphomas	Yes
MRI + gadolinium	Shows promise in delineating extent of disease; pericardial involvement is well demonstrated	Yes
Bipedal lymphography	Most accurate imaging test for evaluating retroperitoneal lymph nodes; provides convenient means for follow-up regarding response to treatment or relapse	Yes
Gallium citrate radionuclide studies	Supradiaphragmatic disease; proper technique is important for quality images	Selected
^{18}F PET	Can identify active foci of Hodgkin's Disease	Investigational

CT = computed tomography; MRI = magnetic resonance imaging; ^{18}F PET = ^{18}F fluorodeoxyglucose positron emission tomography.

B symptoms or clinical stage III or IV disease or if there are blood cell count depressions, an elevated alkaline phosphatase level, or bony abnormalities on imaging.

Biopsy and Surgical Procedure

The largest, most central node in an enlarged group is most likely to be diagnostic. Biopsy of a cervical-supraclavicular node is preferred because chronic inflammatory changes are more commonly present in inguinal or axillary nodes. Although lymph node aspiration may occasionally be sufficient for a diagnosis, biopsy is preferred to provide material for full histopathologic evaluation.

The classic RS cell is a large binucleate or multinucleate cell that is 25 to 30 μm in diameter, with an inclusion body–like macronucleoli in each of the nuclei, prominent euchromatin, spider web–like heterochromatin, and a prominent nuclear membrane with internal heterochromatin deposits. The presence of RS cells is required to establish a diagnosis, but RS-like cells also may be present in virally stimulated lymph nodes. In addition, typical RS cells may be rare in the nodular lymphocyte predominance type of Hodgkin's disease, which more commonly has multilobated (popcorn) cells.[42]

Nowadays, *laparotomy* and *splenectomy* are rarely used for staging Hodgkin's disease. However, in patients in which upstaging alters the treatment plan, laparotomy may be used to exclude occult subdiaphragmatic involvement. Overall, 20% to 30% of patients with clinical stage I or II disease are upstaged at laparotomy, and 90% of these patients have splenic involvement.[43] However, in the absence of laparotomy, disease must be assumed to be present in the abdomen (spleen or upper para-aortic nodes or both), and treatment must accommodate this likelihood.

Classification and Staging

Histopathology

The historically used classification systems for Hodgkin's disease (Jackson and Parker, Lukes and Butler, and the Rye Conference) are listed in Table 18–2.[44, 45] Under the Rye Conference system, four subtypes of Hodgkin's disease were recognized:

- *Nodular sclerosis Hodgkin's disease (NSHD)* is present in about 75% of cases in most series. Cellular nodules, containing plasma cells, neutrophils, and eosinophils, are surrounded by annular bands of polarizable collagen. The RS cells are large and their abundant pale cytoplasm may retract during fixation, leaving lacunar spaces around the nuclei—thus the term *lacunar cells.*
- *Lymphocytic predominance Hodgkin's disease (LPHD)* is present in about 5% of cases. The lymph node architecture may be completely or partially obliterated by a proliferation of benign-appearing lymphocytes, with or without histiocytes. RS cells are few; instead, typical popcorn cells may be present.[42] Nodular and diffuse subtypes are recognized.
- Fifteen to twenty percent of patients have *mixed cellularity Hodgkin's disease (MCHD),* in which a pleocellular infiltrate (plasma cells, neutrophils, eosinophils) and moderate numbers of RS cells are seen.
- *Lymphocyte depletion Hodgkin's disease (LDHD)* is rare, characterized by a predominance of RS cells and few lymphocytes. This aggressive subtype must be carefully distinguished from NSHD and non-Hodgkin's lymphoma (diffuse large cell or anaplastic large cell types).

Of note, immunoperoxidase studies have demonstrated significant differences between nodular LPHD and classic subtypes. Nodular LPHD is CD20+, CD15−, and CD30−, whereas the classic Hodgkin's disease subtypes are CD20−, CD15+, and CD30+.[10]

In 1994, a modification to the Rye Conference system was published by the International Lymphoma Study Group as part of the Revised European-American Lymphoma (REAL) classification system (see Table 18–2).[45] This system classifies Hodgkin's disease through a combination of morphologic, immunophenotypic, genetic, and clinical features, resulting in these subtypes:

1. (nodular) lymphocytic predominance
2. lymphocyte-rich classic Hodgkin's disease (Note:

TABLE 18–2. **Interrelationships of Major Histopathology Classifications of Hodgkin's Disease**

REAL Classification	Jackson and Parker	Rye Conference	Lukes and Butler
Lymphocytic predominance, nodular (with or without diffuse)	Paragranuloma	Lymphocytic predominance, nodular (most cases)	Lymphocytic or histiocytic (nodular diffuse)
Classic Hodgkin's disease			
Lymphocyte-rich classic Hodgkin's disease	Paragranuloma	Lymphocytic predominance, diffuse (most cases) Lymphocytic predominance, nodular (some cases)	Lymphocytic or histiocytic (nodular diffuse)
Nodular sclerosis	Paragranuloma	Nodular sclerosis	Nodular sclerosis
Mixed cellularity	Granuloma	Mixed cellularity (most cases)	Mixed cellularity
Lymphocyte depletion	Sarcoma	Lymphocyte depletion	Diffuse fibrosis Reticular

Numbers 1 and 2 would have been considered to be *lymphocytic predominance* under the Rye Conference scheme.)
3. nodular sclerosis
4. mixed cellularity
5. lymphocyte depletion (acknowledged to be exceedingly rare and often confused with diffuse large cell lymphoma)

The World Health Organization (WHO) has now incorporated this classification system into a new WHO classification of lymphoid neoplasms.[46] The collaborating committees concluded that patient treatment can be determined by the specific lymphoma type in conjunction with tumor grade, if applicable, and clinical prognostic factors, such as the International Prognostic Index.[47]

Staging

The Ann Arbor staging system[48] is used most widely for Hodgkin's disease (Fig. 18–2, Table 18–3),[49] together with the minor modifications that were incorporated into the so-called Cotswolds system in 1989.[50] In the Ann Arbor system, the extent of disease is classified as I through IV, according to the distribution of disease. In addition, the presence of localized extralymphatic disease (such as extension of lymph node involvement to include the pericardium or lung, or isolated bony disease) is acknowledged by the use of the subscript letter *E*. The absence or presence of significant constitutional symptoms (unexplained fever higher than 38°C, drenching night sweats, or weight loss of more than 10% of body weight in the previous 6 months) is designated by the letters *A* or *B*. Thus, an individual who has involvement of the mediastinum, supraclavicular nodes, and para-aortic nodes and a history of unexplained fevers would have stage IIIB disease. An anatomic mapping of common nodes at presentation and staging with patterns of contiguous regional nodal spread is represented in Figure 18–3.[51]

An important deficiency of the Ann Arbor system is its failure to recognize disease bulk. Numerous series have identified bulky or large mediastinal adenopathy (LMA) to be an adverse prognostic factor.[52] The Cotswolds system addressed this issue by using the subscript *X* in the designation of stage for those patients with bulky mediastinal disease. Unfortunately, the measurement employed in the Cotswolds system is the maximum width of the mediastinal mass divided by the intrathoracic diameter at the T5 to T6 interspace, a ratio that results in even modest mediastinal masses being defined as bulky because the thorax is narrower at that level.

The Ann Arbor staging system also incorporates the concept of clinical versus pathologic staging. *Clinical staging (CS)* is defined as the extent of disease identified by the initial biopsy as well as physical examination and imaging studies. The *pathologic stage (PS)* is defined by the information obtained from all additional biopsies (in-

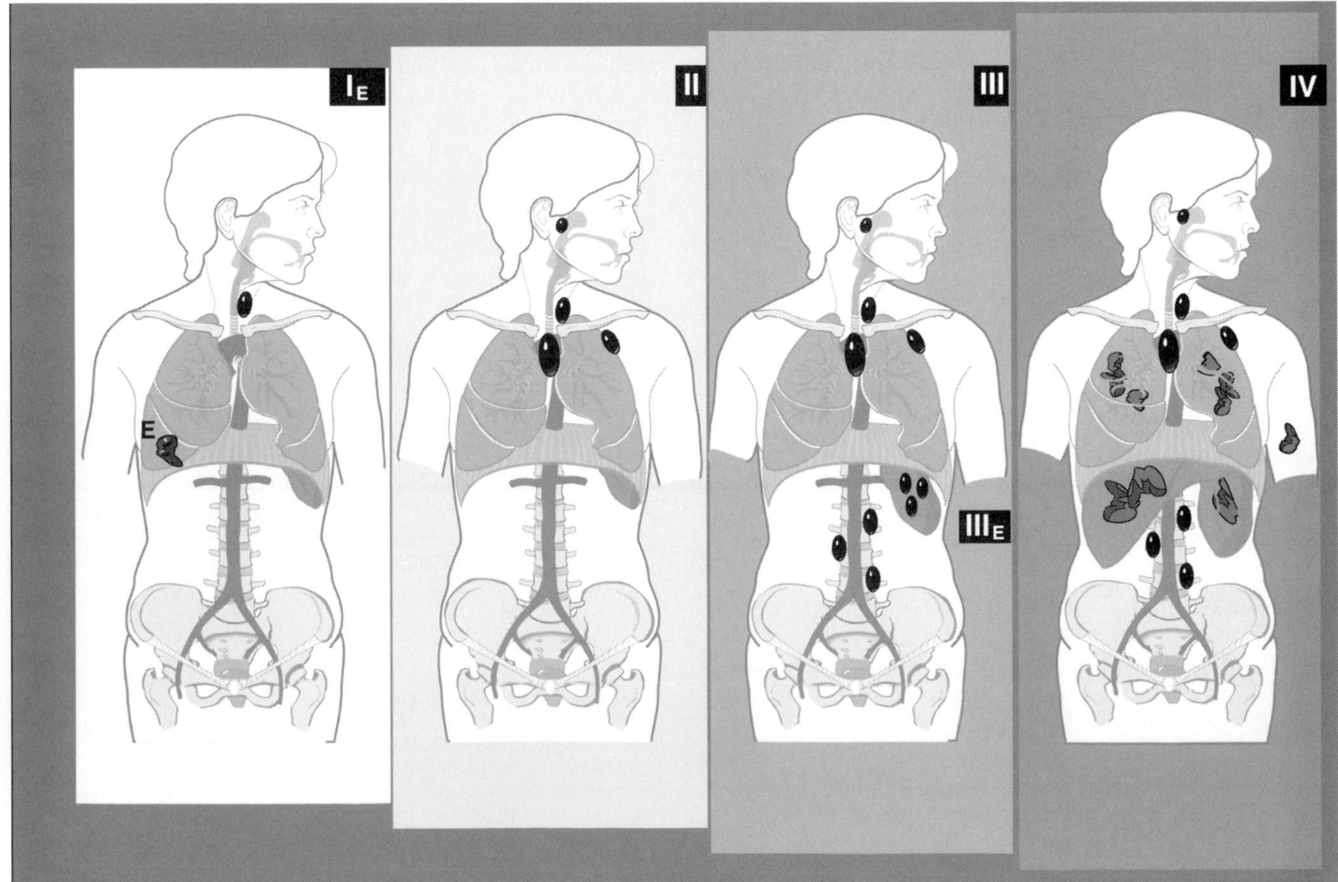

Figure 18–2. Anatomic staging for Hodgkin's disease.

TABLE 18–3. **Ann Arbor Stage and Substage Classification for Hodgkin's Disease**

Stage*	Substage	Descriptor
I	I	Involvement of single node region or lymphoid structure
	I_E	Involvement of single extralymphatic organ/site
II	II	Involvement of two or more node regions; same side of diaphragm
	II_E	Involvement of single node region + localized single extralymphatic organ/site
III	III	Involvement of node regions, both sides of diaphragm
	III_E	± Involvement of localized, single extralymphatic organ/site
	III_S	± Involvement of spleen
	III_{E+S}	± Involvement of both
IV	IV	Diffuse involvement of extralymphatic organ/site ± node regions

E = extralymphatic disease; S = spleen.

*All stages divided: A = without weight loss/fever/sweats; B = with weight loss/fever/sweats.

Used with permission of the American Joint Committee on Cancer (AJCC®), Chicago, Illinois. The original source for this material is the AJCC® Cancer Staging Manual, 5th edition (1997), published by Lippincott-Raven Publishers, Philadelphia, Pennsylvania.

cluding a bone marrow biopsy). Organ involvement is noted with letter symbols: S = spleen, H = liver, L = lung, M = marrow, P = pleura, O = bone (osseous), and D = skin. The concept of CS versus PS was very important in the era when the extent of disease was often defined only after completion of a staging laparotomy and splenectomy. However, because this procedure is no longer performed routinely, it is more reasonable to consider a stage designation that includes the results of physical examination, imaging studies, and bone marrow biopsy only.

Principles of Treatment

Multidisciplinary Treatment Planning

The variety of possible therapeutic strategies for the treatment of patients with Hodgkin's disease and the clear relationship of outcome to appropriate therapy make it imperative that the surgeon, medical oncologist, radiation oncologist, diagnostic radiologist, and pathologist jointly consider the characteristics of each patient in order to devise optimal therapy. Moreover, each participant must have expertise in the respective disciplines because of the complexity of each phase of evaluation and therapy. Stage has a critical role in determining treatment; a concise overview of different treatment modalities by stage of disease is offered in Table 18–4.[53]

Surgery

The primary role of surgery is to obtain tissue diagnosis through biopsy. Radical excision of enlarged nodes is not justified in view of the efficacy of chemotherapy and radiotherapy in treating this disease. For women in whom pelvic irradiation is contemplated, a midline or lateral oophoropexy may be performed as an open procedure, or through laparoscopy.[54]

Radiation Therapy

The responsiveness of Hodgkin's disease to irradiation was first demonstrated within the first decade after the discovery of x-rays in 1896. In the 1950s, Rene Gilbert, a Swiss radiotherapist, laid the foundations for the definitive radiotherapy treatment of Hodgkin's disease,[55, 56] and Vera Peters from the Princess Margaret Hospital in Toronto provided further definition of important principles.[57–59] A systematic study of the role of radiation therapy and the use of supervoltage techniques was subsequently reported by Henry S. Kaplan from Stanford University.[60]

Throughout the 1900s, irradiation has been used as a primary treatment modality for the majority of patients with favorable early-stage Hodgkin's disease and, more recently, together with chemotherapy in combined-modality therapy programs for patients with more advanced disease. The dose required to eradicate Hodgkin's disease in clinically involved nodes is approximately 36 to 44 Gy; the dose required for prophylactic treatment is 25 to 36 Gy. Each treatment fraction delivers 1.5 to 1.8 Gy.

- The use of megavoltage irradiation (linear accelerators) and extended fields to include adjacent (contiguous) clinically uninvolved nodal sites has been considered to be crucial in achieving high cure rates when radiation therapy alone is used to treat Hodgkin's dis-

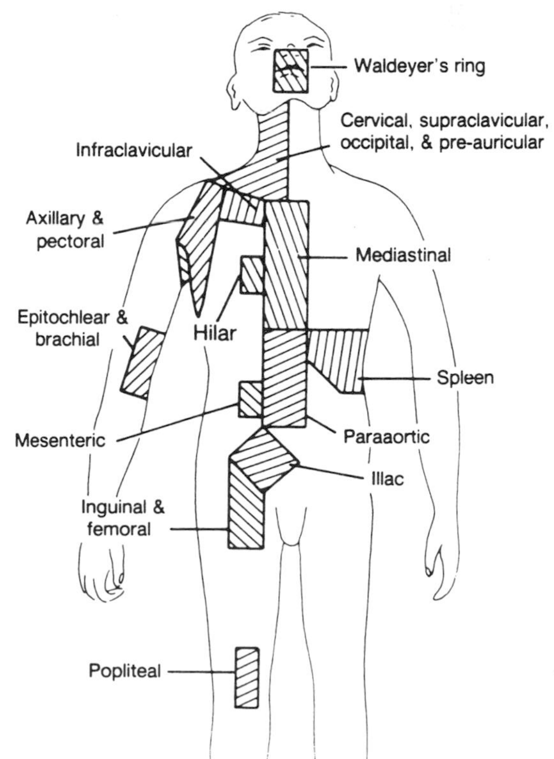

Figure 18–3. Anatomic definition of separate lymph node regions. (From Kaplan HS, Rosenberg SA: The treatment of Hodgkin's disease. Med Clin North Am 1966; 50:1591.)

TABLE 18–4. **Guidelines for Treatment of Hodgkin's Disease in Adults**

Stage	Clinical Presentation	Treatment*
IA or IIA	Supradiaphragmatic, absent or small mediastinal disease	Mantle ± para-aortic-splenic pedicle RT (STNI)
		MAC + IFRT; IC
	Supradiaphragmatic, LMA (>⅓ intrathoracic diameter) or juxtapericardial tumor	MAC + IFRT
	Subdiaphragmatic presentations with laparotomy staging	RT: pelvis + para-aortic
		MAC + IFRT
IB or IIB	Night sweating alone	As for IA, IIA
	Fevers and/or weight loss ± night sweating	MAC + IFRT or IC
IIIA	Favorable: absent or small mediastinal adenopathy, <5 splenic nodules, upper abdominal disease (IIIA1)	MAC + IFRT
		MAC
		Rarely: TNI or STNI ± low dose to liver
	Unfavorable: LMA, >5 splenic nodules, lower abdominal disease (IIIA2)	MAC + IFRT
IIIB		MAC ± IFRT (to sites of bulky or post-ChT residual disease)
IV		MAC ± IFRT (to sites of bulky or post-ChT residual disease)
		IC + BMT
Recurrent	Previous primary RT	MAC
	Previous initial ChT: recurrence <12 mos	BMT + RT
	Previous initial ChT: recurrence >12 mos	Salvage ChT or BMT

LMA = large mediastinal adenopathy; ChT = chemotherapy; RT = radiation therapy; STNI = subtotal nodal irradiation; MAC = multiagent chemotherapy; IFRT = involved field radiation therapy; IC = investigational protocols; TNI = total nodal irradiation; BMT = high dose cytotoxic chemotherapy + hemopoietic stem cell rescue.

*PDQ recommendations: MAC: ABVD = doxorubicin (Adriamycin), bleomycin, vinblastine, dacarbazine; MOPP = mechlorethamine, vincristine, procarbazine, prednisone; MOPP/ABVD; MOPP/ABV.

From Physician Data Query: Adult Hodgkin's Disease. Bethesda, National Cancer Institute, 2000.

ease.[1] However, recognition of high rates of secondary tumors has led many of the more recent clinical trials to abandon the use of extended fields in favor of involved-field treatment.[61]

- *Total nodal irradiation (TNI),* also known as *total lymphoid irradiation (TLI),* includes irradiation to a mantle field above the diaphragm, followed by irradiation of the para-aortic nodes and spleen (or splenic pedicle after splenectomy) and the pelvis, separately or in a single field (an inverted *Y*).
- *Subtotal nodal irradiation (STNI)* refers to a mantle field followed by a para-aortic spleen (or splenic pedicle after splenectomy) field, which has become the most widely used field in patients with stage IA or IIA disease.
- Shielding and field shaping are used to protect the lungs, spinal cord, larynx, heart, humoral and femoral heads, kidneys, gonads, and iliac crest bone marrow. Shaping the field limits the direct radiation dose to the pelvis and spares significant amounts of bone marrow, with only minimal scattered irradiation to the gonads.

Most patients with stage I to IIA supradiaphragmatic disease can be managed effectively with radiation alone.[62, 63] Other series suggest that mantle plus para-aortic and spleen irradiation is a reasonable approach for nearly all patients with stage I to IIA supradiaphragmatic disease, provided there is not massive mediastinal disease.[64] The expected 10-year survival rate is 70% to 80%, and the rate for freedom from relapse is 70% to 80%.[62, 63] In general, the outcome of treatment for patients with subdiaphragmatic disease is similar to that for patients with supradiaphragmatic disease.[65, 66]

Historically, patients with favorable manifestations of stage IIIA disease (i.e., those with anatomic substage III [limited to spleen, splenic hilar, or celiac regions] and an uninvolved spleen or limited splenic involvement [fewer than 5 gross nodules]) could be managed effectively with radiation alone, after staging with laparotomy.[67] However, with the demise of laparotomy, these patients are now managed similarly to patients who present with stage IIIB to IV disease, with an emphasis on the systemic component of management.

Occasionally, favorable presentations may be approached with more limited treatments. One example is CS IA LPHD that is limited to the high neck. If abdominal imaging study results are negative, treatment may be limited to a supramediastinal mantle plus an ipsilateral preauricular field.[68] Another favorable presentation is NSHD that is limited to intrathoracic sites. It is probably safe also to exclude subdiaphragmatic irradiation in these patients. However, despite the success of programs using radiation alone for early-stage disease, there is significant concern regarding late effects, such as second cancers and cardiovascular disease. This has led to many clinical trials in early-stage disease testing programs of combined-modality therapy, which include brief chemotherapy and limited radiation.[69] Others are testing programs of chemotherapy alone.[70]

Late Effects

Complications of radiation therapy include a transient bone marrow suppression in most patients following TNI or STNI, with bone marrow compensatory extension to the femurs for 1 to 5 years and in-field recovery after 5 years.[71] More seriously, but less commonly, symptomatic radiation pneumonitis (5%) and pericarditis (5%) occur.[72] Clinical hypothyroidism is relatively rare (5% to 15%),[73] but subclinical compensatory chemical hypothyroidism is frequent (30% to 60%)[74, 75]; it is detected by an elevation in thyroid-

TABLE 18–5. **Examples of Combinations of Chemotherapeutic Agents Used in the Treatment of Hodgkin's Disease**

Acronym	Agents	Toxicity
MOPP	Mechlorethamine, vincristine (Oncovin), procarbazine, prednisone	Nausea/vomiting, hair loss, myelosuppression, sterility, leukemogenesis
ChlVPP	Chlorambucil, vinblastine, procarbazine, prednisone	Myelosuppression
ABVD	Doxorubicin (Adriamycin), bleomycin, vinblastine, dacarbazine	Cough, dyspnea, pulmonary dysfunction
CBV + ABMT	Cyclophosphamide, carmustine (BCNU), etoposide (VP-16)	Cardiopulmonary complications
Stanford V	Doxorubicin, vinblastine, mechlorethamine, vincristine, bleomycin, etoposide, prednisone	

ABMT = autologous stem cell transplantation.

stimulating hormone and managed with thyroxine replacement.[76] Second malignant tumors are a major risk. The observed and expected ratio is approximately sixfold.[77]

If the pelvis is irradiated, then the gonads receive significant doses, even when appropriate shielding is used. Aspermia may occur with inguinal fields, even with small doses of scattered irradiation. The use of special gonadal shielding can reduce this risk; nevertheless, sperm banking before therapy can be suggested.[78] Menstrual dysfunction in women is common, but recovery usually takes place, and pregnancies producing normal offspring can occur.

Chemotherapy

Since the demonstration in the 1940s that nitrogen mustard has activity against Hodgkin's disease, great progress has been made in the treatment of generalized Hodgkin's disease with combinations of agents. The strategy that has proved to be most effective entails the use of multiple non–cross-resistant agents with additive antitumor effects but without additive host toxicities. A broad choice of agents exists with which to develop such combinations (Tables 18–5 and 18–6).[79–89]

Several three-, four-, or five-drug programs have proved to be effective. The MOPP regimen (see Table 18–5) was the first successful combination demonstrated. DeVita and associates at the National Cancer Institute (NCI) reported complete responses (CRs) in 81% of 194 previously untreated patients with stage III or IV disease who were given the 4-drug combination for 6 months or more.[90] Once the efficacy of MOPP was demonstrated, modifications were developed to decrease the acute toxicities of nausea, vomiting, peripheral neuropathy, constipation, and marrow suppression and the long-term toxicities of sterility and second malignancies. In the early 1970s, doxorubicin was developed and used in several regimens. The most prominent of

TABLE 18–6. **Representative Results of Therapy in the Treatment of Hodgkin's Disease by Stage**

				RFS (%)		OS (%)	
Stage	**Investigator**	**No. of Patients**	**Treatment**	*≥5 Yrs*	*≥10 Yrs*	*≥5 Yrs*	*≥10 Yrs*
IA, IIA	Rosenberg et al[79]	109	STNI or TNI		79		96
IA, IIA	Mauch et al[80]	315	STNI		82		93
IA–IIB	Hughes-Davies et al[81]	47	RT		54		84
		125	MOPP + RT		88		89
IB–IV	Horning et al[82]	47	Stanford V ± RT	85		96	
IB–IV	Radford et al[83]	423	MVPP ± RT	66		71	
			ChlVPP/EVA ± RT	80		80	
IB–IV	Harding et al[84]	60	MVPP	79	65	70	57
II–IV	Hill et al[85]	85	VEEP ± RT	62		89	
IIA–IV	Salvagno et al[86]	133	MOPP/ABVD + RT	83		76	
IIA–IVB	Simmonds et al[87]	83	PACE BOM ± RT	64		90	
IIIB, IV	Ferme et al[88]	418	MOPP/ABV	80		85	
			ABVPP	68		94	
			MOPP/ABV + RT	82		88	
			ABVPP + RT	75		78	
IIIB, IV	Aviles et al[89]	70	EVBD	80		86	
			MVBD	53		58	

RFS = relapse-free survival; OS = overall survival; STNI = subtotal nodal irradiation; TNI = total nodal irradiation; RT = radiation therapy; MOPP = mechlorethamine, vincristine, procarbazine, prednisone; Stanford V = doxorubicin, vinblastine, mechlorethamine, vincristine, bleomycin, etoposide, prednisone; MVPP = mechlorethamine, vinblastine, procarbazine, prednisone; ChlVPP/EVA = chlorambucil, vinblastine, procarbazine, prednisone / etoposide, vincristine, doxorubicin (Adriamycin); VEEP = vincristine, epirubicin, etoposide, prednisolone; ABVD = doxorubicin (Adriamycin), bleomycin, vinblastine, dacarbazine; PACE BOM = prednisolone, doxorubicin (Adriamycin), cyclophosphamide, etoposide, bleomycin, vincristine (Oncovin), methotrexate; ABVPP = doxorubicin (Adriamycin), bleomycin, vinblastine, procarbazine, prednisone; EVBD = epirubicin, vinblastine, bleomycin, dacarbazine; MVBD = mitoxantrone, vinblastine, bleomycin, dacarbazine.

these is the ABVD program (see Table 18–5), which was carefully studied by Bonadonna and associates in Milan and shown to provide a similar CR induction rate when compared with MOPP.[91]

In general, the thrust of clinical research for patients with advanced-stage disease has been twofold. One pathway has been to try to identify the most unfavorable patients in the group and treat them more intensively initially, with a component of high-dose therapy and autologous transplantation. However, the other research question in these patients remains the role of consolidation radiation and its use either as an adjuvant therapy or as an essential component of a combined-modality approach.[92]

Bone Marrow Transplantation

Several different treatment strategies have emerged that require autologous bone marrow transplantation (ABMT) for patients with advanced Hodgkin's disease, whose disease has relapsed or has not responded to initial treatment with multiple drug modalities or chemotherapy regimens.[93] Although ABMT has become a standard treatment approach for these patients, important questions remain related to the timing of the stem cell transplantation, the selection of drug agents, and the role of radiation in these patients.

Combined-Modality Therapy

Historically, chemotherapy was used as an adjuvant after completion of irradiation for patients with early or intermediate stages of disease, and radiation was used as a consolidation treatment for patients with advanced disease who had achieved a CR to chemotherapy.[94] Nowadays, combined-modality therapy is the most frequently used regimen in the management of patients with Hodgkin's disease. Important decisions in the use of combined-modality therapy for Hodgkin's disease include the selection of drug combinations, the sequence of therapy, the dose of irradiation, the fields to be treated, and the potential overlapping toxicities.

In general, treatment is initiated with chemotherapy. This modality has the advantage of treating all sites of disease at the outset, as well as reducing bulky disease to facilitate subsequent irradiation. Most commonly, the entire course of chemotherapy is administered before any irradiation. Occasionally, split-course approaches are used for patients with more limited disease. The extent of radiation fields in combined-modality programs varies from treatment of all initial sites of disease (exclusive of bone marrow) to treatment of bulky sites only (variably defined; larger than 5 cm or visible on imaging). The dose of radiation used varies from 20 to 36 Gy in different series.

Patients with stage I or II bulky mediastinal Hodgkin's disease often have a poor outcome when they are treated with irradiation or chemotherapy alone and are treated best with combined-modality therapy.[95, 96] The rationale for using combined-modality therapy in bulky or advanced-stage disease is that the pattern of failure after treatment with chemotherapy alone is often in initially involved sites, especially bulky sites, and the addition of radiation may reduce that relapse risk. Whether the intensity of chemotherapy can be reduced in the face of the addition of irradiation is not known. One approach that tests this question is the Stanford V regimen (see Table 18–5), which includes a brief (12-week) course of chemotherapy, followed by irradiation to initially bulky (larger than 5 cm) sites of disease.[82]

Recurrent Disease

Relapse after initial therapy occurs most often within 4 years, but late relapses may occur. Approximately 10% to 30% of patients with advanced Hodgkin's disease do not achieve CR with initial treatment, or they have a relapse after initially effective treatment with chemotherapy.[97, 98] The choice of therapy for patients whose disease recurs after primary treatment is dependent on the time to relapse, disease characteristics at the time of relapse, and the initial treatment:

- For patients who were treated initially with radiation therapy alone, the majority who relapse can be treated effectively with combination chemotherapy, such as ABVD, with or without additional radiation.[99]
- Patients who fail to achieve a CR or relapse less than 1 year after initial treatment with chemotherapy are candidates for programs of high-dose chemotherapy with ABMT, with or without complementary radiation.[100, 101, 102] In this group of patients, 40% to 50% of patients have achieved long-term disease-free survival.
- For patients treated with chemotherapy initially and who have a disease-free interval of 1 to 3 years or more, additional chemotherapy with or without irradiation may often achieve durable responses.[103, 104]

Results and Prognosis

When assessing the results of therapy in the treatment of Hodgkin's disease, consideration must be given to the following:

- definitions of disease-free and overall survival
- characteristics of the patients reviewed in terms of staging evaluation and prognostic factors
- treatment regimens and techniques used
- morbidity of therapy

It is of special importance that attention be given to both disease-free and overall survival when interpreting therapy results in early-stage disease, in view of the excellent potential of chemotherapy for salvaging patients treated initially with radiation therapy alone. Representative treatment results are presented in Table 18–6.[4, 105]

Surgery

Until the 1990s, a staging laparotomy was considered to be standard in the evaluation of stage I to IIA patients. That concept was challenged in an EORTC study that randomized patients to undergo the procedure.[106] The H6 trial included patients with only one or two sites of disease and were either asymptomatic with an ESR of lower than 50, or with B symptoms and an ESR of lower than 30. Patients randomized to CS alone were treated to mantle and para-aortic and spleen fields. Patients who underwent

TABLE 18–7. **Survival by Histologic Type and the International Prognostic Index**

Consensus Diagnosis	6-Year OS (%)		5-Year FFS (%)	
	Index 0/1	*Index 4/5*	*Index 0/1*	*Index 4/5*
Follicular	84	17	55	6
Mantle cell	57	0	27	0
Marginal zone B-cell, MALT	89	40	83	0
Marginal zone B-cell, nodal	76	50	30	0
Small lymphocytic	76	38	35	13
Diffuse large B-cell	73	22	63	19
Primary mediastinal large B-cell	77	0	69	0
High-grade B-cell, Burkitt-like	71	0	71	0
Precursor T-lymphoblastic	29	40	29	40
Peripheral T-cell	36	15	27	10
Anaplastic large T-/null cell	61	83	49	83

OS = overall survival; FFS = failure-free survival; MALT = mucosa-associated lymphoid tumor.
Adapted from Armitage JO, Lister TA: Non-Hodgkin's lymphoma. In: American Society of Clinical Oncology Education Booklet, p 338. Alexandria, American Society of Clinical Oncology, 1998, with permission.

laparotomy had treatment defined according to the extent of disease identified by laparotomy. At 7 years of follow-up, there was no difference in either disease-free or overall survival between the groups.

Radiation Therapy

Limited presentations of stage I to IIA supradiaphragmatic disease may be suitable for treatment with mantle irradiation alone. In the H5 trial of the EORTC, patients who were laparotomy-staged PS I or PS II with mediastinal involvement, were younger than 40 years of age, had an ESR of lower than 70, and were lymphocyte-predominant or had nodular-sclerosing histology were randomized to mantle alone versus mantle plus prophylactic treatment to the para-aortic nodes.[107] At 9 years, there was no significant difference in overall survival or freedom from relapse in this favorable group.

Mantle treatment alone has been adopted as a general policy in stage I to IIA patients after a negative result from staging laparotomy at some centers.[108] However, in the absence of laparotomy, even the favorably defined patients of the EORTC H7 trial (women with CS IA disease, without bulky mediastinal masses, younger than age 40, with an ESR of less than 30) fared poorly when the treatment was limited to mantle alone.[109]

Chemotherapy

A lack of cross-resistance was used in the design of programs that alternated three- or four-drug combinations (ABVD following MOPP). Conceptually, this strategy appears to overcome the spontaneous development of multidrug-resistant tumor cells. The Milan group compared alternating cycles of MOPP and ABVD with MOPP treatment alone and showed the combination of MOPP and ABVD to be superior.[91] A large intergroup Cancer and Leukemia Group B study randomized patients with advanced disease to treatment with MOPP, ABVD, or MOPP-ABVD.[97] In this trial, the two doxorubicin-containing regimens proved to be superior to MOPP alone. Largely as a result of this study (as well as the severe toxicity of MOPP), ABVD or MOPP-ABVD have supplanted MOPP alone as the primary first-line regimens used for treatment of this disease.

Combined-Modality Therapy

A large randomized trial of the Southwest Oncology Group evaluated the role of consolidation radiation (20 Gy to initially involved sites) in patients with advanced-stage disease (IIIB to IV) who achieved a CR to MOP-BAP chemotherapy (mechlorethamine, vincristine [Oncovin], procarbazine, bleomycin, doxorubicin [Adriamycin], prednisone).[110] This study demonstrated improvement in disease-free survival, but not overall survival, after consolidation irradiation. A large meta-analysis reported the same conclusion.[111] A similar trial is ongoing in the EORTC, in which the chemotherapy employed is MOPP-ABV (mechlorethamine, vincristine [Oncovin], procarbazine, prednisone, doxorubicin [Adriamycin], bleomycin, vinblastine).[112]

Prognosis

As the therapy for Hodgkin's disease has become increasingly effective, the factors that influence outcome have declined in significance. Nevertheless, several factors, including stage, mediastinal mass, and B symptoms, continue to influence the success and certainly the choice of therapy.

Stage

The stage or extent of disease persists as the most important prognostic variable. Patients with stage IV disease have a 60% to 90% 5-year survival rate compared with 70% to 95% of patients with stages I and II disease (see Table 18–6). Nonetheless, within a given disease stage, other characteristics also influence the success of therapy.

Mediastinal Mass

For patients with limited (stage I or II) disease, contemporary therapies have blurred the impact of prognostic factors. One unfavorable prognostic factor that guides therapeutic decisions is the presence of a large mediastinal mass. LMA, which is defined as a mass that exceeds one third of the transverse diameter of the chest (intrathoracic width measured at the dome of the diaphragm) on a standard posteroanterior chest radiograph, places a patient at a greater risk for disease recurrence if treated with radiation therapy alone. Therefore, these patients are generally treated with combined-modality therapy.[113, 114]

B Symptoms

The presence of B symptoms is another prognostic factor that guides therapy, especially for patients with stage I to II disease.[115] A concordance of both weight loss and fevers is especially ominous.[116] Systemic treatment is generally employed in the presence of B symptoms.

Other factors that have been associated with a less favorable prognosis in stage I and II disease include multiple sites of disease (variably defined, but often more than 2 or 3),[63] measurements of tumor bulk (which include both size of disease and number of sites),[63, 115] older age (older than 40 years in some series, older than 60 in others),[115, 117] unfavorable histology as a function of age (Table 18–7),[118] and an elevation of the ESR.[111, 119] For advanced disease (stage III to IV), a large international study has identified seven independent unfavorable prognostic factors: male sex, patient age of older than 45 years, stage IV disease, hemoglobin of less than 10.5 g/dL, serum albumin of less than 4.0 g/dL, leukocytosis (greater than 15,000/mm^3), and lymphocytopenia (less than 8% of white count or lower than 600 absolute count).[41]

Pediatric Hodgkin's Disease

The biology and natural history of Hodgkin's disease in children is similar to that in adults. However, when irradiation techniques and doses suitable for controlling disease in adults are translated to the pediatric setting, substantial morbidities (primarily musculoskeletal growth inhibition) are produced.[120, 121] In addition, some investigators have shown an increased risk of coronary artery disease and secondary malignant tumors.[122, 123] It is within this context that new strategies for the treatment of pediatric Hodgkin's disease were developed by Donaldson and Link.[124] Indeed, historically, children were thought to have a worse prognosis than adults.[1] However, it is now apparent that the converse is true.[125–127]

This discussion focuses on data that are specific to pediatric Hodgkin's disease. Information common to both pediatric and adult Hodgkin's disease can be found in the previous section (see "Hodgkin's Disease").

Epidemiology and Etiology

Pediatric Hodgkin's disease accounts for 6% of childhood cancers and is epidemiologically distinct from adult Hodgkin's disease. A striking male-to-female predominance exists in the earliest age groups, with a ratio of 4:1 for 3- to 7-year-olds, 3:1 for 7- to 9-year-olds, and 1.3:1 (a ratio more similar to that of adults) for older children.[125, 128] Nonetheless, the disease is uncommon before the age of 5 and, among children, is most common in adolescence.

The role of EBV in the pathogenesis of pediatric Hodgkin's disease is well established. EBV early RNA1 has been shown to be expressed in RS cells in 58% of childhood cases, most commonly under the age of 10.[129] Evidence for a genetic predisposition also exists, which is relevant when counseling families. Parent-child associations have been reported. Siblings have a two- to fivefold increased incidence, and this rate is increased to seven- to ninefold in same sex siblings.[130]

Detection and Diagnosis

Clinical Detection

Clinical presentations fall in rather predictable patterns. Most children are diagnosed on the basis of supradiaphragmatic lymph nodes, with painless cervical adenopathy in 80% of cases. Mediastinal involvement occurs in 76% of adolescents, but it occurs in only 33% of 1- to 10-year-olds. As in adults, mediastinal disease may produce symptoms such as dyspnea, cough, or superior vena cava syndrome. Axillary adenopathy is less common.[1]

Diagnostic Procedures

After pathologic confirmation, the patient undergoes an extensive clinical staging, as is true for adults. This includes a *thorough history* and *physical examination, laboratory testing*, and imaging studies as outlined here:

- Imaging of the thorax should include a *chest radiograph* and *CT scan.*
- Distinguishing normal (or hyperplastic) thymus from nodes in children can be problematic. The usefulness of *gallium scanning* for evaluating supradiaphragmatic nodes in children has not been specifically established, although the procedure is useful in adults.[131]
- Imaging of the abdomen and pelvis should include an *abdominal-pelvic CT scan* and, optimally, a bilateral, lower extremity *LAG.* Of note, in a Pediatric Oncology Group (POG) analysis of 216 children, use of CT scan in discerning intrinsic spleen lesions and abnormal portohepatic and celiac nodal areas were highly predictive of outcome but infrequently observed.[105]
- A report from St. Jude also found *MRI* to be useful for abdominal imaging.[132]

Distinction of reactive lymph node hyperplasia from Hodgkin's disease is problematic; overall, of the 30% of

TABLE 18–8. **Incidence of Stage Change by Laparotomy**

Clinical Stage	No. of Patients	Pathologic Stage				Total Stage Changes	
		I–III	*III_1**	*III_2*	*IV*	*No.*	*%*
I/II	181	13	36	9	3	48	27
III_1	9	2	3	4	—	6	67
III_2	9	—	2	7	—	2	22
IV	4	—	—	—	4	0	0

*Excludes 13 pathologic stage III_1 patients in whom clinical stage was not reported.

Modified from Mendenhall N, Cantor A, Williams J, et al: With modern technique is staging laparotomy necessary in pediatric Hodgkin's disease? A Pediatric Oncology Group study. J Clin Oncol 1993; 11:2218. From Halperin EC, Constine LS, Tarbell NJ, et al: Pediatric Radiation Oncology, 3rd ed. Philadelphia, Lippincott Williams & Wilkins, 1999, with permission.

patients who have an abnormal LAG, approximately 19% have involvement with Hodgkin's disease, whereas 12% have reactive hyperplasia, which is more common in younger children than in adolescents.[133] Older studies have reported CT scanning to be less sensitive than LAG in detecting retroperitoneal Hodgkin's disease, and they have suggested that the accuracy of the abdominal CT scan in children is less than that in adults because of the lack of fat, which provides contrast for the retroperitoneal lymph nodes.[134] However, the quality of CT scanning has improved greatly, increasing its sensitivity and specificity. Moreover, many centers are reluctant to perform LAG in young children because the procedure may require general anesthesia, and at some institutions, expertise in LAG interpretation is lacking.

Of interest is a report from the Dana Farber Cancer Institute on 247 children who presented with supradiaphragmatic Hodgkin's disease and underwent *laparotomy*. Following the laparotomy, it was shown that LAG and CT scan had false-negative result rates of 25% and 22%, respectively, and false-positive result rates of 45% and 14%, respectively.[135] In addition, the study showed that 25% of 202 CS I or II children were upstaged following laparotomy and that 27% of 45 CS III or IV children were downstaged. A review of the POG experience of the impact of laparotomy on stage change is provided in Table 18–8. Complications following staging laparotomy include immediate postoperative morbidity (rare infection, bowel or ureteral obstruction) and a lower than 4% risk of small bowel obstruction owing to adhesion. Nonetheless, postoperative mortality following laparotomy has been essentially unreported in the past 15 years.

Historically, a high rate of postsplenectomy sepsis in children (especially those younger than 5 years old) was reported.[120] Administration of pneumococcal vaccination before surgery and daily prophylactic antibiotics appears to have decreased this risk.[124, 136] In the Dana Farber series, 1% of patients were hospitalized for sepsis, and none died.[135] The risk of infection appears to be related to the intensity of therapy rather than to the splenectomy itself.[120]

Classification and Staging

Histopathology

The histopathology of this disease is described in the adult section (see "Histopathology" in the previous section and Table 18–2). Of interest in pediatric Hodgkin's disease is that the relative distribution of the subtypes in younger children differs from that in adolescents and adults, as shown in an analysis of 2238 patients treated at Stanford University (Table 18–9). LPHD is relatively more common (13%) in younger children (younger than 10 years), whereas LDHD is exceedingly rare. Although NSHD is the most common subtype in all age groups, it is more frequent in adolescents (77%) and adults (72%) than in younger children (44%). Conversely, MCHD is more common in younger children (33%) than in adolescents (11%) or adults (17%).

Staging

For staging techniques and descriptions, consult the adult section (see "Staging" in the previous section, Table 18–3, and Fig. 18–2). Of note, the distribution of stages observed in children is somewhat different than that in adults. Among 2238 consecutive patients with Hodgkin's disease treated at Stanford, 4% were younger than 10 years and 11% were 11 to 16 years old.[125] Stage I or II disease was present in about 60% of children; stage I disease was slightly more common in younger children (18%) than in adolescents (8%), stage II disease occurred in 40% to 50% of all age groups, and stage IV disease was less common in younger children (3%) than in adolescents (15%). B symptoms occurred in 19% of younger children and in 30% of adolescents.

TABLE 18–9. **Distribution of Pathologic Subtypes According to Patient Age**

	≤10 Yrs	11–16 Yrs	≥17 Yrs
Number of patients (%)	91 (4)	235 (11)	1912 (85)
Male-to-female ratio	4:1	1:1	3:2
Histology (%)			
Nodular sclerosis	44	77	72
Mixed cellularity	33	11	17
Lymphocyte predominance	13	8	5
Lymphocyte depletion	0	1	1
Unclassified/interfollicular	10	3	5

Modified from Cleary S, Link M, Donaldson S: Hodgkin's disease in the very young. Int J Radiat Oncol Biol Phys 1994; 28:77, with permission.

Principles of Treatment

Although Hodgkin's disease is one of the few pediatric malignancies that has an adult counterpart with a similar natural history and biology, devising the optimal therapeutic approach for children with this disease is complicated by their increased risk for adverse effects (Table 18–10). In particular, the radiation therapy doses and fields that normally are used in adults can cause profound musculoskeletal retardation, including interclavicular narrowing, shortened sitting height, decreased mandibular growth, and decreased muscle development in the treated volume in children.[121] Thus, whereas adults with early-stage Hodgkin's disease are often treated with full-dose radiation as a single modality, this approach in prepubertal children produces unacceptable sequelae, despite a similar success rate.[137, 138]

Further complicating the treatment of children are gender-specific differences in chemotherapy-induced gonadal injury. The desire to cure young children with minimal side effects has stimulated attempts to reduce staging procedures, the intensity and types of chemotherapy, and the radiation dose and volume. Because of the differences in the age-related developmental status of children and the gender-related sensitivity to chemotherapy, there is no one type of treatment that is ideal for all pediatric patients.

The concept of using combined modality, in the form of chemotherapy and low-dose radiation, in children to effect cure with tolerable sequelae was pioneered at Stanford. Trials for young children with early-stage disease reported excellent local control and survival rates with MOPP and radiation therapy.[124, 139] The radiation doses administered were 15 Gy for patients who were 5 years old, 20 Gy for 6- to 10-year-olds, and 25 Gy for 11- to 14-year-olds. Boosts were given to those who failed to achieve a complete remission or in those with bulky disease (larger than 6-cm nodes or LMA).[124] Although growth deformity was decreased in these particular trials, full course MOPP is associated with a high risk of sterility and secondary leukemia.[140, 141] Thus, alternate regimens were subsequently used.

In general, the use of both radiation and chemotherapy broadens the spectrum of potential toxicities, but it reduces the severity of individual (either drug- or radiation-related) toxicities. Present approaches, discussed in this section, entail chemotherapy in conjunction with reduced radiation doses. The extent of staging should be treatment dependent; the volume of radiation and the intensity and duration of chemotherapy are stage dependent. An outline of our therapeutic recommendations is presented in Table 18–10.

Surgery

The decision to use surgical staging should be considered only when the information obtained at laparotomy is expected to affect the treatment decision. Clearly, this decision depends on the philosophy of treatment or specific therapeutic protocol that must take into account the limitations of clinical staging.[105] This is particularly true if radiation therapy is to be directed only to sites of demonstrable (by surgical sampling) microscopic involvement rather than to gross involvement or to sites of suspected involvement (based on imaging studies). Therefore, the choice of therapy should dictate the extent of staging, rather than staging determining therapy, as in adults:

- For patients with early-stage disease who are treated with radiation therapy alone, both freedom from relapse and overall survival are superior after surgical staging.[142] In addition, if the abdomen is treated, then

TABLE 18–10. **Guidelines for Treatment of Pediatric Hodgkin's Disease**

Stage	Clinical Presentation	Recommendations
IA, IIA	Postpubertal: laparotomy negative, nonbulky mediastinal mass, no juxtapericardial disease	Standard-dose RT (STNI, generally) or low-dose RT (IF)* + ChT
	Prepubertal/pubertal: bulky mediastinal mass or juxtapericardial disease	Low-dose RT (IF)* + ChT
IB, IIB	Postpubertal: laparotomy negative, nonbulky mediastinal mass, no juxtapericardial disease, and night sweats ± fever or weight loss	Standard-dose RT (STNI generally) or low-dose RT (IF)* + ChT
	Prepubertal/pubertal: bulky mediastinal mass or juxtapericardial disease, or fever + weight loss	Low-dose RT (IF)* + ChT
$IIIA_1$, $IIIA_1S+$ (minimal)	Postpubertal: nonbulky mediastinal mass, no juxtapericardial disease	Standard-dose RT (STNI or TNI) or RT + ChT Hepatic RT if spleen is involved and RT only is used
	Prepubertal/pubertal: bulky mediastinal mass or juxtapericardial disease	Low-dose RT (IF) + ChT
$IIIA_1S+$ (extensive), $IIIA_2$, IIIB, IVA, IVB		MAC + low-dose RT (IF) (RT particularly recommended for bulky adenopathy)
Recurrent		ChT, if none previously, otherwise consider BMT (RT ± ChT in selected patients with nodal relapse after ChT alone)

RT = radiation therapy; standard-dose RT = 35–36 Gy ± boost; low-dose RT = ≤25 Gy; STNI = subtotal nodal irradiation; IF = involved field; TNI = total nodal irradiation; MAC = multiagent chemotherapy; BMT = bone marrow transplant; S+ (minimal) based on <5 nodules; S+ (extensive) based on ≥5 nodules; ChT = chemotherapy: 6 ABVD, 6–8 MOPP/ABVD, 6 OPPA/COP(P) or other experimental regimens. Less intensive therapy for early-stage disease is experimental regarding the number of cycles and drug combinations. OPPA = vincristine (Oncovin), prednisone, procarbazine, doxorubicin (Adriamycin); COP(P) = cyclophosphamide, vincristine (Oncovin), procarbazine (prednisone).

*Some institutions always use a mantle field and/or standard dose for bulky mediastinal disease.

the amount of lung, heart, and kidney treated is reduced.

- If a patient has CS III or IV or bulky mediastinal and pericardial disease and surgical staging does not alter the decision to use aggressive chemotherapy, then involved-field radiation therapy based on clinical imaging staging can be considered.
- If the chemotherapeutic regimen is reduced in intensity, then radiation therapy to all sites of known or suspected microscopic involvement must be considered.[121, 124]

On balance, laparotomy with splenectomy has a small rate of morbidity, which argues against its routine use; however, if its results influence the treatment strategy, it remains appropriate.

Radiation Therapy

As discussed for adults, select adolescents with favorable early-stage Hodgkin's disease can be treated with full-dose radiation therapy, reserving chemotherapy for relapse.[128, 138, 143, 144] Children who are appropriate for this approach are pubertal and fully grown, obviating concerns about muscle and bone development. Thus, radiation therapy to mantle and para-aortic fields remains standard for surgically staged adolescents with supradiaphragmatic stage IA to IIA disease.[145] However, data on the association of secondary breast cancer and full-dose (higher than 30 Gy) radiation therapy in females suggest that these patients might best be treated with combined chemotherapy and low-dose radiation therapy.[77, 146]

Patients with LMA or extensive disease involving the pericardium or juxtapericardial nodes usually should not be treated with radiation alone because of an inferior prognosis, as well as the potentially unacceptable pulmonary and cardiac radiation doses. Exceptions include patients with LMA but no juxtapericardial disease in whom sufficient lung and heart can be protected; meticulous technique with successive field reductions are necessary.[147, 148]

Success in the management of patients with Hodgkin's disease with radiation therapy requires excellent technique; select points applicable to children are as follows:

- The mantle field can be simulated with the arms up over the head or down with hands on the hips. Having the arms up over the head pulls the axillary lymph nodes away from the lungs, allowing greater lung shielding. However, the axillary lymph nodes then move into the vicinity of the humeral heads, which should be blocked in growing children. Thus, the position chosen involves weighing concerns regarding lymph nodes, lung, and humeral heads.
- Attempts should be made to position breast tissue under the lung and axillary blocking.
- In a very young child, consideration should be given to treating bilateral areas (e.g., both sides of the neck) to avoid growth asymmetry. However, this is less of a concern with the low radiation doses that are used with chemotherapy.
- Other considerations relate to the risk of second malignant neoplasms. For example, a child with isolated mediastinal disease receiving combined-modality therapy can be treated with shielding of the axilla and thus the breast tissue, and perhaps the thyroid gland.

Clearly, careful planning and judgment are always necessary.

Complications and Late Effects

Acute side effects seen during mantle irradiation include temporary loss of or change in taste, low posterior scalp epilation, xerostomia, skin erythema (particularly on the neck and shoulders), and occasionally, nausea and vomiting that require antiemetics. Mantle irradiation can cause pulmonary, cardiac, and thyroid damage and impair muscle and bone development. However, these effects are less common with the use of modern treatment programs.[122, 149, 150]

Acute effects of para-aortic irradiation are uncommon, but nausea and vomiting can occur. Late effects of para-aortic irradiation are also infrequent. Small bowel obstruction after both surgical staging and irradiation requiring surgical intervention is rare and is related to the total dose given: 1% for doses less than 35 Gy and 3% for doses greater than 35 Gy.[151] Gonadal injuries, including infertility and impaired secretion of sex hormones, are potential but generally preventable complications of pelvic irradiation.

The 15-year actuarial risk of second tumors is approximately 15%.[77, 128, 146] The risk of solid tumors does, however, increase with time. The risk of leukemia is associated primarily with the use of alkylating agents. In addition, several reports on treated pediatric Hodgkin's patients[77, 128, 146] have described an increased observed and expected risk ratio of second tumors for women compared with men, primarily owing to breast cancer.

Chemotherapy

The arguments that favor treatment with chemotherapy alone for all stages contend that it eliminates the need for surgical staging and that the dysmorphic and rare carcinogenic consequences of irradiation are avoided. The disadvantages of the use of chemotherapy alone are the risks of treatment-related fatality, infertility, and leukemogenesis, as well as an increased likelihood of disease recurrence in sites of bulky disease.[152, 153] The longest follow-up data are from the Uganda experience,[154] with only a 67% 9-year survival rate. Subgroups include patients who were CS I to IIIA with a 75% survival rate and patients who were CS IIIB to IV with a 60% and 47% survival rate at 5 and 10 years, respectively.

Combined-Modality Therapy

In 1987, Stanford investigators reported long-term follow-up of patients younger than 14 years of age who were treated with 6 cycles of MOPP chemotherapy and low-dose, involved-field radiation; the actuarial survival rate was 89% with a local control rate of 97%.[124] Long-term side effects included acute leukemias in 3 of 55 children and azoospermia in all 4 boys tested, although inhibition of soft tissue and bone growth was minimal with this approach. Subsequently, the effectiveness of ABVD as the front-line chemotherapy was established.[155–157] Compared with MOPP, second malignancies and sterility were less common.[158] The predominant adverse effects of ABVD are pulmonary toxicity related to bleomycin and cardiovascular toxicity secondary to doxorubicin. These side effects may be exacerbated by the addition of mediastinal or mantle irradiation.[159]

Overall, for children who are prepubescent or have advanced-stage disease, combined-modality therapy, in the form of chemotherapy plus low-dose radiation therapy, appears to be the most appropriate treatment, resulting in excellent long-term survival. Adolescents, particularly if they are male with favorable early-stage disease, may be considered for radiation therapy alone. Future studies will define the optimal chemotherapeutic agents and number of cycles, chemotherapy and radiation therapy scheduling, and the necessary dose and volume of irradiation to maximize cure while decreasing the side effects of chemotherapy and radiation therapy.

Bone Marrow Transplantation for Refractory or Relapsed Disease

Hodgkin's disease may still be cured even after initial treatment programs fail. Relapse occurs most often within 4 years, but late relapse is not rare. The choice of therapy for such patients is dependent on the initial treatment and the disease characteristics at the time of relapse. The data that are specific to children with recurrent Hodgkin's disease are limited. However, it can be noted that an analysis of 81 patients with pediatric Hodgkin's disease, who underwent ABMT and were reported to the European Bone Marrow Transplant Group, did demonstrate a similar outcome to a case-matched group of adults treated similarly (Fig. 18–4).[160]

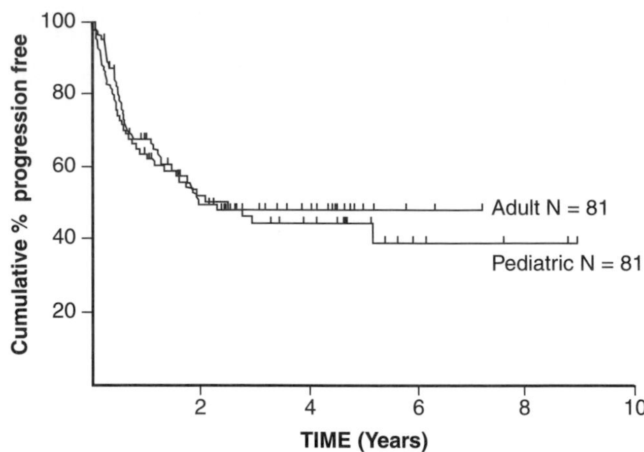

Figure 18–4. Progression-free survival after autologous bone marrow transplantation for Hodgkin's disease: comparison between pediatric and matched adult patients. (χ = 0.2194; p = 0.6395.) (From Williams C, Goldstone A, Pearce R, et al: Autologous bone marrow transplantation for pediatric Hodgkin's disease: a case-matched comparison with adult patients by the European Bone Marrow Transplant Group Lymphoma Registry. J Clin Oncol 1993; 11:2243, with permission.)

Results and Prognosis

The actuarial 10-year survival rate for children with early-stage disease is 85% to 95%; for children with advanced-stage disease, it is 70% to 90% (Tables 18–11, 18–12, and 18–13).* The data for patients with early-stage disease indicate a similar overall survival rate for patients treated with full-dose radiation therapy, combined full-dose radiation therapy and chemotherapy, and combined low-dose radiation therapy and chemotherapy. This similarity was illustrated in a report by Donaldson and associates, comparing results in early-stage disease from Stanford (PS, extended-field radiation therapy alone or combined chemotherapy and involved-field radiation therapy) with those from St. Bartholomew's Hospital (CS, involved- and regional-field full-dose radiation therapy).[161] Overall survival rate from each institution was 91% at 10 years, although the disease-free survival for stage I patients at St. Bartholomew's Hospital was somewhat lower than that at Stanford. However, the toxicities varied greatly among the treatment

*See references 121, 128, 138, 143, 144, 154, 156, 157, 161–171.

TABLE 18–11. **Treatment Results with Radiation Therapy Alone in Children with Early Stage Hodgkin's Disease**

Investigators	No. of Patients	Stage	Mode of Treatment	Survival (%) Overall	Survival (%) Relapse	Follow-up Interval (Yrs)
Donaldson et al[161] (U.K. study)	28	CS* I, II	IF	96	79	10
Donaldson et al[161] (U.S. study)	48	PS† I, II	EF	86	82	10
Gehan et al[138]	39	PS I, II	IF	95	41	5
	58	PS I, II	EF	96	67	5
Jenkin et al[143]	23	CS/PS I	IF‡	95	87	10
	42	PS IIA, IIIA	EF	85	45	10
Maity et al[144]	31	PS IA, IIA	EF	83	64	10
Mauch et al[121] and Tarbell et al[128]	50	PS I, IIA	EF	97	82	11

CS = clinical staging; PS = pathologic staging; IF = involved-field radiation; EF = extended-field radiation.
*Some patients were pathologically staged.
†Some patients were clinically staged.
‡Some patients received chemotherapy.
Modified from Halperin EC, Constine LS, Tarbell NJ, et al: Pediatric Radiation Oncology, 3rd ed, p 214. Philadelphia, Lippincott Williams & Wilkins, 1999, with permission.

TABLE 18–12. **Treatment Results with Chemotherapy Alone in Children with Early- and Advanced-Stage Hodgkin's Disease**

Investigators	No. of Patients	Stage	Mode of Treatment	Survival (%) Overall	Survival (%) Relapse	Follow-up Interval (Yrs)
Olweny et al[154]	38	CS I–II	MOPP × 6	100	100	5
Ekert et al[162]	38	CS IA–IIIA	MOPP or ChlVPP × 6	94	92	4
	8	PS III, IV	MOPP × 6–12	92	80	5
Hutchinson et al[157]	111	PS III–IV	MOPP × 6/ABVD × 6 or ABVD × 6	100	77	3
Lobo-Sanahuja et al[163]	52	CS IA–IIIA	CVPP × 6	100	90	5
	24	PS III–IV	CVPP × 6/EBO × 6	81	60	5
Weiner et al[164]	81	PS IIB, $IIIA_2$	MOPP × 4/ABVD × 4	96	79	5

CS = clinical staging; PS = pathologic staging; MOPP = mechlorethamine, vincristine, procarbazine, prednisone; ChlVPP = chlorambucil, vinblastine, procarbazine, prednisone; ABVD = doxorubicin (Adriamycin), bleomycin, vinblastine, dacarbazine; CVPP = cyclophosphamide, vinblastine, procarbazine, prednisone; EBO = epirubicin, bleomycin, vincristine (Oncovin).

Modified from Halperin EC, Constine LS, Tarbell NJ, et al: Pediatric Radiation Oncology, 3rd ed, p 214. Philadelphia, Lippincott Williams & Wilkins, 1999, with permission.

strategies, underlying the recommendations presented in Table 18–10.

Although relapse-free and overall survival remain excellent for patients with advanced disease when all are analyzed together, patients with stage IV disease continue to fare poorly. This is highlighted by the results from the Stanford group for 57 children (younger than 16 years old) treated with six cycles of chemotherapy (three cycles of ABVD, three cycles of MOPP) and 15- to 25-Gy involved-field radiation therapy.[172] The contrasting results for patients with stage I to III versus stage IV disease are depicted in Figure 18–5.

It is critical to appreciate the extent to which death from causes other than recurrence of Hodgkin's disease compromises overall survival. Although Hodgkin's disease is the main cause of death during the first 10 to 15 years following therapy, other causes of death (e.g., second malignancy or cardiovascular disease) predominate at even longer follow-up times. Of 694 children treated at Stanford for Hodgkin's disease and monitored for 1 to 32 years

TABLE 18–13. **Treatment Results with Combined-Modality Regimens in Children with Early- and Advanced-Stage Hodgkin's Disease**

Investigators	No. of Patients	Stage	Mode of Treatment RT	Mode of Treatment CT	Survival (%) Overall	Survival (%) Relapse	Follow-up Interval (Yrs)
Full-Dose RT + ChT							
Gehan et al[138]	97	PS I, II	IF	MOPP × 6	90	95	5
Donaldson et al[161] (UK)	39	CS* I, II	IF	ChlVPP or MOPP or MVPP × 3–8	86	84	10
Schellong et al[165] (HD78)	73	PS I–IIA	EF	OPPA × 2	97	90	10
Schellong et al[166] (HD82)	100	CS/PS I, IIA	IF	OPPA × 2	100	96	12
Schellong et al[165, 166] (HD85)	53	CS/PS I, IIA	IF	OPA × 2	98	85	5
Low-Dose RT + ChT							
Maity et al[144]	30	CS I, II		COPP × 6 or ABVD × 6 or MOPP × 3/ABVD × 3	90	68	10
Donaldson et al[167]	27	PS I, II		MOPP × 6	100	96	10
Schellong et al[165] (HD87)	104	CS/PS I–IIA	IF	OPA × 2	99	85	5
Schellong[168, 169] (HD90)	274	CS IA, IIA	IF	OPPA × 2 or OEPA × 2		96f/93m	5
Vecchi et al[170]	58	CS IA, IIA	IF	ABVD × 3		95	7
Hudson et al[171]	28	CS I–IIB	IF	COP(P) × 4–5 or ABVD × 3–4	96	96	5
Jenkin et al[143]	27	CS II, III		MOPP × 6	93	89	10
Oberlin et al[156]	67	CS IA, IIA	IF	MOPP × 2/ABVD × 2		89	6
	65	CS IA, IIA	IF	ABVD × 4		.89	6
	133	CS I, II	IF	VBVP × 4 ± OPPA × 2	96	92	3

CS = clinical staging; PS = pathologic staging; IF = involved-field radiation; EF = extended-field radiation; MOPP = mechlorethamine, vincristine (Oncovin), procarbazine, prednisone; ChlVPP = chlorambucil, vinblastine, procarbazine, prednisone; MVPP = mechlorethamine, vinblastine, procarbazine, prednisone; OPPA = vincristine (Oncovin), procarbazine, prednisone, doxorubicin (Adriamycin); OPA = vincristine (Oncovin), prednisone, doxorubicin (Adriamycin); COPP = cyclophosphamide, vincristine (Oncovin), procarbazine, prednisone; ABVD = doxorubicin (Adriamycin), bleomycin, vinblastine, dacarbazine; OEPA = vincristine (Oncovin), etoposide, prednisone, doxorubicin (Adriamycin); VBVP = vinblastine, bleomycin, vincristine, prednisone.

*Some patients were pathologically staged.

Modified from Halperin EC, Constine LS, Tarbell NJ, et al: Pediatric Radiation Oncology, 3rd ed, p 214. Philadelphia, Lippincott Williams & Wilkins, 1999, with permission.

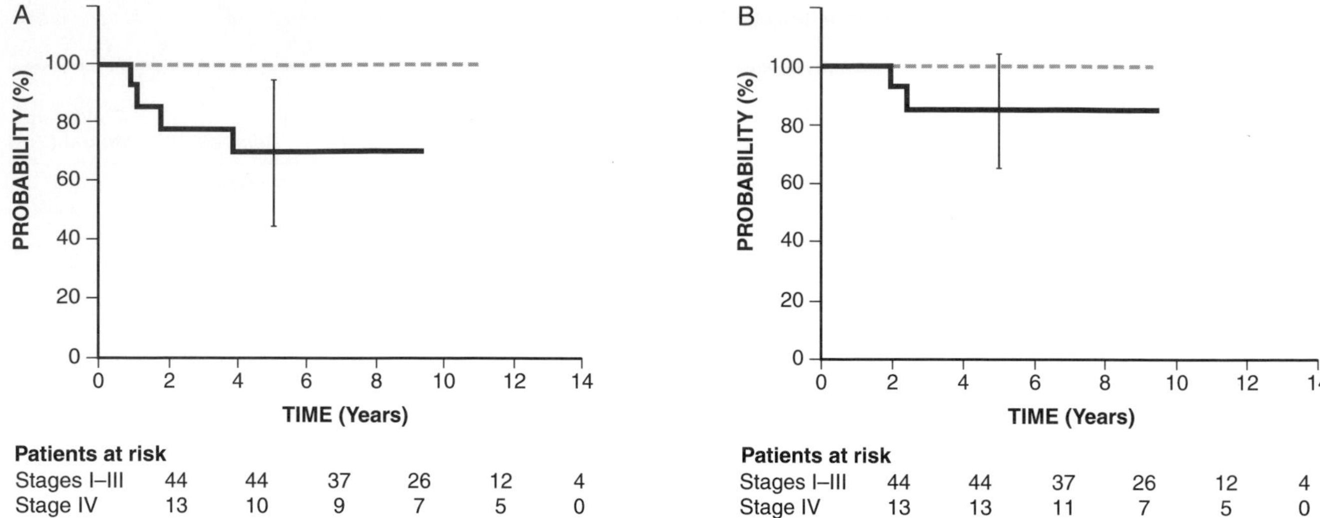

Figure 18–5. Comparison of treatment outcome by stage. (A) Event-free survival and (B) survival for patients with stages I to III disease *(broken line)* versus stage IV disease *(solid line)*. Bars denote 95% confidence intervals rate at 5 years for stage IV. (From Hunger SP, Link MP, Donaldson SS: ABVD/MOPP and low dose involved-field radiotherapy in pediatric Hodgkin's disease: the Stanford experience. J Clin Oncol 1994; 12:2160, with permission.)

(mean 13.1 years), 147 (21%) have died.[146] The causes of death were Hodgkin's disease (54%), second cancers (20%), and accidents or other causes (26%).

Surgery

An important series of studies performed by the German-Austrian Pediatric Hodgkin's Disease Study Group progressively refined the extent of staging and the intensity of chemotherapy and radiation.[165, 166, 168, 169] Staging was reduced from the systematic use of laparotomy (HD-78), to selective laparotomy and splenectomy (HD-82), to infrequent laparotomy without splenectomy (HD-90). In the early studies, OPPA (vincristine [Oncovin], procarbazine, prednisone, and doxorubicin [Adriamycin]) with or without COPP (cyclophosphamide, vincristine [Oncovin], procarbazine, and prednisone) were used. In HD-85 and HD-87, OPA (P = prednisone) was administered to boys in order to reduce testicular toxicity; however, event-free survival declined. In HD-90, girls received OPPA plus COPP (depending on stage), whereas boys received OEPA (adding etoposide to OPA) plus COPP. OEPA was found to be a satisfactory alternative to OPPA, maintaining the reduction in the risk of testicular dysfunction.[173]

Radiation Therapy

Results for children with early-stage Hodgkin's disease are presented in Table 18–11. In the past, extended-field radiation to the mantle and para-aortic regions has been associated with an improved relapse-free survival when compared with more limited volumes in surgically staged patients.[80, 139] However, select patients (e.g., stage IA LPHD with cervical involvement) may be treated to more limited volumes. Radiation therapy alone for patients with CS I and II disease and favorable prognostic factors (female, fewer than 3 sites, low ESR, LPHD or NSHD, no LMA) has been used increasingly, although specific long-term data for children are lacking.[174, 175] In addition, mantle-field irradiation alone has been used for favorable pathologically staged patients, but this approach is still investigational in children.[175]

Chemotherapy

In a report from POG,[164] children treated with four cycles each of MOPP and ABVD had excellent outcomes (see Table 18–12); the addition of radiation therapy to this protocol did not improve disease-free survival or overall survival. However, statistical and quality assurance issues complicate interpretation of these data.[176] Moreover, longer follow-up is necessary to assess the toxicity from eight cycles of chemotherapy. In addition, a beneficial effect with radiation therapy may have been seen if the number of cycles of chemotherapy had been decreased.[177] This is supported by other data from adult patients that demonstrate the appropriateness of combined therapy rather than chemotherapy alone for patients with both early- and advanced-stage disease.[110, 145, 178]

Combined-Modality Therapy

Results for children with both early and advanced disease who were treated with combined-modality regimens are shown in Table 18–13. Reports on the use of combined ABVD and MOPP have documented excellent disease control with diminished toxicity relative to MOPP alone.[148, 157, 179] The intention of all of these investigations was to decrease the number of cycles of MOPP and thus potentially lower the risk of leukemogenesis and sterility, while also diminishing the side effects associated with six cycles of ABVD. In a report on 238 patients from the French Society of Pediatric Oncology, early-stage patients (CS I to IIA) were treated with four cycles of ABVD or two cycles each of MOPP and ABVD plus involved-field, low-dose (20 Gy) radiation therapy.[156] For advanced disease (CS IB to IV), patients were treated with three cycles each of MOPP and ABVD plus extended-field, low-dose radiation therapy. Patients with a poor response to chemotherapy received additional radiation therapy to achieve full dose. The 5-year disease-free survival rate was 86%, and the actuarial survival rate for the entire group was 92%.

The Children's Cancer Study Group also compared alternating MOPP and ABVD (12 cycles) with ABVD (six cycles) and low-dose irradiation (21 Gy) to regions of disease involvement for patients with advanced Hodgkin's disease (stages III and IV).[157] For patients with stage III disease, the 3-year overall survival rate was 90%, whereas the event-free survival rate was 81% (77% for the MOPP-ABVD group and 84% for the ABVD-radiation group). The 3-year event-free survival rate for 111 patients without LMA was 100%. For those with LMA it was 78%, and for patients with stage IV disease it was 60%.

Investigators at Stanford University treated 57 children who were younger than 16 years of age (stage I: 1; stage II: 22; stage III: 21; stage IV: 13) with six cycles of alternating ABVD and MOPP, with involved-field radiation therapy intercalated between cycles.[172] The radiation therapy dose was 15 Gy, with a boost to 25 Gy to sites of bulky disease and to areas that failed to respond completely to two cycles of chemotherapy. Five and 10-year actuarial survival and freedom-from-relapse rates were 96% and 93%. For the stage IV subgroup, the 5-year actuarial survival and freedom-from-relapse rates were 85% and 68%, respectively. A regimen that eliminates dacarbazine while administering ABV-MOPP each month has now been used in children with apparent success.[180]

Prognosis

As with adults, as the treatment of Hodgkin's disease in children has improved, characteristics that influence outcome have diminished in importance. However, several factors continue to influence the success and certainly the choice of therapy. These factors are interrelated; disease stage, bulk, and biologic aggressiveness are frequently co-dependent.[111]

Stage

The stage of disease persists as the most important prognostic variable. Patients with advanced-stage disease, especially stage IV, have an inferior outlook compared with patients with early-stage disease.[153] The bulk of disease is reflected by the disease stage, but more specifically, it is determined by the volume of distinct areas of involvement and the number of disease sites.

Mediastinal Mass

As discussed for adults, LMA places a patient at a greater risk for disease recurrence. For patients with PS I or II disease who are treated with primary radiation therapy, disease-free survival is inferior to that in patients treated with combined-modality therapy. However, overall survival remains high, owing to the effectiveness of salvage chemotherapy.[148] Nevertheless, patients with LMA have a somewhat inferior survival rate. Patients (at least those with a CS not PS classification) with more sites of involvement, which is generally defined as four or more, also fare less well.[181]

B Symptoms

B symptoms reflect biologic aggressiveness and confer a worse prognosis, as discussed for adults. Laboratory studies, including the ESR, serum ferritin, hemoglobin, serum albumen, and serum CD8 antigen levels have been reported to predict a worse outcome.[111] This outcome could reflect disease biology or bulk.

Tumor Histology

Histologic subtype is relevant. A report from the United Kingdom Children's Cancer Study Group that assessed the relevance of histology in 331 children is revealing.[182] Less than 1% had LDHD, obviating any meaningful assessment of its prognostic significance. For patients with other histologies that were treated with combined therapy, no difference in outcome was observed.

Patient Age

Age is significant. Survival rates for children with Hodgkin's disease approach 85% to 95%. In a report from Stanford, the 5- and 10-year survival rates for children younger than 10 years of age with Hodgkin's disease is 94% and 92%, respectively, compared with 93% and 86% for adolescents (aged 11 to 16 years old) and 84% and 73% for adults.[125] Several features of the youngest patient group may influence their improved prognosis, including higher frequency of LP and MP subtypes and of stage I disease, a lower frequency of B symptoms, and the more common use of combined-modality therapy. Multivariate analysis of these data showed that age, stage, histology, and treatment modality (combined radiation and chemotherapy versus radiation alone) were all independent prognostic variables for survival.[125] Although children younger than 4 years of age with Hodgkin's disease are uncommon, even these children would appear to have an excellent prognosis.[127]

Future Clinical Investigations

Devising new strategies for the treatment of children with Hodgkin's disease is problematic because of the overall success of treatment regimens in use at present. However, grouping patients into different risk categories allows investigators to construct protocols that are intended to diminish therapy-induced toxicity for so-called favorable patients, improve treatment effectiveness for so-called unfavorable patients, and aim for both goals in patients with an intermediate prognosis. Unfortunately, the ability to conduct clinical trials in which the differences in survival among treatment arms are likely to be small is compromised by the large numbers of patients necessary to detect such differences. If a reduction in treatment toxicity is the intended goal of a new regimen, then many years of follow-up are necessary to prove effectiveness. Some generalizations regarding ongoing efforts in clinical trials for pediatric Hodgkin's disease are as follows:

- Patients with early-stage disease (I, IIA without bulk disease, and perhaps patients with IIB disease with sweating as the only B symptom) have an excellent prognosis, thus so-called negative questions can be asked: Can the intensity and duration of chemotherapy be decreased, selecting agents that are associated with less severe side effects? Concomitantly, can the volume and, perhaps, dose of radiation therapy be reduced? Can the amount of chemotherapy be based on the response to the initial cycles? Will chemoprotectants and radioprotectants prove to be useful?
- Patients with disease of an intermediate stage or with characteristics indicating that their prognosis is of an intermediate nature (II with bulky disease, IIB with fevers or weight loss, IIIA) are appropriate for study questions that intend to increase efficacy without decreasing toxicity. Generally this entails modification of existing chemoradiation therapy programs.
- Patients with advanced-stage disease (IIIB, IV) require more effective treatment regimens. This might be attainable by increasing dose intensity or the rate of drug delivery and by combining agents into new regimens. The use of hemopoietic growth factors may assist in drug delivery. Definition of the role of radiation therapy in such trials continues to be an important objective.

Of interest are the early-stage and advanced-stage studies in the POG. For patients with IA, IIA, and IIIA disease who do not have large mediastinal disease, two to four cycles of four-drug therapy are being given, dependent on the response to radiation therapy. For other patients (advanced disease), three to five cycles of dose-intensive, six-drug protocols are given, also dependent on response to radiation therapy. Granulocyte-macrophage colony-stimulating factor (GM-CSF) is used, and patients are randomized to a cardioprotectant.

Non-Hodgkin's Lymphoma

Epidemiology and Etiology

Epidemiology

In the year 2000, approximately 55,000 patients in the United States were diagnosed as having non-Hodgkin's lymphoma (NHL), and about 26,000 patients died of this disease.[11] Although each of the NHLs has a characteristic age distribution, the overall peak incidence is in those older than age 50, much later than that for Hodgkin's disease. The incidence is slightly higher in men than in women (1.4:1).[11]

Etiology

- An association of NHL with certain lymphotrophic viral infections (e.g., human T-cell lymphocytic virus–I [HTLV-I] and human immunodeficiency virus [HIV]) has been identified.[183–186] This is highly compatible with a viral etiology or an induced immunologic defect, permitting a malignant clone to proliferate. An increased incidence of NHL in patients who have undergone organ transplantation, people with congenital immune deficiency syndromes, and people infected by the HIV virus also supports this hypothesis.[187]
- Demonstration of the translocation of the c-*MYC* oncogene into the Ig gene locus in Burkitt's lymphoma and a consistent translocation between chromosomes 14 and 18 that results in overproduction of the BCL2 protein have provided a major breakthrough in the study of malignant transformation of lymphoid cells.[188, 189]
- An increased risk of NHL in people exposed to agricultural herbicides, particularly of the phenoxyacetic acid group, has been reported.[190, 191]

Molecular Biology

Advances in molecular genetics have provided new insights into the biology of the lymphoid malignancies. Integral components of these advances include the following:

- assays for markers of lymphoproliferative diseases based on the analysis of antigen receptor gene rearrangements[192, 193]
- recognition of specific oncogenes relevant to the pathogenesis of various lymphoid malignancies[194, 195]

NHLs arise from the transformation of lymphoid cells at specific points in their differentiation, from lymphocyte precursors in the bone marrow and thymus until they become immunocompetent lymphoid cells, capable of participating in an immune response.[183] Normal lymphoid cells undergo specific and irreversible rearrangements of their Ig genes (B-cells) or T-cell receptor genes (T-cells) as they are committed to a specific lineage. These are clone-specific events that can be used to identify clonality, lineage, and degree of differentiation for the individual types (Fig. 18–6).[196] Thus, probes for the T-cell receptor and Ig subunits are used to assign each malignancy to a T-cell or B-cell group, although occasionally even these techniques prove to reveal less than straightforward information about the origin of certain lymphomas. Nevertheless, certain generalizations can be made:

1. *B-cell types:* Small, noncleaved lymphomas, which include Burkitt's and non-Burkitt's subtypes, nearly

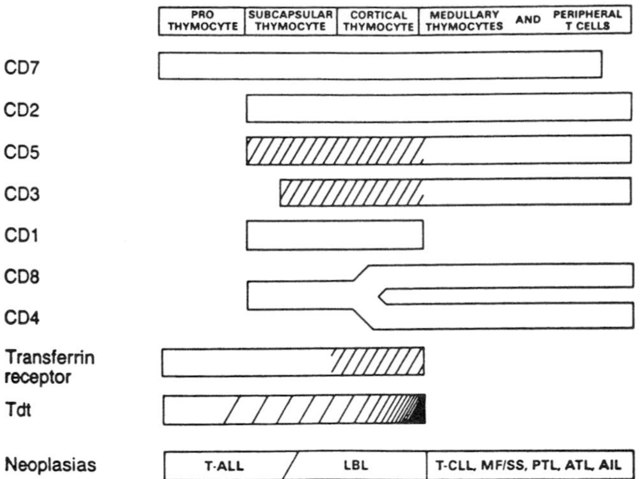

Figure 18–6. Molecular, genetic, and immunophenotypic correlates of normal T-cell differentiation. (From Grignani F, Dalla-Favera R: Molecular biology of lymphoid malignancies. Curr Opin Oncol 1989; 1:4.)

all low-grade (follicular) lymphomas, small lymphocytic lymphomas, mantle zone lymphomas, and most large cell lymphomas are of a B-cell phenotype. Surface Ig (usually of the IgM class) and B-cell–specific antigens (usually detected by the monoclonal antibodies CD19 and CD20) are expressed by these cells and may be used as therapy targets.[189, 197]

Approximately 10% of lymphoblastic lymphomas are considered to be of B-cell origin. They can more appropriately be considered to be derived from stem cells that have an immature phenotype, but they are committed to B-cell differentiation pathways. The Burkitt's subtypes, which include equatorial African and North American forms, have differences in the precise locations of the chromosomal breakpoints associated with the specific translocations that are seen in these tumors.[198]

2. *T-cell types*: Lymphoblastic lymphomas are composed of immature lymphoid cells, which have the phenotype of early or common cortical thymocytes. They almost invariably have the enzyme terminal deoxynucleotidyl transferase, a marker for apoptosis.[199] Most lymphoblastic lymphomas (and some large cell lymphomas) also express T-cell markers. All of the other T-cell lymphomas apparently derive from cells with mature or post-thymic phenotypes. Those that arise from mature cells bear the CD4 antigen and include adult T-cell leukemia or lymphoma, mycosis fungoides, Sézary syndrome, angiocentric T-cell lymphomas, many of the CD30+ anaplastic large cell lymphomas, and most of the peripheral T-cell lymphomas.

   The distinction between lymphoblastic lymphomas and leukemia is generally determined by the percentage of blast cells demonstrated in the bone marrow, with 25% being the most commonly used cutoff point. The biologic correlate to this distinction is not clear, but it appears to involve the degree of differentiation of the neoplastic cell. Malignancies with an immature thymocyte phenotype most frequently present as leukemia, whereas those with a more mature phenotype characteristically present with less marrow involvement, but with accumulations of cells in other areas. Contemporary classification systems acknowledge the identity of these diseases.[45]
3. The growth fraction of the lymphomas varies according to the subtype, and for some aggressive varieties it may approach 100%.[200, 201] For these lymphomas, the doubling times can be extremely short, from 12 hours to a few days. The B-cell tumors have the highest growth fractions, with up to 27% of the cells in S phase.
4. Specific cytogenetic findings distinguish several of the different subtypes of NHL (Table 18–14).[202] Characteristic differences are found not only among different phenotypes but even within an apparently homogeneous phenotype. Because particular genetic abnormalities may correlate with prognosis, such distinctions are important:

   - Most follicular lymphomas carry the t(14;18) chromosomal translocation.[189]
   - Approximately one third of the diffuse large cell lymphomas also carry this translocation, suggesting a pathologic relationship with the follicular lymphomas.[203] However, characteristic karyotypic abnormalities are not found in most of the large cell lymphomas, perhaps owing to the phenotypically heterogeneous types in this category, or because the genetic abnormalities do not involve karyotypic changes.
   - In Burkitt's lymphoma, the proto-oncogene c-*MYC* is translocated from chromosome 8 to the heavy chain locus of chromosome 14.[204] The product of the c-*MYC* oncogene is necessary for cellular proliferation and its abnormal expression may maintain the cell in an inappropriately proliferative state.

Detection and Diagnosis

Clinical Detection

Symptoms and signs of NHL are similar to those in Hodgkin's disease. However, there are some notable differences. Unlike in Hodgkin's disease, noncontiguous spread is common, the mediastinum is often spared, and extranodal

TABLE 18–14. **Common Cytogenetic Alterations in Non-Hodgkin's Lymphoma**

Histologic Subtype	Locus	Abnormality
Mantle cell lymphoma	*BCL1*	t(11;13)
Follicular lymphoma	*BCL2*	t(14;18)
Diffuse large cell lymphoma	*BCL2*	t(14;18)
	MYC	t(8;14)
	BCL6	3q27
Burkitt's lymphoma	*MYC*	t(8;14)
Anaplastic large cell lymphoma	ALK/NPM	t(2;5)

Modified from Smith MR: Non-Hodgkin's lymphoma. Curr Prob Cancer 1996; 20:6.

involvement, such as Waldeyer's lymphoid tissue, skin, the gastrointestinal (GI) tract, and bone, is much more common in NHL. Unsuspected bone marrow involvement occurs much more frequently. In children, initial intra-abdominal manifestations are common, unlike in Hodgkin's disease. Leukemic transformation with a high peripheral lymphocyte count occurs in about 13% of patients with lymphocytic lymphoma.[205]

Diagnostic Procedures

Because of the noncontiguous spread of NHL, most patients have stage III or IV disease.

- *Surgical biopsy* is usually employed to establish the diagnosis. Primary histology, immunophenotyping, and enzymatic and cytogenetic studies are often used to supplement morphologic analysis. The most suspicious node should be selected for excisional biopsy. Frozen sections and needle biopsies are discouraged as a means of establishing the primary diagnosis.
- *Aspiration* of bone marrow or malignant effusions may provide the diagnosis and obviate the need for a lymph node biopsy. The frequent presence of unsuspected bone marrow involvement in NHL has important implications for treatment planning (apparent stage I becomes stage IV). Therefore, *bone marrow biopsy* should be performed in virtually every case. Lymphocytic lymphomas have a high frequency (up to 50%) of bone marrow involvement, whereas large cell lymphomas have a much lower frequency.
- Other biopsies may be indicated in certain situations. For example, sampling of the cerebrospinal fluid is indicated for patients with lymphoblastic or Burkitt's lymphomas, as well as those who have intermediate-grade lymphomas with bone marrow or paranasal sinus disease.
- A complete *physical examination* should be made, including Waldeyer's ring evaluation and a pelvic examination in women.
- Complete *blood cell counts* should be taken, including differential white blood cell and reticulocyte counts. *Blood chemistry analysis*, including lactate dehydrogenase (LDH), alkaline phosphatase, albumin, globulin, Ig, uric acid, and creatinine, should be made.

Imaging work-up for staging includes:

- *Chest x-ray study* (posteroanterior and lateral) and a *CT scan of chest, abdomen,* and *pelvis* are useful in detecting upper retroperitoneal and mesenteric nodes and spleen and liver involvement.
- Additional directed radiographic examinations are appropriate to evaluate specific signs or symptoms. For example, a *head* or *spinal CT scan* or *MRI* may be obtained in the presence of neurologic signs or symptoms, or a *bone scan* in patients with symptomatic bony pain.
- *Gallium whole body scans* may also be useful, especially in patients with intermediate- or high-grade lymphomas.

Classification and Staging

Histopathology

The NHLs are a diverse group of diseases that differ with regard to histology, natural history, and response to therapy. This heterogeneity has led to several histopathologic classifications, which, in turn, have contributed to difficulty in interpreting study results.

In 1982, the NCI appointed a panel of lymphoma pathologists to study the clinical applicability of six major histopathologic classification systems. The panel indicated that all six systems correlated well with clinical outcome and that none was superior to the others. A *Working Formulation* was introduced and recommended for the reporting of results.[206] In this classification, architecture of the gland (follicular versus diffuse) and predominant cell type (small or large lymphocyte) are the two variables that best determine prognosis. A follicular architecture and a small-sized lymphocyte characterize low-grade NHL and predict for a favorable outcome, whereas diffuse and large cell lymphomas are intermediate or high grade and carry a worse prognosis (Table 18–15).

As stated earlier, immunologic studies (immunofluorescence, erythrocyte rosettes, monoclonal antibodies, flow cytometry, Ig, and T-cell gene rearrangement) have begun to clarify these previously poorly understood lymphoproliferative disorders:

- Studies have revealed that all NHLs of nodular type, as well as low-grade mucosa-associated lymphoid tumors (MALT lymphomas), are of B-cell origin.
- Large cell lymphomas are almost always lymphocytic malignancies, usually of B-cell type, but occasionally of T-cell origin.
- Mixed lymphomas are wholly of lymphocytic origin.
- Burkitt's lymphomas demonstrate a surface marker pattern and Ig gene rearrangement characteristic of B-cell origin.
- Mycosis fungoides and Sézary syndrome are of T-lymphocyte origin.
- Angioimmunoblastic lymphadenopathy, lymphomatoid papulosis, and lymphomas arising in patients with celiac disease and sprue are also of T-cell origin.
- Lymphoblastic lymphomas are almost always of T-cell origin, whereas human T-cell leukemia or lymphoma virus-I–associated lymphomas are exclusively T-cell.

The distinction between malignant lymphoma and benign lymphadenopathy can sometimes be difficult. Monoclonality in immunophenotyping and gene rearrangements in such patients are the criteria used to diagnose a neoplastic process.

Based on these newer biologic concepts, an international working group has developed a more functional classification of the NHLs, recognizing newer entities such as MALT lymphomas, mantle cell lymphoma, and monocytoid B-cell lymphoma.[45] Comparisons between this classification and the Working Formulation are seen in Table 18–15.

Staging

The staging system is the same as that used for Hodgkin's disease (see Table 18–3 and Fig. 18–2).

TABLE 18–15. **Comparison of the Working Formulation and the REAL Classification for Non-Hodgkin's Lymphoma**

Grade	Working Formulation	REAL Classification *B-Cell*	REAL Classification *T-Cell*
Low	Small, lymphocytic	B-cell CLL/PLL/SLL Marginal zone/MALT Mantle cell	T-cell CLL/PLL LGL ATL/L
	Follicular, small, cleaved	Follicle center, follicular grade I Mantle cell Marginal zone/MALT	
	Follicular, mixed, small cleaved, and large	Follicle center, follicular grade II Marginal zone/MALT	
Intermediate	Follicular, large cell	Follicle center, follicular grade III	
	Diffuse, small, cleaved	Mantle cell Follicle center, diffuse small cell Marginal zone/MALT	T-cell CLL/PLL LGL ATL/L Angioimmunoblastic Angiocentric
	Diffuse, mixed, small and large	Large B-cell lymphoma Follicle center, diffuse small cell Lymphoplasmacytoid Marginal zone/MALT Mantle cell	Peripheral T-cell, unspecified ATL/L Angioimmunoblastic Angiocentric Intestinal T-cell lymphoma
	Diffuse, large cell	Diffuse large B-cell lymphoma	Peripheral T-cell, unspecified ATL/L Angioimmunoblastic Angiocentric Intestinal T-cell lymphoma
High	Large cell, immunoblastic	Diffuse large B-cell lymphoma	Peripheral T-cell, unspecified ATL/L Angioimmunoblastic Angiocentric Intestinal T-cell lymphoma Anaplastic large cell
	Lymphoblastic	Precursor B-lymphoblastic	Precursor T-lymphoblastic
	Small, noncleaved Burkitt's or non-Burkitt's	Burkitt's High grade B-cell, Burkitt-like diffuse large B-cell	Peripheral T-cell, unspecified

CLL = chronic lymphocytic leukemia; PLL = prolymphocytic leukemia; SLL = small lymphocytic leukemia; MALT = mucosa-associated lymphoid tumor; LGL = large granular lymphocyte leukemia; ATL/L = adult T-cell lymphoma/leukemia.

From Shipp MA, Mauch PM, Harris NL: Non-Hodgkin's lymphoma. In: DeVita VT Jr, Hellman S, Rosenberg SA (eds): Cancer. Principles & Practice of Oncology, 5th ed, p 2165. Philadelphia, Lippincott-Raven, 1997, with permission.

Principles of Treatment for the Common Lymphomas

Multidisciplinary Treatment Planning

Because of the variety of potential staging and treatment options available to patients with NHL, an initial multidisciplinary planning conference is necessary for each patient as soon as the histologic diagnosis is made (Table 18–16). The important issue to be addressed is the optimal therapeutic strategy—primary or adjuvant chemotherapy or radiotherapy—and the sequence of multimodal therapy.

As a general consideration, NHL types can be separated into two distinct prognostic groups: indolent and aggressive. The indolent group responds well to radiation therapy and has a good prognosis in the early stages,[207, 208] although there is a steady rate of relapse in more advanced stages.[209, 210] Indeed, advanced-stage low-grade lymphoma is generally considered to be incurable; if it is indolent and a patient is asymptomatic, treatment may not be initiated.[211] However, these patients are good candidates for novel therapies and clinical trials. When no immediate treatment is selected, these patients must be followed closely, because the majority becomes symptomatic and later requires chemotherapy or radiation therapy. In these patients, the nature of treatment that was initiated at the time of disease progression varies, depending on the symptoms and findings present. If there are B symptoms or findings that are reflective of bone marrow involvement, then systemic therapy is appropriate. If there is locoregional problematic adenopathy, then irradiation to sites of adenopathy is appropriate. Aggressive subtypes of NHL in general have a less favorable prognosis and require more intensive therapy.[207, 212]

Surgery

The primary role of surgery is in establishing diagnosis. Resection of extranodal GI primaries may rarely be curative, although additional treatment for microresidual or macroresidual disease is often indicated.

Radiation Therapy

The role of radiation therapy in the management of NHL has diminished as chemotherapeutic regimens have become

TABLE 18–16. **Guidelines for Treatment of Non-Hodgkin's Lymphoma**

Stage	Characteristics	Treatment
Favorable, Low Grade		
I–II	Nonbulky, 1 or 2 contiguous sites	IFRT IFRT + MAC IFRT + palliative ChT
III–IV	Limited disease burden (<5 sites)	MAC MAC ± IFRT
	Extensive disease (>5 sites)	Observation alone, no cytotoxic therapy for asymptomatic patients MAC ?BMT
Unfavorable, Intermediate or High Grade		
I	Small disease burden (<2.5 cm), no B symptoms, age <60 yrs	MAC ± IFRT Rarely: IFRT
II		MAC ± IFRT
III–IV		MAC
Recurrent		MAC ± BMT ± boost RT (bulky disease)
Special Cases for Treatment		
Head and Neck	Parameningeal evaluation	CNS prophylaxis (intrathecal ChT)
GI	I_E MALT	Antibiotics ± RT
Testes	High-grade I_E	MAC + contralateral testis RT + CNS prophylaxis
CNS	Any	MAC ± RT

IFRT = involved-field radiation therapy; MAC = multiagent chemotherapy; ChT = chemotherapy; BMT = high-dose cytotoxic chemotherapy + hemopoietic stem cell rescue; ? = optional; MALT = mucosa-associated lymphoid tumor.

more effective, yet it remains appropriate as either primary or adjuvant treatment in selected patients. Moreover, its role in these situations continues to be redefined as chemotherapeutic management changes.

Important considerations in the administration of radiation therapy include timing and the volume, dose, and fraction size, each of which depends on whether chemotherapy is being used and the specific agents employed. The radiation therapy portals are designed with knowledge of the common routes of lymphatic spread and the chemotherapy and radiation therapy tolerances of the normal tissues in these regions. The dose and fraction size depend on the assessment of what is necessary for local disease control in light of the potential normal tissue morbidities.

Radiation therapy fields are customarily described according to the lymphoid regions being treated:

- *Involved-field irradiation* denotes treatment limited to the involved nodal regions, according to the Ann Arbor staging system (see Fig. 18–3).
- *Extended-field irradiation* involves treatment of both the involved lymphoid regions and those that are contiguous and presumed to be at a high risk for occult involvement.
- *TNI (or TLI)* includes sequential treatment to all major lymphoid regions, usually in two or three segments.
- *Total body irradiation (TBI)* is treatment of the entire body in each treatment session.

At times, the fields must be designed to treat specific extranodal sites or the whole abdomen when, for example, mesenteric nodes are involved with NHL. Partial transmission lead or cerrobend blocks are appropriate in situations in which lower doses of irradiation are administered to organs concomitant with the treatment of nodal regions.

The dose of radiation necessary to achieve local control depends on the histologic type of the NHL and whether chemotherapy is also used:

- The low-grade and lymphocytic lymphomas may be controlled locally with doses of 30 to 40 Gy in 1.5 to 2 Gy fractions.
- MALT lymphomas may be treated with 20 to 30 Gy.
- Lymphomas with a large cell component require doses of 40 to 50 Gy when radiation alone is being used or 30 to 40 Gy in combined-modality therapy programs.
- When TBI is used without bone marrow transplant for the low-grade lymphomas, daily doses of 0.10 to 0.15 Gy (weekly doses of 0.30 Gy) are administered to a total of only 1.2 to 1.5 Gy.
- TBI as a component of ABMT procedures usually is given in 1.2 to 2.0 Gy fractions to total doses no higher than 13.2 Gy.

Following extensive staging, only 10% to 30% of patients with low-grade lymphoma has localized disease, and most of these patients have follicular subtypes. Radiation therapy is frequently effective for these patients, providing a 10-year disease-free survival rate of 45% to 60% and an actuarial survival rate of 45% to 65%.[213, 214] Patients with nonbulky disease (smaller than 6 to 10 cm), limited to two contiguous sites or less, have a better prognosis.[215] There is no convincing evidence that extended radiation fields are superior to involved fields,[216, 217] yet some patients that are treated with involved-field irradiation do relapse in contiguous nonirradiated sites and, thus, it seems appropriate to include the immediately adjacent clinically uninvolved nodal group or groups.

Occasionally, patients with stage III disease and otherwise favorable characteristics (limited disease burden with fewer than five sites of nonbulky disease and no B symptoms), may be treated effectively with TNI.[218] However, this is a very uncommon extent of disease.

The complications of radiotherapy for NHL are similar to those that occur in the treatment of Hodgkin's disease.

Chemotherapy

Chemotherapy is the mainstay of treatment for the majority of patients with NHL because the majority of NHLs present as systemic disease.[211, 219, 220] The most common drugs used in the management of the NHL include single alkylating agents and CVP (cyclophosphamide, vincristine, prednisone) with or without interferon alfa-2b for the low-grade lymphomas,[221, 222] CHOP (cyclophosphamide, doxorubicin, vincristine, prednisone) for the diffuse large cell and similar lymphomas,[223] and leukemia-like regimens for lymphoblastic and Burkitt's lymphomas.

Adjuvant chemotherapy is of no proven benefit, in terms of disease-free survival, for patients with early-stage, low-grade lymphoma.[224] For the patients with stage III or IV low-grade disease, the prognosis is poorer, with disease-free survival rates of only 20% to 40% at 10 years,[225] despite initial CR rates of 45% to 55%.[222, 226] The overall survival rate of these patients is about 20% to 50% at 10 years.[225] The most effective chemotherapy combination for these lymphomas appears to be CVP.[222, 226, 227] More intensive chemotherapy programs, including those incorporating doxorubicin, do not seem to provide any additional benefit. Alternatively, single alkylating agents such as chlorambucil may be used. Newer agents that hold promise include the purine analogues, fludarabine and 2-chloro-2′-deoxyadenosine (cladribine), used either as single agents or in combinations with cyclophosphamide.[228, 229] Of note, some patients with low-grade lymphomas have been shown to be responsive to interferon alfa. Response rates as high as 62% have been reported[230] and have resulted in an extension in the time to disease progression.[222, 230]

The curative potential of combination chemotherapy in intermediate-grade NHL has been demonstrated clearly. Expected CR and 5-year survival rates are 45% to 70%[220, 231, 232] and 40% to 55%,[233, 234] respectively. Because these tumors have a rapid growth rate, relapses are frequent within 2 years of diagnosis unless a CR has been achieved. CRs are generally durable and, in most patients, are tantamount to cure. However, because of the tendency for early relapse and the potential for cure, prompt and intensive therapy for unfavorable lymphomas is indicated. Several different drug combinations have been used for the intermediate-grade lymphomas (see Table 18–16); a large intergroup study that randomized patients between CHOP,* MACOP-B† and ProMACE-CytaBOM‡ showed no difference in outcome between the different regimens.[220] However, the Australian and New Zealand Lymphoma Group performed a similar study and demonstrated a long-term survival advantage for MACOP-B.[234] Nonetheless, CHOP has been adopted as the standard regimen for these patients in many institutions.[235]

*Cyclophosphamide, doxorubicin (Adriamycin), vincristine (Oncovin), prednisone.

†Methotrexate, doxorubicin (Adriamycin), cyclophosphamide, vincristine (Oncovin), prednisone, bleomycin.

‡Cyclophosphamide, doxorubicin (Adriamycin), etoposide, prednisone—cytarabine, bleomycin, vincristine (Oncovin), methotrexate (with leucovorin rescue).

Aggressive high-grade lymphomas are relatively rare in adult patients, with the exception of human T-cell leukemia or lymphoma virus-I–associated leukemia or lymphoma. The therapies that are effective in intermediate-grade lymphomas give uniformly poor long-term survival rates for these unfavorable lymphomas. Bone marrow and central nervous system (CNS) involvement is frequent in these histologic subtypes and mediastinal predilection in young male adults is an important clinical feature of lymphoblastic lymphoma. Some progress has been made in the treatment of high-grade lymphomas with the use of leukemia-like chemotherapy regimens and CNS prophylaxis.[236–238]

Positive and promising results of a phase II trial that evaluated the effectiveness of rituximab, an anti-CD20 monoclonal antibody, were reported.[239] Researchers found that it was both a safe and successful treatment of follicular B-cell and low-grade bulky, refractory, or relapsed NHL.

Late Effects

Many of the above-mentioned treatment regimens are complex and have a great potential for toxicity. With many of the combinations, patients have profound life-threatening myelosuppression, and most have some degree of mucositis and neurologic dysfunction.[240–242] Therefore, these regimens should be administered only under the supervision of a physician who is experienced in the use of cancer chemotherapeutic agents.

Combined-Modality Therapy

Patients with small lymphocytic lymphomas usually have disseminated or stage IV disease owing to bone marrow involvement; the frequency of marrow involvement is somewhat lower in follicular lymphomas, but disseminated nodal disease is still common. For unfavorable, aggressive histology lymphomas, such as diffuse mixed, diffuse large cell, and immunoblastic subtypes, localized disease is more common and bone marrow involvement is less frequent. However, the prognosis with radiation therapy alone is poor except for selected patients with stage I disease; therefore, a combination of systemic chemotherapy and involved-field irradiation is, at present, the preferred treatment. A large randomized trial by the SWOG randomized patients with nonbulky stage I or II disease to treatment with CHOP chemotherapy alone (eight cycles) or CHOP chemotherapy (three cycles) followed by involved-field irradiation (36 to 50 Gy).[243] The results indicate the superiority of the combined-modality regimen.

Because of the high relapse rate in high-grade lymphomas, some investigators are using high-dose chemotherapy, TBI, and BMT as initial therapy.[244, 245] Follow-up on these studies is too short, at present, to make definitive conclusions. Treatment results for T-cell leukemia and lymphoma have been disappointing because of a high incidence of opportunistic infections during aggressive chemotherapy related to the underlying defect in T-cell function and immunosuppression from chemotherapy.

Special Considerations for Treatment

Extranodal Non-Hodgkin's Lymphoma

With the exception of MALT lymphomas (see "MALT Lymphomas" later in this section), most patients with primary extranodal NHL (stage I_E or II_E) generally have an intermediate-grade histology and are treated similarly to other patients with stage I to II intermediate-grade NHL. Of note, a great deal of success has been demonstrated by some investigators with combined-modality treatments.[246] However, selected extranodal sites require some individualization of therapy.

Paranasal Sinuses

Patients with intermediate- or high-grade NHL involving the paranasal sinuses should receive CNS prophylactic therapy (intrathecal chemotherapy, with or without whole brain irradiation), even if no direct involvement of the CNS can be demonstrated.[247]

Gastrointestinal Tract

This region is the most frequent site of extranodal NHL, and it most commonly involves the stomach. This is a frequent site for MALT lymphomas (see "MALT Lymphomas"), for which specific therapy is indicated. The majority of the remainder are intermediate-grade lymphomas. A complete resection can cure only about one third of patients. A preferable approach is to employ combined-modality therapy with chemotherapy and irradiation, after biopsy documentation of disease.[248] Management programs, at present, emphasize organ preservation in this setting. If a partial gastrectomy has been performed and there is no nodal involvement, treatment with chemotherapy alone following gastrectomy should be sufficient therapy. If regional nodes are involved, both chemotherapy and irradiation should follow. For patients diagnosed with gastric lymphoma before gastrectomy, combined chemotherapy and radiation therapy alone have been reported to provide results similar to that involving gastrectomy, but avoiding the morbidity of that procedure.

Skin

Patients who present with a single, small (smaller than 2.5 cm) lesion and no nodal involvement (stage I_E) may be treated effectively with radiation therapy alone. Chemotherapy should be reserved for patients who subsequently relapse.[249] Patients with more extensive involvement (stage II_E to IV disease) require chemotherapy. Rare patients with mycosis fungoides, a low-grade cutaneous T-cell lymphoma, may be treated with irradiation, topical chemotherapy, or PUVA (psoralen and ultraviolet A) when the disease is limited to the skin.[250] Patients with extracutaneous disease require systemic chemotherapy or interferon or both.

Central Nervous System

Patients who present with primary CNS lymphoma have a poor prognosis; their likelihood of local recurrence is high despite aggressive local radiation therapy, and some patients fail systemically. The frequency of cerebrospinal fluid involvement is low, and for patients with positive cerebrospinal fluid cytology, spinal axis irradiation does not appear to warrant its toxicity. Moreover, the increased use of adjuvant chemotherapy for patients with primary CNS lymphoma contraindicates the use of spinal axis irradiation because of associated bone marrow suppression.[251, 252]

Mucosa-Associated Lymphoid Tumor Lymphomas

MALT lymphomas are usually low-grade lymphomas that originate in extranodal sites and are usually of limited stage (I to II). The most common sites of origin are the GI tract (especially the stomach) and orbit. Less common sites include the salivary glands, lungs, and skin.[225] MALT lymphomas of the stomach have been associated with *Helicobacter pylori* infection,[253] so initial therapy for these patients is usually an antibiotic regimen such as bismuth or omeprazole, amoxicillin, and metronidazole.[254] If there is no associated *H. pylori* infection, or if the MALT lymphoma fails to clear after adequate antibiotic therapy, then moderate-dose irradiation (30 to 36 Gy) may be employed as a primary cytotoxic therapy.[255] Gastrectomy can usually be avoided in this situation, and the role for chemotherapy is unknown.

MALT lymphomas in other locations (orbit, salivary glands, and other sites) may be treated successfully with primary irradiation.[256] When MALT lymphomas are identified as stage III to IV, it is usually associated with transformation to a higher grade lymphoma. At that point, these patients should be treated in a manner similar to other intermediate-grade lymphomas.

Mantle Cell Lymphoma

Mantle cell lymphomas have been identified as being particularly aggressive, usually systemic diseases. Rare cases with stage I to II presentations may be treated with combined-modality therapy, as for intermediate-grade lymphomas. Patients with stage III to IV disease have a poor prognosis after conventional chemotherapy and are considered to be good candidates for clinical trials.[225, 257]

Anaplastic Large Cell Lymphoma

These lymphomas may be confused histologically with Hodgkin's disease. Patients often present with stage III or IV disease. Their management is similar to the more common diffuse large B-cell lymphomas, but their prognosis is somewhat better.[258, 259]

Peripheral T-Cell Lymphoma

Like anaplastic large cell lymphomas, these are usually systemic and require management similar to diffuse large B-cell lymphoma. However, their prognosis is worse.[259, 260]

Results and Prognosis

Chemotherapy

Indolent Lymphomas. Figure 18–7 shows survival curves for low-grade and follicular large cell lymphomas.[261] Heterogeneity among the four curves has borderline significance (p = .07). However, the survival curve for patients with the follicular large cell subtype is significantly worse than the survival curve for those with the follicular small cleaved type. Survival by stage also is shown in Figure 18–7. The survival rate for stage I disease at 10 years is 83%. Survival curves for stages II, III, and IV disease do not differ significantly. Although a substantial proportion of patients with advanced-stage disease are alive at 7 years, the majority of them are not disease free.

Aggressive Lymphomas. The large intergroup phase III trial that established CHOP as the standard regimen for this disease demonstrated an antitumor response rate of 80% and a CR rate of 44% at 3 years.[220, 262] On follow-up to 6 years, the overall survival rates for CHOP are 42%, demonstrating no significant difference with third-generation regimens such as MACOP-B.[262]

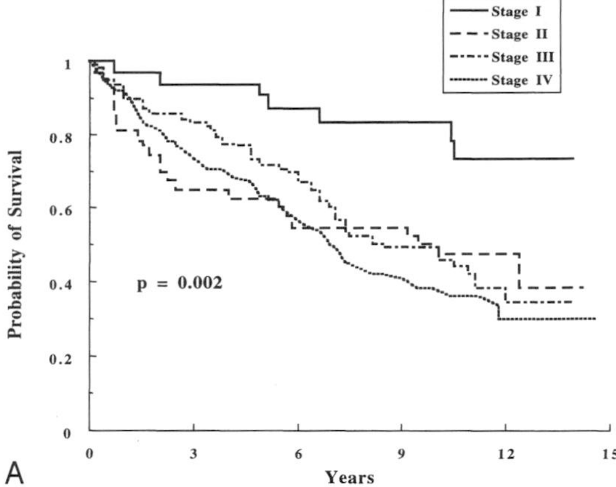

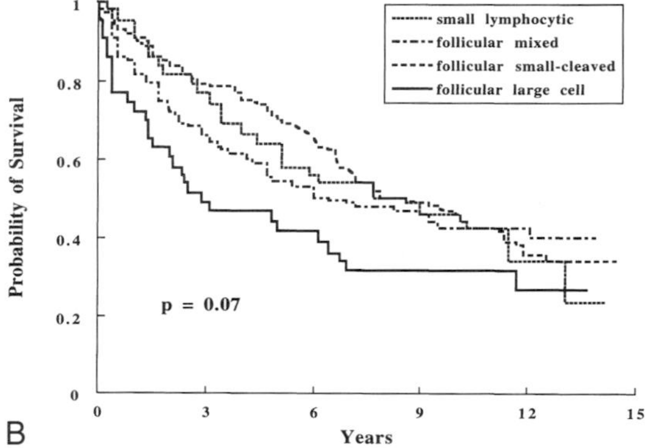

Figure 18–7. Survival results by (A) stage and (B) histology. (Modified from Simon R, Durreleman S, Hoppe RT, et al: The non-Hodgkin's lymphoma pathologic classification project. Long-term follow-up of 1,153 patients with non-Hodgkin's lymphoma. Ann Intern Med 1988; 109:939, with permission.)

Prognosis

- A report with long-term follow-up of 1153 patients has shown that the stage of disease in NHL is less predictive of outcome compared with Hodgkin's disease.[261]
- The histologic subtype of NHL is the most important prognostic determinant. For diffuse large cell lymphomas, an international collaborative study has developed the International Prognostic Index that includes five adverse prognostic factors: impaired performance status, elevated LDH level, stage III or IV, multiple extranodal sites of disease, and age older than 60.[263] Although not a staging system, this index provides help for predicting prognosis and selecting therapy.

Future Clinical Investigations

Presently, patients with intermediate- or high-grade histology and unfavorable features or those who have failed front-line therapy are being treated with high-dose therapy (chemotherapy with or without irradiation) followed by ABMT (with or without bone marrow purging). In a randomized study, the event-free survival rate exceeds 40% at 5 years, compared with 12% for conventional chemotherapy alone.[264] High-dose therapy programs are now being used investigationally as initial treatment for patients with unfavorable prognostic factors,[265] or as consolidation therapy for patients in first remission.[266] Such programs are also employed for some patients with advanced-stage low-grade lymphoma, for which there is presently no curative therapy.[267]

An additional novel approach to the management of patients with B-cell lymphoma is to use anti-CD20 antibodies, because nearly 95% of B-cell lymphomas express this surface phenotype. Trials have been conducted with both so-called cold[268] and radiolabeled antibodies[269] with promising results.

Multiple Myeloma

Epidemiology and Etiology

Epidemiology

Multiple myeloma accounted for 1.1% of estimated new cancer cases in the United States in 2000 and was responsible for 2% of cancer deaths.[11] It constituted 12.7% of new hematologic malignancies and 18.5% of deaths from hematologic malignancies in the United States in the same year. The mean age of affected patients is 62 years and it is the most common lymphoreticular neoplasm in nonwhites.

Etiology

- Survivors of high-dose radiation exposure from atomic bombs in Hiroshima and Nagasaki show a 4.7 times greater incidence of multiple myeloma than the general population. This fact did not become apparent until 20 years after their exposure.[270]

- An increased incidence of multiple myeloma in first-degree relatives and in blacks strongly implicates a genetic susceptibility.[271]
- Although multiple myeloma traditionally has been considered to be a terminally differentiated B-cell malignancy, new evidence suggests that it is an early hematopoietic stem cell disorder that becomes clinically evident at the mature stage of B-cell lineage.[271] Data using cytogenetic and molecular biologic techniques show DNA rearrangements similar to those seen in malignant lymphoma.
- Demonstration of c-*MYC* translocation to an Ig gene location has led to speculation that the *MYC* gene plays a role in the increased B-cell proliferation.[271] The activation of oncogenes presumably occurs, owing to the Ig gene rearrangement and resulting recombination errors. Chromosomal translocations may occasion these events.
- Adhesion molecules mediate binding of multiple myeloma cells to bone marrow stromal cells as the disease progresses; diminished expression of these adhesion molecules facilitates tumor cell mobilization and spread to extramedullary sites and conversion to plasma cell leukemia.[272]
- In addition, there is considerable evidence that IL-6 acts as a paracrine growth factor as well as an inhibitor of apoptosis of tumor cells in this disease.[272]

Detection and Diagnosis

Clinical Detection

Bone pain accompanied by anemia often leads to the diagnosis of multiple myeloma.[273] Pathologic fractures are common and may produce pleurisy-like or radicular pain. In addition, hypercalcemia and renal insufficiency develop in some patients and are more common in patients with Bence Jones proteinuria (homogeneous free light chains of either the κ or λ type).[274] Hypercalcemia is primarily due to increased bone resorption: myeloma cells in culture produce a number of osteoclast-activating factors that are distinct from parathyroid hormone and vitamin D. Other causes of renal impairment include amyloid deposition, uric acid nephropathy, and pyelonephritis.

Patients with multiple myeloma are at an increased risk for severe bacterial infection.[275] Repeated pneumococcal pneumonias and life-threatening meningitis may precede other manifestations of disease. The decreased antibody response seems to result primarily from the increased expression of transforming growth factor–β (TGF-β), secreted by multiple myeloma cells downregulating B-cells, T-cells, and natural killer cells.[272]

Diagnostic Procedures

Diagnosis is based on an association of *osteolytic lesions*, elevated serum or urine *M-protein*, and *marrow plasmacytosis* (more than 10% plasma cells). M-protein can be measured by *serum electrophoresis*. In addition, homogeneous (monoclonal) serum globulins can be detected using paper electrophoresis or immunoelectrophoresis. Immunoelectrophoresis specifically identifies monoclonal increases in IgG (54% of patients with multiple myeloma), IgA, (22%), IgD (less than 1%), and IgE (less than 1%). Serum B-2 microglobulin can be used as a marker of severity of disease.[276]

Definitive diagnosis may be difficult:

- Lytic bone lesions occur with other neoplasms (note that vertebral pedicles are rarely involved in myeloma, but they commonly are in metastatic carcinoma).
- Plasmacytosis of the bone marrow may occur with drug sensitivity, collagen disease (e.g., rheumatoid arthritis), amyloidosis, cirrhosis, and occasionally, with other disseminated neoplasms.
- Homogeneous serum globulins can occur in association with other neoplasms (e.g., of rectosigmoid, prostate, and bile duct), although the significance of the association is unclear.

It is important to identify patients with monoclonal gammopathy of undetermined significance.[277] These are elderly asymptomatic patients with no bone lesions or marrow plasmacytosis and serum M-protein levels of less than 3 g/dL. These patients may remain clinically asymptomatic for many years, although over the course of a decade or more, many develop multiple myeloma or a similar lymphoproliferative disorder.

Classification

The clinical staging of multiple myeloma has evolved based on clinical correlations of outcome with tumor burden (measured with metabolic techniques) and renal function (Table 18–17). Both direct and indirect reflections of the tumor burden include the character and number of bony lesions, hemoglobin and calcium levels, and M-component production rates. These criteria have thus been incorporated into the most widely used staging system for multiple myeloma.

Principles of Treatment

Some patients with multiple myeloma can have an indolent course. For this reason, evidence of progressive or symptomatic disease is usually required to initiate chemotherapy (Fig. 18–8).

Radiation Therapy

Radiation therapy is a useful component of the overall management of patients with plasma cell tumors. The following situations benefit from radiation therapy[278]:

- as primary therapy for patients with solitary plasmacytoma of bone or of isolated extramedullary sites
- as palliative therapy for painful lesions in patients with

TABLE 18–17. **Criteria for Staging Multiple Myeloma**

Stage*	Criteria	Myeloma Cell Mass (cells × $10^{12}/m^2$)
I	All of the following: • Hemoglobin >10 g/dL • Normal serum calcium • Normal bone structure • Low M-protein production as shown by: IgG <5.0 g/dL IgA <3.0 g/dL Urinary κ or λ <4 g/24 hrs	<0.6 (low burden)
II	Fitting neither stage I nor III	0.6–1.2 (intermediate burden)
III	One or more of the following: • Hemoglobin <8.5 g/dL • Serum calcium >12.0 mg/dL • >3 lytic bone lesions • High M-protein production as shown by: IgG >7.0 g/dL IgA >5.0 g/dL Urinary κ or λ >12 g/24 hrs	>1.2 (high burden)

*Subclassification of stages: A = creatinine <2.0 mg/dL; B = creatinine ≥2.0 mg/dL.

multiple myeloma who are no longer responsive to chemotherapy

- as emergency therapy for patients with spinal cord or nerve root compression
- to prevent pathologic fractures in involved weight-bearing bones
- as TBI, particularly in the setting of BMT

Chemotherapy

Without chemotherapy, the median survival time for patients with symptoms is less than 1 year. With presently available treatments, survival can be extended to 3 or 4 years,[279] although treatment strategies that include BMT offer the potential to increase survival duration. Maintenance therapy after initial induction of clinical remission has not been shown to prolong remission or survival duration. Unfortunately, in general, chemotherapy reduces the myeloma cell burden by only one to two logs, and further chemotherapy has not resulted in a further decrease in myeloma cells.

Single Agent

Melphalan is the most commonly used alkylating agent.[280, 281] The addition of prednisone to melphalan improves the response rate, but it has little impact on survival. Melphalan is administered in 4-day, high-dose intermittent courses every 4 to 6 weeks (four courses of 10 mg/m² per day). Prednisone is given concomitantly in doses of 40 to 100 mg/m² per day or 1 to 2 mg/kg per day in four courses. It should be noted that oral melphalan is not consistently absorbed, so it should be given to the point of dose-limiting hematologic toxicity, which is defined as moderate leukopenia (white blood cell count of 2500 to 3000 per mm³). This combination produces a response in 50% to 60% of patients. Median survival of responders is about

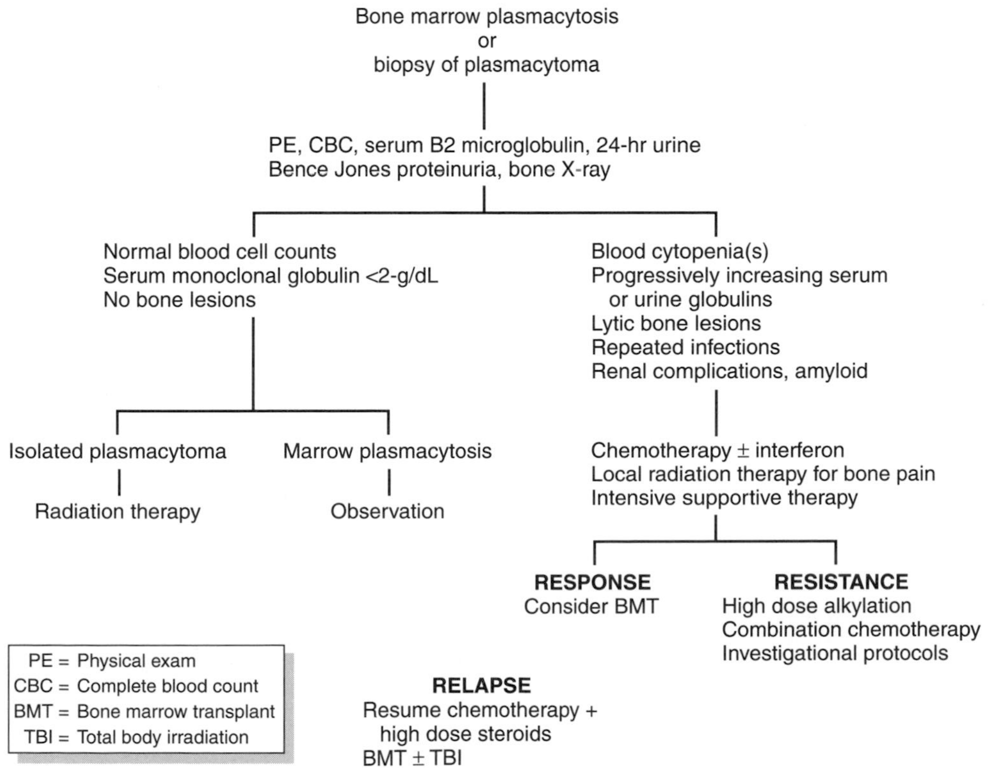

Figure 18–8. Treatment decision tree for multiple myeloma.

two to three times that of nonresponders (3 to 3.5 years versus 1 to 1.5 years).[279]

Interferon. Interferon alfa-2 has been shown to prolong the plateau phase of remission, but, again, without any survival time advantage.[282, 283] After myeloablative therapy supported by stem cell transplant, interferon alfa prolonged both remission duration and survival time in responding patients, although the significance of this effect was lost at long-term follow-up.[284]

Combination Therapy

VAD. Vincristine (0.4 mg per day) and doxorubicin (9 mg/m^2 per day), delivered through a centrally placed catheter by continuous intravenous infusion on days 1 to 4, together with dexamethasone (40 mg per day orally on days 1 to 4, 9 to 12, and 17 to 20), can produce a response rate of up to 67% in untreated patients, but without improvement in overall survival.[285] Responses occur more rapidly than with melphalan and prednisone, so that VAD has become the preferred treatment in patients who are at high risk with greater tumor burden or renal failure or hypercalcemia.

VBCMP. VBCMP therapy (the M2 protocol) is 1.2 mg/m^2 of vincristine intravenously on day 1 (maximum dose 2.0 mg), 20 mg/m^2 of carmustine intravenously on day 1, 400 mg/m^2 of cyclophosphamide intravenously on day 1, 6 mg/m^2 of melphalan orally on days 1 to 4, and 40 mg/m^2 of prednisone orally on days 1 to 7. This regimen, developed at Memorial Sloan-Kettering Cancer Center, gave a response rate of 87% and a median survival of 50 months in a nonrandomized study.[286]

Bone Marrow Transplantation

A prospective randomized study comparing conventional chemotherapy with high-dose therapy supported by ABMT was performed in 200 previously untreated patients.[287] The study showed that high-dose myeloablative therapy was associated with a significantly higher response rate (81% versus 57%; p <.001), 5-year event-free survival rate (28% versus 10%; p = .01) and 5-year overall survival rate (52% versus 12%; p = .03).

A total therapy program, presently being practiced at the University of Arkansas, consists of a series of induction regimens and two cycles of high-dose therapy[288]:

- remission induction with non–cross-resistant combination chemotherapy (two to three cycles of VAD), high-dose cyclophosphamide, GM-CSF with peripheral blood cell collection, and EDAP (etoposide, dexamethasone, cytarabine, cisplatin)
- tandem autotransplantation (200 mg/m^2 of melphalan for two cycles or a second transplant with added TBI or cyclophosphamide in patients not achieving a partial remission after first transplant)
- maintenance therapy with interferon

The median overall survival and event-free survival time were 5.7 and 3.6 years, respectively, and median complete remission duration was close to 4 years.

Patients younger than the age of 70 who are considered to be at high risk with no comorbid illnesses should be given the option of myeloablative treatment with hematopoietic stem cell support.[289] Of note, allogenic transplantation has a high mortality, and emphasis on T-cell depletion while maintaining graft-versus-myeloma effects is being pursued.[290] In addition, early versus late transplant, double versus single transplant, and purging of marrow of myeloma cells are presently under intense investigation.

Supportive Therapies

Bone Disease. Multiple myeloma is characterized by bone reabsorption and increased activity of osteoclast-activating factors, osteopenia, bone pain, and pathologic fractures. The efficacy of pamidronate infusion in reducing bone pain, pathologic fractures, and the need for palliative radiation therapy has been demonstrated in a double-blind placebo-controlled trial.[291] However, in a separate but similar trial, although pamidronate reduced episodes of severe pain and reduced the overall height reduction, there were no other significant effects.[292] Nonetheless, pamidronate in addition to chemotherapy should be considered for all patients with multiple myeloma.

Chronic Anemia. Patients with chronic symptomatic anemia may benefit from a trial of erythropoietin, especially patients with impaired renal function.[293]

Infections. Granulocyte colony-stimulating factor can abbreviate chemotherapy-induced neutropenia.[294] Prophylactic antibiotics, such as TMP-SMX (trimethoprim-sulfamethoxazole), may decrease bacterial infections, but they are similarly expensive and have considerable side effects.[275]

Special Considerations of Treatment

Hypercalcemia. Hypercalcemia should be vigorously managed with hydration, diuretics, corticosteroids, and bisphosphonates. Sixty mg of pamidronate given intravenously over 4 hours with adequate hydration is the initial treatment of choice.[295]

Spinal Cord Compression. If a patient with multiple myeloma has persistent back pain, spinal cord impingement should be suspected until proved otherwise. Extradural compression from myelomatoid involvement of a vertebral body is common. For diagnostic work-up and management, see Chapter 13, Oncologic Emergencies.

Acute Terminal Phase. An acute terminal phase, sometimes resembling acute myeloblastic or myelomonocytic leukemia, has been reported in up to one third of patients.[271] These patients have been generally unresponsive to antileukemic regimens.

Results and Prognosis

The median survival time of patients receiving oral melphalan, with or without prednisone, has ranged from 18 to 36 months, with an overall median of 24 months. Objective response is noted in at least half of the patients treated.

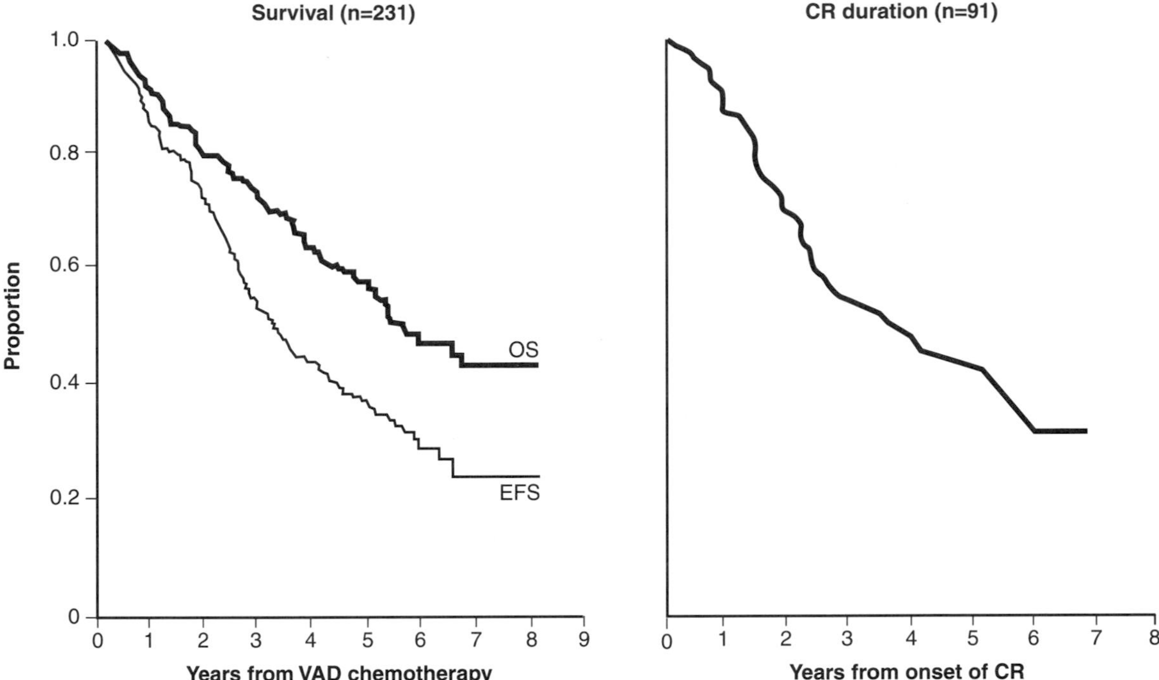

Figure 18–9. The University of Arkansas experience. CR = complete response; OS = overall survival; EFS = event-free survival. (From Mehta J, Singhal S, Desikan R, et al: High dose chemotherapy and stem cell support in myeloma. PPO Updates 1999; 13:1, with permission.)

Initially, multiagent chemotherapy, such as the M2 protocol and VMCP (vincristine, melphalan, cyclophosphamide, prednisone) alternating with VBAP (vincristine, nitrosourea, doxorubicin, prednisone), were reported to give higher response rates (87%) with a median survival of 50 months,[271] but a multicenter randomized trial failed to confirm the better results.[296]

None of these regimens is curative or controls disease for longer than 4 years.[271] Hence, high-dose chemotherapy with hematopoietic stem cell transplant is an active area of clinical investigation.[297] Figure 18–9 reflects the outcome of 231 patients treated at the University of Arkansas with intensive combination chemotherapy, followed by autologous stem cell transplant.[298]

Future Clinical Investigation

Active areas of investigation are in immune modulation, in order to enhance the graft-versus-myeloma effect with prophylactic infusion of T-cells,[299] and to eliminate minimal remedial disease, investigators are looking at infusing idiotypic dendritic cells and idiotypic vaccination to generate cell-mediated and hormonal immunity.[300]

REFERENCES

General

1. Kaplan HS: Hodgkin's Disease, 2nd ed. Cambridge, Harvard University Press, 1980.
2. Canellos GP, Lister TA, Sklar JL (eds): The Lymphomas. Philadelphia, W.B. Saunders, 1998.
3. Mauch PM, Armitage JO, Diehl V, et al: Hodgkin's Disease. Philadelphia, Lippincott Williams & Wilkins, 1999.
4. Halperin EC, Constine LS, Tarbell NJ, et al: Pediatric Radiation Oncology, 3rd ed. Philadelphia, Lippincott Williams & Wilkins, 1999.

Specific

5. Hodgkin T: On some morbid appearances of the absorbent gland and spleen. Medico-Chirurgical Transactions 1832; 17:68.
6. Virchow R: Weisses Blut. Neue notizen aus dem Gebiete der Natur und Heikunde. Froriep's Neue Notizen 1845; 36:151.
7. Kundrat H: Uber Lympho-sarkomatosis. Wien Klin Wochenschr 1893; 6:211.
8. Sternberg C: Uber eine eigenartige unter dem Bilde der Pseudoleukamie verlaufende Tuberculose des lymphatichon Apparates. Ztschr Heilk 1898; 19:21.
9. Reed DM: On the pathologic changes in Hodgkin's disease, with especial reference to its relation to tuberculosis. Johns Hopkins Hosp Rev 1902; 10:133.
10. DeVita VT Jr., Mauch PM, Harris NL: Hodgkin's disease. In: DeVita VT Jr., Hellman S, Rosenberg SA (eds): Cancer: Principles and Practice of Oncology, 5th ed, p 2242. Philadelphia, Lippincott-Raven, 1997.
11. Greenlee RT, Murray T, Bolden S, et al: Cancer statistics, 2000. CA Cancer J Clin 2000; 50:7.
12. Correa P, Conor GT: Epidemiologic patterns of Hodgkin's disease. Int J Cancer 1971; 8:192.
13. Correa P: Hodgkin's disease. International mortality patterns and time trends. World Health Statistics Report 1977; 30:146.
14. Stiller CA, Parkin DM: International variations in the incidence of childhood lymphomas. Paediatr Perinat Epidemiol 1990; 4:303.
15. Beral V, Newton R: Overview of the epidemiology of immunodeficiency-associated cancers. J Natl Cancer Inst 1998; 23:1.
16. Murphy RC, Berdon WE, Ruzal-Shapiro C, et al: Malignancies in pediatric patients with ataxia telangectasia. Pediatr Radiol 1999; 29:225.
17. Tirelli U, Errante D, Dolcetti R: Hodgkin's disease and human immunodeficiency virus infection: clinicopathologic and virologic features of 114 patients from the the Italian cooperative group on AIDS and tumors. J Clin Oncol 1995; 13:1758.
18. Gerold M, Adler R: Hodgkin's disease as an indicator of AIDS. Med Hypotheses 1995; 45:76.
19. Michels KB: The origins of Hodgkin's disease. Eur J Cancer Prev 1995; 4:379.
20. Mueller N, Evans A, Harris N: Hodgkin's disease and Epstein-Barr

virus. Altered antibody pattern before diagnosis. N Engl J Med 1989; 320:689.
21. Chapman AL, Rickson AB: Epstein-Barr virus in Hodgkin's disease. Ann Oncol 1998; 9 (suppl):S5.
22. Jarrett RF, MacKenzie J: Epstein-Barr virus and other candidate viruses in the pathogenesis of Hodgkin's disease. Semin Hematol 1999; 36:260.
23. Westergaard T, Melbye M, Pedersen JB, et al: Birth order, sibship size and risk of Hodgkin's disease in children and young adults: a population-based study of 31 million person-years. Int J Cancer 1997; 72:977.
24. Slivnick DJ, Ellis TM, Nawrocki JF, et al: The impact of Hodgkin's disease on the immune system. Semin Oncol 1990; 17:673.
25. Poppema S, Potters M, Emmens R, et al: Immune reactions in classical Hodgkin's lymphoma. Semin Hematol 1999; 36:253.
26. Poppema S: Immunology of Hodgkin's disease. Baillieres Clin Haematol 1996; 9:447.
27. Lin AY, Kingma DW, Lennette ET, et al: Epstein-Barr virus and familial Hodgkin's disease. Blood 1996; 88:3160.
28. Stein H, Hummel M, Marafioti T, et al: Molecular biology of Hodgkin's disease. Cancer Surv 1997; 30:107.
29. Kuppers R: Identifying the precursors of Hodgkin and Reed-Sternberg cells in Hodgkin's disease: role of the germinal center in B-cell lymphomagenesis. J Acquir Immune Defic Syndr 1999; 21 (suppl):S74.
30. Stein H, Hummel M: Cellular origin and clonality of classic Hodgkin's lymphoma: immunophenotypic and molecular studies. Semin Hematol 1999; 36:233.
31. Marafioti T, Hummel M, Foss HD, et al: Hodgkin and Reed-Sternberg cells represent an expansion of a single clone originating from a germinal center B-cell with functional immunoglobulin gene rearrangements but defective immunoglobulin transcription. Blood 2000; 95:1443.
32. Serrano D, Ghiotto F, Roncella S, et al: The patterns of IL2, IFN-gamma, IL4 and IL5 gene expression in Hodgkin's disease and reactive lymph nodes. Haematologica 1997; 82:542.
33. Kaplan HS, Dorfman RF, Nelsen TS, et al: Staging laparotomy and splenectomy in Hodgkin's disease: analysis of indication and patterns of involvement in 285 consecutive cases, unselected patients. NCI Monograph 1973; 36:291.
34. Kapadia SB, Roman LN, Kingma DW, et al: Hodgkin's disease of Waldeyer's ring. Clinical and histoimmunophenotypic findings and association with Epstein-Barr virus in 16 cases. Am J Surg Pathol 1995; 19:1431.
35. Smitt MC, Stouffer N, Owen JB, et al: Results of the 1988–1989 Patterns of Care Study process survey for Hodgkin's disease. Int J Radiat Oncol Biol Phys 1999; 43:335.
36. Carlsen SE, Bergin CJ, Hoppe RT: MR imaging to detect chest wall and pleural involvement in patients with lymphoma: effect on radiation therapy planning. Am J Roentgenol 1993; 160:1191.
37. Front D, Israel O: The role of Ga-67 scintigraphy in evaluating the results of therapy of lymphoma patients. Semin Nucl Med 1995; 25:60.
38. Zinzani PL, Magagnoli M, Franchi R, et al: Diagnostic role of gallium scanning in the management of lymphoma with mediastinal involvement. Haematologica 1999; 84:604.
39. Bangerter M, Moog F, Buchmann I, et al: Whole-body 2-[18F]-fluoro-2-deoxy-D-glucose positron emission tomography (FDG-PET) for accurate staging of Hodgkin's disease. Ann Oncol 1998; 9:1117.
40. Zinzani PL, Magagnoli M, Chierichetti F, et al: The role of positron emission tomography (PET) in the management of lymphoma patients. Ann Oncol 1999; 10:1181.
41. Hasenclever D, Diehl V: A prognostic score for advanced Hodgkin's disease. International Prognostic Factors Project on Advanced Hodgkin's Disease. N Engl J Med 1998; 339:1506.
42. Mason DY, Banks PM, Chan J, et al: Nodular lymphocyte predominance Hodgkin's disease. A distinct clinicopathological entity. Am J Surg Pathol 1994; 18:526.
43. Leibenhaut MH, Hoppe RT, Efron B, et al: Prognostic indicators of laparotomy findings in clinical stage I–II supradiaphragmatic Hodgkin's disease. J Clin Oncol 1989; 7:81.
44. Lukes RJ, Butler JJ: The pathology and nomenclature of Hodgkin's disease. Cancer Res 1966; 26:1063.
45. Harris NL, Jaffe ES, Stein H, et al: A revised European-American classification of lymphoid neoplasms: a proposal from the International Lymphoma Study Group. Blood 1994; 84:1361.
46. Harris NL, Jaffe ES, Diebold J, et al: Lymphoma classification—from controversy to consensus: the R.E.A.L. and WHO Classification of lymphoid neoplasms. Ann Oncol 2000; 11 (suppl 1):3.
47. The International Non-Hodgkin's Lymphoma Prognostic Factors Project: A predictive model for aggressive non-Hodgkin's lymphoma. N Engl J Med 1993; 329:987.
48. Carbone PP, Kaplan HS, Musshoff K, et al: Report of the committee on Hodgkin's disease staging classification. Cancer Res 1971; 31:1860.
49. American Joint Committee on Cancer: AJCC Cancer Staging Manual, 5th ed. Philadelphia, Lippincott-Raven, 1997.
50. Lister TA, Crowther D, Sutcliffe SB, et al: Report of a committee convened to discuss the evaluation and staging of patients with Hodgkin's disease: Cotswolds meeting. J Clin Oncol 1989; 7:1630.
51. Kaplan HS, Rosenberg SA: The treatment of Hodgkin's disease. Med Clin North Am 1966; 50:1591.
52. Baysogolov GD, Shakhtarina SV, Afanasova NV: Management of Hodgkin's disease patients with mediastinal adenopathy and pulmonary involvement (Stage IIE). Radiother Oncol 1993; 27:107.
53. Physician Data Query: Adult Hodgkin's disease, Bethesda, National Cancer Institute, 2000.
54. Classe JM, Mahe M, Moreau P, et al: Ovarian transposition by laparoscopy before radiotherapy in the treatment of Hodgkin's disease. Cancer 1998; 83:1420.
55. Gilbert R: La roentgentherapie de la granulomatose maligne. J Radiol Electrol 1925; 9:509.
56. Gilbert R: Radiotherapy in Hogkin's disease (malignant granulomatosis): anatomic and clinical foundations; sovereign principles, results. Am J Radiol 1939; 41:198.
57. Peters MV: A study in survivals in Hodgkin's disease treated radiologically. Am J Radiol 1950; 63:299.
58. Peters MV, Middlemiss K: A study of Hodgkin's disease treated by irradiation. Am J Radiol 1958; 79:114.
59. Peters MV: Prophylactic treatment of adjacent areas in Hodgkin's disease. Cancer Res 1966; 26:1232.
60. Kaplan HS: The radical radiotherapy of regionally localized Hodgkin's disease. Radiology 1962; 78:553.
61. Wolf J, Engert A, Diehl V: Issues in the treatment of Hodgkin's disease. Curr Opin Oncol 1998; 10:396.
62. Vlachaki MT, Hagemeister FB, Fuller LM, et al: Long-term outcome of treatment for Ann Arbor Stage I Hodgkin's disease: prognostic factors for survival and freedom from progression. Int J Radiat Oncol Biol Phys 1997; 38:593.
63. Wirth A, Chao M, Corry J, et al: Mantle irradiation alone for clinical stage I–II Hodgkin's disease: long-term follow-up and analysis of prognostic factors in 261 patients. J Clin Oncol 1999; 17:230.
64. Enrici RM, Anselmo AP, Donato V, et al: Relapse and late complications in early-stage Hodgkin's disease patients with mediastinal involvement treated with radiotherapy alone or plus one cycle of ABVD. Haematologica 1999; 84:917.
65. Cutuli B, Petit T, Hoffstetter S, et al: Treatment of subdiaphragmatic Hodgkin's disease: long-term results and side effects. Oncol Rep 1998; 5:1513.
66. Liao Z, Ha CS, Fuller LM, et al: Subdiaphragmatic stage I & II Hodgkin's disease: long-term follow-up and prognostic factors. Int J Radiat Oncol Biol Phys 1998; 41:1047.
67. Hoppe RT, Cox RS, Rosenberg SA, et al: Prognostic factors in pathologic stage III Hodgkin's disease. Cancer Treat Rep 1982; 66:743.
68. Russell K, Hoppe RT, Colby T, et al: Lymphocyte predominant Hodgkin's disease: clinical presentation and results of treatment. Radiother Oncol 1984; 1:197.
69. Wolf J, Tesch H, Parsa-Parsi R, et al: Current clinical trials for the treatment of adult Hodgkin's disease: common strategies and perspectives. Ann Clin Oncol 1998; 9 (suppl 5):S79.
70. van den Berg H, Stuve W, Behrendt H: Treatment of Hodgkin's disease in children with alternating mechlorethamine, vincristine, procarbazine, and prednisone (MOPP) and adriamycin, bleomycin, vinblastine, and dacarbazine (ABVD) courses without radiotherapy. Med Pediatr Oncol 1997; 29:23.
71. Scarantino CW, Rubin P, Constine LS 3rd: The paradoxes in patterns and mechanism of bone marrow regeneration after irradiation. 1. Different volumes and doses. Radiother Oncol 1984; 2:215.

72. Cosset JM, Henry-Amar M, Meerwaldt JH: Long-term toxicity of early stages of Hodgkin's disease therapy: The EORTC experience. EORTC Lymphoma Cooperative Group. Ann Oncol 1991; 2 (suppl):77.
73. Sears JD, Greven KM, Ferree CR, et al: Definitive irradiation in the treatment of Hodgkin's disease. Analysis of outcome, prognostic factors, and long-term complications. Cancer 1997; 79:145.
74. Peerboom PF, Hassink EA, Melkert R, et al: Thyroid function 10–18 years after mantle field irradiation for Hodgkin's disease. Eur J Cancer 1992; 28A:1716.
75. Kuten A, Lubochitski R, Fishman G, et al: Postradiotherapy hypothyroidism: radiation dose response and chemotherapeutic radiosensitization at less than 40 Gy. J Surg Oncol 1996; 61:281.
76. Hancock SL, Cox RS, McDougall IR: Thyroid diseases after treatment of Hodgkin's disease. N Engl J Med 1991; 325:599.
77. Hancock S, Hoppe RT: Long-term complications of treatment and causes of mortality after Hodgkin's disease. Semin Radiat Oncol 1996; 6:225.
78. Hallak J, Hendin BN, Thomas AJ Jr., et al: Investigation of fertilizing capacity of cryopreserved spermatozoa from patients with cancer. J Urol 1998; 159:1217.
79. Rosenberg SA, Kaplan HS: The evoloution and summary results of the Stanford randomized clinical trials of the management of Hodgkin's disease: 1962–1984. Int J Radiat Oncol Biol Phys 1985; 11:5.
80. Mauch PM, Tarbell NJ, Weinstein H, et al: Stage IA and IIA supradiaphragmatic Hodgkin's disease: prognostic factors in surgically staged patients treated with mantle and paraaortic irradiation. J Clin Oncol 1988; 6:1576.
81. Hughes-Davies L, Tarbell NJ, Coleman CN, et al: Stage IA-IIB Hodgkin's disease: management and outcome of extensive thoracic involvement. Int J Radiat Oncol Biol Phys 1997; 39:361.
82. Horning SJ, Williams J, Bartlett NL, et al: Assessment of the Stanford V regimen and consolidative radiotherapy for bulky and advanced Hodgkin's disease: Eastern Cooperative Oncology Group pilot study E1492. J Clin Oncol 2000; 18:972.
83. Radford JA, Crowther D, Rohatiner AZ, et al: Results of a randomized trial comparing MVPP chemotherapy with a hybrid regimen, ChlVPP/EVA, in the initial treatment of Hodgkin's disease. J Clin Oncol 1995; 13:2379.
84. Harding MJ, McNulty LJ, Paul J, et al: Mechlorethamine, vinblastine, procarbazine and prednisolone (MVPP) for advanced Hodgkin's disease. Eur J Cancer 1991; 27:1002.
85. Hill M, Milan S, Cunningham D, et al: Evaluation of the efficacy of the VEEP regimen in adult Hodgkin's disease with assessment of gonadal and cardiac toxicity. J Clin Oncol 1995; 13:1283.
86. Salvagno L, Soraru M, Sotti G, et al: Hybrid MOPP/ABVD and radiotherapy in advanced Hodgkin's disease. Ann Oncol 1995; 6:173.
87. Simmonds PD, Mead GM, Sweetenham JW, et al: PACE BOM chemotherapy: a 12-week regimen for advanced Hodgkin's disease. Ann Oncol 1997; 8:259.
88. Ferme C, Sebban C, Hennequin C, et al: Comparison of chemotherapy to radiotherapy as consolidation of complete or good partial response after six cycles of chemotherapy for patients with advanced Hodgkin's disease: results of the Group d'Etudes des Lymphomes de l'Adulte H89 trial. Blood 2000; 95:2246.
89. Aviles A, Guzman R, Talavera A, et al: Randomized study for the treatment of adult advanced Hodgkin's disease: epirubicin, vinblastine, bleomycin, and dacarbazine (EVBD) versus mitoxantrone, vinblastine, bleomycin, and dacarbazine (MVBD). Med Pediatr Oncol 1994; 22:168.
90. DeVita VT Jr., Simon RM, Hubbard SM, et al: Curability of advanced Hodkin's disease with chemotherapy. Long-term follow-up of MOPP-treated patients at the National Cancer Institute. Ann Intern Med 1980; 92:587.
91. Bonadonna G, Valagussa P, Santoro A: Alternating non-cross-resistant combination chemotherapy or MOPP in stage IV Hodgkin's disease. Ann Intern Med 1986; 104:739.
92. Horning SJ, Rosenberg SA, Hoppe RT, et al: Brief chemotherapy (Stanford V) and adjuvant radiotherapy for bulky or advanced Hodgkin's disease: an update. Ann Oncol 1996; 7 (suppl 4):105.
93. Rodriguez J, Rodriguez MA, Fayed L, et al: ASHAP: a regimen for cytoreduction of refractory or recurrent Hodgkin's disease. Blood 1999; 93:3632.
94. Prosnitz LR, Farber LR, Kapp DS, et al: Combined modality therapy for advanced Hodgkin's disease: long-term followup data. Cancer Treat Res 1982; 66:871.
95. Behar RA, Horning SJ, Hoppe RT: Hodgkin's disease with bulky mediastinal involvement: effective management with combined modality therapy. Int J Radiat Oncol Biol Phys 1993; 25:771.
96. Aviles A, Delgado S: A prospective clinical trial comparing chemotherapy, radiotherapy, and combined therapy in the treatment of early stage Hodgkin's disease with bulky disease. Clin Lab Haematol 1998; 20:95.
97. Canellos GP, Anderson JR, Propert KJ, et al: Chemotherapy of advanced Hodgkin's disease with MOPP, ABVD, or MOPP alternating with ABVD. N Engl J Med 1992; 327:1478.
98. Viviani S, Bonadonna G, Santoro A, et al: Alternating versus hybrid MOPP and ABVD combinations in advanced Hodgkin's disease: ten-year results. J Clin Oncol 1996; 14:1421.
99. Yuen AR, Horning SJ: Hodgkin's disease: management of first relapse. Oncology 1996; 10:233.
100. Nademanee A, O'Donnell MR, Snyder DS, et al: High-dose chemotherapy with or without total body irradiation followed by autologous bone marrow and/or peripheral blood stem cell transplantation for patients with relapsed and refractory Hodgkin's disease: results in 85 patients with analysis of prognostic factors. Blood 1995; 85:1381.
101. Horning SJ, Chao NJ, Negrin RS, et al: High-dose therapy and autologous hematopoietic progenitor cell transplantation for recurrent or refractory Hodgkin's disease: analysis of the Stanford University results and prognostic indices. Blood 1997; 89:801.
102. Sweetenham JW, Carella AM, Taghipour G, et al: High-dose therapy and autologous stem-cell transplantation for adult patients with Hodgkin's disease who do not enter remission after induction chemotherapy: results in 175 patients reported to the European Group for Blood and Marrow Transplantation. Lymphoma Working Party. J Clin Oncol 1999; 17:3101.
103. Viviani S, Santoro A, Negretti E, et al: Salvage chemotherapy in Hodgkin's disease. Results in patients relapsing more than twelve months after first complete remission. Ann Oncol 1990; 1:123.
104. Enblad G, Hagberg H, Gustavsson A, et al: Methyl-GAG, ifosfamide, methotrexate and etoposide (MIME) as salvage therapy for Hodgkin's disease: a prospective study. Eur J Haematol 1998; 60:166.
105. Mendenhall N, Cantor A, Williams J, et al: With modern technique is staging laparotomy necessary in pediatric Hodgkin's disease? A Pediatric Oncology Group study. J Clin Oncol 1993; 11:2218.
106. Carde P, Hagenbeek A, Hayat M, et al: Clinical staging versus laparotomy and combined modality with MOPP versus ABVD in early-stage Hodgkin's disease: the H6 twin randomized trials from the European Organization for Research and Treatment of Cancer Lymphoma Cooperative Group. J Clin Oncol 1993; 11:2258.
107. Carde P, Burgers JM, Henry-Amar M, et al: Clinical stages I and II Hodgkin's disease: a specifically tailored therapy according to prognostic factors. J Clin Oncol 1988; 6:239.
108. Mauch PM, Canellos GP, Shulman LN, et al: Mantle irradiation alone for selected patients with laparotomy-staged IA to IIA Hodgkin's disease: preliminary results of a prospective trial. J Clin Oncol 1995; 13:947.
109. Noordijk EM, Carde P, Mandard AM, et al: Preliminary results of the EORTC-GPMC controlled clincial trial H7 in early-stage Hodgkin's disease. EORTC Lymphoma Cooperative Group. Groupe Pierre-et-Marie-Curie. Ann Oncol 1994; 5 (suppl 2):107.
110. Fabian CJ, Mansfield CM, Dahlberg S, et al: Low-dose involved field radiation after chemotherapy in advanced Hodgkin disease. A Southwest Oncology Group randomized study. Ann Intern Med 1994; 120:903.
111. Specht L: Prognostic factors in Hodgkin's disease. Semin Radiat Oncol 1996; 6:146.
112. Raemaekers J, Burgers M, Henry-Amar M, et al: Patients with stage III/IV Hodgkin's disease in partial remission after MOPP/ABV chemotherapy have excellent prognosis after additional involved-field radiotherapy: interim results from the ongoing EORTC-LCG and GPMC phase III trial. The EORTC Lymphoma Cooperative Group and Groupe Pierre-et-Marie-Curie. Ann Oncol 1997; 8 (suppl):111.
113. Diehl V, Loeffler M, Pfreundschuh M, et al: Further chemotherapy versus low-dose involved-field radiotherapy as consolidation of complete remission after six cycles of alternating chemotherapy in patients with advance Hodgkin's disease. German Hodgkin's Study Group. Ann Oncol 1995; 6:901.

114. Longo DL, Glatstein E, Duffey PL, et al: Alternating MOPP and ABVD chemotherapy plus mantle-field radiation therapy in patients with massive mediastinal Hodgkin's disease. J Clin Oncol 1997; 15:3338.
115. Smolewski P, Robak T, Krykowski E, et al: Prognostic factors in Hodgkin's disease: multivariate analysis of 327 patients from a single institution. Clin Cancer Res 2000; 6:1150.
116. Crnkovich MJ, Leopold K, Hoppe RT, et al: Stage I and IIB Hodgkin's disease: the combined experience at Stanford University and the Joint Center for Radiation Therapy. J Clin Oncol 1987; 5:1041.
117. Canellos GP: Treatment of relapsed Hodgkin's disease: strategies and prognostic factors. Ann Oncol 1998; 9 (suppl 5):S91.
118. Armitage JO, Lister TA: Non-Hodgkin's lymphoma. In: American Society of Clinical Oncology Education Booklet, p 338. Alexandria, American Society of Clinical Oncology, 1998.
119. Friedman S, Henry-Amar M, Cosset JM, et al: Therapeutic implications and sites of relapse predicted by elevated post-therapy erythrocyte sedimentation rate in early stage Hodgkin's disease. Am J Hematol 1991; 37:253.
120. Donaldson SS, Kaplan HS: Complications of treatment of Hodgkin's disease in children. Cancer Treat Rep 1982; 66:977.
121. Mauch PM, Weinstein H, Botnick L, et al: An evaluation of long-term survival and treatment complications in children with Hodgkin's disease. Cancer 1988; 51:925.
122. Hancock SL, Donaldson S, Hoppe RT: Cardiac disease following treatment of Hodgkin's disease in children and adolescents. J Clin Oncol 1993; 11:1208.
123. Boivin JF, Hutchison GB, Zauber AG, et al: Incidence of second cancers in patients treated for Hodgkin's disease. J Natl Cancer Inst 1995; 87:732.
124. Donaldson SS, Link MP: Combined modality treatment with low-dose radiation and MOPP chemotherapy for children with Hodgkin's disease. J Clin Oncol 1987; 5:742.
125. Cleary S, Link M, Donaldson S: Hodgkin's disease in the very young. Int J Radiat Oncol Biol Phys 1994; 28:77.
126. Kennedy BJ, Loeb V, Peterson V, et al: Survival in Hodgkin's disease by stage and age. Med Pediatr Oncol 1992; 20:100.
127. Kung FH: Hodgkin's disease in children 4 years of age or younger. Cancer 1991; 67:1428.
128. Tarbell NJ, Gelber RD, Weinstein HJ, et al: Sex differences in risk of second malignant tumours after Hodgkin's disease in childhood. Lancet 1993; 341:1428.
129. Razzouk B, Gan Y, Mendonca C, et al: Epstein-Barr virus in pediatric Hodgkin disease: age and histiotype are more predictive than geographic region. Med Pediatr Oncol 1998; 28:248.
130. Robertson SJ, Lowman JT, Gutterman S, et al: Familial Hodgkin's disease: a clinical and laboratory investigation. Cancer 1987; 59:1314.
131. Salloum E, Brandt D, Caride V: Gallium scans in the management of patients with Hodgkin's disease: a study of 101 patients. J Clin Oncol 1997; 15:518.
132. Hanna S, Fletcher B, Boulden T, et al: MR imaging of infradiaphragmatic lymphadenopathy in children and adolescents with Hodgkin disease: comparison with lymphography and CT. J Magn Reson Imaging 1993; 3:461.
133. Donaldson SS: Making choices in the staging of children with Hodgkin's disease. Med Pediatr Oncol 1991; 19:211.
134. Castellino RA, Marglin SI: Imaging of abdominal and pelvic lymph nodes: lymphography or computed tomography? Invest Radiol 1982; 17:433.
135. Breuer CK, Tarbell NJ, Mauch PM, et al: The importance of staging laparotomy in pediatric Hodgkin's disease. J Pediatr Surg 1994; 29:1085.
136. Jockovich M, Mendenhall NP, Sombeck MD, et al: Long-term complications of laparotomy in Hodgkin's disease. Ann Surg 1994; 219:615.
137. Barrett A, Crennan E, Barnes J, et al: Treatment of clinical stage I Hodgkin's disease by local radiation therapy alone. A United Kingdom Children's Cancer Study Group study. Cancer 1990; 66:670.
138. Gehan EA, Sullivan MP, Fuller LM, et al: The intergroup Hodgkin's disease in children. A study of stage I and II. Cancer 1990; 65:1429.
139. Donaldson SS, Glatstein E, Rosenberg SA, et al: Pediatric Hodgkin's disease. II. Results of therapy. Cancer 1976; 37:2436.
140. Henry-Amar M, Dietrich PY: Acute leukemia after the treatment of Hodgkin's disease. Hematol Oncol Clin North Am 1993; 7:369.
141. Bokemeyer C, Schmoll HJ, van Rhee J, et al: Long-term gonadal toxicity after therapy for Hodgkin's and non-Hodgkin's lymphoma. Ann Hematol 1994; 68:105.
142. Hudson MM, Donaldson SS: Treatment of pediatric Hodgkin's lymphoma. Semin Hematol 1999; 36:313.
143. Jenkin D, Doyle J, Berry M, et al: Hodgkin's disease in children: treatment with MOPP and low-dose extended field irradiation without laparotomy late results and toxicity. Med Pediatr Oncol 1990; 18:265.
144. Maity A, Goldwein JW, Lange B, et al: Comparison of high-dose and low-dose radiation with and without chemotherapy for children with Hodgkin's disease: an analysis of the experience at the Children's Hospital of Philadelphia and the Hospital of the University of Pennsylvania. J Clin Oncol 1992; 10:929.
145. Mauch PM: Controversies in the management of early stage Hodgkin's disease. Blood 1994; 83:318.
146. Wolden S, Lamborn K, Cleary S, et al: Second cancers following pediatric Hodgkin's disease. J Clin Oncol 1998; 16:536.
147. Behar RA, Hoppe RT: Radiation therapy in the management of bulky mediastinal Hodgkin's disease. Cancer 1990; 66:75.
148. Maity A, Goldwein JW, Lange B, et al: Mediastinal masses in children with Hodgkin's disease. An analysis of the Children's Hospital of Philadelphia and the Hospital of the University of Pennsylvania experience. Cancer 1992; 69:2755.
149. Tarbell NJ, Mauch P, Hellman S: Pulmonary complications of Hodgkin's disease treatment: radiation pneumonitis, fibrosis, and the effect of cytotoxic drugs. In: Lacher M, Redman J (eds): Hodgkin's Disease: The Consequences of Survival, p 296. Philadelphia, Lea & Febiger, 1990.
150. Willman K, Cox R, Donaldson S: Radiation induced height impairment in pediatric Hodgkin's disease. Int J Radiat Oncol Biol Phys 1994; 28:85.
151. Coia LR, Hanks GE: Complications from large field intermediate dose infradiaphragmatic radiation: an analysis of the patterns of care outcome studies for Hodgkin's disease and seminoma. Int J Radiat Oncol Biol Phys 1988; 15:29.
152. Yahalom J, Ryu J, Straus D, et al: Impact of adjuvant radiation on the patterns and rate of relapse in advanced-stage Hodgkin's disease treated with alternating chemotherapy combinations. J Clin Oncol 1991; 9:2193.
153. Bader S, Weinstein H, Mauch P, et al: Pediatric stage IV Hodgkin's disease: long-term survival. Cancer 1993; 72:249.
154. Olweny CLM, Katongole-Mbidde E, Kiire C, et al: Childhood Hodgkin's disease in Uganda—a ten-year experience. Cancer 1978; 42:787.
155. Fryer CJ, Hutchinson RJ, Krailo M, et al: Efficacy and toxicity of 12 courses of ABVD chemotherapy followed by low-dose regional radiation in advanced Hodgkin's disease in children: a report from the Children's Cancer Study Group. J Clin Oncol 1990; 8:1971.
156. Oberlin O, Leverger G, Pacquement M, et al: Low-dose radiation therapy and reduced chemotherapy in childhood Hodgkin's disease: the experience of the French Society of Pediatric Oncology. J Clin Oncol 1992; 10:1062.
157. Hutchinson R, Krailo M, Fryer C: Prognostic factor analysis in advanced Hodgkin's disease (stages III and IV). Results of the CCG 521 trial. Med Pediatr Oncol 1993; 21:61.
158. Santoro A, Bonadonna G, Valagussa P, et al: Long-term results of combined chemotherapy-radiotherapy approach in Hodgkin's disease: superiority of ABVD plus radiotherapy versus MOPP plus radiotherapy. J Clin Oncol 1987; 5:27.
159. Lamonte C, Yeh S, Straus D: Long-term follow-up of cardiac function in patients with Hodgkin's disease treated with mediastinal irradiation and combination chemotherapy including doxorubicin. Cancer Treat Rep 1986; 70:439.
160. Williams C, Goldstone A, Pearce R, et al: Autologous bone marrow transplantation for pediatric Hodgkin's disease: a case-matched comparison with adult patients by the European Bone Marrow Transplant Group Lymphoma Registry. J Clin Oncol 1993; 11:2243.
161. Donaldson SS, Whitaker S, Plowman N, et al: Stage I–II pediatric Hodgkin's disease: long-term follow-up demonstrates equivalent survival rates following different management schemes. J Clin Oncol 1990; 8:1128.
162. Ekert H, Waters KD, Smith PJ, et al: Treatment with MOPP or CHIVPP chemotherapy only for all stages of childhood Hodgkin's disease. J Clin Oncol 1988; 6:1845.

163. Lobo-Sanahuja F, Garcia I, Barrantes JC, et al: Pediatric Hodgkin's disease in Costa Rica: twelve years' experience of primary treatment by chemotherapy alone, without staging laparotomy. Med Pediatr Oncol 1994; 22:398.
164. Weiner M, Leventhal B, Brecher M, et al: Randomized study of intensive MOPP-ABVD with or without low-dose total nodal radiation therapy in the treatment of stages IIB, IIIA2, IIIB, and IV Hodgkin's disease in pediatric patients: a Pediatric Oncology Group study. J Clin Oncol 1997; 15:2769.
165. Schellong G, Bramswig J, Hornig-Franz I, et al: Hodgkin's disease in children: combined modality treatment for stages IA, IB and IIA. Results of 356 patients of the German/Austrian Paediatric Study Group. Ann Oncol 1994; 5:113.
166. Schellong G, Bramswig J, Hornig-Franz I: Treatment of children with Hodgkin's disease: results of the German Pediatric Oncology Group. Ann Oncol 1992; 3:73.
167. Donaldson SS, Link MP: Hodgkin's disease: treatment of the young child. Pediatr Clin North Am 1991; 38:457.
168. Schellong G: The balance between cure and late effects in childhood Hodgkin's lymphoma: the experience of the German-Austrian Study-Group since 1978. Ann Oncol 1996; 7:567.
169. Schellong G: Treatment of children and adolescents with Hodgkin's disease: the experience of the German-Austrian Paediatric Study Group. Baillieres Clin Haematol 1996; 9:619.
170. Vecchi V, Pileri S, Burnelli R, et al: Treatment of pediatric Hodgkin's disease tailored to stage, mediastinal mass, and age. Cancer 1993; 72:2049.
171. Hudson M, Greenwald C, Thompson E: Efficacy and toxicity of multiagent chemotherapy and low-dose involved-field radiotherapy in children and adolescents with Hodgkin's disease. J Clin Oncol 1993; 11:100.
172. Hunger SP, Link MP, Donaldson SS: ABVD/MOPP and low-dose involved-field radiotherapy in pediatric Hodgkin's disease: the Standford experience. J Clin Oncol 1994; 12:2160.
173. Schellong G, Potter R, Bramswig J, et al: High cure rates and reduced long-term toxicity in pediatric Hodgkin's disease: the German-Austrian multicenter trial DAL-HD-90. The German-Austrian Pediatric Hodgkin's Disease Study Group. J Clin Oncol 1999; 17:3736.
174. Gospodarowicz MK, Sutcliffe SB, Clark RM, et al: Analysis of supradiaphragmatic clinical stage I and II Hodgkin's disease treated with radiation alone. Int J Radiat Oncol Biol Phys 1992; 22:859.
175. Jones E, Mauch P: Limited radiation therapy for selected patients with pathological stages IA and IIA Hodgkin's disease. Semin Radiat Oncol 1996; 6:162.
176. Donaldson SS, Lamborn K: Radiation in pediatric Hodgkin's disease. J Clin Oncol 1998; 16:391.
177. Constine LS: Should MOPP-ABVD alone be standard for childhood Hodgkin's? J Clin Oncol 1998; 16:1235.
178. Mendenhall N, Bennett J, Lynch J: Is combined modality therapy necessary for advanced Hodgkin's disease? Int J Radiat Oncol Biol Phys 1997; 38:583.
179. Weiner MA, Leventhal BG, Marcus R, et al: Intensive chemotherapy and low-dose radiotherapy for the treatment of advanced-stage Hodgkin's disease in pediatric patients: a Pediatric Oncology Group study. J Clin Oncol 1991; 9:1591.
180. Khan S, Gilchrist G, Arndt C, et al: Vancouver hybrid: preliminary experience in the treatment of Hodgkin's disease in childhood and adolescence. Mayo Clin Proc 1994; 69:949.
181. Specht L, Nordentoft A, Cold S: Tumor burden as the most important prognostic factor in early stage Hodgkin's disease. Relations to other prognostic factors and implications for choice of treatment. Cancer 1988; 61:1719.
182. Shankar A, Ashley S, Radford M, et al: Does histology influence outcome in childhood Hodgkin's disease? Results from the United Kingdom Children's Cancer Study Group. J Clin Oncol 1997; 15:2622.
183. Shipp MA, Mauch PM, Harris NL: Non-Hodgkin's Lymphomas. In: DeVita VT Jr., Hellman S, Rosenberg SA (eds): Cancer: Principles and Practice of Oncology, 5th ed, p 2165. Philadelphia, Lippincott-Raven, 1997.
184. Knowles DM: Etiology and pathogenesis of AIDS-related non-Hodgkin's. Hematol Oncol Clin North Am 1996; 10:1081.
185. Aboulafia D: Epidemiology and pathogenesis of AIDS-related lymphomas. Oncology 1998; 12:1068.
186. Agape P, Copin MC, Cavrois M, et al: Implication of HTLV-I infection, strongyloidiasis, and P53 overexpression in the development, response to treatment, and evolution of non-Hodgkin's lymphoms in an endemic area (Martinique, French West Indies). J Acquir Immune Defic Syndr 1999; 20:394.
187. Opelz G, Henderson R: Incidence of non-Hodgkin lymphoma in kidney and heart transplant recipients. Lancet 1994; 19:343.
188. Reed JC, Tanaka S: Somatic point mutations in the translocated bcl-2 genes of non-Hodgkin's lymphomas and lymphocytic leukemias: implications for mechanisms of tumor progression. Leuk Lymphoma 1993; 10:157.
189. Whang-Peng J, Knutsen T, Jaffe ES, et al: Sequential analysis of 43 patients with non-Hodgkin's lymphoma: clinical correlations with cytogenetic, histologic, immunophenotyping, and molecular studies. Blood 1995; 85:203.
190. Cantor KP, Blair A, Everett G, et al: Pesticides and other agricultural risk factors for non-Hodgkin's lymphoma among men in Iowa and Minnesota. Cancer Res 1992; 52:2447.
191. Fontana A, Picoco C, Masala G, et al: Incidence rates of lymphomas and environmental measurements of phenoxy herbicides: ecological analysis and case-control study. Arch Environ Health 1998; 53:384.
192. Biemer JJ, Girgenti AJ: Gene rearrangements in malignant lymphomas. Ann Clin Lab Sci 1994; 24:232.
193. Lust JA: Molecular genetics and lymphoproliferative disorders. J Clin Lab Anal 1996; 10:359.
194. Murray PG, Swinnen LJ, Constandinou CM, et al: BCL-2 but not its Epstein-Barr virus-encoded homologue, BHRF1, is commonly expressed in posttransplantation lymphoproliferative disorders. Blood 1996; 87:706.
195. Ye BH: BCL-6 in the pathogenesis of non-Hodgkin's lymphoma. Cancer Invest 2000; 18:356.
196. Grignani F, Dalla-Favera R: Molecular biology of lymphoid malignancies. Curr Opin Oncol 1989; 1:4.
197. Press OW: Prospects for the management of non-Hodgkin's lymphomas with monoclonal antibodies and immunoconjugates. Cancer J Sci Am 1998; 4 (suppl 2):S19.
198. Gaidano G, Dalla-Favera R: Biologic and molecular characteriztion of non-Hodgkin's lymphoma. Curr Opin Oncol 1993; 5:776.
199. Korkolopoulou P, Angelopoulou MK, Kontopidou F, et al: Prognostic relevance of apoptotic cell death in non-Hodgkin's lymphomas: a multivariate survival analysis including Ki67 and p53 oncoprotein expression. Histopathology 1998; 33:240.
200. Schmitt FC, Rabenhorst SH, Maeda SA, et al: Estimation of growth fraction in fine needle aspirates from non-Hodgkin's lymphoma using anti-proliferating cell nuclear antigen: correlation with the Kiel classification. Acta Cytol 1996; 40:199.
201. Winter JN: Prognostic indicators in diffuse, aggressive non-Hodgkin's lymphomas: regulators of growth fraction and programmed cell death. Semin Oncol 1999; 26 (5 suppl 14):26.
202. Smith MR: Non-Hodgkin's lymphoma. Curr Prob Cancer 1996; 20:6.
203. Matolcsy A, Warnke RA, Knowles DM: Somatic mutations of the translocated bcl-2 gene are associated with morphologic transformation of follicular lymphoma to diffuse large-cell lymphoma. Ann Oncol 1997; 8 (suppl 2):119.
204. Akasaka T, Akasaka H, Ueda C, et al: Molecular and clinical features of non-Burkitt's, diffuse large-cell lymphoma of B-cell type associated with the c-MYC/immunoglobulin heavy-chain fusion gene. J Clin Oncol 2000; 18:510.
205. Fiedler W, Weh HJ, Zeller W, et al: Translocation (14;18) and (8;22) in three patients with acute leukemia/lymphoma following centrocytic/centroblastic non-Hodgkin's lymphoma. Ann Hematol 1991; 63:282.
206. The Non-Hodgkin's Lymphoma Pathologic Classification Project: NCI sponsored study of classification of non-Hodgkin's lymphoma: summary and description of a working formulation for clinical usage. Cancer 1982; 49:2112.
207. Fisher RI, Oken MM: Clinical practice guidelines: non-Hodgkin's lymphomas. Cleve Clin J Med 1995; 62 (suppl 1):SI6.
208. Skarin AT, Dorfman DM: Non-Hodgkin's lymphomas: current classification and managment. CA Cancer J Clin 1997; 47:351.
209. Zinzani PL, Magagnoli M, Gherlinzoni F, et al: To what extent can indolent lymphoma be considered? Results of a long term follow-up study from a single center. Haematologica 1998; 83:502.
210. Krackhardt A, Gribben JG: Stem cell transplantation for indolent lymphoma. Curr Opin Hematol 1999; 6:388.

211. Vose JM: Classification and clinical course of low-grade non-Hodgkin's lymphomas with overview of therapy. Ann Oncol 1996; 7 (suppl 6):S513.
212. Mounter PJ, Lennard AL: Management of non-Hodgkin's lymphomas. Postgrad Med J 1999; 75:2.
213. MacManus MP, Hoppe RT: Is radiotherapy curative for stage I and II low-grade follicular lymphoma? Results of a long-term follow-up study of patients treated at Stanford University. J Clin Oncol 1996; 14:1282.
214. Kamath SS, Marcus RB Jr, Lynch JW, et al: The impact of radiotherapy dose and other treatment-related and clinical factors on in-field control in stage I and II non-Hodgkin's lymphoma. Int J Radiat Oncol Biol Phys 1999; 44:563.
215. De Los Santos JF, Mendenhall NP, Lynch JW Jr: Is comprehensive lymphatic irradition for low-grade non-Hodgkin's lymphoma curative therapy? Long-term experience at a single institution. Int J Radiat Oncol Biol Phys 1997; 38:3.
216. Hirota S, Soejima T, Tsurusaki M, et al: Analysis of in-field and marginal relapse in stage I/II non-Hodgkin's lymphoma treated with radiotherapy. Nippon Igaku Hoshasen Gakkai Zasshi 1997; 57:929.
217. Sakata K, Hareyama M, Oouchi A, et al: Treatment of localized non-Hodgkin's lymphomas of the head and neck: focusing on cases of non-lethal midline granuloma. Radiat Oncol Investig 1998; 6:161.
218. Jacobs JP, Murray KJ, Schultz CJ, et al: Central lymphatic irradiation for stage III nodular malignant lymphoma: long-term results. J Clin Oncol 1993; 11:233.
219. Armitage JO: Treatment of non-Hodgkin's lymphoma. N Engl J Med 1993; 328:1023.
220. Fisher RI, Gaynor ER, Dahlberg S, et al: Comparison of a standard regimen (CHOP) with three intensive chemotherapy regimens for advanced non-Hodgkin's lymphoma. N Engl J Med 1993; 328:1002.
221. Arranz R, Garcia-Alfonso P, Sobrino P, et al: Role of interferon alfa-2b in the induction and maintenance treatment of low-grade non-Hodgkin's lymphoma: results from a prospective, multicenter trial with double randomization. J Clin Oncol 1998; 16:1538.
222. Hagenbeek A, Carde P, Meerwaldt JH, et al: Maintenance of remission with human recombinant interferon alfa-2a in patients with stages III and IV low-grade malignant non-Hodgkin's lymphoma. European Organization for Research and Treatment of Cancer Lymphoma Cooperative Group. J Clin Oncol 1998; 16:41.
223. Khaled HM, Zekri ZK, Mokhtar N, et al: A randomized EPOCH vs. CHOP front-line therapy for aggressive non-Hodgkin's lymphoma patients: long-term results. Ann Oncol 1999; 10:1489.
224. Laport GF, Williams SF: The role of high-dose chemotherapy in patients with Hodgkin's disease and non-Hodgkin's lymphoma. Semin Oncol 1998; 25:503.
225. Fisher RI, Dahlberg S, Nathwani BN, et al: A clinical analysis of two indolent lymphoma entities: mantle cell lymphoma and marginal zone lymphoma (including the mucosa-associated lymphoid tissue and monocytoid B-cell subcategories): a Southwest Oncology Group study. Blood 1995; 85:1075.
226. Zucca E, Fontana S, Roggero E, et al: Treatment and prognosis of centrocytic (mantle cell) lymphoma: a retrospective analysis of twenty-six patients treated in one institution. Leuk Lymphoma 1994; 13:105.
227. Bishop JF, Wiernik PH, Wesley MN, et al: A randomized trial of high dose cyclophosphamide, vincristine, and prednisone plus or minus doxorubicin (CVP versus CAVP) with long-term follow-up in advanced non-Hodgkin's lymphoma. Leukemia 1987; 1:508.
228. Cheson BD: New prospects in the treatment of indolent lymphomas with purine analogues. Cancer J Sci Am 1998; 4 (suppl 2):S27.
229. Bocchia M, Bigazzi C, Marconcini S, et al: Favorable impact of low-dose fludarabine plus epirubicin and cyclophosphamide regimen (FLEC) as treatment for low-grade non-Hodgkin's lymphomas. Haematologica 1999; 84:716.
230. Ozer H, Anderson JR, Peterson BA, et al: Combination trial of subcutaneous recombinant alpha 2 b interferon and oral cyclophosphamide in follicular low-grade non-Hodgkin's lymphoma. Med Pediatr Oncol 1994; 22:228.
231. Nair R, Ramakrishnan G, Nair NN, et al: A randomized comparison of the efficacy and toxicity of epirubicin and doxorubicin in the treatment of patients with non-Hodgkin's lymphoma. Cancer 1998; 82:2282.
232. Dreiher J, Shpilberg O, Raanani P, et al: The MACOP-B and VACOP-B combination chemotherapy for young patients with intermediate-grade non-Hodgkin's lymphoma. Leuk Res 1998; 22:997.
233. Shpilberg O, Shiff J, Chetrit A, et al: The cyclophosphamide, vincristine, prednisone, bleomycin, doxorubicin, and procarbazine (COPBLAM-I) regimen for intermediate-grade non-Hodgkin's lymphoma. Long term follow-up in 51 patients. Cancer 1994; 74:3029.
234. Wolf M, Matthews JP, Stone J, et al: Long-term survival advantage of MACOP-B over CHOP in intermediate-grade non-Hodgkin's lymphoma. The Australian and New Zealand Lymphoma Group. Ann Oncol 1997; 8 (suppl 1):71.
235. Tirelli U, Errante D, Van Glabbeke M, et al: CHOP is the standard regimen in patients > or = 70 years of age with intermediate-grade and high-grade non-Hodgkin's lymphoma: results of a randomized study of the European Organization for Research and Treatment of Cancer Lymphoma Cooperative Study Group. J Clin Oncol 1998; 16:27.
236. McMaster ML, Greer JP, Greco FA, et al: Effective treatment of small-noncleaved-cell lymphoma with high-intensity, brief-duration chemotherapy. J Clin Oncol 1991; 9:941.
237. Bouffet E, Frappaz D, Pinkerton R, et al: Burkitt's lymphoma: a model for clinical oncology. Eur J Cancer 1991; 27:504.
238. Tubergen DG, Krailo MD, Meadows AT, et al: Comparison of treatment regimens for pediatric lymphoblastic non-Hodgkin's lymphoma: a Childrens Cancer Group study. J Clin Oncol 1995; 13:1368.
239. Davis TA, White CA, Grillo-Lopez AJ, et al: Single-agent monoclonal antibody efficacy in bulky non-Hodgkin's lymphoma: results of a phase II trial of rituximab. J Clin Oncol 1999; 17:1851.
240. Sparano JA, Wiernik PH, Hu X, et al: Saquinavir enhances the mucosal toxicity of infusional cyclophosphamide, doxorubicin, and etoposide in patients with HIV-associated non-Hodgkin's lymphoma. Med Oncol 1998; 15:50.
241. Itoh K, Igarahi T, Ohtsu T, et al: Toxicity and efficacy of ifosfamide, carboplatin and etoposide (modified ICE) as a salvage chemotherapy in Japanese patients with relapsed or refractory aggressive non-Hodgkin's lymphoma. Int J Hematol 1998; 68:431.
242. Celsing F, Widell S, Merk K, et al: Addition of etoposide to CHOP chemotherapy in untreated patients with high-grade non-Hodgkin's lymphoma. Ann Oncol 1998; 9:1213.
243. Miller TP, Dahlberg S, Cassady JR, et al: Chemotherapy alone compared with chemotherapy plus radiotherapy for localized intermediate- and high-grade non-Hodgkin's lymphoma. N Engl J Med 1998; 339:21.
244. Schenkein DP, Roitman D, Miller KB, et al: A phase II mulitcenter trial of high-dose sequential chemotherapy and peripheral blood stem cell transplantation as initial therapy for patients with high-risk non-Hodgkin's lymphoma. Biol Blood Marrow Transplant 1997; 3:210.
245. Santini G, Salvagno L, Leoni P, et al: VACOP-B versus VACOP-B plus autologous bone marrow transplantation for advanced diffuse non-Hodgkin's lymphoma: results of a prospective randomized trial by the non-Hodgkin's Lymphoma Cooperative Group. J Clin Oncol 1998; 16:2796.
246. van der Maazen RW, Noordijk EM, Thomas J, et al: Combined modality treatment is the treatment of choice for stage I/IE intermediate and high grade non-Hodgkin's lymphoma. Radiother Oncol 1998; 49:1.
247. Cooper DL, Ginsberg SS: Brief chemotherapy, involved field radiation therapy, and central nervous system prophylaxis for paranasal sinus lymphoma. Cancer 1992; 69:2888.
248. Koch P, Grothaus-Pinke B, Hiddenmann W, et al: Primary lymphoma of the stomach: three-year results of a prospective multicenter study. Ann Oncol 1997; 8 (suppl 1):585.
249. Rijlaarsdam JU, Toonstra J, Meijer OWM, et al: Treatment of primary cutaneous B-cell lymphomas of follicle center cell origin: a clinical follow-up study of 55 patients treated with radiotherapy or polychemotherapy. J Clin Oncol 1996; 14:549.
250. Kim YH, Hoppe RT: Mycosis fungoides and the Sezary symdrome. Semin Oncol 1999; 26:276.
251. Ling SM, Roach M 3rd, Larson DA, et al: Radiotherapy of primary central nervous system lymphoma in patients with and without human immunodeficiency virus. Ten years of treatment experience at the University of California San Francisco. Cancer 1994; 73:2570.
252. Abrey LE, DeAngelis LM, Yahalom J: Long-term survival in primary CNS lymphoma. J Clin Oncol 1998; 16:859.
253. Parsonnet J, Hansen S, Rodriguez L, et al: *Helicobacter pylori* infection and gastric lymphoma. N Engl J Med 1994; 330:1267.

254. Roggero E, Zucca E, Pinotti G, et al: Eradication of *Helicobacter pylori* infection in primary low-grade gastric lymphoma of mucosa-associated lymphoid tissue. Ann Intern Med 1995; 122:767.
255. Schecter NR, Portlock CS, Yahalom J: Treatment of mucosa-associated lymphoid tissue lymphoma of the stomach with radiation alone. J Clin Oncol 1998; 16:1916.
256. Smitt MC, Donaldson SS: Radiotherapy is successful treatment for orbital lymphoma. Int J Radiat Oncol Biol Phys 1993; 26:59.
257. Velders GA, Kluin-Nelemans JC, De Boer CJ, et al: Mantle-cell lymphoma: a population-based clinical study. J Clin Oncol 1996; 14:1269.
258. Zinzani PL, Bendandi M, Martelli M, et al: Anaplastic large-cell lymphoma: clinical and prognostic evaluation of 90 adult patients. J Clin Oncol 1996; 14:955.
259. The Non-Hodgkin's Lymphoma Classification Project: A clinical evaluation of the International Lymphoma Study Group Classification of non-Hodgkin's lymphoma. Blood 1997; 89:3909.
260. Lopez-Guillermo A, Cid J, Salar A, et al: Peripheral T-cell lymphomas: initial features, natural history, and prognostic factors in a series of 174 patients diagnosed according to the R.E.A.L. classification. Ann Oncol 1998; 9:849.
261. Simon R, Durreleman S, Hoppe RT, et al: The non-Hodgkin's lymphoma pathologic classification project. Long-term follow-up of 1,153 patients with non-Hodgkin's lymphoma. Ann Intern Med 1988; 109:939.
262. Fisher RI: Cycolphosphamide, doxorubicin, vincristine, and prednisone versus intensive chemotherapy in non-Hodgkin's lymphoma. Cancer Chemother Pharmacol 1997; 40 (suppl):S42.
263. Shipp MA, Harrington DP, Anderson JR, et al: A predictive model for aggressive non-Hodgkin's lymphoma. The international non-Hodgkin's lymphoma prognostic factors project. N Engl J Med 1993; 329:987.
264. Philip T, Guglielmi C, Hagenbeek A, et al: Autologous bone marrow transplantation as compared with salvage chemotherapy in relapses of chemotherapy-sensitive non-Hodgkin's lymphoma. N Engl J Med 1995; 333:1540.
265. Gianni AM, Bregni M, Siena S, et al: High-dose chemotherapy and autologous bone marrow transplantation compared with MACOP-B in aggressive B-cell lymphoma. N Engl J Med 1997; 336:1290.
266. Freedman AS, Takvorian T, Neuberg D, et al: Autologous bone marrow transplantation in poor-prognosis intermediate-grade and high-grade B-cell non-Hodgkin's lymphoma in first remission: a pilot study. J Clin Oncol 1993; 11:931.
267. Bierman PJ, Vose JM, Anderson JR, et al: High-dose therapy with autologous hematopoietic rescue for follicular low-grade non-Hodgkin's lymphoma. J Clin Oncol 1997; 15:445.
268. McLaughlin P, Grillo-Lopez AJ, Link BK, et al: Rituximab chimeric anti-CD20 monoclonal antibody therapy for relapsed indolent lymphoma: half of patients respond to a four-dose treatment program. J Clin Oncol 1998; 16:2825.
269. Kaminski MS, Zasadny KR, Francis IR, et al: Radioimmunotherapy of B-cell lymphoma with [^{131}I] anti-B1 (anti-CD20) antibody. N Engl J Med 1993; 329:459.
270. Cuzick J: Radiation-induced myelomatosis. N Engl J Med 1981; 304:204.
271. Salmon SE, Cassady RJ: Plasma cell neoplasms. In: DeVita VT Jr., Hellman S, Rosenberg SA (eds): Cancer: Principles & Practice of Oncology, 5th ed, p 2344. Philadelphia, Lippincott-Raven, 1997.
272. Anderson KC: Multiple myeloma: advances in disease biology and implication for therapy. In: American Society of Clinical Oncology Educational Booklet, p 135. Alexandria, American Society of Clinical Oncology, 1996.
273. George ED, Sadovsky R: Multiple myeloma: recognition and management. Am Fam Physician 1999; 59:1885.
274. Irish AB, Winears CG, Littlewood T: Presentation and survival of patients with severe renal failure and myeloma. QJM 1997; 90:773.
275. Oken MM, Pomeroy C, Weisdorf D, et al: Prophylactic antibiotics for the prevention of early infection in multiple myeloma. Am J Med 1996; 100:624.
276. Durie BG, Stock-Novack D, Salmon SE, et al: Prognostic value of pretreatment serum beta 2 microglobulin in myeloma: a Southwest Oncology Group Study. Blood 1990; 75:823.
277. Kyle RA, Rajkumar SV: Monoclonal gammopathies of undetermined significance. Hematol Oncol Clin North Am 1999; 13:1181.
278. Wasserman TH: Myeloma and plasmacytomas. In: Perez CA, Brady LW (eds): Principles & Practice of Radiation Oncology, 3rd ed, p 2013. Philadelphia, Lippincott-Raven, 1992.
279. Bataille R, Harousseau JL: Multiple myeloma. N Engl J Med 1997; 336:1657.
280. Alexanian R, Dimopoulos M: Drug therapy: the treatment of multiple myeloma. N Engl J Med 1994; 330:484.
281. Betticher DC, Cerny T, Fey MF: Diagnosis and therapy for multiple myeloma: current aspects. Schweiz Med Wochenschr 1995; 125:541.
282. Cooper MR, Dear K, McIntyer OR, et al: A randomized clinical trial comparing melphalan/prednisone with or without interferon alfa-2b in newly diagnosed patients with multiple myeloma: a Cancer and Leukemia Group B study. J Clin Oncol 1993; 11:155.
283. Westin J, Rodjer S, Turesson I, et al: Interferon alfa-2b versus no maintenance therapy during the plateau phase in multiple myeloma: a randomized study. Cooperative Study Group. Br J Haematol 1995; 89:561.
284. Cunningham D, Powles R, Malpas J, et al: A randomized trial of maintenance interferon following high-dose chemotherapy in multiple myeloma: long-term follow-up results. Br J Hematol 1998; 102:495.
285. Segeren CM, Sonnefeld P, van der Holt B, et al: Vincristine, doxorubicin and dexamethasone (VAD) administered as rapid intravenous infusion for first-line treatment in untreated multiple myeloma. Br J Haematol 1999; 105:127.
286. Case DC Jr, Lee DJ 3rd, Clarkson BD: Improved survival times in multiple myeloma treated with melphalan, prednisone, cyclophosphamide, vincristine and BCNU: M2 protocol. Am J Med 1977; 63:897.
287. Attal M, Harousseau JL, Stoppa AM, et al: A prospective, randomized trial of autologous bone marrow transplantation and chemotherapy in mulitple myeloma. Intergroupe Français du Myelome. N Engl J Med 1996; 335:91.
288. Barlogie B, Jagannath S, Desikan KR, et al: Total therapy with tandem transplants for newly diagnosed multiple myeloma. Blood 1999; 93:55.
289. Powles R, Raje N, Milan S, et al: Outcome assessment of a population-based group of 195 unselected myeloma patients under 70 years of age offered intensive treatment. Bone Marrow Transplant 1997; 20:435.
290. Barlogie B: Advances in mulitple myeloma treatment: biology and therapy. In: American Society of Clinical Oncology Educational Booklet, p 123. Alexandria, American Society of Clinical Oncology, 1996.
291. Berenson JR, Lichtenstein A, Porter L, et al: Efficacy of pamidronate in reducing the skeletal events in patients with advanced mulitple myeloma. N Engl J Med 1996; 334:488.
292. Brincker H, Westin J, Abildgaard N, et al: Failure of oral pamidronate to reduce skeletal morbidity in multiple myeloma: a double-blind placebo-controlled trial. Danish-Swedish cooperative study group. Br J Haematol 1998; 101:280.
293. Goldschmidt H, Lannert H, Bommer J, et al: Multiple myeloma and renal failure. Nephrol Dial Transplant 2000; 15:301.
294. Bociek RG, Armitage JO: Hematopoietic growth factors. CA Cancer J Clin 1996; 46:165.
295. Nussbaum SR, Younger J, Vandepol CJ, et al: Single-dose intravenous therapy with pamidronate for the treatment of hypercalcemia of malignancy comparison of 30-,60-, and 90-mg. dosages. Am J Med 1993; 95:297.
296. Boccadoro M, Marmont F, Tribalto M, et al: Multiple myeloma: VMCP/VBAP alternating combination chemotherapy is not superior to melphalan and prednisone even in high-risk patients. J Clin Oncol 1991; 9:444.
297. Harousseau JL, Attal M, Divine M, et al: Comparison of autologous bone marrow transplantation and peripheral blood stem cell transplantation after first remission induction therapy in multiple myeloma. Bone Marrow Transplant 1995; 15:963.
298. Mehta J, Singhal S, Desikan R, et al: High dose chemotherapy and stem cell support in myeloma. PPO updates. Principles and Practice of Oncology 1999; 13:1.
299. Byrne JL, Carter GI, Ellis I, et al: Autologous GVHD following PBSCT, with evidence for a graft-versus-myeloma effect. Bone Marrow Transplant 1997; 20:517.
300. Reichardt VL, Okada CY, Liso A, et al: Idiotype vaccination using dendritic cells after autologous peripheral blood stem cell transplantation for multiple-myeloma—a feasibility study. Blood 1999; 93:2411.

19 *Pediatric Solid Tumors*

LOUIS S. CONSTINE III, MD, Radiation and Pediatric Oncology
CHARLES PAIDAS, MD, Pediatric Surgery
CINDY L. SCHWARTZ, MD, Pediatric Oncology
DAVID N. KORONES, MD, Medical Oncology

A baby is evidence of God's opinion that life should go on.
CARL SANDBURG

Perspective

Despite, or perhaps as a consequence of, the relative rarity of childhood cancer, its study has provided a greater understanding of the neoplastic process, and served as a paradigm for treatment approaches to responsive cancers. Investigations into the biology of childhood cancer have resulted in the identification of genetic themes relevant to cancer genesis, natural history, prognosis, and therapy. Advances in the treatment of childhood solid tumors have progressed over the past 30 years such that the modalities of surgery, radiation therapy, and chemotherapy are intertwined for maximum efficacy and minimum toxicity (Fig. 19–1).[40, 41]

The appropriate use of these modalities has resulted in an improved outlook for a child diagnosed with either hematologic or solid tumors, and 5-year survival rates have improved from 5% to 10% to greater than 50% to 90%, depending on the histologic subtype.[42, 43] Thus, it is clear that the current issues facing pediatric oncology include identifying high-risk patients, optimizing therapy-to-toxicity ratios for the modalities we use, and minimizing the long-term effects of the diseases and their therapies, particularly for the most favorable patients. Finally, it is estimated that 1 in 900 individuals between the ages of 16 and 40 years is a survivor of childhood cancer,[44] which emphasizes the critical need to address the biologic, psychological, and social consequences of childhood cancer.

General Introduction to Pediatric Tumors

Epidemiology

Neoplastic diseases are second only to accidents as a cause of death in children.[43] The incidence trend by year of childhood malignancies is depicted in Figure 19–2, with the distribution of specific subtypes denoted in Table 19–1. More than half of all childhood malignancies are of the

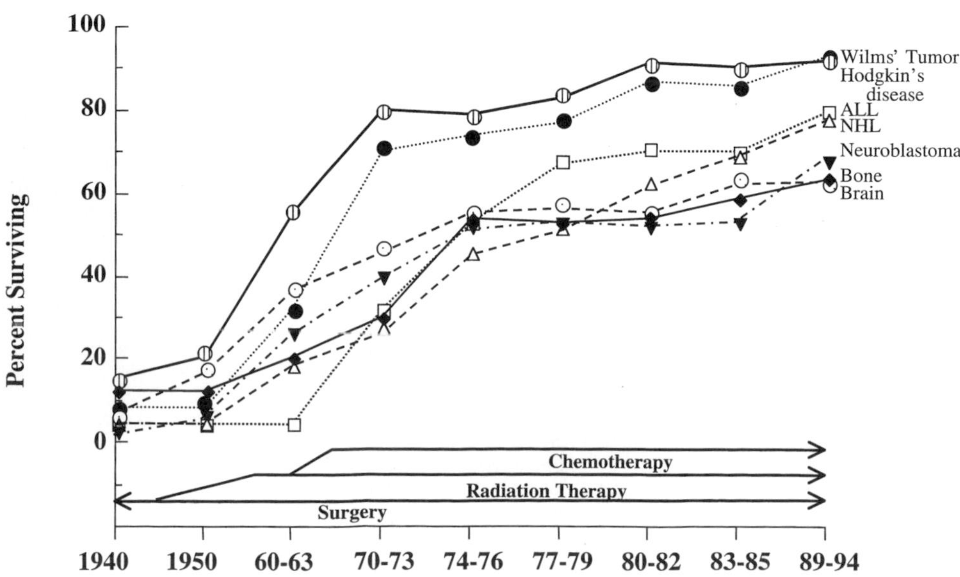

Figure 19–1. Improvement in 2-year survival rates of the principal tumors of children. ALL = acute lymphoblastic leukemia; NHL = non-Hodgkin's lymphoma. (Data from Simone JV, Lyons J: The evolution of cancer care for children and adults. J Clin Oncol 1998; 16:2904, and Landis SH, Murray T, Bolden S, et al: Cancer statistics, 1999. CA Cancer J Clin 1999; 49:8.)

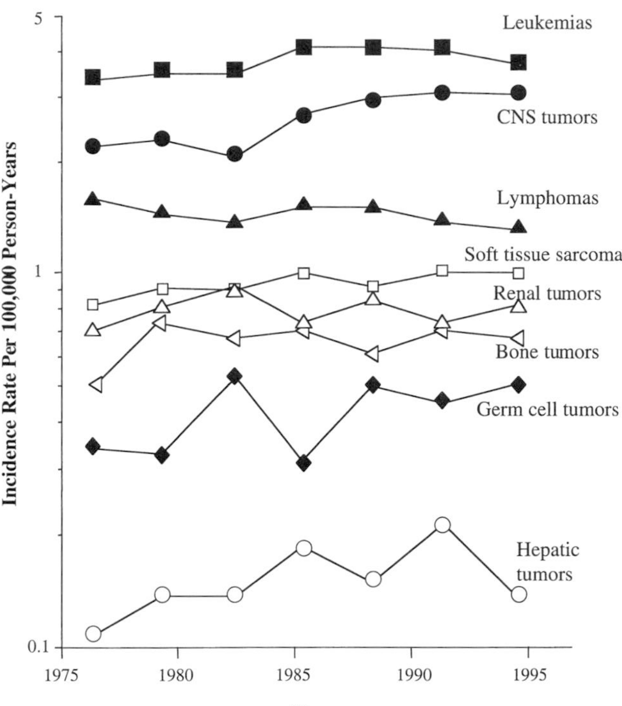

Figure 19–2. The incidence trends for childhood cancers in nine Surveillance, Epidemiology, and End Results (SEER) Program registries from 1975–1977 through 1993–1995. CNS = central nervous system. (Modified from Linet MS, Ries LAG, Smith MA, et al: Cancer surveillance series: recent trends in childhood cancer incidence and mortality in the United States. J Natl Cancer Inst 1999; 91:1051, with permission of Oxford University Press.)

solid tumor variety, with the relative frequencies shown in Figure 19–3.

Etiology

Hereditary Factors

Advances in the field of genetics and molecular biology have dramatically increased our understanding of childhood malignancy. More than 25 years ago, Knudson hypothesized that certain pediatric tumors (retinoblastoma, Wilms') could develop *only* if two independent mutations occurred in a single cell.[48] This "two hit" theory suggested that germinal mutations predispose individuals to heritable tumors because then only one "second hit" would be necessary for tumor development. In his 1997 Karnofsky Memorial Lecture, Knudson listed the cloned hereditary cancer genes of the time (Table 19–2), demonstrating the increasing breadth of knowledge in this field.[49] The nonheritable tumors require two postzygotic mutations and, hence, are less likely to develop in early childhood or be bilateral.

Genetic Events

The recognition that cancer is related to genetic abnormalities, coupled with dramatic advances in cellular biology, particularly recombinant DNA technology, has led to the determination that genetic rearrangements play a significant role in oncogenesis. Rearrangements may result in oncogene activation or loss of tumor suppression genes; examples of the loss of tumor suppressor genes are given in Table 19–3. Understanding such genetic alterations in cancer and host cells may lead to the development of therapeutic modalities that will facilitate cure by directly affecting the genetic abnormality. For example, resistance to drug therapy has been found to be related to expression of the *MDR1* oncogene.[51] Indeed, some molecular markers already are of etiologic significance, whereas others (e.g., amplification of N-*MYC* in neuroblastoma or the related suppression of CD44) predict a poor prognosis.[52]

Therapeutic Advances: Optimization of Multimodal Treatment

Initial advances in the treatment of childhood malignancies were due to the recognition that multiple therapeutic modalities complemented each other:

- Local control was enhanced when surgery was followed by regional irradiation of the tumor bed and nodes.
- The development of multidrug combinations for occult disseminated disease was critical in the evolution of successful therapy.

TABLE 19–1. **Childhood Cancer in the United States: Percent Distribution by Histology, SEER Data 1973–1993**

Cancer	%	Distribution
Leukemias	30.3	
• Acute lymphoblastic leukemia		23.7
• Acute myelogenous leukemia		4.3
• Leukemia, other		2.3
Lymphomas	10.4	
• Hodgkin's disease		4.7
• Non-Hodgkin's disease		5.7
Central nervous system	22.1	
• Ependymoma		1.7
• Astrocytoma		11.3
• Medulloblastoma		6.0
Neuroblastoma	6.1	
Retinoblastoma	1.8	
Kidney/Wilms' tumor	5.9	
Hepatic tumors	1.0	
Bone	5.7	
• Osteosarcoma		2.5
• Ewing's sarcoma		3.0
Soft tissue sarcoma	7.7	
• Rhabdomyosarcoma		5.4
• Other soft tissue sarcomas		2.3
Germ cell, other gonadal neoplasms	3.3	
Histiocytosis	0.6	
Thyroid	1.4	
Melanoma	0.6	

SEER = Surveillance, Epidemiology, and End Results.
From Grovas A, Fremgen A, Rauck A, et al: The National Cancer Data Base report on patterns of childhood cancers in the United States. Cancer 1997; 80:2321.

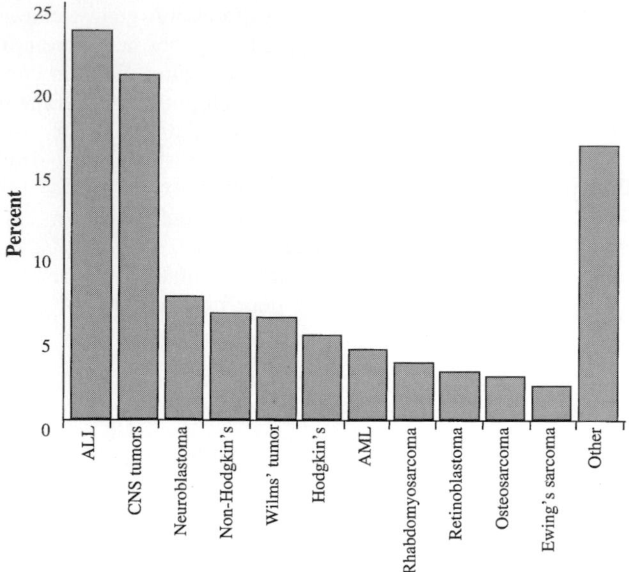

Figure 19–3. Distribution of cancers in children younger than 15 years of age by diagnosis. ALL = acute lymphoblastic leukemia; AML = acute myeloid leukemia; CNS = central nervous system. (Adapted from Gurney JG, Severson RK, Davis S, et al: Incidence of cancer in children in the United States. Sex-, race-, and 1-year age-specific rates by histologic type. Cancer 1995; 75:2186. From Robison LL: General principles of the epidemiology of childhood cancer. In: Pizzo PA, Poplack DG: Principles and Practice of Pediatric Oncology, 3rd ed, p 1. Philadelphia, Lippincott-Raven, 1997, with permission.)

- The effectiveness of radiation therapy and chemotherapy regimens permitted the use of more conservative surgical procedures.
- As successful therapy further evolved, the intensity, duration, and number of treatment modalities could be reduced.

TABLE 19–2. **Cloned Hereditary Cancer Genes**

Gene	Disease
RB1	Hereditary retinoblastoma
TP53	Li-Fraumeni syndrome
WT1	Wilms' tumor
NF1	Neurofibromatosis 1
NF2	Neurofibromatosis 2
APC	Familial adenomatous polyposis
VHL	Von Hippel-Lindau syndrome
TSC2	Tuberous sclerosis 2
CDKN2	Hereditary melanoma 1
PTC	Nevoid basal cell carcinoma syndrome
PTEN	Cowden's disease
MEN1	Multiple endocrine neoplasia 1
RET	Multiple endocrine neoplasia 2
MET	Hereditary papillary renal carcinoma
CDK4	Hereditary melanoma 2
ATM	Ataxia-telangiectasia
HMSH2	Hereditary nonpolyposis colon cancer
HMLH1	Hereditary nonpolyposis colon cancer
HPMS1	Hereditary nonpolyposis colon cancer
HPMS2	Hereditary nonpolyposis colon cancer

From Knudson A: Hereditary cancer: theme and variations. J Clin Oncol 1997; 15:3280, with permission.

Following these advances, a steady reduction in radiation field size and dose for some tumors became possible, as illustrated by the current treatment of Hodgkin's disease and childhood solid tumors. Moreover, radiation therapy now can be more precisely planned and administered using 3D–conformal treatment, permitting either tumor dose escalation or normal tissue sparing; the dose distribution to each structure can be accurately determined. Figure 19–4 displays a typical dose-volume histogram for an abdominal sarcoma that demonstrates this concept. For some drug-sensitive tumors (e.g., non-Hodgkin's lymphomas, neuroblastoma, germ cell tumors), it has become possible to rely

TABLE 19–3. **Examples of Tumor Suppressor Genes and Their Associated Neoplasms**

Gene	Chromosomal Site	Carcinoma	Neuroectodermal and Endocrine Tumor	Other
APC	5q21	Colorectal		
ATM	11q23–24	Breast		Leukemia, lymphoma
BRCA1	17q21	Breast, ovarian		
DCC	18q21	Colorectal		
NF1	17q11		Schwannoma, glioma, melanoma, PNET, neuroblastoma, pheochromocytoma	JCML, sarcoma
NF2	22q12		Vestibular schwannoma, meningioma, melanoma, astrocytoma	
p16^{INK4A}	9p21	Breast, bladder, head and neck, esophageal, lung, ovarian, pancreatic, renal	Astrocytoma, glioma, pheochromocytoma	Mesothelioma, leukemia, osteosarcoma
RB	13q14	Bladder, prostatic, cervical, lung	Retinoblastoma	Sarcoma
TP53	17p13	Breast, colorectal, stomach, lung, esophageal, ovarian, prostatic	Glioma	Sarcoma, leukemia, Burkitt's lymphoma, CML
VHL	3p25.5	Renal	Hemangioblastoma, pheochromocytoma	
WT1	11p13			Wilms' tumor
CDC2L1	1p36		Neuroblastoma, melanoma	

PNET = primitive neuroectodermal tumors; JCML = juvenile chronic myelogenous leukemia; CML = chronic myelogenous leukemia.
Modified from Look TA, Kirsch IR: Molecular basis of childhood cancer. In: Pizzo PA, Poplack DG (eds): Principles and Practices of Pediatric Oncology, 3rd ed, p 37. Philadelphia, Lippincott-Raven, 1997, with permission.

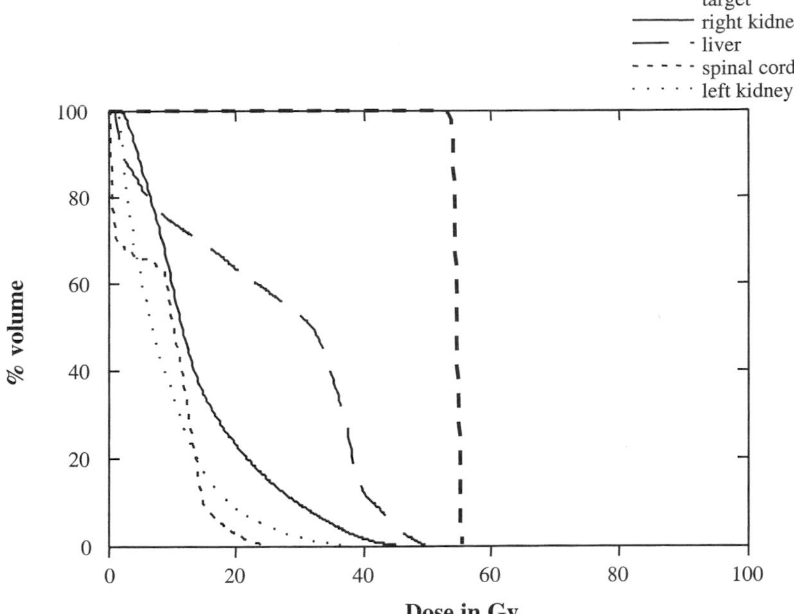

Figure 19–4. A typical dose-volume histogram for an abdominal tumor.

on chemotherapy, with or without surgery, as the sole treatment. In some settings, the duration of chemotherapy has been reduced to a few weeks or months (e.g., for early-stage Wilms' tumor and non-Hodgkin's lymphoma).

Over the past two decades, cure rates have continued to increase as a result of the survival of patients with more advanced or aggressive disease. In some instances, this is a result of newer chemotherapeutic agents (e.g., cisplatin, etoposide), but more often it is a result of the more accurate staging of disease and the use of dose-intensive regimens (including bone marrow transplantation). Advances in other disciplines (particularly diagnostic radiology, infectious disease, blood banking, and surgery) have helped make this possible.

A driving force behind these advances has been the multi-institutional cooperative groups, exemplified in the United States by the Children's Cancer Study Group and the Pediatric Oncology Group, which have recently merged into the Children's Oncology Group. In this setting, investigators have developed treatment strategies with central coordination and peer monitoring systems for an appropriate diagnostic work-up, review of pathology, and acquisition of outcome data. More than 60% of children treated at member institutions have been enrolled in clinical trials, compared with 2% or 3% of adults treated by cooperative group members.[40] For some malignancies, such as leukemia, up to 90% of children are on formal trials. This organized approach to therapy has fostered and encouraged much of the early work on cytogenetics and molecular genetics.

Late Effects and Toxicities Following Multimodal Treatment

Multimodal therapy results in significant toxicity, both acute and long-term. Toxic effects of radiation therapy can be intensified by the use of chemotherapy and vice versa. For example, the addition of chemotherapy may lead to heightened reactions within the radiation field, referred to as a recall phenomenon, that represent independent, but additive, injury to normal tissue cells. For example, actinomycin D can cause a skin reaction that outlines the original radiation field months or even years later.[53] The successful use of multimodal therapy has resulted in a large contingent of long-term survivors who need to be followed closely for late effects (see Chapter 34, Late Effects of Cancer Treatment: Radiation and Chemotherapy Toxicity).

- The chronic sequelae of *radiation therapy* in children include retardation of bone and cartilage growth, intellectual impairments, myelosuppression, nephropathy, hepatopathy, and pneumonitis (Table 19–4).
- Contrary to previously held beliefs, *chemotherapy* can cause late effects, such as infertility (cisplatin) and late cardiac decompensation (anthracyclines). Late effects in other organs, such as lung (bleomycin) and kidney (cisplatin), are being actively studied (Table 19–5).
- Combined-modality therapy has resulted in the enhancement of many of the above-mentioned complications, particularly encephalopathies, pneumonitis, pulmonary fibrosis, cardiomyopathies, hepatopathies, and myelosuppression.

Second malignancies, including leukemias and sarcomas, are of great concern and are attributable more often to combined-modality therapy than to chemotherapy or radiotherapy in isolation. Genetic predispositions to malignancy are relevant in some instances.

Essential Advances in Other Disciplines

Radiology

The revolution in imaging procedures has allowed for a greater accuracy in clinical staging and improved correlations with surgical pathologic evaluations. The impact of

TABLE 19–4. **Long-Term Side Effects of Radiation**

Irradiated Area	Risk
Cranium and nasopharynx	Eyes—cataracts Growth—impaired CNS—learning impairment Hypothalamic dysfunction = decreased growth hormone = decreased gonadotropins, thyroid-stimulating hormones, hyperprolactinemia
Neck and mandible	Hypoplasia of bone/soft tissue Dentition—abnormal formation —abnormal salivary function Thyroid—overt or compensated hypothyroidism
Thorax	Hypoplasia (includes impaired chest wall growth) Lungs—fibrosis, decreased capacity Cardiac—pericardial and valvular thickening Breasts—impaired growth, increased malignancy
Abdomen/pelvis	Hypoplasia (including scoliosis) Liver (if in field)—hepatopathy, veno-occlusive disease, congestive hepatomegaly Kidneys (if in field)—renal failure, atrophy, hypertension Gonads (if in field)—infertility, decreased libido, aspermia, anovulation Gastrointestinal tract—diarrhea, malabsorption, and hemorrhage, obstruction, and perforation due to necrosis
Extremities	Hypoplasia

CNS = central nervous system.

noninvasive methods, preceding and directing the surgical and radiotherapeutic attack, is critical to the design of clinical trials. Ultrasound, a nonionizing mode of imaging, is readily available, and is particularly effective in detecting abdominal or soft tissue masses. Computed tomography (CT) and magnetic resonance imaging (MRI) allow for a more accurate determination of tumor extent. These modalities have the advantage of three-dimensional plan displays. In the future, magnetic resonance spectroscopy may add biochemical information that could be helpful.

Supportive Care

In the past 15 years, the ability to use dose-intensive chemotherapy and radiation therapy has depended on being able to support the patient through periods of marrow aplasia. The development and empiric use of broad-spectrum antibiotics have facilitated the delivery of cytotoxic agents in ways that were not conceivable two decades ago. Hematopoietic colony-stimulating factors, which decrease the duration of myelosuppression after chemotherapy, are now commonly incorporated into treatment regimens. A new era is beginning in which the maximum tolerated doses for many myelosuppressive agents will rise, which will, it is hoped, increase the cure rates.

Advances in transfusion medicine have also been essential in this era of intensive chemotherapeutic regimens:

- Blood products are now relatively free from infectious contamination (e.g., hepatitis, cytomegalovirus, human immunodeficiency virus).
- Platelet products are available, virtually on demand, and can be HLA-matched in instances of alloimmunization.
- Neutrophils may be life saving in the setting of sepsis that is unresponsive to antibiotics.

The administration of multiple chemotherapeutic agents, antibiotics, transfusions, and nutritional support is possible since venous access became assured with the use of tunneled central venous catheters.

Psychosocial Aspects

There has been an increased awareness of the psychosocial aspects critical to pediatric oncology, which include the impact of the disease and its therapy on both the patient and family.[54] Because the majority of children will be cured, an emphasis on maintaining appropriate school achievement, discipline, behavior, and socialization should be stressed. Parents' concerns regarding their role in the occurrence of cancer should be allayed in most instances because childhood cancers are not related to parenting styles (e.g., diet, environment); however, families with potentially heritable malignancies should receive genetic counseling. The ethical rights of the child patient and the impact of cancer on the family, particularly siblings, need special attention. Figure 19–5 displays a schema of potential medical milestones and psychosocial crises associated with childhood cancer.[55]

TABLE 19–5. **Long-Term Side Effects of Chemotherapy**

Drugs	Potential Organ Damage
Doxorubicin	Cardiac—myocardial damage, congestive failure, arrhythmias
Bleomycin	Lungs—fibrosis, impaired diffusion capacity, exacerbated by increased O_2 (e.g., anesthesia) Skin—hyperpigmentation
Cyclophosphamide	Gonadal damage—infertility, sterility, early menopause Bladder—hemorrhagic cystitis, bladder cancer Marrow—secondary acute myeloid leukemia
CCNU/BCNU	Gonadal—infertility Lungs—pulmonary fibrosis, pneumonopathy
Cisplatin	Kidney—decreased glomerular filtration rate Ears—hearing loss (high frequency)
Methotrexate	Liver dysfunction CNS—learning impairment (high dose IV)
6-Mercaptopurine 6-Thioguanine Dactinomycin	Liver dysfunction
Epipodophyllotoxins	Peripheral neuropathy, secondary leukemia
Steroids	Obesity, cataracts, osteoporosis

CNS = central nervous system; CCNU/BCNU = lomustine/carmustine.

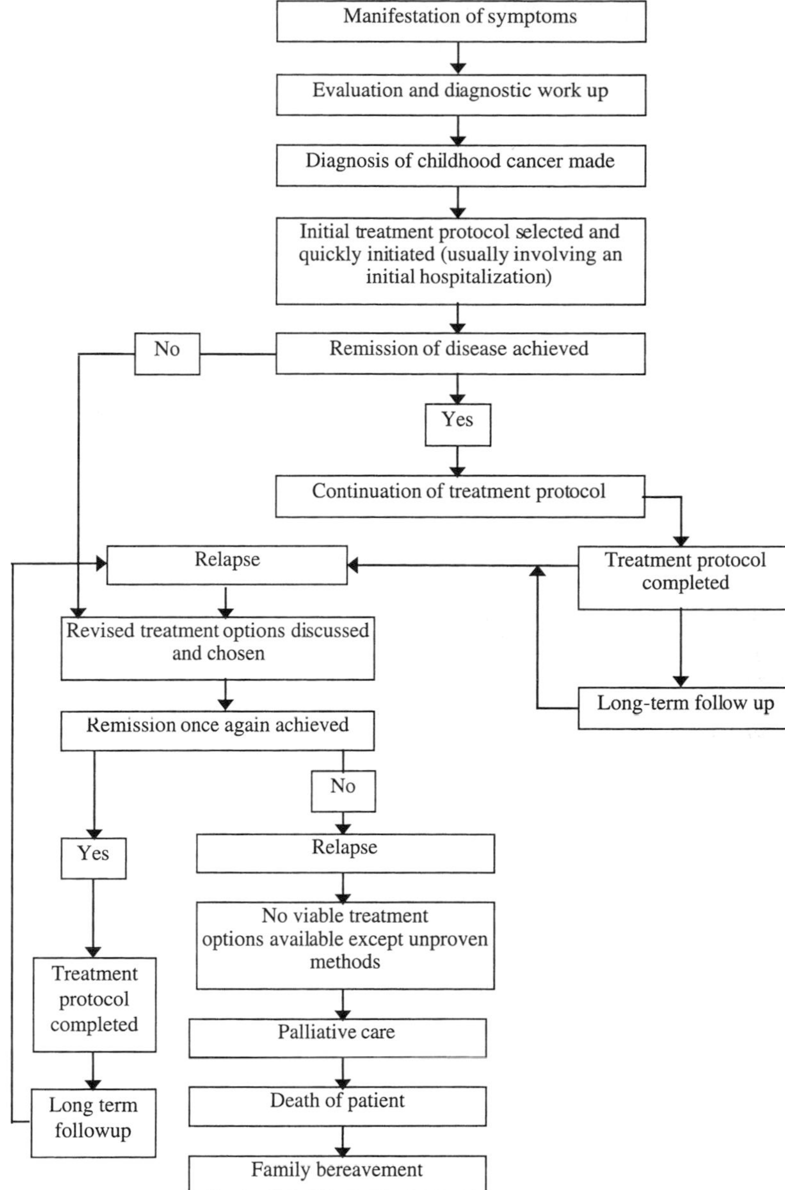

Figure 19–5. A schema of potential medical milestones and psychosocial crises associated with childhood cancer. (From Ruccione KS: Issues in survivorship. In: Schwartz CL, Hobbie WL, Constine LS, et al (eds): Survivors of Childhood Cancer: Assessment and Management. St. Louis, Mosby, 1994, with permission.)

Neuroblastoma

Perspective

Neuroblastoma (NB) is an intriguing and frustrating malignancy. It is biologically complex, with prognoses that range from almost certain cure to almost certain death, depending on patient (and thus biologic) features at diagnosis. NB has a myriad of clinical presentations and paraneoplastic syndromes. These characteristics have led to multiple refinements of staging and pathologic classification systems, as will be seen. NB is also a tumor that may spontaneously regress or mature into a more benign histopathologic type. If we could better understand its biology and genetics and the mechanisms by which either regression or maturation occur, we might be better able to treat this cancer and others.

Epidemiology and Etiology

Epidemiology

Although NB accounts for 7% to 10% of childhood malignancies, it is the most common cancer of infants, accounting for half of all cases.[56] NB is exceedingly rare after age 10 years; conversely, 80% of patients are younger than 4 years at diagnosis, and about one third are infants.[57] Overall, NB occurs in approximately 10.5 white children and 8.8 black children per million in the United States each year.[58] Fifteen percent of childhood cancer deaths are due to NB.

Etiology

NB arises from primitive adrenergic neuroblasts of neural crest tissue in the adrenal medulla, paravertebral sympathetic ganglia, and sympathetic paraganglia (e.g., organ of Zuckerkandl). These tumors presumably arise during fetal or early postnatal life because NB *in situ* is found at autopsy in as many as 1 per 220 adrenal glands of infants who have died for nonmalignant reasons.[59–61] Thus, it is clear that the majority of these lesions involute or spontaneously regress; however, the remainder undergo maturation/differentiation or aggressively proliferate. The malignant transformation may be due to an inappropriate response of these cells to normal signals for morphologic differentiation.

Molecular Biology and Genetics

In rare cases, NB has occurred in multiple siblings[62, 63] and, occasionally, in multiple generations of a family.[64] Knudson and Strong estimated that 2% to 25% of NBs arise in patients with a prezygotic germinal mutation, similar to the mechanism described for familial retinoblastoma.[48] Evidence for this includes the occurrence of bilateral and multifocal disease, for which the median age at presentation is 9 months, in contrast to 22 months for all other patients.[65] NB has been reported to occur with an increased incidence in patients with fetal hydantoin syndrome, von Recklinghausen's disease, Beckwith-Wiedemann syndrome, and Hirschsprung's disease.[64, 66–68]

Chromosomal Changes. Cytogenetic abnormalities have been demonstrated in the tumor cells of many patients with NB. A deletion or rearrangement of the short arm of chromosome 1 (del 1p36.3) is common and may represent deletion of a tumor suppressor gene.[69, 70] More recently, gains of chromosome 17 (segment 17q21–qter) have been found in 54% of tumors; these aberrations were characteristic of advanced disease or older age, or both, and were associated with deletion of 1p and amplification of N-*MYC*.[71, 72]

Proto-Oncogene Amplification. Homogeneous staining regions are long, nonbanding regions of metaphase chromosomes that stain homogeneously, the breakdown of which may result in double minute chromosomes (small paired chromatin bodies of varying size and number). These represent gene amplification from the distal short arms of chromosome 2, which contain the proto-oncogene N-*MYC*, and occur more commonly in patients with advanced-stage disease. The degree of amplification appears to be an intrinsic biologic property of a given NB, which is consistent from the time of diagnosis through periods of progressive disease.[58] Although high N-*MYC* expression is predictive of a poor outcome in older children with NB, it may not have the same significance in infants.[73] It is of interest that overexpression of the gene for multidrug resistance–associated protein (MRP), which has been linked with resistance to chemotherapy, correlates with N-*MYC* oncogene amplification in NB.[74] High levels of MRP are, thus, one possible explanation for the association between N-*MYC* amplification and reduced survival.[75]

DNA Ploidy. The DNA content of NB tumor cells appears to be of prognostic importance, and flow cytometry has been used to determine whether NB cells are pseudodiploid, diploid, or hyperdiploid. For patients with disseminated disease, pseudodiploidy and diploidy have been associated with N-*MYC* amplification and a poor response to therapy, which contrasts with the favorable prognosis for patients with hyperdiploid tumors.[76, 77] In addition, a recent combined retrospective-prospective study by Eckschlager and associates found that individuals with DNA aneuploidy also had a better prognosis.[78]

Biologic Markers

Eighty-five percent to 90% of patients with NB excrete abnormally high levels of catecholamines.[26, 79, 80] Both the catecholamines and their metabolites are used as markers for NB, with vanillylmandelic acid (VMA) and homovanillic acid (HVA) being the most commonly used.[58, 81] While their absolute values are not of prognostic significance, a higher VMA:HVA ratio suggests a better prognosis for patients with disseminated disease. Numata and associates caution, however, that ingestion of banana, a common weaning food, within 24 hours before urine collection can produce a high level of HVA secretion.[81] Although a 24-hour urine collection for catecholamines is most accurate, a single urine collection can be evaluated by comparing the ratio of catecholamine to creatinine present in a sample.[82] Elevated ferritin levels have been noted in approximately half of patients with advanced-stage NB, and these levels also have been associated with a poor prognosis.[83]

Evidence is increasing that the Trk family of neurotrophin receptors are relevant to the biology and clinical behavior of NB. High levels of TrkA mRNA are present in tumors from patients with favorable stage disease, whereas low to undetectable levels are observed in the N-*MYC*–amplified tumors.[84] Recently, TrkC levels have also been shown to correlate with favorable prognosis.[85]

Biologic Behavior

Involution and Spontaneous Regression

NB has an amazing ability to spontaneously regress and mature. This process is characterized by cell death of still immature neuroblasts before complete differentiation.[86] Genetic prerequisites for regression may include an intact chromosome 1 short arm, lack of N-*MYC* amplification, and near-triploidy. Spontaneous regression is noted most commonly in infants younger than 1 year of age. Microscopic residual tumor in these patients rarely results in recurrence.

Maturation

Malignant tumors may spontaneously mature into benign ganglioneuromas. Immunologic mechanisms and maturational processes have been hypothesized to explain these findings. For example, cell- and antibody-mediated cytotoxicity against NB cells has been demonstrated in both healthy and patient volunteers, with consistently low levels observed in patients with advanced disease.[87] Neuroblasts also may differentiate and mature; a variety of substances, such as 5-trifluoromethyl-2-deoxyuridine and papaverine (both of which increase cyclic adenosine monophosphate), interferon-α, and tumor necrosis factor-α, have all been shown to induce neuroblast maturation *in vitro*.[88] In addition, the level of N-*MYC* expression in NB tumor cells has been shown to decrease following *in vitro* differentiation.[89] In fact, the genetic prerequisites for maturation are probably the same as those noted earlier for regression.

Aggressive Proliferation

Most clinically detectable NBs present as advanced tumors. The genetic characteristics of proliferation are the inverse of those for regression and maturation, namely N-*MYC* amplification, del 1;36.3, and diploid/tetraploid content.[86]

Detection and Diagnosis

Infants with localized NB often appear to be healthy, with a mass being the major presenting feature. Conversely, older children (>1 year) often have overtly disseminated disease, and may have systemic manifestations, such as fever, weight loss, general malaise, and fatigue. A reasonable rule is that a child older than 2 years of age with an abdominal mass who appears well is likely to have Wilms' tumor, whereas one who appears chronically ill is more likely to have NB.

Clinical Detection

The clinical presenting features of NB depend on the location of tumor. NB may arise anywhere along the sympathetic nervous system chain. The most common primary site of involvement is in an adrenal gland (35%). Other sites of occurrence include the paraspinal regions of the abdomen (25%), the thorax (15%), the neck (5%), and the pelvis at the organ of Zuckerkandl (5%).

An abdominal mass is frequently the first presenting sign of disease. Such a mass may be large, firm, and irregular and may cross the midline. A child with a persistent cough or respiratory distress may have thoracic masses that can detected by chest x-ray. Cervical masses are often initially diagnosed as lymphadenitis; however, if Horner's syndrome or heterochromia iridis is noted, NB should be suspected. Pelvic masses may cause disturbances of bowel or bladder function as a result of compression.

In some patients, the presenting symptoms are related to secretory products of the tumor. NBs and ganglioneuromas have been shown to produce somatostatin and vasoactive intestinal polypeptide, with vasoactive polypeptide being associated with intractable diarrhea.[90] The syndrome of opsoclonus-myoclonus ("dancing eyes") is an unusual presenting feature of NB: Patients have acute cerebellar ataxia and rapid, dancing, eye movements. Although these patients often have localized disease, they have a tendency for residual neurologic dysfunction, including recurrence of ataxia, mental and extrapyramidal deficits, and behavioral abnormalities.[91, 92] The etiology of this syndrome is unclear, although an autoimmune factor, perhaps an antibody directed against NB that cross-reacts with a cerebellar cell antigen, may cause this damage.

NBs that arise in paravertebral ganglion have a tendency to grow into intervertebral foramina, forming a dumbbell-shaped mass. The intraspinal component may cause spinal cord compression, with paralysis, extremity weakness, or incontinence. Such a situation is an oncologic emergency that has often been treated by surgical decompression or radiation therapy or, more recently, by rapid institution of chemotherapy. Permanent paraplegia may result if this complication is not recognized early.

Sixty percent to 75% of children with NB have metastatic disease at the time of diagnosis.[26, 58] In these children, the presenting features are commonly related to the metastatic tumor rather than to the primary tumor:

- Infants can present with bluish skin nodules.[93, 94] Catecholamines may be released when these nodules are palpated, resulting in an erythematous flush followed by blanching due to vasoconstriction.[93]
- The liver is a common site for metastatic NB in infancy. Rapid hepatic enlargement may result in marked abdominal distention, followed by respiratory compromise.
- NBs may infiltrate the marrow cavity, causing pancytopenia and its resulting complications, such as fever, infection, pallor, lethargy, and bleeding.
- Bone involvement may produce pain, with or without palpable bone masses. Skeletal metastases are usually lytic, and are often seen in the skull, orbit, and proximal long bones. Those patients with bone lesions of the orbit may present with a raccoon-like appearance secondary to proptosis and ecchymoses of the upper and lower eyelids.
- Intracranial metastatic disease is usually meningeal; intracerebral lesions are extremely rare. In infants, meningeal involvement may be manifested by separation of the cranial sutures and can be associated with lytic skull lesions, which allows for a differential diagnosis of leukemia.

Diagnostic Procedures

The diagnosis of NB, as recommended by the second International Neuroblastoma Staging System Conference, includes:

- unequivocal pathologic diagnosis from tumor tissue, or
- a bone marrow aspirate demonstrating unequivocal tumor cells together with the presence of elevated urinary catecholamines[95]

Evaluation of NB requires an examination of the area of primary disease as well as those areas to which NB is known to spread.

- In all instances of suspected NB, a *24-hour urine collection* should be obtained if possible to assess catecholamine (VMA, HVA) secretion. If such collection is not feasible, as may be the case in infants, a urine collection may be analyzed for VMA-to-creatinine and HVA-to-creatinine ratios.

- In addition to the *chest x-ray, CT scan* of the abdomen, pelvis, and chest should be performed. A 1997 multi-institutional retrospective study on imaging of thoracic NB found chest films to be 100% sensitive for diagnosis and *MRI* to be the most effective imaging modality for detection of intraspinal extension, and nodal and chest wall involvement.[96] Patients with cervical masses also should have a CT scan of this area.
- Paravertebral lesions have a propensity to extend into the intervertebral foramina, which may cause spinal cord compression. Therefore, any patient with a paravertebral lesion that appears to be approaching the spinal cord should be further evaluated for possible spinal cord compression. *MRI* is commonly used in this setting.
- A *skeletal survey* and *bone scan* should be performed in all patients to detect bony lesions. Small lytic lesions at the end of long bones may be visible on radiographic scan, but not on bone scan.[97] However, the bone scan is more sensitive in finding lesions of the skull and tubular bones and, in general, is more sensitive than conventional radiographs, although it may be difficult to interpret in infants.[26]
- *Metaiodobenzylguanidine (MIBG) scintigraphy* is a sensitive and specific method for assessing the extent of both the primary tumor and disseminated disease.[98] However, at least one study has suggested that MIBG should be used in conjunction with conventional bone scintigraphy.[99] MIBG also may be useful as a prognostic indicator following treatment.
- Because the bone marrow is a common site of metastatic involvement, *bone marrow aspiration* and *biopsy* should be performed in all patients with NB. Marrow involvement can, at times, be found when monoclonal antibodies to NB are used to detect tumor cells. The prognostic implications of finding marrow tumor cells in this way have not been studied in a prospective manner.
- The liver should be examined by *contrast CT scan* or by a *liver-spleen scan*. In addition, the Pediatric Oncology Group (POG) is currently recommending a liver biopsy for those patients with abdominal disease.

Classification and Staging

Histopathology

Sympathoblasts are the neural crest cells that give rise to the sympathetic nervous system and from which NBs arise. These cells may also differentiate into paraganglionic cells, from which pheochromocytomas and paragangliomas are derived. NBs are composed of small round cells with scant cytoplasm and must be differentiated from similar cell tumors of childhood, such as rhabdomyosarcoma, lymphoma, leukemia, Ewing's sarcoma, and retinoblastoma:

- Neuron-specific enolase may be helpful in differentiating NB from other small round cell tumors that are not of neuroectodermal origin.
- Periodic acid-Schiff staining is usually positive in Ewing's sarcoma and rhabdomyosarcoma, but negative in NB.
- Lymphoid markers can be used to rule out a lymphoma.

NB cells may be densely packed, separated by thin fibrils or bundles, and necrosis and calcification can be seen. The small round cells often form clusters surrounded by pink neurofibrillary material; these "rosettes" are characteristic of NB. With increasing maturation, more fibrillary material is apparent, and ganglionic differentiation may be seen. Electron microscopy can be helpful, particularly if the neurofibrillary material is not distinct. Cytoplasmic structures, consisting of neurofilaments, neurotubules, and neurosecretory granules that contain catecholamines, may be noted.

Recently, the terminology and morphologic criteria of neuroblastic tumors have been revised by the International Neuroblastoma Pathology Committee[86]; the new system is based on a framework of the Shimada classification with minor modifications. It is age linked and dependent on differentiation grade, cellular turnover index, and the presence or absence of schwannian stromal development (Table 19–6). Features of this system include the *mitosis-karyorrhexis index*, which is the number of tumor cells in mitosis and in the process of karyorrhexis; the *mitotic rate*; and *calcification*. A 1999 report by the International Neuroblastoma Pathology Committee supports its reproducibility and prognostic utility.[100]

Staging

Three systems have been used for the staging of NB (Table 19–7), and they require understanding in order to interpret data from various reports. The classic staging system of NB is that of Evans and D'Angio,[101] based on the presurgical extent of disease. This system includes a group called stage IVS NB, which consists of patients who would otherwise be stage IV, but have remote disease confined to selected sites, such as liver, skin, or bone marrow. Most often, these are children younger than 1 year of age and, overall, their prognosis is considerably better than that for others with stage IV disease.[102]

An alternative staging system, used by the POG and derived from St. Jude Children's Research Hospital, is based on the degree of resectability of the primary tumor, as well as metastatic spread,[103] and was an attempt to improve the prognostic value of staging. In particular, lymph node involvement was used as a major criterion in this system, since it was shown that 83% of patients with Evans stage II and stage III tumors without nodal disease survive, compared with 31% of those with nodal disease.[104] However, other reports have questioned the prognostic significance of lymph node involvement.[105, 106]

Two international conferences have finalized a consensus for a new NB staging system (International Neuroblastoma Staging System or INSS), which is postsurgical with reliance on the assessment of tumor resectability and surgical examination of lymph node involvement.[95]

Principles of Treatment

NB is a tumor that is sensitive to both chemotherapy and radiation therapy; nonetheless, for patients with localized

TABLE 19–6. **Prognostic Evaluation of Neuroblastic Tumors According to the International Neuroblastoma Pathology Classification (Shimada System)**

	International Neuroblastoma Pathology Classification	Original Shimada Classification	Prognostic Group
Neuroblastoma	(Schwannian stroma-poor)	Stroma-poor	
Favorable		Favorable	Favorable
<1.5 years	Poor differentiated or differentiating & low or intermediate MKI tumor		
1.5–5 years	Differentiating & low MKI tumor		
Unfavorable		Unfavorable	Unfavorable
<1.5 years	• undifferentiated tumor* • high MKI tumor		
1.5–5 years	a. undifferentiated or poorly differentiated tumor b. intermediate or high MKI tumor		
≥5 years	All tumors		
Ganglioneuroblastoma, intermixed	(Schwannian stroma-rich)	Stroma-rich intermixed (favorable)	Favorable†
Ganglioneuroma	(Schwannian stroma-dominant)		
Maturing		Well differentiated (favorable)	Favorable†
Mature		Ganglioneuroma	
Ganglioneuroblastoma, nodular	(Composite schwannian stroma-rich/ stroma-dominant and stroma-poor)	Stroma-rich nodular (unfavorable)	Unfavorable†

MKI = mitosis-karyorrhexis index.
*Rare subtype, especially diagnosed in this age group. Further investigation and analysis required.
†Prognostic grouping for these tumor categories is not related to patient age.
From Shimada H, Ambros IM, Dehner LP, et al: The International Neuroblastoma Pathology Classification (the Shimada System). Cancer 1999; 86:364, with permission.

disease, surgical therapy alone is frequently sufficient. Although children with disseminated disease will respond to chemotherapy and radiation therapy, permanent disease control has historically been uncommon. It is only through the use of intensive regimens, including bone marrow transplantation (BMT), that the cure rate of those patients with advanced-stage disease appears to be increasing. It has been suggested that NBs can be divided into clinical risk groups based on tumor biology and genetics (Table 19–8).

Surgery

Because of the advances in imaging and early detection, and the improvements in chemotherapeutic regimens and radiation techniques, counterbalanced by the risks involved in neonatal surgery, the role of radical surgical resection in the treatment of NB is currently being debated in some countries.[108, 109] At a minimum, surgery obtains sufficient tissue for the biologic and molecular characterization of the tumor. For those patients with localized disease and easily resectable primary tumors, or conversely, for patients with adverse prognostic factors, such as late age at diagnosis (>2 years), N-*MYC* gene amplification, or unfavorable histopathology, complete removal of the primary tumor offers the best chance of cure.[109, 110] For example, the Children's Cancer Group reported a 98% survival rate for patients with Evans stage I and stage II NB treated with surgery alone.[110]

In some cases, subtotal resection may be sufficient, with or without adjuvant therapy; residual tumor in patients with stage I and stage II disease with favorable prognostic factors may regress spontaneously, or at least not progress.[108, 109, 111] However, patients with advanced disease have infiltrative tumors that cannot be completely resected. Indeed, initial aggressive surgery may be disadvantageous in these patients because of the risk for surgical complications that could delay initiation of chemotherapy.

Radiation Therapy

Although NB is a radiosensitive tumor, radiation therapy is used sparingly in children, a population at high risk for late effects.[112] Nonetheless, radiation therapy is often used for emergency situations, particularly at the time of diagnosis when a large mediastinal mass may produce respiratory symptoms or a dumbbell lesion protruding into the intervertebral foramen may cause cord compression. Patients with early-stage disease can often be treated with surgery alone, or surgery plus a small amount of chemotherapy; thus, the use of radiation therapy in localized disease has been decreasing.

Patients with advanced disease often receive radiation therapy after initial chemotherapy in an attempt to make residual disease surgically resectable or to improve local control. In addition, radiation therapy is a component of conditioning regimens in the setting of autologous or allogeneic BMT. Radiation therapy also may play an important role in the palliative treatment of patients in the terminal stage of NB, for whom bone pain or compression of organs, such as the trachea, bowel, or urinary tract, is causing significant symptoms. Recently, intraoperative radiation has been employed successfully to boost local control rates without incurring the complications and long-term toxicity associated with conventional external beam radiation.[111, 113, 114]

When radiation therapy is used in the initial treatment

TABLE 19–7. **Neuroblastoma Staging Systems***

Evans and D'Angio[101]	Pediatric Oncology Group[26]	INSS[95]
Stage I Tumor confined to the organ or structure of origin.	***Stage A*** Complete gross resection of primary tumor, with or without microscopic residual disease. Intracavitary lymph nodes not adherent to and removed with primary (nodes adherent to or within tumor resection may be positive for tumor without upstaging patient to stage C), histologically free of tumor. If primary in abdomen or pelvis, liver histologically free of tumor.	***Stage 1*** Localized tumor with complete gross excision, without microscopic residual disease; representative ipsilateral lymph nodes negative for tumor microscopically (nodes attached to and removed with the primary tumor may be positive).
Stage II Tumor contiguous beyond the organ or structure of origin, but not crossing the midline. Regional lymph nodes on the ipsilateral side may be involved.	***Stage B*** Grossly unresected primary tumor. Nodes and liver same as in Stage A.	***Stage 2A*** Localized tumor with incomplete gross excision; representative ipsilateral nonadherent lymph nodes negative for tumor microscopically.
Stage III Tumor contiguous beyond the midline. Regional lymph nodes may be involved bilaterally.	***Stage C*** Complete or incomplete resection of primary. Intracavitary nodes not adherent to primary histologically positive for tumor. Liver as in Stage A.	***Stage 2B*** Localized tumor with or without complete gross excision, with ipsilateral nonadherent lymph nodes positive for tumor. Enlarged contralateral lymph nodes must be negative microscopically. ***Stage 3*** Unresectable unilateral tumor infiltrating across the midline† with or without regional lymph node involvement; or localized unilateral tumor with contralateral regional lymph node involvement; or midline tumor with bilateral extension by infiltration (unresectable) or by lymph node involvement.
Stage IV Remote disease involving the skeleton, bone marrow, soft tissue, and distant lymph node groups, etc. (see Stage IV-S).	***Stage D*** Any dissemination of disease beyond intracavitary nodes (e.g., extracavitary nodes, liver, skin, bone marrow, bone).	***Stage 4*** Any primary tumor with dissemination to distant lymph nodes, bone, bone marrow, liver, skin and/or other organs (except as defined for Stage 4S).
Stage IV-S Patients who would otherwise be Stage I or II, but who have remote disease confined to liver, skin, or bone marrow (without radiographic evidence of bone metastases on complete skeletal survey).	***Stage DS*** Infants <1 year of age with Stage IV-S disease (see Evans and D'Angio).	***Stage 4S*** Localized primary tumor as defined for stage 1, 2A, or 2B) with dissemination limited to skin, liver, and/or bone marrow‡ (limited to infants <1 year of age).

INSS = International Neuroblastoma Staging System.

*Multifocal primary tumors (e.g., bilateral adrenal primary tumors) should be staged according to the greatest extent of disease, as defined above, and followed by a subscript letter M (e.g., 3M).

†The midline is defined as the vertebral column. Tumors originating on one side and crossing the midline must infiltrate to or beyond the opposite side of the vertebral column.

‡Marrow involvement in stage 4S should be minimal—i.e., <10% of total nucleated cells identified as malignant on bone marrow biopsy or on marrow aspirate. More extensive marrow involvement would be considered to be stage 4. The metaiodobenzylguanidine scan (if performed) should be negative in the marrow.

From Halperin EC, Constine LS, Tarbell NJ, et al: Pediatric Radiation Oncology, 3rd ed. Philadelphia, Lippincott Williams & Wilkins, 1999, with permission.

of NB, megavoltage equipment and careful attention to sparing normal tissue are necessary. Doses range from 15 to 35 Gy, although no clear dose-response curve has been demonstrated. A 1997 excellent review by Marcus and Tarbell is informative.[115]

Radioimmunotherapy

New studies in the treatment of NB have included investigations into radioisotope treatment. For example, the use of ^{131}I-MIBG therapy has shown promise in specifically targeting NB tumors. A 1999 investigation from the Netherlands found that ^{131}I-MIBG treatment provided the best palliative treatment for recurrent or progressive disease and, when given at diagnosis in unresectable late-stage patients, was as beneficial as combination chemotherapy, while producing less toxicity.[116] Another study, by Garaventa and colleagues, found that the addition of ^{131}I-MIBG to the treatment regimens of patients with late-stage NBs suggested an improvement in the cure rate for stage III patients and the response rate for stage IV patients.[117]

Chemotherapy

Chemotherapy is the major treatment modality for most patients with NB, with the exception of those with favor-

TABLE 19–8. **Clinical/Biologic Types of Neuroblastoma**

Feature	Type 1	Type 2	Type 3
Stage	Usually 1, 2, 4S	Usually 3, 4	Usually 3, 4
N-*MYC*	Normal	Normal	Amplified
DNA ploidy	Hyperdiploid Near triploid	Near diploid Near tetraploid	Near diploid Near tetraploid
1p LOH	Absent	± Present	Usually present
14q LOH	Absent?	± Present	Usually present
Trka expression	High	Variable	Low or absent
Age	Usually <1 year	Usually ≥1 year	Usually 1–5 years
3-year survival	95%	25%–50%	<5%

LOH = loss of heterogeneity.
From Brodeur GM: Molecular basis for heterogeneity in human neuroblastomas. Eur J Cancer 1995; 31A:505, with permission from Elsevier Science.

able, localized disease. The following agents were found to produce the following responses (complete and partial) when used as single agents: cyclophosphamide (59%), doxorubicin (41%), cisplatin (46%), epipodophyllotoxin (30%), vincristine (24%), and actinomycin D (14%).[118] Ifosfamide and carboplatin are also active as single agents.[119, 120]

Nowadays, the most frequent use of chemotherapy is in patients with disseminated disease and, in line with modern trends, the aforementioned agents are used in various combinations with some success. For example, carboplatin-etoposide and vincristine-cyclophosphamide-doxorubicin, in combinations, produced response rates of 71%, with 5-year overall survival and event-free survival rates of 88% and 78%, respectively.[121]

Bone Marrow Transplantation

Despite the clear success of myeloablative therapy and rescue, the advantage of BMT over aggressive non-BMT strategies is unproved. Analyses have suggested a benefit with BMT for patients with high-risk features who do not completely respond to induction chemotherapy.[122] A study of high-risk NB patients by Matthay and colleagues showed that myeloablative therapy with autologous transplant of purged bone marrow resulted in a significantly higher 3-year event-free survival rate than that obtained with treatment by intensive chemotherapy alone—34% versus 22%, respectively.[123] Unfortunately, the 3-year overall survival rates were similar for the two treatments (43% versus 44%, respectively) and, in addition, a separate Japanese report was not able to demonstrate the same advantage.[124]

Autologous BMT is most commonly used, particularly when marrow specimens can be purged of NB tumor cells. Both *in vivo* and *ex vivo* purging methods have been used[125, 126]; in one *ex vivo* method, bone marrow may be incubated with magnetic beads coated with anti-NB antibodies and passed over a magnet to remove tumor cells, although the cost of this method has proved prohibitive in some institutions.[127] Allogeneic BMT has not been shown to be superior to autologous purged BMT.[128, 129]

Special Considerations

As previously stated, NB is a biologically heterogeneous malignancy, and treatment is currently based on a combination of clinical and biologic factors that are predictive of outcome (Table 19–9).[130–132]

Low-Risk Disease

Children with low-risk disease include:

- infants (<1 year of age) and children with either localized resected INSS stage 1 or subtotally resected INSS stage 2A disease
- infants with regional (INSS 2B) or non-N-*MYC*–amplified 4S disease
- older children with 2B disease without N-*MYC* amplification or with favorable histology.

Children with INSS stage 1 disease are appropriately treated with surgery alone, reserving chemotherapy for relapse.[133, 134] Children with INSS 2A disease (Evans-D'Angio stage II) and infants with INSS 2B disease without N-*MYC* amplification are also treated with surgery alone. Any advantage to adjuvant chemotherapy is considered to be controversial at present,[135] and radiation therapy does not appear to improve outcome.[136] In the current POG low-risk study, chemotherapy is reserved for recurrent or progressive disease only.

Intermediate-Risk Disease

Children with intermediate-risk disease include:

- infants with INSS 3 disease, INSS 4 or 4S disease without N-*MYC* amplification
- older children with non-N-*MYC*–amplified INSS 3 disease.

Chemotherapy is moderately aggressive. Children with POG C disease (involved nonadherent lymph nodes) appear to benefit from adjuvant radiation therapy (to the primary and regional lymph nodes) as demonstrated by a randomized POG trial.[137] This approach is supported by a Dana Farber Cancer Institute study of children with subtotally resected Evans-D'Angio stage III disease.[138] However, a 1998 Children's Cancer Group (CCG) study, which included Evans-D'Angio stage III patients (most were INSS 3) who had a favorable biology, did not demonstrate an advantage to irradiation, even for patients with tumors unresectable at second look.[83] Of interest is that this same group of patients also did not benefit from gross total resection.

TABLE 19–9. **Assignment of Risk Group for Neuroblastoma—Guidelines of the Children's Cancer Group and the Pediatric Oncology Group**

INSS Stage	Age	N-*MYC* Status	Shimada Histology Classification	DNA Ploidy	Risk Group
1	0–21 yrs	Any	Any	Any	Low
2A/2B	<1 yr	Any	Any	Any	Low
	≥1 yr to 21 yrs	Nonamplified	Any	NA	Low
	≥1 yr to 21 yrs	Amplified	Favorable	NA	Low
	≥1 yr to 21 yrs	Amplified	Unfavorable	NA	Low
3	<1 yr	Nonamplified	Any	Any	Intermediate
	<1 yr	Amplified	Any	Any	High
	≥1 yr to 21 yrs	Nonamplified	Favorable	NA	Intermediate
	≥1 yr to 21 yrs	Nonamplified	Unfavorable	NA	High
	≥1 yr to 21 yrs	Amplified	Any	NA	High
4	≥1 yr	Nonamplified	Any	Any	Intermediate
	<1 yr	Amplified	Any	Any	High
	≥1 yr to 21 yrs	Any	Any	NA	High
4S	<1 yr	Nonamplified	Favorable	>1	Low
	<1 yr	Nonamplified	Any	=1	Intermediate
	<1 yr	Nonamplified	Unfavorable	Any	Intermediate
	<1 yr	Amplified	Any	Any	High

INSS = International Neuroblastoma Staging System.
Modified from Shimada H, Chatten J, Newton W, et al: Histopathologic prognostic factors in neuroblastic tumors. Definition of subtypes of ganglioneuroblastoma and an age linked classification of neuroblastomas. J Natl Cancer Inst 1984; 73:405; Joshi V, Cantor A, Altshuler G, et al: Recommendations for modification of terminology of neuroblastic tumors and prognostic significance of Shimada classification. A clinicopathologic study of 213 cases from the Pediatric Oncology Group. Cancer 1992; 69:2183; and Look A, Hayes F, Shuster J, et al: Clinical relevance of tumor cell ploidy and N-myc gene amplification in childhood neuroblastoma. A Pediatric Oncology Group Study. J Clin Oncol 1991; 9:581.

In general, children with INSS 4S disease are managed according to their clinical symptoms, with chemotherapy or radiation therapy administered for respiratory or vascular compromise due to hepatomegaly. A 2000 CCG study reported on the positive outcome of patients with stage IV-S (INSS 4S) NB with no N-*MYC* amplification who received minimal treatment (supportive care or low-dose cytotoxic therapy in symptomatic patients).[139] The 5-year survival rate in the supportive care group was 100%, compared with 81% for those requiring cytotoxic therapy. However, the group did recommend intensive early treatment for patients younger than 2 months of age at diagnosis with

TABLE 19–10. **Results of Clinical Trials in Localized Neuroblastoma**

Stage	Treatment	No. Patients	Event-Free Survival (%)	Overall Survival (%)
Node Negative, POG Stage A				
POG[133]	S	101	89	97
CCG[106]	S	87	92	100
ICGN[143]	S + CT	69	90	94
CCG[110]	S*	141	93	99
Node Negative and/or Evans-D'Angio Stage II				
HSC[144]	S ± CT ± RT	25	68	74
Utah[145]	S ± RT	25	NA	84
CCSG[136]	S	75	89[a]	96[b]
	S + RT	66	94[a]	96[b]
SJCRH/POG[146]	S + CT	61	84	87
ICGN[117]	CT ± S	16	74[a]	NA
CCG[106]	S ± CT ± RT	144	76	96
ICGN[143]	S + CT	49	85	96
CCG[110]	S*	233	81	98
Node Positive and/or Evans-D'Angio Stage III				
Utah[145]	S ± RT	13	NA	69
POG[137]	S + CT	28	32	41
	S + CT + RT	29	58	73
ICGN[117]	CT	129	52[a]	NA
Dana-Farber[138]	S + CT	25	72	72
CCG[106]	S + CT + RT	193	63	67
ICGN[143]	S + CT	26	61	87
Duke[147]	S + RT ± CT	146	46[c]	54[c]

*Radiation given to relieve spinal cord compression.
S = surgery; CT = chemotherapy; a = progression-free survival; b = overall survival rate for the whole trial; c = 10-year rates; NA = not available.
Modified from Halperin EC, Constine LC, Tarbell NJ, et al: Pediatric Radiation Oncology, 3rd ed. Philadelphia, Lippincott Williams & Wilkins, 1999.

rapidly progressing abdominal disease. N-*MYC* amplification or adverse histopathologic classification may identify the population that requires cytotoxic therapy.[140, 141]

In the current POG protocol for intermediate-risk patients, chemotherapy includes cyclophosphamide, doxorubicin, carboplatin, and etoposide, with the duration determined by biologic characteristics. Radiation therapy is reserved for persistent tumor despite chemotherapy and second-look surgery.

High-Risk Disease

This group includes children older than 1 year with INSS 3 tumors and an unfavorable biology, and all children with INSS 4 disease (except, perhaps, infants with favorable features). In addition, infants with INSS 3/4S N-*MYC*–amplified disease are also high risk. Based on the observation that chemotherapy dose intensity correlates with response and progression-free survival,[142] high-risk patients are most commonly treated with myeloablative chemotherapy or chemoradiotherapy with stem cell rescue. Following the aggressive chemotherapy regimen, the primary tumor is then resected, if possible, or irradiated if unresectable.

Results and Prognosis

A compilation of the results from a number of trials for the treatment of NB is shown in Table 19–10. Using age and the POG staging system, children with NB can be stratified into three prognostic risk groups: low, intermediate, and high. Survival curves for the low- and high-risk groups, stratified according to age and POG staging at diagnosis, are illustrated in Figure 19–6.

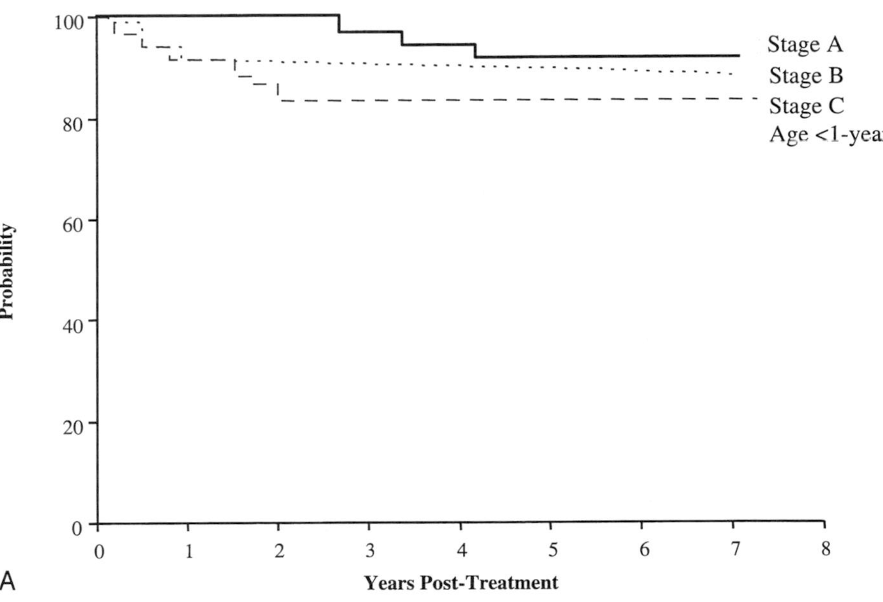

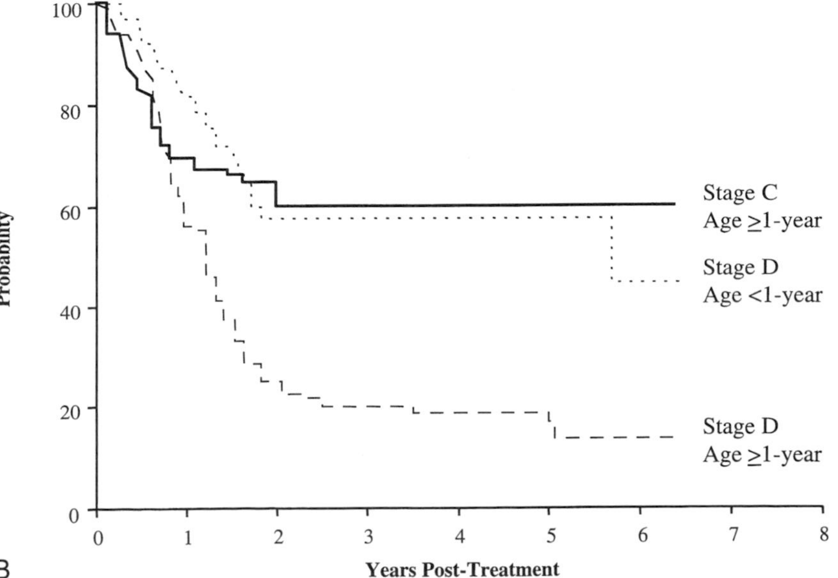

Figure 19–6. Results for children with neuroblastoma according to age and Pediatric Oncology Group stage. (A) Survival in the low-risk group; this group includes patients with complete or partially resected disease and infants with regional disease. (B) Survival in the high-risk group; this group includes children older than 1 year of age with disseminated disease. (From Castleberry RP Jr: Neuroblastoma. Ther Cancer Child 2000; 1:24, with permission.)

In recent years, it has become clear that patients with low-risk disease have a 5-year survival rate of greater than 90%.[134–136] Patients with intermediate-risk disease have a variable outcome, dependent on biologic characteristics, ranging from 55% to a greater than 90% 4-year event-free survival.[83] Children with high-risk disease, treated with dose-intensive chemotherapy and autologous BMT, have a 4-year event-free survival (EFS) of 40% (vs. 19% without BMT).[122]

- Patients with INSS 4S disease with a favorable biology also have a 90% 3-year survival, in contrast to those with N-*MYC* amplification or an adverse histology, who have a 30% to 50% 3-year survival.[140, 141, 149]
- NB in adolescents has different biologic characteristics than in adults and an inferior survival that is less than 30% at 5 years and less than 10% in select subgroups.[150]

Clinical Investigations

Although dose-intensive therapy with stem cell rescue is a clear avenue for progress, toxicity remains a dose-limiting factor. Novel approaches, based on the tumor and host biology, are being pursued, and may enhance the therapeutic ratio.

- *Stimulating NB differentiation*: Agents that mature NB cells, particularly retinoic acid derivatives (e.g., 13-*cis*-retinoic acid, all-*trans*-retinoic acid), are in clinical trials.[123, 151]
- *Reversing MDR and MRP expression*: Expression of the MRP is correlated with N-*MYC* amplification, but is independent of N-*MYC* expression in predicting a poor prognosis.[75] Targeting the expression of this gene may modulate chemotherapy sensitivity.
- *Inducing apoptosis with growth factors*: The neurotrophins (e.g., neurotrophin-3) and their receptors (the Trk family) control the growth and survival of NB. Activation or upregulation of Trk expression with an NB-specific target may inhibit cell growth.[152]
- *Immunologic modulation*: Antibodies (e.g., the anti-ganglioside G[D2] antibody, CH14.18) have demonstrated anti-NB toxicity *in vitro*,[153] and a phase II trial has recently been completed assessing this approach.[154]

Recommended Reading

The current treatment of children with NB is reviewed by Brodeur and Castleberry.[1]

Wilms' Tumor (Nephroblastoma)

Perspective

Wilms' tumor (nephroblastoma) is the most common renal tumor of childhood, and the second most common intra-abdominal tumor in children. Wilms' tumor is an ideal model for the study of childhood cancer:

- The genetic heterogeneity, inherited mutation, and germline mutations seen in Wilms' tumor together suggest that the mechanisms for its tumorigenesis are complex.
- Survival for children with Wilms' tumor increased from 33% in the 1960s to 90% during the 1990s. This remarkable improvement in outcome over the past several decades is illustrated in Table 19–11.[155]
- The clinical trials of the National Wilms' Tumor Study Group (NWTSG), established in 1969, serve as a model of a national cooperative study group. As a result of the work done by NWTSG, indications for radiation therapy and dosing have decreased, the concept of unfavorable histology was introduced, and the delivery of pulse-intensive chemotherapy became commonplace.

The NWTSG is currently in its fifth clinical trial, which began in 1995. The focus of NWTS-5 includes attention to the long-term effects of treatment, the elucidation of the molecular biology of Wilms' tumor, and genetic studies. Moreover, NWTS-5 will closely examine the survivors and their offspring. For further information, the NWTSG web site is www.nwtsg.org.

Epidemiology and Etiology

Epidemiology

Wilms' tumor is the second most common intra-abdominal tumor of childhood (0–19 years) and the most common renal tumor, with an age-adjusted incidence of 6.2 cases per million children in the United States.[155] The incidence rates are slightly higher in U.S. and African black populations than in whites, and significantly lower in several Asian populations.[156, 157] In both the black and white groups, the peak incidence occurs between 2 to 3 years of age, with the mean age at diagnosis being 44 and 31 months for unilateral and bilateral disease, respectively.[58] There has been little change in the age-adjusted U.S. incidence of Wilms' tumor since 1973, and data through 1996 indicate that the 5-year relative survival rate is 90.4%, with a slightly higher survival in females (92.2%) compared with males (88.7%).[155]

Wilms' tumor in the infant is rare among whites and blacks, although in East Asia, 25% to 40% of the cases occur in infants.[156] These variations in incidence along ethnic rather than geographical lines suggest a genetic predisposition. In general, renal tumors in the newborn

TABLE 19–11. **Trends in Survival by Tumor Type for Children Younger Than 15 Years of Age**

	Reported 5-Year Survival Rates by Year of Diagnosis					
Tumor Type/Size	***1960–63***[a]	***1970–73***[a]	***1974–76***[b]	***1977–79***[b]	***1980–85***[b]	***1985–95***[c]
All sites	28%	45%	56%	61.2%	65.2%[d]	72.9%
Acute lymphocytic leukemia	4	34	53.0	68.6	70.7[d]	79.7
Acute myeloid leukemia	3	5	14	24.5[e]	23.2[e]	41.8
Wilms' tumor	33[e]	70[e]	74.1	80.1	80.9	90.6
Brain and nervous system	35	45	54	55.5	57.0	63.3
Neuroblastoma	25	40	48.4	49.7	55.4	66.3
Bones and joints	20[e]	30[e]	54[e]	47.3[e]	50.8[e]	66.4
Hodgkin's disease	52[e]	90	79	84.5	89.3[d]	92.6
Non-Hodgkin's lymphoma	18	26	45	49.6	64.2[d]	74.4

[a]Rates based on Surveillance, Epidemiology and End Results (SEER) data from a series of hospital registries and one population-based registry.
[b]Rates from SEER, based on data from population-based registries in 9 states or areas. Rates are based on follow-up of patients through 1986.
[c]Rates from Ries LAG, Smith MA, Gurney JG, et al (eds): Cancer Incidence and Survival among Children and Adolescents: United States SEER Program 1975–1995. Bethesda, National Cancer Institute, 1999.
[d]The difference in rates between 1974–1976 and 1980–1985 is statistically significant ($p < 0.05$).
[e]The standard error of the survival is between 5 and 10 percentage points.

are most likely to be congenital mesoblastic nephroma or pathologic variants of that tumor. Very rarely, Wilms' tumor may occur in teenagers and adults.[158]

Bilateral Wilms' Tumor

Bilateral Wilms' tumor occurs in 5% of children with Wilms' tumor and tends to occur at an earlier age than that for the peak incidence of Wilms' tumor.[159] These children may have associated anomalies, such as hemihypertrophy and genitourinary anomalies.[160]

Extra-Abdominal Wilms' Tumor

Although extremely rare, extrarenal Wilms' has been described in the retroperitoneum, pelvis, inguinal canal, thorax, cervix, and uterus.[161, 162]

Etiology

Wilms' tumors appear to arise from abnormally persistent clusters of embryonic kidney cells known as nephrogenic rests[163]; these can consist of any of the three renal tissue elements: embryonic blastema, epithelium (tubules), or stroma. Not all tumors contain all three elements.

Hereditary tumors account for approximately 20% to 25% of all Wilms' tumors, sporadic tumors account for 75% to 80%, and the rare familial cases comprise approximately 1% of the total.[164, 165] Hereditary cases are, in general, young children who can have aniridia, genitourinary anomalies and bilateral tumor (4% to 5% of cases).[164, 166]

Hereditary, sporadic, and familial Wilms' tumor appear to be the result of alterations in one or several genes. The most widely studied findings relate to the short arm of chromosome 11.

- Two loci on chromosome 11, the Wilms' tumor (WT) genes *WT1* and *WT2* loci, were initially associated with Wilms' tumor (Fig. 19–7). Deletions in one or both loci are possible; thus, children can present with a picture mimicking associations from both loci.
- *WT1* is found in the 11p13 region, is expressed in the embryonic kidney, and plays a major role in the development of the normal urinogenital system.[167] The loss of DNA-binding activity by this gene, or its inactivation, gives rise to tumor formation—this finding gave rise to the term *tumor suppressor gene*.
- Loss of heterozygosity at the 11p15 locus (*WT2*) is associated with Beckwith-Wiedemann syndrome and the presence of Wilms' tumor.[168] Unfortunately, a gene at the 11p15 locus has yet to be cloned.
- Additional Wilms' tumor loci have been suggested at

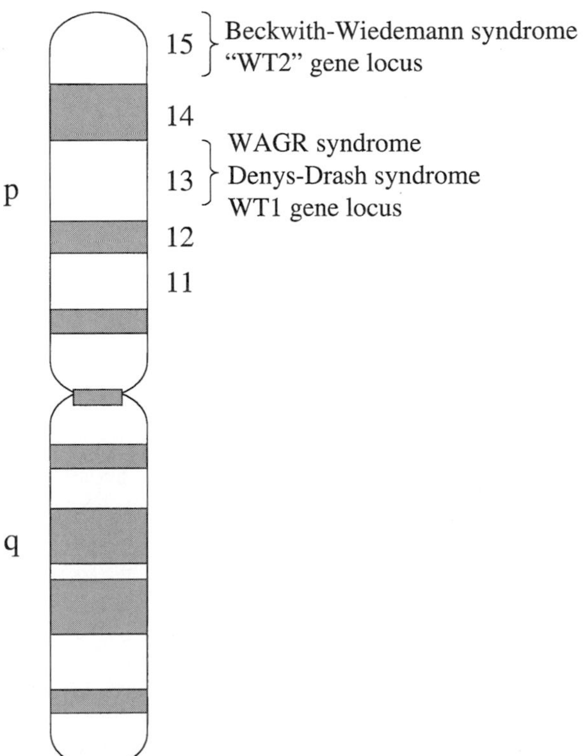

Figure 19–7. The short arm of chromosome 11 contains two loci whose inactivation may contribute to the formation of Wilms' tumor. Moreover, a child can manifest signs from all syndromes associated with both loci.

16q and 1p,[169] in addition to a host of other random and nonrandom abnormalities.[170, 171] These data suggest that several genes are involved in the genesis of Wilms' tumor.

Associated Syndromes

Certain congenital anomalies occur frequently in children diagnosed with Wilms' tumor and are noted more often in patients with bilateral disease.[172, 173]

- Children with *WAGR syndrome* (**W**ilms' tumor, **a**niridia, **g**enitourinary malformations, mental **r**etardation) have a deletion of 11p13.[174, 175]
- *Aniridia* may be either familial or sporadic. One third of patients with aniridia have the sporadic form; Wilms' tumor is associated only with the sporadic form and will develop in one third of those individuals. Mutations of the *PAX6* gene, telomeric with *WT1* on chromosome 11p13, have been shown to be the cause of aniridia.[176, 177] Deletions of chromosome 11p13 that affect both the *PAX6* and *WT1* loci are the basis for the association of aniridia and Wilms' tumor.
- *Denys-Drash syndrome*,[178–180] a condition that involves renal nephropathy, gonadal anomalies, including male pseudohermaphroditism, and a predisposition to Wilms' tumor, also is associated with mutations in the *WT1* gene.[181, 182]
- Rarely, patients with Wilms' may develop *acquired von Willebrand's disease* with significant bruising and bleeding.[183]

Detection and Diagnosis

Clinical Detection

Evaluation begins with an accurate history and physical examination. A family history may reveal other members with Wilms' tumor. In addition, the presence of aniridia and hemihypertrophy must be investigated.

An abdominal mass is the most common presenting sign, and is noted in more than 80% of patients.[58] Abdominal pain and vomiting have been observed in 50% of patients.[184] A smooth, large abdominal mass filling one side of the abdomen is a typical presentation. A more ominous presentation, which may require emergent operation, is the child with rapid abdominal enlargement, fever, hypertension, and anemia. An enlarged liver suggests hepatic metastases. In addition, distended and prominent veins of the anterior abdominal wall may indicate inferior vena caval tumor thrombus. Microscopic hematuria occurs in 20% to 30% of patients; hypertension may be present at diagnosis in 25 to 50% of cases, and is the result of increased renin production.[185, 186]

Diagnostic Procedures

Imaging should be focused on identifying the lesion and its extent of disease. Towards this aim, a chest *x-ray* and CT scan of the abdomen, along with infradiaphragmatic ultrasonography, should suffice.[187] Practically speaking, children with an abdominal mass frequently undergo the following imaging modalities[39a]:

- A plain *radiograph* of the abdomen and chest—coarse calcifications may occur in a Wilms' tumor, but fine-stippled calcifications are noted more frequently in NB.
- *CT* and *MRI* are useful for imaging the location and involvement of the mass with respect to the great vessels, spinal canal, and retroperitoneum.[187] However, although CT of the abdomen is commonly performed to determine exact dimensions and extension of renal mass, some investigators, concerned by the significant radiation dose involved in the use of serial CT on infants, have recommended MRI instead of CT.[188]
- *Abdominal CT* with contrast or *intravenous pyelography* (IVP) will reveal an intrarenal mass displacing and distorting the collecting system of the involved kidney. The opposite kidney should be evaluated for bilateral involvement. Contralateral tumors less than 1 cm in size are frequently difficult to see on CT scan and account for a 7% error rate for incomplete diagnosis. Occasionally, Wilms' tumor is misdiagnosed on IVP when the lesion is actually an NB that has distorted the renal collecting system.[189]
- *Ultrasonography* is especially useful in complementing IVP, but, more specifically, it is essential to look for tumor growth in the renal vein, vena cava, and right side of the heart. Liver metastases may also be demonstrated by ultrasound.
- A *chest x-ray* may reveal pulmonary metastases, the most common site of metastatic spread.[190] *CT of the chest* is a more sensitive method, although one study demonstrated no advantage in obtaining this study at diagnosis in low-risk children.[191] Moreover, the small nodules encountered on CT scan, not visible on plain *x-ray films*, may be benign.
- *Bone scans* are indicated in patients with the clear cell sarcoma variant of Wilms' tumor.
- *Echocardiography* is indicated for children with tumor thrombus extending into the right atrium.

Laboratory Studies

Laboratory evaluation of a child with a suspected Wilms' tumor should include a complete blood cell count, urinalysis, and liver and renal function blood studies. Hypercalcemia has been identified as a paraneoplastic syndrome of Wilms' tumor,[192] but may also suggest a rhabdoid tumor or a congenital mesoblastic nephroma rather than a true Wilms' tumor.[193] An elevated hemoglobin may indicate a rare erythropoietin-secreting Wilms' tumor.[194] In addition, clotting abnormalities can exist due to acquired von Willebrand's disease.

Differential Diagnosis

The most common consideration in the differential diagnosis is NB. The distinction between these two entities should be relatively easy in that an intra-abdominal NB arises from the adrenal gland or the paravertebral ganglia and thus displaces, rather than distorts, the kidney. Multicystic kidneys, hematoma, renal cell carcinoma, and mesoblastic nephroma are other entities that can be confused with Wilms' tumor.

Classification and Staging

Histopathology

Wilms' tumor is, in general, solid and confined by the renal capsule, although it may contain necrotic or cystic areas. However, the tumor frequently infiltrates through the kidney capsule into adjacent structures, and there may be direct extension into the pelvis and ureter or the renal vein and vena cava. Hilar and periaortic lymph node involvement is relatively common, and the lung represents the most common site of distant metastases. Microscopically, the tumor may contain varying amounts of three tissue elements: blastema, epithelia, and stroma. On occasion, skeletal muscle, cartilage, and squamous epithelium have been found.

There are two pathologic entities associated with Wilms' tumor: congenital mesoblastic nephroma and nephroblastomatosis.

- *Congenital mesoblastic nephroma* is a benign mesenchymal tumor of renal origin seen during the first 3 months of life, is distinct from Wilms' tumor, and has a morphology resembling smooth muscle cells or fibroblasts.[195] Cellular variations of this tumor with less benign behavior have been described occasionally.[196, 197] The tumor has a tendency to extend into perirenal tissues and, thus, mandates a radical resection for complete removal.
- The persistence of embryonic renal blastema beyond 36 weeks' gestation is termed *nephroblastomatosis*. Two forms of nephroblastomatosis (nephrogenic rests) have been described, perilobar and intralobar.[163] The more common perilobar form does not enhance with CT scan, but 60% are visible with MRI scan. Intralobar rests, found in the deep cortex and medulla, are less frequent and, when discovered in the nephrectomy specimen, mandate close evaluation of the contralateral kidney. Unfortunately, intralobar rests cannot be identified with CT scan. Thus, when found in a resected kidney or discovered in children with bilateral disease, nephroblastomatosis must be followed closely.

Clear cell sarcomas and rhabdoid tumors of the kidney are considered separate entities from Wilms' tumor. Children with clear cell sarcoma have very high relapse, skeletal metastasis, and mortality rates. Rhabdoid tumors of the kidney are unrelated lesions and of neural crest origin.[26]

Staging

A clinicopathologic staging system has been developed by the NWTSG (Table 19–12).[198] The clinical stage is determined during the operative procedure and confirmed by the pathologist. It is important to remember that staging is the same regardless of the gross appearance or tumor histology. Pediatric Wilms' tumors should always be referred to by their stage and histology (favorable or unfavorable).[198] Accurate staging must include thorough abdominal exploration, including evaluation of the liver and contralateral kidney, presence of peritoneal fluid (especially blood tinged) and grossly enlarged lymph nodes.

TABLE 19–12. **National Wilms' Tumor Study Group—Clinicopathologic Staging System**

Stage 1 (43% of Children)

Tumor limited to the kidney and completely excised. The surface of the renal capsule is intact. The tumor was not ruptured before or during removal. The renal sinus vessels are not involved. There is no evidence of residual tumor beyond the margins of the resection.

Stage II (23% of Children)

Tumor extends beyond the kidney, but is completely excised. There is regional extension; i.e., there is penetration out of the renal capsule into the perirenal soft tissue. Vessels outside the kidney parenchyma either are infiltrated or contain tumor thrombus, or the vessels of the renal sinus are invaded. There is no residual tumor at or beyond the operative margins of resection. There is no evidence of tumor rupture before or during excision, but local spillage to the flank is present. Biopsy of the tumor (except fine-needle aspiration) mandates stage II disease.

Stage III* (20% of Children)

Residual nonhematogenous tumor confined to the abdomen. One or more of the following are found:

- Lymph nodes positive in the hilus, periaortic chain, or beyond (i.e., mesenteric or iliac), confined to the abdomen.
- Penetration of tumor beyond the tumor bed, including peritoneal implants.
- Tumor extends beyond the operative field, either grossly or microscopically.
- Diffuse contamination of the peritoneum before or during resection.
- Unresectable tumor because of local infiltration into structures, such as the colon, duodenum, or inferior vena cava.

Stage IV (10% of Children)

Hematogenous metastasis outside the boundaries described in stage III. Sites of deposits include lung, liver, bone, and brain.

Stage V (4% of Children)

Bilateral involvement at the time of diagnosis.

*Inoperable tumor by imaging alone with or without biopsy is considered stage III disease.

Modified from National Wilms' Tumor Study Committee: Wilms' tumor: status report, 1990. J Clin Oncol 1991; 9:877.

Principles of Treatment

The principles of treatment for Wilms' tumor have evolved from the NWTSG clinical trials (Table 19–13).[160, 199–204] Efforts should be made to treat all children with Wilms' tumor within a clinical trial.

Surgery

The most important requisites for the surgeon are to ensure complete removal without rupture and adequate assessment of the intra-abdominal extent of disease; anything less is inadequate operative decision making. It is recommended that all children undergo initial laparotomy to evaluate the extent of disease and operability and to obtain a biopsy

TABLE 19–13. **NWTSG-5 Treatment Recommendations by Stage for Wilms' Tumor**

Stage	Surgery	Radiation Therapy	Chemotherapy
Stage I* [199]			
Favorable histology/focal or diffuse anaplasia	nephrectomy	NR	18 weeks: V pulse-intensive Ad
Clear cell sarcoma of the kidney	nephrectomy	yes	24 weeks: V A E C + mesna
Rhabdoid tumor of the kidney	nephrectomy	yes	24 weeks: C E Cb + mesna
Stage II [199]			
Favorable histology	nephrectomy	NR	18 weeks: V pulse-intensive Ad
Focal anaplasia	nephrectomy	yes	24 weeks: V A pulse-intensive Ad
Diffuse anaplasia/clear cell sarcoma	nephrectomy	yes	24 weeks: V A E C + mesna
Rhabdoid tumor of the kidney	nephrectomy	yes	24 weeks: C E Cb + mesna
Stage III [200]			
Favorable histology and focal anaplasia	nephrectomy	yes	24 weeks: V A pulse-intensive Ad
Diffuse anaplasia/clear cell sarcoma	nephrectomy	yes	24 weeks: V A E C + mesna
Rhabdoid tumor of the kidney	nephrectomy	yes	24 weeks: C E Cb + mesna
Stage IV [201]			
Favorable histology and focal anaplasia	nephrectomy	yes† + any metastases	24 weeks: V A pulse-intensive Ad
Diffuse anaplasia/clear cell sarcoma	nephrectomy	yes + any metastases	24 weeks: V A E C + mesna
Rhabdoid tumor of the kidney	nephrectomy	yes	24 weeks: C E Cb + mesna
Stage V [160, 202]	bilateral biopsies & lymph node sampling	NR	V Ad A (+ second look) Postop, dependent on response

NWTSG = National Wilms' Tumor Study Group; V = vincristine; Ad = dactinomycin (actinomycin D); A = doxorubicin; C = cyclophosphamide; E = etoposide; Cb = carboplatin; NR = not recommended.

*Tumor weight less than 550 grams and age younger than 24 months is no longer managed with surgery alone.[203, 204]

†Based on local stage.

specimen of the tumor. Gerota's fascia of the contralateral kidney should be opened and the kidney inspected, both anteriorly and posteriorly. Biopsy of the primary tumor is *forbidden*.

Radical nephrectomy is the operative procedure of choice; partial nephrectomy is not routinely recommended for the child with Wilms' tumor. A large transabdominal incision is required to facilitate exploration and excision and, on occasion, a combined thoracoabdominal incision is required. A flank or retroperitoneal approach should never be used because it does not provide adequate visualization of the peritoneal cavity or the contralateral kidney. A review of NWTS-3 disclosed a 20% complication rate following radical nephrectomy. The most frequent complication was intestinal obstruction (7%), followed by intraoperative hemorrhage (6%), and other viscera (1%) and vessel (1%) injuries.[205] Initial unilateral nephrectomy in the presence of bilateral disease predisposes to renal failure.[7] Moreover, there is no difference in survival comparing initial resection followed by chemotherapy with initial bilateral biopsy followed by chemotherapy.[206]

An attempt can be made to ligate the renal vessels early in the resection to reduce the risk of tumor embolus formation; however, early ligation should be abandoned if it increases the risk of tumor rupture, because early renal vein ligation has no effect on survival. The entire ureter, which may have tumor extension, is excised with the specimen. Liver wedge resection for radical and complete tumor excision is acceptable, but formal hepatic lobectomy is rarely indicated. Likewise, partial duodenal resection or colon resection is also acceptable for a complete *en bloc* excision. Aggressive surgical excision is indicated for metastatic disease in certain situations, for example, isolated pulmonary lesions at diagnosis, or metastatic disease not responding to chemotherapy and irradiation.

Thorough inspection of the abdominal cavity should be made for extension or metastatic disease and suspicious sites biopsied. Hilar, periaortic, iliac, and celiac lymph node sampling is mandatory for prognostic determination. In addition, any suspicious nodal basin should be sampled. Titanium clips should be used to mark any suspicious node basins, residual tumor, and margins of resection. Caval thrombus should be identified preoperatively and, if possible, the thrombus should be removed. Caval wall invasion is stage III disease, and any atrial thrombi should be removed under cardiopulmonary bypass.[207] Should preoperative ultrasound reveal tumor extension in the vena cava or right atrium, the surgical excision planning should involve cardiopulmonary bypass, with hypothermia producing good local control in these difficult presentations.[208, 209] Alternatively, preoperative chemotherapy may be used to facilitate removal of tumor,[210] followed 2 weeks later, if necessary, with irradiation if there is no tumor shrinkage.[211] Resection then is usually possible within 6 weeks, and the tumor should then be treated as stage III.

To prevent tumor spillage, involved contiguous tissue should be taken in continuity with the tumor; if spillage occurs, care should be taken to contain it. Local spillage means stage II treatment, but a diffuse peritoneal spillage means stage III disease, requiring total abdominal irradiation and doxorubicin. Bloody peritoneal fluid is a sign of rupture and considered stage III disease. However, if the posterior aspect of the tumor ruptures, in the absence of hematoma or hemorrhage, this condition is considered stage II.

Radiation Therapy

In general, radiation therapy is integrated into a combined-modality protocol with surgery and chemotherapy, and its specific goal is to prevent local and regional recurrences. Ideally, it is given postoperatively and should begin within 10 days after operation because of the increased risk of abdominal recurrence when it is delayed.[212] It should be noted, however, that the relapses that were related to this delay in the aforementioned study occurred primarily in patients with unfavorable histology. Megavoltage apparatus and beam-shaping devices are used to tailor the therapy to the patient, carefully excluding normal tissues beyond the target volume. Daily doses are 1.5 to 1.8 Gy to large and small volumes, respectively. Current total doses and volumes are based on the experience gained from NWTS 1 to 4.

Postoperative radiation therapy is not required for stage I and II favorable histology tumors or stage I anaplastic tumors.[213, 214] However, for patients with stage II anaplastic tumors, stage I to II unfavorable histology tumors including the clear cell or rhabdoid variant, and for all patients with stages III and IV disease, irradiation is necessary.[212] Of note, less radiation therapy is required when doxorubicin is added to vincristine and dactinomycin in treatment of stage III disease.[212] For stage III disease with favorable histology without gross residual disease, radiation therapy is delivered to the tumor bed, defined as the involved kidney and areas of associated disease as imaged preoperatively or defined operatively. The radiation therapy portal always includes the entire width of adjacent vertebrae to avoid scoliosis. The whole abdomen is treated (10 to 12 Gy fractionated for favorable histologic patterns) in patients who experience peritoneal seeding or tumor rupture with diffuse dissemination before or during surgery. Boost doses are administered to sites of residual gross disease.

For stage IV (favorable histology) disease, the primary lesion is treated according to the stage it would be in the absence of metastases. If a chest *x-ray* indicates that the lung is involved, the entire thorax is treated (12 Gy fractionated for favorable histology). Of note, studies have shown that small pulmonary lesions, recognized only on CT scan, may be successfully treated with chemotherapy alone.[215–217] Patients with stage II and stage IV (unfavorable histology) disease are treated as outlined for stage III disease, but with doses based on patient age. An additional boost is given to sites of known residual disease (12 to 38 Gy).

Chemotherapy

In 1966, Farber reported on the utility of dactinomycin as adjuvant chemotherapy for the treatment of Wilms' tumor,[218] closely followed by similar reports on vincristine. NWTS-1 revealed that radiation therapy and either dactinomycin or vincristine could provide approximately 55% relapse-free survival (RFS) in patients in groups II and III, but when the two drugs were used in combination, RFS was 81%.[11] These two drugs have since become the mainstays of therapy for Wilms' tumor.

Current chemotherapy is stage dependent, but should be started 5 days postoperatively. Pulse-intensive regimens for the treatment of stages I to IV are recommended; in the majority of cases, the hematopoietic toxic effects and higher drug dose intensities are well established.[219] Low-stage disease (stage I and II/favorable histology and stage I anaplasia) can be adequately treated with dactinomycin and vincristine without irradiation.[11, 213, 214] Doxorubicin is added to dactinomycin and vincristine in higher stage disease (stage III and IV/favorable histology).[198, 213, 220] The addition of cyclophosphamide to the above-mentioned three-drug regimen has demonstrated a survival benefit for children with stage II to IV diffuse anaplastic histology, but has not done so for those with clear cell sarcoma of the kidney.[211]

In certain cases, when operative resection is risky or questionable, preoperative chemotherapy following percutaneous biopsy is appropriate.[207, 221] In the United States, preoperative chemotherapy has not been used because it limits the ability to accurately determine extent of disease[222, 223]; however, it should be noted that preoperative chemotherapy is commonly used in Europe.[221] Indeed, because of the possibility of tumor rupture, the European consortium, the International Society of Pediatric Oncology (SIOP), favors the preoperative treatment of Wilms' tumor with chemotherapy or radiation therapy. However, the Children's Oncology Group feels that this approach has inherent risks that include potential alteration of the histology, loss of valuable staging information, and the possibility of aggressive multimodal treatment of benign disease. Regardless of the sequence of multimodality therapy, confirmation of the diagnosis of the renal mass should be performed before therapy. There is a 5% to 6% error rate for diagnosis of renal masses when radiography is the sole assessment tool.[224]

Inoperable tumors should be treated with chemotherapy; failure to respond to chemotherapy may necessitate radiation. The drug dosage (vincristine and dactinomycin) must be reduced by 50% in children younger than 1 year of age in order to decrease the serious toxicity rate from 49% to 13% and drug-related deaths from 6% to 0%[225, 226]; this reduction can be performed without compromise in therapeutic effectiveness.

Bilateral Wilms' (stage V) tumors should be treated with chemotherapy after bilateral biopsies and lymph node samplings. Chemotherapy includes vincristine, dactinomycin, and doxorubicin, followed by second-look operation.[202] If bilateral disease is of anaplastic histology, more aggressive chemotherapy and irradiation, as well as an aggressive second-look procedure, are advisable.[198]

Recurrent Wilms' Tumor

Treatment for this group of children depends on several factors, including the site of recurrence, the histology, length of time from nephrectomy to recurrence, and the initial chemotherapy regimen. Children who, after two-drug therapy, demonstrate recurrence in the lungs or brain or in a previously unirradiated abdomen, or any recurrence within 12 months of diagnosis, may benefit from combined-modality treatment.[198, 227, 228] Although histologic confirmation of tumor recurrence in the lung may be required, there does not appear to be any therapeutic benefit to resection of a pulmonary nodule plus radiation therapy or chemotherapy. The other group consists of children with unfavorable histology, post-irradiation abdominal failures, recurrence within 6 months of nephrectomy, or recurrence after three-drug therapy. Overall, the 2-year survival in patients following recurrence is 43%.[229] Combinations of etoposide and carboplatin have been useful, along with autologous BMT.[230, 231]

Results and Prognosis

With the evolution of each NWTSG trial, the control arm of each succeeding protocol was the better outcome of the earlier trial. Comparison of the results from the NWTS-3 clinical trial (summarized in Table 19–14) with the strategies being followed in NWTS-5 (see Table 19–13) provides a concise overview of the development of the multidisciplinary approach that has proved successful in Wilms' tumor.

Two-year relapse-free survival (RFS) or 5-year survival from nephrectomy is considered a cure in Wilms' tumor, although there are isolated reports of recurrences beyond 5 years. These may represent true bilateral Wilms' tumors or nephroblastomatosis. Table 19–14 shows the survival by stage from NWTS-3. Seventy-five percent of relapses occurred within 1 year, and less than 3% occurred after 2 years from the onset of therapy. Some patients with low-stage disease who develop metastases can be cured with intensive chemotherapy and radiation therapy.[232] Unfortunately, patients who develop local abdominal recurrences are rarely cured of their disease, and survival at 2 years is 43%. Children with stage V disease (bilateral disease) have a 3-year survival rate of 92%, even if their most advanced lesion is stage I; if their most advanced lesion is stage III, the survival rate drops to 75% even if there is favorable histology.[196]

Surgical treatment for bilateral Wilms' tumors has varied from secondary partial nephrectomy, to nephrectomy with tumor excision on the more involved side and partial nephrectomy on the opposite side, to bilateral nephrectomy and renal transplantation. Partial nephrectomy after preoperative chemotherapy is a fairly new development in the treatment of Wilms' tumor. This procedure has proved successful in treating nephroblastomatosis[233] and bilateral tumor,[234] although nephron-sparing surgery is not indicated in the case of diffuse anaplasia.

A study of 145 patients with synchronous bilateral Wilms' tumors registered in NWTS-2 and -3 revealed 94 children who underwent initial surgery followed by chemotherapy, with or without irradiation, with a 3-year survival of 82%.[196] The recommended treatment, therefore, for bilateral Wilms' tumor (stage V) is bilateral biopsy, chemotherapy for the most advanced stage, followed by excision of tumor, avoiding bilateral nephrectomy.

Survival rates for NWTS-3 are given in Table 19–14. For anaplastic Wilms' tumor histology, treatment with vincristine, doxorubicin, and cyclophosphamide (VAC) plus abdominal radiation therapy resulted in good disease-free survival and an overall 5-year survival of 87.5% that was not significantly different from that for favorable histology disease.[235]

Prognosis

The prognosis for a child with Wilms' tumor is related to the histology of the tumor, the stage at diagnosis, the child's age, tumor size and, finally, the multimodality treatment used by the pediatric surgeon or urologist, pediatric oncologist, and radiotherapist.[9] Positive prognostic factors are lower stage disease and a favorable histology; negative prognostic factors are unfavorable histology, lymph node involvement, tumor thrombus in the inferior vena cava, and tumor rupture before or during surgery. One exception is that patients with stage I disease with unfavorable histology do as well as those with favorable histology. [198, 236]

TABLE 19–14. **Survival Results from the National Wilms' Tumor Study (NWTS)-3**

Stage	Histology	Regimen	No. of Patients	4-Year Survival Rates (%)	
				Relapse-Free	*Overall*
I	Favorable	V Ad: 10 weeks	306	89	96
		V Ad: 6 months	301	92	97
II	Favorable	V Ad A: 15 months	70	88	94
		V Ad A: 15 months + 20 Gy RT	71	87	90
		Intensive V Ad: 15 months	67	87	91
		Intensive V Ad: 15 months + 20 Gy RT	70	90	95
III	Favorable	V Ad A: 15 months + 10 Gy RT	68	82	91
		V Ad A: 15 months + 20 Gy RT	66	86	87
		Intensive V Ad: 15 months + 10 Gy RT	71	71	85
		Intensive V Ad: 15 months + 20 Gy RT	70	77	85
IV	Favorable	V Ad A: 15 months	64	72	78
		V Ad A C: 15 months	56	78	97
I-III	Unfavorable	V Ad A: 15 months	69	67	68
		V Ad A C: 15 months	61	62	68
IV	Unfavorable	V Ad A: 15 months	12	58	58
		V Ad A C: 15 months	17	53	52
	CCSK	V Ad A: 15 months	25	71	75
		V Ad A C: 15 months	25	60	76
	Rhabdoid	V Ad A: 15 months	13	23	25
		V Ad A C: 15 months	18	27	26

V = vincristine; Ad = dactinomycin (actinomycin D); A = doxorubicin (Adriamycin); C = cyclophosphamide; RT = radiation therapy; CCSK = clear cell sarcoma of the kidney.

From D'Angio GJ, Breslow N, Beckwith JB, et al: The treatment of Wilms' tumor. Results of the Third National Wilms' Tumor Study. Cancer 1989; 64:349.

Tumor Histology

An important contribution by the first NWTS was the recognition that tumor histopathology affected prognosis when certain pathologic categories were defined. Favorable histology includes epithelial differentiation, blastema morphology, and mesenchymal tissue. Anaplasia and sarcomatous changes were noted in a small group of patients (49 out of 427 tumors studied). Twenty-eight (57%) died, as compared with 26 deaths in the remaining 376 patients (6.9%). In this small group, anaplasia[237–239] and sarcomatous changes[211, 240] were termed unfavorable histology. Anaplasia is rarely found in children younger than 2 years of age, with a peak incidence at 5 years of age[241] and an overall incidence of 4.5% in NWTS-3. Succeeding NWTSG data have confirmed the poor prognosis of tumors with unfavorable histology with several exceptions. Stage I anaplastic Wilms' tumors behave clinically like stage I with favorable histology. The 2-year survival for patients with negative lymph nodes is 54% with unfavorable histology and 90% with favorable histology.[214]

Stage

Stage IV and unfavorable histology have similar relapse-free survival rates. The analysis of DNA content has produced useful prognostic information. In stages I and II, patients with DNA aneuploid patterns have significantly lower 2- and 5-year survival rates than those for patients with DNA diploid and DNA tetraploid patterns.[242] However, patients with stage III and stage IV disease are at a high risk of relapse if they have a DNA tetraploid pattern.[243]

Follow-Up

Children with aniridia or hemihypertrophy should be screened with abdominal ultrasound every 3 months until the age of 6. Children with Beckwith-Wiedemann syndrome also should be screened with abdominal ultrasound every 3 months, but until the age of 7.[68, 244, 245] A second Wilms' tumor may develop in the unresected kidney of 1% to 3% of children. The incidence of this metachronous spread is higher if nephrogenic rests were found in the original tumor specimen and the child was younger than 4 years of age. Thus, if nephrogenic rests are found, follow-up is required using the following guidelines:

- If the child is younger than 4 years of age at diagnosis, ultrasound should be performed every 3 months for 6 years.
- If the child is older than 4 years of age at diagnosis, ultrasound should be performed every 3 months for 4 years.
- All other children should be followed every 6 months for 2 years, then yearly for 2 to 3 years.[22, 246]

Long-term follow-up is essential for all patients.[247] Irradiation affects growing cartilage and bone, as well as soft tissues, possibly resulting in scoliosis, shortened height, small or missing ovaries, and slipped epiphyses. Second malignancies also are known to develop in patients treated for Wilms' tumor. Both solid tumors (breast, thyroid, sarcomas) and leukemias have developed.[8, 248] A 2000 article by Paulino and colleagues revealed that 69% of Wilms' tumor patients, treated with radiation therapy at the University of Iowa Children's Hospital between 1968 and 1994, developed late effects, such as muscular hypoplasia, limb length inequality, kyphosis, iliac wing hypoplasia, hypertension, benign neoplasms, second malignancies, scoliosis, and bowel obstruction.[249] Other risk factors include the intensity of therapy (radiation and doxorubicin) and genetic factors.[8]

Clinical Investigations

- Research continues into oncogenes associated with Wilms' tumor, their regulation, ability to control tumor activation, metastatic potential, and refractoriness to chemotherapy.
- Of the newer chemotherapeutic agents, etoposide, cisplatin, and ifosfamide appear to be effective chemotherapeutic agents for recurrent Wilms' tumor; however, their role for improving the prognosis in children with high-stage disease needs to be evaluated.
- Optimization of treatment often means less rather than more treatment, without sacrificing relapse-free survival. Variations in dosage and duration of drug and radiation treatment are being studied to reduce toxicity without compromising results in children whose tumors have a favorable histology and to improve survival in those with unfavorable histology.
- The role of renal sparing for both unilateral and bilateral disease is as yet unclear. Likewise, identifying a subset of children who will benefit from resection only remains to be done. Moreover, the role of pulmonary radiation for metastatic pulmonary disease is under investigation.
- In a 2000 study by Cooper and colleagues, brachytherapy was employed as part of nephron-sparing treatment of Wilms' tumor. Forty-four patients underwent primary chemotherapy followed by partial nephrectomy. The patients with chemoresistant tumors (n = 7) were treated with brachytherapy, and none of the brachytherapy patients had local recurrence.[234]
- Although there are few studies evaluating the usefulness and safety of intraoperative radiation therapy (IORT) in the treatment of Wilms' tumor, the studies that have been done conclude that IORT improves local control, confines radiation to the primary treatment site, and provides complete control of microscopic and gross disease while preserving renal function.[250, 251] The negative aspects of this modality, however, are the complications and late effects associated with radiation in general.

Recommended Reading

Articles giving an overview of Wilms' tumor, its biologic behavior, and how treatment has evolved through coordinated multimodal treatment studies are those written by Beckwith and associates,[2, 163] Grundy and Coppes,[4] Haase,[5] Thomas,[6] Ritchey,[7] Breslow and coworkers,[8, 9] Green and colleagues,[10] and D'Angio and coworkers.[11]

Non-Hodgkin's Lymphoma

Perspective

Childhood non-Hodgkin's lymphomas (NHL) are a heterogeneous group of malignancies that arise from T-cells, B-cells, and their precursors in the lymphoid system. Their systemic nature and the variability in their presentation and patterns of spread reflect their origin from a lineage of cells that migrates throughout the body. Similarly, progress in their treatment mirrors the recognition of their systemic nature and underlying biology. Given the systemic nature of NHL, chemotherapy has become the mainstay of treatment, and specific chemotherapeutic regimens have been developed, based on the underlying cell type of the lymphoma, the primary site, and the extent of disease.

In the past, local therapy resulted in an overall survival of 10% to 30%.[12, 252, 253] Current aggressive multiagent protocols have resulted in overall survival rates of 50% to 90%.[254–256] Of note, childhood NHL differs from adult NHL in the frequencies of immunohistopathologic types and the relative infrequency of nodal as compared with extranodal presentations. There is also a greater propensity for childhood NHL to disseminate noncontiguously, to evolve into leukemia, and to involve the central nervous system.

Epidemiology and Etiology

Epidemiology

Lymphomas comprise 12% of all pediatric cancers, and of these, 55% are non-Hodgkin's and 45% are Hodgkin's disease.[257] NHL is uncommon under the age of 2 years and steadily increases in frequency with age throughout childhood[46]; the male-to-female ratio is 2:1 or 3:1.[46] The frequency of NHL varies markedly in various geographic regions; for example, in equatorial Africa, approximately 50% of childhood cancers are lymphomas, primarily Burkitt's.[13] In addition, the incidence of NHL is increased in patients with disorders associated with abnormal regulation of the immune system.[258] For example, the acquired immunodeficiency syndrome is associated with an increased incidence of NHL.[259] In one study, human immunodeficiency virus–infected children 19 years of age or younger were estimated to have a 360-fold increased risk of developing NHL.[260] The majority of these malignancies are aggressive B-cell, small noncleaved cell, or large cell lymphomas, and they frequently demonstrate evidence of Epstein-Barr virus (EBV) infection.[261]

Etiology

- Immunodeficient states are associated with the development of lymphomas. These are histologically predominantly large cell or immunoblastic, and generally of B-cell origin.[262] A defect in T-cell regulation that permits the expansion of EBV-infected clones of B-cells may explain this association. The X-linked lymphoproliferative syndrome, ataxia-telangiectasia, Wiskott-Aldrich syndrome, and common variable immune deficiency disease are all examples of underlying disorders that place patients at risk of developing NHL.[263]
- Children who receive liver, renal, cardiac, or bone marrow allografts are also at a substantially increased risk of developing NHL because of their immunosuppressive therapy.[264, 265]
- NHL is a relatively uncommon second malignant neoplasm in patients treated for their primary cancer with combined-modality therapy.[266, 267]

Biology

Most childhood NHLs are thought to arise from lymphocyte precursors in the bone marrow and thymus, rather than from immunocompetent lymphoid cells capable of participating in an immune response. The majority of pediatric NHLs can be categorized as small noncleaved cell (Burkitt's) lymphoma, lymphoblastic lymphoma, or large cell lymphoma.[26] The large cell lymphomas are the most heterogeneous group of childhood NHLs: One third are of B-cell origin, a third of T-cell origin, and a third of indeterminate origin. The recently described K_i-1 anaplastic large cell lymphoma comprises approximately 30% to 40% of large cell lymphomas,[268] and the majority are of T-cell origin. In some instances, malignancies which were originally classified as malignant histiocytosis or Hodgkin's disease were subsequently found to be K_i-1 lymphoma.[269]

Specific cytogenetic findings distinguish several of the different subtypes of childhood NHL. Characteristic differences are found not only among different phenotypes, but even within an apparently homogeneous phenotype. Because particular genetic abnormalities may correlate with prognosis, such distinctions are important.[13]

- In Burkitt's lymphoma, the proto-oncogene c-*MYC* is translocated from chromosome 8 to the heavy chain immunoglobulin locus on chromosome 14.[270] Less commonly, c-*MYC* is translocated to chromosome 2, the kappa immunoglobulin light chain locus, or chromosome 22, the lambda immunoglobulin light chain locus.[271]
- Specific chromosomal abnormalities have not been established in lymphoblastic lymphoma, but several translocations have been described. These translocations frequently involve the juxtaposition of T-cell receptor genes and genes encoding transcription factors.[272]
- Characteristic karyotypic abnormalities have not yet been found for most large cell lymphomas, perhaps due to the phenotypically heterogeneous tumors in this category, or because the genetic abnormalities do not involve karyotypic changes. An exception is K_i-1 anaplastic large cell lymphomas, many of which have the chromosomal rearrangement t(2;5)(p23;q35).[273]

Detection and Diagnosis

Clinical Detection

In general, patients present with a limited number of syndromes that tend to correspond to the lymphoma cell type. In one series of 338 children with NHL, 31% of the patients had abdominal tumors, 27% had a mediastinal mass, and 29% had neck primaries (including cervical lymph node primaries).[274] Only 6% had primary lymph node involvement elsewhere, and 8% had miscellaneous extranodal primaries, such as skin, bone, or epidural space. Symptoms are usually of short duration, and relate to location of the primary tumor. Constitutional symptoms, such as fever, weight loss, and night sweats, are unusual in children with NHL.

Children with localized abdominal tumors may present with vomiting, abdominal pain, intussusception, or symptoms mimicking those of appendicitis. A rapidly enlarging abdomen or ascites in an ill child may be indicative of diffuse and massive peritoneal involvement. The majority of these abdominal lymphomas are small noncleaved cell lymphoma (Burkitt's type) and, less commonly, large cell lymphoma. Metastasis to bone marrow[275] or the central nervous system (CNS),[276] or both, is common.

Children with anterior mediastinal masses typically present with cough, wheezing, stridor or shortness of breath. They may have chest pain related to a pleural effusion. Compression of the superior vena cava may cause swelling of the arms and face. There is often associated supraclavicular and cervical adenopathy. These rapidly growing tumors are usually T-cell lymphoblastic lymphomas. They frequently disseminate to the bone marrow, CNS, or testes.

Only a small proportion of children presents with peripheral lymph node involvement outside the head and neck region. A few children present with tumors in unusual extranodal sites such as skin, bone, or the epidural space. These tumors are typically large cell lymphomas and, generally, do not metastasize to the CNS or bone marrow.

Diagnostic Procedures

Surgical biopsy establishes the diagnosis. Although histology remains the primary decision-making criterion, immunophenotyping and enzymatic and cytogenetic studies should supplement morphologic analysis.

- The most suspicious node should be selected for *excisional biopsy.* Needle biopsies are discouraged, although fine-needle aspiration of the nodes has some supporters.[277]
- *Staging laparotomy* is unnecessary because it does not influence treatment or prognosis.[278]
- Aspiration of bone marrow or effusions may provide the diagnosis and obviate the need for a lymph node biopsy.

It is important in these instances to be certain there is sufficient material to perform all tests necessary to confirm the diagnosis. The morphology of cells obtained from effusions can be difficult to interpret and should be used only to make a diagnosis in concert with other studies, such as flow cytometry and immunophenotyping.

- *Laboratory evaluation* should include a complete blood cell count with differential, platelets, erythrocyte sedimentation rate, and reticulocyte count. Electrolytes, uric acid, calcium, phosphorus, lactate dehydrogenase, and tests of renal and liver function should also be obtained. Other studies, such as catecholamines, may be useful in excluding the diagnosis of other tumors.
- *Lumbar puncture* with cytocentrifugation of cerebral spinal fluid (CSF) should be performed.
- Imaging studies include *chest x-ray, CT* or *MRI* of the chest and abdomen (as well as areas of obvious tumor involvement), *bone scan, ultrasound, gallium scintigraphy,* and *plain radiographs,* as indicated.[279, 280]

Classification and Staging

Histopathology

Essentially, all pediatric NHLs are diffuse lymphomas of intermediate or high grade, according to the International Working Formulation. Table 19–15 lists the various histopathologic subtypes.[281] The correlation with immune markers and approximate frequencies are also noted.

Staging

The Ann Arbor staging system for Hodgkin's disease is not appropriate for pediatric NHL because of noncontiguous patterns of involvement and the frequency of extranodal

TABLE 19–15. **Distribution of Histopathologic Types of Non-Hodgkin's Lymphoma with Corresponding Immunophenotype**

Histology	Phenotype	Frequency
Nodular (follicular)		Extremely rare
Diffuse		
Large cell (histiocytic)		25% to 30%
Anaplastic, peripheral	Mostly T-cell	
Diffuse, mediastinal	Mostly B-cell	
Lymphoblastic	Mostly T-cell, but also precursor T-cell, precursor B-cell	30%
Undifferentiated (small noncleaved)	Mature B-cell	40% to 50%
Burkitt's	B-cell (surface Ig chains, usually IgM)	
Non-Burkitt's (pleomorphic)	B-cell (surface Ig chains, usually IgM)	

disease. Several of the systems used for staging[13] are based in some manner on the burden of tumor present at diagnosis, since this correlates with survival.

The system most widely used for pediatric NHL is the St. Jude Children's Research Hospital Staging System for Non-Hodgkin's Lymphoma (Table 19–16).[14] This system can be used for the classification of all pediatric NHLs; furthermore, it takes into account the site, as well as extent, of disease, and can be applied with the use of a minimum number of standard imaging studies and invasive procedures. It also has proved successful in distinguishing children with a favorable prognosis (lower stage, localized disease; stages I and II) from those children with a less favorable prognosis (more extensive or disseminated disease; stages III and IV).[14]

Principles of Treatment

Until the mid-1970s, treatment of NHL with surgery or radiation therapy produced long-term survival in only 10% to 30% of children,[12, 252, 253] the majority of whom had localized disease and favorable presentations. Because the vast majority of patients have occult disseminated disease at diagnosis, intensive, systemic, multiagent chemotherapy regimens now have become an integral part of treatment. Moreover, the improved ability to identify tumor subtypes, together with advances in clinical staging methods, has led to the development of tumor-specific chemotherapy regimens. Optimal initial therapy is essential, because patients whose disease recurs are less likely to benefit from salvage therapy.

TABLE 19–16. **St. Jude Children's Research Hospital Staging System for Non-Hodgkin's Lymphoma**

Stage	Descriptor
I	A single tumor (extranodal) or single anatomic area (nodal), with the exclusion of mediastinum or abdomen
II	A single tumor (extranodal) with regional node involvement, or two or more nodal areas on the same side of the diaphragm, or two single (extranodal) tumors with or without regional node involvement on the same side of the diaphragm, or a primary gastrointestinal tract tumor, usually in the ileocecal area, with or without involvement of associated mesenteric nodes only*
III	Two single tumors (extranodal) on opposite sides of the diaphragm, or two or more nodal areas above and below the diaphragm, or includes all primary intrathoracic tumors (mediastinal, pleural, and thymic), or includes all extensive primary intra-abdominal disease,* or includes all paraspinal or epidural tumors, regardless of other tumor site(s)
IV	Any of the above with initial central nervous system or bone marrow involvement†

*A distinction is made between apparently localized gastrointestinal tract lymphoma and more extensive intra-abdominal disease; their different patterns of survival require appropriate therapy. Stage II disease typically is limited to a segment of the gut, ± associated mesenteric nodes only, and the primary tumor can be completely removed grossly by segmental excision. Stage III disease typically exhibits spread to para-aortic and retroperitoneal areas by implants and plaques in mesentery or peritoneum, or by direct infiltration of structures adjacent to the primary tumor. Ascites may be present, and complete resection of all gross tumor is not possible.

†If marrow involvement is present initially, the proportion of abnormal cells must be ≤25% in an otherwise normal marrow aspirate with a normal peripheral blood picture.

Adapted from Link MP, Donaldson SS: The lymphomas and lymphadenopathy, p 1323. In: Nathan DG, Orkin SH (eds): Nathan and Oski's Hematology of Infancy and Childhood. Philadelphia, W.B. Saunders Co., 1998.

Surgery

Routine staging laparotomy is not indicated because it is unlikely to alter systemic therapy and may, indeed, delay it.[278] In patients with abdominal tumors, laparotomy may be indicated for treatment of an acute abdomen or to establish a diagnosis. However, there have been reports of inadvertent intestinal perforation during tumor biopsy; therefore, this procedure should be performed selectively.[282] Of note, in patients with Burkitt's lymphoma, one can consider debulking, but only if the tumor can be removed with minimal morbidity.[283, 284]

Chemotherapy

NHL is exquisitely sensitive to chemotherapy. Because even children with apparently localized NHL have a high likelihood of having micrometastatic disseminated disease, all children, regardless of stage or histology, should be treated with chemotherapy.[26] Multiagent chemotherapy repeatedly has been demonstrated to be superior to treatment with single agents.[285–287] The precise combination of agents used depends on the subtype of lymphoma.

For children with small noncleaved cell (Burkitt's type) lymphoma, the most effective agents include cyclophosphamide, doxorubicin, vincristine, and prednisone. In patients with advanced-stage disease, a short course of high-dose intensive therapy with these agents, as well as high-dose methotrexate, cytosine arabinoside, etoposide, and, in some instances, ifosfamide, has been proved effective.[288, 289] Because of the high risk of CNS relapse, intrathecal therapy is included in the treatment.

In children with lymphoblastic lymphoma, the LSA2-L2 regimen has been proved effective; this regimen consists of induction, consolidation, and maintenance phases and, in addition to the above-mentioned agents, includes thioguanine, asparaginase, carmustine (BCNU), hydroxyurea, and intrathecal chemotherapy. The optimal duration for children with limited disease is uncertain because it appears that treatment for 6 months or less is associated with a higher rate of relapse.[286, 290] For children with advanced or disseminated disease, more intensive therapy for 15 to 24 months with the same agents is effective.[254]

The treatment for children with large cell lymphoma is less well defined; children with this type of lymphoma have only recently been recognized as having a distinct subtype. Some of the best responses and highest cure rates have been documented in Berlin-Frankfurt-Munster (BFM) protocols, employing methotrexate, cytosine arabinoside, prednisone, cyclophosphamide, etoposide, vincristine, doxorubicin, and ifosfamide.[291]

Radiation Therapy

The role of radiation therapy in the management of NHL has progressively decreased as chemotherapeutic regimens have become more effective. It retains an important role in selected situations, but, in general, does not improve disease-free survival (DFS) and may add unnecessary morbidity. Indeed, reports from the POG[286] and St. Jude Children's Research Hospital[274] have demonstrated successful local and systemic control with chemotherapy alone for children with Murphy/St. Jude stage I and stage II disease, regardless of histology. The addition of localized radiation therapy to chemotherapy has shown no benefit for patients with advanced-stage disease.[274]

Situations in which radiation therapy is appropriate include the following:

- Emergency x-ray radiation therapy is used in the setting of acute airway compromise or spinal cord compression. A hyperfractionated regimen should be considered.
- Some form of presymptomatic treatment of the CNS is warranted in the majority of cases because 30% to 35% of children will develop CNS lymphoma in its absence. Intrathecal chemotherapy alone is effective in most settings without the added morbidity of cranial irradiation. However, patients with CNS involvement, especially those with cranial nerve palsies or spinal cord compression, frequently are treated with radiation therapy and intrathecal chemotherapy given on an urgent basis to prevent permanent neurologic sequelae.[292]
- Radiation therapy is given to selected patients who do not achieve a complete response following initial chemotherapy, with or without surgery.
- Radiation therapy is used to relieve pain associated with uncontrollable disease. It also may be administered as consolidation before BMT in patients with recurrent disease.
- Patients at high risk for meningeal recurrences have been successfully treated with radiation therapy.[293]

Specific indications for cranial radiation therapy include overt leptomeningeal lymphoma at diagnosis, evidence for leukemic transformation (bone marrow involvement with >25% blasts) at diagnosis,[294] and focal cranial nerve deficits.[292] The role of radiation therapy for primary NHL of bone in children is unknown. Excellent local control is afforded by its use; however, there are data that show good outcomes for children with NHL of bone who did not receive local radiation therapy.[295]

Of note, the frequency of second malignancies may be increased following the use of radiation.[296] Indeed, the late effects and toxicities associated with radiation therapy are considerable. Researchers are constantly developing new techniques and protocols in an attempt to limit these effects.[293, 297]

Special Considerations

Treatment of children with NHL can be complicated by a tumor lysis syndrome that can cause severe metabolic derangements and renal failure. Hyperuricemia, hyperkalemia, hyperphosphatemia, and hypocalcemia are associated with this syndrome; it most commonly complicates therapy for Burkitt's lymphoma and T-cell lymphoblastic lymphoma. Careful management is essential, and the temporary use of dialysis may be required. In a study from St. Jude Children's Research Hospital, renal failure in most patients was not attributed to hyperuricemia or hyperphosphatemia; rather, it was more closely associated with oliguria in the 12 hours preceding and 24 hours following initiation of chemotherapy. This finding underscores the importance of careful fluid management.[298]

Children with recurrent NHL should be considered for autologous BMT (high-dose chemotherapy with autologous stem cell rescue).[299, 300]

Results and Prognosis

Results

Prior to 1975, when therapy was primarily directed to the identifiable gross tumor, few children survived this disease (Fig. 19–8).[301] Those children who did well had favorable presentations, including limited resectable abdominal disease, or involvement of a single nodal region or of a single bone. With the current intensive multiagent regimens, survival is excellent for all patients except those with grossly disseminated disease. Most recurrences in NHL occur within 12 months of diagnosis and are uncommon beyond 2 years.[290] Histology is no longer of great prognostic significance for outcome; however, it is the basis for choosing the therapeutic regimen:

- Children with stage I or II disease have an 85% to 90% 2-year DFS.[286, 302] Patients with a nonlymphoblastic histology may fare somewhat better than those with lymphoblastic disease.
- Children with stage III disease have a 60% to 80% 2-year DFS, with follow-up in most studies substantially longer than 2 years.[254, 256, 274]
- The outcome for children with stage IV small noncleaved cell lymphoma or B-cell leukemia has improved to 60% to 80% DFS with short courses of intensive chemotherapy.[261] Those with stage IV lymphoblastic lymphoma (T-cell acute lymphoblastic leukemia) have a 60% to 80% EFS.[256]

Prognosis

- The *tumor burden* at presentation is the principal determinant of outcome.[274] The *clinical stage* assigned to the patient, which is determined by the tumor burden and by disease extent, also predicts outcome.
- The *serum levels* of several substances also appear to correlate with prognosis. It is likely that they reflect tumor bulk, although other biologic explanations are possible. The most predictive substances are lactate dehydrogenase and the interleukin-2 receptor.[303]
- *Bone marrow* or *CNS involvement* at diagnosis has been associated with a poor prognosis.[14] However, newer, more intensive therapies appear to result in significantly improved outcomes for these children with disseminated disease.[289]

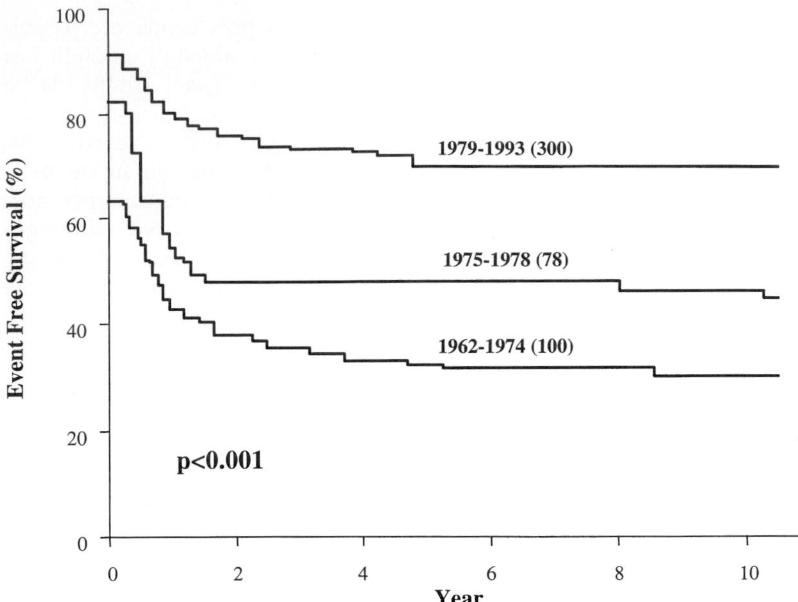

Figure 19–8. Event-free survival of patients with non-Hodgkin's lymphoma treated from 1962 to 1993 at St. Jude Children's Research Hospital. The numbers in parentheses are the total number of patients. Because some patients were not in complete remission at year 0, the curves do not begin at 100%. From 1962 to 1974, a variety of chemotherapy programs were used along with some use of local irradiation. From 1975 to 1978, a single combined-modality protocol was used. From 1979 to 1993, treatment was based on the stage and histologic type of lymphoma. (From Sandlund JT, Downing JR, Crist WM: Non-Hodgkin's lymphoma in childhood. N Engl J Med 1996; 334:1238, with permission. Copyright © 1996 Massachusetts Medical Society. All rights reserved.)

Clinical Investigations

New approaches to diagnosis and therapy are under way that may improve our ability to cure children with NHL.

- A more refined identification of prognostic factors based on biochemistry and molecular genetics could allow a more tailored approach to therapy.
- For patients with particularly poor prognostic factors, such as those with undifferentiated (small noncleaved cell) NHL involving the CNS or bone marrow, more intensive therapies are under investigation.
- New chemotherapeutic agents and monoclonal antibody–targeted immunotoxins are being developed.
- Substances to protect or overcome the adverse effects of therapy may improve the therapeutic ratio by allowing more drug administration (see Chapter 6, Principles of Radiation Oncology and Cancer Radiotherapy). Examples are mesna, to protect the bladder, and hematopoietic growth factors, to ameliorate myelosuppression.
- Advances in delineating the nature of the neoplastic proliferation, for example, chromosomal translocations, c-*MYC* gene activity, may permit therapy that is targeted toward these abnormalities.

Recommended Reading

A historical perspective on NHL is offered by Rosenberg and colleagues.[12] Shad and McGrath[13] and Link and Donaldson[14] provide updated reviews on the treatment of NHL in childhood.

Rhabdomyosarcoma

Perspective

Rhabdomyosarcoma (RMS) is an aggressive malignancy that arises from embryonal mesenchyme, with the potential for differentiating into skeletal muscle.[304, 305] Since Stout's[306] landmark series in 1946, progress in the understanding and treatment of this complex neoplasm has been rapid. RMS can arise in almost any location, is locally invasive, and disseminates early in its course. In the past, the only cures that were accomplished were with radical surgery, and these cures were possible only in the few children who presented without metastases; significant disfigurement and loss of function were common sequelae. High-dose radiation therapy increased the potential for local control but caused a different set of morbidities.[307, 308] As chemotherapy became increasingly effective in both eliminating micrometastatic disease and assisting in local control, the need for aggressive surgery and large-volume irradiation diminished.[309] Overall, survival rates have concomitantly increased from less than about 20% in the 1960s to as high as 70%.[310]

The biologic heterogeneity of this tumor, reflected in its different histologic patterns, and the spectrum of sites involved have made the study of RMS difficult.[311] A paramount role in this progress has been played by investigators as part of the Intergroup Rhabdomyosarcoma Studies (IRSs); this investigational group is now in its fifth generation of protocols. Although IRS-I, -II, and -III were based on a surgically oriented clinical grouping system dependent on the tumor that remained after initial surgery, IRS-IV and -V were based on a more biologically oriented staging system, which is discussed later. Both international and single-institutional studies also have been important, with international studies including those from the SIOP and the Children's Solid Tumor Group in the United Kingdom.

Epidemiology and Etiology

Epidemiology

RMSs account for more than half of childhood soft tissue sarcomas, although these account for only 4% to 8% of childhood malignancies.[26, 312] In the United States, it is the third most common extracranial solid tumor, after NB and Wilms' tumor,[304] with about 250 cases being reported annually.[305] The incidence rate is higher among black children, but this difference is only seen between the females; the male incidences are the same for both ethnic groups.[312] Children aged 2 to 5 years are most commonly affected, and 85% of cases occur before the age of 15 years (Fig. 19–9).[16–18, 313]

Etiology

The etiology of RMS is unknown, but researchers are making progress in terms of discovering environmental factors, heredity, and biology:

- Of interest is a 1993 case control report of 332 children with RMS enrolled on IRS-III, in which an association was detected between RMS and maternal and paternal marijuana and cocaine use.[314]
- An increased frequency of congenital anomalies involving the gastrointestinal (GI), genitourinary, cardiovascular, and central nervous systems exists in children with RMS.[315] RMS is more common in children with neurofibromatosis type I and the Beckwith-Wiedemann syndrome.[316] The pattern of cancers in relatives of children with RMS occasionally has been compared with that in the Li-Fraumeni syndrome, in which germline mutations of *TP53* exist.[317, 318]

Genetics

- In alveolar RMS, 70% of children have a t(2:13)(p35:q14) or t(1:13)(p36:q14) translocation, which may induce cell proliferation via transcriptional

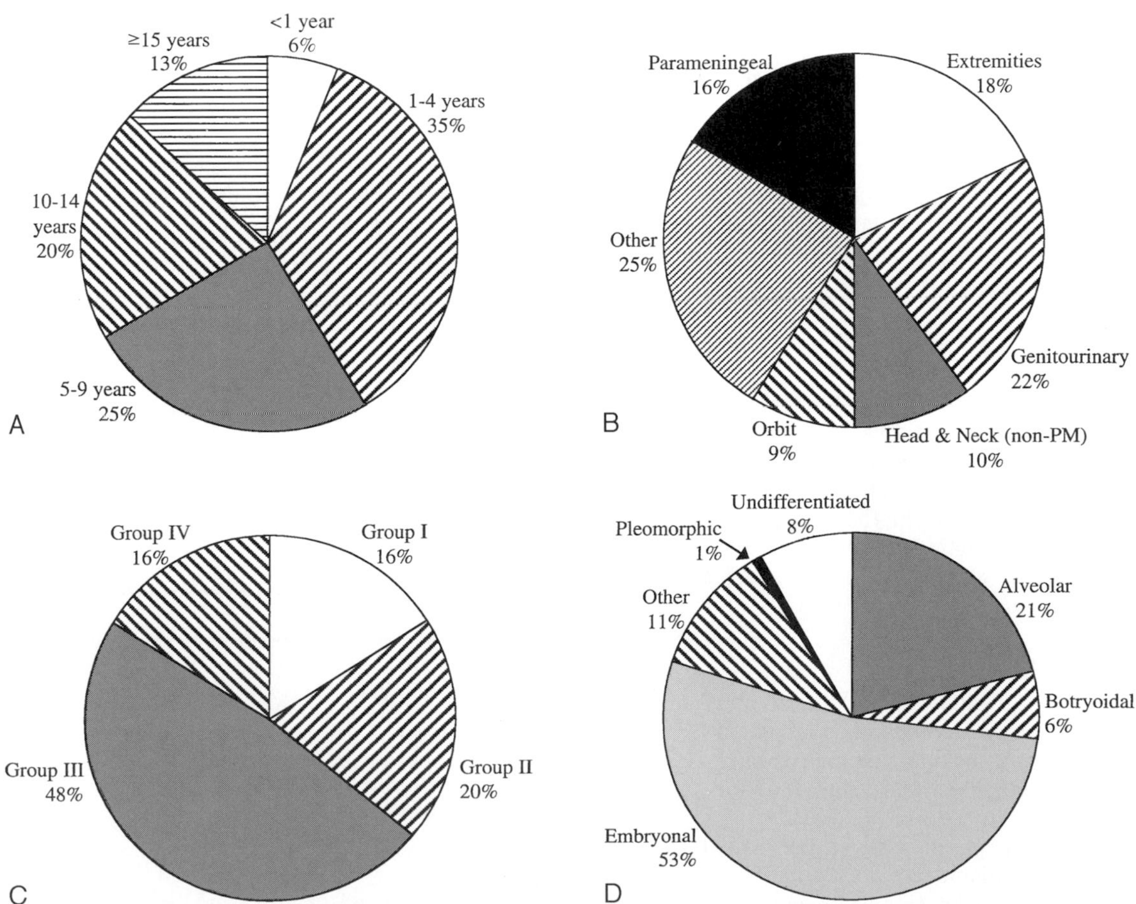

Figure 19–9. Clinical features of rhabdomyosarcoma from URS-I, -II, -III pooled data. (A) Age at presentation. (B) Site of primary tumor. (C) Clinical group. (D) Histology. PM = parameningeal. (Modified from Wexler LH, Helman LJ: Rhabdomyosarcoma and the undifferentiated sarcomas. In: Pizzo PA, Poplack DG (eds): Principles and Practice of Pediatric Oncology, 3rd ed, p 799. Philadelphia, Lippincott-Raven, 1997, with permission.)

deregulation.[319] In embryonal RMS, loss of heterozygosity at the 11p15.5 locus is found.

- The MyoD protein family of gene products control myogenesis and the cessation of cell cycling.[320] MyoD expression can be determined with antibodies, myogenin and MyoD1, and can be used to differentiate RMS from other small blue round cell tumors of childhood.[321, 322]
- N-*MYC* amplification is associated with alveolar RMS and is associated with an inferior prognosis.[323]
- *TP53* mutations can be demonstrated in many RMS tumors and may relate to radiochemotherapy resistance.[324]

Detection and Diagnosis

Clinical Detection

RMS commonly presents as an asymptomatic mass with poorly defined margins. It may infiltrate along fascial planes and into surrounding tissues. The most common sites of metastases are lung, bone, bone marrow, liver, distant muscles, brain, and lymph nodes.[325, 326] Specific presentations relate to the involved site[304]; the frequency of involvement in primary sites is shown in Figure 19–9. The following are primary sites, with the common symptoms at presentation:

- *Orbit*: Swelling, proptosis, discoloration, limitation of extraocular motion.
- *Other head and neck sites*: Hoarseness, polyps, obstruction, dysphagia, decreased hearing, persistent otitis, sinusitis or parotitis, and cranial nerve palsies (particularly the facial nerve). Penetration into the brain can occur with parameningeal sites and mimic an intracranial mass, with headache, vomiting, and diplopia.
- *Retroperitoneum*: GI discomfort or other mass-related symptoms.
- *Genitourinary tract*: Urethral, vaginal, or other perineal masses; hematuria; urinary frequency or retention. Paratesticular RMS can appear as a hydrocele, incarcerated hernia, testicular torsion, or mass.
- *Extremity*: Painful or asymptomatic mass.
- *Trunk*: Mass simulating a hernia or hematoma, or causing a classic superior vena cava syndrome.

Diagnostic Procedures

- *Radiography, CT*, and *MRI* of the involved area and adjacent structures are applied as indicated.[327, 328]
- *Laboratory tests* include complete blood cell count with differential, liver and renal function tests, and urinalysis.
- *Myelography* or *spinal MRI* is performed if spinal cord–related symptoms are present.
- An *arteriogram* or *inferior venacavagram* may assist in determining operability.
- *Biopsy* of the lesion establishes the diagnosis, and should be performed before extensive surgery.
- Evaluation for metastases should include bone marrow biopsy, chest CT, bone scan, liver scan, and abdominal scan.

Specific examinations may include the following:

- *Head and neck*: Skull or dental films, middle ear tomography, lumbar puncture with CSF cytology.
- *Retroperitoneum*: IVP.
- *Genitourinary tract*: Barium enema, IVP, voiding cystourethrogram, ultrasound, cystoscopy, and pelvic examination with the child under anesthesia.

Cytogenetic testing is gaining in importance in increasing diagnostic specificity and formulating tumor-targeted therapy.[329, 330]

Classification and Staging

Histopathology

Most RMS subtypes are soft, fleshy tumors with variations in the extent of invasion and necrosis. Cross-striations and periodic acid-Schiff positivity (from cytoplasmic glycogen) may be seen by light microscopy. Intracytoplasmic filaments and Z-band material may be identified by electron microscopy. Immunohistochemical identifiers include anti-desmin, anti–muscle-specific actin, and the muscle regulatory gene *MyoD1*.[322, 331]

Although the classic four histologic subtypes are embryonal (including botryoidal), alveolar, pleomorphic, and mixed (see Fig. 19–9), the International Classification of Rhabdomyosarcomas project has devised a new system with prognostic relevance and greater reproducibility. Table 19–17 denotes the types, frequencies, and prognoses.[332]

- *Botryoid*: This "grape-like" polypoid variant of embryonal RMS occurs in mucosa-lined organs, including the bladder, vagina, nasopharynx, middle ear, and biliary tree. The stroma is loose with a myxoid character. These tumors are generally localized.
- *Spindle cell*: Spindle-shaped cells and low cellularity characterize this type. It is most commonly paratesticular.
- *Embryonal*: The cells are blastemal and tend to differentiate into striated muscle cells, with cross-striations

TABLE 19–17. **International Classification of Rhabdomyosarcomas**

Histologic Subtype	Frequency (%)	Actuarial 5-yr Survival (%)
I. *Superior prognosis*		
A. Botryoid rhabdomyosarcoma	6	95
B. Spindle cell rhabdomyosarcoma	3	88
II. *Intermediate prognosis*		
A. Alveolar rhabdomyosarcoma	49	66
III. *Poor prognosis*		
A. Alveolar rhabdomyosarcoma	32	54
B. Undifferentiated sarcoma	1	40
IV. *Other*	9	

Data taken from Newton W, Gehan E, Webber B, et al: Classification of rhabdomyosarcomas and related sarcomas. Cancer 1995; 76:1073.

TABLE 19–18. **The IRS Early Grouping System for Rhabdomyosarcomas**

Group	Descriptor
I	Localized disease, completely resected. a. Confined to muscle or organ of origin b. Infiltration outside the muscle or organ of origin
II	Total gross resection with: a. Microscopic residual disease b. Regional lymphatic spread, resected c. Both
III	Incomplete resection with gross residual disease. a. After biopsy only b. After major resection (>50%)
IV	Distant metastatic disease present at onset

IRS = International Rhabdomyosarcoma Studies.
From Halperin EC, Constine LS, Tarbell NJ, et al: Pediatric Radiation Oncology, 3rd ed. Philadelphia, Lippincott Williams & Wilkins, 1999.

present in about one third of cases. The cells are fusiform or stellate, and cellularity is moderate.

- *Alveolar*: The cells tend to line connective tissue septa, reminiscent of alveoli, and may be arranged in strands, clefts, sheets, and clusters. The cells are round and cross-striations are rare. This type is frequent in the extremities of older children.
- *Undifferentiated*: The cells are primitive noncommitted mesenchymal cells arrayed in a diffuse pattern. Because the common antigenic markers are negative, this is a diagnosis of exclusion.

Historically, some patients have been entered into IRS protocols with tumors classified as *extraosseous Ewing's sarcoma* that arise in soft tissue.[333] This tumor is morphologically and cytologically identical to Ewing's sarcoma of bone and is treated accordingly (see section on Ewing's sarcoma).

Staging

The initial system used by the IRS group was a clinicopathologic "grouping" based on the extent of disease at the time of treatment, which essentially corresponded to the completeness of surgery before protocol entry (Table 19–18; see Fig. 19–9). Several weaknesses were inherent in this system: Occasionally, the implied emphasis on maximum surgical debulking led to inappropriately morbid procedures; surgical approaches were not uniformly applied in different institutions; in addition, staging did not reflect tumor biology, such as tumor size, invasiveness, and lymph node involvement.[334, 335]

With the advent of IRS-III, a pretreatment staging system was developed, based on the tumor-node-metastasis–International Union Against Cancer (TNM-UICC) system used by SIOP, which reflected the disease characteristics at diagnosis. This currently used TNM staging system emphasizes tumor size and invasiveness (a/b, T1/T2, respectively), nodal status, and identifiable metastasis. Essentially, stage 1 tumors are in favorable sites (Table 19–19); stage 2 tumors are in unfavorable sites, but they are small (<5 cm) with negative lymph nodes. Stage 3 tumors are in unfavorable sites, and of large size or with positive lymph nodes. Stage 4 tumors are of any size with hematogenous metastasis. This staging system determines the chemotherapeutic regimen to be used, whereas the older IRS clinical grouping system is used to determine the radiotherapeutic guidelines.

Principles of Treatment

The difficulty in eradicating both local and systemic disease while minimizing cosmetic and functional morbidities, further complicated by the varied sites and histologies of RMS, makes its therapy a challenge. With the exception of patients with orbital or bladder primary sites, surgery plus radiation therapy alone has been curative in less than 25% of patients[326]; substantial functional and cosmetic morbidity may result from this approach to therapy. Chemotherapy is oriented toward eradicating micrometastatic disease and reducing the extent of local disease, whereas radiation therapy and surgery must achieve local control. However, the need for aggressive, morbid surgical procedures has diminished, except in selected situations. Nonetheless, the optimal sequencing and intensity of the three modalities are continually evolving.

A summary of the IRS-IV guidelines presents recent

TABLE 19–19. **TNM Pretreatment Staging Classification of Rhabdomyosarcomas for IRS-IV**

Stage	T	T Size	N	M	Tumor Sites
1	T1 or T2	a or b	Any N	M0	Orbit Head and neck (excluding parameningeal) Genitourinary—nonbladder/nonprostate
2	T1 or T2	a	N0 or NX	M0	Bladder/prostate Extremity Head and neck parameningeal Other (including trunk, retroperitoneum, etc.)
3	T1 or T2	a b	N1 Any N	M0	Same as for stage 2
4	T1 or T2	a or b	Any N	M1	All

T1 = tumor confined to anatomic site of origin; T2 = extension; a = ≤5 cm in diameter; b = >5 cm in diameter.
N = regional nodes; NX = clinical status unknown; N0 = not clinically involved; N1 = clinically involved.
M = metastasis; M0 = none; M1 = present.
From Halperin EC, Constine LS, Tarbell NJ, et al: Pediatric Radiation Oncology, 3rd ed. Philadelphia, Lippincott Williams & Wilkins, 1999, with permission.

recommendations for the integration of the three modalities (Table 19–20).[313] Site-specific details follow a general review of the modalities.

Surgery

The role of surgery is to establish the diagnosis and participate with the other modalities in accomplishing local control of the primary tumor. Initial surgery should be an incisional or needle biopsy for diagnosis. Wide resection of the primary tumor, including surrounding normal tissue, offers a reasonable chance for local control. This is site dependent, in terms of both feasibility and associated morbidity. Based on pooled IRS data (see Fig. 19–9), if patients with metastatic disease are excluded, then 16% of patients have minimally invasive disease that can be completely resected (group I), and 20% can undergo subtotal resection leaving microscopic disease (group II).[16–18, 310, 336]

Reoperation for microscopic residual disease following an initial excision is indicated when the first operation is considered suboptimal. This approach is known as *pretreatment re-excision* (PRE) in the IRS guidelines and is site dependent (see "Special Considerations"). Reoperation following chemotherapy as a second-look procedure may

TABLE 19–20. **Therapy Recommendations for IRS-IV, 1991–Present**

Site	TNM Stage	Clinical Group	Operative*/RT Considerations	Radiation Therapy[a]	Chemotherapy[b]
Orbit and eyelid	1	I	Nonexcisional biopsy appropriate.	None	VA
		II	RT to tumor + margin, not whole orbit.	RT	VA
		III		RT vs HFRT	VAC vs VAI vs VIE
Other head and neck lymph (nonparameningeal)	1	I	Biopsy nodes; if positive, consider excision.	None	VAC vs VAI vs VIE
		II		RT	VAC vs VAI vs VIE
		III		RT vs HFRT	VAC vs VAI vs VIE
Paratesticular	1	I	Orchidectomy, resect entire spermatic cord via inguinal incision.	None	VA
		II		RT	VAC vs VAI vs VIE
		III	Sample abdominal/pelvic nodes except Group I.† If scrotal skin involved/violated, area resected + RT.	RT vs HFRT	VAC vs VAI vs VIE
Vulva and vagina	1	I	"Radical" excision *in*appropriate.	None	VAC vs VAI vs VIE
		II	Gross excision often possible at "2nd look" (week 9). Biopsy suspicious nodes; dissection inappropriate. Brachytherapy possible.	RT	VAC vs VAI vs VIE
		III		RT	VAC vs VAI vs VIE
Uterus/cervix	1	I	Hysterectomy only if necessary.	None	VAC vs VAI vs VIE
		II	Preserve ovaries and vagina if possible.	RT	VAC vs VAI vs VIE
		III		RT vs HFRT	VAC vs VAI vs VIE
Cranial parameningeal	2/3	I	Biopsy suspicious nodes; if positive, consider excision. RT day 0 (limited intracranial extension/base of skull erosion/cranial neuropathy) or wk 9.	None for stage 2 RT for stage 3	VAC vs VAI vs VIE
		II		RT	VAC vs VAI vs VIE
		III		RT vs HFRT	VAC vs VAI vs VIE
Extremity	2/3	I	Wide/radical limb-sparing resection. Sample regional nodes. If positive, sample more proximal group.†	None for stage 2 RT for stage 3	VAC vs VAI vs VIE
		II		RT	VAC vs VAI vs VIE
		III	Avoid circumferential RT.	RT vs HFRT	VAC vs VAI vs VIE
Genitourinary (bladder and prostate)	2/3	I	Total resection ± partial cystectomy (diagnosis or "2nd look" after chemo/RT). Node sampling (iliac and para-aortic) only if laparotomy.	None for stage 2 RT for stage 3	VAC vs VAI vs VIE
		II		RT	VAC vs VAI vs VIE
		III		RT vs HFRT	VAC vs VAI vs VIE
Chest wall, trunk, retroperitoneum, and other	2/3	I	Wide excision if feasible (diagnosis, or re-excision pre-chemo or "2nd look"). RT for abdominal tumors usually entails multiple cone-downs.	None for stage 2 RT for stage 3	VAC vs VAI vs VIE
		II		RT	VAC vs VAI vs VIE
		III		RT vs HFRT	VAC vs VAI vs VIE
Any site	4	I	Gross residual disease, RT week 18.5 (except for select parameningeal tumors). Whole lung RT for nodules ± boost. Pulmonary nodules can be resected post chemo/RT if acceptable lung function is preserved.	RT	1. Adr/I, vs
		II		RT	2. V × 6/Mel × 3, vs
		III		RT	3. I/E × 4 followed by VAC ± same drug pair

V = vincristine; A = actinomycin D; C = cyclophosphamide; E = etoposide; I = ifosfamide; Adr = doxorubicin; Mel = melphalan.

*For other head and neck and cranial parameningeal sarcomas, cosmetic and functional outcome determine the extent of surgery, at diagnosis and/or second look.

†Positive inguinal/supraclavicular or iliac/para-aortic nodes denote distant spread, i.e., stage 4.

[a]RT = conventional radiation therapy: group I or II patients = 41.4 Gy; group III patients = 50.4 Gy. HFRT = hyperfractionated radiation therapy; group III patients = 59.4 Gy.

[b]All chemotherapy regimens followed by VAC.

Modified from Wexler LH, Helman LJ: Rhabdomyosarcoma and the undifferentiated sarcomas. In: Pizzo PA, Poplack DG: Principles and Practice of Pediatric Oncology, 3rd ed, p 799. Philadelphia, Lippincott-Raven, 1997, with permission.

be appropriate.[337] Surgery as a salvage procedure, sometimes necessitating an exenteration, is sometimes appropriate with tumors that are otherwise therapy resistant.[338]

The role of lymph node dissection is still being defined. In general, one performs a biopsy on clinically suspicious nodes, but the guidelines for elective dissection are site specific as a result of variability in the frequency of lymph node involvement. For example, routine dissection is performed for patients with extremity tumors, but sampling alone is appropriate for many patients with paratesticular tumors.[339]

Radiation Therapy

The goal of radiation therapy is to provide local-regional control, with or without surgery, but always in conjunction with chemotherapy. Radiation therapy is coordinated with the other modalities so as not to impair surgical healing or drug administration. Major considerations include the primary site (see "Special Considerations"), the suppression of bone marrow, and the interaction of radiation therapy with chemotherapeutic agents.

The problem of local control is highlighted by data from IRS-II.[17, 340] Excluding "special pelvic" sites (whose location restricted the use of radiation therapy), the frequency of local failure was 10% in group II, but was 20% for group III and 41% for group IV. When local relapse was analyzed as a percentage of all relapses, it accounted for 46% of relapses in group I (despite "complete" surgical removal of tumor) and 36%, 53%, and 20% of relapses in groups II, III, and IV, respectively. Patients with tumors with an unfavorable histology or with large tumors fared worse.

RMSs may extensively infiltrate tissues, and radiation portals must encompass the entire extent of the tumor volume. Margins are based on the confidence with which this volume can be identified and on the location of critical normal tissues that should be excluded. For radiation therapy given in conjunction with chemotherapy, a 2-cm margin is generally appropriate. Epiphyses are shielded if this is consistent with adequate tumor coverage. Currently, patients with stage 1 to 2 group I disease do not receive radiation therapy, based on IRS-III data (see Table 19–20).

Aggressive radiation therapy to doses of 50 to 65 Gy can provide local control of gross residual or microscopic disease in 90% of patients[308]; however, the higher dose may result in substantial late effects and morbidity.[341] For example, in IRS-III, the radiation dose for group I and group II patients was 41.4 Gy, but in group III with gross residual disease, 50.4 Gy was given for children 6 years of age or older with tumors 5 cm or larger, and an intermediate dose of 45 Gy was given for children who either were older or had larger tumors, but not both.[15] The local control rate was 90% for groups I and II, but was unacceptably low for group III. In an effort to treat these patients with higher doses without increased normal tissue damage, hyperfractionated radiotherapy is being prospectively tested (1.1 Gy b.i.d. to 59.4 Gy versus 1.8 Gy q.d. to 50.4 Gy) (see Table 19–20); preliminary data support its safety.[336] Data from Memorial Sloan-Kettering[342] and St. Jude[343] support the efficacy of this approach. Current recommendations using single daily fractions are that patients with bulky local RMS should be treated to at least 50 Gy, and postoperative microscopic disease should be treated to at least 40 Gy.[344]

Interstitial radiation therapy will occasionally be advantageous for selected sites and circumstances,[345] and high-dose-rate IORT has been used successfully.[251] However, as always, the improved local control gained should be weighed carefully against the increased risk of late effects associated with high radiation doses.

Chemotherapy

In the 1960s and 1970s, the adjuvant administration of chemotherapy for totally or subtotally resected localized disease was shown to increase survival probability from 10% to 40% to 60% to 80%.[309, 346] Chemotherapy subsequently became a routine part of the therapy of RMS, and several trials were undertaken to establish the optimal drug combinations.

- IRS-I determined that VAC was not superior to VA in group II disease, and "pulse" VAC plus doxorubicin (Adriamycin) was not superior to "pulse" VAC alone in groups II and III disease.[16]
- IRS-II built upon these results and showed no advantage of VAC over VA for group I patients, and no benefit to pulse VAC over cyclic sequential VA for group II patients.[17]
- IRS-III began in 1984 and ended in 1991; it separated patients by histology into either a favorable (embryonal) or unfavorable (alveolar, anaplastic, and monomorphous cell types) category. Several drug pairs (doxorubicin and dacarbazine, dactinomycin and etoposide, dactinomycin and dacarbazine) appear to have been associated with gains in survival.[18]
- IRS-IV began in August 1991 and uses the new staging system to assign drug therapy, as previously discussed (see Table 19–20). The investigators published an initial report on group III patients on the regimen of etoposide, ifosfamide, and vincristine with hyperfractionated radiation therapy.[347] Of the 68 patients enrolled, 73% have achieved a complete response to therapy.

Overall, in addition to VAC, several drugs are shown to be active in RMS. These include dacarbazine, cisplatin, melphalan, methotrexate, etoposide, and ifosfamide; doxorubicin continues to be used in European studies. The challenge remains to identify those drug combinations with the most favorable therapeutic ratio when used in combination with the other modalities, and to determine the optimal sequences, doses, and routes of administration.

Special Considerations

Orbit

Most patients are diagnosed early, and are group III because enucleation (removal of the entire mass without rupture) is avoided. Biopsy, chemotherapy, and radiation therapy constitute the most common approach, and local control is almost uniform. The 10% of patients with alveolar histology have an inferior prognosis, particularly if very young.[348] Chemotherapy alone has been attempted with poor results.[349]

Parameningeal

About 40% of head and neck RMSs are parameningeal and, of these, 80% are embryonal. Complete surgical extirpation with acceptable functional and cosmetic outcome is essentially impossible; in IRS-III, 76% of patients were group III.[18] Intracranial extension and neoplastic meningitis occur in about 35% of patients and, thus, CT or MRI of the head is necessary, as well as CSF assessment.[350] Regional lymph node involvement occurs in less than 20% of patients.[350] Risk factors for subarachnoid involvement include skull base erosion, cranial nerve palsy, and intracranial extension. Patients with any risk factor have an inferior prognosis (about 50% 3-year progression-free survival, vs. 80% for other parameningeal tumor patients).[350]

Although suspicious lymph nodes should be examined, a formal dissection is rarely appropriate. In IRS-IV, the radiation margin has been reduced to 2 cm, and only in patients with diffuse intracranial meningeal extension or multiple sites of brain parenchymal disease is the entire cranial cavity treated. When there is clear evidence of meningeal (including base of skull erosion or nerve palsies) or intracranial extension, radiation therapy is given at the beginning of the treatment course. Otherwise, chemotherapy is given first, with radiation therapy given at week 9. Radiation therapy is omitted only for patients with completely resected small (<5 cm) tumors with negative nodes.

The extent of surgery is determined by the potential cosmetic and functional outcome, and second-look procedures may be effectively performed.[351] Of interest is a 1996 analysis comparing outcomes for parameningeal RMS treated in IRS-III with outcomes in studies from three European cooperative groups.[352] For low-risk patients, 5-year survival was superior in the IRS study, possibly due to early routine radiation therapy, the IRS quality assurance program, and inclusion of patients with smaller tumors without involved lymph nodes.

Other Head and Neck Sites

Parotid region, oral cavity, oropharynx, and larynx RMSs are generally embryonal, whereas cheek and scalp lesions are often alveolar. Superficial lesions may be completely resected with satisfactory cosmesis and function, but deeper lesions routinely require irradiation. Because of the relatively favorable outlook for patients with nonparameningeal head and neck tumors, such patients are classified as having stage I tumors in IRS-IV and, thus, receive less intense chemotherapy than do those with parameningeal tumors. However, if a nonparameningeal head and neck tumor extends to and invades a parameningeal region, it should be treated as a parameningeal RMS. Lymph nodes are involved in 20% of patients, and therefore, all positive nodes should be resected and irradiated.

Bladder

Bladder RMS usually arises as a pedunculated mass in the submucosa and subsequently invades the bladder wall. In boys, the tumor often arises in the bladder neck and invades the prostate, making distinction between these sites problematic. Over 90% are embryonal, of which one third are botryoid; about 15% of patients have overt metastases at diagnosis. The morbidity of excision, when necessitating partial or total pelvic exenteration, is inappropriate in light of the efficacy of radiation therapy and chemotherapy in providing local disease control, and excision should be used only in cases in which all other therapeutic avenues have been exhausted.[338]

Several IRS trials have attempted to define the situations in which surgical excision is appropriate or in which radiation therapy is necessary. In IRS-II, an attempt was made to minimize the use or extent of both surgery and radiation therapy, and radiation therapy was delayed until week 16.[353] At 3 years, the percentage of patients who were alive with a preserved bladder was only 22% as a result of local disease recurrence or persistence, which necessitated cystectomy. In IRS-III, radiation therapy was administered at week 6 except in patients in whom complete removal of the tumor was possible without total cystectomy.[354] The bladder retention rate at 4 years was 60%, and survival for patients without overt metastases was 90%.

In general, tumors in the dome are more commonly resectable at diagnosis than trigone or bladder neck tumors. IRS-IV also recommends bladder-preserving surgery at second look after induction chemoradiotherapy, if possible.[355] However, if viable RMS persists after induction therapy, extirpative surgery may be necessary. Radiation therapy should be designed with consideration for shielding the femoral epiphyseal plates and proximal femurs.

Prostate

Because prostate RMS tends to be locally invasive and disseminates early, radical surgery is rarely possible or indicated. As for bladder tumors, in IRS-II the attempt to avoid or minimize surgery and radiation therapy was unsuccessful.[353] The current therapeutic approach is similar to that for patients with bladder RMS; except for rare patients who had small, completely resected tumors and who are node negative, radiation therapy is given at week 9. Chemotherapy is then continued.

Paratesticular

The spermatic cord is generally the primary site, although it may also be the epididymis or tunics. An orchiectomy is performed through an inguinal incision, with a high ligation of the spermatic cord. Current IRS recommendations also include ipsilateral high and low infrarenal and bilateral iliac node sampling.[356] Radiation therapy is administered to involved lymph nodes and to any violated scrotal tissues, which are also resected.

Vagina and Vulva

Vaginal RMSs are most common in young children (90% younger than 5 years of age), and are frequently botryoidal. The mean age for girls with vulvar lesions is 8 years.[357] Limited surgery (e.g., partial vaginectomy or hemivulvectomy) is preferred,[358] and can be performed as a second-look operation at week 9. Biopsies are performed on suspicious nodes, but dissections are inappropriate.

Radiation therapy is not given if excision is complete. When radiation therapy is required, teletherapy is most common, although intracavitary or interstitial brachytherapy has been used.[359] Either technique should strive to minimize the radiation dose to the ovaries (which at times should be transposed outside the primary radiation volume), hips, and pelvic organs. More than 90% of children are expected to survive.

Uterus and Cervix

Uterine and cervical RMS is much less common than vaginal RMS, and it tends to occur in adolescent girls near the time of puberty. Treatment is intended to preserve pelvic organs when possible. Patients with initially resectable disease are placed in group I or II for treatment by surgery, followed by chemotherapy and then radiation therapy, but only if microscopic residual disease is proved to persist. For those with group III disease, primary chemotherapy is given followed by a second-look laparotomy. If there is gross residual disease that cannot be resected completely, or if microscopic disease is found after resection, the patient receives radiation therapy and continues on chemotherapy. If the second-look exploration shows no demonstrable tumor or tumor that is completely resected, no radiation therapy is given and the patient continues on chemotherapy alone. Survival rates should approximate those for RMS of the vagina and vulva.[360]

Retroperitoneum

RMS in this site is frequently of large bulk at diagnosis, and lymph node involvement occurs in 23% of patients; complete resection is, in general, not feasible. Unfortunately, radiation therapy is limited by normal tissue tolerances, and multiple field reductions are generally necessary. Five-year survival was about 40% in IRS-II.[17]

Extremity

About half of these lesions are alveolar, and the prognosis is relatively unfavorable. In IRS-I and IRS-II, regional lymph node involvement occurred in 15% and 9% of patients with upper and lower extremity lesions, respectively.[325] If substantial morbidity can be avoided, gross excision of the tumor remains superior to biopsy alone. Rarely, amputation may be necessary when radiation therapy will produce unacceptable morbidity and gross excision is not possible.

In IRS-IV, the axillary or inguinal regions are explored, even in the absence of clinically evident nodal involvement. Chemotherapy is always given. Radiation therapy is omitted only for patients with completely resected small (<5 cm) tumors with negative nodes. The tumor is treated with a 2-cm margin, plus regional lymph nodes when involved. One should spare a strip of soft tissue along the extremity to avoid late radiation-induced extremity edema.

Pulmonary Metastasis

Low-dose whole lung irradiation is used as part of the treatment of pulmonary metastasis. If there are a few isolated lung metastases, not encompassing an excessive volume of lung, they may be boosted by a "rifle shot" field. In addition, lung nodules can be resected after chemoradiotherapy if acceptable lung function is preserved.

Results and Prognosis

Results

The overall survival for RMS in IRS-III, according to clinical site and group, is depicted in Figures 19–10 and 19–11, respectively. Table 19–21 provides 5-year survivals for specific subgroups of patients, whereas Table 19–22 provides outcome data for different histopathologic subtypes.

Patients in groups I, II, and III have overall 5-year survivals of 93%, 81%, and 73%, respectively, which validates the overall effectiveness of therapy and the impact of resectability on enhancing outcome. Indeed, a 1999 study by Blakely and associates indicates that surgical debulking of tumors in cases of embryonal RMS improves overall survival rate; this finding will be addressed in IRS-V.[361] Unfortunately, patients with metastatic disease continue to fare poorly, with a 30% 5-year survival; those patients with bone marrow involvement are even less likely to survive.[18] Further discussion of this situation is presented in "Prognosis."

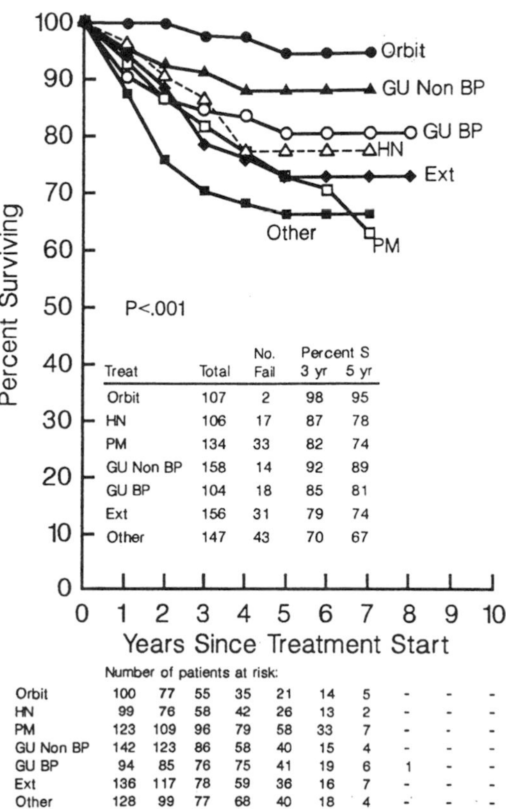

Figure 19–10. Survival by primary site for all patients treated in IRS-III. GU Non BP = genitourinary tract non–bladder/prostate; GU BP = genitourinary tract bladder/prostate; HN = head and neck, nonparameningeal; Ext = extremities; PM = parameningeal sites. (From Crist W, Gehan E, Ragab A, et al: The Third Intergroup Rhabdomyosarcoma Study. J Clin Oncol 1995; 13:610, with permission.)

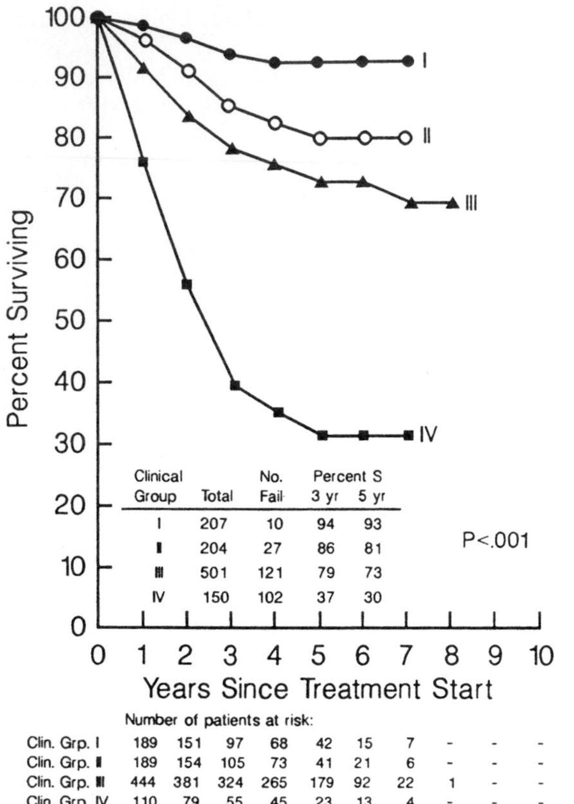

Figure 19–11. Survival by clinical group for all patients treated in IRS-III. (From Crist W, Gehan E, Ragab A, et al: The Third Intergroup Rhabdomyosarcoma Study. J Clin Oncol 1995; 13:610, with permission.)

Prognosis

Implicit in the discussion of the grouping and staging systems for RMSs is the importance of accurately identifying prognostic variables. Most of these variables are interrelated.

Clinical Grouping

Clinical grouping is based on the extent of postsurgical disease at the time that chemotherapy is initiated, and its relevance is supported by data from the three analyzed IRSs (see Table 19–21 and Fig. 19–11).[16–18, 310] The assigned clinical group also reflects the disease site and the biologic invasiveness of the tumor because these two characteristics impact on the resectability of the tumor.

TABLE 19–21. **Percent Survival at 5 Years by Clinical Group and Pretreatment Stage**

	IRS-I	IRS-II	IRS-III
Clinical Group			
I	83	81	93
II	71	80	81
III	52	65	73
IV	21	27	30
All	55	63	71
Pretreatment Stage			
I		91	89
II		73	86
III		52	69
IV		23	30

Data from references 16, 18, 310, 317, and 334.

Primary Site

The association of site and prognosis is shown in Figure 19–10. The primary site in part dictates resectability, which in turn determines the IRS grouping.[16–18, 310] Resectability depends on tumor invasiveness and the morbidity that would attend resection. For example, most orbital lesions are in group III (73.5% in IRS-I, -II, -III),[348] and most extremity tumors are in group I or II. Patients with orbital tumors have a 95% 5-year survival, in contrast to patients with extremity or parameningeal tumors, whose 5-year survival is 74%. Patients with truncal and retroperitoneal tumors have 5-year survivals of 50% and 40%, respectively.[17, 362] The tumor location also determines the presenting signs and symptoms, which generally determine the rapidity of diagnosis; location in turn can affect the size to which the tumor grows.

Tumor Size

The size (≤5 cm vs. >5 cm), by multivariate analysis, is associated with survival time ($p < .001$).[332] Size is also related to tumor site because of presenting symptoms and signs.

Lymphatic Spread

Whereas genitourinary, abdominal/pelvic, and extremity tumors commonly involve regional lymph nodes, tumors in the head and neck, trunk, and female genital organs do not.[325] However, the frequency of lymph node involvement was almost certainly underestimated by previous IRS data because the assessment of nodal status was not systematic. Data from Stanford have shown that 88% of patients presenting with involved nodes had primary tumors that were invasive and extended beyond the site or organ of origin.[363]

Histology

Both IRS and SIOP data confirm the prognostic relevance of a tumor's histology (see Table 19–22). Sarcoma botryoides is the most favorable type, with a 95% survival at 5 years, followed by embryonal 66% and alveolar 54%; rare patients with undifferentiated tumors fare worst, at 45%.[332] However, a 1995 analysis of IRS-III data showed that, *within the different clinical groups*, histology did not exert a prognostic influence.[18] One explanation for this finding is that the distribution of tumor histology also varies by primary site. For example, about 20% of RMSs are alveolar, but this histology is found in approximately half of extremity and perineal tumors and, in addition, more intense chemotherapy is administered to patients with alveolar tumors. Conversely, over 80% of orbital tumors are embryonal, and 90% of genitourinary tumors are embryonal or sarcoma botryoides.[17]

TABLE 19–22. **Therapy and Outcomes for Risk Subgroups in IRS-III, 1984–1991 (1032 Patients)**

Risk Subgroup	Treatment	5-Yr Survival Rates (%) PFS	OS
Group I (favorable histology)	VA × 1 yr	83	93
Group II (favorable histology)	VA × 1 yr + RT	56	54
	VAdrA × 1 yr + RT	77	89
Groups I and II (unfavorable histology)	VAdrC-VAC + P × 1 yr + RT	71	80
Group II (paratesticular)	VA × 1 yr + RT	81	81
Groups II and III (orbit and head)	VA × 1 yr + RT	78	91
Group III (except special pelvic, orbit, and head sites)	VAC × 2 yr + RT	70	70
	VAdrC-VAC + P × 2 yr* + RT	62	63
	VAdrC-VAC + P + E × 2 yr* + RT	56	64
Group III (special pelvic sites)	VAdrAC-VAC + P + E × 2 yr ± RT ± surgery	74	83
Group IV	VAC × 2 yr + RT	27	27
	VAdrAC-VAC + P × 2 yr + RT	27	31
	VAdrAC-VAC + P + E × 2 yr + RT	30	29

V = vincristine; A = actinomycin D; C = cyclophosphamide; Adr = doxorubicin; P = cisplatin; E = etoposide; RT = radiation therapy; PFS = progression-free survival; OS = overall survival.

*Second look surgery was recommended at week 20; if partial response, patients received Adr + imidazole carboxamide (DTIC) or A + E or A + DTIC.

Modified from Pappo A: Rhabdomyosarcoma and other soft tissue sarcomas of childhood. Curr Opin Oncol 1995; 7:361, with permission.

Biology

Briefly, tumor cell ploidy is related to histologic subtype and treatment outcome. Patients with diploid tumors appear to have a worse prognosis than patients with hyperdiploid tumors.[364–366] Cytogenetic findings of note include specific translocations such as t(2;13), and N-*MYC* amplification in alveolar RMS, both of which portend an extremely poor prognosis.[323, 367]

Other

Although younger age is associated with an improved outcome,[368] the specific subgroup of children younger than 1 year of age with alveolar histology have a significantly poorer survival than do older children.[369] Some site-specific variables influence outcome:

- In the head and neck, risk factors that predict tumor access to the cranial subarachnoid space (skull base erosion, cranial nerve palsy, intracranial extension) decrease the likelihood of DFS (51% vs. 81% if no risk factors).[370]
- In extremity sites, the presence of lymph node involvement is strongly associated with a high incidence of metastatic relapse and inferior survival.[371]

Patterns of Relapse

RMS is a systemic disease and essentially all patients are presumed to have at least micrometastatic disease; 16% will have demonstrable metastases at diagnosis. RMS spreads via blood and lymphatics; however, relapse is most frequent locally. Distant spread occurs, in order of decreasing frequency, in the lungs, CNS, lymph nodes, bone, liver, bone marrow, and soft tissues.

Eighty percent of recurrences occur in the first 2 years, following completion of localized therapy in patients having achieved a complete response. If disease recurs while the patient is undergoing primary therapy, median survival is 20 weeks, with long-term survival currently unobtainable. For patients whose disease recurs after having achieved CR and completed therapy, 20% can be successfully salvaged, depending on certain pretreatment characteristics.

Clinical Investigations

IRS-IV was recently implemented, and IRS-V is in various stages of construction. New drug combinations, radiation strategies, and sequencing with surgery are under investigation. BMT continues to be tested in selected patients with metastatic or recurrent disease.

Recommended Reading

A brief but comprehensive overview of childhood RMS is provided by Pappo.[15] For further detailed discussions of IRS-I, -II, and -III, see the reports by Maurer and colleagues[16, 17] and Crist and associates.[18]

Germ Cell Tumors and Teratoma

Germ cell tumors (GCTs) are benign or malignant growths that arise from pluripotential primordial germ cells. Germ cells first appear in the yolk sac endoderm and migrate around the hindgut to the genital ridge of the embryo on the posterior abdominal wall, where they congregate and subsequently become part of the developing gonad.[372] Tumors can arise from these cells, and, independent of the mechanism of origin, the type of tumor that results is determined by the subsequent development of the germ cell. In addition, and for reasons as yet unknown, the abnormal migration of these germ cells results in their presence in locations such as the sacrococcygeal region, the retroperitoneum, the mediastinum, and the cervical and pineal regions.

Those cells that undergo gonadal differentiation become the germinomas, also known as seminomas or gonadoblastomas. Those that maintain their totipotentiality may become embryonal carcinomas. The development of extraembryonic structures results in differentiation to endodermal sinus tumors (yolk sac tumors) or choriocarcinomas (placental tumors). Embryonic differentiation into ectoderm, mesoderm, and endoderm results in teratomas (mature and immature) (Fig. 19–12).[26, 373]

Epidemiology and Etiology

Epidemiology

GCTs account for 2% to 3% of childhood malignancies,[42] and, in general, are more frequent in girls than in boys.[23] The most common sites for GCTs are ovaries and testes, although approximately 40% of childhood GCTs originate in the sacrococcygeal area. Of note, 80% of these tumors are benign and the most common benign form is the sacrococcygeal teratoma; this term is derived from the Greek *teras*, "monster." The remainder of GCTs arise in other locations, including the mediastinum, neck, intracranial region, and retroperitoneum.

Etiology

- Children with sacrococcygeal teratomas have a 12% to 18% incidence of associated anomalies, most often of the anorectal region (e.g., imperforate anus, anal stenosis).[374, 375]
- A triad (Currarino's triad), first described in 1981, is an inherited autosomal dominant pattern consisting of presacral tumors, anal stenosis, and a scimitar sacrum.[376] A high percentage of the presacral masses are teratomas.
- The frequent association of a family history of twinning with the occurrence of sacrococcygeal teratomas resulted in early theories suggesting that teratomas were abortive attempts at the development of twins. It is of interest to note that the common sites of teratomas—the brain, mediastinum, abdomen, and sacrococcygeal regions—are all sites of conjoined twin attachments.

Genetics

Although most GCTs occur in otherwise normal individuals, a genetic tendency for abnormal germ cell development may exist in some families. These findings suggest that abnormal germ cell development may play a role in the ultimate appearance of GCTs:

- Instances of malignant GCTs have been reported in siblings, twins, and up to three generations of individuals in families.[377, 378]
- Gonadal dysgenesis (Swyer syndrome), particularly in phenotypic females with a 46,XY karyotype, has been associated with gonadoblastoma or dysgerminoma.[379] In one family, a phenotypically normal brother of two affected females was diagnosed with a testicular choriocarcinoma containing elements of embryonal carcinoma and seminoma.[380]
- Klinefelter's syndrome is associated with mediastinal GCT.[381, 382]

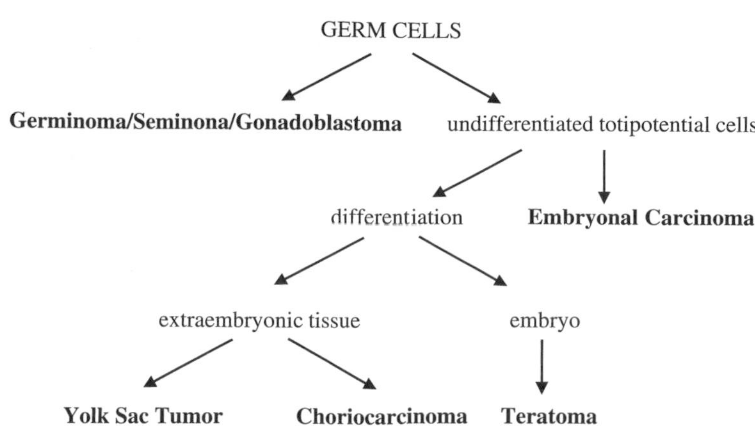

Figure 19–12. Classification of germ cell tumors. (Modified from Halperin EC, Constine LS, Tarbell NJ, et al: Pediatric Radiation Oncology, 3rd ed. Philadelphia, Lippincott Williams & Wilkins, 1999, with permission.)

- In testicular and ovarian tumors, an isochromosome marker of the short arm of chromosome 12, i(12p), has been noted.[383]
- Studies have shown variations in the ploidy of various primary, recurrent, and metastatic tumor specimens[384]; aneuploidy, in particular, may be associated with an unfavorable prognosis.

Detection and Diagnosis

Clinical Detection

Of interest, malignant GCTs with evidence of extraembryonic differentiation often produce proteins commonly elaborated by the corresponding normal extraembryonic structure. These markers have use in the detection and diagnosis of these tumors and subsequent monitoring of the patient. Presence of any of these markers means malignant cells exist.

- *Alpha-fetoprotein* (AFP) is a useful oncologic marker.[385] AFP is present in the serum of human fetuses at 12 to 15 weeks' gestation; however, serum levels of AFP are elevated in patients with GCTs that have endodermal sinus tumor histology (yolk sac origin), as well as in the serum of children with malignant teratomas without detected yolk sac tumor elements. The latter finding suggests that yolk sac tumor elements are present and that more aggressive therapy may be necessary. When evaluating AFP levels, it is important to recognize that the child must reach 9 months of age before the high levels present at birth have fallen to adult levels.[386]

  The rate of disappearance of serum AFP following resection of an AFP-producing tumor correlates with the adequacy of tumor removal.[385] Radiolabeled antibodies to AFP have been developed and may be useful for *in vivo* detection and localization of these neoplasms.
- Beta–human chorionic gonadotropin (β-HCG) is another valuable tumor marker.[387] In addition to GCTs with trophoblastic elements (choriocarcinomas, testicular tumors), hydatidiform moles and pregnancy also produce β-HCG. The finding of an elevated serum β-HCG level in a child whose teratoma does not have histologically recognizable chorionic elements suggests that such elements are nonetheless present within the tumor. Thus, any positive value means malignant cells are present. Usually, choriocarcinoma has the highest elevation of HCG, but embryonal and endodermal sinus tumors also secrete HCG.[387]

However, in general, the presentation and evaluation of a patient depends on the location of the GCT.

Sacrococcygeal

This tumor arises from the anterior portion of the coccyx and, in general, presents as an external mass between the anus and coccyx in infants younger than 2 years old. The appearance varies from a small mass with a dimple to a large pendulous lesion. The overlying skin may be normal or roughened, shiny, hairy, tense, wrinkled, or ulcerated. An intrapelvic component may cause the patient to experience urinary or rectal obstruction. This obstruction may occur in association with an external mass or in the absence of any external tumor. Intradural tumor extension is found in 3% to 5% of the lesions. Polyhydramnios has been associated with sacrococcygeal teratoma in infants.

Evaluation of the patient includes a *physical examination*, with particular attention to the abdominal and rectal examination. Intrapelvic or abdominal extension of an external mass should be sought with a *barium enema*, *ultrasound*, and *IVP* or an *abdominal* and *pelvic CT scan*. *AFP* and *β-HCG* levels should be determined preoperatively. The most frequent alternative diagnosis is meningocele.

Ovarian

In infants, ovarian tumors almost always present as an abdominal mass. Older girls (usually 10 to 15 years old) present with symptoms of abdominal pain (most common), nausea, vomiting, constipation, or urinary tract obstruction; only half will have palpable masses. Acute abdominal pain may be caused by torsion of the tumor on its pedicle or hemorrhage within the tumor. About 5% of the children will have bilateral tumors.[26]

Evaluation consists of a *physical examination* searching for an abdominal mass. An *abdominal x-ray* will reveal calcification in approximately half of the children, most of which will be benign. *Ultrasound* of a teratoma will show both cystic and solid components. Mature elements, such as bone or teeth, may be noted. *CT scans* may be useful in evaluating larger lesions. Preoperative values of *AFP* and *β-HCG* should be obtained.

Testicular

Testicular tumors present as an asymptomatic scrotal mass in boys 1 to 2 years old. Coexisting hydroceles may be present in 15% to 25% of the patients. There is no preponderance of one side over the other and, occasionally, bilateral tumors are noted. Torsion of tumors in undescended testes may present as acute abdominal pain. Malignancy of the testis is 20 to 40 times higher in patients with undescended testes; however, the incidence of cancer is increased not only in the undescended testis of these patients but also in the contralateral testis, suggesting that testicular cancer may result from an intrinsic testicular defect. Neonatal jaundice, maternal disease, and retained placenta also have been indicated as important etiologic factors.[388]

Evaluation consists of a *scrotal examination*, a *CT scan* of the chest and abdomen to look for pulmonary metastases and retroperitoneal adenopathy, a *bone scan*, and preoperative measurements of *AFP* and *β-HCG* serum levels. The differential diagnosis for an intrascrotal mass includes testicular torsion, epididymitis, and testicular infarction. Abdominal, pelvic, and scrotal *ultrasounds* may prove helpful in following patients during treatment.

Mediastinal

This disease is primarily found in young males.[389] Patients with anterior mediastinal masses often have cough, wheezing, dyspnea, and chest pain. Newborns may require immediate intubation for respiratory distress. Intrapericardial tumors can cause congestive heart failure and cardiac tamponade.

Evaluation should include *chest x-ray* and a *CT scan* of the chest; mediastinal teratomas are calcified in approximately 35% of cases. *Echocardiography* is useful for the delineation of intrapericardial tumors. For these tumors, *cardiac catheterization* is necessary to determine whether other cardiac anomalies exist and to evaluate the course of the great blood vessels, as well as the blood supply to the tumor. Serum *AFP* and β-*HCG* values should be obtained preoperatively. All children with mediastinal tumors should have *karyotyping* for Klinefelter's syndrome (XXY).[381]

Abdominal

Most abdominal GCTs are located in the retroperitoneum, although gastric and hepatic tumors have been reported.[390] Retroperitoneal teratomas in children under 2 years of age usually present as asymptomatic abdominal masses; older children may have anorexia, vomiting, and abdominal pain. Rarely, intradural extensions may develop, resulting in neurologic disorders of the lower extremities. Gastric tumors commonly cause abdominal distention and masses. Vomiting and hematemesis may occur.

Evaluation includes *abdominal* and *chest x-rays*. An *ultrasound* or *CT scan* of the abdomen defines the relationship of the tumor mass to adjacent structures[391]; an upper GI series may be necessary, particularly for gastric tumors. A *24-hour urine sample* is collected for catecholamines to distinguish this tumor from the more common NB. Serum samples for *AFP* and β-*HCG* should be obtained.[392]

Head and Neck

GCTs of the head and neck occur most commonly in infants. Cervical teratomas in the newborn present as an obvious neck mass, frequently causing respiratory obstruction; fetal cervical teratomas can result in polyhydramnios and premature labor.[393] Oropharyngeal teratomas usually present as large masses protruding from the mouth, frequently causing respiratory distress and cyanosis.[394]

Management of these tumors consists of an *x-ray of the neck* and *endotracheal intubation* for respiratory distress. In the fetus, the *EXIT procedure* (*ex utero* intrapartum treatment) has shown promising results.[393, 395] Patients with oropharyngeal teratomas should also have *skull films* obtained to detect calcifications and bony abnormalities because calcifications suggest a teratoma. *Ultrasound* will reveal mixed, cystic, or solid tissues. A *CT scan* can reveal the extent of cervical teratomas. Preoperative *thyroid function studies* are required for appropriate evaluation; of note, in patients in whom no residual thyroid tissue is demonstrable after resection, postoperative thyroid function tests should be performed.[396] Serum samples should be obtained preoperatively for the measurement of *AFP* and β-*HCG*.

Intracranial

The pineal region is the most common site of an intracranial GCT, although up to 30% are located in suprasellar or infrasellar regions.[397] Infants present with hydrocephalus and symptoms of increased cranial pressure[398]; in teenagers, headaches are a common presenting complaint. In addition, there may be lethargy, vomiting, visual disturbance, and diabetes insipidus associated with this tumor.[112, 399]

Skull films in the newborn with a teratoma frequently demonstrate calcification[400] that is almost always in a supratentorial location. A *CT scan* may detect or reveal the extent of a tumor and the associated ventricular enlargement. *Arteriography* may be helpful to demonstrate the effect on blood supply and aid in planning the surgical approach. Measurements are made of *AFP* and β-*HCG* in the serum and CSF.[401, 402]

Vaginal

The tumor must be differentiated from an RMS of the vagina (sarcoma botryoides). Girls with vaginal GCT are usually younger than 3 years of age and often present with a bloody vaginal discharge. *Vaginal examination* in such a young child should be performed with the patient under anesthesia. *Chest x-ray*; *CT scan* of the chest, abdomen, and pelvis; and a *bone scan* will be necessary, in addition to serum *AFP* and β-*HCG*.

Classification and Staging

Histopathology

GCTs arise from pluripotential germ cells that can:

- remain in an undifferentiated state (embryonal carcinoma)
- differentiate along a pathway of gonadal differentiation (germinoma)
- differentiate into either embryonic (teratoma) or extraembryonic (endodermal sinus tumor or a choriocarcinoma) structures (see Fig. 19–12)[26]

Germ cell tumors are, thus, a diverse group of tumors with pathologic and clinical characteristics specific to the type of cells involved. Three broad histologic categories are mature and immature teratomas and malignant GCTs.

Teratoma

Teratomas are unusual tumors in that they are composed of all three germ layers: ectoderm, mesoderm, and endoderm. Although all types of germ layer tissues are seen, neural tissues often predominate. They present as a mixture of both cystic and solid elements, and mature structures such as hair, teeth, and bone may be found. Malignancy from any of these tissues may arise, the most common being adenocarcinoma and rhabdomyosarcoma. Extraembryonic tissues may result in endodermal sinus tumor or choriocarcinoma.

Histologically, teratomas have been classified into three main types: mature, immature, and teratoma with malignant components[26]: Mature teratomas with well-differentiated tissues present are benign; immature teratomas have embryonic-appearing neuroglial or neuroepithelial elements, in addition to mature elements. Mature and immature teratomas are most commonly found in infants. Although malignant evolution is more likely to occur in immature teratomas than in mature teratomas, malignancy has occurred years after removal of an apparently benign tumor.[403] Such a malignancy occurs most commonly in the sacrococcygeal area; whether this represents a recurrence or a second primary is unclear. The sacrococcygeal region is also the most common site for a teratoma with malignant components—usually endodermal sinus tumors and embryonal carcinoma.[404] Teratomas display positive staining for AFP or β-HCG only when malignant elements are present.

Malignant Germ Cell Tumors

Endodermal Sinus Tumor. This is the most common malignant GCT in the pediatric age group and usually produces increased levels of AFP.[405, 406] Grossly, the endodermal sinus tumors are pale, tan-yellow, with foci of necrosis and small cystic areas, and are soft and fall apart easily. Microscopically, the cells are pale and resemble those of the yolk sac, with reticular, pseudopapillary, polyvesicular, vitelline, or solid patterns, or a mixture of patterns. Perivascular cuffs of tumor cells, called Schiller-Duval bodies, are characteristic of this type of tumor.

Embryonal Carcinoma. Microscopically these tumors consist of undifferentiated cells, usually densely packed. Embryonal, glandular, papillary, or clear cell adenocarcinomatous patterns are characteristic. Embryonal carcinoma is rarely a pure histologic pattern in infants and children. It is commonly seen in association with teratomas and endodermal sinus tumors.

Choriocarcinoma. Choriocarcinoma has two distinct forms, gestational and nongestational. The gestational form arises within the placenta, and the nongestational form arises from extraplacental tissue of a nonpregnant person. Histologic features are the same for both types, with cells resembling the chorionic layer. The two main components are cytotrophoblasts (large round cells with clear cytoplasm) and syncytiotrophoblasts (syncytia-forming large cells with abundant homogeneous, vacuolated cytoplasm, and dark irregular nuclei). Levels of β-HCG are elevated in children with choriocarcinoma. These tumors are most frequently found in the mediastinum and are associated with metastasis at diagnosis.

Germinoma (Seminoma, Dysgerminoma). These tumors are composed of uniform polyhedral cells with fibrous tissue and infiltrates of lymphocytes. Intracranial tumors are typically called germinomas; *seminoma* is the term for testicular or mediastinal tumors, and *dysgerminoma* for the ovarian tumor. Seminomas are the most common malignancy found in undescended testes. AFP and β-HCG are negative if no other malignant germ cell elements are present.

Staging

Because of the diverse location of these tumors, no satisfactory method of staging appropriate for all tumors has been developed. The staging system described by Brodeur and associates is commonly used.[407] Other staging systems are available for testicular and ovarian tumors, particularly the St. Jude Children's Research Hospital staging system (Table 19–23).[20, 26]

Principles of Treatment

If at all possible, teratomas should be completely removed surgically. Although most are benign, malignancy has been observed to develop in children years after the removal of an apparently benign tumor. Therefore, careful follow-up is necessary for all patients who have had teratomas excised.

In the past, malignant teratomas, embryonal carcinoma, endodermal sinus tumor, and choriocarcinoma were almost uniformly fatal, even with apparently complete surgical resection. The one exception was embryonal carcinoma of the infant testis, in which radical orchiectomy was sometimes curative. In the 1960s, Li and colleagues demonstrated the efficacy of chemotherapy for gestational chorio-

TABLE 19–23. **The St. Jude Children's Research Hospital Staging System for Germ Cell Tumors**

Stage	Descriptor
Testicular Germ Cell Tumors	
I	Limited to one testis (or both), removed by high inguinal orchiectomy; no clinical, radiographic, or histologic evidence of disease beyond the testis; tumor markers normal after appropriate half-life decline*
II	Transscrotal biopsy or scrotal orchiectomy, microscopic disease in scrotum or high in spermatic cord (<5 cm from proximal end), retroperitoneal lymph node involvement <2 cm, and/or increased tumor markers after appropriate half-life decline
III	Retroperitoneal lymph node involvement (>2 cm), but no visceral or extra-abdominal metastases
IV	Visceral abdominal involvement or distant metastases
Ovarian Germ Cell Tumors	
I	Limited to one ovary (or both); negative peritoneal washings; no clinical, radiographic, or histologic evidence of disease beyond the ovaries; tumor markers normal after appropriate half-life decline*
II	Microscopic residual or microscopic positive lymph nodes; negative peritoneal washings; tumor markers positive or negative
III	Gross residual or biopsy only; gross lymph node involvement (>2 cm), but no visceral or extra-abdominal involvement; positive peritoneal washings; tumor markers positive or negative
IV	Visceral abdominal involvement or distant metastases
Malignant Extragonadal Germ Cell Tumors	
I	Complete resection at any site, coccygectomy for sacrococcygeal site, negative tumor margins and adjacent lymph nodes (4 weeks postoperative); tumor markers negative
II	Microscopic residual; microscopic lymph node involvement and/or tumor markers positive
III	Gross residual or biopsy only; gross lymph node involvement (>2 cm); tumor markers positive or negative
IV	Visceral abdominal involvement or distant metastases

*Apha-fetoprotein half-life = 5 days; beta–human chorionic gonadotropin half-life = 16 hours.

From Halperin EC, Constine LS, Tarbell NJ, et al: Pediatric Radiation Oncology, 3rd ed. Philadelphia, Lippincott Williams & Wilkins, 1999, with permission.

carcinomas and testicular GCTs.[408] Subsequently, major advances have been made in the treatment of GCTs.[23, 409–411] Current treatments depend, in part, on histology (Table 19–24).

Surgery

For all GCTs, complete surgical excision should be attempted:

- In general, mature teratomas should be treated with complete surgical resection; immature teratomas may require adjuvant chemotherapy depending on tumor grade. However, at least 85% to 90% of immature teratomas, if completely resected, can be observed without chemotherapy.
- Complete excision of the coccyx is recommended for the surgical treatment of the sacrococcygeal lesions because the coccyx contains pluripotent cells. Failure to remove the coccyx can result in a 40% local recurrence rate. Because operative complications of sacrococcygeal lesions usually involve hemorrhage, control of the tumor vasculature is important. Indications for emergency operation in neonates include bleeding, congestive heart failure, and disseminated intravascular coagulation. Approximately 55% of sacrococcygeal teratomas have an intra-abdominal component, and these are more likely to be malignant. In cases with abdominal and sacral components, the abdominal portion should be done first.
- Cervical GCT diagnosed antenatally with evidence of airway compromise may be delivered using an EXIT procedure. Following cesarean section, the baby remains attached to the placenta for 50 to 60 minutes while the baby's airway is secured.[412]
- Ovarian tumors are typically treated by salpingo-oophorectomy, omentectomy, peritoneal washings, and peritoneal biopsy. It is not necessary to bivalve the contralateral ovary.
- Testicular masses should *never* be approached via a scrotal incision, but rather an inguinal incision should be used. Radical inguinal orchiectomy with high ligation of the spermatic cord is the appropriate procedure.[413] Retroperitoneal lymph node dissection (RPLND) for testicular GCT remains controversial. If the retroperitoneal lymph nodes are enlarged as seen by CT scan, children should undergo RPLND; however, RPLND is currently performed only on protocol, but with some promising results.[414]
- For malignant gonadal and extragonadal lesions, extension along tissue planes may preclude complete removal. Second-look surgery may be of benefit after chemotherapy to completely excise tumor.
- There is a role for surgery in locally recurrent malignant GCT. However, these children should be treated on protocol in conjunction with chemotherapy.

Radiation Therapy

In the past, radiation therapy to the tumor bed was coupled with chemotherapy for malignant GCT. However, in many instances, little effect by radiation therapy was noted and any good responses were counterbalanced by the risk of late side effects; current thinking, as described in Table 19–24, excludes the routine use of radiation therapy. However, in some countries, radiation therapy remains the standard treatment for intracranial GCTs,[415] and a 1999 prospective study found that low-dose radiation therapy produced a complete remission rate of 100%, a 5-year relapse-free survival rate of 91%, and 5-year overall survival rate of 94%.[416] In general, radiation doses of 30 to 50 Gy are used to volumes dependent on the tumor histology, presence of neuraxis disease, age of the patient, and use of chemotherapy.[26] In addition, children with stage I and stage II seminomas are treated with inguinal orchiectomy followed by pelvic and para-aortic nodal irradiation.[417, 418] Radiation therapy also may be beneficial for some patients who do not completely respond to chemotherapy and surgery.[419]

Chemotherapy

For malignant GCT and some immature teratomas, particularly those with increased numbers of neuroglial cells, chemotherapy plays a major role. Responsiveness to chemotherapy was first noted for gestational choriocarcinoma.[420] When gestational choriocarcinoma was treated with methotrexate, a 47% complete response rate was observed; however, nongestational choriocarcinoma was not found to be responsive. Responses to chemotherapy were noted in the 1960s for ovarian tumors, most commonly with drug combinations such as VAC.[421, 422]

TABLE 19–24. **Treatment Strategies for Germ Cell Tumors**

Histology	Primary Site	Stage	Treatment
Teratoma (mature and immature)	All sites	Localized	Surgical resection
Germinomas/dysgerminomas/seminomas	Testicular	I	Surgery
		II	Surgery + PEB*
		III–IV	Surgery + PEB
	All other sites	All stages	Surgery + PEB
Nongerminomatous tumors	Testicular	I	Surgery
		II–IV	Surgery + PEB
	Ovarian	I–IV	Surgery + PEB
	Extragonadal	I–II	Surgery + PEB
		III–IV	Surgery + HD-PEB

PEB = cisplatin, etoposide, bleomycin; HD = high-dose.

*Seminomas in children are rare, and are probably more common in adolescents, in whom the adult guidelines dictating less aggressive therapy should be used. Therefore, treatment with PEB for stage II testicular seminoma might be overtreating. Moreover, radiation therapy may be used in these early-stage patients.

In the 1970s, additional drugs (e.g., vinblastine, cisplatin, bleomycin) were found to have significant single-agent response rates in testicular GCT of young men.[423–425] Einhorn and Donohue used cisplatin, vinblastine, and bleomycin (PVB) to produce a 70% complete response rate and demonstrated a 55% long-term DFS for all patients with testicular carcinoma.[426] Although maintenance therapy was initially used after a period of more intensive therapy, subsequent studies revealed that intensive therapy alone was effective.[427] PVB was shown to be more effective than VAC for patients with ovarian GCT,[422] particularly for those with pure endodermal sinus tumors. Patients with GCT whose disease recurred after PVB were often salvaged using other agents, including ifosfamide, etoposide, and doxorubicin.[428, 429]

More recent treatments have used cisplatin, etoposide, and bleomycin (PEB), as well as high-dose platinum (HD-P) in conjunction with EB.[430, 431] Advanced and recurrent malignant GCT is currently being treated with etoposide, ifosfamide, and cisplatin.[432, 433] In a 2000 study, 81% of patients achieved complete response, and, in the good and intermediate prognostic group, the 3-year survival rate was 100%.[434]

Results and Prognosis

- Children with mature teratomas treated with complete surgical resection have a 100% 5-year survival rate and a 90% to 95% relapse-free survival rate.[435, 436] In addition, approximately 90% of children with immature teratomas will require surgery only and close follow-up.[437, 438]
- EFS rates for malignant GCT also have improved through the addition of chemotherapy. For example, in a study conducted by POG and CCG, children with stage I testicular tumors who had surgical resection alone had a 3-year EFS of 80%.[439] However, those patients with recurrent stage I testicular tumors treated with PEB had a 100% 3-year survival. Moreover, stage II testicular and stage I and stage II ovarian GCT treated with resection and PEB had 3-year EFS of 94%.
- Patients with extragonadal tumors of advanced stages (III and IV) may benefit from HD-PEB. However, ototoxicity with HD-PEB is significant.[440]

Prognosis

Teratomas

- The prognosis for patients with teratomas is dependent primarily on the degree of maturity, the prognosis for mature teratomas being better than that for immature teratomas.
- Malignant teratomas or other forms of malignant GCT are difficult to treat, and prognosis is affected by stage.[407] Because of this situation, age can also be of prognostic significance. Sacrococcygeal teratomas are almost always benign in children younger than 2 months of age, but the likelihood of malignant evolution increases rapidly after this early period. It is thought that later diagnosis explains the increased incidence of malignancy in patients whose teratomas arise within the pelvis or abdomen compared with those with externally visible primaries.
- Mediastinal teratomas behave in a benign manner in children and young teenagers but are more aggressive and often fatal in older patients, requiring aggressive surgical techniques.[441, 442] Similarly, cervical teratomas and intracranial teratomas in infants usually are benign, whereas those presenting in the teenage years or in adult life are frequently malignant.

Malignant Germ Cell Tumors

- Endodermal sinus tumors have been associated with a poor prognosis. However, more recently, survival rates have improved, although they were found to be site specific; testicular tumors fared best, followed by ovarian and sacrococcygeal.[443]
- Embryonal carcinomas continue to have a poor prognosis.[444]
- In general, persistently elevated levels of AFP and β-HCG are indicators of poor prognosis.[445, 446] In addition, serial monitoring of AFP levels can indicate incomplete resection.[447]

Of note, in 1997 the International Germ Cell Cancer Collaborative Group established a prognosis-based staging system for advanced-stage GCTs.[448]

Clinical Investigations

A new international classification of malignant GCT has stratified children into three groups:

- Low risk: all stage I tumors, including stage I immature teratomas
- Intermediate risk: stage II extragonadal and stages II to IV gonadal tumors
- High risk: stages III to IV extragonadal tumors

Through POG, CCG, and SIOP, studies involving the use of multiple chemotherapeutic agents continue. Under consideration is observation alone following surgical resection for all stage I tumors. The roles of PEB and HD-PEB continue to be explored, with attention being given to the ototoxicity. For recurrent malignant GCT, stem cell transplantation and etoposide, ifosfamide, and cisplatin/ifosfamide, carboplatin, and etoposide are under consideration.[449] However, at present the numbers are small, and, thus, cure is difficult to assess.

Recommended Reading

The report of Azizkhan and Caty[19] discusses teratomas with reference to location, age, and incidence of metastases. Ovarian tumors in children and adolescents are reviewed by Cannistra[20] and Lovvorn and colleagues.[21] Testicular cancer in children has been reviewed by Coppes and associates.[22] Several general reviews on GCTs have been written by Rescorla,[23] in addition to one from Europe by Pinkerton.[24]

Langerhans' Cell Histiocytosis

Perspective

Langerhans' cell histiocytosis is a rare and confounding disorder characterized by the proliferation of histiocytes or macrophages called Langerhans' cells.[450] The disease had originally been called histiocytosis X, the "X" chosen to underscore how little was known about this entity.[451] Subsets of histiocytosis X modified by age with common clinical features were designated Letterer-Siwe disease, Hand-Schüller-Christian disease, and eosinophilic granuloma of bone, terms still frequently used today. With the discovery that all subtypes of this disease are characterized by proliferations of Langerhans' cells, the disease is now termed *Langerhans' cell histiocytosis* (LCH).

Although children with this disease are treated by oncologists, it is debatable whether LCH is a true neoplasm. Its behavior in children is quite different from that of a true malignancy, the clinical course being characterized by frequent spontaneous remissions and exacerbations, and the goal of therapy simply being to maintain control over the proliferating cells rather than to completely eradicate an abnormal clone.

Epidemiology and Etiology

Epidemiology

The incidence of LCH is estimated to be 2 to 5 cases per million children per year,[452] with the peak age of onset being 1 to 3 years. Disseminated LCH, previously referred to as Letterer-Siwe disease, is more common in children younger than 2 years of age.

Etiology

The etiology of LCH is unknown.

- Infectious causes have been postulated, but in a 1994 study of potential viral causes of the disease, no virus was detected in the lesions of 56 children with LCH.[453]
- Immunoregulatory imbalance has also been postulated.[454]
- A large epidemiologic study found associations between LCH and thyroid disease, exposure to solvents, and underimmunization.[455]

Biology

The Langherhans' cell is a dendritic, antigen-presenting histiocyte derived from bone marrow CD34-positive stem cells.[456] Although it is found in greatest concentrations in the skin, it is found in many other organs, including lymph nodes. The Langherhans' cell of LCH is phenotypically very similar to the normal Langherhans' cell: both express the surface antigens CD1a and S100, and both contain Birbeck granules, gourd-shaped structures unique to these cells. However, the Langherhans' cell of LCH differs in several respects: It expresses the leukocyte adhesion molecules LFA-3 and ICAM-1,[457] and it has increased expression of interferon-gamma and other cytokines and receptors.[458]

These abnormalities support the hypothesis that immune dysregulation may play a role in the pathogenesis of LCH. For example, many patients with this disorder respond to immunosuppressive agents, such as prednisone, cyclosporine, methotrexate, and 6-mercaptopurine.[27, 459, 460] It also has been postulated that LCH may be caused by a virus or an abnormal host response to the virus, or both. However, numerous exhaustive investigations of possible viral causes (including EBV, cytomegalovirus, human herpesvirus-6, etc.) have failed to detect viruses in the histiocytic lesions with any consistency.[450]

Until recently, histiocytosis had been considered a reactive process and not a malignant one. The prevailing opinion was that LCH is a polyclonal proliferation of histiocytes, but several laboratories have demonstrated conclusively that LCH is a clonal disorder. By using X-linked polymorphic DNA probes, the monoclonality was detected in patients with acute disseminated disease, in those with multifocal disease, and in those with more clinically benign unifocal lesions.[461, 462] Although this monoclonal proliferation raises the possibility that LCH is a neoplasm, this supposition is not yet proved and will require further study. No genetic mutations or cytogenetic abnormalities have been detected in LCH cells.

Detection and Diagnosis

Clinical Detection

The clinical presentation of LCH is highly variable because the disease can involve so many different sites and can mimic so many other maladies. Nonetheless, many children with the disease fall into one of three clinical subsets, each characterized by a well-defined combination of the child's age, signs, symptoms, and imaging and laboratory studies:

- Children younger than 2 years of age are more likely to present with a disseminated form of the disease (formerly called Letterer-Siwe disease). They usually have hepatosplenomegaly, lymphadenopathy, a chronic draining otitis, and cytopenias. They may also have a rash and bone lesions.
- Children aged 2 to 5 years are most likely to have bone involvement and diabetes insipidus (previously referred to as Hand-Schüller-Christian disease).
- Older children typically present with focal bony lesions; this presentation was previously called eosinophilic granuloma of bone.

Table 19–25 summarizes the common signs and symptoms of LCH based on the age of the child.

TABLE 19–25. **Age-Related Patterns of Disease in Children with Langerhans' Cell Histiocytosis**

Group	Symptoms	Physical Examination	Course
<2 years	• Seborrheic or purpuric rash • Anorexia • Failure to thrive • Lymphadenopathy • Organomegaly	• Hepatosplenomegaly • Lymphadenopathy • Hemorrhages	Death may occur from pancytopenia, infection, or organ failure
≥2 years	• Skeletal defects • Diabetes insipidus • Chronic otitis media • Dental problems • Exophthalmos	• Bone tenderness • Swelling over lesions • Exophthalmos	Chronic, fluctuating
Older children	• Solitary or multiple bony lesions	• Bone tenderness • Swelling over lesions	Usually self-limited, may be recurrent

Diagnostic Procedures

- If a patient's physical examination and history are suggestive of LCH, then a surgical *biopsy* must be performed for pathologic confirmation. When possible, biopsies should be performed on easily accessible soft tissue sites, such as skin or mucosal nodules.
- The imaging evaluation to define extent of disease should include a *chest x-ray*, a *skeletal survey* (including skull films), a *bone scan*, and an *abdominal ultrasound* to assess the size of the liver and spleen.
- *MRI* of the head should be obtained in patients with neurologic deficits, exophthalmos, or symptoms of diabetes insipidus.
- Laboratory evaluations should include a complete blood cell count, erythrocyte sedimentation rate, tests of liver function, and prothrombin time/partial prothrombin time.

Staging

There is no uniformly agreed-upon staging system for LCH. In the classic staging of malignancies, disease is classified on the basis of extent of progression—from isolated, resectable, low-stage disease to higher stage, with extensive disease and metastatic spread. Staging in LCH is more akin to grouping; patients are classified on the basis of patterns of disease, which, in turn, are correlated with prognosis.

Several investigators have proposed staging systems for LCH.[463–465] Important prognostic factors incorporated into these staging systems include age at presentation, organ dysfunction, and number of organs involved. One of the more frequently used staging systems is illustrated in Table 19–26.

Principles of Treatment

LCH may not be cancer, but as a disorder of excessive cellular proliferation, it responds to treatment traditionally used for cancer: surgery, radiation therapy, and chemotherapy.[467] Unlike in treatment of cancer, however, the goal in treating LCH is to maintain control over the abnormal proliferation of cells rather than to eradicate all cells. Decisions regarding treatment must incorporate the fact that LCH can be indolent and can even spontaneously remit. Thus, the side effects of therapy should not be greater than those related to the disease itself. Some patients, particularly those children who are asymptomatic and have disease in a single site, may be observed.[468]

Surgery

The role of surgery is limited to obtaining tissue for diagnosis and treatment of single-site bone disease. Aggressive resection of bony lesions is not necessary and should be avoided. Indeed, rates of local recurrence in children with solitary bone lesions are extremely low with biopsy and surgical curettage alone.[469]

Radiation Therapy

Although the lesions of LCH are exquisitely sensitive to small doses of radiation (4.5 to 9 Gy),[470] the role of radiation therapy in the treatment of this disease generally has

TABLE 19–26. **Clinical Staging System for Langerhans' Cell Histiocytosis***

Variable†	Factor	Number of Points
Age at presentation	≥2 years	0
	<2 years	1
Number of organs involved	≤4	0
	>4	1
Presence of organ dysfunction‡	No	0
	Yes	1

*Stage was determined by addition of points for each variable: stage I = 0 points; stage II = 1 point; stage III = 2 points; stage IV = 3 points.

†Patients were staged according to the three prognostic variables derived by Lahey.[463] One point was given for "poorer risk," i.e., age younger than 2 years, involvement of more than four organs, and presence of organ dysfunction.

‡Either hepatic pulmonary, or hematopoietic, as defined by Lahey.[463]

From Osband ME, Lipton JM, Lavin P, et al: Histiocytosis X. Demonstration of abnormal immunity, T-cell histamine H2-receptor deficiency, and successful treatment with thymic extract. N Engl J Med 1981; 304:146, with permission.

been reduced. It should be considered for bone lesions that show no evidence of healing after curettage or excision. Radiation therapy is furthermore indicated in the following situations[26]:

- for local recurrence of a bone lesion after surgery when the relapse site is the sole site of disease
- when curettage is inappropriate because of the risks of fracture (e.g., large femoral lesion)
- when potential compromise of critical structures necessitates a rapid reliable response (e.g., spinal cord or optic nerve compression as a result of a large lesion)
- pain relief

For children with LCH and diabetes insipidus, only 20% to 25% of children have resolution of their diabetes insipidus in response to radiation therapy.[471] Children are more likely to respond if the radiation therapy is instituted within 1 to 2 weeks of onset of symptoms. Therefore, most centers recommend radiation therapy for children with LCH and diabetes insipidus if there is a lesion documented by MRI scanning or patients have had symptoms less than 1 to 2 weeks.[26] The risk of radiation in this setting is panhypopituitarism or growth hormone failure,[472] though the radiation doses used are low and very unlikely to cause such effects.

Chemotherapy

Although multiple chemotherapeutic agents have been proved active against LCH, there is still controversy regarding when to use chemotherapy and which agent or agents to use. Efforts to establish a standard approach to using chemotherapy have been hampered by the rarity of LCH, the tremendous variability in its presentation, and the failure to establish universally agreed-upon risk groups in patients with LCH.

Chemotherapy is indicated for children with disseminated or multifocal disease. Some clinicians take a conservative approach even in this setting, treating only those children who have organ dysfunction or multifocal disease that progresses after observation.[473] The initial treatment in this setting is with prednisone, reserving multiagent therapies, such as vincristine, vinblastine, etoposide, or methotrexate, or a combination, for children in whom the disease progresses or recurs after the treatment with prednisone. Other clinicians advocate prompt, aggressive, multiagent chemotherapy using combinations of prednisone, vinblastine, etoposide, methotrexate, and 6-mercaptopurine (6-MP). The introduction of etoposide, which is particularly potent against LCH, into the multiagent regimens may play a big role in future results. More recent studies are directed at targeting only the highest risk children with disseminated disease to receive aggressive multiagent chemotherapy, while giving less intensive therapy or monotherapy, or both, to children with lower risk disease, that is, those with multifocal bone or soft tissue disease.

Immunotherapy

Based on the premise that LCH may be due in part to immune dysregulation, and that the Langherhans' cell is a component of the immune system, investigators have explored immunotherapy as treatment for LCH. In one of the first studies to suggest a role for this approach, Osband and associates treated children with LCH with calf thymus extract and documented responses in some of the children.[466] However, these results were not reproducible in subsequent studies.[474] A number of children with LCH have responded to the immunosuppressive agent cyclosporine,[475] and prednisone is an effective front-line therapy for disseminated LCH. Other approaches, such as interferon-α or thalidomide, are considered experimental.[476] Overall, immune therapy is not a standard approach for treatment of LCH and is usually reserved for children resistant to standard therapies.

Results and Prognosis

Chemotherapy

McClellan and colleagues adopted a conservative approach in treating 44 children with disseminated LCH: 8 (18%) required no treatment and 17 (39%) responded to prednisone alone.[468] Overall survival was 82% (64% in children with organ dysfunction); however, two thirds of the survivors had permanent sequelae, including diabetes insipidus in 36%.

In one of the largest prospective studies of disseminated LCH, Gadner and associates demonstrated that an aggressive approach resulted in increased survival, fewer recurrences, and fewer long-term complications.[27] They stratified more than 100 children into three risk groups: group A included children with multifocal bone disease; group B children had soft tissue involvement; and group C contained children with organ dysfunction. All children were initially treated with prednisone, vinblastine, and etoposide; children in group B received additional 6-MP and methotrexate; and children in group C received additional 6-MP, methotrexate, and etoposide. Overall survival was 90%: Children with group A and B disease fared particularly well (100% and 90% survival, respectively); survival was 62% in children with organ dysfunction (group C). Thirty-three percent of the children had permanent complications, but only 15% had or developed diabetes insipidus, a considerably lower number than reported in most other series.[468, 472] The results of multiagent chemotherapy in this trial suggest that it boosts cure rates and reduces long-term complications for children with disseminated disease.

A 1999 study focused on the presence of prostaglandin E_2 in bone lesions. Researchers studied the effect of a prostaglandin inhibitor, indomethacin, on 10 children diagnosed with bone LCH.[477] Eight had a complete response to indomethacin treatment, which indicates that further study is merited.

Prognosis

Although the staging systems used by investigators over the past two decades have been as variable as the disease itself, general patterns of disease have been similarly classified, and outcome can be predicted based on these patterns. Children fall into three broad prognostic categories based on the variables described in Table 19–25. Patients with solitary lesions fare the best, with 100% survival[38, 472];

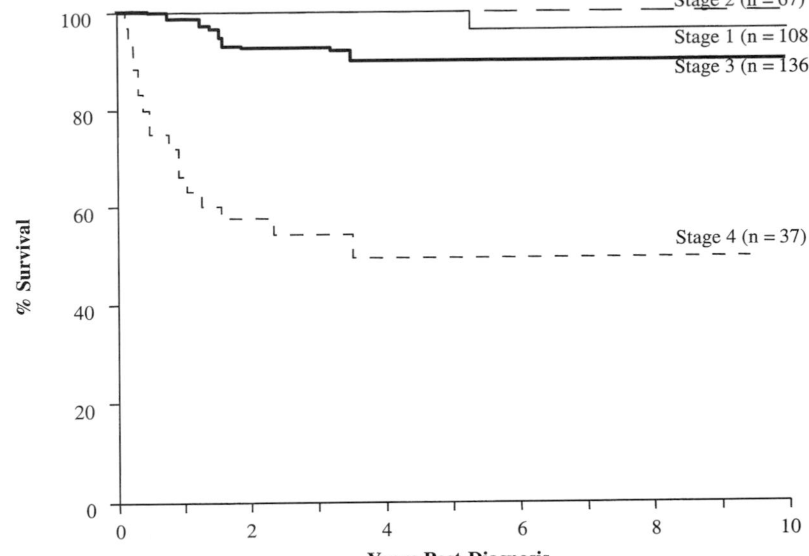

Figure 19–13. Survival of children with Langerhans' cell histiocytosis according to stage. Stage is defined by the DAL HX-83 study (Gadner H, Heitger A, Grois N, et al: Treatment strategy for disseminated Langerhans' cell histiocytosis. Med Pediatr Oncol 1994; 23:72). (From The French Langerhans' Cell Histiocytosis Study Group: A multicenter retrospective survey of Langerhans' cell histiocytosis: 348 cases observed between 1983 and 1993. Arch Dis Child 1996; 75:17, with permission.)

children with disseminated disease but no organ dysfunction do nearly as well, with 82% to 96% survival.[38, 464, 468] Children with disseminated disease and organ dysfunction have the worst survival—33% to 62%.[27, 38, 464, 468, 478] The French Langerhans' Cell Histiocytosis Study Group corroborated this in a retrospective analysis of 348 children with LCH.[478] Although its staging system differed slightly, the Group found the best survival among children with 1 or 2 lesions (100%), and the worst outcome in children with organ dysfunction (49%) (Fig. 19–13). Among children with disseminated disease, younger children, those with organ dysfunction, and those with a poor or brief response to initial chemotherapy had the worst outcome.[27, 478]

Late Effects

The late effects of LCH are considerable. While many are due to the disease itself, some are treatment related, underscoring the importance of carefully selecting therapy for a given child. As many as 33% to 50% of survivors of LCH suffer sequelae.[479] Diabetes insipidus is one of the most common permanent complications of the disease, occurring in 15% to 42% of children with LCH.[27, 468] Other sequelae include orthopedic abnormalities, growth failure, dental problems, cerebellar ataxia, and intellectual deficits.[26, 472, 478] With the exception of diabetes insipidus,[27] there are no data to suggest that treatment can reduce the likelihood of developing these long-term problems.

There is a clear association of second malignancies with LCH.[480] The most common malignancy is leukemia; the majority of cases have occurred following treatment with radiation therapy and/or alkylator-containing chemotherapy regimens, particularly with etoposide,[481, 482] suggesting that most of these secondary malignancies are treatment related.

Recommended Reading

Egeler and D'Angio edited a comprehensive review of the biology and clinical aspects of LCH in a volume of Hematology/Oncology Clinics of North America devoted to LCH.[25] There is an excellent chapter on Langherhans' cell histiocytosis in the textbook *Pediatric Radiation Oncology*.[26] The article by Gadner and colleagues defines the rationale for etoposide-based multiagent chemotherapy for children with disseminated disease.[27]

Pediatric Osteogenic Sarcoma

Perspective

Osteogenic sarcoma is a relatively rare tumor, although it is the most frequently encountered malignant primary tumor of bone.[26] The hallmark of this disease is osteoid or immature bone produced by a malignant proliferating spindle cell stroma. The history of treating this tumor provides insight into the risks inherent in the interpretation of single-arm, nonrandomized clinical trials. In addition, the possibility of evaluating biologic response to therapy has been pioneered in the treatment of osteogenic sarcoma. In the next decade, biologic response to therapy will be correlated with biologic features identifiable at diagnosis. As our understanding of the relationship between tumor biology and response grows, therapy will become increasingly individualized to reflect the unique molecular features of the tumor.

Epidemiology and Etiology

Epidemiology

Osteogenic sarcoma is the most common bone tumor encountered in the first three decades of life and has an incidence rate of 2.6% of all childhood cancers.[257] The male-to-female ratio is approximately 1.5:1. The peak incidence occurs at about the age of 13 for girls and about 14 for boys, corresponding to their respective growth spurts. Taller people appear to be at increased risk, as are individuals with Paget's disease.[483, 484]

Etiology

Osteogenic sarcoma is a rapidly proliferating tumor, the etiology of which is unknown.

- The relatively high incidence of this tumor in adolescents undergoing rapid skeletal growth and in individuals with Paget's disease of the bone suggests that increased bone activity may play a role in the induction of this malignancy.[58] The molecular basis for the phenomenon is unknown.
- Viral induction of osteogenic sarcoma has been noted in animals,[485, 486] and the current evidence in humans for a viral etiology revolves around the detection of simian virus 40 in several human tumors, including osteosarcomas.[487, 488]
- The incidence of osteogenic sarcoma is increased in bones that have previously been irradiated.[489–491] For this reason, radiation has been implicated as causative; however, it must be kept in mind that these patients usually have been treated for a malignancy and, therefore, also may have a genetic basis for increased susceptibility to carcinogenesis.
- Patients with hereditary retinoblastoma, which is associated with a constitutional germline deletion of the *RB1* oncogene, also have an increased incidence of sarcomas as second cancers[492]; more than half of these are osteosarcomas. The *RB1* oncogene is now recognized as a tumor suppressor gene. Loss of heterozygosity at *RB1* was noted in 58% of cases of osteosarcoma in one study, suggesting that this oncogene also plays a significant role in the development of osteosarcoma in those individuals without hereditary predisposition.[493]
- Another tumor suppressor gene that has been associated with osteosarcoma is *TP53* (located on chromosome 17p13.1). Constitutive abnormality at *TP53* is associated with Li-Fraumeni syndrome, a heritable cancer syndrome associated with a number of specific malignancies, including osteosarcoma[494]; loss of heterozygosity at *TP53* has been noted in 54% of patients with osteosarcoma.[493] Studies have shown that 3% to 4% of children with osteosarcoma have constitutive germline mutations of *TP53*.[495]
- *MDM2*, an oncogene localized to 12q13–14, binds to p53. When amplified and overexpressed, it results in functional inhibition of *TP53*[496]; *MDM2* appears to predispose to osteosarcoma.[497, 498]
- P-glycoprotein is an ATP-dependent efflux pump that prevents the accumulation of natural, hydrophobic substances from cells, as well as drugs such as doxorubicin. Recent studies have shown a correlation between the presence of P-glycoprotein in osteosarcomas and poor outcome, with a relative risk of 3.37.[499, 500] However, a recent study that attempted to inhibit P-glycoprotein using cyclosporin A did not show significant benefit (C. Schwartz, personal communication).

Detection and Diagnosis

Clinical Detection

Pain is by far the most common presenting symptom of osteogenic sarcoma, occurring in virtually all patients. Palpable masses, swelling, and limitation of motion are common. Systemic symptoms, such as anorexia and weight loss, are rarely seen; if they are present, one should suspect overt metastatic disease. Patients infrequently present with fractures. Those with pulmonary metastases may have symptoms such as cough, chest pain, or dyspnea.

Diagnostic Procedures

The diagnosis is initially suspected by the presenting symptoms and the radiograph. *Conventional films* of the involved bone characteristically show bone destruction and periosteal new bone formation. When a tumor erupts through the cortex, the formation of new bone produces a "sunburst" appearance, and soft tissue swelling is noted. The diagnosis of osteogenic sarcoma, as with any malignant lesion, rests on an adequate biopsy and histologic examination. To be conclusive, the biopsy must show the presence of osteoid within a sarcomatous tumor.

Other tests may further define the extent of the primary lesion[39a]:

- *CT* or, preferably, *MRI scanning* of the involved region is recommended because the MRI scan can then be used to plan resection and subsequent reconstruction.[501]
- *Arteriography* may be necessary in patients being considered for limb salvage procedures, when the vascular and neurologic integrity of the limb must be assured.
- The lung must be examined by *chest x-ray* and *CT scan* in order to detect metastatic disease.
- Because radionuclides are incorporated into new bone, *technetium-99m bone scans* can outline the primary tumor, multifocal primary lesions, and metastatic lesions.

Classification and Staging

Osteogenic sarcomas have been classified in a number of different ways. Radiologically, they have been classified on the basis of having an osteolytic, sclerosing, or telangiectatic appearance.

Histopathology

Osteogenic sarcomas have been classified by their primary site of origin. Classic osteogenic sarcomas arise from the medullary cavity, usually originating in the metaphyses of the bones. The lower extremities are involved more frequently. Approximately 60% of tumors occur about the knee (40% distal femur and 20% proximal tibia), with 76% occurring in the bones of the upper and lower extremities.[325] Lesions of the sacrum, jaw, and phalanges are much less common. The disease rarely occurs in bones of the skull, but when it does, it is usually a complication of Paget's disease of the bone in adults, or a secondary complication of radiation therapy.[502]

A less aggressive form of osteogenic sarcoma arises in the periosteal area of the bone. It tends to spread along the shaft of the bone, but does not invade the cortex, and is associated with a low incidence of metastasis. Intracortical and extraskeletal osteogenic sarcomas have also been described. Histologically, most osteogenic sarcomas in children are of the classic osteoblastic form, with osteoblasts demonstrating pleomorphism and bizarre mitoses. Necrosis, fibrosis, and calcification may also be noted. Chondroblastic, fibroblastic, telangiectatic, and small cell types have also been described, but are considerably less common in children.

Principles of Treatment

The natural history of osteogenic sarcoma that was treated by surgical resection alone was notable for a rapid appearance of pulmonary metastases 6 to 12 months after diagnosis[503, 504]; 5 years from the time of diagnosis, only 15% to 20% of patients were alive.[503] The results with high-dose radiation therapy alone were worse.[505]

Chemotherapy offered little hope until the early 1970s, when doxorubicin and high-dose methotrexate with leucovorin rescue were found to be effective agents.[506, 507] Early single-arm studies of adjuvant chemotherapy after amputation showed markedly improved survivals (40% to 50%) compared with historical controls treated with amputation alone.[508, 509] However, a subsequent report suggested that these improvements were solely due to improved surgical technique and patient selection.[510] As a result, many patients were not offered adjuvant therapy until controlled randomized studies, performed in the 1980s, showed that adjuvant chemotherapy improves the DFS of patients with osteogenic sarcoma.[28, 511]

Surgery

The mainstay of treatment of osteogenic sarcoma is the attainment of local control. Because the tumor is moderately chemosensitive but radioresistant, the management of the primary tumor requires surgical removal of all gross and microscopic tumor. This removal is achieved most easily by amputation with a wide margin of normal tissue. Instances in which the tumor has recurred in the stump have been attributed to "skip lesions" of tumor in the affected bone, separated from the primary tumor by several centimeters of normal bone.[512] However, with modern scanning techniques, the extent of tumor extension is known and unrecognized skip lesions are extremely rare.[513]

With improvement in the survival of patients with osteogenic sarcoma, limb-sparing surgery has been used in the hope of reducing the functional and psychological morbidity of amputation.[514–516] The portion of bone involved with tumor is removed and replaced by an artificial prosthesis or a bone graft; this procedure can be performed only if the vascular and neurologic integrity of the limb is not compromised. In many instances, preoperative chemotherapy reduces the size of the mass sufficiently to make limb-sparing surgery possible. The DFS of those patients who have had limb-sparing surgery is similar to that of those who have had an amputation.[516] However, young patients with significant limb growth potential may not be ideal candidates for limb salvage of a lower extremity. For patients with lesions of the humerus, any preservation of function in the hand can significantly improve long-term functional results. A 1995 randomized study comparing up-front amputation to limb salvage therapy after induction chemotherapy confirmed the equal efficacy of these approaches.[517]

Tibial turnback procedures have been used, particularly in Europe. After excision of the distal femur, the lower extremity is rotated 180 degrees. Fixation of the distal tibia to the distal end of the remaining femur allows for the ankle to function as a knee joint, effectively converting an above-the-knee amputation to a below-the-knee amputation. The foot remains in place, pointing in the opposite direction.[518] Function is excellent with this approach, which is rarely performed in the United States due to cosmetic acceptance.

Although pulmonary metastases still occur in patients who have received adjuvant chemotherapy, the number of relapses and the number of nodules per relapse are reduced.[519] In many such instances, the number of nodules is sufficiently low that they can be surgically removed. Long-term survival has been documented in patients who have undergone such procedures.[520]

Radiation Therapy

Osteogenic sarcoma is a relatively radioresistant tumor, with the doses required for clinical response often resulting in severe tissue damage and subsequent amputation. For this reason, radiation therapy is not used when surgical resection is possible. However, radiation therapy has been administered to patients whose primary tumor was not amenable to surgical resection; cure with this approach is unusual. Radiation therapy also has been used to prevent and control pulmonary metastases, but, again, is of limited value in this setting. Palliative irradiation for pain or temporary control of metastases is frequently performed.[491]

Chemotherapy

Prior to 1972, chemotherapy for osteogenic sarcoma was ineffective. In 1972, it was shown, almost simultaneously, that doxorubicin or high doses of methotrexate followed by leucovorin rescue produced objective tumor regression in 42% of patients.[506, 507] Since then, these two agents have been the basis for adjuvant chemotherapy. Cisplatin and ifosfamide are other active agents that have become part of standard therapy.[120, 521–523] Ifosfamide, in particular, has been shown to be an effective agent for salvage therapy in those patients who respond poorly to standard regimens.[524]

Although 80% of patients appear to be free of metastases at diagnosis, the rapid onset of pulmonary metastases within a year of diagnosis (despite adequate local control) suggests that micrometastases are often present at diagnosis.[525] Because of this problem, Rosen and colleagues introduced the use of chemotherapy before complete excision of the tumor.[526] Originally designed to allow for preparation of the prosthesis, this approach resulted in earlier treatment of micrometastatic disease and allows for the assessment of the tumor response, as measured by the degree of necrosis in the surgical specimen. A good response is traditionally considered to be at least 90% to 95% necrosis of the tumor.[346] In addition, shrinkage of a large tumor allows limb salvage procedures to become feasible.[527]

Immunotherapy

In past years, in conjunction with surgical resection and, in some instances, chemotherapy, several centers have treated patients with osteogenic sarcoma with various forms of immunotherapy. Attempts to increase or enhance immunologic response to the presence of a tumor have included the use of the bacillus Calmette-Guérin vaccine, interleukin, and the interferons; however, to date, only use of the interferons has demonstrated any advantage over surgically treated controls.[528, 529] More recently, a randomized question in INT-033, a large CCG/POG cooperative group trial, addressed the role of muramyl tripeptide phosphatidylethanolamine as an immunomodulator.[530] This agent stimulates monocyte/macrophage response, resulting in peripheral fibrosis surrounding the tumor with an inflammatory cell infiltration and neovascularization. In patients with relapsed osteosarcoma, 24 weeks of therapy was associated with prolonged survival compared with historic controls.[531] Results of the recently closed study are not yet available.

Results and Prognosis

Surgery

Preoperative chemotherapy allows for the possibility of limb salvage in a number of patients for whom shrinkage of the tumor will make the surgical procedure possible. Studies have shown equivalent outcomes for amputation and limb salvage procedures.[515] The effect of possible delays in therapy as a result of complicated surgical procedures is unknown.

Chemotherapy

The effectiveness of adjuvant chemotherapy in significantly improving the long-term survival of patients with nonmetastatic osteogenic sarcoma has been confirmed in randomized studies.[29] Disease-free and overall survival rates in the order of 65% to 70% can be obtained in patients with nonmetastatic disease at diagnosis who receive adjuvant chemotherapy,[522, 524] while patients treated with surgery alone have only a 20% relapse-free survival rate, unchanged from historical controls.[28, 511]

In the T-10 study, Rosen and colleagues initially reported that outcome could be enhanced for patients with a poor response to bleomycin, cyclophosphamide, dactinomycin (BCD), and methotrexate by deleting methotrexate and substituting cisplatin.[30] Even with a longer follow-up of the T-10 cohort, it was apparent that the absence of an early response continued to predict for significantly inferior outcome.[532] This result was confirmed by a number of groups, including the CCG, which showed an 8-year EFS rate of only 46% in those patients with poor initial responses to therapy, compared with 81% in the good responders, despite the tailoring of therapy.[533, 534]

Tailoring of therapy may improve outcome in poor responders to initial therapy.[535, 536] By adding ifosfamide and etoposide to conventional therapy of poor responders, Bacci and his associates found that outcome in poor responders with good surgical margins was equivalent to that of good responders (71%).[535, 536] Indeed, evaluating the possibility of improving the outcome for those with a poor response to initial therapy by dose intensification has become the focus of a number of studies.[29, 537, 538]

Prognosis

Osteogenic sarcoma in the child or adolescent is almost always high-grade osteoblastic osteogenic sarcoma. Prognostic factors are related to the site of the tumor (patients with distal tumors do better than those with proximal or central axis tumors) and age (prognosis improves with age). Other commonly used prognostic factors include the presence of metastasis and the response to induction therapy. A number of biologic factors are being examined for predictive value in hopes that therapy can eventually be guided by the molecular biology of the individual tumor.

Patients who present with obvious metastatic disease in the lungs have a significantly worse prognosis than that for patients with apparent localized disease; however, with modern chemotherapeutic approaches and aggressive resection of pulmonary nodules, even patients with obvious metastatic disease are potentially curable.[536] A 1998 POG study found that 2-year EFS of newly diagnosed metastatic osteosarcoma was 64% in patients with fewer than eight pulmonary nodules who received intensive chemotherapy and resection of lung metastases when feasible.[539] Meyers and colleagues, however, found that complete surgical excision is necessary for survival in patients with metastatic disease.[540] Patients with multifocal osteogenic sarcoma continue to have an exceedingly poor prognosis, although this prognosis has improved with the use of chemotherapy in combination with aggressive surgery.[541]

Biologic response to therapy has been used to predict eventual outcome of therapy with a given therapeutic regimen. Flow cytometry has suggested that a DNA index suggestive of diploidy predicts for better survival than does an increased DNA index suggestive of hyperdiploidy.[542] In one study, 92 of 96 high-grade osteogenic sarcomas were found to have a hyperdiploid DNA content, whereas low-grade periosteal sarcomas and benign bone tumors had diploid DNA content.[543]

Clinical Investigations

Chemotherapy has improved outcome remarkably for patients with osteosarcoma. Nonetheless, many continue to die of resistant disease. Complete excision of gross disease continues to be an absolute necessity for the achievement of cure in osteogenic sarcoma. Limb salvage is a step along this pathway, but it too is a complicated and traumatic procedure that often results in continual disability for the patients. Improved therapeutic approaches are desperately needed to reduce disability and the risk of recurrence. Newer chemotherapeutic agents being assessed in the phase I/II setting have not, as yet, added to the armamentarium against this tumor.[544, 545] Recent and ongoing trials continue to add agents or to intensify the delivery of chemotherapy known to be effective.

As our knowledge of the biology of this tumor increases, clinical investigations will become increasingly translational. There is hope that further biologic studies will allow classification of patients prognostically by virtue of the tumor biology itself, rather than made entirely on the basis of response to therapies. This type of analysis may allow us to determine which patients will need a more aggressive approach. Approaches designed to overcome the role of multiple drug resistance or those incorporating biologic response modifiers, such as muramyl tripeptide phosphatidylethanolamine, have been attempted. Recent recognition that the ERBB2 receptor is expressed on osteosarcoma cells suggests that Herceptin may be effective in this tumor.[546] Continued translational research, bringing the laboratory findings to the clinical setting, will be necessary to improve the likelihood of curing significantly greater numbers of patients with osteosarcoma.

Recommended Reading

The effect of adjuvant chemotherapy is provided in the articles by Link and colleagues, and Bramwell.[28, 29] Rosen gives a historical perspective on the use of preoperative chemotherapy.[30] Arndt and Christ provide a comprehensive, up-to-date review of our current understanding of the biology and treatment of this tumor.[31]

Pediatric Ewing's Sarcoma/ Primitive Neuroectodermal Tumor

Perspective

In 1921, James Ewing described a tumor that arose in the shaft of long bones but was not associated with bone production.[547] It did, however, diffusely alter bone structure, and was, unlike osteogenic sarcoma, radiosensitive. Now known as Ewing's sarcoma, this is one of the small round cell tumors of childhood, and is similar to the others in its propensity to metastasize and in its responsiveness to chemotherapy. In the past decade, we have come to recognize a characteristic chromosomal translocation, which occurs between the *EWS* gene on chromosome 22 and one of three other genes, as being present in both Ewing's sarcoma and primitive neuroectodermal tumors (PNET).[548, 549] Therefore, these tumors represent a spectrum of disease with similar pathogenesis, but variable expression of neural differentiation, and are sometimes called the *Ewing's sarcoma family of tumors* or *Ewing's/PNET.* Other nomenclature used specifically for PNET includes *Askin tumor, peripheral NB*, and *peripheral neuroepithelioma.*

Over the past two decades, improved treatment with surgery, radiation therapy, and chemotherapy has dramatically changed the outlook for patients with nonmetastatic Ewing's/PNET disease. Recent studies have shown 3- to 5-year EFS rates of 70% to 80%.[550–552] Most deaths occur within 2 years of diagnosis, and late recurrences after 10 to 12 years have been reported.[553, 554]

Epidemiology and Etiology

Epidemiology

Ewing's/PNET is a highly malignant, nonosseous tumor that usually arises in bone but can occasionally occur in soft tissues.[555] It is the most common bone tumor in children younger than 10 years of age, and second only to osteogenic sarcoma in the second decade of life.[58] It accounts for 2% to 3% of childhood cancers, with an annual incidence of 2.8 cases per million children.[257] Although the age at peak incidence of this tumor is between 11 and 17 years, the age range is 5 months to 60 years[32]; 90% of patients are diagnosed before the age of 30 years. The tumor is rare in children younger than the age of 5 years and in children of Asian or African descent.[26]

Etiology

- The cell of origin for Ewing's/PNET has not been unequivocally established. Although Ewing's cells were originally thought to be derived from uncommitted primitive mesenchymal cells,[556] the chromosomal translocation shared with PNET (which has a neural phenotype) suggests a likely neural origin for the entire Ewing's family of tumors.[557] Because the cells are able to synthesize acetylcholine synthetase,[558] they are likely to be derived from postganglionic parasympathetic cells. Even classic Ewing's sarcoma cells, without overt neurologic differentiation, can be induced *in vitro* to undergo neural differentiation.
- The Ewing's sarcoma family of tumors is defined genetically by a specific chromosomal translocation that results in fusion of the *EWS* gene with a member of the *ETS* family of transcription factors, either *FLI1* (90% to 95%) or, less commonly, *ERG, ETV1, E1A-F,* or *FEV.*[559, 560] The *EWS* gene is located at the re-

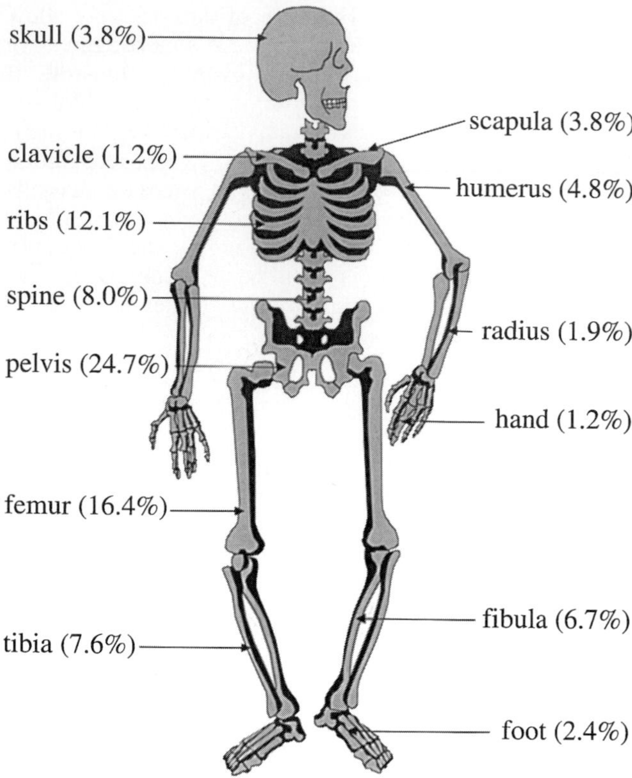

Figure 19–14. Site of primary tumor in 975 patients with Ewing's sarcoma of bone. (From Cotterill SJ, Ahrens S, Paulussen M, et al: Prognostic factors in Ewing's tumor of bone: analysis of 975 patients from the European Intergroup Cooperative Ewing's Sarcoma Study Group. J Clin Oncol 2000; 18:3108, with permission.)

arrangement site on chromosome 22; the site on chromosome 11 is homologous to the *FLI1* locus of the murine Friend leukemia virus. Thus, fusion proteins are formed (commonly, EWS-FLI1) that have been identified as dominant negative transcription factors. Clinical features and outcome may be associated with the specific exons involved in the fusion protein, which may vary with differences in the breakpoints.[561, 562]

- Ewing's/PNET has not been associated with known congenital syndromes, and there is no known evidence for hereditary transmission. Mothers of children with Ewing's/PNET are not at increased risk of malignancy,[563] although one study showed an increase in stomach cancer and neuroectodermal tumors in the families of those with Ewing's/PNET.[564]

Detection and Diagnosis

Clinical Detection

Pain is the most common presenting symptom in patients with Ewing's/PNET[565]; tenderness and swelling are also common. Symptoms are frequently present for several months before diagnosis. Weight loss, fatigue, and fever are frequently noted systemic symptoms that may be accompanied by leukocytosis and an elevated erythrocyte sedimentation rate. In this setting, the diagnosis of osteomyelitis may erroneously be considered.[58] A mass is palpable in many patients, demonstrating the propensity for the tumor to break through the cortex and involve surrounding tissue.[565]

The sites of presentation are illustrated in Figure 19–14; the age distribution for patients with Ewing's sarcoma is shown in Figure 19–15. Overall, the primary lesion occurs in the extremities in 59% of patients (femur 22%, fibula or tibia 21%, humerus 11%), in the pelvis in 22% (ilium 14%), in the ribs in 5%, and elsewhere in 14% (usually in the vertebral bodies). Demonstrable metastatic lesions are present at diagnosis in 14% to 35% of patients. The lesions occur in the lungs, bones, lymph nodes, and bone marrow and, less frequently, in the central nervous system.[58] Neurologic abnormalities occur in 15% of patients, either as spinal cord or peripheral nerve compression.

Diagnostic Procedures

- Biopsy of the lesion establishes the diagnosis and is therefore important. Diagnostic tissue should be obtained from soft tissue and not the cortical bone, if possible. This reduces the potential for pathologic fracture. The scar should be small, easily encompassed by the radiation portal (vertical along the limb), and in a region with a reasonable underlying connective tissue bed, thus reducing the propensity for soft tissue necrosis secondary to irradiation. The usefulness of fine-needle aspiration biopsy for initial evaluation and patient follow-up has been confirmed in a number of studies.[568, 569]
- Radiographs of an involved bone typically demonstrate an expanding destructive lesion in the diaphysis. Periosteal reaction, in the form of periosteal elevation and subperiosteal new bone formation, may occur as the

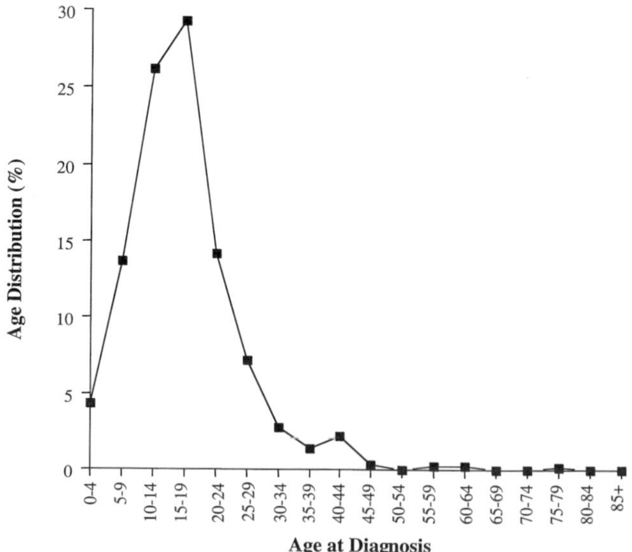

Figure 19–15. Age-specific frequency distribution of Ewing's sarcoma, all races, both sexes, from SEER data 1973–1987. (Modified from Dorfman HD, Czerniak B: Bone cancers. Cancer 1995; 75:203.)

tumor extends through the cortex, producing an "onion skin" appearance. The "sunburst" pattern resulting from radiating spicules occurs more commonly in osteogenic sarcoma. Other radiographic findings in Ewing's/PNET include mottled rarefaction resulting from bone destruction, sclerosis, and cystic loculation.

- The size of the lesion observed on radiographs or by CT scan may underestimate extensive bone marrow space involvement. *MRI* can be helpful in this regard.[570] An associated soft tissue mass is typical,[571] occurring in over 50% of long bone presentations.
- *Chest x-ray* and *CT scan* are obtained to determine if pulmonary metastases are present,[572] whereas MRI is most useful in the determination of disease extent.[570]
- *Radionuclide bone scan* may reveal metastatic lesions, although this technique can exaggerate the linear tumor extent of the primary lesion.
- *Bone marrow biopsy* is needed to determine if there is marrow involvement. Lumbar puncture with cytopathology is obtained in the unusual setting of parameningeal presentations or if neurologic abnormalities are present.[573]
- *Laboratory evaluation* includes complete blood count with differential and renal and liver function tests, including lactate dehydrogenase.[574] The erythrocyte sedimentation rate is frequently elevated.

Classification and Staging

Histopathology

The histologic pattern of Ewing's/PNET is one of monomorphic sheets of small round cells with hyperchromatic nuclei and relatively little cytoplasm. The amount of associated stroma is small, but it can produce a compartmental effect. Tremendous cellularity may be present, with a solidly packed, highly undifferentiated and, at times, dimorphic pattern with large, as well as the previously noted small, cells present. Glycogen in granules with periodic acid-Schiff positivity can usually be demonstrated, but it is not diagnostic.[575] Primitive neural features have been described with less frequency and maturation than in peripheral PNETs. Recent histochemical studies indicate that Ewing's/PNET tumor cells are uniformly vimentin positive and, frequently, cytokeratin positive, indicating origin from epithelial and neuronal elements.[576, 577] The other small round cell tumors of childhood—NB, NHL, and RMS—must be excluded.

Staging

No standard staging system for Ewing's/PNET is accepted. Tumors are classified as localized or disseminated.

Principles of Treatment

Most patients with Ewing's/PNET present with what appears to be localized disease; however, surgery or radiation therapy alone is unlikely to be curative because of the presence of micrometastases. Chemotherapy has become increasingly effective in eliminating these cells, as well as assisting in obtaining local control. This advance has permitted strategies to reduce the need for radical surgery or high-dose, large-volume irradiation.

The goal of therapy is to eradicate all tumor while preserving as much function as possible. However, the optimal integration of the three modalities of therapy in terms of their aggressiveness remains to be determined. Fifteen percent to 35% of patients have demonstrable metastatic disease at diagnosis, and for most of these patients long-term survival is unobtainable, even with aggressive treatment including transplantation.[578, 579]

Surgery

Biopsy using optimal techniques establishes the diagnosis. The nature of the primary tumor resection is determined by the location, extent, and presence or absence of known metastases. Until recently, aggressive surgery was reserved for young patients with the potential for substantial growth impairment as a consequence of radiation therapy or for those with a severe pathologic fracture. Surgical resection of expendable bones was recommended if local control could be achieved without an undue functional deficit.[553] More recently, limb salvage surgery is being used. In other instances, more limited surgery with little normal tissue margin or microscopically positive margins followed by radiation therapy is at least as efficacious in achieving local control. Presurgical chemotherapy is routinely used. In all situations, the expected resulting morbidity should guide the choice inasmuch as local control is excellent either with surgical interventions or with radiation therapy.

Radiation Therapy

The potential for radiation therapy to achieve local control is dependent on the location and extent of the tumor. In general, radiation therapy, together with combination chemotherapy, is successful in approximately 80% of patients with distal extremity lesions, 69% with proximal extremity lesions, and 82% with central lesions, but only 44% of patients with pelvic-sacral tumors, as demonstrated in the 1998 analysis of a POG study.[580] Thus, the use of radiation therapy is considered in light of the surgical procedure deemed appropriate and the associated morbidity with each alone or in combination. Radiation therapy is appropriate for distal extremity lesions in nonexpendable bones and in the setting of subtotal or marginal resection of a bulky tumor. For patients with metastatic Ewing's/PNET, irradiation to the lungs and sites of osseous metastases has been of some value in overall disease control, particularly when part of an intensive myeloablative therapy.[581]

Improvements in chemotherapy, imaging techniques, and information regarding the characteristics of local tumor recurrence have allowed for refinements in the administration of radiation therapy. The traditional treatment volume included a generous margin around the soft tissue component and the entire bone, with successive field reductions to doses of 50 to 55 Gy. Data support the exclusion of one epiphyseal center at the opposite end of the bone from an eccentrically located lesion with peak doses of 55 Gy, depending on the tumor bulk and surgical procedure.[580, 582] Important radiation therapy considerations include treating the surgical scar and shaping fields to maintain lymphatic drainage by sparing a skin strip, preferably located medially.

Chemotherapy

Ewing's/PNET is an extremely chemotherapy-sensitive tumor, with a significant response rate to a number of single agents. Those used in the standard regimens include vincristine, cyclophosphamide, doxorubicin, and ifosfamide.[583] Ifosfamide and etoposide, known to be synergistic in the treatment of Ewing's sarcoma, improved outcome in nonmetastatic tumors in a 1994 pediatric trial in the United States[584]; the toxicity expressed in a recent dose intensification study was considerable.[551] In addition, nonrandomized trials in Italy have revealed a benefit of ifosfamide added to induction chemotherapy for localized Ewing's sarcoma of bone, but not a benefit of ifosfamide and etoposide added to maintenance therapy[585, 586]; differences may relate to dose intensity.

Multiagent chemotherapy has a role in improved systemic and local control, translating into improved overall survival. High-dose intensity use of the more active agents has played a particular role in improving DFS.[587, 588] Although chemotherapy once followed definitive surgery,[589] more recent regimens begin both radiation therapy and surgery after induction chemotherapy.

Bone Marrow Transplantation

Results using autologous BMT or stem cell therapy for patients with metastases at diagnosis or other prognostically poor presentations are promising.[588, 590, 591]

Results and Prognosis

Prior to the use of multiagent chemotherapy, few children with Ewing's/PNET survived, with 85% dying within 2 years of diagnosis.[34] Currently, the overall 5-year DFS is greater than 70%.[592, 593]

Prognosis

The *extent of disease* at diagnosis is the most important prognostic factor. Several variables directly or indirectly relate to this factor, making it difficult to determine the independent significance of any one:

- The presence of grossly metastatic disease at diagnosis is associated with a generally poor outcome.[580] In addition, in earlier studies, patients with bone or bone marrow involvement fared worse than patients with limited pulmonary involvement.[33] Progress in treating patients with metastatic disease is considerable.[589, 590, 594]
- Patients with an *extensive soft tissue component* of the primary tumor have a less favorable prognosis than patients with limited or no soft tissue involvement.[592] The size of the primary as it involves the bone (greater or less than 8 cm) may influence the likelihood of a successful outcome.[58]
- High *serum levels of lactate dehydrogenase* are associated with a poorer outcome, possibly because they reflect the burden or activity of tumor.[574, 595]

The site of involvement is relevant to the likelihood of the success of therapy. Involvement of the pelvis or sacrum is associated with a worse prognosis than is involvement of the proximal extremities (humerus, femur) or central sites such as the rib or vertebrae.[580] These sites are less favorable than is involvement of a distal extremity site. Local recurrence in the primary site occurs in 15% of children with extremity lesions, 47% with rib primaries, and 69% with pelvic tumors.[596]

Clinical Investigations

A further understanding of the molecular pathology and pathologic diversity of Ewing's/PNET will improve the ability to subclassify this tumor and may provide important prognostic information. New radiation therapy techniques, such as hyperfractionation, may enhance the likelihood of local control without increasing local morbidity, although the German trial, CESS 86, did not demonstrate any benefit from a hyperfractionated split-course regimen.[597] Ongoing studies address the possibility of improving outcome by dose intensity. In the long run, improved outcome will derive from an understanding of biologic features that may be of prognostic or therapeutic importance. A focus of future trials will be the biologic studies.

Recommended Reading

Early studies that provide a perspective on the natural history of Ewing's/PNET before modern therapeutic techniques include those by Dahlin and associates[32, 33] and Falk and Albert.[34] Modern approaches to Ewing's/PNET are reviewed by Arndt and Christ.[31] An overall review of the tumor, its biology, presenting features, and appropriate therapy is available in the report by Horowitz and colleagues.[35]

Hepatic Tumors

Perspective

Although primary liver tumors in infancy and childhood are rare, tumors that do occur are frequently malignant.[58] The most common malignant tumors are hepatoblastoma (HBL) and hepatocellular carcinoma (HCC). They comprise the third most common type of intra-abdominal malignant tumor, exceeded only by NB and Wilms' tumor. Only total surgical excision has resulted in long-term survival[26]; however, preoperative chemotherapy can make a previously inoperable tumor operable. In addition, surgical resection, with or without chemotherapy, of pulmonary metastases can produce long-term survival.[598]

Epidemiology and Etiology

Epidemiology

Childhood liver tumors occur at a rate of 1.5 per million per year.[599] HBL is the most frequently noted malignant liver tumor, accounting for 60% to 70% of all such tumors; HCC occurs with the next greatest frequency, 31%.[257] Other less frequently occurring malignant tumors of the liver include rhabdomyosarcoma, leiomyosarcoma, mesenchymoma, and undifferentiated sarcoma.

HBL usually occurs in children younger than 3 years of age, with a mean age of 17 months. The incidence of HCC, however, is relatively constant between 0 to 19 years.[599] Both HBL and HCC have a male predominance of 1.7:1.[26]

Etiology

The incidence of coexisting anomalies in HBL implies that there is a genetic contribution to the pathogenesis of hepatic tumors of childhood.

- There is an increased incidence of HBL in families with familial adenomatous polyposis coli (APC), and a number of authors have suggested that downregulation of the *APC* gene may be involved in the tumorigenesis of HBL.[600, 601]
- Hemihypertrophy has been observed in children with HBL.[602]
- There is an increased risk of developing HBL, as well as Wilms' tumor, NB, and rhabdomyosarcoma, in children with Beckwith-Wiedemann syndrome.[68, 603] Comparative investigations have been made to determine any consistent chromosomal abnormalities; areas on chromosomes 1 and 11 have been identified as possible targets.[604, 605]
- Very low birth weight is also associated with HBL.[606]

With respect to HCC, biologic associations have been more common:

- Hepatic malignancy has been reported in patients with neonatal hepatitis.[607, 608] Because of this association, it has been suggested that vaccination in areas with endemic hepatitis virus may reduce the incidence of HCC.[609]
- The short incubation times from hepatitis B virus infection to HCC carcinogenesis have been associated with somatic mutations of the *MET*/hepatocyte growth factor gene.[610]

In addition, liver tumors are associated with nonviral injury, such as biliary atresia, hereditary tyrosinemia, choledochal cyst, and antitrypsin deficiency.[611, 612]

Detection and Diagnosis

Clinical Detection

Greater than 90% of patients present with an abdominal mass or enlarged abdomen. Less frequently occurring signs and symptoms are abdominal pain, fever, weight loss, and icterus. Occasionally, isosexual precocity may be the presenting sign.[26]

Diagnostic Procedures

Evaluation must determine the magnitude of disease within the liver, the resectability, and the extent of extrahepatic disease.

- An *abdominal and chest x-ray* should be obtained to look for intrahepatic calcifications and metastatic disease. However, plain chest x-ray alone is inadequate for an extent of disease work-up.
- *MRI* will define the lesion in the liver and evaluate the hepatic veins and inferior vena cava for tumor extension.[58]
- A *CT scan* of the abdomen will give additional information regarding size, location, and multiplicity of the tumor. A CT scan of the chest also can be used to determine the presence of pulmonary metastasis.[613]
- *Angiographic studies* of the hepatic and tumor vasculature were, at one time, considered essential to determine resectability and aid in planning the surgical approach.[614] These studies have now largely been superseded by the use of other techniques, including *ultrasound*,[615] although they are still used in specific cases.[616]
- A routine *complete blood count* should be obtained; anemia with a hemoglobin count of less than 10 g/dL is frequently noted.[617] Thrombocytosis (platelet counts greater than 500,000/m^3) is frequent.
- *Liver function tests* should include studies of clotting factors; these values are usually normal unless jaundice is present.
- Serum measurements should be made of *AFP* and *HCG*. Absence of elevated AFP is associated with anaplastic histology and a poor prognosis.[618] HCG

elevation is usually associated with precocious puberty,[619] and, in contrast to AFP, does not parallel management of the tumor.

Classification

Histopathology

Both HBL and HCC arise in hepatocytes. HBL is more frequently isolated to one lobe of the liver with the right lobe predominating,[58] whereas HCC is more likely to occur in both lobes or to be multicentric.[620–622] Vascular invasion occurs frequently, and the lung is the most common organ for metastases.

The histologic classification of HBL is based on the work of Willis,[623] and modified by Ishak and Glunz.[624] The most frequently noted HBL tumor type has an epithelial histology, predominantly of either fetal or embryonal tissue, with the fetal histology having a better prognosis than that for embryonal tumors.[625] Less frequently noted tumor types are mixed epithelial and mesenchymal histology, a small number of an indeterminate type, with the least frequently noted tumor type being of anaplastic histology. Tumors of anaplastic histology are much more cellular and consist of poorly differentiated, small to medium-sized cells.

The histologic pattern for HCC is usually a microtrabecular pattern with neoplastic hepatocytes grouped in clusters, with occasional multinucleated giant cells; HCC, in contrast to HBL, usually arises in an abnormal liver. A less frequently noted pattern is a fibrolamellar type. Found in noncirrhotic livers of children, these tumors are characterized by hyaline bands of collagen, often laminated and interspersed between clumps of plump, polygonal neoplastic cells. Fibrolamellar carcinoma is associated with a more favorable prognosis.[626]

Staging

The staging system is based on both extent of tumor and operative resectability[618, 627, 628]:

- Stage I: complete tumor resection
- Stage II: tumor resection with microscopic residual disease (positive margins, tumor rupture during procedure)
- Stage III: gross residual disease, positive nodes or initially unresectable
- Stage IV: metastatic disease, regardless of magnitude of liver involvement

Principles of Treatment

Childhood liver tumors are rare and, thus, whenever possible, all children and adolescents should be considered candidates for a clinical trial. Total excision of the primary tumor is the major goal of therapy. More than half of HBLs are resectable, mainly because they are unifocal, and resection should be attempted in all children[629, 630]; moreover, preoperative chemotherapy may convert a previously unresectable HBL to an operative resection.[631] Postoperative chemotherapy will improve survival in patients who have had complete operative excision,[630] and there also are reports of survival with chemotherapy in patients with metastases.[632] However, it must be noted that HCC is resectable in less than 30% of children because it is invasive or multicentric. Moreover, liver cirrhosis has been identified in 70% of children with HCC.[633]

Surgery

A preoperative CT or MRI scan should determine resectability and, if necessary, an angiogram can be obtained for further preoperative evaluation. If both lobes are involved, resection is contraindicated. A generous bilateral subcostal incision is made for the celiotomy. Occasionally, the chest must be entered for suprahepatic vena cava control. The liver is inspected, and any invasion of tumor into adjacent viscera is noted. An assessment of the common hepatic artery and its branches and evaluation of the hepatic veins, as well as the portal vein and its tributaries, are mandatory intraoperative maneuvers to determine resectability. Biopsies should be performed on suspicious lymph nodes in the hepatoduodenal ligament.

Lobectomy or extended lobectomy are the operative procedures necessary for complete tumor excision, and *en bloc* resection should be used for extension of tumor. Any metastasis (diaphragm, adjacent organs) should also be removed at primary resection, and a biopsy should be performed on margins of the liver resection to confirm normal liver. Biopsy of the tumor is reserved only for those tumors deemed unresectable. At one time, uncontrolled blood loss was the most common cause of operative mortality; however, surgical techniques have improved over the last two decades.[634, 635] Distant metastases, such as pulmonary metastases, are not contraindications to liver resection, but, rather, pulmonary metastases should be resected.[636, 637]

Liver transplantation is indicated for stage III and stage IV HBL following chemotherapy.[629, 638, 639] Although children with HCC have undergone liver transplantation, their outcome is not as favorable; however, the fibrolamellar histology has a better prognosis.[640]

Radiation Therapy

Radiation has not been shown to affect prognosis, but it has been used in combination with chemotherapy, with some degree of success, for HBL patients with unresectable or microscopic residual disease.[641, 642] However, primary radiation therapy appears to have no defined role in the treatment of HCC.[641–643]

Chemotherapy

In general, for stages I and II HBL and HCC, resection is coupled with chemotherapy. Neoadjuvant agents used have include cisplatin, vincristine, and fluorouracil, followed by resection.[627] Advanced stage III disease can be treated with ifosfamide, cisplatin, and doxorubicin[627]; unresectable stage III HBL also can be treated with etoposide and high-dose cisplatin,[628] hepatic arterial infusions of chemotherapy,[644, 645] radiation therapy,[641] or liver transplantation.[638, 646] Indeed, stage III HBL has a 75% chance of resectability following cisplatin-based chemotherapy.[618] However, for stage III HCC in children, no combination of chemotherapeutic agents has been completely successful, although combination therapy of cisplatin and doxorubicin has been useful.[647, 648]

Stage IV metastatic HBL can be cured in 25% to 30% of children.[627, 628] If the primary tumor is removed, then it is recommended that any pulmonary disease be resected[636, 637]; radiation therapy and multidrug combinations remain under investigation. Again, no effective therapy for HCC in children has been observed. Currently cisplatin and doxorubicin are being used in randomized trials.

Recurrent HBL should be treated on a case-by-case basis. In stage I disease in which pulmonary metastases develop, the chest disease should be resected if the work-up reveals the disease to be localized.[598] In contrast, for HCC, the prognosis is so poor that an appropriate clinical trial is indicated.

Results

Various chemotherapeutic regimens have been used that improve survival in patients with hepatic tumors. These have included doxorubicin and cisplatin.[614, 645, 649] For HBL, other combination therapies that have been used are vincristine, 5-fluorouracil, and cisplatin; this combination has produced results similar to those for doxorubicin and cisplatin, but with less toxicity.[618, 627]

Long-term survival in liver cancer patients has increased from 25% to 70% through the addition of chemotherapy to complete operative excision. In a small series, the preoperative use of chemotherapy shrank the HBL and lowered the AFP levels[614]; this series led to the routine use of preoperative chemotherapy. Of note, preoperative chemotherapy can render a previously inoperable lesion operable.[629, 642] HCC has been shown to respond to resection with cisplatin-based chemotherapy.[626]

Prognosis

- HBL has a more favorable prognosis than HCC. The overall survival rate for HBL is 70%, but only 25% for HCC, regardless of age.[626, 628]
- For stage I and stage II HBL, cure rates are higher than 90%, whereas for children with stage III HBL, the cure rate is 60%, and approximately 20% for stage IV.[618, 626, 628]
- Overall, survival with adjuvant chemotherapy has markedly improved stage I HCC survival, but stage IV HCC in children remains incurable.[626] Nonetheless, the fibrolamellar variant of HCC has a better prognosis, with a 10-year patient survival rate of 47.4% in a 1997 study.[650] Those with the anaplastic type of HCC rarely survive.
- The prognosis has been poor if the primary tumor cannot be completely excised or metastatic dissemination has occurred, with greater than 95% of patients with HCC dying of the disease.[651, 652]

Recommended Reading

Helmberger and associates have examined the modern interaction between imaging and pathology, the advancement of which has improved surgical techniques for the management of hepatic tumors.[36] Bowman and coworkers[37] and Raney and D'Angio[38] discuss the various therapies now available to practitioners. Newman's article is an excellent overall reference, and the bibliography highlights the important role of preoperative chemotherapy for unresectable childhood hepatic malignancies.[39]

REFERENCES

General

1. Brodeur GM, Castleberry RP: Neuroblastoma. In: Pizzo PA, Poplack DG (eds): Principles and Practice of Pediatric Oncology, 3rd ed, p 761. Philadelphia, Lippincott-Raven, 1997.
2. Beckwith JB: New developments in the pathology of Wilms' tumor. Cancer Invest 1997; 194:153.
3. Beckwith JB: National Wilms' Tumor Study: an update for pathologists. Pediatr Dev Pathol 1998; 199:79.
4. Grundy P, Coppes M: An overview of the clinical and molecular genetics of Wilms' tumor. Med Pediatr Oncol 1996; 27:394.
5. Haase GM: Current surgical management of Wilms' tumor. Curr Opin Pediatr Surg 1996; 8:268.
6. Thomas PRM: Radiotherapy in Wilms' tumor. Ann Acad Med Singapore 1996; 25:425.
7. Ritchey ML, Green DM, Thomas PR: Renal failure in Wilms' tumor patients: a report from the National Wilms' Tumor Study Group. Med Pediatr Oncol 1996; 26:75.
8. Breslow NE, Takashima JR, Whitton JA, et al: Second malignant neoplasms following treatment for Wilms' tumor: a report from the National Wilms' Tumor Study Group. J Clin Oncol 1995; 13:1851.
9. Breslow N, Sharples K, Beckwith JB, et al: Prognostic factors in nonmetastastic, favorable history Wilms' tumor: results of the Third National Wilms' Tumor Study. Cancer 1991; 68:2345.
10. Green DM, Breslow NE, Evans I, et al: Relationship between dose schedule and charges for treatment on National Wilms' Tumor Study–4. J Natl Cancer Inst Monogr 1995; 19:21.
11. D'Angio GJ, Breslow N, Beckwith JB, et al: The treatment of Wilms' tumor. Results of the Third National Wilms' Tumor Study. Cancer 1989; 64:349.
12. Rosenberg SA, Diamond HD, Dargeon HW: Lymphosarcoma in childhood. N Engl J Med 1958; 259:505.
13. Shad A, McGrath I: Malignant non-Hodgkin's lymphoma in children. In: Pizzo PA, Poplack DG (eds): Principles and Practice of Pediatric Oncology, 3rd ed, p 545. Philadelphia, Lippincott-Raven, 1997.
14. Link MP, Donaldson SS: The lymphomas and lymphadenopathy. In: Nathan DG, Orkin SH (eds): Nathan and Oski's Hematology of Infancy and Childhood, 5th ed, p 1323. Philadelphia, W.B. Saunders Co., 1998.
15. Pappo A: Rhabdomyosarcoma and other soft tissue sarcomas of childhood. Curr Opin Oncol 1995; 7:361.
16. Maurer HM, Beltangady M, Gehan EA, et al: The Intergroup Rhabdomyosarcoma Study–I: a final report. Cancer 1988; 61:209.
17. Maurer H, Gehan E, Beltangady M, et al: The Intergroup Rhabdomyosarcoma Study–II. Cancer 1993; 71:1904.
18. Crist W, Gehan E, Ragab A, et al: The Third Intergroup Rhabdomyosarcoma Study. J Clin Oncol 1995; 13:610.
19. Azizkhan RG, Caty MG: Teratomas in childhood. Curr Opin Pediatr 1996; 8:287.
20. Cannistra SA: Cancer of the ovary. N Engl J Med 1993; 329:1550.
21. Lovvorn HN III, Tucci LA, Stafford PW: Ovarian masses in the pediatric patient. AORN J 1998; 67:568.
22. Coppes MJ, Arnold M, Beckwith JB, et al: Factors affecting the risk of contralateral Wilms' tumor development: a report from the National Wilms' Tumor Study Group. Cancer 1999; 85:1616.
23. Rescorla FJ, Breitfeld PP: Pediatric germ cell tumors. Curr Prob Cancer 1999; 23:257.
24. Pinkerton C, Pritchard J, Deraker J, et al: ENSG1 randomized study

of high dose melphalan in neuroblastoma. In: Dicke K, Spitzer G, Jaganoth S (eds): Autologous Bone Marrow Transplantation, p 401. Austin, University of Texas Press, 1987.

25. Egeler RM, D'Angio GJ: Langerhans' cell histiocytosis. Hematol Oncol Clin North Am 1998; 12:213.
26. Halperin EC, Constine LS, Tarbell NJ, et al: Pediatric Radiation Oncology, 3rd ed. Philadelphia, Lippincott Williams & Wilkins, 1999.
27. Gadner H, Heitger A, Grois N, et al: Treatment strategy for disseminated Langerhans cell histiocytosis. DAL HX-83 Study Group. Med Pediatr Oncol 1994; 23:72.
28. Link MP, Goorin AM, Horowitz M, et al: Adjuvant chemotherapy of high-grade osteosarcoma of the extremity. Updated results of the Multi-Institutional Osteosarcoma Study. Clin Orthop 1991; 270:8.
29. Bramwell VH: The role of chemotherapy in the management of non-metastatic operable extremity osteosarcoma. Semin Oncol 1997; 24:561.
30. Rosen G, Caparros B, Huvos AG, et al: Preoperative chemotherapy for osteogenic sarcoma. Cancer 1982; 49:1221.
31. Arndt CA, Christ WM: Common musculoskeletal tumors of childhood and adolescence. N Engl J Med 1999; 341:3442.
32. Dahlin DC: Bone Tumors: General Aspects and Data on 6,221 Cases. Springfield, Charles C Thomas, 1978.
33. Dahlin DC, Coventry MP, Scanlon PW: Ewing's/PNET: a critical analysis of 165 cases. J Bone Joint Surg 1961; 43A:185.
34. Falk S, Albert M: Five-year survival of patients with Ewing's/PNET. Surg Gynecol Obstet 1967; 124:319.
35. Horowitz ME, Malaweer MM, Woo SY, et al: Ewing's sarcoma family of tumors. In: Pizzo PA, Poplack DG (eds): Principles and Practice of Pediatric Oncology, 3rd ed, p 831. Philadelphia, Lippincott-Raven, 1997.
36. Helmberger TK, Ros PR, Mergo PJ, et al: Pediatric liver neoplasms: a radiologic-pathologic correlation. Eur Radiol 1999; 9:1339.
37. Bowman L, Hancock M, Santana F, et al: Impact of intensified therapy on clinical outcome in infants and children with neuroblastoma: the St. Jude Children's Research Hospital Experience, 1962–1988. J Clin Oncol 1991; 9:1599.
38. Raney RB, D'Angio GJ: Langerhans' cell histiocytosis (histiocytosis X): experience at the Children's Hospital of Philadelphia, 1970–1984. Med Pediatr Oncol 1989; 17:20.
39. Newman KD: Hepatic tumors in children. Semin Pediatr Surg 1997; 6:38.

39a. Bragg DG, Rubin P, Hricak HH (eds): Oncologic Imaging, 2nd ed. Philadelphia, W.B. Saunders Co., 2001.

Specific

40. Simone JV, Lyons J: The evolution of cancer care for children and adults. J Clin Oncol 1998; 16:2904.
41. Landis SH, Murray T, Bolden S, et al: Cancer statistics, 1999. CA Cancer J Clin 1999; 49:8.
42. Linet MS, Ries LA, Smith MA, et al: Cancer surveillance series: recent trends in childhood cancer incidence and mortality in the United States. J Natl Cancer Inst 1999; 91:1051.
43. Greenlee RT, Murray T, Bolden S, et al: Cancer statistics, 2000. CA Cancer J Clin 2000; 50:7.
44. Bleyer W: The impact of childhood cancer on the United States and the world. CA Cancer J Clin 1990; 40:355.
45. Grovas A, Fremgen A, Rauck A, et al: The National Cancer Data Base report on patterns of childhood cancers in the United States. Cancer 1997; 80:2321.
46. Gurney JG, Severson RK, Davis S, et al: Incidence of cancer in children in the United States. Cancer 1995; 75:2186.
47. Robison LL: General principles of the epidemiology of childhood cancer. In: Pizzo PA, Poplack DG (eds): Principles and Practice of Pediatric Oncology, 3rd ed, p 1. Philadelphia, Lippincott-Raven, 1997.
48. Knudson A, Strong L: Mutations and cancer. Neuroblastoma and pheochromocytoma. Am J Human Genet 1972; 24:514.
49. Knudson A: Hereditary cancer: theme and variations. J Clin Oncol 1997; 15:3280.
50. Look TA, Kirsch IR: Molecular basis of childhood cancer. In: Pizzo PA, Poplack DG (eds): Principles and Practices of Pediatric Oncology, 3rd ed, p 37. Philadelphia, Lippincott-Raven, 1997.
51. Roepe PD: What is the precise role of human MDR 1 protein in chemotherapeutic drug resistance? Curr Pharm Design 2000; 6:241.
52. Comito MA, Savell VH, Cohen MB: CD44 expression in neuroblastoma and related tumors. J Pediatr Hematol Oncol 1997; 19:292.
53. Nixon DW, Pirozzi D, York RM, et al: Dermatologic changes after systemic cancer therapy. Cutis 1981; 27:181.
54. Ruccione KS: Issues in survivorship. In: Schwartz C, Hobbie W, Constine L, et al (eds): Survivors of Childhood Cancer: Assessment and Management, p 329. St. Louis, Mosby, 1994.
55. Schwartz CL, Hobbie WL, Constine LS, et al (eds): Survivors of Childhood Cancer: Assessment and Management. St. Louis, Mosby, 1994.
56. Gale G, D'Angio G, Uri A, et al: Cancer in neonates: the experience at the Children's Hospital of Philadelphia, PA. Pediatrics 1982; 70:409.
57. Bernstein M, Leclerc J, Bunin G, et al: A population-based study of neuroblastoma incidence, survival, and mortality in North America. J Clin Oncol 1992; 10:323.
58. Pappo AS, Rodriguez-Galindo C, Dome JS, et al: Pediatric tumors. In: Abeloff MD, Armitage JO, Lichter AS, et al (eds): Clinical Oncology, 2nd ed, p 2346. New York, Churchill Livingstone, 2000.
59. Beckwith JB, Perrin EV: In situ neuroblastoma: a contribution to the natural history of neural crest tumors. Am J Pathol 1963; 43:1089.
60. Sawada T, Kawakatu H, Horii Y: Incidental neuroblastoma. Lancet 1988; 1:364.
61. Kosloske AM, Bhattacharyya N, Duncan MH: "Incidental" neuroblastoma. Lancet 1987; 2:565.
62. Lemire EG, Chodirker BN, Williams GJ: Familial neuroblastoma: report of a kindred with later age at diagnosis. J Pediatr Hematol Oncol 1998; 20:489.
63. Lo Cunsolo C, Iolascon A, Cavazzana A, et al: Neuroblastoma in two siblings supports the role of 1p36 deletion in tumor development. Cancer Genet Cytogenet 1999; 109:126.
64. Maris JM, Chatten J, Meadows AT, et al: Familial neuroblastoma: a three-generation pedigree and a further association with Hirschsprung disease. Med Pediatr Oncol 1997; 28:1.
65. Kushner BH, Gilbert F, Helson L: Familial neuroblastoma: case reports, literature review, and etiologic considerations. Cancer 1986; 57:1887.
66. Hayflick SJ, Hofman KJ, Tunnessen WW Jr, et al: Neurofibromatosis 1: recognition and management of associated neuroblastoma. Pediatr Dermatol 1990; 7:293.
67. al-Shammri S, Guberman A, Hsu E: Neuroblastoma and fetal exposure to phenytoin in a child without dysmorphic features. Can J Neurol Sci 1992; 19:243.
68. DeBaun MR, Tucker MA: Risk of cancer during the first four years of life in children from The Beckwith-Wiedemann Syndrome Registry. J Pediatr 1998; 132:398.
69. Brodeur G, Azar C, Brother M, et al: Neuroblastoma: effect of genetic factors on prognosis and treatment. Cancer 1992; 70:1685.
70. Caron H, Van Sluis P, de Kraker J, et al: Allelic loss of chromosome 1p as a predictor of unfavorable outcome in patients with neuroblastoma. N Engl J Med 1996; 334:225.
71. Plantz D, Mohapatra G, Matthay K, et al: Gain of the chromosome 17 is the most frequent abnormality detected in neuroblastoma by CGH. Am J Pathol 1997; 150:1.
72. Brown N, Cotterill S, Lastowska M, et al: Gain of chromosome arm 17q and adverse outcome in patients with neuroblastoma. N Engl J Med 1999; 340:1954.
73. Bordow S, Norris M, Haber P, et al: Prognostic significance of MYCN oncogene expression in childhood neuroblastoma. J Clin Oncol 1998; 16:3286.
74. Matsunaga T, Shirasawa H, Hishiki T, et al: Expression of MRP and cMOAT in childhood neuroblastomas and malignant liver tumors and its relevance to clinical behavior. Jpn J Cancer Res 1998; 89:1276.
75. Norris M, Bordow S, Marshall G, et al: Expression of the gene for multidrug-resistance-associated protein and outcome in patients with neuroblastoma. N Engl J Med 1996; 334:231.
76. Kaneko Y, Danda N, Maseki N, et al: Different karyotypic patterns in early and advanced stage neuroblastoma. Cancer Res 1987; 47:311.
77. Bowman L, Castleberry R, Cantor A, et al: Genetic staging of unresectable or metastatic neuroblastoma in infants: a Pediatric Oncology Group Study. J Natl Cancer Inst 1997; 89:373.
78. Eckschlager T, Pilat D, Kodet R: DNA ploidy in neuroblastoma. Neoplasma 1996; 43:23.

79. Laug W, Siegel S, Shaw K, et al: Initial urinary catecholamine metabolite concentrations and prognosis in neuroblastoma. Pediatrics 1978; 62:77.
80. von Studnitz W, Kaser H, Sjoerdsma A: Spectrum of catecholamine biochemistry in patients with neuroblastoma. N Engl J Med 1983; 209:232.
81. Numata K, Kusui H, Kawakatsu H: Increased urinary HVA levels in neuroblastoma screens related to diet, not tumor. Pediatr Hematol Oncol 1997; 14:569.
82. Ishiguro Y, Kato K, Ito T, et al: Nervous system-specific enolase in serum as a marker for neuroblastoma. Pediatrics 1983; 72:696.
83. Matthay KK, Perez C, Seeger RC, et al: Successful treatment of stage III neuroblastoma based on prospective biologic staging: a Children's Cancer Group study. J Clin Oncol 1998; 16:1256.
84. Brodeur G, Nakagawara A, Yamashiro D, et al: Expression of TrkA, TrkB and TrkC in human neuroblastomas. J Neurol Oncol 1997; 31:49.
85. Svensson T, Ryden M, Schilling FH, et al: Coexpression of mRNA for the full-length neurotrophin receptor trk-C and trk-A in favourable neuroblastoma. Eur J Cancer 1997; 33:2058.
86. Shimada H, Ambros I, Dehner L, et al: Terminology and morphologic criteria of neuroblastic tumors: recommendations by the International Neuroblastoma Pathology Committee. Cancer 1999; 86:349.
87. Fukuda M, Nozaki C, Ishiguro Y, et al: Natural antibody against neuroblastoma among Japanese children with or without neuroblastoma. Cancer 1999; 86:2166.
88. Ponzoni M, Casalaro A, Lanciotti M, et al: The combination of gamma-interferon and tumor necrosis factor causes a rapid and extensive differentiation of human neuroblastoma cells. Cancer Res 1992; 52:931.
89. Ihiele CJ, Reynolds CP, Israel MA: Decreased expression of N-myc precedes retinoic acid induced morphological differentiation of human neuroblastoma. Nature 1985; 313:404.
90. Bjellerup P, Theodorsson E, Kogner P: Somatostatin and vasoactive intestinal peptide (VIP) in neuroblastoma and ganglioneuroma: chromatographic characterisation and release during surgery. Eur J Cancer 1995; 31A:481.
91. Koh PS, Raffensperger JG, Berry S, et al: Long-term outcome in children with opsoclonus-myoclonus and ataxia and coincident neuroblastoma. J Pediatr 1994; 125:712.
92. Russo C, Cohn S, Petruzzi M, et al: Long-term neurologic outcome in children with opsoclonus-myoclonus associated with neuroblastoma: a report from the Pediatric Oncology Group. Med Pediatr Oncol 1997; 29:284.
93. Lucky AW, McGuire J, Komp DM: Infantile neuroblastoma presenting with cutaneous blanching nodules. J Am Acad Dermatol 1982; 6:389.
94. Alspaugh CD, Zanolli M: Blue nodules in a newborn. Neuroblastoma. Arch Dermatol 1997; 133:775.
95. Brodeur G, Pritchard J, Berthold F, et al: Revisions of international criteria for neuroblastoma diagnosis, staging and response to treatment. J Clin Oncol 1993; 11:1466.
96. Slovis TL, Meza MP, Cushing B, et al: Thoracic neuroblastoma: what is the best imaging modality for evaluating extent of disease? Pediatr Radiol 1997; 27:273.
97. Kauffman RA, Thrall JH, Keyes JW, et al: False negative bone scans in neuroblastoma metastatic to the ends of long bones. Am J Radiol 1978; 130:131.
98. Okuyama C, Ushijima Y, Sugihara H, et al: ^{123}I-metaiodobenzylguanidine (MIBG) scintigraphy for the staging of neuroblastoma. Kaku Igaku 1998; 35:835.
99. Perel Y, Conway J, Kletzel M, et al: Clinical impact and prognostic value of metaiodobenzylguanidine imaging in children with metastatic neuroblastoma. J Pediatr Hematol Oncol 1999; 21:13.
100. Shimada H, Ambros IM, Dehner LP, et al: The International Neuroblastoma Pathology Classification (the Shimada system). Cancer 1999; 86:364.
101. Evans AE, D'Angio GJ, Randolph J: A proposed staging for children with neuroblastoma. Cancer 1971; 27:374.
102. Evans AE, D'Angio GJ, Propert K, et al: Prognostic factors in neuroblastoma. Cancer 1987; 59:1853.
103. Hayes FA, Green A, Hustu HO, et al: Surgicopathologic staging of neuroblastoma: prognostic significance of regional lymph nodes metastases. J Pediatr 1983; 102:59.
104. Breslow NE, McCann B: Statistical estimation of prognosis of children with neuroblastoma. Cancer Res 1971; 31:2098.
105. Kushner BH, Cheung NK, LaQuaglia MP, et al: Survival from locally invasive or widespread neuroblastoma without cytotoxic therapy. J Clin Oncol 1996; 14:373.
106. Haase GM, Atkinson JB, Stram DO, et al: Surgical management and outcome of locoregional neuroblastoma: comparison of the Children's Cancer Group and the international staging systems. J Pediatr Surg 1995; 30:289.
107. Brodeur G: Molecular basis for heterogeneity in human neuroblastomas. Eur J Cancer 1995; 31A:505.
108. Kaneko M, Iwakawa M, Ikebukuro K, et al: Complete resection is not required in patients with neuroblastoma under 1 year of age. J Pediatr Surg 1998; 33:1690.
109. Granata C, Fagnani AM, Gambini C, et al: Features and outcome of neuroblastoma detected before birth. J Pediatr Surg 2000; 35:88.
110. Perez CA, Matthay KK, Atkinson JB, et al: Biologic variables in the outcome of Stages I and II neuroblastoma treated with surgery as primary therapy: a Children's Cancer Group study. J Clin Oncol 2000; 18:18.
111. Kaneko M, Ohakawa H, Iwakawa M: Is extensive surgery required for treatment of advanced neuroblastoma? J Pediatr Surg 1997; 32:1616.
112. Halperin EC: Neonatal neoplasms. Int J Radiat Oncol Biol Phys 2000; 47:171.
113. Barrientos G, Estelles C, Calvo F, et al: The role of intraoperative radiotherapy in oncological pediatric surgery. Cir Pediatr 1999; 12:136.
114. Haas-Kogan DA, Fisch BM, Wara WM, et al: Intraoperative radiation therapy for high-risk pediatric neuroblastoma. Int J Radiat Oncol Biol Phys 2000; 47:985.
115. Marcus K, Tarbell N: The changing role of radiation therapy in the treatment of neuroblastoma. Semin Radiat Oncol 1997; 7:195.
116. Hoefnagel CA: Nuclear medicine therapy of neuroblastoma. Q J Nucl Med 1999; 43:336.
117. Garaventa A, Bellagamba O, Lo Piccolo MS, et al: ^{131}I-metaiodobenzylguanidine (^{131}I-MIBG) therapy for residual neuroblastoma: a mono-institutional experience with 43 patients. Br J Cancer 1999; 81:1378.
118. Carli M, Green A, Hayes FA; et al: Therapeutic efficacy of single drugs for childhood neuroblastoma: a review. In: Raybaud C, Clement R, LeBreuil G, et al (eds): Pediatric Oncology: Proceedings of the XIIIth Meeting of the International Society of Pediatric Oncology, Marseilles, September 15–19, 1981, p 141. Amsterdam, Excerpta Medica, 1982.
119. Cairo MS: The use of ifosfamide, carboplatin, and etoposide in children with solid tumors. Semin Oncol 1995; 22:23.
120. Voute PA, van den Berg H, Behrendt H, et al: Ifosfamide in the treatment of pediatric malignancies. Semin Oncol 1996; 23:8.
121. Rubie H, Michon J, Plantaz D, et al: Unresectable localized neuroblastoma: improved survival after primary chemotherapy including carboplatin-etoposide. Neuroblastoma Study Group of the Société Française d'Oncologie Pediatrique (SFOP). Br J Cancer 1998; 77:2310.
122. Stram D, Matthay K, O'Leary D, et al: Consolidation chemoradiotherapy and autologous bone marrow transplantation vs continued chemotherapy for metastatic neuroblastoma: a report of two concurrent Children's Cancer Group studies. J Clin Oncol 1996; 14:2417.
123. Matthay KK, Villablanca JG, Seeger RC, et al: Treatment of high-risk neuroblastoma with intensive chemotherapy, radiotherapy, autologous bone marrow transplantation, and 13-cis-retinoic acid. Children's Cancer Group. N Engl J Med 1999; 341:1165.
124. Ohnuma N, Takahashi H, Kaneko M, et al: Treatment combined with bone marrow transplantation for advanced neuroblastoma: an analysis of patients who were pretreated intensively with the protocol of the study group of Japan. Med Pediatr Oncol 1995; 24:181.
125. Lazarus HM, Rowe JM, Goldstone AH: Does in vitro bone marrow purging improve the outcome after autologous bone marrow transplantation? J Hematother 1993; 2:457.
126. Saarinen UM, Wikstrom S, Makipernaa A, et al: In vivo purging of bone marrow in children with poor-risk neuroblastoma for marrow collection and autologous bone marrow transplantation. J Clin Oncol 1996; 14:2791.
127. Ross R, Jeter E, Laver J: Cost analysis of immunomagnetic marrow purging for neuroblastoma: in-house purging versus submission to purging centers. J Hematother 1995; 4:41.
128. Matthay KK, Seeger RC, Reynolds CP, et al: Allogeneic versus

autologous purged bone marrow transplantation for neuroblastoma: a report from the Children's Cancer Group. J Clin Oncol 1994; 12:2382.
129. Philip T, Ladenstein R, Lasset C, et al: 1070 myeloablative megatherapy procedures followed by stem cell rescue for neuroblastoma: 17 years of European experience and conclusions. European Group for Blood and Marrow Transplant Registry Solid Tumour Working Party. Eur J Cancer 1997; 33:2130.
130. Shimada H, Chatten J, Newton W, et al: Histopathologic prognostic factors in neuroblastic tumors. Definition of subtypes of ganglioneuroblastoma and an age linked classification of neuroblastomas. J Natl Cancer Inst 1984; 73:405.
131. Joshi V, Cantor A, Altshuler G, et al: Recommendations for modification of terminology of neuroblastic tumors and prognostic significance of Shimada classification. A clinicopathologic study of 213 cases from the Pediatric Oncology Group. Cancer 1992; 69:2183.
132. Look TA, Hayes F, Shuster J, et al: Clinical relevance of tumor cell ploidy and N-myc gene amplification in childhood neuroblastoma. A Pediatric Oncology Group Study. J Clin Oncol 1991; 9:581.
133. Nitschke R, Smith EI, Shochat S, et al: Localized neuroblastoma treated by surgery: a Pediatric Oncology Group Study. J Clin Oncol 1988; 6:1271.
134. Kushner B, Cheung N, LaQuaglia M, et al: International Neuroblastoma Staging System stage 1 neuroblastoma: a prospective study and literature review. J Clin Oncol 1996; 14:2174.
135. Evans A, Silber J, Arkady S, et al: Successful management of low-stage neuroblastoma without adjuvant therapies: a comparison of two decades, 1972 through 1981 and 1982 through 1992, in a single institution. J Clin Oncol 1996; 14:2405.
136. Matthay KK, Sather HN, Seeger RC, et al: Excellent outcome of stage II neuroblastoma is independent of residual disease and radiation therapy. J Clin Oncol 1989; 7:236.
137. Castleberry RP, Kun LE, Shuster JJ, et al: Radiotherapy improves the outlook for patients older than 1 year with Pediatric Oncology Group stage C neuroblastoma. J Clin Oncol 1991; 9:789.
138. West DC, Shamberger RC, Macklis RM, et al: Stage III neuroblastoma over 1 year of age at diagnosis: improved survival with intensive multimodality therapy including multiple alkylating agents. J Clin Oncol 1993; 11:84.
139. Nickerson HJ, Matthay KK, Seeger RC, et al: Favorable biology and outcome of stage IV-S neuroblastoma with supportive care or minimal therapy: a Children's Cancer Group study. J Clin Oncol 2000; 18:477.
140. Strother D, Shuster J, McWilliams N, et al: Results of Pediatric Oncology Group Protocol 8104 for infants with stages D and DS neuroblastoma. J Pediatr Hematol Oncol 1995; 17:254.
141. Matthay K: Stage 4S neuroblastoma: what makes it special? J Clin Oncol 1998; 16:2003.
142. Cheung N, Heller G: Chemotherapy dose intensity correlates strongly with response, median survival, and median progression-free survival in metastatic neuroblastoma. J Clin Oncol 1991; 9:1050.
143. de Bernardi B, Rogers D, Carli M, et al: Localized neuroblastoma. Surgical and pathologic staging. Cancer 1987; 60:1066.
144. Ninane J, Pritchard J, Morris Jones PH, et al: Stage II neuroblastoma. Adverse prognostic significance of lymph node involvement. Arch Dis Child 1982; 57:438.
145. Jacobson HM, Marcus RB Jr, Thar TL, et al: Pediatric neuroblastoma: postoperative radiation therapy using less than 2000 rad. Int J Radiat Oncol Biol Phys 1983; 9:501.
146. Nitschke R, Cangir A, Crist W, et al: Intensive chemotherapy for metastatic neuroblastoma: a Southwest Oncology Group study. Med Pediatr Oncol 1980; 8:281.
147. Halperin EC: Long-term results of therapy for stage C neuroblastoma. J Surg Oncol 1996; 63:172.
148. Castleberry RP Jr: Neuroblastoma. Therapy of Cancer in Children 2000; 1:24.
149. Katzenstein H, Bowman L, Brodeur G: Prognostic significance of age, MYCN oncogene amplification, tumor cell ploidy, and histology in 110 infants with stage D(s) neuroblastoma: the Pediatric Oncology Group experience. A Pediatric Oncology Group study. J Clin Oncol 1998; 16:2007.
150. Franks L, Bollen A, Seeger R, et al: Neuroblastoma in adults and adolescents. An indolent course with poor survival. Cancer 1997; 79:2028.
151. Villablanca J, Khan A, Avramis V, et al: Phase I trial of 13-cis-retinoic acid in children with neuroblastoma following bone marrow transplantation. J Clin Oncol 1995; 134:894.
152. Ryden M, Sehgal R, Dominici C, et al: Expression of mRNA for the neurotrophin receptor trkC in neuroblastomas with favorable tumor stage and good prognosis. Br J Cancer 1996; 74:773.
153. Batova A, Kamps A, Gillies SD, et al: The Ch14.18-GM-CSF fusion protein is effective at mediating antibody-dependent cellular cytotoxicity and complement-dependent cytotoxicity in vitro. Clin Cancer Res 1999; 5:4259.
154. Yu A, Batova A, Avarado C: Usefulness of a chimeric anti-GD2 (Ch14-18) and GM-CSF for refractory neuroblastoma: a POG Phase II study [abstract]. Proc Am Soc Clin Oncol 1997; 16:513a.
155. Ries LAG, Smith MA, Gurney JG: Cancer Incidence and Survival among Children and Adolescents: United States SEER Program 1975–1995. Bethesda, National Cancer Institute, 1999.
156. Stiller CA, Parkin DM: International variations in the incidence of childhood renal tumours. Br J Cancer 1990; 62:1026.
157. Breslow N, Olshan A, Beckwith JB, et al: Epidemiology of Wilms' tumor. Med Pediatr Oncol 1993; 21:172.
158. Vogelzang NJ, Fremgen AM, Guinan PD, et al: Primary renal sarcoma in adults. A natural history and management study by the American Cancer Society, Illinois Division. Cancer 1993; 71:804.
159. Tomlinson GS, Cole CH, Smith NM: Bilateral Wilms' tumor: a clinicopathologic review. Pathology 1999; 31:12.
160. Shearer P, Parham DM, Fontanesi J, et al: Bilateral Wilms' tumor: review of outcome, associated abnormalities, and late effects in 36 pediatric patients treated at a single institution. Cancer 1993; 72:1422.
161. Benatar B, Wright C, Freinkel AL, et al: Primary extrarenal Wilms' tumor of the uterus presenting as a cervical polyp. Int J Gynecol Pathol 1998; 17:277.
162. Babin EA, Davis JR, Hatch KD: Wilms' tumor of the cervix: a case report and review of the literature. Gynecol Oncol 2000; 76:107.
163. Beckwith JB: Nephrogenic rests and the pathogenesis of Wilms' tumor: development and clinical considerations. Am J Med Genet 1998; 268:79.
164. Breslow NE, Beckwith JB: Epidemiological features of Wilms' tumor: results of the National Wilms' Tumor Study. J Natl Cancer Inst 1983; 68:429.
165. Breslow NE, Olson J, Moksness J, et al: Familial Wilms' tumor: a descriptive study. Med Pediatr Oncol 1996; 27:398.
166. Bonaiti-Pellie C, Chompret A, Tournade MF: Genetics and epidemiology of Wilms' tumor: the French Wilms' tumor study. Med Pediatr Oncol 1992; 20:284.
167. Pritchard-Jones K: The Wilms tumour gene, WT1, in normal and abnormal nephrogenesis. Pediatr Nephrol 1999; 13:620.
168. Schwienbacher C, Angioni A, Scelfo R, et al: Abnormal RNA expression of 11p15 imprinted genes and kidney developmental genes in Wilms' tumor. Cancer Res 2000; 60:1521.
169. Grundy PE, Telzerow PE, Breslow N, et al: Loss of heterozygosity for chromosomes 16q and 1p in Wilms tumors predicts an adverse outcome. Cancer Res 1994; 54:2331.
170. Getman ME, Houseal TW, Miller GA, et al: Comparative genomic hybridization and its application to Wilms' tumorigenesis. Cytogenet Cell Genet 1998; 82:284.
171. Betts DR, Koesters R, Pluss HJ: Routine karyotyping in Wilms tumor. Cancer Genet Cytogenet 1997; 96:151.
172. Li FP, Breslow NE, Morgan JM: Germline WT1 mutations in Wilms' tumor patients: preliminary results. Med Pediatr Oncol 1996; 27:404.
173. Huff V: Genotype/phenotype correlations in Wilms' tumor. Med Pediatr Oncol 1996; 27:408.
174. Coppes MJ, Haber DA, Grundy PE: Genetic events in the development of Wilms' tumor. N Engl J Med 1994; 331:586.
175. Ariel I, Abeliovich D, Bar-ziv J: Renal pathology in WAGR syndrome. Pediatr Pathol Lab Med 1996; 16:1013.
176. Drechsler M, Meijers-Heijboer EJ, Schneider S: Molecular analysis of aniridia patients for deletions involving the Wilms' tumor gene. Human Genet 1994; 94:331.
177. Gronskov K, Rosenberg T, Sand A, et al: Mutational analysis of PAX6: 16 novel mutations including 5 missense mutations with a mild aniridia phenotype. Eur J Human Genet 1999; 7:274.
178. Drash A, Sherman F, Hartmann WIT, et al: A syndrome of pseudohermaphrodism, Wilms' tumor, hypertension, and degenerative renal disease. J Pediatr 1970; 76:585.

179. Friedman AL, Finlay JL: The Drash syndrome revisited: diagnosis and follow-up. Am J Med Genet 1987; 3:293.
180. Gallo GE, Chemes HE: The association of Wilms' tumor, male pseudohermaphroditism and diffuse glomerular disease (Drash syndrome): report of eight cases with clinical and morphologic findings and review of the literature. Pediatr Pathol 1987; 7:175.
181. Little M, Wells C: A clinical overview of WT1 gene mutations. Hum Mutat 1997; 9:209.
182. Patek CE, Little MH, Fleming S: A zinc finger truncation of murine WT1 results in the characteristic urogenital abnormalities of Denys-Drash syndrome. Proc Natl Acad Sci U S A 1999; 96:2931.
183. Jonge Poerink-Stockschlader AB, Dekker I, Risseeuw-Appel IM, et al: Acquired Von Willebrand disease in children with a Wilms' tumor. Med Pediatr Oncol 1996; 26:238.
184. Aron BS: Wilms' tumor: clinical study of 81 patients. Cancer 1974; 637:33.
185. Charlton GA, Sedgwick J, Sutton DN: Anaesthetic management of renin secreting nephroblastoma. Br J Anaesth 1992; 69:206.
186. Steinbrecher HA, Malone PS: Wilms' tumour and hypertension: incidence and outcome. Br J Urol 1995; 76:241.
187. Scott DJ, Wallace WH, Hendry GM: With advances in medical imaging can the radiologist reliably diagnose Wilms' tumours? Clin Radiol 1999; 54:321.
188. Rohrschneider WK, Weirich A, Rieden K, et al: US, CT and MR imaging characteristics of nephroblastomatosis. Pediatr Radiol 1998; 28:435.
189. Rosenfield NS, Leonidas JC, Barwick KW: Aggressive neuroblastoma simulating Wilms' tumor. Radiology 1988; 166:165.
190. Kraker J, de Lemerle J, Voute PA: Wilms' tumor with pulmonary metastases at diagnosis: the significance of primary chemotherapy. J Clin Oncol 1990; 8:1187.
191. Hutchinson RJ: Decision analysis of the expected clinical value of chest computed tomography in children with favorable histology Wilms' tumor. Pediatr Res 1991; 29:4.
192. Coppes MJ: Serum biological markers and paraneoplastic syndromes in Wilms tumor. Med Pediatr Oncol 1993; 21:213.
193. Jayabose S, Iqbal K, Newman L, et al: Hypercalcemia in childhood renal tumors. Cancer 1988; 61:788.
194. Siffring CW, Klein RL, Kastelic JE: The detection of occult renal tumors in children by elevated hematocrit on routine complete blood count: a report of two cases. J Pediatr Surg 1992; 27:1616.
195. Bisceglia M, Carosi I, Vairo M, et al: Congenital mesoblastic nephroma: report of a case with review of the most significant literature. Pathol Res Pract 2000; 196:199.
196. Blute ML, Kelalis PP, Offord KP, et al: Bilateral Wilms' tumor. J Urol 1987; 138:968.
197. Steinfeld AD, Crowley CA, O'Shea PA: Recurrent and metastatic mesoblastic nephroma in infancy. J Clin Oncol 1984; 2:956.
198. National Wilms' Tumor Study Committee: Wilms' tumor: status report, 1990. J Clin Oncol 1991; 9:877.
199. National Wilms' Tumor Study Group: NWTS-5: Phase III multimodality therapy based on histology, stage, age, and tumor size in children with Wilms' tumor, clear cell sarcoma of the kidney, and rhabdoid tumors of the kidney. Seattle, National Wilms' Tumor Study Group, 2000.
200. National Wilms' Tumor Study Group: NWTS-4: Phase III randomized comparison of short- vs long-term maintenance chemotherapy in children with Stages III–IV favorable histology Wilms' Tumor and clear cell sarcoma and comparison of DACT/VCR/DOX vs DACT/VCR/DOX/CTX in patients with Stages II–IV anaplastic Wilms' Tumor. Seattle, National Wilms' Tumor Study Group, 1994.
201. Green DM, Breslow NE, Evans I: Treatment of children with stage IV favorable histology Wilms' tumor: a report from the National Wilms' Tumor Study Group. Med Pediatr Oncol 1996; 26:147.
202. Horwitz JR, Ritchey ML, Moksness J: Renal salvage procedures in patients with synchronous bilateral Wilms' tumors: a report from the National Wilms' Tumor Study Group. J Pediatr Surg 1996; 31:1020.
203. Larsen E, Perez-Atayde A, Green DM: Surgery only for the treatment of patients with stage I (Cassady) Wilms' tumor. Cancer 1990; 66:264.
204. Shamberger RC, Macklis RM, Sallan SE: Recent experience with Wilms' tumor: 1978–1991. Ann Surg Oncol 1994; 1:59.
205. Ritchey ML, Kelalis PP, Breslow NB: Surgical complications after nephrectomy for Wilms tumor: a report from the National Wilms' Tumor Study–3. Surg Gynecol Obstet 1992; 175:507.
206. Shaul DB, Srikanth MM, Ortega JA: Treatment of bilateral Wilms' tumor: comparison of initial biopsy and chemotherapy to initial surgical resection in the preservation of renal mass and function. J Pediatr Surg 1992; 27:1009.
207. Thompson WR, Newman K, Seibel N: A strategy for resection of Wilms' tumor with vena cava or atrial extension. J Pediatr Surg 1992; 17:912.
208. Matthews PN, Evans C, Breckenridge IM: Involvement of the inferior vena cava by renal tumour: surgical excision using hypothermic circulatory arrest. Br J Urol 1995; 75:441.
209. Rodriguez-Rubio FI, Abad JI, Sanz G, et al: Surgical management of retroperitoneal tumors with vena caval thrombus in the inferior cava using cardiopulmonary bypass, arrested circulation and profound hypothermia. Eur Urol 1997; 32:194.
210. Ritchey ML, Kelalis PP, Haase GM, et al: Preoperative therapy for intracaval and atrial extension of Wilms tumor. Cancer 1993; 71:4104.
211. Green DM, Breslow NE, Beckwith JB: Treatment of children with clear-cell sarcoma of the kidney: a report from the National Wilms' Tumor Study Group. J Clin Oncol 1994; 12:2132.
212. Thomas PRM, Tefft M, Compaan PJ: Results of two radiation therapy randomizations in the Third National Wilms' Tumor Study. Cancer 1991; 68:1703.
213. D'Angio GJ, Evans AE, Breslow N: The treatment of Wilms' tumor: results of the National Wilms' Tumor Study. Cancer 1976; 38:633.
214. D'Angio GJ, Evans AE, Breslow N: The treatment of Wilms' tumor: results of the Second National Wilms' Tumor Study. Cancer 1981; 47:2302.
215. deKraker J, Lemerle J, Voute PA: Wilms' tumor with pulmonary metastases at diagnosis. The significance of primary chemotherapy. J Clin Oncol 1990; 8:1187.
216. Wilimas JA, Kaste SC, Kauffman WM, et al: Use of chest computed tomography in the staging of pediatric Wilms' tumor: interobserver variability and prognostic significance. J Clin Oncol 1997; 15:2631.
217. Meisel JA, Guthrie KA, Breslow NE: Significance and management of computed tomography detected pulmonary nodules. a report from the National Wilms Tumor Study Group. Int J Radiat Oncol Biol Phys 1999; 44:579.
218. Farber S: Chemotherapy in the treatment of leukemia and Wilms' tumor. JAMA 1966; 198:826.
219. Green DM, Breslow NE, Beckwith JB: Comparison between single-dose and divided-dose administration of dactinomycin and doxorubicin for patients with Wilms' tumor: a report from the National Wilms' Tumor Study Group. J Clin Oncol 1998; 16:237.
220. D'Angio GJ, Green DM: Primary renal tumors of childhood. In: Holland JF, Frei E (eds): Cancer Medicine, 3rd ed. Philadelphia, Lea & Febiger, 1973.
221. Tournade MF, Com-Nougue C, Voute PA: Results of the Sixth International Society of Pediatric Oncology Wilms' Tumor Trial and Study: a risk-adapted therapeutic approach in Wilms' tumor. J Clin Oncol 1993; 11:1014.
222. Zuppan CW, Beckwith JB, Weeks DA, et al: The effect of preoperative therapy on the histologic features of Wilms' tumor: an analysis of cases from the Third National Wilms' Tumor Study. Cancer 1991; 68:385.
223. Boccon-Gibod LA: Pathological evaluation of renal tumors in children: International Society of Pediatric Oncology approach. Pediatr Develop Pathol 1998; 1:2438.
224. Ritchey ML: The role of preoperative chemotherapy for Wilms' tumor: the NWTSG perspective. Semin Urol Oncol 1999; 17:21.
225. Morgan E, Baum E, Breslow N: Chemotherapy-related toxicity in infants treated according to the Second National Wilms' Tumor Study. J Clin Oncol 1988; 6:51.
226. Corn BW, Goldwein JW, Evans I: Outcomes in low-risk babies treated with half-dose chemotherapy according to the Third National Wilms' Tumor Study. J Clin Oncol 1992; 10:1305.
227. Grundy P, Breslow N, Green DM: Prognostic factors for children with recurrent Wilms' tumor: results from the Second and Third National Wilms' Tumor Study. J Clin Oncol 1989; 7:638.
228. Lowis SP, Foot A, Gerrard MP, et al: Central nervous system metastasis in Wilms' tumor: a review of three consecutive United Kingdom trials. Cancer 1998; 83:2023.
229. Shamberger RC, Guthrie KA, Ritchey ML: Surgery-related factors and local recurrence of Wilms' tumor in National Wilms' Study 4. Ann Surg 1999; 229:292.

230. Pein F, Tournade MF, Zucker JM: Etoposide and carboplatin: a highly effective combination in relapsed or refractory Wilms' tumor—a phase II study by the French Society of Pediatric Oncology. J Clin Oncol 1994; 12:931.
231. Pein F, Michon J, Valteau-Couanet D: High-dose melphalan, etoposide, and carboplatin followed by autologous stem-cell rescue in pediatric high-risk recurrent Wilms' tumor: a French Society of Pediatric Oncology Study. J Clin Oncol 1998; 16:3295.
232. Green DM, Fernbach DJ, Norkool P: The treatment of Wilms' tumor patients with pulmonary metastases detected only with computed tomography: a report from the National Wilms' Tumor Study. J Clin Oncol 1991; 9:1776.
233. Fuchs J, Wunsch L, Flemming P, et al: Nephron-sparing surgery in synchronous bilateral Wilms' tumors. J Pediatr Surg 1999; 34:1505.
234. Cooper CS, Jaffe WI, Huff DS, et al: The role of renal salvage procedures for bilateral Wilms tumor: a 15-year review. J Urol 2000; 163:265.
235. Corey SJ, Anderson JW, Vawter GF: Improved survival for children with anaplastic Wilms' tumor. Cancer 1991; 68:970.
236. Ritchey ML, Haase GM, Shochat S: Current management of Wilms' tumor. Semin Surg Oncol 1993; 9:502.
237. Faria P, Beckwith JB, Mishra K: Focal versus diffuse anaplasia in Wilms' tumor—new definitions with prognostic significance: a report from the National Wilms Tumor Study Group. Am J Surg Pathol 1996; 20:909.
238. Vujanic GM, Harms D, Sandstedt B, et al: New definitions of focal and diffuse anaplasia in Wilms' tumor: the International Society of Paediatric Oncology (SIOP) experience. Med Pediatr Oncol 1999; 32:317.
239. Zuppan CW, Beckwith JB, Luckey DW: Anaplasia in unilateral Wilms' tumor: a report from the National Wilms' Tumor Study Pathology Center. Human Pathol 1988; 19:1199.
240. Weeks DA, Beckwith JB, Mierau GW: Rhabdoid tumor of kidney: a report of 111 cases from the National Wilms' Tumor Study Pathology Center. Am J Surg Pathol 1989; 13:439.
241. Bonadio JF, Storer B, Norkool P: Anaplastic Wilms' tumor: clinical and pathological studies. J Clin Oncol 1985; 3:513.
242. Chen F, Li ZC, Ge RQ, et al: The measurement of DNA content in Wilms' tumor and its clinical significance. J Pediatr Surg 1994; 29:548.
243. Rainwater LM, Hosaka Y, Farrow GM: Wilms' tumors: relationship of nuclear deoxyribonucleic acid ploidy to patient survival. J Urol 1987; 138:974.
244. Green DM, Breslow NE, Beckwith JB: Screening of children with hemihypertrophy, aniridia, and Beckwith-Wiedemann syndrome in patients with Wilms tumor: a report from the National Wilms Tumor Study. Med Pediatr Onocol 1993; 21:188.
245. DeBaun MR, Siegel MJ, Choyke PL: Nephromegaly in infancy and early childhood: a risk factor for Wilms' tumor in Beckwith-Wiedemann syndrome. J Pediatr 1998; 132:401.
246. Paulino AC, Thakkar B, Henderson WG: Metachronous bilateral Wilms' tumor: the importance of time interval to the development of a second tumor. Cancer 1998; 82:415.
247. Evans AE, Norkool P, Evans I: Late effects of treatment for Wilms' tumor. Cancer 1991; 67:331.
248. Hunger SP, Sklar J, Link MP: Acute lymphoblastic leukemia occurring as a second malignant neoplasm in childhood: report of three cases and review of the literature. J Clin Oncol 1992; 10:156.
249. Paulino AC, Wen BC, Brown CK, et al: Late effects in children treated with radiation therapy for Wilms' tumor. Int J Radiat Oncol Biol Phys 2000; 46:1239.
250. Halberg FE, Harrison MR, Salvatierra O Jr, et al: Intraoperative radiation therapy for Wilms' tumor in situ or ex vivo. Cancer 1991; 67:2839.
251. Merchant TE, Zelefsky MJ, Sheldon JM, et al: High-dose rate intraoperative radiation therapy for pediatric solid tumors. Med Pediatr Oncol 1998; 30:34.
252. Bailey RJ, Burgert EL, Dahlin DC: Malignant lymphoma in children. Pediatrics 1961; 28:985.
253. Glatstein E, Kim H, Donaldson SS: Non-Hodgkin's lymphomas. VI. Results of treatment in childhood. Cancer 1974; 34:204.
254. Reiter A, Schrappe N, Parwaresch R: Non-Hodgkin's lymphoma of childhood and adolescence: results of a treatment stratified for biological sub-types and stage—a report of the BFM Group. J Clin Oncol 1995; 13:359.
255. Samuelsson BO, Ridell B, Rockert L: Non-Hodgkin lymphoma in children: a 20-year population-based epidemiologic study in western Sweden. J Pediatr Hematol Oncol 1999; 21:103.
256. Patte C, Kalifa C, Flamant F: Results of the LMB-81 protocol, a modified LSA2-L2 protocol with high dose methotrexate, on 84 children with non-B-cell (lymphoblastic) lymphoma. Med Pediatr Oncol 1992; 21:105.
257. Miller RW, Young JL, Novakovic B: Childhood cancer. Cancer 1994; 75:395.
258. Pozzato G, Mazzaro C, Santini G, et al: Hepatitis C virus and non-Hodgkin's lymphomas. Leuk Lymph 1996; 22:53.
259. Mueller BU: Cancers in children infected with the human immunodeficiency virus. Oncologist 1999; 4:309.
260. Beral V, Peterman T, Berkelman R: AIDS-associated non-Hodgkin's lymphoma. Lancet 1991; 337:805.
261. Mueller BU, Pizzo PA: Pediatric AIDS and childhood cancer. In: Pizzo PA, Poplack DG (eds): Principles and Practice of Pediatric Oncology, 3rd ed, p 1005. Philadelphia, Lippincott-Raven, 1997.
262. Knowles DM: Immunodeficiency-associated lymphoproliferative disorders. Mod Pathol 1999; 12:200.
263. Filipovitch A, Zerbe D, Spector B: Lymphomas in persons with naturally occurring immunodeficiency disorders. In: McGrath I, O'Connor G, Ramot B (eds): Pathogenesis of Leukemias and Lymphomas: Environmental Influences, p 225. New York, Raven Press, 1984.
264. Praghakaran K, Wise B, Chen A: Rational management of posttransplant lymphoproliferative disorder in pediatric recipients. J Pediatr Surg 1999; 34:112.
265. Sheil AG, Disney AP, Matthew TH: Lymphoma incidence, cyclosporine, and the evolution and major impact of malignancy following organ transplantation. Transplant Proc 1997; 29:825.
266. Spurney C, Gorlick R, Meyers PA, et al: Multicentric osteosarcoma, Rothmund-Thomson syndrome, and secondary nasopharyngeal non-Hodgkin's lymphoma: a case report and review of the literature. J Pediatr Hematol Oncol 1998; 20:494.
267. Servitje O, Marti RM, Estrach T: Occurrence of Hodgkin's disease and cutaneous B-cell lymphoma in the same patient: a report of two cases. Eur J Dermatol 2000; 10:43.
268. Murphy SB: Pediatric lymphomas: recent advances and commentary on Ki-1-positive-anaplastic large-cell lymphomas of childhood. Ann Oncol 1994; 5:31.
269. Greer JP, Kinney MC, Collins RD: Clinical features of 31 patients with Ki-1 anaplastic large-cell lymphoma. J Clin Oncol 1991; 9:539.
270. Ambinder RF, Griffin CA: Biology of the lymphomas: cytogenetics, molecular biology, and virology. Curr Opin Oncol 1991; 3:806.
271. McGrath IT: The pathogenesis of Burkitt's lymphoma. Recent Adv Cancer Res 1990; 55:133.
272. Pilozzi E, Muller-Hermelink HK, Falini B, et al: Gene rearrangements in T-cell lymphoblastic lymphoma. J Pathol 1999; 188:267.
273. Hubinger G, Scheffrahn I, Muller E, et al: The tyrosine kinase NPM-ALK, associated with anaplastic large cell lymphoma, binds the intracellular domain of the surface receptor CD30 but is not activated by CD30 stimulation. Exp Hematol 1999; 27:1796.
274. Murphy S, Fairclough D, Hutchison R, et al: Non-Hodgkin's lymphomas of childhood: analysis of the histology, staging, and response to treatment of 338 cases at a single institution. J Clin Oncol 1989; 7:186.
275. McGrath I, Shiramizu B: Biology and treatment of small-cleaved cell lymphoma. Oncology 1989; 3:41.
276. Haddy TB, Adde MA, McGrath IT: CNS involvement in small noncleaved-cell lymphoma: is CNS disease per se a poor prognostic sign? J Clin Oncol 1991; 9:1973.
277. Buchino JJ, Jones VF: Fine needle aspiration in the evaluation of children with lymphadenopathy. Arch Pediatr Adolesc Med 1994; 148:1327.
278. Whalen TV, LaQuaglia MP: The lymphomas: an update for surgeons. Semin Pediatr Surg 1997; 6:50.
279. Hamrick-Turner JE, Saif MF, Powers CI: Imaging of childhood non-Hodgkin lymphoma: assessment by histologic subtype. Radiographics 1994; 14:11.
280. Bangerter M, Griesshammer M, Bergmann L: Progress in medical imaging of lymphoma and Hodgkin's disease. Curr Opin Oncol 1999; 11:339.
281. Kurtzberg J, Graham ML: Non-Hodgkin's lymphoma: biologic clas-

sification and implication for therapy. Pediatr Clin North Am 1991; 38:443.

282. Yanchar NL, Bass J: Poor outcome of gastrointestinal perforations associated with childhood abdominal non-Hodgkin's lymphoma. J Pediatr Surg 1999; 34:1169.
283. Stein JE, Schwenn MR, Jacir NN, et al: Surgical restraint in Burkitt's lymphoma in children. J Pediatr Surg 1991; 26:1273.
284. Miron I, Frappaz D, Brunat-Mentigny M, et al: Initial management of advanced Burkitt lymphoma in children: is there still a place for surgery? Pediatr Hematol Oncol 1997; 14:555.
285. White L, Seigel SE, Duah TC: Non-Hodgkin's lymphoma in children. II Treatment. Crit Rev Oncol Hematol 1992; 1:73.
286. Link MP, Donaldson SS, Berard CW: Results of treatment of childhood localized non-Hodgkin's lymphoma with combination chemotherapy with or without radiotherapy. N Engl J Med 1990; 322:1169.
287. Shimizu H, Kikuchi M, Takaue Y: Improved treatment results of non-Hodgkin's lymphoma in children: a report from the Children's Cancer and Leukemia Study Group of Japan. Int J Hematol 1995; 61:85.
288. Sullivan MP, Brecher M: High-dose cyclophosphamide, high-dose methotrexate with coordinated intrathecal therapy for advanced nonlymphoblastic lymphoma of childhood. Results of a POG study. Am J Pediatr Hematol Oncol 1991; 9:133.
289. Bowman WP, Schuster JJ, Cook B: Improved survival for children with B-cell acute lymphoblastic leukemia and stage IV noncleaved cell lymphoma: a Pediatric Oncology Group study. J Clin Oncol 1996; 14:1252.
290. Meadows A, Sposto R, Jenkin R: Similar efficacy of 6 and 18 months of therapy with four drugs (COMP) for localized non-Hodgkin's lymphoma of children: a report from the Children's Cancer Study Group. J Clin Oncol 1989; 7:92.
291. Reiter A, Schrappe M, Tiemann NM: Successful treatment strategy for Ki-1 anaplastic large cell lymphoma of childhood: a prospective analysis of 62 patients enrolled in 3 consecutive BFM group studies. J Clin Oncol 1994; 12:899.
292. Ingram LC, Fairclough DL, Furman WL: Cranial nerve palsy in childhood acute lymphoblastic leukemia and non-Hodgkin's lymphoma. Cancer 1991; 67:2262.
293. Levy-Piedbois C, Habrand JL: Radiotherapy for leukemias and lymphomas in children. Cancer Radiother 1999; 3:181.
294. Murphy S, Bleyer W: Cranial irradiation is not necessary for central-nervous-system prophylaxis in pediatric non-Hodgkin's lymphoma. Int J Radiat Oncol Biol Phys 1987; 13:467.
295. Haddy T, Keenan A, Jaffee E, et al: Bone involvement in young patients with non-Hodgkin's lymphoma: efficacy of chemotherapy without local radiotherapy. Blood 1988; 72:1141.
296. Loeffler J, Tarbell N, Kozakewich H, et al: Primary lymphoma of bone in children: analysis of treatment results with Adriamycin, prednisone, Oncovin (APL), and local radiation therapy. J Clin Oncol 1986; 4:496.
297. Haddy TB, Adde MA, McCalla J, et al: Late effects in long-term survivors of high-grade non-Hodgkin's lymphomas. J Clin Oncol 1998; 16:2070.
298. Stapleton F, Strother D, Roy S, et al: Acute renal failure at onset of therapy for advanced stage Burkitt's lymphoma and B-cell acute lymphoblastic lymphoma. Pediatrics 1988; 82:863.
299. Philip T, Guglielni C, Hatenbeek A: Autologous bone marrow transplantation as compared with salvage chemotherapy in relapses of chemotherapy-sensitive non-Hodgkin's lymphoma. N Engl J Med 1995; 333:1540.
300. Loiseau HA, Hartmann O, Valteau D, et al: High-dose chemotherapy containing busulfan followed by bone marrow transplantation in 24 children with refractory or relapsed non-Hodgkin's lymphoma. Bone Marrow Transplant 1991; 8:465.
301. Sandlund JT, Downing JR, Crist WM: Non-Hodgkin's lymphoma in childhood. N Engl J Med 1996; 334:1238.
302. Link MP, Shuster JJ, Donaldson SS: Treatment of children and young adults with early-stage non-Hodgkin's lymphoma. N Engl J Med 1997; 337:1259.
303. DeNardo GL, Lamborn KR, DeNardo SJ, et al: Prognostic factors for radioimmunotherapy in patients with B-lymphocytic malignancies. Cancer Res 1995; 55:5893s.
304. Maurer H, Ruymann F, Pochedly C: Rhabdomyosarcoma and Related Tumors in Children and Adolescents. Boca Raton, CRC Press, 1991.
305. Dagher R, Helman L: Rhabdomyosarcoma: an overview. Oncologist 1999; 4:34.
306. Stout A: Rhabdomyosarcoma of the skeletal muscle. Ann Surg 1946; 123:447.
307. Cassady B, Sagerman RH, Tretter P, et al: Radiation therapy for rhabdomyosarcoma. Radiology 1968; 91:116.
308. Tefft M, Lindberg R, Gehan E: Radiation therapy combined with systemic chemotherapy of rhabdomyosarcoma in children: local control in patients enrolled into the Intergroup Rhabdomyosarcoma Study. Natl Cancer Inst Monogr 1981; 56:75.
309. Heyn RM, Holland R, Newton WA Jr, et al: The role of combined chemotherapy in the treatment of rhabdomyosarcoma. Cancer 1974; 34:2128.
310. Crist W, Garnsey L, Beltangady M, et al: Prognosis in children with rhabdomyosarcoma: a report of the Intergroup Rhabdomyosarcoma Studies I and II. J Clin Oncol 1990; 8:443.
311. Womer R: The Intergroup Rhabdomyosarcoma Studies come of age. Cancer 1993; 71:1719.
312. Stiller CA, Parkin DM: International variations in the incidence of childhood soft-tissue sarcomas. Paediatr Perinatol Epidemiol 1994; 8:107.
313. Wexler LH, Helman LJ: Rhabdomyosarcoma and the undifferentiated sarcomas. In: Pizzo PA, Poplack DG (eds): Principles and Practice of Pediatric Oncology, 3rd ed, p 799. Philadelphia, Lippincott-Raven, 1997.
314. Grufferman S, Schwartz A, Ruymann F, et al: Parents' use of cocaine and marijuana and increased risk of rhabdomyosarcoma in their children. Cancer Control Causes 1993; 4:217.
315. Ruymann FB, Maddux HR, Ragab A, et al: Congenital anomalies associated with rhabdomyosarcoma: an autopsy study of 115 cases. A report from the Intergroup Rhabdomyosarcoma Study Committee (representing the Children's Cancer Study Group, the Pediatric Oncology Group, the United Kingdom Children's Cancer Study Group, and the Pediatric Intergroup Statistical Center). Med Pediatr Oncol 1988; 16:33.
316. Yang P, Grufferman S, Khoury MJ, et al: Association of childhood rhabdomyosarcoma with neurofibromatosis type I and birth defects. Genet Epidemiol 1995; 12:467.
317. Birch J, Hartley A, Blair V, et al: Cancer in the families of children with soft tissue sarcoma. Cancer 1990; 66:2239.
318. Cornelis RS, van Vliet M, van de Vijver MJ, et al: Three germline mutations in the TP53 gene. Hum Mutat 1997; 9:157.
319. McManus AP, Gusterson BA, Pinkerton CR, et al: The molecular pathology of small round-cell tumours: relevance to diagnosis, prognosis and classification. J Pathol 1996; 178:116.
320. Zhang JM, Wei Q, Zhao X, et al: Coupling of the cell cycle and myogenesis through the cyclin D1-dependent interaction of MyoD with cdk4. EMBO J 1999; 18:926.
321. Scrable H, Witte D, Shimada H, et al: Molecular differential pathology of rhabdomyosarcoma. Genes Chromosomes Cancer 1989; 1:23.
322. Wang NP, Marx J, McNutt MA, et al: Expression of myogenic regulatory proteins (myogenin and MyoD1) in small blue round cell tumors of childhood. Am J Pathol 1995; 147:1799.
323. Driman D, Thorner P, Greenberg M, et al: MYCN gene amplification in rhabdomyosarcoma. Cancer 1994; 73:2231.
324. Felix CA, Kappel CC, Mitsudomi T, et al: Frequency and diversity of p53 mutations in childhood rhabdomyosarcoma. Cancer Res 1992; 52:2243.
325. Lawrence W Jr, Hays D, Heyn R, et al: Lymphatic metastases with childhood rhabdomyosarcoma: a report from the Intergroup Rhabdomyosarcoma Study. Cancer 1987; 60:910.
326. Donaldson SS, Breneman JC: Rhabdomyosarcoma. In: Perez CA, Brady LW: Principles and Practice of Radiation Oncology, 3rd ed, p 2129. Philadelphia, Lippincott-Raven, 1997.
327. Yang WT, Kwan WH, Li CK: Imaging of pediatric head and neck rhabdomyosarcomas with emphasis on magnetic resonance imaging and a review of the literature. Pediatr Hematol Oncol 1997; 14:243.
328. Mafee MF, Pai E, Philip B: Rhabdomyosarcoma of the orbit. Evaluation with MR imaging and CT. Radiol Clin North Am 1998; 36:1215.
329. Kushner BH, LaQuaglia MP, Cheung NK, et al: Clinically critical impact of molecular genetic studies in pediatric solid tumors. Med Pediatr Oncol 1999; 33:530.
330. Tobar A, Avigad S, Zoldan M, et al: Clinical relevance of molecular diagnosis in childhood rhabdomyosarcoma. Diag Mol Pathol 2000; 9:9.

331. Parham E, Webber B, Holt H, et al: Immunohistochemical study of childhood rhabdomyosarcomas and related neoplasms. Results of an Intergroup Rhabdomyosarcoma Study Project. Cancer 1991; 67:3072.
332. Newton W, Gehan E, Webber B, et al: Classification of rhabdomyosarcomas and related sarcomas. Cancer 1995; 76:1073.
333. Shimada H, Newton WA Jr, Soule EH, et al: Pathologic features of extra-osseous Ewing's sarcoma: a report from the Intergroup Rhabdomyosarcoma Study. Human Pathol 1988; 19:442.
334. Lawrence W, Anderson J, Gehan E, et al: Pretreatment TNM staging of childhood rhabdomyosarcoma. Cancer 1997; 80:1165.
335. Rodary C, Gehan E, Flamant F, et al: Prognostic factors in 951 non-metastatic rhabdomyosarcoma in children: a report from the international rhabdomyosarcoma workshop. Med Pediatr Oncol 1991; 19:89.
336. Donaldson S, Asmar L, Breneman J, et al: Hyperfractionated radiation in children with rhabdomyosarcoma—results of the Intergroup Rhabdomyosarcoma pilot study. Int J Radiat Oncol Biol Phys 1995; 32:903.
337. Wiener E, Lawrence W, Hays D, et al: Survival is improved in clinical group III children with complete response established by second look operations in the Intergroup Rhabdomyosarcoma Study III. Med Pediatr Oncol 1991; 19:399.
338. Michalkiewicz EL, Rao BN, Gross E, et al: Complications of pelvic exenteration in children who have genitourinary rhabdomyosarcoma. J Pediatr Surg 1997; 32:1277.
339. Ferrari A, Casanova M, Massimino M, et al: The management of paratesticular rhabdomyosarcoma: a single institutional experience with 44 consecutive children. J Urol 1998; 159:1031.
340. Wharam MD, Hanfelt JJ, Tefft MC: Radiation therapy for rhabdomyosarcoma: local failure risk for Clinical Group III patients on Intergroup Rhabdomyosarcoma Study II. Int J Radiat Oncol Biol Phys 1997; 38:797.
341. Lombardi F, Navarria P, Gandola L: The evolving role of radiation therapy in the optimal multimodality treatment of childhood cancer. Tumori 1998; 84:270.
342. Merchant T: Delayed-accelerated hyperfractionated radiation therapy for advanced-stage or high-risk rhabdomyosarcoma. Med Pediatr Oncol 1997; 29:45.
343. Regine WF, Fontanesi J, Kumar P, et al: A phase II trial evaluating selective use of altered radiation dose and fractionation in patients with unresectable rhabdomyosarcoma. Int J Radiat Oncol Biol Phys 1995; 31:799.
344. Mandell L, Ghavimi R, Peretz T, et al: Radiocurability of microscopic disease in childhood rhabdomyosarcoma with radiation doses less than 4000 cGy. J Clin Oncol 1990; 8:1536.
345. Nag S, Martinez-Monge R, Ruymann F, et al: Innovation in the management of soft tissue sarcomas in infants and young children: high-dose-rate brachytherapy. J Clin Oncol 1997; 15:3075.
346. Donaldson SS, Castro JR, Wilbur JR, et al: Rhabdomyosarcoma of the head and neck in children: combination treatment by surgery, irradiation and chemotherapy. Cancer 1973; 31:26.
347. Arndt C, Tefft M, Gehan E, et al: A feasibility, toxicity, and early response study of etoposide, ifosfamide, and vincristine for the treatment of children with rhabdomyosarcoma: a report from the Intergroup Rhabdomyosarcoma Study (IRS) IV pilot study. J Pediatr Hematol Oncol 1997; 19:124.
348. Kodet R, Newton W, Hamoudi A, et al: Orbital rhabdomyosarcomas and related tumors in childhood: relationship of morphology to prognosis—an Intergroup Rhabdomyosarcoma Study. Med Pediatr Oncol 1997; 29:51.
349. Rousseau P, Flamant F, Quintana E, et al: Primary chemotherapy in rhabdomyosarcoma and other malignant mesenchymal tumors of the orbit. Results of the International Society of Pediatric Oncology MMT 84 Study. J Clin Oncol 1994; 12:516.
350. Wharam M: Rhabdomyosarcoma of parameningeal sites. Semin Radiat Oncol 1997; 7:212.
351. Blatt J, Synderman C, Wollman M, et al: Delayed resection in the management of non-orbital rhabdomyosarcoma of the head and neck in childhood. Med Pediatr Oncol 1997; 29:294.
352. Benk V, Rodary C, Donaldson S, et al: Parameningeal rhabdomyosarcoma: results of an international workshop. Int J Radiat Oncol Biol Phys 1996; 36:533.
353. Raney RB Jr, Gehan EA, Hays DM, et al: Primary chemotherapy with or without radiation therapy and/or surgery for children with localized sarcoma of the bladder, prostate, vagina, uterus, and cervix. A comparison of the results in Intergroup Rhabdomyosarcoma Studies I and II. Cancer 1990; 66:2072.
354. Heyn R, Newton WA, Raney RB, et al: Preservation of the bladder in patients with rhabdomyosarcoma. J Clin Oncol 1997; 15:69.
355. Hays D, Raney B, Wharam M, et al: Children with vesical rhabdomyosarcoma treated by partial cystectomy with neoadjuvant or adjuvant chemotherapy, with or without radiotherapy. J Pediatr Hematol Oncol 1995; 17:46.
356. Breneman J: Genitourinary rhabdomyosarcoma. Semin Radiat Oncol 1997; 7:217.
357. Hays DM, Shimada H, Raney RB, Jr, et al: Sarcomas of the vagina and uterus: the Intergroup Rhabdomyosarcoma Study. J Pediatr Surg 1985; 20:718.
358. Andrassy RJ, Hays DM, Raney RB: Conservative surgical management of vaginal and vulvar pediatric rhabdomyosarcoma: a report from the Intergroup Rhabdomyosarcoma Study III. J Pediatr Surg 1995; 30:1034.
359. Flamant F, Gerbaulet A, Nihoul-Fekete C, et al: Long-term sequelae of conservative treatment by surgery, brachytherapy, and chemotherapy for vulval and vaginal rhabdomyosarcoma in children. J Clin Oncol 1990; 8:1847.
360. Corpon C, Andrassy R, Hays D, et al: Conservative management of uterine pediatric rhabdomyosarcoma: a report from the Intergroup Rhabdomyosarcoma Study III and IV pilot. J Pediatr Surg 1995; 30:942.
361. Blakely ML, Lobe TE, Anderson JR, et al: Does debulking improve survival rate in advanced-stage retroperitoneal embryonal rhabdomyosarcoma? J Pediatr Surg 1999; 34:736.
362. Ortega J, Wharam M, Gehan E: Clinical features and results of therapy for children with paraspinal soft tissue sarcoma: a report of the Intergroup Rhabdomyosarcoma Study. J Clin Oncol 1991; 9:796.
363. Pedrick R, Donaldson S, Cox R: Rhabdomyosarcoma: the Stanford experience using a TNM staging system. J Clin Oncol 1986; 4:370.
364. Shapiro E, Parham D, Douglass E, et al: Relationship of tumor-cell ploidy to histologic subtype and treatment outcome in children and adolescents with unresectable rhabdomyosarcoma. J Clin Oncol 1991; 9:159.
365. Pappo A, Crist W, Kuttesch J, et al: Tumor-cell DNA content predicts outcome in children and adolescents with clinical group III embryonal rhabdomyosarcoma. J Clin Oncol 1993; 11:1901.
366. Wignaendts LCD, van der Linden JC, van Diest PJ, et al: Prognostic importance of DNA flow cytometric variables in rhabdomyosarcoma. J Clin Pathol 1993; 46:948.
367. Whang-Peng J, Knutsen T, Theil K, et al: Cytogenetic studies in subgroups of rhabdomyosarcoma. Genes Chromosomes Cancer 1997; 5:299.
368. LaQuaglia M, Heller G, Ghavimi F, et al: The effect of age at diagnosis on outcome in rhabdomyosarcoma. Cancer 1994; 73:109.
369. Ragab AH, Heyn R, Tefft M, et al: Infants younger than 1 year of age with rhabdomyosarcoma. Cancer 1986; 58:2606.
370. Mandell L, Massey V, Ghavimi F: The influence of extensive bone erosion on local control in non-orbital rhabdomyosarcoma of the head and neck. Int J Radiat Oncol Biol Phys 1989; 17:649.
371. Mandell L, Ghavimi F, LaQuaglia M, et al: Prognostic significance of regional lymph node involvement in childhood extremity rhabdomyosarcoma. Med Pediatr Oncol 1990; 18:466.
372. Witschi E: Migration of the germ cells of human embryos from the yolk sac to the primitive gonadal fold. Contributions to Embryology 1988; 32:69.
373. Skinner MA: Germ cell tumors. In: Oldham KT, Foglia RP, Colombani PM (eds): Surgery of Infants and Children: Scientific Principles and Practice, p 653. Philadelphia, Lippincott-Raven, 1997.
374. Subbarao P, Bhatnagar V, Mitra DK: The association of sacrococcygeal teratoma with high anorectal and genital malformations. Austral N Z J Surg 1994; 64:214.
375. Ng WT, Ng TK, Cheng PW: Sacrococcygeal teratoma and anorectal malformation. Austral N Z J Surg 1997; 67:218.
376. Lee SC, Chun YS, Jung SE, et al: Currarino triad: anorectal malformation, sacral bony abnormality, and presacral mass—a review of 11 cases. J Pediatr Surg 1997; 32:58.
377. Stettner AR, Hartenbach EM, Schink JC, et al: Familial ovarian germ cell cancer: report and review. Am J Med Genet 1999; 84:43.
378. Heidenreich A, Srivastava S, Moul JW, et al: Molecular genetic parameters in pathogenesis and prognosis of testicular germ cell tumors. Eur Urol 2000; 37:121.

379. Hamers A, de Jong B, Suijkerbuijk RF, et al: A 46,XY female with mixed gonadal dysgenesis and a 48,XY, +7, +i(12p) chromosome pattern in a primary gonadal tumor. Cancer Genet Cytogenet 1991; 57:219.
380. Kingsbury AC, Frost F, Cookson CM: Dysgerminoma, gonadoblastoma and testicular germ cell neoplasia in phenotypically female and male siblings with 46XY genotype. Cancer 1987; 59:288.
381. Bebb GG, Grannis FW Jr, Paz IB, et al: Mediastinal germ cell tumor in a child with precocious puberty and Klinefelter syndrome. Ann Thorac Surg 1998; 66:547.
382. Vilain E, Jaubert F, Fellous M: Pathology of 46,XY pure gonadal dysgenesis; absence of testis differentiation with mutations in the testis-determining factor. Differentiation 1993; 52:151.
383. Heimdal K, Fossa SD: Genetic factors in malignant germ-cell tumors. World J Urol 1994; 12:178.
384. Silver SA, Wiley JM, Perlman EJ: DNA ploidy analysis of pediatric germ cell tumors. Mod Pathol 1994; 7:951.
385. Szmyd K, Chybicka A, Golebiowski W: The evaluation of neoplasm markers in the diagnosis and treatment of germ cell tumors in children. Wiad Lek 1998; 51:193.
386. Wu JT, Book L, Sudan K: Serum alpha fetoprotein (AFP) levels in normal infants. Pediatr Rev 1981; 15:50.
387. Kurisaka M, Saitoh S, Seike M, et al: Gonadotropin, as a tumor marker, in body fluid and tumor tissues of germ cell tumors. No To Shinkei 1989; 41:353.
388. Wanderas EH, Grotmol T, Fossa SD, et al: Maternal health and pre- and perinatal characteristics in the etiology of testicular cancer: a prospective population- and register-based study on Norwegian males born between 1967 and 1995. Cancer Causes Control 1998; 9:475.
389. Weidner N: Germ-cell tumors of the mediastinum. Semin Diag Pathol 1999; 16:42.
390. Satge D, Auge B, Philippe E, et al: Gastric teratoma in newborn children. Ann Pediatr 1990; 37:235.
391. Das DK, Pant CS, Rath B, et al: Fine-needle aspiration diagnosis of intra-thoracic and intra-abdominal lesions: review of experience in the pediatric age group. Diag Cytopathol 1993; 9:383.
392. Tsuchida Y, Terada M, Honna T, et al: The role of subfractionation of alpha-fetoprotein in the treatment of pediatric surgical patients. J Pediatr Surg 1997; 32:514.
393. Larsen ME, Larsen JW, Hamersley SL, et al: Successful management of fetal cervical teratoma using the EXIT procedure. J Matern Fetal Med 1999; 8:295.
394. Papageorgiou C, Papathanasiou K, Panidis D, et al: Prenatal diagnosis of epignathus in the first half of pregnancy: a case report and review of the literature. Clin Exp Obstet Gynecol 2000; 27:67.
395. Liechty KW, Crombleholme TM, Flake AW, et al: Intrapartum airway management for giant fetal neck masses: the EXIT (ex utero intrapartum treatment) procedure. Am J Obstet Gynecol 1997; 177:870.
396. Chowdhary SK, Chitnis M, Perold J, et al: Hypothyroidism in a neonate following excision of a cervical teratoma. Pediatr Surg Int 1998; 14:212.
397. Choi JU, Kim DS, Chung SS: Treatment of germ cell tumors in the pineal region. Childs Nerv Syst 1998; 14:41.
398. Robinson S, Cohen AR: The role of neuroendoscopy in the treatment of pineal region tumors. Surg Neurol 1997; 48:360.
399. Akyuz C, Koseoglu V, Bertan V, et al: Primary intracranial germ cell tumors in children: a report of eight cases and review of the literature. Turk J Pediatr 1999; 41:161.
400. Andze G, Pagbe JJ, Yomi J, et al: Benign giant epignathic teratoma in the newborn. Apropos of an unusual clinical case. J Chirurg 1994; 131:316.
401. Mootha SL, Barkovich AJ, Grumbach MM, et al: Idiopathic hypothalamic diabetes insipidus, pituitary stalk thickening, and the occult intracranial germinoma in children and adolescents. J Clin Endocrinol Metabol 1997; 82:1362.
402. Inamura T, Nishio S, Ikezaki K, et al: Human chorionic gonadotrophin in CSF, not serum, predicts outcome in germinoma. J Neurol Neurosurg Psychiatr 1999; 66:654.
403. Tapper D, Lack EE: Teratomas in infancy and childhood. A 54 year experience at the Children's Hospital Medical Center. Ann Surg 1983; 198:398.
404. Hawkins E, Isaacs H, Cushing B: Occult malignancy in neonatal sacrococcygeal teratomas: a report from a combined pediatric oncology group and children's cancer group study. Am J Pediatr Hematol Oncol 1993; 15:406.
405. Mann JR, Pearson D, Barrett A: Results of the United Kingdom Children's Cancer Study Group's malignant germ cell tumor studies. Cancer 1989; 63:1657.
406. Marina N, Fontanesi J, Kun L: Treatment of childhood germ cell tumors: review of the St. Jude experience from 1979 to 1988. Cancer 1992; 70:2568.
407. Brodeur GM, Howarth CB, Pratt CB: Malignant germ cell tumors in 57 children and adolescents. Cancer 1981; 48:1890.
408. Li MC, Whitmore WR, Golbey RB: Effects of combined drug therapy in metastatic cancer of the testis. JAMA 1960; 174:1291.
409. Siegert W, Beyer J: Germ cell tumors: dose-intensive therapy. Semin Oncol 1998; 25:215.
410. Billmire DF: Germ cell, mesenchymal, and thymic tumors of the mediastinum. Surgery. Semin Pediatr Surg 1999; 8:85.
411. Diez B, Balmaceda C, Matsutani M, et al: Germ cell tumors of the CNS in children: recent advances in therapy. Childs Nerv Syst 1999; 15:578.
412. Shih GH, Boyd GL, Vincent RD, et al: The EXIT procedure facilitates delivery of an infant with a pretracheal teratoma. Anesthesiology 1998; 89:1573.
413. Malogolowkin MH, Mahour GH, Krailo M: Germ cell tumors in infancy and childhood: a 45-year experience. Pediatri Pathol 1990; 10:231.
414. Weissbach L, Bussar-Maatz R, Flechtner H, et al: RPLND or primary chemotherapy in clinical stage IIA/B nonseminomatous germ cell tumors? Results of a prospective multicenter trial including quality of life assessment. Eur Urol 2000; 37:582.
415. Farng KT, Chang KP, Wong TT, et al: Pediatric intracranial germinoma treated with chemotherapy alone. Chin Med J 1999; 62:859.
416. Bamberg M, Kortmann RD, Calaminus G, et al: Radiation therapy for intracranial germinoma: results of the German cooperative prospective trials MAKEI 83/86/89. J Clin Oncol 1999; 17:2585.
417. Sharda NN, Kinsella TJ, Ritter MA: Adjuvant radiation versus observation: a cost analysis of alternate management schemes in early-stage testicular seminomas. J Clin Oncol 1996; 14:2933.
418. Warde P, Gospodarowicz MK, Panzarella T: Stage I testicular seminoma: results of adjuvant irradiation and surveillance. J Clin Oncol 1995; 13:2255.
419. Kersh CR, Constable WC, Hahn SS: Primary malignant extragonadal germ cell tumors: an analysis of the effect of radiotherapy. Cancer 1990; 65:2681.
420. Li MC, Hertz R, Spencer DB: Effect of methotrexate on choriocarcinoma and chorioadenoma. Proc Soc Exp Biol Med 1956; 96:361.
421. Wider FA, Marshall JR, Basridin CAE: Sustained remissions after chemotherapy for primary ovarian cancer containing choriocarcinoma. N Engl J Med 1969; 280:1439.
422. Cangir AL, Smith J, van Eys J: Improved prognosis in children with ovarian cancers following modified VAC (vincristine sulfate, dactinomycin and cyclophosphamide) chemotherapy. Cancer 1978; 42:1234.
423. Samuels ML, Howe CD: Vinblastine in the management of testicular cancer. Cancer 1970; 25:1009.
424. Blum RH, Carter SS, Agre K: A clinical review of bleomycin—a new antineoplastic agent. Cancer 1973; 31:903.
425. Higby DJ, Wallace HJ, Albert D: Diaminodichloro-platinum in chemotherapy of testicular tumors. J Urol 1974; 112:100.
426. Einhorn LH, Donohue JP: Cis-diaminodichloroplatinum, vinblastine, and bleomycin combination chemotherapy in disseminated testicular cancer. Ann Intern Med 1977; 87:293.
427. Einhorn LH, Williams SD, Troner M: The role of maintenance therapy in disseminated testicular cancer. N Engl J Med 1981; 305:727.
428. Einhorn LH, Williams SD: Chemotherapy of disseminated testicular cancer: a random prospective study. Cancer 1980; 46:1339.
429. Loehrer PJ, Einhorn LH, Williams SD: VP-16 plus ifosfamide plus cisplatin as salvage therapy in refractory germ cell cancer. J Clin Oncol 1986; 4:528.
430. Bokemeyer C, Kohrmann O, Tischler J, et al: A randomized trial of cisplatin, etoposide and bleomycin (PEB) versus carboplatin, etoposide and bleomycin (CEB) for patients with "good-risk" metastatic non-seminomatous germ cell tumors. Ann Oncol 1996; 7:1015.
431. Bokemeyer C, Kollmannsberger C, Meisner C, et al: First-line high-dose chemotherapy compared with standard-dose PEB/VIP chemo-

therapy in patients with advanced germ cell tumors: A multivariate and matched-pair analysis. J Clin Oncol 1999; 17:3450.

432. Marina NM, Rodman JH, Murray DJ: Phase I study of escalating targeted doses of carboplatin combined with ifosfamide and etoposide in treatment of newly diagnosed pediatric solid tumors. J Natl Cancer Inst 1994; 86:544.
433. Marina NM, Shema SJ, Bowman LC: Failure of granulocyte-macrophage colony-stimulating factor to reduce febrile neutropenia in children with recurrent solid tumors treated with ifosfamide, carboplatin and etoposide chemotherapy. Med Pediatr Oncol 1994; 23:328.
434. Yoshida T, Yonese J, Kitsukawa S, et al: Treatment results of VIP (etoposide, ifosfamide and cisplatin) chemotherapy as a first-line therapy in metastatic germ cell tumors. Nippon Hinyokika Gakkai Zasshi 2000; 91:55.
435. Gobel U, Calaminus G, Engert J, et al: Teratomas in infancy and childhood. Med Pediatr Oncol 1998; 31:8.
436. Rescorla FJ, Sawin RS, Coran AG, et al: Long-term outcome for infants and children with sacrococcygeal teratoma: a report from the Children's Cancer Group. J Pediatr Surg 1998; 33:171.
437. Cushing B, Giller R, Ablin A, et al: Surgical resection alone is effective treatment for ovarian immature teratoma in children and adolescents: a report of the Pediatric Oncology Group and the Children's Cancer Group. Am J Obstet Gynecol 1999; 181:353.
438. Marina NM, Cushing B, Giller R, et al: Complete surgical excision is effective treatment for children with immature teratomas with or without malignant elements: a Pediatric Oncology Group/Children's Cancer Group Intergroup Study. J Clin Oncol 1999; 17:2137.
439. Cushing B, Giller R, Marina N: Results of surgery alone or surgery plus cisplatin, etoposide and bleomycin (PEB) in children with localized gonadal malignant germ cell tumor (MGCT): a pediatric Intergroup report [abstract]. Proc Am Soc Clin Oncol 1997; 16:511a.
440. Giller R, Cushing B, Lauer S: Comparison of high-dose or standard-dose cisplatin with etoposide and bleomycin (HDPEB vs PEB) in children with stage III and IV malignant germ cell tumors (MGCT) at gonadal primary sites: a pediatric Intergroup trial (POG 9049/ CCG 8882) [abstract]. Proc Am Soc Clin Oncol 1998; 17:525.
441. Parker D, Holford CP, Begent RH, et al: Effective treatment for malignant mediastinal teratoma. Thorax 1983; 38:897.
442. Arai K, Ohta S, Suzuki M, et al: Primary immature mediastinal teratoma in adulthood. Eur J Surg Oncol 1997; 23:64.
443. Davidoff AM, Hebra A, Bunin N, et al: Endodermal sinus tumor in children. J Pediatr Surg 1996; 31:1075.
444. Chraibi Y, Culine S, Terrier-Lacombe MJ, et al: Prognostic factors for extratesticular involvement in stage I testicular cancer. Apropos of 58 cases. Bull Cancer 1994; 81:311.
445. Hanson PR, Belitsky P, Millard OH, et al: Prognostic factors in metastatic nonseminomatous germ cell tumours. Can J Surg 1993; 36:537.
446. Rodabaugh KJ, Bernstein MR, Goldstein DP, et al: Natural history of postterm choriocarcinoma. J Reprod Med 1998; 43:75.
447. Han SJ, Yoo S, Choi SH, et al: Actual half-life of alpha-fetoprotein as a prognostic tool in pediatric malignant tumors. Pediatr Surg Int 1997; 12:599.
448. International Germ Cell Cancer Collaborative Group: International Germ Cell Consensus Classification: a prognostic factor-based staging system for metastatic germ cell cancers. J Clin Oncol 1997; 15:594.
449. Margolin K, Doroshow JH, Ahn C: Treatment of germ cell cancer with two cycles of high-dose ifosfamide, carboplatin, and etoposide with autologous stem-cell support. J Clin Oncol 1996; 14:2631.
450. Willman CL, McClain KL: An update on clonality, cytokines, and viral etiology in LCH. Hematol Oncol Clin North Am 1998; 12:407.
451. Lichtenstein L: Histiocytosis X: integration of eosinophilic granuloma of bone, "Letterer-Siwe disease," and "Schuller-Christian disease" as related manifestations of a single nosologic entity. Arch Pathol 1953; 56:84.
452. Broadbent V, Egeleler RM, Nesbit ME: Langerhans cell histiocytosis: Clinical and epidemiological aspects. Br J Cancer 1994; 70:S11.
453. McLain K, Jin H, Gresik V, et al: Langerhans cell histiocytosis: Lack of a viral etiology. Am J Hematol 1994; 47:16.
454. Osband ME: Immunotherapy of histiocytosis X. Hematol Oncol Clin North Am 1987; 1:131.
455. Bhatia S, Nesbit ME, Egeleler RM, et al: Epidemiologic study of Langerhans cell histiocytosis in children. J Pediatr 1997; 130:774.
456. Caux C, Dezutter-Dambuyant C, Schmitt D, et al: GM-CSF and TNF-α cooperate in the generation of dendritic Langerhans cells. Nature 1992; 360:258.
457. de Graaf JH, Tamminga RYJ, Kamps WA, et al: Langerhans' cell histiocytosis: expression of leukocytic cellular adhesion molecules suggests abnormal homing and differentiation. Am J Pathol 1994; 144:466.
458. Fumihiro F, Hibi S, Imashuku S: Hypercytokinemia in hemophagocytic syndrome. Am J Pediatr Hematol 1993; 15:92.
459. Womer RB, Anunciato KR, Chehrenama M: Oral methotrexate and alternate-day prednisone for low-risk Langerhans cell histiocytosis. Med Pediatr Oncol 1995; 25:70.
460. Korholz D, Janssen G, Gobel U: Treatment of relapsed Langerhans cell histiocytosis by cyclosporin A combined with etoposide and prednisone. Pediatr Hematol Oncol 1997; 14:443.
461. Willman CL, Busque L, Griffith BB: Langerhans' cell histiocytosis (histiocytosis X)—a clonal proliferative disease. N Engl J Med 1994; 331:154.
462. Yu RC, Chu C, Bulwela L, et al: Clonal proliferation of Langerhans' cells in Langerhans' cell histiocytosis. Lancet 1994; 343:767.
463. Lahey ME: Histiocytosis X. Analysis of prognostic factors. J Pediatr 1975; 87:184.
464. Lipton J: The pathogenesis, diagnosis and treatment of histiocytosis syndromes. Pediatr Dermatol 1983; 1:112.
465. Komp DM, Herson J, Starling KA, et al: A staging system for histiocytosis X: a Southwest Oncology Group Study. Cancer 1981; 47:798.
466. Osband ME, Lipton JM, Lavin P, et al: Histiocytosis X. Demonstration of abnormal immunity, T-cell histamine H2-receptor deficiency, and successful treatment with thymic extract. N Engl J Med 1981; 304:146.
467. Ladisch S, Jaffee ES: The histocytoses. In: Pizzo PA, Poplack DG (eds): Principles and Practice of Pediatric Oncology, 3rd ed, p 615. Philadelphia, Lippincott-Raven, 1997.
468. McLellan DJ, Broadvent V, Yeomans E, et al: Langerhans' cell histiocytosis: the case for conservative treatment. Arch Dis Child 1990; 65:301.
469. Berry DH, Gresik M, Maybee D: Histiocytosis in bone only. Med Pediatr Oncol 1990; 18:292.
470. Greenberger JS, Cassady JR, Jaffe N: Radiation therapy in patients with histiocytosis: management of diabetes insipidus and bone lesions. Int J Radiat Oncol Biol Phys 1979; 5:1749.
471. Minehan KJ, Chen MG, Zimmerman D, et al: Radiation therapy for diabetes insipidus caused by Langerhans' cell histiocytosis. Int J Radiat Oncol Biol Phys 1992; 23:19.
472. Willis B, Ablin A, Weinberg V, et al: Disease course and late sequelae of Langerhans' cell histiocytosis: 25 year experience at the University of California, San Francisco. J. Clin Oncol 1996; 14:2073.
473. Broadbent V, Pritchard J, Davies EG, et al: Spontaneous remission of multi-system histiocytosis X. Lancet 1984; 4:253.
474. Ladisch S, Gadner H: Treatment of Langerhans cell histiocytosis—evolution and current approaches. Br J Cancer 1994; 70:S41.
475. Arico M, Colella R, Conter V: Cyclosporine therapy for refractory Langerhans cell histiocytosis. Med Pediatr Oncol 1995; 25:12.
476. Arceci R, Brenner MK, Pritchard J: Controversies and new approaches to treatment of Langerhans cell histiocytosis. Hematol Oncol Clin North Am 1998; 12:339.
477. Munn SE, Olliver L, Broadbent V, et al: Use of indomethacin in Langerhans cell histiocytosis. Med Pediatr Oncol 1999; 32:247.
478. The French Langerhans' Cell Histiocytosis Study Group: A multicenter retrospective survey of Langerhans' cell histiocytosis: 348 cases observed between 1983 and 1993. Arch Dis Child 1996; 75:17.
479. Egeler RM, D'Angio GJ: Medical progress. Langerhans' cell histiocytosis. J Pediatr 1995; 127:1.
480. Greenberger JS, Crocker AC, Vawter G: Results of treatment of 127 patients with systemic histiocytosis. Medicine 1981; 60:311.
481. Haupt R, Fears TR, Rosso P, et al: Increased risk of secondary leukemia after single-agent treatment with etoposide for Langerhans' cell histiocytosis. Pediatr Hematol Oncol 1994; 11:499.
482. Kudo K, Yoshida H, Kiyoi H, et al: Etoposide-related acute promyelocytic leukemia. Leukemia 1998; 12:1171.
483. Gelberg KH, Fitzgerald EF, Hwang S, et al: Growth and develop-

ment and other risk factors for osteosarcoma in children and young adults. Int J Epidemiol 1997; 26:272.
484. Grimer RJ, Carter SR, Tillman RM, et al: Osteosarcoma of the pelvis. J Bone Joint Surg Br 1999; 81:796.
485. Sekiguchi M, Miyazaki S, Fujikawa K, et al: BK virus-induced osteosarcoma (Os515) as a model of human osteosarcoma. Anticancer Res 1996; 16:1835.
486. Schell TD, Knowles BB, Tevethia SS: Sequential loss of cytotoxic T lymphocyte responses to simian virus 40 large T antigen epitopes in T antigen transgenic mice developing osteosarcomas. Cancer Res 2000; 60:3002.
487. Lednicky JA, Stewart AR, Jenkins JJ 3rd, et al: SV40 DNA in human osteosarcomas shows sequence variation among T-antigen genes. Int J Cancer 1997; 72:791.
488. Mendoza SM, Konishi T, Miller CW: Integration of SV40 in human osteosarcoma DNA. Oncogene 1998; 17:2457.
489. Pendlebury SC, Bilous M, Langlands AO: Sarcomas following radiation therapy for breast cancer: a report of three cases and a review of the literature. Int J Radiat Oncol Biol Phys 1995; 31:405.
490. Lustig LR, Jackler RK, Lanser MJ: Radiation-induced tumors of the temporal bone. Am J Otol 1997; 18:230.
491. Tabone MD, Terrier P, Pacquement H: Outcome of radiation-related osteosarcoma after treatment of childhood and adolescent cancer: a study of 23 cases. J Clin Oncol 1999; 17:2789.
492. Wong FL, Boice JD Jr, Abramson DH, et al: Cancer incidence after retinoblastoma. Radiation dose and sarcoma risk. JAMA 1997; 278:1262.
493. Goto A, Kanda H, Ishikawa Y: Association of loss of heterozygosity at the p53 locus with chemoresistance in osteosarcomas. Jpn J Cancer Res 1998; 89:539.
494. Carnevale A, Lieberman E, Cardenas R: Li-Fraumeni syndrome in pediatric patients with soft tissue sarcoma or osteosarcoma. Arch Med Res 1997; 28:383.
495. McIntyre JF, Smith-Sorensen B, Friend SH: Germline mutations of the p53 tumor suppressor gene in children with osteosarcoma. J Clin Oncol 1994; 12:925.
496. Oliner JD, Kinzler KW, Meltzer PS, et al: Amplification of a gene encoding a p53-associated protein in human sarcomas. Nature 1992; 358:80.
497. Ragazzini P, Gamberi G, Benassi MS, et al: Analysis of SAS gene and CDK4 and MDM2 proteins in low-grade osteosarcoma. Cancer Detect Prevent 1999; 23:129.
498. Wunder JS, Eppert K, Burrow SR, et al: Co-amplification and overexpression of CDK4, SAS and MDM2 occurs frequently in human parosteal osteosarcomas. Oncogene 1999; 18:783.
499. Baldini N, Scotlandi K, Barbanti-Brodano G: Expression of P-glycoprotein in high-grade osteosarcomas in relation to clinical outcome. N Engl J Med 1995; 333:1380.
500. Chan HS, Grogan TM, Haddad G: P-glycoprotein expression critical determinant in the response to osteosarcoma chemotherapy. J Natl Cancer Inst 1997; 19:1706.
501. Kumta SM, Chow TC, Griffith J, et al: Classifying the location of osteosarcoma with reference to the epiphyseal plate helps determine the optimal skeletal resection in limb salvage procedures. Arch Orthop Trauma Surg 1999; 119:327.
502. Mancebo-Aragoneses L, Lacambra-Calvet C, Jorge-Blanco A: Paget's disease of the skull with osteosarcoma and neurological symptoms associated. Eur Radiol 1998; 8:1145.
503. Marcove RC, Mike V, Hajek JV, et al: Osteogenic sarcoma in childhood. N Y State J Med 1970; 71:855.
504. Howat AJ, Dickens DR, Boldt DW, et al: Bilateral metachronous periosteal osteosarcoma. Cancer 1986; 58:1139.
505. Taylor WF, Ivins JC, Dahlin DC, et al: Trends and variability in survival from osteosarcoma. Mayo Clin Proc 1978; 53:695.
506. Cortes EP, Holland JF, Wang JJ: Doxorubicin in disseminated osteosarcoma. JAMA 1972; 221:1132.
507. Jaffe N: Recent advance in the chemotherapy of metastatic osteogenic sarcoma. Cancer 1972; 30:1627.
508. Cortes EP, Holland JF, Wang JJ, et al: Amputation and Adriamycin in primary osteosarcoma. N Engl J Med 1974; 291:998.
509. Jaffe N, Frei E, Traggis D, et al: Adjuvant methotrexate and citrovorum-factor treatment of osteogenic sarcoma. N Engl J Med 1974; 291:994.
510. Telander RL, Pairolero PC, Pritchard DJ: Resection of pulmonary metastatic osteogenic sarcoma in children. Surgery 1978; 84:335.
511. Eilber F, Giuliano A, Eckardt J, et al: Adjuvant chemotherapy for osteosarcoma: a randomized prospective trial. J Clin Oncol 1987; 5:21.
512. Wuisman P, Enneking WF: Prognosis for patients who have osteosarcoma with skip metastasis. J Bone Joint Surg Am 1990; 72:60.
513. Bhagia SM, Grimer RJ, Davies AM, et al: Scintigraphically negative skip metastasis in osteosarcoma. Eur Radiol 1997; 7:1446.
514. Marcove RC, Rosen G: En bloc resections for osteogenic sarcoma. Cancer 1980; 45:3040.
515. Sluga M, Windhager R, Lang S, et al: Local and systemic control after ablative and limb sparing surgery in patients with osteosarcoma. Clin Orthop Rel Res 1999; 358:120.
516. Weis LD: The success of limb-salvage surgery in the adolescent patient with osteogenic sarcoma. Adolesc Med 1999; 10:451.
517. Goorin A, Baker A, Geiser P: No evidence for improved event free survival (EFS) with presurgical chemotherapy (pre) for nonmetastatic extremity osteogenic sarcoma. Preliminary results of randomized Pediatric Oncology Group trial 8651 [abstract]. Proc Am Soc Clin Oncol 1995; 14:444.
518. Bridge JA, Schwartz HS, Neff JR: Sarcomas of the bone. In: Abeloff MD, Armitage JO, Lichter AS, et al (eds): Clinical Oncology, 2nd ed, p 2160. New York, Churchill Livingstone, 2000.
519. Bacci G, Ruggieri P, Picci P, et al: Changing pattern of relapse in osteosarcoma of the extremities treated with adjuvant and neoadjuvant chemotherapy. J Chemother 1995; 7:230.
520. Ellis PM, Tattersall MH, McCaughan B, et al: Osteosarcoma and pulmonary metastases: 15-year experience from a single institution. Austral N Z J Surg 1997; 67:625.
521. Jaffe N: Pediatric osteosarcoma: treatment of the primary tumor with intraarterial cis-diaminedichloroplatinum-II (CDP)—advantages, disadvantages, and controversial issues. Cancer Treat Res 1993; 62:75.
522. Uchida A, Myoui A, Araki N, et al: Neoadjuvant chemotherapy for pediatric osteosarcoma patients. Cancer 1997; 79:411.
523. Harris MB, Gieser P, Goorin AM, et al: Treatment of metastatic osteosarcoma at diagnosis: a Pediatric Oncology Group Study. J Clin Oncol 1998; 16:3641.
524. Ferrari S, Mercuri M, Picci P, et al: Nonmetastatic osteosarcoma of the extremity: results of a neoadjuvant chemotherapy protocol (IOR/OS-3) with high-dose methotrexate, intraarterial or intravenous cisplatin, doxorubicin, and salvage chemotherapy based on histologic tumor response. Tumori 1999; 85:458.
525. Kleinerman ES: Biologic therapy for osteosarcoma using liposome-encapsulated muramyl tripeptide. Hematol Oncol Clin North Am 1995; 9:927.
526. Rosen G, Marcove RC, Caparros B, et al: Primary osteogenic sarcoma. Cancer 1979; 43:2163.
527. Kashdan BJ, Sullivan KL, Lackman RD, et al: Extremity osteosarcomas: intraarterial chemotherapy and limb-sparing resection with 2-year follow-up. Radiology 1990; 177:95.
528. Strander H, Bauer HC, Brosjo O, et al: Long-term adjuvant interferon treatment of human osteosarcoma. A pilot study. Acta Oncol 1995; 34:877.
529. Worth LL, Jaffe N, Benjamin RS, et al: Phase II study of recombinant interleukin 1alpha and etoposide in patients with relapsed osteosarcoma. Clin Cancer Res 1997; 3:1721.
530. Kleinerman E: Unique histological changes in lung metastases of osteosarcoma patients following therapy with liposomal muramyl tripeptide (CGP 19835A lipid). Cancer Immunol Immunother 1992; 34:211.
531. Kleinerman ES, Gano JM, Johnston DA: Efficacy of liposomal muramyl tripeptide (CGP 19835A) in the treatment of relapsed osteosarcoma. Am J Clin Oncol 1995; 18:93.
532. Rosen G, Nirenberg A: Neoadjuvant chemotherapy for osteogenic sarcoma: a five year follow-up (T-10) and preliminary report of new studies (T-12). Prog Clin Biol Res 1985; 201:39.
533. Meyers PA, Heller G, Healey J, et al: Chemotherapy for nonmetastatic osteogenic sarcoma: the Memorial Sloan-Kettering experience. J Clin Oncol 1992; 10:2.
534. Provisor AJ, Ettinger LJ, Nachman JB, et al: Treatment of nonmetastatic osteosarcoma of the extremity with preoperative and postoperative chemotherapy: a report from the Children's Cancer Group. J Clin Oncol 1997; 15:76.
535. Bacci G, Picci P, Ferrari S: Primary chemotherapy and delayed surgery for nonmetastatic osteosarcoma of the extremities. Results in

164 patients preoperatively treated with high doses of methotrexate followed by cisplatin and doxorubicin. Cancer 1993; 72:3227.
536. Bacci G, Briccoli A, Ferrari S, et al: Neoadjuvant chemotherapy for osteosarcoma of the extremities with synchronous lung metastases: treatment with cisplatin, Adriamycin and high doses of methotrexate and ifosfamide. Oncol Rep 2000; 7:339.
537. Kawai A, Sugihara S, Kunisada T, et al: The importance of doxorubicin and methotrexate dose intensity in the chemotherapy of osteosarcoma. Arch Orthop Trauma Surg 1996; 115:68.
538. Souhami RL, Craft AW, Van der Eijken JW, et al: Randomised trial of two regimens of chemotherapy in operable osteosarcoma: a study of the European Osteosarcoma Intergroup. Lancet 1997; 350:911.
539. Harris MB, Gieser P, Goorin AM, et al: Treatment of metastatic osteosarcoma at diagnosis: a Pediatric Oncology Group Study. J Clin Oncol 1998; 16:3641.
540. Meyers PA, Heller G, Healey J, et al: Osteogenic sarcoma with clinically detectable metastasis at initial presentation. J Clin Oncol 1993; 11:449.
541. Bacci G, Picci P, Ferrari S, et al: Synchronous multifocal osteosarcoma: results in twelve patients treated with neoadjuvant chemotherapy and simultaneous resection of all involved bones. Ann Oncol 1996; 7:864.
542. Look TA, Douglass EC, Meyer W: Clinical importance of near-diploid tumor stem lines in patients with osteosarcoma of an extremity. N Engl J Med 1988; 318:1567.
543. Bauer H, Kreicberg A, Silfversward C, et al: DNA analysis in the differential diagnosis of osteosarcoma. Cancer 1988; 61:2532.
544. Yu AL, Uttenreuther-Fischer MM, Huang CS, et al: Phase I trial of a human-mouse chimeric anti-disialoganglioside monoclonal antibody ch14.18 in patients with refractory neuroblastoma and osteosarcoma. J Clinl Oncol 1998; 16:2169.
545. Furman WL, Stewart CF, Poquette CA, et al: Direct translation of a protracted irinotecan schedule from a xenograft model to a phase I trial in children. J Clin Oncol 1999; 17:1815.
546. Gorlick R, Huvos AG, Heller G, et al: Expression of HER2/erbB-2 correlates with survival in osteosarcoma. J Clin Oncol 1999; 17:2781.
547. Ewing J: Diffuse endothelioma of bone. Proc N Y Pathol Soc 1921; 21:17.
548. Grier HE: Ewing's sarcoma and primitive neuroectodermal tumors. Pediatr Clin North Am 1997; 44:991.
549. Nagao K, Ito H, Yoshida H, et al: Chromosomal rearrangement t(11;22) in extraskeletal Ewing's sarcoma and primitive neuroectodermal tumour analysed by fluorescence in situ hybridization using paraffin-embedded tissue. J Pathol 1997; 181:62.
550. Evans RG, Nesbit ME, Gehan EA: Multimodal therapy for management of localized Ewing's sarcoma of pelvic and sacral bones: a report from the second intergroup study. J Clin Oncol 1991; 9:1173.
551. Marina NM, Pappo AS, Parham DM, et al: Chemotherapy dose-intensification for pediatric patients with Ewing's family of tumors and desmoplastic small round-cell tumors: a feasibility study at St. Jude Children's Research Hospital. J Clin Oncol 1999; 17:180.
552. Rosito P, Mancini AF, Rondelli R, et al: Italian Cooperative Study for the treatment of children and young adults with localized Ewing sarcoma of bone: a preliminary report of 6 years of experience. Cancer 1999; 86:421.
553. Pritchard D, Dahlin DC, Dauphine RT: Ewing's/PNET: a clinicopathological and statistical analysis of patients surviving 5 years or longer. J Bone Joint Surg Am 1975; 57:10.
554. Sailer S, Harmon D, Mankin H, et al: Ewing's/PNET: surgical resection as a prognostic factor. Int J Radiat Oncol Biol Phys 1988; 15:43.
555. Hadfield MG, Quezado MM, Williams RL, et al: Ewing's family of tumors involving structures related to the central nervous system: a review. Pediatr Develop Pathol 2000; 3:203.
556. Dickman P, Liotta L, Triche T: Ewing's/PNET: characterization in established cultures and evidence of its histogenesis. Lab Invest 1982; 47:375.
557. Dehner LP: Primitive neuroectodermal tumor and Ewing's sarcoma. Am J Surg Pathol 1993; 17:1.
558. O'Regan S, Diebler MF, Meunier FM, et al: A Ewing's sarcoma cell line showing some, but not all, of the traits of a cholinergic neuron. J Neurochem 1995; 64:69.
559. Im YH, Kim HT, Lee C, et al: EWS-FLI1, EWS-ERG, and EWS-ETV1 oncoproteins of Ewing tumor family all suppress transcription of transforming growth factor beta type II receptor gene. Cancer Res 2000; 60:1536.
560. de Alava E, Panizo A, Antonescu CR, et al: Association of EWS-FLI1 type 1 fusion with lower proliferative rate in Ewing's sarcoma. Am J Pathol 2000; 156:849.
561. de Alava E, Kawai A, Healey JH: EWS-FL11 fusion transcript structure is an independent determinant of prognosis in Ewing's sarcoma. J Clin Oncol 1998; 16:1248.
562. Zoubek A, Dockhor-Dworniczak B, Delattre O, et al: Does expression of different EWS chimeric transcripts define clinically distinct risk groups of Ewing tumor patients? J Clin Oncol 1996; 14:1245.
563. Hartley AL, Birch JM, Marsden HB, et al: Malignant disease in the mothers of children with Ewing's tumour. Med Pediatr Oncol 1988; 16:95.
564. Novakovic B, Goldstein AM, Wexler LH, et al: Increased risk of neuroectodermal tumors and stomach cancer in relatives of patients with Ewing's sarcoma family of tumors. J Natl Cancer Inst 1994; 86:1702.
565. Widhe B, Widhe T: Initial symptoms and clinical features in osteosarcoma and Ewing sarcoma. J Bone Joint Surg Am 2000; 82:667.
566. Cotterill SJ, Ahrens S, Paulussen M, et al: Prognostic factors in Ewing's sarcoma of bone: analysis of 975 patients from the European Intergroup Cooperative Ewing's Sarcoma Study Group. J Clin Oncol 2000; 18:3108.
567. Dorfman HD, Czerniak B: Bone cancers. Cancer 1995; 75:203.
568. Kilpatrick SE, Ward WG, Chauvenet AR, et al: The role of fine-needle aspiration biopsy in the initial diagnosis of pediatric bone and soft tissue tumors: an institutional experience. Mod Pathol 1998; 11:923.
569. Collins BT, Cramer HM, Frain BE, et al: Fine-needle aspiration biopsy of metastatic Ewing's sarcoma with MIC2 (CD99) immunocytochemistry. Diag Cytopathol 1998; 19:382.
570. Guyot-Drouot MH, Cotten A, Flipo RM, et al: Contribution of magnetic resonance imaging to the diagnosis of extraskeletal Ewing's sarcoma. Rev Rhum Engl Ed 1999; 66:516.
571. Henk CB, Grampp S, Wiesbauer P, et al: Ewing sarcoma. Diagnostic imaging. Radiologe 1998; 38:509.
572. Giles FJ, Waxman AD, Nguyen KN, et al: Comparison of technetium-99m sestamibi and indium-111 octreotide imaging in a patient with Ewing's sarcoma before and after stem cell transplantation. Cancer 1997; 80:2478.
573. Fouladi M, Gajjar A, Boyett JM, et al: Comparison of CSF cytology and spinal magnetic resonance imaging in the detection of leptomeningeal disease in pediatric medulloblastoma or primitive neuroectodermal tumor. J Clin Oncol 1999; 17:3234.
574. Hannisdal E, Solheim OP, Theodorsen L, et al: Alterations of blood analyses at relapse of osteosarcoma and Ewing's sarcoma. Acta Oncol 1990; 29:585.
575. Banerjee SS, Agbamu DA, Eyden BP, et al: Clinicopathological characteristics of peripheral primitive neuroectodermal tumour of skin and subcutaneous tissue. Histopathology 1997; 31:355.
576. Sinkre P, Albores-Saavedra J, Miller DS, et al: Endometrial endometrioid carcinomas associated with Ewing sarcoma/peripheral primitive neuroectodermal tumor. Int J Gynecol Pathol 2000; 19:127.
577. Gu M, Antonescu CR, Guiter G, et al: Cytokeratin immunoreactivity in Ewing's sarcoma: prevalence in 50 cases confirmed by molecular diagnostic studies. Am J Surg Pathol 2000; 24:410.
578. Hense HW, Ahrens S, Paulussen M, et al: Factors associated with tumor volume and primary metastases in Ewing tumors: results from the (EI)CESS studies. Ann Oncol 1999; 10:1073.
579. Parasuraman S, Langston J, Rao BN, et al: Brain metastases in pediatric Ewing sarcoma and rhabdomyosarcoma: the St. Jude Children's Research Hospital experience. J Pediatr Hematol Oncol 1999; 21:370.
580. Donaldson SS, Torrey M, Link MP, et al: A multidisciplinary study investigating radiotherapy in Ewing's sarcoma: end results of POG 8346. Pediatric Oncology Group. Int J Radiat Oncol Biol Phys 1998; 42:125.
581. Czyzewski EA, Goldman S, Mundt AJ, et al: Radiation therapy for consolidation of metastatic or recurrent sarcomas in children treated with intensive chemotherapy and stem cell rescue. A feasibility study. Int J Radiat Oncol Biol Phys 1999; 44:569.
582. Barbieri E, Emiliani E, Zini G, et al: Combined therapy of localized Ewing's sarcoma of bone: analysis of results in 100 patients. Int J Radiat Oncol Biol Phys 1990; 19:1165.

583. Antman KH: Chemotherapy of advanced sarcomas of bone and soft tissue. Semin Oncol 1992; 19:13.
584. Grier H, Krailo M, Link M, et al: Improved outcome in nonmetastatic Ewing's sarcoma and PNET of bone with the addition of ifosfamide and etoposide to vincristine, Adriamycin, cyclophosphamide, and actinomycin: a Children's Cancer Group and Pediatric Oncology Group report [abstract]. Proc Am Soc Clin Oncol 1994; 13:421.
585. Bacci G, Picci P, Ferrari S: Neoadjuvant chemotherapy for Ewing's sarcoma of bone: no benefit observed after adding ifosfamide and etoposide to vincristine, actinomycin, cyclophosphamide, and doxorubicin in the maintenance phase—results of two sequential studies. Cancer 1998; 82:1174.
586. Ferrari S, Mercuri M, Rosito P, et al: Ifosfamide and actinomycin-D, added in the induction phase to vincristine, cyclophosphamide and doxorubicin improve histologic response and prognosis in patients with nonmetastatic Ewing's sarcoma of the extremity. J Chemother 1998; 10:484.
587. Pape H, Laws HJ, Burdach S, et al: Radiotherapy and high-dose chemotherapy in advanced Ewing's tumors. Strahlenther Onkol 1999; 175:484.
588. Finlay JL: The role of high-dose chemotherapy and stem cell rescue in the treatment of malignant brain tumors: a reappraisal. Pediatr Transplant 1999; 3:87.
589. Jurgens H, Exner U, Gadner H: Multidisciplinary treatment of primary Ewing's/PNET of bone. A 6-year experience of a European Cooperative trial. Cancer 1988; 61:23.
590. Burdach S, Jurgens H, Peters C: Myeloablative radiochemotherapy and hematopoietic stem-cell rescue in poor-prognosis Ewing's sarcoma. J Clin Oncol 1993; 11:1482.
591. Ladenstein R, Lasset C, Pinkeerton R, et al: Impact of megatherapy in children with high-risk Ewing's tumours in complete remission: a report from the EBMT Solid Tumour Registry. Bone Marrow Transplant 1995; 15:697.
592. Givens SS, Woo SY, Huang LY, et al: Non-metastatic Ewing's sarcoma: twenty years of experience suggests that surgery is a prime factor for successful multimodality therapy. Int J Oncol 1999; 14:1039.
593. Carrie C, Mascard E, Gomez F, et al: Nonmetastatic pelvic Ewing sarcoma: report of the French Society of Pediatric Oncology. Med Pediatr Oncol 1999; 33:444.
594. Kushner BH, Meyers PA, Gerald WL: Very-high-dose short-term chemotherapy for poor-risk peripheral primitive neuroectodermal tumors, including Ewing's sarcoma, in children and young adults. J Clin Oncol 1995; 13:2796.
595. Farley F, Healey J, Caparros-Sisson B, et al: Lactase dehydrogenase as a tumor marker for recurrent disease in Ewing's/PNET. Cancer 1987; 59:1245.
596. Brown A, Fixsen J, Plowman P: Local control of Ewing's/PNET: an analysis of 67 patients. Br J Radiol 1987; 60:261.
597. Dunst J, Jurgens H, Sauer R, et al: Radiation therapy in Ewing's sarcoma: an update of the CESS 86 trial. Int J Radiat Oncol Biol Phys 1995; 32:919.
598. Feusner JH, Krailo MD, Haas JE, et al: Treatment of pulmonary metastases of initial stage I hepatoblastoma in childhood. Report from the Children's Cancer Group. Cancer 1993; 71:859.
599. Ries LAG, Kosary CL, Hankey BF: Cancer Incidence and Survival among Children and Adolescents: United States SEER Program 1975–1996. Bethesda, National Cancer Institute, 2000.
600. Blaker H, Hofmann WJ, Rieker RJ, et al: Beta-catenin accumulation and mutation of the CTNNB1 gene in hepatoblastoma. Genes Chromosomes Cancer 1999; 25:399.
601. Jeng YM, Wu MZ, Mao TL, et al: Somatic mutations of beta-catenin play a crucial role in the tumorigenesis of sporadic hepatoblastoma. Cancer Letter 2000; 152:45.
602. Al-Qabandi W, Jenkinson HC, Buckels JA, et al: Orthotopic liver transplantation for unresectable hepatoblastoma: a single center's experience. J Pediatr Surg 1999; 34:1261.
603. Iwama T, Mishima Y: Mortality in young first-degree relatives of patients with familial adenomatous polyposis. Cancer 1994; 73:2065.
604. Simms LA, Reeve AE, Smith PJ: Genetic mosaicism at the insulin locus in liver associated with childhood hepatoblastoma. Genes Chromosomes Cancer 1995; 13:72.
605. Steenman M, Tomlinson G, Westerveld A, et al: Comparative genomic hybridization analysis of hepatoblastomas: additional evidence for a genetic link with Wilms tumor and rhabdomyosarcoma. Cytogenet Cell Genet 1999; 86:157.
606. Ikeda H, Hachitanda Y, Tanimura M: Development of unfavorable hepatoblastoma in children of very low birth weight: results of a surgical and pathologic review. Cancer 1998; 82:1789.
607. Esquivel CO, Gutierrez C, Cox KL, et al: Hepatocellular carcinoma and liver cell dysplasia in children with chronic liver disease. J Pediatr Surg 1994; 29:1465.
608. Moore L, Bourne AJ, Moore DJ, et al: Hepatocellular carcinoma following neonatal hepatitis. Pediatr Pathol Lab Med 1997; 17:601.
609. Chang MH, Chen CJ: Universal hepatitis B vaccination in Taiwan and the incidence of hepatocellular carcinoma in children: for the Taiwan Childhood Hepatoma Study Group. N Engl J Med 1997; 336:1855.
610. Park WS, Dong SM, Kim SY: Somatic mutations is the kinase domain of the Met/hepatocyte growth factor receptor gene in childhood hepatocellular carcinomas. Cancer Res 1999; 59:307.
611. Mieles LA, Esquivel CO, Van Thiel DH: Liver transplantation for tyrosinemia. A review of 10 cases from the University of Pittsburgh. Dig Dis Sci 1990; 35:153.
612. Perlmutter DH: Alpha-1-antitrypsin deficiency. Semin Liver Dis 1998; 18:217.
613. Hatanaka K: CT evaluation of pulmonary metastases: usefulness in comparison with chest radiography. Nippon Igaku Hoshasen Gakkai Zasshi 1999; 59:663.
614. Gauthier F, Valayer J, Thai BL, et al: Hepatoblastoma and hepatocarcinoma in children: analysis of a series of 29 cases. J Pediatr Surg 1986; 21:424.
615. Tschappeler H: Liver tumors in children. Radiologe 1993; 33:679.
616. Perilango G, Sinniah D, Evans AE; et al: Liver tumors. In: D'Angio GJ, Sinniah D, Meadows AT (eds): Practical Pediatric Oncology, p 333. New York, Wiley-Liss, 1992.
617. Giacomantonio M, Ein SH, Mancer K, et al: Thirty years of experience with pediatric primary malignant liver tumors. J Pediatr Surg 1984; 19:523.
618. Ortega JA, Krailo MD, Haas JE: Effective treatment of unresectable or metastatic hepatoblastoma with cisplatin and continuous infusion doxorubicin chemotherapy: a report from the Children's Cancer Study Group. J Clin Oncol 1991; 9:2167.
619. de Monleon JV, Simonin G, Pincemaille O: Precocious puberty secondary to an intramedullary germinoma. Arch Pediatr 1999; 6:46.
620. Exelby PR, Filler RM, Grosfeld JL: Liver tumors in children in the particular reference to hepatoblastoma and hepatocellular carcinoma: American Academy of Pediatrics Surgical Section Survey—1974. J Pediatr Surg 1975; 10:329.
621. Lack EE, Neare C, Vawter GF: Hepatoblastoma: a clinical and pathologic study of 54 cases. Am J Surg Pathol 1982; 6:693.
622. Lack EE, Neave C, Vawter GF: Hepatocellular carcinoma. Review of 32 cases in childhood and adolescence. Cancer 1983; 52:1510.
623. Willis RA: The pathology of the tumours of children. In: Cameron R, Wright GP (eds): Pathological Monographs, 57. London, Oliver and Boyd, 1962.
624. Ishak KG, Glunz PR: Hepatoblastoma and hepatocellular carcinoma in infancy and childhood. Report of 47 cases. Cancer 1967; 20:396.
625. Haas JE, Muczynski KA, Krailo M: Histopathology and prognosis in childhood hepatoblastoma and hepatocarcinoma. Cancer 1989; 64:1082.
626. Douglass E, Ortega J, Feusner J: Hepatocellular carcinoma (HCA) in children and adolescents: results from the Pediatric Intergroup Hepatoma Study [abstract]. Proc Am Soc Clin Oncol 1994; 13:420.
627. Douglass EC, Reynolds M, Finegold M, et al: Cisplatin, vincristine, and fluorouracil therapy for hepatoblastoma: a Pediatric Oncology Group study. J Clin Oncol 1993; 11:96.
628. Ortega JA, Douglass E, Feusner J: A randomized trial of cisplatin (DDP)/vincristine (VCR)/5-fluorouracil (5FU) vs DDP/doxorubicin (DOX) iv continuous infusion (CI) for the treatment of hepatoblastoma (HB): results from the Pediatric Intergroup Hepatoma Study [abstract]. Proc Am Soc Clin Oncol 1994; 13:416.
629. Tagge EP, Tagge DU, Reyes J, et al: Resection, including transplantation, for hepatoblastoma and hepatocellular carcinoma: impact on survival. J Pediatr Surg 1992; 27:292.
630. Fuchs J, Bode U, von Schweinitz D, et al: Analysis of treatment efficiency of carboplatin and etoposide in combination with radical surgery in advanced and recurrent childhood hepatoblastoma: a report of the German Cooperative Pediatric Liver Tumor Study HB 89 and HB 94. Klin Padiatr 1999; 211:305.

631. von Schweinitz D, Burger D, Bode U, et al: Results of the HB-89 Study in treatment of malignant epithelial liver tumors in childhood and concept of a new HB-94 protocol. Klin Padiatr 1994; 206:282.
632. Aramaki M, Kawano K, Kai T, et al: Treatment for extrahepatic metastasis of hepatocellular carcinoma following successful hepatic resection. Hepatogastroenterol 1999; 46:2931.
633. Chen JC, Chen CC, Chen WJ, et al: Hepatocellular carcinoma in children: clinical review and comparison with adult cases. J Pediatr Surg 1998; 33:1350.
634. Hodgson WJ, Morgan J, Byrne D, et al: Hepatic resections for primary and metastatic tumors using the ultrasonic surgical dissector. Am J Surg 1992; 163:246.
635. Okada A, Fukuzawa M, Oue T, et al: Thirty-eight years experience of malignant hepatic tumors in infants and childhood. Eur J Pediatr Surg 1998; 8:17.
636. Passmore SJ, Noblett HR, Wisheart JD: Prolonged survival following multiple thoracotomies for metastatic hepatoblastoma. Med Pediatr Oncol 1995; 24:58.
637. Lam CM, Lo CM, Yuen WK: Prolonged survival in selected patients following surgical resection for pulmonary metastasis from hepatocellular carcinoma. Br J Surg 1998; 85:1198.
638. Koneru B, Flye MW, Busuttil RW: Liver transplantation for hepatoblastoma: the American experience. Ann Surg 1991; 213:118.
639. Superina R, Bilik R: Results of liver transplantation in children with unresectable liver tumors. J Pediatr Surg 1996; 31:835.
640. Venook AP: Treatment of hepatocellular carcinoma: too many options? J Clin Oncol 1994; 12:1323.
641. Habrand JL, Nehme D, Kalifa C, et al: Is there a place for radiation therapy in the management of hepatoblastomas and hepatocellular carcinomas in children? Int J Radiat Oncol Biol Phys 1992; 23:525.
642. von Schweinitz D, Burger D, Mildenberger H: Is laparotomy the first step in treatment of childhood liver tumors?—The experience from the German Cooperative Pediatric Liver Tumor Study HB-89. Eur J Pediatr Surg 1994; 4:82.
643. Broughan TA, Esquivel CO, Vogt DP, et al: Pretransplant chemotherapy in pediatric hepatocellular carcinoma. J Pediatr Surg 1994; 29:1319.
644. Sue K, Ikeda K, Nakagawara A: Intrahepatic arterial injections of cisplatin-phosphatidylcholine-lipiodol suspension in two unresectable hepatoblastoma cases. Med Pediatr Oncol 1989; 17:496.
645. Gerber DA, Arcement C, Carr B, et al: Use of intrahepatic chemotherapy to treat advanced pediatric hepatic malignancies. J Pediatr Gastroenterol Nutr 2000; 30:137.
646. Bilik R, Superina R: Transplantation for unresectable liver tumors in children. Transplant Proc 1997; 29:2834.
647. Pazdur R, Bready B, Cangir A: Pediatric hepatic tumors: clinical trials conducted in the United States. J Surg Oncol 1993; 3:127.
648. Ueno K, Miyazono N, Inoue H: Transcatheter arterial chemoembolization therapy using iodized oil for patients with unresectable hepatocellular carcinoma: evaluation of three kinds of regimens and analysis of prognostic factors. Cancer 2000; 88:1574.
649. Filler RM, Ehrlich PF, Greenberg ML, et al: Preoperative chemotherapy in hepatoblastoma. Surgery 1991; 110:591.
650. Pinna AD, Iwatsuki S, Lee RG, et al: Treatment of fibrolamellar hepatoma with subtotal hepatectomy or transplantation. Hepatol 1997; 26:877.
651. Heifetz SA, French M, Correa M, et al: Hepatoblastoma: the Indiana experience with preoperative chemotherapy for inoperable tumors; clinicopathological considerations. Pediatr Pathol Lab Med 1997; 17:857.
652. Ulmer SC: Hepatocellular carcinoma. A concise guide to its status and management. Postgrad Med J 2000; 107:117.

20 *Tumors of the Head and Neck*

GEORGE E. LARAMORE, MD, PHD, Radiation Oncology
MARC D. COLTRERA, MD, Otolaryngology, Head and Neck Surgery
KAREN J. HUNT, MD, Medical Oncology

The recommended therapy depends to a large extent on which door the patient enters.

R.R. MILLION (Personal communication)

Perspective

The term *head and neck cancer* is in some sense a misnomer. In general usage, *head and neck cancer* does not refer to a single entity but rather to a diverse spectrum of malignancies that arise in a given region of the body. Tumors arising in the head and neck can have a multitude of histologies. In this chapter, we are primarily concerned with those tumors of an epithelial character arising from the mucosal lining of the aerodigestive tract. Tumors such as lymphomas, sarcomas, melanomas, and thyroid carcinomas are discussed elsewhere in this text. We will, however, present short sections on the treatment of salivary gland tumors and chemodectomas.

Even the more common squamous cell carcinomas (SCCs) of the head and neck can have disparate biologic properties depending on their site of origin. In part, this is because of variation in the lymphatic drainage pattern, which can be quite different even for primary sites located only a few centimeters apart. However, distinctions also arise from differences in the average degree of differentiation of tumors from various sites. *Head and neck cancer* thus presents a unique challenge to the clinician.

Management of head and neck tumors is a complex process requiring a multidisciplinary approach. The functional arrangement of the aerodigestive tract is complex, with a variety of anatomic adaptations having evolved to protect the airway from swallowed food and liquid.[18] Malignant processes involving one part of this system can thus have a significant impact on the functionality of other parts as well. Important sensory functions such as vision, hearing, balance, taste, and smell are localized in the head and neck, and the loss of any of these, either owing to a tumor or its treatment, can significantly alter the patient's quality of life. Cosmetic considerations are also important because a person's facial appearance is generally what one notices first when beginning any form of direct social interaction. A final issue relates to communication, which is one of the major distinguishing capabilities between humans and the lower animals. Speaking developed long before the invention of writing in all human societies and continues to be the major vehicle for social intercourse. The loss of the ability to speak always causes significant changes in a patient's lifestyle, and the impact of this loss can be significant.

A "cured" but functionally impaired patient is not the goal of head and neck cancer treatment. Rather, one must interleaf decisions regarding the best approaches to tumor eradication with the goal of optimal, post-treatment rehabilitation. The patient must be brought into the decision-making process because he or she may well decide to select a treatment approach that offers a few percentage points' lower survival probability in return for a better functional or cosmetic result, or both, if the treatment is successful. Organ preservation approaches using various combinations of radiotherapy and chemotherapy, with surgery held in reserve for failure, are examples of this decision. The overall plan of management must be formulated at the outset for these approaches to work effectively. Key individuals on the management team are the head and neck cancer surgeon, the radiation oncologist, the medical oncologist, the diagnostic radiologist, the pathologist, the dental service, the speech therapist, the nutritionist, the oncology nurse, and the social worker. Because the acute side effects of modern therapeutic regimens can be quite severe, placement of a percutaneous gastrostomy (feeding tube) often is required before therapy is even begun. After treatment is completed, combined follow-up clinics involving the various specialty services are essential for optimal care, early diagnosis of recurrences, and management of treatment sequelae.

Epidemiology and Etiology

Epidemiology

In the United States, head and neck cancers account for 3% of all malignancies (excluding nonmelanoma skin cancer). Depending on how one chooses to group the various tumors, head and neck cancers are the seventh and eleventh most common cancers in men and women, respectively. In 2000 the American Cancer Society estimated that these tumors accounted for approximately 40,300 new cases and approximately 11,700 deaths yearly in the United States.[17] Worldwide, they are the sixth most common cancer.

There is a clear association between tobacco and alcohol use and the development of many squamous cell tumors. In the United States, the larynx and mouth are the most common sites, followed by the pharynx and tongue. Tumors are more common with increasing age, poor dental hygiene, low socioeconomic status, and male gender.

In certain regions of India where *pan* (a mixture of betel leaf, lime, catechu, and areca nut) is chewed, squamous cell tumors of the oral cavity (most commonly buccal mucosa) account for approximately 50% of all cancers.[8] Cancer of the nasopharynx is the most common tumor in the Kwantung province of southern China. Both environmental causes and genetic predisposition likely account for this.[19]

Etiology

- *Smoking and high alcohol intake*, particularly in combination, are strikingly common in head and neck cancer patients and are implicated as etiologic factors.[20–22] These agents are also implicated in the development of second malignancies in the subset of patients who are cured of their first head and neck cancer.[23–25]
- *Poor oral hygiene* is another important factor.
- *Epstein-Barr virus* (EBV) is associated with nasopharyngeal carcinoma (NPC) in all races.[26]
- There is a higher frequency of premalignant and malignant oral lesions in young Americans because of the increasing use of *smokeless tobacco*.[8, 27]
- *Carcinoma of the buccal mucosa* is common in India and is associated with the chewing of *pan*[8] and various tobacco-based mixtures.
- *Carcinomas of the nasal cavity* and paranasal sinuses (particularly adenocarcinomas) have shown increased incidence in furniture workers and appear related to wood dust inhalation.[8, 28]
- *Chronic iron deficiency* (Plummer-Vinson syndrome) is an etiologic factor in tongue and postcricoid carcinomas in females.[29] Poor nutrition, typically associated with chronic alcohol ingestion, has been implicated (vitamin A and E deficiencies).
- *Tertiary syphilis* was implicated in tongue carcinoma in the preantibiotic era.[29]
- *Human papillomavirus* (HPV): Based on animal models, it would seem that carcinomas of any squamous epithelium, or any epithelium that may undergo squamous metaplasia, would be potential candidates for being associated with a papillomavirus. HPV DNA has been found in oral papillomas,[30, 31] in leukoplakia lesions, and in oral carcinomas.[31] Laryngeal papillomatosis is associated with HPV-6 and -11, whereas HPV-16 and -18 sequences have been demonstrated in a verrucous carcinoma of the larynx.[11, 32]
- *Ionizing radiation* exposure, particularly in childhood, is implicated in the development of thyroid cancer and salivary gland tumors.[33, 34]

Biology

In the head and neck region, severe dysplasia and carcinoma *in situ* are premalignant lesions that are clearly definable by pathology examination. Although multiple biologic markers have been associated with the development of head and neck cancer, no progressive pathway leading to head and neck cancer has been defined as of yet. It is estimated that SCC of the head and neck requires the accumulation of 8 to 11 mutations, whereas 4 to 7 mutations may be sufficient in salivary gland malignancies.[35]

- *Oncogenes* demonstrating altered expression, amplification, or mutation in head and neck (HN) SCC include *HRAS*, *KRAS*, *NRAS*, *MYC*, *CERB2* and *PRAD1*.[36] With the exception of *PRAD1*, these oncogenes do not appear to play major roles in head and neck cancer development.
- The most commonly mutated *tumor suppressor gene* in HN SCC is *TP53* (47%).[37]
- *Loss of heterozygosity* is most common in 11q, 13q, 6p, 3p, 9p, and 17p.[38]

Detection and Diagnosis

Clinical Detection

Most cancers of the head and neck grow and present as malignant ulcerations of a surface mucosa with raised indurated edges and underlying infiltration-induration. Less commonly, a fungating, elevated, exophytic growth pattern may occur. A tumor with an infiltrative, endophytic growth pattern is thought to be more aggressive and difficult to control than one with an exophytic growth pattern. Palpation may sometimes disclose an endophytic tumor that otherwise is hard to detect.

Symptoms and signs of a presenting tumor depend on location:

- *Oral cavity*: Swelling or ulcer that fails to heal. Local pain may or may not be present. Ipsilateral referred otalgia is not uncommon. Inspection and palpation may reveal an indurated ulcer. Tumors may arise in areas of premalignant change such as leukoplakia (<5%) or erythroplasia (30%).
- *Oropharynx*: Silent (symptoms often delayed) area. Dysphagia, local pain, pain on swallowing, referred otalgia, or a neck mass are common symptoms in more advanced lesions. Inspection, including an indirect mirror examination or fiberoptic examination, should be supplemented with palpation. Topical anesthesia is often helpful.
- *Hypopharynx*: Silent (symptoms often delayed) area. Dysphagia, odynophagia, referred otalgia, or neck mass (node) are common presentations in more advanced tumors. Examination is the same as for the oropharynx.
- *Larynx*: Persistent hoarseness, pain, referred otalgia, dyspnea, and stridor. Indirect mirror examination (lar-

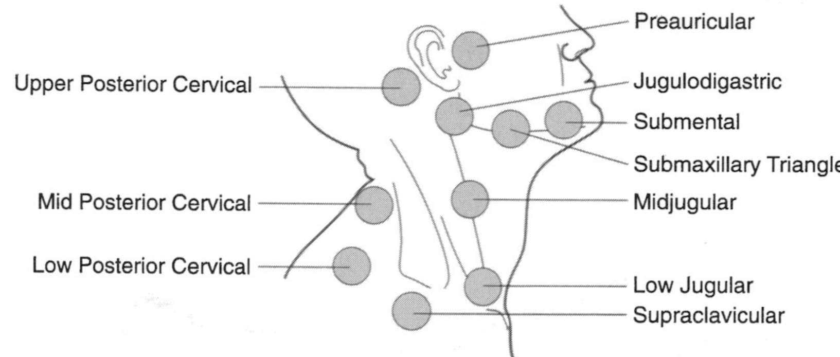

Figure 20–1. Nodal regions of the head and neck. (Redrawn from Fletcher GH, Jesse RH, Lindberg RD, et al: Neck nodes. In: Fletcher GH [ed]: Textbook of Radiotherapy, 3rd ed, pp 249–270. Philadelphia, Lea & Febiger, 1980, with permission.)

yngoscopy) or fiberoptic examination, or both, is essential.

- *Nasopharynx*: Bloody nasal discharge, obstructed nostril, unilateral conductive deafness (eustachian obstruction), and neurologic problems (atypical facial pain, diplopia, hoarseness, Horner's syndrome) resulting from cranial nerve involvement. An otherwise asymptomatic neck mass is also a common presentation. Examination involves indirect nasopharyngoscopy, direct fiberoptic visualization, and cranial nerve assessment.
- *Nose and sinuses:* Bloody nasal discharge, nasal obstruction, facial pain, facial swelling, and diplopia (direct orbital extension). Examination includes anterior rhinoscopy, palpation of orbital margin, and inspection and palpation of roof of mouth and gingivobuccal sulcus.
- *Parotid and submandibular glands*: Local swelling that may or may not be associated with pain; hemifacial paralysis owing to facial nerve involvement.
- A *metastatic cervical node* may be part of the clinical presentation of any of the above-mentioned tumors.

The most common enlarged node is the *jugulodigastric node*, which is just behind the angle of the mandible. Occasionally a neck mass is the sole presenting complaint. Any enlarged cervical node in an adult that persists for more than 1 month is regarded as potentially malignant. In this chapter, we will use the nodal description defined by Fletcher and colleagues,[39] shown in Figure 20–1. For purposes of describing nodal groups sampled at the time of surgery, these are divided by convention into six regions labeled by Roman numerals, as shown in Figure 20–2. Level I includes the submental and submandibular nodes; level II includes the upper jugular nodes that extend from the hyoid bone (carotid bifurcation) superiorly to the base of the skull; level III includes the middle jugular nodes located between the carotid bifurcation and the omohyoid muscle; and level IV includes the lower jugular nodes from the inferior border of the omohyoid muscle to the clavicle. The posterior border of regions II, III, and IV is the posterior border of the sternocleidomastoid muscle, which is the anterior border of the level V group, which includes the spinal accessory group. Level VI denotes the anterior nodal compartment consisting of the pretracheal and paratracheal nodes, the Delphian node, and the perithyroid nodes. Sometimes level VII is used to indicate the upper mediastinal nodes, although this designation is less common.

Diagnostic Procedures

- *Careful inspection*, directly and via mirror, of oral cavity, nasopharynx, oropharynx, larynx, and hypopharynx is necessary. Fiberoptic aerodigestive endoscopy may be invaluable.
- *Palpation,* when performed carefully, often allows one to detect more than by visual examination (particularly for tumor involving the tongue and floor of mouth). A routine for systematic palpation of cervical lymphatics must be followed. Normal cervical nodes are soft, flat, mobile, and less than 1 cm in size. Metastatic cervical nodes become hard, oval or round, and are generally detectable once they grow beyond 1 cm in diameter

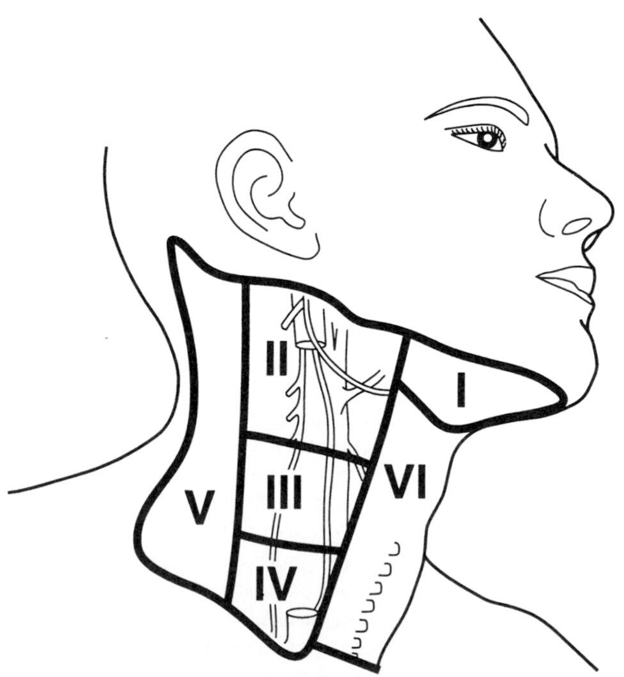

Figure 20–2. Nodal grouping by regions as generally used by the head and neck surgical oncologist. (Redrawn from Suen JY, Stern SJ: Cancer of the neck. In: Myers EN, Suen JY [eds]: Cancer of the Head and Neck, 3rd ed, pp 462–484. Philadelphia, W.B. Saunders, 1996, with permission.)

unless one is dealing with a patient having an obese or muscular neck.

- *Biopsy* of all suspicious lesions is necessary. If clinical suspicion is high but the first report is negative, then repeat the biopsy. Verrucous carcinomas may be easier to diagnose clinically than microscopically.
- *Radiographic studies* are selected according to needs and are essential in the staging work-up.
  - *Plain films*: Skull, sinuses, base of skull, and lateral soft tissue view of neck are not used as much today as they were in the past.
  - *Computed tomography (CT) scans* and *magnetic resonance imaging (MRI)* are being increasingly used in staging evaluation (especially for nasopharynx, oropharynx, larynx, and paranasal sinuses). They are also useful in determining the extent of metastatic disease in the neck[41] and in the retropharyngeal nodes.[42] MRI is particularly useful for detecting tumor infiltration into surrounding soft tissue.
  - *Orthopantomogram of mandible*: Useful to evaluate the degree to which floor of mouth and gingival lesions may have invaded the mandible.
  - *Barium swallow*: Standard and cinefluorography may be useful for pyriform sinus and hypopharynx.
  - *Laryngogram*: May be useful for tumors of the larynx and hypopharynx.
  - *Chest x-ray*: An essential study for detection of metastasis or a second primary.
  - *Bone scan*: For bony metastases in symptomatic patients.
  - *Arteriogram*: May be useful for diagnosis of chemodectomas.
  - *Positron emission tomography (PET)*: This test may be useful in locating occult tumor in the so-called unknown primary setting and in ascertaining tumor recurrence after treatment.[43]
- *Anti-EBV antibody titers*: Immunoglobulin G and immunoglobulin A are fairly specific for nasopharyngeal carcinoma and may aid in the diagnosis of cervical node cancer with unknown primary.

Classification and Staging

Histopathology

More than 80% of cancers arising from the epithelial lining of the aerodigestive tract are SCCs and can be graded as well-differentiated, moderately well-differentiated, or poorly differentiated. Grading has been correlated with prognosis.[41] Several variants of SCCs are recognized, as indicated in Table 20–1. Adenocarcinoma may arise from minor salivary glands in the mucosal lining of the aerodigestive tract, or from major salivary glands—a listing of the various types of these tumors is also given in Table 20–1. In addition to these more common malignancies, a wide variety of nonepithelial malignancies can arise in the head and neck region, including lymphoma, plasmacytoma, melanoma, and sarcomas of soft tissue, cartilage, and bone. These tumors are discussed as the subjects of separate chapters. Thyroid cancer will also be considered elsewhere in this text.

TABLE 20–1. **Histopathology Classification: Common Cancers of the Aerodigestive Tract**

Squamous Cell Carcinoma: Microscopic Variants	Adenocarcinoma—Major or Minor Salivary Gland
Keratinizing well-differentiated; moderately well-differentiated; poorly differentiated	Low-grade adenocarcinoma Acinic cell carcinoma
Nonkeratinizing; anaplastic squamous carcinoma	Adenoid cystic carcinoma
Lymphoepithelioma	Mucoepidermoid (low or high grade)
Transitional cell carcinoma	Carcinoma ex-pleomorphic adenoma
Spindle cell squamous carcinoma	Poorly differentiated adenocarcinoma

Staging

The staging systems presented in this chapter are based on clinical and diagnostic information, using the best possible estimate of the extent of disease before any treatment is given. They use three designations: T stage to define the extent of primary tumor, N stage to define the extent of regional nodal involvement, and M stage to define whether or not distant metastases are present. When surgical treatment is part of the tumor management, additional staging information can be obtained. Such surgical-pathologic staging information may be crucial in deciding the need for, and type of, adjuvant treatment. Staging based on pathologic information is often designated by the subscript "p" after the appropriate TNM staging number. It is important to note that staging systems for cancer have changed over the years. We will use the current definitions of the American Joint Committee on Cancer's *Manual for Staging for Cancer*, 5th edition,[9] and the International Union Against Cancer's *TNM Classification of Malignant Tumors,* 4th edition,[10] in this chapter. The reader should be aware that the staging system for head and neck cancer changed significantly in 1988 and that articles written before that date will most likely use a staging system somewhat different than described herein. The major change in the staging system relates to the nomenclature defining tumor spread to cervical neck nodes. Changes in the staging systems, although important to accurately reflect current information regarding prognosis, make it difficult to compare treatment results from different eras.

Staging Similarities

The head and neck sites are defined anatomically, as are regional nodes. *Tis* refers only to carcinoma *in situ* being documented at the presumed primary site. Situations in which invasive cancer is present are designated T1 to T4, depending on tumor extent. The nodal staging system for all head and neck sites is uniform, except for tumors of the

TABLE 20–2. **Nodal Staging System Common to All Head and Neck Sites Except Nasopharynx**

N Stage	Classification
NX	Regional nodes cannot be assessed
N0	No regional lymph node metastases
N1	Single, ipsilateral involved node ≤3 cm
N2	Single or multiple ipsilateral, contralateral, or bilateral involvement
N2a	Single ipsilateral node >3 cm, but ≤6 cm
N2b	Multiple ipsilateral nodes, none >6 cm
N2c	Bilateral or contralateral nodes, none >6 cm
N3	Involved node >6 cm

Used with permission of the American Joint Committee on Cancer (AJCC®), Chicago, Illinois. The original source for this material is the AJCC® Cancer Staging Manual, 5th ed, 1997, published by Lippincott-Raven Publishers, Philadelphia, Pennsylvania; and International Union Against Cancer (UICC): TNM Classification of Malignant Tumors, 4th ed, New York, Springer-Verlag, 1992.

nasopharynx, and is given in Table 20–2.[9, 10] If the nodal stage cannot be assessed, the stage is NX. Otherwise, the N definitions are based primarily on size. These designations are illustrated schematically in Figure 20–3. As noted earlier, the nodal staging system changed in 1988 and references dated before 1988 use a system in which multiple nodes are categorized as N3 (N3a—a single homolateral node >6 cm, N3b—multiple homolateral nodes, N3c—bilateral or contralateral nodes).

These variables have different impacts on patient prognosis, and in an attempt to simplify matters for the clinician, variables are generally combined into four major stage groups, as indicated in Table 20–3.[9, 10] However, such stage groupings often obscure relevant clinical information. For example, a patient with localized stage IV disease (T4,N0,M0) still has potentially curable disease whereas a patient who is stage IV as a result of the presence of distant metastases generally does not. Such considerations have led to the further subclassifications IVA, IVB, and IVC, as shown in Table 20–3. Stage grouping is somewhat different for nasopharyngeal cancers.

The designation of a particular TNM is not in itself adequate to formulate the best treatment approaches for any given case. Careful attention must be paid to particular routes of local and regional spread and the probability of occult metastatic disease in any given patient in order to optimize the individual treatment. These spread patterns are described in the sections dealing with specific tumor sites.

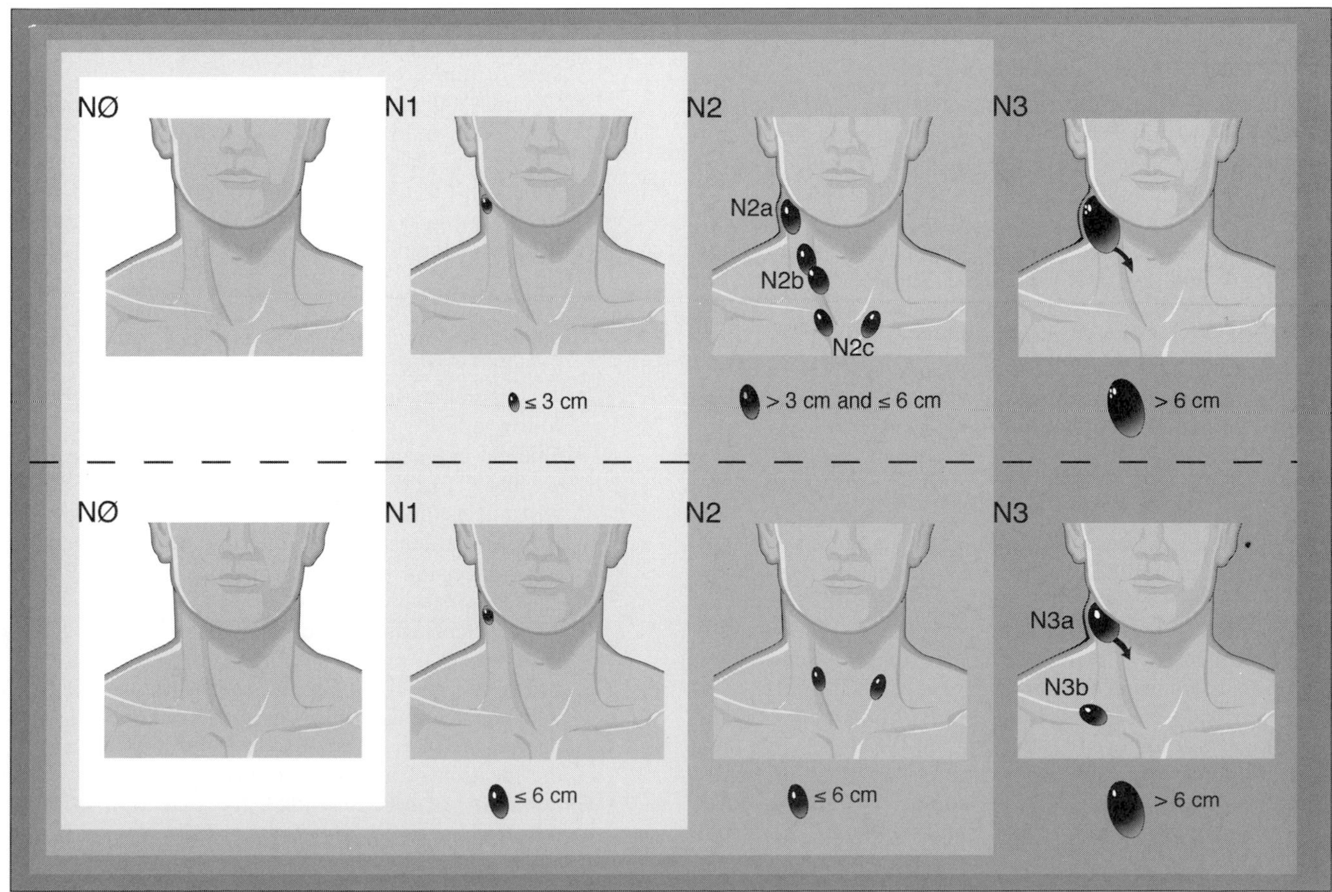

Figure 20–3. The upper set of panels show the staging system for the N category for most head and neck cancers based upon the most recent AJCC/UICC criteria.[9, 10] N0 refers to a clinically negative neck; N1 refers to a single involved ipsilateral node 3 cm or less; N2a refers to a single involved ipsilateral node greater than 3 cm but not more than 6 cm; N2b refers to multiple involved ipsilateral nodes with none greater than 6 cm; N2c refers to contralateral or bilateral nodes with none greater than 6 cm; and N3 refers to at least one involved node being greater than 6 cm. The lower row illustrates the nodal staging system in use for nasopharynx.

TABLE 20–3. **Stage Grouping Common to All Head and Neck Cancers Except Nasopharynx**

Stage Group	T Stage	N Stage	M Stage
Stage 0	Tis	N0	M0
Stage I	T1	N0	M0
Stage II	T2	N0	M0
Stage III	T3	N0	M0
	T1	N1	M0
	T2	N1	M0
	T3	N1	M0
Stage IV			
Stage IVA	T4	N0	M0
	T4	N1	M0
	Any T	N2	M0
Stage IVB	Any T	N3	M0
Stage IVC	Any T	Any N	M1

T = tumor; N = node; M = metastases.

Used with permission of the American Joint Committee on Cancer (AJCC®), Chicago, Illinois. The original source for this material is the AJCC® Cancer Staging Manual, 5th ed, 1997, published by Lippincott-Raven Publishers, Philadelphia, Pennsylvania; and International Union Against Cancer (UICC): TNM Classification of Malignant Tumors, 4th ed, New York, Springer-Verlag, 1992.

Staging Work-Up

The American Joint Committee on Cancer rules for staging classification allow different types of evaluative evidence for classifying the extent of disease at different sites and at different times in a patient's history:

- *Clinical-diagnostic staging (clinical TNM)* includes the standard clinical and radiologic procedures short of surgery. This staging is fundamental and most important.
- *Surgical-pathologic staging (pathologic TNM)* includes surgical exploratory procedures (staging surgery) and consists of biopsy samples of tissue or complete resection of primary site or nodes, or of both, with careful histopathologic study of extent of disease.
- *Retreatment staging (retreatment TNM)* is used for evaluation of recurrent disease or for re-evaluation when additional treatment is necessary.

Recommended Staging Procedures

- *Clinical evaluation* of primary site and cervical lymphatics as outlined earlier is recommended. Re-emphasized are visual inspection, mirror examination, and palpation. The T criteria for each site must be carefully documented, and measurements (three-dimensional if possible) are recommended for all sites.
- *Palpation, mapping*, and *measurement* of cervical nodes are important. Any enlarged, firm cervical node (>1 cm) in an adult must be regarded as malignant until proven otherwise. The number of palpable nodes is an important prognostic factor; however, there is an approximately 15% incidence of false-positive cervical nodes on clinical examination.[44] Mobility is often subjectively evaluated: Reduced mobility may imply escape of the tumor from the confines of the node into tissue planes, although reduced mobility alone does not adversely influence prognosis. Complete fixation (complete immobility of node) may imply invasion of prevertebral muscle, base of skull, or cervical spine and is an objective finding carrying poor prognosis.[44] Size is regarded as a more objective measure than mobility, and studies have shown that nodes greater than 6 cm in diameter are most often unresectable.
- *Examination under anesthesia*, permitting direct inspection of relatively inaccessible sites such as nasopharynx, hypopharynx, and larynx, is an important component of evaluation and should not be omitted. Biopsy of suspicious edges for peripheral extension should be performed.
- *Imaging procedures,* especially contrast-enhanced CT and MRI as outlined previously, are currently recommended:
  - Both CT and MRI can be applied effectively to clinical problems of primary SCC and nodal *metastases*.
  - Iodinated contrast-enhanced CT often can define *tumor size* more accurately than can clinical impressions. With T2-weighted images, MRI can be used to determine tumor extent and offers the advantage of three-dimensional multiplanar images. Gadolinium-enhanced MRI scans are also useful for visualizing tumor extension into surrounding soft tissues.
  - CT and MRI may be useful for finding *occult primary tumors* when enlarged neck nodes are the presenting features. They can direct the surgeon as an alternative to so-called blind biopsies of probable sites of tumor origin.
  - Contrast-enhanced CT and MRI can be particularly useful for *assessing nodes*. The radiologic criteria are size, nodes greater than 1.5 cm, or lymph nodes with central necroses (mixed density on CT or mixed intensity on MRI) regardless of size. Imaging studies change clinical staging 15% to 20% of the time.
  - CT- or ultrasound-guided *biopsy* firmly establishes pathologic diagnosis. False-positive results owing to inflammation can often be ruled out.
  - A *post-treatment baseline scan* can be essential for follow-up.
  - Clinical evaluation can be difficult if there is fibrosis, but CT and MRI can diagnose *recurrent tumor* when it is not possible by direct inspection and palpation at least 25% of the time (e.g., submucosal recurrence and high nodal relapse at base of skull and parapharyngeal area).
  - A *PET scan* can be useful in distinguishing recurrent tumor from post-treatment fibrosis. Tumor actively metabolizes fluorodeoxyglucose (^{18}FDG) whereas necrosis and fibrosis, the common late sequelae, are inert. It can also be helpful in identifying the location of an unknown primary.[43]
- *Chest x-ray* is recommended for detection of lung metastases.
- *Blood cell count* and *liver function* studies are routine.
- *A bone scan* is of value only for symptomatic patients.
- *Arteriography* is diagnostic of chemodectomas (carotid body or glomus jugulare tumors) and also allows the delineation of disease extent. However, contrast-enhanced CT and MRI scans are tending to replace this technique. Appropriate radiologic studies are valuable

when combined otolaryngologic-neurologic resections are contemplated.

Principles of Treatment

General

The goals of treatment in head and neck oncology are to eradicate the cancer, maintain adequate physiologic function, and achieve a socially acceptable cosmetic result.

- *Eradication of cancer* implies both eradication of clinically demonstrable disease (definitive treatment) and eradication of microscopic subclinical disease (elective treatment). The decision to use elective (prophylactic) treatment is based on probability considerations that weigh the likelihood of microscopic disease against the likelihood of treatment complications. One also considers the probability of being able to salvage the patient if the cancer relapses in the site of probable spread if elective treatment is withheld.
- Maintenance of *adequate physiologic function* requires careful evaluation of dysfunction already present and of dysfunction likely to follow treatment in each of the four major functional categories: (1) *special senses* (vision, hearing, balance, taste, smell); (2) *mastication-deglutition* (mandible, teeth, tongue, saliva, palate, pharynx, larynx); (3) *respiration* (larynx, trachea); and (4) *speech* (larynx, tongue). It is hoped that careful evaluation of treatment options will allow one to determine an optimal treatment choice combining a high tumor control probability with minimal functional deficit.
- Acceptable *cosmesis* requires necessary but sufficient surgery, within-tolerance irradiation, and reconstructive surgical and prosthesis rehabilitation. The patient should be informed of treatment outcome and of treatment alternatives. Ultimately, the patient's desires must be respected.

The goals of treatment can only be achieved through a *multidisciplinary approach* involving the head and neck oncologic surgeon, radiation oncologist, medical oncologist, pathologist, radiologist, dentist, nutritionist, nurse oncologist, and social worker. Ideally, each responsible oncologist should evaluate the tumor and the patient before any treatment. After joint consultation, a comprehensive but flexible program is formulated and cooperatively applied. Treatment decisions are primarily based on an appraisal of the patient's tumor, but the patient often plays an important role.[13] Emphasis is given to host factors such as:

- age and general condition
- comorbidity factors
- habits and lifestyle
- occupation
- patient's desires

Surgery and radiation therapy are the *major curative modalities*. Studies have shown the effectiveness of chemotherapy in organ preservation protocols for locally advanced laryngeal[45, 46] and hypopharyngeal tumors,[47] and in augmenting survival in patients with locally advanced nasopharyngeal tumors.[48, 49] However, small primary lesions (T1 and T2) with negative cervical nodes are generally best treated with one modality—either surgery or radiotherapy. Small lesions with involved nodes may need both surgery and irradiation for control of neck disease; the treatment sequence is generally dictated by the choice of therapy for the primary focus. If the primary is to be irradiated definitively, then both sides of the neck may be given 50 Gy before neck dissection. If the primary tumor is to be surgically excised, a neck dissection is also performed and postoperative irradiation may be indicated. The particular radiation dose given depends on the findings at the time of surgery and the pathology report.[50] Large primary lesions (T3 and T4) or extensive cervical node disease, or both, usually need surgery and irradiation. Although optimal sequencing of modalities in this circumstance is still under investigation, many centers favor postoperative irradiation.

Follow-up at regular intervals to detect early recurrence, extension, or complications is important. Patients can often be salvaged if tumor recurrence is detected early. The sequelae of treatment-related complications can often be reduced if appropriate measures are taken early in the course of their development. Late toxicity scoring scales that are most widely used are the Radiation Therapy Oncology Group (RTOG)/European Organization for Radiation Therapy in Cancer (EORTC) abbreviated grades or the more elaborate LENT (Late Effects Normal Tissue) system with ***s***ubjective complaints, ***o***bjective signs and ***m***anagement criteria—SOMA—the A is for more quantitative parameters and studies such as MRI or magnetic resonance spectroscopy.[51]

Surgery

General considerations are listed here. More specific information is covered under the individual sections.

- *Biopsy*: An unequivocal histopathologic diagnosis is mandatory in all cases. Wherever possible fine-needle aspiration of neck masses should be employed rather than incisional biopsy, with its risk of tumor spillage.[52] Any incisions through normal tissue must be well planned and performed only by experienced oncologic surgeons. Injudicious biopsies of cervical nodes performed via poorly situated incisions complicate subsequent therapy and may compromise the patient's outlook.
- *Gross residual disease*: The surgeon should not rely on postoperative radiation to eradicate gross residual disease[53, 54]; potentially curative surgical treatment must remove all gross disease. Piecemeal tumor removal risks recurrence, and adequate wound exposure is required to facilitate total tumor removal. Many standardized operative procedures are described, but each case needs individualization. Technical decisions often need to be made during the surgical procedure and require considerable experience and skill. Although preoperative radiation therapy or chemotherapy may shrink a tumor, any modification of surgical technique must recognize that such shrinkage does not always imply that the scope of the surgical procedure can be reduced.

- *Wide resection margins* improve local control, but practically speaking, resection margins are generally limited to 2 cm in the head and neck region. Inadequate or positive margins require postoperative irradiation rather than waiting for recurrence.[54]
- *Reconstructive procedures* are essential. In the past decade the increasing use of microvascular free flaps has substantially improved reconstruction of the midface, the oral cavity including the mandible, the base of tongue, and the hypopharynx.
- *Flaps*: The most commonly used regional and pedicled flaps are the pectoralis major, the trapezius flaps, and the latissimus dorsi.[55, 56] The most commonly used microvascular free flaps are the radial forearm, fibula, scapula, iliac crest, lateral arm, and jejunal flaps.[57–61] All of these flaps, with the exception of the lateral arm and the jejunum, can include vascularized bone.[62]
- *Neck dissections* without combined therapy can be curative for the occult (N0) neck metastases and the N1 neck. The choice of neck dissection (radical or modified radical neck dissection and more limited selective [functional] neck dissections) depends on the extent of neck disease and the chances for occult malignant spread. The classic radical neck dissection includes removal of all lymphatic tissue in Levels I through V along with the sternocleidomastoid muscle, the internal jugular vein, and the eleventh cranial nerve. A modified radical neck dissection leaves one or more of the nonlymphatic tissue structures mentioned earlier intact. Selective (functional) neck dissections aim to remove just the lymphatic tissue from the neck at all levels or in a selected set of levels.[15]

Radiation Therapy

General Considerations

- *Preservation of function and cosmesis* depends on the selective effect of irradiation to leave muscle, nerves, bones, and major vessels intact. The major advantage of irradiation is its ability to eradicate many cancers without undue complications.
- The *complexity* of modern radical radiation therapy requires that therapy be administered only by specially trained and experienced radiation oncologists who have full dosimetric and physics support facilities.
- A *variety of irradiation techniques* are available and the appropriate choice for a given patient must be made. Customization of treatment techniques is essential. External megavoltage irradiation is the cornerstone of modern treatment in most patients. Interstitial irradiation with selected radioactive isotopes (brachytherapy) is important as a dose-boosting technique for accessible lesions, especially in the oral cavity. Although a variety of isotopes are available, the majority of implants performed today use iridium-192 or iodine-125. Neck nodes can be boosted to high-dose levels with interstitial implants. Although it is arguable, a number of authors have indicated interstitial irradiation increases head and neck radiocurability compared with external irradiation alone for T1 and T2 cancers (92% vs. 65%).[63]

The *electron beam* provides an excellent ancillary technique for boosting doses to superficial regions in the head and neck area. Megavoltage radiation is required for radical treatment although orthovoltage can be used via perioral cones to boost doses to sites of disease. Wang has reported 5-year results using intraoral cones of 75% to 100% depending on site and stage.[64] Intraoperative radiotherapy, using either electron beams or orthovoltage radiation, can be used to deliver tumoricidal doses of radiation to specific regions determined to be at high risk at the time of surgery.[65]

- Radiation *dose selection* is based on tumor size and clinical circumstances. The amount of radiation required depends on the amount of tumor in the target volume.[275] Subclinical microscopic cancer requires 50 Gy in 5 weeks; small lesions (T1) require 60 to 65 Gy; intermediate lesions (T2) require 65 to 70 Gy; and large lesions (T3 and T4) generally need greater than 70 Gy, and even then prospects for permanent control are not great. Dose escalation beyond 75 Gy with external irradiation techniques with standard daily fractionation schedules is fraught with the risk of complications. Such high doses are generally achieved using interstitial irradiation as a component of the treatment plan, but conformal techniques using three-dimensional approaches to treatment planning and delivery also allow one to deliver higher doses to the primary target volume.[66] Altered fractionation schedules, such as twice daily (b.i.d.) hyperfractionation, have been used in clinical trials (see next section). Charged particle radiotherapy offers the ultimate in potential for dose escalation to precisely defined regions.[16]
- The *shrinking field technique*, with dose delivery to each region according to the amount of cancer present, must be used to achieve high doses. The primary site receives the highest dose, peripheral areas at risk for microscopic tumor spread (including neck nodes) receive a lower dose, but never less than 45 to 50 Gy using conventional fractionation schemas.

Fractionation Considerations

It is now generally accepted that *continuous course* radiotherapy is superior to a split-course type of regimen; this is due to an accelerated repopulation of tumor cells during the planned treatment break. Over time, single daily fraction radiotherapy has evolved as the standard radiotherapeutic regimen throughout much of the world, although the specific details of treatment may vary considerably. In the United States, 70 Gy in increments of 1.8 to 2.0 Gy typically is given as definitive therapy, whereas in Canada and much of Great Britain, the standard definitive treatment is 50 to 55 Gy in 2.5-Gy increments. Most recently, the use of hyperfractionated schedules in Europe, based on the successful outcome of EORTC trials, is a favored regimen.[67] Although these regimens produce reasonable results with acceptable acute and late toxicities (as perceived by the physicians using them), there is no reason to believe that they are truly optimal. One can envision tailoring the specific time-dose schedule to take advantage of differences between tumors and normal tissues, in terms of both intrinsic radiosensitivity and repopulation kinetics.[68, 69]

Currently there are two basic approaches that are being investigated. One is termed *hyperfractionation*, which involves reducing the size of the individual treatment fractions to allow for delivery of a greater total radiation dose without significantly increasing normal tissue late effects. To avoid an unacceptably long overall treatment time that would allow the tumor to proliferate, multiple daily fractions are given, generally on a b.i.d. basis; therefore, hyperfractionated courses of radiotherapy tend to be about as long as a course of standard radiotherapy. To allow the normal tissues to recover between the two daily treatments, the time interval must be approximately 4 to 6 hours. Alternatively, one may deliver the same (or perhaps somewhat lower) total dose of radiation over a shorter overall time. This is termed *accelerated fractionation.* Again, multiple daily treatment fractions are used, but the size of the individual treatment fraction is larger than used for hyperfractionation regimens.

Hyperfractionation

Early work in the use of hyperfractionated radiotherapy for head and neck cancer took place at the University of Florida.[70] Treatments were given at 1.2-Gy/fraction b.i.d. to total doses up to 81 Gy. Based on a comparison with historical controls, there was apparent benefit for T2 lesions of the supraglottic larynx and hypopharynx, T3 lesions of the tonsil, and T3 lesions of the hypopharynx. Nodal disease did not appear to influence primary tumor control.[71] On the other hand, Withers and associates[72] present data suggesting that the primary tumor dose needs to be increased if clinically positive nodes are present, even if a hyperfractionated radiotherapy schema is used.

The EORTC conducted a randomized study for patients with advanced oropharyngeal tumors.[67] The standard treatment arm consisted of 2-Gy daily fractions to a total dose of 70 Gy and the experimental arm consisted of 1.15 Gy given b.i.d. to a total dose of 80.5 Gy. A total of 356 patients were entered into the study, and at the 5-year end point, there was a statistically significant improvement in local and regional control with the hyperfractionation arm (59% vs. 40%, $p = 0.02$), but there was no statistically significant improvement in overall survival (40% vs. 32%, $p = 0.08$). The complication rates were comparable between the two treatment arms.

A randomized dose searching study to determine the maximum safe total dose that can be delivered in the head and neck region, using a 1.2-Gy b.i.d. treatment regimen, has been conducted by the RTOG.[73] Patients were randomized to receive total doses of 67.2, 72.0, 76. 8, or 81.6 Gy, using a complex dose-escalation randomization process. A preliminary analysis of 479 patients entered on the three lower dose arms showed a trend toward improved local and regional control at 2 years with increasing radiation dose (25% vs. 37% vs. 42%, $p = 0.08$), although no apparent benefit was noted for overall survival. Even though a final analysis has not yet been published for the 81.6-Gy arm, the RTOG has initiated a randomized trial comparing different fractionation schemes (discussed later in this section).

Accelerated Fractionation

Wang and coworkers have reported on an *accelerated* b.i.d. fractionation scheme that used 1.6-Gy fractions to a total target dose of 67.2 Gy.[74, 75] Because of the larger treatment fraction size, the patients experienced greatly increased acute mucosal reactions and a 2-week break in treatment was required at the 33.6-Gy point. A comparative analysis of the results using this treatment regimen to historical results from the same institution seemed to indicate improved local control for certain classes of tumors, but to date this approach has not been tested in the context of a randomized, clinical trial.

The CHART (continuous, hyperfractionated, accelerated radiotherapy) regimen is perhaps the best known of the more extreme, accelerated schedules that have been used clinically.[76] Three daily treatments of 1.5 Gy each were given to a total dose of 54 Gy, without allowing weekend treatment breaks. As expected, the acute mucosal and skin reactions were quite severe, but of more significance were two cases of cervical cord myelitis that also occurred. A comparative analysis seemed to show some improvement in local tumor control, but, again, no randomized trials have been carried out to date.

Ang and coworkers[77, 78] have developed a *concomitant* b.i.d. boost regimen that delivers the accelerated portion of the radiotherapy only during the last phase of treatment, when the radiation fields have been reduced in size. This is of further theoretical advantage in that the accelerated portion of the radiation is given at a time when the proliferation rate of both the tumor and the normal tissues has been increased in response to the initial portion of irradiation. Typically, the single daily fraction treatments are given to a dose of 54 Gy using standard fields and then during the boost, the first daily treatment is given at 1.8 Gy and the second daily treatment is given at 1.5 Gy. The total dose given to the tumor is in the range of 66 to 74 Gy. Results compared to those with standard fraction radiotherapy are intriguing, and this regimen is one arm of a recently completed RTOG randomized trial. Preliminary results indicate superior local control rates following the concomitant boost.

Although a *meta-analysis* evaluating the use of hyperfractionated radiotherapy in the treatment of human malignancies showed improved local and regional control as well as survival for head and neck cancer patients,[79] it should be noted that one of the four studies analyzed was published only in abstract form. Only the EORTC study had a tightly defined set of site- and stage-specific patient entry criteria.[67] It is also important to note that all of the ongoing studies incorporate a 6-hour interval between daily treatment fractions in order to allow for repair of sublethal and potentially lethal damage in the irradiated normal tissues. When intervals are shortened to less than 6 hours, RTOG investigators have shown that increased toxicity occurs.[80] A recently completed RTOG phase III trial showed improved local control with both hyperfractionation and the concomitant boost compared with standard fractionation for patients with inoperable head and neck cancers.[80a] There was also a trend toward improved survival using these approaches.

Regression Patterns

Analysis of regression patterns after definitive radiotherapy has therapeutic implications with regard to the planning of salvage surgery. It is advisable to wait for a 2- to 3-month postirradiation follow-up for nodes smaller than 6 cm, whereas longer intervals are advised for bulky nodes. This recommendation is based on differences in achieving complete regression at the end of therapy versus waiting 4 to 8 weeks (62% vs. 80% for primaries and 32% vs. 76% for nodes).[81] The significance of regression patterns is not as well established when chemotherapy is added to the treatment regimen.

Chemotherapy

General Considerations

The role of chemotherapy in the treatment of SCC of the head and neck is still evolving. Chemotherapy has been employed before local therapy (i.e., neoadjuvant or induction therapy), as adjuvant therapy after local therapeutic modalities, concurrently with radiation for advanced disease, and as treatment for metastatic or recurrent disease. The probability of response to chemotherapy (defined as a ≥50% reduction in bidimensional tumor measurement) depends on the disease status. The remission rate in patients with untreated head and neck cancers is more than twice that seen when the same agents are given for recurrent or metastatic disease, most likely as a result of changes in the vascular supply after surgery or radiation, or both, or as a result of the presence of more inherently resistant cells. Although chemotherapy for untreated cancers of the head and neck has shown significant activity, use of the currently available agents for treatment of *de novo* tumor presentations is not thought of as a curative modality, but rather as an adjunct to surgery, radiotherapy, or the combination of the two. The most clearly defined role for chemotherapy in head and neck cancer remains as palliative treatment for metastatic or recurrent disease.

Metastatic or Recurrent Disease

Hematogenous metastases from cancers of the head and neck are found in 20% to 40% of patients, especially in those who initially had advanced nodal disease; the most common distant metastatic sites are the lungs, mediastinum, bone, and liver.[82–84] Local recurrence, however, remains the greater problem with these neoplasms, and the majority of patients with distant metastases also have uncontrolled disease in the head and neck region.[82] The development of either unresectable locally recurrent or distant metastatic disease portends a grave prognosis, with median survival times in the 2- to 3-month range without treatment.[85]

Many *single agents* exhibit some degree of activity in head and neck cancer. In studies involving patients with recurrent or metastatic tumors, response rates are in the range of 30% for methotrexate, 30% for cisplatin, 20% for carboplatin, 20% for bleomycin, 15% for 5-fluorouracil (5-FU), 25% for ifosfamide, 39% for hydroxyurea, and 40% for the taxanes paclitaxel and docetaxel, with all agents producing responses lasting 2 to 6 months.[87–91] Methotrexate is the best studied and most commonly used single agent. Doses greater than 200 mg/m^2 add toxicity and cost without significant improvement in survival.[92] The drug is most frequently given in lower doses via escalating weekly intravenous or intramuscular injections; beginning at 40 to 50 mg/m^2, the dose is increased in increments of 10 mg/m^2 per week until toxicity limits further increase in dosage. Mucositis and myelosuppression are the usual dose-limiting side effects with methotrexate administered in this fashion.

Combinations of agents used in the same setting result in higher overall response rates and are more likely to produce CRs, which in turn are associated with a greater prolongation of survival.[93, 94] Cisplatin-containing combinations have produced the highest overall and complete remission (CR) rates. Kish and associates were the first to report on the use of cisplatin in combination with 5-FU by continuous 96-hour infusion for patients with recurrent or metastatic head and neck cancer.[95] Among 30 patients, 27% achieved a CR and 43% a partial remission, for an overall response rate of 70%. The average duration of response was 11.3 months for patients with a CR, but only 6.5 months for patients achieving a partial remission. Subsequent studies (Table 20–4) using this combination have shown overall response rates averaging in the 40% to 50% range, with CRs in the 10% to 15% range. Cisplatin and 5-FU continue to be the most frequently used combination regimen for treatment of patients with head and neck cancer. Cisplatin 100 mg/m^2 is given on the first day of the chemotherapy cycle with 5-FU 1000 mg/m^2 per day given by 96- to 120-hour continuous intravenous infusion; cycles are repeated every 21 to 28 days. Nausea can be a significant side effect from this treatment, requiring the use of serotonin receptor antagonist antiemetics. Painful mucositis (≥ grade 2) occurs in approximately 30% of patients who receive this regimen. Nephrotoxicity, ototoxicity, and grade 3 or 4 myelosuppression occur in less than 30% of patients. The addition of other chemotherapeutic agents such as interferon or leucovorin to the cisplatin and 5-FU combination has no apparent survival benefit.[107–110]

Among the newer multiagent chemotherapeutic regimens are those that combine cisplatin with agents such as the taxanes or ifosfamide, as shown in Table 20–5. Response rates of 30% to 50% are produced by the combination of cisplatin with paclitaxel or docetaxel.[111–115] Shin and colleagues tested the further addition of ifosfamide to paclitaxel and cisplatin in 52 patients, and reported an overall response rate of 58%, with a CR rate of 17%.[118] Although promising, the response rates are similar to those reported in early studies of cisplatin and 5-FU, and it remains to be seen how the taxane-containing regimens will compare with single agents or cisplatin and 5-FU therapy in randomized studies. The addition of ifosfamide or a taxane to cisplatin also adds considerable hematologic toxicity, with 80% to 90% of patients developing severe myelosuppression.

Despite the improved response rates seen with combination chemotherapy, randomized studies to date have shown that combination regimens provide no statistical survival advantage over single agents. Six randomized studies have been performed comparing cisplatin-containing combination chemotherapy with cisplatin alone; although two

TABLE 20–4. **Treatment of Recurrent or Metastatic Squamous Cell Carcinoma of the Head and Neck with Cisplatin and 5-Fluorouracil**

Chemotherapy Regimen	Evaluable Patients	Response Rate % Overall (Complete Remission)	Median Survival	Reference
CDDP: 100 mg/m^2 5-FU: 1 g/m^2/d × 96 hr c.i.	30	70 (27)	27.5 wk	Kish et al[95]
CDDP: 100 mg/m^2 5-FU: 1 g/m^2/d × 96 hr c.i.	20	25 (0)	7.2 mo	Creagan et al[96]
CDDP: 100 mg/m^2 5-FU: 1 g/m^2/d × 96 hr c.i. vs. 600 mg/m^2/d × d1,8 i.v.p.	38	72 (22) 20 (10)	27 wk 20 wk	Kish et al[97]
CDDP: 100 mg/m^2 5-FU: 1 g/m^2/d × 120 hr c.i.	18	11 (0)		Dasmahapatra et al[98]
CDDP: 80 mg/m^2 × 24 hr c.i. 5-FU: 800 mg/m^2/d × 120 hr c.i.	39	46 (18)	5–9 mo	Amrein et al[99]
CDDP: 100 mg/m^2 5-FU: 1 g/m^2/d × 120 hr c.i.	30	60 (17)	9.1 mo	Rowland et al[100]
CDDP: 100 mg/m^2 5-FU: 1 g/m^2/d × 96 hr c.i.	20	35 (5)	6 mo	Mercier et al[101]
CDDP: 20 mg/m^2/d × 5 5-FU: 0.4–0.2 g/m^2/d × 5 i.v.p.	67	52 (21)	8 mo	Merlano et al[102]
CDDP: 100 mg/m^2 5-FU: 1 g/m^2/d × 120 hr c.i.	20	25 (10)	36 wk	Choski et al[103]
CDDP: 120 mg/m^2 5-FU: 1 g/m^2/d × 120 hr c.i. +/− DDTC	56	36 (7)	9–10 mo	Paredes et al[104]
CDDP: 100 mg/m^2 5-FU: 1 g/m^2/d × 120 hr c.i.	49	43 (18)	8 mo	Paccagnella et al[105]
CDDP: 100 mg/m^2 5-FU: 1 g/m^2/d × 96 hr c.i.	20	30 (5)	7 mo	O'Brien et al[106]

CDDP = cisplatin; 5-FU = 5-fluorouracil; DDTC = sodium diethyldithiocarbamate; c.i. = continuous infusion; i.v.p. = bolus.

showed statistically superior response rates with the combination regimen,[120, 121] the overall survival rates with combination therapy were similar to those seen with cisplatin alone.[120–122] When combination chemotherapy was tested against methotrexate, which remains the most commonly used single agent because of its ease of administration and favorable toxicity profile, overall survival rates were again similar, as shown in Table 20–6.

In these randomized studies, median survivals continue to be between 5 and 6 months for all patients. Patients who achieve a CR from chemotherapy have approximately twice the median survival compared with patients who have a partial or no response to treatment. Combination chemotherapy is more likely to produce a CR compared with single-agent therapy, but this advantage needs to be weighed against the added toxicity from combination regimens, particularly in this group of patients, who often have comorbid medical conditions such as emphysema, cardiovascular disease, and poor nutrition. Thus, for patients with head and neck cancer who have distant metastases or local recurrence that is not amenable to further surgery or radiation, the choice of using a single agent versus combination chemotherapy for palliative treatment must be carefully individualized.

TABLE 20–5. **Newer Drug Combinations for Treatment of Recurrent or Metastatic Squamous Cell Carcinoma of the Head and Neck**

Chemotherapy Regimen	Evaluable Patients	Response Rate % Overall (Complete Remission)	Median Survival	Reference
CDDP + paclitaxel	197	34 (8)	7–7.5 mo	Forastiere et al[111]
CDDP + paclitaxel	22	32 (0)		Licitra et al[112]
CDDP + paclitaxel	18	28 (6)		Schilling et al[113]
CDDP + paclitaxel	25	48 (0)	6.5 mo MDR	Thodtmann et al[114]
CDDP + docetaxel	33	52 (9)		Forastiere et al[115]
CDDP + paclitaxel + 5-FU	14	71 (14)		Hussain et al[116]
CDDP + ifosfamide	76	66 (13)	4 mo MDR	Pai et al[117]
CDDP + ifosfamide + paclitaxel	52	58 (17)	8.8 mo	Shin et al[118]
Carboplatin + paclitaxel	35	23	7.3 mo	Fountzilas et al[119]

CDDP = cisplatin; 5-FU = 5-fluorouracil; MDR = median duration of response.

TABLE 20–6. **Randomized Studies Comparing Combination Chemotherapy with Single Agent, Methotrexate**

Reference	Chemotherapy Regimen	Evaluable Patients	Response Rate % Overall (Complete Remission)	Median Survival
Drelichman et al[123]	CDDP + VCR + Bleo	51	40.7 (11.1)	17 wk
	MTx		33.3 (8.3)	24 wk
Vogl et al[124]	CDDP + Bleo + MTx	163	48 (16)*	5.6 mo
	MTx		35 (8) (p = 0.04)	5.6 mo
Williams et al[125]	CDDP + VLB + Bleo	191	24	29 wk
	MTx		16	31.4 wk
Eisenberger et al[126]	Carboplatin + MTx	40	25 (0)	6 mo
	MTx		25 (5)	6 mo
Liverpool Head & Neck[122]	CDDP + 5-FU	200	24 (6)	4–7 mo range
	CDDP + MTx		22 (0)	
	CDDP		28 (2)	(CDDP vs. MTx,* p <0.025)
	MTx		12 (0)	
Forastiere et al[127]	CDDP + 5-FU	277	32 (6)*	6.6 mo
	Carboplatin + 5-FU		21 (2)	5 mo
	MTx		10 (2) (vs. MTx, p <0.001)	5.6 mo

CDDP = cisplatin; VCR = vincristine; Bleo = bleomycin; MTx = methotrexate; VLB = vinblastine; 5-FU = 5-fluorouracil, * = statistically significant.

Neoadjuvant Chemotherapy

The limited benefit from chemotherapy in patients with head and neck cancer who have had previous surgery, radiation therapy, or both, may occur for several reasons:

- The blood supply has been disrupted by the previous treatment.
- The patient may be in poorer overall health as a result of poor nutrition and coexistent lung disease and other medical illness.
- Previous radiation therapy makes patients more susceptible to severe mucositis from treatment with methotrexate, 5-FU, and bleomycin.

These factors have led to investigations of chemotherapy as a first-line modality before surgery or definitive radiation for patients with advanced head and neck cancers. The initial utilization of chemotherapy before local therapy is referred to as *neoadjuvant*, or induction, chemotherapy.

In the neoadjuvant setting, cisplatin-containing combination chemotherapy has produced the best results. As is the case with recurrent disease, the combination of cisplatin and infusional 5-FU is the most frequently used regimen. In the setting of *de novo* cancer, the overall response rate is approximately 80%, and 20% to 60% of patients will achieve a clinical CR, with the maximum response occurring by at least the third cycle of treatment.[98, 99, 128–131] Similar to what is seen with recurrent disease, patients who achieve a CR have the greatest survival benefit.[128, 129, 132, 133]

To further evaluate these encouraging results, many randomized studies have compared local therapy alone with neoadjuvant chemotherapy before local therapy. Twenty of these trials are listed in Table 20–7. In these studies, local therapy most often consisted of radiation alone for inoperable patients and surgery plus radiation for patients with resectable cancers; in some cases, however, local therapy was modified from surgical intervention to radiation alone for patients in remission after chemotherapy. Although two of the trials listed in Table 20–7 did show an overall survival advantage for the chemotherapy arm by subset analysis,[146, 153] the overwhelming majority failed to demonstrate an improved survival with the use of neoadjuvant chemotherapy. In one study, reported in abstract form by DiBlasio and associates, the overall survival was actually worse in the chemotherapy arm, despite a 69% response rate to the neoadjuvant chemotherapy program.[147]

There are other possible explanations for why the trials failed to demonstrate an overall benefit with the use of neoadjuvant chemotherapy. As is the case for most head and neck cancer chemotherapy trials, all but five of these studies evaluated patients who were a heterogeneous group with different subsites of primary disease, which may influence responsiveness to chemotherapy; in addition, patients with resectable and unresectable cancers were often included in the same study. The chemotherapy program was suboptimal in several of these trials, resulting in low response rates before surgical resection. In others, different locoregional therapeutic modalities were employed in the two treatment arms. Many studies included an inadequate number of patients to detect a difference in survival.[154] Patient compliance with treatment was another possible factor; in the study by Schuller and coworkers,[138] only 56% of the patients assigned to preoperative chemotherapy completed the prescribed treatment, and in the Head and Neck Contracts Program,[136] a scant 9% of patients completed the entire neoadjuvant and adjuvant chemotherapy regimen. These issues must be considered when reviewing the negative results from the randomized studies. Although overall survival was not affected by induction chemotherapy in the majority of these trials, several did demonstrate a therapeutic benefit in decreasing the rate of distant metastatic disease.

When Jaulerry and colleagues compared radiation alone, with or without two different neoadjuvant chemotherapy regimens, they observed that the rate of distant metastases in the chemotherapy arms was approximately half that seen in the radiation-alone arm (p <0.03).[144] They also noted that the degree of response to chemotherapy correlated strongly with the subsequent response to radiation therapy, an important observation for future organ preservation ap-

TABLE 20–7. **Randomized Studies Evaluating Neoadjuvant Chemotherapy**

Reference	Chemotherapy Regimen	Evaluable Patients	Local Treatment	Survival	Comments
Stell et al[134]	M, O, B, H, MP, CP	86	R ± S	22%	
	None		R ± S	55% at 30 mo	
Kun et al[135]	B, M, CP, F	83	R ± S	31%	LR increased with CT, p <0.06
	None		R ± S	43% at 2 yr	
HNCP[136]	P, B × 1	443	S + R	37%	DM decreased in arm 2,* OS better in arm 2 for N2 subset*
	Neo P, B + adj P		S + R	45%	
	None		S + R	35% at 5 yr	
Toohill et al[137]	P, F	60	R ± S	56%	
	None		R ± S	70% at 2 yr	
Schuller et al[138]	P, M, B, O	158	S + R	18 mo	DM decreased with CT: 49 vs. 28%
	None		S + R	30 mo MST	
Carugati et al[139]	P, B ± M	120	S + R	38%	
	None		S + R	18% at 5 yr	
Martin et al[140, 141]	P, F	156	S + R or R	38%	
	None		S + R or R	34% at 5 yr	
Jortay et al[142]	B, M, O	226	S + R	35%	Pyriform sinus alone
	None		S + R	35% at 5 yr	
VALCSG[45]	P, F	332	R or S + R	68%	Larynx only LR: 12 vs. 2%.* DM decreased with CT: 11 vs. 17%*
	None		S + R	68% at 2 yr	
Mazeron et al[143]	P, B, M, F	116	R ± S	22 mo	
	None		R ± S	29 mo MST	
Jaulerry et al[144]	P, VN, B, MM, or P	208	R ± S	Equal results	DM decreased with CT*: p <0.03
	F, VN				
	None		R ± S		
Depondt et al[145]	C, F	143	S + R or R	56%	LR worse with CT: 35% vs. 25%
	None		S + R	46% at 4 yr	
Paccagnella et al[146]	P, F	237	S + R or R	29%	DM decreased with CT*
	None		S + R or R	20% at 3 yr; 24 vs. 10%* for inoperable pts	OS and LR better with CT for inoperable pts*
DiBlasio et al[147]	P, F	69	±S ±R		OS better with local therapy: p = 0.04*
	None		NA		
Hasegawa et al[148]	P, F	46	S ± R	61%	
	None		S ± R	68% at 3 yr	
Chan et al[149]	Neo and adj P, F	77	R	80%	Nasopharynx only
	None		R	80.5% at 2 yr	
Dalley et al[150]	P, F	280	NA	60%	
	None			53% at 2 yr	
Lefebvre et al[47]	P, F	194	R or S + R	44 mo	Hypopharynx only. DM decreased with CT: 25% vs. 36%*
	None		S + R	25 mo MST	
El Gueddari et al[151]	B, E, P	339	R	45%	Nasopharynx only. DFS: 41% vs. 30%*
	None		R	43%	
Lewin et al[152]	P, F	461	R ± S	62%	
	None		R ± S	60% DFS	

M = methotrexate; O = vincristine; B = bleomycin; H = hydroxyurea; MP = 6-mercaptopurine; CP = cyclophosphamide; F = 5-fluorouracil; P = cisplatin; VN = vindesine; MM = mitomycin C; C = carboplatin; E = epirubicin; neo = neoadjuvant; adj = adjuvant; R = radiotherapy; S = surgery; CT = chemotherapy; MST = median survival time; DFS = disease-free survival; LR = local recurrence; DM = distant metastases; OS = overall survival; HNCP = Head and Neck Contracts Program; VALCSG = Veterans Affairs Laryngeal Cancer Study Group; NA = not available; * = statistically significant.

proaches to treatment. The two randomized organ preservation studies comparing surgery plus radiotherapy with cisplatin and 5-FU before primary radiotherapy also showed a statistically significant decrease in the number of patients developing distant metastases.[45, 47] The Southwest Oncology Group trial evaluating cisplatin, methotrexate, bleomycin, and vincristine before surgery and radiotherapy showed a reduction in the number of patients developing distant metastases (49% vs. 28%; p = 0.07),[138] as did the Head and Neck Contracts Program study for patients in the neoadjuvant and adjuvant chemotherapy arm (p = 0.011 compared with local therapy alone).[136] By subset analysis, the Head and Neck study also showed an overall survival advantage with the use of neoadjuvant and adjuvant chemotherapy for patients with N2 disease.[153]

The other notable study that showed improved survival by subset analysis is that of Paccagnella and coworkers[146]: Local and regional treatment was individualized to the patient, with operable patients receiving surgery and postoperative radiotherapy, whereas inoperable patients were treated with definitive radiotherapy. Patients on the experimental arm received four cycles of cisplatin and 5-FU before definitive local and regional therapy. Again, there was a statistically significant reduction in distant metastases with the addition of chemotherapy (14% vs. 38%, p = 0.002). More importantly, patients with unresectable tumors had a statistically significant improvement in both local and regional control and survival with the addition of chemotherapy to primary radiotherapy (p = 0.05 and 0.04, respectively). Although six of the studies summarized in

Table 20–7 showed that the distant metastatic rate could be improved by chemotherapy, overall survival has remained unaffected in the majority of these trials, most likely because distant disease is an uncommon site of failure compared with local and regional recurrence. Controlling distant metastases would have little impact on survival for most patients with advanced head and neck cancer.

The overall conclusion from these trials that chemotherapy does not offer a treatment benefit for most patients, at least in terms of survival, is further borne out by two meta-analyses of randomized head and neck cancer trials. An international collaborative group has performed several meta-analyses of chemotherapy in head and neck cancer using published and unpublished individual patient data from these and other randomized trials.[155] The first meta-analysis involved 63 trials that randomized patients to local and regional treatment alone or to chemotherapy plus local therapy. In these studies, chemotherapy was given before local therapy, concurrent with radiation therapy, or after local therapy. The median follow-up time was 6 years. Although there was a small improvement in 5-year survival with the addition of chemotherapy (4%, $p < 0.001$), further analysis showed that an absolute survival benefit was seen only with the concurrent use of chemotherapy (8%, $p < 0.0001$), but not with neoadjuvant or adjuvant administration of chemotherapy (2% and 1%, respectively, values not significant). Subset analysis showed that this outcome was true regardless of tumor stage, tumor site, or type of chemotherapy.

The second meta-analysis from this group[155] evaluated individual patient data from five randomized trials comparing neoadjuvant chemotherapy given preirradiation or concurrent irradiation. This analysis showed an absolute 5-year survival advantage of 4%, again favoring concomitant administration of chemotherapy with radiation. The conclusion from these two meta-analyses was that neoadjuvant chemotherapy offers no survival advantage over local treatment alone, and that the most efficacious method of administering chemotherapy in a multimodality approach for advanced disease is concurrent with radiotherapy. At this time, the main role for induction chemotherapy is as part of an organ preservation approach to avoid debilitating surgery.

Organ Preservation

Another potential use of chemotherapy relates to organ preservation. The basic hypothesis is that response to chemotherapy predicts which patients will do well with a nonsurgical form of therapy. This correlation has been observed in trials employing neoadjuvant chemotherapy before definitive radiation therapy; in one such study, 97.6% of chemotherapy responders subsequently responded to radiation therapy compared with only 5.5% of patients who had not responded to chemotherapy.[156] In this treatment approach, it is vitally important to closely monitor the patient so that those who do not respond adequately can be shifted early to a surgical method of treatment.

Perhaps the best known organ preservation study is the one conducted by the Veterans Administration for patients with advanced laryngeal cancer.[45, 46] Patients were randomized to either a standard treatment arm, consisting of surgery and postoperative radiotherapy, or an experimental arm consisting of induction chemotherapy with cisplatin and 5-FU, with evaluation for response after two chemotherapy cycles. The responders received a third cycle of chemotherapy followed by definitive radiotherapy, whereas the nonresponders went to surgical resection followed by postoperative radiotherapy. With a median follow-up time of 5 years, there was no significant survival difference between the two treatment arms. Furthermore, 66% of surviving patients in the experimental arm maintained an intact, functioning larynx. A Cox regression analysis showed that T stage (T4 vs. other) and prior tracheostomy were significant predictors for laryngeal preservation on the experimental arm. Quality-of-life assessment data indicate that long-term swallowing ability was also better for patients in the experimental arm. In addition, there was a lower rate of distant metastases for patients on the chemotherapy arm (11% vs. 17%; $p = 0.001$).

The EORTC has completed a similar organ preservation study for patients with hypopharyngeal cancer.[47] Patients on the organ preservation arm had the same survival statistics as those on the standard arm. At 3 years, 42% of patients on the experimental arm were alive with an intact, functioning larynx. As with other neoadjuvant studies, distant metastases were significantly decreased in the group receiving chemotherapy.

The aforementioned trials do not address the question of whether the induction chemotherapy added anything to the ultimate tumor control probability or whether equivalent results could have been achieved with radiotherapy alone. This question is being addressed in an ongoing Intergroup trial for laryngeal cancer with three treatment arms: (1) the experimental arm of the VA study is the new standard treatment arm; (2) the second arm uses radiotherapy alone; and (3) the third arm consists of concomitant cisplatin chemotherapy and radiotherapy.

Adjuvant Chemotherapy

An alternate approach to attempt improving outcome for patients with advanced head and neck cancer is to give chemotherapy after surgery, radiation therapy, or both. Adjuvant administration of chemotherapy would avoid delays or other possible compromises in local therapy, which is always a concern with neoadjuvant treatment programs. In addition, there is the theoretical advantage that chemotherapy is more effective in eradicating microscopic disease than grossly evident tumor.

Numerous studies have evaluated chemotherapy given after local treatment. The studies themselves are heterogeneous, evaluating chemotherapy alone after local therapy, concurrent with adjuvant radiation therapy, and in many cases including chemotherapy both before and after the local therapy. The two largest randomized adjuvant trials are the Intergroup IG0034 trial and the Head and Neck Contracts Program study.

The Intergroup study (IG0034) tested the use of adjuvant cisplatin and 5-FU after surgery and before postoperative radiotherapy in 442 patients with operable tumors.[157] Patients were stratified according to tumor site, stage, and margin status. Compliance with regard to the delivery of chemotherapy was only 63%. With a mean time-at-risk of

46 months, there were no differences in terms of local and regional control or survival. However, there was a lower incidence of distant metastases on the chemotherapy arm (15% vs. 23%; p = 0.03). When analyzed according to margin risk factors, patients in the high-risk group (defined as surgical margins <5 mm, extracapsular nodal extension, and/or carcinoma *in situ* at the margin) had improvement with chemotherapy in both local and regional control (72% vs. 66%; p = 0.07) and survival (50% vs. 39%; p = 0.06).

The Head and Neck Contracts Study[136, 153] tested cisplatin and bleomycin in a three-arm study involving 462 patients. One arm was the standard treatment consisting of surgery and postoperative radiotherapy, the second arm was induction chemotherapy with cisplatin and bleomycin before standard treatment, and the third arm consisted of the same induction chemotherapy followed by standard treatment, followed by six monthly doses of cisplatin maintenance chemotherapy. Patient compliance was poor, and only 9% of patients in the third arm received all of their intended chemotherapy. Although there was no difference in local and regional control or survival among the arms, there was a reduction of distant metastases as the site of first relapse for patients on the third arm (9% vs. 19%; p = 0.025). A subsequent multivariate analysis of patient subsets revealed improved disease-free survival in patients with oral cavity primaries, N1 disease, and N2 disease, but improved overall survival only in patients with N2 disease.

Numerous other trials have been carried out, with the majority showing no benefit to chemotherapy given after local treatment, though, as noted in the Intergroup and the Head and Neck Contracts Program studies, the literature suggests that some subsets of patients are more likely to benefit. The lack of overall survival benefit is substantiated by the meta-analyses of chemotherapy in head and neck cancer undertaken by Bourhis and associates that showed that neither induction chemotherapy nor adjuvant chemotherapy improved survival when added to locoregional therapy.[155]

Concomitant Chemotherapy and Radiation Therapy

If chemotherapy is given concomitantly with radiotherapy, then, in addition to its effect on micrometastases, there can also be a potentially synergistic effect in local and regional control.[158, 159] Three general approaches are being used: (1) concomitant chemotherapy with continuous course radiotherapy; (2) concomitant chemotherapy with split-course radiotherapy; and (3) chemotherapy alternating with radiotherapy. Although the acute toxicity associated with the first approach is greater, it offers the advantage of using what is probably the most effective radiotherapy regimen. There are a few trials using concomitant chemotherapy and radiotherapy worth special mention.

An early trial by Guptka and associates[160] compared radiotherapy alone with the combination of radiotherapy along with methotrexate given on days 1 and 14. At 32 months, the group receiving the combination therapy had improved local and regional control and survival, with the differences being most pronounced for the subgroup of patients with oropharyngeal lesions. However, unlike the studies described earlier in this chapter, no difference was noted in terms of the rate of developing distant metastases. Merlano and coworkers[161] compared radiotherapy alone with concomitant radiotherapy and chemotherapy with cisplatin and 5-FU given in an alternating fashion. At the 3-year end point, there was an improvement in both disease-free survival (25% vs. 7%; p <0.009) and overall survival (41% vs. 23%; p <0.05) on the combined treatment arm. Keane and associates[162] tested radiotherapy alone versus split-course radiotherapy with mitomycin C and 5-FU for patients with advanced hypopharyngeal or laryngeal tumors. Toxicity on both arms was comparable, as was local and regional control and survival.

In order to bring out small differences that might not be statistically significant, a meta-analysis of trials using radiotherapy and combinations of various chemotherapeutic agents in the treatment of head and neck cancer was performed by El-Sayed and Nelson.[163] They found that, overall, there was an improvement in survival (22%, confidence interval 8% to 33%), but there was an added cost in terms of increased side effects. The reader is referred to the original paper for details of the analysis and study inclusion criteria.

Combined Modalities

A multimodality assessment of each patient has been emphasized, but it is important to note that every patient does not require a combination of surgery, radiation, and chemotherapy. *Small primary lesions* (T1 and T2) with a clinically negative neck are best managed with one modality (either surgery or radiotherapy) because combining modalities under these conditions can result in overtreatment with an unnecessary risk of increased complications. The cure rates with either modality are the same; therefore, which is used depends largely on the functional outcome and patient preference.

Large primary lesions (T3 and T4) or involvement of cervical lymphatics, on the other hand, generally require a planned combined approach, and currently the most frequent multimodal treatment is radical surgery with adjuvant preoperative or postoperative irradiation. Although surgical techniques may need some modification when radiation therapy is given,[6] the treatment team must guard against imposing "a plurality of minor efforts that may, in themselves, be defeatist."[164] When using a multimodal approach, it is crucial not to de-emphasize each modality to such an extent that the final result fails to achieve the outcome that could be possible with a single modality. Usually at least one modality (surgery or radiotherapy) has to be radical if a combined approach is to succeed.

It has long been recognized that the surgeon should not rely on postoperative radiation to eradicate *gross residual disease*.[165, 166] Potentially curative surgical treatment must remove all gross disease, and in the same way, although preoperative radiation therapy or chemotherapy may shrink a tumor, any modification of surgical technique must recognize that such shrinkage does not always imply that the scope of the surgical procedure can be reduced.

Radiation therapy is highly effective in controlling microscopic, subclinical disease in surgically undisturbed tissues, but at least 50 Gy within 5 weeks is required. Postoperatively, surgically disturbed areas of subclinical disease are thought to require at least 60 Gy and still higher doses are required if there are high-risk features, such as extracapsular nodal extension or positive margins following the surgical resection.[50] There have been no randomized clinical trials that conclusively demonstrate a survival benefit for postoperative radiotherapy. However, a matched-pair analysis comparing surgical treatment of the neck with and without postoperative radiotherapy showed that the addition of this modality reduced the recurrence rate, delayed the development of distant metastases, and reduced the rate of cancer-related death as well as death owing to any cause.[167] The patients involved in this analysis were treated between 1970 and 1990, and the radiation techniques are believed to be suboptimal by modern standards, therefore making its results even more interesting.[168]

Chemotherapy as an adjuvant to radiation, surgery, or to both remains a subject of active clinical investigation.[169] Randomized clinical trials support its use in organ preservation protocols for locally advanced tumors of the larynx[45, 46] and pyriform sinus, or aryepiglottic fold.[47] The concomitant use of chemotherapy and radiotherapy has yielded improved local and regional control in several randomized trials,[169] but at the present time, its routine use appears confined to nasopharyngeal lesions, where a major benefit has been shown in the context of an Intergroup study.[48, 49] Concomitant chemotherapy and radiotherapy results in increased mucositis compared with treatment with radiotherapy alone,[170, 171] but late sequelae appear to be comparable.

In attempts to reduce the acute toxicity, investigators are testing treatment schedules that alternate the two modalities. One such trial showed improved outcome with an alternating radiotherapy-chemotherapy arm, but this outcome may have resulted from an unexpectedly poor rate of local and regional control on the radiotherapy-alone arm.[161] One major trial studied sequential chemotherapy as an adjuvant to surgery and postoperative radiotherapy for patients with operable head and neck tumors.[157] There was no improvement in either local and regional control or survival, but there was a reduction in the incidence of distant metastases (23% vs. 15%, $p = 0.03$). Other studies using chemotherapy have similarly shown a reduced incidence of distant metastases, but this outcome will likely have an impact on survival only when the major causes of death (local and regional failure, intercurrent disease, and second malignant neoplasms) have been adequately addressed. Optimal drug delivery and radiotherapy schedules are yet to be determined.

Special Considerations of Treatment

In general, the first spread of head and neck tumors away from the primary site is to the lymphatics of the neck. Hence, management of the neck is a part of the comprehensive treatment of a patient with head and neck cancer. Table 20–8 shows the approximate incidence of positive neck nodes at the time of presentation for various tumor sites. Also shown are approximate figures for clinically N0 nodes having foci of metastatic tumor, as found during prophylactic neck dissections, as well as the percentage of clinically N0 necks that ultimately develop disease if untreated.

- *Clinically involved nodes* are best managed by radical neck dissection or by modified neck dissection. However, it is recognized that recurrences within the operative field and in the contralateral neck are common and exceed 40% if more than one node is histologically positive and no additional adjuvant therapy is given.[39, 173, 174]
- *Adjunctive radiotherapy* to both sides of the neck significantly reduces this failure pattern and should be considered in all patients with more than one positive node.[2, 50]
- If the primary lesion is managed radiotherapeutically, both sides of the neck receive at least 50 Gy in 5 weeks in the case of an N0 neck at significant risk for occult disease. In the case of clinically positive neck nodes, the neck is either treated with a planned radical neck dissection or modified neck dissection 4 to 6 weeks later, or higher doses in the range of 65 to 75 Gy are given to areas of gross tumor in the neck via a

TABLE 20–8. **Incidence of Lymph Node Metastasis by Site of Primary Tumor in Head and Squamous Cell Carcinoma**

Site	% N+ at Presentation	% N0 Clinically/ N+ Pathologically	% N0–>N+ Without Neck Treatment
Floor of mouth	30–59	40–50	20–35
Gingiva	18–52	19	17
Hard palate	13–24	22	—
Buccal mucosa	9–31	—	16
Oral tongue	34–35	25–54	38–52
Nasopharynx	86–90	—	19*–50
Anterior tonsillar	39–56	—	10–15
Pillar/retromolar trigone	37–56	—	16–25
Soft palate/uvula	58–76	—	22+
Tonsillar fossa	50–83	22	—
Base of tongue	50–71	66	—
Pharyngeal walls	31–54	16–26	33
Supraglottic larynx	52–72	38	—

— = no data; *T1,N0 patients only; + patients received preoperative irradiation; N = nodes.

From Mendenhall WM, Million RR, Cassisi NJ: Elective neck irradiation in squamous cell carcinoma of the head and neck. Head Neck Surg 1980; 3:15–20. Reprinted by permission of John Wiley & Sons, Inc.

shrinking field technique.[2, 50] Use of an electron beam or an interstitial implant may be required to safely achieve an adequate dose.

- If the primary lesion is *resected*, usually a neck dissection is also performed, and at least 60 Gy is given for N2 and above.[2, 175] If significant risk factors such as extracapsular extension are present, higher postoperative doses are warranted.[50]
- *Bilateral neck dissections* may be required for bilateral disease, and all such patients should receive adjunctive irradiation in appropriate doses after the risk factors found at the time of surgery are taken into account.[50]
- Cervical nodes that are *inoperable* owing to fixation to base of skull, cervical spine, or prevertebral muscle, or that are attached to the carotid vessels, should receive preoperative irradiation followed by resection if they become mobile.
- *Retropharyngeal nodes* may be at risk for tumors of the pyriform sinus, nasopharynx, and tumors that involve the posterior pharyngeal wall. In such cases 50 to 55 Gy is given with radiation fields extending up to the base of skull.

Elective (Prophylactic) Treatment

Elective treatment of cervical lymphatics is often controversial as a result of the complexity of factors involved in the treatment decision.[2, 167] One must balance the likelihood of microscopic nodal involvement (depending on primary tumor site, T stage, and macroscopic and microscopic pathology) and the possibility of subsequent salvage (determined by, among other things, closeness of follow-up and patient reliability) against the morbidity-mortality of elective treatment. Radiation therapy is highly effective in eradicating subclinical disease from surgically undisturbed neck lymphatics; 50 Gy in 5 weeks produces minimal long-term sequelae.[39, 176] Selective neck dissection is also effective at controlling subclinical disease and is associated with minimal morbidity.[177]

The primary tumor site is highly important in deciding whether a tumor with a given T stage warrants elective treatment of the neck. In a homogeneous population with nasopharyngeal cancers stage I, Lee and colleagues[178] noted a failure rate of 0% versus 30%, depending on the use of elective neck irradiation or its absence in treatment, respectively. Well-differentiated T1 lesions of the oral cavity that have clear surgical margins do not usually receive elective neck treatment, but a supraomohyoid neck dissection is generally used to provide additional staging information.[177] If the primary is to be treated with definitive radiotherapy, then there is little added morbidity in including the first echelon nodes in the radiation field and then reducing the field after giving 50 Gy. The neck nodes are generally not treated in the case of primary T1 and T2 glottic tumors. For all other situations, consideration should be given to elective cervical node treatment.

Surgical Complications

Rehabilitation, surgical reconstruction, and provision of prostheses are essential when wide resections are performed. Immediate postoperative complications include wound infection, fistula formation, sloughing of skin flaps (especially at trifurcation points), exposure and rupture of carotid artery, aspiration when the airway remains connected to the food passage, peptic ulceration and gastritis with hematemesis, and pulmonary embolism.[12] In experienced hands, the incidence of such complications is low. Many surgeons feel that local complications are more common if preoperative irradiation is used, and surgical techniques (especially skin incisions) need modification in such patients.[177] Delayed surgical problems relate mainly to physiologic problems with deglutition, speech, and tracheitis sicca following laryngectomy. Shoulder disability following radical neck dissection and chronic neck pain also occurs.

Radiation Complications

Dryness of the mouth (xerostomia) is common in patients receiving greater than 35 to 45 Gy to major salivary glands[179] and may last for years. The degree of recovery is dose and volume dependent, but it appears that use of pilocarpine (Saligen) is helpful in reducing side effects.[180, 181] Loss of taste correlates with the onset of salivary dysfunction, and the combined effect of xerostomia and loss of taste put patients at risk for significant weight loss unless vigorous dietary consulting is given. In addition, the decrease in saliva and changes in its chemical constituency put patients at risk for increased incidence of dental caries. These risks can be reduced with comprehensive dental care involving oral hygiene, fluoride treatment, and conservative dental management.[182]

Osteoradionecrosis is a major complication, often precipitated by dental extraction following high-dose irradiation (>60 Gy) to the mandible.[183] The incidence of osteoradionecrosis of the mandible can be reduced if anticipated dental extractions are carried out before beginning radiotherapy and 2 to 3 weeks allowed for adequate healing.[182, 183] Osteoradionecrosis of the mandible may heal with conservative medical management, but most often, hyperbaric oxygen treatments are required.[184] Surgery with flap reconstruction may be necessary and must be coordinated with the hyperbaric oxygen treatments for maximum success. Soft tissue necroses will generally heal if the bone is not exposed, but hyperbaric oxygen treatments are believed by many to be of benefit.

Spinal cord tolerance is generally considered to be 50 Gy and most protocols are even more conservative and recommend not exceeding 45 Gy. Marcus and Million have challenged this tolerance dose after reviewing the records of 1112 patients given a variety of doses to their cervical spinal cord.[185] They feel that the risk is essentially zero, even with doses up to 55 Gy if fractional doses are kept to 1.2 to 2.0 Gy daily. The work of Schultheiss[186] supports the conclusion that 50 Gy in 2-Gy fractions is a conservative estimate of spinal cord tolerance. The generally accepted tolerance doses for selected tissues of importance in the treatment of head and neck cancer are given in Table 20–9 for conventionally fractionated radiotherapy.[1] In the case of hyperfractionated or accelerated fractionated radiotherapy, one additional variable enters. The interval between fractions must be sufficiently long to allow for repair of most damage to normal tissues. An RTOG study by Cox

TABLE 20–9. **Tolerance Doses for Fractionated Radiotherapy for Selected Key Tissues of Importance in the Treatment of Head and Neck Cancer**

Organ System	Complication	TD5/5–TD50/5 (Gy)*
Lens	Cataract	6–12
Salivary gland	Xerostomia	45–150
Thyroid gland	Hypothyroidism	30–45
Cornea	Keratitis	50–60
Middle ear	Serous otitis	50–70
Spinal cord (10 cm)	Myelopathy	50–60
Retina	Retinitis	55–70
Vestibular apparatus	Menière's syndrome	60–70
Mucosa	Ulceration	65–75
Mature bone	Fracture	65–75
Brain (25%)	Encephalopathy	70–80

*The listed radiation doses should be taken only as approximate.

From Laramore GE: General principles of radiation therapy for head and neck cancer. In: Myers EN, Suen JY (eds): Cancer of the Head and Neck, 3rd ed, pp 768–781. Philadelphia, W.B. Saunders Co., 1996, with permission.

and associates[80] demonstrated that interfraction intervals greater than 4.5 hours versus less than 4.5 hours heighten both acute and late effects. Estimates of late toxicity at 1-, 2-, and 3-year intervals were 5.5%, 9.8%, and 15.4%, respectively, with intervals greater than 4.5 hours versus 7.7% at all time periods less than 4.5 hours. For more discussion, see Chapter 34, Late Effects of Cancer Treatment.

Patterns of Failure

Second Malignant Tumors

The development of second malignant tumors (SMTs) in head and neck cancer patients, for whom surgery and irradiation have controlled successfully the locoregional disease, has emerged as a major clinical concern. Second malignant tumors have been reported in as many as 33% of patients with oral cavity, 37% with oropharyngeal, and 21% with laryngeal cancers.[31, 187, 188] An RTOG database analysis of 928 head and neck cancer patients illustrated the risks of developing SMTs: 10% at 3 years, 15% at 5 years, and 28% at 8 years after treatment.[23] This risk appeared to be mainly associated with excessive use of tobacco and alcohol by this patient population. Hence, it is not surprising that the most prevalent sites for SMTs are the upper aerodigestive tract and lung and reflect the diffuse effects of these carcinogens on wide areas of the mucosa. The incidence of SMTs in patients with nasopharyngeal carcinoma, a tumor not associated with tobacco and alcohol, is only about 5% at 5 years—much lower than for other head and neck sites.[189]

Of note is that the incidence of second malignancies does not appear to be influenced by whether the patient received radiation therapy as part of the treatment for the primary tumor. Parker and Enstrom reviewed the records of 2853 patients and found that within the treatment fields that were at increased risk owing to radiation, the incidence of second tumors was 2.2% for patients treated with surgery alone and 2.9% for patients treated with either radiotherapy alone or with surgery and adjuvant radiotherapy.[190]

Patients with early-stage disease have the highest risk of developing SMTs and, because the prognosis for SMTs is poor, endeavors aimed at prevention should be a priority. Pharmacologic intervention (chemoprevention) as an adjunct to smoking cessation programs is under investigation, using vitamin A and its analogues, including the retinoids and carotenoids.[191] In a randomized study of 100 treated head and neck cancer patients, 13-cis-retinoic acid (50 to 100 mg/m^2/d) decreased SMT incidence to 4% versus 24% in the controls at median follow-up of 29 months.[192] There was no impact on overall failure (primary, nodes, and distant metastases), which was slightly over 30% in each arm.

Types of Local-Nodal Recurrence

More than 75% of head and neck cancer patients for whom treatment is ineffective will have a component of failure above the clavicles, either in the primary region, neck nodes, or in both. Some primary sites remain notoriously difficult to control despite aggressive approaches: These include the base of the tongue, pharyngeal walls (lateral and posterior), and the postcricoid regions. Regardless of site, T3 or T4 lesions have a high propensity to recur locally even following multimodal approaches. Recurrence at the primary site re-establishes the potential for cervical lymphatic failure (reseeding) regardless of whether the neck was initially controlled. The single most common failure pattern is the recurrent primary with a neck metastasis.[159, 166]

Metastatic Relapse

It is becoming increasingly apparent that aggressive, locoregional therapy improves disease control above the clavicles, but may have little effect on survival. As extensive T3, T4, N2, and N3 tumors are controlled, the longer survival unmasks an unexpectedly high incidence of hematogenous metastases, most commonly to lung, but also to bone and elsewhere. Patients with large primary lesions and bilateral cervical nodes have an incidence of distant disease as high as 40% to 70% if they survive long enough from their locoregional disease.[173, 193] Adjuvant chemotherapy seems to reduce the probability of distant metastases occurring as a first site of failure.[45, 47, 170]

Intercurrent Disease

Intercurrent disease is also an important factor in ultimate outcome. A high self-destructive element is found in these patients as a group. Most are unable to modify their lifestyle and continue heavy drinking and smoking. Alcohol-related deaths, chronic lung disease, accidents, suicide, and other illnesses account for 10% to 30% of deaths, depending on the reported series.

Results and Prognosis

General Considerations

Five-Year Survival Rates

A comprehensive listing of all head and neck sites offering 5-year determinate survival rates by each stage, based on

TABLE 20–10. **Approximate Determinate* 5-Year Survival in Head and Neck Cancer**

Anatomic Site of Primary Tumor	Overall 5-Year Survival (%)	5-Year Survival According to Stage Grouping (%)			
		I	*II*	*III*	*IV*
Oral cavity					
Mobile tongue	45	80	60	30	15
Floor of mouth	50	80	70	60	30
Buccal mucosa	45	75	65	30	15
Retromolar trigone	60	75	70	60	30
Lower gingiva	65	75	60	50	30
Lip	85	90	85	70	60
Oropharynx					
Tonsil	45	90	60	40	15
Base of tongue	30	60	40	20	10
Pharyngeal wall	20	50	30	20	10
Soft palate	50	85	60	30	15
Nasopharynx	45	60	40	30	15
Larynx					
Glottic	85	95	85	60	35
Supraglottic	55	65	65	55	40
Hypopharynx					
Pyriform sinus	25	30	20	15	5
Postericoid	20	ID	ID	ID	ID
Maxillary sinus	25	35	—	15	—

Excludes patients dead of intercurrent disease; ID = insufficient data.

a review of the literature, can be found in Table 20–10. These rates are independent of modality and are an overview using conventional methods of treatment. A 5-year follow-up is adequate for most sites because recurrences usually occur within the first 2 years and rarely after 4 years. Generally, for most sites, 5-year survival for stage I is 75% to 90%; for stage II, survival is 40% to 70%; for stage III, survival is 20% to 50%; and for stage IV, 10% to 30%.

The Radiation Therapy Oncology Group Experience

The RTOG has a large series of head and neck protocols and registry. Analysis of 1000 cases has allowed the generation of response rate and survival data. For early T stages (T1, T2) and N0 and N1 nodal disease, the CR rate is 80% to 95%, whereas advanced T3 and T4 stages and N2 and N3 nodes have only a 30% to 50% CR rate. Specific details are summarized in Table 20–11.[194]

Surveillance, Epidemiology, and End Result Group Data[17]

For all stages, the 5-year survival rate for oral cavity and pharynx is 55% in whites and 34% in blacks. The majority of 5-year survivors will be alive at 10 years. Of those patients in whom therapy fails, approximately 90% will do so within the first 2 years following treatment. In whites, the 5-year survival rate improved from 43% in the period 1960 to 1963 to 55% in the period 1974 to 1976. However, there has been little change from then until the most recent surveillance period of 1986 to 1993. The adjusted years of life lost decreased from 23.1 in 1970 to 19.9 in 1985.

The Effects of Locoregional Control on Distant Metastatic Dissemination in Carcinoma of the Head and Neck

Leibel and colleagues[195] provide compelling evidence that improved locoregional control decreases dissemination and metastases and translates into better overall survival. Using the large RTOG database in head and neck cancers, they reported the incidence of distant metastases as 24% for patients with no evidence of locoregional disease versus 36% for patients with persistence of cancer at 5 years; the corresponding 5-year survival was 47% compared with 16%. When analyzed by subgroups, this observation applied to early-stage T1–T3,N0 tumors but not the more advanced T3–4,N2–3 lesions, except for hypopharyngeal and nasopharyngeal sites. The probable explanation for this finding is that when cancers are very advanced locally with a high degree of nodal involvement, they are, in all probability, metastatic at the time of presentation. The authors postulated that failure to control earlier primary tumor leads to increased rates of metastatic dissemination because recurrent tumors develop more clonogens that are both phenotypically and genotypically distinct and capable of metastasizing. Based on these biologic considerations, they hypothesized that improved locoregional control at several anatomic sites is likely to decrease the ultimate rate of metastatic disease.

Comorbidity Factors

Comorbidity factors such as diabetes, congestive heart failure, chronic lung disease, and the like adversely impact survival on a stage-for-stage basis.[14]

TABLE 20–11. **Results from Radiation Therapy Oncology Group (RTOG) Registry**

Stage	T,N (AJCC)	Total Evaluation	% CR	% Dead	Estimated Survival Rates		
					1-Yr	*2-Yr*	*3-Yr*
II	T2, N0	249	95	40	83	71	62
III	T1, N1	10	90				
		>48		46	87	63	55
III	T2, N1	38	87				
III	T3, N0	80	79	59	73	48	37
III	T3, N1	38	61	76	45	31	19
IV	T1, N2	9	78				
			>70	60	65	35	31
IV	T2, N2	34	68				
IV	T1, N3	70	57				
			>57	57	54	37	37
IV	T2, N3	23	57				
IV	T3, N2	30	70	83	53	20	11
					55	20	17
IV	T3, N3	33	49	82			
IV	T4, N0	36	75	64	71	48	26
IV	T4, N1	14	64	64	54	27	22
IV	T4, N2	22	41	77	41	13	2
IV	T4, N3	45	31	76	31	22	11

AJCC = American Joint Committee on Cancer; T = tumor; N = node; CR = complete response.
From Marcial VA, Pajak TF, Kramer S, et al: Radiation Therapy Oncology Group (RTOG) studies in head and neck cancer. Semin Oncol 1988; 15:39–60, with permission.

Prognostic Factors

Important prognostic factors are:

- anatomic site of primary tumor
- T stage
- cervical node status
- associated diseases (comorbidity)

Clinical Investigations

The need for predictive assays for tumor radiocurability has been the subject of research since the 1960s, when it was very actively pursued in cervical cancer patients. Interest in this subject has been reawakened by new concepts and techniques developed in the past decade by radiobiologists (see Chapter 5, Basic Principles of Radiobiology). For example, based on the concepts that tumor cells are the target of therapy and that the *in vitro* sensitivity of stem cells reflects their *in vivo* sensitivity, Brock and coworkers[196] developed a special multicellular chamber using a cell-adhesive technique. A survival curve parameter was calculated at 2 Gy (S_2), and when this technique was applied to SCC patients who had been followed for more than 1 year, Peters and associates[196a] showed the recurrence rate to be slightly higher for those patients having an S_2 value greater than 0.4, compared with those with a value less than 0.3. Although this technique has not proved as robust as was desired, nonetheless this was a major clinical-radiobiologic effort, and similar enterprises need to be encouraged because predictive assays are essential in determining the potential biologic basis of combined treatment modalities.

Adjuvant aggressive multiagent chemotherapy is being studied. Past investigations have evaluated the use of sequential chemotherapy as an adjuvant to surgery and radiotherapy, although results to date are significant only in the areas of laryngeal preservation for locally advanced tumors of the hypopharynx and larynx,[45, 47] with no improvement in survival. The simultaneous use of chemotherapy and radiotherapy seems to have the potential of improving locoregional control, and, in addition, a survival advantage has been noted for tumors of the nasopharynx.[48, 49] Although work is continuing on regimens involving cisplatin and its analogues, newer agents such as paclitaxel and its derivatives are the subjects of many current protocols.

Potential improvements in radiation therapy include the use of proton beams, which can be used to deliver higher doses of radiation than can be given with megavoltage photons.[16] High linear energy transfer neutron radiation has been the subject of active investigation for many years, but its only accepted advantage is in the treatment of salivary gland tumors for which there is a much higher relative biologic difference than for the more common SCC.[197, 198] Heavy ion radiotherapy combines the dose distribution advantages of proton beams with the potential biologic advantages of neutron radiation, but trials with this modality are still in the early phases. Conformal three-dimensional treatment planning and delivery is a way of improving the dose distributions that can be achieved with conventional forms of radiotherapy.[66]

Hyperfractionation and accelerated fractionation, with multiple daily doses of radiation, are being studied and the results of several studies appear promising.[67, 69, 72–75, 77, 78, 80a] Most of the randomized clinical trials being performed use twice-daily treatment regimens of 1.1- to 1.2-Gy per fraction. A meta-analysis argues for improved locoregional control and also gives some indication of a survival benefit.[79] The most extreme form of this treatment studied to date is CHART, which involves giving radiotherapy three times a day (8 A.M., 4 P.M., 8 P.M.) on 12 consecutive days at 1.4- to 1.5-Gy fractions to a total dose of 50.4 to

54 Gy.[76] Although a comparative analysis using historical controls showed improved locoregional control for patients with T3 and T4 tumors, there were also two incidents of cervical myelitis, arguing that aggressive treatment regimens need to be thoroughly investigated in a protocol setting before moving into general community use. Unlike epithelial mucosal tissue, spinal cord repair following acute radiation requires 24 hours, not 6 hours, to be completed.

Hyperthermia refers to raising the temperature of tumors in a controlled manner along with the delivery of radiotherapy. Although there are sound biologic reasons why this combination should give a synergistic effect in tumor control,[199] technical difficulties in delivering the heat to deep-seated tumors have prevented it from having a significant clinical impact to date. Even in the setting of interstitial implants, where the heating should be better controlled, no benefit has been found.[200]

Hypoxic cell sensitizers are agents that are preferentially retained in hypoxic cells and act similarly to oxygen in scavenging free electrons, increasing free radical lifetime and stabilizing radiation damage. Misonidazole is the agent that has been most studied to date. Unfortunately, studies in both Europe[201, 202] and the United States[203] have shown no benefit. Because the administration of this agent is limited by neurotoxicity, interest has shifted to other agents such as etanidazole[204] and nimorazole.[205] Nimorazole has a much lower toxicity profile and in a recently completed DAHANCA study showed a 20% therapeutic gain in local control and survival in supraglottic larynx and pharynx cancer,[205] resulting in this agent being adopted in Denmark as standard therapy for head and neck cancers. However, work with PET imaging using [^{18}F]-fluoromisonidazole, a compound that is selectively retained in hypoxic cells, shows that non–small cell lung tumors reoxygenate well during a course of conventionally fractionated radiotherapy, casting some doubt on the clinical importance of the elusive hypoxic cell.[206, 207]

Radioprotective agents, on the other hand, in theory act to protect normal tissues, thus allowing higher doses of radiation to be given to the tumor. The agent that has been most studied to date is a thiophosphate derivative of cysteine known as amifostine (Ethyol, formerly WR-2721).[208, 209] Metabolites of this agent probably act by scavenging free radicals before they can damage the cellular DNA. Because this agent selectively concentrates in the salivary glands, it may be beneficial in preventing xerostomia. There does not appear to be any adverse effect in terms of tumor radioprotection, and ongoing trials are taking place for SCCs.

Specific Head and Neck Sites

The major sites of the subdivisions of head and neck are illustrated in Figure 20–4; tumors arising in these sites are discussed in the remainder of this chapter, along with tumors of the paranasal sinuses, unknown primary sites that present with metastatic neck nodes, chemodectomas, and salivary gland tumors. Anatomic landmarks are approximately indicated by the horizontal and vertical lines.

Certain aspects of evaluation of head and neck tumors are common to all sites. Recommended staging procedures were summarized earlier in this chapter. In determining the information that needs to be obtained on a given patient, it is helpful to think in terms of the TNM staging parameters that need to be ascertained.

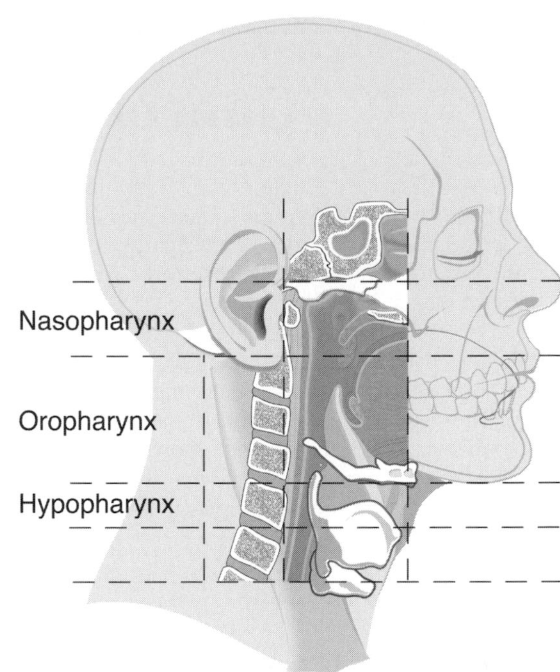

Figure 20–4. Subdivisions of the pharynx. The oral cavity (not shown) lies anterior to the oropharynx and is bounded by the vermilion border of the lips. The lines indicated on this figure can be determined with respect to the following palpable structures: zygomatic arch, external auditory canal, mastoid process, hyoid bone, thyroid cartilage, and cricoid cartilage.

T Work-Up

Careful inspection, palpation, and measurement are the first steps. A CT scan provides important information with regard to tumor extension into deep tissues, bone erosion, or both. Assessment of the mandible by CT scan or orthopantograms, or by both, for invasion is necessary if the lesions approach the mandible. An MRI scan is often helpful in determining changes within soft tissues.

N Work-Up

Bimanual palpation of submental and submandibular regions is necessary. Both sides of the neck should be checked down to the clavicles. The number, size, location, and mobility of enlarged nodes should be noted. CT scanning or MRI is recommended.

M Work-Up

Chest films, complete blood cell count, and a cancer panel that includes liver function tests are routine. Specific symptoms need appropriate work-up (e.g., chest CT, brain CT, bone scan, liver scan).

Cancer of the Oral Cavity

The oral cavity extends from the skin-vermilion junction of the lip to the posterior border of the hard palate superiorly and the circumvallate papillae inferiorly. Subdivisions within the oral cavity include the anterior two thirds of the tongue (anterior to the circumvallate papillae), lip, buccal mucosa, lower alveolar ridge, upper alveolar ridge, retromolar trigone, floor of mouth, and hard palate. Early diagnosis carries good prognosis and it is essential that the general practitioner and the dentist thoroughly examine patients they see in normal follow-up. The areas least commonly examined are the paralingual gutters.

Epidemiology and Etiology

Epidemiology

Oral carcinoma is among the most common of the aerodigestive cancers. The lip is the most common site, followed by the tongue.[17] Cancer of the oral cavity is predominantly a disease of men (80%) and occurs at a median age of 55 to 65 years.

Etiology

- *Cigarette smoking, pipe smoking, tobacco chewing,* and *heavy alcohol intake* are etiologic factors. Daily cigar smokers who do not inhale have approximately a sevenfold increase in oral cavity cancers compared with nonsmokers.[22] It has been estimated that the combination of tobacco and alcohol usage accounts for 75% of all oral and pharyngeal cancers in the United States.[20]
- *Poor oral hygiene* and *chronic trauma* from broken teeth or poorly fitting dentures are common cofactors.
- *Plummer-Vinson syndrome* (iron deficiency anemia, glossitis, achlorhydria, koilonychia) is associated with tongue cancer in females.
- S*unlight* is an important cause of lip cancer.
- *Cultural habits* such as betel nut chewing or reversed smoking in India are strongly associated with oral cancer.

Detection and Diagnosis

Clinical Detection

- Premalignant changes rarely produce symptoms, and diagnosis rests with the physician's or dentist's awareness and examination. Leukoplakia (white patch) occurs mostly on the lower lip, floor of mouth, buccal mucosa, lateral tongue border, and retromolar region. Although more common than erythroplasia, leukoplakia is much less frequently malignant (<2%). Erythroplasia (red patch) tends to occur in the floor of mouth, lateral tongue border, and soft palate. The majority of erythroplasias are invasive carcinoma, carcinoma *in situ*, or severe epithelial dysplasia, and must always be regarded seriously.
- Carcinoma usually presents as a chronic, nonhealing ulcer.
- Pain is paradoxically rare in early lesions. Localized pain is a late symptom indicating deep invasion, perineural involvement, or bone involvement.
- Cervical node presentations are uncommon for early T stages and, when present, the submandibular or jugulodigastric nodes are typically involved.

Diagnostic Procedures

- *Inspection* and *palpation* are important first steps. The malignant ulcer is typically raised, centrally ulcerated, and has indurated edges and an infiltrated base.
- *Biopsy* is mandatory. If the biopsy result is negative, the biopsy should be repeated if clinical index of suspicion is high.
- *Imaging modality*: Both CT and MRI are useful for staging of advanced carcinomas.

Classification and Staging

Histopathology

- *Squamous cell carcinomas (SCCs)* account for 90% to 95% of cancers of the oral cavity and are usually well or moderately well differentiated.[7] Unusual variants of SCC include verrucous carcinoma and spindle cell SCC. Spindle cell SCC is usually a recurrence following unsuccessful radiotherapy. *Adenocarcinomas* of minor salivary gland origin may be encountered. The treatment of these tumors is discussed in the section on salivary gland tumors at the end of this chapter.

Staging

The staging system for carcinomas of the oral cavity is summarized in Table 20–12 and Figure 20–5.

Patterns of Spread

Patterns of Local Spread

- *Tongue* lesions usually arise along the lateral border and infiltrate into the tongue muscle. Extension into the deep tongue musculature and base of tongue carries a worse prognosis. Involvement may extend into floor of mouth, leading in advanced cases to total fixation of the tongue.
- *Floor-of-mouth* cancers typically arise in the anterior region and can spread along the mandibular perios-

TABLE 20–12. **TNM Classification and Stage Grouping for Lip, Oral Cavity, and Oropharynx**

Stage	Grouping	TNM Classification
Stage 0	Tis, N0, M0	Tis: Carcinoma *in situ* N0: No regional lymph node metastasis M0: No distant metastasis
Stage I	T1, N0, M0	T1: Tumor ≤2 cm
Stage II	T2, N0, M0	T2: Tumor >2 cm but ≤4 cm
Stage III	T3, N0, M0 T1, N1, M0 T2, N1, M0 T3, N1, M0	T3: Tumor >4 cm N1: Metastasis in a singular ipsilateral lymph node, <3 cm
Stage IVA	T4, N0,1, M0 Any T, N2, M0	T4: Tumor invaded adjacent structures N2: Metastasis in a single ipsilateral lymph node, >3 cm but ≤6 cm; or, in multiple ipsilateral lymph nodes, none >6 cm; or in bilateral or contralateral lymph nodes, none >6 cm*
Stage IVB	Any T, N3, M0	N3: Metastasis in a lymph node >6 cm
Stage IVC	Any T, any N, M1	M1: Distant metastasis

T = tumor; N = node; M = metastasis.

*N2a: metastasis in single ipsilateral lymph node >3 cm, but not >6 cm; N2b: metastasis in multiple ipsilateral lymph nodes, none >6 cm; N2c: metastasis in bilateral or contralateral lymph nodes, none >6 cm.

Used with permission of the American Joint Committee on Cancer (AJCC®), Chicago, Illinois. The original source for this material is the AJCC® Cancer Staging Manual, 5th ed, 1997, published by Lippincott-Raven Publishers, Philadelphia, Pennsylvania; and International Union Against Cancer (UICC): TNM Classification of Malignant Tumors, 4th ed, New York, Springer-Verlag, 1992.

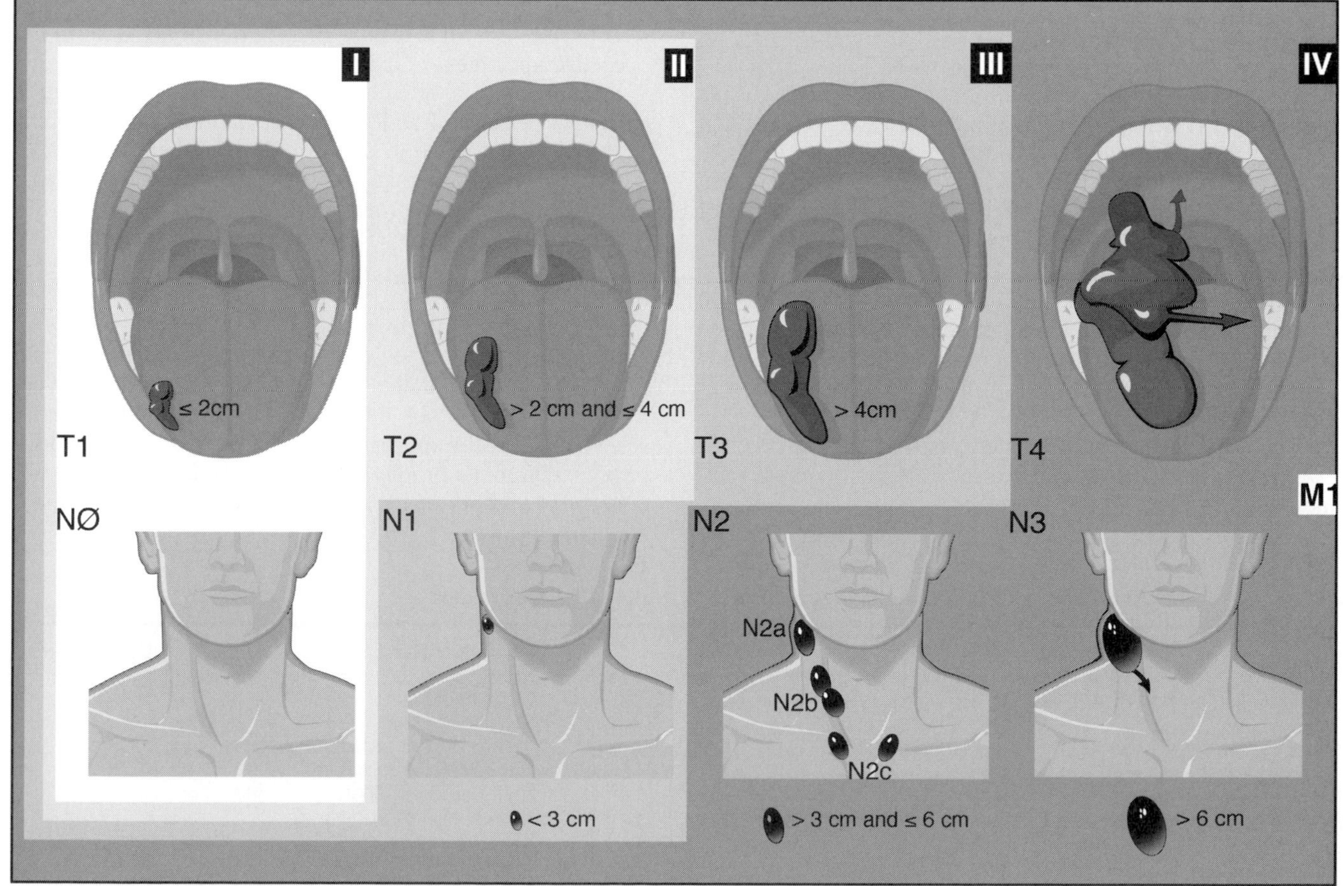

Figure 20–5. Anatomic staging system for tumors of the oral cavity. The primary tumor staging is characterized first by size and then by extension into other sites. For T1, T2, and T3 lesions the cutoff diameters are 2 cm or smaller, larger than 2 cm but 4 cm or smaller, and larger than 4 cm, respectively. Massive tumors extending into contiguous sites or invading the adjacent soft tissues are characterized as T4. The nodal staging is shown in the lower row.

teum without bone invasion, often for significant distances. Actual bone invasion is a serious event.

- *Buccal mucosa* lesions often arise at the occlusal level and typically spread superficially. Deep invasion posteriorly leads to pterygoid muscle involvement and trismus. Verrucous carcinoma—a well-differentiated squamous lesion presenting as a warty mucosal growth—is more common in this region.
- *Alveolar ridge* carcinomas commonly arise from gingival mucosa in the premolar or molar regions, more commonly in the lower jaw. Bone invasion is a relatively early finding.
- *Hard palate* carcinomas are rare and adenocarcinoma is more common than SCC in this area. Spread is along periosteum, and bone invasion may occur.
- Carcinomas of the *lip* usually arise on the lower lip and infiltrate orbicularis oris muscle early. They frequently follow an indolent course with slow progression.

Staging Work-Up

Staging procedures common to all head and neck sites have been discussed earlier in this chapter. Imaging studies of the mandible are particularly important when the lesion appears to be fixed to it.

Metastatic Behavior

With the exception of glottic carcinoma, oral cancers have the lowest incidence of cervical metastases of all head and neck sites. Lip carcinoma produces nodal disease in fewer than 15% of patients and is virtually the only head and neck site to involve submental nodes. The incidence of pathologically positive nodes in patients with tongue tumors who are clinically N0 is in the range of 34%.[210] The remainder of oral cavity carcinomas have nodal disease at diagnosis in 35% to 45% of patients. Submandibular and jugulodigastric are the most commonly affected nodes.[12, 211]

Hematogenous metastases from oral carcinoma occur with a frequency of 15% to 20%, mostly from poorly differentiated, locally advanced lesions having cervical node involvement at presentation.[173] Lung is the most common site.

Principles of Treatment

Principles of treatment for carcinoma of the oral cavity are summarized in Table 20–13. A more detailed discussion follows.

Primary Tumor

Premalignant lesions are best excised and attention directed to removal of inciting factors (smoking, alcohol, poor teeth, denture trauma). A small primary lesion is best managed by either surgery or radiation therapy alone, with the other modality being reserved for salvage. Large lesions (T3 and T4) usually require both modalities, and surgery may have to be radical, especially if mandibular periosteum or bone is involved.

Neck Nodes

Overt nodal disease can be treated surgically with a radical, modified radical, or selective neck dissection. Adjunctive irradiation to the neck is usually indicated if nodes are positive, especially if more than one node is involved, if disease is extranodal, or if a modified dissection was performed. Under these conditions, both sides of the neck should be irradiated, with 60 Gy to the dissected side and 50 Gy to the undisturbed side.[167, 172] If there are high-risk factors such as extracapsular nodal extension found on the operative specimen, at least 63 Gy should be given.[50]

Radiotherapy is often preferred to surgery for elective treatment because of better cosmetic and functional results. If treatment is limited to the primary site, then a review of the literature shows that the subsequent development of disease in the untreated neck is in the range of 5% to 15% for lip cancers, 20% to 50% for tongue cancers, 23% to 30% for floor-of-mouth cancers, 9% to 37% for buccal mucosal tumors, 14% to 19% for gingival tumors, and 15% to 25% for hard palate tumors.[211] These figures cover a wide range of T stages, and many series did not correct for tumor control at the primary site and therefore may include cases in which the neck disease was subsequently seeded by a recurrent primary. Although we do not ordinarily recommend prophylactic neck irradiation for lip cancers or T1 tumors of the buccal mucosa, gingiva, or hard

TABLE 20–13. **Carcinoma of the Oral Cavity/Oropharynx: Principles of Treatment**

Stage	Grouping	Surgery		Radiation Therapy	Chemotherapy
I	T1, N0, M0	Resection	or	DRT: 65–70 Gy	NR
II	T2, N0, M0	Resection	or	DRT: 65–72 Gy	NR
III	T3, N0, M0	Resection	and	ART: preop vs. postop 50–60 Gy	IC III
				HyperFx RT (oropharynx)	CCR
			or	ART: preop vs. postop	
	Any T, N1, M0	Radical resection	and	HyperFx RT (oropharynx)	
			or	DRT: 70–75 Gy	
IV	T4, N2,3, M0	Unresectable		Surgery for RT relapse	IC II
Local relapse		RT for surgery relapse		NR	IC II; CCR
Metastatic		NR			IC II

RT = radiation therapy; DRT = definitive; ART = adjuvant; HyperFx = hyperfractionated; NR = not recommended; IC II = investigational chemotherapy, phase I/II clinical trials; IC III = investigational chemotherapy, phase II/III clinical trials; CCR = concurrent chemotherapy and radiation.

Physicians Data Query: NR except for IC I, II, III, and CCR.

palate, we do in other cases, unless a surgical neck exploration has demonstrated the absence of tumor and that unexplored areas are at low risk in the particular clinical setting in question.

Surgery

Premalignant and small invasive lesions (<1 cm) are generally easiest to treat by local excision. Larger T1 and T2 lesions are also effectively managed by surgery, but resection must be adequate and may include hemiglossectomy for tongue carcinoma or resection of floor of mouth and marginal mandibular resection for a floor-of-mouth carcinoma. Inadequate margins require re-excision or radiotherapy; one should not merely wait for the recurrence before offering this additional treatment. Large primary lesions (T3 and T4) treated surgically require radical procedures that can include hemiglossectomy, hemimandibulectomy, and neck dissection. Frozen section margin checks are important in head and neck surgery, in which margins greater than 2 cm are not always possible. Involved neck nodes are best managed by neck dissection followed by postoperative radiation therapy as described earlier. Fixed nodes should receive preoperative irradiation (50 Gy to both sides of the neck and 60 Gy to the node) in an attempt to mobilize the node and to eradicate extracapsular spread.

Reconstruction of smaller soft tissue defects may be handled by split-thickness skin grafts or local flaps (e.g., tongue).[212] Larger soft tissue defects require pedicled flaps (e.g., pectoralis major[55] or microvascular free flaps). The floor of mouth and tongue can be reconstructed with excellent resultant tongue mobility using a radial forearm microvascular free flap.[58] This flap is especially thin and supple. If mandibular bone must be replaced, then bone and soft tissue can be obtained with scapular, iliac crest, and fibular microvascular free flaps.[59–61]

Radiation Therapy

Radiotherapy is highly effective as a sole modality for T1 and T2 lesions of the oral cavity. For lesions in the anterior oral cavity (oral tongue, floor of mouth, buccal mucosa, lip), radioactive implantation is an integral part of irradiation. Although there have been no randomized clinical trials that directly evaluate the addition of this modality, the general feeling is that brachytherapy improves tumor control when added to standard external beam therapy.[213, 214] A common approach is to combine external irradiation (45–50 Gy to primary and neck) with interstitial implantation (20–30 Gy to primary alone). Permanent eradication of the primary lesions occurs in 80% to 85% of T1 and T2 lesions, with many of the local failures being amenable to surgical salvage.

Combined Modalities

Both surgery and irradiation are commonly required under three circumstances:

1. a large primary (managed surgically) with clinically negative nodes (managed radiotherapeutically)
2. a small primary (managed radiotherapeutically) with positive neck nodes (managed surgically)
3. massive disease in which both modalities are directed to the same region (primary, neck, or both).

In the first circumstance, the treatment sequence is generally surgery followed by radiotherapy; in the second, the sequence is generally radiotherapy followed by surgery; and in the third, the sequence is variable and usually dictated by the nature of the surgery. Many surgeons prefer that radiotherapy does not precede radical surgery because of fears of poor healing and difficult dissections. When both modalities are directed to massive disease, at least one treatment must be radical to maximize the probability of cure.

As a rule, preoperative radiation (up to 30 Gy) does not delay surgery, but doses of 45 to 50 Gy will lead to a 4- to 6-week delay to allow for the radiation reaction to subside. Postoperative radiation will be started when wound healing is usually complete at 1 to 3 weeks after surgery. Immediate combination of surgery and radiation is not advised unless different fields are being treated, such as primary tumor versus neck nodes.

Results and Prognosis

Overall survival for oral cavity carcinoma, except lip, is between 40% and 65%, depending on site and stage. Early primary lesions fare well, but advanced local disease has a poor outlook. For specific details as a function of site and stage, the reader is referred to Table 20–10 and Ingersoll and Goffinet[211] and the literature cited therein. Cervical node status is a significant survival determinant for all sites.

All treatment modalities can produce disability. Surgery may interfere with speech, mastication, and deglutition, and radiotherapy can produce severe xerostomia, dental caries, and mandibular necrosis.

Cancer of the Oropharynx

This anatomic region includes the anterior tonsillar pillar, soft palate, uvula, tonsillar fossa and tonsil, base of tongue (posterior to circumvallate papillae), and pharyngeal walls (lateral and posterior). Tumors in this region, as well as their treatment, can have profound effects on all of the basic aerodigestive functions: mastication, deglutition, respiration, and phonation.

Epidemiology and Etiology

Epidemiology

Tonsil is the most common primary site.[215] Approximately 95% of tonsillar tumors are SCCs, with the majority of the others being lymphomas. Males are affected more often than females in a ratio of 4:1 (although this ratio is declining) and median age is in the range of 55 to 65 years.

Etiology

Smoking and heavy alcohol consumption are especially prevalent in this patient population. Patients with tumors of the oropharynx who survive their first cancer have the highest associated incidence of second primary tumors of the upper aerodigestive tract.

Detection and Diagnosis

Clinical Detection

- Persistent sore throat or pain on swallowing are the most common symptoms. Referred otalgia is also common.
- Enlargement of cervical nodes is a presenting complaint in 20% to 30%.[215]
- Fetor oris, dyspnea, dysphagia, hoarseness, dysarthria, and hypersalivation can be indicators of advanced disease.

Diagnostic Procedures

- *Inspection*, including an indirect mirror examination, is essential.
- *Palpation* should never be omitted. Carcinoma of the base of the tongue may not be apparent visually, but can be obvious on palpation.
- *Biopsy* is essential.
- *Imaging*: CT and MRI may be useful in detecting occult primaries and defining anatomic extensions three-dimensionally. However, base-of-tongue lesions can be difficult to define on CT scan, which cannot easily distinguish between lingual tonsil and cancers.

Classification and Staging

Histopathology

- Overall, approximately 90% of carcinomas are SCCs.[7] Well-differentiated lesions are less common in this site compared with the oral cavity.
- Lymphoepithelioma may occur in tonsil and base of tongue and is a variant of SCC.[7]
- The soft palate may be the site of Queyrat's erythroplasia, a velvety red patch of *in situ* or microinvasive SCC.
- Minor salivary gland carcinomas (usually adenoid cystic or mucoepidermoid) may be encountered, particularly in the base of tongue or soft palate. The treatment of these tumors is discussed in the section on salivary gland tumors at the end of this chapter.
- Lymphoma of Waldeyer's ring is discussed in Chapter 18, Hodgkin's Disease and the Lymphomas.

Staging

The staging system for carcinomas of the oropharynx is summarized in Table 20–12 and Figure 20–6.

Staging Work-Up

Staging procedures common to all head and neck sites have been discussed earlier in this chapter. MRI scans are particularly useful in determining tumor extent for this site.

Patterns of Spread

Local Spread Patterns

- *Carcinoma of the tonsil* commonly extends downward across the glossotonsillar sulcus into the base of the tongue. Such extension should always be ruled out because it carries a relatively poor prognosis, especially if the tongue base is significantly infiltrated. Extension by tonsillar primaries superiorly into soft palate is also common, although less ominous. Trismus indicates deep infiltration into pterygoid muscles.
- *Carcinoma of the base of the tongue* tends to infiltrate anteriorly into the deep tongue muscle. Advanced lesions spread into the anterior two thirds of the tongue and floor of mouth, producing total fixation of the tongue. Downward extension is via the valleculae, epiglottis, and lateral glossoepiglottic ligaments into supraglottic larynx and pyriform sinus.
- *Soft palate carcinomas* tend to infiltrate widely within the soft palate, often involving the uvula and spreading contralaterally. Posterolateral extension into the pterygoid muscles produces trismus.
- *Pharyngeal wall carcinomas* spread longitudinally into nasopharynx and hypopharynx. Anterior extension leads to involvement of tonsillar fossa, base of tongue,

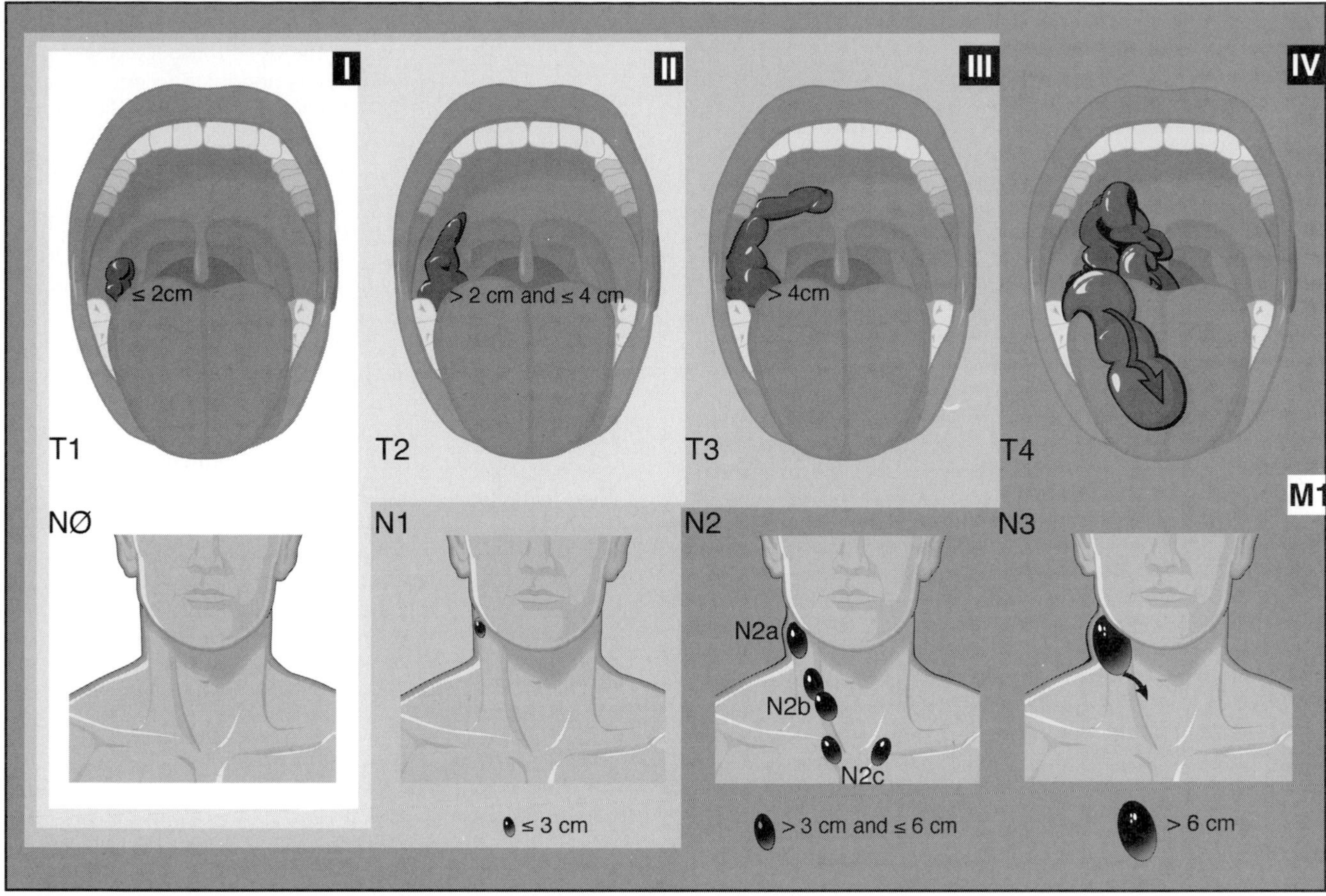

Figure 20–6. Anatomic staging system for tumors of the oropharynx. The primary tumor staging is characterized first by size and then by extension into other sites. For T1, T2, and T3 lesions, the cutoff diameters are 2 cm or smaller, larger than 2 cm but 4 cm or smaller, and larger than 4 cm, respectively. Massive tumors extending into contiguous sites or invading the adjacent soft tissues, or both, are characterized as T4. The nodal staging is shown in the lower row.

pyriform sinus, aryepiglottic folds, and paraglottic larynx. Posterior extension is typically limited by the prevertebral fascia. These lesions may spread laterally and directly into the neck and can involve the carotid sheath.

Metastatic Behavior

Oropharyngeal carcinoma has a high propensity for cervical nodal involvement. Base of tongue tumors may have palpable nodes at the time of diagnosis in the range of 60% to 80%[215] and even if the neck is clinically negative, the incidence of occult metastatic disease has been reported as being approximately 20%.[216] The incidence of bilateral neck disease at the time of presentation may approach 40%. Tonsillar lesions have palpable metastatic nodes at diagnosis in 60% to 70% of cases,[215] whereas pharyngeal wall lesions have involved nodes in 50% to 60%,[215] and soft palate carcinoma has metastasized in 40% to 50%[215]; the most commonly involved nodes are jugulodigastric (Level II). Bilateral nodal disease is relatively frequent and retropharyngeal node involvement is common and should be investigated using CT or MRI scans.

Hematogenous metastases have been documented in tonsillar and base-of-tongue primaries in 10% to 20% of cases.[217] Lung is the most common site. Pharyngeal wall carcinoma metastasizes less often, and soft palate lesions rarely produce hematogenous dissemination. Most hematogenous metastases from oropharyngeal carcinoma occur in patients with massive primary disease, massive or bilateral cervical node deposits, or both.

Principles of Treatment

Principles of treatment for carcinoma of the oropharynx are summarized in Table 20–13. Anatomic and functional considerations favor the use of radiation therapy for single modality treatment of small lesions in this region, with the possible exception of tonsillar primaries, which can be removed transorally with minimal impact on normal function.[217] Surgery combined with radiation therapy offers the best prognosis for more advanced disease (T3 and T4 lesions).[218] Lymphatic dissemination can include surgically inaccessible nodes such as Rouvière's (high retropharyngeal).

Surgery

Small lesions of the tonsillar fossa and soft palate can be approached transorally. Adequate surgical exposure for larger lesions, or those involving the tongue base, can require a median mandibular osteotomy with a paralingual approach. This approach preserves the function of uninvolved structures in the oral cavity and does not interfere with sensation to the chin dependent on an intact mental nerve. Lesions of the posterior pharyngeal wall can be approached via a transhyoid approach, detaching the base of tongue from the hyoid bone, or via a mandibular osteotomy combined with a median glossal split. Both approaches result in normal functioning of the tongue after repair.[219]

If disease involves the mandible or the mandibular periosteum, then a hemimandibulectomy may be necessary. The removed segment of mandible can be readily reconstructed with a bone containing a microvascular free flap, such as a fibula, an iliac crest, or a scapula flap.[59–61] Posterolateral mandibulectomies involving the ramus and posterior body can be left unreconstructed with surprisingly little major disability or cosmetic defect.

Resection of the base of tongue can result in significant swallowing problems. Reconstruction of the base of tongue with a radial forearm microvascular free flap, with or without reinnervation, can restore adequate deglutition.[58] In cases of severe swallowing problems resulting in repeated aspiration, laryngectomy may be necessary to avoid potentially fatal pneumonia. Pharyngeal wall lesions that cannot be closed with a skin graft or that are primarily due to stenosis can be successfully reconstructed with the radial forearm microvascular free flap.[58]

Radiation Therapy

Radiation therapy alone is the treatment of choice for nearly all early oropharyngeal carcinomas (T1 and T2). With the exception of T1,N0 lesions of the tonsil, where only ipsilateral jugulodigastric nodes need to be treated, radiation portals must be large and include not only the primary but all neck lymphatics as well. Pharyngeal wall lesions require irradiation to Rouvière's nodes at the base of skull; lower cervical nodes, down to both clavicles, should be treated prophylactically. Brachytherapy implants can be used to deliver part of the dose to selected lesions.[64]

For T1 lesions, 65 to 70 Gy is adequate to control more than 90% of lesions. T2 disease requires 70 Gy for the same local control; however, more advanced disease is difficult to eradicate with radiation therapy alone. Doses of 75 Gy (or higher) have been reported to control a significant proportion of pharyngeal wall and tonsil T3 and T4 lesions, albeit at fairly high complication rates.[220, 221] Massive base-of-tongue cancer is rarely controlled by any acceptable radiation dose.

A randomized trial has shown hyperfractionated radiotherapy to be more effective than conventionally fractionated radiotherapy for T3 lesions of the oropharynx,[67] although base-of-tongue tumors were excluded from this trial. Elective neck irradiation is recommended for all but the smallest primaries and 50 Gy is adequate; involved nodes need an additional boost with electron beams or radioactive implants to a total of 65 to 75 Gy. If the primary is controlled but nodes fail to regress, then radical or modified neck dissection is necessary.

Results and Prognosis

Overall 5-year survival is in the range of 30% to 60%, depending on site and stage of tumor.[215] Specific data according to anatomic site of primary, T stage, and N stage are summarized in Table 20–10. Tonsil and soft palate have the best prognosis; pharyngeal wall and base of tongue have a very serious outlook. The mortality in oropharyngeal cancer results from regionally recurrent or uncontrollable disease. More radical locoregional treatment results in a greater freedom from disease above the clavicles, but with longer survival, occult metastatic disease becomes evident. Patients also have a high risk of developing other aerodigestive primary carcinomas or bronchogenic carcinoma resulting from epithelial field carcinogenesis secondary to smoking.[23]

Cancer of the Hypopharynx

Anatomically, this area includes the posterior and lateral pharyngeal walls below the base of tongue, the pyriform sinuses, and the postcricoid region. Cancers in this region are among the most lethal of head and neck tumors. Diagnosis is usually late, local disease is advanced, and nodal metastases are common.

Epidemiology and Etiology

Epidemiology

Pyriform sinus is the most common site for a primary lesion in this region. The ratio of disease in males exceeds females by 2:1; the median age is 50 to 60 years.

Etiology

- Heavy tobacco use and alcohol consumption are common antecedent factors.
- Plummer-Vinson syndrome (iron deficiency anemia, glossitis, achlorhydria, koilonychia) is associated with postcricoid cancer in females.

Detection and Diagnosis

Clinical Detection

- Odynophagia (pain on swallowing) is a common presentation. Ipsilateral referred otalgia is also common.

- Dysphagia is a late symptom.
- Hoarseness indicates possible laryngeal involvement through mass effect or paralysis of a vocal cord.
- Fetor oris, difficulty in swallowing saliva, and dyspnea are advanced manifestations.
- An isolated cervical mass can be the only presenting symptom.

Diagnostic Procedures

- *Indirect laryngoscopy* is used to visualize the lesion. If the lesion is located in the pyriform sinus apex (the most inferior aspect), then it may not be visible on indirect laryngoscopy. These lesions can be associated with pooling of secretions in the pyriform sinus or asymmetry.
- *Direct laryngoscopy, esophagoscopy,* and *biopsy* are essential.
- Imaging by *CT* and *MRI* are valuable for diagnosing tumor extensions.

Classification and Staging

Histopathology

Virtually all lesions are SCCs, usually moderately to poorly differentiated.[7]

Staging

The staging system for carcinomas of the hypopharynx is summarized in Table 20–14 and Figure 20–7.

Staging Work-Up

Staging procedures common to all head and neck sites have been discussed earlier in this chapter. Fiberoptic examination and direct examination under anesthesia are especially important for this site.

Patterns of Spread

Patterns of Local Spread

- Pyriform sinus lesions arising on the lateral wall invade thyroid cartilage early. Lesions arising on the medial pyriform sinus are intimately related to larynx, and invade that organ directly through the aryepiglottic fold, entering the paraglottic larynx. Superior spread may lead to invasion of the oropharyngeal wall or base of tongue, and inferior spread may occur into the cervical esophagus.
- Postcricoid carcinoma spreads into the arytenoid region of the larynx, grows circumferentially around the cricopharyngeal region to encircle the upper esophagus, and may spread downward through the esophagus for considerable distances. As a result of its location, it can involve the cricoid cartilage, the only complete ring in the trachea, very early.

Metastatic Behavior

Early cervical node metastases are a hallmark of these lesions. Two thirds to three fourths of all patients have palpable nodes at diagnosis, usually jugulodigastric.[222, 223] Hematogenous metastases are not uncommon. They become manifest in up to 30% of patients, but are usually delayed until the time of local recurrence.

Principles of Treatment

Principles of treatment for hypopharyngeal carcinoma are summarized in Table 20–15. The less common small lesions (T1, early T2) may be adequately managed by radia-

TABLE 20–14. **TNM Classification and Stage Grouping of the Hypopharynx**

Stage	Grouping	TNM Classification
Stage 0	Tis, N0, M0	Tis: Carcinoma *in situ* N0: No regional lymph node metastasis M0: No distant metastasis
Stage I	T1, N0, M0	T1: Tumor at one subsite and ≤2 cm
Stage II	T2, N0, M0	T2: More than one subsite or adjacent site, or tumor >2 cm but ≤4 cm without larynx fixation
Stage III	T3, N0, M0 T1, N1, M0 T2, N1, M0 T3, N1, M0	T3: Tumor >4 cm or with larynx fixation N1: Metastasis in a singular ipsilateral lymph node, ≤3 cm
Stage IVA	T4, N0,1, M0 Any T, N2, M0	T4: Tumor invades cartilage, neck, etc. N2: Metastasis in a single ipsilateral lymph node, >3 cm but ≤6 cm; or, in multiple ipsilateral lymph nodes, none >6 cm; or in bilateral or contralateral lymph nodes, none >6 cm*
Stage IVB	Any T, N3, M0	N3: Metastasis in a lymph node >6 cm
Stage IVC	Any T, any N, M1	M1: Distant metastasis.

T = tumor; N = node; M = metastasis.

*N2a: metastasis in single ipsilateral lymph node >3 cm, but not >6 cm; N2b: metastasis in multiple ipsilateral lymph nodes, none >6 cm; N2c: metastasis in bilateral or contralateral lymph nodes, none >6 cm.

Used with permission of the American Joint Committee on Cancer (AJCC®), Chicago, Illinois. The original source for this material is the AJCC® Cancer Staging Manual, 5th ed, 1997, published by Lippincott-Raven Publishers, Philadelphia, Pennsylvania; and International Union Against Cancer (UICC): TNM Classification of Malignant Tumors, 4th ed, New York, Springer-Verlag, 1992.

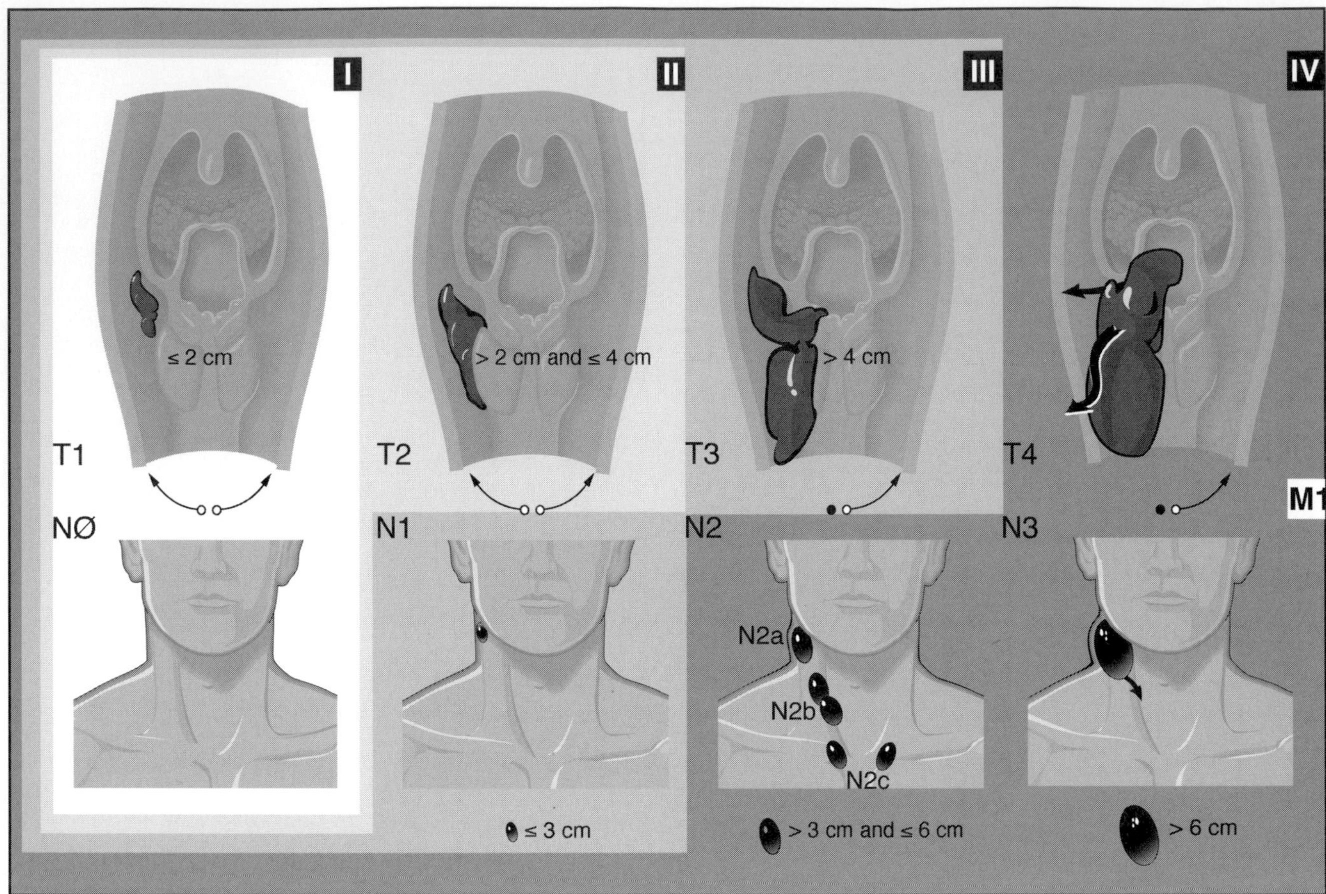

Figure 20–7. Anatomic staging system for tumors of the hypopharynx. The primary tumor staging is characterized both by size and by sites of involvement and vocal cord mobility and then by extension into other anatomic regions. The various sites of the hypopharynx are the postcricoid region (pharyngoesophageal junction), pyriform sinus, and the posterior pharyngeal wall. A T1 tumor involves only one site and is 2 cm or smaller in size; a T2 tumor involves more than one site or is larger than 2 but 4 cm or smaller in size; a fixed vocal cord or size larger than 4 cm makes the tumor a T3; massive tumors invading the adjacent soft tissues or cartilage are characterized as T4. The nodal staging is shown in the lower row.

tion therapy or by surgery. Conservation surgery is possible (partial pharyngectomy, hemilaryngectomy) for superiorly placed lesions. The majority of patients, however, require combined surgery and radiation therapy if they are candidates for a curative approach.[224, 225] An organ preservation protocol involving induction chemotherapy, with patients exhibiting a complete response receiving definitive radiotherapy and the noncomplete responders receiving the standard treatment of surgery and postoperative radiation, has shown equivalent survival when compared with standard treatment of surgery and postoperative radiotherapy.[47] Approximately 40% of patients treated in this manner had an

TABLE 20–15. **Carcinoma of the Hypopharynx: Principles of Treatment**

Stage	Grouping	Surgery		Radiation Therapy	Chemotherapy
I	T1, N0, M0	Partial/total laryngopharyngectomy and ND	or	DRT: 65–74 Gy	NR
II	T2, N0, M0	Partial/total laryngopharyngectomy and ND	or	DRT: 65–74 Gy	RCTO
III	T3, N1, M0	Total laryngopharyngectomy	and	ART: postop	
			or	DRT: 65–74 Gy	RCTO
			or	RT: 65–70 Gy	CCR
IV	T4, N2,3, M0	Total laryngopharyngectomy with reconstructive surgery	and	ART: postop	
			or	DRT: 65–74 Gy	RCTO
			or	RT: 65–70 Gy	CCR
Local relapse		RT for surgery relapse	Surgery for RT relapse		IC II
Metastatic		NR	Occasionally		IC II

DRT = definitive; ART = adjuvant; RT = radiation therapy; NR = not recommended; RCTO = recommend chemotherapy in organ preservation protocol; CCR = concurrent chemotherapy and radiation (experimental); ND = neck dissection; IC II = investigational chemotherapy, phase I/II clinical trials.

intact, functioning larynx at the 3-year end point. Palliation in this region also must be aggressive if it is to be beneficial. Carcinomas of the postcricoid and pyriform apex regions pose serious problems because of direct spread into important adjacent structures and metastasis to tracheoesophageal nodes, often down into superior mediastinum.

Surgery

Small laterally placed lesions can be handled through a lateral pharyngotomy approach and resected with partial pharyngectomy. Depending on the location and defect size, reconstruction can be accomplished through primary closure, skin graft (posterior wall), or radial forearm microvascular free flap.[58] Medially based lesions involving the larynx can be resected with a partial laryngectomy or a total laryngectomy. Reconstruction usually requires only primary closure of the remaining hypopharyngeal mucosa. Large lesions of the hypopharynx or moderate size lesions in the pyriform apex may require total laryngopharyngectomy. Reconstruction options include microvascular jejunal free flaps that can replace the entire cervical esophagus and gastric pull-up.[57]

Radiation Therapy

Small lesions can be treated with definitive radiotherapy. At least 65 to 74 Gy must be given if a standard fractionation scheme is used. If the tumor involves the postcricoid region or the pyriform sinus, then the posterior pharyngeal wall must receive 50 to 55 Gy in order to prophylactically treat the retropharyngeal nodes. The nodes in the supraclavicular region should normally receive prophylactic radiation to approximately 50 Gy. Advanced tumors may be treated using induction chemotherapy according to an organ preservation protocol developed by the EORTC.[47] Concomitant chemotherapy and radiotherapy offer the potential of increased tumor control compared with their being used sequentially in an organ preservation protocol, but, at present, this technique must be regarded as experimental.

Results and Prognosis

Early lesions with negative nodes have 5-year survival rates higher than 70%.[223, 226] The majority of cases are, however, advanced and overall survival rarely exceeds 25% in any series (see Table 20–10). Postcricoid carcinomas and pyriform apex lesions fare more poorly than superiorly based pyriform sinus lesions. Super-radical measures above the clavicles achieve better locoregional control, but longer median survival times unmask hematogenous metastases, and 5-year outcomes are little improved compared with conservative measures. A randomized trial using an organ preservation protocol for patients with Stages T2 to T4, N0 to N2b tumors has shown equivalent local control (71%) and survival (30%) compared with radical resection and postoperative irradiation.[47] Nonetheless, better systemic therapy is needed to improve the grim prognosis.

Cancer of the Larynx

Carcinomas of the larynx are the most common malignant tumors encountered in head and neck oncology, with approximately 10,100 new cases estimated for 2000.[17] They arise from the epithelial lining of the laryngeal mucous membrane; a clear distinction must be made between lesions arising in the supraglottic larynx (epiglottis, aryepiglottic folds, arytenoids, false cords) and in the glottic larynx (true vocal cords), the carcinomas arising in the supraglottic larynx being rare. Carcinomas of the larynx, especially glottic lesions, usually are not immediately life threatening, and major therapeutic decisions revolve around preservation of laryngeal function. The larynx is an organ of phonation and serves as an air passage and as a sphincter guarding the airway. Conservation laryngeal surgery has emphasized the importance of the larynx as an airway and a sphincter. Loss of voice owing to disease or treatment is a serious handicap, but an ineffective airway or an inefficient sphincter may be fatal.

Epidemiology and Etiology

Epidemiology

Glottic carcinoma accounts for 60% to 65% of all laryngeal cancer; 30% to 35% arise in the supraglottis, and 5% or less arise in subglottic sites.[227] The male-to-female ratio is approximately 4.5 to 1, with a peak incidence in the sixth and seventh decades.[17, 227]

Etiology

Heavy tobacco use and alcohol consumption are common antecedent factors. Someone who smokes 30 cigarettes per day has approximately an 18 times higher risk of developing laryngeal cancer than someone who has never smoked.[228] A daily cigar smoker who does not inhale may have a 10-fold greater risk of developing laryngeal cancer than a nonsmoker.[22]

Detection and Diagnosis

Clinical Detection

- Hoarseness that persists is the cardinal manifestation of glottic carcinoma; it is much less common with supraglottic carcinoma.
- Sore throat is a common presentation for supraglottic carcinoma.

- Referred otalgia is not uncommon with supraglottic lesions.
- Dyspnea occurs with advanced exophytic carcinomas.
- Dysphagia implies advanced disease involving the hypopharynx.
- Cervical lymphadenopathy, especially jugulodigastric, may be a presentation of supraglottic carcinoma, but virtually never of glottic carcinoma.

Diagnostic Procedures

- *Indirect laryngoscopy* is essential in all cases of persistent (>1 month) hoarseness.
- *Direct laryngoscopy, cervical esophagoscopy,* and *biopsy* are essential.
- Imaging by *CT* and *MRI* are valuable for diagnosing tumor extensions.

Classification and Staging

Histopathology

More than 95% of laryngeal carcinomas are SCCs.[7] Leukoplakia of the laryngeal mucosa often accompanies carcinoma, and a wide spectrum of borderline, premalignant epithelial changes may be encountered, sometimes without clear evidence of invasion. Most SCCs of the true cord are well differentiated or moderately well differentiated; supraglottic carcinomas tend to be less differentiated. Verrucous carcinoma is a clinicopathologic variant of squamous carcinoma and is characterized by a warty growth showing an extremely well-differentiated pattern. Occasionally adenoid cystic carcinomas of minor salivary gland origin or lymphomas are encountered.

Staging

The staging system for carcinomas of the larynx is summarized in Table 20–16 and Figures 20–8 and 20–9. Note that the criteria vary according to the subsite of tumor origin.

Staging Work-Up

Staging procedures common to all head and neck sites have been discussed earlier in this chapter. For this tumor site, special attention must be paid to careful evaluation via direct laryngoscopy. Fine-cut CT scanning provides important information with regard to tumor extension beyond the larynx. Evaluation of thyroid cartilage invasion on CT can be difficult because of the variability of cartilage calcification.

Patterns of Spread

Patterns of Local Spread

SUPRAGLOTTIC CARCINOMA

Whole larynx coronal section studies disclose a variety of typical intralaryngeal spread patterns determined to a significant degree by various anatomic subcompartments within the organ (epilarynx, paraglottic space, pre-epiglottic space, Reinke's space, anterior subglottic triangle, anterior commissure tendon). Common patterns include:

- epiglottis to pre-epiglottic space
- epiglottis to aryepiglottic fold
- aryepiglottic fold to pyriform sinus
- false cord to paraglottic space to pre-epiglottic space
- false cord to ventricle to true cord

TABLE 20–16. **TNM Classification and Stage Grouping of the Larynx**

		TNM Classification	
Stage	**Grouping**	***Glottis***	***Supra- or Subglottis***
Stage 0	Tis, N0, M0	Tis: Carcinoma *in situ* N0: No regional lymph node metastasis M0: No distant metastasis	Tis: Carcinoma *in situ* N0: No regional lymph node metastasis M0: No distant metastasis
Stage I	T1, N0, M0	T1: Tumor limited to TVC with mobility T1a: One cord; T1b: both cords	T1: One subsite with mobility
Stage II	T2, N0, M0	T2: Extends to supra- or subglottis and/or impaired mobility	T2: Tumor extends to more than 1 subsite/glottis, without fixation
Stage III	T3, N0, M0	T3: Cord fixation	T3: Cord fixation, and/or postcricoid or pre-epiglottic space
	T1–3, N1, M0	N1: Metastasis in a single ipsilateral lymph node, ≤3 cm in greatest dimension	N1: Metastasis in a single ipsilateral lymph node, ≤3 cm in greatest dimension
Stage IVA	T4, N0–N1, M0	T4: Tumor extends beyond larynx, invades cartilage, neck, etc	T4: Tumor extends beyond larynx, cartilage invasion
	Any T, N2, M0	N2: Metastasis in a single ipsilateral lymph node, >3 cm but ≤6 cm in greatest dimension; or, in multiple ipsilateral lymph nodes, none >6 cm in greatest dimension; or, in bilateral or contralateral lymph nodes, none >6 cm	N2: Metastasis in a single ipsilateral lymph node, >3 cm but ≤6 cm in greatest dimension; or, in multiple ipsilateral lymph nodes, none >6 cm in greatest dimension, or, in bilateral or contralateral lymph nodes, none >6 cm
Stage IVB	Any T, N3, M0	N3: Metastasis in a lymph node, >6 cm in greatest dimension	N3: Metastasis in a lymph node, > 6 cm in greatest dimension
Stage IVC	Any T, any N, M1	M1: Distant metastasis	M1: Distant metastasis

T = tumor; N = node; M = metastasis.

Used with permission of the American Joint Committee on Cancer (AJCC®), Chicago, Illinois. The original source for this material is the AJCC® Cancer Staging Manual, 5th ed, 1997, published by Lippincott-Raven Publishers, Philadelphia, Pennsylvania; and International Union Against Cancer (UICC): TNM Classification of Malignant Tumors, 4th ed, New York, Springer-Verlag, 1992.

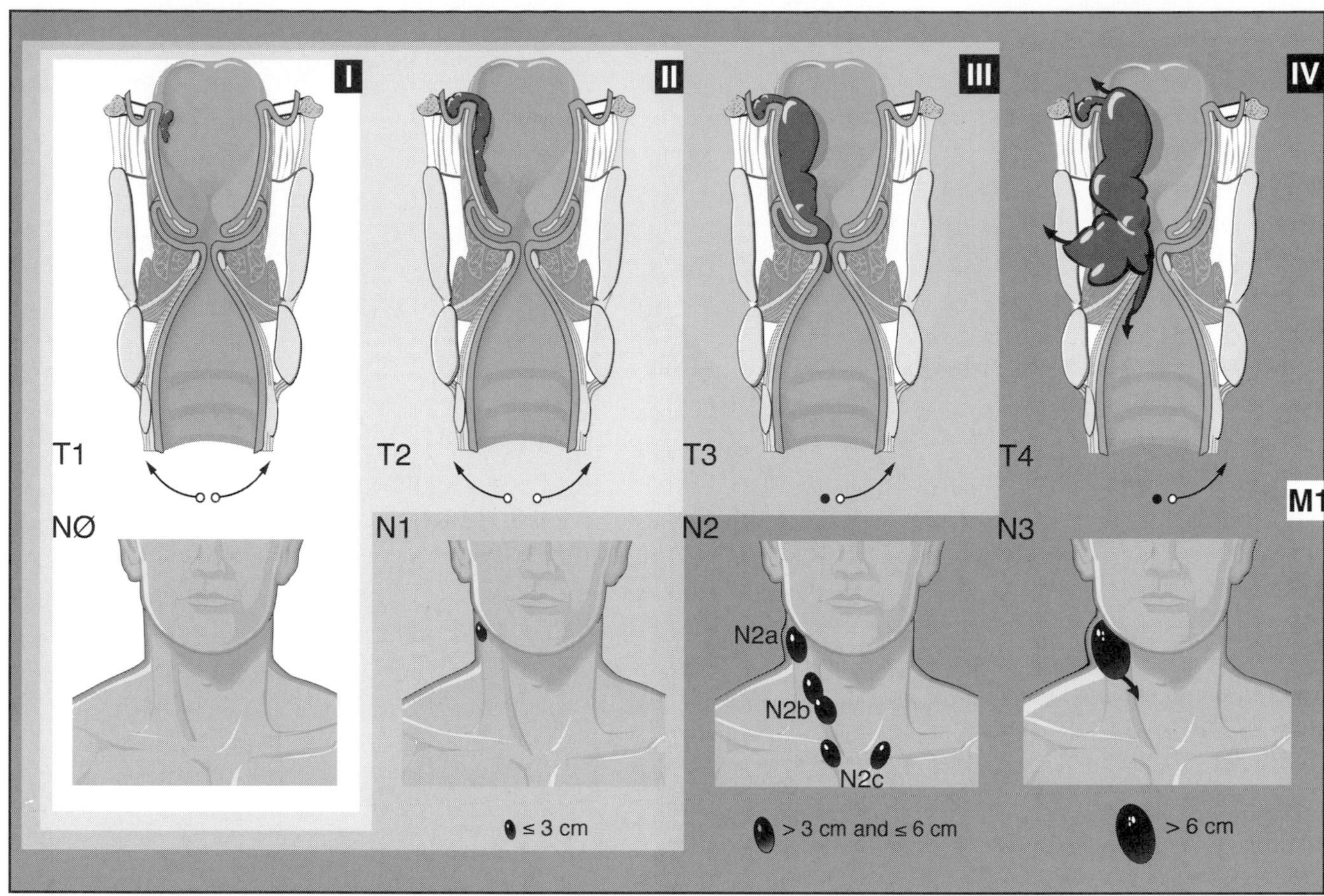

Figure 20–8. Anatomic staging system for tumors of the supraglottic larynx. The primary tumor staging is characterized first by sites of involvement and vocal cord mobility and then by extension into other anatomic regions. The various sites of the supraglottis are the false cords (ventricular bands), arytenoids, epiglottis, and aryepiglottic folds. A T1 tumor involves only one site; a T2 tumor involves more than one site or extends to the vocal cords without impairing their mobility; a T3 tumor has cord fixation; a T4 tumor extends beyond the larynx or invades the adjacent cartilage or soft tissues of the neck. The nodal staging is shown in the lower row.

Extension to the anterior commissure at the origin of the thyroepiglottic ligament may lead to thyroid cartilage invasion.

GLOTTIC CARCINOMA

One half of all true cord cancers involve only the anterior third of the cord, and 75% occur in the anterior two thirds of the cord.[227] The anterior commissure is involved in about 15% of cancers. Anterior subglottic extension may be difficult to detect.

Several mechanisms may be responsible for cord fixation and all imply deep invasion. Most commonly, thyroarytenoid muscle invasion is responsible for a fixed cord, but other mechanisms include lateral cricoarytenoid muscle invasion, cricoarytenoid joint involvement, transverse arytenoid muscle invasion, and perineural infiltration.

Metastatic Behavior

Cervical node involvement is rare with glottic carcinoma (less than 10% incidence) and occurs only when the disease spreads from the cord into the supraglottic region.[227] Primary supraglottic carcinoma has a significant propensity to cervical metastases, and 45% to 55% of patients have nodal disease at presentation.[227] The first node involved is usually the jugulodigastric.

Principles of Treatment

Treatment selection depends on the site and extent of the lesion. Early lesions (T1 or T2,N0,M0) are curable by surgery or radiation alone, and the selection of modality includes considerations such as voice preservation and the desire to reserve radiation therapy for future second primary treatment.

Supraglottic Carcinoma

Principles of treatment for supraglottic carcinoma are summarized in Table 20–17. Treatment must be directed at the primary lesion and at cervical lymphatics. Small primary lesions (T1 or T2) are treated equally well by radiation or supraglottic laryngectomy (horizontal partial laryngectomy). Large primary lesions may be managed with total laryngectomy, generally with adjuvant radiation therapy.

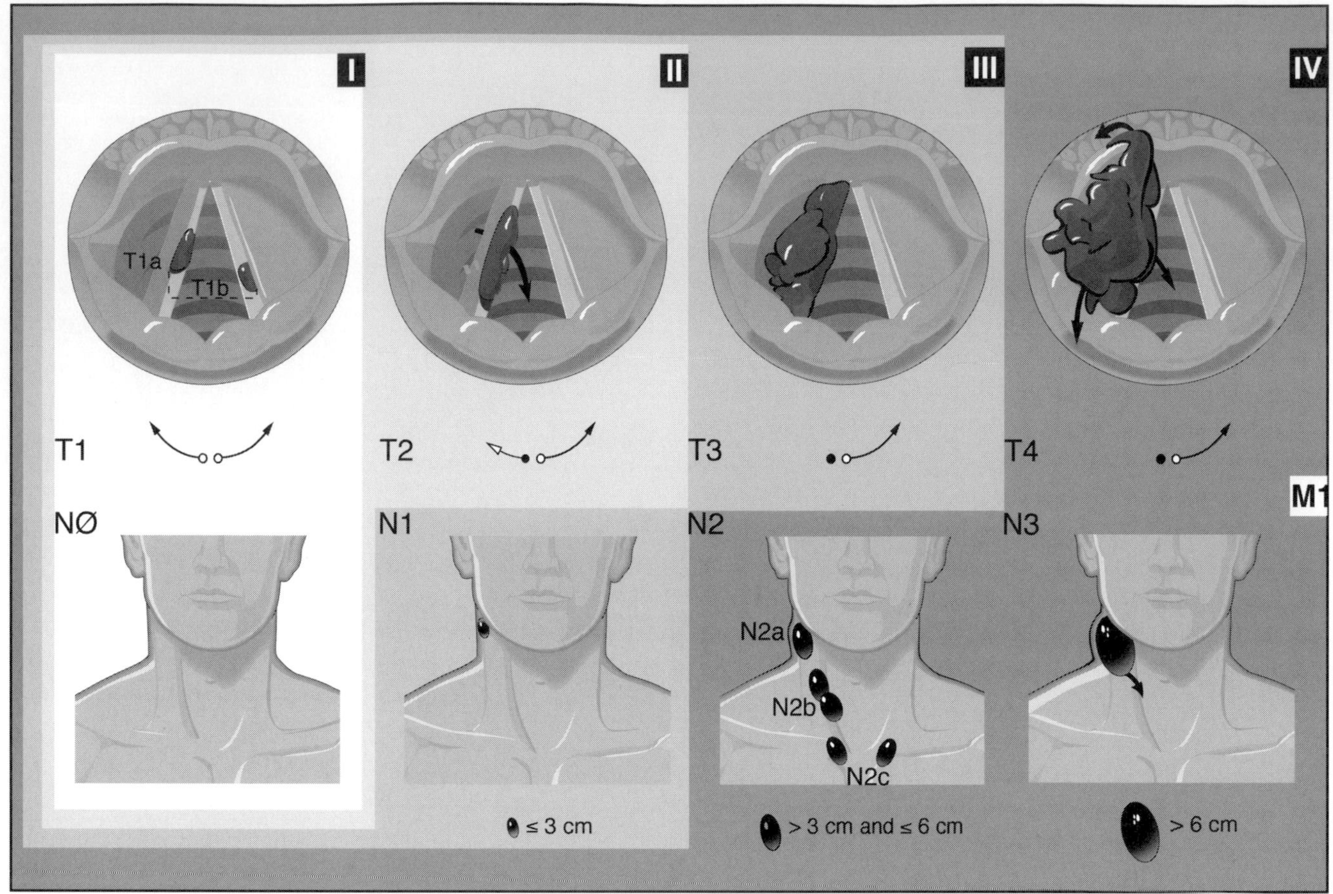

Figure 20–9. Anatomic staging system for tumors of the glottic larynx. The primary tumor staging is characterized first by sites of involvement and vocal cord mobility, and then by extension into other anatomic regions. A T1 tumor involves one or both cords; a T2 tumor either extends to the supraglottis or subglottis or is associated with impaired (not fixed) cord mobility; a T3 tumor has cord fixation; a T4 tumor extends beyond the larynx or invades the adjacent cartilage or soft tissues of the neck. The nodal staging is shown in the lower row.

Patients with stage III or IV lesions, for whom primary surgical treatment involves a total laryngectomy, may be treated via an organ preservation protocol.[45, 46] Elective neck treatment can be given either by neck dissection or radiation therapy. The large number of treatment options requires careful evaluation of each patient's suitability for any procedure and a cooperative interaction between members of the treatment team.

Surgery by supraglottic laryngectomy controls more than 80% of T1 and T2 supraglottic carcinomas, but the surgeon and patient must be prepared for total laryngectomy should the partial procedure prove technically impossible. Positive margins require postoperative radiation. T3 or T4 primary lesions usually need total laryngectomy with adjuvant radiotherapy.[229, 230]

Radiation therapy is a highly effective treatment for T1 and T2 lesions.[229, 230] Doses ranging from 66 to 70 Gy are necessary. Local control is in the range of 85% to 95% for T1 lesions and in the range of 75% to 80% for T2 lesions. Patients who relapse following irradiation may be salvaged by total laryngectomy, only occasionally by horizontal laryngectomy.[231] More advanced supraglottic carcinomas are rarely controlled at the primary site by irradiation alone, though selected cases with more exophytic lesions have been reported to achieve 50% to 70% local control.[232] More often, these patients have respiratory distress and cervical metastases, and are managed surgically. Radiation therapy is often added preoperatively or postoperatively.[229, 230] The treatment of choice for subclinical neck disease is radiation therapy.

Organ preservation protocols involving induction chemotherapy are the preferred approach in patients with stage III and IV tumors who are able to withstand the rigors of this treatment and who wish to keep their larynx.[45, 46] This approach has yielded equivalent survival to standard surgery and postoperative radiotherapy with approximately two thirds of surviving patients maintaining an intact, functioning larynx. Speech communication profiles were clearly better in the patients treated on the laryngeal preservation arm of the protocol.[233] Careful patient monitoring for failure is critical in this approach.

Glottic Carcinoma

Principles of treatment for glottic carcinoma are summarized in Table 20–17. Glottic carcinoma only rarely requires treatment directed to the cervical lymphatics. Early glottic carcinomas (Tis, T1, or T2) are equally well treated by

TABLE 20–17. **Carcinoma of the Supraglottic Larynx and Glottic Larynx: Principles of Treatment**

Stage	Grouping	Surgery		Radiation Therapy		Chemotherapy
Supraglottic Larynx						
I	T1, N0, M0	Supraglottic/partial laryngectomy; spare vocal cord	or	DRT: 65–70 Gy		NR
II	N0–1, T2, N0, M0	Supraglottic laryngectomy and ND	or	DRT: 65–70 Gy		NR
III	T1–3, N0–1, M0	Total laryngectomy	and	ART: postop		
			or	DRT: 70 Gy	and	RCTO induction
IV	T4, N1–3, M0	Total laryngectomy plus pharyngectomy with	and	DRT: 70 Gy	or	RCTO
				ART: postop		
		reconstructive surgery if needed	or	DRT: 70 Gy	and	RCTO
Local relapse		RT for surgery relapse		Surgery for RT relapse		IC II
Metastatic		NR		Occasionally		IC II
Glottic Larynx						
I	T1, N0, M0	Cordectomy/hemilaryngectomy		DRT preferred: 63–66 Gy		NR
II	T2, N0, M0	Hemilaryngectomy or total laryngectomy		DRT preferred: 66–70 Gy		NR
III	T1–3, N0–1, M0	Total laryngectomy and ND		ART		RCTO
			or	DRT: 70–72 Gy		
IV	T4, N1–3, M0	Total laryngectomy and ND		ART		
			or	DRT: 70–72 Gy		RCTO
Local relapse		RT of surgery relapse		Surgery for RT relapse		IC II
Metastatic		NR		Possibly		IC II

ND = neck dissection; DRT = definitive; ART = adjuvant; RT = radiation therapy; NR = not recommended; RCTO = recommended chemotherapy organ preservation protocol; IC II = investigational chemotherapy, phase I/II clinical trials.

radiation therapy or by various conservation surgical procedures (cord stripping, cordectomy, or vertical hemilaryngectomy, as indicated). It is generally believed that radiotherapy results in a better functional voice. Fixed cord lesions do less well with irradiation, though local control has been achieved in selected patients. Cartilage invasion reduces the probability of tumor control with primary radiation therapy, although it is not an absolute contraindication to a laryngeal sparing approach with surgery held in reserve for salvage.

Surgery may be used as single modality therapy for T1 and selected T2 lesions with local control and cure rates of over 90%.[234, 235] In selected cases, endoscopic chordectomy procedures can result in excellent voice preservation equivalent to radiation therapy.[236] Advanced lesions involving fixation of the true vocal cord, subglottic extension, or extension into the hypopharynx typically require total laryngectomy or near total laryngectomy. The patient is at increased risk for a postsurgical stomal recurrence if there is subglottic extension, and postoperative radiation therapy is recommended. Total laryngectomy may also be indicated for situations in which reconstruction may lead to intractable aspiration. Acceptable speech can be regained after total laryngectomy via a variety of methods including electrolarynx devices, esophageal speech, and a surgically created tracheoesophageal fistula fitted with a one-way valve. Hemilaryngectomy is possible for selected lesions.

Radiation therapy is highly effective in achieving local control in early-stage glottic tumors.[229, 230] Local control is in the range of 85% to 95% for Tis and T1 tumors and in the range of 75% to 80% for T2 lesions. Doses in the range of 65–70 Gy are given, and it has been shown that treating at 2 Gy per fraction results in better local control than treating at 1.8 Gy per day.[237–239] Impaired cord mobility lowers the tumor control probability for T2 lesions. Selected T3 cases may be irradiated,[229, 230] but cartilage destruction indicating extensive disease (T4) is rarely controlled with radiation alone. Care must be taken not to underdose the anterior commissure region when it is involved.

Organ Preservation Protocols

See earlier discussion of "Supraglottic Carcinoma."

Subglottic Carcinoma

Tumors arising in the subglottic larynx can spread to both cervical lymph nodes and nodes in the upper paratracheal chain. The overall incidence of positive nodes at the time of presentation is in the range of 10% to 20%. Radiation, whether given definitively or as an adjuvant to surgery, must include the upper mediastinal nodes.[229, 230]

Surgery will typically require a total laryngectomy because the cricoid cartilage, the single complete cartilaginous ring in the upper airway, is in close proximity.

Radiation therapy is a viable treatment modality for early-stage (T1, T2) tumors, with surgery held in reserve for salvage.

Organ preservation protocols would have to be regarded as experimental because too few patients with subglottic tumors were included in the randomized trial to permit one to draw any conclusions regarding efficacy.[45, 46]

Results and Prognosis

Prognosis in supraglottic carcinoma is mainly determined by cervical node status and in glottic carcinoma by cord mobility. Supraglottic carcinoma without cervical metastases has a 5-year survival of 70% to 80%, but with cervical node disease the survival falls to 30% to 50%.[229, 230] Glottic carcinoma has a 5-year survival of 80% to 90% in the absence of cord fixation, but falls to 50% to 60% with cord fixation. Organ preservation protocols involving induction chemotherapy constitute a new standard of care for patients with locally advanced tumors who wish to maintain their larynx.[45, 46] In institutions following a policy of radiation therapy for early laryngeal cancer, significantly more T1 and T2 patients retain a functional larynx (70% to 80%) than if surgery is the first line of treatment.[229, 230, 240]

Cancer of the Nasopharynx

Nasopharyngeal carcinoma (NPC) accounts for only a small percentage of head and neck cancers in the United States. Because its protean clinical manifestations can lead to misdiagnosis, a high index of suspicion is required. Anatomically, this area includes the posterior and lateral pharyngeal walls above the soft palate and the superior surface of the soft palate extending to the posterior choanae. Even with large lymph nodes, it is generally among the more radioresponsive of head and neck tumors. Unlike other head and neck tumors, adjuvant chemotherapy seems to improve both local control and survival.[48, 49] Patients who are cured of their primary tumor do not exhibit the same high incidence of second primary neoplasms as occurs for other head and neck sites.[189]

Epidemiology and Etiology

This disease is uncommon in white populations (2% of all head and neck cancer in the United States).[19] The age distribution is bimodal, with a small peak in adolescence and young adulthood and the major peak occurring between 50 and 70 years of age. This disease is not associated with tobacco or alcohol consumption. A strikingly high incidence of NPC is found among the southern Chinese, where it accounts for 13% to 20% of all cancer and up to 57% of all head and neck cancer.[241] There is also a high incidence in Middle Eastern countries.[242] Nitrosamines from salted fish may contribute to the high incidence of tumors found in southern China.[243] EBV is a possible carcinogen or cocarcinogen in patients having World Health Organization types 2 and 3 tumors.[244] High titers of IgG and IgA antibodies to EBV antigens are present in the vast majority of NPC patient sera.[245]

Detection and Diagnosis

Clinical Detection

- Common presentations are lymphadenopathic (cervical node with an initially unknown primary), otologic (owing to eustachian obstruction), and nasal (posterior choanae obstruction).
- Atypical facial pain resulting from trigeminal involvement or base of skull destruction can be a perplexing diagnostic problem.
- Cranial nerve involvement occurs in 15% to 25% of cases and most commonly involves nerve VI.[163, 181] There are two principal cranial nerve syndromes: the retroparotidian syndrome owing to Rouvier's nodes involving IX, X, XI, and XII (with, occasionally, Horner's syndrome resulting from involvement of the sympathetic chain) and the petrosphenoidal syndrome involving III, IV, V, and VI via extension through the foramen lacerum into the middle cranial fossa. Very rarely, the II nerve can be involved.

Diagnostic Procedures

- *Nasopharyngoscopy* with a nasopharyngeal mirror or via fiberoptic nasopharyngoscope is mandatory whenever the diagnosis of NPC is a possibility.
- *Biopsy* is necessary to confirm an NPC.
- Imaging is best performed by contrast-enhanced *CT* and *MRI*. CT is superior for bone destruction and MRI for soft tissue extensions.
- *Anti-EBV antibody titers* may be helpful in suggesting a nasopharyngeal tumor in an occult primary work-up.

Classification and Staging

Histopathology

Ninety percent of these lesions are SCC or its variants. Minor salivary gland tumors and lymphomas can also occur, but they are discussed in other sections of this text. NPC has a tendency toward poor differentiation and unusual growth patterns. The World Health Organization recommends the following nomenclature:

Type 1: keratinizing SCC (30% of cases)
Type 2: nonkeratinizing carcinoma (50% to 70% of cases)
Type 3: lymphoepithelioma (25% of cases)

Nonkeratinizing carcinoma and lymphoepithelioma are variants of SCC.

Staging

The staging system for carcinomas of the nasopharynx is summarized in Table 20–18 and Figure 20–10.

TABLE 20–18. **TNM Classification and Stage Grouping of the Nasopharynx**

Stage	Grouping	TNM Classification
Stage 0	Tis, N0, M0	Tis: Carcinoma *in situ*
Stage I	T1, N0, M0	T1: Tumor confined to nasopharynx N0: no regional lymph nodes T2: Extends to oropharynx and/or nasal fossa
Stage IIA	T2a, N0, M0	T2a: No parapharyngeal extension
Stage IIB	T2b, N0, M0 T1, N1, M0 T2a,b, N1, M0	T2b: Parapharyngeal extension N1: Unilateral lymph node(s), 6 cm or less, above SCF
Stage III	T3, N0–2, M0 T1, N2, M0 T2a,b, N2, M0	T3: Invades bony structures and/or paranasal sinuses N2: Bilateral lymph node(s), 6 cm or less, above SCF
Stage IVA	T4, N0–2, M0	T4: Tumor invades skull, cranial nerve, orbit, or hypopharynx
Stage IVB	Any T, N3, M0	N3a: Lymph nodes greater than 6 cm; N3b: lymph nodes extending to SCF
Stage IVC	Any T, any N, M1	M1: Distant metastasis

T = tumor; N = node; M = metastasis.

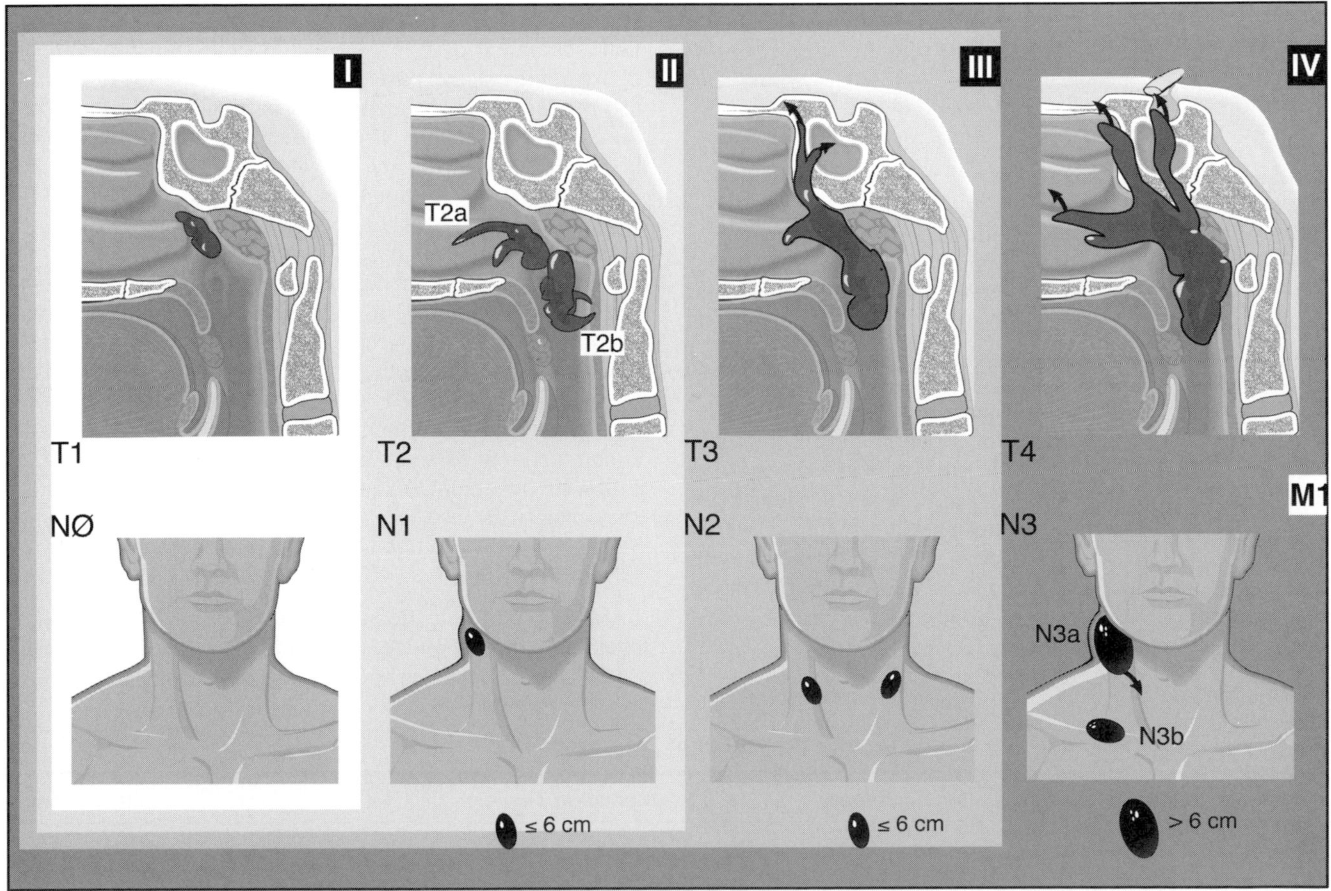

Figure 20–10. Anatomic staging system for tumors of the nasopharynx. The primary tumor staging is characterized first by sites of involvement and then by extension into other anatomic regions, such as the oropharynx, base of skull, and cranial nerve involvement. The sites of the nasopharynx are posterosuperior wall, lateral wall (including Rosenmüller's fossa), and the inferior wall, which is the upper surface of the soft palate. A T1 tumor is confined to the nasopharynx; a T2 tumor extends into the soft tissues of the oropharynx and/or nasal fossa; a T3 tumor invades bony structures or paranasal sinuses, or both; a T4 tumor invades the base of skull or involves cranial nerves, orbit, or hypopharynx. The nodal staging is shown in the lower row.

Staging Work-Up

Staging procedures common to all head and neck sites have been discussed earlier in this chapter. For this tumor site, special attention must be paid to fine-cut CT scans to evaluate the base of skull. The value of anti-EBV antibody titers in staging has not been delineated, but higher titers may correlate with more advanced disease. Dysphagia, hoarseness, and hemiatrophy of the tongue (Horner's syndrome), can indicate Rouvière's node involvement.

Patterns of Spread

- *Superior*: via the foramen lacerum into the cavernous sinus (the petrosphenoidal crossway) with involvement of cranial nerves II to VI and erosion of skull base.
- *Anterosuperior*: into the infratemporal fossa and foramen ovale to involve the mandibular division of nerve V.
- *Lateral*: into the medial ostium of the eustachian tube, producing obstruction and secondary serous otitis media with conductive deafness (actual spread along the eustachian tube is exceptionally rare).
- *Posterior*: into the prevertebral musculature, producing pain on flexion or extension of the head.
- *Anterior*: into the nasal cavity and the paranasal sinuses.
- *Inferior*: into the oropharyngeal wall and soft palate.

Metastatic Behavior

NPC is notorious for early and extensive cervical node disease, especially if the histology is lymphoepithelioma. Seventy percent to 85% of NPC patients have palpable nodes at diagnosis.[246] Nodal disease is bilateral or contralateral in 40% to 50% of all cases. The most common nodal group is the jugulodigastric, followed by the upper posterior cervical group deep to the upper end of the sternomastoid. Retropharyngeal nodes of Rouvière are commonly affected but can be difficult to detect.[42] Nodal disease can be extensive while the primary lesion is small. Hematogenous metastases are a significant problem, with an overall incidence of 25% in most series.[193, 246, 247] Patients with bilateral cervical nodes have up to a 40% to 70% likelihood of developing distant disease. Bone and lung are the most common sites of metastases.

Principles of Treatment

Principles of treatment for carcinoma of the nasopharynx are summarized in Table 20–19. The inaccessibility of the nasopharynx, the proximity of the tumors to the skull base and to cranial nerves, and the widespread lymphatic involvement dictate radiation therapy rather than surgery as the procedure of choice. Radiation techniques for NPC are especially complex and should only be undertaken by experienced radiation therapists. Concomitant chemotherapy added to radiotherapy improves outcome for patients with stage III and IV tumors.[48, 49] The acute toxicity associated with this form of treatment is appreciable, and one must be prepared to aggressively support the patient nutritionally.

Surgery

Surgical resection is reserved for cases of persistent or recurrent disease that are resectable without requiring sacrifice of the major neurologic or vascular structures.[248] Neck dissection may be indicated for persistent lymphadenopathy following radiation therapy.

Radiation Therapy

There is no place for small-volume irradiation in the primary treatment of NPC. Radiation fields must encompass structures from the base of the skull to the clavicles, and use is made of a shrinking field pattern to deliver highest doses to gross disease. Prophylactic irradiation to the neck is required even for stage I lesions.[178] Keratinizing and nonkeratinizing carcinomas require 65 Gy for T1 and T2 lesions, and 70 Gy for T3 and T4 disease. Lymphoepithelioma needs 60 to 65 Gy for T1 or T2, and 65 to 70 Gy for T3 and T4.[19] Neck nodes may require electron beam or interstitial boosts, but in the case of lymphoepitheliomas, even large nodes may respond amazingly rapidly.

Concomitant chemotherapy should be used along with radiation for stage III and IV (localized) tumors. Retreatment of local failures with radiation is feasible using a combination of external beam radiotherapy to 40 Gy followed by an intracavitary brachytherapy boost of approximately 20 Gy.[3]

Chemotherapy

Intergroup 0099 has demonstrated a survival benefit when chemotherapy was added to radiotherapy for patients with

TABLE 20–19. **Carcinoma of the Nasopharynx: Principles of Treatment**

Stage	Grouping	Surgery	Radiation Therapy	Chemotherapy
I	T1, N0, M0	NR	DRT: 65–70 Gy	NR
II	T2, N0, M0	NR	DRT: 65–70 Gy	NR
III	T1–3, N1, M0 T3, N0, M0	NR	DRT: 70–75 Gy	CT/RT with CT
IV	T4, N0–3, M0	NR	DRT: 70–75 Gy	CT/RT with CT
	T, any N, any M1	NR	RT: 50 Gy	IC II
	N1–3	NR	DRT: 60–70 Gy	IC II
Relapse and recurrence		Selected cases	Occasional PRT with intracavitary source	IC II

RT = radiation therapy; DRT = definitive; PRT = palliative; NR = not recommended; CT/RT with CT = concomitant chemotherapy and radiation therapy followed by consolidation chemotherapy; IC II = investigational chemotherapy, phase I/II clinical trials.

stage III and IV disease.[48, 49] The protocol was concomitant cisplatin at 100 mg/m^2 given on days 1, 22, and 43 during the radiotherapy. In addition, postradiation chemotherapy has been used, giving cisplatin at 80 mg/m^2 on day 1 and 5-FU at 1 g/m^2 per day on days 1 through 4 every 4 weeks for 3 courses.

Results and Prognosis

The overall 5-year survival is 45%.[19, 193, 247] Prognosis is related to both the T and N stages and histology, with survival decreasing from 50% to 60% for T1 lesions to 10% to 20% for T4 lesions treated with radiation alone (see Table 20–6). Overall, lymphoepithelioma has a better prognosis (60% to 65%) than SCC (40% to 45%). As radiation techniques have improved, local control has also improved; however, hematogenous metastases have been unmasked. With radiation alone, approximately 40% of all failures relapse at the primary site only, whereas 60% are metastatic failures.[19] With chemotherapy, according to Intergroup 0099,[48, 49] the 3-year survival for patients with stage III and IV tumors improved from 46% to 76%. The incidence of distant failure also was reduced from 35% to 13%.

Cancer of Nasal Vestibule, Nasal Cavity, and Paranasal Sinuses

Cancer in this area progresses insidiously, masquerading as chronic sinusitis. Diagnosis is often delayed until the lesion is well advanced. Anatomically, the nasal vestibule is the entrance to the nasal cavity and tumors arising here are usually considered separately from those arising elsewhere in the nasal cavity. The remainder of the nasal cavity includes the septum, floor, choanae, and the inferior, middle and superior turbinates. The paranasal sinuses include the maxillary, ethmoid, sphenoid, and frontal sinuses.

■ NASAL VESTIBULE

Epidemiology and Etiology

The nasal vestibule is lined by skin having numerous hair follicles and glands. The majority of nasal vestibule tumors are squamous cell in nature and are generally moderately to well differentiated. Tobacco usage is common, and the median age at presentation is about 60 years with a male predominance.

Detection and Diagnosis

- Presenting complaints often are a unilateral, persistent nodule. Physical findings may consist of only a crusting or a scab.
- Diagnostic procedures include direct inspection with *nasal speculum, fiberoptic nasal examination,* and *biopsy.*

Classification and Staging

Histopathology

Squamous cell tumors dominate, with other histologies being extremely rare.

Staging

No widely recognized staging system exists for the nasal vestibule. Some older series report results using the same staging system as for skin cancer.[249]

Staging Work-Up

Staging procedures common to all head and neck sites have been discussed earlier in this chapter. Both nasal cavities must be carefully assessed. CT and MRI scans are important to evaluate the degree of tissue infiltration by the tumor. Axial and coronal reconstructions should be obtained.

Patterns of Spread

Patterns of Local Spread

Spread is by direct invasion of contiguous structures. The septal or alar cartilages can be involved, and the tumor can cause perforation of the nasal septum. Growth posteriorly into the nasal cavity can confuse the site of origin. The tumors can spread inferiorly to involve the upper lip and columella.

Metastatic Behavior

Cervical nodes are typically involved in less than 10% of cases, with another 10% to 20% of patients developing nodal metastases at some point in their clinical course.[250, 251] The ipsilateral submandibular node is most commonly involved but the facial nodes are also at risk.

Principles of Treatment

Surgery and irradiation are equally effective as single modalities for smaller lesions. The cosmetic outcome often dictates the choice of therapy. Large lesions require a combined approach.

- *Surgery* is used for lesions invading the bone.
- *Radiation therapy* is preferred for some small lesions because of better cosmetic results. Often a brachytherapy implant can be used.[252] Superficially penetrating electron beams can reduce the attendant side effects.
- *Postoperative radiation* is frequently required after surgical resection of the larger lesions.

Results and Prognosis

Local control rates may approach 100% for smaller lesions treated with brachytherapy implants[250, 251]; in larger tumors, the control rate drops to 50% to 60%.

■ NASAL CAVITY

Epidemiology and Etiology

The nasal cavity begins at the limen nasi, that is, the transition from skin to mucosa, and ends at the posterior choanae, where the nasopharynx begins. Nasal cavity tumors are quite rare in the United States; males are affected more commonly than females (3:2) and median age is 50 to 60 years.[250, 251] Chronic sinusitis, nasal polyps, or both precede the disease in 10% to 20% of cases. Inverting papilloma, although technically a benign lesion, is associated with invasive squamous cell tumors in about 10% to 15% of cases.

A higher-than-expected incidence of adenocarcinoma is found in furniture workers, and workers in the nickel industry have a risk factor approximately 40 times greater than that of the general population.[253]

Detection and Diagnosis

- Presenting symptoms are unilateral nasal obstruction or epistaxis.
- Diagnostic procedures include direct inspection with *nasal speculum, fiberoptic nasal examination,* and *biopsy.*

Classification and Staging

Histopathology

Eighty-five percent of carcinomas in the nasal fossa are SCCs; transitional cell carcinoma is a poorly differentiated variant of SCC. Tumors may have either an ulcerative or a fungating appearance. Minor salivary gland adenocarcinomas may occur (adenoid cystic or mucoepidermoid), but these tumors are considered in a separate section of this chapter. Lymphomas, malignant melanomas, and the rare esthesioneuroblastoma (which arise from the olfactory epithelium) may also be encountered. Such tumors are discussed elsewhere in this text.

Staging

No widely recognized staging system exists for SCC nasal cavity tumors, although staging systems do exist for certain specific lesions such as esthesioneuroblastoma.

Staging Work-Up

Staging procedures common to all head and neck sites have been discussed earlier in this chapter. Both nasal cavities and all paranasal sinuses must be carefully assessed. Radiologic assessment is crucial. Sinonasal CT or MRI scans should be performed in both axial and coronal sections.

Patterns of Spread

Patterns of Local Spread

The most common site of origin is the middle or inferior turbinate, which is attached to the lateral nasal wall. The septum, vestibule, floor, and choanae may also be primary sites. Spread is typically along the walls of the nasal cavity with ready access to the maxillary sinus. Tumors may spread posteriorly, into the nasopharynx, and anteriorly, where they may protrude from the nose. Tumors arising from the roof of the nasal cavity may spread into the anterior cranial fossa; for example, esthesioneuroblastomas arise and invade the skull via the olfactory nerve. Subarachnoid seeding is possible.

Metastatic Behavior

Cervical nodes are rarely involved (8% to 15%) and usually only with locally advanced disease.[250, 251] Jugulodigastric and submandibular are the common nodal sites with retropharyngeal nodes being involved on rare occasions. Hematogenous spread is exceptionally rare.

Principles of Treatment

Surgery and irradiation are equally effective for smaller lesions, whereas large lesions require a combined approach.[250, 251]

- *Surgical approaches* to the nasal cavities include lateral rhinotomy and midface degloving procedures.[254] The mid-face degloving procedure involves no incisions on the external face and offers excellent cosmesis; it also allows for a wider resection compared with lateral rhinotomy.
- *Radiation therapy* typically involves 45 to 50 Gy given to a fairly generous volume followed by a boost to 65 to 70 Gy.[255, 256] Lesions of the septum may be treated with brachytherapy implants.

Results and Prognosis

Reported 5-year survivals are usually between 55% and 85%,[250, 251] depending on stage. Nasal septal tumors have been reported to have a better prognosis than tumors arising elsewhere within the nasal cavity—79% versus 58% determinate 5-year survival.[257] Small lesions limited to one region (e.g., turbinate) have cure rates in excess of 90%.

■ PARANASAL SINUS TUMORS

The paranasal sinuses develop embryologically as diverticuli from the nasal cavity and consist of the maxillary, ethmoid, frontal, and sphenoid sinuses. The cavities are lined with pseudostratified, columnar epithelium and contain mucous glands. Adenocarcinomas are considered of minor salivary gland origin and are discussed elsewhere in this chapter. Squamous cell tumors of the maxillary sinus account for 80% to 90% of all paranasal sinus cancers and are the main topic of the following discussion. Lesions of the ethmoid, frontal, and sphenoid sinuses are mentioned only briefly.

Epidemiology and Etiology

There is approximately a 2:1 male predominance for maxillary sinus cancers, with 95% of cases occurring in patients over 40 years and 75% occurring in the seventh or eighth decades of life.[250] Workers in the nickel and wood working industries have an increased risk of tumors of the maxillary and ethmoid sinuses. In addition, exposure to thorium in Thorotrast is associated with cancers in the maxillary antrum.[250, 251, 253]

Detection and Diagnosis

Clinical Detection

Maxillary and Ethmoid Sinuses

Early lesions masquerade as sinusitis. Any unilateral sinusitis showing bone destruction should be fully investigated. Typical presentations include nasal obstruction, bloody nasal discharge, unilateral sinusitis, loosening of teeth, poor fitting of dental plates, and paresthesia of the anterior cheek (V3). Diplopia, epiphora, or proptosis indicates orbital invasion.

Inspection of the oral cavity may demonstrate tumor extension into the upper alveolus and hard palate. Palpation of the infraorbital ridge for irregularity is important.

Sphenoid Sinus

Cranial nerve palsies and headaches are common presenting symptoms.

Diagnostic Procedures

- *Biopsy* is essential.
- *Imaging*: Plain sinus x-rays have been largely supplanted by screening sinus CT scanning for the evaluation of chronic sinusitis. As such, the diagnosis of an incidental finding of sinus cancer has been improved. *CT* and *MRI* scans should be performed in both axial and coronal planes to show adjacent parasinus invasion.

Classification and Staging

Histopathology

More than 85% of these lesions are SCCs with various degrees of differentiation.

Staging

Only the maxillary and ethmoid sinuses have commonly accepted staging systems as summarized, respectively, in Tables 20–20 and 20–21. The staging system for tumors of the maxillary sinus is shown schematically in Figure 20–11. Previous staging systems for the maxillary sinus were based on dividing it into an anteroinferior portion (the infrastructure) and a posterosuperior portion (the suprastructure) via Ohngren's line, which joins the medial canthus of the eye with the angle of the mandible. This designation is still useful for discussion of therapeutic options.

Staging Work-Up

Staging procedures common to all head and neck sites have been discussed earlier in this chapter. Especially important for this site is *nasal endoscopy. Fine-cut CT* scanning provides important information with regard to tumor extension beyond the sinus.

TABLE 20–20. **TNM Classification and Stage Grouping of the Maxillary Sinus**

Stage	Grouping	TNM Classification
Stage 0	Tis, N0, M0	Tis: Carcinoma *in situ* N0: No regional lymph node metastasis M0: No distant metastasis
Stage I	T1, N0, M0	T1: Antral mucosa, no bone involvement
Stage II	T2, N0, M0	T2: Bone erosion or destruction, except for posterior wall
Stage III	T3, N0–1, M0	T3: Cheek, floor of orbit, ethmoid, posterior wall of sinus, pterygoids, infratemporal fossa
	T1, N1, M0 T2, N1, M0	N1: Metastasis in a singular ipsilateral lymph node, ≤3 cm
Stage IVA	T4, N0–1, M0	T4: Orbital contents and other adjacent structures
Stage IVB	Any T, N2–3, M0	N2: Metastasis in a single ipsilateral lymph node, >3 cm but ≤6 cm; or, in multiple ipsilateral lymph nodes, none >6 cm; or in bilateral or contralateral lymph nodes, none >6 cm* N3: Metastasis in a lymph node >6 cm
Stage IVC	Any T, any N, M1	M1: Distant metastasis

T = tumor; N = node; M = metastasis.

*N2a: metastasis in single ipsilateral lymph node >3 cm; but not >6 cm; N2b: metastasis in multiple ipsilateral lymph nodes, none >6 cm; N2c: metastasis in bilateral or contralateral lymph nodes, none >6 cm.

TABLE 20–21. **TNM Classification and Stage Grouping of the Ethmoid Sinus**

Stage	Grouping	TNM Classification
Stage 0	Tis, N0, M0	Tis: Carcinoma *in situ* N0: No regional lymph node metastasis M0: No distant metastasis
Stage I	T1, N0, M0	T1: Tumor confined to ethmoids
Stage II	T2, N0, M0	T2: Tumor extends into nasal cavity
Stage III	T3, N0–1, M0 T1, N1, M0 T2, N1, M0	T3: Tumor extends to anterior orbit and/or maxillary sinus N1: Metastasis in a singular ipsilateral lymph node, ≤3 cm
Stage IVA	T4, N0–1, M0	T4: Tumor has intracranial extension involving sphenoid or frontal sinuses, extension into orbital apex and/or skin of nose
Stage IVB	Any T, N2–3, M0	N2: Metastasis in a single ipsilateral lymph node, >3 cm but not >6 cm; or, in multiple ipsilateral lymph nodes, none >6 cm; or in bilateral or contralateral lymph nodes, none >6 cm* N3: Metastasis in a lymph node >6 cm
Stage IVC	Any T, any N, M1	M1: Distant metastasis

T = tumor; N = mode; M = metastasis.

*N2a: metastasis in single ipsilateral lymph node >3 cm, but not >6 cm; N2b: metastasis in multiple ipsilateral lymph nodes, none >6 cm; N2c: metastasis in bilateral or contralateral lymph nodes, none >6 cm.

Used with permission of the American Joint Committee on Cancer (AJCC®), Chicago, Illinois. The original source for this material is the AJCC® Cancer Staging Manual, 5th ed, 1997, published by Lippincott-Raven Publishers, Philadelphia, Pennsylvania; and International Union Against Cancer (UICC): TNM Classification of Malignant Tumors, 4th ed, New York, Springer-Verlag, 1992.

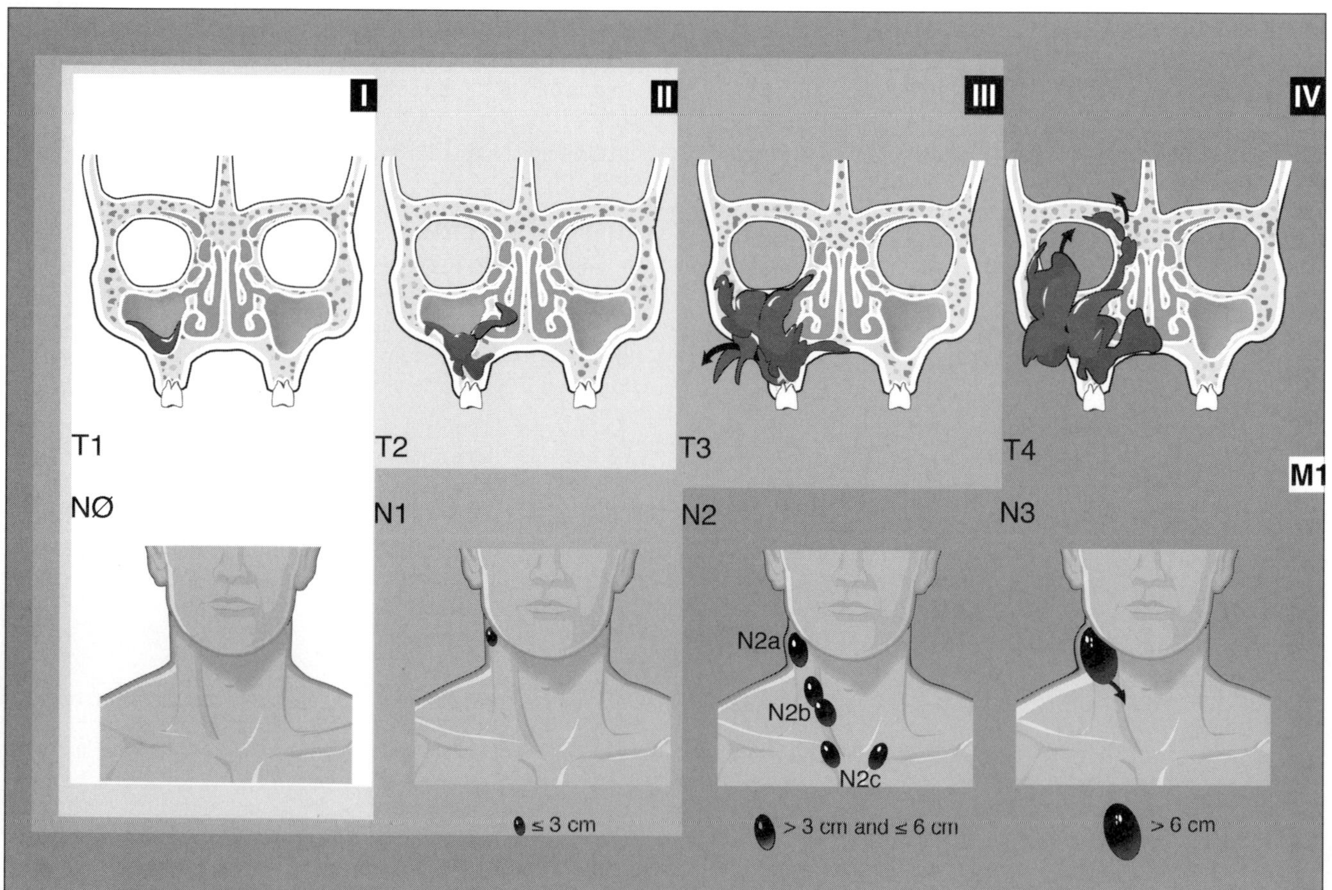

Figure 20–11. Anatomic staging system for tumors of the maxillary sinus. The primary staging system is characterized by depth of tumor penetration and extension to adjacent structures. A T1 tumor is confined to the antral mucosa; a T2 tumor erodes bone or extends into the hard palate or middle nasal meatus; a T3 tumor invades the floor of the orbit, ethmoid sinus, cheek, or the posterior wall of the sinus; a T4 tumor invades the orbital contents and/or extends intracranially or to other structures. The nodal staging is shown in the lower row.

Patterns of Spread

Patterns of Local Spread

Maxillary sinus: Lesions of the suprastructure tend to break through the floor of the orbit, involve infraorbital nerve, and displace the eye, causing diplopia. Extension superomedially leads to involvement of the ethmoid sinus. Posterior extension leads to involvement of the pterygoid plates, muscles, infratemporal fossa, and skull base. Infrastructure lesions erode through the floor of the sinus and appear as fungations on the superior maxillary alveolus, gingivobuccal sulcus, and hard palate. Anterior extension erodes through the bone to involve the skin of the cheek.

Ethmoid sinus: Spread may be intracranial superiorly, into the orbit laterally and into the nasal cavity or maxillary sinus inferiorly.

Sphenoid sinus: Spread may be intracranially or into the nasopharynx anteriorly.

Metastatic Behavior

Cervical node involvement is uncommon (10% to 15%); when it occurs, it is usually to the ipsilateral submandibular node.[258] Spread into the subcutaneous tissues of the cheek puts the facial node at risk. During follow-up an additional 14% to 29% of patients in whom the neck is untreated may develop nodal metastases.[250, 259] Distant metastases are uncommon and usually appear with massive locally recurrent disease.

Principles of Treatment

Maxillary Sinus

Principles of treatment for carcinoma of the maxillary sinus are summarized in Table 20–22.

- Although it is possible to cure a portion of early lesions with surgery or radiation alone, the most fruitful approach for most cases is a *combined surgical-radiotherapeutic* program.[250, 251] This combined approach is clearly required for more advanced tumors.
- Although investigational, concomitant chemotherapy along with radiotherapy seems to aid in local control, particularly for the more poorly differentiated tumors.

Surgery

Surgery alone can be used for lesions restricted to the antral mucosa. Medially located lesions can be resected with a medial maxillectomy. Total maxillectomy can be performed with or without orbital exenteration for orbital extension. In cases in which radiation therapy or combined chemoradiation are the primary modalities, before initiating radiotherapy, limited drainage procedures may be necessary to deal with tumor necrosis and infection. A neck dissection is added for involved nodes.

Reconstruction is important for appearance, speech, and eating. The majority of maxillectomy procedures spare the overlying facial skin. Obturator inserts are commonly attached to denture plates and fill out the area behind the cheek. The mid-face can also be reconstructed with bone and soft tissue using a scapular or iliac crest microvascular free flap.[59, 61]

Radiation Therapy

Radiation is usually given as an adjuvant to surgery. It may be given either preoperatively or postoperatively, and 60 to 70 Gy is given depending on the tumor burden left behind after surgery. The radiation fields must encompass the entire maxillary sinus, adjacent nasal cavity and ethmoids, and a portion of the orbit, and orbital shielding must be used carefully to avoid blocking areas at risk for residual disease. If residual disease remains following surgery, then additional radiotherapy may be given via brachytherapy molds inserted into the surgical defect. Definitive radiotherapy to maximum doses requires careful treatment planning and delivery.

Although it is generally not believed to be necessary to treat the N0 neck, data suggest that this should be performed for more advanced tumors.[259] Extending the treatment fields in this manner adds considerable morbidity.

Ethmoid Sinus

A surgical resection must be *en bloc* and a cranial-facial approach may be required. Radiation is given postoperatively except for completely resected early-stage tumors. Definitive radiotherapy is given when surgery is not an option.

TABLE 20–22. **Carcinoma of the Maxillary Sinus: Principles of Treatment**

Stage		Surgery	Radiation Therapy	Chemotherapy
I	T1, N0	Limited resection of maxillary sinus	ART: optional postop	NR
II	T2, N0	Limited or complete resection of maxillary sinus	ART: 50–60 Gy pre- or postop	NR
III	T3, N0	Total maxillectomy with or without orbital exenteration	ART: 50–60 Gy pre- or postop	IC II
IV	T4, N3	If resectable, total maxillectomy with or without orbital exenteration and radical ND, if possible	DRT: 70 Gy incl. to foci BT boost 10–20 Gy	IC II
Relapse after Rx				
		Selected cases	NR	IC II
For N0		NR	NR	NR
For N1,2		Radical ND if primary controlled	Postop RT	IC II

ND = neck dissection; RT = radiation therapy; DRT = definitive; ART = adjuvant; BT = brachytherapy mold; NR = not recommended; ICII = investigational chemotherapy, phase I/II clinical trial.

From Kramer TS: Nasal vestibule, nasal cavity, and paranasal sinuses. In: Laramore GE (ed): Radiation Therapy of Head and Neck Cancer, pp 145–170. Berlin, Springer-Verlag, 1989; and Parsons JT, Stringer SP, Mancuso AA, et al: Nasal vestibule, nasal cavity, and paranasal sinuses. In: Million, RR, Cassisi, NJ (eds): Management of Head and Neck Cancer: A Multidisciplinary Approach, 2nd ed, pp 551–598. Philadelphia, J. B. Lippincott, 1994; with permission.

Sphenoid Sinus

Tumors in this area are generally treated with definitive radiotherapy in the same manner as nasopharyngeal tumors.

Results and Prognosis

Overall 5-year survival is typically 20% to 30%, but with combined therapy survival may approach 75% for early-stage lesions of the maxillary sinus.[250, 251] The mortality of this disease is largely owing to locally recurrent disease leading to base of skull and intracranial invasion. A report by Waldron and coworkers[260] describes 29 cases of ethmoid sinus tumors, of which only 12 were SCC. Although the overall local failure rate for the entire group of 29 patients was 48%, the local failure rate was 75% for the SCC group. Data are lacking on treatment results for SCCs of the sphenoid sinus, which may be hard to distinguish from advanced nasopharyngeal tumors.

Unknown Primary Tumors

Unknown primary refers to the situation in which a patient presents with metastatic disease and careful evaluation fails to reveal a primary site. Herein we are concerned with the specific situation in which a patient develops a cervical lymph node metastasis that is histologically proven to be SCC; such cases represent approximately 3% to 5% of all head and neck cancer cases. Although it is possible for an adenocarcinoma of the head and neck (e.g., thyroid or salivary gland) to present in this manner, the overwhelming majority of adenocarcinomas that are metastatic to the cervical nodes originate below the clavicles. The location of the lymph node may give a clue as to the probable site of origin.[261] Definitive treatment in this setting can yield 5-year survival in the range of 30% to 50%.[262–264]

Epidemiology and Etiology

The classic presentation is a single, solitary neck mass that is discovered by the patient. Location is critical in prognosis: high jugular or midjugular nodes versus supraclavicular (Virchow's nodes). About 15% of cases have multiple unilateral masses and 10% have bilateral neck masses.[262] The age, sex, and racial background of the patient can provide clues as to the possible primary site. Pain may indicate the presence of necrosis in the node. Cranial nerve abnormalities are uncommon but may occur. Most patients in whom the neck mass is confirmed to be a carcinoma will have a history of excessive tobacco or alcohol use, or both.

Detection and Diagnosis

A careful history and physical examination may reveal clues to the primary site of origin.[261, 265] In children a neck mass is generally of infectious etiology. A thyroid carcinoma is more likely to occur in females, and nasopharyngeal carcinoma is more likely in patients with an Asian or Aleut ethnic background. It is important to determine whether a skin cancer has been previously removed from the head and neck region.

A history of earaches, particularly with swallowing, suggests a primary site in the hypopharynx or oropharynx, with the pain being referred via branches of the IX and X nerves. Hoarseness may indicate a primary in the larynx or hypopharynx, but could also indicate a mediastinal tumor involving the recurrent laryngeal nerve. Nasal stuffiness can result from tumors in the nasopharynx or paranasal sinuses. Serous otitis or cranial nerve symptoms are often suggestive of nasopharyngeal tumors.

High jugular nodes suggest a nasopharyngeal, oropharyngeal, or hypopharyngeal primary, whereas midjugular nodes suggest a laryngeal, hypopharyngeal, or thyroid primary. Metastatic disease in the posterior cervical chain is most suggestive of a nasopharyngeal primary. Low cervical nodes suggest thyroid, cervical esophagus, or lung primaries. It must be kept in mind that the jugulodigastric node is the most commonly involved node for most sites in the head and neck.

Diagnostic Procedures

- Repeated *physical examinations* by different physicians can often determine the primary site.
- Contrast-enhanced *CT* or *MRI* scans, or both, are key studies.
- *PET* imaging shows promise in identifying the primary site.[43]
- A *chest radiograph* will rule out either a lung primary or further metastatic spread of tumor.
- *Examination under anesthesia* with particular attention to the nasopharynx, base of tongue, and pyriform sinus is helpful. Directed biopsies of any suspicious areas are indicated.
- Elective random *biopsies* of the nasopharynx may be indicated.
- *EBV titers*, if elevated, may suggest a nasopharyngeal primary.[26]
- Either a *needle biopsy* or an *excision* of the node may be necessary to establish a diagnosis if the primary site is not found.

Classification and Staging

The great majority of neck masses (other than in supraclavicular locations) turn out to be a result of benign conditions.[266] Malignant conditions can include lymphomas, carotid body tumors, malignant melanoma, plasmacytoma, and adnexal skin cancers. In the Johnson and Newman series,[266] only about 5% of cases turned out to be of squamous cell origin without an identifiable primary site.

Principles of Treatment

We recommend treating the mucosal sites of likely primary tumor origin as well as the neck itself. If the neck mass alone is addressed, with surgery or ipsilateral neck irradiation, or both, then the incidence of subsequent development of a mucosal primary is in the range of 20% to 44%.[261–265, 267] If an occult primary develops after treatment, then the 5-year survival probability is in the range of 20% to 30%.[262, 264]

Surgery

Surgery is important in treating the involved neck in the case of advanced nodal disease. Although there is some debate regarding a limited excision versus a neck dissection, it is generally believed that a neck dissection is warranted in situations in which the nodal mass is greater than 3 cm (e.g., nodal stage >N1). Reddy and Marks[264] found that the disease-free 5-year survival was 61% for those patients who had a neck dissection before radiotherapy, compared with 37% for those patients who had only a nodal biopsy before radiotherapy.

Radiation Therapy

Radiation fields should cover the whole neck, the supraclavicular fossa, and the probable primary sites. The uninvolved neck and supraclavicular fossa should receive 50 Gy, whereas the involved neck and probable mucosal sites should receive 55 to 60 Gy. If specific high-risk factors are present in the involved neck after a surgical dissection, then this area should receive 63 to 65 Gy.[50] The treatment fields should cover the nasopharynx, tonsillar fossa, base of tongue, Waldeyer's ring, and pyriform sinus. Because the principal side effect of treatment is xerostomia, patients should have adequate dental prophylaxis before therapy.

Results and Prognosis

If the probable mucosal primary sites are treated with radiotherapy, the subsequent development of a primary head and neck lesion is in the range of 6% to 8%, compared with 20% to 40% in patients in which the mucosal surfaces at risk were not treated.[261–265, 267] Overall 5-year survivals are in the range of 30% to 50%.[262–264]

Tumors of the Ear

Tumors of the external and middle ear complex are rare but pose serious management problems. The lesions often masquerade as chronic inflammatory or degenerative diseases, which results in delayed diagnosis. In this section, we will discuss only carcinomas, leaving the discussion of chemodectomas to the next section.

Classification and Staging

No universally accepted classification has been proposed. A useful subdivision classified these lesions in terms of their site of origin:

- carcinoma of the auricle
- carcinoma of the external auditory canal
- carcinoma of the petromastoid (origin in the middle ear—mastoid complex)

Carcinoma of the auricle is a variant of skin cancer, with a correspondingly excellent outlook. Carcinomas of the auditory canal and the petromastoid have a poorer prognosis, largely owing to delay in diagnosis, their proximity to vital structures, and a tendency toward conservative, rather than radical, therapeutic measures. More than 85% of the mortality of ear cancer results from local recurrence leading to intracranial extension.[268]

Principles of Treatment

Small lesions limited to the auditory canal can be managed by surgery or radiation therapy. However, most patients require an aggressive combined surgical-radiotherapeutic approach.

Surgery

Lesions of the external auditory canal, limited to the cartilaginous portion, can be removed with a sleeve resection. Lesions that encroach on the bony canal can be removed *en bloc* by a lateral temporal bone resection.[269] The approach is via the mastoid and all structures lateral to the middle ear ossicles are removed. If uninvolved by tumor, then the facial nerve is left undisturbed. Larger tumors may require complete temporal bone resections that include dissection down to the level of the carotid artery.[270] Reconstruction requires attention to the resulting facial nerve paralysis.

Radiation Therapy

Radiation fields should be localized to the primary unless lymph nodes are clinically or radiographically involved. Either a photon wedge pair (often oriented superiorly-inferiorly) or a combination of electrons and photons may be used.[271, 272] The target dose should be in the range of 65 to 70 Gy, with careful attention to field shaping and beam entry directions, so that adjacent areas of the central nervous system do not exceed tolerance doses.

Results and Prognosis

Control for early-stage lesions is in the range of 90%, whereas local control is in the range of 30% to 50% for more advanced tumors.[270–272]

Chemodectoma

Chemodectomas arise from collections of neuroepithelial cells that are distributed throughout the body.[273] They are most commonly found in the temporal bone (glomus jugulare tumors) or in the cervical region (carotid body, intravagale, or ganglion nodosum). Histologically, they resemble the glomus bodies from which they arise. They tend to be highly vascular, and those arising in the temporal bone may be locally destructive. Only a very small percentage of these tumors undergo a malignant degeneration. No universally accepted staging classification exists.

Detection and Diagnosis

Temporal Bone Tumors

Clinical presentations include deafness, pulsatile tinnitus, otalgia, facial paralysis, and otorrhea. Symptoms are usually of several years' standing. The female-to-male ratio is approximately 5 to 1 and the median age is 50 to 60 years.[274]

Diagnosis demands a high index of suspicion:

- *Otoscopy* is abnormal in 90% of patients, revealing a pulsating red eardrum or a polypoid mass in the external canal.
- *CT scans* are essential to evaluate bone destruction.
- *Carotid arteriography* is diagnostic in most cases and reveals a characteristic vascular blush, best visualized with subtraction techniques.
- *Biopsy* may be hazardous because of extreme bleeding and is not necessary in most cases.

Carotid Body Tumors

Clinical presentations are most generally a painless mass at the bifurcation of the common carotid artery. Although uncommon, cranial nerve palsies involving IX, X, and XII may be present. The female-to-male ratio is approximately 1:1 and the average age at onset is 40 to 50 years, although the range of presentation is wide.

Diagnosis similarly requires a high index of suspicion:

- *CT* or *MRI scan* with contrast is usually sufficient for diagnosis.
- *Angiography* reveals the characteristic high degree of vascularity associated with these tumors.
- *Biopsy* may be hazardous because of extreme bleeding and is not necessary in most cases.
- In the absence of hypertension, urinary catecholamine metabolite testing is probably not necessary but needs to be considered.

Principles of Treatment

Temporal Bone Tumors

Treatment for early lesions arising in the tympanic cavity (glomus tympanicum) without significant extension is surgical excision.[275] Lesions arising in the jugular bulb (glomus jugulare) or extensive lesions of the tympanic cavity can be managed with surgery or radiation therapy. Although formal dose response data are lacking, it is generally believed that doses of 45 to 50 Gy produce prolonged growth delay and probably permanent control in most patients.[276–278] These tumors generally do not regress markedly but rather stabilize in size and do not regrow in 80% to 90% of irradiated patients. Radiation therapy will usually improve tinnitus, otalgia, and otorrhea; hearing is rarely restored and cranial nerve palsies are usually permanent. Surgical resection for glomus jugulare lesions is performed in some centers, and although good results have been reported with this formidable procedure in terms of tumor control, the complication rate approaches 20%.[276]

Carotid Body Tumors

When resection is possible, surgery is the treatment of choice for these lesions. These tumors can become locally invasive and as they become more advanced, the incidence of operative complications increases. Although the majority of these lesions have been treated surgically, there is evidence that radiation is effective as well. Doses in the range of 45 to 50 Gy provide long-term control.[279]

Results and Prognosis

Prognosis for survival is excellent; fewer than 10% of patients die from this disease within 5 years of diagnosis. However, very long-term recurrences occur often, delayed by 10 or more years. Nonetheless, most patients will die with their disease rather than because of it.

Tumors of the Salivary Glands

Salivary gland tumors are relatively rare, constituting about 5% to 7% of all head and neck malignancies. There are approximately 2000 to 2500 such tumors occurring each year in the United States; about 85% of salivary gland tumors arise in the parotid glands and about 75% of these are benign. The majority of these benign growths are pleomorphic adenomas (also known as benign mixed tumors); less frequently occurring benign tumors are monomorphic adenomas and Warthin's tumors.

With respect to the other major salivary glands, about 50% of submandibular tumors are malignant and approximately 100% of tumors arising in the sublingual glands are malignant. There are also between 600 and 1000 minor nests of glandular cells scattered throughout the upper aerodigestive tract, and about 75% of tumors arising in these minor salivary glands are malignant. The relatively long natural history of many of these tumors makes it difficult to accurately assess the impact of new treatment modalities.

Epidemiology and Etiology

Except for tumors of Warthin's duct, for which there is approximately a 5:1 male-to-female ratio, there is no sexual predilection. Although these tumors can occur at any age, the median age of occurrence is 40 to 50 years.[7] Radiation exposure is the only known etiologic factor.[33] Some studies indicate an association between salivary gland tumors and breast cancer.[280, 281]

Detection and Diagnosis

Clinical Detection

Parotid lesions present as a swelling in the parotid area. Clinical features suggestive of parotid malignancy include rapid growth of lesion, local pain, facial palsy, tenderness, attachment to surrounding structures, trismus, and palpable cervical nodes. Submandibular and sublingual lesions generally present as a painless, firm mass.

Minor salivary lesions may occur anywhere along the mucosa of the aerodigestive tract and usually present as nodular surface growths, often without ulceration. The hard palate is the most common site, but the base of tongue is another frequent location.

Diagnostic Procedures

- Tumor may masquerade as acute infection; the character of salivary discharge should be noted and a *culture* taken.
- *Bimanual examination* should be performed for parotid, submandibular, and sublingual lesions to locate site of primary and exclude calculi.
- *Imaging*: Plain x-ray studies and sialograms may be helpful in major gland lesions but have been largely supplanted by CT or MRI, or by both.
- *Needle aspiration cytology* is accurate in a high proportion of cases and may be used for diagnosis.
- *Incisional biopsies* are generally not performed. Parotid lesions can be diagnosed by *superficial lobectomy*—frozen section examination. Submandibular or sublingual gland lesions need excision and frozen section evaluation.
- Minor salivary gland tumors are generally diagnosed by *standard biopsy.*

Classification and Staging

Histopathology

The most detailed classification of salivary gland malignancies was performed by Batsakis and Regezi.[282] As a working model, one can group these tumors into two major categories:

- *Low grade,* consisting of low-grade mucoepidermoid tumors, acinic cell carcinomas, and the occasional low-grade adenocarcinoma
- *High grade,* consisting of high-grade mucoepidermoid carcinomas, most adenocarcinomas, carcinomas, pleomorphic adenomas, adenoid cystic carcinomas, malignant mixed tumors, and squamous cell tumors

In a patient with a squamous cell tumor of the parotid, care must be take to rule out a periparotid metastasis from a squamous cell skin cancer of the head or facial region. Histology is an important factor in survival.[283]

Staging

The T-staging system for major salivary gland tumors is defined in Table 20–23 and illustrated in Figure 20–12. The nodal staging system is the same as for other head and neck sites as indicated in Table 20–2 and Figure 20–3. Stage grouping differs from other head and neck sites, as indicated in Table 20–23. There is no commonly accepted staging system for tumors of minor salivary gland origin, but some papers report results using the same staging system as for SCCs arising in the same sites.

Staging Work-Up

Staging procedures common to all head and neck sites have been described earlier in this chapter. Procedures of particular note for salivary gland tumors include cranial nerve evaluation and CT or MRI scans, or both, to evaluate local tumor extension. Sialograms may be indicated for parotid or submandibular lesions.

TABLE 20–23. **TNM Classification and Stage Grouping of the Major Salivary Glands**

Stage	Grouping	TNM Classification
Stage I	T1, N0, M0	T1: Tumor ≤2 cm N0: No regional lymph node metastasis M0: No distant metastasis
	T2, N0, M0	T2: Tumor >2 cm, but ≤4 cm
Stage II	T3, N0, M0	T3: >4 cm, but ≤6 cm and/or having extraparenchymal extension
Stage III	T1, N1, M0 T2, N1, M0	N1: Metastasis in a singular ipsilateral lymph node, ≤3 cm
Stage IV	T3, N1–3, M0 T4, any N, M0 Any T, any N, M1 Any T, N2–3, M0	N2: Metastasis in a single ipsilateral lymph node, >3 cm but not >6 cm; or, in multiple ipsilateral lymph nodes, none >6 cm; or in bilateral or contralateral lymph nodes, none >6 cm* N3: Metastasis in a lymph node >6 cm T4: >6 cm and/or invades VII nerve or base of skull M1: Distant metastasis

T = tumor; N = node; M = metastasis.

*N2a: metastasis in single ipsilateral lymph node >3 cm, but not >6 cm; N2b: metastasis in multiple ipsilateral lymph nodes, none >6 cm; N2c: metastasis in bilateral or contralateral lymph nodes, none >6 cm.

Used with permission of the American Joint Committee on Cancer (AJCC®), Chicago, Illinois. The original source for this material is the AJCC® Cancer Staging Manual, 5th ed, 1997, published by Lippincott-Raven Publishers, Philadelphia, Pennsylvania; and International Union Against Cancer (UICC): TNM Classification of Malignant Tumors, 4th ed, New York, Springer-Verlag, 1992.

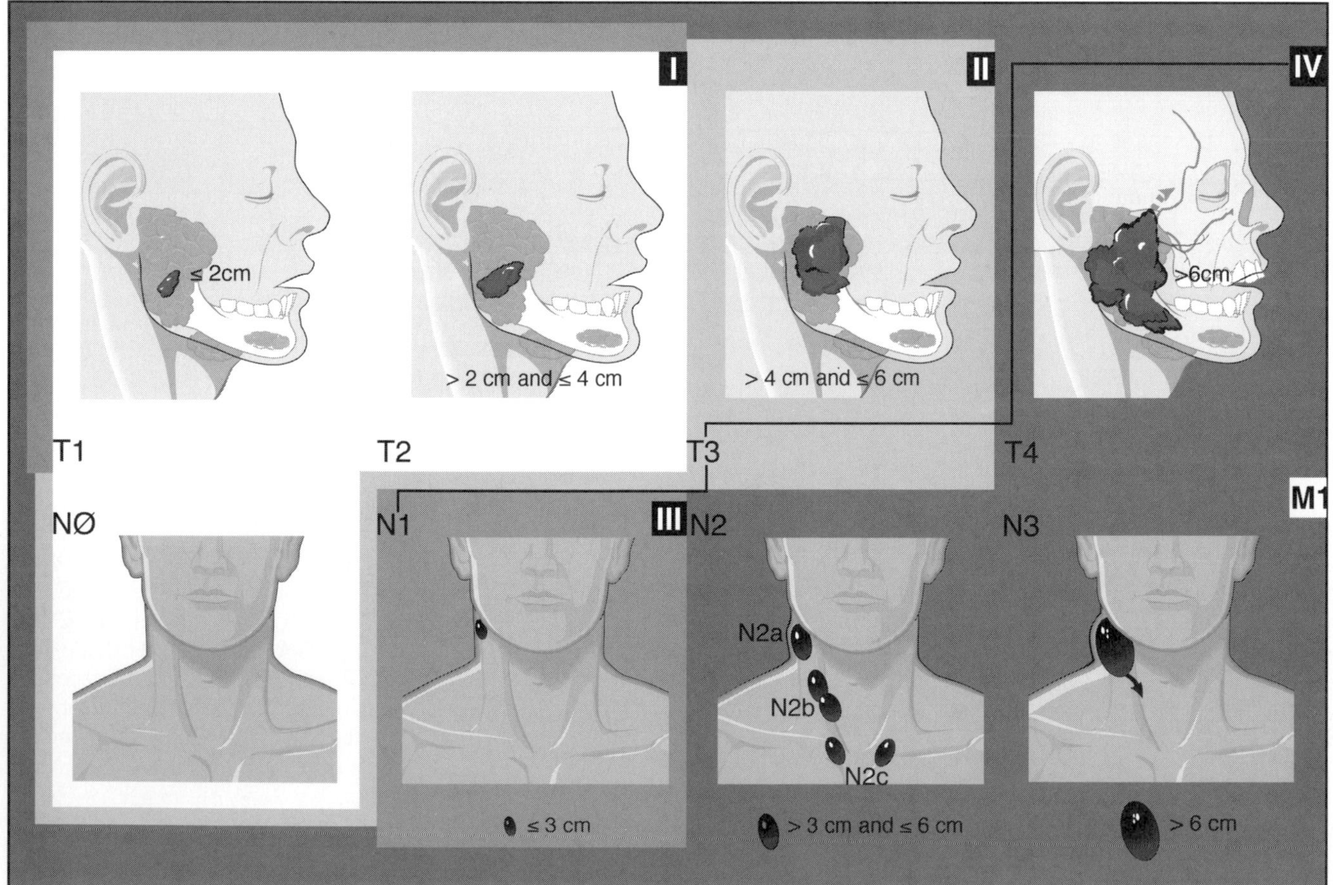

Figure 20–12. Anatomic staging system for major salivary gland tumors (parotid gland is illustrated). The primary staging system is characterized first by size and then by extension to adjacent structures. For T1 and T2 lesions, the cutoff diameters are 2 cm or smaller and larger than 2 cm but 4 cm or smaller, respectively. A T3 tumor is larger than 4 cm but 6 cm or smaller and/or has extraparenchymal extension. Massive tumors >6 cm and/or invading the VII nerve or base of skull are characterized as T4. The nodal staging is shown in the lower row.

Patterns of Spread

Patterns of Local Spread

Parotid gland cancers arise in the superficial lobe (lateral to the facial nerve) in 90% of cases. Local growth is by expansion and infiltration of parotid gland, and pain or facial nerve paralysis are highly indicative of malignancy. Large lesions involve skin and may erode the mandible. Deep lobe lesions may present as an oropharyngeal growth or with cranial nerve involvement. Submandibular and sublingual growths spread beyond the gland early and enter surrounding tissues. Tumors of minor salivary glands have a variable local growth pattern depending on the specific site of origin. Adenoid cystic carcinoma, in all sites, has a tendency to involve peripheral nerves and to spread centrally in a perineural pattern.

Metastatic Behavior

The incidence of cervical node metastases varies according to histologic subtype.[284] For parotid tumors, the incidence at presentation is approximately 44% for high-grade mucoepidermoid, 21% for malignant mixed tumor, 37% for squamous cell, 13% for acinic cell, and 5% for adenoid cystic. Hematogenous metastases are common and range from about 13% for acinic cell carcinoma to 41% for adenoid cystic carcinoma.[284] Lung metastases from adenoid cystic carcinomas may lie quiescent for years after presentation and the patient may not require immediate treatment; some patients can live asymptomatically with their metastases.

TABLE 20–24. **Effect of Postoperative Radiation Therapy on Local Control of Salivary Gland Tumors**

Reference	Surgery	Surgery & Radiation Therapy
Fu et al[286]	39/52 (75%)	24/29 (83%)
Shidnia et al[287]	22/38 (58%)	21/30 (70%)
Tran et al[288]	36/68 (53%)	43/57 (75%)
Fitzpatrick and Theriault[289]	30/110 (27%)	174/239 (73%)
Borthne et al[290]	51/96 (53%)	34/52 (66%)
Miglianico et al[291]	17/38 (44%)	33/43 (78%)
Reddy and Marks[292]	0/12 (0%)	6/8 (75%)
Bisset and Fitzpatrick[293]	9/30 (30%)	37/54 (68%)
North et al[294]	13/23 (58%)	62/67 (92%)
Armstrong et al[295]	30/46 (66%)	36/46 (73%)
Frankenthaler et al[296]	73/91 (80%)	56/64 (88%)
Molinari et al[297]	31/36 (85%)	22/32 (68%)
OVERALL	**351/640 (55%)**	**548/721 (76%)**

Numbers indicate the number of patients in the various series; percentages indicate local control probability.

Principles of Treatment

Malignant Tumors

Surgery

In general, surgery is the primary treatment for patients with operable, localized tumors, regardless of histology. For parotid tumors, one generally attempts to spare the facial nerve, but nerve graft procedures can restore reasonable cosmesis if its sacrifice is required.[285] For low-grade tumors, the neck is generally dissected only if there is indication of metastatic disease. In the case of high-grade tumors, neck dissection or other treatment is recommended as a prophylactic measure in N0 necks.

Radiation Therapy

Although salivary gland tumors were once considered to be radioresistant, it is now recognized that radiation therapy has a role to play, both in an adjuvant setting for operable tumors and also in the treatment of inoperable lesions. Table 20–24 shows the effect of adjuvant radiotherapy in reducing the rate of local and regional recurrence following surgery. Unfortunately, a similar analysis does not point to a corresponding increase in patient survival.

Postoperative radiotherapy is indicated:

- whenever the tumor is high grade (any histology except low-grade mucoepidermoid, low-grade adenocarcinoma, or acinic cell carcinoma with clear margins), or is metastatic squamous cell carcinoma regardless of the surgical margins
- when the surgical margins are "close" or microscopically positive (which will include most deep lobe tumors in which the facial nerve was not sacrificed) regardless of the grade of the lesion
- when the resection has been performed for recurrent disease regardless of the margin status or tumor histology
- when tumor has invaded skin, bone, nerve, or extraglandular tissue
- when regional nodes are confirmed positive on a neck dissection
- when there is gross residual or unresectable disease

In the postoperative setting, the primary resection bed is generally given 60 to 63 Gy if the margins are clear; higher doses in the range of 70 to 75 Gy are used if there is gross residual disease. For any histology except low-grade mucoepidermoid tumors and the occasional low-grade adenocarcinoma, the clinically N0 neck is generally treated to 50 Gy. In the case of adenoid cystic carcinomas that have a propensity to spread along cranial nerves, the initial radiation fields must cover the courses of the cranial nerves adjacent to (or traversing) the tumor to the point where they enter the base of skull.

In the case of unresectable tumors, local control with conventionally fractionated radiotherapy is only about 25%.[197] High linear energy transfer neutron radiation seems to be more effective than conventional photon radiotherapy in this setting. A randomized, clinical trial conducted by the RTOG and the Medical Research Council of Great Britain has shown a highly significant improvement in locoregional control for major salivary gland tumors using fast neutron radiotherapy.[198] Unfortunately, as a result of distant metastases, there was no corresponding improvement in long-term survival.

Minor salivary gland tumors also seem to respond well

to fast neutrons, with local control rates approaching 60% for tumors in which there were no dose-limiting neural tissues.[298] Modern, hospital-based, neutron radiotherapy facilities allow precise shaping of the beam and thus cause fewer side effects than occurred with the older, laboratory-based facilities. In addition, use of conventional photon radiotherapy in an accelerated fractionation regimen may improve the results over those achieved using a conventional fractionation schema. Wang and Goodman showed 5-year actuarial local control rates of 100% for 9 parotid tumors and 78% for 15 minor salivary gland tumors treated with an accelerated, twice-a-day fractionation schema.[263] Although these results are intriguing, a randomized clinical trial is required to truly evaluate this approach.

Pleomorphic Adenomas

Pleomorphic adenomas of the parotid gland are a special topic in themselves and are the most common parotid gland tumor. They rarely infiltrate the facial nerve and so may generally be treated with a superficial parotidectomy. Long-term local control rates with surgery alone are in the range of 95% or better.[300]

A more limited excision followed by postoperative radiotherapy can achieve equivalent success, but there may be a small risk of a malignant transformation.[301] Barton and associates[302] argued that postoperative radiotherapy should be used in situations in which there is tumor spillage or gross residual disease left behind at surgery and noted that recurrences may take place beyond 20 years. This points out the necessity for long-term follow-up to evaluate both response and complications. In such settings, a dose to approximately 60 to 65 Gy in 1.8- to 2.0-Gy increments to the resection bed would be appropriate. In situations in which one is dealing with a large, recurrent tumor after one or more previous surgeries and the next surgery would be fraught with morbidity, fast neutron radiotherapy might be an option.[303]

Recommended Reading

A basic discussion of the principles of radiation therapy as they apply to the treatment of head and neck tumors is given in the book chapter by Laramore.[1] The texts by Million and Cassisi[2] and Wang[3] provide excellent, detailed descriptions of head and neck cancer and its treatment. The text by Laramore[4] gives a clinically oriented discussion of the role of radiotherapy in the treatment of head and neck cancer and provides a good summary of expected outcomes using standard techniques before the advent of concomitant chemotherapy-radiotherapy and hyperfractionated radiotherapy trials. The classic text by Fletcher[5] is always relevant. For more on the surgical perspective, the single volume surgical atlas by Bailey and colleagues[6] includes explanations of standard head and neck oncologic extirpative and reconstructive procedures along with their indications. A comprehensive review of the pathology of head and neck neoplasms is presented by Gnepp.[7] The book chapter by Clayman and associates[8] provides an overview of the problem of second malignant tumors in the head and neck tumor patient population and approaches to their prevention.

REFERENCES

General References

1. Laramore GE: General principles of radiation therapy for head and neck cancer. In: Myers EN, Suen JY (eds): Cancer of the Head and Neck, 3rd ed, pp 768–781. Philadelphia, W.B. Saunders Co., 1996.
2. Million RR, Cassisi NJ (eds): Management of Head and Neck Cancer: A Multidisciplinary Approach, 2nd ed. Philadelphia, Lippincott, 1994.
3. Wang CC: Radiation Therapy for Head and Neck Neoplasms: Indications, Techniques, and Results. Boston, John Wright–PSG Inc., 1983.
4. Laramore GE (ed): Radiation Therapy of the Head and Neck Cancer. Berlin, Springer-Verlag, 1989.
5. Fletcher GH (ed): Textbook of Radiotherapy. Philadelphia, Lea & Febiger, 1980.
6. Bailey BJ, Calhoun KH, Coffey AR, et al (eds): Atlas of Head & Neck Surgery—Otolaryngology. Philadelphia, Lippincott-Raven, 1996.
7. Gnepp DR: Pathology of the Head and Neck. New York: Churchill Livingstone, 1988.
8. Clayman GL, Lippman SM, Laramore GE, et al: Head and neck cancer. In: Holland JF, Frei E III, Bast RC Jr, et al (eds): Cancer Medicine, 4th ed, pp 1645–1710. Philadelphia, Lea & Febiger, 1997.
9. American Joint Committee on Cancer: Manual for Staging for Cancer, 5th ed. Philadelphia, Lippincott-Raven Publishers, 1997.
10. International Union Against Cancer (UICC): TNM Classification of Malignant Tumors, 4th ed. New York: Springer-Verlag, 1992.
11. Kashina HK: Epidemiology and carcinogens in head and neck cancer. In: Fee WE, Goepfert H, Johns ME, et al (eds): Head and Neck Cancer, pp 39–43. Philadelphia, B.C. Decker, 1990.
12. Koch WM: Complications of surgery of the neck. In: Eisele DW (ed): Complications in Head and Neck Surgery, pp 393–413. St. Louis, Mosby, 1993.
13. Patow C, Gaare R: Ethics and the otolaryngologist. In: Cummings CW, Fredrickson JM, Harker LA, et al (eds): Otolaryngology—Head & Neck Surgery, 3rd ed, pp 369–380. St. Louis, Mosby, 1998.
14. Piccirillo JF, Pugliano FA: Evaluation, classification, and staging. In: Myers EN, Suen JY (eds): Cancer of the Head and Neck, 3rd ed, pp 33–49. Philadelphia, W.B. Saunders Co., 1996.
15. Robbins KT: Neck Dissection Classification and TNM Staging of Head and Neck Cancer. Alexandria, VA, American Academy of Otolaryngology Head and Neck Surgery Foundation, Inc., 1991.
16. Thornton AF, Laramore GE: Particle radiation therapy. In: Gunderson LL, Tepper JE (eds): Clinical Radiation Oncology. New York, Churchill Livingston, 2000.

17. Greenlee RT, Murray T, Bolden S, et al: Cancer statistics, 2000. CA Cancer J Clin 2000; 50:7–33.

Specific References

18. Lederman M: The anatomy of cancer with special reference to tumors of the upper air and food passages. J Laryngol Otol 1964; 78:181–208.
19. Griem ML, Chiang DTC: Nasopharynx. In: Laramore GE (ed): Radiation Therapy of Head and Neck Cancer, pp 89–105. Berlin, Springer-Verlag, 1989.
20. Blot WJ, McLaughlin JK, Winn DM, et al: Smoking and drinking in relation to oral and pharyngeal cancer. Cancer Res 1988; 48:3282–3287.
21. Lippman SM, Bassfor TL, Meyskens FL: A quantitatively scored cancer-risk assessment tool: its development and use. J Cancer Educ 1992; 7:15–36.
22. Nelson NJ: "Big smoke" has big risks: daily cigar use causes cancer, heart disease. J Natl Cancer Inst 1998; 90:562–564.
23. Cooper JS, Pajak TF, Rubin P, et al: Second malignancies in patients who have head and neck cancers: incidence, effect on survival, and implications for chemoprevention based on the RTOG experience. Int J Radiat Oncol Biol Phys 1989; 17:449–456.
24. Schwartz LH, Ozsahin M, Zhang GM, et al: Synchronous and metachronous head and neck carcinomas. Cancer 1994; 74:1933–1938.
25. Day GL, Blot WJ, Shore RE, et al: Second cancers following oral and pharyngeal cancers: role of tobacco and alcohol. J Natl Cancer Inst 1994; 86:131–137.
26. Coates HL, Pearson GR, Neel HB, et al: Epstein-Barr virus–associated antigens in nasopharyngeal carcinoma Arch Otolaryngol 1978; 104:427–430.
27. Squier CA: Smokeless tobacco and oral cancer: a cause for concern? CA Cancer J Clin 1984; 34:242–247.
28. Brinton LA, Blot WJ, Becker JA, et al: A case-control study of cancer of the nasal cavity and paranasal sinuses. Am J Epidemiol 1984; 119:896–906.
29. Thawley SE, Panje WR, Batsakis JG, et al (eds): Comprehensive Management of Head and Neck Tumors, vols I and II. Philadelphia, W.B. Saunders Co., 1987.
30. Jenson AB, Lancaster WD, Hartman DP, et al: Frequency and distribution of papillomavirus structural antigens in verrucae, multiple papillomas, and condylomata of the oral cavity. Am J Pathol 1982; 107:212–218.
31. Licciardello JTW, Spitz MR, Hong WK: Multiple primary cancers in patients with cancer of the head and neck: second cancer of the head and neck, esophagus and lung. Int J Radiat Oncol Biol Phys 1989; 17:467–476.
32. Brandsma JL, Steinberg BM, Abramson AL, et al: Presence of human papillomavirus type 16 related sequences in verrucous carcinoma of the larynx. Cancer Res 1986; 46:2185–2188.
33. Shore-Freedman E, Abrahams C, Recant W, et al: Neurilemomas and salivary gland tumors of the head and neck following childhood irradiation. Cancer 1983; 51:2159–2163.
34. Shore RE, Woodward ED, Hemplemannn LH: Radiation induced thyroid cancer. In: Boice JD, Fraumeni JF Jr (eds): Radiation Carcinogenesis: Epidemiology and Biological Significance, pp 131–138. New York, Raven Press, 1984.
35. Renan MJ: How many mutations are required for tumorigenesis? Implications from human cancer data. Mol Carcinog 1993; 7:139–146.
36. Irish JC, Bernstein A: Oncogenes in head and neck cancer. Laryngoscope 1993; 103:42–52.
37. Brennan JA, Boyle JO, Koch WM, et al: Association between cigarette smoking and mutation of the p53 gene in head and neck squamous carcinoma. N Engl J Med 1995; 332:712–717.
38. Nawroz H, van der Reit P, Hruban RH, et al: Allelotype of head and neck squamous cell carcinoma. Cancer Res 1994; 54:1152–1155.
39. Fletcher GH, Jesse RH, Lindberg RD, et al: Neck nodes. In: Fletcher GH (ed): Textbook of Radiotherapy, 3rd ed, pp 249–270. Philadelphia, Lea & Febiger, 1980.
40. Suen JT, Stern SJ: Cancer of the neck. In: Myers EN, Suen JY (eds): Cancer of the Head and Neck, 3rd ed, pp 462–484. Philadelphia, W.B. Saunders Co., 1996.
41. Williams DW III: Imaging of laryngeal cancer. Otolaryngol Clin North Am 1997; 30:35–58.
42. Chong VF, Fan YF, Khoo JB: Retropharyngeal lymphadenopathy in nasopharyngeal carcinoma. Eur J Radiol 1995; 21:100–105.
43. Rege S, Maass A, Chaiken L, et al: Use of positron emission tomography with fluorodeoxyglucose in patients with extracranial head and neck cancers. Cancer 1994; 73:3047–3058.
44. Spiro RH, Alfonso AE, Farr HW, et al: Cervical node metastasis from epidermoid carcinoma of the oral cavity and oropharynx. A critical assessment of current staging. Am J Surg 1974; 128:562–567.
45. The Department of Veterans Affairs Laryngeal Cancer Study Group: Induction chemotherapy plus radiation compared with surgery plus radiation in patients with advanced laryngeal cancer. N Engl J Med 1991; 324:1685–1690.
46. Wolf G, Hong WK, Fisher SG: Neoadjuvant chemotherapy for organ preservation: current status. In: Shah JP, Johnson JT (eds): Proceedings of 4th International Conference on Head and Neck Cancer, pp 89–97. Arlington, VA, Society of Head and Neck Surgeons, 1996.
47. Lefebvre JL, Chavalier D, Lubonski B, et al: Larynx preservation in pyriform sinus cancer: preliminary results of a European Organization for Research and Treatment of Cancer phase III trial. J Natl Cancer Inst 1996; 88:890–899.
48. Al-Sarraff M, Leblanc M, Giri PGS, et al: Superiority of chemoradiotherapy (CT-RT) vs. radiotherapy (RT) in patients with locally advanced nasopharyngeal cancer (NPC). Preliminary results of intergroup (0099) (SWOG 8892.RTOG 8817.ECOG 2388) randomized study [Abstract]. Proceedings of the American Society of Clinical Oncology 1996; 15:313.
49. Al-Sarraf M, Le Blanc M, Giri PGS, et al: Chemo-radiotherapy vs. radiotherapy in patients with advanced nasopharyngeal cancer: phase III randomized Intergroup Study 0099. J Clin Oncol 1998; 16:1310–1317.
50. Peters LJ, Goepfert H, Ang KK, et al: Evaluation of the dose for postoperative radiation therapy of head and neck cancer: first report of a prospective randomized trial. Int J Radiat Oncol Biol Phys 1993; 26:3–11.
51. Cooper JS, Fu K, Marks J, et al: Late effects of radiation therapy in the head and neck region. Int J Radiat Oncol Biol Phys 1995; 31:1141–1164.
52. Patt BS, Schaefer SD, Vuitch F: Role of fine-needle aspiration in the evaluation of neck masses. Med Clin North Am 1993; 77:611–623.
53. Amdur RJ, Parsons JT, Mendenhall WM, et al: Postoperative irradiation for squamous cell carcinoma of the head and neck: an evaluation of treatment results and complications. Int J Radiat Oncol Biol Phys 1989; 16:25–36.
54. Laramore GE, Scott CB, Schuller DE, et al: Is a surgical resection leaving positive margins of benefit to the patient with locally advanced squamous cell carcinoma of the head and neck? A comparative study using the Intergroup Study 0034 and the Radiation Therapy Oncology Group head and neck database. Int J Radiat Oncol Biol Phys 1993; 27:1011–1016.
55. Ariyan S: The pectoralis major myocutaneous flap. A versatile flap for reconstruction in the head and neck. Plast Reconstr Surg 1979; 63:73–81.
56. Maves MD, Panje WR, Shagets FW: Extended latissimus dorsi myocutaneous flap reconstruction of major head and neck defects. Otolaryngol Head Neck Surg 1984; 92:551–558.
57. Biel MA, Maisel RH: Free jejunal autograft reconstruction of the pharyngoesophagus: review of a ten year experience. Arch Otolaryngol Head Neck Surg 1987; 96:369–375.
58. Muldowney JB, Cohen JI, Porto DP, et al: Oral cavity reconstruction using the free radial forearm flap. Arch Otolaryngol Head Neck Surg 1987; 113:1219–1224.
59. Baker SR, Sullivan MJ: Osteocutaneous free scapular flap for one-stage mandibular reconstruction. Arch Otolaryngol Head Neck Surg 1988; 114:267–277.
60. Hidalgo, D: Fibula free flap: a new method of mandible reconstruction. Plast Reconstr Surg 1989; 84:71–79.
61. Urken ML, Vickery C, Weinberg H, et al: The internal oblique-iliac crest osseomyocutaneous free flap in oromandibular reconstruction. Arch Otolaryngol Head Neck Surg 1989; 118:339–349.
62. Urken ML: Composite free flaps in oromandibular reconstruction: review of the literature. Arch Otolaryngol Head Neck Surg 1991; 117:724–732.
63. Wendt CD, Peters LJ, Delclos L, et al: Primary radiotherapy in the

treatment of stage I and II oral tongue cancers: importance of the proportion of therapy delivered with interstitial therapy. Int J Radiat Oncol Biol Phys 1990; 18:1287–1292.
64. Wang CC: How essential is interstitial radiation therapy to curability of head and neck cancer? Int J Radiat Oncol Biol Phys 1990; 18:1529–1530.
65. Freeman SB, Hamaker RC, Singer MI, et al: Intraoperative radiotherapy of head and neck cancer. Arch Otolaryngol Head Neck Surg 1990; 116:165–168.
66. Leibel SA, Ling CC, Kutcher GJ, et al: The biological basis for conformal three-dimensional radiation therapy. Int J Radiat Oncol Biol Phys 1991; 21:805–811.
67. Horiot J, Le Fur R, N'Guyen T, et al: Hyperfractionation versus conventional fractionation in oropharyngeal cancer: final analysis of a randomized trial of the EORTC cooperative group of radiotherapy. Radiother Oncol 1993; 25:231–241.
68. Peters L, Ang K: The role of accelerated fractionation in head and neck cancers. Semin Radiat Oncol 1992; 2:180–194.
69. Fowler JF, Harair PM: Hyperfractionation promise in cancer treatment. Contemp Oncol 1993; 1:14–25.
70. Parsons JT, Mendenhall WM, Stringer SP: Twice-a-day radiotherapy for squamous cell carcinoma of the head and neck: the University of Florida experience. Head Neck 1993; 15:87–96.
71. Freeman DE, Mendenhall WM, Parsons JT, et al: Does neck stage influence local control in squamous cell carcinomas of the head and neck? Int J Radiat Oncol Biol Phys 1992; 23:733–736.
72. Withers HR, Peters LJ, Taylor JMG, et al: Local control of carcinoma of the tonsil by radiation therapy: an analysis of patterns of fractionation in nine institutions. Int J Radiat Oncol Biol Phys 1995; 33:549–562.
73. Cox JD, Pajak TF, Marcial VA, et al: Dose-response for local control with hyperfractionated radiation therapy in advanced carcinomas of the upper aerodigestive tracts: preliminary report of Radiation Therapy Oncology Group Protocol 83–13. Int J Radiat Oncol Biol Phys 1990; 18:515–521.
74. Wang CC, Suit HD, Blitzer, PH: Twice-a-day radiation therapy for supraglottic carcinoma. Int J Radiat Oncol Biol Phys 1986; 12:3–7.
75. Wang CC: Local control of oropharyngeal carcinoma after two accelerated hyperfractionation radiation therapy schemes. Int J Radiat Oncol Biol Phys 1988; 14:1143–1146.
76. Saunders MI, Dische S, Grosch EJ, et al: Experience with CHART. Int J Radiat Oncol Biol Phys 1991; 21:871–878.
77. Ang KK, Peters LJ, Weber RS, et al: Concomitant boost schedules in the treatment of carcinoma of the oropharynx and nasopharynx. Int J Radiat Oncol Biol Phys 1990; 19:1339–1345.
78. Mak AC, Morrison WH, Garden AS, et al: Base-of-tongue carcinoma: treatment results using concomitant boost radiotherapy. Int J Radiat Oncol Biol Phys 1995; 33:289–296.
79. Stuschke M, Thames HD: Hyper-fractionated radiotherapy of human tumors: overview of the randomized clinical trials. Int J Radiat Oncol Biol Phys 1997; 37:259–267.
80. Cox JD, Pajak YF, Marcial VA, et al: ASTRO plenary: interfraction interval is a major determinant of late effects, with hyperfractionated radiation therapy of carcinomas of upper respiratory and digestive tracts: results from Radiation Therapy Oncology Group Protocol 8313. Int J Radiat Oncol Biol Phys 1991; 20:1191–1196.
80a. Fu KK, Pajak TF, Trotti A, et al: A Radiation Therapy Oncology Group (RTOG) phase III randomized study to compare hyperfractionation and two variants of accelerated fractionation to standard fractionation radiotherapy for head and neck squamous cell carcinomas: first report of RTOG 9003. Int J Radiat Oncol Biol Phys 2000; 48:7–16.
81. Bataini J-P: The ESTRO Regaud lecture: Head and neck cancer and the radiation oncologist. Radiother Oncol 1991; 21:1–10.
82. Kotwall C, Sako K, Razack MS, et al: Metastatic patterns in squamous cell cancer of the head and neck. Am J Surg 1987; 154:439–442.
83. Cerezo L, Millan I, Torre A, et al: Prognostic factors for survival and tumor control in cervical lymph node metastases from head and neck cancer. A multivariate study of 492 cases. Cancer 1992; 69:1224–1234.
84. Leemans CR, Tiwari R, Nauta JJP, et al: Regional lymph node involvement and its significance in the development of distant metastases in head and neck carcinoma. Cancer 1993; 71:452–456.
85. Stell PM: Survival times in end-stage head and neck cancer. Eur J Surg Oncol 1989; 15:407–410.
86. Catimel G, Verweij J, Mattijssen V, et al: Docetaxel (Taxotere): an active drug for the treatment of patients with advanced squamous cell carcinoma of the head and neck. Ann Oncol 1994; 5:533–537.
87. Verweij J: Docetaxel: an interesting new drug for the treatment of head and neck cancers and soft tissue sarcomas. Anticancer Drugs 1995; 6:19–24.
88. Smith RE, Thorton DE, Allen J: A phase II trial of paclitaxel in squamous cell carcinoma of the head and neck with correlative laboratory studies. Semin Oncol 1995; 22:41–46.
89. Dreyfuss AI, Clark JR, Norris CM, et al: Docetaxel: an active drug for squamous cell carcinoma of the head and neck. J Clin Oncol 1996; 14:1672–1678.
90. Schantz SP, Harrison LB, Forastiere AA: Cancer of the head and neck. In: DeVita VT, Hellman S, Rosenberg SA (eds): Cancer: Principles & Practice of Oncology, 5th ed, pp 741–801. Philadelphia, Lippincott, 1997.
91. Forastiere AA, Shank D, Neuberg D, et al: Final report of a phase II evaluation of paclitaxel in patients with advanced squamous cell carcinoma of the head and neck. Cancer 1998; 82:2270–2274.
92. Taylor SG IV, McGuire WP, Hauck WW, et al: A randomized comparison of high-dose infusion methotrexate versus standard-dose weekly therapy in head and neck squamous cell cancer. J Clin Oncol 1984; 2:1006–1011.
93. Urba SG, Forastiere AA: Systemic therapy of head and neck cancer: most effective agents, areas of promise. Oncology 1989; 3:79–88.
94. Khanuja PS, Kish JA, Ensley JF: The significance and improved disease-free interval and survival for patients with recurrent head and neck cancer who achieve complete response to effective chemotherapy [Abstract]. Proc Am Soc Clin Oncol 1991; 10:205.
95. Kish JA, Weaver A, Jacobs J, et al: Cisplatin and 5-fluorouracil infusion in patients with recurrent and disseminated epidermoid cancer of the head and neck. Cancer 1984; 53:1819–1824.
96. Creagan ET, Ingle JN, Schutt AJ, et al: A phase II study of cis-diaminedichloroplatinum and 5-fluorouracil in advanced upper aerodigestive neoplasms. Head Neck Surg 1984; 6:1020–1023.
97. Kish JA, Ensley JF, Jacobs J, et al: A randomized trial of cisplatin (CACP) and 5-fluorouracil (5-FU) infusion and CACP + 5-FU bolus for recurrent and advanced squamous cell carcinoma of the head and neck. Cancer 1985; 15:2740–2744.
98. Dasmahapatra KS, Citrin P, Hill GJ, et al: A prospective evaluation of 5-fluorouracil plus cisplatin in advanced squamous cell carcinoma of the head and neck. J Clin Oncol 1985; 3:1486–1489.
99. Amrein PC, Weitzman SA: Treatment of squamous-cell carcinoma of the head and neck with cisplatin and 5-fluorouracil. J Clin Oncol 1985; 3:1632–1639.
100. Rowland KM Jr, Taylor SG IV, Spiers AS, et al: Cisplatin and 5-FU infusion chemotherapy in advanced, recurrent cancer of the head and neck: an Eastern Cooperative Oncology Group pilot study. Cancer Treat Rep 1986; 70:461–464.
101. Mercier RJ, Neal GD, Mattox DE, et al: Cisplatin and 5-fluorouracil chemotherapy in advanced or recurrent squamous cell carcinoma of the head and neck. Cancer 1987; 60:2609–2612.
102. Merlano M, Grimaldi A, Brunetti I, et al: Simultaneous cisplatin and 5-fluorouracil as second-line treatment of head and neck cancer. Cancer Treat Rep 1987; 71:485–488.
103. Choski AJ, Hong WK, Dimery IW, et al: Continuous cisplatin (24-hour) and 5-fluorouracil (120-hour) infusion in recurrent head and neck squamous cell carcinoma. Cancer 1988; 61:909–912.
104. Paredes J, Hong WK, Felder TB, et al: Prospective randomized trial of high-dose cisplatin and fluorouracil infusion with or without sodium diethyldithiocarbamate in recurrent and/or metastatic squamous cell carcinoma of the head and neck. J Clin Oncol 1988; 6:955–962.
105. Paccagnella A, Pappagallo GL, Segati R, et al: Response and toxicity of cisplatin and 120-h 5-fluorouracil infusion in pretreated and untreated patients with advanced epidermoid cancer of the head and neck. Am J Clin Oncol 1990; 13:194–198.
106. O'Brien M, Schofield JB, Lorentzos A, et al: The use of cisplatin plus 5-fluorouracil chemotherapy in an unselected group of patients with recurrent squamous cell carcinoma of the head and neck. Eur J Cancer B Oral Oncol 1994; 30B:265–267.
107. Vokes EE, Schilsky RL, Weichselbaum RR, et al: Cisplatin, 5-fluorouracil, and high-dose leucovorin for advanced head and neck cancer. Cancer 1989; 63:1048–1053.
108. Amrein PC, Fabian RL: Treatment of recurrent head and neck cancer

with cisplatin and 5-fluorouracil vs. the same plus bleomycin and methotrexate. Laryngoscope 1992; 102:901–906.

109. Hussain M, Benedetti J, Smith RE, et al: Evaluation of 96-hour infusion fluorouracil plus cisplatin in combination with alpha interferon for patients with advanced squamous cell carcinoma of the head and neck. Cancer 1995; 76:1233–1237.
110. Schrijvers D, Johnson J, Jiminez U, et al: Phase III trial of modulation of cisplatin/fluorouracil chemotherapy by interferon alfa-2b in patients with recurrent or metastatic head and neck cancer. J Clin Oncol 1998; 16:1054–1059.
111. Forastiere AA, Leong T, Murphy B: A phase III trial of high-dose paclitaxel + cisplatin + G-CSF versus low-dose paclitaxel + cisplatin in patients with advanced squamous cell carcinoma of the head and neck: an Eastern Cooperative Group trial [Abstract]. Proc Am Soc Clin Oncol 1997; 16:384a.
112. Licitra L, Capri G, Fulfaro F, et al: Biweekly paclitaxel and cisplatin in patients with advanced head and neck carcinoma. A phase II trial. Ann Oncol 1997; 8:1157–1158.
113. Schilling T, Heinrich B, Kau R, et al: Paclitaxel administered over 3 h followed by cisplatin in patients with advanced head and neck squamous cell carcinoma: a clinical phase I study. Oncology 1997; 54:89–95.
114. Thodtmann F, Theiss F, Kemmerich M, et al: Clinical phase II evaluation of paclitaxel in combination with cisplatin in metastatic or recurrent squamous cell carcinoma of the head and neck. Ann Oncol 1998; 9:335–337.
115. Forastiere A, Glisson B, Murphy B, et al: A phase II study of docetaxel and cisplatin in patients with locally advanced, recurrent and/or metastatic squamous cell carcinoma of the head and neck, not curable by standard therapy [Abstract]. Proc Am Soc Clin Oncol 1998; 17:399a.
116. Hussain M, Salwen W, Kucuk O, et al: Paclitaxel, cisplatin and 5-fluorouracil in patients with advanced or recurrent squamous cell carcinoma of the head and neck: a preliminary report. Semin Oncol 1997; 24(suppl 19):43–45.
117. Pai VR, Parikh DM, Mazumdar AT, et al: Phase II study of high-dose ifosfamide as a single agent and in combination with cisplatin in the treatment of advanced and/or recurrent squamous cell carcinoma of the head and neck. Oncology 1993; 50:86–91.
118. Shin DM, Glisson BS, Khuri FR, et al: Phase II trial of paclitaxel, ifosfamide, and cisplatin in patients with recurrent head and neck squamous cell carcinoma. J Clin Oncol 1998; 16:1325–1330.
119. Fountzilas G, Skarlos D, Athanassiades A, et al: Paclitaxel by three-hour infusion and carboplatin in advanced carcinoma of nasopharynx and other sites of the head and neck. A phase II study conducted by the Hellenic Cooperative Oncology Group. Ann Oncol 1997; 8:451–455.
120. Jacobs C, Lyman G, Velez-Garcia E, et al: A phase III randomized study comparing cisplatin and fluorouracil as single agents and in combination for advanced squamous cell carcinoma of the head and neck. J Clin Oncol 1992; 10:257–263.
121. Clavel M, Vermorken JB, Cognetti F, et al: Randomized comparison of cisplatin, methotrexate, bleomycin and vincristine (CABO) versus cisplatin and 5-fluorouracil (CF) versus cisplatin (C) in recurrent or metastatic squamous cell carcinoma of the head and neck. A phase III study of the EORTC Head and Neck Cancer Cooperative Group. Ann Oncol 1994; 5:521–526.
122. Liverpool Head and Neck Oncology Group: A phase III randomised trial of cisplatinum, methotrexate, cisplatinum + methotrexate, and cisplatinum + 5-FU in end stage squamous cell carcinoma of the head and neck. Br J Cancer 1990; 61:311–315.
123. Drelichman A, Cummings G, Al-Sarraf M: A randomized trial of the combination of cis-platinum, oncovin and bleomycin (COB) versus methotrexate in patients with advanced squamous cell carcinoma of the head and neck. Cancer 1983; 52:399–403.
124. Vogl SE, Schoenfeld DA, Kaplan BH, et al: A randomized prospective comparison of methotrexate with a combination of methotrexate, bleomycin, and cisplatin in head and neck cancer. Cancer 1985; 56:432–442.
125. Williams SD, Velez-Garcia E, Essessee I, et al: Chemotherapy for head and neck cancer. Comparison of cisplatin + vinblastine + bleomycin versus methotrexate. Cancer 1986; 57:18–23.
126. Eisenberger M, Krasnow S, Ellenberg S, et al: A comparison of carboplatin plus methotrexate versus methotrexate alone in patients with recurrent or metastatic head and neck cancer. J Clin Oncol 1989; 7:1341–1345.
127. Forastiere AA, Metch B, Schuller DE, et al: Randomized comparison of cisplatin plus fluorouracil and carboplatin plus fluorouracil versus methotrexate in advanced squamous-cell carcinoma of the head and neck: a Southwest Oncology Group study. J Clin Oncol 1992; 10:1245–1251.
128. Rooney M, Kish J, Jacobs J, et al: Improved complete response rate and survival in advanced head and neck cancer after three-course induction therapy with 120-hour 5-FU infusion and cisplatin. Cancer 1985; 55:1123–1128.
129. Thyss A, Schneider M, Sanitini J, et al: Induction chemotherapy with cis-platinum and 5-fluorouracil for squamous cell carcinoma of the head and neck. Br J Cancer 1986; 54:755–760.
130. Teatani G, Meloni F, Bisail M, et al: Neoadjuvant chemotherapy with cisplatinum and 5-fluorouracil in advanced head and neck cancer. J Chemother 1990; 2:394–396.
131. Boni C, Moretti G, Savoldi L, et al: Neoadjuvant chemotherapy with continuous infusion of cisplatin and fluorouracil in stage II–IV, M0 squamous cell carcinoma of the head and neck. Tumori 1996; 82:567–572.
132. Al-Kourainy K, Kish J, Ensley J, et al: Achievement of superior survival for histologically negative versus histologically positive complete responders to cisplatin combination in patients with locally advanced head and neck cancer. Cancer 1987; 59:233–238.
133. Spaulding MB, Fischer SG, Wolf GT, et al: Tumor response, toxicity, and survival after neoadjuvant organ-preserving chemotherapy for advanced laryngeal carcinoma. J Clin Oncol 1994; 12:1592–1599.
134. Stell PM, Dalby JE, Strickland P: et al: Sequential chemotherapy and radiotherapy in advanced head and neck cancer. Clin Radiol 1983; 34:463–467.
135. Kun LE, Toohill RJ, Holoye PY, et al: A randomized study of adjuvant chemotherapy for cancer of the upper aerodigestive tract. Int J Radiat Oncol Biol Phys 1986; 12:173–178.
136. Head and Neck Contracts Program: Adjuvant chemotherapy for advanced head and neck squamous carcinoma. Final report of the Head and Neck Contracts Program. Cancer 1987; 60:301–311.
137. Toohill RJ, Anderson T, Byhardt RW, et al: Cisplatin and fluorouracil as neoadjuvant therapy in head and neck cancer. Arch Otolaryngol Head Neck Surg 1987; 113:758–761.
138. Schuller DE, Metch B, Stein DW, et al: Preoperative chemotherapy in advanced resectable head and neck cancer: final report of the Southwest Oncology Group. Laryngoscope 1988; 98:1205–1211.
139. Carugati A, Pracher R, de la Torre A: Combination chemotherapy pre-radical treatment for head and neck squamous cell carcinoma [Abstract]. Proc Am Soc Clin Oncol 1988; 7:152.
140. Martin M, Hazan A, Vergnes L, et al: Randomized study of 5-fluorouracil and cisplatin as neoadjuvant therapy in head and neck cancer: a preliminary report. Int J Radiat Oncol Biol Phys 1990; 19:973–975.
141. Martin M, Malaurie E, Langlet PM, et al: A randomized prospective study of CDDP and 5FU as neoadjuvant chemotherapy in head and neck cancer: a final report [Abstract]. Proc Am Soc Clin Oncol 1995; 14:294.
142. Jortay A, Demard F, Dalesio O, et al: A randomized EORTC study on the effect of preoperative polychemotherapy in pyriform sinus carcinoma treated by pharyngolaryngectomy and irradiation. Results from 5 to 10 years. Acta Chir Belg 1990; 90:115–122.
143. Mazeron JJ, Martin M, Brun B, et al: Induction chemotherapy in head and neck cancer: results of a phase III trial. Head Neck 1992; 14:85–91.
144. Jaulerry C, Rodriguez J, Brunin F, et al: Induction chemotherapy in advanced head and neck tumors, results of two randomized trials. Int J Radiat Oncol Biol Phys 1992; 23:483–489.
145. Depondt J, Gehanno P, Martin M, et al: Neoadjuvant chemotherapy with carboplatin/5-fluorouracil in head and neck cancer. Oncology 1993; 50:23–27.
146. Paccagnella A, Orlando A, Marchiori C, et al: Phase III trial of initial chemotherapy in stage III or IV head and neck cancers: a study by the Gruppo di Studio sui Tumori della Testa e del Collo. J Natl Cancer Inst 1994; 86:265–272.
147. DiBlasio B, Barbieri W, Bozzetti A, et al: A prospective randomized trial in resectable head and neck carcinoma: loco-regional treatment with and without neoadjuvant chemotherapy [Abstract]. Proc Am Soc Clin Oncol 1994; 13:279.
148. Hasegawa Y, Matsuura H, Fukushima M, et al: A randomized trial of neoadjuvant chemotherapy with cisplatin and 5-FU in advanced

head and neck cancer [Abstract]. Proc Am Soc Clin Oncol 1994; 13:286.

149. Chan AT, Teo PM, Leung TW, et al: A prospective randomized study of chemotherapy adjunctive to definitive radiotherapy in advanced nasopharygeal carcinoma. Int J Radiat Oncol Biol Phys 1995; 33:569–577.
150. Dalley D, Beller E, Aroney R, et al: The value of chemotherapy prior to definitive local therapy in patients with locally advanced squamous cell carcinoma of the head and neck [Abstract]. Proc Am Soc Clin Oncol 1995; 14:297.
151. El Gueddari B: Final results of the VUMCA I randomized trial comparing neoadjuvant chemotherapy plus radiotherapy to RT alone in undifferentiated nasopharyngeal carcinoma [Abstract]. Proc Am Soc Clin Oncol 1998; 17:385a.
152. Lewin F, Damber L, Jonsson H, et al: Neoadjuvant chemotherapy with cisplatin and 5-fluorouracil in advanced squamous cell carcinoma of the head and neck: a randomized phase III study. Radiother Oncol 1997; 1997;43:23–28.
153. Jacobs C, Makuch R: Efficacy of adjuvant chemotherapy for patients with resectable head and neck cancer: a subset analysis of the Head and Neck Contracts Program. J Clin Oncol 1990; 8:838–847.
154. Forastiere AA: Randomized trials of induction chemotherapy. A critical review. Hematol Oncol Clin North Am 1991; 5:725–736.
155. Bourhis J, Pignon JP: Meta-analysis in head and neck squamous cell carcinoma. What is the role of chemotherapy? Hematol Oncol Clin North Am 1999; 13:769–775.
156. Ensley JF, Jacobs JR, Weaver A, et al: Correlation between response to cisplatinum-combination chemotherapy and subsequent radiotherapy in previously untreated patients with advanced squamous cell cancers of the head and neck. Cancer 1984; 54:811–814.
157. Laramore GE, Scott CB, Al-Sarraf M, et al: Adjuvant chemotherapy for resectable squamous cell carcinomas of the head and neck: report on Intergroup Study 0034. Int J Radiat Oncol Biol Phys 1992; 23:705–713.
158. Vokes EE, Weichselbaum, RR: Concomitant chemotherapy: Rationale and clinical experience in patients with solid tumors. J Clin Oncol 1990; 8:911–934.
159. Fu KK, Phillips TL: Biologic rationale of combined radiotherapy and chemotherapy. Hematol Oncol Clin North Am 1991; 5:737–751.
160. Guptka NK, Pointon RCS, Wilkinson PM: A randomized clinical trial to contrast radiotherapy with radiotherapy and chemotherapy given synchronously in head and neck cancer. Clin Radiol 1987; 38:575–581.
161. Merlano M, Vitale V, Rosso R, et al: Treatment of advanced squamous cell carcinomas of the head and neck with alternating chemotherapy and radiotherapy. N Engl J Med 1992; 327:1115–1121.
162. Keane TJ, Cummings BJ, O'Sullivan B, et al: A randomized trial of radiotherapy compared with split course radiotherapy combined with mitomycin C and 5-fluorouracil as an initial treatment for advanced laryngeal and hypopharyngeal squamous cell carcinoma. Int J Radiat Oncol Biol Phys 1993; 25:613–618.
163. El-Sayed S, Nelson N: Adjuvant and adjunctive chemotherapy in the management of squamous cell carcinoma of the head and neck region: a meta-analysis of prospective and randomized trials. J Clin Oncol 1996; 14:838–847.
164. del Regato JA, Spjut HJ, Cox JD: Ackerman and del Regato's Cancer: Diagnosis, Treatment and Prognosis, 6th ed. St. Louis. C.V. Mosby, 1985.
165. Jaram B, Strong EW, Shah J, et al: Elective postoperative radiation therapy in stages III and IV epidermoid carcinoma of the head and neck. Am J Surg 1980; 149:580–584.
166. Suen JY, Newman RK, Hannahs K, et al: Evaluation of the effectiveness of postoperative radiation therapy for the control of local disease. Am J Surg 1980; 140:577–579.
167. Lundahl RE, Foote RL, Bonner JA, et al: Combined neck dissection and postoperative radiation therapy in the management of the high-risk neck: a matched-pair analysis. Int J Radiat Oncol Biol Phys 1998; 40:529–534.
168. Peters LJ: The efficacy of postoperative radiotherapy for advanced head and neck cancer: quality of the evidence. Int J Radiat Oncol Biol Phys 1998; 40:527–528.
169. Fu KK: Combined-modality therapy for head and neck cancer. Oncology 1997; 11:1781–1796.
170. Adelstein DJ, Saxton JP, Lavertu P, et al: Concurrent radiation and chemotherapy (CT) versus (vs) radiotherapy (RT) alone in resectable stage III and IV squamous cell head and neck cancer (SCHNC): a phase III randomized trial [Abstract]. Proc Am Soc Clin Oncol 1996; 15:26.
171. Brizel DM, Albers ME, Fisher SR, et al: Hyperfractionated irradiation with or without concurrent chemotherapy for locally advanced head and neck cancer. N Engl J Med 1998; 338:1798–1804.
172. Mendenhall WM, Million RR, Cassisi NJ: Elective neck irradiation in squamous cell carcinoma of the head and neck. Head Neck Surg 1980; 3:15–20.
173. Kalnins IK, Leonard AG, Sako K, et al: Correlation between prognosis and degree of lymph node involvement in carcinoma of the oral cavity. Am J Surg 1977; 134:450–454.
174. Chu W, Strawitz JG: Results in suprahyoid, modified radical, and standard radical neck dissections for metastatic squamous cell carcinoma: recurrence and survival. Am J Surg 1978; 136:512–515.
175. Kramer S, Gelber RD, Snow JB, et al: Combined radiation therapy and surgery in the management of advanced head and neck cancer: final report of the Radiation Therapy Oncology Group. Head Neck Surg 1987; 10:19–30.
176. Laramore GE: Treatment of nodes in the clinically N0 neck. In: Laramore GE (ed): Radiation Therapy of the Head and Neck Cancer, pp 37–40. Berlin, Springer-Verlag, 1989.
177. Spiro RH, Morgan GJ, Strong EW, et al: Supraomohyoid neck dissection. Am J Surg 1996; 172:650–653.
178. Lee AWM, Sham JST, Poon YF, et al: Treatment of stage I nasopharyngeal carcinoma: analysis of the patterns of relapse and the results of withholding elective neck irradiation. Int J Radiat Oncol Biol Phys 1989; 17:1183–1190.
179. Mossman KL: Quantitative radiation dose-response relationships for normal tissues in man. II: response of the salivary glands during radiotherapy. Radiat Res 1983; 95:392–398.
180. Johnson JT, Ferretti GA, Nethery WJ, et al: Oral pilocarpine for post-irradiation xerostomia in patients with head and neck cancer. N Engl J Med 1993; 329:390–395.
181. Rieke JW, Hafermann MD, Johnson JT, et al: Oral pilocarpine for radiation-induced xerostomia: integrated efficacy and safety results from two prospective randomized clinical trials. Int J Radiat Oncol Biol Phys 1995; 31:661–669.
182. Rothwell BR: Prevention and treatment of the orofacial complications of radiotherapy. J Am Dent Assoc 1987; 114:316–322.
183. Marx RE, Johnson RP: Studies in the radiobiology of osteoradionecrosis and their clinical significance. Oral Surg Oral Med Oral Pathol 1987; 64:379–390.
184. Marx RE, Johnson RP, Kline SN: Prevention of osteoradionecrosis: a randomized prospective clinical trial of hyperbaric oxygen versus penicillin. J Am Dent Assoc 1985; 111:49–54.
185. Marcus RB, Million RR: The incidence of myelitis after irradiation of the cervical spinal cord. Int J Radiat Oncol Biol Phys 1990; 19:3–8.
186. Schultheiss TE: Spinal cord radiation "tolerance": doctrine versus data. Int J Radiat Oncol Biol Phys 1990; 19:219–221.
187. Lippman SM, Hong WK: Second malignant tumors in head and neck squamous cell carcinoma: the overshadowing threat for patients with cancer of the head and neck: second cancer of the head and neck, esophagus and lung. Int J Radiat Oncol Biol Phys 1989; 17:691–694.
188. McDonald S, Haie C, Rubin P, et al: Second malignant tumors in patients with laryngeal carcinoma: diagnosis, treatment and prevention. Int J Radiat Oncol Biol Phys 1989; 17:457–465.
189. Cooper JS, Scott CB, Marcial V, et al: The relationship of nasopharyngeal carcinomas and second independent malignancies based on the Radiation Therapy Oncology Group experience. Cancer 1991; 67:1673–1677.
190. Parker RG, Enstrom JE: Second primary cancers following initial treatment of patients with head and neck cancers. Int J Radiat Oncol Biol Phys 1988; 14:561–564.
191. Lippman SM, Spitz MR, Huber MH, et al: Strategies for chemoprevention of premalignancy and second primary tumors in the head and neck. Curr Opin Oncol 1995; 7:234–241.
192. Hong WK, Lippman SM, Itri LM, et al: Prevention of second primary tumors with isotretinoin in squamous cell carcinoma of the head and neck. N Engl J Med 1990; 323:795–801.
193. Laramore GE, Clubb B, Quick C, et al: Nasopharyngeal carcinoma in Saudi Arabia: a retrospective study of 166 cases treated with curative intent. Int J Radiat Oncol Biol Phys 1988; 15:1119–1127.

194. Marcial VA, Pajak TF, Kramer S, et al: Radiation Therapy Oncology Group (RTOG) studies in head and neck cancer. Semin Oncol 1988; 15:39–60.
195. Leibel SA, Scott CB, Mohiuddin M, et al: The effect of local-regional control on distant metastatic dissemination in carcinoma of the head and neck: results of an analysis from the RTOG head and neck database. Int J Radiat Oncol Biol Phys 1991; 21:549–556.
196. Brock WA, Baker FL, Wike JL, et al: Cellular radiosensitivity of primary head and neck squamous cell carcinomas and local tumor control. Int J Radiat Oncol Biol Phys 1990; 18:1283–1287.
196a. Peters LJ, Brock WA, Chapman JD, et al: Predictive assays of tumor radiocurability. Am J Clin Oncol 1988; 1:275–287.
197. Laramore GE: Radiotherapy as the primary treatment for malignant salivary gland tumors. In: Johnson JT, Didolkar MS (eds): Head and Neck Cancer, vol III, pp 599–605. Amsterdam, Elsevier Science Publishers, 1993.
198. Laramore GE, Krall JM, Griffin TW, et al: Neutron versus photon irradiation for unresectable salivary gland tumors: final report of an RTOG-MRC randomized clinical trial. Int J Radiat Oncol Biol Phys 1993; 27:235–240.
199. Hall EJ: Radiobiology for the Radiologist, 4th ed, pp 257–288. Philadelphia, J.B. Lippincott, 1994.
200. Emami B, Scott C, Perez CA, et al: Phase III study of interstitial thermoradiotherapy compared with interstitial radiotherapy alone in the treatment of recurrent or persistent human tumors: a prospectively controlled randomized study by the Radiation Therapy Oncology Group. Int J Radiat Oncol Biol Phys 1996; 34:1097–1104.
201. Overgaard J, Hansen HS, Andersen AP, et al: Misonidazole combined with split course radiotherapy in the treatment of invasive carcinoma of the larynx and pharynx: report from the DAHANCA study. Int J Radiat Oncol Biol Phys 1989; 16:1065–1068.
202. Van den Bogaert W, van der Schueren E, Horiot JC, et al: The EORTC randomised trial on three fractions per day and misonidazole (trial no. 22811) in advanced head and neck cancer: long-term results and side effects. Radiother Oncol 1995; 35:91–99.
203. Fazekas J, Pajak TF, Wasserman T, et al: Failure of misonidazole-sensitized radiotherapy to impact on outcome among stage III–IV squamous cancers of the head and neck. Int J Radiat Oncol Biol Phys 1987; 13:1155–1160.
204. Eschwege F, Sancho-Garnier H, Chassagne D, et al: Results of a European randomized trial of etanidazole combined with radiotherapy in head and neck carcinomas. Int J Radiat Oncol Biol Phys 1997; 39:275–281.
205. Overgaard J, Hansen HS, Overgaard M, et al: A randomized double-blind phase III study of nimorazole as a hypoxic radisensitizer of primary radiotherapy in supraglottic larynx and pharynx carcinoma. Results of the Danish Head and Neck Cancer Study (DAHANCA) Protocol 5-85. Radiother Oncol 1998; 46:135–146.
206. Koh WJ, Bergman KS, Rasey JS, et al: Evaluation of oxygenation status during fractionated radiotherapy in human nonsmall cell lung cancers using [F-18] fluoromisonidazole positron emission tomography. Int J Radiat Oncol Biol Phys 1992; 22:199–212.
207. Koh WJ, Griffin TW, Rasey JS, et al: Positron emission tomography: a new tool for characterization of malignant disease and selection of therapy. Acta Oncol 1994; 33:323–327.
208. Tannehill SP, Mehta MP: Amifostine and radiation therapy: past, present, and future. Semin Oncol 1996; 23:69–77.
209. Savoye C, Swenberg C, Hugot S, et al: Thiol WR-1065 and disulphide WR-33278, two metabolites of the drug ethyol (WR-2721), protect DNA against fast neutron-induced strand breakage. Int J Radiat Oncol Biol Phys 1997; 71:193–202.
210. Decroix Y, Ghossein NA: Experience of the Curie Institute in treatment of cancer of the mobile tongue. II. Management of the neck nodes. Cancer 1981; 47:503–508.
211. Ingersoll I, Goffinet DR: Oral cavity. In: Laramore GE (ed): Radiation Therapy of Head and Neck Cancer, pp 45–68. Berlin, Springer-Verlag, 1989.
212. Panje WR, Morris MR: Oral cavity and oropharyngeal reconstruction. In: Cummings CW, Fredrickson JM, Harker LA, et al (eds): Otolaryngology—Head & Neck Surgery, pp 1635–1653. St. Louis, Mosby, 1998.
213. Bachaud JM, Delannes M, Allouache N, et al: Radiotherapy of stage I and II carcinomas of the mobile tongue and/or floor of mouth. Department of Radiotherapy, Centre Claudius Regaud, Toulouse, France. Radiother Oncol 1994; 31:199–206.
214. Beitler JJ, Vikram B, Levendag PC: Brachytherapy for cancer of the head and neck. In: Nag S (ed): Principles and Practice of Brachytherapy, pp 269–290. Armonk, NY, Futura Publishing, 1997.
215. Wisbeck W, Laramore GE: Oropharynx. In: Laramore GE (ed): Radiation Therapy of Head and Neck Cancer, pp 69–87. Berlin, Springer-Verlag, 1989.
216. Oruga JH, Biller HF, Wette R: Elective neck dissection for pharyngeal and laryngeal cancers: an evaluation. Ann Otol Rhinol Laryngol 1971; 80:646–651.
217. Lee WR, Mendenhall WM, Parsons JT, et al: Carcinoma of the tonsillar region: a multi-variate analysis of 243 patients treated with radical radiotherapy. Head Neck 1993; 15:283–288.
218. Shrewsbury D, Adams GL, Duvall AJ III, et al: Carcinoma of the tonsillar region: a comparison of radiation therapy with combined preoperative radiation and surgery. Otolaryngol Head Neck Surg 1981; 89:979–985.
219. Genden EM, Thawley SE, O'Leary MJ: Malignant neoplasms of the oropharynx. In: Cummings CW, Fredrickson JM, Harker LA, et al (eds): Otolaryngology—Head & Neck Surgery, pp 1463–1511. St. Louis, Mosby, 1998.
220. Seydel AG, Scholl H: Carcinoma of the soft palate and uvula. Am J Roentgenol 1974; 120:603–607.
221. Kaplan R, Million RR, Cassisi NJ: Carcinoma of the tonsil: results of radical irradiation with surgery reserved for radiation failures. Laryngoscope 1977; 87:600–607.
222. Byhardt RW, Cox JD: Patterns of failure and results of preoperative irradiation vs. radiation alone in carcinoma of the pyriform sinus. Int J Radiat Oncol Biol Phys 1980; 6:1135–1141.
223. Martin SA, Marks JE, Lee JY, et al: Carcinoma of the pyriform sinus: predictors of TNM relapse and survival. Cancer 1980; 46:1974–1981.
224. Elias MM, Hilgers FJ, Keus RB, et al: Carcinoma of the pyriform sinus: a retrospective analysis of treatment results over a 20-year period. Clin Otolaryngol Allied Sci 1995; 20:249–253.
225. Zelefsky MJ, Kraus DH, Pfister DG, et al: Combined chemotherapy and radiotherapy versus surgery and postoperative radiotherapy for advanced hypopharyngeal cancer. Head Neck 1996; 18:405–411.
226. Million RR, Cassisi NJ: Radical irradiation for carcinoma of the pyriform sinus. Laryngoscope 1981; 91:439–450.
227. Lederman M: Cancer of the larynx, part I: Natural history in relation to treatment. Br J Radiol 1971; 44:569–578.
228. Wynder EL, Covey LS, Mauchi K, et al: Environmental factors in cancer of the larynx—a second look. Cancer 1976; 38:1591–1601.
229. Laramore GE: Larynx. In: Laramore GE (ed): Radiation Therapy of Head and Neck Cancer, pp 125–143. Berlin, Springer-Verlag, 1989.
230. Million RR, Cassisi NJ, Mancuso AA: Larynx. In: Million RR, Cassisi NJ (eds): Management of Head and Neck Cancer: A Multidisciplinary Approach, 2nd ed, pp 431–497. Philadelphia, Lippincott, 1994.
231. Sorensen H, Hansen HS, Thomsen KA: Partial laryngectomy following irradiation. Laryngoscope 1980; 90:1344–1349.
232. Harwood AR, Beale FA, Cummings BJ, et al: Supraglottic laryngeal carcinoma: an analysis of dose-time-volume factors in 410 patients. Int J Radiat Oncol Biol Phys 1983; 9:311–319.
233. Hillman RE, Walsh MJ, Wolf GT, et al: Functional outcomes following treatment for advanced laryngeal cancer: part I—voice preservation in advanced laryngeal cancer & part II—laryngectomy rehabilitation: the state of the art in the VA system. Ann Otol Rhinol Laryngol 1998; S172:2–27.
234. Johnson JT, Myers EN, Hao SP, et al: Outcome of open surgical therapy for glottic carcinoma. Ann Otol Rhinol Laryngol 1993; 102:752–755.
235. Thomas JV, Olsen KD, Neel HB III, et al: Early glottic carcinoma treated with open laryngeal procedures. Arch Otolaryngol Head Neck Surg 1994; 120:264–268.
236. Cragle SP, Brandenburg JH: Laser chordectomy or radiotherapy: cure rates, communications and cost. Otolaryngol Head Neck Surg 1993; 108:648–654.
237. Kim RY, Marks ME, Salter MM, et al: Early stage glottic cancer: importance of dose fractionation in radiation therapy. Radiology 1992; 182:273–275.
238. Ricciardelli EJ, Weymuller EA, Koh WJ, et al: Effect of radiation fraction size on local control rates for early glottic cancer. Arch Otolaryngol Head Neck Surg 1994; 120:737–742.
239. Franchin G, Minatel E, Gobitti C, et al: Radiation treatment of

glottic squamous cell carcinoma, stage I and II: analysis of factors affecting prognosis. Int J Radiat Oncol Biol Phys 1998; 40:541–548.

240. Pfister DG, Strong E, Harrison L, et al: Larynx preservation with combined chemotherapy and radiation therapy in advanced but resectable head and neck cancer. J Clin Oncol 1991; 9:850–859.
241. Ho JH: An epidemiologic and clinical study of nasopharyngeal carcinoma. Int J Radiat Oncol Biol Phys 1978; 4:183–198.
242. Clubb B, Quick C, Amer M, et al: Nasopharyngeal carcinoma in Saudi Arabia: selected clinical and epidemiological aspects. Ann Saudi Med 1990; 10:171–175.
243. Yu MC, Ho JHC, Lai SH, et al: Cantonese-style salted fish as a cause of nasopharyngeal carcinoma: report of a case-control study in Hong Kong. Cancer Res 1986; 46:956–961.
244. Faggioni A, Corradini C, Venanzoni M, et al: Nasopharyngeal carcinoma: the diagnostic value of the antibody-dependent, cellular cytotoxicity test and of EBV serology. J Exp Pathol 1987; 3:471–477.
245. Levine PH: Immunologic markers for Epstein-Barr virus in the control of nasopharyngeal carcinoma and Burkitt lymphoma. Cancer Detect Prev (Suppl) 1987; 1:217–223.
246. Dickson RI: Nasopharyngeal carcinoma: an evaluation of 209 patients. Laryngoscope 1980; 91:333–354.
247. Lee AWM, Poon YF, Foo W, et al: Retrospective analysis of 5037 patients with nasopharyngeal carcinoma treated during 1976–1985: overall survival and patterns of failure. Int J Radiat Oncol Biol Phys 1992; 23:261–270.
248. Fee WE Jr, Gilmer PA, Goffinet DR: Surgical management of recurrent nasopharyngeal carcinoma after radiation failure at the primary site. Laryngoscope 1988; 98:1220–1226.
249. Mendenhall NP, Parsons JT, Cassisi NJ, et al: Carcinoma of the nasal vestibule. Int J Radiat Oncol Biol Phys 1984; 10:627–637.
250. Kramer TS: Nasal vestibule, nasal cavity, and paranasal sinuses. In: Laramore GE (ed): Radiation Therapy of Head and Neck Cancer, pp 145–170. Berlin, Springer-Verlag, 1989.
251. Parsons JT, Stringer SP, Mancuso AA, et al: Nasal vestibule, nasal cavity, and paranasal sinuses. In: Million RR, Cassisi NJ (eds): Management of Head and Neck Cancer: A Multidisciplinary Approach, 2nd ed, pp 551–598. Philadelphia, J.B. Lippincott, 1994.
252. Pop LA, Kaanders JH, Heinerman EC: High dose intracavitary brachytherapy of early and superficial carcinoma of the nasal vestibule as an alternative to low dose rate interstitial radiation therapy. Radiother Oncol 1993; 27:69–72.
253. Roush GC: Epidemiology of cancer of the nose and paranasal sinuses—current concepts. Head Neck Surg 1979; 2:3–11.
254. Bingham BJ, Griffiths MV: Sublabial rhinotomy with septal transfixation as an approach to the nasal fossa, paranasal sinuses and nasopharynx. J Laryngol Otol 1989; 103:661–663.
255. Karim AB, Kralendonk JH, Njo KH, et al: Ethmoid and upper nasal cavity carcinoma: treatment, results and complications. Radiother Oncol 1990; 19:109–120.
256. Antonello M, Polico R, Botner F, et al: Radiation treatment in the carcinoma of paranasal sinuses and nasal cavity. Acta Otorhinolaryngol Ital 1996; 16:347–354.
257. McNicoll W, Hopkin N, Dalley VM, et al: Cancer of the paranasal sinuses and nasal cavities. Part II: Results of treatment. J Laryngol Otol 1984; 98:707–718.
258. Kent SE, Majumdar B: Metastases of malignant diseases of the nasal cavity and paranasal sinuses. J Laryngol Oncol 1984; 98:471–474.
259. Paulino AC, Fisher SG, Marks JE: Is prophylactic neck irradiation indicated in patients with squamous cell carcinoma of the maxillary sinus? Int J Radiat Oncol Biol Phys 1997; 39:283–289.
260. Waldron JN, O'Sullivan B, Warde P, et al: Ethmoid sinus cancer: twenty-nine cases managed with primary radiotherapy. Int J Radiat Oncol Biol Phys 1998; 41:361–369.
261. Haas JS, Cox JD: Cervical nodal metastasis from an unknown primary carcinoma. In: Laramore GE (ed): Radiation Therapy of Head and Neck Cancer, pp 211–218. Berlin, Springer-Verlag, 1989.
262. Jesse RH, Perez CA, Fletcher GH: Cervical lymph node metastasis: unknown primary cancer. Cancer 1973; 31:854–859.
263. Harper CS, Mendenhall WM, Parsons JT, et al: Cancer in neck nodes with unknown primary site: role of mucosal radiotherapy. Head Neck 1990; 12:463–469.
264. Reddy SP, Marks JE: Metastatic carcinoma in the cervical lymph nodes from an unknown primary site: results of bilateral neck plus mucosal irradiation vs. ipsilateral neck irradiation. Int J Radiat Oncol Biol Phys 1997; 37:797–802.
265. Million RR, Cassisi NJ, Mancuso AA: The unknown primary. In: Million RR, Cassisi NJ (eds): Management of Head and Neck Cancer: A Multidisciplinary Approach, 2nd ed, pp 311–320. Philadelphia, Lippincott, 1994.
266. Johnson JT, Newman RK: The anatomic location of neck metastasis from occult squamous cell carcinoma. Otolaryngol Head Neck Surg 1981; 89:54–58.
267. Freeman D, Mendenhall WM, Parsons JT, et al: Unknown primary squamous cell carcinoma of the head and neck: is mucosal irradiation necessary? Int J Radiat Oncol Biol Phys 1992; 23:889–890.
268. Conley J, Schuller DE: Malignancies of the ear. Laryngoscope 1976; 86:1147–1163.
269. Kinney SE, Wood BG: Malignancies of the external ear canal and temporal bone: surgical techniques and results. Laryngoscope 1987; 97:158.
270. Prasad S, Janecka IP: Efficacy of surgical treatments for squamous cell carcinoma of the temporal bone: a literature review. Otolaryngol Head Neck Surg 1994; 110:270–280.
271. Korzeniowski S, Pszon J: The results of radiotherapy of cancer of the middle ear. Int J Radiat Oncol Biol Phys 1990; 18:631–633.
272. Million RR, Cassisi NJ, Mancuso AA: Temporal bone. In: Million RR, Cassisi NJ (eds): Management of Head and Neck Cancer: A Multidisciplinary Approach, 2nd ed, pp 751–764. Philadelphia, Lippincott, 1994.
273. Olson LE, Cox JD: Chemodectomas. In: Laramore GE (ed): Radiation Therapy of Head and Neck Cancer, pp 171–179. Berlin, Springer-Verlag, 1989.
274. Gulya AJ: The glomus tumor and its biology. Laryngoscope 1993; 103:7–15.
275. Brammer RE, Graham MD, Kemink JL: Glomus tumors of the temporal bone: contemporary evaluation and therapy. Otolaryngol Clin North Am 1984; 17:499–512.
276. Springate SC, Haraf D, Weichselbaum RR: Temporal bone chemodectomas—comparing surgery and radiation therapy. Oncology 1991; 5:131–137.
277. Powell S, Peters N, Harmer C: Chemodectoma of the head and neck: results of treatment in 84 patients. Int J Radiat Oncol Biol Phys 1992; 22:919–924.
278. Schild SE, Foote RL, Buskirk SJ, et al: Results of radiotherapy for chemodectomas. Mayo Clin Proc 1992; 67:537–540.
279. Mendenhall WM, Million RR, Parsons JT, et al: Chemodectoma of the carotid body and ganglion nodosum treated with radiation therapy. Int J Radiat Oncol Biol Phys 1986; 12:2175–2178.
280. Abbey LM, Schwab BH, Landau GC, et al: Incidence of second primary breast cancer among patients with a first primary salivary gland tumor. Cancer 1984; 54:1439–1442.
281. Wick MR, Ockner DM, Mills SE, et al: Homologous carcinomas of the breast, skin, and salivary glands. A histologic and immunohistochemical comparison of ductal mammary carcinoma, ductal sweat gland carcinoma, and salivary duct carcinoma. Am J Clin Pathol 1998; 109:75–84.
282. Batsakis JG, Regezi JA: The pathology of head and neck tumors: salivary glands, part I. Head Neck Surg 1978; 1:59–68.
283. Spiro RH: Management of malignant tumors of the salivary glands. Oncology 1998; 12:671–680.
284. Hanna EY, Suen JY: Neoplasms of the salivary glands. In: Cummings CW, Fredrickson JM, Harker LA, et al (eds): Otolaryngology—Head and Neck Surgery, pp 1255–1302. St. Louis, Mosby, 1998.
285. Calhoun KH: Management of the facial nerve in parotid malignancies. In: Shah JP, Johnson JT (eds): Proceedings of 4th International Conference on Head and Neck Cancer, pp 712–718. Arlington, VA, Society of Head and Neck Surgeons, 1996.
286. Fu KK, Leibel SA, Levine ML, et al: Carcinoma of the major and minor salivary glands: analysis of treatment results and sites and causes of failures. Cancer 1977; 40:2882–2890.
287. Shidnia H, Hornback NB, Hamaker R, et al: Carcinoma of major salivary glands. Cancer 1980; 45:693–697.
288. Tran L, Sadeghi A, Hanson D, et al: Major salivary gland tumors: treatment results and prognostic factors. Laryngoscope 1986; 96:1139–1144.
289. Fitzpatrick PJ, Theriault C: Malignant salivary gland tumors. Int J Radiat Oncol Biol Phys 1986; 12:1743–1747.
290. Borthne A, Kjellevold K, Kaalhus O, et al: salivary gland malignant neoplasms: treatment and prognosis. Int J Radiat Oncol Biol Phys 1986; 12:747–754.
291. Miglianico L, Eschwege F, Marandas P, et al: Cervico-facial adenoid cystic carcinoma: study of 102 cases. Influence of radiation therapy. Int J Radiat Oncol Biol Phys 1987; 13:673–678.

292. Reddy SP, Marks JE: Treatment of locally advanced, high-grade, malignant tumors of major salivary glands. Laryngoscope 1988; 98:450–454.
293. Bissett RJ, Fitzpatrick PJ: Malignant submandibular gland tumors. A review of 91 patients. Am J Clin Oncol 1988; 11:46–51.
294. North CA, Lee DJ, Piantadosi S, et al: Carcinoma of the major salivary glands treated by surgery or surgery plus postoperative radiotherapy. Int J Radiat Oncol Biol Phys 1990; 18:1319–1326.
295. Armstrong JG, Harrison LB, Spiro RH, et al: The role of postoperative radiation in malignant tumors of major salivary gland origin: a matched pair analysis using historical controls. Arch Otolaryngol Head Neck Surg 1990; 116:290–293.
296. Frankenthaler RA, Luna MA, Lee SS, et al: Prognostic variables in parotid gland cancer. Arch Otolaryngol Head Neck Surg 1991; 117:1251–1256.
297. Molinari R, Guzzo M, Mattavelli F, et al: Indications and efficacy of postoperative radiation therapy for salivary gland cancer. In: Johnson JT, Didolkar MS (eds): Head and Neck Cancer, vol. III, pp 607–617. Amsterdam, Elsevier Science Publishers, 1993.
298. Douglas JG, Laramore GE, Austin-Seymour M, et al: Neutron radiotherapy for adenoid cystic carcinoma of minor salivary glands. Int J Radiat Oncol Biol Phys 1996; 36:87–93.
299. Wang CC, Goodman M: Photon irradiation of unresectable carcinomas of salivary glands. Int J Radiat Oncol Biol Phys 1991; 21:569–576.
300. Stevens KL, Hobsley M: The treatment of pleomorphic adenomas by formal parotidectomy. Br J Surg 1982; 69:1–3.
301. Dawson AK, Orr JA: Long-term results of local excision and radiotherapy in pleomorphic adenoma of the parotid. Int J Radiat Oncol Biol Phys 1985; 11:451–455.
302. Barton J, Slevin NJ, Gleave EN: Radiotherapy for pleomorphic adenoma of the parotid gland. Int J Radiat Oncol Biol Phys 1992; 22:925–928.
303. Buchholz TA, Laramore GE, Griffin TW: Fast neutron irradiation of recurrent pleomorphic adenomas of the parotid gland. Am J Clin Oncol 1992; 15:441–445.

21 *Gynecologic Tumors*

CARLOS A. PEREZ, MD, Radiation Oncology
PERRY W. GRIGSBY, MD, Radiation Oncology
DAVID G. MUTCH, MD, Gynecologic Oncology
K. S. CLIFFORD CHAO, MD, Radiation Oncology
JACK BASIL, MD, Gynecologic Oncology

So absolute she seems
And in herself complete

JOHN MILTON (1608–1674),
Paradise Lost

Perspective

Gynecologic cancers include malignant tumors of the cervix, endometrium (uterine sarcomas and gestational trophoblastic tumors), ovary, fallopian tube, vagina, and vulva. The most frequent gynecologic cancer before the age of 50 is carcinoma of the cervix; in older women it is carcinoma of the endometrium. Although carcinoma of the ovary does not occur as frequently, certainly it is the most lethal (Table 21–1). After the reproductive years and menopause, the incidence of endometrial cancer and epithelial ovarian cancer rises sharply. These two malignancies have quite different biologic behavior despite a close anatomic and functional relationship. Cancers of the endometrium usually present early in the history of the disease with irregular bleeding, which often results in early diagnosis and high cure rates. On the other hand, although ovarian cancer presents in the same general age group, it has no early symptoms, is difficult to detect, and is diagnosed in late stages, when cure is difficult to achieve.[11]

In 1930, uterine cancer (endometrial and cervical) was the most common cause of death in women. Since then, death rates have dropped more than two thirds, and now are roughly equivalent to those for ovarian cancer because of the availability of the Papanicolaou (Pap) smear and the accessibility of the endometrial cavity to diagnostic curettage. However, cancer of the ovary, without a clear means of early diagnosis, remains the fourth leading cause of cancer deaths in women, causing more than 14,000 deaths in the United States in 2000.[12]

The Pap smear[13, 14] provides a means of early detection of practically all cervical carcinomas, as well as those in a preneoplastic process; almost all cases would be preventable or curable if every woman had an annual Pap smear. Unfortunately, in the 1992 National Heath Interview Survey, only 43% of women reported that they had a Pap smear in the previous year.[15] Nonetheless, most gynecologic cancers are curable. The role of surgery, central to the management of most gynecologic neoplasias, has been greatly enhanced since the first operations for cervical cancer and ovarian neoplasia in the mid- to late 1800s. The technologic developments of radiation oncology and knowledge of radiation biology have enhanced the role of this modality. In the 1950s, chemotherapy for gynecologic malignancies made a dramatic entrance with the discovery that methotrexate could cure metastatic choriocarcinoma. Since then, a broad experience in the use of chemotherapy in gynecologic cancer has developed.[11]

Although there are similarities in cancer detection, diagnosis, and treatment, each of these cancers behaves quite differently from one another in a number of ways. Therefore, each patient requires optimal individualization of management. A multidisciplinary and integrated approach to the management of these patients, with optimal use of each modality, has substantially improved outcome and enhanced the quality of life of many women affected by these neoplasias.

TABLE 21–1. **Incidence and Mortality of Gynecologic Cancer in the United States, 2000**

Site	Incidence	Mortality
Cervix		
Carcinoma *in situ*	65,000	—
Invasive	12,800	4600
Endometrium	36,100	6500
Ovary	23,100	14,000
Vulva	3400	800
Vagina	2100	600

Data from American Cancer Society: 2000 Facts and Figures. Atlanta, American Cancer Society, 2000.

Carcinoma of the Uterine Cervix

Epidemiology and Etiology

Epidemiology

In the United States, it is estimated that there were 12,800 new cases of invasive cervical cancer in the year 2000 and 4600 deaths from the disease,[12] in addition to over 65,000 cases of carcinoma *in situ* or premalignant disease.[10] Although the mean age at diagnosis is 52 years, cervical cancer can be found in women between the ages of 17 and 90 years.[16] Elderly postmenopausal women (age >60 years) who have become less active or sexually inactive and are not being annually screened by Pap smears account for an increasing percentage of advanced-stage (IIB and III) cervical cancer patients.[3] In addition, the incidence of cervical carcinoma is substantially higher among women in low socioeconomic groups.[17] Carcinoma of the cervix is most common in Latin American and Western European women[12]; the role played by male circumcision in cervical carcinogenesis, previously suggested by low incidences in Jewish women, now is considered debatable.[18]

Of the several histologic subtypes of cervical carcinoma, squamous cell (epidermoid) carcinoma is the most frequent and accounts for 85% to 90% of invasive cervical cancers. Epidermoid carcinoma occurs more frequently in women who had first intercourse at an early age, have had multiple partners (or their partners have had multiple partners), or have had a large number of pregnancies.[19, 20] Agarwal and coworkers,[18] in a case control study in India, documented an increased risk for cervical cancer when the husband had sexual relations before marriage and when the husband had three or more extramarital sexual partners. A history of sexually transmitted disease was an important risk factor, as was lack of circumcision of the husband. In fact, cervical cancer is often associated with a history of sexually transmitted diseases, including gonorrhea, syphilis, herpes simplex, and *Trichomonas* or *Chlamydia* infections. In addition, if a woman or her partner has ever had genital warts, then she is at increased risk of developing human papillomavirus (HPV)–related cervical cancer.[21] Of note, there now is some degree of evidence that links the use of oral contraceptives with carcinoma of the uterine cervix.[22, 23]

Etiology

- Cervical carcinomas are often seen in women who have a history of sexually transmitted diseases. The identification of herpes simplex virus type II (HSV-2) and the presence of high antibody titers against this virus have been reported, and a correlation was suggested with cervical cancer.[24] However, although a cause-and-effect relationship has not been proven, HSV-2 may act as a cofactor.[25, 26]
- HPV plays an important role in the pathogenesis of cervical carcinoma.[27, 28] More than 120 different genotypes of HPV have been identified,[29] and nearly all degrees of cervical intraepithelial neoplasia and invasive cancers have been associated with HPV infections. HPV types 6 and 11 are usually found in benign condylomata acuminata, low-grade dysplasias, and laryngeal papillomas. HPV types 16, 18, 31, 33, 35, and 39 are associated with high-grade dysplasias and carcinomas. Bosch and associates,[30] in an analysis of 1000 histologic sections, noted more than 20 different genital HPVs associated with cervical cancer. In squamous cell carcinoma, HPV 16 predominated (51% of specimens), but in adenocarcinoma and adenosquamous carcinoma (56% and 39% of solid tumors, respectively), HPV 18 was more common.
- In addition to its effects on women alone, Boon and colleagues[31] have suggested that HPV, estimated to be present in over 75% of the Balinese Hindu population with genital carcinomas, may be a cofactor in genital carcinogenesis in both sexes. In contrast, in the Netherlands, where men are usually circumcised, the man is exclusively a vector of the HPV and not a victim as in Bali.
- Of interest with respect to the role of the man, several authors have noted a significantly higher incidence of carcinoma of the cervix in the wives of men with penile carcinoma.[32, 33] Boon and colleagues[31] pointed out that, even when the spouse does not have penile carcinoma, he may have contributed to the development of cervical carcinoma by being a vector of HPV.

Detection and Diagnosis

Screening

The Pap smear uses exfoliative cytology as a method for screening cervical carcinoma. Optimal cytologic samples include a cervical scrape, endocervical sampling with a brush (which provides superior samples),[34] and collecting cells from the "posterior vaginal pool." The technique for obtaining the Pap smear has been described in many standard textbooks.[4]

Pap smears have proven very effective in diagnosing preclinical cervical disease, yet certain pitfalls may occur. Over the past decade, improvements in screening techniques have led to false-negative rates of less than 10% to 20%,[35, 36] as a result of physician sampling error, inadequate screening methods, and inaccurate interpretation by the cytopathologist.[37] However, in an invasive carcinoma, the malignant cells may be masked by cellular debris and inflammatory cells. If a gross lesion is seen, cervical biopsy (not cytology) should be performed. The National Institutes of Health has published consensus guidelines for screening, prevention, and treatment of cervical carcinoma[38]; it is now strongly recommended that women obtain Pap smears on an annual basis (Table 21–2).

Because of its role in cervical cancer etiology, there is increasing interest in developing screening methods for HPV. Molecular techniques for identification of HPV DNA

TABLE 21–2. **ACOG Suggested Frequency of Cytologic Screening for Cervical Cancer**

Patient Population	Frequency
≥18 years or any age sexually active	Initial smear
High risk: Early sexual intercourse, multiple partners	Annually
Low risk: Late sexual intercourse, single partners	After two successive negative smears, 3- to 5-year risk of abnormality is small; decision of patient and physician
Diethylstilbestrol exposed	Onset of menstruation or 14 years old or symptomatic (whichever occurs first) every 6 months—annually
S/P hysterectomy	Vaginal smears 3 to 5 per year
S/P therapy for preinvasive/ invasive malignancy	Every 3 months for 2 years, then every 6 months
Postmenopausal	
Sexually active	Annually
Sexually inactive	Every other year

ACOG = American College of Obstetrics and Gynecology; S/P = salpingo-oophorectomy.

From DuBeshter B, Lin J, Angel C, et al: Gynecologic tumors. In: Rubin P (ed): Clinical Oncology: A Multidisciplinary Approach for Physicians and Students, 7th ed, pp 363–418. Philadelphia, W.B. Saunders Co., 1993.

are highly sensitive and specific; however, their usefulness in the diagnosis and management of squamous cell carcinoma of the cervix is reliant on health resource availability and local policies.[39, 40]

Clinical Detection

Cervical intraepithelial neoplasia and early invasive carcinomas of the cervix are usually asymptomatic and discovered only with routine screening. An abnormal Pap smear should be followed by colposcopy because neoplastic epithelium has patterns of growth that are distinct from disease regression that may be recognized under the magnification of the colposcope[41]; cervical biopsy may be guided by the colposcopic findings. However, at times, the abnormal epithelium is not evident on the cervical portio and colposcopy is inadequate. In these situations, diagnostic cone biopsy may be required.

The most common presenting complaint is abnormal vaginal bleeding, including postcoital bleeding, irregular menses, or postmenopausal bleeding. As the tumor increases in size, the patient may complain of yellowish, bloody, or foul-smelling vaginal discharge. In more advanced cases, the patient can have pelvic or back pain or urinary symptoms. Examination of the patient with cervical cancer may reveal a friable ulcerated lesion, or the cervix may be replaced with an exophytic tumor. Sometimes the cervix appears normal on speculum examination, but palpation reveals an expanded, firm, barrel-shaped cervix. The tumor may completely ulcerate the cervix, which may be impossible to identify, and a crater may be found at the top of the vagina, extending out onto the vaginal fornices.

Local spread beyond the cervix to the parametrial tissues is best appreciated on bimanual rectovaginal examination. The tumor may involve the vaginal walls. In more advanced stages, it invades the base of the bladder or rectum. Low back pain suggests the possibility of periaortic lymph node involvement with extension into the lumbosacral roots, or hydronephrosis should be considered.

Diagnostic Procedures

- Every patient with carcinoma of the cervix should be jointly evaluated by the radiation and gynecologic oncologist. After a *general physical examination* with special attention to the supraclavicular (nodal) areas, abdomen, and liver, a careful pelvic examination should be carried out with as little discomfort as possible; it should include inspection of the external genitalia, vagina, and uterine cervix, rectal examination, and bimanual palpation of the pelvis. Cystoscopy or rectosigmoidoscopy should be performed in all patients with stage IIB, III, and IVA disease or in those with earlier stages who have a history of urinary or lower gastrointestinal tract disturbances. An outline of the diagnostic procedures for carcinoma of the cervix is presented in Table 21–3.[42]
- *Colposcopy* may adequately evaluate the exocervix and a portion of the endocervix adjacent to the transition of the squamous and columnar epithelium (T zone). This examination, performed with a colposcope, provides a 10- to 15-fold magnification view of the cervix.
- *Conization* must be performed in specific situations, such as when no gross lesion of the cervix is noted and endocervical tumor is suspected, diagnosis of microinvasive carcinoma is made on biopsy, or the pa-

TABLE 21–3. **Diagnostic Work-Up for Carcinoma of the Uterine Cervix**

General
History
Physical examination, including bimanual pelvic and rectal examinations
Diagnostic Procedures
Cytologic smears (Papanicolaou) if not bleeding
Colposcopy
Conization (subclinical tumor)
Punch biopsies (edge of gross tumor, four quadrants)
Dilatation and curettage
Cytoscopy rectosigmoidoscopy (stages IIB, III, and IVA)
Radiographic Studies
Standard
Chest radiography
Intravenous pyelography
Barium enema (stages III and IVA and earlier stages if there are symptoms referable to colon or rectum)
Complementary
Lymphangiography
Computed tomography or magnetic resonance
Laboratory Studies
Complete blood count
Blood chemistry
Urinalysis

From Perez CA: Uterine cervix. In: Perez CA, Brady LW (eds): Principles and Practice of Radiation Oncology, 3rd ed, pp 1733–1834. Philadelphia, Lippincott-Raven, 1998.

tient is not reliable for continuous follow-up. When a gross lesion of the cervix is present, multiple punch biopsies should be obtained from the margin of any suspicious area, as well as in all four quadrants of the cervix and from any suspicious areas in the vagina.

- *Fractional curettage* of the endocervical canal and the endometrium is recommended at the time of initial evaluation or during the first intracavitary radioisotope insertion (if the patient is treated with radiation therapy).
- For invasive carcinoma, patients should have complete peripheral blood evaluation, including hemogram, white blood cell count, differential, and platelet count, and SMA-12, with particular attention to blood urea nitrogen, creatinine, uric acid, liver function values, and urinalysis.
- Chest radiographs and intravenous pyelograms (IVPs) should be obtained in all patients for staging purposes. Currently, it is common practice at some institutions to obtain a computed tomography (CT) scan of the pelvis and abdomen with contrast material; this study is a substitute for the IVP. A barium enema study should be performed in patients with stage IIB, III, and IVA disease, as well as those with earlier stages who have symptoms referable to the colon and rectum.

Classification and Staging

Histopathology

- Squamous cell lesions are seen most frequently (Table 21–4).[43] Within this group are keratinizing and nonkeratinizing cancers. There is no difference in prognosis between the two types.
- Adenocarcinoma occurs in about 10% of cases; however, there is evidence that the incidence is increasing.[44, 45] These cancers originate in the endocervical canal and often are of greater volume at diagnosis. In some reports, the survival is equivalent to that of squamous cell carcinoma[46]; in others, a lower survival for patients with adenocarcinoma has been described.[47]
- Clear cell carcinomas of the vagina and cervix have been associated with diethylstilbestrol (DES) exposure *in utero*, initially described in 1971.[48] The risk of developing cancer is small—estimated to be in the upper range of 1 in 1000 to 1 in 10,000.[49] More commonly, benign abnormalities such as adenosis (glandular epithelium located in the vagina) and cervical changes (transverse ridges, "cock's comb") are seen.
- Small cell carcinomas of the cervix are of neuroendocrine origin. These cancers are very aggressive and are often widely disseminated at the time of diagnosis.[50] The prognosis for patients treated with conventional therapy, even at an early stage, is dismal.
- Other rare cervical malignancies include verrucous carcinoma, adenoid basal cell carcinoma, adenoid cystic carcinoma, and glassy cell carcinoma. Primary cervical sarcomas or lymphomas are rare.

TABLE 21–4. **Histologic Classification of Uterine Cervix Carcinoma**

Type	Incidence (%)
Squamous Carcinoma	
Large cell nonkeratinizing	57
Large cell keratinizing	22
Small cell nonkeratinizing	6
Adenocarcinoma	
Endocervical	10
Endometrioid	2
Clear cell	2
Others	1
Mixed Epithelial Carcinoma	
Adenosquamous	2–5
Glassy cell	1
Neuroendocrine	
Carcinoid	<1
Small cell	1

Modified from Bragg DG, Rubin P, Youker JE (eds): Oncologic Imaging. Philadelphia, W.B. Saunders Co., 1985.

Staging

It is imperative that the gynecologic, medical, and radiation oncologists jointly stage the tumor in every patient, with bimanual pelvic and rectal examination under general anesthesia. Ideally, staging should be performed before the institution of therapy. However, on occasion, after an initial evaluation, the final staging is postponed because of logistic and economic reasons until the time of a surgical procedure or the first intracavitary radioisotope insertion (which should be performed within 2 weeks from initiation of external irradiation, if the patient is treated with this modality). In surgically treated patients, the clinical staging can be performed under anesthesia immediately before the radical hysterectomy is performed.

The International Federation of Gynecology and Obstetrics (FIGO) staging recommendations were last published in 1999.[51] Differences between these and earlier recommendations involve a change in stage IB to include all clinically visible tumors limited to the cervix and preclinical cancers larger than IA2. The staging of stage IB lesions (confined to the cervix) is subdivided into IB1 (clinical lesions less than 4 cm in size) and IB2 (lesions greater than 4 cm in size). A parallel TNM staging system has been proposed by the American Joint Committee on Cancer (AJCC).[5] The current criteria for the various stages are defined in Table 21–5 and Figure 21–1. When staging is performed, all histologic types should be included, and when there is a disagreement regarding staging, the earlier stage should be selected for statistical purposes.

The FIGO staging system is based on clinical evaluation (inspection, palpation, colposcopy); x-ray examination of the chest, kidneys, and skeleton; and endocervical curettage and biopsies. Lymphangiograms, arteriograms, CT and magnetic resonance imaging (MRI) findings, and laparoscopy or laparotomy findings are of value in planning, but they should not be used for clinical staging. Suspected invasion of the bladder or rectum should be confirmed by biopsy. Bullous edema of the bladder and swelling of the mucosa of the rectum are not accepted as definitive criteria

TABLE 21–5. **Staging of Carcinoma of the Uterine Cervix**

Stage	Grouping	FIGO Staging	Descriptor
I	T1	I	T1: Cervical carcinoma confined to uterus (extension to corpus should be disregarded)
	T1a	IA	T1a: Preclinical invasive carcinoma, diagnosed by microscopy only
IA1	T1a1,N0,M0	IA1	T1a1: Minimal microscopic stromal invasion (≤3 mm in depth)
IA2	T1a2,N0,M0	IA2	T1a2: Tumor with invasive component ≤5 mm taken from base of epithelium and ≤7 mm in horizontal spread
	T1b	IB	T1b: Clinical lesions confined to the cervix or preclinical lesions greater than IA
IB1	T1b1,N0,M0	IB1	T1b1: Clinical lesions ≤4 cm in size
IB2	T1b2,N0,M0	IB2	T1b2: Clinical lesions >4 cm in size N0: No regional lymph node metastasis M0: No distant metastasis
II	T2	II	T2: Cervical carcinoma invades beyond uterus, but not to pelvic wall or to lower third of vagina
IIA	T2a,N0,M0	IIA	T2a: Tumor without parametrial invasion
IIB	T2b,N0,M0	IIB	T2b: Tumor with parametrial invasion
III	T3	III	T3: Cervical carcinoma extends to pelvic wall and/or involves lower third of vagina and/or causes hydronephrosis or nonfunctioning kidney
IIIA	T3a,N0,M0	IIIA	T3a: Tumor involves lower third of vagina, with no extension to pelvic wall
IIIB	T1,N1,M0 T2,N1,M0 T3a,N1,M0 T3b,Any N,M0	IIIB	T3b: Tumor extends to pelvic wall and/or causes hydronephrosis or nonfunctioning kidney N1: Regional lymph node metastasis
IVA	T4,Any N,M0	IVA	T4: Tumor invades mucosa of the bladder or rectum and/or extends beyond the true pelvis
IVB	Any T,Any N,M1	IVB	M1: Distant metastasis

FIGO = International Federation of Gynecology and Obstetrics.

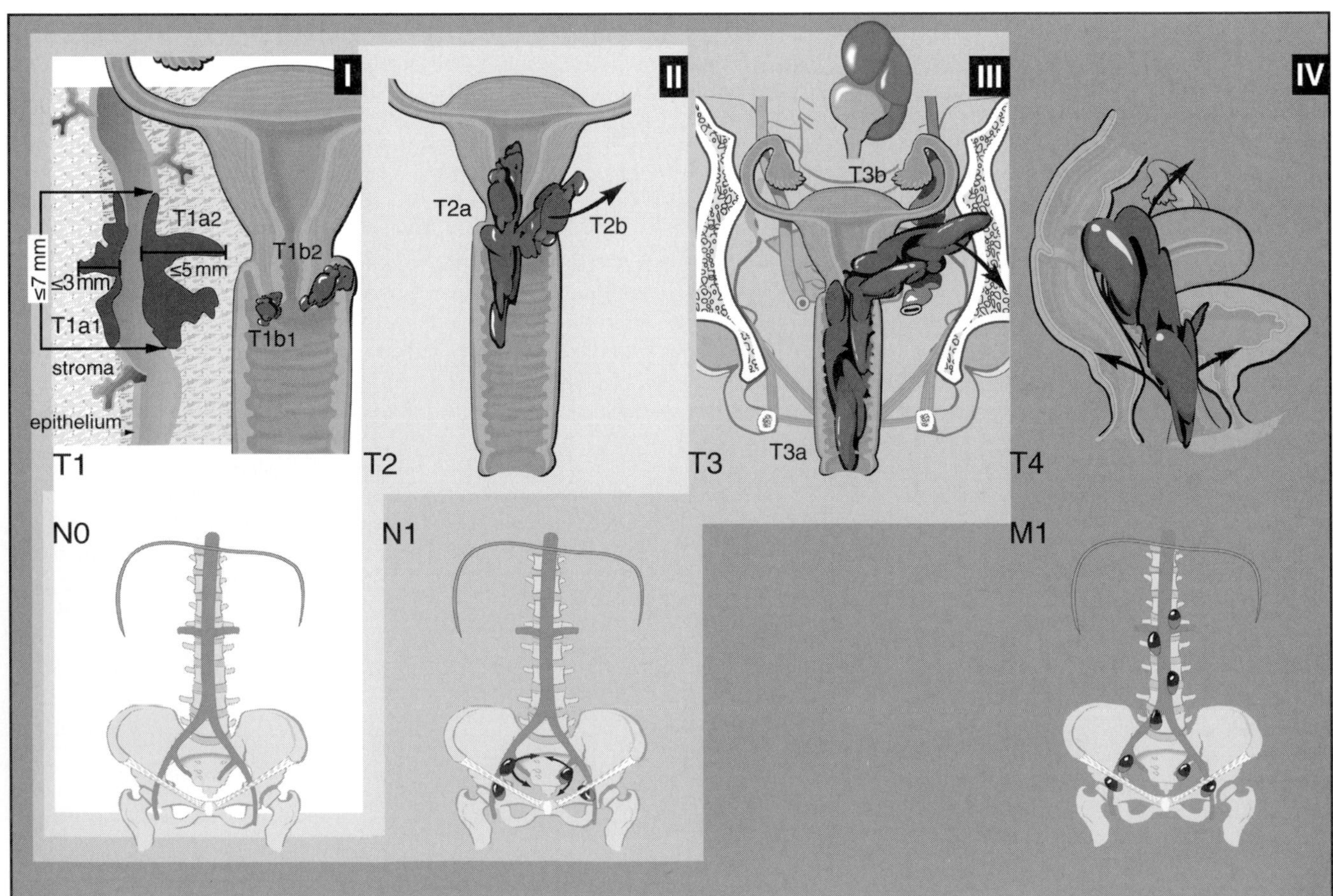

Figure 21–1. Anatomic staging for carcinoma of the uterine cervix.

for staging. Some gynecologists have advocated the use of pretherapy laparotomy, particularly to evaluate the presence of para-aortic lymph nodes, and studies have demonstrated a clinical benefit with this procedure.[52, 53]

Principles of Treatment

A multidisciplinary approach with close cooperation between the various members of the oncology team is mandatory for optimal management of these patients, and an integrated team approach should be vigorously pursued. The controversy continues, however, between those who advocate either radical surgery or radiation therapy for the treatment of early carcinoma of the uterine cervix. In general, there has been a decline in the use of irradiation that may be related to earlier tumor detection because of greater awareness by physicians and patients, the widespread use of Pap smear screening, and greater use of surgery in the treatment of these patients. Table 21–6 summarizes the treatment decisions by stage.[42, 54] Participation in clinical trials is strongly advised.

Cervical intraepithelial neoplasia (CIN; grades 1–3) is usually treated with cryotherapy, loop electrosurgical excision procedure (LEEP), conization, or laser therapy. The recurrence rate following cold-knife conization treatment is approximately 3%,[55] although it is less successful in HIV-positive women.[56] Hysterectomy also has been used to treat cervical dysplasias and carcinoma *in situ* in the postreproductive age group. In addition, patients with carcinoma *in situ*, which may include those with severe dysplasia, are usually treated with a total abdominal hysterectomy, with or without a small vaginal cuff. The decision to remove the ovaries depends on the age of the patient and the status of the ovaries. Occasionally, when the patient wishes to have more children, carcinoma *in situ* may be treated conservatively with a therapeutic conization, laser, or cryotherapy. Irradiation also can be useful for the treatment of *in situ* carcinoma, particularly in patients with strong medical contraindications for surgery or when there is multifocal carcinoma *in situ* in both the cervix and the vagina.[57]

Surgery generally is limited to cancers in stages I and IIA. It also may be used in previously irradiated patients with recurrent disease. The different types of total abdominal hysterectomy are intrafascial, extrafascial type I, modified radical type II, and radical type III (Table 21–7). The choice of definitive irradiation or radical surgery for stage IB and IIA carcinoma of the cervix remains highly controversial, and the preference of one procedure over the other depends on the oncologist involved, the general condition of the patient, and the characteristics of the lesion.

Surgery

The risk of lymph node metastases in lesions that have less than 3 mm of invasion is less than 1%.[58] Therefore, patients with stage IA disease who fulfill the Society of Gynecologic Oncologists criteria for microinvasion (neoplastic epithelium invades the stroma to a depth of less than or equal to 3 mm beneath the basement membrane, while lymphovascular involvement is not demonstrated) can be treated with extrafascial hysterectomy without pelvic lymphadenectomy.[59] Because the incidence of lymph node metastases has a greater significance in lesions with 3 to 5 mm invasion, a modified radical hysterectomy and pelvic lymphadenectomy are recommended in these patients. Cone biopsy (with clear margins) also can be used if childbearing potential is desired; however, this conservative treatment has not been extensively evaluated.[60] Any stage IA patient who is a poor surgical candidate may be treated with radiation therapy (one or two intracavitary insertions for 6500 to 8000 milligram-hours [mgh]).[57]

Patients with stage IB tumors may be treated with radical hysterectomy and pelvic lymphadenectomy or radiation therapy. During a radical hysterectomy, the uterus, cervix, surrounding parametrial tissues, cardinal ligaments, and upper vagina are removed. The ovaries may be left *in situ* in young women. Many gynecologic oncologists limit radical hysterectomy as primary treatment to patients with cervical tumors less than 4 cm in size. Patients with bulky (>4 cm) or barrel-shaped tumors are then treated with preoperative external beam and intracavitary irradiation followed by an extrafascial hysterectomy, or with higher doses of irradiation alone. Nonetheless, at least one study has shown that tumor size is of less importance than tumor stage in predicting survival.[61]

Surgical treatment for stage IIA cervical carcinoma is

TABLE 21–6. **Multidisciplinary Treatment Decisions by Stage for Cervical Carcinoma**

Stage	Surgery		Radiation Therapy	Chemotherapy
IA (T1a,N0) microinvasive	Total hysterectomy Conization in select groups	or	Intracavitary RT mainly Pt. A: 70 Gy; Pt. B: 50 Gy	NR
IB* invasive (T1b,N0)	Radical hysterectomy plus pelvic node dissection		Combined intracavitary and external RT	CCR
IIA (T2a,N0)	Extrafascial	and/or	Pt. A: 75 Gy, Pt. B: 55 Gy Para-aortic 45 Gy	
IIB (T2b,N0)	NR, surgical staging		Combined external, intracavitary, and vaginal RT	CCR
IIIA,B (T3,N1,M0)	NR, surgical staging			IC II
IV (T4,N0,M0)	Exenteration for central locations		Pt. A: 80 Gy, Pt. B: 60 Gy Para-aortic: 45 Gy	
IV (Any T,Any N,M+)	NR		Palliative radiation therapy	IC II

*Bulky or barrel-shaped cervix, stages I–IIA: preoperative irradiation and extrafascial hysterectomy.
RT = radiation therapy; NR = not recommended; CCR = concurrent chemotherapy and irradiation; IC II = investigational chemotherapy, phase I/II trials.

TABLE 21–7. **Types of Abdominal Hysterectomy**

	Intrafascial	Extrafascial Type I	Modified Radical Type II	Radical Type III
Cervical fascia	Partially removed	Completely removed	Completely removed	Completely removed
Vaginal cuff removal	None	Small rim removed	Proximal 1–2 cm removed	Upper third to half removed
Bladder	Partially mobilized	Partially mobilized	Partially mobilized	Mobilized
Rectum	Not mobilized	Rectovaginal septum partially mobilized	Rectovaginal septum partially mobilized	Mobilized
Ureters	Not mobilized	Not mobilized	Unroofed in ureteral tunnel	Completely dissected to bladder entry
Cardinal ligaments	Resected medial to ureters	Resected medial to ureters	Resected at level of ureter	Resected at pelvic sidewall
Uterosacral ligaments	Resected at level of cervix	Resected at level of cervix	Partially resected	Resected at postpelvic insertion
Uterus	Removed	Removed	Removed	Removed
Cervix	Partially removed	Completely removed	Completely removed	Completely removed

Type IV, extended radical hysterectomy (partial removal of bladder and/or ureter), in addition to type III.

From Perez CA: Uterine cervix. In: Perez CA, Brady LW (eds): Principles and Practice of Radiation Oncology, 3rd ed, pp 1733–1834. Philadelphia, Lippincott-Raven, 1998.

radical hysterectomy with pelvic–para-aortic lymphadenectomy. An alternative is definitive irradiation. Lesion size and the patient's medical condition may influence the choice of treatment.

Radiation Therapy

Radiation therapy has been very effective in the treatment of all stages of cervical carcinoma. Approximate cure rates include 85% for stage I, 65% for stage II, 45% for stage III, and 25% for stage IV. Treatment plans are designed individually, based on the clinical (and surgical) stage of the disease. Most commonly, patients are treated with combinations of external beam and intracavitary radiation therapy. We advocate the customization of radiation dose to extent or stage of disease, as described in the Mallinckrodt Institute of Radiology guidelines for treatment.[42] In addition, a fine review paper by Lanciano describes many of the current treatment techniques and discusses possible means of optimization.[62]

External Beam Irradiation

External beam radiation therapy is used to treat the pelvis, including tissues between the obturator foramina and the lower common iliac lymph nodes and, as indicated, the para-aortic lymph nodes. Various portals for external beam irradiation can be designed. Extended-field irradiation (including the para-aortic lymph nodes) may be used if initial evaluation reveals para-aortic metastases or when occult disease is suspected.[63] The total irradiation dose given is usually described in relation to two reference points according to International Commission on Radiation Units and Measurements Report No. 38.[64] Point A is 2 cm lateral and 2 cm superior to the lateral vaginal fornix or external cervical os and, theoretically, represents the area where the uterine artery crosses the ureter. Point B is 3 cm lateral to point A and corresponds to the location of the obturator lymph nodes. In general, with low-dose-rate (LDR) treatment, 75 to 90 Gy is delivered to point A and 50 to 65 Gy is delivered to point B, depending on the stage and volume of the tumor.[42] Computer-generated isodose curves for both internal and external radiation sources allow more accurate determination of effective tumor doses and tolerable normal tissue doses and volumes (Fig. 21–2). The standard radiation therapy for cervical neoplasms of stage IB and higher is now accepted as external beam to the pelvis in combination with intracavitary application(s); radiation therapy is also used in the preoperative, postoperative, and adjuvant settings.[65] Of note, a 1997 survey of major academic centers showed that the majority of facilities use some form of central block for delivering homogenous radiation.[66] The study demonstrated that use of a standard—compared with an individualized—shield resulted in potential dose inhomogeneity, and the authors advised further investigation into techniques of shield construction.

Intracavitary Irradiation

Intracavitary irradiation has become essential in the treatment of cervical carcinoma. A hollow, metal tube (tandem) is inserted into the endocervical canal and uterus. Two vaginal colpostats (ovoids) are also placed in the vaginal fornices, and radioactive sources are inserted in the devices. The dose distribution is generally pear shaped, with the largest dose in the area of the upper vagina, cervix, and parametria (Fig. 21–3). The importance of intracavitary irradiation in enhancing the results in cervical cancer has been emphasized.[62, 67, 68]

In the early 1990s, the increasing use of high-dose-rate (HDR) brachytherapy versus LDR intracavitary radiation therapy prompted reviews by Fu and Phillips[69] and Orton and associates,[70] and there still is an ongoing debate as to which is more efficacious. More recent reviews have shown that, even today, techniques used at different institutions vary considerably; fraction sizes range from 5 to 7 Gy, with a median of 5 fractions.[71] In general, nonrandomized studies and one randomized clinical trial suggest that similar survival and local tumor control are achieved using

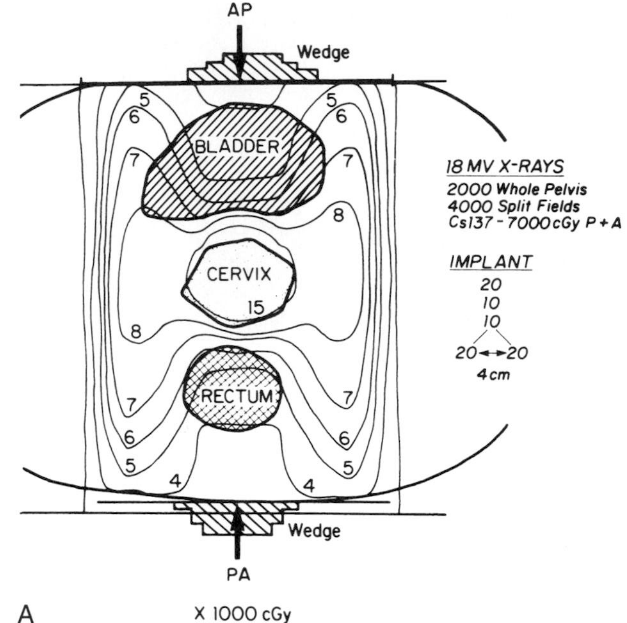

Figure 21–2. (A) Composite isodose curves through point A for patient with stage IIB carcinoma of the uterine cervix treated with external irradiation and two intracavitary insertions. Doses and source arrangement are shown. High doses can be delivered to the cervix and parametrial tissues with relative sparing of the bladder and rectum. (B) Composite isodose curves through point A using 40 Gy whole pelvis dose and reduced brachytherapy dose (46 Gy to point A). (From Perez CA: Uterine cervix. In: Perez CA, Brady LW [eds]: Principles and Practice of Radiation Oncology, 3rd ed, pp 1733–1834. Philadelphia, Lippincott-Raven, 1998, with permission.)

fractionated HDR compared with protracted LDR therapy for stage IB and II, but with lower complication rates.[72, 73] Nonetheless, a 1999 retrospective study has suggested that poorer rates are seen in patients with stage IIIB using HDR brachytherapy.[74]

Interstitial Irradiation

Interstitial implants also may be of benefit in the treatment of cervical carcinoma when adequate radiation therapy cannot be obtained with standard intracavitary applicators, depending on the geometry of the tumor and surrounding tissues.[75, 76] With interstitial therapy, a template is placed on the vulva, and hollow needles are inserted through the template into the tumor and surrounding tissues. After adequate placement is confirmed, a ^{192}Ir source is inserted into the needles. This device is particularly useful in patients with bulky parametrial disease, as well as in those who have vaginal recurrences after surgical therapy for cervical carcinoma.

Persistent or Recurrent Disease

If carcinoma recurs after treatment with radiation therapy, the patient may be a candidate for surgery. The recurrence must be central and confined to the cervix, uterus, bladder, and rectum. However, patients with disease that extends to the sidewall or patients with distant metastases cannot be salvaged by surgery. Pelvic exenteration (removal of uterus, cervix, bladder, rectum, with subsequent urostomy and colostomy) may be performed. In selected cases, an anterior exenteration (removal of bladder, anterior vagina, cervix, and uterus) may be acceptable if the tumor is confined to the cervix and upper vagina. Although reasonable cure

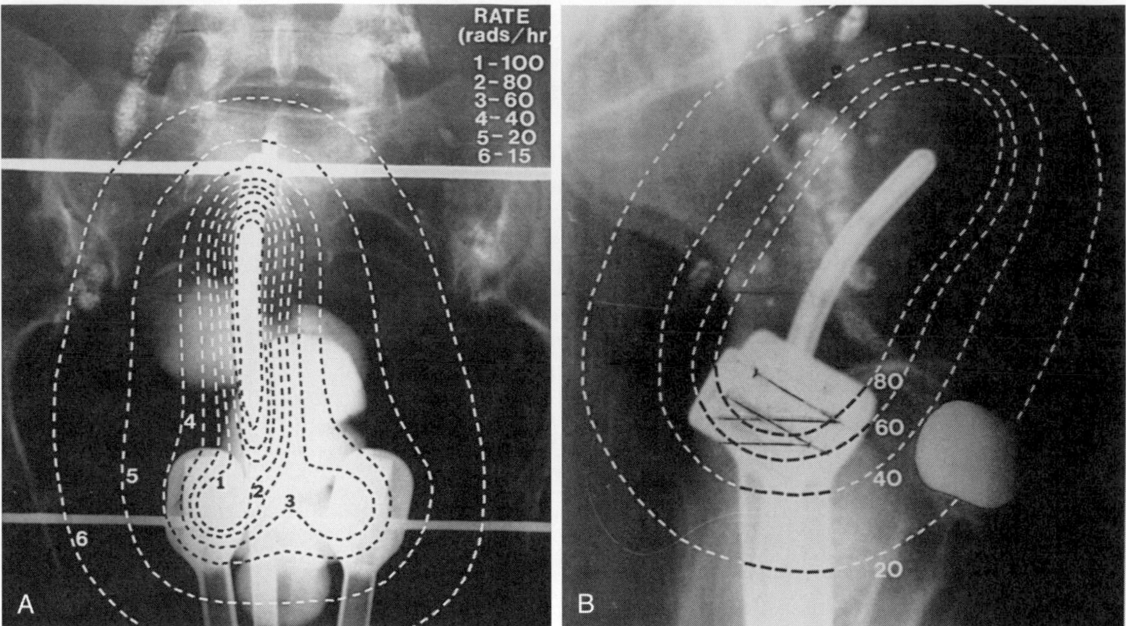

Figure 21–3. (A) Anteroposterior and (B) lateral radiographs of standard intracavitary insertion with afterloading Fletcher-Suit tandem and ovoids. Slight deviation of the tandem to the left is apparent. However, there is good symmetry between the tandem and the ovoids. On the lateral projection, the tandem is crossing the ovoids near the center of the long axis. Radiopaque marker is placed on the anterior lip of the cervix. A Foley balloon with Hypaque outlines the bladder neck. (From Perez CA: Uterine cervix. In: Perez CA, Brady LW [eds]: Principles and Practice of Radiation Oncology, 3rd ed, pp 1733–1834. Philadelphia, Lippincott-Raven, 1998, with permission.)

rates are obtainable in patients undergoing exenterative surgery (20% to 40%), this procedure remains relatively rare because of high mortality and morbidity rates.[77]

Palliative Irradiation

Frequently the radiation oncologist is faced with the challenge of treating a patient with stage IVB or recurrent carcinoma who requires palliation of pelvic pain or bleeding. If vaginal bleeding is the main concern, a single intracavitary insertion with tandem and colpostats for about 6000 mgh (55 Gy to point A) suffices. If irradiation was delivered previously, lower intracavitary doses should be prescribed (4000 to 5000 mgh).

Spanos and associates[78] reported a 6% complication rate in 290 patients treated in Radiation Therapy Oncology Group protocol 85-02. Irradiation consisted of 3.7 Gy per fraction given twice daily for 2 consecutive days, repeated at 3- to 6-week intervals for a total of three courses, aiming to a total tumor dose of 44.4 Gy. No patient receiving less than 30 Gy developed late toxicity. There was no significant difference in the incidence of complications for patients with a 2- or 4-week rest ($p = 0.47$).

Chemotherapy

Primary (first-line) chemotherapy is used chiefly in patients with advanced or disseminated disease and generally takes the form of combination protocols including cisplatin.[79–81] However, there is increasing use of concomitant chemotherapy with irradiation for stages IIB, III, and IVA.[82, 83] Indeed, for patients with bulky stage IB, combination protocols of radiation therapy with cisplatin, or cisplatin and 5-fluorouracil (5-FU) may become the recommended standard of care.[84, 85]

Multiple agents have been evaluated for efficacy in patients with advanced or recurrent disease (Table 21–8). Administered as single agents, response rates of at least 19 agents have varied from 15% to 25%,[97] and one agent, cisplatin, has been studied in great detail.[84, 98, 99] Although an early randomized trial by the Southwest Oncology Group showed no advantage of combination drugs over cisplatin alone,[100] combination regimens containing cisplatin now demonstrate improved rates of survival and progression.[101, 102]

Combined Modalities

Radiation Therapy and Chemotherapy

In an attempt to improve survival, investigators added chemotherapeutic agents, initially as radiosensitizers, to the standard radiation treatment. For example, the addition of hydroxyurea has been shown to minimally improve response and survival rates.[103, 104] Other agents, such as mitomycin C, etoposide, 5-FU, and cisplatin, have been investigated, and combinations of the last two compounds in particular have generated studies with increased response rates and improved survival over irradiation alone.[83, 105]

Results from several cooperative oncology groups show that cisplatin-based chemotherapy, when given at the same time as radiation therapy, prolongs survival in women with locally advanced cervical cancers, as well as in women with stage I–IIA disease who have metastatic disease in

TABLE 21–8. **Neoadjuvant Chemotherapy in Cervical Cancer: Review of the Literature**

Author	No. of Patients	FIGO Stage	Study Design Chemotherapy	CR + PR (%)	CR (%)	Comments
Eddy et al[86]	15	IB	CT-Sx, PO	82	6	2-year DFS, 76%
Leone et al[87]	57	IIB–IVA	CT-RT/Sx, PI	53	7	
Serur et al[88]	20	IB2	CT-Sx, BOP/PBM	90	10	
Benedetti-Panici et al[89]	128	IB2–III	CT-Sx, PB/PBM	83	15	10-year DFS: 91% and 44% for stage IB2–IIB and III
Zanetta et al[90]	34	IB2–IIIB	CT-Sx, PITax	34	16	
Sugiyama et al[91]	23	IB2–IIIB	CT, P CPT-11	78	13	
Randomized Trials						
Souhami et al[92]	107	IIIB	BODP	—	CT-RT = 47; RT = 33	5-year survival in CT-RT 23% vs. 39% in RT group; p = 0.02
Kumar et al[93]	CT-RT = 80; RT = 88	IIB–IVA	BIP	CT-RT = 70; RT = 69.3	—	2-year survival in CT-RT 38% vs. 36% in RT group; p = 0.59
Sundfør et al[94]	CT-RT = 47; RT = 47	IIIB–IVA	P-5FU	CT-RT = 80; RT = 82	CT-RT = 53; RT= 57	5-year DFS in CT-RT 70% vs. 57% in RT group; p = NS
Sardi et al[95]	CT-Sx-RT = 41; (Sx)-RT = 47	IB1	BOP	CT-Sx-RT = 90%	—	8-year survival in CT-Sx-RT 82% vs. 77% in Sx-RT group; p = NS
	CT-Sx-RT = 41; (Sx)-RT = 47	IB2	BOP	CT-Sx-RT = 83%	—	9-year survival in CT-Sx-RT 80% vs. 61% in Sx-RT group; p <0.01
Kumar et al[96]	CT-RT = 36; RT = 36	IIIB	BIP	—	CT-RT = 68; RT = 58	Estimated survival in CT-RT 71% vs. 69% in RT group; p = NS

CT = chemotherapy; Sx = surgery; RT = radiation therapy; PO = cisplatin and vincristine; PI = cisplatin and ifosfamide; BOP = bleomycin, vincristine, and cisplatin; PBM = cisplatin, bleomycin, and methotrexate; PB = cisplatin and bleomycin; PITax = cisplatin, ifosfamide, and paclitaxel (Taxol); P CPT-11 = cisplatin and irinotecan; BODP = bleomycin, vincristine, mitomycin, and cisplatin; BIP = bleomycin, ifosfamide-mesna, and cisplatin; P-5FU = cisplatin and 5-fluorouracil; CR = complete response; PR = partial response; DFS = disease-free survival; NS = not statistically significant.

Adapted from Kumar L, Kaushal R, Nandy M, et al: Chemotherapy followed by radiotherapy versus radiotherapy alone in locally advanced cervical cancer: a randomized study. Gynecol Oncol 1994; 54:307–315.

the pelvic lymph nodes, positive parametrial disease, or positive surgical margins at the time of primary surgery.

Southwest Oncology Group 8797 was a study for women with FIGO stage IA2, IB, or IIA carcinoma of the cervix with metastatic disease in the pelvic lymph nodes, positive parametrial involvement, or positive surgical margins at the time of primary radical hysterectomy combined with total pelvic lymphadenectomy.[106] Patients had confirmed negative para-aortic lymph nodes; if the para-aortic lymph nodes were not sampled, the patients had confirmed negative common iliac lymph nodes. One hundred twenty-seven patients were randomized to be treated with pelvic external beam irradiation along with 5-FU and cisplatin, and 116 were treated with pelvic external beam irradiation alone. The median follow-up for survivors was 43 months. The 3-year survival rate for women treated with the chemotherapy-irradiation combination was 87%, compared with 77% for women receiving pelvic irradiation only.

The Gynecologic Oncology Group (GOG) conducted a randomized study (Protocol No. 85) in which patients with clinical stage IIB, III, and IVA carcinoma of the cervix and negative para-aortic nodes were treated with external pelvic and intracavitary irradiation alone or combined with 5-FU and cisplatin (177 patients); 191 received hydroxyurea.[107] With a median follow-up for survivors of 8.7 years, the 5-year survival rate for patients receiving cisplatin and 5-FU was 60% compared with 47% for women treated with hydroxyurea (p = 0.03).

GOG Protocol No. 120 for the same patient population was a three-arm randomized trial comparing (1) irradiation plus hydroxyurea versus (2) irradiation plus weekly cisplatin versus (3) irradiation plus hydroxyurea, cisplatin, and 5-FU.[102] In an analysis of 526 patients, the 4-year survival rate for women in the weekly cisplatin and irradiation group and in the irradiation, 5-FU, cisplatin, and hydroxyurea group was 69% compared with 37% for women treated with hydroxyurea and irradiation (p <0.001). Overall survival was significantly better in the two groups receiving cisplatin alone or cisplatin combined with 5-FU and hydroxyurea compared with the group receiving hydroxyurea. Hematologic toxicity was greater in the group treated with the three drugs compared with cisplatin or hydroxyurea alone.

The Radiation Therapy Oncology Group reported a randomized study of 388 patients with stage IB and IIA cervix tumors larger than 5 cm who had positive pelvic lymph nodes or stage IIB to IVA disease.[83] Patients were treated with either pelvic and para-aortic irradiation or pelvic irradiation and three cycles of concurrent chemotherapy consisting of cisplatin and a 4-day infusion of 5-FU. With a median follow-up of 43 months for survivors, the 5-year overall survival rate for women in the irradiation and cisplatin and 5-FU group was 73% compared with 58% for women in the irradiation-only group (p = 0.004). Disease-free survival was 67% with chemotherapy and irradiation and 40% with irradiation alone (p = 0.001). There were no significant differences in late complications in the treatment groups.

GOG Protocol No. 123 included women with bulky (4 cm or greater) stage IB carcinoma of the cervix with negative pelvic and para-aortic nodes.[84] In this study, 183 patients were randomized to be treated with pelvic external beam and intracavitary irradiation followed by extrafascial hysterectomy, and 186 received external beam (pelvic) and intracavitary radiation therapy along with weekly cisplatin followed by extrafascial hysterectomy. With a median follow-up for survivors of 35.7 months, the progression-free survival rate for women treated with irradiation with cisplatin chemotherapy was 79%, compared with 63% for those treated with irradiation alone ($p < 0.001$). The overall 3-year survival rates were 83% with combination therapy and 74% with irradiation alone ($p = 0.0008$).

Adjuvant or definitive radiation therapy is widely used to treat women with cervical cancer. Strong consideration should be given to the use of concurrent chemotherapy with radiation therapy in women with locally advanced stage IB–IVA cervical cancer, as well as in women with stage I–IIA disease who have metastatic disease in the pelvic lymph nodes, positive parametrial disease, or positive surgical margins at the time of primary surgery.

The optimal chemotherapy regimen has not been established. Although information about long-term complications is incomplete for some of these trials, to date all of these regimens appear tolerable. Continued clinical research is necessary to identify further improvements in radiation therapy and chemotherapy for women with locally advanced cervical carcinoma.

Postoperative Combination Therapy with Radical Hysterectomy

Patients who have undergone radical hysterectomy should be considered for postoperative irradiation (with or without chemotherapy)[108] if they have high-risk prognostic factors, giving them an intermediate risk of failure.[109] These factors include positive pelvic lymph nodes or microscopic positive or close (<3 mm) margins of resection, deep stromal invasion, or vascular-lymphatic permeation. When metastatic pelvic lymph nodes are present, treatment consists of 50 Gy to the whole pelvis delivered with a four-field technique. Patients with positive common iliac or para-aortic node metastases should also receive 50 Gy to the periaortic region.

In patients receiving postoperative irradiation, extreme care should be exercised in designing treatment techniques, including intracavitary insertions; because of the surgical extirpation of the uterus, the bladder and rectosigmoid may be closer to the radioactive sources than in the patient with an intact uterus. Furthermore, vascular supply may be affected by the surgical procedure, and adhesions can prevent mobilization of the small bowel loops that occasionally may be fixed in the pelvis.

Special Considerations of Treatment

Small Cell Carcinoma of the Cervix

At Washington University, patients with small cell carcinoma of the cervix are treated with the same irradiation techniques as those outlined for other histologic varieties of cervical carcinoma in combination with multiagent chemotherapy. The most frequently prescribed drugs are cyclophosphamide (1000 mg/m^2), doxorubicin (Adriamycin) (50 mg/m^2), and vincristine (1 mg/m^2) given every 3 or 4 weeks. Etoposide (VP16) is being incorporated more frequently into some of the regimens.[110, 111] Depending on age and tolerance to therapy, the doses of irradiation may be decreased by approximately 10%.

Cervical Cancer in Pregnancy

The concurrent presence of carcinoma *in situ* or invasive carcinoma of the uterine cervix and pregnancy, although rare, poses a therapeutic dilemma to the gynecologic and radiation oncologists. In late pregnancy, if the tumor is small, definitive therapy is postponed and delivery is allowed.[112, 113] However, because generally there is believed to be a need to institute therapy as soon as possible, the accepted method of treatment in patients in the first 6 months of pregnancy is to carry out definitive surgery or radiation therapy, as indicated by the stage of the disease. In the third trimester of pregnancy, when the fetus may be salvaged, a cesarean section combined with a radical hysterectomy and lymphadenectomy or followed by definitive treatment postpartum is preferred by most gynecologic oncologists.[114] Although it has not been clinically proven that vaginal delivery deleteriously affects the treatment prognosis, some authors have suggested that it may be a factor in recurrent disease.[115]

If a radical hysterectomy is performed and positive pelvic lymph nodes are found, the usual postoperative irradiation, including external beam with or without intracavitary insertion, should be carried out. If it is decided to terminate the pregnancy and treat the patient with external irradiation, then initially the whole pelvis is irradiated (40 Gy in 4 weeks). Usually an abortion occurs, and there is some involution of the uterus. After this dose of irradiation, careful evacuation of the uterus and an intracavitary insertion may be performed under general anesthesia. Two intracavitary insertions for a total of 6500 mgh (55 Gy to point A) and an additional 10 or 20 Gy are delivered to the parametria with a midline block. If surgery is to be carried out, then approximately 4000 mgh is given.

Cervical Stump Carcinoma

Subtotal hysterectomy is rarely performed today because these patients are then at risk to develop carcinoma of the uterine cervix[116, 117]; however, there are still many women who retain a cervical stump. Because the natural history of carcinoma of the cervical stump is similar to that of the cervix in the intact uterus, the diagnostic work-up, clinical staging, and basic principles of therapy are the same. However, because of the previous surgical procedures and the presence of adhesions in the pelvis, surgery becomes somewhat more problematic. In addition, the lack of a uterine cavity into which a tandem containing two or three sources is inserted makes intracavitary therapy more difficult. As many sources as are technically feasible may be inserted into the remaining cervical canal, but the achievable dose of intracavitary therapy depends on the number of sources that can be placed (1000 to 3000 mgh for one to three sources). These complications increase the importance of delivery of a higher whole-pelvis irradiation dose, and, in general, patients with stage I disease are treated with a

TABLE 21–9. **Survival Rates for Patients with Stages I and II Carcinoma of the Uterine Cervix Treated with Radical Hysterectomy**

Study	Stage	No. of Patients	5-Year Survival Rate (%)	10-Year Survival Rate (%)	Comments
Hopkins and Morley[121]	IB	213	92	—	Lesions <3 cm, survival 94%
Averette et al[122]	IB & IIA	978	90.1	—	Wertheim-Meigs
Massi et al[123]	IB	283	83	—	Schauta
	IB	175	78	—	Wertheim-Meigs
Alvarez et al[124]	IB & IIA	48	73.6	60.6	Type III
Bissett et al[125]	IB	123	86.3	—	
Landoni et al[126]	IB & IIA	169	83	—	
Magrina et al[127]*	IA & IB	56	96.4	—	Tumor ≤2 cm
			94.6	—	Tumor >2 cm

*Modified radical hysterectomy.

combination of 20 Gy to the whole pelvis and 30 Gy to the parametria with midline shielding combined with two intracavitary insertions. More advanced stages should be treated with 40 Gy to the whole pelvis and 20 Gy to the parametria with midline shielding, combined with the same intracavitary doses. With care as to the length of external beam treatment, carcinoma of the cervical stump can be treated with irradiation with 5-year survival rates similar to those of patients with intact uteri.[118, 119]

Results of Treatment

When therapeutic results in invasive carcinoma of the cervix are evaluated, a direct comparison of surgically treated or irradiated patients is fraught with many uncertainties, including patient selection, reporting of surgical cases using staging determined by laparotomy findings, and different treatment techniques. A review of 152 papers published at the end of the 1980s[120] concluded that the existing literature of the time was of limited help in deciding the best treatment for patients with cervical carcinoma and that properly designed, prospectively randomized studies with careful consideration of relevant end points were necessary to elucidate existing areas of controversy. The situation has not shown much improvement since that time.

For patients with stage IA disease, the standard treatment of care is surgery, although where this is contraindicated, at least one study has shown a 100% 10-year progression-free survival rate with irradiation alone.[57] Both surgery and adequate irradiation are equally effective in the treatment of stage IB and IIA carcinoma of the cervix; numerous noncontrolled studies support the merits of either modality, with no significant difference in survival or pelvic tumor control (Tables 21–9 and 21–10). The main advantage of surgical treatment is the preservation of ovarian function in women younger than 40 years of age.

Surgery

Radical surgery has been effective in the treatment of *in situ*, stage I, and stage IIA cervical carcinomas. For stage I disease, cure rates are about 85%.[9] With improved anesthesia, surgical techniques, and antibiotic therapy, the mortality rate for radical hysterectomy with pelvic lymphadenectomy has decreased to 0.5% or less.[130] The most frequent sequela after radical hysterectomy is urinary dysfunction as a result of partial denervation of the detrusor muscle.[131] Patients may have various degrees of loss of bladder sensation, inability to initiate voiding, residual urine retention, and incontinence. Other complications, as observed by Magrina and associates[132] following a modified radical hysterectomy, include wound infection (4%), hematoma (2%), ileus or intestinal obstruction (5%), enterocutaneous or rectovaginal fistula (0.8%), vesicovaginal or ureterovaginal fistula (0.6%), hydronephrosis (3.3%), and stress urinary incontinence or decreased bladder sensation (21%). Pneumonia was noted in 5.8% of patients, pulmo-

TABLE 21–10. **Survival Rates of Patients with Stages I and II Carcinoma of the Uterine Cervix Treated with Radiation Therapy**

Study	Stage	No. of Patients	5-Year Survival Rate (%)	Comments
Coia et al[128]	IB	168	74	Patterns of Care Study
Hopkins and Morley[121]	IB	97	86	Lesions <3 cm, survival = 88%; >3 cm = 73%
Lowrey et al[129]	IB, IIA–B	130	81	
Perez[42]	IB–IIB	394	85	
Eifel et al[97]	IB	1494	88	Tumor <5 cm
			69	Tumor 5–7.9 cm
Rotman et al[63]	IB–IIB	367	44*	Pelvic field
			55*	Pelvic + para-aortic nodes
Morris et al[83]	IB & IVA	193	58	

*10-year overall survival.

nary embolism in 2.1%, myocardial infarction in 4.3%, and lymphedema or lymphocyst in approximately 20%.

In the same study,[132] the incidence of morbidity in patients treated with radical hysterectomy, compared with a modified radical hysterectomy, was somewhat higher. Patients who had a pelvic lymphadenectomy experienced a greater incidence of lower extremity lymphedema than those who did not undergo this procedure. Preoperative or postoperative pelvic irradiation was a significant predisposing factor for urinary tract infection, lymphedema, and bowel obstruction in comparison with patients who did not receive pelvic irradiation. In another study following radical hysterectomy, some loss of defecatory urge associated with chronic rectal dysfunction was observed.[133] Manometric studies have suggested that this loss was due to a disruption of the spinal arcs controlling defecation.[134] Other complications of surgery include hemorrhage, infection, stricture and fibrosis of the intestine or rectosigmoid colon, and bladder and rectovaginal fistulae. Nonetheless, it must be stated that postsurgical complications are generally more amenable to correction than are late complications after irradiation.

Recurrent Disease Following Surgery

It is relatively easy to treat surgical recurrences with irradiation, which can salvage about 20% to 60% of patients with localized pelvic recurrences after surgery alone.[135, 136] A combination of whole-pelvis external irradiation and additional parametrial dose with midline shielding, together with chemotherapy, is needed.[108, 137] In addition, one or two intracavitary insertions can be used to boost the dose to the vaginal vault or the parametrium or paravaginal tissues, depending on tumor volume.[138, 139] Finally, phase II studies have been completed that demonstrate a role for first-line chemotherapy for recurrent cancer of the cervix.[102, 140, 141]

Radiation Therapy

Radiation therapy is effective in the treatment of cervical carcinoma and is superior to a surgical approach in more locally advanced stages. With combined external beam irradiation and brachytherapy, the 5-year survival rate for stage IB is 86% to 92% and, for stage IIA, is about 75%. The overall pelvic failure rate in stage IB is approximately 5% to 35%, depending on size, and in stage IIA, 15% to 25%.[142] Until recently, most patients with stage IIB tumors were treated with irradiation alone, and the 5-year survival rate was 60% to 65%. The pelvic failure rate ranges from 32% to 50%, depending on the degree of parametrial involvement.[128, 142]

In stage IIIB carcinoma, the 5-year survival rate following radiation therapy alone ranges from 25% to 48%, and the pelvic failure rate ranges from 38% to 50%. Komaki and associates,[67] in an analysis of the Patterns of Care Study data, reported a significant increase in local/pelvic tumor control (69%) in patients with stage III carcinoma of the cervix treated in 1983, compared with 37% and 49% in earlier periods ($p = 0.03$). Five-year survival increased from 25% to 47% ($p = 0.02$). The authors suggested that the improvement in pelvic tumor control may be associated with higher external beam doses, but more likely it was related to the substantial increase in the percentage of patients receiving brachytherapy (96%) and more careful dosimetry and dose calculations for intracavitary therapy. The authors also noted a decrease in major complications from 15% in 1973 and 13% in the 1978 Patterns of Care Survey to 7% in 1983.

In an analysis of more than 1200 cervical cancer patients monitored for a minimum of 5 years, Perez and coworkers[143] noted that severe small bowel, rectosigmoid, and bladder injury, together, rarely exceeded a 10% complication rate, and major sequelae were usually less than 5%. However, these complications were found to be dose related; the rectosigmoid complications were 2% to 4% for 60 to 80 Gy, 7% to 8% for 80 to 95 Gy, and 13% for more than 95 Gy. The authors suggested a revision of tolerance doses ($T_{5/5}$) for the small bowel to less than 60 Gy, rectosigmoid to less than 75 Gy, and bladder to less than 80 Gy, provided small volumes are irradiated. A previous analysis by the same group had shown that patients who developed sequelae of therapy had a slightly better survival than patients who did not develop any complications; this finding was thought to be related to improved tumor control with higher doses of irradiation.[144]

Lanciano and associates,[145] in 95 tandem and ovoid insertions performed for cervical cancer in 91 patients and for endometrial cancer in 4, observed two uterine perforations and a vaginal laceration in 2 patients. Twenty-four percent of implants in 16 patients were associated with temperatures higher than 100.5°F; only one patient required implant removal because of fever. The use of antibiotics preoperatively and intraoperatively did not reduce the risk of perioperative temperature elevation. Five implants (5%) were removed because of presumed sepsis, pulmonary disease, arterial hypotension, change in mental status, and myocardial infarction. Deep vein thrombosis or pulmonary embolism was not observed.

Low-Dose-Rate Versus High-Dose-Rate Brachytherapy

Only a few randomized studies have been published comparing HDR and LDR brachytherapy for carcinoma of the cervix.[146–148] Teshima and associates[146] reported on a prospective randomized study of 430 patients with carcinoma of the uterine cervix treated with either LDR (171 patients) or HDR (259 patients) brachytherapy combined with external irradiation. Cause-specific and overall survival were comparable for each clinical stage with either modality. Similar results were reported by Patel and associates.[147]

Postoperative Radiation Therapy

To date, no controlled studies have shown improved survival with postoperative pelvic irradiation after radical surgery in the presence of positive pelvic nodes. However, in general, the selection of high-risk patients (lymph node metastases) has made analysis of the significance of this adjuvant treatment difficult. For example, Kinney and coworkers[149] compared results of therapy in 82 patients with stage IB and IIA carcinoma of the cervix found to have pelvic lymph node metastases at the time of hysterectomy and bilateral lymphadenectomy with 103 similar patients who received 50 Gy to the pelvis postoperatively. Although the incidence of pelvic recurrences was 67% and 27%, respectively, the 5-year survival rate was 72% for the surgery-only patients and 64% for the group receiving adjuvant irradiation. This lack of impact on overall survival, which was also seen in a later report by the same group,[150] has been ascribed to high-risk patient selection in the irradiated group.

When postoperative radiation therapy is given to selected patients, further complications of the additional therapy are expected because of intestinal adhesions to denuded surfaces in the pelvis. Enteric complications, such as obstruction, fistula, or dysfunction, were observed in 30% of patients so treated by Barter and associates[151] and in 24% of patients reported by Fiorica and associates.[152] Other investigators, however, have reported no increase in the incidence of severe complications in patients treated with postoperative irradiation.[109, 153]

Montz and coworkers[154] evaluated bowel obstruction in 98 patients undergoing radical hysterectomy for a nonadnexal gynecologic malignancy. Patients were separated into three groups: those treated with radical hysterectomy alone (n = 60), those receiving postoperative pelvic irradiation (n = 20), and those receiving preoperative pelvic irradiation (n = 18). Postoperative small bowel obstruction occurred in three patients (5%) in the first group, all of whom required surgical management. The incidence of small bowel obstruction was significantly higher ($p < 0.05$) in the groups that received concomitant radiation therapy (20% and 22%, respectively).

Recurrent Disease Following Radiation

Reirradiation of previously irradiated patients must be undertaken with extreme caution. It is very important to analyze the techniques used in the initial treatment (beam energy, volume, doses delivered with external or intracavitary irradiation). Also, the period of time between the two treatments must be taken into consideration because it is postulated that some repair of the initial damage may take place in the interval. In general, external irradiation for recurrent tumor is given to limited volumes (40 to 45 Gy, 1.8 Gy tumor dose per fraction, preferentially using lateral portals). Occasionally, intracavitary or interstitial irradiation can be used to treat relatively circumscribed recurrences.

Chemotherapy

In 1993, Thomas[155] summarized the rationale and potential limitations of neoadjuvant chemotherapy in stage IB carcinoma of the cervix. She pointed out that early randomized trials of neoadjuvant chemotherapy and irradiation had been reported in patients with stage IIB and III cervical cancer.[92, 156, 157] Although response rates to the chemotherapy were between 30% and 85%, none of the studies had shown an advantage for pelvic tumor control or survival. However, in a 2000 update,[85] Thomas noted that a number of trials now have begun to demonstrate improved survival (30% to 50% reduction) with the use of concurrent chemotherapy in the regimens.[83, 84, 102, 107]

HYDROXYUREA

Following a prospective, double-blind, randomized trial, Piver and coworkers[103] reported on women with untreated stage IIB cervical cancer randomized to be treated with irradiation and placebo or with a combination of similar irradiation and hydroxyurea (80 mg/kg every third day starting on the first day of radiation therapy and continuing for 12 weeks). The 5-year survival rates were significantly higher for the hydroxyurea group than for the placebo group. In another larger randomized trial by the GOG, reported by Stehman and associates,[104] 296 surgically staged patients with stage IIB through IVA disease and negative para-aortic nodes were randomized to irradiation plus either hydroxyurea (139 patients) or misonidazole (157 patients). The median progression-free survival was 42.9 months for the patients treated with hydroxyurea and 40.4 months with misonidazole. Survival was not statistically different between the regimens, with 33.8% deaths in the hydroxyurea and 38.9% deaths in the misonidazole groups ($p = 0.25$). However, a 1999 study by Rose and colleagues[102] demonstrated a significant improvement using cisplatin-based regimens over hydroxyurea alone, although the method of hydroxyurea administration in that study has been criticized.[159]

CISPLATIN

Cisplatin has been studied in a variety of doses and schedules,[97] and it has demonstrated activity both as a single agent and in combination. However, its value has been disputed when compared with irradiation, particularly with respect to survival. For example, one study randomized 107 patients with stage IIIB carcinoma of the cervix to treatment with irradiation alone or combined with bleomycin, vincristine, mitomycin, and cisplatin (BOMP).[92] The overall 5-year survival rate for the neoadjuvant-treated patients was 23%, in contrast to 39% for those treated with irradiation alone ($p = 0.02$). Locoregional and distant failures were similar in both groups. In another study, Tattersall and associates[160] reported on a randomized trial of 260 patients with stage IIB to IVA cervical cancer; 131 patients were treated with pelvic irradiation (45 to 55 Gy in 4 to 5 weeks followed by 30 to 35 Gy intracavitary insertion), and 129 received chemotherapy (cisplatin [60 mg/m^2] and epirubicin [110 mg/m^2] administered at 3-week intervals for three cycles) followed by similar pelvic irradiation. Patients who received primary chemotherapy had a significantly higher pelvic failure rate (29%) than those who received radiation therapy alone (19%) ($p < 0.003$). Patients who received chemotherapy had significantly inferior 3-year disease-free survival (40%) compared with those who received radiation therapy alone (50%) ($p = 0.02$).

Other combined-modality trials have not shown this discrepancy in survival. Kumar and associates[93] reported on 94 patients with stage IIB to IV carcinoma of the cervix randomized to be treated with chemotherapy (two cycles of bleomycin, ifosfamide-mesna, and cisplatin) followed by radiation therapy, and 90 patients randomized to be treated with the same irradiation alone. In the chemoirradiation group, the 32-month survival rates were 63% for IIB, 50% for IIIB, and 23% for IVA tumors. The corresponding survival rates in patients treated with irradiation alone were 59% for IIB and 27% for IIIB tumors, although differences were not statistically significant. In a Swedish study,[94] 47 patients with stage IIB to IVA carcinoma of the cervix were randomized to be treated with external irradiation alone (64.8 Gy, 1.8-Gy fractions, box technique), and 47 patients were treated with a combination of three cycles of cisplatin (100 mg/m² IV) and 5 days of 5-FU (1 g/m² per day, IV continuous infusion) administered every third week, followed by the same pelvic external irradiation. The 5-year disease-free survival rates were 70% with chemoirradiation and 57% with irradiation alone ($p = 0.07$). However, the incidence of pelvic recurrence was 60% and 47%, respectively, although distant metastasis was 19% and 35%, respectively. Two patients in the chemoirradiation group and one in the irradiation-alone group died as a consequence of therapy.

Prognostic Factors

Tumor Stage and Size

A number of studies have shown that the survival rate decreases as the tumor stage increases with increasing tumor size (Fig. 21–4).[142, 161, 162] Eifel and associates,[163] in a review of 1526 patients with stage IB squamous cell carcinoma of the uterine cervix treated with irradiation alone, noted pelvic tumor control in 97% of tumors less than 5 cm and 84% for those 5 to 7 cm. In addition, several retrospective studies have demonstrated decreased survival and a greater incidence of distant metastases in patients with endometrial extension of a primary cervical carcinoma (endometrial stroma invasion or replacement of the endometrium by tumor only).[164, 165]

In a separate retrospective study,[61] the group analyzed results from patients who had received preoperative irradiation plus surgery, and these data indicated that, for this mode of treatment, tumor size was of less importance than clinical stage, irradiation dose, and pelvic node status at the time of surgery.

Histology

Few reports have shown a significant correlation of survival or tumor behavior with the degree of differentiation of squamous cell carcinoma or adenocarcinoma of the cervix. Several groups have reported similar survival for comparable stages of adenocarcinoma or squamous cell carci-

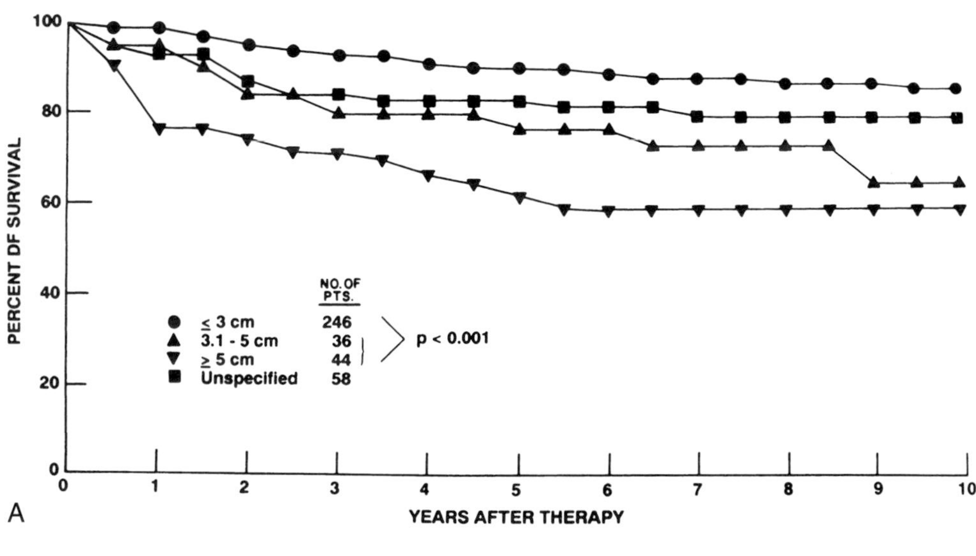

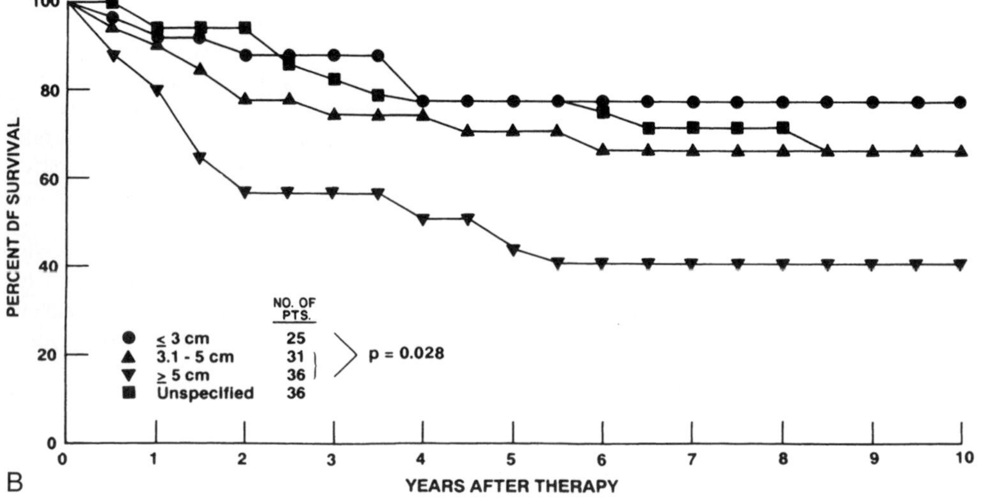

Figure 21–4. Carcinoma of the uterine cervix (1959–1986): disease-free survival correlated with tumor size. (A) Stage IB. (B) Stage IIA. Bulky tumors are larger than 5 cm. (From Perez CA, Grigsby PW, Nene SM, et al: Effect of tumor size on the prognosis of carcinoma of the uterine cervix treated with irradiation alone. Cancer 1992; 69:2796–2806, with permission.)

noma.[46, 166] In contrast, Eifel and associates,[47] in an analysis of 1767 patients with stage IB carcinoma of the cervix, identified 229 (13%) who had adenocarcinoma; the others had squamous cell carcinoma. The 5-year survival rates were 72% and 81%, respectively. The incidence of pelvic recurrence was similar (17% for adenocarcinoma and 13% for squamous cell carcinoma). However, the incidence of distant metastases was greater for patients with adenocarcinoma (37% versus 21%) ($p < 0.01$). In a large surgicopathologic staging study of clinical stage IB patients, adverse prognostic factors were capillary-lymphatic space involvement, larger tumor size, and increasing depth of stromal invasion.[161]

Age, Race, and Socioeconomic Status

According to some reports, prognosis is the same in younger and older patients,[167] although other authors have noted decreased survival in women younger than 35 who have a greater frequency of poorly differentiated tumors.[168] Several authors also have noted a correlation between race or socioeconomic characteristics of patients, or both, and outcome of therapy.[169, 170]

General Host Factors

In addition to stage, tumor volume, and vascular[171] or lymphatic invasion, other host factors may affect the prognosis of patients with cervical carcinoma:

- Dusenbery and coworkers,[172] in 20 patients with carcinoma of the cervix who had hemoglobin of less than 12.5 g/dL, noted that erythropoietin induced a prompt reticulocyte response by the beginning of radiation therapy in comparison with concurrent controls.
- Decreased survival in 260 patients with an oral temperature higher than 100°F was reported by Van Herik.[173] Kapp and Lawrence[174] have published similar observations.

Cellular Oncogenes

Alterations in either the expression or function of cellular genes that control cell growth and differentiation in cervical cancer have, to date, shown no clear-cut usefulness as prognostic markers.[134] The *MYC* oncogene is amplified from 3 to 30 times in approximately 20% of squamous cell carcinomas; however, the relevance of this observation to clinical outcome is unknown.[175]

Prolongation of Treatment Time

Several studies have described lower pelvic tumor control and survival rates in invasive carcinoma of uterine cervix when the overall time in a course of irradiation is prolonged.[176–178] Fyles and associates[176] first reported an approximately 1% loss of tumor control per day of prolongation of treatment time beyond 30 days in 830 patients with cervical carcinoma treated with irradiation alone. Lanciano and associates,[178] in an analysis of 837 patients treated with irradiation for squamous cell carcinoma of the uterine cervix, also described a 4-year actuarial in-field recurrence increase from 6% to 20% when total treatment time increased from 6 weeks or less to 10 weeks ($p = 0.0001$). This translated into a significantly decreased survival rate.

Perez and coworkers,[179] in 1330 patients treated with definitive irradiation, noted a strong correlation between overall treatment time and pelvic tumor control in stages IB, IIA, and IIB. In stage III, although pelvic failure was higher with prolongation of treatment time, the difference was not statistically significant. There was also a strong correlation between overall treatment time and survival in stages IB, IIA, and IIB. The 10-year cause-specific survival rates in stage IB were 86% with overall treatment time of 7 weeks or less, 78% for 7.1 to 9 weeks, and 55% for more than 9 weeks ($p \leq 0.01$) (Fig. 21–5A). The corresponding rates in stage IIA were 73%, 41%, and 43%, respectively ($p \leq 0.01$) (Fig. 21–5B).

Therefore, in patients treated with radiation therapy, overall treatment time should be as short as possible, and any planned or unplanned interruptions or delays should be avoided. Timely integration of external beam and intracavitary irradiation in patients with carcinoma of the uter-

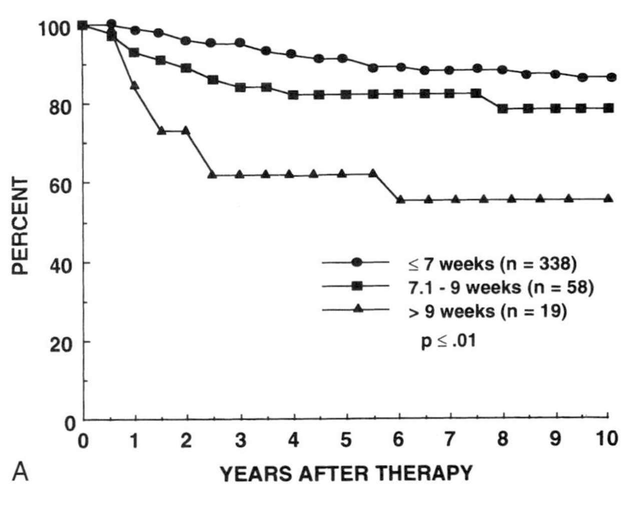

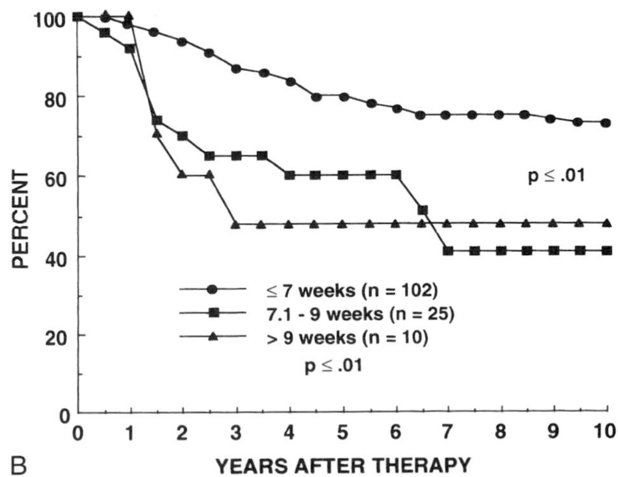

Figure 21–5. Cause-specific survival correlated with overall treatment time in (A) stage IB and (B) IIA carcinoma of the uterine cervix. (From Perez CA, Grigsby PW, Castro-Vita H, et al: Carcinoma of the uterine cervix. I. Impact of prolongation of treatment time and timing of brachytherapy on outcome of radiation therapy. Int J Radiat Oncol Biol Phys 1995; 32:1275–1288, with permission.)

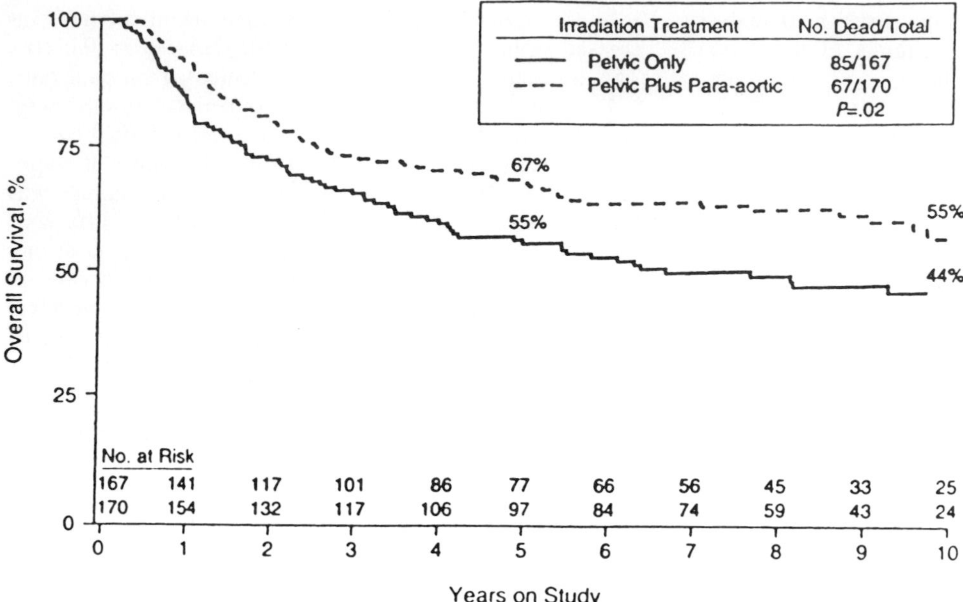

Figure 21–6. Overall probability of survival by assigned treatment group. *No. at Risk* indicates the number of patients in each irradiation arm (presented with data for pelvic only on top) for whom information was complete at each year. (From Rotman M, Pajak TF, Choi K, et al: Prophylactic extended-field irradiation of para-aortic lymph nodes in stages IIB and bulky IB and IIA cervical carcinomas: ten-year treatment results of RTOG 79-20. J Am Med Assoc 1995; 274:387–393, with permission.)

ine cervix is an important factor in improving pelvic tumor control.

Metastatic Para-Aortic Lymph Nodes

Para-aortic lymph node metastases are frequently combined with distant dissemination but are clinically apparent in only 10% to 20% of patients who have recurrences. In the 1970s, Nelson and coworkers[180] reported on 104 patients with stage II and III cervical carcinoma who had exploratory laparotomy and para-aortic lymph node biopsies; 12.5% of patients with stage IIA disease, 14.9% with stage IIB, and 38.4% with stage III had metastatic para-aortic lymph nodes. They were later treated with 60 Gy to the para-aortic region. Within 4 years, 50% of these patients had distant metastases. In 1994, Grigsby and associates[181] observed a 30% actuarial survival rate at 5 years and 25% at 10 years in 31 patients with histologically confirmed metastatic para-aortic lymph nodes from carcinoma of the cervix treated with irradiation (45–50 Gy in 5 to 6 weeks). The 5- and 10-year survival rate was 45% for clinical stage IB disease. At 5 years, the survival rates were 30% for stage II and 22% for stage III; there were no survivors after 7 years.

In order to reduce this failure rate, some groups have looked at elective para-aortic lymph node irradiation. Rotman and the Radiation Therapy Oncology Group[63] updated the results of a randomized study of 337 evaluable patients with stage IIB carcinoma of the uterine cervix with no clinical or radiographic evidence of para-aortic lymphadenopathy. These patients, in addition to receiving standard pelvic irradiation, were randomized to electively receive 45 Gy to the para-aortic region (1.6 to 1.8 Gy fractions). The 10-year survival was 55% for patients receiving elective para-aortic irradiation, and 44% for those receiving treatment to the pelvis only ($p = 0.02$) (Fig. 21–6). The locoregional tumor control rate was similar (69% in the para-aortic irradiation group and 65% in the pelvic-irradiated group). The 10-year grade 4 or 5 (major) complication rate was 8% in the group receiving para-aortic irradiation compared with 4% in patients treated with pelvic irradiation alone ($p = 0.06$).

Endometrial Carcinoma

Epidemiology and Etiology

Epidemiology

Endometrial cancer is the most prevalent cancer of the female genital tract in the United States. The American Cancer Society estimates that 36,100 new cases were diagnosed in the year 2000[12]; the incidence rate was about 21 per 100,000. There were about 6500 deaths from endometrial cancer in 2000; the mortality rate was about 3 per 100,000. Therefore, endometrial cancer accounts for 6% of all cancers and 2% of cancer deaths in women.

The majority of women diagnosed with endometrial cancer are postmenopausal, and their ages range from 50 to 70 years. The mean age at diagnosis is 63 years,[183] and the peak occurs at about 70 to 74 years[184]; nonetheless, the incidence rate still is about 4 per 100,000 in women younger than 40 years of age.[185] From 1986 to 1990, the incidence in white women younger than 50 years was 2.19 times higher compared with black women; as the age at diagnosis rose, the ratio declined but remained elevated in whites.[184] Over the same time period, the age-adjusted mortality rates were reversed.

Etiology

Most of the risk factors for the development of endometrial cancer relate to estrogen levels.[186]

- *Obesity* is a risk factor[187] and is believed to be due to a relative increase in circulating free estrogen through an increased conversion of circulating androgens into estrone.[186]
- Other factors include diabetes mellitus,[188] hypertension,[189] anovulation,[190] nulliparity,[191] unopposed estrogen replacement therapy,[192] and tamoxifen therapy.[193, 194]
- Obesity, hypertension, and diabetes mellitus constitute a triad that occurs frequently in women with endometrial cancer.[195]
- Low-dose oral contraceptives may be used in healthy, nonsmoking older women as a treatment modality in the premenopausal years to reduce the risk factors from estrogen replacement therapy.[196, 197]
- Although, in general, endometrial cancer is a disease of postmenopausal women, when it appears in younger patients, a positive family history can indicate a hereditary association. One such association is with hereditary nonpolyposis colorectal cancer[198, 199]; endometrial cancer is the second most common malignancy found with this disease.[200] Hereditary nonpolyposis colorectal cancer is an autosomal dominant disease caused by known mutations in mismatch repair genes, in particular *MLH1*, *MSH2*, and *MSH6*. However, the spectrum of mutations that can occur varies on a country-to-country basis; this has confounded, to date, the use of these and similar mutations for screening.[201, 202]

Detection and Diagnosis

Clinical Detection

The most common symptom in patients with endometrial cancer is abnormal uterine bleeding, which occurs in more than 90% of patients; in premenopausal patients, menometrorrhagia is usually noted. However, the majority of women with endometrial cancer are postmenopausal, and postmenopausal bleeding is always abnormal and, therefore, is usually reported early. A dilatation and curettage (D&C), endometrial biopsy, or aspiration curettage is indicated in postmenopausal women with vaginal spotting. An abnormal Pap smear may suggest the presence of endometrial carcinoma because endometrial cells may appear in the vaginal pool. However, the diagnosis should be confirmed from a sample of endometrial tissue. Patients may present with symptoms of a pelvic mass, but a pelvic mass rarely occurs in the absence of bleeding.

The growth pattern and spread of endometrial cancer are unpredictable. Typically, if undiagnosed, the cancer spreads by direct invasion into the myometrium. The tumor may extend into the lower uterine segment and eventually into the endocervix and ectocervix. Other sites of involvement may then include the pelvic and para-aortic lymph nodes, fallopian tubes, ovaries, and uterine serosa; it may also spread intraperitoneally to the upper abdomen. However, because the spread of the disease is unpredictable, there can be dissemination to sites outside the uterus without having deep myometrial invasion by the tumor. Also, it is not uncommon for patients to have positive para-aortic lymph node involvement without having pelvic lymph node involvement.

There is no accepted standard for routine screening of women for endometrial carcinoma; the Pap smear has not been found to be reliable, although a retrospective study did find that a positive cervical cytology correlated with a risk of high-grade, more advanced stage disease.[203] The American Cancer Society recommends that endometrial sampling of asymptomatic women at high risk of developing endometrial cancer should begin at menopause[204] and may be indicated at various intervals thereafter, depending on the degree of risk and other factors determined by the physician.

Diagnostic Procedures

The standard method for diagnosing endometrial carcinoma has been the fractional D&C. The first part of this procedure is to obtain four-quadrant cervical biopsies, followed by curettage of the endocervical canal. The cervix is dilated, and systematic curetting of the entire endometrial cavity is performed. All three specimens should be maintained separately for pathologic evaluation.

Other outpatient procedures that may be performed are endometrial biopsy or fluid hysteroscopy, and some investigators advocate that hysteroscopy and directed endometrial biopsies and curettage are more accurate than a fractional D&C.[205, 206]

The usual diagnostic work-up of patients with endometrial carcinoma comprises a history and physical examination. A complete blood count, serum chemistries, and a chest x-ray are performed. A barium enema may be performed if there are gastrointestinal symptoms. A CT scan of the abdomen and pelvis can be performed to evaluate possible lymphadenopathy and a pelvic mass. An MRI scan is capable of predicting the depth of myometrial invasion (Table 21–11).[43]

Classification and Staging

Histopathology

- The proliferation of endometrial glands with a relative decrease in endometrial stroma can be identified as endometrial hyperplasia. Simple hyperplasia is distinguished from atypical hyperplasia by the presence of nuclear atypia.
- Endometrial carcinoma occurs with a variety of histologic subtypes (Table 21–12). The most common endometrial cell type is endometrioid adenocarcinoma, which occurs in about 80% of cases. This type is composed of malignant glandular epithelial cells, and an admixture of squamous metaplasia is not uncom-

TABLE 21–11. **Imaging Procedures for Detection and Diagnosis of Endometrial Carcinoma for Primary Tumor and Regional Lymph Nodes**

Method	Capability	Recommended for Use
Computed tomography (CT)	Accurate staging information; assesses myometrial invasion; not known to be accurate in detecting lymph node spread	All patients except those with clinical stage I, grade 1 tumor, or clinical stage IV
Magnetic resonance imaging	Not yet investigated; potentially useful in local tumor staging	Unknown
Urography	Detects ureteral obstruction, bladder invasion; screens for unsuspected renal anomaly	All operative candidates
Barium enema	Detects serosal implantation of peritoneal spread; screens for diverticulosis, adenomatous polyps	Patients with colonic symptoms or guaiac-positive stool
Biopsy	Confirms lesions detected by radionuclide scan, CT scans, or lymphangiogram	Patients with suspicious lesions

Adapted from Bragg DG, Rubin R, Youker JE (eds): Oncologic Imaging. Philadelphia, W.B. Saunders Co., 1985.

mon. The criterion for distinguishing well-differentiated endometrial adenocarcinoma from atypical hyperplasia is that the carcinoma is characterized by an infiltrating cellular or glandular pattern that produces a desmoplastic response in the stroma. Other characteristics of carcinoma include confluent glandular bridges, aggregates of glands lacking intervening stroma, and branching, complex papillary epithelial-lined processes.[208] Histologic grading of endometrial adenocarcinoma is based on architectural criteria and reflects the amount of non–gland-forming tumor (see Table 21–12). Tumor grade is based on the proportion of solid sheets of tumor cells relative to the glandular pattern. For papillary serous and clear cell tumors, the grade is based on nuclear criteria rather than the architectural pattern.

- Adenosquamous tumors contain malignant elements of both the glandular and the squamous epithelium.
- Large, anaplastic cells with clear cytoplasm characterize clear cell carcinomas. Clear cell carcinoma is histologically similar to tumors of the ovary and fallopian tube. This type occurs in about 4% of cases.[209]
- Uterine papillary serous carcinoma of the endometrium is histologically similar to papillary serous carcinoma of the ovary. This subtype, which occurs in about 5% to 10% of patients, tends to metastasize to the upper abdomen, as does papillary serous carcinoma of the ovary.[210]
- Other histologic subtypes that may occur are mucinous adenocarcinoma, squamous cell carcinoma, mixed types, undifferentiated carcinoma, and metastatic carcinoma from other primary sites.

TABLE 21–12. **Histologic Classification of Endometrial Tumors**

Histologic Classification	Incidence (%)
Endometrioid	75–80
• Ciliated adenocarcinoma • Secretory adenocarcinoma • Papillary or villoglandular • Adenocarcinoma with squamous differentiation • Adenocanthoma • Adenosquamous	
Clear cell carcinoma	4
Uterine papillary serous	<10
Squamous cell	<1
Mucinous	1
Mixed	10
Undifferentiated	—

Modified from Physicians' Data Query: Endometrial Cancer. Bethesda, National Cancer Institute, May 1999.

Staging

For many years the FIGO staging for endometrial cancer was based on a clinical examination and a D&C. However, clinical staging underestimates the extent of disease found at surgery; therefore, the current FIGO staging system for endometrial cancer is based on surgical-pathologic findings (Fig. 21–7). The surgical staging procedure includes sampling of the peritoneal fluid for cytologic evaluation and abdominal and pelvic exploration with biopsy of suspicious areas. This procedure is followed by a pelvic and para-aortic lymph node dissection.[211] A total extrafascial hysterectomy and bilateral salpingo-oophorectomy are performed. The FIGO and American Joint Committee staging systems are compared in Table 21–13.

Principles of Treatment

A summary of the multidisciplinary treatment decisions for patients with endometrial carcinoma is presented in Table 21–14. Most cases are treated with irradiation or surgery or both. Chemotherapy and hormonal therapy are still considered to be experimental.

Surgery

Total abdominal hysterectomy and bilateral salpingo-oophorectomy is the standard treatment for most women with endometrial carcinoma, and surgery represents the primary treatment for 92% to 96% of women with endometrial cancer.[186] Pelvic and, if indicated, para-aortic lymph node sampling or pelvic lymphadenectomy are frequently performed, although the impact of these procedures on survival has not been established (careful exploration of the entire abdominal cavity and peritoneal washings for

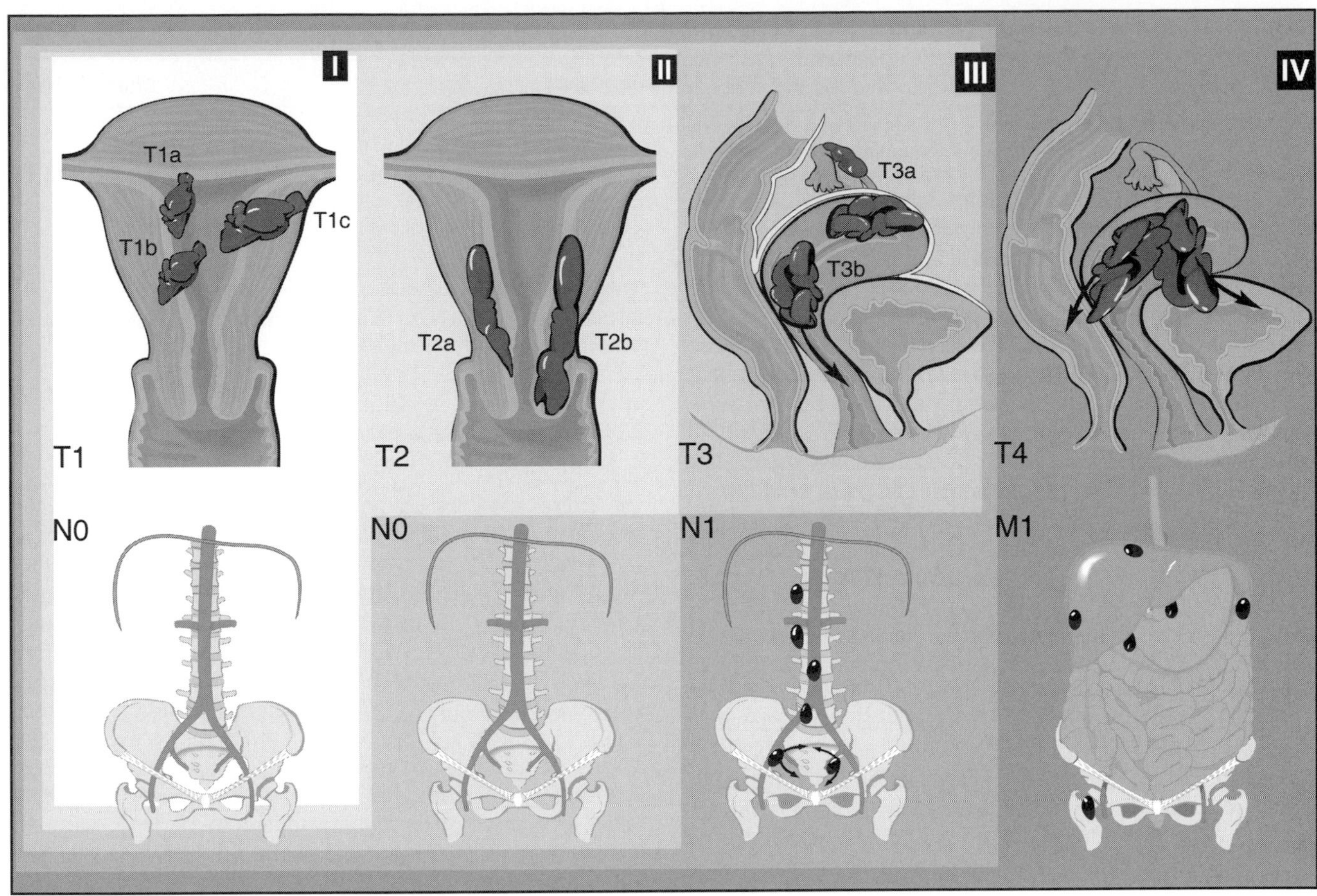

Figure 21–7. Anatomic staging for endometrial carcinoma.

cytology assessment are routinely performed). In stage I endometrial cancer, if the tumor is well differentiated and the nodes are negative, the benefit of further postoperative treatment is disputed.[212, 213] However, for most other stages of disease, the best results are obtained with either surgery alone, or surgery combined with irradiation. Some patients have regional or distant metastasis that may respond to chemotherapy or hormonal therapy.

TABLE 21–13. **Staging of Carcinoma of the Corpus Uteri***

Stage	Grouping	FIGO Staging	Descriptor
I	T1	I	T1: Tumor confined to corpus uteri
IA	T1a,N0,M0	IA	T1a: Tumor limited to endometrium
IB	T1b,N0,M0	IB	T1b: Tumor invades up to or less than one half of myometrium
IC	T1c,N0,M0	IC	T1c: Tumor invades to more than one half of myometrium
			N0: No regional lymph node metastasis
			M0: No distant metastasis
II	T2	II	T2: Tumor invades cervix, but does not extend beyond uterus
IIA	T2a,N0,M0	IIA	T2a: Endocervical glandular involvement only
IIB	T2b,N0,M0	IIB	T2b: Cervical stromal invasion
III	T3	III	T3: Local and/or regional spread as specified in T3a, b, and/or N1
IIIA	T3a,N0,M0	IIIA	T3a: Tumor involves serosa and/or adnexa (direct extension or metastasis) and/or cancer cells in ascites or peritoneal washings
IIIB	T3b,N0,M0	IIIB	T3b: Vaginal involvement (direct extension or metastasis)
IIIC	T1–3b,N1,M0		N1: Regional lymph node metastasis
IVA	T4,Any N,M0	IVA	T4: Tumor invades bladder mucosa and/or bowel mucosa
IVB	Any T,Any N,M1	IVB	M1: Distant metastasis

FIGO = International Federation of Gynecology and Obstetrics.
*Endometrium, myometrium, etc.
Used with the permission of the American Joint Committee on Cancer (AJCC®), Chicago, Illinois. The original source for this material is the AJCC® Cancer Staging Manual, 5th edition (1997), published by Lippincott-Raven Publishers, Philadelphia, Pennsylvania.

TABLE 21–14. **Multidisciplinary Treatment Decisions by Stage for Endometrial Carcinoma**

Stage	Surgery		Radiation Therapy		Chemotherapy
I (T1,N0)	TAH BSO; selected pelvic and para-aortic nodal sampling	and/or	ART preop or postop 45–50 Gy; intracavitary or external RT		NR
II (T2,N0)	TAH BSO; pelvic and para-aortic nodal sampling	and/or	ART preop or postop 45–50 Gy external plus intracavitary 20–40 Gy to vagina		NR
III (T3,N0)	TAH BSO; pelvic and para-aortic nodal sampling	and	ART postop or DRT; intracavitary and external to higher doses; 60–65 Gy if only RT	and/or	HT; IC II
IV (Any T,N1,M+)	NR		PRT	and	HT; IC II

TAH BSO = total abdominal hysterectomy, bilateral salpingo-oophorectomy; NR = not recommended; ART = adjuvant; RT = radiation therapy; DRT = definitive; PRT = palliative; HT = hormonal therapy; IC II = investigational chemotherapy, phase I/II clinical trials.

Modified from DuBeshter B, Lin J, Angel C, et al: Gynecologic tumors. In: Rubin P (ed): Clinical Oncology: A Multidisciplinary Approach for Physicians and Students, 7th ed, pp 363–418. Philadelphia, W.B. Saunders Co., 1993.

Radiation Therapy

Primary treatment with irradiation is reserved for patients who are medically inoperable. These patients tend to be older than the average patient population and, in general, have several severe comorbid conditions, which may have led to the reduced cure rates seen with irradiation alone.[214, 215] The overall survival of these patients is limited, but their disease-specific survival is comparable to that of patients treated with surgery when appropriate prognostic factors are taken into account.[216]

Radiation therapy is an important adjuvant in the treatment of patients with endometrial carcinoma. Adjuvant pelvic radiation therapy may be administered either preoperatively or postoperatively, and can consist of external irradiation, brachytherapy, or both. When external radiation therapy is administered, it is delivered to the pelvis from the region of the bifurcation of the aorta to the introitus of the vagina. At some institutions, preoperative irradiation is administered to patients with less well differentiated tumors or cervical involvement.[217, 218] Currently, postoperative irradiation is used frequently,[219–221] and, particularly for stage I, is administered based on features found at the time of surgery; indications include tumor grade (G2 or G3), 50% or more depth of myometrial invasion, extrauterine spread, lymph node involvement, and status of surgical margins.

Chemotherapy

Cytotoxic chemotherapy as treatment for patients with endometrial carcinoma is under investigation. Nonetheless, several chemotherapy agents have been used as single agents or in combination regimens in patients with advanced, recurrent, or metastatic disease. The first single agent that was identified as having significant activity in patients with endometrial cancer was doxorubicin, with a total response rate of up to 37% and a complete response rate of about 20%.[222] However, it was found subsequently that combination doxorubicin-based therapy offered a greater advantage over single-agent administration, though frequently at the cost of greater toxicity.[223, 224]

Cisplatin has been administered as a single agent, at doses of 50 to 80 mg/m^2 every 3 weeks, and has resulted in response rates of about 20%.[225] Other platinum-based compounds (e.g., carboplatin) have been considered because of their reduced toxicity compared with cisplatin; carboplatin has been given at doses of 300 to 400 mg/m^2 every 4 weeks as a substitute for cisplatin and has demonstrated similar efficacy.[226, 227]

Paclitaxel (Taxol) was used in a recent phase II GOG study to treat patients with advanced or recurrent endometrial cancer.[228] Patients were treated with 200 to 250 mg/m^2 of paclitaxel every 3 weeks. The overall response rate for the 28 patients in the study was 35.7%. In general, however, the majority of chemotherapy regimens under trial at present are multidrug combinations used in the treatment of advanced or recurrent disease. Although they are deemed experimental at present, many of these regimens appear to offer an advantage to patients with an otherwise poor prognosis; Table 21–15 lists a few of the multidrug regimens that have been used for patients with endometrial carcinoma.

Hormonal Therapy

Progestational agents are known to be effective in reversing endometrial hyperplasia, especially in younger women,[235, 236] and also may have a role in treating patients with advanced or recurrent endometrial cancer.[237] Standard progestational agents include hydroxyprogesterone, medroxyprogesterone, and megestrol.[238, 239] Hormonal therapy may be the treatment of choice for advanced or recurrent disease that is not amenable to surgery or radiation or has highly positive receptor levels[240]; however, the use of progestational agents as an adjuvant therapy recently has come under some dispute.[241]

Results of Treatment

- Because of the heterogeneous nature of endometrial cancer, the 5-year survival rates for patients with surgical stage I disease range from 36% to 95%.[186] This improvement over reported rates from pre-1988 results, in all probability, from patients with extrauterine disease being allocated to a different stage rather than remaining within the same stage grouping as patients who are clinically staged.
- Patients who are surgically staged and have occult cervical involvement without extrauterine disease (stage II) have survival rates similar to those of pa-

TABLE 21–15. **Chemotherapy in Endometrial Cancer**

Author	No. of Patients	Stage	Study Design	CR + PR (%)	CR (%)	Mean Response (mos)	Mean Survival (mos)	Toxicity
Alberts et al[229]	42	III–IV/ recurr	PA VBL	30.9	7.1	8	10	Leukopenia (1–4) 88% Thrombocytopenia 20% Deaths—0
Burke et al[230]	87	I–IV/ recurr	PAC	45	14	4.8	10.5	Neutropenia 92% Thrombocytopenia 20% Deaths—0
Thigpen et al[225]	276	Adv/ recurr	A	17	5	3.2	6.9	Leukopenia 75%
			A + C	17	13	3.9	7.3	Thrombocytopenia 17% Deaths—7
Long et al[231]	30	Adv/ recurr	PA Mtx-VBL	67	27	7.2	9.9	Neutropenia Deaths—2
Cornelison et al[232]	50	Adv/ recurr	PAV-M	48	20	7.0	9.4	Neutropenia 8% Thrombocytopenia 12% Deaths—1
Pierga et al[233]	49	Adv/ recurr	PV 5-FU	41	14.3	7	14	Leukopenia 15% Thrombocytopenia 14% Deaths—0
Lissoni et al[234]	49	Adv/ recurr	ETP	73	—	—	—	Neutropenia 61% Deaths—?1

PA VBL = cisplatin, doxorubicin, and vinblastine; PAC = cisplatin, doxorubicin, and cyclophosphamide; A = doxorubicin; A + C = doxorubicin and cyclophosphamide; PA Mtx-VBL = cisplatin, doxorubicin, methotrexate, and vinblastine; PAV-M = cisplatin, doxorubicin, etoposide, and megestrol acetate; PV 5-FU = cisplatin, etoposide, and 5-fluorouracil; ETP = epirubicin, paclitaxel, and cisplatin.

tients with surgical stage I disease (about 90%). However, those with gross cervical involvement have survival rates of 50% to 80%.[242]

- Surgical stage III cancer includes involvement of the uterine serosa, adnexal involvement, positive peritoneal cytology, vaginal metastasis, and positive pelvic or para-aortic lymph nodes. Despite the highly varied sites of involvement for patients with either surgical or clinical stage III disease, the 5-year survival rates are about 40% to 50%.
- It is uncommon for patients with stage IV disease to have tumor limited to the pelvis. Overall, the 5-year survival rate for patients with stage IV endometrial cancer is about 15%.[243]

Prognostic Factors

Tumor Histology and Grade

Histologic and pathologic factors for cancer of the endometrium have been studied in great detail. Since the 1980s, it has been recognized that both serous and clear cell adenocarcinomas have a poor prognosis, associated with a high relapse rate and poor survival.[244, 245] A 2000 study from Japan has confirmed that the poor prognosis of these tumor types is independent of other histologic factors and lymph node status.[246]

Prognosis also has been correlated with tumor histology grade. The grades are assessed on the degree of differentiation, with well-differentiated tumors being grade 1 (G1) and poor or undifferentiated tumors being grade 3 or 4 (G3–4). A study by Reisinger and coworkers[247] concluded that tumor grade was the greatest predictor of survival, with 37% of grade 3 patients having a 5-year survival.

Lymph Node Status

A detailed study from the GOG showed that the greatest risk for recurrent disease was associated with metastasis to the pelvic or para-aortic lymph nodes, intraperitoneal involvement, and positive lymph–vascular space invasion.[248] Possession of two or more risk factors increased the risk of recurrence. Corn and colleagues[249] noted a higher distant failure rate and lower survival in patients who had a pelvic recurrence.

Myometrial Invasion

The depth of myometrial invasion has been shown to be an independent prognostic indicator.[250, 251] Nonetheless, the independence of this factor may not be clear cut because at least one study has shown that myometrial invasion was always accompanied by lymph–vascular space invasion.[252]

Sarcoma of the Uterus

Epidemiology and Etiology

Epidemiology

Sarcomas constitute less than 1% of gynecologic malignancies and represent about 1% to 3% of all malignant tumors of the uterus.[253] These tumors are derived from pure mesenchymal tissue or mixtures of epithelial and mesenchymal tissue. The mean patient age at diagnosis is about 60 years; women with endometrial stromal sarcomas and leiomyosarcomas tend to be younger than those with mixed mesodermal tumors.[254] Some studies also have demonstrated the possibility of a racial component.[255]

Etiology

- Previous pelvic irradiation, often administered for benign uterine bleeding 5 to 25 years earlier, is one of the few known etiologic factors for uterine sarcomas; about 2.4% to 17% of women with uterine sarcomas have a history of previous pelvic irradiation.[256, 257] Of the different types of uterine sarcomas, mixed mesodermal tumors are most often associated with previous irradiation.
- As with endometrial carcinomas, at least one study has shown an association between uterine sarcomas and endogenous estrogen use[258] and marital status,[259] but it is not known to be associated with nulliparity or obesity.

Detection and Diagnosis

- Common presenting symptoms and signs are abnormal uterine bleeding, abdominal pain, tumor prolapse through the cervical os, or a pelvic mass; the diagnostic evaluation of patients for uterine sarcomas is the same as that for endometrial carcinoma.
- The Pap smear is rarely diagnostic, and an endometrial biopsy or D&C is performed for diagnosis.
- It is not uncommon for the D&C to reveal copious amounts of tissue from the endometrial cavity, and this material is often diagnostic. When small amounts of tissue are obtained or only an endometrial biopsy is performed, only 4% of stromal sarcomas and leiomyosarcomas are identified correctly, compared with 91% of mixed mesodermal tumors.[260]

Classification and Staging

Histopathology

Histology is an important prognostic factor in uterine sarcoma, and mitotic activity and grade strongly influence the natural history of the tumor. The histologic classification used most often is that of the GOG (Table 21–16). It should be noted that the uterine neoplasm classification of the International Society of Gynecologic Pathologists uses the term *carcinosarcoma* for all primary uterine neoplasms containing malignant elements of both epithelial and stromal light microscopic appearance, regardless of whether malignant heterologous elements are present.[261]

- Pure leiomyosarcomas constitute about 20% to 50% of uterine sarcomas.[262, 263] These tumors often occur in premenopausal women and are not associated with prior pelvic irradiation. The leiomyosarcoma frequently is diagnosed after a hysterectomy is performed for a presumed leiomyomatous uterus. Histologically, the smooth muscle cells have increased atypia, pleomorphism, and cellularity. The degree of atypia and mitotic activity are used to differentiate leiomyosarcomas from benign smooth muscle tumors. Leiomyosarcomas that have more than 10 mitoses per 10 high-power fields are classified as malignant.[9]
- Mixed mesodermal tumors represent about 30% to 50% of all uterine sarcomas.[264] These tumors are composed of an admixture of a sarcomatous stromal component and malignant epithelium. The epithelial component frequently is adenocarcinoma; however, squamous carcinoma also may be present. The mesenchymal component may be a fibrosarcoma, rhabdomyosarcoma, or an endometrial stromal sarcoma component. Carcinosarcoma (malignant mixed müllerian tumor, homologous type) is the most common type.
- Endometrial stromal sarcoma occurs in about 15% to 20% of patients with uterine sarcomas. Histologically, increased numbers of endometrial stromal cells are seen with varying degrees of atypia and pleomorphism. High-grade stromal sarcomas have 10 or more mitotic figures per 10 high-power fields, whereas low-grade stromal sarcomas have fewer than 10. Low-grade tumors were formerly termed *endolymphatic stromal myosis*, which is descriptive of their predilection to extend into lymphatic or vascular channels within the uterus. These low-grade sarcomas have a protracted natural history, and may recur many years after the initial diagnosis. High-grade tumors have a poor prognosis.

TABLE 21–16. **Uterine Sarcoma Classification Proposed by the Gynecologic Oncology Group**

Mesenchymal

- Leiomyosarcoma
- Endometrial stromal sarcoma: low and high grade
- Mixed differentiated sarcomas with epithelial elements
- Other uterine sarcomas

Mixed Epithelial-Stromal

- Adenocarcinoma without heterologous elements
- Carcinosarcoma with heterologous elements

Staging

Uterine sarcomas are generally staged by the FIGO system for carcinoma of the endometrium (see Table 21–13). A thorough abdominal exploration, including inspection of peritoneal surfaces and pelvic and para-aortic lymph node sampling, is an important determinant of the exact disease extent. In stage I and II disease, lymph node metastases occur in 15% to 45%[265]; tumor extent at initial diagnosis is the most important predictor of prognosis, and patients with lymph node metastases have a poor outlook.

Principles of Treatment

Uterine sarcomas are relatively rare tumors, but they are characterized by aggressive growth and by a poor overall prognosis. The rarity of these tumors has not allowed for the standardization of either diagnostic or therapeutic techniques,[266] but, in general, the standard treatment can be considered to be surgery for stage I; surgery and radiation therapy for stage II; and surgery and radiation, with or without chemotherapy for stage III. Of note, few if any studies have identified any therapeutic advantage to adjuvant therapy in stage I patients.[264, 267]

Surgery

Medically suitable patients with a preoperative diagnosis of uterine sarcoma are candidates for surgical evaluation of the pelvis and abdomen with removal of the uterus, fallopian tubes, and ovaries. Pelvic and para-aortic lymph node sampling, omental biopsy, and peritoneal washings are also performed. More extensive surgery, such as exenteration, has been proposed for locally advanced disease, but few data exist regarding this approach; exenteration for select patients with local pelvic recurrence may be an option. Hysterectomy for advanced disease is largely palliative but can control hemorrhage from the uterine tumor. Excision of a pelvic recurrence is unlikely to be successful because distant metastases occur in more than 80% of cases with a pelvic recurrence.

Extent of disease at presentation is a major prognostic factor. In one retrospective study of uterine sarcoma (stages I–IV), 25 of the surviving 26 patients had presented with stage I disease. The authors noted that adjuvant therapy had not influenced either survival or local tumor control and concluded that the treatment of choice remained total abdominal hysterectomy.[268]

Radiation Therapy

Adjuvant postoperative pelvic irradiation has been used to decrease pelvic failure for patients with uterine sarcomas. In some reports, postoperative pelvic irradiation does not appear to improve absolute survival,[264, 267] but this therapeutic strategy has not been tested in a prospective, randomized clinical trial. However, a number of nonrandomized trials have identified a therapeutic advantage to postoperative irradiation.[269–271] In a California retrospective study of 66 patients with uterine sarcoma, the 2- and 5-year actuarial survival rates were 50% and 25% for surgery alone compared with 61% and 44% for surgery plus irradiation.[269] There was also a 33% locoregional failure rate in the surgery-alone group; this was 0% in the combined-modality group. Two reports from the late 1990s have confirmed the benefit of adjuvant postoperative radiation therapy for disease-specific survival and locoregional control.[270, 271]

The treatment approach advocated at the Mallinckrodt Institute of Radiology is to use a preoperative intracavitary implant for patients with stage I malignant mixed mesodermal tumors, followed within 3 days by a total abdominal extrafascial hysterectomy, bilateral salpingo-oophorectomy, and pelvic and para-aortic lymph node sampling. In addition, adjuvant postoperative external radiation therapy is administered to patients with poor risk factors. Patients with stage II disease undergo preoperative external irradiation and brachytherapy, and a total abdominal extrafascial hysterectomy and bilateral salpingo-oophorectomy are performed in 4 to 6 weeks. This rationale was supported by Larson and coworkers,[272] who demonstrated that therapy with surgery combined with external irradiation and brachytherapy resulted in a higher local tumor control rate and better overall survival than surgery in combination with either brachytherapy or external radiation therapy. Other groups similarly follow this treatment protocol, though noting the high degree of morbidity.[273]

Chemotherapy

Because most patients are at a substantial risk for recurrence, chemotherapy has often been used following surgery. In the 1980s, Omura and coworkers[274] reported the results of a randomized clinical trial of adjuvant doxorubicin in patients with stage I and II uterine sarcomas. Postoperatively, the patients were randomized to receive doxorubicin or no further therapy; there was no difference in the two arms of the study for recurrence rates, progression-free intervals, or survival. However, two later prospective trials showed that doxorubicin, either as a single agent or in combination chemotherapy, demonstrated improved survival rates, although the small numbers of patients in the studies negated any statistical significance.[275, 276]

Newer agents, such as ifosfamide, have been used in phase II trials for advanced or recurrent tumor and produced total response rates of 31%, 27%, and 17% in mixed mesodermal tumors, endometrial stromal sarcomas, and leiomyosarcomas, respectively.[277] Cisplatin also has been used to treat advanced or recurrent tumors, with a total response rate of 19% with mixed mesodermal tumors; the response rate with leiomyosarcomas was only 3%.[278]

There is a general opinion that adjuvant chemotherapy brings some degree of survival benefit by controlling subclinical distant disease in patients with uterine sarcoma. However, to date, this supposition has not been supported by any large, randomized clinical trials. Indeed, the largest prospective trial of adjuvant combination chemotherapy for stage I uterine sarcomas failed to show any impact on long-term survival.[279]

Prognosis

The majority of the identified prognostic factors are related to histologic features.

- In a large study of 310 cases of uterine sarcomas of mixed pathology, survival was found to be best in those patients with either leiomyosarcomas or endometrial stromal sarcomas and worst with carcinosarcomas or mixed mesodermal sarcomas.[280]
- Larson and associates[281] studied 143 patients with uterine leiomyosarcomas and demonstrated that the 5-year survival rate was 65% for cases with a low mitotic rate (>10 mitotic figures per 10 high-power fields) compared with 17% for those with a higher mitotic rate.
- Major and coworkers[282] evaluated 453 cases of stage I and II uterine sarcomas and demonstrated that the recurrence rates were 53% for mixed müllerian tumors and 71% for leiomyosarcomas.

Other reported factors are similar to those identified with endometrial carcinomas (i.e., deep myometrial invasion, lymphatic or vascular space invasion, involvement of the isthmus or cervix, and high-grade, serous, and clear cell carcinomatous components).[261]

Gestational Trophoblastic Neoplasms

Perspective

Gestational trophoblastic neoplasms (GTNs) have a number of distinguishing features that have fascinated physicians for centuries. Tumors of this type were rarely curable before the advent of effective chemotherapy, and they were particularly tragic because they afflicted young women in their reproductive years. Fortunately, today, the vast majority of patients with GTN can be cured because both effective treatment and a reliable tumor marker for monitoring treatment, human chorionic gonadotropin (hCG), are available. Indeed, during the last half of the century, highly effective chemotherapy regimens were developed that made GTN a success story in oncology.[283] Currently available treatment can cure all but patients in the high-risk group, characterized by metastasis to the brain or liver or a history of prior chemotherapy, and even this group demonstrates an 80% cure rate.[284] Nevertheless, because of the rarity of this type of tumor, some confusion still exists regarding its appropriate classification and management.

Epidemiology and Etiology

Epidemiology

The spectrum of GTN includes molar pregnancy (both complete and partial), invasive mole, placental site trophoblastic tumor, and choriocarcinoma. The single most important risk factor for development of the disease is a prior history of a molar gestation. There are wide geographic and ethnic variations in the incidence of molar pregnancy. Some of the highest rates are found in Asia, India, and Africa; rates of 1 in 150 and 1 in 100 pregnancies have been reported in China and Indonesia, respectively. The lowest rates are found in Europe and North America (1:1000).[285] In the United States, molar pregnancy is one half as frequent among black women as among other women.[286]

Etiology

Evaluations of the clinical and pathologic factors have shown that the most significant risk factors are trophoblastic hyperplasia, maternal age, and history of molar pregnancy.[287]

- As stated earlier, the most important risk factor for development of GTN is a prior molar gestation. Approximately one half of patients with choriocarcinoma develop the disease after a molar gestation, with the remaining cases occurring after a nonmolar pregnancy.
- Maternal age is an important risk factor for molar pregnancy. The highest risk is for women at the extremes of reproductive age (i.e., older than 40 years of age and younger than age 20); the risk may be 100 times greater for women over 50 years of age.[285]
- The chromosomal aberrations identified with molar gestations eventually may give important insight into the etiology of this disease. Complete moles are most frequently diploid with a 46,XX karyotype, the entire genome being composed of paternal chromosomes[288]; women younger than 20 years and older than 36 years have an increased risk of complete mole.[289] In contrast, partial moles have a triploid karyotype (69,XXY)[290]; no association with parental age has been identified.[291]

Detection and Diagnosis

After evacuation of a molar pregnancy, persistent GTN may develop in 20% of women with a complete mole and 4% with a partial mole.[292]

Complete Mole

Complete molar pregnancy is characterized by diffuse swelling of the chorionic villi and diffuse trophoblastic hyperplasia in the absence of embryonic or fetal tissues. Although excessive uterine size is a classic feature, it occurs in only 50% of patients with complete moles. However, abnormal vaginal bleeding occurs in virtually all patients with molar pregnancy. Therefore, most patients are diagnosed when bleeding or uterine enlargement with absent fetal heart tones prompts investigation by ultrasound, the most reliable diagnostic method of choice.

Other presenting signs associated with complete molar pregnancies include large ovarian cysts (theca-lutein), hyperemesis, and pre-eclampsia; occurrence of pre-eclampsia in the first trimester of pregnancy is virtually pathognomonic of a molar gestation. Although it is not diagnostic of molar gestations, the hCG level is usually higher in molar than in nonmolar gestations.

Partial Mole

In contrast to complete molar pregnancies, partial molar pregnancies display focal swelling of the chorionic villi and trophoblastic hyperplasia; embryonic or fetal tissues may be present. Vaginal bleeding is a common symptom, but excessive uterine size and large ovarian cysts are distinctly uncommon with partial moles, so that the diagnosis is seldom suspected. Most cases are diagnosed after pathologic review following evacuation of what was presumed to be an incomplete abortion.[293]

Invasive Mole

Invasive mole is most frequently diagnosed during gonadotropin follow-up of a molar gestation.[294] Human chorionic gonadotropin is a weak thyrotropin agonist that reaches a peak in normal pregnancy at 10 to 12 weeks, when it suppresses serum thyrotropin levels.[295] However, trophoblastic tumors, hydatidiform mole, and choriocarcinoma secrete very large amounts of hCG; therefore, a diagnosis is made when either a plateau or increase in serum hCG level (>300 mIU/mL) occurs at approximately 4 weeks postevacuation together with cytologic abnormalities.[296] Another factor that may be useful in the diagnosis of invasive GTN that is currently under study is early pregnancy factor, which has shown a 91% accuracy at diagnosing malignancy.[297]

Importantly, patients with molar gestations can be stratified into low- and high-risk categories on the basis of clinical and laboratory parameters. Those who have large-for-dates uteri or a pre-evacuation serum hCG level higher than 100,000 mIU/mL (high-risk molar pregnancy) have about a 50% risk of developing invasive mole. Patients without these and other high-risk features have less than a 5% risk. Invasive mole also can occur after spontaneous abortion, tubal pregnancy, or any gestational event. In these cases, the diagnosis is usually made when a serum hCG level is obtained in conjunction with ultrasound to evaluate abnormal vaginal bleeding, the most frequent presenting symptom.

Metastatic Gestational Trophoblastic Neoplasms

Although invasive mole occasionally can be found in metastatic sites such as the lung, generally when metastases occur, the histology, if obtained, is choriocarcinoma. The most frequent symptoms in patients with metastatic gestational trophoblastic disease are abnormal vaginal bleeding and abdominal pain. Because this tumor can spread hematogenously, the lung, liver, and brain can be involved by tumor. Persistent cough, hemoptysis, stroke, hemianopsia, and other symptoms reflecting the metastatic sites can occur as the initial symptoms. A serum hCG level should be obtained in any woman of reproductive age who has a metastatic tumor without a known primary tumor if histology is unavailable.

Classification and Staging

Histopathology

- Complete mole is characterized histologically by hydropic villi, trophoblastic hyperplasia, and the absence of fetal vessels.[298] In contrast, partial moles often have evidence of fetal development, and there is an admixture of villi, some with hydropic change and some without.
- Invasive mole appears similar to complete mole histologically, but, in addition, it invades the myometrium.
- Choriocarcinoma consists predominantly of cytotrophoblast and syncytiotrophoblast and does not have chorionic villi.
- Placental site tumors are composed of intermediate trophoblast; there are no villi. These tumors are notable for low hCG production not reflective of tumor burden.

Staging

The number of staging systems that have been developed for gestational trophoblastic tumors is reflective of differing views regarding the best method to classify these tumors. Older systems (e.g., the previous FIGO system) were elegant in their simplicity but failed to take into account a number of known risk factors; therefore, in the early 1990s,[299] FIGO added prognostic risk factors to the classic staging system (Table 21–17). Nonetheless, many investigators describe difficulties with regard to the best way to apply the existing staging systems, and attempts are still being made to resolve scoring systems.[300]

Principles of Treatment

Surgery

A patient with low-risk gestational trophoblastic disease desirous of further childbearing may receive surgery in the form of suction D&C of the uterus as primary therapy[301]; spontaneous regression rates of greater than 60% have been reported after D&C alone.[302] However, in a patient with a large uterus, this procedure can be formidable and accompanied by excessive blood loss. In patients who have completed childbearing, a hysterectomy may be performed with the mole left *in situ*. Theca-lutein cysts should be left intact at the time of hysterectomy unless removal is otherwise indicated because they invariably involute over several months after removal of the molar pregnancy.

A key role for surgery is in the treatment of patients with

TABLE 21–17. **International Federation of Gynecology and Obstetrics (FIGO) Staging of Gestational Trophoblastic Tumors**

Stage	Grouping	Risk Factors*	Descriptor
I			I: Disease confined to the uterus
IA	T1,M0	without	IA: Disease confined to the uterus with no risk factors
IB	T1,M0	1	IB: Disease confined to the uterus with one risk factor
IC	T1,M0	2	IC: Disease confined to the uterus with two risk factors
II			II: GTT extends outside the uterus, but is limited to the genital structures (ovary, tube, vagina)
IIA	T2,M0	without	IIA: GTT involving genital structures with no risk factors
IIB	T2,M0	1	IIB: GTT involving genital structures with one risk factor
IIC	T2,M0	2	IIC: GTT involving genital structures with two risk factors
III			III: GTT extends to the lungs, with or without known genital tract involvement
IIIA	Any T,M1a	without	IIIA: GTT extends to the lungs, with or without known genital tract involvement with no risk factors
IIIB	Any T,M1a	1	IIIB: GTT extends to the lungs, with or without known genital tract involvement with one risk factor
IIIC	Any T,M1a	2	IIIC: GTT extends to the lungs, with or without known genital tract involvement with two risk factors
IV			IV: All other metastatic sites
IVA	Any T,M1b	without	IVA: All other metastatic sites with no risk factors
IVB	Any T,M1b	1	IVB: All other metastatic sites with one risk factor
IVC	Any T,M1b	2	IVC: All other metastatic sites with two risk factors

GTT = gestational trophoblastic tumors.

*Risk factors affecting staging: 1. hCG levels >100,000 IU/24-hour urine; 2. Detection of the disease more than 6 months from termination of the antecedent pregnancy.

Used with the permission of the American Joint Committee on Cancer (AJCC®), Chicago, Illinois. The original source for this material is the AJCC® Cancer Staging Manual, 5th edition (1997), published by Lippincott-Raven Publishers, Philadelphia, Pennsylvania.

high-risk metastatic disease, especially in those patients demonstrating foci of chemoresistant tumor. In some reports, hysterectomy, with or without thoracotomy, combined with salvage chemotherapy resulted in cure rates of 98% in this high-risk group.[303, 304] In addition, craniotomy may be required in the treatment of central nervous system metastases to control bleeding and to alleviate intracranial pressure.[305]

Radiation Therapy

Like surgery, the role of radiation therapy in the management of patients with GTN is, in general, limited to the high-risk group with metastases, particularly with metastases to the central nervous system. In these patients, whole-brain irradiation (30 Gy) is recommended, although intrathecal chemotherapy alone also has been used successfully.[304, 305] The dose of whole-brain irradiation is critical in achieving metastatic control; doses of less than 22 Gy have demonstrated a 5-year actuarial survival rate of 24% compared with 91% with doses of 22 Gy or more.[306]

Chemotherapy

GTNs are exquisitely sensitive to a variety of chemotherapeutic agents, with the exception of placental site tumors, which have a variable response.[307] Nonmetastatic and low-risk metastatic GTNs can be managed successfully with single-agent chemotherapy,[308, 309] using either methotrexate or actinomycin D. However, use of single agents should be restricted to those patients who have not failed first-line chemotherapy, have a low World Health Organization score,[310] and have no evidence of choriocarcinoma. Intuitively, failure rates with the use of single agents are higher in those patients with metastatic disease.

High-risk metastatic GTN should be treated aggressively with combination chemotherapy. Until the last decade, the standard regimen consisted of methotrexate, actinomycin D, and cyclophosphamide (or chlorambucil) (MAC) [311]; this regimen induced a remission rate of about 50%.[294] However, the standard of care is now considered to be EMA-CO (alternating cycles of etoposide, methotrexate, actinomycin D with cyclophosphamide, vincristine), which demonstrates a remission rate of about 70% in these patients.[312–315] The major complications of this regimen are related to myelosuppression, which tends to be dose-limiting; addition of granulocyte colony-stimulating factor has been shown to assist in maintaining the treatment schedule.[316] Late sequelae are uncommon.[315] Relapse may be treated with cisplatin-based therapy; tumors that are refractory to platinum-based therapy have shown a good response to ifosfamide, alone or in combination.[317, 318] For those patients who develop drug resistance, salvage surgery is also important.

Follow-Up, Results, and Prognosis

Follow-Up

Surveillance of patients treated for gestational trophoblastic disease is mandatory. Fortunately, these tumors produce large amounts of hCG (with the exception of placental site tumor), which can be measured accurately in the serum and is close to an ideal tumor marker. Patients with either a complete or partial mole should undergo weekly serum β-hCG measurement until a normal level is reached. After three normal levels, serum hCG measurements may be obtained at longer intervals. The follow-up for patients with invasive mole or choriocarcinoma is similar to that for patients with a molar pregnancy. However, in cases in which remission was difficult to achieve (requiring more than three or four courses of chemotherapy), the period of serum hCG follow-up should be extended to 2 years because late recurrences are possible.

Results and Prognosis

Currently, patients undergoing evacuation of a molar pregnancy have an excellent prognosis, both in terms of their outlook for future fertility and with respect to the available treatment should an invasive mole or choriocarcinoma develop. Most patients (80%) with a molar pregnancy have no further sequelae after evacuation of the mole; the remaining 20% develop either nonmetastatic or metastatic GTN that requires chemotherapy. However, virtually all patients with nonmetastatic disease are cured, although some (<5%) may require hysterectomy or uterine resection to remove a focus of resistant tumor. Patients with low-risk metastatic GTN also have an excellent prognosis.

Currently, about 5% of patients with high-risk metastatic GTN die of the disease.[313, 315] Poor prognostic factors have been identified as the presence of liver or brain metastases, or both,[315, 319] an interval of more than 24 months since the antecedent pregnancy,[315] patient age, and previous inadequate chemotherapy.[319] In patients with two or more poor prognostic factors, the survival rates are 82% and 43%, respectively.[319] Of some concern, a small but significant increase in the risk of secondary malignant tumors has been reported following treatment with sequential or combination therapy.[315, 320]

Carcinoma of the Fallopian Tube

Epidemiology and Etiology

Carcinoma of the fallopian tube is an uncommon malignancy that accounts for 0.3% to 1.1% of all female genital tract cancers.[321, 322] The most common form of this cancer is a papillary serous carcinoma, but only about 300 cases of these are reported each year in the United States[323]; the paucity of information makes its natural history and management unfamiliar. In most series, the median patient age at diagnosis is between 55 and 60 years. The clinical course of fallopian tube carcinoma is often similar to that of epithelial ovarian carcinoma, although there are several significant differences.

Detection and Diagnosis

Clinical Detection

Unlike epithelial ovarian carcinoma, fallopian tube carcinoma is often symptomatic. The three most common symptoms and signs are abnormal vaginal bleeding, a pelvic mass, and abdominal or pelvic pain.[324] Pelvic pain is more common in tubal carcinoma than in ovarian carcinoma; as the tumor in the fallopian tube enlarges, pain results from the peristaltic contractions of a hollow viscus. The lack of specificity of these findings and the rarity of tubal carcinoma make accurate preoperative diagnosis very difficult.

Diagnostic Procedures

Fallopian tube carcinoma often may be mistaken for an ovarian neoplasm, uterine leiomyomata, hydrosalpinx, or a tubo-ovarian abscess—all of which are more common than tubal carcinoma. Therefore, the diagnosis of fallopian tube carcinoma is considered before surgery in only 0% to 15% of patients[325, 326]; the majority are identified during surgery or by pathologic examination.

- Rarely, fallopian tube carcinoma is detected on Pap smear,[327] but in general the positivity of this method is only 25% to 50%. Cytologic findings play the greatest role in staging.
- Pelvic ultrasound may demonstrate tubal carcinoma,[324] but it is often mistaken for an ovarian tumor because tubal carcinoma appears frequently as a complex fusiform mass on ultrasound. A number of studies have shown that contrast-enhanced MRI demonstrates superior characterization and differentiation over ultrasound.[328, 329]
- Although laparotomy is necessary for definitive diagnosis of primary tubal carcinoma, there still can be uncertainty on gross examination.

Classification and Staging

Histopathology

- Benign neoplasms can arise from the fallopian tube and are usually of mesodermal origin. These tumors include leiomyomata, adenomatoid tumors, and teratomas.
- Malignant neoplasms resemble serous adenocarcinoma of the ovary and may assume papillary, alveolar, or medullary growth patterns; Hu's criteria for diagnosing tubal carcinoma specified that most of the tumor must be in the fallopian tube, with involvement of the tubal mucosa in a papillary pattern.[330]
- These tumors rarely contain mucin, but they may have associated benign or malignant squamous components.[331]
- There must be a clearly defined transition between normal and malignant epithelium in the tube.

- Tubal carcinomas spread transmurally; the tumor gradually extends from the tubal mucosa to serosa and may also occur via the ostia into the endometrial or intraperitoneal cavity.
- Lymphatic spread is common to both para-aortic and pelvic lymph nodes; however, the exact frequency of nodal spread at initial diagnosis is unclear because surgical staging has not been performed uniformly.

No uniform grading system exists, but most incorporate assessment of architectural abnormalities and nuclear atypia.

Staging

Staging for fallopian tube carcinoma is by a surgical-pathologic system (Table 21–18). Because carcinoma *in situ* in the fallopian tube is a defined entity, it is included in stage 0.[5]

Principles of Treatment

Primary treatment of adenocarcinoma of the fallopian tube is surgical resection at the time of initial diagnosis. Recent reports advocate lymph node sampling because nodal involvement may occur early in the course of disease spread, and they may occur even earlier than the extent of pelvic spread may indicate. Some investigators have reported satisfactory results with conservative surgical treatment (unilateral salpingectomy only) in cases in which tumor has not invaded beyond the mucosa.[332] Most patients, however, require some form of adjuvant treatment (chemotherapy, irradiation) postoperatively to combat bulky residual disease or to treat assumed microscopic involvement.

Deciphering the literature in search of the most favorable treatment regimens is fraught with difficulties resulting from the relative rarity of this disease. Most studies reporting results of adjuvant therapy cover a time span of several decades, are without prospective randomization of patients or use of consistent staging schema, and, therefore, were poorly reported.

Surgery

Exploratory laparotomy with total abdominal hysterectomy, bilateral salpingo-oophorectomy, omentectomy, tumor resection (as complete as possible), peritoneal washings with a thorough evaluation of all peritoneal surfaces, and pelvic and para-aortic lymph node sampling should be performed. Surgical cytoreduction to minimize residual tumor may be of benefit in prolonging mean survival, although not in patients with advanced disease.[333] In general, most investigators suggest that stage I and II patients have a good prognosis with primary surgical treatment, but the majority support adjuvant therapy following extensive debulking in all stages.[325, 334, 335]

Second-Look Laparotomy

Although the value of second-look laparotomy has not been well defined, in some series, it has provided useful prognostic information in the assessment of response to chemotherapy.[336, 337] The likelihood of being free of disease at second-look laparotomy has been related to the initial stage and amount of residual disease remaining after initial surgery.[336, 338] However, the predictive value in remaining disease free appears to be limited, and several authors have reported relapse rates of 19% to 40% after a negative second-look operation.[337, 338]

Radiation Therapy

Postoperative radiation therapy has been a traditional form of therapy for fallopian tube carcinoma dissemination and recurrence. However, although its use has been recommended by some authors, it has been questioned by oth-

TABLE 21–18. **Staging of Carcinoma of the Fallopian Tube**

Stage*	Grouping	Descriptor
0	Tis	Tis: Carcinoma *in situ* (limited to tubal mucosa)
I	T1	T1: Tumor confined to fallopian tube(s)
IA	T1a,N0,M0	T1a: Tumor limited to one tube without penetrating serosal surface; no ascites
IB	T1b,N0,M0	T1b: Tumor limited to both tubes without penetrating serosal surface; no ascites
IC	T1c,N0,M0	T1c: Tumor limited to one or both tubes with extension onto or through tubal serosa, or with malignant cells in ascites or peritoneal washings
		N0: No regional lymph node metastasis
		M0: No distant metastasis
II	T2	T2: Tumor involves one or both fallopian tubes with pelvic extension
IIA	T2a,N0,M0	T2a: Extension and/or metastasis to uterus and/or ovaries
IIB	T2b,N0,M0	T2b: Extension to other pelvic structures
IIC	T2c,N0,M0	T2c: Pelvic extension with malignant cells in ascites or peritoneal washings
III	T3 and/or N1	T3: Tumor involves one or both fallopian tubes with peritoneal implants outside pelvis
IIIA	T3a,N0,M0	T3a: Microscopic peritoneal metastasis outside pelvis
IIIB	T3b,N0,M0	T3b: Macroscopic peritoneal metastasis outside pelvis ≤2 cm in greatest dimension
IIIC	T3c and/or N1,M0	T3c: Peritoneal metastasis outside pelvis >2 cm in greatest dimension
		N1: Regional lymph node metastasis
IV	Any T,Any N,M1	M1: Distant metastasis

*American Joint Committee on Cancer/International Union Against Cancer/International Federation of Gynecology and Obstetrics stages.

Used with the permission of the American Joint Committee on Cancer (AJCC®), Chicago, Illinois. The original source for this material is the AJCC® Cancer Staging Manual, 5th edition (1997), published by Lippincott-Raven Publishers, Philadelphia, Pennsylvania.

TABLE 21–19. **Survival in Fallopian Tube Carcinoma**

			Postoperative Treatment				
Author	**No. of Cases**	**Stage**	***RT***	***Single CT***	***Combo CT***	***RT & CT***	**Survival (%)**
Schray et al[341]	21	I & II	17	—	—	4	42–78
	12	III & IV	4	—	—	2	33
Peters et al[346]	65	I & II	33	6	1	4	29–61
	29	III & IV	5	6	14	2	0–17
Kaya et al[355]	30	I–IV	20		3	5	36.7*
Pectasides et al[349]	14	I–IV	—	—	14	—	48*
Klein et al[344]	42	I & II	22	—	20	—	RT—53*
	31	III & IV	2		29		CT—27*
Jereczek et al[340]	26	I–IV	14	—	4	—	33*
Cormio et al[337]	38	I–II	—	—	38	—	29*

RT = radiation therapy; CT = chemotherapy.
*5-year survival rate.

ers.[325, 332, 339, 340] Early small studies observed promising results using techniques similar to those used in treatment of ovarian carcinoma, such as whole-abdominal external beam irradiation or intraperitoneal administration of radioactive nuclides (e.g., ^{32}P, ^{198}Au).[341, 342] Nonetheless, the small patient numbers in these studies demand that future investigations explore the usefulness of these techniques, especially whole-abdominal irradiation,[343] although at least one study has shown no advantage.[344]

A study using the FIGO staging system for fallopian tube carcinoma compared outcome in carcinoma *in situ* versus stage I following the use of either irradiation or cisplatin-based chemotherapy[332]; the stage I patients treated with irradiation showed a significantly better prognosis than patients treated with chemotherapy ($p = 0.17$). However, little information exists regarding combination or concomitant use of chemotherapy and irradiation as postoperative treatment. Because both modalities have shown a response used together or separately, a prospective, randomized study may be of help in this regard, although some consideration should always be given to the potential for increased toxicity as a result of the combination therapy.[345]

Chemotherapy

In the late 1980s, reports of treatments using CAP (cyclophosphamide, doxorubicin, and cisplatin) combination chemotherapy demonstrated response rates and 5-year survival superior to those with single-agent therapy and non–cisplatin-based combination chemotherapy regimens[346]; response rates in patients with advanced or recurrent disease were as high as 81%.[347] In a prospective trial, 18 patients receiving at least 6 to 12 cycles of CAP achieved an overall response rate of 53%, similar to that seen in ovarian carcinoma.[348] In the 1990s, despite the limitations of small patient numbers, further investigations have continued to support the use of platinum-based multiagent chemotherapy.[336, 349–351]

Because the normal fallopian tube epithelium exhibits cyclic changes in response to hormonal variations of the menstrual cycle, progesterones were studied for possible use in treatment of fallopian tube malignancies, but with no success.[352–354]

Results and Prognosis

Overall, 5-year survival for fallopian tube carcinoma is 30% to 50% (Table 21–19). However, because most series include patients treated over a 10- to 20-year span, current data supporting the modern trend toward adjuvant therapy with combined-modality therapy require clinical trials.

Prognostic Factors

In most series, about 60% of patients with tubal carcinoma present with disease confined to the pelvis (stage I or II), with only 40% in stage III or IV[343, 356, 357]; with ovarian cancer the ratio is reversed.[358] On a univariate analysis, a number of prognostic factors have emerged:

- postoperative adjuvant therapy[343, 346, 356]
- optimal debulking surgery[346, 356, 357]
- absence of closure of the fimbriated end of the tube[359]
- nulliparity[356]
- age[343, 346, 359]
- stage,[342, 346, 356, 357, 359] particularly stage I versus II/III/IV[343]
- tumor differentiation[356, 357]

However, in the few studies with sufficient numbers to allow for a multivariate analysis, stage at presentation is the only consistent factor.[343, 346, 357, 359] In addition, the presence of vascular or lymphatic invasion with early-stage disease has been shown in one study to decrease 5-year survival rates to 29% versus 83% for those who do not have such invasion.[360]

Ovarian Cancer

Epidemiology and Etiology

Epidemiology

Ovarian cancer is the most lethal type of gynecologic malignancy,[361] resulting in approximately 14,000 deaths per year.[12] In the year 2000, there was an estimated 23,100 cases of ovarian cancer newly diagnosed in the United States.[12] Of considerable import to the outcome of this disease is that, in the majority of cases (>70%), ovarian cancer presents as advanced stage III or IV disease; this finding is, in all probability, due to patients tending to be asymptomatic until metastatic disease is present.

The incidence of ovarian cancer increases with age[362]; the majority of cancers occur in postmenopausal women, and the average patient age at diagnosis is about 65 years.[362] Most ovarian cancers are of epithelial cell origin, but in the less than 1% of epithelial ovarian cancers that occur in women 20 years of age and younger, the majority are of germ cell origin.[363]

Etiology

The exact etiology of ovarian cancer remains unknown, but studies have identified endocrine, environmental, and genetic risk factors:

- An increased risk for ovarian cancer has been associated with nulliparity[364, 365]; suggested protective effects against development of ovarian cancer include multiparity,[366] oral contraceptive use,[367] breast feeding,[368] early first pregnancy,[366] and previous hysterectomy.[369] Some of these protective effects support the incessant ovulation theory, which is based on the hypothesis that ovarian cancer develops from a genetic error made during repair of surface epithelium; another hypothesis frequently discussed involves excessive gonadotropin secretion.[370]
- Use of talcum powder[371] and exposure to asbestos[372] have been suggested as risk factors, although definitive associations have not been established.
- Most epithelial ovarian cancers occur sporadically, but genetic factors may play a role in up to 10% of ovarian malignancies.[373]

Ovarian cancer that is inherited tends to affect women 10 to 20 years earlier than sporadic ovarian cancer. The mode of inheritance in ovarian cancer is consistent with autosomal dominance with variable penetrance. Three distinct hereditary ovarian cancer syndromes have been described: familial site-specific ovarian cancer, Lynch II syndrome, and hereditary breast-ovarian cancer syndrome.

- The relative risk of hereditary ovarian cancer in a first-degree relative is approximately 4[374]; the risk range varies from 1 (for mothers of cases) to 4 (for sisters) to 6 (for daughters).[375] This risk increases further when more than one first-degree family member is affected.[375, 376]
- Lynch II syndrome is a family cancer syndrome that includes multiple adenocarcinomas. It is characterized by nonpolyposis colon cancer in conjunction with endometrial, breast, and ovarian cancer.[377, 378]
- Hereditary breast-ovarian cancer syndrome has been linked in some families to a mutation in the *BRCA1* gene, located on chromosome 17q, and, possibly, to the *BRCA2* gene, located on 13q[379]; these genes are involved in pathways associated with DNA repair.[380] Genetic testing for mutations in the *BRCA1*, *BRCA2*, and other similarly associated genes (*hMLH1*, *hMLH2*, *hPMS1*, and others) is available; however, the majority of ovarian cancer patients with possible hereditary disease test negative, suggesting that there are other predisposing factors.[381, 382]

Detection and Diagnosis

Clinical Detection

Currently no reliable screening test exists for ovarian cancer in the general population.[383]

- *Routine pelvic examination* is the current recommendation for women over the age of 40, but its benefit as a primary screen for ovarian cancer is limited, and it needs to be performed in combination with other tests.[384]
- Multiple studies have assessed *ultrasonography*, both transabdominal and more recently transvaginal, as a screening tool for ovarian cancer. Transvaginal sonography, in particular, has proved to have high sensitivity, although its specificity improves when used in combination with other screening methods.[385]
- Addition of *color flow Doppler* to detect ovarian vasculature changes has been advocated by some, but further study is needed to assess the accuracy of this adjunctive tool.[386]
- CA-125 is a cell surface glycoprotein that has been studied as a screening test for ovarian cancer. This glycoprotein is shed from the surface of damaged cells and can be elevated in a number of benign and malignant conditions. In many patients with ovarian cancer, CA-125 is used as a tumor marker to assess response to treatment and as a marker for recurrent disease; however, its role in a screening test is still under investigation.[387]

Use of a combination of routine pelvic examination, transvaginal ultrasound, and CA-125 improves both the sensitivity and specificity in screening for ovarian cancer[384, 388]; however, this approach is not cost effective for the general population, especially premenopausal women. In combination, these tests have a more practical application when used to screen a select population, such as women with a family history of ovarian cancer.

Diagnostic Procedures

Characteristics suggesting ovarian malignancy include a complex adnexal mass with ascites, cul-de-sac nodularity, pelvic or para-aortic lymphadenopathy, a pleural effusion, or a combination of these characteristics. Early-stage ovarian cancer usually has few symptoms, but if symptoms are present, they are nonspecific; they can include irregular menses, abdominal or pelvic pain, dyspareunia, or changes in bowel or bladder habits. Advanced-stage ovarian cancer is more likely to manifest symptoms, but, again, these complaints are usually nonspecific. Abdominal bloating, abdominal distention, early satiety, nausea, constipation, and dyspnea are more suggestive of advanced ovarian cancer.

An adnexal mass on pelvic examination is the most common sign of ovarian cancer. This finding is clearly abnormal in postmenopausal women because ovaries become atrophic and are nonpalpable in most postmenopausal women. Points to be considered when a pelvic mass is palpated on manual examination are size, consistency, and mobility of the mass and age of the patient. A schematic diagram of the management of an adnexal mass is shown in Figure 21–8.

Ultimately, the diagnosis of ovarian cancer depends on histologic confirmation of ovarian cancer at the time of exploratory surgery. Routine preoperative evaluation should include a complete history and physical examination, including Pap smear, chest x-ray, mammogram, complete blood count, blood chemistries, and liver function tests.

- A *transvaginal ultrasound* may provide useful information about the pelvic mass, such as size and differentiation between a cystic and solid mass.
- A *barium enema* or *colonoscopy*, or both, and IVP are often recommended in patients 40 to 45 years of age and older to exclude primary colonic and bladder involvement.
- Other radiologic studies, such as CT and MRI, provide little additional information and rarely change management in patients with a pelvic mass.

Classification and Staging

Histopathology

Ovarian tumors are classified based on their histologic origin within the ovary. Between 80% and 90% of ovarian tumors are of epithelial cell origin. These tumors are histologically classified as benign, borderline (low malignant potential), or malignant. They are composed of a variety of histologic subtypes.

- Borderline (low malignant potential) tumors of the ovary represent about 10% to 15% of epithelial ovarian tumors. Histologically, these tumors exhibit greater cellular proliferation and cytologic atypia than those seen in benign ovarian tumors, without the destructive stromal invasion associated with malignant ovarian tumors. Histologic types include serous, mucinous, endometrioid, clear cell, and Brenner tumors. These tumors have the ability to recur after many years because of their indolent growth patterns.
- Serous carcinomas are the most common histologic subtype, comprising approximately 50% of epithelial ovarian cancers. These tumors are usually cystic and solid, and frequently are bilateral; a bilateral condition may reflect a monoclonal origin.[389] Microscopically, they contain papillary or glandular elements and often contain calcium concretions called psammoma bodies.
- Fifteen percent of epithelial ovarian cancers are of the mucinous subtype; 5% to 10% may be bilateral. These tumors are usually large, cystic, and multilobulated and are filled with mucinous material. Pseudomyxoma peritonei is a condition associated with mucinous tumors of the ovary, bowel, or appendix in which mucinous material coats the peritoneal cavity.

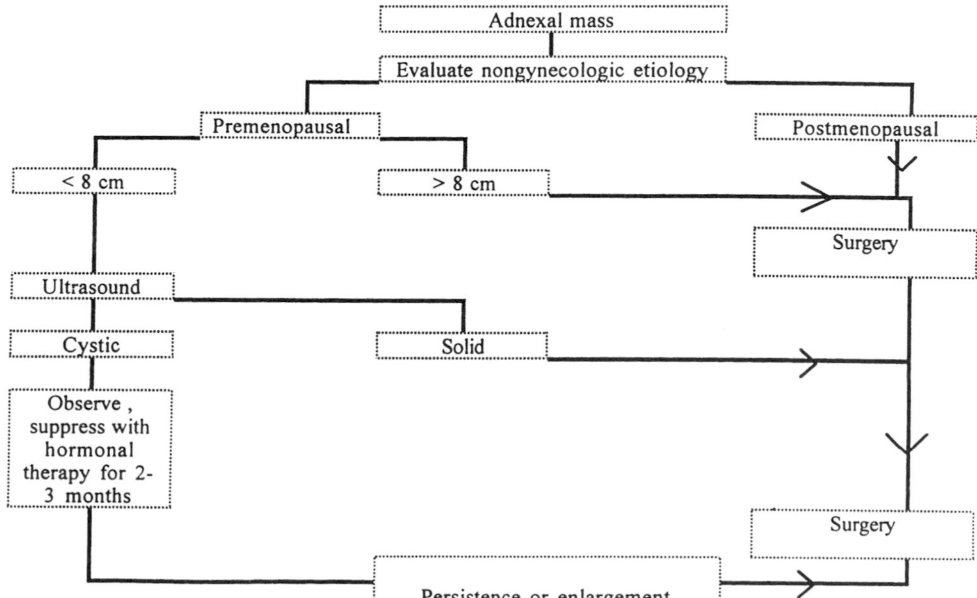

Figure 21–8. Preoperative evaluation of a patient with an adnexal mass. (Modified from Berek JS, Hacker NF [eds]: Practical Gynecologic Oncology, 3rd ed, p 332. Baltimore, Lippincott Williams & Wilkins, 2000.)

TABLE 21–20. **Classification of Germ Cell Tumors of the Ovary**

A. Dysgerminoma
B. Endodermal sinus tumor
C. Embryonal carcinoma
D. Teratoma
  1. Immature teratoma
  2. Mature teratoma
    a. Solid
    b. Cystic (dermoid)
  3. Monodermal/highly specialized
    a. Carcinoid
    b. Stroma ovarii
    c. Others
E. Choriocarcinoma
F. Polyembryona
G. Mixed

Adapted from Serov SF, Scully RE, Sobin LH: Histological Typing of Ovarian Tumours: International Histological Classification of Tumours, No. 9. Geneva, World Health Organization, 1973.

- Endometrioid cancers of the ovary resemble cancer of the endometrium, and they account for about 10% to 20% of epithelial ovarian cancers. These tumors can coexist with a synchronous primary cancer of the endometrium in up to one third of cases, and they may also arise in the setting of endometriosis.
- Clear cell cancers of the ovary account for only 5% of epithelial ovarian cancers, and they are not associated with DES exposure, as are clear cell cancers of the vagina. They are commonly bilateral, and many are found in stage I. There is disagreement on whether clear cell cancers of the ovary have a worse stage-for-stage prognosis when compared with other epithelial ovarian cancer subtypes.[390, 391] Microscopically, these tumors contain hobnail cells and cells with abundant glycogen.
- Brenner tumors of the ovary are rare and, when present, are usually benign. These tumors are most often unilateral and stage I. Histologically, they are characterized by transitional epithelium within fibrous stroma.

Tumors arising from primitive germ cells of the embryonic gonad are referred to as germ cell tumors. They are classified as both benign and malignant; some benign variants can degenerate into malignant types. Germ cell tumors of the ovary account for approximately 10% of all ovarian tumors and, in contrast to tumors of epithelial origin, tend to affect younger women and grow more rapidly. A modification of the World Health Organization classification of germ cell tumors of the ovary is shown in Table 21–20.[392] Other histologic types of ovarian tumors found are sex cord stromal tumors derived from the sex cords or the mesenchyme of the embryonic gonad, granulosa cell tumors, thecomas, fibromas, Sertoli-Leydig cell tumors, and gynandroblastomas.

Staging

The revised surgical staging system for ovarian cancer is shown in Table 21–21 and illustrated in Figure 21–9. Surgical stage of disease is based on the extent of disease present at the time of diagnosis. Because treatment and prognosis of ovarian cancer depend on the stage of disease, thorough surgical staging is important and should be performed by someone skilled in pelvic surgery and familiar with the staging procedure.

If an ovarian malignancy is suspected preoperatively, a vertical midline incision affords optimal exposure to the upper abdomen. When the peritoneal cavity is entered, ascites or pelvic washings should be collected and sent for cytologic examination. The remainder of the staging

TABLE 21–21. **Staging of Cancer of the Ovary**

Stage	Grouping	FIGO Staging	Descriptor
I	T1	I	T1: Tumor limited to ovaries (one or both)
IA	T1a,N0,M0	IA	T1a: Tumor limited to one ovary; capsule intact, no tumor on ovarian surface, no malignant cells in ascites or peritoneal washings
IB	T1b,N0,M0	IB	T1b: Tumor limited to both ovaries; capsules intact, no tumor on ovarian surface, no malignant cells in ascites or peritoneal washings
IC	T1c,N0,M0	IB2	T1c: Tumor limited to one or both ovaries with any of the following: capsule ruptured, tumor on ovarian surface, malignant cells in ascites or peritoneal washings
			N0: No regional lymph node metastasis
			M0: No distant metastasis
II	T2	II	T2: Tumor involves one or both ovaries with pelvic extension
IIA	T2a,N0,M0	IIA	T2a: Extension and/or implants on uterus and/or tube(s); no malignant cells in ascites or peritoneal washings
IIB	T2b,N0,M0	IIB	T2b: Extension to other pelvic tissues; no malignant cells in ascites or peritoneal washings
IIC	T2c,N0,M0	IIC	T2c: Pelvic extension (2a or 2b) with malignant cells in ascites or peritoneal washings
III	T3 and/or N1	III	T3: Tumor involves one or both ovaries with microscopically confirmed peritoneal metastasis outside pelvis and/or regional lymph node metastasis
IIIA	T3a,N0,M0	IIIA	T3a: Microscopic peritoneal metastasis beyond pelvis
IIIB	T3b,N0,M0	IIIB	T3b: Macroscopic peritoneal metastasis beyond pelvis, ≤2 cm in greatest dimension
IIIC	T3c,N0,M0	IIIC	T3c: Peritoneal metastasis beyond pelvis, >2 cm in greatest dimension
	Any T,N1,M0		N1: Regional lymph node metastasis
IV	Any T,Any N,M1	IV	M1: Distant metastasis

FIGO = International Federation of Gynecology and Obstetrics.

Used with the permission of the American Joint Committee on Cancer (AJCC®), Chicago, Illinois. The original source for this material is the AJCC® Cancer Staging Manual, 5th edition (1997), published by Lippincott-Raven Publishers, Philadelphia, Pennsylvania.

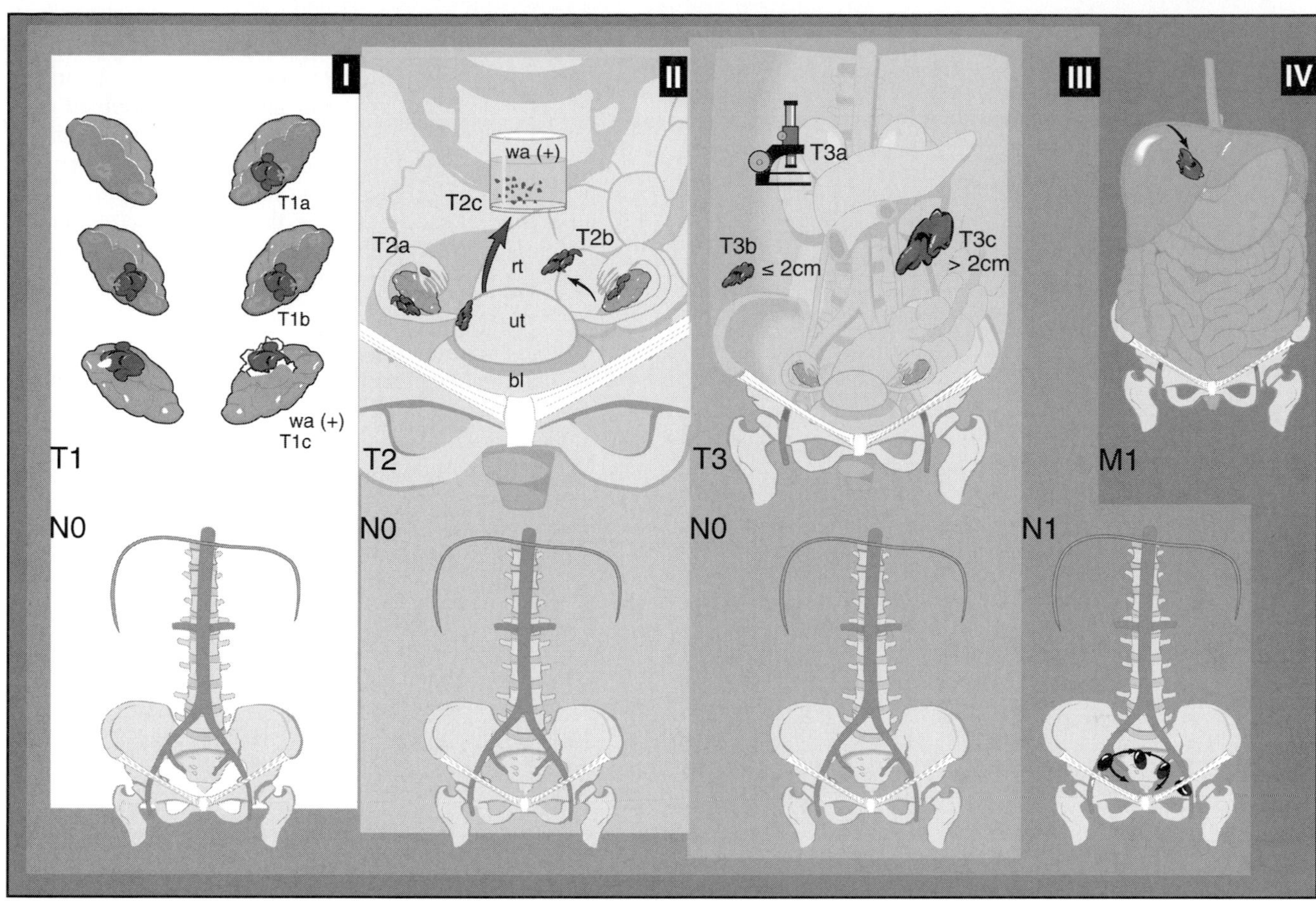

Figure 21–9. Anatomic staging for ovarian cancer.

procedure for ovarian cancer consists of careful inspection of the pelvis and abdomen, including the upper abdomen, with biopsy of any suspicious areas. If no gross disease is evident, several biopsy specimens are obtained. The areas for which biopsies should be performed include the peritoneal surface of the cul-de-sac, the vesicouterine peritoneum, the paracolic gutters, the lateral sidewalls, and the subdiaphragmatic space. An infracolic omentectomy should be performed, as well as retroperitoneal lymph node sampling and removal of any enlarged nodes.[393] Complete surgical staging should be performed if a frozen section of the mass reveals malignancy but it appears to be confined to the ovaries or pelvis. If widespread metastatic disease is present, diagnosis should be confirmed histologically, followed by cytoreductive surgery.

Principles of Treatment

Surgery

Surgery plays a significant role in the treatment of patients with ovarian cancer in stages I to III. As stated earlier, surgical staging of ovarian cancer is imperative because it confirms histologic diagnosis and measures the extent of disease, which guides further therapy and provides important prognostic information.[394] The subsequent surgery should be tailored to the individual patient and is commonly followed by adjuvant chemotherapy or irradiation.

Complete surgical resection is adequate treatment for patients with early-stage (stages I and II) borderline (low malignant potential) tumors of the ovary.[395] Conservative surgery with unilateral cystectomy or adnexectomy is advocated for patients who wish to retain childbearing capability[396]; partial oophorectomy may also be employed.[397] If childbearing is no longer an issue, a total abdominal hysterectomy and bilateral salpingo-oophorectomy are recommended. To date, no data show that adjuvant therapy improves survival in early-stage tumors, although long-term follow-up is recommended.[398] The prognosis for patients with more advanced-stage borderline tumors is relatively poor, leading some authors to support postoperative therapy for these patients; however, this recommendation remains controversial.[399, 400]

After complete surgical staging for ovarian cancer, about 10% to 15% of patients are diagnosed with early-stage disease. The standard surgical procedure for all patients with epithelial ovarian cancer is total abdominal hysterectomy and bilateral salpingo-oophorectomy with complete surgical staging. However, if there is no evidence of tumor spread beyond the ovary at the time of staging laparotomy and a grade 1 lesion is noted on frozen section, the uterus and contralateral ovary may be left *in situ* to preserve childbearing capability.[401] This treatment does not preclude the surgeon from performing a complete staging procedure; further therapy in patients with stage IA grade 1 disease is of no proven benefit.[402] After the patient completes childbearing, a second surgical procedure to remove the uterus and other ovary is recommended. Many studies have examined patients with more advanced stage I disease and those with moderate or poorly differentiated tumors[403–405]; further therapy with cytotoxic drugs or radiation therapy is recommended for these patients.

The majority of patients diagnosed with ovarian cancer have advanced disease and undergo cytoreductive surgery with postoperative therapy. Primary cytoreductive surgery is defined as the removal of as much of the tumor burden as possible. The potential benefits include a more enhanced response to chemotherapy and irradiation, an increase in patient immunocompetence, and symptomatic relief to the patient by reduction in tumor burden. In experienced hands, about 80% of patients with advanced ovarian cancer can undergo optimal debulking of the disease.[406]

Standard surgery includes total abdominal hysterectomy, bilateral salpingo-oophorectomy, omentectomy, and tumor debulking. The last may consist of surgery to resect tumor involving the gastrointestinal tract, the urinary tract, the retroperitoneal lymphatics, the subdiaphragmatic space, or the spleen. Optimal tumor debulking refers to tumor resection in which no residual disease greater than 1 cm exists; several studies have shown an inverse relationship between the amount of residual disease and survival.[407, 408]

Second-Look Laparotomy

Second-look laparotomy is a controversial procedure performed on a patient who has no clinical evidence of disease after adjuvant treatment with chemotherapy; it has been used frequently in the management of patients with advanced ovarian cancer. The procedure consists of exploratory surgery with pelvic washings, multiple biopsies, and resection of any residual tumor. Biopsies are taken from any suspicious areas, areas where disease was present initially, and any adhesions. Some studies have shown that microscopic disease may be found in one third of patients with no gross evidence of disease.[409]

Second-look laparotomy is the most sensitive and specific method to detect residual or recurrent disease. It provides information regarding response to various chemotherapeutic agents and comparisons of the number of chemotherapeutic cycles needed to achieve a complete response. It also enables the surgeon to resect any residual tumor that may be present. However, because of the incumbent surgical morbidity rate, this procedure was reviewed by the GOG, which recommended its use in specific patient populations (e.g., those with incompletely resected tumor).[410]

Secondary Cytoreductive Surgery

Controversy surrounds secondary cytoreduction as a planned therapeutic modality. This procedure is usually reserved for patients with recurrent or persistent disease after primary therapy, and the goal of secondary cytoreduction is to remove as much gross disease as possible. Despite the controversy, a survival advantage has been shown for patients who have undergone complete secondary resection of their disease.[411, 412]

Radiation Therapy

The use of radiation therapy as an adjuvant treatment modality for epithelial ovarian cancer has declined over the past two decades, although it still serves as part of some combined-modality approaches, as a salvage therapy for patients with persistent disease, and in palliation.[413–415] Because ovarian cancer spreads throughout the abdominal cavity, radiation therapy must encompass the entire peritoneal cavity to be effective. This goal can be accomplished by a variety of techniques.

- Whole-abdominal irradiation can be administered by an open-field technique or by a moving strip technique. Studies have compared adjuvant whole-abdominal irradiation with different chemotherapeutic agents, with and without pelvic irradiation, and both have been found to be effective in the treatment of ovarian cancer.[416] However, intestinal complication rates as high as 30% have been reported with whole-abdominal irradiation.[417] No randomized trial has been performed that compares whole-abdominal irradiation and platinum-based combination chemotherapy, the standard adjuvant chemotherapy regimen currently used in the United States, although a small phase II trial showed no survival benefit and increased delayed toxicity.[418]
- Radiocolloids have been given intraperitoneally to treat early-stage ovarian cancer. ^{32}P, ^{198}Au, and ^{212}Pb have been used, and ^{32}P, which emits β-rays, appears to be the safest. In a large, randomized trial, adjuvant cisplatin demonstrated a significant improvement in relapse rate compared with ^{32}P, although the relative effects on survival were less obvious.[419] In addition, in one limited randomized trial, high complication rates were reported with the use of ^{32}P.[420]

Chemotherapy

With the exception of patients with borderline tumors of the ovary and those with stage IA grade 1 disease, chemotherapy is used in almost all patients with epithelial ovarian cancer. Since the 1950s, ovarian tumors have been known to be chemosensitive. During the 1970s, the use of cisplatin in combination chemotherapy was found to be efficacious in combating ovarian cancer. More recently, paclitaxel in combination with a platinum compound has been adopted as the standard adjuvant chemotherapeutic regimen for treating metastatic epithelial ovarian cancer.

Infusion of chemotherapeutic agents into the peritoneal cavity via an intraperitoneal catheter has been used in the treatment of ovarian cancer in an attempt to deliver cytotoxic drugs in a large volume directly to the tumor. Agents used for the intraperitoneal method have included cisplatin, 5-FU, etoposide, and mitoxantrone; cisplatin appears to be the most effective agent used in intraperitoneal administration of chemotherapy. A number of studies have demonstrated a survival advantage using this treatment.[421–423]

Immunotherapy has been studied for the treatment of ovarian cancer, but this modality has not been demonstrated to be effective as a primary treatment. Bacillus Calmette-Guérin and *Corynebacterium parvum*, both with and without chemotherapeutic agents, have shown no survival advantages.[424] Radioimmunotherapy also is under investigation, with some limited success.[425, 426] In addition, the use of cytokines, such as interferon-alfa, interferon-γ, interleukin-2, and tissue necrosis factor, has been evaluated; the response rates ranged from 25% to 50%.[427, 428] The current use of immunotherapy is limited to research studies and should be considered experimental.

Special Considerations of Treatment

Nonepithelial Ovarian Cancers

Tumors of germ cell origin are uncommon but aggressive tumors that present a therapeutic challenge because they tend to affect women in their reproductive years. Treatments differ based on histologic subtype, stage of disease, and the reproductive wishes of the patient.

Dysgerminomas should be treated with surgical resection and a staging procedure; the staging procedure is the same as that performed for epithelial ovarian cancer. If the patient wishes to preserve fertility, a unilateral oophorectomy along with surgical staging is performed. The conservative surgical approach may be used[429] even in the presence of metastatic disease because of tumor sensitivity to adjuvant chemotherapy. If childbearing is completed, it is appropriate to perform a total abdominal hysterectomy, bilateral salpingo-oophorectomy, and staging procedure. Dissemination via the lymphatics is not uncommon; therefore, evaluation of the lymph nodes should not be excluded from the staging procedure. Patients with stage IA disease may be followed with close surveillance because adjuvant therapy has no proven benefit.

Dysgerminomas are highly radiosensitive, but because adjuvant chemotherapy is effective and preservation of fertility is a concern in the reproductive age group, radiation therapy is not considered a first-line treatment option unless chemotherapy is not used. The treatment of choice for advanced-stage (stage II–IV) dysgerminomas is combination chemotherapy. Bleomycin, etoposide, and cisplatin (BEP) and cisplatin, vinblastine, and bleomycin (PVB) are two chemotherapy regimens that have been successful, and cure rates of up to 90% have been reported for advanced-stage disease.[430, 431]

Treatment of all patients with endodermal sinus tumors includes chemotherapy. Initial treatment consists of exploratory surgery with unilateral oophorectomy. After the diagnosis is established, all gross disease should be resected, but total abdominal hysterectomy and bilateral salpingo-oophorectomy with surgical staging are not necessary. After surgery, a combination chemotherapeutic regimen containing cisplatin such as BEP or PVB should be administered. Ninety percent survival rates have been reported in stage I disease and up to 80% survival rates in advanced disease.[432] Embryonal carcinomas are treated in the same manner as endodermal sinus tumors.[430, 431]

Immature teratomas are treated similarly to dysgerminomas. Stage IA grade 1 disease is treated by surgical therapy followed by close surveillance. More advanced disease is treated by surgical resection followed by adjuvant chemotherapy. The BEP regimen has an 86% relapse-free survival rate.[433] Radiation therapy is not a component of first-line therapy, but it can be used in patients with persistent disease after chemotherapy.

Treatment of granulosa cell tumors of the ovary depends on the stage of disease and age of the patient. A staging laparotomy with unilateral adnexectomy should be performed in patients with no gross evidence of metastatic disease who wish to preserve fertility. Other patients should undergo total abdominal hysterectomy, bilateral salpingo-oophorectomy, and staging. An evaluation of the endometrium should be undertaken when conservative therapy is performed because of the concomitant risk of endometrial cancer. Metastatic and recurrent disease can be treated by adjuvant chemotherapy with VAC (vincristine, actinomycin D, cyclophosphamide) or by radiation therapy, but because advanced-stage disease is uncommon, data are limited. The prognosis for granulosa cell tumors is good, although late recurrence is not uncommon.

Sertoli-Leydig cell tumors of the ovary are managed much the same as granulosa cell tumors of the ovary. Tumor resection with surgical staging is performed, with the use of adjuvant chemotherapy or irradiation reserved for patients with metastatic or persistent disease.

Results and Prognosis

Surgery

The GOG performed a retrospective analysis on a randomized trial to study the effects of cytoreductive surgery on the outcome of trials.[434] They showed that, of those patients with suboptimal debulking (i.e., residual tumor of >1 cm), the patients whose residual tumors were smaller than 2 cm had a significant improvement in survival over those with more than 2 cm of residual disease. Since that time, other groups have gone on to look at how radical the debulking should be, and at least two groups have demonstrated that complete cytoreduction is possible in advanced-disease patients.[435, 436]

Radiation Therapy

A 1998 randomized trial compared high- and low-dose whole-abdomen radiation therapy in stage I to III ovarian cancer patients.[437] Results at 5 years showed that both overall and disease-free survival were slightly higher in the low-dose groups (83% vs. 72% and 74% vs. 67%, respectively). However, in general, the use of radiation therapy has been reduced during the 1990s because a number of randomized trials demonstrated that it provided no benefit as either an adjuvant or consolidation treatment modality.[438–440]

Chemotherapy

In the 1950s, single-agent chemotherapy for ovarian cancer was first popularized. Alkylating agents, such as chlorambucil, melphalan, and cyclophosphamide, were primarily used, and response rates were 35% to 65%. However, studies were retrospective, and patient populations were not well defined.[441] When used alone, these agents had minimal side effects; however, with long-term therapy of more than 2 years, the total doses of the alkylating agents were found to cause an increased risk of acute nonlymphocytic leukemia.[442]

In the late 1970s, the heavy metal cisplatin was found to be the most active single agent against ovarian cancer.[443] It was tested in a series of studies as a component of combination chemotherapy for ovarian cancer. Following these trials, a number of meta-analyses have suggested that platinum-based therapies are better than nonplatinum and that platinum-based combinations are more effective than the single agent.[444, 445] Multiple combinations have been examined for the best components; for example, investigators have looked at the roles of cyclophosphamide,[446, 447] bleomycin,[448, 449] epirubicin,[447] doxorubicin,[446] etoposide,[449] and vinblastine.[448] Meta-analyses of the doxorubicin studies in particular demonstrated benefit as a result of a three-drug platinum-based combination.[450, 451] Although cisplatin has proved to be the most active agent, its optimal use is yet to be decided.[452–454]

Cisplatin has a spectrum of toxicity that includes ototoxicity, peripheral neuropathy, renal toxicity, myelosuppression, hypomagnesemia, nausea, and vomiting. Carboplatin, an alternative to cisplatin, is a second-generation platinum analogue that has a more favorable toxicity profile. Studies comparing carboplatin plus cyclophosphamide to cisplatin plus cyclophosphamide show survival to be equivalent in both groups, although patients treated with carboplatin plus cyclophosphamide experienced less toxicity.[455, 456] The possible factors that may affect selection of carboplatin over cisplatin include tumor type, treatment intention, and the other drugs being used.[457]

The combination of paclitaxel plus a platinum compound is considered by most to be the first-line adjuvant chemotherapeutic regimen in patients with advanced ovarian cancer.[458, 459] This finding resulted from a phase III prospective, randomized trial comparing paclitaxel plus cisplatin with the previous standard combination therapy of cyclophosphamide plus cisplatin. The paclitaxel-cisplatin group showed a survival advantage of 38 months to 24 months over the cyclophosphamide-cisplatin group.[460] Several phase II studies that examined the use of paclitaxel in previously treated ovarian cancer patients revealed a 30% to 40% response rate.[461, 462]

Prognostic Factors

Histology

One of the main factors of prognostic significance is the grade of tumor differentiation, especially in early-stage disease.[394, 463] Patients with clear cell carcinoma also have a significantly worse prognosis than those with other histologic types.[390, 464]

Residual Disease

The amount of residual tumor present after cytoreductive surgery is important in the prognosis of disease. Patients with minimal residual disease have a better prognosis and a better response to chemotherapy than patients with suboptimally debulked disease.[393, 465] Patients with optimally debulked stage IV disease have a survival advantage.[466]

Age

Patient age also has been found by some authors to be a prognostic factor.[391]

Vaginal Carcinoma

Epidemiology and Etiology

Vaginal cancer is a rare gynecologic malignancy, constituting only 1% of malignant neoplasms of the female genital tract.[12] Indeed, metastatic involvement of the vagina, particularly by cervical or vulvar carcinoma, occurs much more frequently than primary vaginal cancer. This fact has led to the FIGO staging system requiring that tumors involving both the vagina and cervix or the vagina and vulva be classified as primary cervical or vulvar carcinoma, respectively.

In the United States, it is estimated that only 2100 cases of vaginal cancer were diagnosed, and 600 patients died of the tumor in the year 2000.[12] Of the possible involved histologic types, primary squamous cell carcinoma of the vagina has a peak incidence in the 50- to 70-year-old age group, with a mean age of 60 to 65 years.[467] In contrast, clear cell vaginal carcinoma, which has been linked to maternal diethylstilbestrol (DES) exposure, occurs in young women, with a peak incidence at age 19 years.[468]

Etiology

- In the past 30 years, interest has focused on an increased incidence of clear cell adenocarcinoma of the vagina in young women, which, in 1971, was found to be related to the administration of DES to their mothers during pregnancy.[469, 470] The incidence of clear cell adenocarcinoma in women exposed prenatally to DES is estimated to be about 1 per 1000[468, 470]; it has been observed that the risk was greatest for those exposed during the first 18 weeks *in utero*.[471] As summarized by Hanselaar and associates[471] and Hicks and Piver,[472] the most recent findings of registries of these patients are as follows:

    1. Sixty percent of registered patients had been exposed to DES or similar synthetic estrogens *in utero*.
    2. Sixty percent of the registered lesions were vaginal, and 40% were cervical primary tumors.
    3. Age at diagnosis has two incidence peaks: one at

age 19 to 26 years, and a second later peak at about 70 years of age.

4. The risk of developing adenocarcinoma of the cervix or vagina in the exposed female population was approximately 1 case per 1000 women, which implies that these tumors are extremely rare among DES-exposed women, and that DES is not a complete carcinogen.

- About 90% of patients had early-stage adenocarcinoma (stage I or II) at the time of diagnosis.
- Although vaginal intraepithelial neoplasia (VaIN) is a precursor of invasive carcinoma, the risk of progression is low in patients treated appropriately.[473]
- The role of HPV in the genesis of vaginal cancer, as well as cancer of the cervix and vulva, is a focus of current research.[474, 475]

Detection and Diagnosis

Clinical Detection

Abnormal vaginal bleeding is the presenting symptom in 50% to 75% of patients with primary vaginal tumors, either as dysfunctional bleeding or postcoital spotting. Vaginal discharge is also common. Less frequent presenting complaints are dysuria and pelvic pain, which occur when the tumor has spread to adjacent organs. Symptoms referable to the gastrointestinal or genitourinary tract may reflect involvement by vaginal cancer.

Diagnostic Procedures

In addition to a complete history and physical examination, speculum examination and palpation of the vagina are essential components of the diagnostic work-up (Table 21–22). Most vaginal cancers are located in the upper one third of the vagina on the posterior wall. Because this site can be hidden by the speculum blade, careful inspection of all vaginal surfaces is mandatory during examination. In addition, the speculum must be rotated as it is withdrawn so that anterior or posterior wall lesions, which occur frequently, are not overlooked. Bimanual pelvic and rectal examinations are integral elements in the clinical evaluation of these patients.

- *Exfoliative cytology* studies may detect early squamous cell lesions of the vagina, but this is not true for clear cell adenocarcinomas, which often grow in submucosal locations. Routine cytologic Pap smear of the vagina should be continued even for patients who have previously undergone hysterectomy.[476, 477]
- *Schiller's test* (with Lugol's solution) and *colposcopy* are particularly useful for directed biopsies in abnormal sites in the vagina.
- A metastatic evaluation including cytoscopy and proctosigmoidoscopy should be performed on patients with pathologically confirmed invasive vaginal carcinoma.
- In addition to the chest x-ray, IVP, and barium enema, CT and MRI increasingly have been used to evaluate patients with tumors of the vagina. Lesions are better seen on T2-predominant images using transverse planes 5 mm thick.
- *Biopsy* is the cornerstone of diagnosis and usually can be performed in the office without anesthesia.

TABLE 21–22. **Diagnostic Work-Up for Carcinoma of the Vagina**

General

- History
- Physical, including careful bimanual pelvic examination
- Special studies
- Exfoliative cytology (clear cell adenocarcinomas may not be detected)
- Colposcopy and directed biopsies (including Schiller's test)
- Biopsies and examination under anesthesia to determine extent
- Cytoscopy
- Proctosigmoidoscopy (as indicated)
- Radiographic studies

Radiographic Studies

Standard

- Chest radiographs
- Intravenous pyelogram

Complementary

- Barium enema
- Lymphangiogram
- Computed tomography or magnetic resonance imaging scans of pelvis and abdomen

Laboratory Studies

- Complete blood count
- Blood chemistry
- Urinalysis

From Perez CA, Garipagaoglu M: Vagina. In: Perez CA, Brady LW (eds): Principles and Practice of Radiation Oncology, 3rd ed, pp 1891–1914. Philadelphia, Lippincott-Raven, 1998.

Classification and Staging

Histopathology

- Squamous cell carcinoma accounts for 85% of primary vaginal cancers (most nonkeratinizing), with adenocarcinoma, melanoma, and other histologic subtypes making up the remainder (Table 21–23).
- The majority of nonsquamous vaginal cancers are adenocarcinomas and comprise approximately 5% of primary vaginal tumors; endometrioid, mucinous, papil-

TABLE 21–23. **Histologic Classification of Malignant Tumors of the Vagina**

Metastatic (e.g., cervical, endometrial, ovarian)
Squamous cell carcinoma
Adenocarcinoma—clear cell
Endodermal sinus tumor
Malignant melanoma
Sarcoma botryoides
Lymphomas
Carcinoid
Rhabdomyosarcoma

From DuBeshter B, Lin J, Angel C, et al: Gynecologic tumors. In: Rubin P (ed): Clinical Oncology: A Multidisciplinary Approach for Physicians and Students, 7th ed, pp 363–418. Philadelphia, W.B. Saunders Co., 1993.

lary, and clear cell variants have been reported. Vaginal adenocarcinomas occur in younger patients than do squamous cell carcinomas, and they usually arise from the Bartholin or Skene submucosal glandular epithelium. Most of these tumors are polypoid or nodular.

- Adenoid cystic carcinoma of the vagina is extremely rare. Until 1996, only 45 cases of adenoid cystic carcinoma of Bartholin's gland had been reported in the world literature.[478]
- Neuroendocrine small cell carcinoma may occur in the vagina, either in pure form or associated with squamous or glandular elements. A high proportion show ultrastructural or immunohistochemical evidence of neuroendocrine differentiation. The tumor tends to be aggressive, with a propensity for early spread.[479]
- Sarcoma botryoides occurs primarily in children younger than 5 years old, and it is characterized grossly by a polypoid mass resembling a bunch of grapes and microscopically by crowded rhabdomyoblasts in a distinct subepithelial cambium layer.[2]
- Melanoma accounts for only 3% of vaginal malignancies; it is usually located in the distal third of the vagina. Microscopy demonstrates pleomorphic cells laden with melanin, although pigmentation may be absent in the amelanotic variety. Progression of preexisting melanosis to malignant melanoma of the vagina has been reported.[480, 481]
- Endodermal sinus tumor of the vagina is similar histologically to its ovarian counterpart, with typical Schiller-Duval bodies.
- Most primary malignant lymphomas involving the vagina are the diffuse large cell type, but nodular lymphomas also occur. Characteristically, the mucosa is intact; a submucosal mass is frequently seen. Marker studies are useful in equivocal cases of lymphoma-like lesions.

Staging

Tumors are staged using the FIGO or AJCC staging system (Table 21–24 and Fig. 21–10). Staging studies for evaluation of a patient with vaginal carcinoma include pelvic/rectal examination under anesthesia, cystoscopy, proctoscopy, chest x-ray, CT scan of the abdomen and pelvis, barium enema, vaginal biopsies, and endocervical, endometrial, and, if indicated, vulva biopsies. A thorough search should be performed to exclude metastatic involvement of the vagina from another site.

TABLE 21–24. **Staging of Cancer of the Vagina**

Stage*	Grouping	Descriptor
I	T1,N0,M0	T1: Tumor confined to vagina N0: No regional lymph node metastasis M0: No distant metastasis
II	T2,N0,M0	T2: Tumor invades paravaginal tissue, but not to pelvic wall
III	T1,N1,M0 T2,N1,M0 T3,N0,1,M0	T3: Tumor extends to pelvic wall N1: Regional lymph node metastasis
IVA	T4,Any N,M0	T4†: Tumor invades mucosa of bladder or rectum and/or extends beyond the true pelvis
IVB	Any T,Any N,M1	M1: Distant metastasis

*American Joint Committee on Cancer/International Union Against Cancer/International Federation of Gynecology and Obstetrics stages.

†If bladder is not involved, then tumor is Stage III.

Principles of Treatment

Surgery

Laser surgery may be appropriate treatment, particularly in patients with localized intraepithelial disease and in young patients in whom there is a desire to preserve ovarian function.[482] In general, if performed in patients with stage I tumors in the middle or upper third of the vagina, surgical treatment consists of a radical hysterovaginectomy and pelvic lymph node dissection. Anterior vaginal lesions may be difficult to excise with an adequate margin of healthy tissue without injury to the urethra or bladder, and, in posterior lesions, special attention should be given to the anterior rectal wall. For lesions in the lower third of the vagina that may encroach on the vulva, radical vulvovaginectomy and bilateral groin lymph node dissection may be carried out. Adjuvant radiation therapy should be considered in stage I patients.[483]

Surgery for stage I clear cell adenocarcinoma may have the advantage of ovarian preservation and better vaginal function after skin graft. However, surgery for vaginal clear cell adenocarcinoma requires removal of most of the vagina followed by reconstructive procedures because a radical hysterectomy and lymph node dissection are necessary to encompass the area from the parametria and paracolpium to the side walls of the pelvis. Para-aortic nodes should be sampled before the procedure to determine if there is lymphatic disease beyond the pelvis.

Vaginal melanomas are sometimes treated primarily with radical surgical resection (vaginectomy, hysterectomy, and pelvic lymphadenectomy) because these tumors are aggressive.[484] Radical surgery also has been used for the treatment of localized malignant lymphomas of the vagina. However, some authors[485, 486] believe that radical surgery should be avoided in relatively young women (49 years, mean age), and preference should be given to partial surgery combined with radiation therapy and multiagent chemotherapy.

Radiation Therapy

Several authors have discussed the complex management of patients with carcinoma of the vagina and the need for individualized radiation therapy techniques.[487–489] For locally extensive tumors, a combination of irradiation and surgery has been suggested to improve therapeutic results,[483] although more complications may be seen from combined therapy.

External Beam Therapy

Use of external beam irradiation for stage I disease should be reserved for bulkier lesions to supplement intracavitary

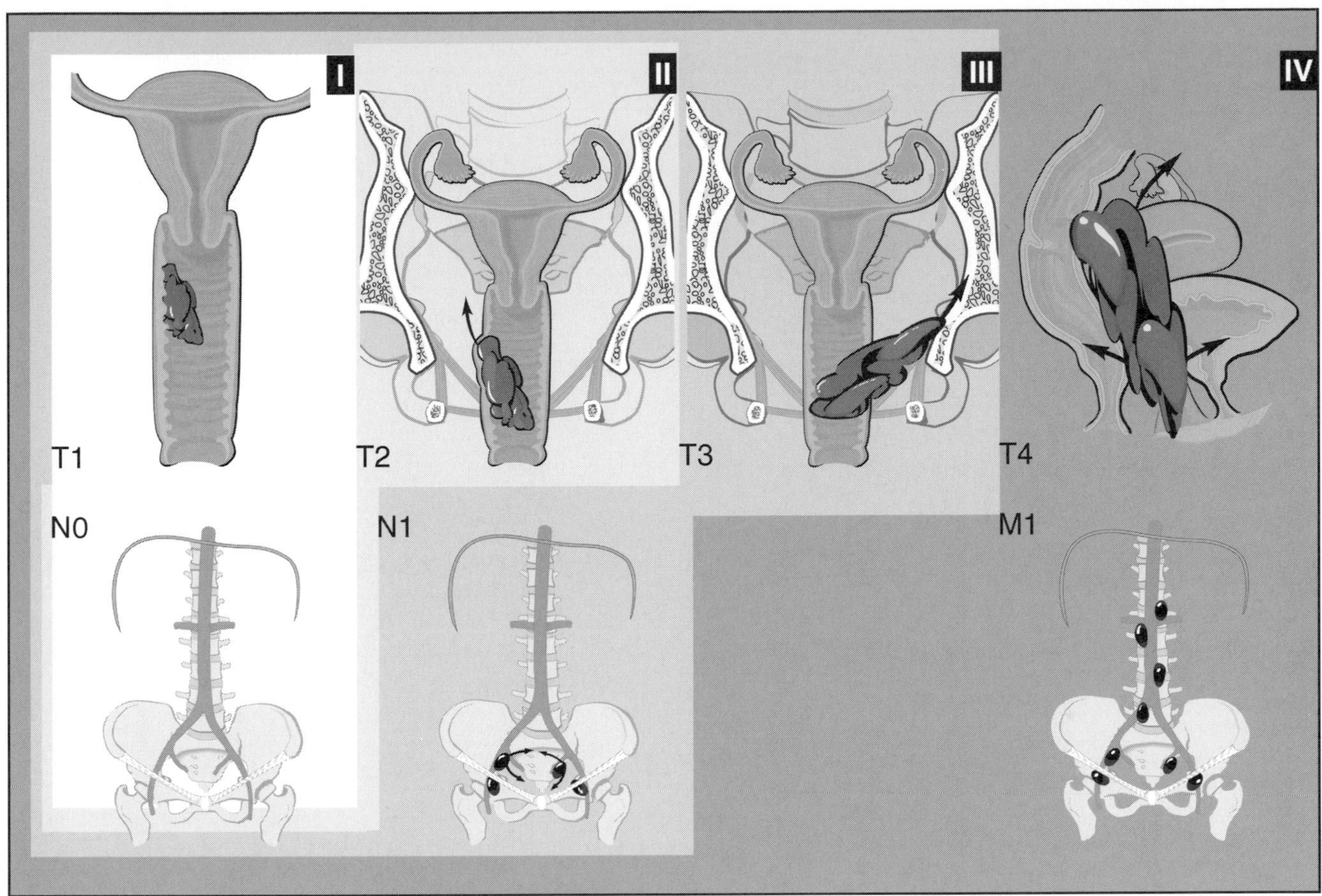

Figure 21–10. Anatomic staging for vaginal carcinoma.

and interstitial therapy. Because patients with stage II tumors have more advanced paravaginal disease, they should be treated with an external irradiation dose (20 Gy to the whole pelvis and an additional parametrial dose with a midline block [5 half-value layer] for a total of 45 to 50 Gy), in combination with interstitial and intracavitary irradiation for a total dose of 70 to 80 Gy.

For advanced tumors, 40 Gy whole pelvis and 55 to 60 Gy total parametrial dose (with midline shielding) have been given in combination with interstitial and intracavitary insertions to deliver a total tumor dose of 75 to 80 Gy to the vaginal tumor and 65 Gy to parametrial and paravaginal extensions.

Intracavitary Radiation Therapy

An intracavitary LDR application delivering 60 to 70 Gy to the involved vaginal mucosa is usually sufficient to control carcinoma *in situ* lesions, although some recent investigators have advocated the use of HDR.[490, 491] Because vaginal carcinoma tends to be multicentric, the entire vaginal mucosa should be treated to a dose of 50 to 60 Gy.

Superficial (0.5- to 1-cm thick) stage I tumors may be treated with an intracavitary cylinder covering the entire vagina (60 Gy LDR mucosal dose) and an additional 20 to 30 Gy mucosal dose to the tumor area. If the lesion is thicker and localized to one wall, then 60 to 70 Gy is delivered to the entire vaginal mucosa with an intracavitary cylinder and an additional 15 to 20 Gy to the gross tumor with an interstitial implant.

Interstitial Radiation Therapy

Paravaginal or parametrial interstitial implants or both should be considered if residual tumor is present after the planned external and intracavitary therapy is completed.[492] Additional doses of 20 to 30 Gy to a limited volume are usually well tolerated.[139] An interstitial implant boost of 20 to 25 Gy is sometimes given to patients with extensive parametrial infiltration.

Recurrent Disease

Postirradiation local failure of vaginal carcinoma can be effectively treated with surgery or with interstitial brachytherapy.[493] The surgical procedure may range from wide local excision or partial vaginectomy to posterior or total pelvic exenteration.

Chemotherapy

Minimal data exist on the use of chemotherapy in malignant vaginal neoplasias; generally, it is used only as salvage therapy. Drugs in which phase I/II evaluation in squamous

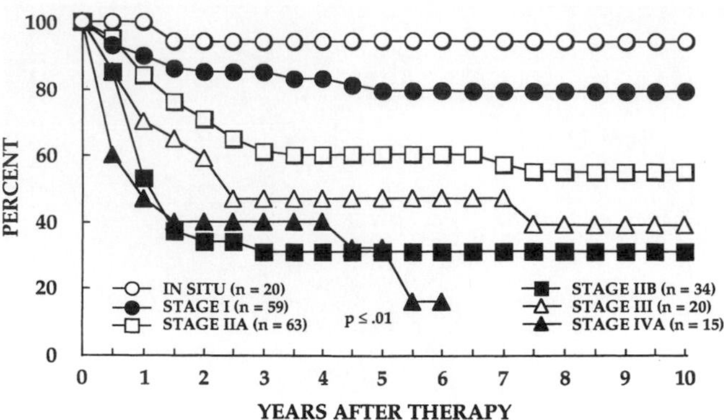

Figure 21–11. Disease-free survival for all patients with primary carcinoma of the vagina (stages 0 through IVA). (From Perez CA, Garipagaoglu M: Vagina. In: Perez CA, Brady LW [eds]: Principles and Practice of Radiation Oncology, 3rd ed, pp 1891–1914. Philadelphia, Lippincott-Raven, 1998, with permission.)

cancer of the vagina has been reported include cisplatin,[494–496] mitoxantrone,[497] and 5-FU.[498, 499] Rhabdomyosarcoma of the vagina is generally treated with a combination of surgical resection and systemic chemotherapy.[500, 501]

Results of Treatment

Surgery

As stated earlier, surgery is used principally in patients with early-stage vaginal cancer, and only in stage 0 or superficial stage I is it used as the sole modality of treatment. In one group of 23 patients who underwent upper vaginectomy for grade 3 vaginal intraepithelial neoplasia, there was a 83% 3-year disease-free survival rate.[502]

Radiation Therapy

With adequate and timely therapy, the survival rates of patients with carcinoma of the vagina are comparable to those reported for carcinoma of the cervix, ranging from 35% to 95% at 5 years, depending on stage of disease[503, 504] (Fig. 21–11). Perez and associates[489] noted that 19 of 20 patients (95%) with stage 0 carcinoma of the vagina treated by various techniques had tumor control in the pelvis 5 years after initial irradiation. In stage I, the pelvic tumor control rate was 86% (51 of 59 patients treated). In patients with more advanced tumors, pelvic control decreased significantly (40% to 50%, depending on tumor extent and technique used) (Table 21–25). Similar results were reported by Chyle and associates.[506]

Table 21–26 summarizes local tumor control data reported by several authors. Chyle and associates[506] updated the results in 301 patients with primary vaginal carcinoma (271 squamous cell and 30 adenocarcinoma) treated with radiation therapy. The 10-year local recurrence rate was 17% in 37 stage 0 patients, 15% in 59 stage I patients, 18% in 104 stage II patients, 35% in 55 stage III patients, and 60% in 16 patients with stage IVA disease. The 10-year local recurrence was 22% in 80 patients with a history of previous gynecologic malignancy and 22% in 191 without such a history. Ten-year survival rates were 78% in stage 0, 55% in stage I, 51% in stage II, 37% in stage III, and 40% in stage IVA disease. The 10-year survival rate was 59% in patients with a history of previous gynecologic malignancy, and 49% in those without such a history ($p = 0.15$).

Prognostic Factors

- The most significant factor influencing prognosis is the clinical stage of the tumor, which reflects size and depth of penetration into the vaginal wall or surrounding tissues.[245]
- In comparing patients with adenocarcinoma with those with squamous cell carcinoma, Chyle and associates[506] noted a significant difference in incidence rates of local recurrence (52% and 20%, respectively, at 10 years) and distant metastases (48% and 10%, respec-

TABLE 21–25. **Carcinoma of the Vagina: Anatomic Sites of Failure (MIR, 1953–1984)**

Stage	No.	Local/Parametrial Only	Local/Parametrial Plus Distant Metastases	Distant Metastases Only	Dead of Intercurrent Disease
0	20	1 (5%)	0	0	8 (40%)
I	59	5 (8%)	3 (5%)	5 (8%)	23 (39%)
		14%			
IIA	64	11 (17%)	11 (17%)	8 (13%)	17 (27%)
		34%			
IIB	34	5 (15%)	10 (29%)	8 (24%)	7 (21%)
		44%			
III	20	1 (5%)	6 (30%)	4 (20%)	5 (25%)
		35%			
IVA	15	4 (27%)	7 (47%)	0	3 (20%)
		73%			

MIR = Mallinckrodt Institute of Radiology.
From Perez CA, Garipagaoglu M: Vagina. In: Perez CA, Brady LW (eds): Principles and Practice of Radiation Oncology, 3rd ed, pp 1891–1914. Philadelphia, Lippincott-Raven, 1998.

TABLE 21–26. **Five-Year Local Tumor Control for Carcinoma of the Vagina Correlated with Stage**

Author	No. of Patients	Percent Local Tumor Control by Stage				
		I	*II*	*III*	*IVA*	*Total*
Peters et al[506]	81	—	—	—	—	35
Stock et al[507]	49	50	47	40	0	39
Leung and Sexton[508]	84	77	67	57	50	68
Chyle et al[505]	301	84	82	60	69	77
Perez et al[488]	211	86	62	65	26	70

Modified from Chyle V, Zagars GK, Wheeler JA, et al: Definitive radiotherapy for carcinoma of the vagina: outcome and prognostic factors. Int J Radiat Oncol Biol Phys 1996; 35:891–905.

tively), as well as a lower 10-year survival rate (20% vs. 50%). Patients with nonepithelial tumors (sarcoma, melanoma) have a poor prognosis, with a high incidence of local failure and distant metastasis.

- In addition, overexpression of *HER2-NEU* oncogenes in squamous cell cancer of the lower genital tract is a rare event that may be associated with aggressive biologic behavior.[510]

Vulvar Carcinoma

Perspective

The vulva is prone to a number of malignancies, which, because of their location, should be amenable to early diagnosis and treatment. Unfortunately, the extensive lymphatics in this region contribute to nodal metastases even with early lesions. Over the past two decades, significant advances have been made in the management of vulvar malignancy. The predominant approach to therapy of vulvar carcinomas has been surgical, but more individualized surgical treatment and the increasing use of radiation therapy and chemotherapy have reduced treatment morbidity in both early and advanced vulvar malignancies.[511, 512]

Epidemiology and Etiology

Epidemiology

Carcinoma of the vulva is infrequent, accounting for just over 1% of female genital malignancies and 0.6% of all cancers in the United States in women. Approximately two women per 100,000 per year in the United States are afflicted, with an estimated 3400 new cases having occurred in the year 2000.[12]

Over 70% of vulvar malignancies arise in the labia majora and minora, 10% to 15% in the clitoris, and 4% to 5% in the perineum and fourchette. The vestibule, Bartholin's gland, and the clitoral prepuce are unusual primary sites, each accounting for less than 1% of vulvar cancers. Carcinomas arising in the vulvar area ordinarily follow a predictable pattern of spread to the regional lymphatic nodes. Superficial inguinofemoral lymph nodes are involved first, followed by the deep inguinofemoral nodes. Metastasis to the contralateral inguinal or pelvic lymph nodes is very unusual (1%) in the absence of ipsilateral inguinofemoral node metastasis. Invasive carcinoma occurs more frequently in postmenopausal women, with a peak incidence in the sixth and seventh decades of life. However, the median patient age for carcinoma *in situ* is considerably younger, and the incidence appears to be rising in Western countries.[513, 514]

Etiology

The etiology of cancer of the vulva involves a history of genital neoplasia, smoking, compromised immunity, and genital infections, particularly HPV.[515] A 1996 review suggested that vulvar carcinoma has, in fact, two etiologies, only one of which is related to HPV.[516]

- Previously suspected associations with obesity and heart disease, which commonly afflict patients in this age group, have not been confirmed in recent case control studies.
- A strong association has been suggested between HPV and herpes simplex virus with vulvar neoplasia.[517–519] HPV type 16 appears to be the most common type, but a number of others also have been identified.[520, 521] There has been the suggestion by a number of authors that cofactors may be required in the development of HPV-related vulvar carcinoma: the most important of these may be smoking.[515, 517, 518]
- Mitchell and associates[522] noted that second genital squamous neoplasms occurred in 13% of women with invasive vulvar cancers. The risk of a second primary tumor was significantly increased in patients with HPV DNA, intraepithelioid growth pattern, or dysplasia.

Detection and Diagnosis

The most common complaint of patients with vulvar carcinoma is a mass in the vulva; pruritus, bleeding, and pain also may be noted, although up to 20% of patients are asymptomatic. A high index of suspicion and judicious use of biopsies contribute to an early diagnosis of these tumors. Metastatic disease in the groin lymph nodes or at distant sites also may be symptomatic.

Diagnostic Procedures

Clinical history and a complete physical examination, including a careful bimanual pelvic examination, is mandatory (Table 21–27). In addition to the vulvar and anal areas and perineum, the physical examination should include the vagina and cervix, which should be thoroughly inspected. Besides accurate determination of the extent and depth of the primary lesion (size, fixation), an essential part of the physical examination is assessment of the regional lymph nodes.

- A *Pap smear* of the cervix and vagina should be performed.[204]
- *Chest radiographs* should be routinely obtained. CT or MRI may aid in the outline of tumor extent and in evaluating the inguinal, pelvic, and para-aortic lymph nodes.
- Other studies include cystoscopy, proctosigmoidoscopy, barium enema, and IVP when indicated.
- *Biopsy* is easily performed under local anesthesia in the office[524]; a biopsy is warranted with virtually all ulcerated, discolored (red, white, pigmented), or exophytic lesions of the vulva.
- Careful inspection of the vulva with a colposcope or a magnifying glass after application of 3% acetic acid has, to a certain extent, replaced the use of toluidine blue in assessing preclinical vulvar lesions,[525] although toluidine blue is an inexpensive method of differentiating between vulvar intraepithelial neoplasia (VIN) and hyperplasia.[526]

TABLE 21–27. **Diagnostic Work-Up for Vulvar Tumors**

General

- History
- Physical examination, including careful bimanual pelvic examination

Special Studies

- Exfoliative cytology of cervix and vagina
- Colposcopy and directed biopsies (including Schiller's test)
- Biopsies and examination under anesthesia to determine tumor extent
- Cytoscopy
- Proctosigmoidoscopy (as indicated)

Radiographic Studies

Standard

- Chest radiographs
- Intravenous pyelogram

Complementary

- Barium enema
- Lymphangiogram
- Computed tomography or magnetic resonance imaging scans of pelvis and abdomen

Laboratory Studies

- Complete blood count
- Blood chemistry
- Urinalysis

From Perez CA, Grigsby PW, Chao KSC, et al: Vulva. In: Perez CA, Brady LW (eds): Principles and Practice of Radiation Oncology, 3rd ed, pp 1915–1942. Philadelphia, Lippincott-Raven, 1998.

Classification and Staging

Histopathology

- Preinvasive forms of vulvar malignancy include carcinoma *in situ* (Bowen's disease or erythroplasia of Queyrat and Paget's disease). Clinically these lesions may be flat, raised (maculopapular), or ulcerated, and they can be white (leukoplakia), red (erythroplastic), or hyperpigmented.
- Squamous cell carcinoma constitutes over 90% of invasive lesions of the vulva. These tumors are ulcerated and endophytic in one third of the cases; the remainder are exophytic. Histologically, most of these tumors are well differentiated with keratin formation. Tumors less than 2 cm in diameter and invading less than 5 mm of the basal membrane are often classified as microinvasive carcinoma, and should be separated from more invasive tumors because of their excellent prognosis. Two variants of squamous cell carcinoma infrequently described are adenosquamous and basaloid carcinoma; these tumors may invade locally, but they rarely metastasize.
- Adenocarcinoma may originate from the periurethral Skene's glands, but the majority arise either in Bartholin's gland or from bulboadnexal structures associated with Paget's disease. Occasionally Bartholin's gland carcinoma may be squamous cell when it originates near the orifice of the duct, papillary if it arises from the transitional epithelium of the duct, or adenocarcinoma when it arises from the gland itself.
- Melanoma represents 2% to 9% of vulvar malignancies. A number of varieties are described: mucosal lentiginous, nodular, and superficial spreading melanoma.[527]

Staging

FIGO adopted a modified surgical staging system for vulvar cancer in 1989.[528, 529] Staging errors led to acceptance of the current surgical evaluation of the inguinal lymph nodes. Tumor assessment is based on physical examination with endoscopy in cases of bulky disease. Nodal status is determined by surgical evaluation of the groins. The combined AJCC and FIGO staging systems are shown in Table 21–28 and Figure 21–12.

Principles of Treatment

An evolving philosophy has affected the treatment of women with vulvar cancer as a result of a greater emphasis on prognostic factors and organ preservation.[530]

TABLE 21–28. **Staging of Cancer of the Vulva**

Stage*	Grouping	Descriptor
I	T1	T1: Tumor confined to the vulva or vulva and perineum, ≤2 cm in greatest dimension
IA	T1a,N0,M0	T1a: Tumor confined to vulva or vulva and perineum, ≤2 cm in greatest dimension, with stromal invasion ≤1 mm†
IB	T1b,N0,M0	T1b: Tumor confined to vulva or vulva and perineum, ≤2 cm in greatest dimension, with stromal invasion >1 mm†
		N0: No regional lymph node metastasis
		M0: No distant metastasis
II	T2,N0,M0	T2: Tumor confined to vulva or vulva and perineum, >2 cm in greatest dimension
III	T1,N1,M0	T3: Tumor of any size with adjacent spread to the lower urethra and/or vagina or anus
	T2,N1,M0	N1: Unilateral regional lymph node metastasis
	T3,N0,M0	
	T3,N1,M0	
IVA	T1–3,N2,M0	T4: Tumor invades any of the following: upper urethral mucosa, bladder mucosa, rectal mucosa, or is fixed to the pubic bone
	T4,Any N,M0	N2: Bilateral regional lymph node metastasis
IVB	Any T,Any N,M1	M1: Distant metastasis

*American Joint Committee on Cancer/International Union Against Cancer/International Federation of Gynecology and Obstetrics stages.
†Depth of invasion is measured from the epithelial-stromal junction of the adjacent dermal papilla to the deepest point of invasion.
Used with the permission of the American Joint Committee on Cancer (AJCC®), Chicago, Illinois. The original source for this material is the AJCC® Cancer Staging Manual, 5th edition (1997), published by Lippincott-Raven Publishers, Philadelphia, Pennsylvania.

Surgery

The preinvasive forms of vulvar malignancies (carcinoma *in situ* and Paget's disease) and microinvasive tumors can be treated in a variety of ways, including topical chemotherapy, cryosurgery, laser beam therapy, or surgical resection. The preferred method of treatment is surgery, which varies from wide local excision to partial vulvectomy, depending on the extent and multiplicity of intraepithelial lesions and the patient's wish to preserve the vulva. Burke and associates have summarized this subject.[531]

Wide local excision is appropriate for most stage 0

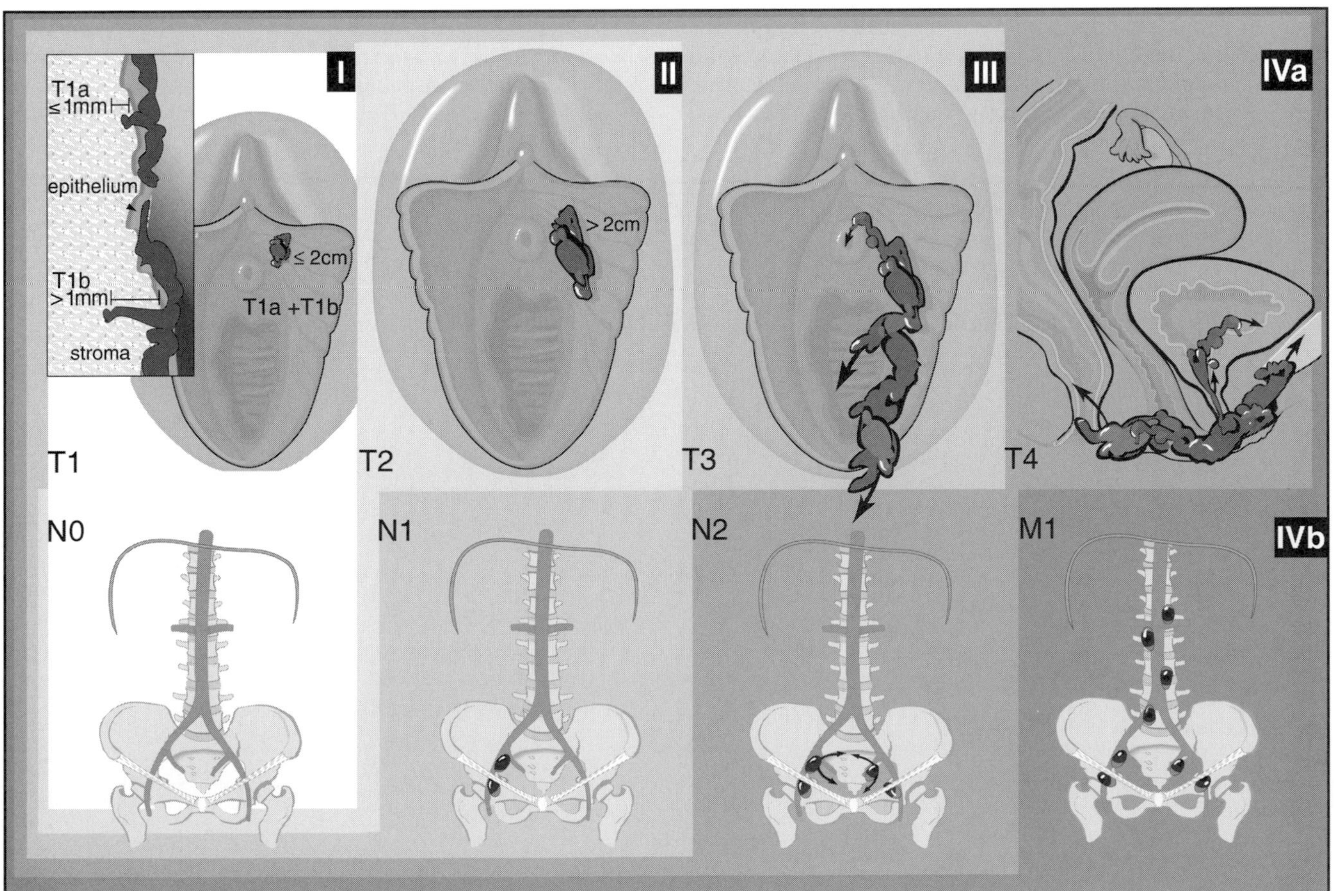

Figure 21-12. Anatomic staging for carcinoma of the vulva.

lesions. However, because VIN is multifocal in more than one half of patients, even wide local excision can involve most of the vulva. Therefore, skinning vulvectomy with skin grafting has been used for widespread multifocal lesions.[532] Of importance is the finding of occult early foci of invasion, usually less than 1 mm, in up to 20% of patients being treated for VIN.[533] The carbon dioxide excisional laser also has been used with success.[534]

The traditional management of patients with invasive stage I and II carcinoma of the vulva consisted of radical vulvectomy with inguinofemoral lymphadenectomy.[535, 536] However, because of the morbidity associated with radical vulvectomy and to enhance psychosexual rehabilitation, there is increasing use of wide local excision with ipsilateral groin dissection in patients with well-lateralized superficial tumors less than 3 mm thick. A modified radical vulvectomy, which leaves normal structures intact but removes the tumor with a wide margin, also has been used by several investigators with equally effective and less disfiguring results.[537–539] Individualized vulvectomy is associated with outcomes and survival similar to radical vulvectomy but with fewer postoperative complications.

Because of the importance of lymph node status as a prognostic factor, it is the extent of lymphadenectomy or the role of groin irradiation, or both, that has created the greatest controversy. Some investigators have advocated omitting lymph node dissection in patients with invasion less than 1 mm[540]; because metastases, although rare, have been reported in this situation,[541] we currently omit groin dissection only in patients with tumors less than 0.75 mm thick without multifocal invasion. In general, patients with positive nodes undergo additional nodal dissection of the deep nodes and the contralateral groin, are treated with postoperative irradiation, or both. The use of separate groin incisions has dramatically reduced the morbidity associated with *en bloc* radical vulvectomy and groin dissection. Treatment guidelines for lateralized or centrally operable tumors are summarized in Figure 21–13. In patients with pathologically negative inguinal nodes, no further dissection or postoperative therapy needs to be used.

Some stage III and IV tumors can be completely resected by radical vulvectomy or some variation of pelvic exenteration and vulvectomy. However, radical surgery is frequently ineffective in curing patients with bulky tumors or positive groin nodes, and most recent therapeutic efforts have focused on preoperative multimodality treatment that combines radiation therapy or chemoirradiation with less radical surgery.[531]

Radiation Therapy

The role of radiation therapy alone in the primary management of carcinoma of the vulva remains controversial, primarily because of a lack of long-term data on the results of treatment with modern techniques and because of the traditional belief that vulvar tissues could not tolerate high doses of irradiation (over 60 Gy). Nevertheless, vulvar cancers are radioresponsive, and function-sparing operations are feasible in some patients with advanced disease. Radical radiation therapy has been used successfully in some patients when surgery is not an option.[535, 542, 543]

Patients with clinically positive inguinal nodes may benefit from a course of preoperative irradiation (45 to 50 Gy), as suggested by Boronow and associates.[544] However, in general, following bilateral inguinofemoral lymphadenectomy and the discovery of positive nodes—particularly more than one positive node—postoperative irradiation to the groin and pelvis is performed.[545, 546] The role of postoperative irradiation in patients with negative nodes is still in dispute.[547, 548]

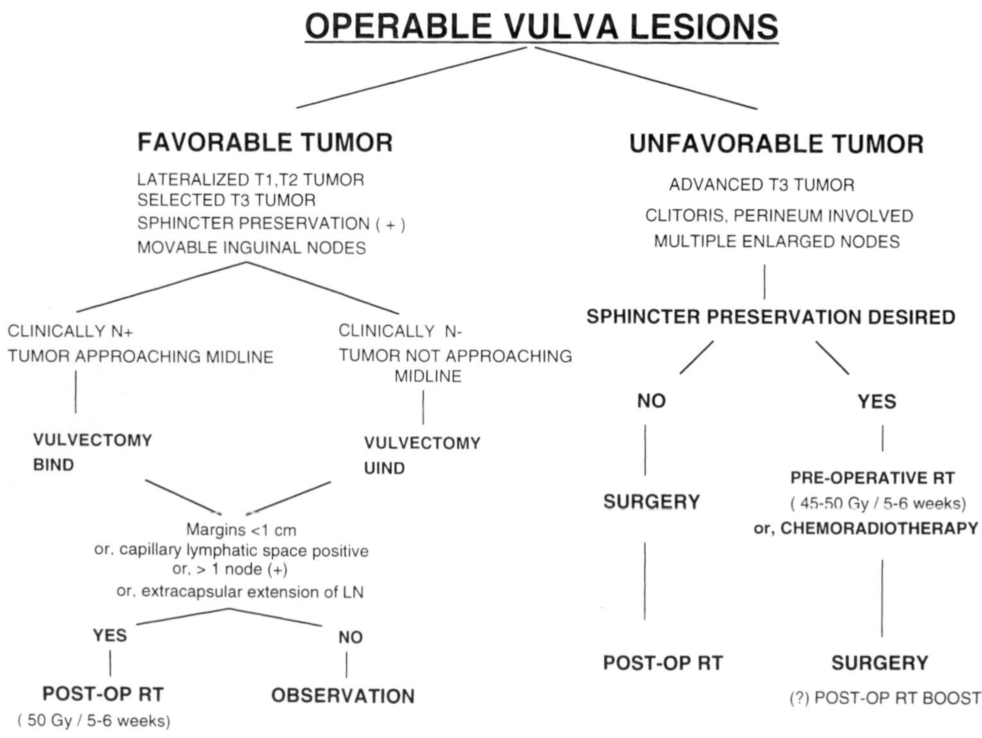

Figure 21–13. Algorithm illustrating the various therapeutic options for patients with favorable or unfavorable operable carcinoma of the vulva. BIND = bilateral inguinal node dissection; UIND = unilateral inguinal node dissection. (From Perez CA, Grigsby PW, Chao KSC, et al: Vulva. In: Perez CA, Brady LW [eds]: Principles and Practice of Radiation Oncology, 3rd ed, pp 1915–1942. Philadelphia, Lippincott-Raven, 1998, with permission.)

Radical surgery is frequently ineffective in curing patients with bulky tumors, and most recent therapeutic efforts have focused on the use of adjuvant irradiation or preoperative multimodality treatment that combines radiation therapy or chemoirradiation with less radical surgery. The use of adjuvant radiation therapy in one study demonstrated lower local recurrence rates.[549] The experience with preoperative chemoirradiation involves small numbers of patients, and results are preliminary. To date, results look promising,[550–552] although reports of high toxicity have been made.[550, 553]

Chemotherapy

Several drug regimens have been used in squamous cell vulvar cancer, most frequently incorporating bleomycin, vincristine, cisplatin, mitomycin C, or methotrexate in various three- or four-agent combinations with limited activity in phase II studies.[531] However, to date, the most promising success has been seen in chemoirradiation regimens.

Results and Prognosis

Surgery

For vulvar carcinoma *in situ* and early cancers, the results with limited resection as outlined here have been good. VIN is 100% curable. For invasive cancers, prognosis is best determined by lesion size and whether there is metastatic involvement of lymph nodes.

As stated previously, attempts have been made to combine surgery with radiation therapy to improve therapeutic results. Snijders-Keilholz and coworkers[554] performed a retrospective analysis of 44 patients with squamous carcinoma of the vulva; 39 were treated with curative intent with surgery alone or with surgery combined with irradiation. The 5-year cancer-specific survival rate was 65%. Although this analysis involved a group of elderly patients, it was concluded that curative therapy should be aggressive. All irradiated patients suffered from moist desquamation as an acute side effect, but serious late side effects did not occur.

Mariani and associates[555] described the results in 58 patients with vulvar carcinoma who underwent radical vulvectomy and unilateral inguinal lymphadenectomy; 16 patients with inguinal node metastases received ^{60}Co irradiation as an alternative to pelvic node dissection. The overall 5-year actuarial survival rate in patients without nodal involvement was 84%; in patients with positive inguinal nodes treated with the combined approach, it was 64%. Patients with one involved node had a 74% survival rate, and those with two or more metastatic nodes had a survival rate of 49%.

Radiation Therapy

Stehman and associates[556] published results of a GOG protocol that randomized 58 patients with squamous carcinoma of the vulva and nonsuspicious (N0 or N1) inguinal nodes to receive either groin dissection or groin irradiation, each in conjunction with radical vulvectomy. The study was closed prematurely because of an excessive number of groin relapses in the irradiation group, and the groin dissection regimen had a significantly better progression-free interval ($p = 0.03$) and survival ($p = 0.04$). However, this study was vehemently criticized, and was followed by a study that compared inguinofemoral irradiation to lymphadenectomy for N0 and N1 vulvar carcinoma.[557]

Forty-eight patients underwent radical vulvectomy followed by either lymphadenectomy (25 patients) or inguinofemoral irradiation (23 patients).[557] Actuarial nodal tumor control was 100% in the first group and 91% in the group that received inguinofemoral irradiation ($p = 0.14$). In addition, there was no difference in cause-specific survival at 3 years (96% and 90%, respectively) ($p = 0.47$). The morbidity of lymphadenectomy included lymphedema (16%), seroma (16%), infection (44%), and wound separation (68%). In the irradiated patients, 16% developed lymphedema, and only 9% had a significant skin reaction. Thus, irradiation of the N0 or N1 inguinofemoral nodes was confirmed as an alternative to lymphadenectomy for squamous cell carcinoma of the vulva if the proper irradiation technique and dose are used. The acute and late morbidities were less than those with lymphadenectomy.

Perez and coworkers[558] reported on 68 patients with primary and 18 with recurrent tumors. The rates for tumor control in each patient group are given in Table 21–29. The actuarial 5-year disease-free survival rates were 87% for patients with T1,N0 disease, 62% for those with T2–3,N0 disease, 30% for those with T1–3,N1 disease, and 11% for those with recurrent tumors (Fig. 21–14). There was no significant impact of type of vulvectomy on outcome. There were no long-term survivors with T4 or N2–3 disease. Four of 17 patients treated for postvulvectomy recurrent disease remain disease-free after local tumor excision and radiation therapy.

A few reports have described outcome after interstitial irradiation. Pohar and coworkers[559] reported on 34 patients treated with ^{192}Ir brachytherapy for vulvar cancer (21 at first presentation, when surgery was contraindicated or declined); 12 patients had FIGO stage III or IV disease, 8 had stage II, 1 had stage I, and 1 had stage 0. Thirteen patients were treated for recurrent disease. With a median follow-up of 31 months, 10 of 34 patients (29%) were alive. Actuarial 5-year local tumor control was 47%, and locoregional tumor control was 45%; 5-year disease-specific survival was 56% and overall survival was 29%.

TABLE 21–29. **Primary Tumor Control in Patients Treated with Definitive Surgery and/or Radiation Therapy**

Stage	Biopsy Only	Wide Excision	Partial/ Simple Vulvectomy	Radical Vulvectomy
T1–2,N0	4/4 (100%)	8/9 (89%)	0/1	4/4 (100%)
T3,N0	4/5 (80%)	—	5/6 (83%)	1/3 (33%)
T1–3,N1–3	4/5 (80%)	3/4 (75%)	3/3 (100%)	12/17 (71%)
T4,Any N	0/4	—	1/1 (100%)	—

From Perez CA, Grigsby PW, Chao KSC, et al: Irradiation in carcinoma of the vulva: factors affecting outcome. Int J Radiat Oncol Biol Phys 1998; 42:335–344.

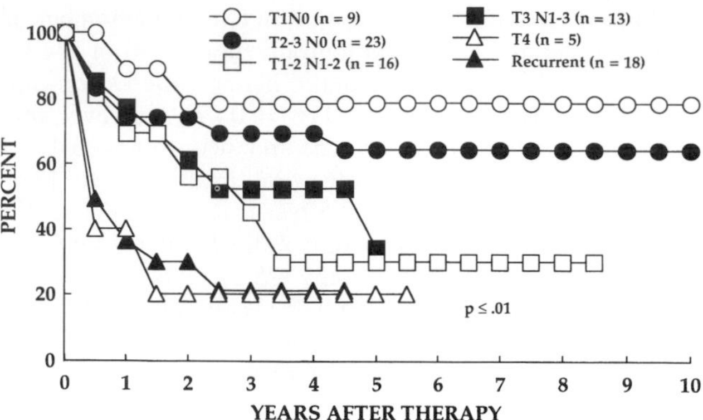

Figure 21–14. Disease-free survival correlated with stage for 66 patients with primary vulvar tumors and 18 with recurrent tumors treated at the Washington University Medical Center. (From Perez CA, Grigsby PW, Chao KS, et al: Irradiation in carcinoma of the vulva: factors affecting outcome. Int J Radiat Oncol Biol Phys 1998; 42:335–344, with permission.)

Subset analysis disclosed higher actuarial 5-year locoregional tumor control in patients treated at first presentation (80% vs. 16%) ($p = 0.01$).

Chemotherapy and Chemoirradiation

Thomas and associates[560] described the results in 33 patients with vulvar cancer treated with 5-FU, with or without mitomycin C. Nine patients with primary disease received chemotherapy and irradiation as definitive management; five of them had clinically suspicious inguinal lymph nodes. All nine patients received irradiation to the vulva, and four of five with positive nodes also were treated in the inguinal areas. Six of nine patients were disease free with follow-up of 5 to 43 months. Six of nine had an initial complete response of the vulvar tumor, although three later had relapses in the vulva. No patient developed nodal or distant metastases.

Russell and coworkers[561] observed 16 complete responses in 25 women with locally advanced or recurrent squamous cell carcinoma of the vulva. The patients received 5-FU continuous infusion for 96 hours (in 11 patients combined with three doses of cisplatin at 100 mg/m^2) and pelvic irradiation (median dose, 54 Gy). Twelve of 18 previously untreated patients were cancer-free at 2 to 52 months; 3 patients developed intermittent urinary incontinence, and four developed leg edema.

Forty-two patients with advanced squamous cell carcinoma of the vulva were treated with a combination regimen of bleomycin (180 mg) and external irradiation (30 to 45 Gy)[562]; 20 patients had primary and 22 had recurrent disease. Of 15 patients with primary disease, 5 showed complete and 10 had partial responses; 4 underwent surgery. Of these, 1 was alive after 60 months with no evidence of disease, 2 died of unrelated causes without signs of recurrence, and 17 relapsed and died of carcinoma of the vulva.

Wahlen and coworkers[563] described 19 patients with locally advanced vulvar cancer (4 stage II and 15 stage III); all but 2 had clinically negative inguinal lymph nodes. The patients received 45 to 50 Gy to the pelvis and inguinal nodes with concurrent chemotherapy (5-FU in a 96-hour continuous infusion, 1000 mg/m^2/day, during weeks 1 and 5 of radiation therapy). Ten patients received boosts with implants or electrons, and six others underwent local excision. With a median follow-up of 34 months, combined therapy resulted in a local tumor control rate of 75% (14 of 19); all five failures occurred within 6 months of treatment. Four of these patients were rendered disease free by radical vulvectomy or exenteration, or both, for an overall local control rate of 95% (18 of 19).

Prognostic Factors

The main prognostic factor for cancer of the vulva is, without doubt, the presence of lymph node metastasis.[245, 537, 564, 565] In addition, the size, depth of invasion, and histologic subtype of the primary tumor, as well as degree of lymphatic and vascular invasion, correlate closely with the incidence of regional lymph node involvement and prognosis.[566–568] In patients with vulvar carcinoma, Origoni and associates[569] showed that extracapsular extension was of prognostic value, even in patients with a single positive lymph node. This observation has been confirmed by others.[570]

Kurzl and Messerer,[571] in a multivariate analysis of 124 patients with various stages of vulvar carcinoma treated with simple vulvectomy and local or inguinal irradiation (40 Gy), found that age, dissociated growth, lymphatic spread, tumor thickness, and ulceration were relevant prognostic factors. In addition, local recurrence is related to the adequacy of the surgical resection margins. Heaps and coworkers,[572] in an analysis of formalin-fixed tissue specimens, demonstrated a sharp rise in the incidence of local recurrence for tumors with microscopic margins less than 8 mm (margin of 1 cm in fresh, unfixed tissue).

Sequelae of Therapy

- Common sequelae associated with radical surgery are those related to wound problems, primarily infection, and necrosis. Although the reported incidence of wound infection varies greatly, attempts have been made to improve wound healing following radical vulvectomy.[573, 574]
- Leg edema is a serious complication of nodal dissection or radiation treatment, or both.[575]
- With a tumor at the skin or mucosal surface, which requires that the peak dose be at the surface, it is to be expected that literally all patients have a significant acute cutaneous and mucosal reaction to radiation therapy. Of more concern, however, is the incidence of late (chronic) sequelae, some of which can be attributed to the fractionation scheme used.
- Occasionally necrosis and fracture of the femoral head/neck may be observed; Grigsby and coworkers[576] reported a 5% actuarial 5-year incidence of fractures in patients receiving doses of 50 Gy or higher.

Cosmetic results with conservation surgery and irradiation may be very rewarding if appropriate surgical and irradiation techniques are applied (Fig. 21–15).

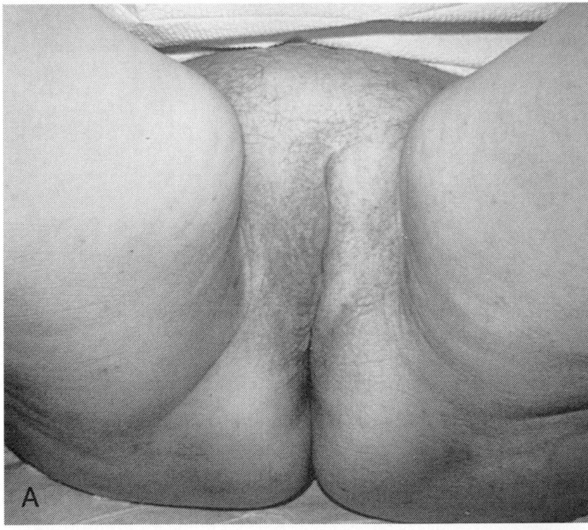

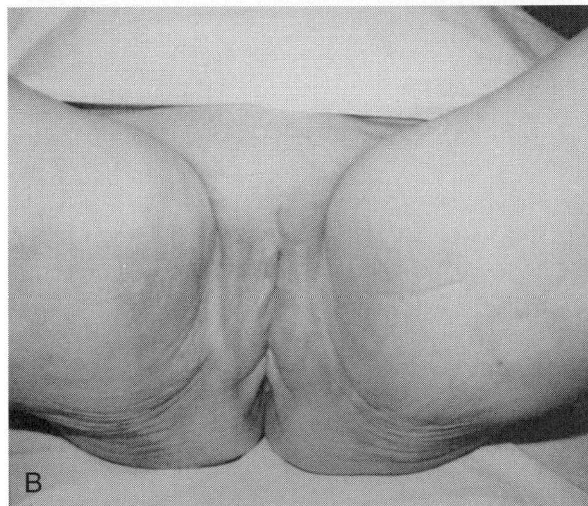

Figure 21-15. (A and B) Cosmetic results that can be achieved if appropriate surgical and irradiation techniques are applied. (From Perez CA, Grigsby PW, Chao KS, et al: Vulva. In: Perez CA, Brady LW [eds]: Principles and Practice of Radiation Oncology, 3rd ed, pp 1915–1942. Philadelphia, Lippincott-Raven, 1998, with permission.)

Recommended Reading

In addition to recently updated classic textbooks by DiSaia and Creasman[3] and Morrow and Curtin,[6] several multiauthored textbooks provide a comprehensive view of gynecologic oncology for the student. The texts by Knapp and Berkowitz,[1] Hoskins, Perez, and Young,[4] and Berek and Hacker[9] provide a timely and thorough review of the field. Several other textbooks deal with the pathologic,[2] radiotherapeutic,[7] and chemotherapeutic[8] aspects of this field and are highly recommended.

REFERENCES

General

1. Knapp RC, Berkowitz RS (eds): Gynecologic Oncology, 2nd ed. New York, McGraw-Hill, 1992.
2. Kurman RJ, Blaustein A (eds): Blaustein's Pathology of the Female Genital Tract, 4th ed. New York, Springer-Verlag, 1994.
3. DiSaia PJ, Creasman WT: Clinical Gynecologic Oncology, 5th ed. St Louis, Mosby, 1997.
4. Hoskins WJ, Perez CA, Young RC (eds): Principles and Practice of Gynecologic Oncology, 3rd ed. Philadelphia, Lippincott Williams & Wilkins, 2000.
5. American Joint Committee on Cancer: AJCC Cancer Staging Manual, 5th ed. Philadelphia, Lippincott-Raven, 1997.
6. Morrow CP, Curtin JP (eds): Synopsis of Gynecologic Oncology, 5th ed. New York, Churchill Livingstone, 1998.
7. Perez CA, Brady LW (eds): Principles and Practice of Radiation Oncology, 3rd ed. Philadelphia, Lippincott-Raven, 1998.
8. Deppe G, Baker VV (eds): Gynecologic Oncology: Principles and Practice of Chemotherapy. New York, Oxford University Press, 1999.
9. Berek JS, Hacker NF (eds): Practical Gynecologic Oncology, 3rd ed. Philadelphia, Lippincott Williams & Wilkins, 2000.

Specific

10. American Cancer Society: 2000 Facts and Figures. Atlanta, American Cancer Society, 2000.
11. DuBeshter B, Lin J, Angel C, et al: Gynecologic tumors. In: Rubin P (ed): Clinical Oncology: A Multidisciplinary Approach for Physicians and Students, 7th ed, pp 363–418. Philadelphia, W.B. Saunders Co., 1993.
12. Greenlee RT, Murray T, Bolden S, et al: Cancer statistics, 2000. CA Cancer J Clin 2000; 50:7–33.
13. Vilos GA: Dr. George Papanicolaou and the birth of the Pap test. Obstet Gynecol Surv 1999; 54:481–483.
14. Foulks MJ: The Papanicolaou smear: its impact on the promotion of women's health. J Obstet Gynecol Neonatal Nurs 1998; 27:367–373.
15. Martin LM, Calle EE, Wingo PA, et al: Comparison of mammography and Pap test use from the 1987 and 1992 National Health Interview Surveys: are we closing the gaps? Am J Prev Med 1996; 12:82–90.

Carcinoma of the Uterine Cervix

16. Lawson HW, Lee NC, Thames SF, et al: Cervical cancer screening among low-income women: results of a national screening program, 1991–1995. Obstet Gynecol 1998; 92:745–752.
17. Segnan N: Socioeconomic status and cancer screening. IARC Sci Publ 1997; 138:369–376.
18. Agarwal SS, Sehgal A, Sardana S, et al: Role of male behavior in cervical carcinogenesis among women with one lifetime sexual partner. Cancer 1993; 72:1666–1669.
19. Gawande V, Wahab SN, Zodpey SP, et al: Parity as a risk factor for cancer of the cervix. Indian J Med Sci 1998; 52:147–150.
20. Parazzini F, Chatenoud L, La Vecchia C, et al: Determinants of risk of invasive cervical cancer in young women. Br J Cancer 1998; 77:838–841.
21. Beutner KR, Reitano MV, Richwald GA, et al: External genital warts: report of the American Medical Association Consensus Conference. AMA Expert Panel on External Genital Warts. Clin Infect Dis 1998; 27:796–806.
22. La Vecchia C, Tavani A, Franceschi S, et al: Oral contraceptives and cancer. A review of the evidence. Drug Safety 1996; 14:260–272.
23. Beral V, Hermon C, Kay C, et al: Mortality associated with oral contraceptive use: 25 year follow up of cohort of 46,000 women from Royal College of General Practitioners' oral contraception study. BMJ 1999; 318:96–100.
24. Menczer J, Yaron-Schiffer O, Leventon-Kriss S, et al: Herpesvirus type 2 in adenocarcinoma of the uterine cervix: a possible association. Cancer 1981; 48:1497–1499.
25. Jones C: Cervical cancer: is herpes simplex virus type II a cofactor? Clin Microbiol Rev 1995; 8:549–556.
26. Balbi C, Di Grazia F, Piscitelli V, et al: Retrospective study of cervical papillomavirus lesions: early Herpes simplex virus proteins as markers of risk for progression. Minerva Ginecol 1996; 48:175–179.
27. Lazo PA: The molecular genetics of cervical carcinoma. Br J Cancer 1999; 80:2008–2018.
28. Stoler MH: Human papillomaviruses and cervical neoplasia: a model for carcinogenesis. Int J Gynecol Pathol 2000; 19:16–28.
29. Mougin C, Humbey O, Gay C, et al: Human papillomaviruses, cell cycle and cervical cancer. J Gynecol Obstet Biol Reprod 2000; 29:13–20.
30. Bosch FX, Manos MM, Muñoz N, et al: Prevalence of human papillomavirus in cervical cancer: a worldwide perspective. The

International Biological Study of Cervical Cancer (IBSCC) Study Group. J Natl Cancer Inst 1995; 87:796–802.
31. Boon ME, Susanti I, Tasche MJA, et al: Human papillomavirus (HPV)-associated male and female genital carcinomas in a Hindu population: the male as vector and victim. Cancer 1989; 64:559–565.
32. Graham S, Priore R, Graham M, et al: Genital cancer in wives of penile cancer patients. Cancer 1979; 44:1870–1874.
33. Iversen T, Tretli S, Johansen A, et al: Squamous cell carcinoma of the penis and of the cervix, vulva and vagina in spouses: is there a relationship? An epidemiological study from Norway, 1960–92. Br J Cancer 1997; 76:658–660.
34. Kristen GB, Holund B, Grinsted P: Efficacy of the cytobrush versus cotton swab in true collection of endocervical cells. Acta Cytol 1989; 33:849–851.
35. Labbe S, Petitjean A: False negatives and quality assurance in cervico-uterine cytology. Ann Pathol 1999; 19:457–462.
36. Renshaw AA, Bellerose B, DiNisco SA, et al: False negative rate of cervical cytologic smear screening as determined by rapid re-screening. Acta Cytol 1999; 43:344–350.
37. Spitzer M: Cervical screening adjuncts: recent advances. Am J Obstet Gynecol 1998; 179:544–556.
38. National Institutes of Health: Consensus Development Conference Statement on Cervical Cancer. Gynecol Oncol 1997; 66:351–361.
39. Jacobs MV, Snijders PJ, Voorhorst FJ, et al: Reliable high risk HPV DNA testing by polymerase chain reaction: an intermethod and intramethod comparison. J Clin Pathol 1999; 52:498–503.
40. Womack SD, Chirenje ZM, Gaffikin L, et al: HPV-based cervical cancer screening in a population at high risk for HIV infection. Int J Cancer 2000; 85:206–210.
41. Brewer CA, Wilczynski SP, Kurosaki T, et al: Colposcopic regression patterns in high-grade cervical intraepithelial neoplasia. Obstet Gynecol 1997; 90:617–621.
42. Perez CA: Uterine cervix. In: Perez CA, Brady LW (eds): Principles and Practice of Radiation Oncology, 3rd ed, pp 1733–1834. Philadelphia, Lippincott-Raven, 1998.
43. Bragg DG, Rubin P, Youker JE (eds): Oncologic Imaging. Philadelphia, W.B. Saunders Co., 1985.
44. Quinn MA: Adenocarcinoma of the cervix. Ann Acad Med 1998; 27:662–665.
45. Bergstrom R, Sparen P, Adami HO: Trends in cancer of the cervix uteri in Sweden following cytological screening. Br J Cancer 1999; 81:159–166.
46. Grigsby PW, Perez CA, Kuske RR, et al: Adenocarcinoma of the uterine cervix: lack of evidence for a poor prognosis. Radiother Oncol 1988; 12:289–296.
47. Eifel PJ, Burke TW, Morris M, et al: Adenocarcinoma as an independent risk factor for disease recurrence in patients with stage IB cervical carcinoma. Gynecol Oncol 1995; 59:38–44.
48. Herbst AL, Cole P, Colton T, et al: Age-incidence and risk of diethylstilbestrol-related clear cell adenocarcinomas of the vagina and cervix. Am J Obstet Gynecol 1977; 12:43–50.
49. Hatch EE, Palmer JR, Titus-Ernstoff L, et al: Cancer risk in women exposed to diethylstilbestrol in utero. JAMA 1998; 280:630–634.
50. Sykes AJ, Shanks JH, Davidson SE: Small cell carcinoma of the uterine cervix: a clinicopathological review. Int J Oncol 1999; 14:381–386.
51. Pecorelli S, Benedet JL, Creasman WT, et al: FIGO staging of gynecologic cancer. Int J Gynecol Obstet 1999; 64:5–10.
52. Holcomb K, Abulafia O, Matthews RP, et al: The impact of pretreatment staging laparotomy on survival in locally advanced cervical carcinoma. Eur J Gynaecol Oncol 1999; 20:90–93.
53. Goff BA, Muntz HG, Paley PJ, et al: Impact of surgical staging in women with locally advanced cervical cancer. Gynecol Oncol 1999; 74:436–442.
54. Physicians' Data Query: Cervical Cancer. Bethesda, National Cancer Institute, December 1999.
55. Favalli G, Lomini M, Schreiber C, et al: The use of carbon-dioxide laser surgery in the treatment of intraepithelial neoplasia of the uterine cervix. Przegl Lek 1999; 56:58–64.
56. Holcomb K, Matthews RP, Chapman JE, et al: The efficacy of cervical conization in the treatment of cervical intraepithelial neoplasia in HIV-positive women. Gynecol Obstet 1999; 74:428–431.
57. Grigsby PW, Perez CA: Radiotherapy alone for medically inoperable carcinoma of the cervix: Stage IA and carcinoma *in situ*. Int J Radiat Oncol Biol Phys 1991; 21:375–378.
58. Simon NL, Gore H, Shingleton HM, et al: Study of superficially invasive carcinoma of the cervix. Obstet Gynecol 1986; 68:19–24.
59. Jones WB, Mercer GO, Lewis JL Jr, et al: Early invasive carcinoma of the cervix. Gynecol Obstet 1993; 51:26–32.
60. Okamato Y, Ueki K, Ueki M: Pathological indications for conservative therapy in treating cervical cancer. Acta Obstet Gynecol Scand 1999; 78:818–823.
61. Grigsby PW, Perez CA, Chao KS, et al: Lack of effect of tumor size on the prognosis of carcinoma of the uterine cervix Stage IB and IIA treated with preoperative irradiation and surgery. Int J Radiat Oncol Biol Phys 1999; 45:645–651.
62. Lanciano R: Optimizing radiation parameters for cervical cancer. Semin Radiat Oncol 2000; 10:36–43.
63. Rotman M, Pajak TF, Choi K, et al: Prophylactic extended-field irradiation of para-aortic lymph nodes in stages IIB and bulky IB and IIA cervical carcinomas: ten-year treatment results of RTOG 79–20. JAMA 1995; 274:387–393.
64. ICRU Report No. 38: Dose and volume specification for reporting intracavitary therapy in gynecology. Bethesda, International Commission on Radiation Units and Measurements, 1985.
65. Wolfson AH: Conventional radiation therapy of cervical cancer. Semin Surg Oncol 1999; 16:242–246.
66. Wolfson AH, Abdel-Wahab M, Markoe AM, et al: A quantitative assessment of standard vs. customized midline shield construction for invasive cervical carcinoma. Int J Radiat Oncol Biol Phys 1997; 37:237–242.
67. Komaki R, Brickner TJ, Hanlon AL, et al: Long-term results of treatment of cervical carcinoma in the United States in 1973, 1978, and 1983: Patterns of Care Study. Int J Radiat Oncol Biol Phys 1995; 31:973–982.
68. Eifel PJ: Intracavitary brachytherapy in the treatment of gynecologic neoplasms. J Surg Oncol 1997; 66:141–147.
69. Fu KK, Phillips TL: High-dose-rate versus low-dose-rate intracavitary brachytherapy for carcinoma of the cervix. Int J Radiat Oncol Biol Phys 1990; 19:791–796.
70. Orton CG, Seyedsadr M, Somnay A: Comparison of high and low dose rate remote afterloading for cervix cancer and the importance of fractionation. Int J Radiat Oncol Biol Phys 1991; 21:1425–1434.
71. Nag S, Orton C, Young D, Erickson B: The American Brachytherapy Society survey of brachytherapy practice for carcinoma of the cervix in the United States. Gynecol Oncol 1999; 73:111–118.
72. Sarkaria JN, Petereit DG, Stitt JA, et al: A comparison of the efficacy and complication rates of low dose-rate versus high dose-rate brachytherapy in the treatment of uterine cervical carcinoma. Int J Radiat Oncol Biol Phys 1994; 30:75–82.
73. Orton CG: High and low dose-rate brachytherapy for cervical carcinoma. Acta Oncol 1998; 37:117–125.
74. Petereit DG, Sarkaria JN, Potter D, et al: High-dose-rate versus low-dose-rate brachytherapy in the treatment of cervical cancer: analysis of tumor recurrence—the University of Wisconsin experience. Int J Radiat Oncol Biol Phys 1999; 45:1267–1274.
75. Keys H, Gibbons SK: Optimal management of locally advanced cervical carcinoma. J Natl Cancer Inst Monogr 1996; 21:89–92.
76. Monk BJ, Tewari K, Burger RA, et al: A comparison of intracavitary versus interstitial irradiation in the treatment of cervical cancer. Gynecol Oncol 1997; 67:241–247.
77. Houvenaeghel G, Martino M, Bladou F, et al: Value of surgery in the treatment of advanced cervical cancers. Ann Chir 1998; 52:425–433.
78. Spanos WJ, Clery M, Perez CA, et al: Late effect of multiple daily fraction palliation schedule for advanced pelvic malignancies (RTOG 8502). Int J Radiat Oncol Biol Phys 1994; 29:961–967.
79. Rose PG, Blessing JA, Gerhenson DM, et al: Paclitaxel and cisplatin as first-line therapy in recurrent or advanced squamous cell carcinoma of the cervix: a Gynecologic Oncology Group study. J Clin Oncol 1999; 17:2676–2680.
80. Sugiyama T, Yakushiji M, Noda K, et al: Phase II study of irinotecan and cisplatin as first-line chemotherapy in advanced or recurrent cervical cancer. Oncology 2000; 58:31–37.
81. Burnett AF, Roman LD, Garcia AA, et al: A phase II study of gemcitabine and cisplatin in patients with advanced, persistent, or recurrent squamous cell carcinoma of the cervix. Gynecol Oncol 2000; 76:63–66.
82. Nguyen HN, Nordqvist SR: Chemotherapy of advanced and recurrent cervical carcinoma. Semin Surg Oncol 1999; 16:247–250.

83. Morris M, Eifel PJ, Lu J, et al: Pelvic radiation with concurrent chemotherapy compared with pelvic and para-aortic radiation for high-risk cervical cancer. N Engl J Med 1999; 340:1137–1143.
84. Keys HM, Bundy BN, Stehman FB, et al: Cisplatin, radiation, and adjuvant hysterectomy compared with radiation and adjuvant hysterectomy for bulky stage IB cervical carcinoma. N Engl J Med 1999; 340:1154–1161.
85. Thomas GM: Concurrent chemotherapy and radiation for locally advanced cervical cancer: the new standard of care. Semin Radiat Oncol 2000; 10:44–50.
86. Eddy GL, Manetta A, Alvarez RD, et al: Neoadjuvant chemotherapy with vincristine and cisplatin followed by radical hysterectomy and pelvic lymphadenectomy for FIGO stage IB bulky cervical cancer: a Gynecologic Oncology Group pilot study. Gynecol Oncol 1995; 57:412–416.
87. Leone B, Vallejo C, Perez J, et al: Ifosfamide and cisplatin as neoadjuvant chemotherapy for advanced cervical carcinoma. Am J Clin Oncol 1996; 19:132–135.
88. Serur E, Mathews RP, Gates J, et al: Neoadjuvant chemotherapy in stage IB2 squamous cell carcinoma of the cervix. Gynecol Oncol 1997; 65:348–356.
89. Benedetti-Panici P, Greggi S, Scambia G, et al: Long-term survival following neoadjuvant chemotherapy and radical surgery in locally advanced cervical cancer. Eur J Cancer 1998; 34:341–346.
90. Zanetta G, Lissoni A, Pellegrino A, et al: Neoadjuvant chemotherapy with cisplatin, ifosfamide and paclitaxel for locally advanced squamous-cell cervical cancer. Ann Oncol 1998; 9:977–980.
91. Sugiyama T, Nishida T, Kumagai S, et al: Combination therapy with irinotecan and cisplatin as neoadjuvant chemotherapy in locally advanced cervical cancer. Br J Cancer 1999; 81:95–98.
92. Souhami L, Gil RA, Allan SE, et al: A randomized trial of chemotherapy followed by pelvic radiation therapy in stage IIIB carcinoma of the cervix. J Clin Oncol 1991; 9:970–977.
93. Kumar L, Kaushal R, Nandy M, et al: Chemotherapy followed by radiotherapy versus radiotherapy alone in locally advanced cervical cancer: a randomized study. Gynecol Oncol 1994; 54:307–315.
94. Sundfør K, Tropé CG, Högberg T, et al: Radiotherapy and neoadjuvant chemotherapy for cervical carcinoma: a randomized multicenter study of sequential cisplatin and 5-fluorouracil and radiotherapy in advanced cervical carcinoma stage IIIB and IVA. Cancer 1996; 77:2371–2378.
95. Sardi JE, Giaroli A, Sananes C, et al: Long-term follow-up of the first randomized trial using neoadjuvant chemotherapy in stage Ib squamous cell carcinoma of the cervix: the final results. Gynecol Oncol 1997; 67:61–69.
96. Kumar L, Grover R, Pokharel YH, et al: Neoadjuvant chemotherapy in locally advanced cervical cancer: two randomized studies. Aust N Z J Med 1998; 28:387–390.
97. Eifel PJ, Berek JS, Thigpen JT: Cancer of the cervix, vagina, and vulva. In: DeVita VT Jr, Hellman S, Rosenberg SA (eds): Cancer: Principles and Practice of Oncology, 5th ed, pp 1433–1478. Philadelphia, Lippincott-Raven, 1997.
98. Giardina G, Richiardi G, Danese S, et al: Weekly cisplatin as neoadjuvant chemotherapy in locally advanced cervical cancer: a well-tolerated alternative. Eur J Gynaecol Oncol 1997; 18:173–176.
99. de Wit R, van der Zee J, van der Burg ME, et al: A phase I/II study of combined weekly systemic cisplatin and locoregional hyperthermia in patients with previously irradiated recurrent carcinoma of the uterine cervix. Br J Cancer 1999; 80:1387–1391.
100. Alberts DS, Kronmal R, Baker LH, et al: Phase II randomized trial of cisplatin chemotherapy regimens in the treatment of recurrent or metastatic squamous cell cancer of the cervix: a Southwest Oncology Group study. J Clin Oncol 1987; 5:1791–1795.
101. Kumar L, Pokharel YH, Kumar S, et al: Single agent versus combination chemotherapy in recurrent cervical cancer. J Obstet Gynaecol Res 1998; 24:401–409.
102. Rose PG, Bundy BN, Watkins EB, et al: Concurrent cisplatin-based radiotherapy and chemotherapy for locally advanced cervical cancer. N Engl J Med 1999; 340:1144–1153.
103. Piver MS, Barlow JJ, Vongtama V, et al: Hydroxyurea: A radiation potentiator in carcinoma of the uterine cervix. Am J Obstet Gynecol 1983; 147:803–808.
104. Stehman FB, Bundy BN, Thomas G, et al: Hydroxyurea versus misonidazole with radiation in cervical cancer: long-term follow-up of a Gynecologic Oncology Group trial. J Clin Oncol 1993; 11:1523–1528.
105. Kaern J, Trope C, Sundfor K, Kristensen GB: Cisplatin/5-fluorouracil treatment of recurrent cervical carcinoma: a phase II study with long-term follow-up. Gynecol Oncol 1996; 60:387–392.
106. Peters WA III, Liu PY, Barrett RJ II, et al: Concurrent chemotherapy and pelvic radiation therapy compared with pelvic radiation therapy alone as adjuvant therapy after radical surgery in high-risk early-stage cancer of the cervix. J Clin Oncol 2000; 18(8):1606–1613.
107. Whitney CW, Sause W, Bundy BN, et al: Randomized comparison of fluorouracil plus cisplatin versus hydroxyurea as an adjunct to radiation therapy in stage IIB-IVA carcinoma of the cervix with negative para-aortic lymph nodes: a Gynecologic Oncology Group and Southwest Oncology Group study. J Clin Oncol 1999; 17:1339–1348.
108. Wang CJ, Lai CH, Huang HJ, et al: Recurrent cervical carcinoma after primary radical surgery. Am J Obstet Gynecol 1999; 181:518–524.
109. Hart K, Han I, Deppe G, et al: Postoperative radiation for cervical cancer with pathologic risk factors. Int J Radiat Oncol Biol Phys 1997; 37:833–838.
110. Morris M, Gershenson DM, Eifel P, et al: Treatment of small cell carcinoma of the cervix with cisplatin, doxorubicin, and etoposide. Gynecol Oncol 1992; 47:62–65.
111. Chang TC, Hsueh S, Lai CH, et al: Phase II trial of neoadjuvant chemotherapy in early-stage small cell cervical cancer. Anticancer Drugs 1999; 10:641–646.
112. van Vliet W, van Loon AJ, ten Hoor KA, et al: Cervical carcinoma during pregnancy: outcome of planned delay in treatment. Eur J Obstet Gynecol Reprod Biol 1998; 79:153–157.
113. Steiner RA: Gynecologic neoplasms in pregnancy. Ther Umsch 1999; 56:616–623.
114. Sood AK, Sorosky JI: Invasive cervical cancer complicating pregnancy. How to manage the dilemma. Obstet Gynecol Clin North Am 1998; 25:343–352.
115. Cliby WA, Dodson MK, Podratz KC: Cervical cancer complicated by pregnancy: episiotomy site recurrences following vaginal delivery. Obstet Gynecol 1994; 84:179–182.
116. Hannoun-Levi JM, Peiffert D, Hoffstetter S, et al: Carcinoma of the cervical stump: retrospective analysis of 77 cases. Radiother Oncol 1997; 43:147–153.
117. Farley JH, Taylor RR: Cervical carcinosarcoma occurring after subtotal hysterectomy, a case report. Gynecol Oncol 1997; 67:322–324.
118. Kovalic JJ, Grigsby PW, Perez CA, et al: Cervical stump carcinoma. Int J Radiat Oncol Biol Phys 1991; 20:933–938.
119. Barillot I, Horiot JC, Cuisenier J, et al: Carcinoma of the cervical stump: a review of 213 cases. Eur J Cancer 1993; 29A:1231–1236.
120. Zola P, Volpe T, Castelli G, et al: Is the published literature a reliable guide for deciding between alternative treatments for patients with early cervical cancer? Int J Radiat Oncol Biol Phys 1989; 16:785–797.
121. Hopkins MP, Morley GW: Radical hysterectomy versus radiation therapy for stage IB squamous cell cancer of the cervix. Cancer 1991; 68:272–277.
122. Averette HE, Nguyen HN, Donato DM, et al: Radical hysterectomy for invasive cervical cancer. A 25-year prospective experience with the Miami technique. Cancer 1993; 71(suppl):1422–1437.
123. Massi G, Savino L, Susini T: Schauta-Amreich vaginal hysterectomy and Wertheim-Meigs abdominal hysterectomy in the treatment of cervical cancer: a retrospective analysis. Am J Obstet Gynecol 1994; 171:928–934.
124. Alvarez RD, Gelder MS, Gore H, et al: Radical hysterectomy in the treatment of patients with bulky early stage carcinoma of the cervix uteri. Surg Gynecol Obstet 1993; 176:539–542.
125. Bissett D, Lamont DW, Nwabineli NJ, et al: The treatment of stage I carcinoma of the cervix in the west of Scotland, 1980–1987. Br J Obstet Gynaecol 1994; 101:615–620.
126. Landoni F, Maneo A, Colombo A, et al: Randomised study of radical surgery versus radiotherapy for stage Ib-IIa cervical cancer. Lancet 1997; 350:535–540.
127. Magrina JF, Goodrich MA, Lidner TK, et al: Modified radical hysterectomy in the treatment of early squamous cervical cancer. Gynecol Oncol 1999; 72:183–186.
128. Coia L, Won M, Lanciano R, et al: The Patterns of Care Outcome Study for cancer of the uterine cervix: results of the Second National Practice Survey. Cancer 1990; 66:2451–2456.
129. Lowrey GC, Mendenhall WM, Million RR: Stage IB or IIA-B

carcinoma of the intact uterine cervix treated with irradiation: a multivariate analysis. Int J Radiat Oncol Biol Phys 1992; 24:205–210.
130. Lee YN, Wang KL, Lin MH, et al: Radical hysterectomy with pelvic lymph node dissection for treatment of cervical cancer: a clinical review of 954 cases. Gynecol Oncol 1989; 32:135–142.
131. Sekido N, Kawai K, Akaza H: Lower urinary tract dysfunction as persistent complication of radical hysterectomy. Int J Urol 1997; 4:259–264.
132. Magrina JF, Goodrich MA, Weaver AL, et al: Modified radical hysterectomy: Morbidity and mortality. Gynecol Oncol 1995; 59:277–282.
133. Barnes W, Waggoner S, Delgado G, et al: Manometric characterization of rectal dysfunction following radical hysterectomy. Gynecol Oncol 1991; 42:116–119.
134. Stehman FB, Perez CA, Kurman RJ, et al: Uterine cervix. In: Hoskins WJ, Perez CA, Young RC (eds): Principles and Practice of Gynecologic Oncology, 2nd ed, pp 785–858. Philadelphia, Lippincott-Raven, 1997.
135. Lanciano R: Radiotherapy for the treatment of locally recurrent cervical cancer. J Natl Cancer Inst Monogr 1996; 21:113–115.
136. Ijaz T, Eifel PJ, Burke T, et al: Radiation therapy of pelvic recurrence after radical hysterectomy for cervical carcinoma. Gynecol Oncol 1998; 70:241–246.
137. Maneo A, Landoni F, Cormio G, et al: Concurrent carboplatin/5-fluorouracil and radiotherapy for recurrent cervical carcinoma. Ann Oncol 1999; 10:803–807.
138. Jobsen JJ, Lee JWH, Cleton FJ, et al: Treatment of locoregional recurrence of carcinoma of the cervix by radiotherapy after primary surgery. Gynecol Oncol 1989; 33:368–371.
139. Gupta AK, Vicini FA, Frazier AJ, et al: Iridium-192 transperineal interstitial brachytherapy for locally advanced or recurred gynecological malignancies. Int J Radiat Oncol Biol Phys 1999; 43:1055–1060.
140. Piver MS, Ghamande SA, Eltabbakh GH, et al: First-line chemotherapy with paclitaxel and platinum for advanced and recurrent cancer of the cervix—a phase II study. Gynecol Oncol 1999; 75:334–337.
141. Lhomme C, Fumoleau P, Fargeot P, et al: Results of a European Organization for Research and Treatment of Cancer/Early Clinical Studies Group phase II trial of first-line irinotecan in patients with advanced or recurrent squamous cell carcinoma of the cervix. J Clin Oncol 1999; 17:3136–3142.
142. Perez CA, Grigsby PW, Chao KSC, et al: Tumor size, irradiation dose, and long-term outcome of carcinoma of uterine cervix. Int J Radiat Oncol Biol Phys 1998; 41:307–317.
143. Perez CA, Fox S, Lockett MA, et al: Impact of dose in outcome of irradiation alone in carcinoma of the uterine cervix: analysis of two different methods. Int J Radiat Oncol Biol Phys 1991; 21:885–898.
144. Perez CA, Breaux S, Bedwinek JM, et al: Radiation therapy alone in the treatment of carcinoma of the uterine cervix. II. Analysis of complications. Cancer 1984; 54:235–246.
145. Lanciano RM, Corn B, Martin E, et al: Perioperative morbidity of intracavitary gynecologic brachytherapy. Int J Radiat Oncol Biol Phys 1994; 29:969–974.
146. Teshima T, Inoue T, Ikeda H, et al: High-dose rate and low-dose rate intracavitary therapy for carcinoma of the uterine cervix: final results of Osaka University Hospital. Cancer 1993; 72:2409–2414.
147. Patel PD, Sharma SC, Negi PS, et al: Low dose rate vs. high dose rate brachytherapy in the treatment of carcinoma of the uterine cervix: a clinical trial. Int J Radiat Oncol Biol Phys 1994; 28:335–341.
148. el-Baradie M, Inoue T, Inoue T, et al: HDR and MDR intracavitary treatment for carcinoma of the uterine cervix. A prospective randomized study. Strahlenther Onkol 1997; 173:155–162.
149. Kinney WK, Alvarez RD, Reid GC, et al: Value of adjuvant whole-pelvis irradiation after Wertheim hysterectomy for early-stage squamous carcinoma of the cervix with pelvic nodal metastasis: A matched-control study. Gynecol Oncol 1989; 34:258–262.
150. Kinney WK, Hodge DO, Egorshin EV, et al: Surgical treatment of patients with stages IB and IIA carcinoma of the cervix and palpably positive pelvic lymph nodes. Gynecol Oncol 1995; 57:145–149.
151. Barter JF, Soong SJ, Shingleton HM, et al: Complications of combined radical hysterectomy-postoperative radiation therapy in women with early stage cervical cancer. Gynecol Oncol 1989; 32:292–296.
152. Fiorica JV, Roberts WS, Greenberg H, et al: Morbidity and survival patterns in patients after radical hysterectomy and postoperative adjuvant pelvic radiotherapy. Gynecol Oncol 1990; 36:343–347.
153. Mitsuhashi N, Takahashi M, Yamakawa M, et al: Results of postoperative radiation therapy for patients with carcinoma of the uterine cervix: evaluation of intravaginal cone boost with an electron beam. Gynecol Oncol 1995; 57:321–326.
154. Montz FJ, Holschneider CH, Solh S, et al: Small bowel obstruction following radical hysterectomy: risk factors, incidence, and operative findings. Gynecol Oncol 1994; 53:114–120.
155. Thomas GM: Is neoadjuvant chemotherapy a useful strategy for the treatment of stage IB cervix cancer? Gynecol Oncol 1993; 49:153–155.
156. Chauvergne J, Rohart J, Heron JF, et al: Randomized phase III trial of neoadjuvant chemotherapy (CT) and radiotherapy (RT) versus RT in stage IIB, III carcinoma of the cervix (CACX): a cooperative study of the French Oncology Centres [abstract]. Proc Am Soc Clin Oncol 1988; 7:524.
157. Cardenas J, Olguin A, Figueroa F, et al: Randomized neoadjuvant chemotherapy in cervical carcinoma stage IIB: PEC + RT versus RT [abstract]. Proc Am Soc Clin Oncol 1991; 10:620.
158. Tattersall MHN, Ramirez C, Coppleson M: A randomized trial comparing platinum-based chemotherapy followed by radiotherapy vs. radiotherapy alone in patients with locally advanced cervical cancer. Int J Gynecol Oncol 1992; 2:244–251.
159. Piver MS: Treatment of high-risk cervical cancer. N Engl J Med 1999; 341:696–697.
160. Tattersall MH, Loorvidhaya V, Vootiprux V, et al: Randomized trial of epirubicin and cisplatin chemotherapy followed by pelvic radiation in locally advanced cervical cancer: Cervical Cancer Study Group of the Asian Oceanian Clinical Oncology Association. J Clin Oncol 1995; 13:444–451.
161. Delgado G, Bundy B, Zaino R, et al: Prospective surgical-pathological study of disease-free interval in patients with stage IB squamous cell carcinoma of the cervix: A Gynecologic Oncology Group study. Gynecol Oncol 1990; 38:352–357.
162. Finan MA, DeCesare S, Fiorica JV, et al: Radical hysterectomy for stage IB1 vs IB2 carcinoma of the cervix: Does the new staging system predict morbidity and survival? Gynecol Oncol 1996; 62:139–147.
163. Eifel PJ, Morris M, Wharton JT, et al: The influence of tumor size and morphology on the outcome of patients with FIGO stage IB squamous cell carcinoma of the uterine cervix. Int J Radiat Oncol Biol Phys 1994; 29:9–16.
164. Grimard L, Genest P, Girard A, et al: Prognostic significance of endometrial extension in carcinoma of the cervix. Gynecol Oncol 1988; 31:301–309.
165. Perez CA, Grigsby PW, Camel HM, et al: Irradiation alone or combined with surgery in stage IB, IIA, and IIB carcinoma of the uterine cervix: update of a nonrandomized comparison. Int J Radiat Oncol Biol Phys 1995; 31:703–716.
166. Kilgore LC, Soong S-J, Gore H, et al: Analysis of prognostic features in adenocarcinoma of the cervix. Gynecol Oncol 1988; 31:137–148.
167. Brewster WR, DiSaia PJ, Monk BJ, et al: Young age as a prognostic factor in cervical cancer: results of a population-based study. Am J Obstet Gynecol 1999; 180:1464–1467.
168. Gerbaulet A, Lartigau E, Haie-Meder C, et al: Cervical cancer in young women. Contracept Fertil Sex 1994; 22:405–409.
169. Chen F, Trapido EJ, Davis K: Differences in stage at presentation of breast and gynecologic cancers among whites, blacks, and Hispanics. Cancer 1994; 73:2838–2842.
170. Weiss LK, Kau TY, Sparks BT, et al: Trends in cervical cancer incidence among young black and white women in metropolitan Detroit. Cancer 1994; 73:1849–1854.
171. Cooper RA, West CM, Wilks DP, et al: Tumour vascularity is a significant prognostic factor for cervix carcinoma treated with radiotherapy: independence from tumour radiosensitivity. Br J Cancer 1999; 81:354–358.
172. Dusenbery KE, McGuire WA, Holt PJ, et al: Erythropoietin increases hemoglobin during radiation therapy for cervical cancer. Int J Radiat Oncol Biol Phys 1994; 29:1079–1084.
173. Van Herik M: Fever as a complication of radiation therapy for carcinoma of the cervix. Am J Roentgenol Radium Ther Nucl Med 1965; 43:104–109.

174. Kapp DS, Lawrence R: Temperature elevation during brachytherapy for carcinoma of the uterine cervix: adverse effect on survival and enhancement of distant metastases. Int J Radiat Oncol Biol Phys 1984; 10:2281–2292.
175. Kersemaekers AM, Fleuren GJ, Kenter GG, et al: Oncogene alterations in carcinomas of the uterine cervix: overexpression of the epidermal growth factor receptor is associated with poor prognosis. Clin Cancer Res 1999; 5:577–586.
176. Fyles A, Keane TJ, Barton M, et al: The effect of treatment duration in the local control of cervix cancer. Radiother Oncol 1992; 25:273–279.
177. Girinsky T, Rey A, Roche B, et al: Overall treatment time in advanced cervical carcinomas: A critical parameter in treatment outcome. Int J Radiat Oncol Biol Phys 1993; 27:1051–1056.
178. Lanciano RM, Pajak TF, Martz K, et al: The influence of treatment time on outcome for squamous cell cancer of the uterine cervix treated with radiation: a Patterns of Care Study. Int J Radiat Oncol Biol Phys 1993; 25:391–397.
179. Perez CA, Grigsby PW, Castro-Vita H, et al: Carcinoma of the uterine cervix. I. Impact of prolongation of overall treatment time and timing of brachytherapy on outcome of radiation therapy. Int J Radiat Oncol Biol Phys 1995; 32:1275–1288.
180. Nelson JH, Boyce J, Macasaet M, et al: Incidence, significance and follow-up of para-aortic lymph node metastases in late invasive carcinoma of the cervix. Am J Obstet Gynecol 1977; 128:336–340.
181. Grigsby PW, Vest ML, Perez CA: Recurrent carcinoma of the cervix exclusively in the paraaortic nodes following radiation therapy. Int J Radiat Oncol Biol Phys 1994; 28:451–455.
182. Perez CA, Grigsby PW, Nene SM, et al: Effect of tumor size on the prognosis of carcinoma of the uterine cervix treated with irradiation alone. Cancer 1992; 69:2796–2806.

Endometrial Carcinoma

183. Platz CE, Benda JA: Female genital tract cancer. Cancer 1995; 75(suppl):270–294.
184. Schottenfeld D: Epidemiology of endometrial neoplasia. J Cell Biochem 1995; 23(suppl):151–159.
185. SEER Cancer Statistics Review 1973–1997. Bethesda, National Cancer Institute, 2000.
186. Rose PG: Medical progress: endometrial carcinoma. N Engl J Med 1996; 335:640–649.
187. Pettigrew R, Hamilton-Fairley D: Obesity and female reproductive function. Br Med Bull 1997; 53:341–358.
188. Parazzini F, La Vecchia C, Negri E, et al: Diabetes and endometrial cancer: an Italian case-control study. Int J Cancer 1999; 81:539–542.
189. Soler M, Chatenoud L, Negri E, et al: Hypertension and hormone-related neoplasms in women. Hypertension 1999; 34:320–325.
190. Meirow D, Schenker JG: The link between female infertility and cancer: epidemiology and possible aetiologies. Human Reprod Update 1996; 2:63–75.
191. Farquhar CM, Lethaby A, Sowter M, et al: An evaluation of risk factors for endometrial hyperplasia in premenopausal women with abnormal menstrual bleeding. Am J Obstet Gynecol 1999; 181:525–529.
192. Beral V, Banks E, Reeves G, et al: Use of HRT and the subsequent risk of cancer. J Epidemiol Biostat 1999; 4:191–210.
193. Suh-Bergmann EJ, Goodman A: Surveillance for endometrial cancer in women receiving tamoxifen. Ann Intern Med 1999; 131:127–135.
194. Treilleux T, Mignotte H, Clement-Chassagne C, et al: Tamoxifen and malignant epithelial-nonepithelial tumours of the endometrium: report of six cases and review of the literature. Eur J Surg Oncol 1999; 25:477–482.
195. Weiderpass E, Personn I, Adami HO, et al: Body size in different periods of life, diabetes mellitus, hypertension, and risk of postmenopausal endometrial cancer. Cancer Causes Control 2000; 11:185–192.
196. Sulak PJ: Endometrial cancer and hormone replacement therapy: appropriate use of progestins to oppose endogenous and exogenous estrogen. Endocrinol Metabol Clin North Am 1997; 26:399–412.
197. Van Winter JT, Bernard ME: Oral contraceptive use during the perimenopausal years. Am Fam Physician 1998; 58:1373–1377.
198. Gruber SB, Thompson WD: A population-based study of endometrial cancer and familial risk in younger women: Cancer and Steroid Hormone Study Group. Cancer Epidemiol Biomarkers Prev 1996; 5:411–417.
199. Berends MJ, Kleibuker JH, de Vries EG, et al: The importance of family history in young patients with endometrial cancer. Eur J Obstet Gynecol Reprod Biol 1999; 82:139–141.
200. Parc YR, Halling KC, Burgart LJ, et al: Microsatellite instability and hMLH1/hMSH2 expression in young endometrial carcinoma patients: associations with family history and histopathology. Int J Cancer 2000; 86:60–66.
201. Planck M, Koul A, Fernebro E, et al: hMLH1, hMSH2 and hMSH6 mutations in hereditary non-polyposis colorectal cancer families from southern Sweden. Int J Cancer 1999; 83:197–202.
202. Park JG, Park YJ, Wijnen JT, et al: Gene-environment interaction in hereditary nonpolyposis colorectal cancer with implications for diagnosis and genetic testing. Int J Cancer 1999; 82:516–519.
203. DuBeshter B, Warshal DP, Angel C, et al: Endometrial carcinoma: the relevance of cervical cytology. Obstet Gynecol 1991; 77:458–462.
204. Hall KL, Dewar MA, Perchalski J: Screening for gynecologic cancer: Vulvar, vaginal, endometrial, and ovarian neoplasms. Primary Care 1992; 19:607–620.
205. Larson DM, Johnson KK, Broste SK, et al: Comparisons of D&C and office endometrial biopsy in predicting final histopathologic grade in endometrial cancer. Obstet Gynecol 1995; 86:38–42.
206. Obemair A, Geramou M, Gucer F, et al: Does hysteroscopy facilitate tumor cell dissemination? Incidence of peritoneal cytology from patients with early stage endometrial carcinoma following dilatation and curettage (D&C) versus hysteroscopy and D&C. Cancer 2000; 88:139–143.
207. Physicians' Data Query: Endometrial Cancer. Bethesda, National Cancer Institute, May 1999.
208. Kurman RJ, Norris HJ: Evaluation of criteria for distinguishing atypical endometrial hyperplasia from well-differentiated carcinoma. Cancer 1982; 49:2547–2559.
209. Christopherson WM, Alberhasky RC, Connelly PJ: Carcinoma of the endometrium. I. A clinicopathologic study of clear-cell carcinoma and secretory carcinoma. Cancer 1982; 49:1511–1523.
210. Gallion HH, Van Nagell JR Jr, Powell DF, et al: Stage I serous papillary carcinoma of the endometrium. Cancer 1989; 63:2224–2228.
211. Boronow RC: Surgical staging of endometrial cancer: evolution, evaluation, and responsible challenge: a personal perspective. Gynecol Oncol 1997; 66:179–189.
212. Eltabbakh GH, Piver MS, Hempling RE, et al: Excellent long-term survival and absence of vaginal recurrences in 332 patients with low-risk stage I endometrial adenocarcinoma treated with hysterectomy and vaginal brachytherapy without formal staging lymph node sampling: report of a prospective trial. Int J Radiat Oncol Biol Phys 1997; 38:373–380.
213. Irwin C, Levin W, Fyles A, et al: The role of adjuvant radiotherapy in carcinoma of the endometrium: results in 550 patients with pathologic stage I disease. Gynecol Oncol 1998; 70:247–254.
214. Fishman DA, Roberts KB, Chambers JT, et al: Radiation therapy as exclusive treatment for medically inoperable patients with stage I and II endometrioid carcinoma with endometrium. Gynecol Oncol 1996; 61:189–196.
215. Petereit DG, Sarkaria JN, Chappell RJ: Perioperative morbidity and mortality of high-dose-rate gynecologic brachytherapy. Int J Radiat Oncol Biol Phys 1998; 42:1025–1031.
216. Grigsby PW, Kuske RR, Perez CA, et al: Medically inoperable stage I adenocarcinoma of the endometrium treated with radiotherapy alone. Int J Radiat Oncol Biol Phys 1987; 13:483–488.
217. Higgins RV, van Nagell JR Jr, Horn EJ, et al: Preoperative radiation therapy followed by extrafascial hysterectomy in patients with stage II endometrial carcinoma. Cancer 1991; 68:1261–1264.
218. Reisinger SA, Staros EB, Feld R, et al: Preoperative radiation therapy in clinical stage II endometrial carcinoma. Gynecol Oncol 1992; 45:174–178.
219. Ahamd NR, Lanciano RM, Corn BW, et al: Postoperative radiation therapy for surgically staged endometrial cancer: impact of time factors (overall treatment time and surgery-to-radiation interval) on outcome. Int J Radiat Oncol Biol Phys 1995; 33:837–842.
220. Algan O, Tabesh T, Hanlon A, et al: Improved outcome in patients treated with postoperative radiation therapy for pathologic stage I/II endometrial cancer. Int J Radiat Oncol Biol Phys 1996; 35:925–933.
221. Calvin DP, Connell PP, Rotmensch J, et al: Surgery and postoperative radiation therapy in stage II endometrial carcinoma. Am J Clin Oncol 1999; 22:338–343.

222. Thigpen JT, Buchsbaum WJ, Mangan C, et al: Phase II trial of Adriamycin in the treatment of advanced or recurrent endometrial cancer: a Gynecologic Oncology Group study. Cancer Treat Rep 1979; 63:21–27.
223. Campora E, Vidali A, Mammoliti S, et al: Treatment of advanced or recurrent adenocarcinoma of the endometrium with doxorubicin and cyclophosphamide. Eur J Gynecol Oncol 1990; 11:181–183.
224. Thigpen JT, Blessing JA, DiSaia PJ, et al: A randomized comparison of doxorubicin alone versus doxorubicin plus cyclophosphamide in the management of advanced or recurrent endometrial carcinoma: a Gynecologic Oncology Group study. J Clin Oncol 1994; 12:1408–1414.
225. Thigpen JT, Vance RB, Khansur T: The platinum compounds and paclitaxel in the management of carcinomas of the endometrium and uterine cervix. Semin Oncol 1995; 22(suppl):67–75.
226. Green JB, Green S, Alberts DS, et al: Carboplatin therapy in advanced endometrial cancer. Obstet Gynecol 1990; 75:696–700.
227. Burke TW, Munkarah A, Kavanagh JJ, et al: Treatment of advanced or recurrent endometrial carcinoma with single-agent carboplatin. Gynecol Oncol 1993; 51:397–400.
228. Ball H, Blessing JA, Lentz S, et al: A phase II trial of paclitaxel in patients with advanced or recurrent adenocarcinoma of the endometrium: a Gynecologic Oncology Group study. Gynecol Oncol 1996; 62:278–281.
229. Alberts DS, Mason NL, O'Toole RV, et al: Doxorubicin-cisplatin-vinblastine combination chemotherapy of advanced endometrial carcinoma: a Southwest Oncology Group Study. Gynecol Oncol 1987; 26:193–201.
230. Burke TW, Stringer CA, Morris M, et al: Prospective treatment of advanced or recurrent endometrial carcinoma with cisplatin, doxorubicin, and cyclophosphamide. Gynecol Oncol 1991; 40:264–267.
231. Long HJ III, Langdon RM Jr, Cha SS, et al: Phase III trial of methotrexate, vinblastine, doxorubicin and cisplatin in advanced/recurrent endometrial carcinoma. Gynecol Oncol 1995; 58:240–243.
232. Cornelison TL, Baker TR, Piver MS, et al: Cisplatin, Adriamycin, etoposide, megestrol acetate versus melphalan, 5-fluorouracil, medroxyprogesterone acetate in the treatment of endometrial carcinoma. Gynecol Oncol 1995; 59:243–248.
233. Pierga JY, Dieras V, Paraiso D, et al: Treatment of advanced or recurrent endometrial carcinoma with combination of etoposide, cisplatin, and 5-fluorouracil: a phase II study. Gynecol Oncol 1996; 60:59–63.
234. Lissoni A, Gabriele A, Gorga G, et al: Cisplatin-, etoposide- and paclitaxel-containing chemotherapy in uterine adenocarcinoma. Ann Oncol 1997; 8:969–972.
235. Randall TC, Kurman RJ: Progestin treatment of atypical hyperplasia and well-differentiated carcinoma of the endometrium in women under age 40. Obstet Gynecol 1997; 90:434–440.
236. Kim YB, Holschneider CH, Ghosh K, et al: Progestin alone as a primary treatment of endometrial carcinoma in premenopausal women: Report of seven cases and review of the literature. Cancer 1997; 79:320–377.
237. Lentz SS: Advanced and recurrent endometrial carcinoma: hormonal therapy. Semin Oncol 1994; 21:100–106.
238. Lentz SS: Endocrine therapy of endometrial cancer. Cancer Treat Res 1998; 94:89–106.
239. Crespo C, Gonzalez-Martin A, Lastra E, et al: Metastatic endometrial cancer in lung and liver: complete and prolonged response to hormonal therapy with progestins. Gynecol Oncol 1999; 72:250–255.
240. Vishnevsky AS, Tsyrlina EV, Sofroniy DF, et al: Criteria of endometrial carcinoma sensitivity to hormone therapy: pathogenetic type of the disease and the tumor reaction to tamoxifen. Eur J Gynaecol Oncol 1993; 14:139–143.
241. Martin-Hirsch PL, Lilford RJ, Jarvis GJ: Adjuvant progestagen therapy for the treatment of endometrial cancer: review and meta-analyses of published randomised controlled trials. Eur J Obstet Gynecol Reprod Biol 1996; 65:201–207.
242. Grigsby PW, Perez CA, Camel HM, et al: Stage II carcinoma of the endometrium: results of therapy and prognostic factors. Int J Radiat Oncol Biol Phys 1985; 11:1915–1923.
243. Cook AM, Lodge N, Blake P: Stage IV endometrial carcinoma: a 10 year review of patients. Br J Radiol 1999; 72:485–488.
244. Nieberg RK, Hirschowitz SL: Malignant endometrial pathology. Curr Opin Obstet Gynecol 1992; 4:594–600.
245. Kosary CL: FIGO stage, histology, histologic grade, age and race as prognostic factors in determining survival for cancers of the female gynecological system: an analysis of 1973–87 SEER cases of cancers of the endometrium, cervix, ovary, vulva, and vagina. Semin Surg Oncol 1994; 10:31–46.
246. Sakuragi N, Hareyama H, Todo Y, et al: Prognostic significance of serous and clear cell adenocarcinoma in surgically staged endometrial carcinoma. Acta Obstet Gynecol Scand 2000; 79:311–316.
247. Reisinger SA, Staros EB, Mohiuddin M: Survival and failure analysis in stage II endometrial cancer using the revised 1988 FIGO staging system. Int J Radiat Oncol Biol Phys 1991; 21:1027–1032.
248. Morrow CP, Bundy BN, Kurman RJ, et al: Relationship between surgical-pathological risk factors and outcome in clinical stage I and II carcinoma of the endometrium: a Gynecologic Oncology Group study. Gynecol Oncol 1991; 40:55–65.
249. Corn BW, Lanciano RM, D'Agostino R Jr, et al: The relationship of local and distant failure from endometrial cancer: defining a clinical paradigm. Gynecol Oncol 1997; 66:411–416.
250. Zaino RJ, Kurman RJ, Diana KL, et al: Pathologic models to predict outcome for women with endometrial adenocarcinoma: the importance of the distinction between surgical stage and clinical stage—a Gynecologic Oncology Group study. Cancer 1996; 77:1115–1121.
251. Hirai M, Hirono M, Oosaki T, et al: Prognostic factors relating to survival in uterine endometrioid carcinoma. Int J Gynaecol Obstet 1999; 66:155–162.
252. De Gois NM, Martins NV, Abrao FS, et al: Peritumorous lymph-vascular invasion, grade of histologic differentiation, and myometrial infiltration as prognostic factors of endometrial carcinoma. Rev Paul Med 1993; 111:385–390.

Sarcoma of the Uterus

253. Meden H, Meyer-Rath D, Schauer A, et al: Endometrial stromal sarcoma of the uterus. Anticancer Drugs 1991; 2:35–37.
254. Podczaski ES, Woomert CA, Stevens CW, et al: Management of malignant mixed mesodermal tumors of the uterus. Obstet Gynecol 1989; 32:240–244.
255. Arrastia CD, Fruchter RG, Clark M, et al: Uterine carcinosarcomas: incidence and trends in management and survival. Gynecol Oncol 1997; 65:158–163.
256. George M, Pejovic MH, Kramar A: Uterine sarcomas: prognostic factors and treatment modalities: study of 209 patients. Gynecol Oncol 1986; 24:58–67.
257. Meredith RF, Eisert DR, Kaka Z, et al: An excess of uterine sarcomas after pelvic irradiation. Cancer 1986; 58:2003–2007.
258. Schwartz SM, Weiss NS, Daling JR, et al: Exogenous sex hormone use, correlates of endogenous hormone levels, and the incidence of histologic types of sarcoma of the uterus. Cancer 1996; 77:717–724.
259. Schwartz SM, Weiss NS: Marital status and the incidence of sarcomas of the uterus. Cancer Res 1990; 50:1886–1890.
260. Wheelock JB, Krebs HB, Schneider V, et al: Uterine sarcoma: analysis of prognostic variables in 71 cases. Am J Obstet Gynecol 1985; 151:1016–1022.
261. Silverberg SG, Major FJ, Blessing JA, et al: Carcinosarcoma (malignant mixed mesodermal tumor) of the uterus: a Gynecologic Oncology Group pathologic study of 203 cases. Int J Gynecol Pathol 1990; 9:1–19.
262. Rose PG, Piver MS, Tsukada Y, et al: Patterns of metastasis in uterine sarcoma: An autopsy study. Cancer 1989; 63:935–938.
263. Gonzalez-Bosquet E, Martinez-Palones JM, Gonzalez-Bosquet J, et al: Uterine sarcoma: a clinicopathological study of 93 cases. Eur J Gynaecol Oncol 1997; 18:192–195.
264. Ayhan A, Tuncer ZS, Tanir M, et al: Uterine sarcoma: the Hacettepe Hospital experience of 88 consecutive patients. Eur J Gynaecol Oncol 1997; 18:146–148.
265. Chen SS: Propensity of retroperitoneal lymph node metastasis in patients with stage I sarcoma of the uterus. Gynecol Oncol 1989; 32:215–217.
266. Melilli GA, Di Gesu G, Loizzi V, et al: Clinical experience with uterine sarcoma. Minerva Ginecol 1998; 50:291–295.
267. Hornback NB, Omura G, Major FJ: Observations on the use of adjuvant radiation therapy in patients with stage I and II uterine sarcoma. Int J Radiat Oncol Biol Phys 1986; 12:2127–2130.
268. Tinkler SD, Cowie VJ: Uterine sarcoma: a review of the Edinburgh experience from 1974 to 1992. Br J Radiol 1993; 66:998–1001.

269. Echt G, Jepson J, Steel J, et al: Treatment of uterine sarcomas. Cancer 1990; 66:35–39.
270. Knocke TH, Kucera H, Dorfler D, et al: Results of postoperative radiotherapy in the treatment of sarcoma of the corpus uteri. Cancer 1998; 83:1972–1979.
271. Ferrer F, Sabater S, Farrus B, et al: Impact of radiotherapy on local control and survival in uterine sarcoma: a retrospective study from the Grup Oncologic Catala-Occita. Int J Radiat Oncol Biol Phys 1999; 44:47–52.
272. Larson B, Silfversward C, Nilsson B, et al: Mixed Mullerian tumours of the uterus: prognostic factors: a clinical and histopathological study of 147 cases. Radiother Oncol 1990; 17:123–132.
273. Monk BJ, Solh S, Johnson MT, et al: Radical hysterectomy after pelvic irradiation in patients with high risk cervical cancer or uterine sarcoma: morbidity and outcome. Eur J Gynaecol Oncol 1993; 14:506–511.
274. Omura GA, Blessing JA, Major F, et al: A randomized clinical trial of adjuvant Adriamycin in uterine sarcomas: a Gynecologic Oncology Group study. J Clin Oncol 1985; 3:1240–1245.
275. Piver MS, Lele SB, Marchetti DL, et al: Effect of adjuvant chemotherapy on time to recurrence and survival of stage I uterine sarcoma. J Surg Oncol 1988; 38:233–239.
276. Peters WA III, Rivkin SE, Smith WR, et al: Cisplatin and Adriamycin combination chemotherapy for uterine stromal sarcomas and mixed mesodermal tumors. Gynecol Oncol 1989; 34:323–327.
277. Sutton GP, Blessing JA, Manetta A, et al: Gynecologic Oncology Group studies with ifosfamide. Semin Oncol 1992; 19(suppl):31–34.
278. Thigpen JT, Blessing JA, Beecham J, et al: Phase II trial of cisplatin as first-line chemotherapy in patients with advanced or recurrent uterine sarcomas: a Gynecologic Oncology Group study. J Clin Oncol 1991; 9:1962–1966.
279. Hempling RE, Piver MS, Baker TR: Impact on progression-free survival of adjuvant cyclophosphamide, vincristine, doxorubicin (Adriamycin), and dacarbazine (CYVADIC) chemotherapy for stage I uterine sarcoma: a prospective trial. Am J Clin Oncol 1995; 18:282–286.
280. Nickie-Psikuta M, Gawrychowski K: Different types and different prognosis: study of 310 uterine sarcomas. Eur J Gynaecol Oncol 1993; 14(suppl):105–113.
281. Larson B, Silfversward C, Nilsson B, et al: Prognostic factors in uterine leiomyosarcoma: a clinical and histopathological study of 143 cases: the Radiumhemmet series 1936–1981. Acta Oncol 1990; 29:185–191.
282. Major FJ, Blessing JA, Silverberg SG, et al: Prognostic factors in early-stage uterine sarcoma: a Gynecologic Oncology Group study. Cancer 1993; 71:1702–1709.

Gestational Trophoblastic Neoplasms

283. Seckl MJ, Newlands ES: Treatment of gestational trophoblastic disease. Gen Diag Pathol 1997; 143:159–171.
284. Lewis JL Jr: Diagnosis and management of gestational trophoblastic disease. Cancer 1993; 71(suppl):1639–1647.
285. Di Cintio E, Parazzini F, Rosa C, et al: The epidemiology of gestational trophoblastic disease. Gen Diag Pathol 1997; 143:103–108.
286. Hayashi K, Bracken MB, Freeman DH Jr, et al: Hydatidiform mole in the United States (1970–1977): a statistical and theoretical analysis. Am J Epidemiol 1982; 115:67–77.
287. Ayhan A, Tuncer ZS, Halilzade H, et al: Predictors of persistent disease in women with complete hydatidiform mole. J Reprod Med 1996; 41:591–594.
288. Kajii T, Ohama K: Androgenetic origin of hydatidiform mole. Nature 1977; 268:633–634.
289. Parazzini F, La Vecchia C, Pampallona S: Parental age and risk of complete and partial hydatidiform mole. Br J Obstet Gynaecol 1986; 93:582–585.
290. Lawler SD, Fisher RA, Dent J: A prospective genetic study of complete and partial hydatidiform moles. Am J Obstet Gynecol 1991; 164:1270–1277.
291. Berkowitz RS, Bernstein MR, Harlow BL, et al: Case-control study of risk factors for partial molar pregnancy. Am J Obstet Gynecol 1995; 173:788–794.
292. Goldstein DP, Berkowitz RS: Current management of complete and partial hydatidiform molar pregnancy. J Reprod Med 1994; 39:139–146.
293. Zalel Y, Dgani R: Gestational trophoblastic disease following the evacuation of partial hydatidiform mole: a review of 66 cases. Eur J Obstet Gynecol Reprod Biol 1997; 71:67–71.
294. Berkowitz RS, Goldstein DP: Gestational trophoblastic disease. Cancer 1995; 76(suppl):2079–2085.
295. Hershman JM: Human chorionic gonadotropin and the thyroid: hyperemesis gravidarum and trophoblastic tumors. Thyroid 1999; 9:653–657.
296. Balaram P, John M, Rajalekshmy TN, et al: A multivariate analysis of prognostic indicators in complete hydatidiform mole. Eur J Obstet Gynecol Reprod Biol 1999; 87:69–75.
297. Fan X, Yan L, Jia S, et al: A study of early pregnancy factor activity in the sera of women with trophoblastic tumor. Am J Reprod Immunol 1999; 41:204–208.
298. Hancock BW, Newlands ES, Berkowitz RS: Gestational trophoblastic disease. London, Chapman & Hall Medical, 1997.
299. Einhorn N: Evolution and current status of gynecologic cancer staging. Curr Prob Obstet Gynecol Fertil 1992; 15:251–268.
300. Kohorn EI: Staging and assessing trophoblastic tumors: A possible solution to an intractable problem. J Reprod Med 1998; 43:33–36.
301. Soper JT: Surgical therapy for gestational trophoblastic disease. J Reprod Med 1994; 39:168–174.
302. Horn LC, Bilek K: Clinicopathologic analysis of gestational trophoblastic disease: report of 158 cases. Gen Diag Pathol 1997; 143:173–178.
303. Sablinska B, Kietlinska Z, Zielinski J: Chemotherapy combined with surgery in the treatment of gestational trophoblastic disease (GTD). Eur J Gynaecol Oncol 1993; 14(suppl):146–151.
304. Lurain JR: High-risk metastatic gestational trophoblastic tumors: current management. J Reprod Med 1994; 39:217–222.
305. Evans AC Jr, Soper JT, Clarke-Pearson DL, et al: Gestational trophoblastic disease metastatic to the central nervous system. Gynecol Oncol 1995; 59:226–230.
306. Schechter NR, Mychalczak B, Jones W, et al: Prognosis of patients treated with whole-brain radiation therapy for metastatic gestational trophoblastic disease. Gynecol Oncol 1998; 68:183–192.
307. Newlands ES, Bower M, Fisher RA, et al: Management of placental site trophoblastic tumors. J Reprod Med 1998; 43:53–59.
308. DuBeshter B, Berkowitz RS, Goldstein DP, et al: Management of low risk metastatic gestational trophoblastic tumors. J Reprod Med 1991; 36:36–39.
309. Homesley HD: Development of single-agent chemotherapy regimens for gestational trophoblastic disease. J Reprod Med 1994; 39:185–192.
310. World Health Organization Scientific Group on Gestational Trophoblastic Diseases: Technical Report Series No. 692. Geneva, WHO, 1983.
311. Berkowitz RS, Goldstein DP, Bernstein MR: Modified triple chemotherapy in the management of high-risk metastatic gestational trophoblastic tumors. Gynecol Oncol 1984; 19:173–181.
312. Newlands ES, Bagshawe KD, Begent RH, et al: Results with the EMA/CO (etoposide, methotrexate, actinomycin D, cyclophosphamide, vincristine) regimen in high risk gestational trophoblastic tumours, 1979 to 1989. Br J Obstet Gynaecol 1991; 98:550–557.
313. Schink JC, Singh DK, Rademaker AW, et al: Etoposide, methotrexate, actinomycin D, cyclophosphamide, and vincristine for the treatment of metastatic, high-risk gestational trophoblastic disease. Obstet Gynecol 1992; 80:817–820.
314. Soper JT, Evans AC, Clarke-Pearson DL, et al: Alternating weekly chemotherapy with etoposide-methotrexate-dactinomycin/cyclophosphamide-vincristine for high-risk gestational trophoblastic disease. Obstet Gynecol 1994; 83:113–117.
315. Newlands ES, Bower M, Holden L, et al: The management of high-risk gestational trophoblastic tumours (GTT). Int J Gynaecol Obstet 1998; 60(suppl):S65–S70.
316. Hartenbach EM, Saltzman AK, Carter JR, et al: A novel strategy using G-CSF to support EMA/CO for high-risk gestational trophoblastic disease. Gynecol Oncol 1995; 56:105–108.
317. Sutton GP, Soper JT, Blessing JA, et al: Ifosfamide alone or in combination in the treatment of refractory malignant gestational trophoblastic disease. Am J Obstet Gynecol 1992; 167:489–495.
318. Lotz JP, Andre T, Donsimoni R, et al: High dose chemotherapy with ifosfamide, carboplatin, and etoposide combined with autologous bone marrow transplantation for the treatment of poor-prognosis germ cell tumors and metastatic trophoblastic disease in adults. Cancer 1995; 75:874–885.

319. Kim SJ, Bae SN, Kim JH, et al: Risk factors for the prediction of treatment failure in gestational trophoblastic tumors treated with EMA/CO regimen. Gynecol Oncol 1998; 71:247–253.
320. Rustin GJ, Newlands ES, Lutz JM, et al: Combination but not single-agent methotrexate chemotherapy for gestational trophoblastic tumors increases the incidence of second tumors. J Clin Oncol 1996; 14:2769–2773.

Carcinoma of the Fallopian Tube

321. Nikrui N, Duska LR: Fallopian tube carcinoma. Surg Oncol Clin North Am 1998; 7:363–373.
322. Ng P, Lawton F: Fallopian tube carcinoma: a review. Ann Acad Med Singapore 1998; 27:693–697.
323. Thigpen JT: Ovaries and fallopian tubes. In: Abeloff MD, Armitage JO, Lichter AS, et al (eds): Clinical Oncology, 2nd ed. New York, Churchill Livingstone, 2000.
324. Granberg S, Jansson I: Early detection of primary carcinoma of the fallopian tube by endovaginal ultrasound. Acta Obstet Gynecol Scand 1990; 69:667–668.
325. Butler DF, Bolton ME, Spanos WJ Jr, et al: Retrospective analysis of patients with primary fallopian tube carcinoma treated at the University of Louisville. J Ky Med Assoc 1999; 97:154–164.
326. Baalbaky I, Vinatier D, Leblanc E, et al: Clinical aspects of primary cancer of the fallopian tube. A retrospective study of 20 cases. J Gynecol Obstet Biol Reprod 1999; 28:225–231.
327. Warshal DP, Burgelson ER, Aikins JK, et al: Post-hysterectomy fallopian tube carcinoma presenting with a positive Papanicolaou smear. Obstet Gynecol 1999; 94:834–836.
328. Yamashita Y, Torashima M, Hatanaka Y, et al: Adnexal masses: accuracy of characterization with transvaginal ultrasound and precontrast and postcontrast MR imaging. Radiology 1995; 194:557–565.
329. Outwater EK, Siegelman ES, Chiowanich P, et al: Dilated fallopian tubes: MR imaging characteristics. Radiology 1998; 208:463–469.
330. Hu CY, Taylor ML, Hertz AT: Primary carcinoma of the fallopian tube. Am J Obstet Gynecol 1950; 59:58–67.
331. Moore DH, Woosley JT, Reddick RL, et al: Adenosquamous carcinoma of the fallopian tube: a clinicopathologic case report with verification of the diagnosis by immunohistochemical and ultrastructural studies. Am J Obstet Gynecol 1987; 157:903–905.
332. Klein M, Rosen A, Graf A, et al: Primary fallopian tube carcinoma: a retrospective survey of 51 cases. Arch Gynecol Obstet 1994; 255:141–146.
333. Cass I, Resnik E, Chambers JT, et al: Combination chemotherapy with etoposide, cisplatin, and doxorubicin in mixed mullerian tumors of the adnexa. Gynecol Oncol 1996; 61:309–314.
334. Nordin AJ: Primary carcinoma of the fallopian tube: a 20-year literature review. Obstet Gynecol Surv 1994; 49:349–361.
335. Ben-Hur H, Dgani R, Ben-Arie A, et al: Diagnostic dilemmas and current therapy of fallopian tube cancer. Eur J Gynaecol Oncol 1999; 20:108–109.
336. Barakat RR, Rubin SC, Saigo PE, et al: Second-look laparotomy in carcinoma of the fallopian tube. Obstet Gynecol 1993; 82:748–751.
337. Cormio G, Gabriele A, Maneo A, et al: Second-look laparotomy in the management of fallopian tube carcinoma. Acta Obstet Gynecol Scand 1997; 76:369–372.
338. Rubin SC, Hoskins WJ, Hakes TB, et al: Recurrence after negative second-look laparotomy for ovarian cancer: analysis of risk factors. Am J Obstet Gynecol 1988; 159:1094–1098.
339. Frigerio L, Pirondini A, Pileri M, et al: Primary carcinoma of the fallopian tube. Tumori 1993; 79:40–44.
340. Jereczek B, Jassem J, Kobierska A: Primary cancer of the fallopian tube: report of 26 patients. Acta Obstet Gynecol Scand 1996; 75:281–286.
341. Schray MF, Podratz KC, Malkasian GD: Fallopian tube cancer: the role of radiation therapy. Radiother Oncol 1987; 10:267–275.
342. Rauthe G, Vahrson HW, Burkhardt E: Primary cancer of the fallopian tube: treatment and results of 37 cases. Eur J Gynaecol Oncol 1998; 19:356–362.
343. Wolfson AH, Tralins KS, Greven KM, et al: Adenocarcinoma of the fallopian tube: results of a multi-institutional retrospective analysis of 72 patients. Int J Radiat Oncol Biol Phys 1998; 40:71–76.
344. Klein M, Rosen A, Lahousen M, et al: Evaluation of adjuvant therapy after surgery for primary carcinoma of the fallopian tube. Arch Gynecol Obstet 1994; 255:19–24.
345. Higgins RV, Myers VT, Hall JB: Radiation myelopathy after chemotherapy and radiation therapy for fallopian tube carcinoma. Gynecol Oncol 1997; 64:285–287.
346. Peters WA III, Andersen WA, Hopkins MP: Results of chemotherapy in advanced carcinoma of the fallopian tube. Cancer 1989; 63:836–838.
347. Peters WA III, Andersen WA, Hopkins MP, et al: Prognostic features of carcinoma of the fallopian tube. Obstet Gynecol 1988; 71:757–762.
348. Morris M, Gershenson DM, Burke TW, et al: Treatment of fallopian tube carcinoma with cisplatin, doxorubicin, and cyclophosphamide. Obstet Gynecol 1990; 76:1020–1024.
349. Pectasides D, Barbounis V, Sintila A, et al: Treatment of primary fallopian tube carcinoma with cisplatin-containing chemotherapy. Am J Clin Oncol 1994; 17:68–71.
350. Cormio G, Maneo A, Gabriele A, et al: Treatment of fallopian tube carcinoma with cyclophosphamide, Adriamycin, and cisplatin. Am J Clin Oncol 1997; 20:143–145.
351. Silver DF, Piver MS: Gemcitabine salvage chemotherapy for patients with gynecologic malignancies of the ovary, fallopian tube, and peritoneum. Am J Clin Oncol 1999; 22:450–452.
352. Eddy GL, Copeland LJ, Gershenson DM, et al: Fallopian tube carcinoma. Obstet Gynecol 1984; 64:546–552.
353. Podratz KC, Podczaski ES, Gaffey TA, et al: Primary carcinoma of the fallopian tube. Am J Obstet Gynecol 1986; 154:1319–1326.
354. Yoonessi M, Leberer JP, Crickard K: Primary fallopian tube carcinoma: treatment and spread pattern. J Surg Oncol 1988; 38:97–100.
355. Kaya S, Grillo M, Gent HJ: Therapy of primary fallopian tube cancer: a retrospective study of 30 cases. Zentral Gynakol 1992; 114:254–258.
356. Wang PH, Yuan CC, Chao HT, et al: Prognosis of primary fallopian tube adenocarcinoma: report of 25 patients. Eur J Gynaecol Oncol 1998; 19:571–574.
357. Rosen AC, Klein M, Hafner E, et al: Management and prognosis of primary fallopian tube carcinoma: Austrian Cooperative Study Group for Fallopian Tube Carcinoma. Gynecol Obstet Invest 1999; 47:45–51.
358. Chang J, Sharpe JC, A'Hern RP, et al: Carcinosarcoma of the ovary: incidence, prognosis, treatment and survival of patients. Ann Oncol 1995; 6:755–758.
359. Alvarado-Cabrero I, Young RH, Vamvakas EC, et al: Carcinoma of the fallopian tube: a clinicopathological study of 105 cases with observations on staging and prognostic factors. Gynecol Oncol 1999; 72:367–379.
360. Pfeiffer P, Mogensen H, Amtrup F, et al: Primary carcinoma of the fallopian tube: a retrospective study of patients reported to the Danish Cancer Registry in a 5-year period. Acta Oncol 1989; 28:7–11.

Ovarian Cancer

361. Herrin VE, Thigpen JT: Chemotherapy for ovarian cancer: current concepts. Semin Surg Oncol 1999; 17:181–188.
362. Yancik R: Ovarian cancer: age contrasts in incidence, histology, disease stage at diagnosis and mortality. Cancer 1993; 71:517–523.
363. Kozlowski KJ: Ovarian masses. Adolesc Med 1999; 10:337–350.
364. Thompson SD: Ovarian cancer screening: a primary care guide. Lippincott's Prim Care Pract 1998; 2:244–250.
365. Unkila-Kallio L, Tiitinen A, Wahlstrom T, et al: Reproductive features in women developing ovarian granulosa cell tumour at a fertile age. Human Reprod 2000; 15:589–593.
366. Adami HO, Hsieh CC, Lambe M, et al: Parity, age at first childbirth, and risk of ovarian cancer. Lancet 1994; 344:1250–1254.
367. Hulka BS: Epidemiologic analysis of breast and gynecologic cancer. Prog Clin Biol Res 1997; 396:17–29.
368. Siskind V, Green A, Bain C, et al: Breastfeeding, menopause, and epithelial ovarian cancer. Epidemiology 1997; 8:188–191.
369. Beard CM, Hartmann LC, Atkinson EJ, et al: The epidemiology of ovarian cancer: a population-based study in Olmsted County, Minnesota, 1935–1991. Ann Epidemiol 2000; 10:14–23.
370. Risch HA: Hormonal etiology of epithelial ovarian cancer, with a hypothesis concerning the role of androgens and progesterone. J Natl Cancer Inst 1998; 90:1774–1786.
371. Gertig DM, Hunter DJ, Cramer DW, et al: Prospective study of talc use and ovarian cancer. J Natl Cancer Inst 2000; 92:249–252.
372. Heller DS, Gordon RE, Katz N: Correlation of asbestos fiber burden in fallopian tubes and ovarian tissue. Am J Obstet Gynecol 1999; 181:346–347.

373. Ponder BAJ, Waring MJ: The Genetics of Cancer. Boston, Dordrecht, 1995.
374. Kerber RA, Slattery ML: The impact of family history on ovarian cancer risk: The Utah Population Database. Arch Intern Med 1995; 155:905–912.
375. Stratton JF, Pharoah P, Smith SK, et al: A systematic review and meta-analysis of family history and risk of ovarian cancer. Br J Obstet Gynaecol 1998; 105:493–499.
376. Piver MS, Baker TR, Jishi MF, et al: Familial ovarian cancer: a report of 658 families from the Gilda Radner Familial Ovarian Cancer Registry 1981–1991. Cancer 1993; 71(suppl):582–588.
377. Langston AA, Ostrander EA: Hereditary ovarian cancer. Curr Opin Obstet Gynecol 1997; 9:3–7.
378. Lin KM, Shashidharan M, Thorson AG, et al: Cumulative incidence of colorectal and extracolonic cancers in MLH1 and MSH2 mutation carriers of hereditary nonpolyposis colorectal cancer. J Gastrointest Surg 1998; 2:67–71.
379. Boyd J: Molecular genetics of hereditary ovarian cancer. Oncology (Huntingt) 1998; 12:399–406.
380. Chen JJ, Silver D, Cantor S, et al: BRCA1, BRCA2, and Rad51 operate in a common DNA damage response pathway. Cancer Res 1999; 59(suppl):1752s–1756s.
381. Rubin SC, Blackwood MA, Bandera C, et al: BRCA1, BRCA2, and hereditary nonpolyposis colorectal cancer gene mutations in an unselected ovarian cancer population: relationship to family history and implications for genetic testing. Am J Obstet Gynecol 1998; 178:670–677.
382. Santarosa M, Dolcetti R, Magri MD, et al: BRCA1 and BRCA2 genes: role in hereditary breast and ovarian cancer in Italy. Int J Cancer 1999; 83:5–9.
383. MacDonald ND, Rosenthal AN, Jacobs IJ: Screening for ovarian cancer. Ann Acad Med Singapore 1998; 27:676–682.
384. Schutter EM, Sohn C, Kristen P, et al: Estimation of probability of malignancy using a logistic model combining physical examination, ultrasound, serum CA 125, and serum CA 72-4 in postmenopausal women with a pelvic mass: an international multicenter study. Gynecol Oncol 1998; 69:56–63.
385. DePriest PD, Gallion HH, Pavlik EJ, et al: Transvaginal sonography as a screening method for the detection of early ovarian cancer. Gynecol Oncol 1997; 65:408–414.
386. Buckshee K, Temsu I, Bhatla N, et al: Pelvic examination, transvaginal ultrasound and transvaginal color Doppler sonography as predictors of ovarian cancer. Int J Gynaecol Obstet 1998; 61:51–57.
387. Verheijen RH, von Mensdorff-Pouilly S, van Kamp GJ, et al: CA 125: fundamental and clinical aspects. Semin Cancer Biol 1999; 9:117–124.
388. Jacobs I, Davies AP, Bridges J, et al: Prevalence screening for ovarian cancer in postmenopausal women by CA 125 measurement and ultrasonography. Br Med J 1993; 306:1030–1034.
389. Kupryjanczyk J, Thor AD, Beauchamp R, et al: Ovarian, peritoneal, and endometrial serous carcinoma: clonal origin of multifocal disease. Mod Pathol 1996; 9:166–173.
390. Tammela J, Geisler JP, Eskew PN Jr, et al: Clear cell carcinoma of the ovary: poor prognosis compared to serous carcinoma. Eur J Gynaecol Oncol 1998; 19:438–440.
391. Kennedy AW, Markman M, Biscotti CV, et al: Survival probability in ovarian clear cell adenocarcinoma. Gynecol Oncol 1999; 74:108–114.
392. Serov SF, Scully RE, Sobin LH: Histological Typing of Ovarian Tumours: International Histological Classification of Tumours, No. 9. Geneva, World Health Organization, 1973.
393. Hoskins WJ: Surgical staging and cytoreductive surgery of epithelial ovarian cancer. Cancer 1993; 71(suppl):1534–1540.
394. Zanetta G, Rota S, Chiari S, et al: The accuracy of staging: an important prognostic determinator in stage I ovarian carcinoma: a multivariate analysis. Ann Oncol 1998; 9:1097–1101.
395. Trope C, Kaern J, Vergote IB, et al: Are borderline tumors of the ovary overtreated both surgically and systemically? A review of four prospective randomized trials including 253 patients with borderline tumors. Gynecol Oncol 1993; 51:236–243.
396. Morris RT, Gershenson DM, Silva EG, et al: Outcome and reproductive function after conservative surgery for borderline ovarian tumors. Obstet Gynecol 2000; 95:541–547.
397. Rice LW, Berkowitz RS, Marks SD, et al: Epithelial ovarian tumors of borderline malignancy. Gynecol Oncol 1990; 39:195–198.
398. Buttini M, Nicklin JL, Crandon A: Low malignant potential ovarian tumors: a review of 175 consecutive cases. Austral N Z J Obstet Gynaecol 1997; 37:100–103.
399. Gershenson DM, Silva EG: Serous ovarian tumors of low malignant potential with peritoneal implants. Cancer 1990; 65:578–585.
400. Barakat RR, Benjamin I, Lewis JL Jr, et al: Platinum-based chemotherapy for advanced-stage serous ovarian carcinoma of low malignant potential. Gynecol Oncol 1995; 59:390–393.
401. Gonzalez-Lira G, Escudero-De Los Rios P, Salazar-Martinez E, et al: Conservative surgery for ovarian cancer and effect on fertility. Int J Gynaecol Obstet 1997; 56:155–162.
402. Zanetta G, Chiari S, Rota S, et al: Conservative surgery for stage I ovarian carcinoma in women of childbearing age. Br J Obstet Gynaecol 1997; 104:1030–1035.
403. Young RC, Walton CA, Ellenberg SS, et al: Adjuvant therapy in stage I and stage II epithelial ovarian cancer: results of two prospective randomized trials. N Engl J Med 1990; 322:1021–1027.
404. Monga M, Carmichael JA, Shelley WE, et al: Surgery without adjuvant chemotherapy for early epithelial ovarian carcinoma after comprehensive surgical staging. Gynecol Oncol 1991; 43:195–197.
405. Ahmed FY, Wiltshaw E, A'Hern RP, et al: Natural history and prognosis of untreated stage I epithelial ovarian carcinoma. J Clin Oncol 1996; 14:2968–2975.
406. Piver MS, Balcer T: The potential for optimal (<2 cm) cytoreductive surgery in advanced ovarian cancer at a tertiary medical center: a prospective study. Gynecol Oncol 1986; 24:1–8.
407. Le T, Krepart GV, Lotocki RJ, et al: Does debulking surgery improve survival in biologically aggressive ovarian carcinoma? Gynecol Oncol 1997; 67:208–214.
408. Scarabelli C, Gallo A, Franceschi S, et al: Primary cytoreductive surgery with rectosigmoid colon resection for patients with advanced epithelial ovarian carcinoma. Cancer 2000; 88:389–397.
409. Hempling RE, Wesolowski JA, Piver MS: Second-look laparotomy in advanced ovarian cancer: a critical assessment of morbidity and impact on survival. Ann Surg Oncol 1997; 4:349–354.
410. Williams SD, Blessing JA, DiSaia PJ, et al: Second-look laparotomy in ovarian germ cell tumors: the Gynecologic Oncology Group experience. Gynecol Oncol 1994; 52:287–291.
411. Cormio D, di Vagno G, Cazzolla A, et al: Surgical treatment of recurrent ovarian cancer: report of 21 cases and review of the literature. Eur J Obstet Gynecol Reprod Biol 1999; 86:185–188.
412. Eisenkop SM, Friedman RL, Spirtos NM: The role of secondary cytoreductive surgery in the treatment of patients with recurrent epithelial ovarian carcinoma. Cancer 2000; 88:144–153.
413. Sedlacek TV, Spyropoulos P, Cifaldi R, et al: Whole-abdomen radiation therapy as salvage treatment for epithelial ovarian carcinoma. Cancer J Sci Am 1997; 3:358–363.
414. Gelblum D, Mychalczak B, Almadrones L, et al: Palliative benefit of external-beam radiation in the management of platinum refractory epithelial ovarian carcinoma. Gynecol Oncol 1998; 69:36–41.
415. Cardenes H, Randall ME: Integrating radiation therapy in the curative management of ovarian cancer: current issues and future directions. Semin Radiat Oncol 2000; 10:61–70.
416. Sell A, Bertelsen K, Anderson JE, et al: Randomized study of whole abdomen irradiation versus pelvic irradiation plus cyclophosphamide in treatment of early ovarian cancer. Gynecol Oncol 1990; 37:367–373.
417. Potter ME, Partridge EE, Shingleton HM, et al: Intraperitoneal chromic phosphate in ovarian cancer: risks and benefits. Gynecol Oncol 1989; 32:314–318.
418. Reid GC, Roberts JA, Hopkins MP, et al: Primary treatment of stage III ovarian carcinoma with sequential chemotherapy and whole abdominal radiation therapy. Gynecol Oncol 1993; 49:333–338.
419. Bolis G, Colombo N, Pecorelli S, et al: Adjuvant treatment for early epithelial ovarian cancer: results of two randomized clinical trials comparing cisplatin to no further treatment or chromic phosphate (^{32}P). G.I.C.O.G.: Gruppo Interregionale Collaborativo in Ginecologia Oncologica. Ann Oncol 1995; 6:887–893.
420. Vergote IB, Vergote-De Vos LN, Abeler VM, et al: Randomized trial comparing cisplatin with radioactive phosphorus or whole-abdomen irradiation as adjuvant treatment of ovarian cancer. Cancer 1992; 69:741–749.
421. Barakat RR, Almadrones L, Venkatraman ES, et al: A phase II trial of intraperitoneal cisplatin and etoposide as consolidation therapy in patients with stage II–IV epithelial ovarian cancer following negative surgical assessment. Gynaecol Oncol 1998; 69:17–22.

422. Morgan RJ Jr, Braly P, Cecchi G, et al: Phase II trial of intraperitoneal cisplatin with intravenous doxorubicin and cyclophosphamide in previously untreated patients with advanced ovarian cancer: long-term follow-up. Gynecol Oncol 1999; 75:419–426.
423. Gadducci A, Carnino F, Chiara S, et al: Intraperitoneal versus intravenous cisplatin in combination with intravenous cyclophosphamide and epidoxorubicin in optimally cytoreduced advanced epithelial ovarian cancer: a randomized trial of the Gruppo Oncologico Nord-Ovest. Gynecol Oncol 2000; 76:157–162.
424. Creasman WT, Omura GA, Brady MF, et al: A randomized trial of cyclophosphamide, doxorubicin, and cisplatin with and without bacillus Calmette-Guérin in patients with suboptimal stage III and IV ovarian cancer: a Gynecologic Oncology Group study. Gynecol Oncol 1990; 39:239–243.
425. Meredith RF, Partridge EE, Alvarez RD, et al: Intraperitoneal radioimmunotherapy of ovarian cancer with lutetium-177-CC49. J Nucl Med 1996; 37:1491–1496.
426. Juweid M, Swayne LC, Sharkey RM, et al: Prospects of radioimmunotherapy in epithelial ovarian cancer: results with iodine-131-labeled murine and humanized MN-14 anti-carcinoembryonic antigen monoclonal antibodies. Gynecol Oncol 1997; 67:259–271.
427. Willemse PHB, DeVries EGE, Mulder NH, et al: Intraperitoneal human recombinant interferon alpha in minimal residual ovarian cancer. Eur J Cancer 1990; 26:353–358.
428. Edwards RP, Gooding W, Lembersky BC, et al: Comparison of toxicity and survival following intraperitoneal recombinant interleukin-2 for persistent ovarian cancer after platinum: twenty-four-hour versus 7-day infusion. J Clin Oncol 1997; 15:3399–3407.
429. Casey AC, Bhodauria S, Shapter A, et al: Dysgerminoma: the role of conservative surgery. Gynecol Oncol 1996; 63:352–357.
430. Gershenson DM: Update on malignant ovarian germ cell tumors. Cancer 1993; 71(suppl):1581–1590.
431. Williams SD, Blessing JA, Liao SY, et al: Adjuvant therapy of ovarian germ cell tumors with cisplatin, etoposide, and bleomycin: a trial of the Gynecologic Oncology Group. J Clin Oncol 1994; 12:701–706.
432. Willemse PH, Aalders JG, Bouma J, et al: Long-term survival after vinblastine, bleomycin, cisplatin treatment in patients with germ cell tumors of the ovary: an update. Gynecol Oncol 1987; 28:268–297.
433. Loehrer PJ, Johnson D, Elson P, et al: Importance of bleomycin in favorable-prognosis disseminated germ cell tumors: an Eastern Clinical Oncology Group study. J Clin Oncol 1995; 13:470–476.
434. Hoskins WJ, McGuire WP, Brady MF, et al: The effect of diameter of largest residual disease on survival after primary cytoreductive surgery in patients with suboptimal residual epithelial ovarian carcinoma. Am J Obstet Gynecol 1994; 170:979–980.
435. van Dam PA, Tjalma W, Weyler J, et al: Ultraradical debulking of epithelial ovarian cancer with the ultrasonic surgical aspirator: a prospective randomized trial. Am J Obstet Gynecol 1996; 174:943–950.
436. Eisenkop SM, Friedman RL, Wang HJ: Complete cytoreductive surgery is feasible and maximizes survival in patients with advanced epithelial ovarian cancer: a prospective study. Gynecol Oncol 1998; 69:103–108.
437. Fyles AW, Thomas GM, Pintilie M, et al: A randomized study of two doses of abdominopelvic radiation therapy for patients with optimally debulked stage I, II, and III ovarian cancer. Int J Radiat Oncol Biol Phys 1998; 41:543–549.
438. Lawton F, Luesley D, Blackledge G, et al: A randomized trial comparing whole abdominal radiotherapy with chemotherapy following cisplatinum cytoreduction in epithelial ovarian cancer: West Midlands Ovarian Cancer Group Trial II. Clin Oncol (Royal Coll Radiol) 1990; 2:4–9.
439. Lambert HE, Rustin GJ, Gregory WM, et al: A randomized trial comparing single-agent carboplatin with carboplatin followed by radiotherapy for advanced ovarian cancer: a North Thames Ovary Group study. J Clin Oncol 1993; 11:440–448.
440. Chiara S, Conte P, Franzone P, et al: High-risk early-stage ovarian cancer: Randomized clinical trial comparing cisplatin plus cyclophosphamide versus whole abdominal radiotherapy. Am J Clin Oncol 1994; 17:72–76.
441. Tobias JS, Griffiths CT: Management of ovarian cancer: current concepts and future prospects. N Engl J Med 1976; 294:818–822.
442. Greene MH, Boice JD Jr, Greer BE, et al: Acute nonlymphocytic leukemia after therapy with alkylating agents for ovarian cancer: a study of five randomized clinical trials. N Engl J Med 1982; 307:1416–1421.
443. Wiltshaw E, Subramarian S, Alexopoulos C, et al: Cancer of the ovary: a summary of experience with cis-dichloro-diamineplatinum (II) at the Royal Marsden Hospital. Cancer Treat Rep 1979; 63:1545–1548.
444. Advanced Ovarian Cancer Trialists' Group: Chemotherapy in advanced ovarian cancer: an overview of randomized clinical trials. Br Med J 1991; 303:884–893.
445. Aabo K, Adams M, Adnitt P, et al: Chemotherapy in advanced ovarian cancer: four systematic meta-analyses of individual patient data from 37 randomized trials: Advanced Ovarian Cancer Trialists' Group. Br J Cancer 1998; 78:1479–1487.
446. Gruppo Interregionale Collaborativo in Ginecologia Oncologica: Long-term results of a randomized trial comparing cisplatin with cisplatin and cyclophosphamide with cisplatin, cyclophosphamide, and Adriamycin in advanced ovarian cancer. Gynecol Oncol 1992; 45:115–117.
447. Wils J, van Geuns H, Stoot J, et al: Cyclophosphamide, epirubicin and cisplatin (CEP) versus epirubicin plus cisplatin (EP) in stage Ic-IV ovarian cancer: a randomized phase III trial of the Gynecologic Oncology Group of the Comprehensive Cancer Center Limburg. Anticancer Drugs 1999; 10:257–261.
448. Tokuhashi Y, Kikkawa F, Tamakoshi K, et al: A randomized trial of cisplatin, vinblastine, and bleomycin versus cyclophosphamide, aclacinomycin, and cisplatin in epithelial ovarian cancer. Oncology 1997; 54:281–286.
449. Homesley HD, Bundy BN, Hurteau JA, et al: Bleomycin, etoposide, and cisplatin combination therapy of ovarian granulosa cell tumors and other stromal malignancies: A Gynecologic Oncology Group study. Gynecol Oncol 1999; 72:131–137.
450. The Ovarian Cancer Meta-Analysis Project: Cyclophosphamide plus cisplatin versus cyclophosphamide, doxorubicin, and cisplatin chemotherapy of ovarian carcinoma: a meta-analysis. J Clin Oncol 1991; 9:1668–1674.
451. Fanning J, Bennett TZ, Hilgers RD: Meta-analysis of cisplatin, doxorubicin, and cyclophosphamide versus cisplatin and cyclophosphamide chemotherapy of ovarian carcinoma. Obstet Gynecol 1992; 80:954–960.
452. Marth C, Trope C, Vergote IB, et al: Ten-year results of a randomised trial comparing cisplatin with cisplatin and cyclophosphamide in advanced, suboptimally debulked ovarian cancer. Eur J Cancer 1998; 34:1175–1180.
453. Bolis G, Favalli G, Danese S, et al: Weekly cisplatin given for 2 months versus cisplatin plus cyclophosphamide given for 5 months after cytoreductive surgery for advanced ovarian cancer. J Clin Oncol 1997; 15:1938–1944.
454. Cocconi G, Bella M, Lottici R, et al: Mature results of a prospective randomized trial comparing a three-weekly with an accelerated weekly schedule of cisplatin in advanced ovarian carcinoma. Am J Clin Oncol 1999; 22:559–567.
455. Alberts DS, Green S, Hannigan EV, et al: Improved therapeutic index of carboplatin plus cyclophosphamide versus cisplatin plus cyclophosphamide: final report by the Southwest Oncology Group of a phase III randomized trial in stages III (suboptimal) and IV ovarian cancer. J Clin Oncol 1992; 10:706–717.
456. Swenerton K, Jeffrey J, Stuart G, et al: Cisplatin-cyclophosphamide versus carboplatin-cyclophosphamide in advanced ovarian cancer: a randomized phase III study of the National Cancer Institute of Canada Clinical Trials Group. J Clin Oncol 1992; 10:718–726.
457. Lokich J, Anderson N: Carboplatin versus cisplatin in solid tumors: an analysis of the literature. Ann Oncol 1998; 9:13–21.
458. Schink JC: Current initial therapy of stage III and IV ovarian cancer: challenges for managed care. Semin Oncol 1999; 26(suppl):2–7.
459. Muggia FM, Braly PS, Brady MF, et al: Phase III randomized study of cisplatin versus paclitaxel versus cisplatin and paclitaxel in patients with suboptimal stage III or IV ovarian cancer: a Gynecologic Oncology Group study. J Clin Oncol 2000; 18:106–115.
460. McGuire WP, Hoskins WJ, Brady MF, et al: Cyclophosphamide and cisplatin compared with paclitaxel and cisplatin in patients with stage III and stage IV ovarian cancer. N Engl J Med 1996; 334:1–6.
461. Einzig AI, Wiernik PH, Sasloff J, et al: Phase II study and long term follow-up of patients treated with Taxol for advanced ovarian adenocarcinoma. J Clin Oncol 1992; 10:1748–1753.
462. Thigpen JT, Blessing JA, Ball H, et al: Phase II trial of paclitaxel

in patients with progressive ovarian carcinoma after platinum-based chemotherapy: a Gynecology Oncology Group study. J Clin Oncol 1994; 12:1748–1753.
463. Villa A, Parazzini F, Acerboni S, et al: Survival and prognostic factors of early ovarian cancer. Br J Cancer 1998; 77:123–124.
464. Goff BA, Sainz de la Cuesta R, Muntz HG, et al: Clear cell carcinoma of the ovary: a distinct histologic type with poor prognosis and resistance to platinum-based chemotherapy in stage III disease. Gynecol Oncol 1996; 60:412–417.
465. Tamakoshi K, Kikkawa F, Nakashima N, et al: Clinical behavior of borderline ovarian tumors: a study of 150 cases. J Surg Oncol 1997; 64:147–152.
466. Curtin JP, Malik R, Venkatraman ES, et al: Stage IV ovarian cancer: impact of surgical debulking. Gynecol Oncol 1997; 64:9–12.

Vaginal Carcinoma

467. Herbst AL, Green TH Jr, Ulfelder H: Primary carcinoma of the vagina. Am J Obstet Gynecol 1970; 106:210–218.
468. Melnick S, Cole P, Anderson D, et al: Rates and risks of diethylstilbestrol-related clear-cell adenocarcinoma of the vagina and cervix: an update. N Engl J Med 1987; 316:514–516.
469. Herbst AL, Ulfelder H, Poskanzer DC: Adenocarcinoma of the vagina: association of maternal stilbestrol therapy with tumor appearance in young women. N Engl J Med 1971; 284:878–881.
470. Herbst AL, Anderson D: Clear cell adenocarcinoma of the vagina and cervix secondary to intrauterine exposure to diethylstilbestrol. Semin Surg Oncol 1990; 6:343–346.
471. Hanselaar A, van Loosbroek M, Schuurbiers O, et al: Clear cell adenocarcinoma of the vagina and cervix: an update of the central Netherlands registry showing twin age incidence peaks. Cancer 1997; 79:2229–2236.
472. Hicks ML, Piver MS: Conservative surgery plus adjuvant therapy for vulvovaginal rhabdomyosarcoma, diethylstilbestrol clear cell adenocarcinoma of the vagina, and unilateral germ cell tumors of the ovary. Obstet Gynecol Clin North Am 1992; 19:219–233.
473. Aho M, Vesterinen E, Meyer B, et al: Natural history of vaginal intraepithelial neoplasia. Cancer 1991; 68:195–197.
474. Sugase M, Matsukura T: Distinct manifestations of human papillomaviruses in the vagina. Int J Cancer 1997; 72:412–415.
475. van Beurden M, ten Kate FW, Tjong-A-Hung SP, et al: Human papillomavirus DNA in multicentric vulvar intraepithelial neoplasia. Int J Gynecol Pathol 1998; 17:12–16.
476. McIntosh DG: Pap smear screening after hysterectomy. Compr Ther 1998; 24:14–18.
477. Davila RM, Miranda MC: Vaginal intraepithelial neoplasia and the Pap smear. Acta Cytol 2000; 44:137–140.
478. DePasquale SE, McGuinness TB, Mangan CE, et al: Adenoid cystic carcinoma of Bartholin's gland: a review of the literature and report of a patient. Gynecol Oncol 1996; 61:122–125.
479. Joseph RE, Enghardt MH, Doering DL, et al: Small cell neuroendocrine carcinoma of the vagina. Cancer 1992; 70:784–789.
480. Lee RB, Buttoni L Jr, Dhru K, et al: Malignant melanoma of the vagina: a case report of progression from preexisting melanosis. Gynecol Oncol 1984; 19:238–245.
481. Kerley SW, Blute ML, Keeney GL: Multifocal malignant melanoma arising in vesicovaginal melanosis. Arch Pathol Lab Med 1991; 115:950–952.
482. Sopracordevole F, Parin A, Scarabelli C, et al: Laser surgery in the conservative management of vaginal intraepithelial neoplasms. Minerva Ginecol 1998; 50:507–512.
483. Stock RG, Chen AS, Seski J: A 30-year experience in the management of primary carcinoma of the vagina: analysis of prognostic factors and treatment modalities. Gynecol Oncol 1995; 56:45–52.
484. Irvin WP Jr, Bliss SA, Rice LW, et al: Malignant melanoma of the vagina and locoregional control: radical surgery revisited. Gynecol Oncol 1998; 71:476–480.
485. Prévot S, Hugol D, Audouin J, et al: Primary non-Hodgkin's malignant lymphoma of the vagina: report on three cases and review of the literature. Pathol Res Pract 1992; 188:78–85.
486. Perren T, Farrant M, McCarthy K, et al: Lymphomas of the cervix and upper vagina: a report of five cases and a review of the literature. Gynecol Oncol 1992; 44:87–95.
487. Woodburn R, Randall ME: Advances in gynecologic radiation oncology. Curr Opin Oncol 1997; 9:471–477.
488. Perez CA, Gersell DJ, McGuire WP, et al: Vagina. In: Hoskins WJ, Perez CA, Young RC (eds): Principles and Practice of Gynecologic Oncology, 2nd ed, pp 753–784. Philadelphia, Lippincott-Raven, 1997.
489. Perez CA, Grigsby PW, Garipagaoglu M, et al: Factors affecting long-term outcome of irradiation in carcinoma of the vagina. Int J Radiat Oncol Biol Phys 1999; 44:37–45.
490. MacLeod C, Fowler A, Dalrymple C, et al: High-dose-rate brachytherapy in the management of high-grade intraepithelial neoplasia of the vagina. Gynecol Oncol 1997; 65:74–77.
491. Ogino I, Kitamura T, Okajima H, et al: High-dose-rate intracavitary brachytherapy in the management of cervical and vaginal intraepithelial neoplasia. Int J Radiat Oncol Biol Phys 1999; 40:881–887.
492. Nag S, Martinez-Monge R, Selman AE, et al: Interstitial brachytherapy in the management of primary carcinoma of the cervix and vagina. Gynecol Oncol 1998; 70:27–32.
493. Charra C, Roy P, Coquard R, et al: Outcome of treatment of upper third vaginal recurrences of cervical and endometrial carcinomas with interstitial brachytherapy. Int J Radiat Oncol Biol Phys 1998; 40:421–426.
494. Long HJ III, Cross WG, Wieand HS, et al: Phase II trial of methotrexate, vinblastine, doxorubicin, and cisplatin in advanced/recurrent carcinoma of the uterine cervix and vagina. Gynecol Oncol 1995; 57:235–239.
495. Behbakht K, Massad LS, Yordan EL, et al: A bleomycin/ifosfamide/cisplatin regimen exhibits poor activity against persistent or recurrent squamous gynecologic cancers. Eur J Gynaecol Oncol 1996; 17:7–12.
496. Zanetta G, Lissoni A, Gabriele A, et al: Intense neoadjuvant chemotherapy with cisplatin and epirubicin for advanced or bulky cervical and vaginal adenocarcinoma. Gynecol Oncol 1997; 64:431–435.
497. Muss HB, Bundy BN, Christopherson WA: Mitoxantrone in the treatment of advanced vulvar and vaginal carcinoma: a Gynecologic Oncology Group study. Am J Clin Oncol 1989; 12:142–144.
498. Roberts WS, Hoffman MS, Kavanagh JJ, et al: Further experience with radiation therapy and concomitant intravenous chemotherapy in advanced carcinoma of the lower female genital tract. Gynecol Oncol 1991; 43:233–236.
499. Mundt AJ, Rotmensch J, Waggoner S, et al: Phase I trial of concomitant chemoradiotherapy for cervical cancer and other advanced pelvic malignancies. Gynecol Oncol 1999; 72:45–50.
500. Raney RB Jr, Gehan EA, Hays DM, et al: Primary chemotherapy with or without radiation therapy and/or surgery for children with localized sarcoma of the bladder, prostate, vagina, uterus, and cervix: A comparison of the results in Intergroup Rhabdomyosarcoma Studies I and II. Cancer 1990; 60:2072–2081.
501. Andrassy RJ, Wiener ES, Raney RB, et al: Progress in the surgical management of vaginal rhabdomyosarcoma: a 25-year review from the Intergroup Rhabdomyosarcoma Study Group. J Pediatr Surg 1999; 34:731–734.
502. Hoffman MS, DeCesare SL, Roberts WS, et al: Upper vaginectomy for *in situ* and occult, superficially invasive carcinoma of the vagina. Am J Obstet Gynecol 1992; 166:30–33.
503. Lee WR, Marcus RB Jr, Sombeck MD, et al: Radiotherapy alone for carcinoma of the vagina: the importance of overall treatment time. Int J Radiat Oncol Biol Phys 1994; 29:983–988.
504. Creasman WT, Phillips JL, Menck HR: The National Cancer Data Base report on cancer of the vagina. Cancer 1998; 83:1033–1040.
505. Perez CA, Garipagaoglu M: Vagina. In: Perez CA, Brady LW (eds): Principles and Practice of Radiation Oncology, 3rd ed, pp 1891–1914. Philadelphia, Lippincott-Raven, 1998.
506. Chyle V, Zagars GK, Wheeler JA, et al: Definitive radiotherapy for carcinoma of the vagina: outcome and prognostic factors. Int J Radiat Oncol Biol Phys 1996; 35:891–905.
507. Peters WA, Kumar NB, Morley GW: Carcinoma of the vagina: factors influencing outcome. Cancer 1985; 55:892–897.
508. Stock RG, Mychalczak B, Armstrong JG, et al: The importance of brachytherapy technique in the management of primary carcinoma of the vagina. Int J Radiat Oncol Biol Phys 1992; 24:747–753.
509. Leung S, Sexton M: Radical radiation therapy for carcinoma of the vagina: impact of treatment modalities on outcome: Peter MacCallum Cancer Institute experience 1970–1990. Int J Radiat Oncol Biol Phys 1993; 25:413–418.
510. Berchuck A, Rodriguez G, Kamel A, et al: Expression of epidermal growth factor receptor and HER-2/neu in normal and neoplastic cervix, vulva, and vagina. Obstet Gynecol 1990; 76:381–387.

Vulvar Carcinoma

511. Thomas GM, Dembo AJ, Bryson CP, et al: Changing concepts in the management of vulvar cancer. Gynecol Oncol 1991; 42:9–21.
512. Hacker NF: Radical resection of vulvar malignancies: a paradigm shift in surgical approaches. Curr Opin Obstet Gynecol 1999; 11:61–64.
513. Giles GG, Kneale BL: Vulvar cancer: the Cinderella of gynaecological oncology. Austral N Z J Obstet Gynaecol 1995; 35:71–75.
514. Jones RW, Baranyai J, Stables S: Trends in squamous cell carcinoma of the vulva: the influence of vulvar intraepithelial neoplasia. Obstet Gynecol 1997; 90:448–452.
515. Ansink AC, Heintz AP: Epidemiology and etiology of squamous cell carcinoma of the vulva. Eur J Obstet Gynecol Reprod Biol 1993; 48:111–115.
516. Trimble CL, Hildesheim A, Brinton LA, et al: Heterogenous etiology of squamous carcinoma of the vulva. Obstet Gynecol 1996; 87:59–64.
517. Hildesheim A, Han CL, Brinton LA, et al: Human papillomavirus type 16 and risk of preinvasive and invasive vulvar cancer: results from a seroepidemiological case-control study. Obstet Gynecol 1997; 90:748–754.
518. Madeleine MM, Daling JR, Carter JJ, et al: Cofactors with human papillomavirus in a population-based study of vulvar cancer. J Natl Cancer Inst 1997; 89:1516–1523.
519. Basta A, Adamek K, Pitynski K: Intraepithelial neoplasia and early stage vulvar cancer: Epidemiological, clinical and virological observations. Eur J Gynaecol Oncol 1999; 20:111–114.
520. Kurman RJ, Trimble CL, Shah KV: Human papillomavirus and the pathogenesis of vulvar carcinoma. Curr Opin Obstet Gynecol 1992; 4:582–585.
521. Iwasawa A, Nieminen P, Lehtinen M, et al: Human papillomavirus in squamous cell carcinoma of the vulva by polymerase chain reaction. Obstet Gynecol 1997; 89:81–84.
522. Mitchell MF, Prasad CJ, Silva EG, et al: Second genital primary squamous neoplasms in vulvar carcinoma: viral and histopathologic correlates. Obstet Gynecol 1993; 81:13–18.
523. Perez CA, Grigsby PW, Chao KSC, et al: Vulva. In: Perez CA, Brady LW (eds): Principles and Practice of Radiation Oncology, 3rd ed, pp 1915–1942. Philadelphia, Lippincott-Raven, 1998.
524. Taylor PT Jr: Biopsy of lesions of the female genital tract. Surg Oncol Clin North Am 1995; 4:121–135.
525. Heinzl S: The value of colposcopy in assessment of intraepithelial neoplasia of the lower genital tract. Arch Gynecol Obstet 1995; 257; 425–430.
526. Joura EA, Zeisler H, Losch A, et al: Differentiating vulvar intraepithelial neoplasia from nonneoplastic epithelial disorders: the toluidine blue test. J Reprod Med 1998; 43:671–674.
527. Ragnarsson-Olding BK, Kanter-Lewensohn LR, Lagerlof B, et al: Malignant melanoma of the vulva in a nationwide, 25-year study of 219 Swedish females: clinical observations and histopathologic features. Cancer 1999; 86:1273–1284.
528. Shepherd JH: Revised FIGO staging for gynecological cancer. Br J Obstet Gynaecol 1989; 96:889–892.
529. Creasman WT: New gynecologic cancer staging. Obstet Gynecol 1990; 75:287–288.
530. Cavanagh D: Vulvar cancer: continuing evolution in management. Gynecol Oncol 1997; 66:362–367.
531. Burke TW, Eifel PJ, McGuire WP, et al: Vulva. In: Hoskins WJ, Perez CA, Young RC (eds): Principles and Practice of Gynecologic Oncology, 2nd ed, pp 717–752. Philadelphia, Lippincott-Raven, 1997.
532. Ayhan A, Tuncer ZS, Dogan L, et al: Skinning vulvectomy for the treatment of vulvar intraepithelial neoplasia 2–3: a study of 21 cases. Eur J Gynaecol Oncol 1998; 19:508–510.
533. Chafe W, Richards A, Morgan L, et al: Unrecognized invasive carcinoma in vulvar intraepithelial neoplasia (VIN). Gynecol Oncol 1988; 31:154–162.
534. Sideri M, Spinaci L, Spolti N, et al: Evaluation of CO_2 laser excision or vaporization for the treatment of vulvar intraepithelial neoplasia. Gynecol Oncol 1999; 75:277–281.
535. Anderson JM, Cassady JR, Shimm DS, et al: Vulvar carcinoma. Int J Radiat Oncol Biol Phys 1995; 32:1351–1357.
536. Burger MP, Hollema H, Emanuels AG, et al: The importance of the groin node status for the survival of T1 and T2 vulval carcinoma patients. Gynecol Oncol 1995; 57:327–334.
537. Farias-Eisner R, Cirisano FD, Grouse FD, et al: Conservative and individualized surgery for early squamous carcinoma of the vulva: the treatment of choice for stage I and II (T1-2N0-1M0) disease. Gynecol Oncol 1994; 53:55–58.
538. Carramaschi F, Ramos ML, Nisida AC, et al: V-Y flap for perineal reconstruction following modified approach to vulvectomy in vulvar cancer. Int J Gynaecol Obstet 1999; 65:157–163.
539. Magrina JF, Gonzalez-Bosquet J, Weaver AL, et al: Squamous cell carcinoma of the vulva, stage IA: long-term results. Gynecol Oncol 2000; 76:24–27.
540. Gomez Rueda N, Vighi S, Garcia A, et al: Histologic predictive factors: Therapeutic impact in vulvar cancer. J Reprod Med 1994; 39:71–76.
541. Hicks ML, Hempling RE, Piver MS: Vulvar carcinoma with 0.5 mm of invasion and associated inguinal lymph node metastasis. J Surg Oncol 1993; 54:271–273.
542. Kumar PP, Good RR, Scott JC: Techniques for management of vulvar cancer by irradiation alone. Radiat Med 1988; 6:185–191.
543. Perez CA, Grigsby PW, Galakatos A, et al: Radiation therapy in management of carcinoma of the vulva with emphasis on conservation therapy. Cancer 1993; 71:3707–3716.
544. Boronow RC, Hickman BT, Regan MT, et al: Combined therapy as an alternative to exenteration for locally advanced vulvovaginal cancer. II. Results, complications, and dosimetric and surgical considerations. Am J Clin Oncol (CCT) 1987; 10:171–181.
545. Hacker NF: Current management of early vulvar cancer. Ann Acad Med Singapore 1998; 27:688–692.
546. Morgan MA, Mikuta JJ: Surgical management of vulvar cancer. Semin Surg Oncol 1999; 17:168–172.
547. Kucera H, Vavra N, Kucera E: Inguinal irradiation versus no lymph node therapy in small vulvar carcinoma with clinically negative lymph nodes (T1, N0-1). Gynakol Geburtshilfliche Rundsch 1995; 35:209–214.
548. Manavi M, Berger A, Kucera E, et al: Does T1, N0-1 vulvar cancer treated by vulvectomy but not lymphadenectomy need inguinofemoral radiation? Int J Radiat Oncol Biol Phys 1997; 38:749–753.
549. Faul CM, Mirmow D, Huang O, et al: Adjuvant radiation for vulvar carcinoma: improved local control. Int J Radiat Oncol Biol Phys 1997; 38:381–389.
550. Lupi G, Raspagliesi F, Zucali R, et al: Combined preoperative chemoradiotherapy followed by radical surgery in locally advanced vulvar carcinoma: A pilot study. Cancer 1996; 77:1472–1478.
551. Cunningham MJ, Goyer RP, Gibbons SK, et al: Primary radiation, cisplatin, and 5-fluorouracil for advanced squamous carcinoma of the vulva. Gynecol Oncol 1997; 66:258–261.
552. Moore DH, Thomas GM, Montana GS, et al: Preoperative chemoradiation for advanced vulvar cancer: a phase II study of the Gynecologic Oncology Group. Int J Radiat Oncol Biol Phys 1998; 42:79–85.
553. Grigsby PW, Graham MV, Perez CA, et al: Prospective phase I/II studies of definitive irradiation and chemotherapy for advanced gynecologic malignancies. Am J Clin Oncol 1996; 19:1–6.
554. Snijders-Keilholz T, Trimbos JB, Hermans J, et al: Management of vulvar carcinoma radiation toxicity: results and failure analysis in 44 patients (1980–1989). Acta Obstet Gynecol Scand 1993; 72:668–673.
555. Mariani L, Lombardi A, Atlante M, et al: Radiotherapy for vulvar carcinoma with positive inguinal nodes: adjunctive treatment. J Reprod Med 1993; 38:429–436.
556. Stehman FB, Bundy BN, Thomas G, et al: Groin dissection versus groin radiation in carcinoma of the vulva: a Gynecologic Oncology Group study. Int J Radiat Oncol Biol Phys 1992; 24:389–396.
557. Petereit DG, Mehta MP, Buchler DA, et al: Inguinofemoral radiation of N0, N1 vulvar cancer may be equivalent to lymphadenectomy if proper radiation technique is used. Int J Radiat Oncol Biol Phys 1993; 27:963–967.
558. Perez CA, Grigsby PW, Chao KSC, et al: Irradiation in carcinoma of the vulva: factors affecting outcome. Int J Radiat Oncol Biol Phys 1998; 42:335–344.
559. Pohar S, Hoffstetter S, Peiffert D, et al: Effectiveness of brachytherapy in treating carcinoma of the vulva. Int J Radiat Oncol Biol Phys 1995; 32:1455–1460.
560. Thomas G, Dembo A, DePetrillo A, et al: Concurrent radiation and chemotherapy in vulvar carcinoma. Gynecol Oncol 1989; 34:263–267.
561. Russell AH, Mesic JB, Scudder SA, et al: Synchronous radiation and

cytotoxic chemotherapy for locally advanced or recurrent squamous cancer of the vulva. Gynecol Oncol 1992; 47:14–20.

562. Scheistroen M, Trope C: Combined bleomycin and irradiation in preoperative treatment of advanced squamous cell carcinoma of the vulva. Acta Oncol 1993; 32:657–661.
563. Wahlen SA, Slater JD, Wagmer RJ, et al: Concurrent radiation therapy and chemotherapy in the treatment of primary squamous cell carcinoma of the vulva. Cancer 1995; 75:2289–2294.
564. Garcia Iglesias A, Tejerizo Lopez LC, Garcia Sanchez MH, et al: Prognosis factors in cancer of the vulva. Eur J Gynaecol Oncol 1993; 14:386–391.
565. van der Velden J, Hacker NF: Prognostic factors in squamous cell cancer of the vulva and the implications for treatment. Curr Opin Obstet Gynecol 1996; 8:3–7.
566. Malfetano JH, Piver S, Tsukada Y, et al: Univariate and multivariate analyses of 5-year survival, recurrence, and inguinal node metastases in stage I and II vulvar carcinoma. J Surg Oncol 1985; 30:124–131.
567. Woolcott RJ, Henry RJW, Houghton CRS: Malignant melanoma of the vulva. J Reprod Med 1988; 33:699–702.
568. Ayhan A, Tuncer R, Tuncer ZS, et al: Risk factors for groin metastasis in squamous carcinoma of the vulva: a multivariate analysis of 39 cases. Eur J Obstet Gynecol Reprod Biol 1993; 48:33–36.
569. Origoni M, Sideri M, Garsia S, et al: Prognostic value of pathological patterns of lymph node positivity in squamous cell carcinoma of the vulva, stage III and IVA FIGO. Gynecol Oncol 1992; 45:313–316.
570. van der Velden J, van Lindert AC, Lammes FB, et al: Extracapsular growth of lymph node metastases in squamous cell carcinoma of the vulva: the impact on recurrence and survival. Cancer 1995; 75:2885–2890.
571. Kurzl R, Messerer D: Prognostic factors in squamous cell carcinoma of the vulva: a multivariate analysis. Gynecol Oncol 1989; 32:143–150.
572. Heaps JM, Fu YS, Montz FJ, et al: Surgical-pathologic variables predictive of local recurrence in squamous cell carcinoma of the vulva. Gynecol Oncol 1990; 38:309–314.
573. Reedy MB, Capen CV, Baker DP, et al: Hyperbaric oxygen therapy following radical vulvectomy: an adjunctive therapy to improve wound healing. Gynecol Oncol 1994; 53:13–16.
574. van Lindert AC, Symons EA, Damen BF, et al: Wound healing after radical vulvectomy and inguino-femoral lymphadenectomy: experience with granulocyte colony stimulating factor (filgastrim, r-metHuG-CSF). Eur J Obstet Gynecol Reprod Biol 1995; 62:217–219.
575. Slavin JD Jr, Engin IO, Spencer RP, et al: "Elephantine" calf swelling after groin resection and radiation therapy for vulvar carcinoma. Clin Nucl Med 1999; 24:278–279.
576. Grigsby PW, Roberts HL, Perez CA: Femoral neck fracture following groin irradiation. Int J Radiat Oncol Biol Phys 1995; 32:63–67.

22 *Urologic and Male Genital Cancers*

MACK ROACH III, MD, Radiation Oncology, Medical Oncology, and Urology
ERIC SMALL, MD, Medical Oncology and Urology
DAVID M. REESE, MD, Medical Oncology and Urology
PETER CARROLL, MD, Urology

He who masters the two sciences of the pulse and the urine will possess almost all that is necessary for diagnosis and prognosis. Conversely, he who knows only one of these two sciences will be prone to a thousand errors, for in the study of disease, the science of urine is as valuable as that of the pulse.

JOHANNES ACUTARIUS

Perspective

Since the last edition of this textbook was released, there have been a number of advances in the management of urologic malignancies. The use of modern surgical techniques has resulted in a reduction in morbidity, including impotence, incontinence, infection, and blood loss, as well as a reduction in the duration of hospitalization and the costs associated with radical prostatectomies. Also, improved computer-based imaging and delivery systems have allowed for the more accurate administration of higher doses of radiation with reduced toxicity. In addition, radioactive seed implants have begun to gain widespread popularity with the hope of further reducing morbidity while delivering higher doses of radiation.

The recognition of the high rate of failure among patients with high-grade prostate cancer who have been treated with surgery or radiation alone has prompted studies including combined-modality therapy. Using data from these trials, we have learned how to predict the risk of death as a result of prostate cancer at 5, 10, and 15 years with radiation therapy alone. More importantly, we now can define the subsets of patients who would benefit from the use of either short-term or long-term hormonal therapy combined with radiation therapy. Prospective trials have also tested the use of neoadjuvant hormonal therapy before surgery in an attempt to address this group of patients. Unfortunately, all of these trials have shown negative results in terms of improvement in survival rate thus far. This may reflect differences in patient selection, but further studies are required to resolve this question.

Progress has also been made in our understanding of other urologic tumors. Renal tumors, previously believed to be resistant to chemotherapy, have begun to respond to biologic response modifiers. Tumor markers, such as p53, have been validated as important factors for patients with bladder cancer, and the incorporation of these markers into the management of patients will surely form the basis for further studies. For the first time, gene therapy has been shown to be feasible. For these reasons and more, the future of the treatment of urologic tumors is bright.

Kidney Cancer

Epidemiology and Etiology

Epidemiology

It is estimated that there were 31,200 new cases of kidney cancer in the United States in the year 2000 and 11,900 deaths from the disease.[5] Approximately 85% of malignant kidney tumors are adenocarcinomas (renal cell carcinoma [RCC]). It should be noted that the incidence of RCC is higher in developed countries; rates in the United States have increased approximately 2% per year since 1970.

RCC most commonly occurs in adults between the ages of 50 and 70 years, although cases in children and infants have been reported.[6] The current male-to-female ratio is 1:4.

Etiology

The cause of RCC is unknown. However, smoking is a major identified risk factor and confers a two-fold elevation in relative risk for the development of the disease. Other risk factors include obesity (especially in females), hypertension, analgesic abuse, and acquired cystic kidney disease in dialysis patients. Specific dietary factors or exposure to radiation have not been consistently linked to an increased risk, although consumption of fruits and vegetables may be protective.[7] Exposure to asbestos or cadmium has been associated with the development of RCC in some series.

Patients with von Hippel–Lindau syndrome have a 40% chance of developing RCC. Mutations in the *VHL1* tumor suppressor gene, located on chromosome 3p25, are associated with this syndrome and the development of sporadic RCC, in particular the clear cell type.[8] Other heritable syndromes associated with RCC include tuberous sclerosis and polycystic kidney disease. In addition to the *VHL1* gene, additional loci on chromosome 3p may be involved in the development and progression of RCC.[9] Other potential pathogenetic alterations in RCC include overexpression of growth factors and their receptors, alterations in cell cycle proteins, and expression of angiogenesis factors.

Detection and Diagnosis

Clinical Detection

Owing to its protean clinical signs and symptoms, RCC has been called the *internist's tumor.* However, small tumors rarely produce symptoms and the diagnosis is often delayed until the disease is advanced. The most common clinical presentations include hematuria (50% to 60%), abdominal or flank pain (40%), and a palpable mass (30% to 40%). This classic triad occurs as a combination in less than 10% of patients. RCC is increasingly being diagnosed as an incidental kidney mass (20% to 40% of patients), owing to the widespread use of computed tomography (CT), magnetic resonance imaging (MRI), and ultrasonography for other indications.[10]

Approximately 30% of patients will have detectable metastases at the time of initial presentation, and they may have symptoms referable to organ involvement. The most common sites of metastasis are lung (50% to 60%), bone (30% to 40%), liver (30% to 40%), and brain (5% to 10%).[11] RCC may metastasize to virtually any site, however, including the thyroid, skin, vagina, pancreas, retina, prostate, and skeletal muscle.[12]

Paraneoplastic Syndromes

A large number of paraneoplastic syndromes have been associated with RCC, including hypercalcemia (owing to tumor production of parathyroid hormone–related protein), fever, erythrocytosis (owing to tumor erythropoietin production), hepatic dysfunction in the absence of metastases (Stauffer's syndrome), amyloidosis, and dermatomyositis.[13] In addition, anemia occurs in 20% to 30% of patients with newly diagnosed RCC.

Diagnostic Procedures

- *Urinalysis* discloses microscopic hematuria in more than half of RCC cases, but this finding is nonspecific.
- *Urine cytology* has a low yield.

Imaging

Intravenous urography, angiography, ultrasonography, and CT scanning are all used to evaluate renal masses.

- *CT scan* is the most sensitive and specific of these imaging techniques, with 90% accuracy in defining tumor extent.[14]
- *Ultrasonography* is most helpful in differentiating solid from cystic lesions.
- *Angiography* is used selectively to assess tumor vascularity before embolization or nephron-sparing surgery.
- *MRI* can be used to determine the extent of inferior vena cava involvement[15]; it is particularly useful in patients allergic to contrast material.

The diagnosis of RCC is often made on clinical grounds, but it ultimately requires obtaining tissue, which is usually performed at surgery for localized tumors. In general, all masses that are potentially RCC should be resected. CT- or ultrasound-guided fine-needle aspiration biopsy and core biopsy may be useful, but making a definitive diagnosis on the basis of cytology alone is often difficult. Simple cysts, angiomyolipomas, and renal pseudotumors have characteristic radiologic appearances, and they do not require a tissue diagnosis because of the sensitivity and specificity of imaging, unless the diagnosis is in doubt.

Classification and Staging

Histopathology

Most RCCs arise from the renal cortex and originate in the proximal convoluted tubule cell. They have traditionally been classified according to cell type (clear, granular, or spindle) and growth pattern (acinar, papillary, or sarcomatoid), with the clear cell type accounting for 75% of cases. In 1997, an international consensus conference developed a classification system that divides renal cell carcinomas into the following categories:

- conventional (clear cell) (70%)
- papillary (10% to 15%)
- chromophobe (5%)
- collecting duct (<1%)
- unclassified (5%)

These categories constitute the preferred histopathologic classification system.[16]

Tumors smaller than 3 cm have sometimes been called renal adenomas, but the biologic distinction (if any) between these lesions and carcinomas is unclear, and they should be managed in a similar fashion to larger cancers. Other unusual malignant tumors of the kidney include neuroendocrine neoplasms, juxtaglomerular cell tumors, sarcomas, and lymphomas. Transitional cell tumors of the renal pelvis are similar to cancers of the bladder, ureter, and urethra. Oncocytomas are uncommon benign tumors with a characteristic radiologic, gross, and histologic appearance. Angiomyolipomas, leiomyomas, and lipomas represent other benign kidney tumors that are very uncommon.

Staging

The tumor, node, metastasis (TNM) system has been revised for renal cell carcinoma (Figure 22–1 and Table 22–1).[17, 18] T1 and T2 tumors are defined on the basis of size, but both are limited to the kidney. T3 tumors invade the adrenal gland, perinephric tissue, or the renal vein or vena cava below the level of the diaphragm, whereas T4 tumors extend beyond Gerota's fascia. Regional lymph nodes are no longer classified on the basis of size but on the number of nodes involved.

The stage groupings of the new classification system have changed because of the above-mentioned changes in the T and N categories (see Table 22–1). Stage I and II tumors are T1 and T2 cancers without nodal disease, whereas stage III tumors may be T1 to T3 lesions with a single (N1) involved regional lymph node. Stage IV tumors are either locally extensive (T4), have multiple involved regional nodes (N2), or distant metastases (M1).

The primary goals of the staging evaluation are to define the local disease extent for potential surgical resection and to evaluate the patient for the presence of metastases. Laboratory tests are useful to evaluate organ function and diagnose possible paraneoplastic syndromes:

- *Standard blood tests* include a complete blood count, electrolytes, blood urea nitrogen, creatinine, liver enzymes, alkaline phosphatase, and serum calcium.
- *CT scan* of the abdomen and pelvis is generally the imaging modality of choice because it defines tumor size, extrarenal tumor extension, regional adenopathy, and possible vascular invasion. *MRI* is superior, however, in defining the extent of vena cava involvement and tumor extension into the liver.
- *Chest x-ray film or CT scan* is obtained to evaluate possible lung metastases.
- *Bone scan* is usually obtained if potentially curative nephrectomy is planned or the patient has bony pain, an elevated alkaline phosphatase, or known metastases in other sites.

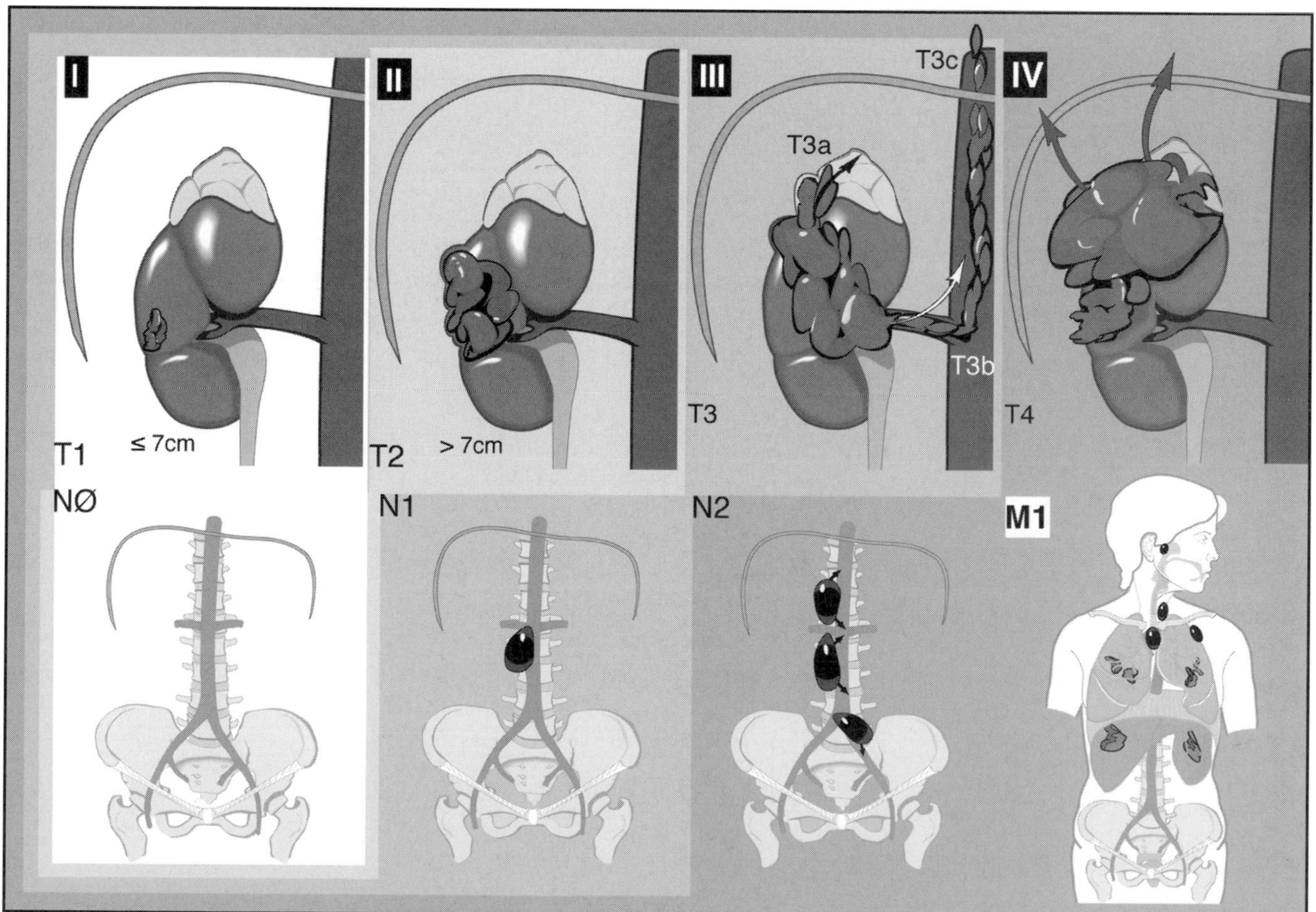

Figure 22–1. Anatomic staging for renal cell carcinoma (see Table 22–1).

TABLE 22–1. **Staging Table for Renal Cell Carcinoma**

Stage	Grouping	Descriptor
I	T1 N0 M0	T1: Tumor ≤7 cm in greatest dimension, limited to kidney N0: No regional lymph node metastasis M0: No distant metastasis
II	T2 N0 M0	T2: Tumor >7 cm in greatest dimension, limited to kidney
III	T1,2 N1 M0	N1: Metastasis in single regional lymph node
	T3a N0,N1 M0	T3a: Tumor invades adrenal gland or perinephritic tissues; not beyond Gerota's fascia
	T3b N0,1 M0	T3b: Tumor grossly extends into renal veins or vena cava below diaphragm
	T3c N0,1 M0	T3c: Tumor grossly extends into renal veins or vena cava above diaphragm
IV	T4 N0,1 M0	T4: Tumor invades Gerota's fascia
	Any T N2 M0	N2: Metastases in more than 1 regional lymph node
	Any T Any N M1	M1: Distant metastasis

TX: primary tumor cannot be assessed; T0: no evidence of primary tumor.
Used with permission of the American Joint Committee on Cancer (AJCC®), Chicago, Illinois. The original source for this material is the AJCC® Cancer Staging Manual, 5th ed, 1997, published by Lippincott-Raven Publishers, Philadelphia, Pennsylvania.

- Occasionally useful tests include an *arteriograph* and *venacavogram.*

Principles of Treatment

The natural history of RCC can be unpredictable. It is one of the rare solid tumors that is capable of growing to a massive size without metastasizing, yet metastases may occur from tumors less than 3 cm in size. Despite these extremes of tumor behavior, some general observations can be made (Table 22–2).

In the vast majority of patients with locally advanced or metastatic disease, tumor progression (and, ultimately, patient death) will occur if the cancer is left untreated. In addition, no known therapy is consistently curative for metastatic RCC, although rare patients who are treated with immunotherapy may have longlasting complete responses (cure). These results are confounded by the possibility of spontaneous regression of metastatic RCC occurring after resection of the primary tumor. In the past, it was presumed that spontaneous regression was quite rare (<1% of patients),[19] but recent placebo-controlled trials of new immunotherapeutic agents have documented complete responses in up to 3% of patients treated with placebo,[20, 21] suggesting that spontaneous tumor regression may be more common than realized. These observations must be kept in mind when evaluating new therapeutics for RCC.

The prognosis for patients with RCC is related to both tumor and host factors. Important patient-related adverse prognostic factors include poor performance status, presence of symptoms, such as pain or anorexia, and significant weight loss. In addition, the presence of hypercalcemia, an elevated erythrocyte sedimentation rate, and an elevated alkaline phosphatase level correlate with poor outcome. Tumor-related prognostic factors of importance include the tumor stage, grade, histologic type (clear cell and collecting duct carcinomas have a worse prognosis), and for metastatic tumors, number and resectability of metastases.[22] A large number of molecular markers are being evaluated as prognostic factors in RCC, but no markers have consistently demonstrated clinical use.

Surgery

Surgical resection is the only curative therapy for RCC. The cure rate for RCC is highly dependent on the pathologic tumor stage.[23]

- *Radical nephrectomy,* removal of the kidney and Gerota's fascia, is the cornerstone of RCC treatment. This may be performed using a thoracoabdominal, anterior, or extraperitoneal approach, depending on tumor anatomy and the experience of the surgeon. Early ligation of the renal artery and vein are important to prevent tumor embolization.[24]
- *Regional lymphadenectomy* and removal of the ipsilateral adrenal gland are routinely performed and aid in tumor staging, but the evidence is unclear about whether lymphadenectomy improves overall survival. In addition, adrenalectomy may be omitted during radical nephrectomy that is performed for smaller renal

TABLE 22–2. **Multidisciplinary Treatment for Renal Cell Carcinoma**

Stage	Surgery	Radiation Therapy	Chemotherapy
T1/T2 N0 M0	Simple/radical nephrectomy	NR	NR
T3a N0 M0	Radical nephrectomy ± RLND	PRT	Arterial embolization
T3b N0 M0	Radical nephrectomy (including involved veins) ± RLND		IM (αIFN)
Any T N1-3 M0	Radical nephrectomy + RLND	PRT	Arterial embolization IM (αIFN)
T4 N0 M0	Radical nephrectomy	PRT	IM (αIFN)
Any T Any N M1	Palliative resection + radical nephrectomy	PRT	IL-2, αIFN IC I/II
Recurrence	Palliative resection where appropriate	NR, PRT	NR

RLND: regional lymph node dissection; NR: not recommended; PRT: palliative radiation therapy; IM: immunotherapy; IC I/II: investigational clinical trials (phase I/II).

cancers originating in the lower pole, in which the adrenal appears normal both by imaging and intraoperative inspection.

- *Nephron-sparing surgery* (*partial nephrectomy*) may be appropriate in some patients, for example, those with small tumor or indeterminate lesions. In addition, nephron-sparing surgery should be considered in those with single kidneys, bilateral renal cancers, or renal insufficiency. Despite the concern that RCC is often multifocal, local recurrence after partial nephrectomy is rare, occurring in 4.8% to 11.6% of patients who undergo the procedure.[25–27] Not surprisingly, local recurrence is more common in those with higher stage (i.e., T2 or T3) disease compared with those with T1 disease. There appears to be no significant differences in cancer biology or recurrence rates in cancers located peripherally compared with those located centrally.[28]
- *Nephrectomy* is often used as a palliative measure in patients with severe pain, intractable bleeding (hematuria), symptoms as a result of compression of adjacent organs, or heart failure from arteriovenous shunting within the tumor. Such patients, however, are also candidates for angioinfarction.
- The role of nephrectomy in patients who present with metastatic disease is unclear. Advantages of nephrectomy include a reduction in tumor burden, a decrease in the risk of complications during systemic therapy, and the removal of the primary tumor, which could trap trafficking lymphocytes.[29] However, any potential benefits should be balanced against the possible morbidity of surgery and that some patients, despite undergoing nephrectomy, will not receive systemic therapy because of early cancer progression. Some have argued that surgery should follow systemic therapy in those who have responded to it.[30, 31] Performing nephrectomy solely to promote spontaneous regression of metastases is inappropriate, but when it is used to reduce tumor burden, nephrectomy may play a role when systemic immune therapy is planned as part of the overall treatment program.[32]

Radiation Therapy

Radiotherapy has been used both in the preoperative setting and as postoperative adjuvant treatment for patients at high risk of relapse. However, delivery of adequate radiation doses is hampered by the tolerance of the small bowel, stomach, liver, spinal cord, and contralateral kidney. There is a paucity of well-conducted randomized trials evaluating preoperative or postoperative radiotherapy in patients with high-risk (T3, T4, N1–2) tumors, and consequently, adjunctive radiation therapy is not routinely recommended for the treatment of RCC.

Radiation therapy does play a role in the palliative treatment of metastases, particularly those involving the brain or bone. Satisfactory relief of symptoms can usually be obtained in over 50% of patients with symptomatic metastases.[33]

Chemotherapy

The results of using systemic chemotherapy for metastatic RCC have been disappointing.[34] Most single agents that have been examined have not had significant anticancer activity, and the use of single-agent chemotherapy outside of the investigational setting is not justified. Agents that may have modest activity include vinblastine and floxuridine.[35] Because of the poor results with available agents, the study of new drugs and regimens in patients who have not received chemotherapy is appropriate.

Hormonal therapy, in particular progestational agents, has been used to treat metastatic RCC. However, the proportion of patients responding to these maneuvers is low, and if responses do occur, they are generally of short duration.[36]

Biologic Response Modifiers

The occurrence of occasional spontaneous regressions, very late relapses (>10 years) after nephrectomy, and prolonged disease stabilization despite no systemic therapy all suggest that immune factors are capable of regulating tumor growth and metastasis. These observations have led to the intense investigation of the use of immunotherapy for this tumor type in the last decade. Available immunotherapeutic modalities currently can be categorized broadly into three treatment strategies:

Interleukin-2

Interleukin-2 (IL-2) is a naturally occurring hormone that has multiple immunoregulatory properties. IL-2 stimulates and enhances lymphocyte proliferation, enhances lymphocyte cytotoxicity, induces killer cell activity, and induces interferon-γ (γIFN) and tumor necrosis factor (TNF) production. Although it has no direct antitumor activity, IL-2 affects tumor growth by activating lymphoid cells *in vivo,* including killer cells, lymphokine-activated killer cells, and tumor-infiltrating lymphocytes.[37]

IL-2 therapy has been administered in several ways. In the original National Cancer Institute studies, IL-2 was administered in high doses as a short bolus infusion.[38] This regimen requires patient hospitalization and has substantial toxicity, including hypotension and a vascular leak syndrome. In a review of 255 patients treated on seven clinical studies with high-dose IL-2, 5% of patients had a complete response and 9% had a partial response, but the rate of therapy-related deaths was 4%.[39] Therefore, high-dose IL-2 should only be administered by physicians experienced in its use, and careful clinical and hemodynamic monitoring is required.

In an effort to reduce side effects and simplify delivery, IL-2 also has been administered in a low-dose, subcutaneous fashion.[40] Programs have reported response rates comparable to bolus IL-2 and generally result in lower toxicity, but whether durable responses occur with these regimens is not known. There is no generally accepted standard approach to IL-2–based therapy, and further investigation is ongoing, including combining IL-2 with chemotherapeutic agents.

IL-2 also has been combined with other biologically active agents, including interferon-α (αIFN), retinoids, and cellular products, but it does not appear to improve survival rate.[41] These strategies need to be assessed further in clinical studies.

TABLE 22–3. **Five-Year Survival Rates for Radical Nephrectomy Assessed by Robson's Stage**

Reference	Years	*n*	Stage 1	Stage 2	Stage 3 (3A,3B)	Stage 4	All	Notes
Robson et al[48]	1949–1964	88	66	64	42	11	52	Crude
Skinner et al[49]	1935–1965	203	68	50	49	—	57	Crude
Middleton et al[50]	1950–1967	61	59	48	—	—	59	Crude
Waters et al[51]	1957–1977	130	51	59	(53, 12)	0	—	Majority are RN
Boxer et al[52]	1956–1976	96	56	100	50	8	37	RN and PN
Siminovitch et al[53]	1968–1978	175	82	58	(31, 11)	—	—	NED rates
Medeiros et al[54]	1960–1978	121	82	50	46	0	—	90/121 are RN
Selli et al[55]	1970–1981	115	93	63	80	13	73	Includes 20 patients with DM
Giuliani et al[56]	1970–1987	200	80	70	(5, 52)	0–7	—	All RN
Sene et al[57]	1965–1985	155	81	65	39	6	—	
Rabinovitch et al[58]	1978–1988	172	—	—	—	—	87	

RN: radical nephrectomy; PN: partial nephrectomy; NED: no evidence of disease; DM: distant metastases.

From Rabinovitch RA: Renal cell cancer. In Leibel SA, Phillips TL (eds): Textbook of Radiation Oncology, pp 711–724. Philadelphia, W.B. Saunders, 1998, with permission.

Interferon

Interferons have direct tumor antiproliferative activity and modulate host immune responses, including activating mononuclear cells, inducing the expression of major histocompatibility complex antigens, and enhancing cytotoxic lymphocyte activity.[42] αIFN induces responses in approximately 10% of patients with metastatic RCC,[43] with the most common side effects being impairment of performance status and flulike symptoms. γIFN, in contrast, has minimal antitumor activity.[21, 44]

Cellular Therapy

Adoptive immunotherapy is the transfer to the host of cellular products intended to modulate antitumor effects, either directly or indirectly. Clinical trials of adoptive immunotherapy have involved the administration of lymphokine-activated killer cells or tumor-infiltrating lymphocytes in conjunction with cytokines, typically IL-2. However, randomized trials comparing IL-2 alone with IL-2 and cellular products have not demonstrated an improvement in response rates or survival rates.[45, 46] The use of adoptive immunotherapy is an area of active investigation, but it is not yet performed outside the setting of a clinical trial.

Results and Prognosis

The most important factor influencing survival is the pathologic stage of the tumor. Patients with disease confined to the kidney have survival rates of 45% to 90%, whereas those with locally extensive disease have a greater than 50% rate of mortality at 5 years.[47] The 5-year survival rates for a number of clinical trials of patients undergoing nephrectomy are shown in Table 22–3.

Stages I and II

For patients with stage I tumors, 5-year survival rates are 65% to 90%, with very high rates for those with small (<3 cm) tumors. Five-year survival rates for stage II tumors are 45% to 80%. No additional therapy beyond radical nephrectomy is indicated. The majority of recurrences in these patients are distant metastases, typically occurring within 3 years of diagnosis.[58]

Stage III

The outcome for patients with stage III cancers may vary substantially, and survival rates range from 10% to 45%. Patients with tumor invasion into the renal vein or vena cava have an improved prognosis compared with those with nodal metastases.[59] Despite these suboptimal outcomes, adjunctive therapies beyond radical nephrectomy have not improved survival rates, although well-performed trials are lacking.

Stage IV

Five-year survival rates in those with advanced disease remain poor (0% to 10%). The major obstacle to cure is the lack of uniformly effective systemic therapies, and all patients with advanced RCC should be considered candidates for appropriate clinical trials.

Clinical Investigations

Because response rates for available agents remain poor, the continued evaluation of new treatment programs is a high priority for laboratory and clinical investigation in advanced RCC. Gene therapy, novel cytokine treatment strategies, and new chemotherapeutic agents are all being tested, and all patients should be treated in the context of a clinical trial when possible.

Bladder Cancer

Epidemiology and Etiology

Epidemiology

Bladder cancer ranks as the sixth most common cancer and the ninth leading cause of cancer deaths in the United States of America[5]; it is estimated that there were 53,200 new cases of bladder cancer diagnosed in the United States in the year 2000. Roughly 38,300 of these tumors were diagnosed in the male population, compared with 14,900 in the female population, and approximately 8,100 men and 4,100 women were expected to die of bladder cancer. Survival rates tend to be better in men than in women, perhaps because of the infrequency of unexplained bleeding from the genitalia in the male population compared with the female population. Bladder cancer rarely presents before age 40 and the median age at diagnosis is 65 years.

The relatively high survival rate compared with mortality reflects that the majority of these tumors are superficial. In addition, it is commonly believed that the predominance of bladder cancer among men is a result of occupational exposures to industrial carcinogens and a higher incidence of smoking, although some studies question this assertion.[60] Another possible explanation is that being male is a risk factor per se because androgenic hormones appear to stimulate carcinogenesis in bladder tissue, whereas estrogenic hormones block it.[61] Bladder cancer is reported to be nearly twice as common among white men compared with black men, but it is unclear how much of this reflects a failure to make an early diagnosis in black men.

Etiology

Smoking Tobacco

Bladder cancer has been strongly associated with the smoking of tobacco. Nearly one half of the cases occurring in men and one third of the cases occurring in women have been attributed to tobacco use[62]; smoking appears to increase the risk of developing bladder cancer by two to three times the rate in nonsmokers. Smoking black tobacco, unfiltered cigarettes, or more than two packs daily, and early age of smoking appear to confer a much higher risk of developing bladder cancer.[62–67]

Occupational Carcinogens

Numerous occupational factors have been associated with the development of bladder cancer.[68] Most noteworthy of these factors are aromatic amines and polycyclic aromatic hydrocarbons[69]; for example, polycyclic aromatic hydrocarbon exposure resulting from work as a chimney sweep or the production of aluminum and gasoline is associated with a high risk. Exposure to 2-naphthylamine, 4-aminobiphenyl, and benzidine resulting from dyestuff or rubber manufacturing also is strongly associated with the development of bladder cancer,[70] as well as occupations that increase exposure to diesel exhaust, such as truck drivers and delivery workers. Chlorinated aliphatic hydrocarbons (used in dry cleaning and shoe making) and benzenes are two types of solvents commonly associated with bladder cancer.[71, 72]

Dietary and Other Factors

A number of dietary and other factors have been associated with the increased risk of bladder cancer. For example, chlorinated municipal drinking water and water contaminated by fertilizers have been associated with a higher risk.[73, 74] The chronic use of phenacetin, treatment with cyclophosphamide, and radiation exposure all have been implicated as iatrogenic causative agents.[75–77] Some studies also have suggested a modest association between coffee consumption and the risk of bladder cancer.[78, 79] However, most studies have failed to prove an association between coffee or artificial sweeteners and bladder cancer.[80–82]

Schistosoma haematobium is associated with the development of endemic squamous cell carcinoma. This relatively common entity, found in countries such as Egypt, tends to occur 10 to 20 years earlier than transitional cell carcinoma in this country.[83, 84] The mechanism for its ontogeny is unknown but is believed to be related to chronic trauma, although genetic mechanisms are being considered. Similar mechanisms are proposed for patients with chronic urinary tract infections or catheterizations secondary to spinal cord injury.[85, 86]

Detection and Diagnosis

Clinical Detection

Hematuria is the most common presenting sign for patients with bladder cancer.[87] Usually painless, it may sometimes be associated with irritative symptoms, including urgency or burning on urination. Hematuria may be characterized by more than three to five cells per high-power field on microscopy, or it may be grossly evident. With respect to hematuria, there may be a role for screening urine to detect bladder cancer in asymptomatic individuals; however, there have been too few well-performed studies to be certain at this point.[88]

On rare occasions, a diagnosis has been made incidentally as a result of a *transrectal ultrasound* conducted during the assessment or treatment of prostate cancer.

Diagnostic Procedures

Cystoscopic examination with deep biopsies of abnormalities is essential for making the diagnosis and following the progression of bladder cancer.[89] If a lesion is noted, then the patient should undergo a *transurethral resection of bladder* (TURB) to confirm the diagnosis and define the extent of disease. TURB is performed under anesthesia to allow for resection of the visible tumor and sampling of muscle within the area of the tumor. Diagrams of the suspicious areas should be prepared to ensure that the regions previously involved could be monitored for the regrowth or persistence of disease and response to therapy. If a large papillary tumor is found, then multiple resections may be required.

If the tumor appears to be solid or invasive, then a CT scan before the TURB is recommended by some authorities.[89] CT scans of the abdomen and pelvis are frequently used to identify lymph node involvement, as well as bony, hepatic, and drop metastases (Figure 22–2)[90]; occasionally, biopsy of a metastatic focus combined with CT imaging confirms a diagnosis. *Urinary cytology* may be helpful, but it tends only to localize disease to the urinary tract. In addition, urinary cytology has a poor sensitivity for low-grade tumors and is more predictive of the presence of high-grade transitional cell cancer.[91]

Imaging

- *Ultrasonography* may be useful in excluding upper tract disease and distinguishing calcifications and stones from soft-tissue masses. Although ultrasonography can generally detect tumors larger than 1.5 cm, it is not adequate or necessary for staging.
- *Intravenous pyelography* is most useful at defining defects in the calyces and the renal pelvis and for identifying obstruction of ureters. In addition, intravenous pyelograms are used to identify obstruction of the ureters and local extension and to exclude the presence of unexpected pathology. Bladder tumors have similar urographic characteristics to those of the upper urinary tracts (Figure 22–3).
- *CT and MRI scans* can define the pelvic anatomy in some detail, but they are unnecessary for patients with superficial tumors.[89] Kim and coworkers compared the accuracy of contrast material–enhanced CT with MR imaging in the staging of 36 patients with bladder cancer.[92] Images were evaluated in a blinded fashion and staging was found to be correct in 16 of 29 patients (55%) with CT and 27 of 36 patients (75%) with MR imaging. Overstaging was the most common error, and both CT and MR imaging were more accurate for higher staged tumors. In particular, MRI has a relatively high specificity in patients with invasive disease but a very low sensitivity in patients with superficial disease.[92] However, this type of imaging is also critical for the management of patients with locally advanced disease (i.e., T2 to T4).
- *Chest x-ray films* are usually obtained, justified in part by the strong association between smoking and bladder cancer.
- *Bone scans* are probably only indicated for symptomatic disease or in patients with advanced or high-grade disease.[89] However, Davey and colleagues reported their experience with the use of routine bone

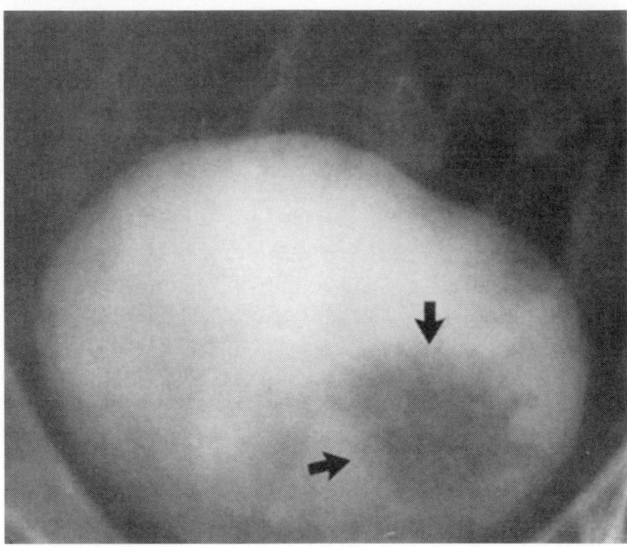

Figure 22–3. A coned view of the bladder from an intravenous urogram, demonstrating a mass lesion as a filling defect *(arrows)* with a frondlike surface representing transitional cell carcinoma of the bladder. (From Badalament RA, Ryan PR, Bahn DK: Imaging for transitional cell carcinomas. In: Vogelzang NJ, Scardino PT, Shipley WU, et al [eds]: Comprehensive Textbook of Genitourinary Oncology, 2nd ed, pp 356–366. Philadelphia, Lippincott Williams & Wilkins, 2000, with permission.)

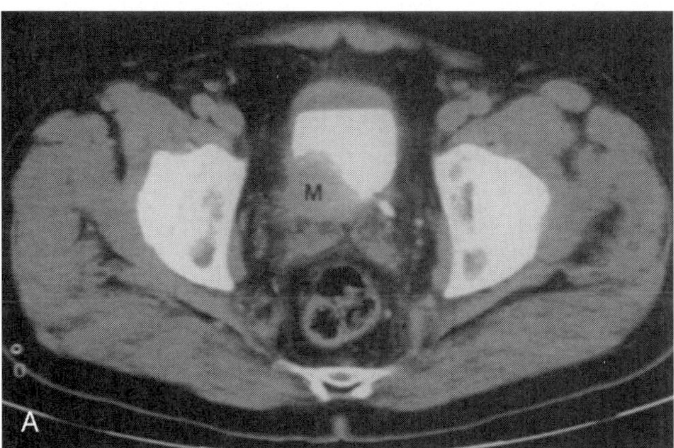

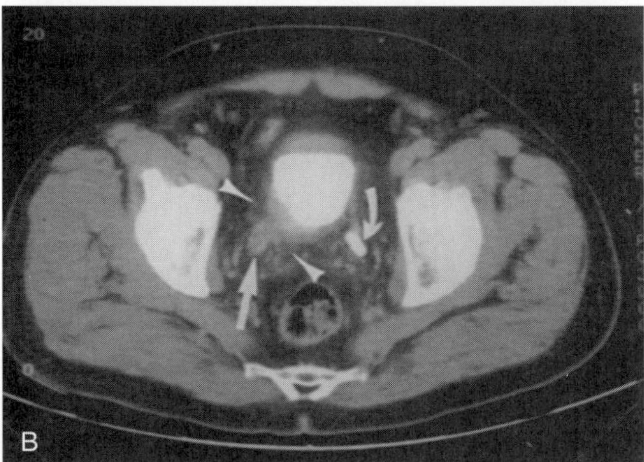

Figure 22–2. (A) Enhanced CT scan of the pelvis, demonstrating a mass lesion (M) from transitional cell carcinoma in the posterior aspect of the bladder in the region of the right ureterovesical orifice. (B) A superior CT section, showing the obstructed ureter *(arrow)* and extension into the perivesicular fat *(arrowheads)*. The normal ureter *(curved arrow)* is seen on the patient's left. (From Badalament RA, Ryan PR, Bahn DK: Imaging for transitional cell carcinomas. In: Vogelzang NJ, Scardino PT, Shipley WU, et al [eds]: Comprehensive Textbook of Genitourinary Oncology, 2nd ed, pp 356–366. Philadelphia, Lippincott Williams & Wilkins, 2000, with permission.)

scintigraphy for staging 221 patients with invasive bladder cancer.[93] The incidence of detectable metastases was 12% and the sensitivity was only 38%.

In general, bone scans (see earlier comments), chest x-ray films, and a complete blood cell count (blood urea nitrogen, creatinine, calcium, and serum alkaline phosphatase) are generally considered baseline studies for patients with invasive disease.

Classification and Staging

Histopathology

- The vast majority of bladder cancers occurring in adults in this country are classified as transitional cell carcinomas (TCC)[68] (Figure 22–4)[94]; in children, rhabdomyosarcomas are the most common. A patient with TCC with areas of squamous or adenocarcinoma is believed to have a similar prognosis to patients with TCC alone. TCCs are usually classified as grade 1 (well differentiated), grade 2 (moderately well differentiated), or grade 3 (poorly differentiated), based on the degree of differentiation.
- Squamous carcinomas (endemic to Egypt) may make up 8% of bladder tumors.
- Adenocarcinomas are the next most common and tend to occur in the urachus or, frequently, the trigone of the bladder.

A variety of other tumor types, including sarcomas, lymphomas, and small cell carcinomas, make up the remaining cases.

Staging

The current American Joint Commission on Cancer (AJCC) TNM staging system is summarized in Table 22–4 and illustrated in Figure 22–5. The stage assigned is dependent on an assessment of the depth of penetration of the bladder wall; management recommendations for bladder cancer are dependent on the stage.[89] As a result of this requirement, muscle *must* be contained in the biopsy specimen for the biopsy to be considered adequate.

Principles of Treatment

Bladder cancer is usually classified as (1) superficial, (2) invasive, or (3) metastatic. At presentation, approximately 75% of cases are superficial, 20% are invasive, and 5% are metastatic.

Superficial bladder cancer, by definition, is confined to the mucosa, and patients are usually controlled for long

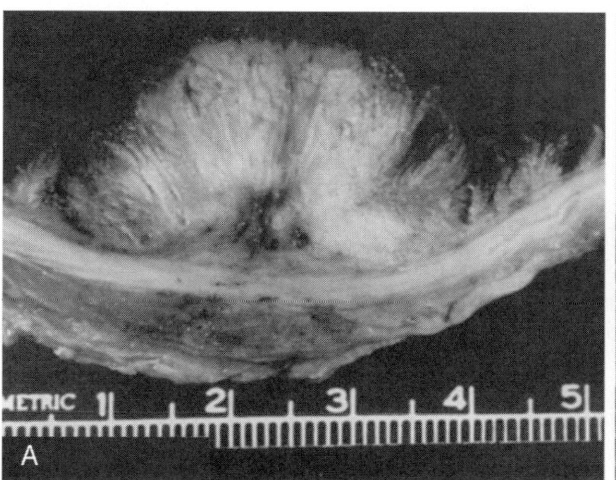

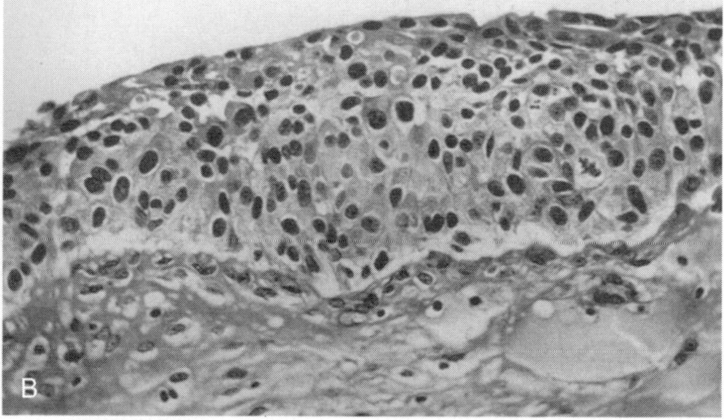

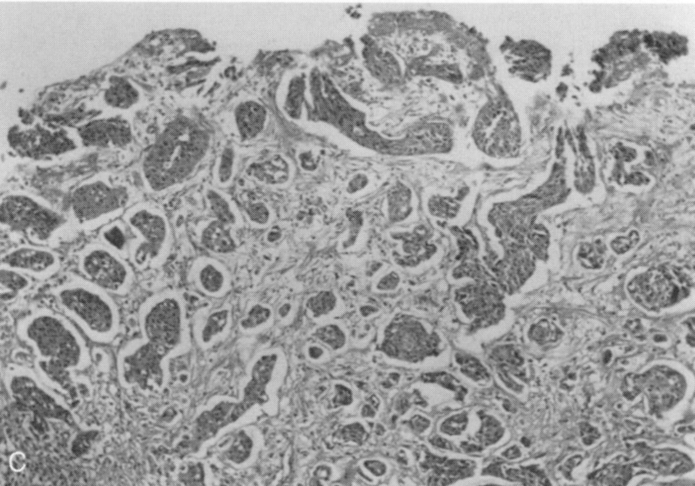

Figure 22–4. Histology of transitional cell carcinomas: (A) A papillary noninvasive transitional cell carcinoma. (B) A transitional cell carcinoma *in situ*. There is marked variability in size of the nuclei, which are hyperchromatic and exhibit loss of polarity. (C) Invasive transitional cell carcinoma. The tumor cells are growing in irregular clusters of varying sizes and shapes, and as single cells in a focally desmoplastic stroma. (From Holzbeierlein JM, Smith JA Jr: Natural history and surgical management. In: Vogelzang NJ, Scardino PT, Shipley WU, et al [eds]: Comprehensive Textbook of Genitourinary Oncology, 2nd ed, pp 384–394. Philadelphia, Lippincott Williams & Wilkins, 2000, with permission.)

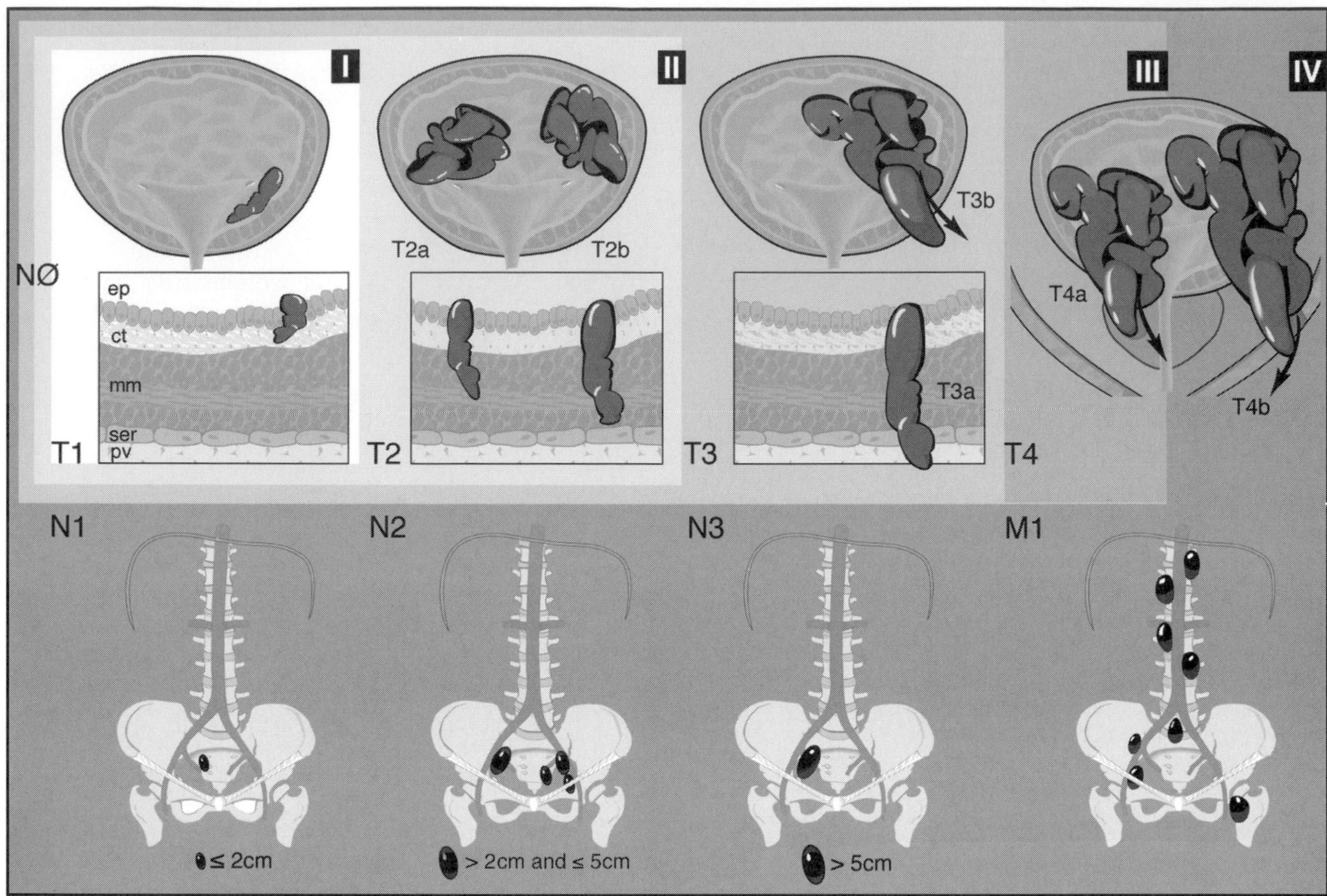

Figure 22–5. Anatomic staging for transitional cell carcinoma of the bladder (see Table 22–4).

periods of time or cured with local therapies. Seventy percent of superficial bladder cancers are Ta, whereas 30% are T1 and less than 10% are Tis. These cancers are usually low grade and they rarely become invasive (10%). However, these tumors do recur locally in approximately 50% of cases within 6 to 12 months, although most of these recurrences are similarly of low stage and grade.

Nearly 95% of patients presenting with Ta lesions have grade 1 disease and two thirds have unifocal disease. If a patient with what appears to be a Ta lesion does not have a low-grade tumor, then suspect undiagnosed invasive disease. Patients with stage T1 disease are just as likely to have unifocal disease, but the vast majority has stage T2 or T3 disease. Fifty percent of patients with T1 disease have a recurrence if the disease arose from a single focus and 70% do when multiple foci were found. Extensive Tis is associated with an 85% risk of local recurrence and a 30% chance of progressing to invasive cancer. Patients with diffuse patchy disease often have so-called field changes within the bladder, and they may have superficial or invasive disease. These cytologic changes can involve the entire urothelial tract, including the urethra, bladder, ureters, and renal pelvis.

Superficial Disease

Patients with stage Ta (grade 2 or 3) disease are most often managed with TURB and careful follow-up with cystoscopy (Table 22–5).[89] These patients are typically advised to undergo cystoscopy, urine cytology, and repeat TURB (as indicated) at 3-month intervals. If no recurrences are noted in the first year, then follow-up intervals are extended. Patients with stage Tis disease or T1 tumors require more aggressive local therapy, consisting of TURB and intravesical chemotherapy.

Bacille Calmette-Guérin (BCG) has been established as the gold standard of intravesical treatment because of higher complete response rates (70%) compared with other drugs, as well as lower cost.[89, 95] Intravesical BCG reduces recurrences and progression to invasive disease. BCG is administered by instillation directly into the bladder through a urethral catheter and drained out 1 to 2 hours later. Complete response rates can be increased from the expected 73% to 87% with three additional BCG instillations given at 3 months.[95] In complete responders, maintenance BCG, using three weekly treatments at 6-month intervals, improves long-term complete response rates from 65% to nearly 90%. Side effects include allergic reactions, bladder infection, irritability, and, rarely, systemic mycobacterial infection. Thiotepa, mitomycin C, and doxorubicin have been used as alternatives, but they are no more effective and more costly. These agents may also cause systemic myelosuppression because they can be absorbed from the bladder. Some studies have suggested that *TP53* may be a prognostic indicator of tumors that may prove unresponsive to intravesical BCG,[96] whereas others suggest

TABLE 22–4. **Staging Table for Transitional Cell Carcinoma of the Urinary Bladder**

Stage	Grouping	Descriptor
I	T1 N0 M0	T1: Tumor invades subepithelial connective tissue N0: No regional lymph node metastasis M0: No distant metastasis
II	T2a,b N0 M0	T2a: Tumor invades superficial muscle (inner half) T2b: Tumor invades deep muscle (outer half)
III	T3a,b N0 M0	T3: Tumor invades perivesical tissue T3a: microscopically; T3b: macroscopically (extravesical mass)
IV	T4a N0 M0	T4a: Tumor invades prostate, uterus, vagina
	T4b N0 M0	T4b: Tumor invades pelvic wall, abdominal wall
	Any T N1 M0	N1: Metastasis in one lymph node, ≤2 cm in greatest dimension
	Any T N2 M0	N2: Metastasis in one lymph node, >2 cm but ≤5 cm in greatest dimension or multiple lymph nodes, none <5 cm
	Any T N3 M0	N3: Metastasis in a lymph node >5 cm in greatest dimension
	Any T Any N M1	M1: Distant metastasis

TX: primary tumor cannot be assessed; T0: no evidence of primary tumor; Ta: noninvasive papillary carcinoma; Tis: carcinoma *in situ*: flat tumor.

Used with permission of the American Joint Committee on Cancer (AJCC®), Chicago, Illinois. The original source for this material is the AJCC® Cancer Staging Manual, 5th ed, 1997, published by Lippincott-Raven Publishers, Philadelphia, Pennsylvania.

that *TP53* does not predict the response to BCG therapy.[97, 98]

The impact of adjuvant therapy for Ta or T1 disease on survival remains controversial. In a combined analysis from the European Organization for Research and Treatment of Cancer (EORTC) and the Medical Research Council (MRC) using randomized clinical trials,[99] a statistically significant benefit of adjuvant treatment as opposed to no adjuvant treatment was found in terms of the disease-free interval; no effect was seen on either survival or progression-free survival. However, the means and choice of therapy are likely to have a major impact on such an analysis, and despite such study results, many practitioners believe that adjuvant therapy prolongs survival.

Invasive Bladder Cancer

Invasive bladder cancer, by definition, involves extension of TCC into the detrusor muscle. Once it gets through the muscle, the tumor has access to fat, surrounding structures, and regional lymph nodes. Up to 50% of these patients may die of distant metastases. The major treatment options for invasive bladder cancer include (1) radical cystectomy, (2) preoperative irradiation and cystectomy, (3) chemotherapy followed by cystectomy, (4) definitive irradiation, (5) chemotherapy, followed by radiation, or (6) concurrent chemotherapy and radiation. Adjuvant chemotherapy can be added to any of these options. Regardless of treatment type, the major recognized prognostic factors include T stage, grade, tumor size, tumor growth characteristics (papillary versus solid), ureteral obstruction, anemia, age, and tumor *TP53* status.

Surgery

The standard treatment for invasive bladder cancer in this country is *radical cystoprostatectomy.* Historically, the 5-year survival rate with surgery alone has been approximately 50%, with patients with pathologic stage T2 doing better (60%) and pathologic stage T3a faring worse (30%). In selected cases, *partial cystectomy* has been shown to be adequate therapy.[100] Patients selected for this procedure usually have small tumors (<4 cm) and no evidence of multicentricity, dysplasia, or carcinoma *in situ* in the bladder mucosa distant from the tumor, assessed on multiple random punch biopsies; it is generally confirmed intraoperatively that the patients selected for partial cystectomy have tumor-free margins. In these highly selected patients, the overall actuarial survival rate has been shown to be 80% at 5 years[100]; however, given current techniques of bladder replacement surgery, partial cystectomy is performed less commonly than it was previously.

Radical cystectomy includes removal of the prostate in men and removal of the uterus, ovaries, and anterior vaginal vault in women. In addition, the urethra is removed in men and women who are at high risk of urethral recurrence; men with cancers in the prostate or at the bladder neck are more likely to have urethral disease, either initially or in a delayed fashion. Although prostatic urethral disease is a risk factor for urethral recurrence, recent evidence suggests that *orthotopic diversion* may be considered in those patients with only proximal prostatic urethral involvement.[101]

TABLE 22–5. **Multidisciplinary Treatment for Bladder Cancer**

Stage	Surgery	Radiation Therapy	Chemotherapy
Tis/Ta N0 M0	TURBT	NR	IV: BCG or CT
T1 N0 M0	TURBT	NR	IV: BCG or CT
T2a,2b N0 M0	Radical cystectomy/segmental cystectomy/TURBT (+ ACT ± ART)	ART: 60–70 Gy	ACT: MVC
T3a,3b,4a N0 M0	Radical cystectomy/TURBT (+ ACT ± ART)	ART: 60–70 Gy	ACT: MVC
T4b N0 M0	Radical cystectomy	ART: 60–70 Gy	NCT: cisplatin-based
Any T N1–3 M0	Radical cystectomy + urinary diversion		
Any T Any N M1	NR	PRT	CT: cisplatin-based

TURBT: transurethral resection of the bladder tumor; ACT: adjuvant chemotherapy; ART: adjuvant radiation therapy; NR: not recommended; PRT: palliative radiation therapy; IV: intravesical therapy; BCG = bacille Calmette-Guérin; CT: thiotepa, mitomycin C, doxorubicin; MVC: methotrexate, vinblastine, cisplatin; NCT: neoadjuvant chemotherapy followed by radical cystectomy or RT.

It is interesting that urethral recurrence may actually be lower in patients who undergo bladder substitution compared with those who undergo either conduit urinary diversion or construction of a continent urinary reservoir, and have their urethra left in place.[102]

Urinary diversion may be accomplished using a variety of techniques. Many patients undergo urinary diversion using single segments of small and large intestine into which the ureters are implanted. These conduits are attached to the anterior abdominal wall and an appliance is attached. Alternatively, continent urinary reservoirs may be fashioned and either attached to the urethra (orthotopic bladder replacement) or to the anterior abdominal wall (continent urinary reservoir). Such reservoirs are composed of three segments: an efferent mechanism that protects the upper urinary tract from high-pressure reflux, a compliant urinary reservoir, and an efferent continence mechanism. As mentioned earlier, the efferent continence mechanism may be composed of the urethra or, in those who require urethrectomy, the appendix, small intestine, or ileocecal valve, which are refashioned into catheterizable abdominal stomas.[103–105] Potential complications of radical cystectomy include impotence, incontinence, infection, psychologic trauma, and inconveniences associated with the management of an ileal loop.

Radiation Therapy

Preoperative and Postoperative Radiation Therapy

Although some experts have made a strong argument for planned preoperative radiotherapy, few patients are offered this strategy today. For example, Parsons and Million and Swanson and associates have concluded that preoperative radiation followed by cystectomy is superior to surgery alone.[106, 107] Unfortunately, the randomized trials evaluating preoperative radiotherapy for TCC of the bladder have not answered this question.[108] Surgery followed by postoperative radiotherapy is not favored because of the impression of a higher risk of pelvic recurrences and post-treatment complications.[109, 110] In addition, a combination of both preoperative and postoperative radiotherapy demonstrates improved 5-year survival rates, but they are at the cost of unacceptably high bowel toxicity.[111]

Definitive Radiation Therapy

External beam irradiation is the most common definitive primary treatment for carcinoma of the urinary bladder in the United Kingdom and many places in Europe and Canada, and the Edinburgh series is one of the largest to evaluate the efficacy of definitive radiotherapy alone.[112] In this series, the complete response rate to definitive radiotherapy for all T stages was 45% and the 5-year local control rate was 25% for T1 to T3 and 16% for T4.[112, 113] Response and local control rates were higher with high-grade lesions, but because of the high rate of distant metastases, the survival rate was lower.

It has been shown that locoregional control may be dependent on overall treatment time. Local control was worse for patients treated by split-course radiotherapy with a gap of approximately 1 month.[114] For patients treated with continuous course radiotherapy, a difference could not be found in local control rates between patients treated in 44 days or less and those treated in 45 to 74 days.

Combined-Modality Therapy

Because of the results of numerous encouraging pilot studies and some randomized trials, combined radiation and chemotherapy has replaced radiotherapy alone as the preferred approach for bladder-sparing treatment. An example of the results from this kind of approach was updated by Shipley and associates.[115] In this trial, patients with T2 to T4 lesions underwent a complete transurethral resection of the bladder tumor (when possible), followed by two cycles of methotrexate, vinblastine, and cisplatin chemotherapy (MVC) and then whole pelvic irradiation to 40 Gy. Patients who responded completely or who were unsuitable for surgery received an additional cycle of cisplatin and a booster dose of radiation to a portion of the bladder, for a total dose of 68.4 Gy. Patients who failed to have a complete response underwent a radical cystectomy. In more than half of the patients the bladder was preserved, and the 5-year survival rate was similar to that expected by surgery alone during the same time period.

Some patients who are not considered suitable for one of these very aggressive regimens may still be candidates for radical radiotherapy combined with a milder form of chemotherapy, such as 5-fluorouracil (5-FU), in an attempt to take advantage of synergism between these modalities.[116] Of note, age alone probably should not be considered a contraindication for aggressive chemoradiation.[117]

Neoadjuvant or Adjuvant Chemotherapy

Several prospective randomized trials have tested the use of chemotherapy before definitive local therapy (neoadjuvant chemotherapy).[118–122] Although the use of neoadjuvant chemotherapy before radiotherapy or surgery increases local control, there appears to be no increased survival. For example, the National Cancer Institute of Canada conducted a prospective randomized trial to determine whether the addition of concurrent cisplatin to preoperative or definitive radiation therapy in patients with muscle-invasive bladder cancer improved local control or survival.[123] Patients and their physicians selected either definitive radiotherapy or precystectomy radiotherapy. Patients were then randomly allocated to receive intravenous cisplatin 100 mg/m^2 at 2-week intervals for three cycles concurrent with pelvic radiation, or to receive radiation without chemotherapy. Concurrent cisplatin was associated with an improved pelvic control of locally advanced bladder cancer with preoperative or definitive radiation, but it did not improve overall survival or distant metastases. Shipley and associates have also reported the experience of the Radiation Therapy Oncology Group Trial 89–03.[115] Patients were randomized to receive either concurrent radiotherapy (control arm) or neoadjuvant MCV chemotherapy. There appeared to be no advantage to the use of MCV chemotherapy in this setting.

Patients initially managed with radical cystectomy who are found to be at an increased risk of systemic relapse because of the presence of lymph node metastases or regionally advanced disease may benefit from adjuvant chemotherapy.[124, 125] However, other trials have failed to show a definitive survival benefit with the use of adjuvant chemotherapy, and its routine use following definitive local therapy remains controversial.[126, 127] The major criticisms of adjuvant chemotherapy trials have cited "major flaws of execution," including small numbers of treated patients and protocol violations. Despite these controversies, most oncologists consider adjuvant chemotherapy for patients at very high risk of relapse, such as those with T3b tumors or positive pelvic lymph nodes.[89] It is hoped that ongoing randomized trials will determine the true usefulness of adjuvant therapy in reducing systemic relapse rates.

Results and Follow-Up

Surgery

In addition to the use of partial cystectomy alone, incorporating TURB or partial cystectomy with neoadjuvant chemotherapy, a *bladder-sparing approach,* has been pioneered by investigators at Memorial Sloan-Kettering.[128] These investigators have described the results of such an approach in 60 patients who achieved a complete response (T0) on TURB after the fourth cycle of combination chemotherapy with methotrexate, vinblastine, doxorubicin, and cisplatin. Twenty-eight of these patients refused surgery and only underwent a TURB, whereas 15 had a partial cystectomy and 17 underwent radical resection. The overall survival rates of patients were 75%, 73%, and 65% for patients treated with TURB, partial cystectomy, and radical resection, respectively. Sixty-one percent and 53% of patients treated with TURB and partial resection, respectively, had intact bladders at 10 years. These patients were highly selected, however, and it is unclear what proportion of patients would be suitable for such an approach.

Of note, although orthotopic bladder replacement was once reserved for men only, clinical and laboratory experience suggests that it also may be an acceptable procedure in women.[129] Women with bladder cancer whose cancers are not located at the bladder neck and have a clear urethral margin at the time of cystectomy are candidates for this procedure, and approximately 66% of women undergoing radical cystectomy for the management of bladder cancer fall into this group.[130–132] Intraoperative inspection and frozen section assessment of the bladder neck limits the risk of urethral recurrence.

With respect to urinary diversion, Gburek and associates have summarized the Mayo Clinic experience, comparing neobladder with the Studer technique with the ileal conduit diversion by the same group of surgeons over the same time period.[133] For both procedures, the perioperative complication rate was 18% and the reoperation rate was roughly 5%. The late complication rate was 21% for neobladder compared with 12% for conduits. Late reoperations were required in 11% and 8% of cases for neobladder and conduit patients, respectively.

One study has suggested that the use of a neobladder may be associated with a better outcome because of fewer delays.[134] In this study, Hautmann and Paiss evaluated 135 patients who underwent an ileal neobladder procedure and 78 who underwent conduit diversion to assess whether orthotopic bladder replacement had an impact on the decision to perform cystectomy. In the neobladder and conduit groups, an average of 2.1 and 4.1 transurethral bladder resections were performed, respectively. The interval from the primary diagnosis to cystectomy was 11.8 months in the neobladder and 16.7 months in the conduit group. Cystectomy was performed 4.1 months after the diagnosis of invasive cancer in the neobladder group, whereas radical surgery was delayed for 15.4 months in the conduit group. It was found that cancer-specific 5-year survival rates were 76.6% and 28.35% in the two groups, respectively, and delayed cystectomy was a risk factor only in advanced disease stages. The authors concluded that the use of an ileal neobladder may decrease physician reluctance to perform cystectomy early in the disease process, increasing the survival rate. It is premature to assume that the observations made by these authors apply to other doctors and patients. However, of particular concern is the very low survival rate among the patients treated with conduits.

Radiation Therapy

Investigators from the University of Texas M. D. Anderson Cancer Center conducted a retrospective comparison of patients treated with preoperative radiotherapy and radical cystectomy ($n = 338$), or radical cystectomy alone ($n = 232$).[135] For those with T3b disease, the actuarial 5-year local control rate was 91% for the group who received combined therapy compared with 72% for the arm who received cystectomy alone. Patients with T3b disease who received preoperative radiotherapy also fared slightly better at 5 years in terms of freedom from distant metastasis (67% versus 54%), disease freedom (59% versus 47%), and overall survival (52% versus 40%). The authors concluded that because the patients treated with cystectomy were operated on using modern surgical techniques and that 80% of those with stage T3b disease received multiagent chemotherapy, the benefits of preoperative radiation might be underestimated. Despite the views of these and other investigators, preoperative radiotherapy is not widely used in this country.

Combined-Modality Therapy

Zietman and associates have reported on contemporary experience with a phase I-II bladder preservation protocol.[136] The investigators combined twice-daily radiation with 5-FU and cisplatin chemotherapy in 18 patients post-TURB. The 3-year overall and native bladder survival rates were approximately 80%. This type of treatment approach is likely to form the basis for the next generation of bladder-sparing phase III protocols. However, only prospective randomized trials are likely to definitively answer the question of optimal treatment. Chemoradiotherapy with possible bladder sparing should be considered a treatment option, but it has not yet been proven, to the satisfaction of most urologists, to be comparable to immediate radical surgery. Therefore, this approach is only recommended in the setting of a clinical trial or for selected patients refusing surgery.

The addition of chemotherapy appears to improve the results expected from radiotherapy alone. For example, investigators from the University Hospital of Erlangen reported their experiences with 333 patients with TCC of the bladder, treated with either radiotherapy alone or cisplatin-based chemoradiation following TURB.[137] The treatment-related mortality rate was less than 1% and complete responses occurred in 57% of patients treated with radiotherapy alone, compared with 70% for carboplatin-based and 85% for cisplatin-based chemoradiation. Five-year survival rates after radiotherapy alone or with carboplatin- or cisplatin-based chemoradiation were 47%, 57%, and 69%, respectively. However, following a multivariate analysis, the only significant factor that correlated with survival was the resection status following TURB.

Follow-Up

The standard follow-up for patients who have had treatment for superficial or invasive disease involves repeated cystoscopies accompanied by periodic urine cytology. However, the optimal method of follow-up of postoperative patients is controversial. Some authorities recommend routine follow-up with intravenous pyelography and ultrasonography[89]; however, some investigators disagree. From 1987 to 1988, Holmang and coworkers studied 680 patients in western Sweden with an initial diagnosis of bladder carcinoma.[138] All carcinomas of the kidney, renal pelvis, and ureter and all surgically treated cases of ureteral stricture were included in this analysis. They noted "a low annual incidence" of malignant upper urinary tract and renal tumors and ureteral strictures. During follow-up, renal pelvic or ureteral carcinoma developed in 16 patients, renal cell carcinoma was diagnosed in two, and six underwent surgery for benign obstruction of the distal ureter. Thus, assuming that 50% of the patients were cured and all 24 patients with one of these complications belonged to these survivors, only approximately 7% of these patients would have been identified on routine follow-up. Based on this observation, the authors discouraged the practice of routinely imaging the upper urinary tract during the follow-up of patients with bladder carcinoma. They recommended urography only at the time of diagnosis, when tumor progression occurs, and when signs or symptoms of upper tract pathology are present.

In an effort to simplify the follow-up of these patients, various noninvasive strategies have been investigated:

- *Bladder tumor antigen:* Studies have demonstrated that the bladder tumor antigen (BTA) assay might be useful in diagnosing transitional cell carcinoma (TCC) of the bladder.[139] However, BTA does not appear to be useful in detecting upper urinary tract TCC.[140] The addition of karyotyping appears to improve the sensitivity of predicting recurrences; however, these tests do not appear to be reliable enough to abandon cystoscopy, although they may act as a complement.[141, 142]
- *Ki-67:* The Ki-67 labeling index may be an independent predictive factor for recurrence of superficial bladder cancer.[143]
- *VEGF:* Tumor angiogenesis, as determined by microvessel density measurement, also appears to be an independent prognostic indicator for patients with invasive TCC of the bladder.[144] As another means of measurement, tumor angiogenesis may be dependent on vascular endothelial growth factor (VEGF), and high expression of VEGF mRNA in superficial bladder cancers appears to be associated with earlier recurrence and progression.[145]
- *Telomerase:* The detection of the activity of the enzyme telomerase may also have potential clinical use in evaluating voided urine samples of patients with bladder cancer.[146, 147]
- *NMP22:* NMP22, an immunoassay for a urinary nuclear matrix protein, has been evaluated as an indicator for TCC of the urinary tract. In one study, patients with active TCC had significantly higher urinary NMP22 levels than those with no evidence of disease.[148] Of note, there was no effect from tumor grade, extent of disease, or exposure to intravesical therapy on urinary NMP22 levels.

Landman and colleagues have reported a comparison of some of these various assays for 47 patients with bladder cancer.[149] NMP22 and the telomerase assays gave similar sensitivity and specificity for the detection of bladder cancer, and they appeared to offer a greater sensitivity than the BTA assay or conventional cytology, or both. The detection of stage I tumors was relatively poor for all assays used, being 69% with NMP22, 65% with telomerase, 13% with BTA, and 6% with cytology. Stage II tumors were detected at a higher rate of 86% with NMP22, 72% with telomerase, 36% with BTA, and 36% with cytology. A relatively high detection rate was noted for stage III tumors, at 93% with NMP22, 93% with telomerase, 79% with BTA, and 79% with cytology. In 30 patients with hematuria but without bladder cancer, they reported an overall specificity of 77% for NMP22, 80% for telomerase, 73% for BTA, and 94% for cytology alone.

Thus, the routine use of these assays outside the setting of a clinical trial cannot be recommended. In addition, despite the apparent correlation between these various markers and the aggressiveness of TCC, alterations of *TP53,* Ki-67 proliferative index, microvascular counts, or ploidy may not be strongly predictive of lymph node status in patients affected with high-stage, high-grade bladder cancer.[150]

Prognostic Factors

Defining which patients are likely to progress after treatment for superficial or invasive disease is one of the most important issues involved in managing patients with TCC of the bladder. Not only does this problem impact the decision of patients considering very aggressive therapy but it also impacts the design of clinical trials. Of the factors considered important, *tumor grade* (Figure 22–6), *tumor size,* and *previous recurrence rates* per year have been the best described.[151] In addition to these factors, how therapy is delivered may also have a substantial impact on the risk of recurrence. For example, patients managed with delayed resection or without maintenance chemotherapy appear to be at an increased risk for recurrences.[152]

Among the best studied predictors of a reduced survival

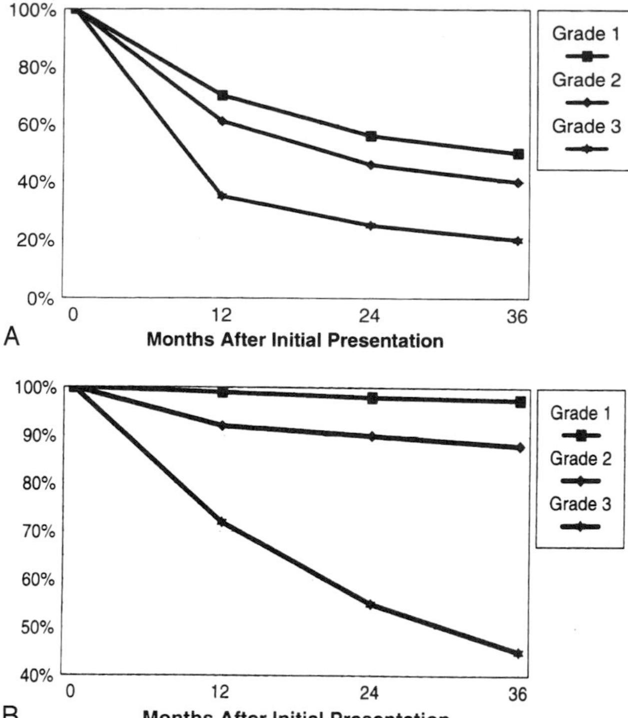

Figure 22–6. Importance of tumor grade on (A) disease-free survival and (B) progression-free survival. (Adapted from Heney NM, Ahmed S, Flanagan MJ, et al: Superficial bladder cancer; progression and recurrence. J Urol 1983; 130:1083–1086; From Holzbeierlein JM, Smith JA Jr: Natural history and surgical management. In: Vogelzang NJ, Scardino PT, Shipley WU, et al [eds]: Comprehensive Textbook of Genitourinary Oncology, 2nd ed, pp 384–394. Philadelphia, Lippincott Williams & Wilkins, 2000, with permission.)

is the overexpression of the tumor suppressor gene *TP53*. *TP53* is a crucial regulator of the cell cycle and apoptosis (programmed cell death), and is usually undetectable in normal cells. Its overexpression typically implies the accumulation of aberrant forms of the protein. Esrig and associates used immunohistochemistry to detect p53 in histologic specimens from 243 patients with TCC of the bladder treated by radical cystectomy for stages pTa (noninvasive disease) to pT4.[153] The detection of nuclear p53 was significantly associated with an increased risk of recurrence of bladder cancer ($p < 0.001$) and with decreased overall survival ($p < 0.001$) (Figure 22–7). Among patients with cancer confined to the bladder and no detectable nuclear p53, approximately 10% recurred at 5 years compared with 60% to 80% for tumors that had p53 immunoreactivity. In a multivariate analysis (stratifying for grade, pathologic stage, and the lymph node status), nuclear p53 status was the only independent predictor of recurrence and overall survival for patients who had cancer confined to the bladder ($p < 0.001$).

Investigators from Memorial Sloan-Kettering Cancer Center made similar observations concerning the significance of *TP53* in 90 patients treated with neoadjuvant methotrexate, vinblastine, doxorubicin, and cisplatin (MVAC).[154] These investigators reported that the impact of *TP53* overexpression on survival was predominantly in T2 and T3a tumors, and they noted a long-term survival rate of 41% in patients with *TP53* overexpression compared with 77% in patients whose *TP53* was not overexpressed. Nonetheless, in general, *TP53* overexpression is considered to be a weak prognostic indicator for invasive tumors.[155, 156]

The *retinoblastoma protein* (pRB) is another tumor suppressor that regulates progression through the cell cycle. Statistically significant associations have been observed for both patients who are *TP53* positive and pRB negative with disease progression and reduced survival.[157] The most marked increase in progression and decreased overall survival was observed in patients whose tumors had both alterations. These data suggest that aberrant *TP53* and pRB

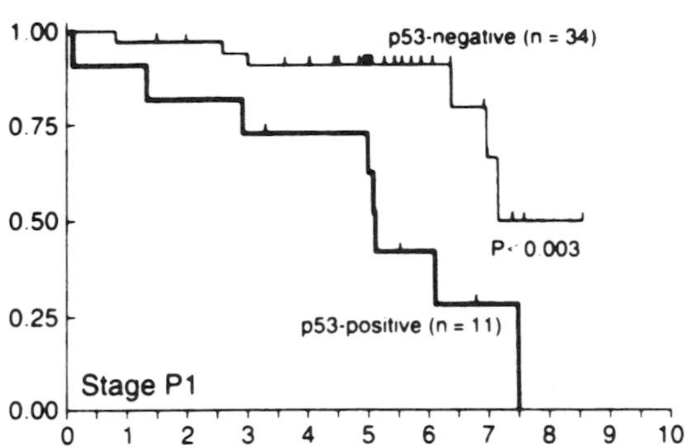

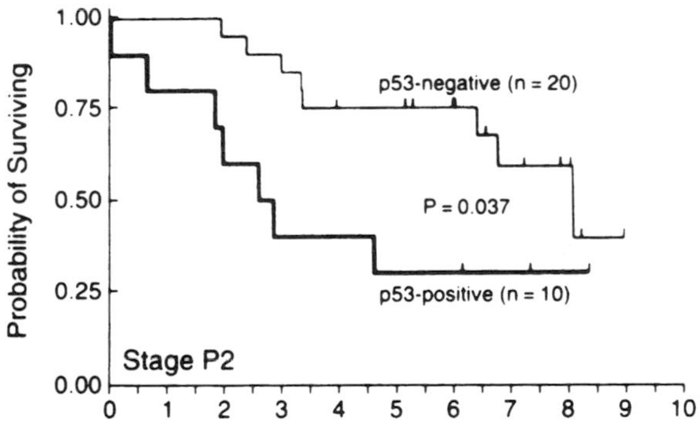

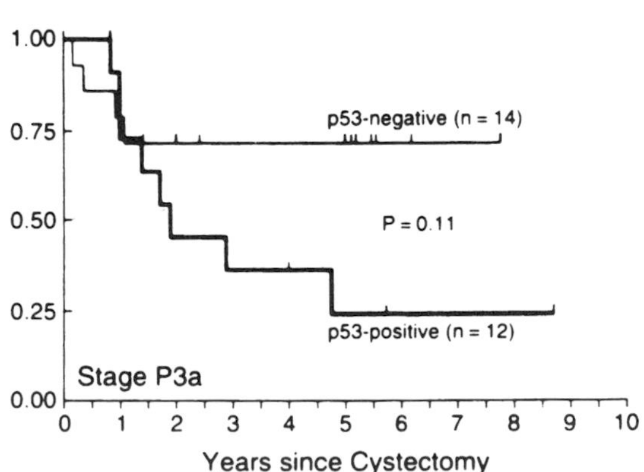

Figure 22–7. Probability of survival following radical cystectomy according to pathologic stage and stratified by p53 immunoreactivity for patients with node-negative P1, P2, or P3a transitional cell carcinoma. (From Esrig D, Elmajian D, Groshen S, et al: Accumulation of nuclear p53 and tumor progression in bladder cancer. N Engl J Med 1994; 331:1259–1264, with permission.)

expression may deregulate cell cycle control at the G_1 checkpoint, resulting in tumor cells with reduced responsiveness to programmed cell death.

Metastatic Disease

Patients with unresectable or metastatic disease are generally treated with chemotherapy, although long-term survival is unusual with available regimens; in most series, the median survival for patients with metastatic bladder cancer is approximately 1 year. Patients with a good performance status, absence of liver, lung, or bone metastases, and a normal alkaline phosphatase have the greatest chance of long-term survival.[89]

The specific chemotherapy program chosen depends on an assessment of the patient's general medical condition (renal and cardiac function) and extent of disease. Cisplatin-containing regimens, such as MVAC or CMV, have been used most commonly, and they produce responses in 30% to 70% of patients. However, there is substantial toxicity with these regimens, especially in elderly patients. Alternative programs have been investigated. The taxanes (paclitaxel and docetaxel) have shown activity as first-line and salvage therapies, both alone and in combination with other agents such as carboplatin or cisplatin. Gemcitabine, a new antimetabolite, has also demonstrated promising single-agent activity against bladder cancer and is being evaluated as a component of combination regimens. One of the most important research tasks for the future will be to identify new systemic regimens with enhanced efficacy and tolerability.

Prostate Cancer

Perspective

Prostate cancer is an enigma. For no other common malignancy is there less agreement among experts on whether men should be screened or how they should be treated. The confusion and controversy have peaked during a revolution in men's attitudes toward their health in general and the prostate in particular. This revolution has been fostered and threatened by use of the Internet. Patients who do their own research in an attempt to resolve these issues frequently find that the more they learn, the more confused they are about what is the right thing to do. As more information becomes available, more questions are generated than answers are provided.

The impact of screening on survival is one of the most difficult issues to resolve. Both the urologist and the radiation oncologist potentially stand to benefit directly from the theory that early local treatment is important. Conversely, skeptics, including epidemiologists and bureaucrats whose job it is to keep medical costs down, seem to be the most difficult to convince of the benefits of local therapy. These unspoken truths further compromise our ability to reach a consensus.

The one item on which most experts agree is that a multidisciplinary approach is key to the optimal management of prostate cancer. Obtaining tissue for diagnosis requires the input of the urologist *and* the pathologist. If the tumor is missed with the first biopsy, then the diagnosis is delayed. Determining the aggressiveness of the tumor is most accurately determined by the appearance of the tumor under a microscope, as assessed by the pathologist. If the pathologist is not familiar with the intricacies of accurately defining prostate cancer tumor grades, then the patient may not receive the appropriate treatment.

Treatment of localized disease is most frequently administered by a urologist or radiation oncologist. When these first two experts disagree (as they frequently do), it has become increasingly common for a medical oncologist to be consulted for a less biased perspective. As more research dollars have become available, researchers whose interests previously excluded prostate cancer have become more interested. These researchers add a fresh perspective and new tools not previously used. For these reasons and more, there is great optimism that, over the next 10 years, we will provide answers where we once had only questions, and fewer men will die unnecessarily or suffer therapy-related toxicities.

Epidemiology and Etiology

Epidemiology

Prostate cancer is the most commonly diagnosed noncutaneous malignancy, and the second leading cancer killer in men living in the United States. The incidence of prostate cancer peaked in 1992 at approximately 300,000 new cases per year,[158] but it has subsequently fallen to an estimated 180,400 cases for the year 2000.[5] The rapid rise in the incidence of prostate cancer occurred as a consequence of widespread prostate specific antigen (PSA)–based screening in the early 1990s. In addition, there has been a recent decline in mortality due to prostate cancer[159]; the decline reflects in part the so-called harvest phenomenon that occurs when screening results in the identification of prevalent cases not previously diagnosed. It also is likely that early detection has resulted in a substantial reduction in prostate cancer–related mortality, although this has not been proven definitively.

Prostate cancer is generally considered a disease of older men, although in 1992, 44% of newly diagnosed men were younger than 70 years of age.[160] The lifetime risk of being diagnosed with prostate cancer peaked as high as 1 in 5 (SEER data, 1992–94), but it is likely to be lower by more recent statistics. For the year 2000, it is estimated that prostate cancer made up 29% of newly diagnosed cancers in men and accounted for 11% of all cancer deaths, with 31,900 men expected to die of this disease.[5]

Prostate cancer in black Americans continues to be diagnosed at a more advanced stage and, therefore, the disease-specific survival in this population is lower than for whites. The issues of race and good science have not been as closely linked as they should be. Although most urologists and many epidemiologists seem to believe that there is a strong relationship between outcome and race, most data from prospective randomized trials do not support this assertion.[161] Recent studies seem to suffer from the lack of understanding that SEER data do not provide sufficient detail or control of differences in the initial evaluation, staging, and treatment to allow the issue of the independent prognostic significance of race to be assessed.[162, 163]

Although the incidence of occult (latent) prostate cancer appears to be similar around the world, mortality rates from prostate cancer vary widely. Scandinavian countries have the highest mortality rates, whereas Asian and developing countries have the lowest (Figure 22–8).[164, 165] The high mortality rates in Scandinavian countries are of interest because so-called watchful waiting or deferred treatment appears to be more commonly used in these countries, although PSA screening is widely available. Men who migrate from low risk areas of the world (e.g., Japan) seem to acquire a risk approaching that of the higher risk regions of the world (e.g., United States).

Etiology

- Men castrated early in life rarely develop prostate cancer, implicating the male hormone *testosterone* as a requirement for prostate cancer tumorigenesis.
- *Age* appears to be a major risk factor, with the incidence of prostate cancer climbing steeply in men older than 60 years of age. By the age of 80, most men have at least microscopic prostate cancer (although this may not be clinically relevant).
- *Family history* is a risk factor, based on case-control studies among first-degree family members. There have been suggestions that hereditary prostate cancer is linked to a locus on chromosome 1 *(HPC1),* but an abnormality at this locus occurs in a very small percentage of men (~9%) and appears to be linked to a subset of early-onset cancers.[166] Recent studies have not been universally confirmatory, however, and the search for familial prostate cancer genes continues. In addition, familial prostate cancer has been associated with a worse prognosis in some studies, but not in others.[167, 168]
- *Race* has been implicated as a risk factor for developing prostate cancer. The incidence of prostate cancer among blacks in the United States is nearly twice that of whites and 40 times that of the native Japanese male. However, these major differences may be a result of diet or other lifestyle changes, because the risk increases among Asian men who adopt a western lifestyle.
- Of the *dietary factors,* fat is most often implicated, although to date none of the studies have been considered definitive. A diet high in beta-carotene and low in fat may be protective,[169, 170] as may be exercise.[171] Diets high in selenium, vitamin E, soy (genistein) and lycopenes (tomatoes) also have been associated with a reduced risk of prostate cancer.[172–176] Use of tobacco has been associated with an increased risk, but definitive studies are lacking.[177]
- Although an early study suggested an association between vasectomy and prostate cancer, more recent studies have not.[177–179]
- Benign prostatic hypertrophy is not associated with prostate cancer.[180]

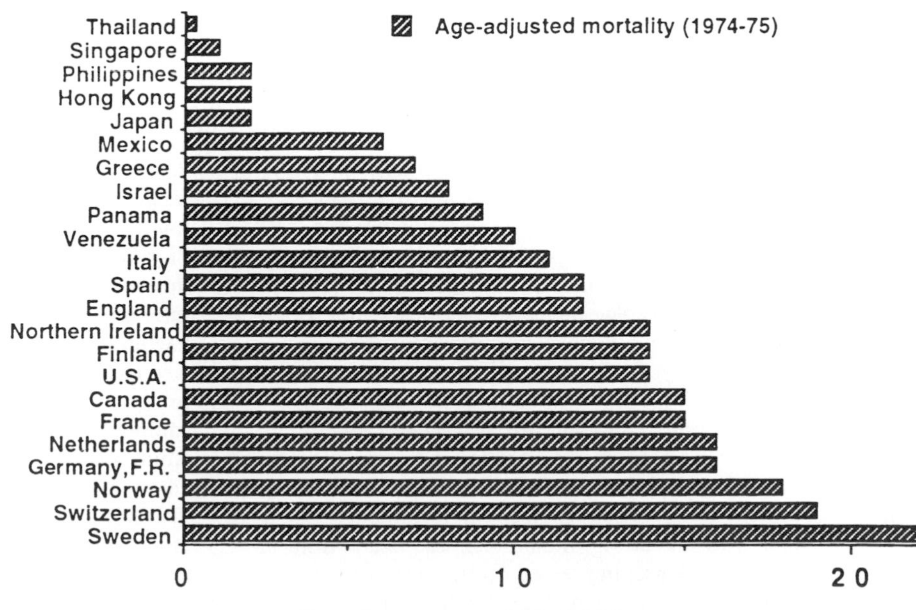

Figure 22–8. International prostate cancer mortality rates. (Modified from Silverberg E: Cancer statistics, 1980. CA Cancer J Clin 1980; 30:23–38; From Roach M III, Wallner K: Prostate cancer. In: Leibel SA, Phillips TL [eds]: Textbook of Radiation Oncology, pp 741–784. Philadelphia, W.B. Saunders, 1998.)

Detection and Diagnosis

Clinical Detection

The biologic behavior of prostate cancer is, in many ways, similar to that of breast cancer. Both are primarily adenocarcinomas that tend to spread to lymph nodes and the bone marrow. Both promote fears of loss of sexual function and both appear to be associated with a prolonged survival following castration. As with breast cancer, screening is capable of detecting disease at early stage, even when the disease is not palpable.

Most men are asymptomatic and diagnosed with prostate cancer solely because of an elevated PSA level (>60%). The next most common presentation is a palpable abnormality noted on digital rectal exam (DRE). Even in this setting, the positive biopsy may arise from a portion of the gland not originally noted on DRE. Much less frequently, a diagnosis is made incidentally following a transurethral resection of the prostate (TURP) for obstructive symptoms. Rarely, patients with locally advanced disease present with obstructive symptoms due to bulky tumor. After adjustment for the extent of disease and tumor grade, survival does not appear to be adversely affected by the presence of obstructive symptoms; some men develop advanced disease without ever manifesting obstructive symptoms.[181]

Screening

Screening for prostate cancer remains a controversial topic. Some investigators believe that screening might actually result in poorer health outcomes and increased cost[182]; other investigators believe that screening can be cost-effective.[183] In addition, screening has generally been advocated by the American Cancer Society (ACS) but not the National Cancer Institute (NCI). Despite the controversies surrounding screening, it is possible that at least some portion of the recent drop in the age-adjusted mortality rates can be attributed to screening, which resulted in earlier treatment.[184] In fact, a recent prospective randomized trial from Canada suggests that prostate cancer mortality can be substantially reduced with widespread PSA screening,[185] although methodological flaws in this study may render the results inconclusive. For example, the decrease in mortality observed in such reports is likely to reflect the identification of men with locally advanced high-grade prostate cancer who received earlier hormonal therapy as a component of local therapy or at the time of a rising PSA level after failing local therapy, rather than the treatment of very early prostate cancer.[186–188] The men with very early disease detected by screening have such a low mortality rate that a decrease in mortality from local treatment would not likely be significant until nearly 10 years following screening.[189] If a patient is not a candidate for any type of therapy, then he should not be screened. Unfortunately, this is not usually a straightforward decision. A more practical solution is to screen even marginally acceptable patients, but only treat men who are at significant risk for death from prostate cancer.[165, 189] Screening based on the serum marker PSA is the most cost-effective method for the detection of early disease.

The DRE lacks sensitivity and specificity, with roughly 50% of suspicious nodules turning out to be cancer; however, many prostate cancers are not palpable. In addition, many cancers detected by DRE are locally advanced and probably not curable. At least 25% to 50% of patients have extracapsular extension that is missed by DRE, and nearly an equal number have a false-positive reading.[190] Evaluation of the seminal vesicles by palpation is also inaccurate. Approximately 10% of the men believed not to have seminal vesicle involvement by the cancer actually do (and 40% of patients identified as having seminal vesicle involvement do not), identified when the gland is subsequently examined pathologically.

The most commonly used serum assays have a normal PSA range of 0 to 4.0 ng/mL. However, patients with a PSA reading in the range of 2.6 to 4.0 ng/mL should be considered at high risk[191]; a consistently rising PSA level may be associated with the presence of cancer, even if it is within the normal range.[192–194] Nonetheless, it is advisable to be cautious when deciding that a PSA level is in fact rising because significant interassay variations and fluctuations are commonly observed over short periods of observation.[195] A DRE performed before obtaining a PSA reading has very little impact on PSA values in men without prostate cancer, but if the PSA level is elevated, the exam may increase the PSA slightly.[196] Therefore, it is probably prudent to do the PSA screening before obtaining a DRE. Prostatitis, urinary tract infections, and benign prostatic hypertrophy also may cause an elevation of PSA and must be considered in each patient.

The so-called PSA density (PSA per unit volume of prostate tissue) uses transrectal ultrasonography to adjust for PSA levels resulting from benign prostatic hypertrophy; however, the utility of this approach remains controversial.[197, 198] Recent studies have shown that cancer is associated with a lower ratio of free-to-total serum PSA.[199–201] Incorporating the use of the free-to-total PSA ratio may increase specificity without compromising sensitivity.[201, 202] Age-specific reference ranges also may make PSA a more useful marker, although the use of age-specific reference ranges has not been universally adopted.[201]

Diagnostic Procedures

- *Transrectal ultrasound* (TRUS) with biopsy is recommended when the PSA level is elevated or an abnormality is discovered on DRE. The number of positive biopsies is considered by some authorities to have independent prognostic significance, and consequently, the number of samples typically obtained in the 1990s has increased substantially.[203, 204] Usually, sextant biopsies (both bases, midglands, and apices) are taken, but in high-risk patients, the seminal vesicles may also be sampled.[205]
- Routine chest x-ray films or cystoscopies are not indicated unless there is a smoking history or urinary symptoms.[206]
- Bone scans are not justified if the PSA is ≤10 ng/mL.[207]
- Neither abdominal nor pelvic CT or MRI appears to be warranted if the PSA level is less than 20 ng/mL.[208]

Based on the pretreatment clinical stage, pretreatment PSA levels, and the Gleason score, a patient's risk of positive lymph nodes, seminal vesicle involvement, and the extracapsular extension can be roughly estimated[209]; neither CT nor MRI is sensitive enough to replace pelvic lymphadenectomy for identifying such patients. However, one study suggests that ^{111}In-based scans may be helpful in identifying lymph node involvement in selected high-risk patients.[210]

Classification and Staging

The normal anatomy of the prostate is considered to be made up of zones, a concept first put forward by McNeal[211] and now widely accepted.[212] Under this system of classification, the prostate consists of four zones (Figure 22–9)[213, 214]:

- *The peripheral zone*—this zone makes up the bulk of the normal adult gland (70% of the glandular tissue) and is the region most prone to the development of carcinomas.
- *The central zone*—this is a cone-shaped volume of tissue encompassing 20% of the glandular tissue.
- *The transition zone*—this zone, found in the midprostate, consists of two equal portions of glandular tissue (5% to 10% of total glandular tissue) and is the site of a small percentage of clinical carcinomas.
- *The nonglandular anterior fibromuscular stroma.*

Histopathology

More than 95% of all prostate cancers are adenocarcinomas,[215] and the most widely used grading system was first described by Gleason and Mellinger.[216] The so-called Gleason score is a sum of the two most common histologic patterns. Using this approach, the Gleason score (GS) may range from 2 to 10. Five major categories, 2–4, 5, 6, 7, and 8–10, appear to be optimal for segregating prognostic risk groups based on their GS, and numerous studies have demonstrated that GS correlates with pathologic stage and survival.[217–220] Of note, some pathologists divide histologic subtypes into well differentiated, moderately differentiated, or poorly differentiated. This practice compromises the predictive value of tumor grade because moderately differentiated tumors usually include tumors with Gleason scores of 5 through 7 (Table 22–6): patients with a GS of 5 have a significantly better outcome than patients with a GS of 7.[217, 218, 220]

Small cell (anaplastic) tumors and lymphomas are occasionally identified and are usually treated with chemotherapy, with or without radiotherapy. Sarcomas are frequently managed by surgery with or without postoperative radiotherapy.

Staging

The major clinical staging system has been changed several times over the last 10 years. The most recent staging system in use at the time of publication is described in Table 22–7 and is illustrated in Figure 22–10.[17] Patients diagnosed incidentally as having prostate cancer following TURP are considered to have stage T1a or T1b (formerly A1 or A2), signifying focal and diffuse disease, respectively. The designation T1c is used if a patient has nonpalpable disease not detected by imaging (i.e., detected through PSA screening alone). Palpable tumor contained within the gland and limited to one lobe is stage T2a (previously, B1 or B2) and T2b, if both lobes are involved. Once the cancer has extended through the capsule, the stage is T3a (C1), if involvement is focal or T3b if either seminal vesicle is involved. Involvement of the lymph nodes is classified as N1–3 (depending on size).

Tumor Grading

Most patients are diagnosed by needle biopsy, which is highly specific (0% to 2% false positive)[223]; for low-grade

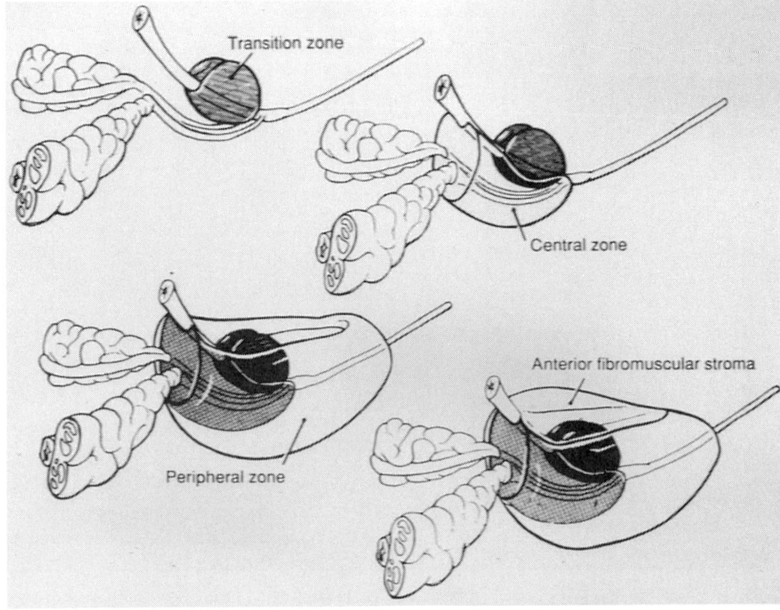

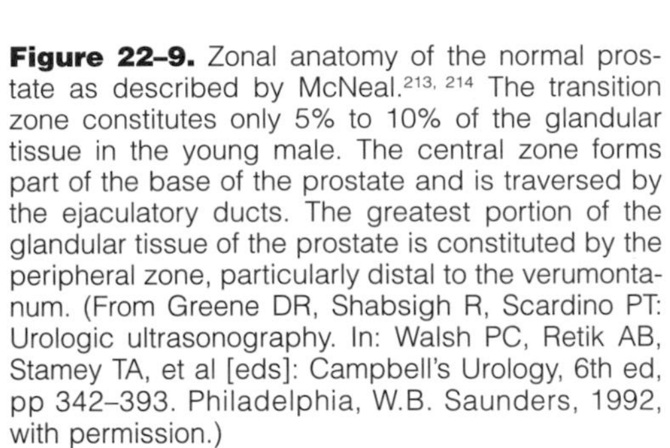

Figure 22–9. Zonal anatomy of the normal prostate as described by McNeal.[213, 214] The transition zone constitutes only 5% to 10% of the glandular tissue in the young male. The central zone forms part of the base of the prostate and is traversed by the ejaculatory ducts. The greatest portion of the glandular tissue of the prostate is constituted by the peripheral zone, particularly distal to the verumontanum. (From Greene DR, Shabsigh R, Scardino PT: Urologic ultrasonography. In: Walsh PC, Retik AB, Stamey TA, et al [eds]: Campbell's Urology, 6th ed, pp 342–393. Philadelphia, W.B. Saunders, 1992, with permission.)

TABLE 22–6. **Relationship Between Biopsy Stage and Final Pathologic Stage**

	Pathologic Gleason Score			
Biopsy Grade	***2–4****	***5–7****	***8–10****	***No. of Patients†***
Well (2–4)	50%	**48%**	2%	122
Moderate (5–7)	10%	74%	**15%**	258
Poor (8–10)	1%	25%	74%	81

*Modified from review by Johnstone and associates[221] and Benson.[222]

†Number of patients in series from Benson and review of five series by Johnstone and associates. Underlined figures reflect understaging and boldface numbers reflect overstaging.

From Roach M III, Wallner K: Prostate cancer. In Leibel SA, Phillips TL (eds): Textbook of Radiation Oncology, pp 741–784. Philadelphia, W.B. Saunders, 1998, with permission.

and intermediate-grade tumors (Gleason score 2–4) there is roughly a 50% probability of overgrading and a 15% chance of undergrading; for intermediate tumors there is a 10% chance of overgrading; for high-grade tumors there is roughly a 25% chance of overgrading. The likelihood of undergrading increases as the PSA level increases, with undergrading uncommon in patients with a normal PSA reading.[224]

Predictive Index (PSA)

The serum PSA level tends to increase as the volume of cancer within the gland increases. This probably reflects greater leakage of PSA into the circulation or disruption of normal prostate parenchyma.[193] However, very poorly differentiated cancers can be associated with a normal PSA reading. Because of this complex interaction between PSA and tumor grade, PSA screening alone cannot be relied on to predict tumor volume. Pretreatment PSA screening, tumor grade (Gleason score), and clinical stage have been combined to generate nomograms that predict the likelihood of finding organ-confined disease, extracapsular extension, seminal vesicle involvement, and lymph node involvement (Table 22–8).[209, 218] Of note, lymph node involvement by prostate cancer is associated with a poor long-term survival; it is rare that such patients are disease free at 10 years if treated with locoregional therapy alone.[225]

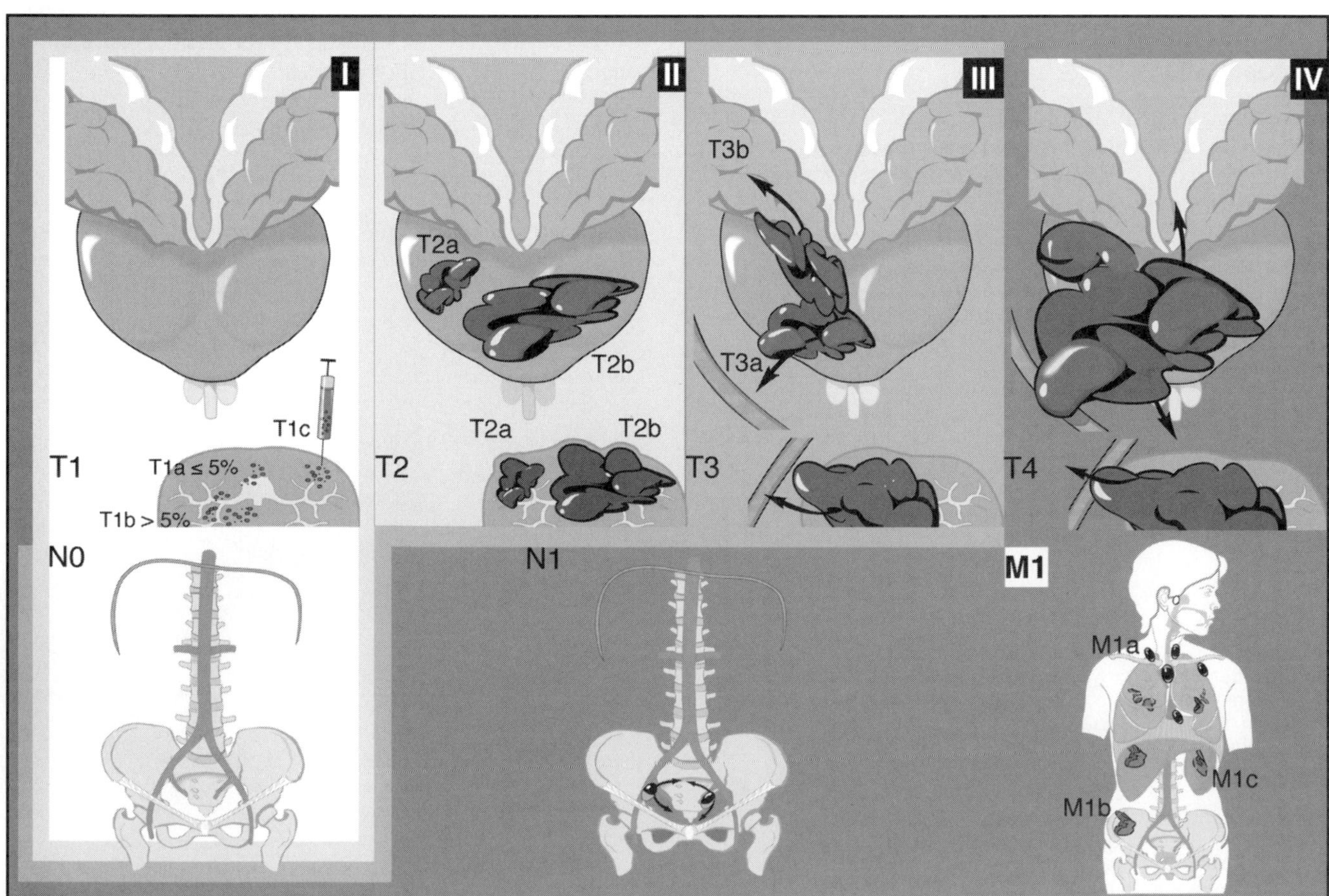

Figure 22–10. Anatomic staging for prostate cancer (see Table 22–7).

TABLE 22–7. **Staging Table for Prostate Cancer**

Stage	Grouping	Grading	Descriptor
I	T1a N0 M0	G1	T1a: Tumor incidental histologic finding in ≤5% of tissue resected N0: No regional lymph node metastasis M0: No distant metastasis
II	T1a N0 M0	G2–4	T1: Clinically inapparent tumor, not palpable or visible on imaging T1b: Tumor incidental histological finding in >5% of tissue resected
	T1b,c N0 M0	Any G	T1c: Tumor identified by needle biopsy
	T2* N0 M0	Any G	T2: Tumor confined within prostate
III	T3† N0 M0	Any G	T3: Tumor extends through the prostate capsule
IV	T4 N0 M0	Any G	T4: Tumor is fixed or invades adjacent structures other than seminal vesicles: bladder neck, external sphincter, rectum, levator muscles, or pelvic wall
	Any T N1 M0	Any G	N1: Metastasis in regional lymph node or nodes
	Any T Any N M1‡	Any G	M1: Distant metastasis

G1 = well differentiated (slight anaplasia); G2 = moderately differentiated (moderate anaplasia); G3–4 = poorly differentiated or undifferentiated (marked anaplasia).

*T2 is further defined: T2a = tumor involves one lobe; T2b = tumor involves both lobes.

†T3 is further defined: T3a = extracapsular extension (unilateral or bilateral); T3b = tumor invades seminal vesicles.

‡M1 is further defined: M1a = nonregional lymph nodes; M1b = bones; M1c = other sites.

Used with permission of the American Joint Committee on Cancer (AJCC®), Chicago, Illinois. The original source for this material is the AJCC® Cancer Staging Manual, 5th ed, 1997, published by Lippincott-Raven Publishers, Philadelphia, Pennsylvania.

TABLE 22–8. **Nomogram for the Prediction of Final Pathologic Stage**

	PSA (ng/mL)																							
	0.0–4.0						*>4.0–10*						*>10–20*						*>20*					
Score	*Clinical Stage*						*Clinical Stage*						*Clinical Stage*						*Clinical Stage*					
	T1a	*T1b*	*T2a*	*T2b*	*T2c*	*T3a*	*T1a*	*T1b*	*T2a*	*T2b*	*T2c*	*T3a*	*T1a*	*T1b*	*T2a*	*T2b*	*T2c*	*T3a*	*T1a*	*T1b*	*T2a*	*T2b*	*T2c*	*T3a*
Prediction of organ-confined disease (%)																								
2–4	100	85	88	76	82	—	100	78	83	67	71	—	100	—	61	52	—	—	—	—	20	7	—	—
5	100	75	81	67	73	—	100	70	73	56	64	43	100	49	58	43	37	26	—	—	32	—	3	—
6	100	68	72	54	60	42	100	53	62	44	48	33	—	36	44	28	37	19	—	—	14	11	4	5
7	—	54	61	41	46	—	100	39	51	32	37	26	—	24	36	19	24	14	—	—	18	4	5	3
8–10	—	—	48	31	—	—	—	32	39	22	25	12	—	11	29	14	15	9	—	—	3	1	2	2
Prediction of established capsular penetration (%)																								
2–4	0	15	14	26	17	—	0	22	19	34	27	—	0	—	40	49	—	—	—	—	80	94	—	—
5	0	22	20	34	26	—	0	29	28	45	34	58	0	49	43	58	61	75	—	—	68	—	97	—
6	0	30	29	46	38	59	0	45	38	56	49	68	—	62	56	73	59	82	—	—	86	90	96	95
7	—	43	39	59	50	—	0	58	49	68	59	75	—	73	64	81	73	86	—	—	80	96	95	98
8–10	—	—	50	68	—	—	—	64	59	77	71	87	—	87	70	86	82	92	—	—	97	99	97	98
Prediction of seminal vesicle involvement (%)																								
2–4	0	1	1	2	2	—	0	2	1	3	3	—	0	—	3	4	—	—	—	—	12	30	—	—
5	0	3	2	4	4	—	0	4	3	6	6	5	0	7	5	8	12	11	—	—	11	—	29	—
6	0	6	5	9	9	8	0	9	6	11	12	11	—	15	11	19	17	18	—	—	35	40	53	31
7	—	12	9	17	17	—	0	18	12	22	23	18	—	28	19	33	33	31	—	—	31	73	62	55
8–10	—	—	17	29	—	—	—	29	22	38	40	40	—	55	29	50	53	49	—	—	81	93	73	65
Prediction of lymph node involvement (%)																								
2–4	0	2	1	2	4	—	0	2	1	2	5	—	0	—	1	3	—	—	—	—	2	7	—	—
5	0	4	2	4	8	—	0	4	2	5	10	8	0	5	2	6	13	11	—	—	3	—	29	—
6	0	8	3	9	17	15	0	9	4	11	19	16	—	11	5	13	22	20	—	—	9	18	53	31
7	—	15	7	18	31	—	0	18	8	20	34	28	—	21	9	24	39	35	—	—	11	44	62	55
8–10	—	—	13	32	—	—	—	30	15	35	53	50	—	41	17	40	59	54	—	—	35	76	73	65

Dash represents lack of sufficient data to calculate probability.

From Partin AW, Yoo J, Carter B, et al: The use of prostate specific antigen, clinical stage and Gleason score to predict pathological stage in men with localized prostate cancer. J Urol 1993; 150:110–114, with permission.

Principles of Treatment

Multidisciplinary Treatment (Table 22–9)

The major locoregional treatment options for men with clinically localized prostate cancer are as follows:

- retropubic or perineal radical prostatectomy, with or without postoperative radiotherapy
- external beam radiotherapy
- permanent radioactive seed implants (usually ^{125}I or ^{108}Pd) with or without external beam radiotherapy
- temporary radioactive seed implants (usually ^{192}Ir) combined with external beam radiotherapy
- androgen deprivation
- deferred treatment, sometimes called watchful waiting

Additional local treatment options include cryosurgery (freezing the prostate) and thermal ablation (destroying the prostate using very high temperatures). Neither of these last two modalities has gained widespread support, and definitive data regarding efficacy are lacking. Based simply on the physics of dosimetric control (i.e., the ability to focus the modality), thermal ablation is likely to hold the most promise.

Comparing possible modes of treatment highlights an interesting finding. When compared with age-matched controls, patients treated with surgery have a higher survival rate than men who do not have prostate cancer at all. This observation suggests that men undergoing radical prostatectomies are healthier than are men in the general population. In addition, it should be noted that patients treated with surgery are usually younger and healthier, tend to have lower PSA levels, Gleason scores, and earlier stage disease than patients treated with radiation, thus making it difficult to compare outcomes.[165] Despite these observations, the survival results at 10 to 15 years appear to be similar for comparably staged patients treated with either surgery or radiation.[165, 217, 225, 226] One early prospective randomized trial compared radiotherapy with surgery, but because of its small size and the unusually poor outcome in irradiated patients, this trial has largely been ignored.[227]

Most studies suggest that pretreatment PSA screening is the major predictor of treatment failure.[201, 228] To date, however, PSA has not been shown to predict death from prostate cancer. Early failures correlate with the risk of distant failures, so it is likely that with longer follow-up, PSA will be shown to correlate with late deaths.[229] However, the Gleason score, clinical stage, and lymph node status have been shown to predict death from prostate cancer, and they can be combined to predict disease-specific survival.[220, 230] This is particularly true for lymph node involvement, as noted previously.

Surgery

Radical Prostatectomy

In the early 1990s, the percentage of patients treated with radical prostatectomy increased from 11.4% to 29.1%, reflecting the belief by most urologists that surgery is more likely to be curative than radiotherapy.[160, 231] Because the patient's first contact is generally with a urologist, this belief is commonly conveyed to the patient early in the decision-making process. However, over the last few years, there has been a resurgence in the use of radiotherapy, particularly when accompanied by radioactive seed implants.[232, 233] Whether this trend will continue remains to be seen.

Radical prostatectomy involves removing the prostate from the space below the bladder, in front of the rectum, and immediately above the external sphincter (which controls urinary continence). Following a radical prostatectomy, the PSA should become (and remain) undetectable; a detectable PSA implies the presence of cancer cells, either locally or at a metastatic site. Because PSA can be used in this way, the failure rates following surgery are now higher than before the availability of PSA assaying. Stein and colleagues were among the first to report PSA results at 10 years following prostatectomy.[234] In this series, only 40% of patients with clinical stages T1 and T2 and pathologic N0 had an undetectable PSA at 10 years. Some contemporary prostatectomy series with shorter follow-up (2 to 4 years) show even higher PSA failure rates.[235, 236] In this study, the rates reflect that only half of patients under-

TABLE 22–9. **Multidisciplinary Treatment for Prostate Cancer**

Prognostic Group*	Surgery	Radiation Therapy	Chemotherapy
Low risk			
Gleason score: 2–6 PSA: ≤10 ng/mL T1-2	Watchful waiting Radical prostatectomy ± nerve sparing	RT: ~70 Gy	No HT
Intermediate risk			
Gleason score >6 **or** PSA >10 ng/mL **or** T3+	Radical prostatectomy ± lymphadenectomy	RT: 70–80 Gy	Short-term HT
High risk			
Gleason score >8 **and/or** PSA >10 ng/mL **and/or** T3+	Radical prostatectomy ± lymphadenectomy	RT: 72–80 Gy	Long-term HT

RT = radiation therapy; as risk group increases, radiation dose increases; HT = hormonal therapy.
*For further explanation of risk groups, see Table 22–10.

going surgery have organ-confined disease; however, even among those patients with organ-confined disease, 10% to 25% will fail within 5 to 10 years.[237]

The higher-than-expected failure rates after surgery can be explained, in part, by some patients failing because of the development of distant metastases. However, the relatively high incidence of late failures in some series suggests that some of these patients could be detected as a result of a slowly rising PSA, which is typical in local tumor recurrence.[238] Based on a series of patients undergoing TRUS-directed biopsies for a rising PSA level following radical prostatectomy, as many as 50% of such patients demonstrated local failure.[239] The likelihood of a local recurrence did not appear to depend on whether the surgical margins were reported as positive or negative. The possibility that local recurrences were a result of contamination of the surgical bed is supported by studies that demonstrate that in 91% of cases, RT-PCR–positive cells can be identified in the circulation, and in 33% there is cytological evidence of cancer cells in the tumor bed.[240, 241]

Radiation Therapy

External Beam Radiation Therapy (Conventional and Three-Dimensional Conformal)

During the early 1990s, the use of radiation therapy increased from 27.6% to 31% for patients with prostate cancer, somewhat lower than the rise in the use of surgery.[160, 231] A number of studies have supported the long-term efficacy of radiation therapy in the management of clinically localized prostate cancer. Based on DRE alone, the local control rate following external beam irradiation has been estimated to be between 70% and 90%.[217, 220, 226, 242] However, it should be noted that using a rising PSA level to define failure, DRE is now known to underestimate the incidence of local failure.

Early conventional external beam radiation therapy series typically used doses of 60 to 70 Gy, because it was believed that this dose was sufficient and close to the maximum dose tolerated by normal tissues.[242] In the late 1980s, computer-based treatment planning ushered in the use of three-dimensional conformal radiation therapy (3D-CRT). The term *conformal* was used to reflect that blocks could be designed and placed in the field, resulting in a radiation dose distribution that conformed to the shape of the target.

Several retrospective studies have suggested a reduction in acute toxicity with the use of 3D-CRT compared with historical controls.[243–247] Of interest, two prospective randomized trials have been completed, but neither demonstrated a reduction in acute toxicity,[248, 249] although in one, a higher dose of radiation was given to the patients treated with 3D-CRT (78 Gy versus 70 Gy).[227] However, and probably of greater importance, at least one of the trials demonstrated a reduction in late complications.[250]

Several academic centers have reported an improvement in the disease-free survival based on PSA outcomes when high-dose 3D-CRT is compared with conventional techniques and doses.[226, 251–253] The Radiation Therapy Oncology Group (RTOG) is planning to begin a phase III trial to address this question. A new and higher level of sophistication involves the use of even more complex technology to allow the delivery of higher doses of radiation. This next generation of radiation therapy allows greater dose inhomogeneity and is called *intensity modulated radiotherapy.*[254, 255]

Prostate Brachytherapy (Radioactive Seed Implants)

Prostate brachytherapy involves the permanent or temporary placement of radioactive sources directly into the prostate, but there appears to be greater interest in permanent implants. Prostate brachytherapy was first reported in 1917, but it first became a popular therapy in the 1970s.[256, 257] Until the availability of modern imaging, a retropubic approach was required to place ^{125}I radioactive seeds into the prostate under direct visualization. This technique lost popularity in the 1980s because of inferior local control rates compared with some external beam radiation therapy series.[258, 259] A transperineal ultrasound–based approach was adopted and refined by investigators from the Northwest Tumor Institute in Seattle in the mid- to late 1980s.[260] Seven- and eight-year data using this approach have been published,[261] and based on these favorable outcomes, it is likely that enthusiasm for this treatment approach will not wane in the near future.

Prostate brachytherapy can be used as a sole modality or in combination with external beam radiation therapy. Because of rapid dose fall-off, brachytherapy alone can adequately treat only intracapsular disease and minimal transcapsular extension. If brachytherapy is used in patients with a higher risk of extraprostatic disease, then it should be combined with external beam radiation therapy to allow for wider coverage of the periprostatic tissues and seminal vesicles. Iridium-192 is the only widely used isotope for temporary prostate implants, although the use of palladium-108 is increasing.[262] Temporary implants incorporate afterloading techniques, based on postimplant CT scans, which allow adjustments to be made for suboptimal needle placement. Temporary ^{192}Ir implants are generally combined with external beam radiation therapy allowing for a wider margin around the prostate to compensate for extracapsular extension.

Postoperative Radiation Therapy

Although the impact of postoperative radiation on survival remains unproven, it seems reasonable to assume that patients whose only remaining burden consists of microscopic residual disease might benefit from adjuvant rather than so-called salvage radiation treatment. External beam irradiation reduces the local recurrence of essentially all solid tumors with positive margins, and tumors of the prostate appear to be no exception.[263–265] Patients who are treated before demonstrating a clinical local recurrence appear to have an improvement in freedom from PSA failure than those undergoing salvage treatment. In addition, only 50% of patients who receive salvage radiation therapy for biopsy-proven recurrences are considered successfully treated at 3 years.[266]

Hormonal Therapy

Hormonal Therapy and Radiation Therapy (Locally Advanced)

Based on the results of several prospective randomized trials, androgen suppression is frequently added to radiation therapy for the treatment of locally advanced prostate cancer. To date, four prospective randomized trials have shown an improvement in local control with the use of hormonal therapy with radiation therapy.[187, 188, 267–269] Three of these trials have demonstrated an improvement in disease-free survival,[187, 188, 269] and two trials have suggested an improved overall survival and disease-specific survival with the use of longterm hormonal therapy control.[187, 188] The conclusions from these studies are consistent with the recent pseudo–meta-analysis of RTOG trials reported by Roach and associates,[270] and they are summarized in Table 22–10. Based on this analysis, it appears that even a short course of androgen suppression (4 months) can enhance the survival of relatively low-risk patients, whereas high-risk patients require long-term hormonal therapy after radiation.

Rationale for using androgen ablation and radiation can be found in both experimental and clinical observations. These latter observations include:

- evidence of synergistic interactions between hormonal ablation and radiation
- evidence of shrinking or debulking of the tumor based on surgical series
- observations from clinical trials combining radiation with hormonal therapy[271]

Both androgen ablation and radiation independently have been shown to be capable of inducing apoptosis in cell lines.[272, 273] In addition, synergistic interactions between radiation and hormone suppression have been observed for a number of cancer cell lines and animal models.[274, 275] Thus, in a tumor composed of both androgen-dependent and androgen-independent cells, it is not surprising to find enhanced killing when radiation and hormonal ablation are combined.

It is also common practice to use androgen suppressive therapy alone for the treatment of prostate cancer. This approach is supported by a randomized trial conducted by the Medical Research Council (MRC) demonstrating that early androgen ablative therapy improved outcome in patients with M0 disease when they received early (compared with delayed) hormonal therapy.[186] This philosophy is further supported by a European study that demonstrated that despite the opportunity for hormonal therapy salvage, those patients receiving early hormonal therapy had a higher survival rate than patients treated initially with radiation therapy alone.[188] However, a note of caution must be made concerning both of these studies. Firstly, the MRC trial had 29 patients on the observation arm that apparently died of prostate cancer without ever receiving hormonal therapy. This raises questions about whether this trial was actually a study of treatment versus no treatment. Secondly, in the EORTC trial, patients were generally not offered hormonal therapy until they became symptomatic, and it is not known whether the control arm would have done much better if treated at the time of PSA failure.

Metastatic Disease and Hormonal Therapy

The mainstay of treating metastatic prostate cancer is androgen deprivation therapy. Although numerous other drugs have been tried, none have been proven to match the biologic activity of androgen suppression.[271] Fortunately, due to the modern widespread use of PSA screening, fewer men are being diagnosed with metastatic disease and the mortality rate appears to be dropping.[159]

There are a number of ways to block the physiologic effects of the androgen hormone testosterone, including orchiectomy, diethylstilbestrol, and the use of luteinizing hormone–releasing hormone (LHRH) agonists, such as goserelin acetate and leuprolide. All of these modalities appear to be equally effective in producing castrate levels of testosterone (<50 ng/mL). Although most experts believe that all of these approaches are roughly equal, there continues to be controversy surrounding the need to add antiandrogenic agents, such as flutamide, bicalutamide and

TABLE 22–10. **Combined Results of Disease-Specific Survival from 5 RTOG Prospective Randomized Trials of Patients with Prostate Cancer (RTOG 75–06, 77–06, 83–07, 85–31, and 86–10)**

	RT Alone		RT + Short-Term HT*		RT + Long-Term HT	
Risk Group	*5-Year Survival (%)*	*8-Year Survival (%)*	*5-Year Survival (%)*	*8-Year Survival (%)*	*5-Year Survival (%)*	*8-Year Survival (%)*
2	94	83	100	98	93	89
3	83	70	80	67	93	88
4	64	42	64	49	81	69

RT = radiation therapy; HT = hormonal therapy.
Risk Group 2: Gleason score 2–6, T3Nx or Gleason score 2–6, N+ or Gleason score 7, T1–2Nx.
Risk Group 3: Gleason score 7, T3Nx or Gleason score 7, N+ or Gleason score 8–10, T1–2Nx.
Risk Group 4: Gleason score 8–10, T3Nx or Gleason score 8–10, N+.
*Goserelin acetate and flutamide, 2 months before and 2 months after RT.
Modified from Roach M III, Lu J, Pilepich MV, et al: Predicting long term survival and the need for hormonal therapy: a meta-analysis of RTOG prostate cancer trials. Int J Radiat Oncol Biol Phys 2000; 47:617–627.

nilutamide. When one of these antiandrogens is added to an LHRH agent or orchiectomy, it is usually called *combined androgen blockade* (CAB).

The rationale for using CAB exists, in part, because adrenal androgens are capable of producing the androgen precursors dihydroepiandrosterone (DHEA) and androstenedione, which can be converted into dihydrotestosterone (DHT) within both the prostate and, potentially, the tumor.[276] DHT is the most active form of testosterone but only represents as much as 5% of the normal serum testosterone. Therefore, despite medical or surgical castration, circulating levels of testosterone resulting from adrenal precursors may be clinically significant.[277, 278]

Prospective randomized trials have produced mixed conclusions regarding the advantage of CAB compared with monotherapy. A National Cancer Institute trial (NCI 0036) comparing an LHRH agent alone with an LHRH agent plus an antiandrogen demonstrated a survival advantage for the men receiving CAB.[279] An even larger study, conducted by the Southwest Oncology Group (SWOG), compared orchiectomy with orchiectomy plus CAB and showed better PSA responses, but there was no statistically significant difference in survival.[280] Some investigators have explained this discrepancy by noting that LHRH agents can cause a paradoxical flare in prostate cancer that will be blocked by antiandrogens; the flare does not occur with orchiectomy alone.[281] Thus, antiandrogens might be beneficial when combined with LHRH agents but not with orchiectomy.

Roughly 90% of patients with metastatic prostate cancer will respond to hormonal therapy. Unfortunately, within 18 months of beginning such therapy, the majority of these men will manifest evidence of failure and will develop what is commonly called *hormone refractory prostate cancer* (HRPC). The survival of patients with HRPC is usually 10 to 12 months. Despite this poor prognosis, patients with HRPC may respond to several alternative therapies, including antiandrogen withdrawal, secondary hormonal manipulations, and chemotherapy. It is now well recognized that approximately 25% of patients with a rising PSA level who are receiving CAB may experience PSA decline or objective improvement with the discontinuation of antiandrogen[282–284]; the mechanism for this phenomenon is unknown, but it may involve acquired mutations in the androgen receptor. The use of adrenolytic agents, such as high-dose ketoconazole or aminoglutethimide, or steroids, such as prednisone or hydrocortisone, may also produce clinical benefit in some men with HRPC. However, the response to secondary hormonal manipulations is generally transient (4 to 6 months). Among the standard chemotherapeutic programs, regimens combining antimicrotubule agents with estramustine have shown the most promise.[283, 285, 286] The treatment of HRPC is an area of intense clinical investigation, and novel drugs such as suramin (an anti–growth factor agent) may eventually find a role in the management of hormone refractory disease.[287]

Special Considerations

Rising PSA Level without Evidence of Metastatic Disease

Although the incidence of metastatic prostate cancer appears to be decreasing, nearly half of all men treated for localized disease with radical prostatectomy or radiation therapy will manifest biochemical evidence of progressive disease. If these men live long enough, then it is likely that they will eventually develop metastatic disease. For selected patients with local recurrences, a local salvage therapy may render them free of disease. For the remaining patients, watchful waiting or androgen-suppressive therapy are the remaining options.

Before the availability of the serum marker PSA, hormonal therapy was generally reserved for patients with symptoms of progressive disease. With the awareness that a rising PSA level is evidence of progression, many men are treated to delay the time to clinical progression. There are no prospective clinical trials directly testing the merits of early hormonal therapy for a rising PSA; however, studies demonstrating that early androgen ablative therapy improves survival compared with delayed treatment in men with localized disease provides support for this strategy.[186, 188, 270] It is likely that selected patients will benefit (in terms of quality of life and overall survival) with the use of early hormonal therapy, but it is also likely that some men are being castrated unnecessarily.

An alternative means of selecting relapsed patients for further treatment is based on the doubling time of PSA levels when plotted from their nadirs.[288] When PSA levels rise slowly (i.e., doubling time >1 year) from less than 1 μg toward 10 μg, a decision to treat local recurrence includes MRI or magnetic resonance spectroscopy of the prostate gland, identification of a positive foci, and needle biopsy confirmation with TRUS guidance. If the patient is a good surgical risk, then surgical salvage is possible; an alternate salvage therapy is localized seed implants with ^{125}I or ^{108}Pd, with attention to minimizing the radiation dose to the smallest achievable volume of the anterior rectal wall. Encouraging results have been reported by Grado and associates.[233] The greatest challenge in managing prostate cancer patients with rising PSA levels continues to be deciding who needs what and when.

Results and Prognosis

Outcomes Following Radical Surgery and Radiation Therapy Treatment

A summary of the characteristics of patients and outcomes from selected surgical series from several major institutions is provided in Table 22–11. The gold standard for any cancer treatment should be long survival. Data suggest that by combining Gleason score and clinical stage, overall and disease-specific survivals can be estimated to 15 years.[220] However, the majority of the trials on which these estimates were made were conducted before the widespread use of PSA screening and probably represent a worst-case scenario. Table 22–12 summarizes the results of long-term survivals based on an analysis of patients treated with radiation therapy on prospective randomized trials. More recent series have included patients who may have benefited from PSA screening, and earlier end points have been adopted to assess the efficacy of treatment. Prostate biopsies and post-treatment PSA levels have become the most common intermediate surrogates for long-term survival.

TABLE 22–11. **Data from Selected Surgical Series; Outcomes by Clinical Stage, PSA Level, and Gleason Score**

Series	Clinical Stage	*n*	PSA NED %		PSA Level (ng/mL)	*n*	PSA NED %		Gleason Score	*n*	PSA NED%	
			5-yr	*10-yr*			*5-yr*	*10-yr*			*5-yr*	*10-yr*
Partin et al[289]	T1a	48	100	100	0–4.0	284	92	NA	2–4	91	98	82
	T1b	90	91	91	4.1–10.0	237	83	NA	5	219	92	88
	T1c	23	100	NA	10.1–20.0	105	56	NA	6	391	85	70
	T2a	438	87	76	>20.1	40	45	NA	7	128	62	50
	T2b	240	71	52					8–10	65	46	15
	T2c	55	69	60								
Catalona et al[290]	T1a	21	74	NA	0–4.0	117	95	NA				
	T1b	60	74	NA	4.1–9.9	394	93	NA				
	T1c	119	98	NA	≥10.0	253	71	NA				
	T2a	270	56	NA								
	T2b	455	56	NA								
	T2c											
Zietman et al[291]	T1	11	57*		≤15 (≈10)	37	55	NA				
	T2a	23			>15 (≈>10)	23	25	NA				
	T2b-c	20										
	T2 (nos)	8										
Zincke et al[292]	T1a	47	NA	NA					2–3	292	83	71
	T1b	177	76	70					4–6	2096	74	53
	T2a	887	76	56					7–10	782	51	35
	T2b-c	2059	66	47								
D'Amico et al[293]					0–10	182	<80	NA	2–4	102	<75	NA
					10–20	101	<50	NA	5–7	202	<60	NA
					>20	64	<20	NA	8–10	43	<20	NA

NED = no evidence of disease.
*Excludes patients of longer follow-up and patients with undetectable PSA postoperatively.
Modified from Roach M III, Wallner K: Prostate cancer. In: Leibel SA, Phillips TL (eds): Textbook of Radiation Oncology, pp 741–784. Philadelphia, W.B. Saunders, 1998.

TABLE 22–12. **Data from Selected Radiation Therapy Series; Outcomes by Clinical Stage, PSA Level, and Gleason Score**

Series	Clinical Stage	*n*	PSA NED %		PSA Level (ng/mL)	*n*	PSA NED %		Gleason Score	*n*	PSA NED%	
			5-yr	*10-yr*			5-yr	10-yr			*5-yr*	*10-yr*
Kaplan et al[294]	T1	44	≈48	NA	<10	32	≈65	NA	2–5	33	≈70	NA
	T2	35	≈60	NA	10–20	26	≈75	NA	6–7	54	≈40	NA
	T3-4	37	≈15	NA	>20–50	31	≈25	NA	8–10	29	10	NA
					>50	28	≈15	NA				
Zagars et al[295]	T1a	18	NA	NA	0–4.0	90	86	NA	2–4	112	75	NA
	T1b	57	NA	NA	4.1–10.0	82	67	NA	5–6	95	60	NA
	T1c	47	NA	NA	10.1–30.0	78	45	NA	7	41	63‡	NA
	T2a	42	NA	NA	>30	19	20	NA	8–10	16	32‡	NA
	T2b	81	NA	NA								
	T2c	24	NA	NA								
Kuban et al[296]	T1b	27	72	35	0–4.0	43	69	59	2–4	113	74	42
	T2a	60	63	18	4.1–10.0	125	57	18	5–7	211	48	11
	T2b-c	62	60	21	10.1–20.0	89	56	0	8–10	64	33	9
	T3-4	246	34	11	>20.1	138	20	0				
Zietman et al[297]	T1-T2a	220	66	47	<4.0	29	80	NA	2–4	36	26*	NA
	T2b-c	284	51	29	4–10	42	42	NA	5–6	73		NA
	T3-4	540	42	18	10–20	28	30	NA	7–10	33		NA
					20–50	36	0	NA				
					>50	22	0	NA				
Roach et al[298]	T1b-c	90	60	NA	0–<4.0	73	90†	NA	2–5	160	60	NA
	T2	272	50	NA	4.1–<10.0	146	60	NA	6–7	223	50	NA
	T3-4	128	30	NA	10.1–20.0	110	35	NA	8–10	60	30	NA
					>20.1	146	30	NA				

NED = no evidence of disease.
*4-year PSA >1 ng/mL.
†At 4-year follow-up.
‡At 3-year follow-up.
Modified from Roach M III, Wallner K: Prostate cancer. In: Leibel SA, Phillips TL (eds): Textbook of Radiation Oncology, pp 741–784. Philadelphia, W.B. Saunders, 1998.

Biopsies obtained following radiation therapy are the most accurate method of defining local control following radiation therapy but they are not routinely performed. Palpable regrowth is associated with persistent disease in 90% of patients.[299] Post-treatment biopsies show a much higher incidence of residual tumor than palpation, although biopsies acquired less than 2 or 3 years after irradiation may continue to reflect resolving disease.[300] This potential source of ambiguity, cost, and lack of sensitivity has discouraged investigators from routinely recommending post-treatment biopsies.

Prostate irradiation usually results in a 90% or higher reduction in the serum PSA level within 6 to 12 months. Lack of such a decline suggests inadequate local treatment or metastatic disease; a rapidly rising PSA level usually reflects distant metastases. Most investigators seem to believe that the risk of relapse rises progressively as nadir values increase to higher than 1.0 ng/mL.[301, 302] Other investigators have suggested that the nadir should be below 0.5 ng/mL.[303, 304] Nonetheless, a rising PSA level appears to be the most agreed-upon measure of progression.

Considering the obvious differences between patients treated with surgery compared with radiation therapy, the freedom from PSA failure at 5 years suggests similar efficacies for both surgery and radiation therapy (Table 22–13).

Complications of Therapy

Surgery

Based on national statistics, the mortality rate associated with radical prostatectomy approaches 2%, but when it is performed by experts, that is, urologic surgeons who limit their practice to oncology, particularly prostate cancer, the risk is generally much lower.[231]

- *Pelvic pain* and *transient incontinence* are the most common immediate short-term complications.
- *Urinary stress incontinence* is reported by experts to occur in 5% to 14% of patients or less, but it appears more common when patients are surveyed.
- *Thromboembolytic events, myocardial infarctions,* and *wound infections* occur in approximately 1% of patients. However, among men aged 65 years and older, nearly 8% suffered major myocardial infarctions within 30 days of surgery.[231]
- *Impotence* is the most common long-term complication with radical prostatectomy. Impotence appears to depend, in part, on the expertise of the surgeon and the preoperative sexual function of the patient. Following a standard radical prostatectomy, 90% to 100% of men are reported to be impotent. Following a nerve-sparing prostatectomy, as many as 70% of men younger than 60 years of age may maintain some degree of potency in the hands of some experts. Older men fair far less well despite this nerve-sparing procedure.[305, 306]

External Beam Radiation Therapy

Treatment-related mortality, severe complications, and incontinence rates are reported to occur following radiation therapy in 0.2%, 1.9%, and 0.9% of patients, respectively.[307] Urethral strictures, hematuria, and late, moderately severe rectal bleeding occur in roughly 5.4%, 5.1%, and 5.4% of patients, respectively.

TABLE 22–13. **Summary of PSA Results for Selected Surgical and Radiation Therapy Series**

Prognostic Factor	Surgical Series PSA NED (%*) 5 yrs	Surgical Series PSA NED (%*) 10 yrs	RT Series PSA NED (%†) 5 yrs	RT Series PSA NED (%†) 10 yrs	Comments
Clinical Stage					
T1a	74–100	100	NA	NA	In addition to differences in T stage, a larger percentage of surgical patients have lower PSAs (<10 ng/mL: average 67% versus 51%) and lower tumor grades (Gleason score ≥7: 27% versus 42%) and patients with positive nodes are frequently excluded.
T1b	74–91	70–91	66–72	32–47	
T1c	100	NA	NA	NA	
T2a	56–87	56–76	63	18–47	
T2b-2c	56–70	47–60	60	21–29	
T3-4	NA	NA	30‡–34	10–21	
PSA Level					
0–4	85–95	NA	80–86	NA	Patients treated by surgery tend to have lower T stage tumors (≈ ⅓ T3).
4.1–10.0	55–93	NA	42–67	NA	
10.1–20.0	56	NA	30–75	NA	
Gleason Score					
2–4	<75–98	82	68–75	NA	Patients treated by surgery tend to have lower T stage tumors (≈ ⅓ T3).
5–6	85–92	53–88	60	NA	
7	62	50	63§	NA	
8–10	<20–46	15§	10‖–33	9	

NED = no evidence of disease; RT = radiation therapy.
*PSA failure defined as 0.2 to 0.6 ng/mL.
†PSA failure defined as 1.0 to 4.0 ng/mL.
‡>1 ng/mL at 4 years.
§Excludes node patients who are positive.
‖At 3 years.
From Roach M III, Wallner K: Prostate cancer. In: Leibel SA, Phillips TL: Textbook of Radiation Oncology, pp 741–784. Philadelphia, W.B. Saunders, 1998.

- During the delivery of radiation, most patients note increased *frequency* and *dysuria*, and some patients, particularly those receiving pelvic irradiation, report mild *diarrhea*.[251] Urinary incontinence following radiotherapy is usually related to prior TURP.
- *Rectal bleeding* occurs in up to 10% of patients during treatment, but it does not necessarily correlate with late bleeding. It appears to be dose- and volume-related and is largely preventable.[250, 308, 309]
- *Fecal incontinence* is rare, but rectal urgency and a reduction in rectal storage capacity may be bothersome in as many as 10% of patients.[310]

Loss of potency is the most common, permanent morbidity resulting from radiation therapy. Based on mailed questionnaires, potency is preserved in roughly 80% of patients at 15 to 20 months after treatment.[217] However, there is a further loss of potency with time as a result of aging and late radiation-induced periprostatic fibrosis. When potency is maintained, the frequency and quality of intercourse and the volume of the ejaculate tend to be reduced.[309] The high likelihood of at least partial loss of erectile function should be conveyed to patients before treatment.

Brachytherapy

Acute toxicity tends to be somewhat greater following brachytherapy than following external beam irradiation.

- Acute obstruction occurs in 2% to 25% of patients and urinary incontinence may occur in up to 50% of patients if they previously had a TURP.
- Rectal injury is uncommon with TRUS-based techniques.

Maintenance of potency with brachytherapy has generally been reported to be higher (~80%) than that following prostatectomy or external beam radiation therapy.[311, 312] However, because it is commonly believed that implants result in less impotence, potent and sexually active patients are more likely to seek an implant. This bias makes it difficult to compare the risk of impotence following brachytherapy with that for external beam radiation therapy or surgery.

Germ Cell Tumors of the Testes

Epidemiology and Etiology

Epidemiology

Germ cell tumors (GCTs) account for 1% of all male malignancies, with 6900 new cases diagnosed annually in the United States.[5] Despite its overall curability, approximately 300 to 500 men die each year as a consequence of these tumors. It is the most common malignancy among men aged 15 to 35. Seminoma accounts for 40% of all germ cell tumors, whereas nonseminoma germ cell tumors (NSGCT) account for 60%. By and large, GCT is a malignancy of early adulthood, with the incidence of seminoma peaking in the 25-to-45-year-old group; the highest incidence of nonseminoma occurs in a slightly younger group of men (15-to-30-year-old group).[313]

Etiology

A history of cryptorchidism appears to be related to the development of GCT, with the risk being 10- to 40-fold higher in cryptorchid testes. Approximately 5% to 20% of GCTs arising in patients with a history of cryptorchidism occur in the normal, descended testicle, suggesting that systemic sequelae of cryptorchidism (e.g., testicular atrophy) are of greater etiologic importance than local or anatomic abnormalities.[314] Men with undescended testis located in the abdomen are more likely to develop testis cancer compared with those with testis located in the inguinal region.

Molecular Biology

The isochromosome of the short arm of chromosome 12, i(12p), has been reported to be present in up to 90% of GCT patients.[315] The presence of i(12p) has been used diagnostically in patients with midline carcinomas of unknown origin, allowing, in one series, a definitive diagnosis of GCT in 28% of patients, and also serving as a marker of chemotherapy sensitivity.[316] The presence of three or more copies of i(12p) has been correlated with poor prognosis of GCT.[317] The gene or genes on i(12p) that may be involved in carcinogenesis have not been identified.[318] Nonetheless, cyclin D2, a member of the D cyclins, important in the regulation of the G_1 checkpoint of the cell cycle, is encoded by a gene on 12p and is overexpressed in nearly all GCTs. Therefore, aberrant cyclin D2 expression may be important in germ cell tumorigenesis.[319]

Detection and Diagnosis

Clinical Detection

In addition to malignancy, the differential diagnosis of a testicular mass includes testicular torsion, hydroceles, varicoceles, spermatoceles, and epididymitis. Signs and symptoms indistinguishable from acute epididymitis have been observed in up to one fourth of patients with testicular neoplasms.

- Up to 70% of patients with testicular cancer present with testicular swelling.
- Testicular pain is a presenting feature of 18% to 46%

of patients with GCT. Acute pain may be associated with torsion of the neoplasm, infarction, or bleeding in the tumor, as well as with epididymitis.
- Less commonly presenting symptoms will include gynecomastia in human chorionic gonadotropin (HCG)–producing tumors such as choriocarcinoma (10%), back or flank pain from metastatic disease (10%), and infertility in less than 5% of tumors. Approximately 25% of patients with advanced disease have symptoms referable to their metastases, such as back pain.

Diagnostic Procedures

- *Testicular ultrasonography* is a sensitive and specific test that can discriminate between a testicular neoplasm and nonmalignant processes. The obvious presence of a testicular mass on physical examination does not obviate the need for careful bilateral sonography, given the 2% to 4% incidence of bilateral lesions.[320]
- *Transinguinal orchiectomy* is the definitive procedure for both pathologic diagnosis and local control of testicular carcinoma and, in some cases, may be a curative procedure. The removal of a suspicious testicle by inguinal orchiectomy should be undertaken even in patients in whom a diagnosis of disseminated GCT has been made by biopsy of a metastatic site, because the testes appear to be chemotherapy sanctuaries for cancer cells.[321]
- *Transscrotal biopsy* or orchiectomy should *not* be performed because both are associated with an increased risk of local recurrence or spread to inguinal lymph nodes.[322]

Imaging

All patients with GCT should undergo CT of the chest, abdomen, and pelvis. In patients with NSGCT, abdominopelvic CT understaging (false negatives) occurs in as high as 50% of patients. The incidence of occult retroperitoneal lymph node metastases in patients with seminoma who have a normal CT scan is estimated to be 10% to 25%.

Classification and Staging

Histopathology

Two major histologic types of GCT are recognized: pure seminoma and nonseminomatous germ cell tumors. NSGCT are either pure tumors (yolk sac, embryonal, choriocarcinoma, teratocarcinoma) or of mixed (seminoma + NSGCT) composition. Any nonseminomatous component, no matter how limited, changes the histopathologic classification to NSGCT.[323]

Staging

Stage I (or A) refers to tumors confined to the testis with no evidence of nodal or pulmonary parenchymal involvement

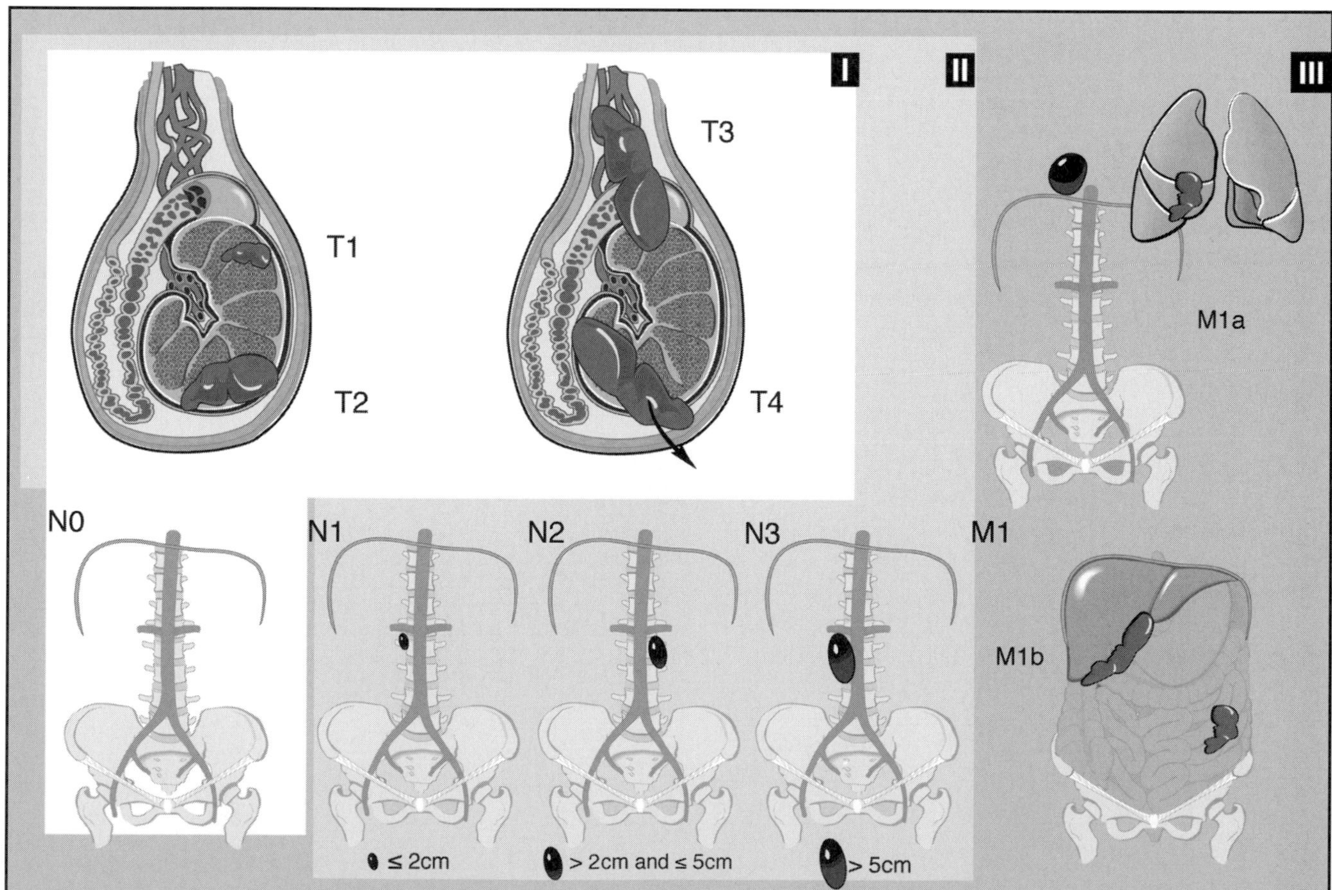

Figure 22–11. Anatomic staging for germ cell carcinoma (see Table 22–14).

(Figure 22–11; Table 22–14). Stage II (or B) denotes tumors with retroperitoneal lymph node metastases. Stage II patients are further subdivided by the relative tumor burden. In seminoma patients, tumor burden is clinically defined by the size of nodal involvement detected by imaging studies, whereas in NSGCT this is usually, but not always, a pathologic diagnosis. Stage IIA (or B1) implies minimal but definite nodal involvement, generally of a microscopic nature; IIB (or B2) refers to macroscopic disease or a larger number of microscopic metastases, whereas IIC (or B3) indicates bulky retroperitoneal nodal disease. Stage III (or C) refers to disease that has spread beyond the retroperitoneum, usually to supradiaphragmatic lymph nodes, pulmonary parenchyma, or other sites, including liver, bone, or brain.

Staging Evaluation

Tumor Markers

Tumor markers have become a fundamental component of the laboratory evaluation of patients with suspected testicular neoplasms, offering diagnostic, staging, and prognostic information, as well as measuring disease progression and response to therapy. Thus, along with the usual laboratory studies obtained on patients with suspected GCT, preorchiectomy levels of HCG alpha-fetoprotein (AFP) and lactate dehydrogenase (LDH) are mandatory.

- In germ cell tumors, HCG is produced by syncytiotrophoblastic cells in embryonal carcinoma, choriocarcinoma, and seminoma. Extremely high levels of HCG are generally associated with choriocarcinoma. While seminomas are generally believed to be marker negative, the incidence of HCG-positive seminoma varies from 5% to 40%. However, in general, these HCG elevations do not exceed a level of 100 mIU/mL, and they probably do not connote a worse prognosis.[324]
- AFP elevations are most commonly seen in embryonal carcinoma and yolk sac tumors. Pure seminomas and pure choriocarcinomas do not produce AFP. Thus, in the absence of hepatitis or other causes of AFP, the presence of an elevated AFP in a histologically pure seminoma *by definition* identifies the presence of nonseminomatous elements and mandates that the management proceed accordingly.
- LDH is a nonspecific marker that appears to be related to tumor burden and can serve as both an indicator of response to treatment and as a predictor of prognosis.

Approximately 85% of NSGCTs will have an elevation of either AFP or β-HCG. AFP elevation alone is seen in 40% of cases, and HCG elevation alone is seen in 50% to 60% of cases. It is important to note that up to 30% of patients with early-stage NSGCT will have normal serum markers, so the absence of marker elevation should not influence the decision to perform an orchiectomy.

Principles of Treatment

Germ Cell Tumor (Seminoma)

The natural history of GCT is largely defined by lymphatic spread to the retroperitoneal lymph nodes early in the disease, with hematogenous dissemination developing later. Thus, virtually all GCTs with pulmonary or visceral metastases will have concomitant retroperitoneal lymph node involvement. Pure choriocarcinoma is an exception, characterized by early hematogenous dissemination to lungs, brain, and viscera.

Whereas nodal involvement is less common in semi-

TABLE 22–14. **Staging Table for Cancer of the Testis**

Stage	Grouping	Serum Tumor Marker (S)	Descriptor
I	pT1–4 N0 M0	SX	N0: No regional lymph node metastasis M0: No distant metastatis
IA	pT1 N0 M0	S0	pT1: Tumor limited to testis and epididymis without vascular invasion; tumor may invade into tunica albuginea but not tunica vaginalis
IB	pT2 N0 M0	S0	pT2: Tumor limited to testis and epididymis with vascular invasion or tumor extending through tunica albuginea involving tunica vaginalis
	pT3 N0 M0	S0	pT3: Tumor invades spermatic cord with or without vascular or lymphatic invasion
	pT4 N0 M0	S0	pT4: Tumor invades scrotum with or without vascular or lymphatic invasion
IIA	pT/Tx any N1 M0	S0-1	N1: Metastasis with a lymph node mass ≤2 cm in greatest dimension; or multiple lymph node masses, no one >2 cm in greatest dimension
IIB	pT/Tx any N2 M0	S0-1	N2: Metastasis with lymph node mass >2 cm but ≤5 cm; or multiple lymph node masses, any one >2 cm but ≤5 cm in greatest dimension
IIC	pT/Tx any N3 M0	S0-1	N3: Metastasis with a lymph node mass >5 cm in greatest dimension
IIIA	pT/Tx any Any N M1a	S0-1	M1a: Nonregional nodal or pulmonary metastasis
IIIB	pT/Tx any N1–3 M0	S2	
	pT/Tx any Any N M1a	S2	
IIIC	pT/Tx any N1–3 M0	S3	
	pT/Tx any Any N M1a	S3	
	pT/Tx any Any N M1b	Any S	M1b: Distant metastasis other than to non-regional lymph nodes and lungs

pTx = primary tumor cannot be assessed; pT0 = no evidence of primary tumor; pTis = intratubular germ cell neoplasia; SX = marker studies not available.
S1 = lactate dehydrogenase (LDH) <1.5 × N and human chorionic gonadotropin (HCG) <5000 mIU/mL and alpha-fetoprotein (AFP) <1000 ng/mL.
S2 = LDH <1.5–10 × N or HCG <5000–50,000 mIU/mL or AFP <1000–10,000 ng/mL.
S3 = LDH >10 × N or HCG >50,000 mIU/mL or AFP >10,000 ng/mL.

noma than in NSGCT, ureteral obstructions seem to occur more commonly than in NSGCTs because of either bulky disease or more diffuse sheetlike spreading. It is extremely unusual for seminomas to present with hepatic or pulmonary metastases; when they do, it is virtually always in the setting of retroperitoneal nodal involvement.

Clinical Stage I Seminoma

Cancer confined to the testis is the most common presentation of seminoma, accounting for nearly 70% of all patients with this diagnosis. However, approximately 15% of clinical stage I seminoma patients will, in fact, have occult retroperitoneal disease; therefore, many practitioners recommend elective postoperative radiation of the lymph nodes.

Surgery

The standard form of treatment for stage I GCT is radical inguinal orchiectomy, with or without radiation therapy (Table 22–15). Retroperitoneal lymphadenectomy is not recommended for patients with seminomas. In a surveillance study, Warde and coworkers assessed various prognostic factors predictive of disease progression in patients with clinical stage I seminoma following orchiectomy.[325] With a median follow-up of 6.1 years, 31 patients had relapse, for an actuarial 5-year relapse-free rate of 84.9%. The 5-year actuarial survival rate was 97.1% and the cause-specific survival rate was 99.5%. On multivariate analysis, age and tumor size were predictive of relapse. The risk of relapse in 57 patients with none of the three adverse prognostic factors (age 34 years or older, tumor 6 cm or smaller, and no small vessel invasion) was only 6%. Ninety percent of the recurrences were in the para-aortic nodes and very close follow-up with CT scans was required. These investigators continue to recommend prophylactic para-aortic irradiation outside of a study setting.

Radiation Therapy

Because of the very great radiosensitivity of seminomas and the risk of occult nodal spread, the standard of practice has been to follow inguinal orchiectomy for stage I testicular seminomas with adjuvant radiation to the para-aortic and ipsilateral pelvic and inguinal lymph nodes. Doses of 25 to 30 Gy are considered adequate by most authorities. After adjuvant radiation, the cause-specific 5-year survival rate is 97% or higher.

Chemotherapy

Although surveillance and adjuvant chemotherapy results are encouraging, these therapies must still be considered experimental because decades of experience have proved radiation therapy to be extremely efficacious and relatively nonmorbid.[326]

Clinical Stage II Seminoma

Surgery

Patients with limited stage IIA GCT are candidates for retroperitoneal lymph node dissection (RPLND). After orchiectomy, patients with serologic disease should be treated only with chemotherapy, because failure after lymphadenectomy alone is common. It is interesting that approximately 23% of patients with presumed stage II GCT will have pathologic stage I disease noted at the time of lymphadenectomy. Patients with more significant stage II GCT are best managed with primary chemotherapy followed by selective surgery.

Radiation Therapy

Over 90% of seminoma patients with masses smaller than 5 cm (stage IIA and IIB) will be cured with standard abdominal radiation therapy alone. The use of salvage chemotherapy in patients with masses smaller than 5 cm who relapse after initial radiation therapy results in a cause-specific survival rate of 95% to 100%. Therefore, radiation therapy is recommended for small-volume (<5 cm) retroperitoneal disease. In contrast, higher failure rates are reported in patients with masses between 5 and 10 cm in size, and the relapse rate after radiation therapy alone in patients with masses larger than 10 cm is unacceptably high, at approximately 35%. It is generally recommended that patients with stage IIC seminoma (masses >5 cm), and especially patients with masses larger than 10 cm, be treated initially with chemotherapy. This approach results in cure rates ranging from 85% to 95%.[326]

Prophylactic mediastinal and supraclavicular irradiation

TABLE 22–15. **Multidisciplinary Treatment for Cancer of the Testis**

Stage	Surgery	Radiation Therapy	Chemotherapy
Seminoma			
I	Radical inguinal orchiectomy	Postop RT: 25–30 Gy	NR
IIA	Radical inguinal orchiectomy ± RPLND	<5 cm: postop RT: 25–30 Gy	
IIB	Radical inguinal orchiectomy ± RPLND	NR	MCT: PEB
III	Radical inguinal orchiectomy	NR	MCT: PEB
Non-Seminoma			
I	Radical inguinal orchiectomy	NR	NR
II	Radical inguinal orchiectomy + RPLND	NR	MCT: PEB
III	NR	NR	MCT: PEB

RPLND = retroperitoneal lymph node dissection; NR = not recommended; postop = postoperative; MCT = multidrug chemotherapy; PEB = cisplatin + etoposide + bleomycin.

is no longer recommended by most authorities, and it is only given on the rare occasions in which there is isolated progression of the disease following chemotherapy.[327] In addition, the International Consensus Conference in Leeds in 1989 recommended that inguinoscrotal irradiation also be omitted even when scrotal interference has occurred.[328]

Nonseminomatous Germ Cell Tumor

The more aggressive biology of NSGCT is evidenced by the 60% to 70% of patients with NSGCT who will have nodal or other metastatic involvement at presentation, compared with 25% in patients with pure seminoma. The distribution of retroperitoneal lymph node metastases in NSGCT is well known and provides the basis for specific surgical approaches (Figure 22–12). The paracaval, interaortocaval, and right common iliac lymph nodes are considered primary landing sites for right-sided tumors. The interaortocaval, left para-aortic, and common iliac lymph nodes are the primary landing sites for left-sided cancers. Suprahilar nodal involvement does not occur in patients with microscopic or low-burden infrahilar disease, whereas 25% of patients with gross infrahilar disease have been found to have positive suprahilar nodes.[329]

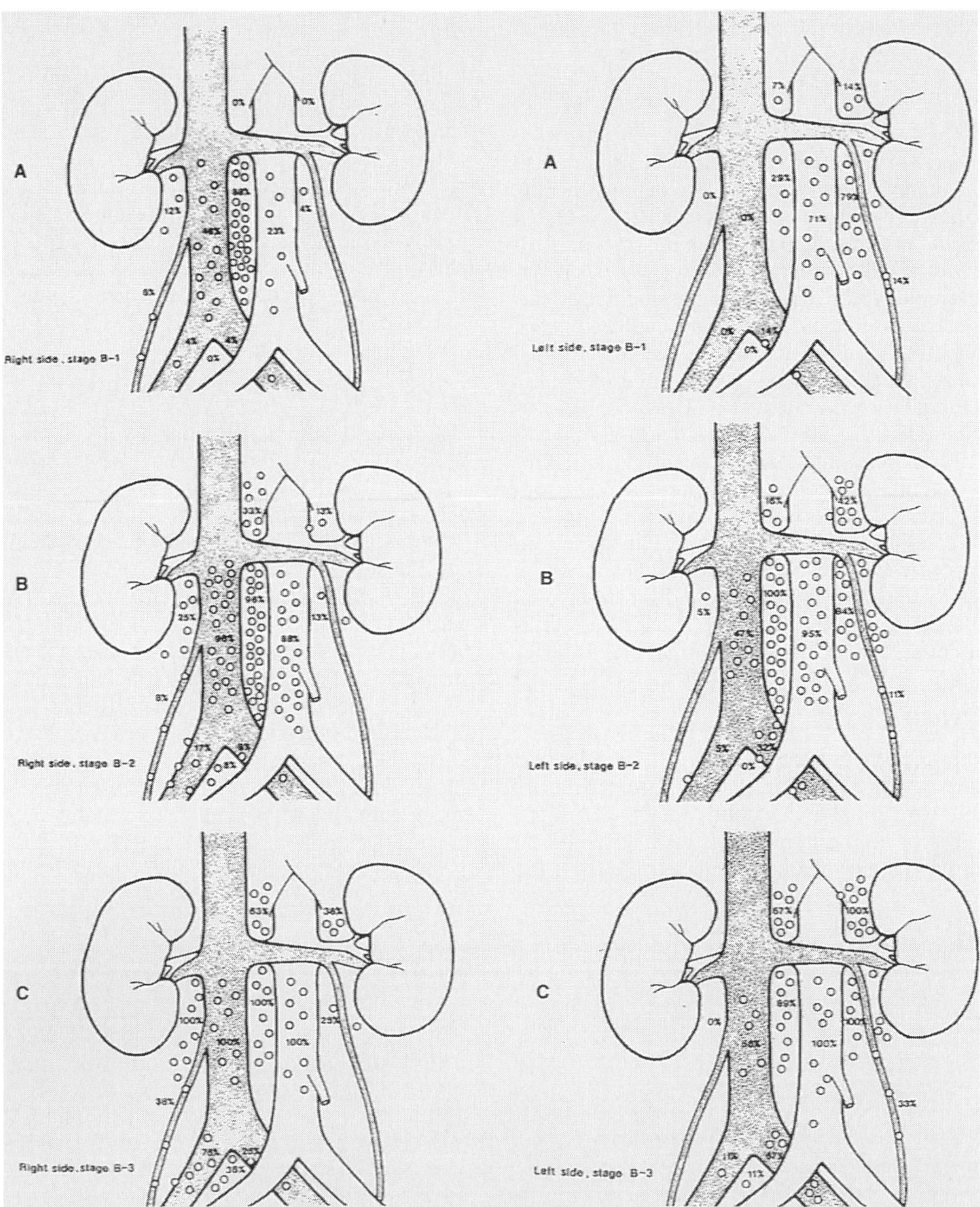

Figure 22–12. Mapping of metastatic landing sites for right-sided tumors and left-sided tumors. (From Donohue JP, Sachary FM, Maynard BR: Distribution of nodal metastases in nonseminomatous testis cancer. J Urol 1982; 128:315–320, with permission.)

Clinical Stage I NSGCT

Surgery

Clinical stage I NSGCT accounts for approximately 50% of all NSGCTs. The diagnostic use of RPLND lies in its ability to detect occult nodal metastases that occur in 20% to 40% of all clinical stage I NSGCTs. Additionally, it is well established that surgical cures with RPLND alone can be achieved in patients with clinical stage I NSGCT. After RPLND, clinical stage I NSGCT patients are restaged as either pathologic stage I or pathologic stage IIA (microscopic nodal involvement). Despite a 10% relapse rate for stage I NSGCT patients, the efficacy of salvage chemotherapy results in a long-term survival rate approaching 100%.

Either a modified or template dissection may be performed, in which only the primary and secondary nodal landing sites are removed, thereby sparing sympathetic fibers on the contralateral side. Alternatively, a nerve-sparing approach can be performed, whereby the sympathetic nerve supply can be preserved, even on the ipsilateral side. Use of either technique will allow for maintenance of antegrade ejaculation in greater than 90% of patients with stage I disease undergoing such procedures.[320, 330]

Fourteen trials of surveillance for stage I nonseminomatous testis cancer have been conducted, encompassing 1337 patients.[331] The median follow-up in these trials was 40 months. Three hundred and seventy-nine relapses (28%) have been documented; relapse rates have varied from 13% to 35%. Read and colleagues summarized the Medical Research Council's prospective study of surveillance for stage I testicular teratoma.[332] The 2-year actuarial relapse-free rate after orchiectomy was 75%; the rate at 5 years was 71%. Five patients died of cancer or treatment-related complications that resulted in a 98% 5-year survival rate. Of those that relapsed, 13% had elevated serum tumor markers as their only evidence of disease. Of those patients with metastatic disease, retroperitoneal relapse was detected in 61%. Other sites of relapse included the lung (25%), the mediastinum (7%), and the supraclavicular nodes (3%). Of patients with relapse in the supraclavicular nodes, markers were elevated in 55%. Therefore, 68% of those who relapsed had elevated serum tumor markers. Of the 100 patients who relapsed, 63 had small to moderate disease (i.e., <IIB).

Although most recurrences occurred within the first 2 years, continued follow-up is necessary because late recurrences have been reported. Several factors have been assessed for their ability to help predict relapse in these patients: T stage, vascular invasion, lymphatic invasion, the extent of embryonal carcinoma, and marker status before orchiectomy. Friedman and colleagues retrospectively pooled the Medical Research Council surveillance population and examined histologic variables and 2-year relapse rates.[333] Four variables correlated with relapse: invasion of testicular veins, invasion of testicular lymphatics, absence of yolk sac elements, and the presence of undifferentiated elements. The number of factors correlated with risk of recurrence.

These data have been interpreted to suggest that the strategy of surveillance yields equivalent results to RPLND in carefully selected clinical stage I NSGCT patients.[330, 334] As long as staging, treatment, and surveillance guidelines are strictly observed, nearly 100% of clinical stage I NSGCT patients can be cured, whether surveillance or RPLND with or without adjuvant chemotherapy is used. Each patient with clinical stage I NSGCT must be informed of these alternatives and be allowed to choose the methods of management most suited to his wishes and needs.

Chemotherapy

Up to 50% of patients with high-risk clinical stage I NSGCT are subsequently found to have nodal involvement. It has been suggested that chemotherapy might serve as effective primary adjunctive therapy after orchiectomy, thereby sparing patients an RPLND. Several investigators have used two cycles of chemotherapy and have reported very low relapse rates (generally less than 5%) in patients with median follow-ups as long as 4 to 6 years. These results must be balanced with the concern that the use of primary chemotherapy exposes at least 50% of patients to unnecessary chemotherapy. Adjuvant chemotherapy for stage I NSGCT in lieu of an RPLND is generally not undertaken in the United States.

The development of extraordinarily effective chemotherapy for disseminated NSGCT has also resulted in an effort to minimize so-called up-front treatment for clinical stage I NSGCT. The strategy of surveillance after orchiectomy, followed by systemic therapy at the first sign of relapse, is based on the observation that only 20% to 40% of clinical stage I patients have occult nodal involvement, the belief that the majority of these patients can thus be spared the morbidity associated with RPLND, and the confidence in chemotherapy as a curative salvage modality for those patients who do relapse.

Clinical Stage II NSGCT

Surgery

Patients with stage IIA or IIB NSGCT have minimal or moderate retroperitoneal lymphadenopathy. This category includes patients with clinical stage I NSGCT who are found to harbor occult nodal involvement at RPLND (pathologic stage IIA). The standard primary treatment for patients with clinical stage IIA or B disease is RPLND.

Chemotherapy

In an international study, patients with stage IIA or IIB disease after RPLND were randomized to either immediate adjuvant chemotherapy or no adjuvant therapy (followed by chemotherapy at the time of relapse). With a median follow-up of 4 years, 49% of the patients in the observation arm relapsed, compared with 6% in the adjuvant therapy arm. Patients in the observation arm who relapsed were treated with salvage chemotherapy. Because of effective salvage therapy, the overall survival rate (97%) was the same in both arms.[335] Most centers recommend adjuvant chemotherapy over surveillance in patients with moderate retroperitoneal lymph node involvement, that is, stage IIB disease (because a relapse rate of 40% to 50% can be predicted), but an option for patients with minimal microscopic disease is surveillance after RPLND, because patients with true pathologic stage IIA disease are at a very low risk of relapse (0% to 10%).

Advanced Disease

The functional definition of advanced GCT includes those stages of tumor in which locally directed therapy (radiation therapy for seminoma, RPLND for NSGCT) offers unacceptably poor results. Thus, for most investigators, lymph nodes larger than 2 cm in patients with NSGCT define advanced disease, whereas bulky IIC disease (generally, masses >5 cm) in patients with seminoma is considered advanced disease. A variety of chemotherapy regimens will result in approximately 80% of patients with advanced GCT achieving a complete response, with 70% achieving long-term apparent cures (so-called good prognosis patients). However, 20% to 30% of patients carry a poor prognosis and will ultimately die from their disease. Studies of pretreatment clinical characteristics have sought to identify prognostic features that can be prospectively used to segregate this diverse group of advanced GCT patients into poor and good prognostic subsets.

A common classification system has been developed. In this system, NSGCT patients with a good prognosis have a testis or retroperitoneal primary, no nonpulmonary visceral metastases, and low serum tumor markers. Patients with intermediate prognosis are the same as those with a good prognosis, but they have intermediate serum tumor markers. Patients with poor prognosis have a mediastinal primary, nonpulmonary visceral metastases (liver, bone, brain) or high levels of serum tumor markers. Five-year overall survival rates for the good, intermediate, and poor prognosis categories with current regimens is 92%, 80%, and 48%, respectively.

By definition, seminomas are never poor-prognosis cases. Seminomas are segregated into good-prognosis cases (any primary site, but no nonpulmonary visceral metastases), with an 86% 5-year survival rate, and intermediate-prognosis cases (any primary site, but with the presence of nonpulmonary visceral metastases), with a 72% 5-year survival rate.[336]

Chemotherapy

Standard chemotherapy consists of treatment with the PEB regimen: cisplatin, etoposide, and bleomycin. Because it is not likely that the extraordinarily high cure rate for patients with good risk can be improved, most efforts in the treatment of those patients have been aimed at optimizing treatment with less toxic regimens that will have equal efficacy. Trials evaluating (1) the elimination of bleomycin, (2) a reduction in the number of chemotherapy cycles administered, or (3) the substitution of carboplatin for cisplatin have been undertaken.[337]

The outlook for patients who are poor risk is grim, with only 38% to 62% of patients achieving a complete response. Thus, whereas the major concern in patients with good risk has been the reduction of toxicity, the major objective of clinical investigation in patients with poor risk has been to improve efficacy, with less concern for reducing toxicity. Clinical trials in patients with a poor prognosis have generally relied on either or both of two approaches:

- The first has been to exploit agents that have been demonstrated to be efficacious in the salvage setting.
- The second has evaluated the role of dose escalation.

There is a lack of consensus regarding the optimal management of high-risk GCT. Every effort should be made to enroll and treat patients with poor-prognosis GCTs on clinical trials.[338]

Residual Masses and Recurrent Disease

Residual masses after systemic therapy for advanced seminoma are observed in 60% to 85% of patients, although only 20% to 25% of these patients will have residual malignancy. Nearly half (42%) of patients with residual abnormalities larger than 3 cm in size have been found to have viable malignancy, whereas no patient with a normal imaging study or residual mass smaller than 3 cm who then underwent exploratory surgery has been found to have viable tumor.[339] Thus, surgery is recommended in seminoma patients with residual masses larger than 3 cm.

Forty percent of patients with advanced-stage NSGCT will have residual masses appear on a CT scan after chemotherapy. Malignancy (viable GCT) is found in the surgical specimens of approximately 15% to 20% of these patients, whereas fibrosis and necrosis or teratoma are found in the remaining 75% to 80% of patients in roughly equal proportions. No single variable or group of variables appears to be consistently and sufficiently predictive to allow the identification of patients in whom RPLND can be avoided. Patients with residual carcinoma in their specimens have an overall long-term survival rate of approximately 50%, whereas the survival rate for patients with fibrosis and necrosis is in the 85% to 90% range. Although teratoma in the residual mass may be histologically benign, the rationale for aggressive and complete early debulking of teratomas includes the following:

- the risk of local complications as well as growth into unresectable lesions
- the risk of late recurrence
- the risk of malignant transformation into non–germ cell malignancies such as sarcomas and carcinomas

Thus, resection of residual masses in patients with NSGCT treated with chemotherapy is generally recommended.[340]

Most investigators have recommended the resection of residual pulmonary nodules. From 10% to 30% of specimens have been reported as malignant, teratoma has been observed in 26% to 60% of specimens, and the fraction of specimens containing only fibrosis and necrosis has ranged from 14% to 64%. Thus, whereas as few as 10% of residual pulmonary nodules may harbor malignancy, the 25% to 60% incidence of teratoma and the inability to predict which nodules will contain only fibrosis and necrosis mandate surgical removal of all postchemotherapy residual masses, if it is technically feasible.[341] Larger initial node size, the presence of teratomatous elements in the primary tumor, and the extent of pretreatment marker elevation correlate with the risk of residual disease following chemotherapy.

For patients with residual disease in multiple sites, simultaneous resection can be performed by an experienced surgeon with a low risk of complications. There is a high concordance between the histologic findings identified in the retroperitoneum and lung (54% to 75%). Although the histology of the retroperitoneum predicts pathology in the lung, the converse is not as true. If the primary tumor fails to contain teratoma and the retroperitoneum contains necrosis only, then there is an approximately 90% likelihood of necrosis in the lung. Some would argue that such patients might undergo serial imaging of the chest rather than thoracotomy.

Salvage Chemotherapy

Salvage combination chemotherapy regimens result in durable complete response rates of only approximately 20%. The use of high-dose chemotherapy with peripheral stem cell transplant or bone marrow transplant may increase these numbers slightly.

Complications of Therapy

Surgery

The acute surgical morbidity of orchiectomy is minimal, similar to that seen with simple inguinal hernia repair. The surgical complications specific to retroperitoneal lymphadenectomy (apart from any usual complications of major intra-abdominal surgery) include retrograde ejaculation, although as noted, nerve-sparing procedures in patients with nonextensive disease dramatically decrease the risk of ejaculatory dysfunction.

Radiation Therapy

Acute complications associated with low-dose para-aortic irradiation include mild nausea, slight reddening of the skin, and a transient reduction in spermatogenesis.[327] Late complications are uncommon, but they include impaired contralateral spermatogenesis, second malignancies, and an increased risk of gastrointestinal complications (peptic ulcer disease or hemorrhagic gastritis intestinal obstruction).[342] The risk of major gastrointestinal complications appears to be dose related, with the incidence being 0%, 2%, and 6% for less than 25 Gy, 25 to 35 Gy, and 40 to 45 Gy, respectively.[320] The risk of secondary malignancies is relatively low, with the risk ratio of 2.5 for malignancies of the lung and bladder, but the risk is probably increased for gastrointestinal primaries (although less well documented).[327]

Chemotherapy

Acute toxicities associated with chemotherapy for GCTs largely represent the toxicities anticipated from the individual chemotherapeutic agents composing these regimens. However, there exist also unique chronic toxicities with the treatment of GCT:

- The potential for chronic renal insufficiency or ototoxicity in up to 20% of patients mandates careful monitoring of renal function.
- The acute pulmonary toxicity of bleomycin is manifested as noninfectious pneumonitis. Up to 20% of patients with GCT treated with bleomycin-containing regimens will develop clinically apparent pneumonitis, and 3% to 4% of patients have died from pulmonary toxicity in some series. This is a dose-related complication, with a markedly increased incidence at cumulative doses greater than 400 units, although toxicity may occur at lower doses.[343]
- Chronic vascular toxicities associated with chemotherapy include Raynaud's phenomenon, vascular occlusive events, and potential alterations in cholesterol metabolism.
- The chronic reproductive toxicities associated with chemotherapeutic treatment of GCT include oligospermia, azoospermia, and Leydig cell dysfunction. In one study, azoospermia was seen in 27% of patients and Leydig cell dysfunction in 86% of patients after treatment with chemotherapy. Sperm counts generally increase in the second and third year after therapy, and return to normal in about 50% of men. Approximately 25% of men are permanently azoospermic, and it appears that Leydig cell dysfunction may persist at 3 to 9 years after therapy.[343]

Survivors of testis cancer experience 30% more tumors than are expected for a general population, with the highest relative risk for developing a second non–germ cell tumor seen in patients treated with either radiation alone or with radiation plus chemotherapy. Secondary malignancies are an expected late occurrence in patients with treated testicular cancer, with a relative risk of between 1.38 and 2.0. Radiation-containing treatment regimens may have a higher association with secondary solid tumors, whereas chemotherapy (etoposide) may be more likely to result in secondary leukemias (<1% incidence overall). These risks, although they are quite small compared with the impact of not undergoing therapy, must nevertheless be considered in the therapeutic decision-making process and be discussed with each patient.[343]

Recommended Reading

Two recently published texts provide an all-encompassing view of the field of genitourinary oncology: Vogelzang and associates'[1] *Comprehensive Textbook of Genitourinary Oncology,* now in its 2nd edition, and Raghaven and colleagues'[2] *Principles and Practice of Genitourinary Oncology.* Excellent chapters also may be found in Leibel and Phillips'[3] *Textbook of Radiation Oncology* and De Vita and coworkers'[4] *Cancer. Principles & Practice of Oncology.*

REFERENCES

General

1. Vogelzang NJ, Scardino PT, Shipley WU, et al (eds): Comprehensive Textbook of Genitourinary Oncology, 2nd ed. Philadelphia, Lippincott Williams & Wilkins, 2000.
2. Raghaven D, Scher H, Leibel SA, et al (eds): Principles and Practice of Genitourinary Oncology. Philadelphia, Lippincott-Raven, 1997.
3. Leibel SA, Phillips TL (eds): Textbook of Radiation Oncology. Philadelphia, W.B. Saunders, 1998.
4. DeVita VT Jr, Hellman S, Rosenberg SA (eds): Cancer. Principles & Practice of Oncology, 5th ed. Philadelphia, Lippincott-Raven, 1997.

Specific

Kidney

5. Greenlee R, Murray T, Bolden S, et al: Cancer statistics, 2000. CA Cancer J Clin 2000; 50:7–33.
6. Linehan WM, Shipley WU, Parkinson DR: Cancer of the kidney and ureter. In: DeVita VT Jr, Hellman S, Rosenberg SA (eds): Cancer. Principles & Practice of Oncology, 5th ed, pp 1271–1299. Philadelphia, Lippincott-Raven, 1997.
7. Tavani A, La Vecchia C: Epidemiology of renal cell carcinoma. J Nephrol 1997; 10:93–106.
8. Gnarra JB, Lerman MI, Zbar B, et al: Genetics of renal-cell carcinoma and evidence for a critical role for von Hippel–Lindau in renal tumorigenesis. Semin Oncol 1995; 22:3–8.
9. Erlandsson R: Molecular genetics of renal cell carcinoma. Cancer Genet Cytogenet 1998; 104:1–18.
10. Porena M, Vespasiani G, Rosi P, et al: Incidentally detected renal cell carcinoma: role of ultrasonography. J Clin Ultrasound 1992; 20:395–400.
11. Ritchie AWS, Chisolm GD: The natural history of renal carcinoma. Semin Oncol 1983; 10:390–400.
12. Motzer RJ, Bander NH, Nanus DM: Renal-cell carcinoma. N Engl J Med 1996; 335:865–875.
13. Gold PJ, Fefer A, Thompson JA: Paraneoplastic manifestations of renal cell carcinoma. Semin Urol Oncol 1996; 14:216–222.
14. Johnson CD, Dunnick NR, Cohan RH, et al: Renal adenocarcinoma: CT staging of 100 tumors. American Journal of Roentgenology 1987; 148:59–63.
15. Semelka RC, Shoenut JP, Magro CM, et al: Renal cancer staging: comparison of contrast-enhanced CT and gadolinium-enhancing fat-suppressed spin-echo and gradient-echo MR imaging. J Magn Reson Imaging 1993; 3:597–602.
16. Storkel S, Eble J, Adlakha K, et al: Classification of renal cell carcinoma. Cancer 1997; 80:987–989.
17. American Joint Committee on Cancer: AJCC Cancer Staging Manual, 5th ed. Philadelphia, Lippincott-Raven, 1997.
18. Guinan P, Sobin LH, Algaba F, et al: TNM staging of renal cell carcinoma. Cancer 1997: 80:992–993.
19. Lokich J: Spontaneous regression of renal cell cancer: case report and review of the literature. Am J Clin Oncol 1997; 20:416–418.
20. Oliver RT, Nethersell AB, Bottomley JM: Unexplained spontaneous regression and alpha-interferon as treatment for metastatic renal cell carcinoma. Br J Urol 1989; 63:128–131.
21. Gleave ME, Elhilali M, Fradet Y, et al: Interferon gamma-1b compared with placebo in metastatic renal cell carcinoma. N Engl J Med 1998; 338:1265–1271.
22. Gelb A: Renal cell carcinoma: current prognostic factors. Cancer 1997; 80:981–986.
23. Giberti C, Oneto F, Martorana G, et al: Radical nephrectomy for renal cell carcinoma: long-term results and prognostic factors in a series of 328 cases. Eur Urol 1997; 31:40–48.
24. Robson CJ: Radical nephrectomy for renal cell carcinoma. J Urol 1963; 89:37–42.
25. Thrasher JB, Robertson JE, Paulson D: Expanding indications for conservative renal surgery in renal cell carcinoma. Urology 1994; 43:160–168.
26. Polascik TJ, Pound CR, Meng MV, et al: Partial nephrectomy: technique, complications and pathological findings. J Urol 1995; 154:1312–1318.
27. Hafez KS, Novick AC, Campbell SC: Patterns of tumor recurrence and guidelines for followup after nephron sparing surgery for sporadic renal cell carcinoma. J Urol 1997; 157:2067–2070.
28. Hafez KS, Novick AC, Butler BP: Management of small solitary unilateral renal cell carcinomas: impact of central versus peripheral tumor location. J Urol 1998; 159:1156–1160.
29. Walther MM, Yang JC, Pass HI, et al: Cytoreductive surgery before high dose interleukin-2 based therapy in patients with metastatic renal cell carcinoma. J Urol 1997; 158:1675–1678.
30. Bennett RT, Lerner S, Taub HC, et al: Cytoreductive surgery for stage IV renal cell carcinoma. J Urol 1995; 154:32–34.
31. Levy DA, Swanson DA, Slaton JW, et al: Timely delivery of biological therapy after cytoreductive nephrectomy in carefully selected patients with metastatic renal cell carcinoma. J Urol 1998; 159:1168–1173.
32. Wolf JS, Aronson FR, Small EJ, et al: Nephrectomy for metastatic renal cell carcinoma: a component of systemic treatment regimens. J Surg Oncol 1994; 55:7–13.
33. Halperin EC, Harisiadis L: The role of radiation therapy in the management of metastatic renal cell carcinoma. Cancer 1983; 51:614–617.
34. Yagoda A, Abi-Rached B, Petrylak D: Chemotherapy for advanced renal-cell carcinoma: 1983–1993. Semin Oncol 1995; 22:42–60.
35. Small EJ, Frye JW, Wilkinson MJ, et al: A phase I/II study of alternating constant rate infusion floxuridine with constant rate infusion vinblastine for the treatment of metastatic renal cell carcinoma. Cancer 1994; 73:2803–2807.
36. Kjaer M: The role of medroxyprogesterone acetate (MPA) in the treatment of renal adenocarcinoma. Cancer Treat Rev 1988; 15:195–209.
37. Gitlitz BJ, Belldegrun A, Figlin R: Immunotherapy and gene therapy. Semin Urol Oncol 1996; 14:237–243.
38. Rosenberg SA, Yang YC, Topalian SI, et al: Treatment of 283 consecutive patients with metastatic melanoma or renal cell cancer using high-dose bolus interleukin-2. J Am Med Assoc 1994; 271:907–913.
39. Fyfe G, Fisher RI, Rosenberg SA, et al: Results of treatment of 255 patients with metastatic RCC who received high-dose recombinant interleukin-2 therapy. J Clin Oncol 1995; 13:688–696.
40. Bukowski RM: Natural history and therapy of metastatic renal cell carcinoma: the role of interleukin-2. Cancer 1997; 80:1198–1220.
41. Negrier S, Escudier B, Lasset C, et al: Recombinant human interleukin-2, recombinant human interferon alfa-2a, or both in metastatic renal-cell carcinoma. N Engl J Med 1998; 338:1272–1278.
42. Agarwala SS, Kirkwood JM: Interferons in the treatment of solid tumors. Oncology 1994; 51:129–136.
43. Wirth MP: Immunotherapy for metastatic renal cell carcinoma. Urol Clin North Am 1993; 20:283–295.
44. Small EJ, Weiss GR, Malik UK, et al: The treatment of metastatic renal cell carcinoma patients with recombinant human gamma interferon. Cancer J Sci Am 1998; 4:162–167.
45. Law TM, Motzer RJ, Mazumdar M, et al: Phase III randomized trial of interleukin-2 with or without lymphokine-activated killer cells in the treatment of patients with advanced renal cell carcinoma. Cancer 1995; 76:824–832.
46. Figlin R, Thompson J, Roudet C, et al: Multicenter randomized placebo-controlled trial of CD8(+) tumor infiltrating lymphocyte therapy (CD8(+) TIL)/recombinant interleukin-2 (IL-2) in metastatic renal cell carcinoma (MRCC) [Abstract]. Proceedings of the American Society of Clinical Oncology 1998; 17:318.
47. Nativ O, Sabo E, Raviv G, et al: The impact of tumor size on clinical outcome in patients with localized renal cell carcinoma treated by radical nephrectomy. J Urol 1997; 158:729–732.
48. Robson CJ, Churchill BM, Anderson W: The results of radical nephrectomy for renal cell carcinoma. J Urol 1969; 101:297–301.
49. Skinner DG, Colvin RB, Vermillion CD, et al: Diagnosis and management of renal cell carcinoma. A clinical and pathologic study of 309 cases. Cancer 1971; 28:1165–1167.
50. Middleton RG, Presto AJ III: Radical thoracoabdominal nephrectomy for renal cell carcinoma. J Urol 1973; 110:36–37.
51. Waters WB, Richie JP: Aggressive surgical approach to renal cell carcinoma: review of 130 cases. J Urol 1979; 122:306–309.
52. Boxer RJ, Waisman J, Lieber MM, et al: Renal carcinoma: computer analysis of 96 patients treated by nephrectomy. J Urol 1979; 122:598–601.
53. Siminovitch JMP, Montie JE, Straffon RA: Prognostic indicators in renal adenocarcinoma. J Urol 1983; 130:20–23.
54. Medeiros LJ, Gelb AB, Weiss LM: Renal cell carcinoma. Prognostic significance of morphologic parameters in 121 cases. Cancer 1988; 61:1639–1651.
55. Selli C, Hinshaw WM, Woodard BH, et al: Stratification of risk factors in renal cell carcinoma. Cancer 1983; 52:899–903.
56. Giuliani L, Gilberti C, Martorana G, et al: Radical extensive surgery for renal cell carcinoma: long-term results and prognostic factors. J Urol 1990; 143:468–473.
57. Sene AP, Hunt L, McMahon RFT, et al: Renal carcinoma in patients undergoing nephrectomy: analysis of survival and prognostic factors. Br J Urol 1992; 70:125–134.
58. Rabinovitch RA, Zelefsky MJ, Gaynor JJ, et al: Patterns of failure following surgical resection of renal cell carcinoma: implications for adjuvant local and systemic therapy. J Clin Oncol 1994; 12:206–212.

59. Thrasher JB, Paulson DF: Prognostic factors in renal cell carcinoma. Urol Clin North Am 1993; 20:247–262.

Bladder

60. Hartge P, Harvey EB, Linehan WM, et al: Unexplained excess risk of bladder cancer in men. J Natl Cancer Inst 1990; 82:1636–1640.
61. Imada S, Akaza H, Ami Y, et al: Promoting effects and mechanisms of action of androgen in bladder carcinogenesis in male rats. Eur Urol 1997; 31:360–364.
62. Hartge P, Silverman D, Hoover R, et al: Changing cigarette habits and bladder cancer risk: a case-controlled study. J Natl Cancer Inst 1987; 78:1119–1125.
63. D'Avanzo B, Negri E, La Vecchia C, et al: Cigarette smoking and bladder cancer. Eur J Cancer 1990; 26:714–718.
64. Lopez-Abente G, Gonzalez CA, Errezola M, et al: Tobacco smoke inhalation pattern, tobacco type, and bladder cancer in Spain. Am J Epidemiol 1991; 134:830–839.
65. Vineis P: Black (air-cured) and blond (flue-cured) tobacco and cancer risk. I: Bladder cancer. Eur J Cancer 1991; 27:1491–1493.
66. Momas I, Daures JP, Festy B, et al: Bladder cancer and black tobacco cigarette smoking. Some results from a French case-control study. Eur J Epidemiol 1994; 10:599–604.
67. Hashmi AH, Naqvi AA, Rizvi AH: Analysis of known risk factors for bladder cancer in Pakistani population. Journal of the Pakistan Medical Association 1995; 45:41–42.
68. Scher HI, Shipley WU, Herr HW: Cancer of the bladder. In: De Vita VT Jr, Hellman S, Rosenberg SA (eds): Cancer. Principles & Practice of Oncology, 5th ed, pp 1300–1322. Philadelphia, Lippincott-Raven, 1997.
69. Ronneberg A, Haldorsen T, Romundstad P, et al: Occupational exposure and cancer incidence among workers from an aluminum smelter in western Norway. Scand J Work Environ Health 1999; 25:207–214.
70. Straif K, Weiland SK, Werner B, et al: Workplace risk factors for cancer in the German rubber industry: Part 2. Mortality from non-respiratory cancers. Occup Environ Med 1998; 55:325–332.
71. Smith EM, Miller ER, Woolson RF, et al: Bladder cancer risk among laundry workers, dry cleaners, and others in chemically-related occupations. J Occup Med 1985; 27:295–297.
72. Tremblay C, Armstrong B, Theriault G, et al: Estimation of risk of developing bladder cancer among workers exposed to coal tar pitch volatiles in the primary aluminum industry. Am J Ind Med 1995; 27:335–348.
73. Morales S-VM, Llopis GA, Tejerizo PML, et al: Concentration of nitrates in drinking water and its relationship with bladder cancer. J Environ Pathol Toxicol Oncol 1993; 12:229–236.
74. Cantor KP, Lynch CF, Hildesheim ME, et al: Drinking water source and chlorination byproducts. I. Risk of bladder cancer. Epidemiology 1998; 9:21–28.
75. Johansson SL, Cohen SM: Epidemiology and etiology of bladder cancer. Semin Surg Oncol 1997; 13:291–298.
76. Drake MJ, Nixon PM, Crew JP: Drug-induced bladder and urinary disorders. Incidence, prevention and management. Drug Saf 1998; 19:45–55.
77. McCredie M, Stewart J, Smith D, et al: Observations on the effect of abolishing analgesic abuse and reducing smoking on cancers of the kidney and bladder in New South Wales, Australia, 1972–1995. Cancer Causes Control 1999; 10:303–311.
78. Vena JE, Freudenheim J, Graham S, et al: Coffee, cigarette smoking, and bladder cancer in western New York. Ann Epidemiol 1993; 3:586–591.
79. Donato F, Boffato P, Fazioli R, et al: Bladder cancer, tobacco smoking, coffee and alcohol drinking in Brescia, northern Italy. Eur J Epidemiol 1997; 13:795–800.
80. Elcock M, Morgan RW: Update on artifical sweeteners and bladder cancer. Regul Toxicol Pharmacol 1993; 17:35–43.
81. Viscoli CM, Lachs MS, Horwitz RI: Bladder cancer and coffee drinking: a summary of case-control research. Lancet 1993; 341:1432–1437.
82. Stensvold I, Jacobsen BK: Coffee and cancer: a prospective study of 43,000 Norwegian men and women. Cancer Causes Control 1994; 5:401–408.
83. Warren W, Biggs PJ, el-Baz M, et al: Mutations in the p53 gene in schistosomal bladder cancer: a study of 92 tumours from Egyptian patients and a comparison between mutational spectra from schistosomal and non-schistosomal urothelial tumours. Carcinogenesis 1995; 16:1181–1189.
84. Shaw ME, Elder PA, Abbas A, et al: Partial allelotype of schistosomiasis-associated bladder cancer. Int J Cancer 1999; 80:656–661.
85. Warren JW: Catheter-associated urinary tract infections. Infect Dis Clin North Am 1997; 11:609–622.
86. West DA, Cummings JM, Longo WE, et al: Role of chronic catheterization in the development of bladder cancer in patients with spinal cord injury. Urology 1999; 53:292–297.
87. Hall RR: Superficial bladder cancer. BMJ 1994; 308:910–913.
88. Messing EM, Young TB, Hunt VB, et al: Comparison of bladder cancer outcome in men undergoing hematuria home screening versus those with standard clinical presentations. Urology 1995; 45:387–396.
89. Scher H, Bahnson R, Cohen S, et al: NCCN urothelial cancer practice guidelines. National Comprehensive Cancer Network. Oncology (Huntingt) 1998; 12:225–271.
90. Badalament RA, Ryan PR, Bahn DK: Imaging for transitional cell carcinomas. In: Vogelzang NJ, Scardino PT, Shipley WU, et al (eds): Comprehensive Textbook of Genitourinary Oncology, 2nd ed, pp 356–366. Philadelphia, Lippincott Williams & Wilkins, 2000.
91. Badalament RA, Fair WR, Whitmore WF Jr, et al: The relative value of cytometry and cytology in the management of bladder cancer: the Memorial Sloan-Kettering Cancer Center experience. Semin Urol 1988; 6:22–30.
92. Kim B, Semelka RC, Ascher SM, et al: Bladder tumor staging: comparison of contrast-enhanced CT, T1- and T2-weighted MR imaging, dynamic gadolinium-enhanced imaging, and late gadolinium-enhanced imaging. Radiology 1994; 193:239–245.
93. Davey P, Merrick MV, Duncan W, et al: Bladder cancer: the value of routine bone scintigraphy. Clin Radiol 1985; 36:77–79.
94. Holzbeierlein JM, Smith JA Jr: Natural history and surgical management. In: Vogelzang NJ, Scardino PT, Shipley WU, et al (eds): Comprehensive Textbook of Genitourinary Oncology, 2nd ed, pp 384–394. Philadelphia, Lippincott Williams & Wilkins, 2000.
95. Lamm DL: BCG immunotherapy for transitional-cell carcinoma in situ of the bladder. Oncology (Huntingt) 1995; 9:947–952.
96. Caliskan M, Turkeri LN, Mansuroglu B, et al: Nuclear accumulation of mutant p53 protein: a possible predictor of failure of intravesical therapy in bladder cancer. Br J Urol 1997; 79:373–377.
97. Pages F, Flam TA, Viellefond A, et al: p53 status does not predict initial clinical response to bacillus Calmette-Guerin intravesical therapy in T1 bladder tumors. J Urol 1998; 159:1079–1084.
98. Pfister C, Flaman JM, Dunet F, et al: p53 mutations in bladder tumors inactivate the transactivation of the p21 and Bax genes, and have a predictive value for the clinical outcome after bacillus Calmette-Guerin therapy. J Urol 1999; 162:69–73.
99. Pawinski A, Sylvester R, Kurth KH, et al: A combined analysis of European Organization for Research and Treatment of Cancer, and Medical Research Council randomized clinical trials for the prophylactic treatment of stage TaT1 bladder cancer. European Organization for Research and Treatment of Cancer Genitourinary Tract Cancer Cooperative Group and the Medical Research Council Working Party on Superficial Bladder Cancer. J Urol 1996; 156:1934–1940.
100. Dandekar NP, Tongaonkar HB, Dalal AV, et al: Partial cystectomy for invasive bladder cancer. J Surg Oncol 1995; 60:24–29.
101. Iselin CE, Robertson CN, Webster GD, et al: Does prostate transitional cell carcinoma preclude orthotopic bladder reconstruction after radical cystoprostatectomy for bladder cancer? J Urol 1997; 158:2123–2126.
102. Freeman JA, Tarter TA, Esrig D, et al: Urethral recurrence in patients with orthotopic ileal neobladders. J Urol 1996; 156:1615–1619.
103. Lampel A, Fisch M, Stein R, et al: Continent diversion with the Mainz pouch. World J Urol 1996; 14:85–91.
104. Bihrle R: The Indiana Pouch continent urinary reservoir. Urol Clin North Am 1997; 24:773–779.
105. Hautmann RE, de Petriconi RD, Gottfried HW, et al: The ileal neobladder: complications and functional results in 363 patients after 11 years of followup. J Urol 1999; 161:422–427.
106. Parsons JT, Million RR: The role of radiation therapy alone or as an adjunct to surgery in bladder carcinoma. Semin Oncol 1990; 17:566–582.
107. Swanson DA, Liles A, Zagars GK: Preoperative irradiation and radical cystectomy for stages T2 and T3 squamous cell carcinoma of the bladder. J Urol 1990; 143:37–40.

108. Huncharek M, Muscat J, Geschwind JF: Planned preoperative radiation therapy in muscle invasive bladder cancer: results of a meta-analysis. Anticancer Res 1998; 18:1931–1934.
109. Maulard-Durdux C, Dufour B, Hennequin C, et al: Postoperative radiation therapy in 26 patients with invasive transitional cell carcinoma of the upper urinary tract: no impact on survival? J Urol 1996; 155:115–117.
110. Hall MC, Womack JS, Roehrborn CG, et al: Advanced transitional cell carcinoma of the upper urinary tract: patterns of failure, survival and impact of postoperative adjuvant radiotherapy. J Urol 1998; 160:703–706.
111. Reisinger SA, Mohiuddin M, Mulholland SG: Combined pre- and postoperative adjuvant radiation therapy for bladder cancer—a ten-year experience. Int J Radiat Oncol Biol Phys 1992; 24:463–468.
112. Duncan W, Quilty PM: The results of a series of 963 patients with transitional cell carcinoma of the urinary bladder primarily treated by radical megavoltage x-ray therapy. Radiother Oncol 1986; 7:299–310.
113. Quilty PM, Kerr GR, Duncan W: Prognostic indices for bladder cancer: an analysis of patients with transitional cell carcinoma of the bladder primarily treated by radical megavoltage x-ray therapy. Radiother Oncol 1986; 7:311–321.
114. De Neve W, Lybeert ML, Goor C, et al: Radiotherapy for T2 and T3 carcinoma of the bladder: the influence of overall treatment time. Radiother Oncol 1995; 36:183–188.
115. Shipley WU, Winter KA, Kaufman DS, et al: Phase III trial of neoadjuvant chemotherapy in patients with invasive bladder cancer treated with selective bladder preservation by combined radiation therapy and chemotherapy: initial results of Radiation Therapy Oncology Group 89–03. J Clin Oncol 1998; 16:3576–3583.
116. Rotman M, Aziz H, Porrazzo M, et al: Treatment of advanced transitional cell carcinoma of the bladder with irradiation and concomitant 5-fluorouracil infusion. Int J Radiat Oncol Biol Phys 1990; 18:1131–1137.
117. Raghavan D: Management of advanced bladder cancer in the elderly. Urol Clin North Am 1992; 19:797–806.
118. Schultz PK, Herr HW, Zhang ZF, et al: Neoadjuvant chemotherapy for invasive bladder cancer: prognostic factors for survival of patients treated with M-VAC with 5-year follow-up. J Clin Oncol 1994; 12:1394–1401.
119. Scher HI: Neoadjuvant chemotherapy for invasive bladder cancer: prognostic factors for survival of patients treated with M-VAC with 5-year follow-up. J Urol 1995; 153:545–546.
120. Martinez-Pineiro JA, Gonzalez Martin M, Arocena F, et al: Neoadjuvant cisplatin chemotherapy before radical cystectomy in invasive transitional cell carcinoma of the bladder: a prospective randomized phase III trial. J Urol 1995; 153:964–973.
121. Malmstrom PU, Rintala E, Wahlqvist R, et al: Five-year followup of a prospective trial of radical cystectomy and neoadjuvant chemotherapy: Nordic Cystectomy Trial I. The Nordic Cooperative Bladder Cancer Study Group. J Urol 1996; 155:1903–1906.
122. Anonymous: Phase III trial of neoadjuvant chemotherapy in patients with invasive bladder cancer treated with selective bladder preservation by combined radiation therapy and chemotherapy: initial results of Radiation Therapy Oncology Group 89–03. J Urol 1999; 162:623–624.
123. Coppin CM, Gospadarowicz MK, James K, et al: Improved local control of invasive bladder cancer by concurrent cisplatin and preoperative or definitive radiation. The National Cancer Institute of Canada Clinical Trials Group. J Clin Oncol 1996; 14:2901–2907.
124. Stockle M, Meyenburg W, Wellek S, et al: Adjuvant polychemotherapy of nonorgan-confined bladder cancer after radical cystectomy revisited: long-term results of a controlled prospective study and further clinical experience. J Urol 1995; 153:47–52.
125. Freiha F, Reese J, Torti FM, et al: A randomized trial of radical cystectomy versus radical cystectomy plus cisplatin, vinblastine and methotrexate chemotherapy for muscle invasive bladder cancer. J Urol 1996; 155:495–499.
126. McCaffrey JA, Herr HW: Adjuvant and neoadjuvant chemotherapy for urothelial carcinoma. Surg Oncol Clin N Am 1997; 6:667–681.
127. Dimopoulos MA, Moulopoulos LA: Role of adjuvant chemotherapy in the treatment of invasive carcinoma of the urinary bladder. J Clin Oncol 1998; 16:1601–1612.
128. Herr HW, Bajorin DF, Scher HI: Neoadjuvant chemotherapy and bladder-sparing surgery for invasive bladder cancer: ten-year outcome. J Clin Oncol 1998; 16:1298–1301.
129. Stein JP, Grossfeld GD, Freeman JA, et al: Orthoptic lower urinary tract reconstruction in women using the Kock ileal neobladder: updated experience in 34 patients. J Urol 1997; 158:400–405.
130. Stein JP, Cote RJ, Freeman JA, et al: Indications for lower urinary tract reconstruction in women after cystectomy for bladder cancer: a pathological review of female cystectomy specimens. J Urol 1995; 154:1329–1333.
131. Stenzl A, Draxl H, Posch B, et al: The risk of urethral tumors in female bladder cancer: can the urethra be used for orthotopic reconstruction of the lower urinary tract? J Urol 1995; 153:950–955.
132. Stein JP, Esrig D, Freeman JA, et al: Prospective pathologic analysis of female cystectomy specimens: risk factors for orthotopic diversion in women. Urology 1998; 51:951–955.
133. Gburek BM, Lieber MM, Blute ML: Comparison of studer ileal neobladder and ileal conduit urinary diversion with respect to perioperative outcome and late complications. J Urol 1998; 160:721–723.
134. Hautmann RE, Paiss T: Does the option of the ileal neobladder stimulate patient and physician decision toward earlier cystectomy? J Urol 1998; 159:1845–1850.
135. Pollack A, Zagars GZ: Radiotherapy for stage T3b transitional cell carcinoma of the bladder. Semin Urol Oncol 1996; 14:86–95.
136. Zietman AL, Shipley WU, Kaufman DS, et al: A phase I/II trial of transurethral surgery combined with concurrent cisplatin, 5-fluorouracil and twice daily radiation followed by selective bladder preservation in operable patients with muscle invading bladder cancer. J Urol 1998; 160:1673–1677.
137. Birkenhake S, Martus P, Kuhn R, et al: Radiotherapy alone or radiochemotherapy with platin derivatives following transurethral resection of the bladder. Organ preservation and survival after treatment of bladder cancer. Strahlenther Onkol 1998; 174:121–127.
138. Holmang S, Hedelin H, Anderstrom C, et al: Long-term followup of a bladder carcinoma cohort: routine followup urography is not necessary. J Urol 1998; 160:45–48.
139. Pode D, Shapiro A, Wald M, et al: Noninvasive detection of bladder cancer with the BTA stat test. J Urol 1999; 161:443–446.
140. Zimmerman RL, Bagley D, Hawthorne C, et al: Utility of the Bard BTA test in detecting upper urinary tract transitional cell carcinoma. Urology 1998; 51:956–958.
141. Van der Poel HG, Van Balken MR, Schamhart DH, et al: Bladder wash cytology, quantitative cytology, and the qualitative BTA test in patients with superficial bladder cancer. Urology 1998; 51:44–50.
142. Thomas L, Leyh H, Marberger M, et al: Multicenter trial of the quantitative BTA TRAK assay in the detection of bladder cancer. Clin Chem 1999; 45:472–477.
143. Asakura T, Takano Y, Iki M, et al: Prognostic value of Ki-67 for recurrence and progression of superficial bladder cancer. J Urol 1997; 158:385–388.
144. Bochner BH, Cote RJ, Weidner N, et al: Angiogenesis in bladder cancer: relationship between microvessel density and tumor progression. J Natl Cancer Inst 1995; 87:1603–1612.
145. Crew JP, O'Brien T, Bicknell R, et al: Urinary vascular endothelial growth factor and its correlation with bladder cancer recurrence rates. J Urol 1999; 161:799–804.
146. Landman J, Kavaler E, Droller MJ, et al: Applications of telomerase in urologic oncology. World J Urol 1997; 15:120–124.
147. Kavaler E, Landman J, Chang Y, et al: Detecting human bladder carcinoma cells in voided urine samples by assaying for the presence of telomerase activity. Cancer 1998; 82:708–714.
148. Carpinito GA, Stadler WM, Briggman JV, et al: Urinary nuclear matrix protein as a marker for transitional cell carcinoma of the urinary tract. J Urol 1996; 156:1280–1285.
149. Landman J, Chang Y, Kavaler E, et al: Sensitivity and specificity of NMP-22, telomerase, and BTA in the detection of human bladder cancer. Urology 1998; 52:398–402.
150. Lianes P, Charytonowicz E, Cordon-Cardo C, et al: Biomarker study of primary nonmetastatic versus metastatic invasive bladder cancer. National Cancer Institute Bladder Tumor Marker Network. Clin Cancer Res 1998; 4:1267–1271.
151. Kurth KH, Denis L, Bouffioux C, et al: Factors affecting recurrence and progression in superficial bladder tumours. Eur J Cancer 1995; 31A:1840–1846.
152. Bouffioux C, Kurth KH, Bono A, et al: Intravesical adjuvant chemotherapy for superficial transitional cell bladder carcinoma: results of 2 European Organization for Research and Treatment of Cancer randomized trials with mitomycin C and doxorubicin comparing

early versus delayed instillations and short-term versus long-term treatment. European Organization for Research and Treatment of Cancer Genitourinary Group. J Urol 1995; 153:934–941.

153. Esrig D, Elmajian D, Groshen S, et al: Accumulation of nuclear p53 and tumor progression in bladder cancer. N Engl J Med 1994; 331:1259–1264.
154. Sarkis AS, Bajorin DF, Reuter VE, et al: Prognostic value of p53 nuclear overexpression in patients with invasive bladder cancer treated with neoadjuvant MVAC. J Clin Oncol 1995; 13:1384–1390.
155. Jinza S, Takano Y, Iki M, et al: Prognostic significance of p53 protein overexpression in transitional cell carcinoma of the renal pelvis and ureter. Urol Int 1998; 60:147–151.
156. Plastiras D, Moutzouris G, Barbatis C, et al: Can p53 nuclear overexpression, Bcl-2 accumulation and PCNA status be of prognostic significance in high-risk superficial and invasive bladder tumours? Eur J Surg Oncol 1999; 25:61–65.
157. Cordon-Cardo C, Sheinfeld J, Dalbagni G: Genetic studies and molecular markers of bladder cancer. Semin Surg Oncol 1997; 13:319–327.

Prostate

158. Stephenson RA, Smart CR, Mineau GP, et al: The fall in incidence of prostate carcinoma. On the down side of a prostate specific antigen induced peak in incidence—data from the Utah Cancer Registry. Cancer 1996; 77:1342–1348.
159. Brawley OW: Prostate carcinoma incidence and patient mortality. Cancer 1997; 80:1857–1863.
160. Mettlin C: Changes in early detection of prostate cancer in the United States. Ann NY Acad Sci 1995; 768:68–72.
161. Roach M: Is race an independent prognostic factor for survival from prostate cancer? J Natl Med Assoc 1998; 90(suppl):S713–S719.
162. Roach M, Alexander M: The prognostic significance of race and survival from breast cancer. A model for assessing the reliability of reported survival differences. J Natl Med Assoc 1995; 87:214–219.
163. Robbins AS, Whittemore AS, Van Den Eeden SK, et al: Race, prostate cancer survival, and membership in a large health maintenance organization. J Natl Cancer Inst 1998; 90:986–990.
164. Silverberg E: Cancer statistics, 1980. CA Cancer J Clin 1980; 30:23–38.
165. Roach M III, Wallner K: Prostate cancer. In: Leibel S, Phillips TL (eds): Textbook of Radiation Oncology, pp 741–784. Philadelphia, W.B. Saunders, 1998.
166. Gronberg H, Isaacs SD, Smith JR, et al: Characteristics of prostate cancer in families potentially linked to the hereditary prostate cancer 1 (HPC1) locus. J Am Med Assoc 1997; 278:1251–1255.
167. Kupelian PA, Kupelian VA, Witte JS, et al: Family history of prostate cancer in patients with localized prostate cancer: an independent predictor of treatment outcome. J Clin Oncol 1997; 15:1478–1480.
168. Hanus MC, Zagars GK, Pollack A: Familial prostate cancer: outcome following radiation therapy with or without adjuvant androgen ablation. Int J Radiat Oncol Biol Phys 1999; 43:379–383.
169. Daviglus ML, Dyer AR, Persky V, et al: Dietary beta-carotene, vitamin C, and risk of prostate cancer: results from the Western Electric Study. Epidemiology 1996; 7:114–115.
170. Schuurman AG, van der Brandt PA, Dorant E, et al: Association of energy and fat intake with prostate carcinoma risk: results from The Netherlands Cohort Study. Cancer 1999; 86:1019–1027.
171. Gallagher RP, Fleshner N: Prostate cancer. 3. Individual risk factors. CMAJ 1998; 159:807–813.
172. Nelson MA, Porterfield BW, Jacobs ET, et al: Selenium and prostate cancer prevention. Semin Urol Oncol 1999; 17:91–96.
173. Moyad MA, Brumfield SK, Pienta KJ: Vitamin E, alpha- and gamma-tocopherol, and prostate cancer. Semin Urol Oncol 1999; 17:85–90.
174. Moyad MA: Soy, disease prevention, and prostate cancer. Semin Urol Oncol 1999; 17:97–102.
175. Zackheim HS: Tomatoes, tomato-based products, lycopene, and epidemiologic literature. J Natl Cancer Inst 1999; 91:1331.
176. Fleshner NE, Klotz LH: Diet, androgens, oxidative stress and prostate cancer susceptibility. Cancer Metastasis Rev 1998–1999; 17:325–330.
177. Hiatt RA, Armstrong MA, Klatsky AL, et al: Alcohol consumption, smoking, and other risk factors and prostate cancer in a large health plan cohort in California (United States). Cancer Causes Control 1994; 5:66–72.
178. Giovannucci E, Ascherio A, Rimm EB, et al: A prospective cohort study of vasectomy and prostate cancer in US men. J Am Med Assoc 1993; 269:873–877.
179. Lesko SM, Louik C, Vezina R, et al: Vasectomy and prostate cancer. J Urol 1999; 161:1848–1852.
180. Hutchison GB: Incidence and etiology of prostate cancer. Urology 1981; 17 (suppl):4–10.
181. Brawn PN, Johnson EH, Speights VO, et al: Incidence, racial differences, and prognostic significance of prostate carcinomas diagnosed with obstructive symptoms. Cancer 1994; 74:1607–1611.
182. Krahn MD, Mahoney JE, Eckman MH, et al: Screening for prostate cancer. A decision analytic view. J Am Med Assoc 1994; 272:773–780.
183. Benoit RM, Naslund MJ: The economics of prostate cancer screening. Oncology (Huntingt) 1997; 11:1533–1543.
184. Landis SH, Murray T, Bolden S, et al: Cancer statistics, 1998. CA Cancer J Clin 1998; 48:6–29.
185. Labrie F, Candas B, Dupont A, et al: Screening decreases prostate cancer death: first analysis of the 1988 Quebec prospective randomized controlled trial. Prostate 1999; 38:83–91.
186. Anonymous: Immediate versus deferred treatment for advanced prostatic cancer: initial results of the Medical Research Council Trial. The Medical Research Council Prostate Cancer Working Party Investigators Group. Br J Urol 1997; 79:235–246.
187. Pilepich MV, Caplan R, Byhardt RW, et al: Phase III trial of androgen suppression using goserelin in unfavorable-prognosis carcinoma of the prostate treated with definitive radiotherapy: report of Radiation Oncology Group Protocol 85–31. J Clin Oncol 1997; 15:1013–1021.
188. Bolla M, Gonzalez D, Warde P, et al: Improved survival in patients with locally advanced prostate cancer treated with radiotherapy and goserelin. N Engl J Med 1997; 337:295–300.
189. Albertsen PC, Hanley JA, Gleason DF, et al: Competing risk analysis of men aged 55 to 74 years at diagnosis managed conservatively for clinically localized prostate cancer. J Am Med Assoc 1998; 280:975–980.
190. Byar DP, Mostofi FK: Carcinoma of the prostate: prognostic evaluation of certain pathologic features in 208 radical prostatectomies. Examined by step-section technique. Cancer 1972; 30:5–13.
191. Smith DS, Carvalhal GF, Mager DE, et al: Use of prostate specific antigen cutoffs for prostate cancer screening in black and white men. J Urol 1998; 160:1734–1738.
192. Smith DS, Catalona WJ, Herschman JD: Longitudinal screening for prostate cancer with prostate-specific antigen. J Am Med Assoc 1996; 276:1309–1315.
193. Jacobsen SJ, Bergstrahl EJ, Guess HA, et al: Predictive properties of serum-prostate-specific antigen testing in a community-based setting. Arch Intern Med 1996; 156:2462–2468.
194. Smith DS, Bullock AD, Catalona WJ, et al: Racial differences in a prostate cancer screening study. J Urol 1996; 156:1366–1369.
195. Kadmon DWA, Williams RH, Pavlik VN, et al: Pitfalls in interpreting prostate specific antigen velocity. J Urol 1996; 155:1655–1657.
196. Crawford ED, Schutz MJ, Clejan S, et al: The effect of digital rectal examination on prostate-specific antigen levels. J Am Med Assoc 1992; 267:2227–2228.
197. Filella X, Alcover J, Molina R, et al: Clinical usefulness of free PSA fraction as an indicator of prostate cancer. Int J Cancer 1995; 63:780–784.
198. Effert PBR, Handt S, Wolff JM, et al: Metabolic imaging of untreated prostate cancer by positron emission tomography with ^{18}fluorine-labeled deoxyglucose. J Urol 1996; 155:994–998.
199. Oesterling JE, Jacobsen SJ, Klee GG, et al: Free, complexed, and total serum prostate specific antigen: the establishment of appropriate reference ranges for their concentrations and ratios. J Urol 1995; 154:1090–1095.
200. Pannek J, Partin AW: The role of PSA and percent free PSA for staging and prognosis prediction in clinically localized prostate cancer. Semin Urol Oncol 1998; 16:100–105.
201. Catalona WJ, Partin AW, Slawin KM, et al: Use of the percentage of free prostate-specific antigen to enhance differentiation of prostate cancer from benign prostatic disease: a prospective multicenter clinical trial. J Am Med Assoc 1998; 279:1542–1547.
202. McCormack RT, Rittenhouse HG, Finlay JA, et al: Molecular forms of prostate-specific antigen and the human kallikrein gene family: a new era. Urology 1995; 45:729–744.

203. Narayan PGV, Taylor SP, Tewari A, et al: The role of transrectal ultrasound-guided biopsy-based staging, preoperative serum prostate-specific antigen, and biopsy Gleason score in prediction of final pathologic diagnosis in prostate cancer. Urology 1995; 46:205–212.
204. Lewis P, Bloemers M, Weinberg V, et al: Prognostic value of biopsy extent and era on the outcome of patients with prostate cancer treated with radiotherapy [Abstract]. Int J Radiat Oncol Biol Phys 1998; 42 (suppl):308.
205. Guillonneau B, Debras B, Veillon B, et al: Indications for preoperative seminal vesicle biopsies in staging of clinically localized prostate cancer. Eur Urol 1997; 32:160–165.
206. Ranparia DJ, Hart L, Assimos DG: Utility of chest radiography and cystoscopy in the evaluation of patients with localized prostate cancer. Urology 1996; 48:72–74.
207. Vijayakumar V, Vijayakumar S, Quadri SF, et al: Can prostate-specific antigen levels predict bone scan evidence of metastases in newly diagnosed prostate cancer? Am J Clin Oncol 1994; 17:432–436.
208. Huncharek M, Muscat JK: Serum prostate-specific antigen as a predictor of radiographic staging studies in newly diagnosed prostate cancer. Cancer Invest 1995; 13:31–35.
209. Partin AW, Kattan MW, Subong EN, et al: Combination of prostate-specific antigen, clinical stage, and Gleason score to predict pathological stage of localized prostate cancer: a multi-institutional update. J Am Med Assoc 1997; 277:1445–1451.
210. Polascik TJ, Manyak MJ, Haseman MK, et al: Comparison of clinical staging algorithms and ^{111}indium-capromab pendetide immunoscintigraphy in the prediction of lymph node involvement in high risk prostate carcinoma patients. Cancer 1999; 85:1586–1592.
211. McNeal JE: Anatomy of the prostate: an historical survey of divergent views. Prostate 1980; 1:3–13.
212. Wheeler TM: Anatomy of the prostate and the pathology of prostate cancer. In: Vogelzang NJ, Scardino PT, Shipley WU, et al (eds): Comprehensive Textbook of Genitourinary Oncology, 2nd ed, pp 587–604. Philadelphia, Lippincott Williams & Wilkins, 2000.
213. McNeal JE: Normal and pathologic anatomy of prostate. Urology 1981; 17 (suppl):11–16.
214. McNeal JE: Normal histology of the prostate. Am J Surg Pathol 1988; 12:619–633.
215. Vera-Donoso CD, Vidal J, Gomez S, et al: Carcinoma of prostatic ducts. Eur Urol 1991; 19:8–11.
216. Gleason DF, Mellinger GT: Prediction of prognosis for prostatic adenocarcinoma by combined histological grading and clinical staging. J Urol 1974; 111:58–64.
217. Bagshaw MA, Cox RS, Ray GR: Status of radiation treatment of prostate cancer at Stanford University. NCI Monogr 1988; 7:47–60.
218. Partin AW, Yoo J, Carter HB, et al: The use of prostate specific antigen, clinical stage and Gleason score to predict pathologic stage in men with localized prostate cancer. J Urol 1993; 150:10–14.
219. Ohori M, Goad JR, Wheeler TM, et al: Can radical prostatectomy alter the progression of poorly differentiated prostate cancer? J Urol 1994; 152:1843–1849.
220. Roach M III, Lu J, Pilepich MV, et al: Long-term survival after radiotherapy alone: Radiation Therapy Oncology Group prostate cancer trials. J Urol 1999; 161:864–868.
221. Johnstone PAS, Riffenburgh R, Saunders EL, et al: Grading inaccuracies in diagnostic biopsies revealing prostatic adenocarcinoma: implications for definitive radiation therapy. Int J Radiat Oncol Biol Phys 1995; 32:479–482.
222. Benson MC: Application of flow cytometry and automated image analysis to the study of prostate cancer. NCI Monogr 1988; 7:25–29.
223. Benson MC: Fine-needle aspiration of the prostate. NCI Monogr 1988; 7:19–24.
224. Kojima M, Troncoso P, Babaian RJ: Use of prostate-specific antigen and tumor volume in predicting needle biopsy grading error. Urology 1995; 45:807–812.
225. Hanks GE, Buzydlowski J, Sause WT, et al: Ten-year outcomes for pathologic node-positive patients treated in RTOG-7506. Int J Radiat Oncol Biol Phys 1998; 40:765–768.
226. Hanks GE: Long-term control of prostate cancer with radiation. Past, present, and future. Urol Clin North Am 1996; 23:605–616.
227. Paulson DF, Lin GH, Hinshaw W, et al: Radical surgery versus radiotherapy for adenocarcinoma of the prostate. J Urol 1982; 128:502–504.
228. Kupelian P, Katcher J, Levin H, et al: External beam radiotherapy versus radical prostatecomy for clinical stage T1–2 prostate cancer: therapeutic implications of stratification by pretreatment PSA levels and biopsy Gleason scores. Cancer J Sci Am 1997; 3:78–87.
229. Lee WR, Hanks GE, Hanlon A: Increasing prostate-specific antigen profile following definitive radiation therapy for localized prostate cancer: clinical observations. J Clin Oncol 1996; 15:230–238.
230. Oefelein MG, Smith ND, Grayhack JT, et al: Long-term results of radical retropubic prostatectomy in men with high grade carcinoma of the prostate. J Urol 1997; 158:1460–1465.
231. Lu-Yao GL, McLerran D, Wassan J, et al: An assessment of radical prostatectomy. Time trends, geographic variation, and outcomes. The Prostate Patient Outcomes Research Team. JAMA 1993; 269:2633–2636.
232. Ragde H, Elgamal AA, Snow PB, et al: Ten-year disease free survival after transperineal sonography-guided iodine-125 brachytherapy with or without 45-Gray external beam irradiation in the treatment of patients with clinically localized, low to high Gleason grade prostate carcinoma. Cancer 1998; 83:989–1001.
233. Grado GL, Larson TR, Balch CS, et al: Actuarial disease-free survival after prostate cancer brachytherapy using interactive techniques with biplane ultrasound and fluoroscopic guidance. Int J Radiat Oncol Biol Phys 1998; 42:289–298.
234. Stein A, deKernion JB, Dorey F, et al: Adjuvant radiotherapy in patients post-radical prostatectomy with tumor extending through capsule or positive seminal vesicles. Urology 1992; 39:59–62.
235. Frazier HA, Robertson JE, Humphrey PA, et al: Is prostate specific antigen of clinical importance in evaluating outcome after radical prostatectomy? J Urol 1993; 149:516–518.
236. Smitt MC, Heltzel M: The results of radical prostatectomy at a community hospital during the prostate specific antigen era. Cancer 1996; 77:928–933.
237. Lerner SE, Blute ML, Zincke H: Risk factors for progression in patients with prostate cancer treated with radical prostatectomy. Semin Urol Oncol 1996; 14 (suppl):12–20.
238. Partin AW, Pearson JD, Landis PK, et al: Evaluation of serum prostate-specific antigen velocity after radical prostatectomy to distinguish local recurrence from distant metastases. Urology 1994; 43:649–659.
239. Connolly JA, Shinohara K, Presti JC Jr, et al: Local recurrence after radical prostatecotomy: characteristics in size, location, and relationship to prostate-specific antigen and surgical margins. Urology 1996; 47:225–231.
240. Ward JF, Nowacki M, Sands JP, et al: Malignant cytological washings from radical prostatectomy specimens: a possible mechanism for local recurrence of prostate cancer following surgical treatment of organ confined disease. J Urol 1996; 156:1381–1384.
241. Oefelein MG, Kaul K, Herz B, et al: Molecular detection of prostate epithelial cells from the surgical field and peripheral circulation during radical prostatectomy. J Urol 1996; 155:238–242.
242. Leibel SA, Hanks GE, Kramer S: Patterns of care outcome studies: results of the national practice in adenocarcinoma of the prostate. Int J Radiat Oncol Biol Phys 1984; 10:401–409.
243. Soffen EM, Hanks GE, Hunt MA, et al: Conformal static field radiation therapy treatment of early prostate cancer versus non-conformal techniques: a reduction in acute morbidity. Int J Radiat Oncol Biol Phys 1992; 24:485–488.
244. Sandler HM, Perez-Tamayo C, Ten Haken RK, et al: Dose escalation for stage C (T3) prostate cancer: minimal rectal toxicity observed using conformal therapy. Radiother Oncol 1992; 23:53–54.
245. Vijayakumar S, Awan A, Karrison T, et al: Acute toxicity during external-beam radiotherapy for localized prostate cancer: Comparison of different techniques. Int J Radiat Oncol Biol Phys 1993; 25:359–371.
246. Bermudez M-A, Roach M, Rosenthal S, et al: The impact of age and conformal technique on acute toxicity in patients receiving radiation therapy for clinically localized prostate cancer [Abstract]. Int J Radiat Oncol Biol Phys 1995; 32 (suppl):1061.
247. Fukunaga-Johnson N, Sandler HM, McLaughlin PW, et al: Results of 3D conformal radiotherapy in the treatment of localized prostate cancer. Int J Radiat Oncol Biol Phys 1997; 38:311–317.
248. Pollack A, Zagars GK, Starkschall G, et al: Conventional vs. conformal radiotherapy for prostate cancer: preliminary results of dosimetry and acute toxicity. Int J Radiat Oncol Biol Phys 1996; 34:555–564.
249. Tait DM, Nahum AE, Meyer LC, et al: Acute toxicity in pelvic radiotherapy; a randomized trial of conformal versus conventional treatment. Radiother Oncol 1997; 42:121–136.
250. Dearnaley DP, Khoo VS, Norman AR, et al: Comparison of radiation

side-effects of conformal and conventional radiotherapy in prostate cancer: a randomized trial. Lancet 1999; 353:267–272.
251. Roach M, Pickett B, Rosenthal SA, et al: Defining treatment margins for six field conformal irradiation of localized prostate cancer. Int J Radiat Oncol Biol Phys 1994; 28:267–275.
252. Pollack A, Zagars G: External beam radiotherapy dose-response of prostate cancer. Int J Radiat Oncol Biol Phys 1997; 39:1011–1018.
253. Horwitz EM, Hanlon AL, Hanks GE: Update on the treatment of prostate cancer with external beam irradiation. Prostate 1998; 37:195–206.
254. Pickett B, Vigneault E, Kurhanewicz J, et al: Static field intensity modulation to treat a dominant intra-prostatic lesion to 90 Gy compared to seven field 3-dimensional radiotherapy. Int J Radiat Oncol Biol Phys 1999; 44:921–929.
255. Fraass BA, Kessler ML, McShan DL, et al: Optimization and clinical use of multisegment intensity-modulated radiation therapy for high-dose conformal therapy. Semin Radiat Oncol 1999; 9:60–77.
256. Barringer BS: Radium in the treatment of carcinoma of the bladder and prostate. JAMA 1917; 68:1227–1230.
257. Whitmore WF, Hilaris B, Grabstald H: Retropubic implantation of iodine 125 in the treatment of prostate cancer. J Urol 1972; 108:918–920.
258. Kuban DA, el-Mahdi AM, Schellhammer PF: I-125 interstitial implantation for prostate cancer. What have we learned 10 years later? Cancer 1989; 63:2415–2420.
259. Fuks Z, Leibel SA, Wallner KE, et al: The effect of local control on metastatic dissemination in carcinoma of the prostate: long-term results in patients treated with ^{125}I. Int J Radiat Oncol Biol Phys 1991; 21:537–547.
260. Blasko JC, Ragde H, Grimm PD: Transperineal ultrasound-guided implantation of the prostate: morbidity and complications. Scand J Urol Nephrol 1991; 137:113–118.
261. Ragde H, Blasko JC, Grimm PD, et al: Brachytherapy for clinically localized prostate cancer: results at 7- and 8-year follow-up. Semin Surg Oncol 1997; 13:438–443.
262. Mate TP, Gottesman JE, Hatton J, et al: High dose-rate afterloading ^{192}Iridium prostate brachytherapy: feasibility report. Int J Radiat Oncol Biol Phys 1998; 41:525–533.
263. Schild SE, Wong WW, Grado GL, et al: Radiotherapy for isolated increases in serum prostate-specific antigen levels after radical prostatectomy. Mayo Clin Proc 1994; 69:613–619.
264. Wu JJ, King SC, Montana GS, et al: The efficacy of postprostatectomy radiotherapy in patients with an isolated elevation of serum prostate-specific antigen. Int J Radiat Oncol Biol Phys 1995; 32:317–323.
265. Anscher MS, Robertson CN, Prosnitz R: Adjuvant radiotherapy for pathologic stage T3/4 adenocarcinoma of the prostate: ten-year update. Int J Radiat Oncol Biol Phys 1995; 33:37–43.
266. Rogers R, Grossfeld GD, Roach M III, et al: Radiation therapy for the management of biopsy-proven, local recurrence following radical prostatectomy. J Urol 1998; 160:1748–1753.
267. Pilepich MV, Krall JM, al-Saraf M, et al: Androgen deprivation with radiation therapy compared with radiation therapy alone for locally advanced prostatic carcinoma: a randomized comparative trial of the Radiation Therapy Oncology Group. Urology 1995; 45:616–623.
268. Lawton CA, Winter K, Byhardt R, et al: Androgen suppression plus radiation versus radiation alone for patients with D1 (pN+) adenocarcinoma of the prostate (results based on a national prospective randomized trial, RTOG 85–31). Int J Radiat Oncol Biol Phys 1997; 38:931–939.
269. Laverdiere J, Gomez JL, Cusan L, et al: Beneficial effect of combination therapy administered prior and following external beam radiation therapy in localized prostate cancer. Int J Radiat Oncol Biol Phys 1997; 37:247–252.
270. Roach M III, Lu J, Pilepich MV, et al: Predicting long term survival and the need for hormonal therapy: a meta-analysis of RTOG prostate cancer trials. Int J Radiat Oncol Biol Phys 2000; 47:609–615.
271. Roach M III: Neoadjuvant total androgen suppression and radiotherapy in the management of locally advanced prostate cancer. Semin Urol Oncol 1996; 14:32–38.
272. Sklar G: Combined antitumor effect of suramin plus irradiation in human prostate cancer cells: The role of apoptosis. J Urol 1993; 150:1526–1532.
273. Rupnow BA, Murtha AD, Alarcon RM, et al: Direct evidence that apoptosis enhances tumor responses to fractionated radiotherapy. Cancer Res 1998; 58:1779–1784.
274. Widmark A, Damber J-E, Bergh A, et al: Estramustine potentiates the effects of irradiation on the Dunning (R3327) rat prostatic adenocarcinoma. Prostate 1994; 24:79–83.
275. Zietman AL, Nakfoor BM, Prince EA, et al: The effects of androgen deprivation and radiation therapy on an androgen-sensitive murine tumor: an *in vitro* and *in vivo* study. Cancer J Sci Am 1997; 3:31–36.
276. Geller J, Candari C: Comparison of dihydrotestosterone levels in prostatic cancer metastases and primary prostate cancer. Prostate 1989; 15:171–175.
277. Geller J: Rationale for blockade of adrenal as well as testicular androgens in the treatment of advanced prostate cancer. Semin Oncol 1985; 12 (suppl):28–35.
278. Geller J: Basis for hormonal management of advanced prostate cancer. Cancer 1993; 71 (suppl):1039–1045.
279. Crawford ED, Blumenstein BA, Goodman PJ, et al: Leuprolide with and without flutamide in advanced prostate cancer. Cancer 1990; 66:1039–1044.
280. Eisenberger MA, Blumenstein BA, Crawford ED, et al: Bilateral orchiectomy with or without flutamide for metastatic prostate cancer. N Engl J Med 1998; 339:1036–1042.
281. Roach M III: Current status of androgen suppression and radiotherapy for patients with prostate cancer. J Steroid Biochem Mol Biol 1999; 69:239–245.
282. Small EJ, Srinivas S: The antiandrogen withdrawal syndrome. Experience in a large cohort of unselected patients with advanced prostate cancer. Cancer 1995; 76:1428–1434.
283. Scher HI, Mazumdar M, Kelly WK: Clinical trials in relapsed prostate cancer: defining the target. J Natl Cancer Inst 1996; 88:1623–1634.
284. Kelly WK, Slovin S, Scher HI: Steroid hormone withdrawal syndromes. Pathophysiology and clinical significance. Urol Clin North Am 1997; 24:421–431.
285. Schmidt JD, Gibbons RP, Murphy GP, et al: Adjuvant therapy for localized prostate cancer. Cancer 1993; 71 (suppl):1005–1013.
286. Roessler W, Hinke A, Wieland WF: Experience in advanced prostatic cancer: orchiectomy and flutamide versus orchiectomy and estramustine phosphate. Urology 1994; 43 (suppl):57–60.
287. Beedassy A, Cardi G: Chemotherapy in advanced prostate cancer. Semin Oncol 1999; 26:428–438.
288. Pruthi RS, Johnstone I, Tu IP, et al: Prostate-specific antigen doubling times in patients who have failed radical prostatectomy: correlation with histologic characteristics of the primary cancer. Urology 1997; 49:737–742.
289. Partin AW, Pound CR, Clemens JQ, et al: Serum PSA after anatomic radical prostatectomy: the Johns Hopkins experience after 10 years. Urol Clin North Am 1993; 20:713–725.
290. Catalona WJ, Smith DS: 5-year tumor recurrence rates after anatomical radical prostatectomy for prostate cancer. J Urol 1994; 152:1837–1842.
291. Zietman AL, Edelstein RA, Coen JJ, et al: Radical prostatectomy for adenocarcinoma of the prostate: the influence of preoperative and pathologic findings on biochemical disease-free outcome. Urology 1994; 43:828–833.
292. Zincke H, Oesterling JE, Blute ML, et al: Long-term (15 years) results after radical prostatectomy for clinically localized (stage T2c or lower) prostate cancer. J Urol 1994; 152:1850–1857.
293. D'Amico A, Whittington R, Malkowicz SB, et al: A multivariate analysis of clinical and pathological factors that predict for prostate specific antigen failure after radical prostatectomy for prostate cancer. J Urol 1995; 154:131–138.
294. Kaplan ID, Cox RS, Bagshaw MS: Prostate specific antigen after external beam radiotherapy for prostate cancer: follow-up. J Urol 1993; 149:519–522.
295. Zagars GK, Pollack A: Radiation therapy for T1 and T2 prostate cancer: prostate-specific antigen and disease outcome. Urology 1995; 45:476–483.
296. Kuban DA, el-Mahdi AM, Schellhammer PF: Potential benefit of improved local tumor control in patients with prostate carcinoma. Cancer 1995; 75:2373–2382.
297. Zietman AL, Coen JJ, Dallow KC, et al: The treatment of prostate cancer by conventional radiation therapy: an analysis of long-term outcome. Int J Radiat Oncol Biol Phys 1995; 32:287–292.
298. Roach M III, Burton E, Kroll S, et al: 501 men irradiated for clinically localized prostate cancer (1987–1995): preliminary analysis of experience at UCSF and affiliated facilities [Abstract]. Int J Radiat Oncol Biol Phys 1996; 36 (suppl):248.
299. Kabalin JN, Hodge KK, McNeal JE, et al: Identification of residual

cancer in the prostate following radiation therapy: role of transrectal ultrasound guided biopsy and prostate specific antigen. J Urol 1989; 142:326–331.

300. Crook JM, Perry GA, Robertson S, et al: Routine prostate biopsies following radiotherapy for prostate cancer: results for 226 patients. Urology 1995; 45:624–632.
301. Zagars GK: The prognostic significance of a single serum prostate-specific antigen value beyond six months after radiation therapy for adenocarcinoma of the prostate. Int J Radiat Oncol Biol Phys 1993; 27:39–45.
302. Kavadi VS, Zagars GK, Pollack A: Serum prostate-specific antigen after radiation therapy for clinically localized prostate cancer: prognostic implications. Int J Radiat Oncol Biol Phys 1994; 30:279–287.
303. Critz FA, Tarlton RS, Holladay DA: Prostate specific antigen-monitored combination radiotherapy for patients with prostate cancer. I-125 implant followed by external beam irradiation. Cancer 1995; 75:2383–2391.
304. Zietman AL, Tibbs MK, Dallow KC, et al: Use of PSA nadir to predict subsequent biochemical outcome following external beam radiation therapy for T1–2 adenocarcinoma of the prostate. Radiother Oncol 1996; 40:159–162.
305. Catalona WJ, Basler JW: Return of erections and urinary continence following nerve sparing radical retropubic prostatectomy. J Urol 1993; 150:905–907.
306. Catalona WJ, Carvalhal GF, Mager DE, et al: Potency, continence and complication rates in 1870 consecutive radical retropubic prostatectomies. J Urol 1999; 162:433–438.
307. Shipley WU, Zietman AL, Hanks GE, et al: Treatment related sequelae following external beam radiation for prostate cancer: a review with an update in patients with T1 and T2 tumor. J Urol 1994; 152:1799–1805.
308. Schultheiss TE, Hanks GE, Hunt MA, et al: Incidence of and factors related to late complications in conformal and conventional radiation treatment of cancer of the prostate. Int J Radiat Oncol Biol Phys 1995; 32:643–649.
309. Roach M III, Chinn DM, Holland GP, et al: A pilot survey of sexual function and quality of life following 3D conformal radiotherapy for clinically localized prostate cancer. Int J Radiat Oncol Biol Phys 1996; 35:869–874.
310. Litwin M: Measuring health related quality of life in men with prostate cancer. J Urol 1994; 152:1882–1887.
311. Stock RG, Stone NN, Iannuzzi C: Sexual potency following interactive ultrasound-guided brachytherapy for prostate cancer. Int J Radiat Oncol Biol Phys 1996; 35:267–272.
312. Zelefsky MJ, Wallner KE, Ling CC, et al: Comparison of the 5-year outcome and morbidity of three-dimensional conformal radiotherapy versus transperineal permanent iodine-125 implantation for early-stage prostatic cancer. J Clin Oncol 1999; 17:517–522.

Germ Cell Tumors of the Testes

313. Oliver RTD: A comparison of the biology and prognosis of seminoma and nonseminoma. In: Horwich A (ed): Testicular Cancer: Clinical Investigation and Management, pp 95–124. New York, Chapman & Hall, 1991.
314. Bosl GJ, Bajorin DF, Sheinfeld J, et al: Cancer of the testis. In: De Vita VT Jr, Hellman S, Rosenberg SA (eds): Cancer. Principles & Practice of Oncology, 5th ed, pp 1397–1425. Philadelphia, Lippincott-Raven, 1997.
315. Kurie JM, Bosl GJ, Dmitrovsky E: Genetic and biologic aspects of treatment response and resistance in male germ cell cancer. Semin Oncol 1992; 19:197–205.
316. Motzer RJ, Rodriguez E, Reuter VR, et al: Molecular and cytogenetic studies in the diagnosis of patients with poorly differentiated carcinomas of unknown primary site. J Clin Oncol 1995; 13:274–282.
317. Bosl GJ, Ilson DH, Rodriguez E, et al: Clinical relevance of the I(12p) chromosome in germ cell tumors. J Natl Cancer Inst 1994; 86:349–355.
318. Sandberg AA, Meloni AM, Suijkerbuijk RF: Reviews of chromosome studies in urological tumors. III. Cytogenetics and genes in testicular tumors. J Urol 1996; 155:1531–1556.
319. Houldsworth J, Reuter V, Bosl GJ, et al: Aberrant expression of cyclin D2 is an early event in male germ cell tumorigenesis. Cell Growth Differ 1997; 8:293–299.
320. Fung CY, Garnick MB: Clinical stage I carcinoma of the testis: A review. J Clin Oncol 1988; 6:734–750.
321. Leibovitch I, Little JS Jr, Foster RS, et al: Delayed orchiectomy after chemotherapy for metastatic nonseminomatous germ cell tumors. J Urol 1996; 155:952–954.
322. Markland C: Special problems in managing patients with testicular cancer. Urol Clin North Am 1977; 4:427–451.
323. Mostofi FK, Price EB: Tumors of the male genital system. In: Atlas of Tumor Pathology. 2nd ser, fasc 8. Washington D.C., Armed Forces Institute of Pathology, 1973.
324. Klein EA: Tumor markers in testis cancer. Urol Clin North Am 1993; 20:67–73.
325. Warde P, Gospodarowicz M, Banerjee K, et al: Prognostic factors for relapse in stage I testicular seminoma treated with surveillance. J Urol 1997; 157:1705–1709.
326. Horwich A, Dearnaley DP: Treatment of seminoma. Semin Oncol 1992; 19:171–180.
327. Thomas GM, Williams SD: Testis. In: Perez CA, Brady LW (eds): Principles and Practice of Radiation Oncology, 3rd ed, pp 1695–1715. Philadelphia, Lippincott-Raven, 1998.
328. Thomas GM: Consensus statement on the investigation and management of testicular seminoma: EORTC Genito-Urinary Group Monograph 7. In: Newling DW, Jones WG (eds): Prostate Cancer and Testicular Cancer. New York, Wiley-Liss, 1990.
329. Donohue JP, Sachary FM, Maynard BR: Distribution of nodal metastases in nonseminomatous testis cancer. J Urol 1982; 128:315–320.
330. Rorth M: Therapeutic alternatives in clinical stage 1 nonseminomatous disease. Semin Oncol 1992; 19:190–196.
331. Stenberg C: Role of primary chemotherapy in stage I and low-volume stage II nonseminomatous testis tumors. Urol Clin North Am 1993; 20:93–109.
332. Read G, Stenning SP, Cullen MH, et al: Medical Research Council prospective study of surveillance for stage I testicular teratoma. J Clin Oncol 1992; 10:1762–1768.
333. Friedman LS, Parkinson MC, Jones WG, et al: Histopathology in the prediction of relapse of patients with stage I testicular teratoma treated by orchiectomy alone. Lancet 1987; 2:294–298.
334. Foster RS, Roth BJ: Clinical stage I nonseminoma: surgery versus surveillance. Semin Oncol 1998; 25:145–153.
335. Williams SD, Birch R, Einhorn LH, et al: Treatment of disseminated germ cell tumors with cisplatin, bleomycin, and either vinblastine or etoposide. N Engl J Med 1987; 316:1435–1440.
336. International Germ Cell Cancer Collaborative Group: International Germ Cell Consensus Classification: a prognostic factor-based staging system for metastatic germ cell cancers. J Clin Oncol 1997; 15:594–603.
337. Garrow GC, Johnson DH: Treatment of "good risk" metastatic testicular cancer. Semin Oncol 1992; 19:159–165.
338. Dodd PM, Motzer RJ, Bajorin DF: Poor-risk germ cell tumors. Recent developments. Urol Clin North Am 1998; 25:485–493.
339. Bajorin DF, Herr H, Motzer RJ, et al: Current perspectives on the role of adjunctive surgery in combined modality treatment for patients with germ cell tumors. Semin Oncol 1992; 19:148–158.
340. Donohue JP, Leviovich I, Foster RS, et al: Integration of surgery and systemic therapy: results and principles of integration. Semin Urol Oncol 1998; 16:65–71.
341. Brenner PC, Herr HW, Morse MJ, et al: Simultaneous retroperitoneal, thoracic and cervical resection of postchemotherapy residual masses in patients with metastatic nonseminomatous germ cell tumors of the testis. J Clin Oncol 1996; 14:1765–1769.
342. Coia LR, Hanks GE: Complications from large field intermediate dose infradiaphragmatic radiation: An analysis of the patterns of care outcome studies for Hodgkin's disease and seminoma. Int J Radiat Oncol Biol Phys 1988; 15:29–35.
343. Grossfeld GD, Small EJ: Long-term side effects of treatment for testis cancer. Urol Clin North Am 1998; 25:503–515.

23 *The Leukemias*

EILEEN SCIGLIANO, MD, Hematology
ADRIANNA VLACHOS, MD, Pediatric Hematology/Oncology
VESNA NAJFELD, PhD, Hematology
BRENDA SHANK, MD, PhD, Radiation Oncology

Clay lies still, blood's a rover; Breath's a ware that will not keep. Up lad; when the journey's over there'll be time enough to sleep.

A. E. HOUSMAN

Perspective

Leukemia was first recognized as a distinct entity in the early 1800s by Bennett, who described a series of patients with "purulent material" in their blood, and introduced the term *leukocythemia*.[1] This report was followed by Virchow, who described the microscopic appearance of the blood of a similar patient as having "the same colorless or white bodies which also occur in normal blood," and coined the term *weisses blut* (white blood) to describe the condition.[2] He later introduced the word *leukemia*, which he derived from the Greek, meaning *white blood*.[3] The subsequent understanding of the origin of these white cells from the bone marrow gave rise to the term *myeloid*, meaning *marrow derived*,[4] and the further classification of this disorder into myelocytic and lymphocytic types by Naegeli[5] led to the modern classification of myeloid and lymphoid leukemias. The leukemias are clonal disorders characterized by uncontrolled proliferation of cells. In the acute leukemias, there is a block in differentiation of hematopoietic or lymphopoietic cells leading to the accumulation of immature "blast forms" in the blood, bone marrow, and sometimes, extramedullary sites. In the chronic leukemias, the accumulating cells are differentiated and mature, but are part of the leukemic clone.

Advances in molecular techniques have enabled the identification of leukemia-specific cytogenetic and molecular abnormalities, the cloning of many of the genes involved in these abnormalities, and the biochemical characterization of the gene products, leading to a greater understanding of the pathogenesis of the leukemias.[6] It has become apparent from clinical trials that specific cytogenetic and molecular abnormalities are associated with leukemias that share common clinicopathologic manifestations, including their response to treatment (all-*trans*-retinoic acid [ATRA] for t[15;17]-positive acute promyelocytic leukemia [APL]; high-dose cytarabine consolidation for t[8;21]-, or inv 16–positive leukemia) and prognosis (leukemias with "poor prognosis": cytogenetic abnormalities such as t[9;22], del 5, del 7). A molecular classification of leukemias may lead to the development and use of specific therapies that target a specific molecular event. Another important outcome of these advances has been the ability to detect minimal residual disease (MRD) with increasing sensitivity. This ability will enable the detection of patients who have not achieved molecular remissions, as well as the identification of patients at earlier stages of relapse.

Advances in therapy for the leukemias have relied increasingly on the use of dose intensification, primarily in the form of high-dose chemotherapy with stem cell transplantation. Allogeneic stem cell transplantation is the only curative therapy for patients with relapsed or refractory acute myeloid leukemia (AML), and it may be the treatment of choice in selected patients with first remission AML. Stem cell transplantation is the only curative therapy for chronic myelogenous leukemia (CML). Advances in stem cell transplantation include:

- the use of selected grafts (CD34+ selection, T-cell depletion) to ameliorate transplant-related complications such as graft-versus-host disease (GVHD)
- adoptive immunotherapy via donor buffy coat infusions to treat relapse following transplantation
- the use of alternative sources of stem cells, including unrelated donors; mismatched, related donors; and umbilical cord blood

Acute Myeloid Leukemia

The AMLs are a group of clonal, hematopoietic stem cell disorders characterized by arrested differentiation of stem cells, resulting in a block in their development into mature, functioning blood cells. The leukemic cells retain the ability to proliferate, and the accumulation of these immature, poorly functioning cells in the bone marrow inhibits the development of normal hematopoietic cells. Suppression of normal hematopoiesis gives rise to cytopenias that result in the clinical signs and symptoms characteristic of this disease: anemia, hemorrhage, and infection. This block in differentiation may occur in any of the hematopoietic lineages (granulocytic/monocytic, erythrocytic, megakaryocytic), and, in some cases, before lineage commitment occurs (mixed lineage or biphenotypic leukemias), as well as during different developmental stages within a given hematopoietic lineage (myeloblastic leukemia, promyelocytic leukemia). The acute myeloid leukemias are a heterogeneous group of diseases that differ with respect to morphologic appearance, histochemical staining patterns, immunophenotypic expression, cytogenetic abnormalities, clinical features, and response to therapy.

Epidemiology and Etiology

Epidemiology

The incidence of AML is 2.6 per 100,000 persons.[7] Incidence rates are slightly higher for males than females, and for whites than nonwhites. The incidence rises with age, occurring rarely before age 40 (<1 in 100,000), and increasing to an incidence of 16 cases per 100,000 by age 75.[7] The median age at diagnosis is 65 years. In adults, AML represents about 90% of all acute leukemias.

Etiology

The etiology of AML is still largely unknown. Although numerous genetic, drug, environmental, and occupational factors have been identified as potentially leukemogenic, the vast majority of patients presenting with *de novo* AML have not been exposed to an antecedent risk factor.

Environmental Factors

Of the environmental exposures, only three have been well documented to be associated with the development of AML: benzene exposure,[8] ionizing radiation,[9] and prior exposure to chemotherapy.[10]

BENZENE

Chronic exposure to benzene, as seen in leather and rubber industry workers and painters, has been associated with a significantly increased incidence of AML. Benzene inhibits DNA synthesis, introduces DNA strand breaks, and can result in chromosomal abnormalities following chronic exposure. AML, as well as bone marrow failure (aplastic anemia), can occur decades following exposure.

IONIZING RADIATION

Evidence of an increased risk of AML following exposure to ionizing radiation has come from a number of fields: studies of atomic bomb survivors; patients receiving radiation therapy for benign conditions (e.g., for ankylosing spondylitis[11]); patients exposed to Thorotrast (a radioactive contrast agent[12]); and early cohorts of radiologists, in whom AML developed at a greater-than-expected rate. Survivors of the atomic bomb explosions in Hiroshima had a 30-fold increase in the incidence of AML,[13] with the risk being directly related to dose. There is less certainty about the increased risk of leukemia with respect to diagnostic radiation, *in utero* exposure, background radiation, radon, and other sources of low-dose exposure. Those who work in the nuclear industry are exposed to protracted low-dose ionizing radiation and may have an increased risk of leukemia.[14]

CHEMOTHERAPY

An increased incidence of AML is associated with prior exposure to chemotherapy for treatment of both malignant and nonmalignant disorders. The drugs with the greatest leukemogenic potential include alkylating agents (Cytoxan, mechlorethamine, bis-chloroethyl-nitroso-urea [BCNU], chlorambucil, busulfan), procarbazine, and topoisomerase II inhibitors (etoposide, teniposide, daunomycin, and doxorubicin).[15,16] The incidence of AML in patients treated with alkylating agents for Hodgkin's disease increases steadily from the time of treatment and plateaus at about 10 years, with a cumulative risk of about 13%.[17] The incidence of AML is greatest in those patients receiving combined-modality therapy with radiation and alkylating agent chemotherapy, and is smallest (<1%) in those patients who receive radiation alone, or a nonalkylator-containing chemotherapy regimen.

Other environmental exposures, including cigarette smoking,[18] hair dyes,[19] and nonionizing radiation (particularly, electromagnetic radiation[20]), have been linked to an increased leukemia risk, although there are conflicting reports in the literature. A 1997 study comparing residential magnetic field exposure in children with acute lymphoblastic leukemia and the same exposure in a control group found no increased risk of acute lymphoblastic leukemia (ALL).[21]

Genetic Factors

There is an increased incidence of AML in individuals with constitutional genetic defects, including Down and Klinefelter's syndromes,[22,23] as well as in individuals with genetic disorders associated with chromosomal instability and increased chromosome breakage, such as Fanconi's anemia,[24] Bloom's syndrome,[25] ataxia telangiectasia,[26] and germline *TP53* mutations.[27] The high rate of concordance for AML in monozygotic twins may reflect a common genetic event, an *in utero* leukemogenic event, or metastasis of leukemic cells from one fetus to the other. This increased risk of leukemia (1 in 5) in monozygotic twins is most pronounced during early infancy, and drops to that of a nonidentical sibling (1 in 800) within 6 months of age.[28]

PRIOR CLONAL DISEASE

AML may develop from the progression of other clonal disorders of the hematopoietic stem cell, including the myeloproliferative disorders (chronic myelogenous leukemia, polycythemia vera, essential thrombocythemia, agnogenic myeloid metaplasia), paroxysmal nocturnal hemoglobinuria,[29] aplastic anemia,[30] and myelodysplasia. In some cases, the risk of progression to AML is increased by treatment of the disorder, such as the use of ^{32}P, or the use of chlorambucil in patients with polycythemia vera.[31]

VIRUSES

RNA viruses have been strongly implicated in the etiology of leukemia in experimental animals,[32] and the human retrovirus HTLV-1 has been identified as the cause of a T-cell lymphoma/leukemia in humans.[33] In addition, the Epstein-Barr virus (EBV) has been associated with oncogenesis in acute B-cell leukemias, endemic Burkitt's lymphomas, and human immunodeficiency virus–associated lymphomas.[34]

Pathogenesis

AML is believed to result from the malignant transformation of a single hematopoietic stem cell. Clonal proliferation and a block in normal differentiation and maturation are characteristic features. Studies of patients with AML, who are heterozygous for the enzyme glucose-6-phosphate dehydrogenase (G6PD), have demonstrated the clonal nature of this disease[35] by showing that the leukemic cells all contain a single enzyme type, whereas normal tissues are composed of mixtures of cells with both enzyme types. In about 30% of patients who enter clinical remission following treatment, clonal hematopoiesis persists.[36] The persistence of these preleukemic cells suggests that the pathogenesis of AML is, in fact, a multistep process, with an initial transformation event in a hematopoietic stem cell followed by additional genetic abnormalities in descendants of clonally derived cells.[37]

Leukemic hematopoiesis gives rise to red cells, platelets, and granulocytes, which are all part of the leukemic clone. Leukemic transformation may occur at the level of a committed stem cell (progenitor cell leukemia), resulting in only cells of the granulocyte/monocyte/macrophage lineage being involved in the leukemic clone,[38] but such an occurrence is rare. The development of leukemias that are characterized by either two populations of leukemic cells (biclonal or bilineage leukemia), with one expressing myeloid markers and one expressing lymphoid markers, or by a single population of leukemic cells simultaneously expressing both myeloid and lymphoid markers (mixed lineage, biphenotypic or hybrid leukemia), suggests that leukemic transformation may occur at the level of a pluripotent stem cell.[39] The phenotype of the resulting leukemia reflects both the differentiation commitment and degree of maturation that occurs. Phenotypic variants have distinctive clinical and cytogenetic associations.

Oncogenes and anti-oncogenes are believed to have a critical role in the pathogenesis of acute leukemia.[40] Mutations of the *RAS* oncogene are the most commonly detected molecular abnormalities in AML, affecting 20% to 30% of cases with a predominance of *NRAS* activation.[41] *RAS* gene products are involved in controlling the proliferation and differentiation of many types of cells. A study of AML patients found that those employed in industries in which there was a strong likelihood of exposure to solvents had a substantially increased risk for AML associated with a *RAS* mutation, whereas there was no risk for *RAS*-negative AML.[42]

It is likely that leukemogenesis is a multistep process involving a susceptible hematopoietic cell, a genetic event (oncogenes, chromosomal translocations), and environmental influences (chemical, viral, radiation). The increasing use of cytogenetic and molecular techniques to characterize leukemias may improve our understanding of the etiology of leukemia and lead to the identification of preventable risk factors.

Detection and Diagnosis

History/Clinical Symptoms

The clinical manifestations of AML reflect the decrease in production of normal hematopoietic cells and the proliferation and accumulation of leukemic cells in the bone marrow, blood, and in extramedullary sites. Common presenting symptoms are

- weakness, dyspnea on exertion, and fatigue reflecting anemia
- easy bruising, gum or nose bleeding, excessive bleeding following minor injuries or dental procedures, secondary to thrombocytopenia or coagulopathy
- pustules and pyogenic skin infections, secondary to neutropenia

In addition, pulmonary infections with gram-positive and gram-negative organisms are seen. Constitutional symptoms, such as fever, occur in about 50% of patients.[43] Malaise and anorexia are also common presenting symptoms, but weight loss is unusual, reflecting the acute onset of this disease.

Up to 20% of patients may present with markedly elevated white blood cell (WBC) counts (usually exceeding 100,000/mm^3), and may develop a hyperleukocytosis syndrome.[44] Clinical manifestations including dizziness, stupor, dyspnea, priapism, pulmonary insufficiency, and intracerebral and pulmonary hemorrhage result from leukocyte microthrombi. Myeloblast levels in excess of 100,000/mm^3 represent a medical emergency, requiring prompt reduction in the blast count by leukapheresis. Prompt institution of chemotherapy should be undertaken.

Neurologic symptoms resulting from central nervous system involvement are uncommon presenting features;

however, about 5% of all patients will have asymptomatic central nervous system (CNS) involvement based on cerebrospinal fluid cytology.[45] The risk of CNS involvement in AML is highest in patients with high circulating blast counts, elevated lactate dehydrogenase activity, and the monocytic variants of AML, particularly myelomonocytic leukemia with eosinophilia (M4Eo).[46]

Physical Examination

The physical examination may reveal pallor and signs of hemorrhage (oral hemorrhagic bullae, petechiae in the mouth and, on extremities, ecchymoses). Gingival hyperplasia, lymphadenopathy, hepatosplenomegaly, and skin infiltration (leukemia cutis) are more common in the monocytic subtypes of AML.[47] Chloromas, extramedullary tumors formed by collections of myeloblasts and granulocytes, may present as subcutaneous masses.[48] Sweet's syndrome (neutrophilic dermatitis), a cutaneous paraneoplastic syndrome associated with AML characterized by painful red-brown nodules, represents a dense dermal infiltrate of neutrophils.[49]

Peripheral Blood Findings

The majority of patients with AML present with pancytopenia. Decreased production of normal blood cells is generally considered to be a result of crowding out of normal hematopoietic cells by an infiltration of the bone marrow with leukemic cells; however, there is some evidence suggesting that normal hematopoiesis may be directly inhibited by leukemic cells.[50]

The total WBC count usually ranges from 5000 to 30,000/mm^3, but nearly 50% of patients will have leukopenia (WBC <5000/mm^3) and absolute neutropenia (absolute neutrophil count <1000/mm^3). About 5% to 20% of patients will present with markedly elevated WBC counts (greater than 100,000 cells/mm^3). Examination of the peripheral smear nearly always reveals the presence of blast forms, although a small percentage of patients may present without circulating leukemic cells. Leukemic blasts are typically agranular cells with a high nuclear-to-cytoplasmic ratio, basophilic cytoplasm, uncondensed chromatin, and prominent nucleoli. Auer rods, rodlike cytoplasmic inclusions formed by aggregated lysosomes, are present in about 30% to 50% of cases,[51] and are considered to be pathognomonic of myeloid leukemia.

Anemia and reticulocytopenia, secondary to inadequate red blood cell production, is almost always present. Thrombocytopenia, with platelet counts usually less than 50,000/mm^3, is also a constant feature at presentation and is secondary to inadequate platelet production as well as shortened platelet survival. The presence of disseminated intravascular coagulation (DIC) in patients with the acute promyelocytic subtype of AML may contribute to thrombocytopenia.

Bone Marrow Findings

Aspiration of bone marrow, usually from the posterior iliac crest, is routinely performed to confirm the diagnosis of acute leukemia. Bone marrow aspirate smears stained with Giemsa allow for a qualitative assessment of bone marrow cell morphology. Aspirate samples are also sent for histocytochemical, immunophenotypic, cytogenetic, and molecular analysis to enable classification of the type of leukemia.

Characteristically, the bone marrow of a patient with AML is hypercellular, and megakaryocytes are decreased or absent. Normal hematopoietic cells are replaced by a monotonous infiltration of blasts. By definition, the diagnosis of acute leukemia is made when 30% or more of bone marrow nucleated cells are blasts. Occasionally, it may be difficult or even impossible to aspirate marrow from a patient with AML, a so-called dry tap. This situation can result when the marrow space is packed with blasts or when there is an increase in reticulin fibrosis, as seen with acute megakaryoblastic leukemia.[52] In this case, a bone marrow biopsy should be performed.

Cytochemistry

Histocytochemical staining of bone marrow aids in distinguishing myeloid from lymphoid leukemias and helps to distinguish among the subtypes of AML:

- Cells of the granulocytic/monocytic lineage stain with myeloperoxidase (MPO), Sudan black B (SBB), and chloroacetate esterase (CAE).
- Nonspecific esterase (NSE) staining is characteristic of monocytes alone.
- Periodic acid–Schiff reaction (PAS) stains lymphoid and erythroid cells.
- Terminal deoxynucleotidyltransferase (TdT) is a nuclear enzyme detected by immunofluorescence or immunoperoxidase techniques. TdT is expressed by most lymphoblasts; however, about 20% of myeloblasts may be TdT positive.[53]

Immunophenotyping

Immunophenotyping of bone marrow cells is performed using monoclonal antibodies that recognize myeloid- and lymphoid-specific glycoprotein antigens (referred to as clusters of differentiation or CDs) on the surface of normal and leukemic hematopoietic cells. AMLs usually express CD13, CD15, CD33, and, if monocytoid, CD14. Lymphoid-associated antigens include the common ALL antigen (CALLA or CD10), CD19, CD20, and the T-cell receptor antigen, CD3. CD34 may be expressed by blasts of all lineages, particularly primitive cells.

Cytogenetics

Cytogenetic analysis of bone marrow is a crucial part of the evaluation of a patient with leukemia because chromosomal abnormalities are associated with specific subtypes, response to therapy, and prognosis. The abnormalities identified may influence therapy both by guiding specific drug therapy (e.g., ATRA in patients with t[15;17]), and by identifying patients with worse prognoses who might be candidates for more aggressive therapy, earlier stem cell transplantation, or experimental therapies. Nonrandom chromosomal abnormalities are found in up to 90% of *de novo* AML cases.[54] Although many of the translocated genes have been cloned and their products identified, how they participate in leukemogenesis is not completely understood. The most common cytogenetic abnormalities are described in the following sections.

t(8;21)(q22;q22) AML1/ETO

Translocation (8;21) occurs in about 15% of AML cases, most commonly French-American-British (FAB) Cooperative Group subtypes M1 and M2, and is associated with a more favorable response to chemotherapy. This translocation results in the fusion of the *ETO* gene on chromosome 8, and the *AML1* gene on chromosome 21.[55]

t(15;17)(q22;q21) PML/RARA

The molecular basis of t(15;17) is the fusion of the retinoic acid receptor alpha gene (*RARA*) on chromosome 17 with the *PML* gene on chromosome 15 forming a chimeric *PML/RARA* gene. This fusion can be detected by reverse transcriptase polymerase chain reaction (RT-PCR), Southern blotting, and fluorescence *in situ* hybridization (FISH).[56] Detection of t(15;17) by these sensitive methods may assist diagnosis when cytogenetic analysis is inadequate, and these methods have been used to monitor disease and identify relapse. Patients with APL and t(15;17) have a high rate of response to differentiation therapy with ATRA.[57] The protein products of the chimeric gene have been shown to inhibit myeloid cell differentiation in the absence of retinoic acid; in the presence of retinoic acid, the chimeric products induce terminal differentiation. The development of a leukemia similar to APL in *PML/RARA* transgenic mice supports the pathogenic role of the fusion protein in the development of APL.[58]

inv(16)(p13q22) AND t(16;16)(p13;q22) CBF/MYH11

Inversions and translocations of chromosome 16 have been identified in AML FAB subtype M4, with either eosinophilia or abnormal eosinophils, and identify a subgroup of patients with a more favorable prognosis.[54] These rearrangements result in the fusion of the *CBF* gene on 16p13 with *MYH11* gene on 16q22.

t(9;22)(q34;q11) BCR/ABL

About 2% to 5% of patients with AML have the Philadelphia chromosome (Ph^1) translocation, which is associated with lower complete remission rates and shorter median survival.[54]

Laboratory Features

Hyperuricemia, the most common biochemical abnormality seen, results from the high turnover rate of the proliferating leukemic cells. It can lead to urate precipitation, obstructive uropathy, and acute renal failure.[59] Tumor lysis syndrome may occur with initiation of treatment as a complication of intensive cytotoxic chemotherapy or in patients with rapidly rising or very high blast counts, and it results in potentially life-threatening metabolic complications, including hyperkalemia, hyperphosphatemia, hypocalcemia, and hyperuricemia.[60] All patients should receive vigorous intravenous hydration and therapy with allopurinol prior to institution of chemotherapy.

Falsely decreased glucose levels and arterial oxygen saturation can be seen in patients with high blast counts. This so-called *leukocyte larceny* is an *in vitro* phenomenon that results from utilization of glucose and oxygen by leukocytes when a blood sample is allowed to stand prior to separation of plasma.[61, 62]

Coagulation studies are usually normal unless DIC, commonly associated with APL, is present and results in prolongation of the prothrombin and partial thromboplastin times and decreased fibrinogen levels.

Classification

In 1976, Bennett and associates proposed the first uniform classification system for AML, which is based on morphologic and cytochemical characteristics identified by review of peripheral blood and bone marrow films from more than 200 cases of acute leukemia by seven French, American and British hematologists.[63] The FAB classification has evolved over the past 20 years, and additional subtypes identified through the use of nonmorphologic methods, including immunophenotyping (M0, M7), electron microscopy (M7), and cytogenetics (M4Eo) have been identified.[64–66] The current FAB classification divides AML into eight subtypes.

Subtypes

M0: Acute Myeloid Leukemia Without Differentiation or Maturation

Minimally differentiated AML represents about 1% to 3% of AML cases.[68] Previously classified as undifferentiated, most of these leukemias can be shown to be myeloid in origin by ultrastructural cytochemistry, or the use of antimyeloperoxidase monoclonal antibodies.[69] The M0 subtype is associated with a higher incidence of cytogenetic abnormalities (including trisomy 8, monosomy 5, monosomy 7, and trisomy 13), frequent expression of the multidrug-resistance P-glycoprotein (P-170), a lower complete remission rate following conventional induction chemotherapy, and a shorter median survival.[70]

M1: Acute Myeloid Leukemia Without Maturation

The M1 subtype, which accounts for 15% to 20% of AML, is characterized by the presence of poorly differentiated blast cells, which constitute 90% or more of the nonerythroid cells found in the bone marrow. Up to 10% of cells may be maturing granulocytic cells or monocytes. Granules and Auer rods are rarely seen.

M2: Acute Myeloid Leukemia With Maturation

M2 represents the most common subtype of AML, accounting for 25% to 30% of AML cases. Myeloblasts constitute between 30% and 90% of the nonerythroid cells in the bone marrow, and more than 10% of the nonerythroid cells are maturing granulocytes. The blasts have prominent azurophilic granules, and Auer rods are commonly seen. About 46% of patients with this subtype of AML have a translocation between chromosomes 8 and 21 (t[8;21]).[71] These patients have significantly longer remission and survival rates compared with patients with normal cytogenetics or those with abnormalities of 5, 7, or 11.[72] A subtype of M2, M2Baso, characterized by myeloblasts with distinct basophilic granules, has been identified.[73]

M3: Acute Promyelocytic Leukemia

APL accounts for about 10% of AML cases. In APL, the bone marrow contains more than 30% promyelocytes, characterized by the presence of heavy azurophilic granulation. Auer rods are almost always present, and sometimes appear in bundles, referred to as *faggot cells*. Patients with APL have a distinct clinical syndrome characterized by younger age at presentation, frequent association with a bleeding diathesis, the presence of a balanced translocation involving chromosomes 15 and 17 in 80% to 100% of cases, and a unique response to treatment with the differentiating agent ATRA.

M4: Acute Myelomonocytic Leukemia

Acute myelomonocytic leukemia (AMML) represents about 20% to 25% of AML cases. This subtype morphologically resembles M2, except that cells of the monocytic lineage, monoblasts, promonocytes, and monocytes constitute more than 20% of the nonerythroid cells in the bone marrow. Extramedullary disease, including gingival infiltration, leukemia cutis, and meningeal leukemia are more common in this subtype. A subset of M4, M4Eo, is associated with increased (10% to 50%) numbers of marrow and peripheral blood eosinophils and with abnormalities of chromosome 16.[74] Complete remission rates, remission duration, and overall survival are improved in patients with the M4Eo variant and inversion 16 compared with patients with M4 without inversion 16.[75]

M5: Acute Monocytic Leukemia

Acute monocytic leukemia represents 10% of AML cases. In monocytic leukemia, 80% or more of all the nonerythroid cells in the bone marrow are made up of monoblasts, promonocytes, and monocytes. Monocytic leukemia is more commonly associated with extramedullary involvement, hepatosplenomegaly, lymphadenopathy, and hyperleukocytosis than with other AML subtypes.

M6: Erythroleukemia

Erythroleukemia represents about 5% of AML cases. The diagnosis of erythroleukemia is made when at least 50% of nucleated bone marrow cells are erythroblasts, and at least 30% are myeloblasts. Dyserythropoiesis is a characteristic feature of the erythroid precursors and consists of giant multinucleated forms, nuclear lobulation, nuclear fragmentation, megaloblastosis, and cytoplasmic vacuolization. Dysplastic features are seen in both myeloid cells and megakaryocytes. Ringed sideroblasts may be present. Peripheral blood examination reveals anisocytosis, poikilocytosis, anisochromia, basophilic stippling, and the presence of nucleated red blood cells. Patients with erythroleukemia tend to be older at the time of diagnosis, and the disease is frequently preceded by a myelodysplastic phase. Cytogenetic abnormalities, particularly deletions of 5q and 7q, are commonly seen.[76] These features are likely to be responsible for the poor response to therapy and short remission duration seen in this subtype of AML.

M7: Acute Megakaryoblastic Leukemia

Acute megakaryoblastic leukemia constitutes 5% to 10% of adult AML cases. The blasts are undifferentiated, pleomorphic cells, sometimes resembling maturing megakaryocytes. The diagnosis is made when at least 30% of bone marrow cells are undifferentiated, SBB-negative, MPO-negative blasts, and there is either ultrastructural evidence of platelet peroxidase or immunologic detection of platelet-specific proteins, including platelet glycoproteins Ib, IIb/IIIa, IIIa, or a factor VIII–related antigen.[77, 78] Marked marrow fibrosis is a common feature caused by fibroblast proliferation, secondary to the secretion of platelet-derived growth factor by the leukemic cells, and often results in an inaspirable marrow, or *dry tap*.[79] Megakaryocytic fragments and megakaryoblasts circulate in the peripheral blood. The M7 variant of AML is the subtype most prevalent in leukemias arising in patients with Down syndrome, accounting for up to 50% of AML cases in those patients.[80] M7 has a poor prognosis compared with other subtypes of AML, and remission rates are typically less than 50%. However, children with Down syndrome and AML have a remarkably good prognosis (including those with the M7 variant), with event-free survival rates of 77% to 100%.[81]

Secondary Leukemias

Secondary leukemias account for about 10% to 15% of all cases of AML and usually arise following treatment with cytotoxic drugs or radiation therapy, or with both, for a prior malignancy. They are typically preceded by a myelodysplastic phase of variable duration (months to years) characterized by refractory cytopenias, dysplastic changes in the hematopoietic cells of the blood and bone marrow, and an increased number of immature cells (5% to 25% myeloblasts) in the bone marrow. Nonrandom, clonal cytogenetic abnormalities are found in about 50% of cases, and usually involve chromosomes 5, 7, or 8.[82] The mechanisms of leukemogenesis in therapy-related leukemias remain to be defined; however, genes responsible for myeloid cell growth and differentiation have been localized to the long arm of chromosome 5.[83] Therapy-related AML is usually refractory to conventional induction therapy for AML, and the overall prognosis for these patients is poor.

AML developing in patients who have received prior therapy with topoisomerase II inhibitors forms a distinct subgroup among the therapy-related AMLs. It is typically not preceded by a myelodysplastic phase, is characterized by more rapid onset, and is associated with chromosomal rearrangements involving chromosomes 11 and 21.[84]

Preleukemia or Myelodysplastic Syndromes

The myelodysplastic syndromes (MDS) are a group of clonal, stem cell disorders characterized by refractory cytopenias, which are associated with dysplastic changes in the bone marrow, and a propensity to evolve to acute leukemia. The incidence is approximately half that of AML, and increases with age such that the prevalence in persons older than age 65 has been estimated to be about 0.1%.[85] The median age at diagnosis is 70.

Risk factors associated with the development of MDS mimic those of AML and include ionizing radiation, benzene, cigarette smoke, and chemotherapeutic drugs, particularly alkylating agents.[86] High-dose chemotherapy or total-body irradiation, which is used as the preparative regimen for patients undergoing stem cell transplantation, is associated with a significant risk of patients developing MDS or AML (11% to 18% over a 5- to 6-year period).[87]

The FAB morphologic classification divides the myelodysplastic syndromes into five subtypes: refractory anemia (RA), refractory anemia with ringed sideroblasts (RARS), refractory anemia with excess of blasts (RAEB), refractory anemia with excess blasts in transformation (RAEB-T), and chronic myelomonocytic leukemia (CMML). The RAEB subtype is characterized by a bone marrow having 5% to 20% blasts, and the RAEB-T by a marrow with 20% to 30% blasts. CMML is characterized by splenomegaly, monocytosis, neutrophilia, and less than 20% blasts in the bone marrow.

The median survival and rate of transformation to acute leukemia correlate with the FAB subtype. Patients with RAEB and RAEB-T have median survivals of 5 to 12 months, and 25% to 55% will progress to AML within 1 year. In contrast, patients with RA and RARS have median survivals of 3 to 6 years, and in one study only 5% of RA patients progressed to AML at 1 year, and none of the RARS patients underwent leukemic transformation within 2 years of follow-up.[88]

CLINICAL SIGNS

The clinical manifestations of MDS reflect the consequences of pancytopenia: anemia, bleeding, and infection. Peripheral smear analysis reveals dysplastic changes in all three cell lines: hypogranulation and hyposegmentation (Pelger-Huët) of neutrophils; anisocytosis, poikilocytosis and macrocytosis of red cells; large, abnormally granular or hypogranular platelets. Bone marrow evaluation typically reveals a hypercellular marrow with dysplastic features, including features of dyserythropoiesis: megaloblastic erythroid maturation, nuclear budding, ringed sideroblasts, and micromegakaryocytes. Cytochemical and immunophenotypic analysis of blasts usually reveals them to be myeloid in origin (SBB or MPO positive, CD13 and CD33 positive). Splenomegaly and a peripheral blood monocyte count greater than 1×10^9/L are features of CMML. Chromosomal abnormalities are seen in up to 60% of cases of *de novo* MDS and more than 80% of cases of secondary MDS.[89] The most common abnormalities involve chromosomes 5, 7, 8, and 20.

TREATMENT

Supportive care in the form of antibiotics, transfusion of blood and platelets, and chelation therapy (for iron overload) is the mainstay of therapy because the majority of patients affected are older individuals who are less tolerant of chemotherapy. In addition, the disease is often refractory to even intensive chemotherapy.[90] Low dose cytosine arabinoside (ara-C), hematopoietic growth factors, differentiating agents such as 5-azacytidine, and retinoic acid have all been evaluated but found not to affect survival.[91–93] Allogeneic bone marrow transplantation has resulted in overall disease-free survival rates of 30% to 40%, with better outcomes in younger patients (less than 40 years old) who have better prognostic features (RA or RARS, *de novo* vs. secondary MDS).[94, 95]

Principles of Treatment

The goal of therapy for AML is eradication of the leukemic clone, and restoration of normal hematopoiesis. This goal is usually accomplished using myelosuppressive chemotherapy and, if successful, results in a period of bone marrow aplasia with subsequent recovery of normal, polyclonal hematopoiesis. Achievement of complete remission (CR), defined as the presence of less than 5% blasts in the bone marrow and restoration of normal blood counts, is a prerequisite for curing AML. The length of patient survival directly correlates with attainment and duration of CR. Patients who do not achieve complete remission generally die within 2 to 4 months of infection or bleeding complications.

Current treatment strategies are divided into induction therapy, intended to induce a CR, and postremission therapy, intended to prevent relapse. Postremission therapy may consist of consolidation (chemotherapy regimens in similar doses to that given during induction), intensification (chemotherapy regimens at higher doses), or maintenance (lower doses of chemotherapy given over extended periods of time).

Median survival for untreated AML is approximately 2 months. Spontaneous remissions are extremely rare, and in most cases, short lived, but approximately 100 cases have been reported in the literature.[96] Even with the best induction and postremission chemotherapy regimens available, the majority of patients will relapse and die of acute leukemia. Approximately 25% to 40% of patients with AML treated with chemotherapy are alive 5 years after diagnosis.[97, 98]

Decision to Treat

The median age at diagnosis of AML is 65 years. Although older age alone is not a contraindication to treatment, patients older than 60 years of age have lower remission rates compared with younger patients, and the presence of concomitant medical problems may increase treatment-related morbidity and mortality. Discussions with the patient and family members regarding the diagnosis, treatment plan, anticipated adverse side effects, and prognosis should be undertaken. If definitive therapy is decided on, treatment should be initiated promptly because most patients are symptomatic at diagnosis, and the risk of complications from pancytopenia will not be eliminated until normal hematopoiesis is restored.

General Principles

Patients are generally treated in single, isolation rooms to provide privacy during periods of intensive care and discomfort and to decrease the risk of exogenously acquired infection during the period of neutropenia. Hand washing before and after contact with the patient, along with meticulous care of indwelling catheters, is important for decreasing pathogen exposure. The use of protected environments such as laminar air flow and the use of nonabsorbable antibiotics for gut and skin decontamination have not been shown to decrease consistently the incidence of infection and are not used routinely.[99]

Placement of an indwelling central venous catheter will facilitate administration of chemotherapy, antibiotics, blood products, other medications, and fluids as well as permit easy access for blood drawing. Hydration with intravenous fluids and treatment with allopurinol should be started before instituting chemotherapy in order to lessen the risk of tumor lysis syndrome.

Laboratory assessment, in addition to blood counts, review of the peripheral smear, and bone marrow aspirate, should include serum chemistries (to identify electrolyte disturbances) and coagulation studies (to determine if DIC is present). Human leukocyte antigen (HLA) typing may be helpful in the event that HLA-matched platelets are required because of the development of alloimmunization. In addition, HLA typing should be performed on potential candidates for bone marrow transplantation in order to identify bone marrow donors.

Supportive Care

Successful induction therapy hinges on the ability to support a patient through a lengthy period of bone marrow aplasia and pancytopenia. The increased success in treating patients with acute leukemia over the past 20 years is largely the result of improvements in supportive care.

Antibiotics

Infection is the leading cause of death in patients undergoing induction chemotherapy for AML, and, therefore, the rapid institution of broad-spectrum antibacterial therapy in the febrile, neutropenic (absolute neutrophil count <500/mm^3) patient significantly reduces mortality from gram-negative infections.[100] Commonly used regimens include a beta-lactam antibiotic plus an aminoglycoside, or monotherapy with a third-generation cephalosporin, such as ceftazidime. Empiric antibiotic therapy is safe and effective, and should be continued until resolution of neutropenia. The use of vancomycin as part of the initial, empiric antibiotic regimen has not been shown to alter survival; however, vancomycin should be included in institutions in which methicillin-resistant *Staphylococcus aureus* or *Streptococcus mitis* are known to be a problem.[101] Gram-positive bacteremia, caused by streptococci, *S. aureus*, and *Staphylococcus epidermidis*, has increased in frequency with the use of indwelling venous catheters, and vancomycin should be added if a catheter infection is suspected. Empiric antifungal therapy with amphotericin should be instituted if a neutropenic patient remains febrile after a 4 to 7 days of broad-spectrum antibiotic therapy or has recurrent fever.[102]

Hematopoietic Growth Factors

Several randomized, placebo-controlled trials have evaluated the use of granulocyte-macrophage colony–stimulating factor (GM-CSF) and granulocyte colony–stimulating factor (G-CSF) in patients with newly diagnosed AML,[103–110] or refractory or relapsed AML.[111] Although the trials vary with respect to patient age, induction regimen, timing, dose, and kind of growth factor administered, they consistently show a significant reduction in the duration of severe neutropenia in growth factor–treated patients. However, the impact of growth factor administration on the incidence of severe infections, antibiotic usage, and duration of hospitalization varies from study to study. Only one study has shown an improvement in survival for patients receiving growth factor following chemotherapy.[103] Importantly, there does not appear to be an increase in the incidence of drug-resistant leukemia, or leukemic relapse with the use of GM-CSF or G-CSF based on the results of these studies. The use of myeloid growth factors prior to chemotherapy (cytokine priming) to enhance leukemic cell kill by increasing the proportion of proliferating leukemic cells present during the administration of cell cycle–specific chemotherapy has not been shown to improve complete remission rates or survival.[112, 113]

Transfusions

Red blood cell transfusions should be administered to maintain a hemoglobin level of above 8 g/dL to 9 g/dL in patients with symptomatic coronary artery disease or active bleeding. Platelet transfusions should be given prophylactically when the platelet count falls below 5000 to 10,000/mm^3, or at higher levels when bleeding is present.[114] A 1998 prospective, multicenter study showed that a prophylactic platelet transfusion threshold of 10,000/mm^3 was not associated with a higher bleeding risk than the more generally used threshold of 20,000/mm^3.[115] A higher threshold for prophylactic platelet transfusion was indicated in patients with fever, sepsis, coagulation abnormalities, or for those on anticoagulant therapy.[116] Random donor platelets may be used initially, but single donor or HLA-matched platelets may be tried if the patient becomes refractory.[117] Patients who may be candidates for allogeneic bone marrow transplantation should not receive blood products from family members because this action may increase the risk of graft rejection.

Leukocyte transfusions have become more feasible now that large numbers of neutrophils can be collected from G-CSF–treated normal donors, and some studies have shown them to be beneficial.[118] However, these transfusions may be complicated by the transmission of infection (particularly cytomegalovirus), alloimunization, and pulmonary toxicity.[119]

Management of Coagulopathy

DIC, characterized by thrombocytopenia, prolongation of the prothrombin, activated partial thromboplastin, and thrombin times, increased levels of fibrin degradation products, and hypofibrinogenemia occurs in about 30% of patients with AML, most commonly in patients with the acute promyelocytic subtype (M3).[120] The bleeding diathesis associated with APL is often exacerbated by cytotoxic chemotherapy and is associated with a high rate of early mortality, primarily from intracranial hemorrhage. The development of DIC in patients with APL has been attributed both to the release of procoagulants from the abnormal promyelocytes during chemotherapy-induced cell lysis[121] and to excessive fibrinolytic activity.[122, 123]

The use of heparin in the management of these patients remains controversial. Although a number of small, retrospective studies have suggested that the use of prophylactic heparin decreases fatal hemorrhage,[124–127] in the largest, retrospective study published, no benefit with respect to the incidence of hemorrhagic deaths, complete remission rate, or survival could be attributed to the use of heparin.[128] Management strategies include

- the use of cryoprecipitate to maintain the fibrinogen level above 100 mg/dL
- platelet transfusions to maintain the platelet count above 20,000/mm^3 in the absence of active bleeding
- platelet transfusions to maintain the platelet count above 50,000/mm^3 in the presence of active bleeding
- fresh frozen plasma in patients with active bleeding and prolonged prothrombin and partial thromboplastin times

Heparin therapy may be initiated if monitoring of the aforementioned laboratory parameters suggests ongoing consumption despite the earlier listed maneuvers.[129] The use of ATRA does not appear to have altered the risk of hemorrhagic death from APL.[130]

Treatment and Results

Induction Chemotherapy

Conventional Induction Therapy

The standard induction regimen for newly diagnosed AML consists of ara-C plus an anthracycline, and it results in CR rates of 50% to 90%. The results from randomized clinical trials have identified several major tenets of therapy:

- Continuous infusion of ara-C at 100 mg/m^2/day for 7 days is used with a bolus infusion of daunorubicin at 45 mg/m^2/day for 3 days. This regimen of "7 + 3" has become the most widely used regimen for treatment of AML and is the standard against which new regimens are tested.[131]
- Continuous infusion ara-C is superior to every-12-hour bolus infusions. This finding is likely due to the very short, 15-minute half-life of ara-C.
- Adding other agents such as 6-thioguanine or etoposide to the "7 + 3" regimen has not been found to improve complete remission rates, but has been found to improve relapse-free survival.[132]

Three randomized studies comparing the anthracyclines idarubicin and daunorubicin for induction showed improved CR rates in the idarubicin arm.[133–135] In two of these studies, remission duration and survival were also improved in the idarubicin arm.[134, 135]

HIGH DOSE ARA-C

Based on the observation of a steep dose-response curve for ara-C, increasing doses of this agent have been used in an attempt to overcome ara-C resistance in leukemic blasts and improve remission rates and survival.[136] Ara-C, given in doses of 1 to 3 g/m^2, results in CR in up to 50% of patients with relapsed and refractory AML.[137, 138] Moderate increases in the ara-C dose, from 100 mg/m^2 to 500 mg/m^2, have not been shown to improve remission rates or survival.[139, 140]

Randomized studies comparing high-dose ara-C (HDAC) with conventional-dose ara-C for induction in patients with newly diagnosed AML have shown equivalent CR rates; however, disease-free survival was significantly improved in patients receiving HDAC.[141, 142] The more intensive induction regimens using HDAC may result in improved disease-free survival, despite similar clinical CR rates by actually inducing true molecular remissions.

Postremission Therapy

Despite CR rates of up to 90% following standard induction chemotherapy, median remission durations are relatively short (12 to 15 months), and long-term survival is achieved in only 10% to 15% of patients. The majority of patients will relapse and die of acute leukemia. The goal of postremission therapy is to eradicate residual leukemic cells, prevent relapse, and improve survival. Postremission strategies include consolidation chemotherapy, high-dose chemotherapy with autologous bone marrow transplantation, and allogeneic bone marrow transplantation. The best postremission therapy for an individual patient may depend on various prognostic factors including patient age; phenotypic, cytogenetic, and molecular characteristics of the leukemia; and the availability of a suitably matched stem cell donor.

Consolidation Chemotherapy

Low-dose maintenance chemotherapy following induction can prolong CR duration compared with no further therapy.[143] Prolonging the duration of maintenance therapy does not appear to improve survival; however, increasing the intensity of postremission therapy may improve outcome. In the largest study evaluating the role of HDAC consolidation for postremission therapy, patients entering remission following standard induction were randomized to receive four cycles of consolidation with one of three doses of ara-C: 100 mg/m^2 $\times$ 5 doses, 400 mg/m^2 $\times$ 5 doses, or 3 g/m^2 $\times$ 6 doses.[144] For patients 60 years of age or younger, the 4-year disease-free survival rate was significantly better in the high-dose arm (44%) compared with the lower dose arms (24% in 100 mg/m^2 arm and 29% in 400 mg/m^2 arm). However, for patients older than 60 years of age, the 4-year disease-free survival was 16% or less for all dose arms. In this study, the survival benefit of HDAC was not seen in patients with unfavorable cytogenetics.[145] These results suggest that for patients younger than 60 with favorable cytogenetics (t[8;21], inv 16), consolidation using repetitive cycles of HDAC yields the best disease-free survival results.

Allogeneic Bone Marrow Transplantation

Allogeneic bone marrow transplantation (allo-BMT) was first demonstrated to be an effective antileukemic therapy when it was shown to induce long-term remissions in about 10% of patients with chemotherapy-resistant, relapsed leukemia.[146] It remains the only curative therapy for patients with relapsed or refractory AML. More recently, allo-BMT has been used as postremission therapy, resulting in long-term, disease-free survival rates of 45% to 75% when HLA-identical siblings are used as donors. Table 23–1 summarizes the results of several trials of allo-BMT for AML in first remission.

There are several mechanisms by which allo-BMT may cure AML. Supralethal doses of marrow-ablating chemoradiotherapy, delivered to the patient during the preparative regimen, have the potential to eradicate the leukemic clone. Patients are rescued from the consequences of marrow ablation by infusion of normal hematopoietic cells from the allogeneic donor. In addition, an immunologic effect, referred to as graft-versus-leukemia (GVL), contributes to cure by harnessing the immune cells of the infused donor marrow, which then contribute to leukemic cell kill. GVHD and GVL appear to go hand-in-hand, although there is some evidence that they may be mediated by different subsets of T-cells in the donor graft. Relapse rates are inversely correlated with the degree of GVHD,[159] and there is an increased relapse rate in identical twin transplants where no GVHD occurs,[160] and in patients undergoing allo-BMT in which T-cells have been removed from the donor marrow in an effort to ameliorate GVHD.[161]

Despite promising results, there remains considerable controversy regarding the use of allo-BMT for patients in first remission because some patients may already be cured and the transplant-related mortality is considerable. Table 23–2 summarizes the results of several randomized studies comparing conventional postremission chemotherapy with allo-BMT. These studies have consistently demonstrated a decreased relapse rate and a trend towards improved disease-free survival for patients undergoing allo-BMT in first remission, but most have shown equivalent rates of overall survival. In part, this is due to the higher rate of transplant-related mortality, primarily from GVHD and interstitial pneumonia. In some studies, however, patients who relapsed following conventional postremission chemotherapy were successfully treated with allo-BMT.

ALTERNATIVE DONORS

PARTIALLY MATCHED, RELATED DONORS

The results using related donors, mismatched at only a single HLA locus, appear to be equivalent to transplants between HLA-identical siblings.[169] For greater degrees of mismatch, T-cell depletion has been used to ameliorate GVHD; however, it is associated with increased rates of relapse and graft failure. More recently, transplants have been performed between haploidentical, related individuals with encouraging results.[170, 171]

UNRELATED DONORS

Fewer than 35% of patients will have a suitable, HLA-matched family donor. Increasingly, alternative donors are being used. In 1986, the National Marrow Donor Program (NMDP) was created in the United States to facilitate the identification and procurement of bone marrow from unrelated donors for patients lacking related donors. The NMDP has established a registry network of more than 3 million HLA-typed volunteers, and the probability of finding an HLA-A, -B, or -DR–matched donor within the NMDP has increased from less than 10% in 1987 to 64% in 1995.[172] Allo-BMT for AML using matched, unrelated donors is associated with a 60% to 80% incidence of acute GVHD, and disease-free survival varies according to status of leukemia at time of transplant. For patients with high-risk leukemia (greater than first remission, secondary leukemia, primary induction failure, or poor-risk cytogenetics), disease-free survival is about 20%.[173] For good-risk patients, disease-free survival is about 40%.[174]

UMBILICAL CORD BLOOD

The newest source of hematopoietic stem cells used for transplantation is umbilical cord blood. The relative immaturity of lymphocytes in cord blood could theoretically reduce the risk and severity of GVHD, which would allow transplants to be performed across greater degrees of HLA mismatch.[175] In fact, results from related and unrelated cord-blood transplants have shown relatively low rates of

TABLE 23–1. **Allogeneic Bone Marrow Transplantation for Acute Myeloid Leukemia in First Remission**

Study	No. of Patients	Time Period	% Relapse	% TRM	% LFS	Comments
Adults						
Zittoun et al[147]	144	1986–1993	24	17	55	Prospective randomized study
Blaise et al[148]	101	1987–1990	14	8	75	Prospective randomized study (Cy TBI data shown)
Schiller et al[149]	28	1982–1990	32	32	45	Single-center study
Carella et al[150]	104	1983–1991	29	24	52	Prospective randomized study
Weaver et al[151]	184	1987–1990	—	—	42–52	Single-center long-term follow-up
Mehta et al[152]	85	1978–1987	25	33	48	Single-center long-term follow-up
Gorin et al[153]	566	1987–1992	25	26	55	Multicenter analysis
IBMTR[154]	2247	1989–1995	24 ± 2	—	59 ± 2	Multicenter analysis
Jourdan et al[155]	109	1987–1992	26	25	55	Multicenter analysis
Children						
Wells et al[156]	54	1986–1989	—	—	54	Multicenter prospective study
Michel et al[157]	32	1987–1990	25	3	72	Multicenter prospective study

TRM = transplant-related mortality; LFS = leukemia-free survival; Cy TBI = cyclophosphamide and total body irradiation; IBMTR = International Bone Marrow Transplant Registry.

From Warrell RP, Barrett AJ, Pandolfi PP, et al: Acute myelocytic leukemia, p 125. Education Program, American Society of Hematology 39th Annual Meeting, 1997.

TABLE 23–2. **Allogeneic Bone Marrow Transplantation Versus Chemotherapy for Acute Myeloid Leukemia in First Remission**

		Relapse		Actuarial Rates* Disease-Free Survival		Survival		
Study	**No. of Patients**	***Chemo (%)***	***Trans (%)***	***Chemo (%)***	***Trans (%)***	***Chemo (%)***	***Trans (%)***	**Statistically Significant Differences ($p < 0.05$)**
Cassileth et al[162]	54 Trans 29 Chemo	—	—	30	42	43	42	None
Cassileth et al[163]	113 Trans 117 Chemo	61	29	35	43	52	46	Relapse rate Overall survival
Schiller et al[149]	28 Trans 54 Chemo	60	32	38	48	53	45	Relapse rate
Reiffers et al[164]	23 Trans 20 Chemo	82	22	16	66	—	—	Relapse rate, disease-free survival rate
Appelbaum et al[165]	44 Trans 46 Chemo	—	—	20	40	30	40	None
Conde et al[166]	14 Trans 25 Chemo	78	10	17	70	—	—	Relapse rate
Champlin et al[167]	23 Trans 44 Chemo	70	40	—	—	27	40	Relapse rate

*At 5 years in studies by Schiller,[149] Appelbaum,[165] and Champlin[167]; at 4 years in studies by Cassileth[162, 163]; at 3 years in study by Conde[166]; at 2 years in study by Reiffers.[164]

Adapted from Estey EH, Kantarjian H, Keating MJ: Therapy for acute myeloid leukemia. In: Hoffman R, Benz EJ, Shattil S, et al (eds): Hematology Basic Principles and Practice, 2nd ed, p 1014. New York, Churchill-Livingstone, 1995.

acute and chronic GVHD, even in mismatched transplants.[176]

Autologous Bone Marrow Transplantation

Despite efforts to expand the pool of allogeneic donors, and because of older age at diagnosis, only about 10% to 15% of patients with AML will be candidates for allo-BMT. Autologous transplantation (auto-BMT) offers a way to harness the antileukemic efficacy of ablative doses of radiation and chemotherapy, while avoiding the morbidity and mortality of GVHD. In auto-BMT, hematopoietic recovery from high-dose chemoradiation is provided by an infusion of the patient's own bone marrow or peripheral blood stem cells previously collected during a period of remission. The transplant-related mortality for patients undergoing auto-BMT is generally less than 10%, compared with a mortality rate of 25% to 30% for patients undergoing allo-BMT; however, relapse rates are significantly higher (50% to 60%). When auto-BMT is performed in first remission, 3- to 5-year disease-free survival rates of 25% to 75% have been reported. Table 23–3 summarizes the results of trials of auto-BMT for AML.

The disadvantages of auto-BMT include the potential for reinfusion of contaminating leukemic cells in the infused marrow, as well as the absence of an immune GVL effect. Gene marking studies, in which the neomycin-resistance gene, *NEO,* was transferred into harvested bone marrow cells, have demonstrated that leukemic cells in the reinfused marrow do, in fact, contribute to relapse, by documenting the presence of the genetic marker in leukemic cells at the time of relapse.[185]

MARROW PURGING

Methods designed to purge marrow of leukemic cells prior to reinfusion have included *ex vivo* treatment of marrow with cytotoxic drugs, such as 4-hydroperoxycyclophosphamide or mafosfamide,[186, 187] or with leukemia-specific

TABLE 23–3. **Autologous Bone Marrow Transplantation for Acute Myeloid Leukemia**

Author	N	CR	Purging	%DFS	F/U (mo)
Burnett et al[177]	90	CR1	No	48	12
Korbling et al[178]	22	CR1	Yes	61	31
	30	CR2	Yes	34	19
Santos et al[179]	17	CR1	Yes	47	21
	71	CR2	Yes	28	21
Gorin et al[180]	263	CR1	26%	48	28
McMillan et al[181]	82	CR1	No	48–67	31
Chao et al[182]	30	CR1	Yes	57	31
	20	CR1	No	32	54
Linker et al[183]	32	CR1	Yes	76	22
	26	CR2	Yes	56	22

CR = complete remission, DFS = disease-free survival, F/U = follow-up.

From Antin JH, Lee SJ, Chao NJ, et al: Bone marrow transplantation for hematologic malignancies, p 151. Education Program, American Society of Hematology 39th Annual Meeting, 1997.

monoclonal antibodies.[188] Retrospective analyses of data from both the European Cooperative Group for Bone Marrow Transplantation and the Autologous Blood and Marrow Transplant Registry of North America show decreased relapse rates in patients receiving purged marrows compared with recipients of unpurged marrows, with the greatest benefit seen in patients transplanted within the first 6 months of complete remission.[189, 190] The clinical benefit of purging, however, remains unproven, and, to date, no prospective, randomized studies comparing purged versus unpurged auto-BMT for AML have been conducted.

Peripheral Blood Stem Cell Transplants

The use of G-CSF–mobilized peripheral blood stem cells results in shorter engraftment times compared with the use of bone marrow.[190] In addition, it has been hypothesized that peripheral blood stem cell harvests may have less leukemic cell contamination and may, therefore, lead to lower rates of relapse. Controlled trials of autologous bone marrow versus autologous peripheral blood stem cell transplants will need to be conducted to answer this question.

Results

Table 23–4 summarizes the results of several randomized trials comparing auto-BMT with allo-BMT for patients in first CR. Although most trials consistently show higher relapse rates in patients undergoing auto-BMT, survival is not always better in the allo-BMT arm because transplant-related mortality is higher.

Two large, randomized trials of postremission therapy for patients with AML were reported in the 1990s.[147, 163] In the Zittoun study,[147] patients 45 years old or younger with an HLA-identical sibling underwent allo-BMT, whereas the remaining patients were randomized to receive an unpurged auto-BMT, or consolidation with HDAC. The relapse rate was higher in the chemotherapy group (57%) compared with those undergoing autologous (40%) or allogeneic transplant (24%). Five-year disease-free survival was significantly improved for those patients undergoing either allogeneic or autologous transplantation (55% and 48% respectively) compared with those receiving chemotherapy (30%). Overall survival, however, was similar in the three groups, and was believed to be due to the better salvage rates with secondary auto-BMT in patients who relapsed after chemotherapy. In the Cassileth study,[163] there was no significant difference in disease-free survival among the three groups of patients with a median follow-up of 4 years. The impact of lower relapse rates seen in the autologous and allogeneic arms was neutralized by the higher transplant-related mortality in these two groups compared with patients receiving chemotherapy alone.

Prognostic Factors in AML

The decision regarding the optimal postremission therapy for an individual patient should take into account patient and disease-related prognostic factors (Table 23–5):

- The use of allo-BMT is limited by patient age and is generally not performed in patients older than 55 years of age because of the increased transplant-related morbidity and mortality. Similarly, consolidation using HDAC does not improve survival in patients older than 60 years of age.
- Prognostic features that are associated with resistance to chemotherapy include certain cytogenetic abnormalities (5q-, monosomy 7, trisomy 8, Philadelphia chromosome, 11q23 rearrangements, and t[6;9]), antecedent hematologic disorder, secondary AML, CD34 expression, TdT expression, and *MDR* expression.[54, 195, 196]
- Patients with "good-risk" cytogenetic abnormalities, such as inv 16 and t(8;21), have improved survival when treated with HDAC consolidation. A strategy of consolidation with HDAC, and salvage with allo-BMT or auto-BMT should relapse occur, may be a reasonable approach in this group. For younger patients with poor-risk cytogenetic abnormalities, allo-BMT in first remission may be the best approach.

TABLE 23–4. **Allogeneic Versus Autologous Bone Marrow Transplantation (BMT) for Acute Myeloid Leukemia in First Remission**

		Relapse		Actuarial Rates* Disease-Free Survival (DFS)		Survival		
Study	**No. of Patients**	***Auto-BMT %***	***Allo-BMT %***	***Auto-BMT %***	***Allo-BMT %***	***Auto-BMT %***	***Allo-BMT %***	**Statistically Significant Differences ($p < 0.05$)**
Cassileth et al[163]	113 Allo 116 Auto	48	29	35	43	43	46	None
Cassileth et al[191]	19 Allo 39 Auto	—	—	54	41	—	—	None
Lowenberg et al[192]	21 Allo 32 Auto	60	34	35	51	37	66	Relapse and survival rates
Rieffers et al[164]	20 Allo 15 Auto	59	22	41	61	—	—	Relapse and DFS rates
Amadori et al[193]	22 Allo 35 Auto	78	45	21	51	—	—	Relapse and DFS rates

*At 5 years in study by Amadori[193]; at 3–4 years in studies by Cassileth[163, 191] and Lowenberg[192]; at 2.5 years in study by Reiffers.[164]

Modified from Estey EH, Kantarjian H, Keating MJ: Therapy for acute myeloid leukemia. In: Hoffman R, Benz EJ, Shattil S, et al (eds): Hematology Basic Principles and Practice, 2nd ed, p 1014. New York, Churchill-Livingstone, 1995.

TABLE 23–5. **Prognostic Factors in Acute Myeloid Leukemia**

Factor	Favorable	Unfavorable
Clinical		
Age	<40 years	>60 years
Leukemia	*De novo*	Secondary
WBC count	<10,000/mm³	>100,000/mm³
DIC	Absent	Present
LDH	Normal	High
Serum albumin	Normal	Low
FAB type	M3, M4Eo	M0, M5a, M5b, M6, M7
Cytogenetics	inv 16, t(8;21) normal	5q−, 7, +8
Auer rods	Present	Absent
In vitro		
Clonogenic assay	Normal growth	Autonomous growth
Labeling index	High	Low
Bone marrow		
Fibrosis	Absent	Present
Cytoreduction	Rapid	Slow
Courses to complete remission	Single	Multiple
Pronormoblasts	Rare	Many
Eosinophils	Present	Absent

WBC = white blood cell; DIC = disseminated intravascular coagulation; LDH = lactate dehydrogenase; FAB = French-American-British.
From Miller KB: Clinical manifestations of acute myeloid leukemia. In: Hoffman R, Benz EJ, Shattil S, et al (eds): Hematology Basic Principles and Practice, 3rd ed, p 1025. New York, Churchill-Livingstone, 1998.

- For patients older than age 55, the risk-benefit ratio would favor chemotherapy.

With improved understanding of other prognostic variables and the molecular classification of leukemias, as well as the use of sensitive techniques to identify MRD in patients in clinical remission, it may be possible to select patients for whom more aggressive therapy in first remission, such as allo-BMT, is appropriate versus waiting for relapse.

Treatment of Relapsed or Refractory Leukemia

Relapsed Disease

Once leukemic relapse occurs, outcome is generally poor. Salvage therapy with regimens containing HDAC may result in CR in about 60% of patients, but remission duration is usually short and long-term disease-free survival after relapse is rare.[197] The probability of achieving a second remission is strongly correlated with the duration of first remission, approaching 60% in those patients who relapse after 6 to 12 months compared with 20% to 30% in those with shorter remission durations.[198] However, second remissions are invariably shorter than first remissions, and only about 15% of patients achieving a second remission are expected to be alive at 5 years.[197] Reinduction, for those patients who have relapsed more than 1 year following remission, may be attempted using the initial induction regimen. For those with earlier relapse, other investigational approaches should be tried.

Allo-BMT for patients in first relapse or second remission results in long-term disease-free survival in 20% to 30% of patients.[199, 200] Patients who are transplanted during early relapse (<30% blasts in bone marrow) may have improved survival compared with those transplanted after receiving reinduction chemotherapy to induce a second remission because they avoid the morbidity and mortality associated with exposure to additional chemotherapy. In the absence of a matched, related donor, consideration should be given to the use of a matched, unrelated donor, particularly in patients younger than 45 years of age.

Harvesting autologous bone marrow or peripheral blood stem cells from patients in first remission should be considered strongly, particularly for those patients who lack a suitable allogeneic donor, or are not otherwise candidates for allo-BMT. High-dose chemotherapy and auto-BMT result in long-term survival in 30% of patients who have relapsed.[201, 202]

Refractory Disease

Patients are considered to have primary refractory disease when CR is not obtained after two adequate attempts at induction. In these patients, allo-BMT is the treatment of choice and may result in long-term disease-free survival in 15% to 20% of patients.[203]

Relapse Following Allo-BMT

Induction of a GVL effect by infusion of donor leukocytes has been shown to induce remission in patients relapsing after allo-BMT.[204] This approach has been most successful for patients with CML who relapse following transplant, but it also has been tried for patients with acute leukemia.

Special Management Issues

Treatment of Acute Promyelocytic Leukemia

APL is a clinically, biologically, and molecularly distinct subtype of AML, characterized by a bleeding diathesis, younger age at presentation, the presence of a balanced translocation between chromosomes 15 and 17, and a unique response to the differentiating agent ATRA. The coagulopathy associated with APL is exacerbated with initiation of conventional induction chemotherapy, and peri-induction mortality is higher in APL than in other subtypes of AML. The risk of fatal hemorrhage (CNS and pulmonary) is associated with high circulating blast and promyelocyte counts, low platelet count, older age, and anemia,[127] and has not been diminished by the use of heparin or antithrombolytic therapy.[128]

ATRA causes terminal differentiation and the eventual apoptotic death of leukemic cells, and has been shown to result in complete clinical remissions in up to 90% of patients with APL.[205] Because complete remission is achieved through maturation and differentiation of the leukemic cell, the characteristic period of marrow aplasia and the toxicities seen with conventional chemotherapy do not occur with ATRA. The coagulopathy associated with APL reverses more quickly following initiation of ATRA therapy compared with conventional chemotherapy; however, a 1997 trial comparing induction with ATRA versus conventional chemotherapy showed no difference in the rate of severe or fatal hemorrhage.[130] Remissions following ATRA therapy usually occur at 5 to 6 weeks.

Although ATRA is highly successful in inducing complete remission, if maintained on ATRA alone, most patients will relapse within a few months. Thus, current treatment strategies of APL include the use of ATRA in conjunction with anthracycline/ara-C–based chemotherapy as either part of the induction regimen or as postremission therapy. Two prospective, randomized trials have shown that relapse rates were significantly lower and disease-free survival was significantly better in patients receiving ATRA plus chemotherapy compared with those receiving chemotherapy alone.[130, 206]

A unique and potentially fatal toxicity associated with the use of ATRA is the retinoic acid syndrome, which has been reported to occur in about 25% of patients within the first 3 weeks of initiation of ATRA therapy.[207] The retinoic acid syndrome consists of fever, dyspnea, hypotension, edema, weight gain, pulmonary interstitial infiltrates, and pleural and pericardial effusions. This syndrome is often, but not uniformly, preceded by a leukocytosis, and some investigators have recommended initiating chemotherapy, along with ATRA, if the initial WBC count is greater than $5000/mm^3$ or if there is a rapid rise in WBC count following initiation of ATRA. The institution of high-dose corticosteroid therapy early in the course of the retinoic acid syndrome results in symptomatic improvement and recovery in most patients.

Recently, arsenic trioxide has been shown to induce complete morphologic and molecular remissions in patients with acute promyelocytic leukemia who have relapsed following conventional therapy.[208] This agent appears to induce cytodifferentiation and apoptosis in leukemic cells.

Treatment of the Elderly

Approximately 60% of patients with AML are older than 60 years of age at diagnosis. Although older age alone is not a contraindication to treatment, remission rates progressively decline with increasing age, and poorer outcomes, as well as shorter survival are more common[209, 210]; mortality rates during induction chemotherapy for patients older than 60 years of age are 40% to 65%. There is an increased incidence of treatment-related leukemias and antecedent myelodysplastic syndromes in elderly patients, both of which are associated with greater refractoriness to induction chemotherapy. The higher incidence of poor-risk cytogenetic abnormalities in elderly patients with AML, including monosomy 5 and 7, also contributes to poorer outcome.[211] Because of comorbid medical conditions, in addition to age-related chronic cardiac, pulmonary, or renal dysfunction, elderly patients are less able to withstand the acute toxicities of intensive chemotherapy. Finally, older patients may have less bone marrow regenerative capacity.

Low dose ara-C (10 mg/m^2) can be used in older patients who are not candidates for more intensive chemotherapy. Studies comparing low-dose ara-C with conventional induction chemotherapy showed no difference in survival despite higher CR rates in the conventional chemotherapy arm because the early death rate was also greater in this arm.[212] Otherwise healthy elderly patients with AML, particularly those without poor prognostic features, should be offered conventional induction chemotherapy. Using this approach, investigators have reported remission rates approaching 50%.[213]

Several controlled trials have incorporated the use of hematopoietic growth factors in an attempt to shorten the duration of neutropenia and improve outcome in elderly patients receiving induction chemotherapy for AML. A randomized, placebo-controlled study of GM-CSF in AML patients 55 to 70 years of age who received conventional induction chemotherapy demonstrated decreased treatment-related toxicity and improved median survival in patients receiving GM-CSF compared with placebo.[102] However, three other randomized, placebo-controlled studies using GM-CSF[103] or G-CSF[106, 109] failed to show any difference in survival. Although modest decreases in the duration of neutropenia were achieved, it is not clear that routine use of G-CSF in the setting of induction is of sufficient benefit. Similarly, the benefits of dose intensification that have been demonstrated for induction and postremission therapy appear to be confined to younger patients, with the major trials of HDAC for postremission therapy showing no advantage in patients older than 55 to 60 years of age.[144]

Treatment of Pregnant Women

Leukemia is the second leading cause of cancer-related death in women younger than 35 years of age, and it occurs in about 1 in 75,000 pregnancies.[214] A successful pregnancy can still be achieved even when total body irradiation has been used as part of therapy;[215] however, cytotoxic chemotherapy administered during the first trimester of pregnancy is associated with an increased risk of fetal abnormalities.[216] Chemotherapy administered during the second and third trimesters has not been associated with an increased risk to fetal development, although there is an increase in premature delivery, higher perinatal mortality, and lower birth weight;[217] marrow hypoplasia and cytopenia in the newborn may result from exposure to chemotherapy at the time of delivery.[218] Maternal to fetal transmission of AML has been reported.[219]

Future Directions

Peripheral Blood Stem Cell Transplants

Increasingly, peripheral blood stem cells pheresed from normal donors following treatment with G-CSF or GM-

CSF are being used in allogeneic transplant. Peripheral blood stem cell transplants are associated with more rapid engraftment, equivalent rates of acute GVHD, but a greater incidence of chronic GVHD.[220, 221] Prospective studies comparing bone marrow and peripheral blood transplants will be needed to determine if outcome is improved using peripheral blood as a source of stem cells.

Graft Manipulation

The increase in understanding and characterization of the cellular components of bone marrow and peripheral blood grafts has led to various manipulations designed to improve engraftment across HLA barriers, ameliorate GVHD, improve immune recovery, and prevent relapse. These maneuvers have included transplantation of very large numbers of CD34+ cells ("mega dose") to aid engraftment in haplo-identical transplants,[171] partial T-cell depletion to lessen GVHD, and delayed "add back" of T-cells to harness a GVL effect and hasten immune recovery.[222]

Minitransplants

Recognizing the increased transplant-related mortality from the preparative regimen, particularly in older (>55 years) individuals, transplants have been performed using less toxic, nonmyeloablative regimens, in conjunction with peripheral blood stem cells, to ameliorate transplant-related mortality yet preserve the GVL effect. These minitransplants have met with some success, but leukemic relapse remains a problem, and future investigations are focusing on enhancing GVL through the use of donor lymphocyte infusions.[223]

Minimal Residual Disease Detection

At diagnosis of AML, there are approximately 10^{12} leukemic cells in the body. Conventional induction chemotherapy results in a 2- to 3-log reduction in the number of leukemic cells, resulting in a morphologic CR; however, it is likely that, in most patients, billions of residual leukemic cells remain. Methodologies, including multiparameter flow cytometry and PCR, have enabled the sensitive detection and quantitation of residual leukemic cells. Monitoring patients for MRD may guide therapy by detecting relapse early, or by identifying those patients who are not truly in remission.

Chronic Myelogenous Leukemia

Chronic myelogenous leukemia (CML) is a clonal disorder of the hematopoietic stem cell, associated with marked expansion of progenitor, precursor, and mature hematopoietic cells and their premature release into the peripheral blood. Clinically, the disease is characterized by granulocytosis, thrombocytosis, basophilia, and splenomegaly, and typically evolves from an indolent, chronic phase of variable duration to a rapidly fatal phase of acute leukemia.

Epidemiology and Etiology

Epidemiology

CML accounts for about 20% of all leukemias, and occurs in about 1.3 per 100,000 population, with a slightly increased incidence in males.[224] The median age of patients at diagnosis is 50 years. Patients under the age of 10 years usually develop the juvenile variant, a similar but clinically distinct illness known as *juvenile CML.*

Etiology

Exposure to ionizing radiation is associated with the development of CML, as demonstrated by the significantly increased incidence of CML in survivors of the atomic bomb explosions at Hiroshima and Nagasaki[225] and in patients given radiotherapy for ankylosing spondylitis.[11] No other physical or chemical risk factors have been identified. Identical twin studies suggest that CML is not hereditary.[226]

Pathogenesis

In 95% of cases of CML, the hematopoietic cells contain a reciprocal translocation between the long arms of chromosomes 9 and 22, resulting in two derivative chromosomes, 9q+ and 22q−, the latter referred to as the Philadelphia chromosome (Ph^1).[227, 228] This translocation results in the fusion of the cellular oncogene, *ABL*, on chromosome 9 with the breakpoint cluster region gene, *BCR*, on chromosome 22.[229] The identification of this characteristic translocation in granulocytic, erythrocytic, megakaryocytic, and lymphocytic cells provides one line of evidence that CML arises from a single, multipotent stem cell.[230] G6PD enzyme studies further confirm the clonal origin of this malignancy by identifying a single isoenzyme type in neutrophils, monocytes, eosinophils, basophils, platelets, erythrocytes, B-lymphocytes, and sometimes T-lymphocytes from women with CML who were heterozygous for the G6PD enzyme.[231] Studies with B-lymphoblastoid cell lines derived from G6PD-heterozygous patients with CML led to the hypothesis of a multistep pathogenesis for Ph^1-positive CML in which the Ph^1 chromosome in some patients with CML was the result of subclonal evolution from an antecedent, clonally proliferating Ph^1-negative stem cell.[232]

The chimeric *BCR-ABL* gene encodes a hybrid protein of 210 kDa with increased tyrosine kinase activity, is found in all CML patients,[233] and is believed to be central to the pathogenesis of CML. The *BCR-ABL* gene product has been shown to induce cell proliferation, transform hematopoietic cells, and suppress apoptosis *in vitro*. A CML-like disease has been induced in mice by introduction of the *BCR-ABL* gene into bone marrow progenitors.[234]

The adaptor molecule, CRKL, is a cytoplasmic signaling protein and a major *in vivo* substrate of the deregulated *BCR-ABL* tyrosine kinase. CRKL functions as a molecular link with other signaling proteins; specifically, it acts as a mediator between *BCR-ABL* and its SH3 domain, and, via its SH2 domain, can interact with other tyrosine phosphorylated proteins. Therefore, *BCR-ABL* may include a formation of multimeric complexes of signaling proteins. In addition, mutational analysis has indicated that autophosphorylation sites on *BCR-ABL* play a critical role in its transforming ability.[235, 236]

Detection and Diagnosis

Chronic Phase

Clinically, CML is characterized by a biphasic or triphasic course. Patients typically present in the first (or chronic) phase with symptoms related to the hypermetabolic state associated with this disease, including fatigue, malaise, fever, night sweats, and weight loss. Splenomegaly is seen in up to 80% to 90% of cases, and patients may present with complaints of abdominal fullness, left upper quadrant pain, or early satiety related to an enlarging spleen. Hepatomegaly is seen in about half of patients. Patients may complain of sternal tenderness or bone pain related to an expanding marrow cavity. Complications secondary to leukostasis may occur when the WBC count exceeds 300,000/mm^3. Impaired circulation in the lung, CNS, sensory organs, and penis may result in dyspnea, tachypnea, cyanosis, dizziness, slurred speech, blurred vision, tinnitus, hearing loss, and priapism. These symptoms can be treated with leukapheresis and the institution of myelosuppressive therapy.

Increasingly, CML is being diagnosed in asymptomatic patients found to have elevated blood counts during routine health screening. Patients in chronic phase are generally well, and elevated blood counts, splenomegaly, and symptoms are easily controlled with myelosuppressive agents such as hydroxyurea or busulfan, or with interferon alfa (αIFN).

Accelerated Phase

In all patients with CML, there is an inevitable progression to a more aggressive stage of disease that may be characterized by fever, night sweats, weight loss, bone pain, increasing splenomegaly, progressive anemia, thrombocytopenia, basophilia, and increased numbers of blasts in the blood and bone marrow. The accelerated and blast phases of CML are characterized by increased karyotypic instability and the development of additional chromosomal abnormalities including a double Ph^1 chromosome, trisomy 8, and an isochromosome for the long arms of chromosome 17 and trisomy 19.[237] The hallmark feature of this transforming phase is the failure of previously successful therapy to control blood counts, splenomegaly, and symptoms. Patients in this stage comprise a heterogeneous group, with some progressing rapidly to blastic phase over several months, whereas others have a slower course. Average survival is approximately 1 year. In some patients, disease control may be re-established with a change in chemotherapy.

Blast Phase

The terminal, or blastic, phase of CML is characterized by blood and bone marrow findings indistinguishable from acute leukemia. The majority of acute leukemias are myeloblastic; however, in 25% to 30% of cases, the leukemic cells are morphologically, cytochemically, and immunophenotypically lymphoid.[238] The majority of lymphoid blast crises involve cells of B-cell lineage,[240] although a T-lymphocyte phenotype is occasionally seen.[238, 240] Patients with acute lymphoblastic transformation appear to have a better response to treatment and have longer survival than those with myeloid transformation.[241] Survival in blastic phase is uniformly short, with a median duration of 4 to 6 months.[242] Interestingly, patients presenting in blastic phase appear to have longer survivals than those who undergo blastic transformation from a preceding chronic stage.[243]

Diagnosis

Blood

- *Leukocytosis*, the hallmark of CML, is usually in the range of 100 to 300 × 10^9/L, with granulocytes from all stages of maturation present in the peripheral blood. In the chronic phase, blasts usually comprise less than 10% of the peripheral blood leukocytes. There is a marked increase in eosinophils and basophils.[244] The degree of basophilia does not usually exceed 10% to 15% during chronic phase, but may reach 30% to 80% of the total leukocyte count, and has been designated Ph^1-positive basophilic CML.[245] A dramatic rise in the basophil count may be seen in the terminal blastic transformation phase and gives rise to acute basophilic leukemia.
- *Anemia* is frequently present, and nucleated red blood cells are often seen in the peripheral blood.
- *Thrombocytosis* occurs in about half of patients, and platelet counts exceeding 1,000,000/μL are not uncommon.
- Functional abnormalities of both neutrophils (defective adhesion, migration, and phagocytosis) and platelets (decreased aggregation in response to epinephrine) have been identified.[246]

Bone Marrow

- The bone marrow aspirate and biopsy are hypercellular with marked granulocytic hyperplasia.
- The myeloid-to-erythroid ratio is typically increased to between 10:1 and 25:1 from the normal ratio of 3:1.
- Eosinophils and basophils are increased.
- Megakaryocytes may be increased in number and dysplastic in appearance; they are sometimes seen in clusters.

- Gaucher-like cells may be seen and represent lipid-laden macrophages.
- Reticulin fibrosis is usually increased.

Laboratory Features

- Leukocyte alkaline phosphatase activity is characteristically decreased or absent in CML, in contrast to other disorders associated with granulocytosis.[247] Leukocyte alkaline phosphatase activity may normalize with treatment or rise in response to infection or progression to blast crisis.
- Increased production of uric acid, secondary to a high rate of cell turnover, results in hyperuricemia and hyperuricosuria, and is commonly seen in CML; this condition may cause gouty arthritis and urate nephropathy.
- Pseudohyperkalemia, secondary to the release of potassium from WBCs during clotting, spurious hypoxemia, and pseudohypoglycemia from *in vitro* utilization of oxygen and glucose by granulocytes are *in vitro* artifacts that may occur in CML.

Cytogenetics and Molecular Analysis

There are several methods available for detecting the Ph[1] chromosome: conventional cytogenetics, Southern blot analysis for detection of *BCR-ABL* rearrangements, RT-PCR, immunoprecipitation for detection of abnormal proteins, and fluorescence in-situ hybridization (FISH). FISH enables detection of the molecular translocation in nondividing cells and thus has the advantage of allowing identification of this abnormality in peripheral blood samples.

Chronic Myelogenous Leukemia Variants

Ph[1] CHROMOSOME–NEGATIVE CHRONIC MYELOGENOUS LEUKEMIA

Approximately 5% to 10% of patients with a clinical picture identical to that of Ph[1]-positive CML are Ph[1] negative by cytogenetic analysis.[248] The majority of these patients are found to have the *BCR-ABL* rearrangement and have a clinical course and response to therapy that is indistinguishable from that of patients with Ph[1]-positive CML.[249] In a small number of patients who have phenotypic characteristics of CML and are Ph[1] negative, the *BCR-ABL* rearrangement has not been detected. This subgroup may be a heterogeneous mix of patients with a disease more like myelodysplasia or chronic myelomonocytic leukemia. In these patients, progression of the disease is characterized by progressive leukocytosis, organomegaly, extramedullary infiltrates, and eventual bone marrow failure, in contrast to the evolution to acute leukemia as seen in Ph[1]-negative, *BCR*-positive CML patients.[250]

JUVENILE CHRONIC MYELOGENOUS LEUKEMIA

Juvenile chronic myelogenous leukemia (JCML) is a rare disorder seen in young children.[251] Patients present with fever, night sweats, weight loss, marked hepatosplenomegaly, and lymphadenopathy. Leukocytosis may be present with granulocytes and blasts in the peripheral smear. Eosinophilia and basophilia are not usually seen, as with adult CML. Cytogenetic analysis is usually normal.

Mutations of the *NRAS* oncogene have been identified in up to 30% of patients with JCML[252] but are only rarely detected in CML.[253] This finding further distinguishes JCML from CML and suggests a potential role for *NRAS* in the pathogenesis of JCML.

Prognosis

Survival for patients with CML has improved over the past few decades, secondary to more effective therapy and earlier diagnosis, with a median survival of about 4 to 5 years.[254] Death during the chronic phase from complications related to hyperleukocytosis and leukostasis, splenic infarction or rupture, and thrombosis or hemorrhage has essentially been eliminated by the use of myelosuppressive therapy, interferon, and better supportive care. Unfortunately, survival after transformation to the blastic phase remains short. Thus, overall survival in this disease is determined by time to disease transformation from chronic to blast phase. The duration of chronic phase is variable, but it may last as long as 10 to 20 years.

Numerous prognostic models and staging systems have been proposed to identify patients at greater or lesser risk of transformation.[255–258] Although the time to transformation cannot be predicted in an individual patient, risk during a particular period can be defined by the identification of good and poor prognostic factors (Table 23–6). Using a synthesis staging system based on the most consistent prognostic characteristics identified in their analysis of the cur-

TABLE 23–6. **Poor Prognostic Factors in Chronic Myelogenous Leukemia**

Clinical
Older age
Symptoms at diagnosis
Significant weight loss
Hepatomegaly
Splenomegaly
Poor performance
Black race
Laboratory
Anemia
Thrombocytosis, thrombocytopenia, megakaryocytopenia
Increased blasts, or blasts + promyelocytes in blood or marrow
Increased basophils in blood or marrow
Collagen or reticulin fibrosis grades 3–4
Treatment associated
Longer time to achieve hematologic remission with busulfan chemotherapy
Short remission duration
Total dose of busulfan or hydroxyurea therapy required in the first year to control the disease
Lack of significant suppression of Ph[1]-positive metaphases with intensive chemotherapy or αIFN therapy
Poor initial response to αIFN therapy

αIFN = interferon alfa.

From Kantarjian HM, Deisseroth A, Kurzrock R, et al: Chronic myelogenous leukemia: a concise update. Blood 1993; 82:691.

rently published staging systems, Kantarjian and colleagues[260] segregated patients into better, intermediate, and poor-risk groups, with median survivals of 5, 3.5, and 2.5 years, respectively. However, because the risk of transformation occurs randomly within each prognostic group, there will be patients in the higher risk population who have long survival and those in the good-risk group who will transform early. Prognostic factors should be taken into account when making treatment decisions, but their ultimate value in predicting outcome in an individual patient is limited.

Principles of Treatment

The initial objective of treatment for CML is amelioration of symptoms. This is usually accomplished by decreasing the WBC count through the use of myelosuppressive agents. Therapeutic interventions that may improve survival include hydroxyurea and interferon. Allogeneic bone marrow transplantation is the only curative therapy for CML.

Radiation Therapy

Splenic irradiation was used with some success in controlling signs and symptoms of CML from the early 1900s until the 1950s, when chemotherapy was introduced[261]; however, early studies comparing the outcome of patients receiving radiation therapy with those left untreated showed no difference in survival.[262] Currently, radiation therapy is reserved for palliative treatment in patients unresponsive to chemotherapy, with marked splenomegaly or splenic pain, or with both, and for treatment of extramedullary tumors.[263]

Chemotherapy

Busulfan

Busulfan, an oral alkylating agent that exerts its antileukemic effect by suppressing early progenitor cells, was shown to be more effective than radiation therapy in the treatment of CML.[264] Busulfan is given in doses of 4 to 8 mg/day until the WBC count falls to 20,000 to 30,000/mm³. Because the leukocyte count may continue to fall for weeks after cessation of the drug, it is important that busulfan be discontinued before the WBC count falls into the normal range. Therapy may be reinstituted when the leukocyte count rises above 50,000/mm³, and it is not uncommon for patients to require maintenance doses. Unpredictable, prolonged myelosuppression may occur in 5% to 10% of patients treated with busulfan and may take months to years to resolve.[265]

Hydroxyurea

Hydroxyurea is a ribonucleotide reductase inhibitor that exerts its antileukemic effect by inhibiting DNA synthesis in late progenitor cells and has not been associated with the prolonged myelosuppression seen with busulfan.[266] A prospective, randomized trial comparing the use of hydroxyurea with busulfan in patients with CML showed a significant survival advantage in those patients treated with hydroxyurea; they had a median survival of 58 months, compared with 45 months for those treated with busulfan.[267]

Hydroxyurea is given orally at a dose of 1 to 5 g/day initially, depending on the degree of leukocytosis. Its effect is more rapid but less sustained than that of busulfan; thus, blood counts need to be monitored frequently (2 to 3 times/week) following initiation of therapy and the dose adjusted as the WBC count falls. Patients usually require daily maintenance doses of 500 mg to 2 g/day to maintain a WBC count of about 20,000/mm³. Long-term studies of the leukemogenic potential of hydroxurea in patients with polycythemia vera have not shown an increase in the incidence of acute leukemia.[268]

Radiation therapy and chemotherapeutic agents such as busulfan and hydroxyurea are successful in controlling blood counts, inducing hematologic remissions, decreasing splenomegaly, and controlling symptoms in most patients in the chronic phase of CML. However, these therapies have not been successful in eliminating the Ph¹ chromosome, delaying onset of blast crisis, or significantly prolonging survival. Prolonged remission with loss of the Ph¹ chromosome has been reported in some patients who survive busulfan-induced marrow aplasia[269] and in some patients receiving high-dose hydroxyurea.[270]

Intensive chemotherapy regimens such as those used to induce remission in patients with AML have been tried in patients with CML and result in transient cytogenetic responses in about 30% of patients.[271] However, the use of intensive chemotherapy increases morbidity and has not resulted in significant prolongation of survival or a decrease in transformation to blast phase.

Interferon

Interferons are a family of cell-regulatory glycoproteins with antiviral, antiproliferative, immunomodulatory, and differentiation-inducing effects.[272] Interferon alfa was shown to have a cytoreductive effect and induce hematologic remissions in patients with CML in the early 1980s[273] and was first reported to induce a decrease in Ph¹ chromosome–positive cells in patients with CML in 1986.[274]

The mechanism by which αIFN restores Ph¹ chromosome–negative hematopoiesis is not completely understood. The abnormal proliferation of CML progenitors may be related to their lack of responsiveness to normal, negative regulatory influences from the marrow environment,[275] which may be a consequence of their reduced adhesion to bone marrow stroma.[276] Studies have demonstrated that αIFN treatment of CML progenitors results in restoration of adhesion and inhibition of progenitor proliferation.[277]

αIFN induces complete hematologic responses, defined as normalization of blood counts, absence of immature cells and eradication of signs and symptoms of disease, including palpable splenomegaly, in about 70% to 80% of patients with chronic phase CML.[278] The degree of cytogenetic response has been classified as complete (0% Ph¹-positive cells), partial (1% to 34% Ph¹-positive cells), and minor (35% to 90% Ph¹-positive cells). Major cytogenetic responses include complete and partial responses (Ph¹ <35%)[274] and have been reported in 15% to 40% of patients following treatment with αIFN. The ability of αIFN

TABLE 23–7. **Results of Interferon Alfa (αIFN) Therapy in Early Chronic-Phase Chronic Myelogenous Leukemia**

Study	Therapy	No. of Patients	αIFN (MU/m²) Median Daily Dose: *Planned*	αIFN (MU/m²) Median Daily Dose: *Delivered*	CHR	Cytogenetic Response (%): *Any*	Cytogenetic Response (%): *Major*	Cytogenetic Response (%): *Complete*	Median Survival (mo)
MDACC[280]	αIFN	274	5	5	80	56	38	26	89
Mahon et al[281]	αIFN	52	5	5	81	—	44	38	—
ICSG-CML[282]	αIFN	218	5	4.3	62	55	19	8	72
	Chemotherapy	104	—	—	53	34	1	0	52
Ohnishi et al[283]	αIFN	80	5	4.0	39	44	7.5	9	65+
	Busulfan	79	—	—	54	29	2.5	2.5	50
Alimena et al[284]	αIFN	65	1–2.5	—	46	55	12	—	—
Ozer et al[285]	αIFN	107	5	3.2	59	—	29	13	66
Allan et al[286]	Wellferon	293	3–12	2 (3.2)	68	22	11	6	61
	Busulfan or hydroxyurea	294	—	—	—	—	—	—	41
Hehlmann et al[287]	αIFN	133	5	2	31	18	10	7	66
	Busulfan	186	—	—	23	4	1	0	45
	Hydroxyurea	194	—	—	39	5	1.5	1	56

MU = million units; CHR: complete hematologic response; MDACC = M.D. Anderson Cancer Center; ICSG-CML = Italian Cooperative Study Group on Chronic Myeloid Leukemia.

From Kantarjian HM, O'Brien S, Anderlini P, et al: Treatment of myelogenous leukemia: current status and investigational options. Blood 1996; 87:3069.

to induce a major cytogenetic response appears to correlate with the stage of disease and the time from diagnosis, with the greatest degree of response occurring in patients in early chronic phase (<12 months from diagnosis).[279]

Table 23–7 summarizes the results of clinical trials of αIFN in patients with chronic phase CML. A meta-analysis by the Chronic Myeloid Leukaemia Trialists Collaborative Group of seven randomized trials comparing αIFN with cytotoxic drugs concluded that the 5-year survival rate was significantly better with αIFN (57%) than with either hydroxyurea or busulfan (42%).[288] Most trials of αIFN have shown that survival is directly correlated with the degree of cytogenetic response as illustrated in Figure 23–1; however, some studies have shown improvement in survival for interferon-treated patients even in cytogenetic nonresponders.[285, 286]

The optimal dose schedule of αIFN remains to be determined. There is some evidence suggesting that higher doses of 5 million units (U)/m² daily lead to higher rates of hematologic and cytogenetic responses[284]; however, the use of low-dose αIFN has been reported to show similar rates of hematologic and major cytogenetic responses.[290, 291] An initial cytogenetic response may not be seen until 6 to 9 months following initiation of therapy, and major responses may take much longer to achieve, with a median time of 12 to 18 months.[280, 281] Some patients who ultimately achieve a major response may not do so until after 3 to 5 years of therapy.[282] Thus, the optimal duration of therapy with αIFN is unknown.

INTERFERON PLUS CYTOSINE ARABINOSIDE

Ara-C can decrease Ph¹ chromosome–positive cells[292] and appears to have a synergistic effect when used with αIFN.[293] A randomized trial comparing αIFN with αIFN plus ara-C in patients with newly diagnosed CML showed significantly higher rates of hematologic remission (67% vs. 54%), major cytogenetic responses (39% vs. 22%), and improved survival at 3 years (88% vs. 76%) in patients receiving both drugs.[294] In both groups, patients who achieved a major cytogenetic response had longer survival.

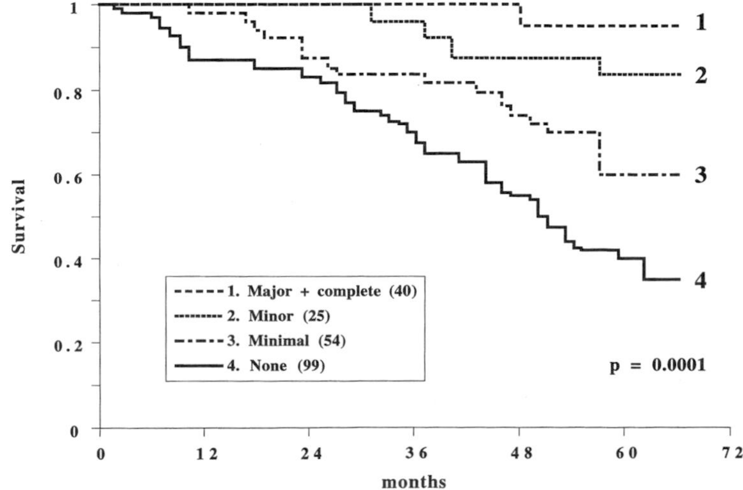

Figure 23–1. Prospective study of the Italian Cooperative Study Group on CML. Survival rate of the patients who were assigned to receive interferon (IFN, Roferon-A) according to the degree of karyotypic response. (From Greenberg P, Tura S, Gilliland DG: Myeloproliferative disorders and myelodysplastic syndromes: cytokine treatment and clonality analyses, p 29. Education Program, American Society of Hematology 35th Annual Meeting, 1993, with permission.)

TOXICITY OF INTERFERON

Interferon therapy is associated with considerable toxicity, including fatigue, weight loss, myalgias, insomnia, depression, and neurotoxicity. Immune-mediated complications have been identified, and include hemolysis, thrombocytopenia, hypothyroidism, and collagen vascular disorders.[295] About 15% to 25% of patients are intolerant of therapy and must discontinue, and another 30% to 50% of patients require dose reductions.

Minimal Residual Disease in Chronic Myelogenous Leukemia

Despite promising results with αIFN, it remains unproven whether interferon can cure patients with CML. Most patients who become Ph[1] chromosome negative after treatment with αIFN continue to have detectable *BCR-ABL* transcripts in their blood, as demonstrated by RT-PCR analysis.[296, 297] The consequence of persistent *BCR-ABL* positivity in patients in continuous clinical and cytogenetic remission is unknown.

Allogeneic Bone Marrow Transplant

The first successful allogeneic bone marrow transplant (allo-BMT) for CML was performed in 1970[298]; since then, allo-BMT has evolved as the only curative therapy for CML resulting in long-term, disease-free survival in up to 70% of patients.[299, 300] CML is the most common disease for which allo-BMT is currently performed. Table 23–8 summarizes the results of allo-BMT for CML in chronic phase.

Factors affecting transplant outcome include patient age, stage of disease, prior therapy, interval from diagnosis to transplant, and source of stem cells.

- Age: Patients older than age 55 are generally not considered candidates for allo-BMT because transplant-related mortality, primarily secondary to GVHD, increases with age. However, the Seattle group has transplanted patients up to 60 years of age with disease-free survival rates of over 70%.[307]
- Stage of disease: International Bone Marrow Transplant Registry (IBMTR) data for 2231 recipients of HLA-identical sibling transplants for CML between 1987 and 1994 show 3-year leukemia-free survival rates of 57%, 41%, and 18% for patients transplanted in first chronic phase, accelerated phase, and blast phase respectively.[301] The 3-year actuarial probability of relapse is 13% for transplants performed in first chronic phase, 26% in accelerated phase, and 58% in blast phase.
- Prior therapy: Patients treated with busulfan before transplant have been shown to have higher transplant-related mortality and significantly worse leukemia-free survival than those treated with hydroxyurea.[303] There are conflicting data regarding the impact of prior treatment with αIFN. In one study, treatment with αIFN for more than 1 year before transplant was associated with a significantly higher transplant-related mortality secondary to infections and worse 5-year survival rates compared with patients receiving interferon for less than 12 months.[308] However, several other studies have not found an adverse affect on outcome for patients receiving interferon prior to transplant.[309–311]
- Interval from diagnosis to transplant: Several studies have shown that patients transplanted within 1 year of diagnosis have lower transplant-related mortality and improved leukemia-free survival compared with those transplanted later.[303, 304]
- Type of transplant: The immune effects of GVL appear to be particularly important in CML. Patients undergoing transplant using bone marrow depleted of T-cells have much higher relapse rates than those receiving unmanipulated bone marrow.

Transplant Versus Interferon

A retrospective analysis comparing the survival of 548 patients with chronic phase CML receiving HLA-identical sibling transplants with the survival of 196 patients treated

TABLE 23–8. **Allogeneic Bone Marrow Transplantation (BMT) in Chronic-Phase Chronic Myelogenous Leukemia**

Study Group	No. of Patients	EFS % (at x year)	Unfavorable Prognostic Factors for Disease-Free Survival (relative risk)
IBMTR[301]	2231	57 (3)	T-cell depletion (5.4) Age > 20 yr (2.6)
EBMT[302]	2942	42 (5)	Age > 20 yr (1.5) T-cell depletion (1.4) Male recipient/female donor (1.2)
Goldman et al, IBMTR[303]	450	No busulfan: 61 (3) Prior busulfan: 45 (3)	Prior busulfan therapy (1.5) Time to BMT > 1 yr (1.7)
Biggs et al[304]	62	58 (3)	Time to BMT > 1 yr (2.7) Male recipient/female donor (2.5) Prior busulfan therapy (2.2)
Clift et al[305]	325	75 (5)	Not stated
Snyder et al[306]	94	64 (5)	Older age (1.1) Longer time to BMT (1.48; ≥ 1 yr: 1.26)

EFS = event-free survival; IBMT = International Bone Marrow Transplant Registry; EBMT = European Group for Blood and Marrow Transplantation.
Adapted from Kantarjian HM, O'Brien S, Anderlini P, et al: Treatment of chronic myelogenous leukemia: current status and investigational options. Blood 1996; 87:3069.

with hydroxyurea or interferon was performed by the IBMTR.[312] As expected, the study confirmed the higher early mortality for patients undergoing allo-BMT, but there was a long-term survival advantage of HLA-identical sibling transplants over both hydroxyurea and interferon. The survival advantage for transplant was greatest if the transplant was performed soon after diagnosis (within 1 year) and if the patients had intermediate-risk or high-risk prognostic factors.

Alternative Donors

Only 25% to 30% of patients with CML will have a related, histocompatible donor. Transplantation from HLA-matched, unrelated donors has had moderate success with disease-free survival rates of 30% to 40%; however, this technique has been associated with higher rates of graft failure and an increased incidence of acute and chronic GVHD.[313] The use of alternative sources of allogeneic stem cells for transplantation, including peripheral blood progenitor cells and umbilical cord blood cells, is being explored.[314, 315]

Relapse Following Bone Marrow Transplantation

Patients who relapse after allo-BMT can often be reinduced into a second cytogenetic remission using donor leukocyte infusions.[316, 317] The efficacy of this strategy relies on the induction of a GVL effect mediated by the infused donor T-cells, resulting in suppression of the Ph[1]-positive clone, and allowing recovery of residual donor hematopoiesis. Donor leukocyte infusions have been very successful in patients who relapse following allo-BMT for CML, with hematologic and cytogenetic remission rates of 70% to 80%.[204] Response rates are greater in patients treated at the time of molecular or cytogenetic relapse compared with those who have progressed to hematologic relapse. Complications of this adoptive immunotherapy are considerable, with a 50% incidence of marrow suppression, 60% to 80% incidence of acute GVHD, and a nearly 20% mortality rate.[318]

Future directions in this area may rely on the preemptive use of donor leukocyte infusions in patients at increased risk for relapse. Patients who relapse in chronic phase have been treated with a second allo-BMT and have a 4-year survival rate of about 30%.[319]

Minimal Residual Disease

Increasingly, molecular monitoring for the presence of MRD or for evidence of early relapse is being employed in patients undergoing allo-BMT for CML. Studies using the PCR have identified *BCR-ABL*–positive cells in more than 50% of patients following allogeneic bone marrow transplantation.[320, 321] In these studies, the risk of relapse was associated with multiple PCR assays being positive, and with the persistence of *BCR-ABL* positive cells more than 6 months following transplantation.

Autologous Transplantation for Chronic Myelogenous Leukemia

The majority of patients with CML may not be candidates for allo-BMT because they lack a suitable donor or because of advanced patient age. For these patients, initial treatment with αIFN may be the optimal approach. It has been shown that normal, Ph[1]-negative, hematopoietic progenitors coexist with their malignant counterparts in the bone marrow of patients with CML, and that high-dose chemotherapy may transiently restore Ph[1]-negative hematopoiesis.[322] The use of high-dose chemotherapy, together with an infusion of autologous progenitor cells collected during chronic phase, has resulted in complete and partial cytogenetic responses in up to 60% of patients.[323] In the majority of patients, however, the responses are transient, and Ph[1]-positive hematopoiesis recurs. Despite these findings, autologous bone marrow transplantation (auto-BMT) may be associated with prolonged survival when compared with conventional chemotherapy. In a review of 200 autologous transplants performed in 8 transplant centers in Europe and North America, the median survival was 42 months.[324] In a study from the Hammersmith group, the 5-year survival of patients autografted with unpurged progenitor cells was significantly higher than age-matched controls treated with conventional chemotherapy (56% vs. 28%).[325]

Genetic marker studies have demonstrated that the presence of Ph[1]-positive cells in the infused marrow contributes to relapse.[326] Methods to remove Ph[1]-positive cells have included *ex vivo* purging with chemotherapeutic agents,[327, 328] use of gamma interferon (γIFN),[329] tyrosine kinase inhibitors,[330] and antisense oligodeoxynucleotides directed against the *BCR-ABL* gene[331, 332] and the proto-oncogene *MYB*.[333] Other strategies have focused on the isolation of normal, Ph[1]-negative cells by the use of long-term liquid cultures, which results in a selective loss of Ph[1]-positive progenitors.[334]

The role of auto-BMT in the management of CML remains to be defined, and randomized studies addressing this issue are under way.

New Therapies in CML

STI-571 (*S*ignal *T*ransduction *I*nhibitor) is a new agent that inhibits the activity of the *BCR-ABL* tyrosine kinase. It has been shown to inhibit the growth of *BCR-ABL*–positive cells, resulting in death by apoptosis.[334a] Phase I trials of STI-57 in patients with chronic phase CML who failed αIFN therapy showed rapid (within 3 to 4 weeks of initiation of therapy) and complete hematologic responses in 100% of patients when doses of at least 300 mg per day were used. There was no dose-limiting toxicity. Overall, cytogenetic responses were seen in 55% of patients at 5 months, with 10% of responses being complete.* Phase II and III trials of this novel agent are currently under way.

What Is the Best Therapy for CML?

The optimal therapy for CML in chronic phase remains controversial. Interferon and hydroxyurea prolong survival

*Information obtained from a Hematology Grand Rounds lecture given by Dr. Brian Druker.

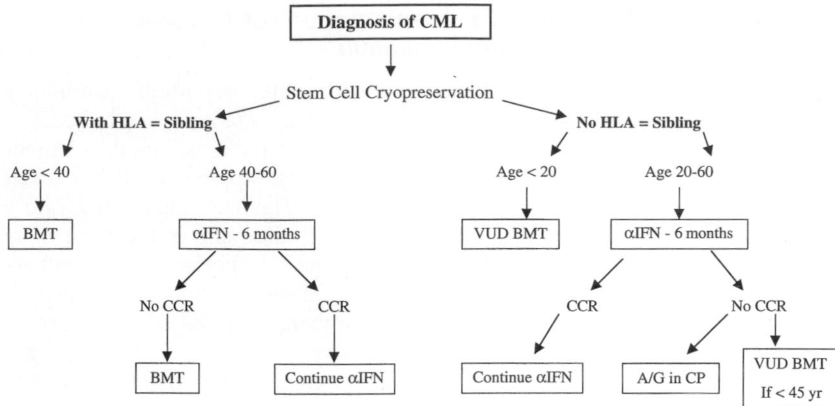

Figure 23–2. Algorithm for planning treatment of newly diagnosed CML patient 60 years old or younger. (From Goldman JM: Chronic myeloid leukemia: New strategies for cure, p 3. Education Program, American Society of Hematology 39th Annual Meeting, 1997, with permission.)

and have little treatment-related mortality. However, prolongation of survival with interferon correlates with cytogenetic response to treatment, which only occurs in a minority of patients. In addition, even in patients who have complete cytogenetic responses, *BCR-ABL* transcripts persist and, thus, it is not clear if interferon can ultimately cure patients with CML. Some studies have shown that prolonged therapy with interferon prior to allogeneic transplant has a negative impact on transplant outcome, yet the median time to exhibit a response to interferon may be 1 to 2 years. Thus, an approach of trying interferon indefinitely until a cytogenetic response occurs may compromise the outcome of transplant.

Allogeneic transplantation, on the other hand, may cure 50% to 60% of patients with chronic phase CML, although treatment-related mortality is high, and outcome is worse if transplant is delayed for more than a year following diagnosis. In addition, morbidity and mortality increase with age, and only 25% to 30% of patients may have an HLA-matched donor. The use of matched, unrelated donors is associated with higher transplant mortality.

For patients not entered into clinical trials, the algorithm outlined in Figure 23–2 suggests a reasonable approach for managing patients presenting in chronic phase. Prognostic variables should also be taken into account when making decisions regarding therapy because patients with intermediate-risk and high-risk prognostic features may have better survival if transplanted earlier.

Acute Lymphoblastic Leukemia

Epidemiology and Etiology

Epidemiology

The past 50 years are marked by extraordinary advances in the treatment of childhood cancer. At the forefront of this progress is the remarkable improvement in the cure rates for children with acute lymphoblastic leukemia (ALL). ALL comprises approximately 80% of the 2500 annual cases of childhood leukemia in the United States.[336] Fortunately, this disease has gone from a fatal diagnosis in the early 1950s to one with a cure rate approaching 80%.[337] Because leukemia represents half of the 5000 new childhood cancer cases per year in the United States, this rise in cure rate demonstrates significant progress in the battle to overcome this disease.

The study of the epidemiology of this rare disorder, with an incidence of only 110 cases per million U.S. children younger than 15 years of age per year, reveals some important observations. Patients with ALL are most commonly male, and it is predominantly (80%) a pre–B-cell–lineage disease. In the developed world, the frequency of childhood leukemia increases rapidly after birth, peaks before 5 years of age, and then declines. The incidence declines rapidly to the point that acute nonlymphoblastic leukemia (ANLL) predominates in adolescence. ALL represents only 20% of adult leukemias.

The study of ALL and ANLL in children with Down syndrome offers a special challenge, with a 10-fold increased risk of these diseases during the first decade of life. An understanding of its pathophysiology will increase our understanding of the etiology of leukemia.

Etiology

ALL is the result of the clonal proliferation and accumulation of leukemic lymphoblasts in the bone marrow and other lymphoid tissue. Proliferation of immature precursors, at any stage of hematopoietic development, can arise from "defective" progenitors that lack the capacity to differentiate. This may be the result of growth factor dysregulation by activated growth factor genes, or by blast production of excess growth factors. Alternatively, leukemia may result from a single damaged progenitor cell that gives rise to malignant progeny by a process of uncontrolled self-renewal.[336] Early studies of immunoglobulin

(Ig) heavy chain gene rearrangement in the leukemic cells from patients with ALL showed that this disease is of B-cell lineage and has clonal origins.[338] Later studies based on PCR methodology confirmed the clonal origin of almost 100% of childhood B-lineage ALL.[339, 340] Therefore, the most common and phenotypically unclassifiable ALL results from the proliferation of cells blocked in the early stage of B-cell differentiation before the immunoglobulins are synthesized. In comparison, the leukemic event in B-cell ALL occurs at a later stage of B-cell differentiation when the cell can already synthesize immunoglobulins. Studies of clonality during remission revealed that, in some patients, nonclonal hematopoiesis was restored (i.e., the bone marrow was repopulated with normal cells), but in others, the remission marrow was characterized by the same clonal product as found at diagnosis.[341] Detection of clonal hematopoiesis in remission was associated with ultimate relapse in 89% of these cases; however, the clonal cytogenetic abnormalities detected at relapse may be different from those originally observed at diagnosis.[342]

With advancements in molecular biology, a genetic basis has been postulated for many of the leukemias. Two mechanisms act in the pathogenesis of human leukemias; acquired genetic lesions can activate cellular proto-oncogenes or inactivate tumor suppressor genes (anti-oncogenes), both leading to loss of control and subsequent, unchecked proliferation of the leukemic cell.[343] These genetic alterations may take the form of point mutations, gene amplifications, gene deletions, or chromosomal translocations. Chromosomal translocations are present in many cases of acute leukemia; a translocation may reposition a gene to a new site, causing the new proto-oncogene to act as a promoter or enhancer element on another distinct gene. For example, in the translocation t(8;14) abnormality, the enhancer for the immunoglobulin heavy chain gene is juxtaposed near the *MYC* gene, resulting in Burkitt's lymphoma. A translocation can also occur within two genes, leading to a subsequent fusion gene and a chimeric protein, as seen in the t(9;22) abnormality found in ALL and CML.[344] Thirman and coworkers[345] have shown multiple rearrangements in 20 different cases of acute leukemia, all involving chromosome band 11q23.

The observation that mixed-lineage leukemia (MLL) gene rearrangements and 11q23 abnormalities may occur in lymphoid as well as in myeloid disorders, as well as the presence of the Ph^1 chromosome in myeloid and erythroid progenitor cells of two patients with Ph^1-positive ALL,[346] indicates that, in some patients with ALL, the disease may involve a multipotential stem cell. With advances in molecular genetic analysis, these abnormalities may be more common than previously represented by standard cytogenetic techniques, and molecular genetics may be able to direct more specific therapy by risk group stratification. In addition, molecular techniques will offer greater sensitivity for detecting MRD. The section on "Classification" will further delineate chromosomal translocations as they are related to disease prognosis and treatment.

Detection and Diagnosis

Clinical Detection

Clinical manifestations of ALL result from the accumulation of leukemic blast cells in bone marrow, leading to a reduction in normal hematopoietic cells, and from infiltration of lymph nodes, liver, and spleen. Two thirds of patients have signs and symptoms for less than 6 weeks prior to diagnosis. Many cases exhibit nonspecific viral-type symptomatology with low-grade fever, malaise, anorexia, lethargy, and abdominal discomfort. Fifty percent of the patients present with specific signs of bleeding, bruising, and pallor associated with thrombocytopenia and anemia. Petechiae, gingival bleeding, and epistaxis are often reported. Various infections are present, secondary to decreased neutrophil counts. One third of the patients, more common than with other leukemias, will present with bony tenderness as a result of periosteal invasion and subperiosteal hemorrhage. This tenderness can manifest as painful bones or joints, or, occasionally, as a limp. Splenomegaly is more common than hepatomegaly. Lymphadenopathy may be present, but is not unusually prominent. In males, testicular involvement may be manifest by unilateral or, rarely, bilateral, painless enlargement. This enlargement is rare as the initial presenting symptom, but may be the first sign of relapse. Patients may present acutely with severe bleeding, infection, or respiratory distress, or may be serendipitously detected on a routine complete blood count in an asymptomatic patient.

Less than 5% of the patients will have CNS disease at diagnosis.[347] It is more common in patients who are younger than 2 years of age, and in those with T-cell ALL. Leukemic cells can be present in the CNS at diagnosis through perivascular invasion or deposition from hemorrhage, or at relapse by invasion of the leptomeninges from the periphery. CNS leukemia usually manifests with headache, vomiting, lethargy, and papilledema on physical exam. Cranial nerve palsies, nuchal rigidity, and seizures may be present, but such symptoms are rare.

Diagnosis

A *complete blood count* may be abnormal, or may have some elements that are normal in a patient suspected of having leukemia. Only 50% of the patients will have a WBC count greater than 10,000/mm^3, 20% with WBC above 50,000/mm^3. The other patients may have normal or decreased WBC counts. Normochromic, normocytic anemia may be present from decreased production secondary to marrow invasion, but only 25% of patients will have severe anemia (hemoglobin <6 g/dL). Thrombocytopenia is noted in the majority of patients; however, 25% will have a platelet count above 100,000. *Blood chemistries* may show an abnormally high lactate dehydrogenase level and hyperuricemia. A *chest x-ray* should be performed because mediastinal masses can be seen, especially in T-cell ALL, and may need emergent care.

A definitive diagnosis is made by a *bone marrow aspirate* that usually is significant for a homogenous population of cells, or "sheets" of lymphoblasts, with a paucity of normal elements. Greater than 25% leukemic blast cells define leukemia; less than 25% blasts are seen in lymphomas. A *bone marrow biopsy* should be performed because a "packed" or hypoplastic marrow is difficult to diagnose from an aspirate. A biopsy also differentiates leukemic infiltration from myelofibrosis or bone infarction, which can be found in adults.

The diagnosis of ALL is classically made by morphology; however, cytochemical staining techniques can aid in differentiating ALL from myeloid leukemias. NSE, MPO, and SBB are usually negative in ALL. TdT staining is important and is positive in most cases of ALL. Immunophenotyping of the malignant cells will assist in the classification of the leukemia. Chromosomal analysis, along with molecular studies, should be performed to further define the cells. A *lumbar puncture* must also be performed to document whether there is CNS involvement with leukemia cells. Cytocentrifugation of the spinal fluid may reveal a pleocytosis, with CNS leukemia defined as fewer than 5 leukocytes/μL.

The specific diagnosis of ALL is made after obtaining a thorough history, physical examination, and supporting peripheral blood and bone marrow laboratory results. Ten percent of cases need more detailed evaluations to differentiate ALL from other diseases. Various systemic disorders may mimic symptoms found in ALL:

- Patients with bone or joint pain associated with juvenile rheumatoid arthritis may also present with fever, pallor, decreased WBC, or splenomegaly, or a combination of these signs.
- Infectious mononucleosis can present with fever, lymphadenopathy, and hepatosplenomegaly along with immature lymphocytes on the peripheral blood smear. Occasionally, patients may also be thrombocytopenic and anemic. The immature lymphocytes are atypical, classic for the EBV infection, but the bone marrow aspirate will show normal elements along with the viral lymphocytes or monocytoid cells.
- Other viral infections, such as cytomegalovirus, can behave similarly.
- Pertussis can be associated with a WBC count of above 50,000/mm^3, but the clinical "whooping" cough should differentiate the infection from ALL.
- Leukemoid reactions can be seen with other infections such as tuberculosis, histoplasmosis, as well as granulomatous diseases such as sarcoid.
- Acute hemolytic syndrome can be noted to have associated elevated WBC counts.
- Sepsis can also be seen with leukocytosis, or with the reverse (i.e., neutropenia with a "maturation arrest" of myeloid precursors), and toxic granulations of the cells.
- Down syndrome patients can have leukemoid reactions in the neonatal period; however, this is rarely a congenital leukemia presentation.

Other hematologic and oncologic disorders should also be differentiated from ALL. The most common cause of thrombocytopenia, especially in children, is idiopathic or immune thrombocytopenic purpura. The usual presenting symptom is bruising, most often after an antecedent viral illness. Occasional excessive bleeding may also lead to anemia. The WBC count and differential are usually normal. The bone marrow is remarkable for an excess number of megakaryocytes, with other normal elements. The peripheral blood smear may show large, "young" platelets. Aplastic anemia can present with fever, infections, and pancytopenia; however, the bone marrow aspirate will be hypocellular, without evidence of blast cells. Bone marrow failure syndromes may have myelodysplastic or hypocellular bone marrows, or, occasionally, hypercellular ones with a paucity of one cell line only. Malignant cell infiltration of the bone marrow, as seen with neuroblastoma, retinoblastoma, rhabdomyosarcoma, or Ewing's sarcoma, rarely leads to pancytopenia. In these entities, the bone marrow is noted to have clumps of malignant cells, or rosettes.

Specific diagnosis of ALL is very important, particularly for those diseases listed earlier whose treatment can involve the use of glucocorticoids. Revesz and associates[348] reported the adverse effect of prednisolone pretreatment in children subsequently diagnosed with ALL. The CR rate was similar in the pretreated patients as in the controls, but the continuous CR rate at 36 months was only 15% in the former group, as compared with 43% in the latter. This continuous CR rate was similar to patients with relapsed ALL. Therefore, pretreating patients with prednisolone decreases the possibility of a cure, and a definitive diagnosis must be made first.

Classification

Initially, the terms *acute* and *chronic* referred to the natural history of the leukemia, prior to the intervention of chemotherapy; currently, leukemias are classified morphologically. Chronic leukemia is characterized by an expansion of mature marrow precursors, whereas acute leukemias are named according to the predominant cell line involved. In children, ALL comprises 80% of the cases, whereas AML is rare, encompassing only 15% of all cases. Acute undifferentiated leukemias make up the remaining 5% of the cases; these leukemias are being reclassified as molecular genetic techniques improve.

Morphologic Classification

The hallmark of acute leukemias is the blast cell. A stained bone marrow smear shows the lymphoblast to be an undifferentiated cell with homogenous, diffusely distributed nuclear chromatin with one or more indistinct nucleoli, and a thin rim of basophilic cytoplasm, usually without granules. Normal bone marrow has less than 5% blasts, and usually these cells are not evident in the peripheral blood. Myeloblasts are larger, with more cytoplasm, along with cytoplasmic granules and larger distinct nucleoli.

In 1976, the FAB Cooperative Group published a uniform system of classification and nomenclature of the acute leukemias, thus providing a standardized way of clinically studying patients and chemotherapy trials.[63] This system is based on the morphologic appearance of bone marrow and peripheral blood in Romanowsky-stained smears and is supplemented by cytochemical testing. ALL is subdivided into three types, L1, L2, and L3, according to individual cytologic features and the degree of heterogeneity in the distribution among the leukemic population. The individual features that are incorporated in this system are cell size, nuclear chromatin, nuclear shape, presence of nucleoli, and the amount of cytoplasm together with its degree of basophilia:

- L1 leukemia cells are predominantly small cells, about twice the size of a small lymphocyte. The cells are homogeneous with a finely dispersed nuclear chromatin and a regular shaped nucleus. Some folding of the nucleus can occur. Nucleoli are rare and, if present, are small. The cytoplasm is scanty and mildly basophilic.

- L2 cells are larger than L1, and their size can be more heterogeneous. The nuclear chromatin is also more heterogeneous, and the nuclear shape may have deep clefting. Nucleoli are usually present and can be large. The cytoplasm is more basophilic and more abundant than in L1 cells.
- L3 cells are the classic Burkitt's type cells and are homogeneously large with a regular shaped nucleus and one or more prominent nucleoli. The cytoplasm is very abundant and intensely basophilic, with many classic cytoplasmic vacuoles. These cells are highly mitotic, and dividing cells are often evident.

Most childhood ALL is of the L1 subtype. Burkitt's lymphoma with bone marrow involvement or B-cell ALL will have L3 type cells. L2 cells are often difficult to differentiate from myeloblasts, and the previously stated cytochemical reactions need to be performed for clarification.

Phenotypic Classification

The lineage of the leukemic cell is also important, especially as it is related to prognosis. This identification has been used in type-specific treatment to improve outcome. B-cell ALL, or Burkitt's type, expresses characteristic cell surface immunoglobulin. T-cell ALL is defined by the rosetting of the cells in the presence of sheep red blood cells, or, currently, it is characterized by a positive reaction with monoclonal antibodies that recognize T-cell antigens. Non T-cell, non B-cell ALL defines those leukemic cells whose origin is unclear. Molecular studies have shown these cells to have immunoglobulin gene rearrangements, usually of the Ig heavy chain. The undifferentiated leukemic cells are immature and uncommitted, retaining all immunoglobulin and T-cell receptor genes in the germline form.

Surface antigens have been used to delineate lymphoid from myeloid leukemia, as well as to define the precursor stage of the B-lineage leukemic cell. Lineage infidelity or mixed-lineage expression appears in leukemic cells in which there is a simultaneous expression of myeloid-associated antigens on ALL cells. Wiersma and associates[349] used dual-fluorescence analysis to demonstrate mixed-lineage expression in 22% of 236 studied ALL cases. By FAB criteria, myeloid-antigen positivity was distributed among low-risk, intermediate-risk, and high-risk patients, as was negativity. However, the prognosis was much worse in those patients with positive expression. In a univariate analysis for B-lineage ALL, myeloid-antigen expression was a significant predictor of relapse.

Through immunophenotyping, it is clear that the most common form of ALL is the CALLA-positive pre–B-cell ALL; CALLA represents the common ALL antigen and is now defined as the CD10 surface antigen. CALLA is a neutral endopeptidase 24.11 (neprilysin) with normal enzymatic function on blasts.[350, 351] Pre–B-cell ALL usually has L1 blasts, which may or may not express cytoplasmic immunoglobulin heavy chains, but have no surface immunoglobulin. B-cell ALL is rare, comprising only 1% to 2% of all cases. This type of ALL is characterized by L3 blasts, which express surface immunoglobulin (usually IgM), and is synonymous with Burkitt's lymphoma. B-cell ALL is associated with positivity for CD20, CD19, HLA-DR, but not CALLA.[352] T-cell ALL has a classic phenotypical presentation. TdT is a marker enzyme that is present in pre-B and T-lymphoblasts, and can help differentiate between ALL and AML.[353] *Biphenotypic leukemia* is a term used for leukemic cells that express both myeloid and lymphoid antigens and may result from the clonal expansion of a malignant progenitor cell that is capable of bilineage differentiation; this uncommon acute leukemia has a poor prognosis.[354]

Molecular and Cytogenetic Classification

Abnormalities in chromosome number and structure can be identified in 60% to 90% of patients with ALL. Numerical chromosome abnormalities can be assessed by conventional cytogenetics, by flow cytometry, and by interphase FISH using a panel of probes to detect multiple hybridization targets (chromosomes). Flow cytometry estimates ploidy to within two to four chromosomes. The current recommendation is *to perform all three tests* in newly diagnosed patients.

MYC and Burkitt's Lymphoma Translocations

In 8% of patients, the distal end of the long arm of chromosome 8 translocates to the long arm of chromosome 14, producing the t(8;14)(q24.1;q32.3) translocation, whereas the variant translocations t(8;22)(q24.1;q11.2) and t(2;8)(p11.2;q24.1) occur in 15% and 5% of the patients, respectively.[355, 356] In each translocation, juxtaposition of *MYC* on 8q24.1 with one of the immunoglobulin loci causes *MYC* dysregulation. In patients with t(8;14), the breakpoint on chromosome 8 leaves the *MYC* coding sequences intact,[355, 357] whereas in the variant translocations, the breakpoint regions are at variable distances from the *c-MYC* coding region.[358] The critical event in these rearrangements is that the *c-MYC* gene is displaced, and is under the influence of transcription-stimulating sequences in each of the Ig loci, leading to a high level of transcription. B-cell ALL is defined when cells with elevated levels of *c-MYC* expression and increased proliferation rates comprise greater than 25% of the bone marrow.

12p Rearrangement

Rearrangements and deletions of the short arm of chromosome 12 occur in 5% to 10% of children with *de novo* and relapsed ALL,[359, 360] representing one of the most common chromosomal abnormalities in childhood ALL.[342, 361] Cytogenetic abnormalities of 12p, when reanalyzed with FISH, result in at least three different molecular changes: deletion of *KIP1* (localized on 12p12), amplification of *CCND2* (localized on 12p13), and rearrangements or deletion of *TEL* (localized on 12p12).[362, 363] Cytogenetic deletions of 12p were confirmed by finding loss of heterozygosity in 15% to 33% of patients with ALL.[364, 365]

t(12;21)(p13;q22) TEL-AML1 (ETV6-CBFA2)

In t(12;21), the 5′ region of *TEL* (*ETV6*) is juxtaposed to the *AML1* (*CBFA2*) gene located on 21q22, resulting in a fusion transcript *TEL-AML1* (*ETV6-CBFA2*).[366, 367] Cytogenetic identification of t(12;21) is not as accurate as detection by FISH or other molecular methods because the translocated portions of 12p and 21q are virtually identical by G-banding; therefore, the incidence of t(12;21) reported by conventional cytogenetics to be less than 0.05% is probably an underestimate.[361] FISH and PCR methods have detected 15% to 39% of pediatric patients with *TEL-AML1* fusion, this representing the most frequent gene rearrangement in childhood cancer. In addition, up to 3% of adult ALL patients have *TEL-AML1* fusion. Almost exclusively, t(12;21) is detected in patients ages 1 to 12, with associated pre–B-cell lineage (CD10+, CD19+); as many as 25% of these patients may coexpress at least two myeloid antigens.[368, 369]

Importantly, patients with *TEL-AML1* fusion have a significantly lower rate of relapse when compared with *TEL-AML1–* negative patients ($p = 0.004$); thus, detection of the fusion transcript by PCR methodology confers a favorable prognosis.[368] Rearrangements of the *TEL* gene are also associated with improved survival among patients treated with antimetabolite-based therapy.[370] In patients with *TEL-AML1* fusion, the reciprocal *AML1-TEL* fusion transcript was found in 45%,[368] suggesting that the *TEL-AML1* chimeric protein may be biologically relevant.

t(1;19)(q23;p13.2) E2A/PBX

The t(1;19) is found in 25% of childhood pre-B ALL, and has been reported in some cases of adult ALL and in rare patients with T-cell ALL and AML.[371, 372] This translocation may be present in two forms: as a balanced translocation and as its variant, an unbalanced form der(19)t(1;19).[373] For patients of all ages, prognosis of der(19) is better than t(1;19); however, the overall prognosis is poor.

It has been suggested that survival may improve with intensive treatment.[374] Over 85% of patients with t(1;19) express the identical breakpoint on chromosome 19, within the single intron of the *E2A* gene that encodes Ig enhancer transcription factors, and on chromosome 1q23, which interrupts the homeobox gene *PBX1*.[371, 375] Molecular detection of the t(1;19) is now possible with PCR analysis[376, 377]; further, monoclonal antibodies specific for the common form of the *E2A/PBX1* chimeric protein have been developed, and their initial clinical utility has been demonstrated.[378]

11q23 Rearrangements

The frequent involvement of band q23 on the long arm of chromosome 11 was found in 10% to 15% of patients with ALL revealing the translocations t(4;11)(q21;q23), t(10;11)(p14;15;q23), t(14;11)(q21;q23), t(11;19)(q23;p13), and t(1;11)(p32;q23).[21, 58, 107] These translocations occur more frequently in children regardless of the phenotype, and account for two thirds of the acute leukemic chromosomal abnormalities in patients younger than 1 year of age. The 11q23 rearrangements are also observed in therapy-related leukemia, especially in patients treated with inhibitors of topoisomerase II.[84, 381] These translocations confer a very poor prognosis.

The *MLL* gene, also referred to as *ALL1*, *HRX*, and *HTRX* (because of its shared homology with the *Drosophila* trithorax protein) is located on 11q23 and is rearranged in the great majority of patients with 11q23 translocations.[345, 382] Translocations of 11q23 were found in 20 different reciprocal chromosomal exchanges and, to date, a description of the *MLL* gene with 7 other genes has been characterized. The breakpoints within the *MLL* gene are clustered within a restricted 8-kilobase region.[383] The *MLL* gene is also rearranged in patients without visible chromosomal translocations.[384, 385] DNA probes from this region can be used with Southern blot analysis to detect the *MLL* rearrangements.[339, 340, 386] In the clinical setting, molecular detection of *MLL* rearrangements is more frequent in patients with t(4;11)(q21;q23). These infant ALL patients usually have mixed lymphoid and myeloid features and a very poor prognosis.

The identification of the translocation is important because more aggressive chemotherapy or allo-BMT (in first remission) is often recommended for these patients.[361] Furthermore, the specific translocation, such as t(4;11) and not a 11q23 breakpoint *per se*, is associated with the poor prognosis of these infants.[387] In adults, 23% of patients have *MLL* rearrangements[388] and some investigators have reported adverse prognosis for any patients with *MLL* gene rearrangements.[389] Four balanced translocations were found in therapy-related acute leukemia, including t(9;11)(p22;q23) or t(11;19)(q23;p13) in AML, t(4;11)(q21;q33) in ALL, and t(11;16)(q23;p13.3) in both ALL and AML.[390, 391]

t(9;22)(q34;11) BCR-ABL

The Ph[1] chromosome t(9;22)(q34;q11.1) occurs in 2% to 6% of children, and in 17% to 25% of adults with ALL,[392, 393] with more cases reported as more sensitive molecular techniques are developed and used. When the Ph[1] chromosome is found in children at diagnosis, it is present as a single abnormality in about 50% of the cases; pseudodiploidy is the most frequent model number.[361] Approximately 25% of children, as well as a small percentage of adults, have partial or complete monosomy 7 in Ph[1] cells.[394] Historically, the Ph[1] chromosome is detected cytogenetically, but higher sensitivity is provided by molecular methods such as Southern blot analysis, RT-PCR and, more recently, by FISH. The Ph[1] chromosome found in ALL is cytogenetically indistinguishable from the Ph[1] chromosome in CML. As a result of this translocation, most of the *ABL* oncogene on 9q34 is juxtaposed next to the *BCR* gene on 22q11.1, creating a new *BCR-ABL* hybrid gene.[395, 396] The fusion gene encodes for one of two abnormal proteins, $P210^{BCR\text{-}ABL}$ and $P190^{BCR\text{-}ABL}$, which have strong tyrosine kinase activities.[397] In both childhood and adult ALL, the Ph[1] chromosome is associated with poor prognosis and is independent of age and WBC count; therefore, identifying the Ph[1] chromosome is of crucial importance because allo-BMT in first remission may be the proposed treatment of choice.[398]

14q11 Rearrangements

Five major translocation groups in T-cell ALL involve the q11 region of the long arm of chromosome 14, where the

T-cell receptor (TCR) alpha and delta reside. The most frequent of these translocations is the t(11;14)(p13;q11), detected in about 7% of childhood T-cell ALL; the breakpoint is within the alpha-delta locus of the *TCR* gene. The t(11;14)(p15;q11) and t(10;14)(q24;q11) are found in about 1% and 5% to 10% of T-cell malignancies, respectively, and they also disrupt this locus. The t(8;14)(q24;q11) is found in 2% of T-cell leukemia, but is not restricted to this lineage. On the molecular level, the *TCR*-alpha gene is rearranged with the *c-MYC* oncogene resulting in transcriptional dysregulation. Finally, t(1;14)(p32-34;q11) has been identified in 3% of T-cell ALL. As a consequence of this translocation, the *TAL1* gene on chromosome 1 is inactivated. *TAL1* deletions are not detected cytogenetically, but molecular methods have shown that 30% of patients with T-cell ALL have *TAL1* rearrangements, making this abnormality the most frequent genetic lesion in this form of leukemia.[399, 400]

Prognostic Factors

Prognostic factors become important as clinical features become predictors of outcome. These factors place patients in designated risk categories; this allows high-risk patients to be put on intensive treatments, while not adding the excess toxicity to standard-risk patients. However, prognostic factors can change as chemotherapy advances are made, equalizing those factors that were once thought to be the most predictive of outcome. Immunologic classification of the leukemic blasts has helped to define treatments. Division of patients into T, B, pre-B, and early pre-B ALL better defines risk. Another prognostic factor identified was the genetic characteristic of the cell: Ploidy, or the total chromosome number, affects prognosis,[401] because an increased number identifies patients with a better prognosis. The worst prognosis is seen with pseudodiploidy: a normal number of chromosomes, but with structural abnormalities.[402] The underlying basis of the effect of these translocations may be explained by the genes encoded at the breakpoints. However, the clinical relevance of identifying genetic lesions in ALL is not only to identify patients at diagnosis who may benefit from a more aggressive therapy such as BMT but also to use these genetic markers to monitor minimal residual disease after therapy.

Principles of Treatment and Results

The purpose of therapy in ALL is to eradicate invading leukemia cells and restore hematopoiesis. This is accomplished through a process beginning with remission induction, in which a 99% leukemic cell kill is attempted, followed by intensification and CNS treatment, and completed with consolidation and maintenance treatment.

Historically, achieving leukemic eradication has been a stepwise attempt. The natural history of ALL demonstrates a median survival of 2 months from time of diagnosis.[403] This began to change when, in 1947, Farber and associates noted the importance of folic acid to leukemic cell production and saw improvement in patients treated with the antimetabolite of folic acid, aminopterin.[404] In 1952, Elion and Hitchings[405] found nucleic acid synthesis to be important in cell turnover and, subsequently, thiopurines to be active in murine leukemia. Burchenal and coworkers[406] then showed 6-mercaptopurine to be effective in human leukemia and, at the same time, Pearson and Farber[407] independently discovered steroids to be lymphocytotoxic (lympholytic), resulting in transient ALL remissions. In 1955, the first clinical trial[408] randomized selected patients into stratified groups and qualitatively defined CR as "bone marrow clear of recognizable leukemia cells and resolution of leukemic infiltration of other organs and tissues, with reestablishment of normal hematopoietic elements in both the peripheral blood and bone marrow."

It became clear that the most significant factor for improved survival is achieving CR[409]; patients who achieved CR had an extended median survival of 10 months. The Acute Leukemia Group B[410] conducted the first combination trial comparing methotrexate (MTX) and 6-mercaptopurine, alone and in combination, and found an improvement in response but with an undesirable increase in toxicity. The toxicity was such that the doses had to be reduced, with a subsequent reduction in efficacy. Therefore, chemotherapeutic agents with different dose-limiting toxicities were postulated to provide better results without unacceptable side effects. In 1962, vincristine was introduced and found to be effective without bone marrow suppression and, in concert with steroid therapy, was synergistic.[411] Combination therapy was postulated to decrease drug resistance of leukemic cells by targeting multiple sites of action.[412]

Continued development of new agents, such as asparaginase and doxorubicin, increased the CR rate to over 95%[413]; however, most patients continued to relapse. Cytogenetic studies showed relapse to result from recurrent disease, not new disease: CNS disease was responsible for 50% to 60% of the relapses, frequently with normal bone marrow, and it was theorized that the drugs used had not penetrated the blood-brain barrier. Therefore, any leukemia cells in the CNS at diagnosis could be treated briefly with intrathecal MTX, but would soon relapse, occasionally reseeding the bone marrow, leading to subsequent bone marrow disease. Therefore, low-dose brain radiation therapy was used in conjunction with intrathecal MTX, which decreased meningeal leukemic relapse to less than 10%.[414] By the early 1960s, supportive care in the form of transfusions and antibiotics allowed for the possible cure of ALL, and with improved CR rates, CNS prophylaxis, and maintenance therapy, the overall cure rate increased to 40%.

As leukemic cell classification became possible by the mid-1970s, researchers noted that patients with T-cell ALL had an increased incidence of CNS disease. Radiation was found to be effective in prophylaxis as well as treatment of CNS relapse; however, minor atrophy was noted on brain imaging studies, along with a deficit in cerebral function, prompting questions of whether another means of prophylaxis could be used. Investigators[415, 416] studied systemic, intermediate-dose MTX compared with cranial irradiation, both with intrathecal MTX, as a CNS prophylaxis for ALL. Both arms provided a decrease in the risk of CNS relapse as compared with no CNS prophylaxis, but radiation therapy was deemed better. However, it was noted that, in the chemotherapy group, fewer patients had systemic and testicular relapses. Many protocols were subsequently conducted with regard to drug dosages and scheduling, aiming for less toxicity, while preserving the efficacy, as well as testing new agents.[417] Standard-risk and high-risk patient groups were also defined, stratified, and treated accordingly.[418] The standard-risk patients were treated with an attempt to increase efficacy while sparing toxicity, whereas high-risk patients were more intensively treated because of the high probability of relapse, accepting the increased toxicity. In treating these patients, a statistically significant difference in event-free survival (EFS) emerged, with the most important prognostic factor being the risk group assignment.

Niemeyer and colleagues[419] analyzed 17 large clinical studies and found the essential components of curative therapy to include intensive early therapy (consisting of three or more drugs) and adequate CNS prophylaxis. High-risk patients received a further increase in therapy with a second or reinduction course, after the initial induction and consolidation phases, and EFS improved to 70%. The addition of epipodophyllotoxins and higher dose single agents were also proposed with varying results.[420, 421] The various EFSs obtained were difficult to evaluate and compare because the criteria for standard and high risk were not uniform and the methods of data analysis were also different, with varying follow-up durations. A collaboration in the mid-1990s produced a uniform risk classification system so that these variables will be accounted for in future studies, thus making them more accessible to comparison.[422]

The 30-year experience at St. Jude's Children's Research Hospital, as delineated by Rivera and associates,[423] exemplifies the pediatric experience with ALL. Figure 23–3 demonstrates an EFS from 1962 to 1966 of 9±3%; by 1967 to 1979, the EFS increased to 36±2% with the realization of the need for CNS prophylaxis. As further systemic advances were made from 1979 to 1983, the EFS further rose to 53±2%, and with further intensification and the knowledge of non–cross-resistant drug pairs, the overall EFS was reported at 71±4% by 1984 to 1988. Problems with deaths from infection during remission improved from 33% to less than 1% with the advent of *Pneumocystis carinii* pneumonia prophylaxis. However, at this time a new entity emerged, namely secondary leukemia.

As investigators attempted to intensify therapy and increase survival, they noted that this, in turn, increased morbidity. The Berlin-Frankfurt-Munster (BFM) protocol used by the French and Belgian groups[424] increased the disease-free survival of moderate-risk and high-risk patients to the level of the standard-risk patients; however, there was an associated high toxicity during the early phases of treatment. The subsequent BFM protocol[425] had a CR rate of 98.7% and a 6-year EFS of 72±2%, and the benefit of intensive reinduction was confirmed even in the standard-risk patients. The Dutch Childhood Leukemia Study Group[426] also reported an EFS at 6 years of 82±2.8% in non–high-risk patients; most of the relapses were isolated to the bone marrow. The major advantage of this protocol was the excellent EFS without the use of anthracyclines, alkylating agents, or cranial radiation therapy in this specific group of patients, thus potentially decreasing the post-treatment long-term sequelae without compromising efficacy.

Supportive Care

As previously stated, with the advancements in chemotherapeutic protocols, the overall EFS for children with ALL is 70%. However, certain groups still have an EFS of less than 50%, thus warranting an intensification of treatment in these patients. With the increase in myelosuppressive agents, patients have longer periods of neutropenia and a subsequent increase in infectious episodes. Also, prolonged periods of neutropenia result in increases in time between chemotherapy treatments and an inability to give the patients the intensification proposed. As a result of this problem, the availability of specific colony-stimulating factors and their role in preventing neutropenia and its problems have been studied.

Welte and colleagues[427] randomized patients with high-risk ALL who would receive intensive chemotherapy to

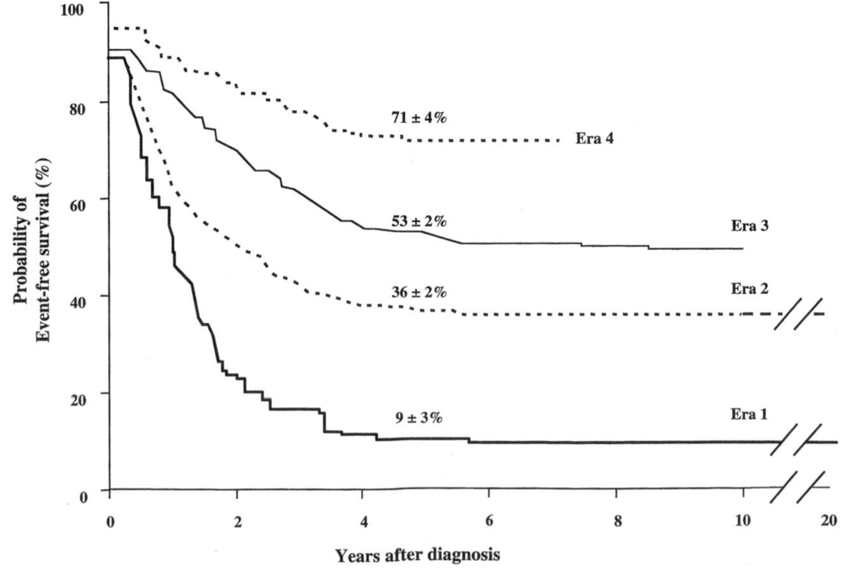

Figure 23–3. Kaplan-Meier estimates (±SE) of event-free survival rate among 1702 children with acute lymphoblastic leukemia, according to treatment era. Event-free survival was significantly improved from each era to the next (p <0.001 by the log-rank test). (From Rivera GK, Pinkel D, Simone JV, et al: Treatment of acute lymphoblastic leukemia: 30 years' experience at St. Jude Children's Research Hospital. N Engl J Med 1993; 329:1289, with permission.)

receive or not receive prophylactic G-CSF. Fever and neutropenia were documented for each group, with 17% noted in the G-CSF–treated group and 40% in the untreated group ($p = 0.007$). Statistically significant differences were also noted in the number of days of neutropenia (17.4 days vs. 61.6 days; $p < 0.001$), the percentage of chemotherapy delays (29% vs. 51%; $p = 0.007$), the incidence of fever (29% vs. 46%) and bacterial infections (8% vs. 15%; $p = 0.04$), and mucositis (2% vs. 8%, $p = 0.07$). There were no differences in severe infections, pneumonias, and septicemias. Overall treatment outcome, however, was not affected. Pui and coworkers[428] studied G-CSF in children with ALL treated on a randomized, double-blind, placebo-controlled trial. The G-CSF–treated group demonstrated a more rapid recovery from neutropenia (6.1 days vs. 14 days; $p = 0.007$); however, the rate of hospitalization and median hospital days were not statistically different. Once again, there was a significant difference in documented infections (12% vs. 27%; $p = 0.009$), but not a difference in severe infections. There was no difference in treatment or treatment outcome; however, a postulated difference in quality of life may be made.

Bone Marrow Transplantation

With new chemotherapeutic agents introduced over the past 20 years, well-implemented protocols, and better definition of high-risk versus standard-risk patients, more patients with ALL survive beyond 5 years and proceed to lead healthy lives. Unfortunately, the patients who relapse become a more difficult group of patients to treat and ultimately cure.[429, 430] Patients who do not respond to induction chemotherapy or who relapse while on therapy or within 6 months of the completion of therapy have a very poor prognosis[431]; thus, many proceed to BMT as an alternative treatment. Late relapses in these patients may have a more favorable prognosis.[432]

BMT, also called stem cell transplantation, is a means of administering very-high-dose chemotherapy or radiation therapy, or both, to manage the relapsed disease while rescuing the patient by infusion of his or her own previously harvested stem cells (autologous, auto-BMT) or the stem cells of a healthy compatible related or unrelated donor (allogeneic, allo-BMT). BMT has been used in patients with selected high-risk ALL in first complete remission with better results compared with chemotherapy alone. In Ph^1-positive ALL and infant t(4;11) ALL, for example, BMT in first remission has shown improved results compared with BMT performed after relapse. A City of Hope study found a disease-free survival (DFS) of 61% for those high-risk patients transplanted in first remission.[433, 434] An update, with a 10-year follow-up, continued to show these results (46% vs. 28%); however, the difference was no longer statistically significant.[435]

BMT has long been used for relapsed leukemia with varying success. The Italian BMT group published their 10-year experience comparing allo-BMT and chemotherapy in a relapsed group.[436] The 5-year DFS for the allo-BMT group was 41.1%, whereas that for the chemotherapy group was 21.7%. Furthermore, it was noted that patients who relapsed within 30 months of initial CR did better with allo-BMT compared with chemotherapy alone (3-year DFS of 33.4% vs. 16.1%, respectively, $p = 0.002$). The difference in outcome with chemotherapy in those patients relapsing early versus late was statistically significant ($p = 0.0001$), with those relapsing after 30 months faring much better.

As the science of allo-BMT has improved, alternative donors have been used for high-risk patients. These sources include partially mismatched related donors, as well as both matched and mismatched unrelated donors. Szydlo and colleagues published a review of the results of allo-BMT for leukemia reported to the International Bone Marrow Transplant Registry (IBMTR).[437] There were more than 2000 patients with BMT with data available for analysis: 20% of HLA-identical sibling BMT, 32% of HLA-mismatched related BMT, and 19% of unrelated donor BMT were performed for ALL. Overall, it was noted that patients who underwent alternative donor BMT had more advanced disease and lower pretransplant performance scores than patients receiving sibling transplants. This may result from the fact that patients who had unrelated donor BMT also had the longest time from initial diagnosis to BMT. An increase in transplant-related mortality and a decrease in leukemia-free survival were seen with alternative donor BMT, as compared with sibling BMT, but the relapse rate was the same. The increase in transplant-related mortality was ascribed to more graft failures, and an increased risk of acute and chronic GVHD.

Special Groups

Infant Leukemia

Infant ALL requires specific mention because it carries a significantly poorer prognosis and poses a considerable challenge to the treating physician. The clinical presentation and response to treatment of infant ALL have placed this entity in a distinct group. Neonates (<30 days of age) and infants (<365 days of age) may present with nonspecific symptoms, such as fever, feeding problems, and failure to thrive, or with systemic signs including significant hepatosplenomegaly and bleeding, associated with increased WBC and decreased platelets, respectively. Most infants present with CNS disease at diagnosis. The most significant finding is the genetic translocation of t(4:11)(q21;q23) in cells of early B-cell lineage, which are usually HLA-DR positive, CD19 positive, but CALLA (CD10) negative.

Chen and associates[438] reviewed 30 cases of infant ALL by molecular, genetic, and normal cytogenetic analyses. Overall, 70% of infants were found to have 11q23 rearrangements, some of which required molecular analysis for detection. This result correlated with poor prognosis, with an EFS at 46 months of 15% in those patients with the 11q23 rearrangement and 80% in patients with the normal germline 11q23. Cimino and coworkers[439] studied 15 infants with ALL and reported that of those 12 patients with *HRX* rearrangements, 11 died of progressive disease whereas the 3 patients with germline *HRX* were alive and in complete remission. From these data, the Pediatric Oncology Group (POG) conducted a retrospective analysis of bone marrows from patients with infant ALL.[440] *HRX* (*MLL*) rearrangements were detected in 81% of the cases, two thirds found by standard cytogenetic analysis alone, whereas one third required molecular techniques. Molecular analysis is vital to defining these rearrangements and should be done in concert with standard cytogenetic techniques. Hilden and colleagues[441] compared MLL gene rearrangements and fusion transcripts in infants with ALL, using Southern blot analysis and RT-PCR, respectively. Southern blotting most often detected unusual rearrangements, whereas RT-PCR was not adequate for those unusual fusion transcripts formed from uncommon breakpoints. RT-PCR should not, therefore, be used alone, but should be combined with Southern blotting.

The poor outcome in infant ALL is usually due to early treatment failure, with both bone marrow and CNS relapses, despite aggressive systemic chemotherapy and CNS treatment. The POG[442] documented a poor 4-year EFS of $27 \pm 6\%$ using an intensive therapeutic protocol. An elevated WBC of greater than 50,000/mm^3 was found in 56% of the patients; 55% were CALLA negative and 26% had CNS disease at diagnosis. Chromosome 11 abnormality was found in one third of the patients evaluated, and the majority of these had t(4;11)(q21;q23). Ninety-three percent entered CR, but 60% relapsed. The factors found to be significant for improved survival were diagnosis at greater than 274 days of age (57% vs. 18%) and an initial WBC of less than 50,000/mm^3 ($p = 0.007$). Similar studies reported by Reaman and associates[443] from the Children's Cancer Group revealed an overall EFS of 23% at 4 years. In reviewing the outcome of three POG studies, Rubnitz and coworkers[440] found an estimated EFS of 19% for those patients with a rearranged *HRX* versus 46% for those with germline *HRX*. The patients with the rearranged *HRX* had a younger median age at diagnosis and an increased initial WBC. Unlike the previously mentioned reports by Chen and Cimino, both of these groups had a poorer survival compared with older children with ALL. Infants with ALL, therefore, require more aggressive, innovative therapies, including bone marrow transplantation to increase their survival.

Down Syndrome and Acute Lymphoblastic Leukemia

Children with Down syndrome have historically demonstrated an increased risk of acute leukemia[444]; it has been noted to be in the range of a 10- to 30-fold increase in incidence from the general population. In a POG study,[445] these patients were found to be older than other diagnosed children and to have slightly higher hemoglobin levels. The patients had an improved CR rate with intensive therapy; however, this was associated with increased toxicity. Down syndrome patients tend to have other inherent medical problems on presentation, making chemotherapy treatment more precarious. The overall mortality was not increased, but morbidity was elevated compared with normal children. These patients can be cured of ALL, but must be closely monitored for adverse side effects.

Adult Acute Lymphoblastic Leukemia

Unlike ALL in children, ALL in adults portends a poor prognosis. The rate of CR is 70% to 80%, with long-term DFS of only 25% to 30%.[446, 447] New chemotherapeutic trials have attempted to improve survival. Understanding the differences in immunophenotyping and genetic abnormalities between adults and children may lead to advancements by individualizing therapy.

In a French multicenter trial,[448] it was noted that T-lineage (26% of patients) and B-lineage (63%) ALL were statistically different, both at presentation and after treatment. The T-lineage ALL adult patients were younger in age (77% <35 years of age vs. 50%; $p = .001$), had a male predominance (75% vs. 55%), presented with an increased WBC (WBC >30,000/mm^3 in 55% vs. 30.5%; $p < 0.001$) and, more commonly, had CNS involvement (10.5% vs. 5%; $p < 0.04$). In treating these patients, an overall 78% CR rate was achieved (81% for T-lineage and 74% for B-lineage ALL). Age was the most important favorable prognostic factor for T-lineage ALL; a 3-year DFS of 54.1% if younger than 35 years of age, compared with 27.2% if older than 35 years of age. In B-lineage ALL, initial WBC was most indicative, with a DFS of 36% if WBC lower than 30,000/mm^3, and 15.2% if above 30,000/mm^3. Overall, T-lineage ALL had a more favorable prognosis, unlike that noted in children. Patients were not stratified by cytogenetic characteristics, so the decrease in B-lineage ALL survival may have been secondary to Ph^1-positive ALL, which has a very poor prognosis.

The Groupe Français de Cytogenetique Hematologique[449] examined ploidy and translocations in adult ALL patients. Clonal chromosomal abnormalities were found in 85% of those tested. The most common abnormality was the Ph^1 chromosome. It was found in older patients (median age 38 years) and correlated with a shorter EFS duration of 6 months and a 3-year EFS of 0%. Those patients without the Ph^1 chromosome had a median age of 21 years and a median EFS duration of 46 months, with a 3-year EFS of 52%. Rearrangements involving chromosome 11q23 were also found to correlate with a poor prognosis. Of the T-lineage patients, 26% had rearrangements of chromosome 14, 14% with t(10;14). The t(10;14) conferred a favorable prognosis with a 3-year EFS of 75%, whereas the other chromosome 14 abnormalities had an EFS of 42%.

The principles of treatment for adult ALL[450] are similar to those for childhood ALL, but poorer outcomes warrant innovative changes. Weiss and coworkers[451] attempted to intensify induction remission, with the addition of high-dose ara-C and mitoxantrone and the support of G-CSF. The incidence of CR increased and time to CR (a presumed prognostic indicator) decreased significantly, but the slight increase in median survival was not statistically significant. Attal and colleagues[452] attempted to improve survival by incorporating BMT into ALL consolidation protocols. Allo-BMT demonstrated a 3-year DFS of 68%, whereas auto-BMT had a DFS of 26%. However, the toxicity of allo-BMT was significant, with transplant-related deaths reaching 12% (vs. 2% with auto-BMT), and increased incidences of acute and chronic GVHD of 37% and 17%, respectively. In addition, the relapse rate with allo-BMT was 12%, very low compared with the 62% seen with auto-BMT. Data from the IBMTR reported by Horowitz and associates[453] confirmed the lower relapse rate (26% for BMT vs. 59% for chemotherapy-treated patients), but the high toxic death rate (38% vs. 4%, respectively) had its impact on DFS (44% vs. 38%, respectively). Improvements with allo-BMT may decrease the toxicity rate and eventually result in an increase in overall DFS.

CNS prophylaxis is also key to the prevention of CNS relapse and subsequent bone marrow relapse in adult ALL. As the results from childhood ALL have demonstrated, CNS prophylaxis with intrathecal or systemic chemotherapy, or both, has resulted in decreases in CNS leukemia. This decrease is more pronounced in high-risk patients.[454]

Elderly patients (>60 years of age) deserve special mention and consideration. They are usually excluded from clinical trials because of their decreased tolerance to chemotherapy and because of coexisting medical conditions.[450] They also have more adverse biologic features, with a higher incidence of Ph^1-positive ALL and a lower incidence of T-lineage ALL. In sequential studies,[455, 456] the CR rate was 65%, but the median survival was only 4 months with an overall 3-year survival of 21%.

To further investigate the poor outcomes in adult ALL, Brisco and coworkers[457] have examined MRD and its correlation to outcome. Other investigators[458, 459] showed the level of MRD at the end of induction to correlate with long-term survival in childhood ALL. These Australian studies found MRD to be greater in adults than in children, and increased in patients who relapsed. The authors postulated that adult ALL was more drug resistant than childhood ALL. Thus, advances such as new chemotherapeutic agents, immunomodulatory agents, and BMT must be explored to win the battle against adult ALL.

Complications of Therapy

Long-Term Sequelae

With an incidence of approximately 7800 new cases per year and a 5-year overall survival rate of 70%, there are 5400 patients per year who will become long-term survivors.[460] By the year 2010, one of every 250 adults between the ages of 15 and 45 years will be a survivor of childhood cancer.[461] As this circumstance occurs, long-term sequelae become a major concern. Some children may have complications secondary to the disease itself or to the treatment of the disease, namely side effects of chemotherapy and radiation therapy. Of note are the effects of anthracycline-induced cardiotoxicity, chemotherapy- and radiation-associated neurotoxicity, various endocrine deficiencies, and the risk of secondary malignancies.

CARDIOTOXICITY

Anthracyclines, specifically doxorubicin, have been shown to be very active in the treatment of ALL, and some protocols reportedly used up to 550 mg/m^2 of doxorubicin as a total dose. Lipshultz and associates[462] reported that 10% of the evaluated patients had acute congestive heart failure: Half responded to medications, whereas half had recurrent heart failure; two patients required cardiac transplantation. On echocardiograph evaluation, the only significant finding was decreased left ventricular posterior wall thickness in these patients as compared with controls. Impaired function occurred when the total anthracycline dose was greater than 227 mg/m^2 ($p < 0.0001$). In fact, 65% of patients who received more than this amount had increased afterload, decreased contractility, or both. Fractional shortening was also significantly decreased in these patients.

Analysis revealed the risk factors for cardiac abnormality to be higher doses of doxorubicin, a longer time between completion of doxorubicin treatment and echocardiogram, and younger than 4 years of age at the time of treatment. However, most of the patients were asymptomatic. Arrhythmias were uncommon, and even decreased left ventricular exercise tolerance did not correlate with ventricular abnormalities. The median length of time from completion of the chemotherapy to this study was 6.4 years, with a median age of 13.5 years at study and 4.8 years at diagnosis. In a subsequent analysis, Lipshultz and coworkers[463] found decreased left ventricular contractility and mass to be more pronounced in females. A younger age at diagnosis continued to be significant.

NEUROTOXICITY

Many chemotherapeutic agents have associated neurotoxicity, such as vincristine-associated sensorimotor peripheral neuropathy, myelopathy from MTX, and demyelination or even necrosis from MTX and cranial radiation therapy.[464, 465] Patients can present with a variety of symptoms during treatment. The symptoms can be mild and reversible, and they include areflexia, sensory impairment, muscle weakness to eventual atrophy, pain, and delays in nerve conduction that may be permanent. Harila-Saari and colleagues[466] reported decreases in amplitudes of median nerve somatosensory evoked potentials of patients compared with controls. These amplitudes were more affected after CNS therapy. Treatment produced some recovery, but, in less successful cases, amplitudes did not return to normal.

Neurotoxicity is more common in women and children who receive CNS therapy in the treatment of ALL.[467–469] Various forms of treatment have been used in the place of radiation therapy, namely intrathecal agents with intermediate to high doses of systemic therapy, in order to prevent CNS relapse. However, the long-term neurotoxicity is reportedly equal to that of radiation therapy.

SECOND MALIGNANCIES

Chemotherapeutic agents are mutagenic, and they can lead to the development of secondary neoplasms. A retrospective analysis of close to 10,000 patients by the Children's Cancer Study Group[470] found 43 second malignancies, occurring 3 months to 13.2 years after the diagnosis of ALL. Fifty-six percent were CNS tumors, whereas 23% were new leukemias or lymphomas. The actuarial estimated cumulative proportion of patients with secondary malignancies increased with time, from 0.3% to 1.52% to 2.53% at 5, 10, and 15 years from diagnosis, respectively. The group found no association between sex, race, or the doses of cyclophosphamide or anthracycline and the occurrence of a second malignancy. However, a significant 3.3-fold reduction of risk occurred in patients who were diagnosed with ALL after the age of 5 years. Those patients who received radiation therapy, either with initial treatment or at relapse, had an increased risk, at 10 years after diagnosis, of having a second tumor (1.6% in the radiation group vs. 0.3% in the nonradiation group). All of the CNS tumors occurred in irradiated patients. Unfortunately, no plateau was noted in the occurrence of secondary tumors in irradiated patients. No epipodophyllotoxins were used in the aforementioned patients. However, more recently, epipodophyllotoxins have been implicated in second malignancies, most commonly leukemias, and these malignancies have been noted to occur within a shorter time from the completion of chemotherapy.

Chronic Lymphocytic Leukemia

Epidemiology and Etiology

Epidemiology

Chronic lymphocytic leukemia (CLL) is the most common type of leukemia in the western hemisphere, accounting for approximately 30% of leukemias, but is rare in Asia.[471] CLL is a disease primarily of the elderly (≥70 years of age), with an incidence of about 20 to 30 cases per 100,000.[472] The disease is rarely seen before the age of 40.[473] In a more recent period, from 1989 to 1993, the diagnosis was made at a later age (71.0 years), compared with 1980 to 1989, when it was diagnosed at 65.8 years.[474] In this later period, the disease was also diagnosed more often in a low-risk clinical stage, and the survival had markedly improved, which led the authors to suggest that the natural history of CLL had changed. The male-to-female ratio has been described as approximately 2:1,[473, 475] although in a study of 137 patients at a London hospital, the ratio was about 1.3:1.[476]

Etiology

In a study of workers in the petroleum distribution industry, the risk of CLL was most closely related to duration of employment; the highest risk occurred in white collar workers with long service.[477] However, these workers had received only background levels of benzene exposure, the known industry-associated carcinogen. In a meta-analysis of all cohort studies of petroleum workers in the United States and the United Kingdom, there was no increase in CLL (or in chronic myeloid or acute lymphocytic leukemias).[478]

CLL is the only leukemia that has not been associated with radiation.[225] Although some support has been offered in the literature for a relationship between exposure to magnetic fields and leukemia, especially for CLL, a review of the latest studies indicates that no firm conclusions can be drawn because of inconsistencies between and within studies, which weakened the evidence.[476] CLL has a family occurrence rate that is 2-fold to 7-fold higher than in control populations,[480] and families may also have an increased risk of other leukemias or lymphomas.[481, 482]

Pathogenesis

The use of the G6PD chromosome–linked marker demonstrated that a single G6PD enzyme type was found in neoplastic B-cells of patients with CLL, but granulocytes, erythrocytes, platelets, and some lymphocytes displayed enzyme variants in proportions similar to that in skin.[483, 484] This observation provided the initial evidence that CLL has a clonal origin, arising from a progenitor cell after the B-cell pathway has diverged from the myeloid and T-lymphocyte pathways. More recent molecular studies of Ig heavy chain gene rearrangements have confirmed these earlier findings.[485]

The observation that cells in most patients with CLL synthesize a monoclonal immunoglobulin with the same light chain and the same variable region was further evidence that, at the time of diagnosis, all CLL cells are descended from a single progenitor. Confirming this origin of CLL is the lack of t(14;18) chromosomal rearrangement in CD34+/CD19+ cells[486] and the presence of the same clone in CLL and in the transformed cells of high-grade lymphoma in patients with Richter's syndrome.[487, 488] A 1997 finding, which awaits confirmation, is that trisomy 12 and Rb deletion (retinoblastoma gene) may occur in CD34+ cells in a subset of patients with CLL, indicating that a less committed hematopoietic cell may be a target for malignant transformation in B-cell CLL.[489]

Chromosomal Abnormalities

CYTOGENETICS

Approximately 40% to 50% of patients have clonal chromosomal abnormalities identified by conventional cytogenetics. This may be an underestimation because chromosomal changes may occur in one or more cell subsets of the malignant clone. Historically, trisomy 12 was described as the most common chromosomal rearrangement in CLL[490, 491]; however, advances in conventional cytogenetics and the application of interphase FISH have demonstrated that deletion of part of the long arms of chromosomes 11 and 13 might be more frequent chromosomal rearrangements in CLL.[492–494]

TRISOMY 12

Trisomy 12 may be present as the sole abnormality or in combination with other chromosomal rearrangements; it is detected by classic cytogenetics in 5% to 36% of patients with CLL and by FISH in 11% to 55% (Table 23–9). FISH studies are more representative of the true incidence of trisomy 12 because the interphase FISH methodology provides information on cells independent of their cycling

TABLE 23–9. **Incidence of Trisomy 12 Detected by Classic Cytogenetics and Interphase FISH**

No. of Patients Studied	Trisomy 12 (%)		Reference
	Cytogenetics	*FISH*	
979	36	N/A	Reviewed in Juliusson and Gahrton[491]*
42	5	14.2	Döhner et al[495]
183		11.5	Que et al[496]
117		35.0	Escudier et al[497]
50		16.0	Reinening et al[498]
85		20.0	Witzig et al[499]
50		14.0	Knauf et al[500]
42	9.5	19.0	Arif et al[501]
20		55.0	Lishner et al[502]
26	27.0	31.0	Finn et al[503]
340	9	20.0	Garcia-Marco et al[504]
61	6.5	11.4	Woessner et al[505]
200		14.0	Döhner et al[506]

FISH = fluorescence *in situ* hybridization.
*This review includes data from 16 centers, including results from the International Working Party on Chromosomes in CLL.

status. Because only a fraction of the cells are trisomic, either normal cells or disomic neoplastic B-cells are also present. The prevalence of trisomic cells varies among individual patients from 6% to 70%.[507–509]

It is generally believed that patients with trisomy 12 have an unfavorable prognosis when compared with a normal karyotype or patients demonstrating other chromosomal abnormalities.[490] Evidence from the late 1990s has documented that in patients with CLL and typical B-cell morphology, trisomy 12 was the most common abnormality.[500, 505, 509, 510] In a study of 544 patients, trisomy 12 was found to be characteristic of a subgroup of CLL with a more advanced disease stage and, possibly, worse prognosis[511]; follow-up analysis over a 4-year period demonstrated a clonal expansion of cells with trisomy 12 as the disease progressed.[509] These observations suggest that trisomy 12 might be relevant in the cell activation process in CLL.[504, 512, 513] In addition, the survival of patients with trisomy 12 (assessed by FISH) or with an abnormal karyotype (assessed by conventional chromosome banding analysis) was significantly shorter than the survival of patients with diploid karyotypes (7.8 years vs. 5.5 years vs. 14.4 years).[497] The observations that trisomy 12 was documented in B-cells but was absent from T-cells[508] and CD34+ cells in the majority of patients[489] again confirms that trisomy 12 occurs in a committed B-cell progenitor.

REARRANGEMENTS OF 13q

Structural rearrangements involving the long arms of chromosome 13 were found, through cytogenetics, to be the second most common chromosomal abnormality in CLL, and they are associated with a better prognosis than other clonal aberrations.[491, 514–516] The incidence has been estimated to range between 10% and 45%.[494, 509] FISH analysis documented deletion of 13q14 in 63% of patients, whereas Southern blot analysis of highly purified malignant cells indicated that the loss of this region may occur in more than 95% of malignant cells.[506, 517, 518] Allelic deletions of 13q12.3, encompassing the *BRCA2* gene, were found by interphase FISH in 80% of 35 patients with CLL, indicating that the loss of this region might represent the most frequent genetic event at chromosome 13q in CLL.[518] Although trisomy 12 or 13q rearrangements are found separately in a substantial proportion of cases with CLL, they coexist in only 2% to 5% of patients, implying that each change may play a distinct pathogenetic role.[519]

REARRANGEMENTS OF 11q

In CLL, the frequency of deletions of the long arm of chromosome 11 by conventional cytogenetics has been reported to be between 1% and 9%.[490, 520, 521] An interphase FISH study identified a clinical subset of B-cell CLL that is defined by deletion of 11q22.3–q23.1 in about 20% of B-cells, representing the second most frequent aberration following 13q12–14 deletions.[506] In a study of 214 patients with CLL, those with 11q deletions had a more rapid disease progression, and in those who were younger than 55 years old, the median survival time was significantly shorter.[506]

OTHER CHROMOSOMAL ABNORMALITIES

Three translocations involving the Ig heavy chain gene on the long arm of chromosome 14 occur sporadically in B-cell CLL, but the number of patients with these abnormalities is low. Three putative cellular oncogenes, *BCL1*, *BCL2*, and *BCL3*, have been found to be rearranged by these translocations.[502, 522, 523]

Detection and Diagnosis

Clinical Detection

CLL is an indolent disorder in which increased proliferation and prolonged survival of mature-looking lymphocytes can lead to an accumulation of lymphocytes in bone marrow, blood, lymph nodes, spleen, liver, and extralymphatic sites. Most cases are of the B-cell phenotype but also coexpress CD5.[524] Surface immunoglobulin is present, frequently of the IgM isotype or, less often, IgM and IgD, or IgD alone.[525] There is also a rare CLL with a T-cell phenotype (1% to 2%), which appears to be a distinct clinicopathologic entity from other T-cell lymphoproliferative diseases. It has an indolent course[526] and may be defined as having a systemic proliferation of CD3+, CD4+, CD8−, post-thymic T-lymphocytes.[527] Positive staining for CD23 may distinguish CLL from the more aggressive entity known as mantle cell lymphoma.

Clinical presentation may be very subtle, with discovery often being incidental, triggered by a finding of lymphocytosis on a routine blood count. Symptoms that may bring a patient to a physician's attention include lymphadenopathy, which may be very bulky in some cases. Other symptoms include fatigue, malaise, weight loss, and excessive sweating. Abdominal distention or discomfort from splenomegaly or hepatomegaly, or from both, may be present. Physical findings are usually lymph node enlargement and organomegaly. Infection is common as the disease progresses, most likely a result of a defective B-cell population, which can no longer produce an appropriate antibody response to infectious agents.

Diagnosis

Diagnosis may be made with a persistent lymphocytosis of greater than 10 × 10^3/mm^3.[524] If the lymphocyte count is between 5 and 10 × 10^3/mm^3, additional studies to establish clonality are necessary for diagnosis. For lymphocyte counts less than 5 × 10^3/mm^3, a relative lymphocytosis (>50% of peripheral white count) and evidence of monoclonality may establish the diagnosis.[528] Surface immunoglobulins and other B-cell markers are usually present.[525] The bone marrow is usually hypercellular with 20% to 30% of nucleated cells being mature-appearing lymphocytes; lymph nodes, when involved, are diffusely infiltrated by a monotonous population of small lymphocytes.[525] Thrombocytopenia and anemia may be present; if severe, these are poor prognostic signs. Hypogammaglobulinemia may be present in up to 40% of cases.

Classification

There are two common staging systems for CLL, the Rai and Binet classifications (Table 23–10). The consensus for absolute lymphocyte count threshold level is less than 5 × 10^3/mm^3, and bone marrow lymphocytosis must be greater than 30%.[532] The median duration of survival in patients with Rai stage 0 or Binet stage A disease exceeds 10 years. In a review of 745 cases of CLL, clinical staging by either of these classifications was valuable in discriminating patients with different survival prognoses.[533] Subdividing further by nodal size offered no additional advantage.

In the Revised European-American Lymphoma Classification, B-cell CLL is described as B-cell CLL/prolymphocytic leukemia/small lymphocytic lymphoma (CLL/SLL) under peripheral B-cell neoplasms.[534] The Revised European-American Lymphoma Classification group's lymphoid neoplasms are well defined by morphologic, immunophenotypic, and genotypic characteristics. Morphologically, CLL/SLL cells are uniform, slightly larger than normal lymphocytes, with a round, smooth nucleus. Immunophenotypically, they express pan–B-cell antigens (CD19, CD20, CD22), and the T-cell antigen CD5 in fresh tissue. Surface immunoglobulin is present, and is frequently an IgM or IgM and IgD isotype. Rearrangement of the heavy-chain and light-chain genes is found in the majority of cases, and trisomy 12 occurs in approximately one third.

Another prognostic factor, in addition to stage, appears to be lymphocyte doubling time. Patients with shorter doubling times (<1 year) have a significantly lower survival rate than those with doubling times greater than 1 year.[535] Age and sex may also alter prognosis, with patients 70 years of age or older faring worse than younger patients, and women doing better than men in a multivariate analysis.[536] However, the significance of these variables is less than the stage variables of hemoglobin level, hepatomegaly, number of lymphoid areas involved, and lymphocytosis. In an Italian study of 264 patients, 53 patients who were younger than 50 years of age did better than the 201 patients who were 50 years of age or older.[537] In another multivariate analysis of 137 patients, older age again yielded a significantly worse prognosis, as did the presence of fever, in addition to higher stage (Binet or Rai) and the stage variables of lymphadenopathy, hemoglobin level, and platelet count.[476] In this study, the number of nodal sites was not a statistically significant prognostic factor on multivariate analysis. Hallek offers an excellent review of prognostic factors.[538]

Principles of Treatment

Observation

Observation alone is sufficient for many patients in the early stage of their disease. A randomized French study of 612 patients compared treatment versus no treatment in patients with Binet stage A disease.[535] There was no difference in 5-year survival between the treated (75%) and untreated groups (82%). In a review of the experience at one institution in London, it was found that 48% of their patients were deemed not to need treatment at presentation, and 36% never received any specific therapy, despite the

TABLE 23–10. **Staging of Chronic Lymphocytic Leukemia**

Rai Classification[471, 529, 530]		
Modified Stage	***Stage***	***Definition***
Low risk	0	Lymphocytosis in blood and bone marrow
Intermediate risk	I	Lymphocytosis and lymphadenopathy
	II	Lymphocytosis and hepatomegaly, splenomegaly, or both; ± lymphadenopathy
High risk	III	Lymphocytosis and anemia (Hb < 11 g/dL); ± lymphadenopathy, splenomegaly, hepatomegaly
	IV	Lymphocytosis and thrombocytopenia (platelets < 100 × 10^3/mm^3); ± anemia and organomegaly

Binet Classification[530, 531]	
Stage	***Definition***
A	Hb ≥ 10 g/dL and platelets ≥ 100 × 10^3/mm^3; < 3 enlarged areas*
B	Hb ≥ 10 g/dL and platelets ≥ 100 × 10^3/mm^3; ≥ 3 enlarged areas
C	Hb < 10 g/dL and/or platelets < 10^3/mm^3; any number of enlarged areas

*Areas: head and neck (including Waldeyer's ring), axillary, inguinal (unilateral or bilateral for these are still one area), liver, spleen.

fact that their study covered patients spanning a 24-year period (1966 to 1990).[476] However, treatment should be instituted if patients develop significant anemia or thrombocytopenia (e.g., Rai stage III or IV, or Binet stage C).

Chemotherapy

Chlorambucil and prednisone combined have been the mainstay of first-line treatment of CLL patients. Although this combination has a higher response rate than chlorambucil alone, survival rates were not significantly improved in two early, small, randomized studies.[536, 539] Two later randomized trials did not show an improvement in response rate with the combination,[540, 541] whereas a third trial showed an improvement in response rate for Binet stage B patients, but not in overall survival.[542]

Prednisone increases CLL patients' susceptibility to infections, which are more severe and difficult to control after prednisone therapy.[543] A variety of polychemotherapy regimens have been compared with chlorambucil-prednisone, such as COP (cyclophosphamide, vincristine, and prednisone) or CHOP (cyclophosphamide, doxorubicin, vincristine, and prednisone); however, no regimen has consistently been shown to be better than chlorambucil-prednisone.[544] In a French randomized trial of Binet stage C patients, the addition of MTX to CHOP did not improve survival over CHOP alone.[542]

High-dose chlorambucil therapy (15 mg/day for a maximum of 6 months, followed by maintenance of 5 to 15 mg chlorambucil twice per week) has been compared with Binet's modified CHOP regimen in a large randomized trial.[545] The high-dose chlorambucil regimen was found to be superior for both response rate and for median survival (Table 23–11).

Fludarabine, a purine analogue, has shown significant activity in CLL, both in previously treated[546] and in untreated patients,[547–549] although overall survival was no different from other regimens, such as CHOP or CAP (cyclophosphamide, doxorubicin, prednisone).[547, 549] In the large French prospective randomized trial of fludarabine versus CAP, there was a significantly improved progression-free interval with fludarabine and a trend towards improved overall survival in previously untreated patients.[549] Response rates were high (>70%) in untreated patients,[547–550] and toxicity was low in most studies.[551] The addition of prednisone to fludarabine did not offer any additional benefit, as shown in a large clinical trial,[552] but did appear to increase the risk of infection. Although use of fludarabine as a first-line intervention, alone or in combination with 2-chlorodeoxyadenosine (another purine analogue with similar efficacy), is gaining acceptance, both are still considered second-line therapies at present, until results are available on studies in progress.[553]

TABLE 23–11. **Results of International Trial of High-Dose (HD) Chlorambucil Versus CHOP Regimen**

	% CR*	% CR + PR*	Median Survival (mo)	% 5-Yr Survival
HD Chlorambucil	61	89	68	61
CHOP	32	75	47	36

CHOP = cyclophosphamide, doxorubicin, vincristine, and prednisone; CR = complete remission; PR = partial remission.

*As percent of evaluable cases.

From Jaksic B, Brugiatelli M, Krc I, et al: High-dose chlorambucil versus Binet's modified cyclophosphamide, doxorubicin, vincristine, and prednisone regimen in the treatment of patients with advanced B-cell chronic lymphocytic leukemia: results of an international multicenter randomized trial. Cancer 1997; 79:2107–2114.

Radiation Therapy

There has been a long history of using radiation therapy in the treatment of CLL, either in standard daily treatment to local sites of bulky disease or to the entire body with low doses of external irradiation given intermittently over several weeks. Specialized techniques, such as extracorporeal irradiation of lymphocytes, endolymphatic irradiation, subtotal body irradiation, thymic irradiation, or splenic irradiation, have also been tried, as described in comprehensive reviews.[554, 555]

A small randomized trial (26 patients) compared chlorambucil and prednisone with two low-dose total body irradiation (TBI) regimens: 10 cGy/day, 3 days/wk × 5 wks, up to 3 courses (4.5 Gy total dose) or, later in the study, 5 cGy/day × 5 days/wk × 2 wks, up to 3 courses (1.5 Gy total dose).[556] There was a comparable median survival duration in the two groups (136 weeks in the TBI arms, and 135 weeks in the chemotherapy arm), but there was considerable hematologic toxicity and an inability to complete all planned courses in the TBI groups. A larger, randomized prospective trial with 108 consecutive patients who had a variety of indolent lymphoproliferative diseases, including CLL (41 patients), demonstrated that TBI was as effective as chlorambucil and prednisone in each of the diseases.[557] Median survival for CLL patients was 48 months with chemotherapy and 51 months with TBI (15 cGy/day, 2 days/wk × 5 wks, to a total dose of 1.5 Gy).

Splenic irradiation has been used effectively to decrease the lymphocyte load in patients with CLL, as well as to decrease spleen size and the pain associated with splenomegaly.[558, 559] Fraction sizes have been 0.25 to 1 Gy, given one to three times a week, to total doses from 1 to 12 Gy. Total doses greater than 5 Gy appear to be more effective in reducing spleen size.[559] However, this treatment is rarely used because it induces severe cytopenia.

Splenectomy

When an enlarged spleen contributes to thrombocytopenia or anemia, splenectomy may be helpful, although any contribution to increased survival has been in doubt because most studies reported in the past have been small and have not been controlled for prognostic factors. A 1997 study compared 55 patients who underwent splenectomy over a 22-year period with fludarabine-treated patients matched for age, serum albumin level, sex, hemoglobin level, Rai stage, number of prior therapies, and time from diagnosis.[560] There were major hematologic benefits in most post-splenectomy patients, with highly significant increases in hemoglobin and platelet concentration, as well as neutrophil concentration, which is not addressed generally in other studies. Overall survival was equivalent in the two

TABLE 23–12. **Results of Allogeneic Bone Marrow Transplantation (BMT) Trials in Chronic Lymphocytic Leukemia Patients**

Study	No. Pts.	Median Age/Range (yrs)	Conditioning Regimen	Status at BMT	Toxic Deaths	No. Pts. Alive in CR/Duration in Mos.
Rabinowe et al[561]	8	40/31–54	Cy/TBI	7 MD; 1 CR	1	7/6–18+
Bartlett-Pandite et al[562]	13	45/27–57*	Cy/TBI	—	2	8
Michallet et al[563]	54	41/21–58	Cy/TBI†	7 responsive 19 stable 21 progressive	25	24/5–80+
Khouri et al[564]	15	43/25–55	Cy/TBI	Relapse or refractory	2	8/3–60+

MD = minimal disease; CR = complete remission; TBI = total body irradiation; Cy = cyclophosphamide; Bu = busulfan.
*In overall group, which included 32 autologous BMT patients.
†Nineteen patients received ≥1 additional drugs; three patients received Bu/Cy only.

groups, although there was a nonsignificant increase in overall survival in the 29 patients with Rai stage IV disease who had splenectomy when compared with the 26 control patients with this stage.

Bone Marrow Transplantation

Although CLL is an indolent disease of older patients, and relatively nontoxic and effective chemotherapy exists, there is an emerging role for BMT as newer techniques (e.g., the use of stem cells and growth factors) make transplantation less toxic and, thus, more feasible for such patients. Table 23–12 is a summary of published results for CLL patients who have received an allo-BMT.[561–564] In most of these studies,[561–563] T-cell depletion was performed on the donor marrow for some or all of the patients. It is clear from these data that some patients have achieved remissions for more than 5 years.

The experience with auto-BMT is similar, as summarized in Table 23–13, although fewer patients have been reported.[561, 562–565] As seen in Tables 23–12 and 23–13, transplantation for CLL is usually performed in patients who are younger than 50 years, who will be able to tolerate this aggressive treatment. At present, high-dose therapy with transplantation is the only treatment that has the potential for actual cure of CLL. Longer follow-up in a larger number of patients will be necessary to assess the role of this experimental therapy in this disease.[566]

Special Considerations of Treatment

Prevention of Infection

Infections, primarily bacterial, are a major cause of morbidity and mortality in CLL patients. The principal factor responsible is hypogammaglobulinemia; patients with progressive disease and decreasing IgG levels are most susceptible to death from infections. It has been demonstrated in a randomized study that high-dose intravenous IgG levels protect against major bacterial infections,[567] but the cost is high in comparison with treatment of infections with antibiotics.[568] One study has shown that low-dose immunoglobulins for 6 or 12 months are effective as prophylaxis against infection, although this regimen was not cost effective.[569]

Biologic Therapy

Targeting antigens of CLL, with or without a conjugated radioisotope, is a theoretically attractive therapy option, but its use is still in its infancy. Promising results have been seen with iodine-131-Lymph-1, an anti-HLA-DR; adenopathy decreased in five of five patients, and lymphocytes also decreased in two of the five patients.[570] Other antibodies that have shown promise include CAMPATH-1[571, 572] and anti-CD20 antibody (IDEC C2B8 or rituximab)[569, 572, 573]; however, tumor lysis syndrome may occur in patients with high numbers of circulating lymphocytes treated with anti-CD20 antibody.[573]

Results and Prognosis

The disease may transform into an acute leukemia[574] or Richter's syndrome, which is a malignant large cell lymphoma that appears to arise from the original B-cell CLL, having the same immunoglobulin isotype and light chain type.[575] However, most patients die from the effects of the tumor directly, or from immunosuppression and infection.

TABLE 23–13. **Results of Autologous Bone Marrow Transplantation (BMT) Trials in Chronic Lymphocytic Leukemia Patients**

Study	No. Pts.	Median Age/Range (yrs)	Conditioning Regimen	Status at BMT	Toxic Deaths	No. Pts. Alive in CR/Duration in Mos.
Rabinowe et al[561]	12	45/27–54	Cy/TBI	10 MD; 2 CR	1	5/6–31+; 5—too early
Bartlett-Pandite et al[562]	32	45/27–57*	Cy/TBI	—	3	26
Khouri et al[565]	11	59/37–66	Cy/TBI	5 CR	2	6/2–29+

MD = minimal disease; CR = complete remission; Cy = cyclophosphamide; TBI = total body irradiation.
*In overall group, which included 13 allogeneic BMT patients.

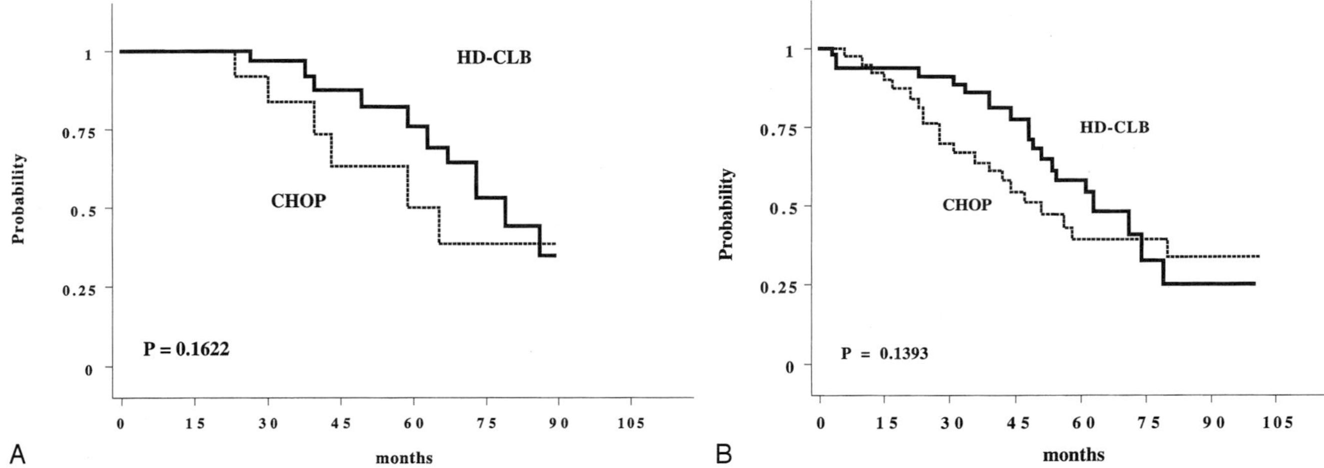

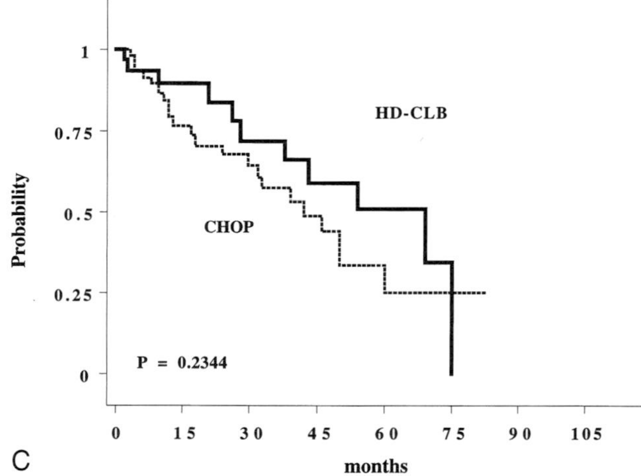

Figure 23–4. High-dose chlorambucil versus Binet's modified CHOP schedule according to Binet stage. (A) Stage A (46 patients). (B) Stage B (98 patients). (C) Stage C (78 patients). (From Jaksic B, Brugiatelli M, Krc I, et al: High-dose chlorambucil versus Binet's modified cyclophosphamide, doxorubicin, vincristine, and prednisone regimen in the treatment of patients with advanced B-cell chronic lymphocytic leukemia: results of an international multicenter randomized trial. Cancer 1997; 79:2107.)

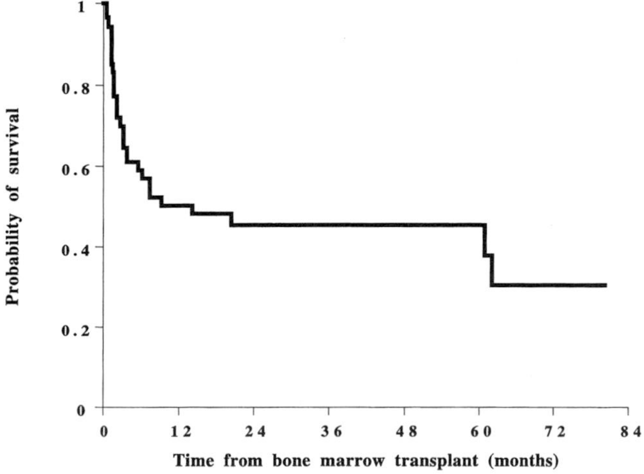

Figure 23–5. Survival probability after HLA-identical sibling bone marrow transplantation in 54 patients with chronic lymphocytic leukemia. At 12 months, 23 patients are considered to be at risk of dying: 24 months, 16 patients; 36 months, 9 patients; 48 months, 7 patients; 60 months, 6 patients; 72 months, 2 patients; 84 months, 0 patients. (From Michallet M, Archimbaud E, Bandini G, et al: HLA-identical sibling bone marrow transplantation in younger patients with chronic lymphocytic leukemia. Ann Int Med 1996; 124:311.)

Survival rates by Binet stage as a function of therapy (high-dose chlorambucil vs. CHOP) in the large randomized study previously cited[545] are shown in Figure 23–4. High-dose chlorambucil resulted in a significantly higher response rate than CHOP (see Table 23–11) and longer overall survival for the group as a whole, although survival differences were not significant within each stage.

Bone marrow transplantation results are still early, that is, patient numbers are small and follow-up is relatively short for this slowly progressing disease, but early results are promising (Figure 23–5).

Clinical Investigations

The most useful clinical trials in the future will be randomized trials involving fludarabine and other purine analogues, and stem cell transplantation studies in larger numbers of patients followed for long intervals. The role of monoclonal antibodies alone, or in combination with chemotherapy, still needs to be defined.

REFERENCES

General

1. Bennett JH: Two cases of hypertrophy of the spleen and liver, in which death took place from suppuration of the blood. Edinburgh Med Surg J 1845; 64:413.
2. Virchow R: Weisses Blut. Froriep's Notizen 1845; 30:151.
3. Virchow R: Die Leukemia. In: Virchow R (ed): Cesammelte Abhandlunge zur Wissenschaftlichen Medizin, p 190. Frankfurt, Meidinger, 1856.
4. Neumann E: Ein Fall von Leukamie mit Erkrankung des Knochenmarkes. Archiv fur Kinderheilkunde 1970; 11:1.
5. Naegeli O: Uber richt Knochenmark und Myeloblasten. Deutsch Medizinische Wochenschrift 1900; 26:287.
6. Cline MJ: The molecular basis of leukemia. N Engl J Med 1994; 330:328.

Specific

Acute Myeloid Leukemia

7. Ries LAG, Kosary C, Hankey B, et al (eds): SEER Cancer Statistics Review, 1973–1994. Bethesda, National Institutes of Health, 1994.
8. Smith MT: The mechanism of benzene-induced leukemia: a hypothesis and speculations on the causes of leukemia. Environ Health Perspect 1996; 104(suppl)6:1219–1225.
9. Greaves MF: Aetiology of acute leukaemia. Lancet 1997; 349:344–349.
10. Quesnel B, Kantarjian H, Bjergaard JP, et al: Therapy-related acute myeloid leukemia with t(8;21), inv(16), and t(8;16): a report on 25 cases and review of the literature. J Clin Oncol 1993; 11:2370–2379.
11. Toolis F, Potter B, Allan NC, et al: Radiation-induced leukemia in ankylosing spondylitis. Cancer 1981; 48:1582–1585.
12. Andersson M, Carstensen B, Visfeldt J: Leukemia and other related hematological disorders among Danish patients exposed to thorotrast. Radiat Res 1993; 132:224.
13. Ichimaru M, Ishimaru T, Belsky JL: Incidence of leukemia in atomic bomb survivors belonging to a fixed cohort in Hiroshima and Nagasaki, 1950–71: radiation dose years after exposure, age at exposure, and type of leukemia. J Radiat Res 1978; 1:262.
14. IARC Study Group: Direct estimates of cancer mortality due to low doses of ionizing radiation: an international study. Lancet 1994; 344:1039.
15. Kyle R: Second malignancies associated with chemotherapeutic agents. Semin Oncol 1982; 9:133.
16. Pedersen-Bjergaard J, Phillip P: Balanced translocations involving chromosome bands 11q23 and 21q22 are highly characteristic of myelodysplasia and leukemia following therapy with cytostatic agents targeting at DNA-topoisomerase II. Blood 1991; 78:1147.
17. Pedersen-Bjergaard J, Larsen SO: Incidence of acute nonlymphocytic leukemia, preleukemia and acute myeloproliferative syndrome up to 10 years after treatment of Hodgkin's disease. N Engl J Med 1984; 307:955.
18. Siegel M: Smoking and leukemia: evaluation of a causal hypothesis. Am J Epidemiol 1993; 138:1.
19. Mele A, Szklo M, Visani G, et al and the Italian Leukemia Study Group: Hair dye use and other risk factors for acute leukemia and pre-leukemia: a case-control study. Am J Epidemiol 1994; 139:609.
20. Sahl JD, Kelsh MA, Greenland S: Cohort and nested case-control studies of hematopoietic cancers and brain cancer among electric utility workers. Epidemiology 1993; 4:104.
21. Linet MS, Hatch EE, Kleinerman RA, et al: Residential exposure to magnetic fields and acute lymphoblastic leukemia in children. N Engl J Med 1997; 337:1.
22. Fong C, Brodeur GM: Down's syndrome and leukemia: epidemiology, genetics, cytogenetics and mechanisms of leukemogenesis. Cancer Genet Cytogenet 1987; 28:55.
23. Miller OJ, Berg WR, Schmike RN, et al: A family with XXXXY male, a leukaemic male, and two 21 trisomic mongoloid females. Lancet 1961; 2:78.
24. Auerbach AD, Allen RG: Leukemia and preleukemia in Fanconi anemia patients. Cancer Genet Cytogenet 1991; 51:1.
25. Shiraishi Y, Kobuchi H, Utsumi K, et al: Levels of sister-chromatid exchanges in hybrids between Bloom syndrome B-lymphoblastoid cells and various cell lines with lymphoid malignancy. Mutat Res 1990; 243:13–20.
26. Taylor AM, Metcalfe JA, Thick J, et al: Leukemia and lymphoma in ataxia telangectasia. Blood 1996; 87:423–438.
27. Greaves M: A natural history for pediatric acute leukemia. Blood 1993; 82:1043.
28. Miller RN: Deaths from childhood leukemia and solid tumors among twins and other sibs in the United States, 1960–67. J Natl Cancer Inst 1971; 56:203.
29. Devine DV, Gluck WL, Rosse WF, et al: Acute myeloblastic leukemia in paroxysmal nocturnal hemoglobinuria. J Clin Invest 1987; 79:314.
30. de Planque MM, Kluin-Nelemans HC, van Krieken HJM, et al: Evolution of acquired severe aplastic anemia to myelodysplasia and subsequent leukemia in adults. Br J Haematol 1988; 70:55.
31. Kwong YL: Leukemic risk in polycythaemia vera and essential thrombocytopenia. Eur J Haematol 1996; 56:90–92.
32. Spiegelman S, Axel R, Baxt W, et al: The relevance of RNA tumor viruses to human cancer. Johns Hopkins Med J 1973; 2(suppl):282–312.
33. Feuer G, Chen IS: Mechanisms of human T-cell leukemia virus-induced leukemogenesis. Biochim Biophys Acta 1992; 1114:223–233.
34. Knecht H, Berger C, al-Homsi AS, et al: Epstein-Barr virus oncogenesis. Crit Rev Oncol Hematol 1997; 26:117–135.
35. Fialkow PJ, Singer JW, Adamson JW, et al: Acute nonlymphocytic leukemia: heterogeneity of stem cell origin. Blood 1981; 57:1068.
36. Fialkow P, Janssen J, Bartram C: Clonal remissions in acute nonlymphocytic leukemia: evidence for a multistep pathogenesis of the malignancy. Blood 1990; 77:1415.
37. Fialkow PJ, Singer JW, Raskind WH, et al: Clonal development, stem cell differentiation and clinical remissions in acute nonlymphocytic leukemia. N Engl J Med 1987; 317:468.
38. Fialkow P, Singer J, Adamson J, et al: Acute nonlymphocytic leukemia: expression in cells restricted to granulocytic differentiation. N Engl J Med 1979; 301:1.
39. Mirro J, Kitchingman GR, Williams DL, et al: Mixed lineage leukemia: the implication for hemopoietic differentiation. Blood 1986; 68:597.
40. Wolff L: Contribution of oncogenes and tumor suppressor genes to myeloid leukemia. Biochim Biophys Acta 1997; 1332(3):F67–F104.
41. Radich JP, Kopecky KJ, Williams CL, et al: N-ras mutations in adult de novo acute myelogenous leukemia: prevalence and clinical significance. Blood 1990; 76:801.
42. Taylor JA, Sandler DP, Bloomfield CD, et al: Ras oncogene activation and occupational exposures in acute myeloid leukemia. J Natl Cancer Inst 1992; 84:1626.
43. Burke PJ, Braine HG, Rathbun HK et al: The clinical significance of fever in acute myelocytic leukemia. John Hopkins Med J 1976; 139:1.
44. Murray JC, Dorfman SR, Brandt ML, et al: Renal venous thrombosis complicating acute myeloid leukemia with hyperleukocytosis. J Pediatr Hematol Oncol 1996; 18(3):327–330.
45. Dekker AW, Elderson A, Punt K, et al: Meningeal involvement in

patients with acute nonlymphocytic leukemia. Cancer 1985; 56:2078.
46. Holmes R, Keating MJ, Cork A: A unique pattern of central nervous system leukemia in acute myelomonocytic leukemia associated with inv(16) (p13q22). Blood 1985; 65:1071.
47. Jaffe ES, Blattner WA, Blayney DW, et al: The pathologic spectrum of adult T-cell leukemia/lymphoma in the United States. Human T-cell leukemia/lymphoma virus-associated lymphoid malignancies. Am J Surg Pathol 1984; 8(4):263–275.
48. Byrd JC, Weiss RB: Recurrent granulocytic sarcoma. An unusual variation of acute myelogenous leukemia associated with 8;21 chromosomal translocation and blast expression of the neural cell adhesion molecule. Cancer 1994; 73(8):2107–2112.
49. Ferrandiz C, Ribera M, Flores A, et al: Sweet's syndrome and acute myelogenous leukemia. Int J Dermatol 1990; 29:209.
50. Rosti V, Bergamaschi G, Ponchio L, et al: c-abl function in normal and chronic myelogenous leukemia hematopoiesis: in vitro studies with antisense oligomers. Leukemia 1992; 6(1):1–7.
51. Glick AD, Paniker K, Flexner JM, et al: Acute leukemia of adults: Ultrastructural, cytochemical, and histological observations in 100 cases. Am J Pathol 1980; 73:459.
52. Wu CD, Medeiros LJ, Miranda RN, et al: Chronic myeloid leukemia manifested during megakaryoblastic crisis. South Med J 1996; 89(4):422–427.
53. Painetta E, Van Ness B, Bennett J: Lymphoid lineage associated features in acute myeloid leukemia: phenotypic and genotypic correlations. Br J Haematol 1992; 82:324.
54. Mrøzek K, Heinonen K, de la Chapelle A, et al: Clinical significance of cytogenetics in acute myeloid leukemia. Semin Oncol 1997; 24:17.
55. Erikson P, Gao J, Chang K-S, et al: Identification of breakpoint in t(8;21) acute myelogenous leukemia and isolation of a fusion transcript AML1/ETO, with similarity to drosophila segmentation gene, runt. Blood 1992; 81:1832.
56. Kakizuka A, Miller WH, Umesono K, et al: Chromosomal translocation t(15;17) in human acute promyelocytic leukemia fused RAR with a novel putative transcription factor, PML. Cell 1991; 66:663.
57. Grignani F, Fagiuli M, Alcalay M, et al: Acute promyelocytic leukemia: from genetics to treatment. Blood 1994; 83:10.
58. He LZ, Tribioli C, Rivi R, et al: Acute leukemia with promyelocytic features in PML/RARalpha transgenic mice. Proc Natl Acad Sci U S A 1997; 94:5302.
59. Zhang SF, Wang HL, Guo BY: A clinicopathological study of leukemic kidney. Chung Hua Nei Ko Tsa Chih 1992; 31(3):149–151.
60. Van der Hoven B, Thunnissen PL, Sizoo W: Tumour lysis syndrome in haematological malignancies. Neth J Med 1992; 40(1–2):31–35.
61. Salomon J: Spurious hypoglycemia and hyperkalemia in myelomonocytic leukemia. Am J Med Sci 1974; 267:359.
62. Sacchetti A, Grynn J, Pope A, et al: Leukocyte larceny: spurious hypoxemia confirmed with pulse oximetry. J Emerg Med 1990; 8(5):567–569.
63. Bennett JM, Catovsky D, Daniel MT, et al: Proposals for the classification of the acute leukemias. French-American-British (FAB) Cooperative Group. Br J Haematol 1976; 33:451.
64. Bennett JM, Catovsky D, Daniel MT, et al: Proposed revised criteria for the classification of acute myeloid leukemia. Ann Intern Med 1985; 103:626.
65. Bennett JM, Catovsky D, Daniel MT, et al: Criteria for the diagnosis of acute leukaemia of megakaryocyte lineage (M7). Ann Intern Med 1985; 103:460.
66. Bennett JM, Catovsky D, Daniel MT, et al: Proposals for the recognition of minimally differentiated acute myeloid leukaemia. Br J Haematol 1991; 78:325.
67. Carr JH, Rodak BF (eds): Clinical Hematology Atlas. Philadelphia, W.B. Saunders Co., 1999.
68. Lee EJ, Pollak A, Leavitt RD, et al: Minimally differentiated acute nonlymphocytic leukemia: A distinct entity. Blood 1987; 70:1400.
69. Matutes E, Pombo de Oliveira M, Foroni L et al: The role of ultrastructural cytochemistry and monoclonal antibodies in clarifying the nature of undifferentiated cells in acute leukemia. Br J Haematol 1988; 69:205.
70. Cuneo A, Ferrant A, Michaux JL, et al: Cytogenetic profile of minimally differentiated (FAB M0) acute myeloid leukemia: correlation with clinicobiologic findings. Blood 1995; 85:3688.
71. Nucifora G, Rowley JD: The AML1 and ETO genes in acute myeloid leukemia with a t(8;21). Leuk Lymphoma 1994; 14(5–6):353–362.
72. Schiffer CA, Lee EJ, Romiyasu T, et al: Prognostic impact of cytogenetic abnormalities in patients with de novo acute nonlymphocytic leukemia. Blood 1989; 73:263.
73. Catovsky D, Matutes E, Buccheri V, et al: A classification of acute leukaemia for the 1990's. Ann Hematol 1991; 62:16.
74. Liu PP, Hajra A, Wijmenga C, et al: Molecular pathogenesis of the chromosome 16 inversion in the M4Eo subtype of acute myeloid leukemia. Blood 1995; 85(9):2289–2302.
75. Haferlach T, Gassmann W, Loffler H, et al: Clinical aspects of acute myeloid leukemias of the FAB types M3 and M4Eo. Ann Hematol 1993; 66:165.
76. Olopade OI, Thangavelu M, Larson RA, et al: Clinical morphologic and cytogenetic characteristics of 26 patients with acute erythroblastic leukemia. Blood 1992; 80:2873.
77. Gassmann W, Loffler H: Acute megakaryoblastic leukemia. Leuk Lymphoma 1995; 18(suppl 1):69–73.
78. Helleberg C, Knudsen H, Hansen PB, et al: CD34+ megakaryoblastic leukaemic cells are CD38−, but CD61+ and glycophorin A+: improved criteria for diagnosis of AML-M7? Leukemia 1997; 11:830–834.
79. Imbert M, Nguyen D, Sultan C: Myelodysplastic syndromes (MDS) and acute myeloid leukemias (AML) with myelofibrosis. Leuk Res 1992; 16(1):51–54.
80. Zipursky A, Poon A, Doyle J: Leukemia in Down syndrome: a review. Pediatr Hematol Oncol 1992; 9:139.
81. Ravindranath Y, Abella E, Krischer JP, et al: Acute myeloid leukemia (AML) in Down's syndrome is highly responsive to chemotherapy: experience on Pediatric Oncology Group AML Study 9498. Blood 1992; 80:2210.
82. Pedersen-Bjergaard J, Phillip P, Larsen SO, et al: Chromosome aberrations and prognostic factors in therapy-related myelodysplasia and acute nonlymphocytic leukemia. Blood 1990; 76:1083.
83. Westbrook CA, LeBeau MM: Deletions of 5q in myeloid leukemia. In: Kirsch IR (ed): Causes and Consequences of Chromosomal Aberrations, p 223. Boca Raton, CRC Press, 1995.
84. Ratain MJ, Rowley JD: Therapy-related acute myeloid leukemia secondary to inhibitors of topoisomerase II: from bedside to the target genes. Ann Oncol 1992; 3:107.
85. Cartwright RA: Incidence and epidemiology of the myelodysplastic syndromes. In: Mufti GJ, Galton DAG (eds): The Myelodysplastic Syndromes. New York, Churchill Livingstone, 1992.
86. Rodella S, Ciccone G, Rege-Cambrin G, et al: Cytogenetics and occupational exposures in acute nonlymphocytic leukemia and myelodysplastic syndrome. Working Group on the Epidemiology of Hematolymphopoietic Malignancies in Italy. Scand J Work Environ Health 1993; 19(6):369–374.
87. Darrington DL, Vose JM, Anderson JR: et al: Incidence and characterization of secondary myelodysplastic syndrome and acute myelogenous leukemia following high dose chemoradiotherapy and autologous stem-cell transplantation for lymphoid malignancies. J Clin Oncol 1994; 12:2527.
88. Sanz GF, Sanz MA, Vallespi T, et al: Two regression models and a scoring system for predicting survival and planning treatment in myelodysplastic syndromes: a multivariate analysis of prognostic factors in 370 patients. Blood 1989; 74:395.
89. Mecucci C, van den Berghe H: Cytogenetics. Hematol Oncol Clin North Am 1992; 6:522.
90. Hiddemann W, Jahns-Streubel G, Verbeek W, et al: Intensive therapy for high-risk myelodysplastic syndromes and the biological significance of karyotype abnormalities. Leuk Res 1998; 22(suppl):S23–S26.
91. Seng JE, Peterson BA: Low dose chemotherapy for myelodysplastic syndromes. Leuk Res 1998; 22(6):481–484.
92. Boogaerts MA: Stem cell transplantation and intensified cytotoxic treatment for myelodysplasia. Curr Opin Hematol 1998; 5(6):465–471.
93. Estey EH: Incorporating new modalities into guidelines. Topotecan for myelodysplastic syndromes. Oncology 1998; 12:81–86.
94. Anderson JE, Appelbaum FR, Fisher LD, et al: Allogeneic bone marrow transplantation for patients with myelodysplastic syndrome. Blood 1993; 82:677.
95. Sutton L, Chastang C, Ribaud P, et al for the Societe Francaise de Greffe de Moelle: Factors influencing outcome in de novo myelodys-

plastic syndromes treated by allogeneic bone marrow transplantation: a long-term study of 71 patients. Blood 1996; 88:358.
96. Mitterbauer M, Fritzer-Szekeres M, Mitterbauer G, et al: Spontaneous remission after acute myeloid leukemia after infection and blood transfusion associated with hypergammaglobulinaemia. Ann Hematol 1996; 73(4):189–193.
97. Ino T, Hirano M, Kojima H, et al: Treatment results for unselected patients with acute myelogenous leukemia. During a 10-year period, August 1984 to July 1994. Rinsho Ketsueki 1996; 37(9):817–824.
98. Bassan R, Raimondi R, Lerede T, et al: Outcome assessment of age group-specific (± 50 years) post-remission consolidation with high-dose cytarabine or bone marrow autograft for adult acute myelogenous leukemia. Haematologica 1998; 83(7):627–635.
99. Bodey GP, McCredie KB, Keating MJ, et al: Treatment of acute leukemia in protected environment units. Cancer 1979; 44(2):431–436.
100. Daenen S, Erjavec Z, Uges DR, et al: Continuous infusion of ceftazidime in febrile neutropenic patients with acute myeloid leukemia. Eur J Clin Microbiol Inf Dis 1995; 14(3):188–192.
101. Karp JE, Dick JD, Angelopulos C, et al: Empiric use of vancomycin during prolonged treatment-induced granulocytopenia: randomized, double-blind, placebo-controlled clinical trial in patients with acute leukemia. Am J Med 1986; 81:237.
102. Freifeld A, Marchigiani D, Walsh T, et al: A double-blind comparison of empirical oral and intravenous antibiotic therapy for low-risk febrile patients with neutropenia during cancer chemotherapy. N Engl J Med 1999; 341(5):305–311.
103. Rowe JM, Andersen JW, Mazza JJ, et al: A randomized placebo-controlled phase III study of granulocyte-macrophage colony-stimulating factor in adult patients (>55 to 70 years of age) with acute myelogenous leukemia: a study of the Eastern Cooperative Oncology Group (E1490). Blood 1995; 86:457.
104. Stone RM, Berg DT, George SL, et al: Granulocyte-macrophage colony-stimulating factor after initial chemotherapy for elderly patients with primary acute myelogenous leukemia. N Engl J Med 1995; 332:1671.
105. Witz F, Harousseau JL, Cahn JY, et al: GM-CSF during and after remission induction treatment for elderly patients with acute myeloid leukemia (AML) [abstract]. Blood 1995; 86:512a.
106. Zittoun RA, Mandelli F, de Witte T, et al: Recombinant human granulocyte-macrophage colony stimulating factor (GM-CSF) during induction treatment of acute myelogenous leukemia (AML). A randomized trial from EORTC-GIMEMA leukemia cooperative groups [abstract]. Blood 1994; 84:231a.
107. Dombret H, Chastang C, Fenaux P, et al: A controlled study of recombinant human granulocyte colony-stimulating factor in elderly patients after treatment for acute myelogenous leukemia. N Engl J Med 1995; 332:1678.
108. Buchner T, Hiddemann W, Wormann B, et al: GM-CSF multiple course priming and long-term administration in newly diagnosed AML: hematologic and therapeutic effects [abstract]. Blood 1994; 84:27a.
109. Heil G, Hoelzer D, Sanz M, et al: A randomized, double-blind, placebo-controlled, phase III study of Filgrastim in remission induction and consolidation therapy for adults with de novo acute myeloid leukemia. Blood 1997; 90:4710.
110. Godwin JE, Kopecky KJ, Head DR, et al: A double-blind placebo-controlled trial of granulocyte colony-stimulating factor in elderly patients with previously untreated acute myelogenous leukemia: a Southwest Oncology Group Study (9031). Blood 1998; 91:3607.
111. Ohno R, Tomonaga M, Kobayashi T, et al: Effect of granulocyte colony-stimulating factor after intensive induction therapy in relapsed or refractory acute leukemia. N Engl J Med 1990; 323:871.
112. Ohno R, Naoe T, Kanamaru A, et al: The Kohseisho Leukemia Study Group: A double blind controlled study of granulocyte colony-stimulating factor started two days before induction chemotherapy in refractory acute myeloid leukemia. Blood 1994; 83:2086.
113. Peterson BL, Bhalla GK, Slabama NYH, et al: A phase III trial with or without GM-CSF administered before and during high dose cytarabine in patients with relapsed or refractory acute myelogenous leukemia. CALGB 9021. Proc Am Soc Clin Oncol 1996; 15(suppl):3.
114. Webb IJ, Anderson KC: Transfusion support in acute leukemias. Semin Oncol 1997; 24:141.
115. Wandt H, Frank M, Ehninger G, et al: Safety and cost effectiveness of a 10×10^9/l trigger for prophylactic platelet transfusions compared with the traditional 20×10^9/l trigger: a prospective comparative trial in 105 patients with acute myeloid leukemia. Blood 1998; 91:3601.
116. Gmur J, Burger J, Schanz U, et al: Safety of stringent prophylactic platelet transfusion policy for patients with acute leukemia. Lancet 1991; 338:1223.
117. Schiffer CA: Prevention of alloimmunization against platelets. Blood 1991; 77:1.
118. Vamvaka EC, Pineda AA: Meta-analysis of clinical studies of the efficacy of granulocyte transfusions in the treatment of bacterial sepsis. J Clin Apheresis 1996; 11:1.
119. Kumar L: Leukemia: management of relapse after allogeneic bone marrow transplantation. J Clin Oncol 1994; 12(80):1710–1717.
120. Neame PB, Soamboonsrup P, Leber B, et al: Morphology of acute promyelocytic leukemia with cytogenetic or molecular evidence for the diagnosis: characterization of additional microgranular variants. Am J Hematol 1997; 56(3):131–142.
121. Gralnick HR, Abrell E: Studies of the procoagulant and fibrinolytic activity of promyelocytes in acute promyelocytic leukemia. Br J Haematol 1973; 24:89.
122. Bennett B, Booth A, Croll A, et al: The bleeding disorder in acute promyelocytic leukemia: fibrinolysis due to u-PA rather than defibrination. Br J Haematol 1989; 71:511.
123. Sakata Y, Murakami T, Noro A, et al: The specific activity of plasminogen activator inhibitor-1 in disseminated intravascular coagulation with acute promyelocytic leukemia. Blood 1991; 77:1949.
124. Drapkin RL, Gee TS, Dowling MD, et al: Prophylactic heparin therapy in acute promyelocytic leukemia. Cancer 1978; 41:2484.
125. Cordonnier C, Vernant JP, Brun B, et al: Acute promyelocytic leukemia in 57 previously untreated patients. Cancer 1985; 55:18.
126. Kantarjian HM, Keating MJ, Walters RS, et al: Acute promyelocytic leukemia: M.D. Anderson Hospital experience. Am J Med 1986; 80:789.
127. Cunningham I, Gee TS, Reich LM, et al: Acute promyelocytic leukemia: treatment results during a decade at Memorial Hospital. Blood 1989; 73:116,
128. Rodeghiero F, Avvisati G, Castaman G, et al: Early deaths and anti-hemorrhagic treatments in acute promyelocytic leukemia: a GIMEMA retrospective study in 268 consecutive patients. Blood 1990; 75:2112.
129. Tallman MS, Kwaan HC: Reassessing the hemostatic disorder associated with acute promyelocytic leukemia. Blood 1992; 79:543.
130. Tallman MS, Andersen JW, Schiffer CA, et al: All-trans-retinoic acid in acute promyelocytic leukemia. N Engl J Med 1997; 337:1021.
131. Hansen OP, Pedersen-Bjergaard J, Ellegaard J, et al: Aclarubicin plus cytosine arabinoside versus daunorubicin plus cytosine arabinoside in previously untreated patients with acute myeloid leukemia: a Danish national phase III trial. The Danish Society of Hematology Study Group on AML, Denmark. Leukemia 1991; 5(6):510–516.
132. Bishop JF, Matthews JP, Young GA, et al: Intensified induction chemotherapy with high dose cytarabine and etoposide for acute myeloid leukemia: a review and updated results of the Australian Leukemia Study group. Leuk Lymph 1998; 28(3–4):315–327.
133. Wiernik PH, Banks PL, Case DC Jr, et al: Cytarabine plus idarubicin or daunorubicin as induction and consolidation therapy for previously untreated adult patients with acute myeloid leukemia. Blood 1992; 79:313.
134. Berman E, Heller G, San Torsa J, et al: Results of a randomized trial comparing idarubicin and cytosine arabinoside with daunorubicin and cytosine arabinoside in adult patients with newly diagnosed acute myelogenous leukemia. Blood 1991; 77:1666.
135. Vogler WR, Velez-Garcia E, Weiner RS, et al: A phase III trial comparing idarubicin and daunorubicin in combination with cytarabine in acute myelogenous leukemia: a Southwestern Cancer Study Group Study. J Clin Oncol 1992; 10:1103.
136. Plunkett W, Iacoboni S, Keating MJ: Cellular pharmacology and optimal therapeutic concentrations of 1-beta-D-arabinofuranosylcytosine 5'-triphosphate in leukemic blasts during treatment of refractory leukemia with high dose 1-beta-D-arabinofuranosylcytosine. Scand J Haematol 1986; 44:51.
137. Herzig RH, Wolff SN, Lazarus HM, et al: High dose cytosine arabinoside therapy for refractory leukemia. Blood 1983; 62:361.
138. Hiddemann W, Kreutzmann H, Straif K, et al: High dose cytosine arabinoside and mitoxantrone: a highly effective regimen in refractory acute myeloid leukemia. Blood 1987; 69:744.

139. Dillman RO, Davis RB, Green MR, et al: A comparative study of two different doses of cytarabine for acute myeloid leukemia: a Phase III trial of Cancer and Leukemia Group B. Blood 1991; 78:2520.
140. Schiller G, Gajewski J, Mimers S, et al: A randomized study of intermediate versus conventional-dose cytarabine as intensive induction for acute myelogenous leukemia. Br J Haematol 1992; 81:170.
141. Bishop JF, Matthews JP, Young GA, et al: A randomized study of high-dose cytarabine in induction in acute myeloid leukemia. Blood 1996; 87:1710.
142. Weick J, Kopecky J, Appelbaum F, et al: A randomized investigation of high dose versus standard dose cytosine arabinoside with daunorubicin in patients with previously untreated acute myeloid leukemia: a Southwest Oncology Group Study. Blood 1996; 88:2841.
143. Cassileth PA, Harrington DP, Hines JD, et al: Maintenance chemotherapy prolongs remission duration in adult acute nonlymphocytic leukemia. J Clin Oncol 1988; 6:583.
144. Mayer RJ, Davis RB, Schiffer CA, et al: Intensive post-remission chemotherapy in adults with acute myeloid leukemia. N Engl J Med 1994; 331:896.
145. Bloomfield CD, Lawrence C, Arthur DC, et al: Curative impact of intensification with high-dose cytarabine (hiDAC) in acute myeloid leukemia (AML) varies by cytogenetic group [abstract]. Blood 1994; 84(suppl 1):111a.
146. Thomas ED, Buckner CD, Banaji M, et al: One hundred patients with acute leukemia treated by chemotherapy, total body irradiation, and allo-BMT. Blood 1977; 49:511.
147. Zittoun RA, Mandelli F, Willemze R, et al: Autologous or allogeneic bone marrow transplantation compared with intensive chemotherapy in acute myelogenous leukemia. European Organization for Research and Treatment of Cancer (EORTC) and the Gruppo Italiano Malattie Ematologiche Maligne dell'Adulto (GIMEMA) Leukemia Cooperative Groups. N Engl J Med 1995; 332:217.
148. Blaise D, Maraninchi D, Archimbaud E, et al: Allogeneic bone marrow transplantation for acute myelogenous leukemia in first remission. Busulfan-Cytoxan versus Cytoxan-total body irradiation as preparative regimens: a report from the Groupe d'Etudes de la Greffe de Moelle Osseuse. Blood 1992; 79:2578.
149. Schiller GJ, Nimer SDF, Territo MC, et al: Bone marrow transplantation versus high-dose cytarabine-based combination chemotherapy for acute myelogenous leukemia in first remission. J Clin Oncol 1992; 10:41.
150. Carella AM, Frassoni F, Damasio E, et al: Allogeneic versus autologous marrow transplantation for patients with acute myelogenous leukemia in first remission. An update of the Genoa experience with 159 patients. Leukemia 1992; 6(suppl 4):78.
151. Weaver CH, Clift RA, Deeg HJ: Effect of graft-versus-host disease prophylaxis on relapse in patients transplanted for acute myelogenous leukemia. Bone Marrow Transplant 1994; 14:8851.
152. Mehta J, Powles R, Treleaven JG, et al: Long-term follow-up of patients undergoing allogeneic bone marrow transplantation for acute myeloid leukemia in first complete remission after cyclophosphamide total body irradiation and cyclosporine. Bone Marrow Transplant 1996; 18:741.
153. Gorin NC, Labopin M, Fouillard L, et al: Retrospective evaluation of autologous bone marrow transplantation vs. allogeneic bone marrow transplantation from an HLA identical related donor in acute myelocytic leukemia. A study of the European Cooperative Group for Bone Marrow Transplantation (EBMT). Bone Marrow Transplant 1996; 18:111.
154. ABMTR Newsletter: 1996 summary slides show current use and outcome of blood and marrow transplantation. Milwaukee, IBMTR/ABMTR Statistical Center 1996; 3:10.
155. Jourdan E, Maraninchi D, Reiffers J, et al for the Societe Francaise des Greffes de Moelle (SFGM): Early allogeneic transplantation favourably influences the outcome of adult patients suffering from acute myeloid leukemia. Bone Marrow Transplant 1997; 90:875.
156. Wells RJ, Woods WG, Buckley JD, et al: Treatment of newly diagnosed children and adolescents with acute myeloid leukemia: a Children's Cancer Group Study. J Clin Oncol 1994; 12:2367.
157. Michel G, Leverger G, Leblanc T, et al: Allogeneic bone marrow transplantation for children with acute myeloid leukemia in first complete remission: a prospective study from the French Society of Pediatric Hematology and Immunology (SHIP). Bone Marrow Transplant 1996; 18:455.
158. Warrell RP, Barrett AJ, Pandolfi PP, et al: Acute Myelocytic Leukemia, p 120. Paper presented at 39th Annual Meeting of the American Society of Hematology, December 6, 1997.
159. Sullivan KM, Weiden PL, Storb R, et al: Influence of acute and chronic graft-versus-host disease on relapse and survival after bone marrow transplantation from HLA-identical siblings as treatment of acute and chronic leukemia. Blood 1989; 73:1720.
160. Gale RP, Horowitz MM, Ash RC, et al: Identical-twin bone marrow transplants for leukemia. Ann Intern Med 1994; 120:646.
161. Marmon A, Horowitz MM, Gale RP, et al: T-cell depletion of HLA-identical transplants in leukemia. Blood 1991; 78:2120.
162. Cassileth PA, Lynch E, Hines JD, et al: Varying intensity of postremission therapy in acute myeloid leukemia. Blood 1992; 79:1924.
163. Cassileth PA, Harrington DP, Appelbaum FR, et al: Chemotherapy compared with autologous or allogeneic bone marrow transplantation in the management of acute myeloid leukemia in first remission. N Engl J Med 1998; 339:1649.
164. Reiffers J, Gaspard MH, Maraninchi D, et al: Comparison of allogeneic or autologous bone marrow transplantation and chemotherapy in patients with acute myeloid leukemia in first remission: a prospective controlled trial. Br J Haematol 1989; 72:57.
165. Appelbaum FR, Fisher LD, Thomas ED, and the Seattle Marrow Transplant Team: Chemotherapy v marrow transplantation for adults with acute non-lymphocytic leukemia: a five-year follow-up. Blood 1988; 72:179.
166. Conde E, Iriondo A, Rayon C, et al: Allogeneic bone marrow transplantation versus intensification chemotherapy for acute myelogenous leukemia in first remission: a prospective controlled trial. Br J Haematol 1988; 68:219.
167. Champlin RE, Ho WG, Gale RP, et al: Treatment of acute myelogenous leukemia, a prospective controlled trial of bone marrow transplantation versus consolidation chemotherapy. Ann Intern Med 1985; 102:285.
168. Estey EH, Kantarjian H, Keating MJ: Therapy for acute myeloid leukemia. In: Hoffman R, Benz EJ, Shattil S, et al (eds): Hematology Basic Principles and Practice, 2nd ed, p 1014. New York, Churchill Livingstone, 1995.
169. Beatty PG, Clif RA, Mickleson E, et al: Marrow transplantation from related donors other than HLA-identical siblings. N Engl J Med 1985; 313:765.
170. Aversa F, Tabilio A, Terenzi A: et al: Successful engraftment of T-cell-depleted haploidentical "three-loci" incompatible transplants in leukemia patients by addition of recombinant human granulocyte colony-stimulating factor-mobilized peripheral blood progenitor cells to bone marrow inoculum. Blood 1994; 84:3948.
171. Reisner Y, Martelli M: Bone marrow transplantation across HLA barriers by increasing the number of transplanted cells. Immunol Today 1995; 16:437.
172. Sierra J, Anasetti C: Marrow transplantation from unrelated donors. Curr Opin Hematol 1995; 2:444.
173. Sierra J, Storer B, Hansen JA, et al: Transplantation of marrow cells from unrelated donors for treatment of high-risk acute leukemia: the effect of leukemic burden, donor HLA-matching, and marrow cell dose. Blood 1997; 89:4226.
174. Hansen JA, Henslee-Downey J, McCullough J, et al: Analysis of 462 transplantations from unrelated donors facilitated by the National Marrow Donor Program. N Engl J Med 1993; 328:593.
175. de La Selle V, Gluckman E, Bruley-Rosset M: Newborn blood can engraft adult mice without inducing graft-vs-host disease across non H-2 antigens. Blood 1996; 87:3977.
176. Gluckman E, Rocha V, Boyer-Chammard A, et al: Outcome of cord-blood transplantation from related and unrelated donors. N Engl J Med 1997; 337:373.
177. Burnett AK, Tansey P, Watkins R, et al: Transplantation of unpurged autologous bone-marrow in acute myeloid leukaemia in first remission. Lancet 1984; 2:1068.
178. Korbling M, Hunstein W, Fliedner TM, et al: Disease-free survival after autologous bone marrow transplantation in patients with acute myelogenous leukemia. Blood 1989; 74:1898.
179. Santos GW, Yaeger AM, Jones RJ, et al: Autologous bone marrow transplantation. Ann Rev Med 1989; 40:99.
180. Gorin NC, Aegerter P, Auvert B, et al: Autologous bone marrow transplantation for acute myelocytic leukemia in first remission: a European survey of the role of marrow purging. Blood 1990; 75:1606.

181. McMillan AK, Goldstone AH, Linch DC, et al: High-dose chemotherapy and autologous bone marrow transplantation in acute myeloid leukemia. Blood 1990; 76:480.
182. Chao NJ, Stein AS, Long GD, et al: Busulfan/etoposide: initial experience with a new preparatory regimen for autologous bone marrow transplantation in patients with acute nonlymphoblastic leukemia. Blood 1993; 81:319.
183. Linker CA, Ries CA, Damon LE, et al: Autologous bone marrow transplantation for acute myeloid leukemia using busulfan plus etoposide as a preparative regimen. Blood 1993; 81:311.
184. Antin JH, Lee SJ, Chao NJ, et al: Bone marrow transplantation for hematologic malignancies, p 151. American Society of Hematology 39th Annual Meeting, December 6, 1997.
185. Brenner MK, Rill DR, Moen RC, et al: Gene-marking to trace origin of relapse after autologous bone-marrow transplantation. Lancet 1993; 341:85.
186. Murgo AJ, Weinberger BB: Pharmacological bone marrow purging in autologous transplantation: focus on the cyclophosphamide derivatives. Crit Rev Oncol Hematol 1993; 14(1):41–60.
187. Olivieri A, Poloni A, Montanari M, et al: Pharmacologic bone marrow purging: is there any place for etoposide? In vitro comparison with mafosfamide. J Hematother 1997; 6(2):137–144.
188. Hammert LC, Ball ED: Purging autologous bone marrow with monoclonal antibodies for transplantation in acute myelogenous leukemia. Blood Rev 1997; 11(2):80–90.
189. Miller CB, Rowlings PA, Jones RJ, et al: Autotransplants for acute myelogenous leukemia (AML): effect of purging with 4-hydroperoxycyclophosphamide (4HC). Blood 1995; 86:100a.
190. To LB, Roberts MM, Haylock DN, et al: Comparison of haematological recovery times and supportive care requirements of autologous recovery phase peripheral blood stem cell transplants, autologous bone marrow transplants and allogeneic bone marrow transplants. Bone Marrow Transplant 1992; 9:277.
191. Cassileth PA, Andersen J, Lazarus HM, et al: Autologous bone marrow transplant in acute myeloid leukemia in first remission. J Clin Oncol 1993; 11:314.
192. Lowenberg B, Verdonck LJ, Dekker AW, et al: Autologous bone marrow transplantation in acute myeloid leukemia in first remission: results of a Dutch prospective study. J Clin Oncol 1990; 8:287.
193. Amadori S, Testi AM, Arico M, et al for the Associazione Italiana Ematologia ed Oncologia Pediatrica Cooperative Group: prospective comparative study of bone marrow transplantation and postremission chemotherapy for childhood acute myelogenous leukemia. J Clin Oncol 1993; 11:1046.
194. Miller KB: Clinical manifestations of acute myeloid leukemia. In: Hoffman R, Benz EJ, Shattil S, et al (eds): Hematology Basic Principles and Practice, 3rd ed, pp 1025–1042. New York, Churchhill Livingstone, 1998.
195. Marosi C, Koller U, Koller-Weber E, et al: Prognostic impact of karyotype and immunologic phenotype in 125 adult patients with de novo acute nonlymphocytic leukemia. Cancer Genet Cytogenet 1992; 61:14.
196. Lee EJ, Yang J, Leavitt RD, et al: The significance of CD34 and TdT determinations in patients with untreated de novo acute myeloid leukemia. Leukemia 1992; 6:1203.
197. Keating MJ, Kantarjian H, Smith TL, et al: Response to salvage therapy and survival after relapse in acute myelogenous leukemia. J Clin Oncol 1989; 7:1071.
198. Hiddemann W, Martin WR, Sauerland CM, et al: Definition of refractoriness against conventional chemotherapy in acute myeloid leukemia: a proposal based on the results of retreatment by thioguanine, cytosine arabinoside, and daunorubicin (TAD 9) in 150 patients with relapse after standardized first line therapy. Leukemia 1990; 4:184.
199. Appelbaum FR, Clift RA, Buckner D, et al: Allogeneic marrow transplantation for acute nonlymphoblastic leukemia after first relapse. Blood 1983; 61:949.
200. Clift RA, Buckner CD, Appelbaum FR, et al: Allogeneic marrow transplantation during untreated first relapse of acute myeloid leukemia. J Clin Oncol 1992; 10:1723.
201. Chopra R, Goldstone AH, McMillan AK, et al: Successful treatment of acute myeloid leukemia beyond first remission with autologous bone marrow transplantation using busulfan/cyclophosphamide and unpurged marrow: the British autograft group experience. J Clin Oncol 1991; 9:1840.
202. Petersen FB, Lynch MHF, Clift RA, et al: Autologous marrow transplantation for patients with acute myeloid leukemia in untreated first relapse or in second complete remission. J Clin Oncol 1993; 11:1353.
203. Biggs JC, Horowitz MM, Gale RP, et al: Bone marrow transplants may cure patients with acute leukemia never achieving remission with chemotherapy. Blood 1992; 80:109.
204. Kolb HJ, Schattenberg A, Goldman JM, et al: Graft-versus-leukemia effect of donor lymphocyte transfusions in marrow grafted patients. Blood 1995; 86:2041.
205. Warrell RP Jr: Differentiation therapy of acute promyelocytic leukemia with Tretinoin (all-trans-retinoic acid). N Engl J Med 1991; 324:1385.
206. Fenaux P, Le Deley MC, Castaigne S, et al: Effect of all-transretinoic acid in newly diagnosed acute promyelocytic leukemia. Results of a multicenter randomized trial. Blood 1993; 82:3241.
207. Frankel SR, Eardley A, Lauwers G, et al: The "retinoic acid syndrome" in acute promyelocytic leukemia. Ann Intern Med 1992; 117:292.
208. Soignet SL, Maslak P, Wang Z-G, et al: Complete remissions after treatment of acute promyelocytic leukemia with arsenic trioxide. N Engl J Med 1998; 339:1341.
209. Manoharan A: Acute myeloblastic leukaemia in the elderly: biology, prognostic factors and treatment. Int J Hematol 1998; 68(3):235–243.
210. Harousseau JL: Acute myeloid leukemia in the elderly. Blood Rev 1998; 12(3):145–153.
211. Swansbury GJ, Lawler SD, Alimena G, et al: Long-term survival in acute myelogenous leukemia: a second follow-up of the Fourth International Workshop on Chromosomes in Leukemia. Cancer Genet Cytogenet 1994; 73:1.
212. Tilly H, Castaigne S, Bordessoule D, et al: Low dose cytarabine versus intensive chemotherapy in the treatment of acute nonlymphocytic leukemia in the elderly. J Clin Oncol 1990; 8:272.
213. Mayer RJ, Davis RB, Schiffer CA, et al: Comparative evaluation of intensive post-remission therapy with different dose schedules of Ara-C in adults with acute myeloid leukemia: initial results of a CALGB phase III study [abstract]. Proc Am Soc Clin Oncol 1992; 11:261.
214. Baer MR: Management of unusual presentations of acute leukemia. Hematol Oncol Clin North Am 1993; 7(1):275–292.
215. Wang WS, Tzeng CH, Hsieh RK, et al: Successful pregnancy following very high-dose total body irradiation (1575 cGy) and bone marrow transplantation in a woman with acute myeloid leukemia. Bone Marrow Transplant 1998; 21(4):415–417.
216. Doll DC, Rigenberg QS, Yarbro JW: Management of cancer during pregnancy. Arch Intern Med 1988; 148:2058.
217. Caligiuri MA, Mayer RJ: Pregnancy and leukemia. Semin Oncol 1989; 16:388.
218. Okun DB, Groncy PK, Sieger L, et al: Acute leukemia in pregnancy: transient neonatal myelosuppression after combination chemotherapy in the mother. Med Pediatr Oncol 1979; 7:315,
219. Osada S, Horibe K, Oiwa K, et al: A case of infantile acute monocytic leukemia caused by vertical transmission of the mother's leukemic cells. Cancer 1990; 65:1146.
220. Majohno I, Sagli G, Scimi R, et al: High incidence of chronic graft-vs-host disease after primary allogeneic peripheral blood stem cell transplants for patients with hematological malignancies. Bone Marrow Transplant. 1996; 17:555.
221. Appelbaum FR: Allogeneic hematopoietic stem cell transplants for acute leukemia. Semin Oncol 1997; 24:114.
222. Naparstek E, Or R, Nagler A, et al: T-cell depleted allogeneic bone marrow transplantation for acute leukaemia using Campath-1 antibodies and post-transplant administration of donor's peripheral blood lymphocytes for prevention of relapse. Br J Haematol 1995; 89:506.
223. Giralt S, Estey E, Albitar M, et al: Engraftment of allogeneic hematopoietic progenitor cells with purine analog containing chemotherapy: harnessing graft-versus-leukemia without myeloablative therapy. Blood 1997; 89:4531.

Chronic Myeloid Leukemia

224. Boring CC, Squires TS, Tong T: Cancer statistics. CA Cancer J Clin 1993; 43:18.
225. Preston DL, Kusumi S, Tomonaga M, et al: Cancer incidence in

atomic bomb survivors. Part III: leukemia, lymphoma and multiple myeloma. Radiat Res 1994; 137(suppl 2):S68–S97.
226. Goh K, Swisher SN, Herman EC Jr: Chronic myelocytic leukemia in identical twins: Additional evidence of the Philadelphia chromosome as postzygotic abnormality. Arch Intern Med 1967; 120:214.
227. Pasternak G, Hochhaus A, Schultheis B, et al: Chronic myelogenous leukemia: molecular and cellular aspects. J Cancer Res Clin Oncol 1998; 124(12):643–660.
228. Faderl S, Talpaz M, Estrov Z, et al: Chronic myelogenous leukemia: biology and therapy. Ann Intern Med 1999; 131(3):207–219.
229. DeKlein A, Van Kessel AG, Grosveld G, et al: A cellular oncogene is translocated to the Philadelphia chromosome in chronic myelocytic leukemia. Nature 1982; 300:765.
230. Nolte M, Koto Y, Strife A, et al: Demonstration of the Philadelphia translocation by fluorescence in situ hybridization in paraffin sections and identification of aberrant cells by a combined FISH/immunophenotyping approach. Histopathology 1995; 26:433.
231. Barr RD, Fialkow PJ: Clonal origin of chronic myelocytic leukemia. N Engl J Med 1973; 289:307.
232. Fialkow PJ, Martin PJ, Najfeld V, et al: Evidence for a multistep pathogenesis of chronic myelogenous leukemia. Blood 1981; 58:158.
233. Warmuth M, Danhauser-Riedl S, Hallek M: Molecular pathogenesis of chronic myeloid leukemia: implications for new therapeutic strategies. Ann Hematol 1999; 78(2):49–64.
234. Daley GQ, Van Etten RA, Baltimore D: Induction of chronic myelogenous leukemia in mice by the $p210^{bcr/abl}$ gene of the Philadelphia chromosome. Science 1990; 247:824.
235. Salgia SM, Okuda K, Uemura N, et al: The proto-oncogene product p120ABL and adaptor proteins CRKL and c-CRK link c-abl, p190BCR/ABL and p210BCR/ABL to the phosphatidylinositol-3' kinase pathway. Oncogene 1996; 15:839.
236. Bai RY, Jahn T, Schrem S, et al: The SH2 containing adapter protein GRB10 interacts with BCR-ABL. Oncogene 1998; 27:941.
237. Salles MT, Cervantes G, Guarner J, et al: Chronic myelocytic leukemia in accelerated phase with I(17)(q10) and loss of p53 gene. Case report. Arch Med Res 1997; 28(2):293–296.
238. Cervantes F, Villamor N, Esteve J, et al: 'Lymphoid' blast crisis of chronic myeloid leukaemia is associated with distinct clinicohaematological features. Br J Haematol 1998; 100(1):123–128.
239. Attias D, Grunberger T, Vanek W, et al: B-lineage lymphoid blast crisis in juvenile chronic myelogenous leukemia: II: Interleukin-1-mediated autocrine growth regulation of the lymphoblasts. Leukemia 1995; 9(5):884–888.
240. Jacobs P, Greaves M: Ph^1 positive T lymphoblastic transformation. Leuk Res 1984; 8:737.
241. Janossy G, Woodruff RK, Pippard MJ, et al: Relation of "lymphoid" phenotype and response to chemotherapy incorporating vincristine-prednisolone in the acute phase of Ph^1 positive leukemia. Cancer 1979; 43:426.
242. Alimena G, Dallapiccola B, Gastaldi R, et al: Chromosomal, morphological and clinical correlations in blastic crisis of chronic myeloid leukemia. A study of 69 cases. Scand J Haematol 1982; 28:103.
243. Kanda Y, Chiba S, Hinda H, et al: Long-term third chronic phase of chronic myelogenous leukemia maintained by interferon-alpha and methotrexate. Leuk Lymph 1999; 33(1–2):193–197.
244. Khouri I, Kantarjian H, Talpaz M, et al: Chronic myeloid leukemia. In: Abeloff MD, Armitage JO, Lichter AS, et al (eds): Clinical Oncology, p 2035. New York, Churchill Livingstone, 1995.
245. Crisan D, Mattson JC, al-Saadi A: Chronic granulocytic leukemia: reassessment of morphologic and cytogenetic characteristics in Ph1-positive and Ph1-negative cases. Eur J Haematol 1991; 46(2):77–84.
246. Mayani H: Composition and function of the hematopoietic microenvironment in human myeloid leukemia. Leukemia 1996; 10(6):1041–1047.
247. DePalma L, Delgado P, Werner M: Diagnostic discrimination and cost effective assay strategy for leukocyte alkaline phosphatase. Clin Chim Acta 1996; 244(1):83–90.
248. Costello R, Sainty D, Lafage-Pochitaloff M, et al: Clinical and biological aspects of Philadelphia-negative/BCR-negative chronic myeloid leukemia. Leuk Lymph 1997; 25(3–4):225–232.
249. Aurich J, Duchayne E, Huguet-Rigal F, et al: Clinical, morphological, cytogenetic and molecular aspects of a series of Ph-negative chronic myeloid leukemias. Hematol Cell Ther 1998; 40(4):149–158.
250. Montefusco E, Alimena G, Lo Coco F, et al: Ph-negative and bcr-negative atypical chronic myelogenous leukemia: biological features and clinical outcome. Ann Hematol 1992; 65(1):17–21.
251. Berg SL, Phebus CK, Wenger SL: Juvenile chronic myelogenous leukemia with abnormalities of chromosomes 4 and 5. Cancer Genet Cytogenet 1990; 44(1):55–59.
252. Miyauchi J, Asada M, Sasaki M, et al: Mutations of the N-ras gene in juvenile chronic myelogenous leukemia. Blood 1994; 83:2248.
253. Collins SJ, Howard M, Andrews DF, et al: Rare occurrence of N-ras point mutations in Philadelphia chromosome positive chronic myeloid leukemia. Blood 1989; 73:1028.
254. Giralt S, Kantarjian H, Talpaz M: The natural history of chronic myelogenous leukemia in the interferon era. Semin Hematol 1995; 32:152.
255. Hasford J, Ansari H, Pfirrmann M, et al: Analysis and validation of prognostic factors for CML: German CML Study Group. Bone Marrow Transplant 1996; 17(suppl 3):S49–S54.
256. Braga GW, Chauffaille ML, Moncau JE, et al: Chronic myeloid leukemia (CML): prognostic factors and survival analysis. Revista Paul Med 1996; 114(1):1083–1190.
257. Devergie A, Apperley JF, Labopin M, et al: European results of matched unrelated donor bone marrow transplantation for chronic myeloid leukemia. Impact of HLA class II matching. Chronic Leukemia Working Party of the European Group for Blood and Marrow Transplantation. Bone Marrow Transplant 1997; 20(1):11–19.
258. Hasford J, Pfirrmann M, Hehlmann R, et al: A new prognostic score for survival of patients with chronic myeloid leukemia treated with interferon alfa. J Natl Cancer Inst 1998; 90(11):850–858.
259. Kantarjian HM, Deisseroth A, Kurzrock R, et al: Chronic myelogenous leukemia: a concise update. Blood 1993; 82:691.
260. Kantarjian HM, Keating MJ, Smith TL, et al: Proposal for a simple synthesis prognostic staging system in chronic myelogenous leukemia. Am J Med 1990; 88:1.
261. Pusey W: Report of cases treated with roentgen rays. JAMA 1902; 38:911.
262. Minot G, Buckman T, Isaacs R: Chronic myelogenous leukemia. JAMA 1924; 82:1489.
263. Koc Y, Miller KB, Schenkein DP, et al: Extramedullary tumors of myeloid blasts in adults as a pattern of relapse following autologous bone marrow transplantation. Cancer 1999; 85(3):608–615.
264. Medical Research Council Working Party: Chronic granulocytic leukemia: Comparison of radiotherapy and busulfan therapy. Br Med J 1968; 1:201.
265. Kitagawa S, Saito M, Miura Y: Recombinant human erythropoietin at high doses stimulates thrombopoiesis: treatment for protracted severe myelosuppression complicating interferon-alpha and busulphan therapy for chronic myelogenous leukaemia. Eur J Haematol 1995; 55(4):285–286.
266. Gandhi V, Plunkett W, Kantarjian H, et al: Cellular pharmacodynamics and plasma pharmacokinetics of parenterally infused hydroxyurea during a phase I clinical trial in chronic myelogenous leukemia. J Clin Oncol 1998; 16(7):2321–2331.
267. Hehlmann R, Heimpel H, Hasford J, et al: Randomized comparison of busulfan and hydroxyurea in chronic myelogenous leukemia: prolongation of survival by hydroxyurea. Blood 1993; 82:398.
268. Fruchtman SM, Mack K, Kaplan ME, et al: From efficacy to safety: a Polycythemia Vera Study Group report on hydroxyurea in patients with polycythemia vera. Semin Hematol 1997; 34:17.
269. Finney R, McDonald GA, Baikie AG, et al: Chronic granulocytic leukaemia with Ph^1 negative cells in bone marrow and a ten year remission after busulfan hypoplasia. Br J Haematol 1972; 23:283.
270. Kolitz JE, Kempin SJ, Schluger A, et al: A phase II trial of high-dose hydroxyurea in chronic myelogenous leukemia. Semin Oncol 1992; 19(suppl): 27.
271. Cunningham I, Gee T, Dowling M, et al: Results of treatment of Ph^1+ chronic myelogenous leukemia with an intensive treatment regimen (L5 protocol). Blood 1979; 53:375.
272. Urabe A: Interferons for the treatment of hematological malignancies. Oncology 1994; 51(2):137–141.
273. Talpaz M, McCredie KB, Mavligit GM, et al: Leukocyte interferon-induced myeloid cytoreduction in chronic myelogenous leukemia. Blood 1983; 62:689.
274. Talpaz M, Kantarjian HM, McCredie K, et al: Hematologic remission and cytogenetic improvement induced by recombinant human interferon alpha in chronic myelogenous leukemia. N Engl J Med 1986; 314:1065.

275. Eaves AC, Cashman JD, Gaboury LA, et al: Unregulated proliferation of primitive chronic myelogenous leukemia progenitors in the presence of normal marrow adherent cells. Proc Natl Acad Sci U S A 1986; 83:5306.
276. Gordon MY, Dowding CR, Riley GP, et al: Altered adhesive interactions with marrow stroma of haematopoietic progenitor cells in chronic myeloid leukemia. Nature 1987; 328:342.
277. Bhatia R, McCarthy JB, Verfaillie CM: Interferon-alpha restores normal beta-1 integrin-mediated inhibition of hematopoietic progenitor proliferation by the marrow microenvironment in chronic myelogenous leukemia. Blood 1996; 87:3883.
278. Talpaz M, Kantarjian HM, Kurzrock R, et al: Interferon-alpha produces sustained cytogenetic responses in chronic myelogenous leukemia Philadelphia chromosome positive patients. Ann Intern Med 1991; 114:532.
279. Kantarjian HM, O'Brien S, Anderlini P, et al: Treatment of chronic myelogenous leukemia: current status and investigational options. Blood 1996; 87:3069.
280. Kantarjian H, Smith T, O'Brien S, et al: Prolonged survival in chronic myelogenous leukemia following cytogenetic response to alpha interferon therapy. Ann Intern Med 1995; 122:254.
281. Mahon F, Montastruc M, Faberes C, et al: Predicting complete cytogenetic response in chronic myelogenous leukemia patients treated with recombinant interferon alpha. Blood 1994; 84:3592.
282. Tura S, Baccarani M, Zuffa E, for the Italian Cooperative Study Group on Chronic Myeloid Leukemia: Interferon alfa-2a as compared with conventional chemotherapy for the treatment of chronic myeloid leukemia. N Engl J Med 1994; 330:820.
283. Ohnishi K, Ohno R, Tomonaga M, et al: A randomized trial comparing interferon-alfa with busulfan for newly diagnosed chronic myelogenous leukemia in chronic phase. Blood 1995; 86:906.
284. Alimena G, Morra E, Lazzarino M, et al: Interferon alpha-2b as therapy for Ph1-positive chronic myelogenous leukemia: a study of 82 patients treated with intermittent or daily administration. Blood 1988; 72:642.
285. Ozer H, George S, Schiffer C, et al: Prolonged subcutaneous administration of recombinant alfa-2b interferon in patients with previously untreated Philadelphia chromosome-positive chronic phase chronic myelogenous leukemia: effect on remission duration and survival: Cancer and Leukemia Group B Study 8583. Blood 1993; 82:2975.
286. Allan NC, Richards SM, Shepherd PC: UK Medical Research Council randomized, multicenter trial of interferon-alpha for chronic myeloid leukaemia: improved survival irrespective of cytogenetic response. The UK Medical Research Council's Working Parties for Therapeutic Trials in Adult Leukaemia. Lancet 1995; 345:1392.
287. Hehlmann R, Heimpel H, Hasford J, et al: Randomized comparison of interferon-alfa with busulfan and hydroxyurea in chronic myelogenous leukemia. Blood 1994; 84:4064.
288. Chronic Myeloid Leukemia Trialists' Collaborative Group: Interferon alfa versus chemotherapy for chronic myeloid leukemia: a meta-analysis of seven randomized trials. J Natl Cancer Inst 1997; 89:1616,
289. Gilliland DG, Silverstein MN, Anderson JE, et al: Myeloproliferative disorders and myelodysplastic syndromes: cytokine treatment and clonality analyses, p 29. American Society of Hematology 39th Annual Meeting, December 6, 1997.
290. Schofield JR, Robinson WA, Murph JR, et al: Low doses of interferon-alfa are as effective as higher doses in inducing remissions and prolonging survival in chronic myeloid leukemia. Ann Intern Med 1994; 121:736.
291. Benelux CML Study Group: Randomized study on hydroxyurea alone versus hydroxyurea combined with low-dose interferon-A2b for chronic myeloid leukemia. Blood 1998; 91:2713.
292. Robertson MJ, Tantravahi R, Griffin JD, et al: Hematologic remission and cytogenetic improvement after treatment of stable-phase chronic myelogenous leukemia with continuous infusion of low-dose cytarabine. Am J Hematol 1993; 43:95.
293. Guilhot F, Dreyfus B, Brizard A, et al: Cytogenetic remissions in chronic myelogenous leukemia using interferon alpha 2a and hydroxyurea with or without low-dose cytosine arabinoside. Leuk Lymphoma 1991; 4:49.
294. Guilhot F, Chastang C, Michallet M, et al for the French Chronic Myeloid Leukemia Study Group: interferon alfa-2b combined with cytarabine versus interferon alone in chronic myelogenous leukemia. N Engl J Med 1997; 337:223.
295. Sacchi S, Kantarjian H, O'Brien S, et al: Immune-mediated and unusual complications during interferon alfa therapy in chronic myelogenous leukemia. J Clin Oncol 1995; 13:2401.
296. Lee M, Kantarjian H, Talpaz M: Detection of minimal residual disease by polymerase chain reaction in Philadelphia chromosome-positive chronic myelogenous leukemia following interferon therapy. Blood 1992; 79:1920.
297. Hochhaus A, Lin F, Reiter A, et al: Quantification of residual disease in chronic myelogenous leukemia patients on interferon alfa therapy by competitive polymerase chain reaction. Blood 1996; 87:1549.
298. Fefer A, Cheever MA, Thomas ED: Disappearance of Ph-pos cells in four patients with chronic myelogenous leukemia following chemotherapy, irradiation and marrow transplantation from an identical twin. N Engl J Med 1979; 300:33.
299. Thomas ED, Clift RA, Fefer A, et al: Marrow transplantation for the treatment of chronic myelogenous leukemia. Ann Intern Med 1986; 104:155.
300. Enright H, McGlave P: Bone marrow transplantation for chronic myelogenous leukemia. Curr Opin Oncol 1998; 10(2):100–107.
301. Horowitz MM, Rowlings PA, Passweg JR: Allogeneic bone marrow transplantation for CML: a report from the International Bone Marrow Transplant Registry. Bone Marrow Transplant 1996; 17(suppl 3):S5.
302. Gratwohl A, Hermans J, for the Working Party Chronic Leukemia of the European Group for Blood and Marrow Transplantation (EBMT): Allogeneic bone marrow transplantation for chronic myeloid leukemia. Bone Marrow Transplant 1996; 17(suppl 3):S7.
303. Goldman JM, Szydlo R, Horowitz MM, et al for the Advisory Committee of the IBMTR: choice of pretransplant treatment and timing of transplants for chronic myelogenous leukemia in chronic phase. Blood 1993; 82:2235.
304. Biggs JC, Szer J, Crilley P, et al: Treatment of chronic myeloid leukemia with allogeneic bone marrow transplantation after preparation with BuCy2. Blood 1992; 80:1352.
305. Clift RA and Storb R: Marrow transplantation for CML: the Seattle experience. Bone Marrow Transplant 1996; 17(suppl 3):S1.
306. Snyder DS, Negrin R, O'Donnell M, et al: Fractionated total-body irradiation and high dose etoposide as a preparatory regimen for bone marrow transplantation for 94 patients with chronic myelogenous leukemia in chronic phase. Blood 1994; 84:1672.
307. Clift RA, Appelbaum FR, Thomas ED: Treatment of chronic myeloid leukemia by marrow transplantation. Blood 1993; 82:1954.
308. Beelen DW, Graeven U, Almaagacli AH, et al: Prolonged administration of interferon-alpha in patients with chronic phase Philadelphia chromosome-positive chronic myelogenous leukemia before allogeneic bone marrow transplantation may adversely affect transplant outcome. Blood 1995; 85:2981.
309. Giralt SA, Kantarjian HM, Talpaz M, et al: Effect of prior interferon alfa therapy on the outcome of allogeneic bone marrow transplantation for chronic myelogenous leukemia. J Clin Oncol 1993; 11:1055.
310. Shepherd P, Richards S, Allan N: Survival after allogeneic bone marrow transplantation in patients randomized into a trial of IFN-alfa versus chemotherapy: no significant adverse effect of prolonged IFN-alfa administration [abstract]. Blood 1995; 86(suppl 1):94.
311. Horowitz MM, Giralt S, Szydlo R, et al: Effect of prior interferon therapy on outcome of HLA-identical sibling bone marrow transplants for chronic myelogenous leukemia in first chronic phase [abstract]. Blood 1996; 88(suppl 1):682a.
312. Gale RP, Hehlmann R, Zhang MJ, et al: Survival with bone marrow transplantation versus hydroxyurea or interferon for chronic myelogenous leukemia. Blood 1998; 91:1810.
313. McGlave P, Bartsch G, Anasetti C, et al: Unrelated donor marrow transplantation therapy for chronic myelogenous leukemia: initial experience of the national marrow donor program. Blood 1993; 81:543.
314. Korbling M, Przepiorka D, Huh YO, et al: Allogeneic blood stem cell transplantation for refractory leukemia and lymphoma: potential advantage of blood over marrow allografts. Blood 1995; 85:1659.
315. Laporte JP, Gorin NC, Rubinstein P, et al: Cord-blood transplantation from an unrelated donor in an adult with chronic myelogenous leukemia. N Engl J Med 1996; 335:167.
316. Kolb HJ, Mittermuller J, Clemm C, et al: Donor leukocyte transfusions for treatment of recurrent chronic myelogenous leukemia in marrow transplant patients. Blood 1990; 76:2462.
317. Porter DL, Roth MS, McGarigle C, et al: Induction of graft-versus-

host disease as immunotherapy for relapsed chronic myeloid leukemia. N Engl J Med 1994; 330:100.
318. Drobyski WR, Keever CA, Roth MS, et al: Salvage immunotherapy using donor leukocyte infusions as treatment for relapsed chronic myelogenous leukemia after allogeneic bone marrow transplantation: efficacy and toxicity of a defined T-cell dose. Blood 1993; 82:2310.
319. Arcese W, Goldman JM, D'Arcangelo E, et al: Outcome for patients who relapse after allogeneic bone marrow transplantation for chronic myeloid leukemia. Blood 1993; 82:3211.
320. Roth MS, Antin JH, Ash R, et al: Prognostic significance of Philadelphia chromosome-positive cells detected by the polymerase chain reaction after allogeneic bone marrow transplant for chronic myelogenous leukemia. Blood 1992; 79:276.
321. Radich JP, Gehly G, Gooley T, et al: Polymerase chain reaction detection of the BCR-abl fusion transcript after allogeneic marrow transplantation for chronic myeloid leukemia: results and implications in 346 patients. Blood 1995; 85:2632.
322. Coulombel L, Kalousek DK, Eaves CJ, et al: Long term marrow culture reveals chromosomally normal hematopoietic progenitor cells in patients with Philadelphia chromosome-positive chronic myelogenous leukemia. N Engl J Med 1983; 306:1493.
323. Butturini A, Keating A, Goldman J, et al: Autotransplants in chronic myelogenous leukaemia: strategies and results. Lancet 1990; 335:1255,
324. McGlave PB, DeFabritiis P, Deisseroth A, et al: Autologous transplants for chronic myelogenous leukaemia: results from eight transplant groups. Lancet 1994; 343:1486.
325. Hoyle C, Gray R, Goldman J: Autografting for patients with CML in chronic phase: an update. Br J Haematol 1994; 86:76.
326. Deisseroth AB, Zhifei Z, Claxton D, et al: Genetic marking shows that Ph positive cells present in autologous transplants of chronic myelogenous leukemia (CML) contribute to relapse after autologous bone marrow in CML. Blood 1994; 83:3068.
327. Degliantoni G, Mangoni N, Rizzoli V. In vitro restoration of polyclonal hematopoiesis in a chronic myelogenous leukemia after in vitro treatment with 4-hydroperoxycyclophosphamide. Blood 1985; 65:753.
328. Carlo-Stella C, Mangoni L, Almicic C, et al: Autologous transplant for chronic myelogenous leukemia using marrow treated ex vivo with mafosfamide. Bone Marrow Transplant 1994; 14:425.
329. McGlave P, Miller J, Miller W, et al: Autologous marrow transplant therapy for CML using marrow treated ex vivo with human recombinant interferon gamma [abstract]. Blood 1994; 84:537.
330. Druker BJ, Tamura S, Buchdunger E, et al: Effects of a selective inhibitor of the abl tyrosine kinase on the growth of bcr-abl positive cells. Nat Med 1996; 2:561.
331. Szczylik C, Skorski T, Nicolaides NC, et al: Selective inhibition of leukemia cell proliferation by BCR-ABL antisense oligodeoxynucleotides. Science 1991; 253:562.
332. de Fabritiis P, Amadori S, Petti MC, et al: In vitro purging with BCR-ABL antisense oligodeoxynucleotides does not prevent haematological reconstitution after autologous bone marrow transplantation. Leukemia 1995; 9:662.
333. Calabretta B, Sims RB, Valiteri M, et al: Normal and leukemic hematopoietic cells manifest differential sensitivity to inhibitory effects of c-myb antisense oligonucleotides: an in vitro study relevant to bone marrow purging. Proc Natl Acad Sci USA 1991; 88:2351.
334. Barnett MJ, Eaves CJ, Phillips GL, et al: Autografting with cultured marrow in chronic myelogenous leukemia: results of a pilot study. Blood 1994; 84:724.
334a. Gambacorti-Passarini C, le Coutre P, Mologni L, et al: Inhibition of the ABL kinase activity blocks the proliferation of BCR/ABL+ leukemic cells and induces apoptosis. Blood Cells Mol Dis 1997; 23:380.
335. Goldman JM: Chronic myeloid leukemia: new strategies for cure, p 3. American Society of Hematology 39th Annual Meeting, December 1997.

Acute Lymphoblastic Leukemia

336. Niemeyer CM, Sallan SE: Acute lymphoblastic leukemia. In: Nathan DG, Oski FA (eds): Hematology of Infancy and Childhood, 5th ed, p 1245. Philadelphia, W.B. Saunders Co., 1998.
337. Pui CH: Recent advances in the biology and treatment of childhood acute lymphoblastic leukemia. Curr Opin Hematol 1998; 5:292.
338. Korsmeyer SJ, Arnold A, Bakshi A, et al: Immunoglobulin gene rearrangement and cell surface antigen expression in acute/lymphocytic leukemia of T-ce11 and B-cell precursor origins. Proc Natl Acad Sci U S A 1983; 80:301.
339. Potter MN, Steward CG, Maitiand NJ, et al: Detection of clonality in childhood acute lymphoblastic leukemia by the polymerase chain reaction. Leukemia 1992; 6:289.
340. Januszkiewicz DA, Nowak JS: Detection of clonality of polymerase chain reaction in childhood B lineage acute lymphoblastic leukemia. Ann Hematol 1994; 68:107.
341. Brisco MJ, Condon J, Hughes E, et al: Prognostic significance of monoclonality in remission marrow in acute lymphoblastic leukemia in childhood. Leukemia 1993; 7:1514.
342. Raimondi SC, Pui C-H, Head D, et al: Cytogenetically different clones at relapse of childhood acute lymphoblastic leukemia. Blood 1993; 82:576.
343. Cleary ML: A promiscuous oncogene in acute leukemia. N Engl J Med 1993; 329:958.
344. Thandla S, Aplan PD: Molecular biology of acute lymphobastic leukemia. Semin Oncol 1997; 24:45.
345. Thirman MJ, Gill HJ, Burnett RC, et al: Rearrangements of the MLL gene in acute lymphoblastic and acute myeloid leukemias with 11 q23 chromosomal translocations. N Engl J Med 1993; 329:909.
346. Tachibana N, Raimondi SC, Laner SJ, et al: Evidence for a multipotential stem ceil disease in some childhood Philadelphia chromosome-positive acute lymphoblastic leukemia. Blood 1987; 70:1458.
347. Tomura N, Hirano H, Kato K, et al: Central nervous system involvement of leukemia and systemic lymphoma in children: CT and MRI findings. No To Shinkei 1997; 49:993.
348. Revesz T, Kardos G, Kajtar P, et al: The adverse effect of prolonged prednisolone pretreatment in children with acute lymphoblastic leukemia. Cancer 1985; 55:1637.
349. Wiersma S, Ortega J, Sobel E, et al: Clinical importance of myeloid-antigen expression in acute lymphoblastic leukemia of childhood. N Engl J Med 1991; 324:800.
350. Tran-Paterson R, Boileau G, Giguere V, et al: Comparative levels of CALLA/neutral endopeptidase on normal granulocytes, leukemic cells, and transfected COS-1 cells. Blood 1990; 76:775.
351. Sato Y, Itoh F, Hinoda Y, et al: Expression of CD10/neutral endopeptidase in normal and malignant tissues of the human stomach and colon. J Gastroenterol 1996; 31:12.
352. Small TN, Keever CA, Weiner-Fedus S, et al: B-cell differentiation following autologous, conventional, or T-cell depleted bone marrow transplantation: a recapitulation of normal B-cell ontogeny. Blood 1990; 76:1647.
353. Meenan B, Heavey C, Lichtenstein A, et al: Terminal transferase expression in the differential diagnosis of acute leukemias. Eastern Cooperative Oncology Group. Leuk Lymphoma 1996; 22;265.
354. Matutes E, Morilla R, Farahat N, et al: Definition of acute biphenotypic leukemia. Haematologica 1997; 82:64.
355. Croce CM, Nowell PC: Molecular basis of human B cell neoplasia. Blood 1985; 65:1.
356. Ganwersky CE, Croce CM: Chromosomal translocations in leukemia. Semin Cancer Biol 1993; 4:330.
357. Saglio G, Grazia Borrello M, Guerrasio A, et al: Preferential clustering of chromosomal breakpoints in Burkitt's lymphomas and L3 type acute lymphoblastic leukemias with a t(8;14). Genes Chromosomes Cancer 1993; 8:1–7.
358. Kornblau SM, Goodacre A, Cabanillas F: Chromosomal abnormalities in adult non-endemic Burkitt's lymphoma and leukemia: 22 new reports and a review of 148 cases from the literature. Hematol Oncol 1991; 9:63–78.
359. Secker-Walker LM, Chessels JM, Steward EL, et al: Chromosomes and the other prognostic factors in acute lymphoblastic leukemia: a long-term follow up. Br J Haematol 1989; 72: 336.
360. van der Plas DC, Dekker I, Hagemeijer A, et al: 12p chromosomal aberrations in percursor B childhood acute lymphoblastic leukemia predict an increased risk of relapse in the central nervous system and are associated with typical blast cell morphology. Leukemia 1994; 8:2041.
361. Raimondi SC: Current status of cytogenetic research in childhood acute lymphoblastic leukemia. Blood 1993; 81: 2237.
362. Sato Y, Suto Y, Pietenpol J, et al: *TEL* and *KIP1* define the smallest region of deletions on 12p13 in hematopoietic malignancies. Blood 1995; 86:1525.
363. Hoglund M, Johansson B, Pedersen-Bjergaard J, et al: Molecular

characterization of 12p abnormalities in hematological malignancies: deletion of *KIP1*, rearrangement of *TEL* and amplification of *CCND2*. Blood 1996; 87:324.

364. Cave H, Gerard B, Martin E, et al: Loss of heterozygosity in the chromosomal region 12p12-13 is very common in childhood acute lymphoblastic leukemia and permits precise localization of a tumor-suppressor gene distinct from p7KIP1. Blood 1995; 86:3869.
365. Takenchi S, Bartram CR, Miller CW, et al: Acute lymphoblastic leukemia in childhood: identification of two distinct regions of deletions on the short arm of chromosome 12 in the region of *TEL* and *KIP1*. Blood 1996; 87:3368.
366. Golub TR, Barker GF, Bohlander SK, et al: Fusion of *TEL* gene on 12p13 the AML-1 gene on 21q22 in acute lymphoblastic leukemia. Proc Natl Acad Sci U S A 1995; 92:4917.
367. Romana SP, Manchauffe M, LeConiat M, et al: The t(12;21) of acute lymphoblastic leukemia results in a *TEL-AML1* gene fusion. Blood 1995; 85:3662.
368. McLean TW, Ringold S, Neuberg D, et al: *TEL/AML-1* dimerizes and is associated with a favorable outcome in childhood acute lymphoblastic leukemia. Blood 1996; 88:4254.
369. Borkhardt A, Cazzaniga O, Viehmann S, et al: Incidence and clinical relevance of *TEL-AML* fusion gene in children with acute lymphoblastic leukemia enrolled in the German and Italian multicenter therapy trails. Blood 1997; 90:571.
370. Rubnitz JE, Shuster JJ, Land VJ, et al: Case control study suggests a favorable impact of *TEL* rearrangement in patients with B lineage acute lymphoblastic leukemia treated with antimetabolite-based therapy: a Pediatric Oncology Group study. Blood 1997; 89:1143.
371. Kamps MP, Murre C, Sun X-H, et al: A new homeobox gene contributes the DNA binding domain of the t(1;19) translocation protein in pre-B ALL. Cell 1990; 60:547.
372. Vagner-Capodano AM, Moziconacci MJ, Zattaro-Cannoni H, et al: t(1;19) in a M4-ANLL. Cancer Genet Cytogenet 1994; 73:86.
373. Skikano T, Kaneko Y, Takazawa M, et al: Balanced and unbalanced 1;19 translocation-associated acute lymphoblastic leukemias. Cancer 1986; 58:2239.
374. Secker-Walker LM, Berger R, Fenaux P, et al: Prognostic significance of the balance t(1;19) and unbalance der(19)t(1;19) translocations in acute lymphoblastic leukemia. Leukemia 1992; 5:363.
375. Nourse J, Mellentin JD, Galili N, et al: Chromosomal translocation t(1;19) results in synthesis of a homeobox fusion mRNA that codes for a potential chimeric transcription factor. Cell 1990; 60:535.
376. Hunger SP, Galili N, Caroll AJ, et al: The t(1;19)(q23;p13) result in consistent fusion of *E2A* and *PBX1* coding sequences in acute lymphoblastic leukemia. Blood 1991; 77:687.
377. Privatera E, Kamps MP, Hayashi Y, et al: Different molecular consequences of the 1;19 chromosomal transiocation in childhood B cell precursor acute lymphoblastic leukemia. Blood 1992; 79:1781.
378. Sang B-C, Shi L, Dias P, et al: Monoclonal antibodies specific to the acute lymphoblastic leukemia t(1;19)-associated *E2A/pbx1* chimeric protein: characterization and diagnostic utility. Blood 1997; 89:2909.
379. Mitelman F, Kaneko Y, Trent J: Report of the committee on chromosome changes in neoplasia. Cytogenet Cell Genet 1991; 58:1053.
380. Pui C-H, Frankel LS, Carroll AJ, et al: Clinical characteristics and treatment outcome of childhood acute lymphoblastic leukemia with the t(4;11)(q21;q23): a collaborative study of 40 cases. Blood 1991; 77:440.
381. Hunger SP, Tkachuck DC, Amylon MD, et al: *HRX* involvement in de novo and secondary leukemia with diverse chromosome 11q23 abnormalities. Blood 1993; 81:3197.
382. Cimino G, Moir DT, Cananni E, et al: Cloning of *ALL-1* the locus involved in leukemia with the t(4;11)(q21;q23), t(9;11)(p22;q23) and t(11;19)(q23;p13) chromosome translocations. Cancer Res 1991; 51:6712.
383. Gu Y, Alder H, Nakamura T, et al: Sequence analysis of the breakpoint cluster region on the *ALL-1* gene involved in acute leukemia. Cancer Res 1994; 54:2327.
384. Schichiwan SA, Caliguri NA, Gu Y, et al: *ALL-1* partial duplication in acute leukemia. Proc Natl Acad Sci U S A 1994; 91:6230.
385. Scihiman SA, Caliguri MA, Strout MP, et al: *ALL-1* tandem duplication in acute myeloid leukemia with a normal karyotype involve homologous recombination between *A/u* elements. Cancer Res 1994; 54:4277.
386. Super HJ, Rothberg PG, Kobayashi H, et al: Clonal, nonconstitutional rearrangements of the MLL gene in infant twins with acute lymphoblastic leukemia: in utero chromosome rearrangement of 11 q23. Blood 1994; 83:641.
387. Heerema NA, Arthur DC, Sather H, et al: Cytogenetic features of infants less than 12 months of age at diagnosis of acute lymphoblastic leukemia: impact of the 11q23 breakpoint on outcome: a report of the children cancer group. Blood 1994; 83:2274.
388. Bower M, Parry P, Carter M, et al: Prevalence and clinical correlations of MLL gene rearrangements in AML-M4/M5. Blood 1994; 84:3776.
389. Behm FG, Raimondi SC, Frestedt JL, et al: Rearrangement of the *MLL* gene confers a poor prognosis in childhood acute lymphoblastic leukemia, regardless of presenting age. Blood 1996; 87:2870.
390. Rowley JD, Reshami S, Sobulo O, et al: All patients with t(11;16)(q23;p13.3) that involves *MLL* and *CBP* have treatment-related hematologic disorders. Blood 1997; 90:535.
391. Taki T, Sako M, Tsuchida M, et al: The t(11;16) (q23;p13) translocation in myelodysplastic syndrome fuses the *MLL* gene to the *CBP* gene. Blood 1997; 89:3945.
392. Ribiero RC, Abromowitch M, Raimondi SC, et al: Clinical and biological hallmarks of the Philadelphia chromosome in childhood acute lymphoblastic leukemia. Blood 1987; 70:948.
393. Christ W, Caroll A, Schuster J, et al: Philadelphia chromosome positive childhood acute lymphoblastic leukemia: clinical and cytogenetic characteristics and treatment outcome. A Pediatric Oncology Group study. Blood 1990; 76:489.
394. Russo C, Caroil A, Kohlers S, et al: Philadelphia chromosome and monosomy 7 in childhood acute lymphoblastic leukemia. A Pediatric Oncology Group study. Blood 1991; 77:1050.
395. Heisterkamp N, Stephenson JR, Grofen J, et al: Localization of the Gabl oncogene adjacent to a translocation breakpoint in chronic myelogenous leukemia. Nature 1983; 303:239.
396. Hermans A, Heisterkamp N, von Lindern M, et al: Unique fusion of *bcr* and *c-abl* genes in Philadelphia chromosome positive acute lymphoblastic leukemia. Cell 1987; 51:33.
397. Ilaria RL Jr, Van Etten RA: P210 and P190 (bcr/abl) induce the tyrosine phosphorylation and DNA binding activity of multiple specific STAT family members. J Biol Chem 1996; 271:31704.
398. Lestingi TM, Hooberman AL: Philadelphia chromosome-positive acute lymphoblastic leukemia. Hematol Oncol Clin North Am 1993; 7:161.
399. Brown L, Cheng JT, Chen Q, et al: Site-specific recombination of the *TAL1* gene is a common occurrence in human T cell leukemia. EMBO J 1990; 9:3343.
400. Aplan PD, Lambardi DP, Reaman GH, et al: Involvement of the putative hematopoietic transcription factor SCL in T cell acute lymphoblastic leukemia. Blood 1992; 79:1327.
401. Williams DL, Tsiatis A, Brodeur GM, et al: Prognostic importance of chromosome number in 136 untreated children with acute lymphoblastic leukemia. Blood 1982; 60:864.
402. Micallef-Eynaud PD, Eden OB, Grace E, et al: Cytogenetic abnormalities in childhood acute lymphoblastic leukemia. Pediatr Hematol Oncol 1993; 10:25.
403. Frei E III: Acute leukemia in children. Cancer 1984; 53:2013.
404. Farber S, Diamond LK, Mercer RD, et al: Temporary remissions in acute leukemia produced by folic acid antagonist, 4-aminopteroyl-glutamic acid (aminopterin). N Engl J Med 1948; 238:787.
405. Elion GB, Hitchings GH: Metabolic basis for the actions of analogs of purines and pyrimidines. Adv Chemother 1965; 2:91.
406. Burchenal JH, Murphy ML, Ellison RB, et al: Clinical evaluation of a new antimetabolite: 6 mercaptopurine in the treatment of leukemia and allied diseases. Blood 1953; 8:965.
407. Henderson ES: Acute lymphoblastic leukemia. In: Gunz FW, Henderson ES (eds): Leukemia, 4th ed, p 575. New York, Grune and Stratton, 1983.
408. Frei E III, Holland JF, Schneiderman MA, et al: A comparative study of two regimens of combination chemotherapy in acute leukemia. Blood 1958; 13:1126.
409. Freireich EJ, Gehan EA, Sulman D, et al: The effect of chemotherapy on acute leukemia in the human. J Chron Dis 1961; 14:593.
410. Frei E III, Freireich EJ, Gehan E, et al: Studies of sequential and combination antimetabolite therapy in acute leukemia: 6-mercaptopurine and methotrexate. Blood 1961; 18:431.
411. Karon MR, Freireich EJ, Frei E III: A preliminary report on vincristine sulfate: a new agent for the treatment of acute leukemia. Pediatrics 1962; 30:791.

412. Frei E III: Combination cancer therapy: Presidential Address. Cancer Res 1972; 32:2593.
413. Steinherz PG, Gaynon P, Miller DR, et al: Improved disease-free survival of children with acute lymphoblastic leukemia at highrisk for early relapse with the New York regimen—a new intensive therapy protocol: a report from the Children's Cancer Study Group. J Clin Oncol 1986; 4:744.
414. Aur RJA, Simone JV, Husto HO, et al: A comparative study of central nervous system irradiation and intensive chemotherapy early in remission in childhood acute lymphoblastic leukemia. Cancer 1972; 29:381.
415. Freeman AI, Weinberg V, Brecher ML, et al: Comparison of intermediate-dose methotrexate with cranial irradiation for the post-induction treatment of acute lymphoblastic leukemia in children. N Engl J Med 1983; 308:477.
416. Steinherz PG: Radiotherapy vs intrathecal chemotherapy for CNS prophylaxis in childhood ALL: Oncology 1989; 3:47–53.
417. Furman L, Camitta BM, Jaffe N, et al: Development of an effective treatment program for childhood acute lymphoblastic leukemia: a preliminary report. Med Pediatr Oncol 1976; 2:157.
418. Clavell LA, Gelber RD, Cohen HJ, et al: Four-agent induction and intensive asparaginase therapy for treatment of childhood acute lymphoblastic leukemia. N Engl J Med 1986; 315:657.
419. Niemeyer CM, Hitchcock-Bryan S, Sallan SE: Comparative analysis of treatment programs for childhood acute lymphoblastic leukemia. Semin Oncol 1985; 12:122.
420. Rivera GK, Mauer AM: Controversies in the management of childhood acute lymphoblastic leukemia: treatment intensification, CNS leukemia, and prognostic factors. Semin Hematol 1987; 24:12.
421. Dahl GV, Rivera GK, Look AT, et al: Teniposide (VM-26) plus cytarabine improves outcome in childhood acute lymphoblastic leukemia presenting with a leukocyte count greater or equal to 100 × 10(9)/L. J Clin Oncol 1987; 5:1015.
422. Smith M, Arthur D, Camitta B, et al: Uniform approach to risk classification and treatment assignment for children with acute lymphoblastic leukemia. J Clin Oncol 1996; 14:18.
423. Rivera GK, Pinkel D, Simone JV, et al: Treatment of acute lymphoblastic leukemia: 30 years'experience at St. Jude Children's Research Hospital. N Engl J Med 1993; 329:1289.
424. Boilletot A, Behar C, Benoit Y, et al: Treatment of acute lymphoblastic leukemia in children with the BFM protocol: a cooperative pilot study. Am J Pediatr Hematol Oncol 1987; 9:317.
425. Reiter A, Schrappe M, Ludwig WD, et al: Chemotherapy in 998 unselected childhood acute lymphoblastic leukemia patients. Results and conclusions of the multicenter trial ALL-BFM 86. Blood 1994; 84:3122.
426. Veerman AJP, Hahlen K, Kamps WA, et al: High cure rate with a moderately intensive treatment regimen in non-high-risk childhood acute lymphoblastic leukemia: results of protocol ALL Vl from the Dutch Childhood Leukemia Study Group. J Clin Oncol 1996; 14:911.
427. Welte K, Reiter A, Mempel K, et al: A randomized phase III study of the efficacy of granulocyte colony-stimulating factor in children with high-risk acute lymphoblastic leukemia. Berlin-Frankfurt-Munster Study Group. Blood 1996; 87:3143.
428. Pui C-TL, Boyett-JM, Hughes WT, et al: Human granulocyte colony stimulating factor after induction chemotherapy in children with acute lymphoblastic leukemia. N Engl J Med 1997; 336:1781.
429. Bezwoda WR, Bernasconi C, Hutchinson RM, et al: Mitoxantrone for refractory and relapsed acute leukemia. Cancer 1990; 66:418.
430. Bernstein ML, Abshire TC, Pollock BH, et al: Idarubicin and cytosine arabinoside reinduction therapy for children with multiple recurrent or refractory acute lymphoblastic leukemia: a Pediatric Oncology Group study. J Pediatr Hematol Oncol 1997; 19:68.
431. Bleyer WA, Sather H, Hammond GD: Prognosis and treatment after relapse of acute lymphoblastic leukemia and non-Hodgkin's lymphoma 1985: a report from the Children's Cancer Study group. Cancer 1986; 58:590.
432. Rivera GK, Hudson MM, Liu Q, et al: Effectiveness of intensified rotational combination chemotherapy for late hematologic relapse of childhood acute lymphoblastic leukemia. Blood 1996; 88:831.
433. Chao NJ, Forman SJ, Schmidt GM, et al: Allogeneic bone marrow transplantation for high-risk acute lymphoblastic leukemia during first complete remission. Blood 1991; 78:1923.
434. Snyder DS, Chao NJ, Amylon MD, et al: Fractionated total body irradiation and high-dose etoposide as a preparatory regimen for bone marrow transplantation for 99 patients with acute leukemia in first complete remission. Blood 1993; 82:2920.
435. Chao NJ, Blume KG, Forman SJ, et al: Long-term follow-up of allogeneic bone marrow recipients for Philadelphia chromosome-positive acute lymphoblastic leukemia. Blood 1995; 85:3353.
436. Uderzo C, Valsecchi MG, Bacigalupo A, et al: Treatment of childhood acute lymphoblastic leukemia in second remission with allogeneic bone marrow transplantation and chemotherapy: ten-year experience of the Italian Bone Marrow Transplantation Group and the Italian Pediatric Hematology Oncology Association. J Clin Oncol 1995; 13:352.
437. Szydlo R, Goldman JM, Klein JP, et al: Results of allogeneic bone marrow transplants for leukemia using donors other than HLA-identical siblings. J Clin Oncol 1997; 15:1767.
438. Chen C-S, Sorensen PHB, Domer PH, et al: Molecular rearrangements on chromosome 11 q23 predominate in infant acute lymphoblastic leukemia and are associated with specific biologic variables and poor outcome. Blood 1993; 81:2386.
439. Cimino G, LoCoco F, Biondi A, et al: ALL-1 gene at chromosome 11 q23 is consistently altered in acute leukemia of infancy. Blood 1993; 82:544.
440. Rubnitz JE, Link MP, Shuster JJ, et al: Frequency and prognostic significance of HRX rearrangements in infant acute lymphoblastic leukemia: a Pediatric Oncology Group study. Blood 1994; 84:570.
441. Hilden JM, Frestedt JL, Moore RO, et al: Molecular analysis of infant acute lymphoblastic leukemia: MLL gene rearrangement and reverse transcriptase-polymerase chain reaction for t(4;11)(q21;q23). Blood 1995; 86:3876.
442. Frankel LS, Ochs J, Shuster JJ, et al: Therapeutic trial for infant acute lymphoblastic leukemia: the Pediatric Oncology Group experience (POG 8493). J Pediatr Hematol Oncol 1997; 19:35.
443. Reaman G, Zeltzer P, Bleyer WA, et al: Acute lymphoblastic leukemia in infants less than one year of age: a cumulative experience of the Children's Cancer Study Group. J Clin Oncol 1985; 3:1513.
444. Miller RW: Persons at exceptionally high risk of leukemia. Cancer Res 1967; 27:2420.
445. Ragab AH, Abdel-Mageed A, Shuster JJ, et al: Clinical characteristics and treatment outcome of children with acute lymphoblastic leukemia and Down's syndrome. A Pediatric Oncology Group study. Cancer 1991; 67:1057.
446. Hoeizer D, Thiel E, Loffler H, et al: Prognostic factors in a multicenter study for the treatment of acute lymphoblastic leukemia in adults. Blood 1988; 71:123.
447. Berman E, Weiss M, Kempin S, et al: Intensive therapy for adult acute lymphoblastic leukemia. Semin Hematol 1991; 28:72.
448. Boucheix C, David B, Sebban C, et al: Immunophenotype of adult acute lymphoblastic leukemia, clinical parameters, and outcome: an analysis of a prospective trial including 562 tested patients (LALA87). Blood 1994; 84:1603.
449. The Groupe Francais de Cytogenetique Hematologique: Cytogenetic abnormalities in adult lymphoblastic leukemia: correlations with hematologic findings and outcome. A collaborative study of the Groupe Francais de Cytogenetique Hematologique. Blood 1996; 87:3135.
450. Laport GF, Larson IRA: Treatment of adult acute lymphoblastic leukemia. Semin Oncol 1997; 24:70.
451. Weiss M, Maslak P, Feldman E, et al: Cytarabine with high-dose mitoxantrone induces rapid complete remissions in adult acute lymphoblastic leukemia without the use of vincristine or prednisone. J Clin Oncol 1996; 14:2480.
452. Attal M, Blaise D, Marit G, et al: Consolidation treatment of adult acute lymphoblastic leukemia: a prospective, randomized trial comparing allogeneic versus autologous bone marrow transplantation and testing the impact of recombinant interleukin-2 after autologous bone marrow transplantation. Blood 1995; 86:1619.
453. Horowitz MM, Messerer D, Hoelzer D, et al: Chemotherapy compared with bone marrow transplantation for adults with acute lymphoblastic leukemia in first remission. Ann Intern Med 1991; 115:13.
454. Cortes J, O'Brien SM, Pierce S, et al: The value of high-dose systemic chemotherapy and intrathecal therapy for central nervous system prophylaxis in different risk groups of adult acute lymphoblastic leukemia. Blood 1995; 86:2091.
455. Larson RA, Dodge RK, Burns CP, et al: A five-drug remission

induction regimen with intensive consolidation for adults with acute lymphoblastic leukemia. Cancer and Leukemia Group B Study 8811. Blood 1995; 85:2025.
456. Larson RA, Linker CA, Dodge RK, et al: Granulocyte-colony stimulating factor (filgrastim; G-CSF) reduces the time to neutrophil recovery in adults with acute lymphoblastic leukemia receiving intensive remission induction chemotherapy: Cancer and Leukemia Group B Study 9111 [abstract]. Proc Am Soc Clin Oncol 1994; 13:305.
457. Brisco MJ, Hughes E, Neoh SH, et al: Relationship between minimal residual disease and outcome in adult acute lymphoblastic leukemia. Blood 1996; 87:5251.
458. Wasserman R, Galili N, Ito Y, et al: Residual disease at the end of induction therapy as a predictor of relapse during therapy in childhood B-lineage acute lymphoblastic leukemia. J Clin Oncol 1992; 10:1879.
459. Brisco MJ, Condon J, Hughes E, et al: Outcome prediction in childhood acute lymphoblastic leukemia by molecular quantification of residual disease at the end of induction. Lancet 1994; 343:196.
460. Laudis SH, Murray T, Bolden S, et al: Cancer statistics, 1999. CA Cancer J Clin 1999; 49:8.
461. Bleyer WA: The impact of childhood cancer on the United States and the world. CA Cancer J Clin 1990; 40:355.
462. Lipshultz SE, Colan SD, Gelber RD, et al: Late cardiac effects of doxorubicin therapy for acute lymphoblastic leukemia in childhood. N Engl J Med 1991; 324:808.
463. Lipshultz SE, Lipsitz SR, Mone SM, et al: Female sex and drug dose as risk factors for late cardiotoxic effects of doxorubicin therapy for childhood cancer. N Engl J Med 1995; 332:1738.
464. Casey EB, Jellife AM, Le Quesne PM, et al: Vincristine neuropathy. Clinical and electrophysiological observations. Brain 1973; 96:69.
465. Vainionpaa L: Clinical neurological findings of children with acute lymphoblastic leukaemia at diagnosis and during treatment. Eur J Pediatr 1993; 152:115.
466. Harila-Saari AH, Vainionpaa LK, Kovala TT, et al: Nerve lesions after therapy for childhood acute lymphoblastic leukemia. Cancer 1997; 82:200.
467. Bleyer WA, Fallavollita J, Robison L, et al: Influence of age, sex, and concurrent intrathecal methotrexate therapy on intellectual function after cranial irradiation during childhood. Pediatr Hematol Oncol 1990; 7:329.
468. Waber DP, Urion DK, Tarbell NJ, et al: Late effects of central nervous system treatment of acute lymphoblastic leukemia in childhood are sex-dependent. Dev Med Child Neurol 1990; 32:238.
469. Schriock EA, Schell MJ, Carter M, et al: Abnormal growth pattern and adult short stature in 115 long-term survivors of childhood leukemia. J Clin Oncol 1991; 9:400.
470. Neglia JP, Meadows AT, Robison LL, et al: Second neoplasms after acute lymphoblastic leukemia in childhood. N Engl J Med 1991; 325:1330.

Chronic Lymphocytic Leukemia

471. Foon KA, Rai KR, Gale RP: Chronic lymphocytic leukemia: new insights into biology and therapy. Ann Int Med 1990; 113:525–539.
472. Rai KR: Chronic lymphocytic leukemia in the elderly population. Clin Geriatr Med 1997; 13:245–249.
473. SEER Cancer Statistics Review, 1973–1995. NIH Publication No. 98-2789. Bethesda, National Cancer Institute, 1998.
474. Rozman C, Bosch F, Montserrat E: Chronic lymphocytic leukemia: a changing natural history. Leukemia 1997; 11:775–778.
475. Henderson ES, Han T: Current therapy of acute and chronic leukemia in adults. CA Cancer J Clin 1986; 36:322–350.
476. Karmiris T, Rohatiner AZ, Love S, et al: The management of chronic lymphocytic leukemia at a single centre over a 24-year period: prognostic factors for survival. Hematol Oncol 1994; 12:29–39.
477. Rushton L, Romaniuk H: A case-control study to investigate the risk of leukaemia associated with exposure to benzene in petroleum marketing and distribution workers in the United Kingdom. Occup Environ Med 1997; 54:152–166.
478. Raabe GK, Wong O: Leukemia mortality by cell type in petroleum workers with potential exposure to benzene. Environ Health Perspect 1996; 104(suppl 6):1381–1392.
479. Feychting M: Occupational exposure to electromagnetic fields and adult leukaemia: a review of the epidemiological evidence. Radiat Environ Biophys 1996; 35:237–242.
480. Shah AR, Maeda K, Deegan MJ, et al: A clinicopathologic study of familial chronic lymphocytic leukemia. Am J Clin Path 1992; 97:184.
481. Linet MS, Van Natta MLV, Brookmeyer R, et al: Familial cancer history and chronic lymphocytic leukemia. A case control study. Am J Epidemiol 1989; 130:655–664.
482. Cuttner J: Increased incidence of hematologic malignancies in first-degree relatives of patients with chronic lymphocytic leukemia. Cancer Invest 1992; 10:103–109.
483. Najfeld V, Fialkow PJ, Karande A, et al: Chromosome analysis of lymphoid cell lines derived from patients with chronic lymphocytic leukemia. Int J Cancer 1980; 26:543–544.
484. Solanki DL, McCurdy PR, MacDermott RP: Chronic lymphocytic leukemia: a monoclonal disease. Am J Hematol 1982; 13:159–162.
485. Lenormand B, Ghanem N, Tilly H, et al: Rearrangement of immunoglobulin light and heavy chain genes and correlation with phenotypic markers in B cell chronic lymphocytic leukemia. Leukemia 1991; 5:928–936.
486. Voso MT, Hohaus S, Moos M, et al: Lack of t(14;18) polymerase chain reaction-positive cells in highly purified CD34+ cells and their CD19 subsets in patients with follicular lymphoma. Blood 1997; 89:3763–3768.
487. Michiels JJ, van Dongen JJM, Hagemijer A, et al: Richter syndrome with identical immunoglobulin gene rearrangements in the chronic lymphocytic leukemia and the supervening non Hodgkin lymphoma. Leukemia 1989; 3:819–824.
488. Cherepakhin V, Baird SM, Meisenholder GW, et al: Common clonal origin of chronic lymphocytic leukemia and high grade lymphoma of Richter's syndrome. Blood 1993; 82:3141–3147.
489. Gahn B, Schafer C, Neef J, et al: Detection of trisomy 12 and Rb-deletion in CD34-positive cells of patients with B cell chronic lymphocytic leukemia. Blood 1997; 89:4275–4281.
490. Juliusson G, Oscier DG, Fitchett M, et al: Prognostic subgroups in B cell chronic lymphocytic leukemia defined by specific chromosomal abnormalities. N Engl J Med 1990; 323:720–724.
491. Juliusson G, Gahrton G: Chromosome aberrations in B cell chronic lymphocytic leukemia. Cancer Genet Cytogenet 1990; 45:143–160.
492. Liu Y, Szekely L, Grander D, et al: Chronic lymphocytic leukemia cells with allelic deletions at 13q14 commonly have one intact RB1 gene: evidence for a role of an adjacent locus. Proc Nat Acad Sci 1993; 90:8697–8701.
493. Chapman RM, Corcoran MM, Gardiner A, et al: Frequent homozygous deletions of the D13S25 locus in chromosome region 13q14 defines the location of a gene critical in leukemogenesis in chronic B-cell lymphocytic leukemia. Oncogene 1994; 9:1289–1293.
494. Döhner H, Stilgenbauer S, James MR, et al: 11q deletions identify a new subset of B-cell chronic lymphocytic leukemia characterized by extensive nodal involvement and inferior prognosis. Blood 1997; 89:2516–2522.
495. Döhner H, Pohl S, Bulgay-Morschel M, et al: Trisomy 12 in chronic lymphocytic leukemia—a metaphase and interphase cytogenetic analysis. Leukemia 1993; 7:516–520.
496. Que TH, Marco JG, Ellis J, et al: Trisomy 12 in chronic lymphocytic leukemia detected by fluorescence in situ hybridization: analysis by stage, immunophenotype and morphology. Blood 1993; 82:571–575.
497. Escudier SM, Pereira-Leahy JM, Drach JW, et al: Fluorescent in situ hybridization and cytogenetic studies of trisomy 12 in chronic lymphocytic leukemia. Blood 1993; 81:2702–2707.
498. Reinening G, Clodi K, Koning M, et al: Detection of trisomy 12 in chronic lymphocytic leukemia: comparison of a polymerase chain reaction based technique with fluorescence in situ hybridization. Br J Haematol 1994; 87:843–845.
499. Witzig TE, Borell TJ, Herath JF, et al: Detection of trisomy 12 by FISH in untreated B-chronic lymphocytic leukemia: correlation with stage and CD20 antigen expression intensity. Leuk Lymphoma 1994; 14:447–451.
500. Knauf WU, Knuutila S, Zeigmeister B, et al: Trisomy 12 in B cell chronic lymphocytic leukemia: correlations with advanced disease, atypical morphology, high level of sCD25 and with refractoriness to treatment. Leuk Lymphoma 1995; 19:289–294.
501. Arif M, Tanaka K, Asov H, et al: Independent clones of trisomy 12 and retinoblastoma gene deletion in Japanese B cell chronic lymphocytic leukemia, detection by fluorescence in situ hybridization. Leukemia 1995; 9:1822–1827.
502. Lishner M, Lalkin A, Klein A, et al: The BCL-1, BCL-2, and

BCL-3 oncogenes are involved in chronic lymphocytic leukemia. Detection by fluorescence in situ hybridization. Cancer Genet Cytogenet 1995; 85:118–123.
503. Finn WG, Thangvelu M, Yelavarthy KK, et al: Karyotype correlates with peripheral blood morphology and immunophenotype in chronic lymphocytic leukemia. Am J Clin Pathol 1996; 105:458–467.
504. Garcia-Marco JA, Price CM, Ellis J, et al: Correlation of trisomy 12 with proliferating cells by combined immunocytochemistry and fluorescence in situ hybridization in chronic lymphocytic leukemia. Leukemia 1996; 10:1705–1711.
505. Woessner S, Sole F, Perez-Losada A, et al: Trisomy 12 is a rare cytogenetic finding in typical chronic lymphocytic leukemia. Leuk Res 1996; 20:369–374.
506. Döhner H, Stilgenbauer S, Fischer K, et al: Cytogenetic and molecular cytogenetic analysis of B cell chronic lymphocytic leukemia: specific chromosome aberrations identify prognostic subgroups of patients and point to loci of candidate genes. Leukemia 1997; 11(suppl 2):S19–S24.
507. Raghoebier S, van Kriekan JHHM, Kok F, et al: Mosaicism of trisomy 12 in chronic lymphocytic leukemia detected by nonradioactive in situ hybridization. Leukemia 1992; 6:1220–1226.
508. Garcia-Marco JA, Matutes E, Morila R, et al: Trisomy 12 in B cell chronic lymphocytic leukemia. Assessment of lineage restriction by simultaneous analysis of immunophenotype and genotype in interphase cells by fluorescence in situ hybridization. Br J Haematol 1994; 87:44–50.
509. Garcia-Marco JA, Price CM, Catovsky D: Interphase cytogenetics in chronic lymphocytic leukemia. Cancer Genet Cytogenet 1997; 94:52–58.
510. Criel A, Verhoef G, Vlietinck R, et al: Further characterization of morphologically defined typical and atypical CLL: a clinical, immunophenotypic, cytogenetic and prognostic study on 390 cases. Br J Haematol 1997; 97:383–391.
511. Matutes E, Oscier D, Garcia-Marco J, et al: Trisomy 12 defines a group of CLL with atypical morphology: correlation between cytogenetics, clinical and laboratory features in 544 patients. Br J Haematol 1996; 92:382–388.
512. Gerdes J, Lemke H, Baisch H, et al: Cell cycle analysis of a cell proliferation-associated human nuclear antigen defined by the monoclonal antibody Ki-67. J Immunol 1984; 133:1710–1715.
513. Cordone I, Matutes E, Catovsky D: Characterization of normal peripheral blood cells in cycle identified by monoclonal antibody Ki-67. J Clin Pathol 1992; 45:201–205.
514. Fitchett M, Griffith MJ, Oscier DG, et al: Chromosome abnormalities involving band 13q14 in hematological malignancies. Cancer Genet Cytogenet 1987; 24:143–150.
515. Oscier DG: Cytogenetic and molecular abnormalities in chronic lymphocytic leukemia. Blood Rev 1994; 8:88–97.
516. Döhner H, Pilz T, Fischer K, et al: Molecular cytogenetic analysis of RB-1 deletions in chronic B-cell leukemias. Leuk Lymphoma 1994; 16:97–103.
517. Jabbar SAB, Ganeshaguru K, Wickremasinghe RG, et al: Deletion of chromosome 13(band q14) but no trisomy 12 is a clonal event in B cell chronic lymphocytic leukemia (CLL). Br J Haematol 1995; 90:476–478.
518. Garcia-Marco J, Caldes C, Price CM, et al: Frequent somatic deletions of the 13q12.3 locus encompassing BRCA2 in chronic lymphocytic leukemia. Blood 1996; 88:1568–1575.
519. Oscier DG, Thompsett A, Fischer K, et al: Differential rates of somatic hypermutation in VH genes among subsets of chronic lymphocytic leukemia defined by chromosomal abnormalities. Blood 1997; 89:4153–4160.
520. Fegan C, Robinson H, Thompson P, et al: Karyotypic evolution in CLL: identification of a new subgroup of patients with deletions of 11q and advanced or progressive disease. Leukemia 1995; 9:2003–2008.
521. Hernandez JM, Mecucci C, Criel A, et al: Cytogenetic analysis of B cell chronic lymphoid leukemias classified according to morphologic and immunophenotyping (FAB) criteria. Leukemia 1995; 9:2140–2146.
522. Dyer JM, Zani VJ, Lu WZ, et al: BCL2 translocations in leukemias of mature B cells. Blood 1994; 83:3682–3688.
523. Michauz L, Dierlamm J, Wlodarska I, et al: t(14;19)/BCL3 rearrangements in lymphoproliferative disorders: a review of 23 cases. Cancer Genet Cytogenet 1997; 94:36–43.
524. Bennett JM, Catovsky D, Daniel MT, et al and the French-American-British (FAB) Cooperative Group: proposals for the classification of chronic (mature) B and T lymphoid leukemias. J Clin Pathol 1989; 42:567–584.
525. Kroft SH, Finn WG, Peterson LC: The pathology of the chronic lymphoid leukaemias. Blood Rev 1995; 9:234–250.
526. Phyliky RL, Li C-Y, Yam LT: T-cell chronic lymphocytic leukemia with morphologic and immunologic characteristics of cytotoxic/suppressor phenotype. Mayo Clin Proc 1983; 58:709–720.
527. Wong KF, Chan JKC, Sin VC: T-cell form of chronic lymphocytic leukaemia: a reaffirmation of its existence. Br J Haematol 1996; 93:157–159.
528. Batata A, Shen B: Chronic lymphocytic leukemia with a low lymphocyte count. Cancer 1993; 71:2732–2738.
529. Rai KR, Sawitsky A, Cronkite EP, et al: Clinical staging of chronic lymphocytic leukemia. Blood 1975; 46:219–234.
530. Cheson BD, Bennett JM, Grever M, et al: National Cancer Institute-sponsored Working Group guidelines for chronic lymphocytic leukemia: revised guidelines for diagnosis and treatment. Blood 1996; 87:4990–4997.
531. Binet JL, Auquier A, Dighiero G, et al: A new prognostic classification of chronic lymphocytic leukemia derived from a multivariate survival analysis. Cancer 1981; 48:198–206.
532. Tefferi A, Phyliky RL: A clinical update on chronic lymphocytic leukemia. I: Diagnosis and prognosis. Mayo Clin Proc 1992; 67:349–353.
533. Skinnider LF, Tan L, Schmidt J, et al: Chronic lymphocytic leukemia: a review of 745 cases and assessment of clinical staging. Cancer 1982; 50:2951–2955.
534. Harris NL, Jaffe ES, Stein H, et al: A revised European-American classification of lymphoid neoplasms: a proposal from the International Lymphoma Study Group. Blood 1994; 84:1361–1392.
535. French Cooperative Group on Chronic Lymphocytic Leukemia: Effects of chlorambucil and therapeutic decision in initial forms of chronic lymphocytic leukemia (stage A): results of a randomized clinical trial on 612 patients. Blood 1990; 75:1414–1421.
536. Mandelli F, DeRossi G, Mancini P, et al: Prognosis in chronic lymphocytic leukemia: a retrospective multicentric study from the GIMEMA group. J Clin Oncol 1987; 5:398–406.
537. Molica S, Brugiatelli M, Callea V, et al: Comparison of younger versus older B-cell chronic lymphocytic leukemia patients for clinical presentation and prognosis. Eur J Haematol 1994; 52:216–221.
538. Hallek M, Kuhn-Hallek I, Emmerich B: Prognostic factors in chronic lymphocytic leukemia. Leukemia 1997; 11(suppl 2):S4–S13.
539. Sawitsky A, Rai KR, Glidewell O, et al for the CALGB: Comparison of daily vs intermittent chlorambucil and prednisone therapy in the treatment of patients with chronic lymphocytic leukemia. Blood 1977; 50:1049–1059.
540. Spanish Cooperative Group on CLL (PETHEMA): Treatment of chronic lymphocytic leukemia: a preliminary report of Spanish (PETHEMA) trials. Leuk Lymphoma 1991; 5(suppl):89–91.
541. Catovsky D, Richards S, Fooks J, et al: CLL trials in the United Kingdom. Leuk Lymphoma 1991; 5(suppl):105–112.
542. French Cooperative Group on Chronic Lymphocytic Leukemia: Is the CHOP regimen a good treatment for advanced CLL? Results from two randomized clinical trials. Leuk Lymphoma 1994; 13:449–456.
543. Shaw R, Boggs DR, Silberman HR, et al: A study of prednisone therapy in chronic lymphocytic leukemia. Blood 1961; 17:182–195.
544. Wilhelm M, Tony H-P, Rueckle-Lanz H, et al: First-line therapy of advanced chronic lymphocytic leukemia. Leukemia 1997; 11(suppl 2):S14–S18.
545. Jaksic B, Brugiatelli M, Krc I, et al: High-dose chlorambucil versus Binet's modified cyclophosphamide, doxorubicin, vincristine, and prednisone regimen in the treatment of patients with advanced B-cell chronic lymphocytic leukemia: results of an international multicenter randomized trial. Cancer 1997; 79:2107–2114.
546. Keating MJ, Kantarjian H, Talpaz M, et al: Fludarabine: a new agent with major activity against chronic lymphocytic leukemia. Blood 1989; 74:19–24.
547. Binet JL, Chastang C, Chevret S, et al: Comparison of fludarabine (FDB), CAP and CHOP in advanced previously untreated chronic lymphocytic leukemia (CLL) [abstract]. Blood 1993; 84(suppl 1):140a.
548. Rai KR, Peterson B, Kolitz J, et al: Fludarabine induces a

high complete remission rate in previously untreated patients with active chronic lymphocytic leukemia [abstract]. Blood 1995; 86(suppl):607.

549. French Cooperative Group on CLL, Johnson S, Smith AG, et al: Multicentre prospective randomised trial of fludarabine versus cyclophosphamide, doxorubicin, and prednisone (CAP) for treatment of advanced-stage chronic lymphocytic leukaemia. Leukemia 1996; 347:1432–1438.
550. Keating MJ, Kantarjian H, O'Brien S, et al: Fludarabine: a new agent with marked cytoreductive activity in untreated chronic lymphocytic leukemia. J Clin Oncol 1991; 9:44–49.
551. Wright SJ, Robertson LE, O'Brien S, et al: The role of fludarabine in hematological malignancies. Blood Rev 1994; 8:125–134.
552. O'Brien S, Kantarjian H, Beran M, et al: Results of fludarabine and prednisone therapy in 264 patients with chronic lymphocytic leukemia with multivariate analysis-derived prognostic model for response to treatment. Blood 1993; 82:1695–1700.
553. Bergmann L: Present status of purine analogs in the therapy of chronic lymphocytic leukemias. Leukemia 1997; 11(suppl 2):S29–S34.
554. Paule B, Cosset JM, Bourgeois JPL: The possible role of radiotherapy in chronic lymphocytic leukaemia: a critical review. Radiother Oncol 1985; 4:45–54.
555. Kempin S, Shank B: Radiation in chronic lymphocytic leukemia. In: Gale RP, Rai KR (eds): Chronic Lymphocytic Leukemia: Recent Progress and Future Direction, pp 337–352. New York, Alan R. Liss, Inc., 1987.
556. Rubin P, Bennett JM, Begg C, et al: The comparison of total body irradiation vs chlorambucil and prednisone for remission induction of active chronic lymphocytic leukemia: an ECOG study. Part I: total body irradiation-response and toxicity. Int J Radiat Oncol Biol Phys 1981; 7:1623–1632.
557. Jacobs P, King HS: A randomized prospective comparison of chemotherapy to total body irradiation as initial treatment for the indolent lymphoproliferative diseases. Blood 1987; 69:1642–1646.
558. Chisesi T, Capnist G, Dal Fior S: Splenic irradiation in chronic lymphocytic leukemia. Eur J Haematol 1991; 46:202–204.
559. Paulino AC, Reddy SP: Splenic irradiation in the palliation of patients with lymphoproliferative and myeloproliferative disorders. Am J Hosp Palliat Care 1996; 13:32–35.
560. Seymour JF, Cusack JD, Lerner SA, et al: Case/control study of the role of splenectomy in chronic lymphocytic leukemia. J Clin Oncol 1997; 15:52–60.
561. Rabinowe SN, Soiffer RJ, Gribben JG, et al: Autologous and allogeneic bone marrow transplantation for poor prognosis patients with B-cell chronic lymphocytic leukemia. Blood 1993; 82:1366–1376.
562. Bartlett-Pandite L, Soiffer R, Gribben JG, et al: Autologous and allogeneic bone marrow transplantation for B-cell CLL: balance between toxicity and efficacy [abstract]. Blood 1994; 84(suppl 1):536a.
563. Michallet M, Archimbaud E, Bandini G, et al: HLA-identical sibling bone marrow transplantation in younger patients with chronic lymphocytic leukemia. Ann Int Med 1996; 124:311–315.
564. Khouri IF, Przepiorka D, van Besien K, et al: Allogeneic blood or marrow transplantation for chronic lymphocytic leukaemia: timing of transplantation and potential effect of fludarabine on acute graft-versus-host disease. Br J Haematol 1997; 97:466–471.
565. Khouri IF, Keating MJ, Vriesendorp HM, et al: Autologous and allogeneic bone marrow transplantation for chronic lymphocytic leukemia: preliminary results. J Clin Oncol 1994; 12:748–758.
566. Dreger P, Schmitz N: The role of stem cell transplantation in the treatment of chronic lymphocytic leukemia. Leukemia 1997; 11(suppl 2):S42–S45.
567. Cooperative Group for the Study of Immunoglobulin in Chronic Lymphocytic Leukemia: Intravenous immunoglobulin for the prevention of infection in chronic lymphocytic leukemia. N Engl J Med 1988; 319:902–907.
568. Weeks JC, Tierney MR, Weinstein MC: Cost effectiveness of prophylactic intravenous immune globulin in chronic lymphocytic leukemia. N Engl J Med 1991; 325:81–86.
569. Molica S, Musto P, Chiurazzi F, et al: Prophylaxis against infections with low-dose intravenous immunoglobulins (IVIG) in chronic lymphocytic leukemia. Haematologica 1996; 81:121–126.
570. DeNardo GL, Lewis J, DeNardo SJ, et al: Effect of Lym-1 radioimmunoconjugate on refractory chronic lymphocytic leukemia. Cancer 1994; 73:1425–1432.
571. Lim SH, Hale G, Marcus RE, et al: CAMPATH-1 monoclonal antibody therapy in severe refractory autoimmune thrombocytopenic purpura. Br J Haematol 1993; 84:542–544.
572. Maloney DG: Advances in immunotherapy of hematologic malignancies. Curr Opin Hematol 1998; 5:237–243.
573. Jensen M, Winkler U, Manzke O, et al: Rapid tumor lysis in a patient with B-cell chronic lymphocytic leukemia and lymphocytosis treated with an anti-CD20 monoclonal antibody (IDEC-C2B8, rituximab). Ann Hematol 1998; 77:89–91.
574. Frenkel EP, Ligler FS, Graham MS, et al: Acute lymphocytic leukemia transformation of chronic lymphocytic leukemia. Am J Hematol 1981; 10:391–398.
575. Harousseau JL, Flandrin G, Tricot G, et al: Malignant lymphoma supervening in chronic lymphocytic leukemia and related disorders. Richter's syndrome: a study of 25 cases. Cancer 1981; 48:1302–1308.

24 *Soft Tissue Sarcoma*

IRA J. SPIRO, MD, PhD, Radiation Oncology
HERMAN D. SUIT, MD, DPhil, Radiation Oncology
RANDY N. ROSIER, MD, PhD, Orthopedic Oncology
DEEPAK M. SAHASRABUDHE, MD, Medical Oncology

For extreme diseases, extreme methods of cure.

HIPPOCRATES

Perspective

Soft tissue sarcomas are a class of malignant tumors that arise largely, though not exclusively, from mesenchymal connective tissues. Their distinction from carcinomas is based on their origin from connective rather than epithelial tissues. However, some types of epithelia arise from the mesoderm, and tumors derived from these tissues are also considered to be sarcomas. Consequently, tumors classified as sarcomas are characterized by a common morphology and clinical behavior; therefore, they are dealt with as a group as well as individually.

Soft tissue sarcomas are uncommon neoplasms that represent approximately 0.7% of all malignancies in men and 0.6% in women.[1] Perhaps because of their rarity and tendency to evolve with few early symptoms, diagnosis and treatment are often delayed. Therefore, patients with suspicious soft tissue masses should undergo biopsy immediately, especially if the masses have recently changed in size or become symptomatic. However, care must be taken not to compromise later curative resection and to maintain tissue planes, as much as possible, in order to limit tumor dissemination.

It is clear that sarcomas require a therapeutic approach that establishes local control and, thereby, eliminates the potential for metastasis in patients with truly limited disease. Although soft tissue sarcomas were generally treated in the past by surgery alone, increasingly surgery is being replaced by a combined-modality approach. Exciting advances have taken place in the 1980s and 1990s in our understanding of the genetic determinants of this disease. Together with the continuing refinement in treatment techniques, there should be improvement in the management of patients with soft tissue sarcoma.[2]

Epidemiology and Etiology

Epidemiology

Sarcomas are relatively rare mesenchymal tumors, with an estimated 8100 arising in soft tissue and 2500 in bones and joints in the year 2000.[1] It has been estimated also that there are approximately 100 benign tumors for each malignant tumor of soft tissue.[3] The male-to-female ratio is approximately 1.15:1.[1] For some time, the incidence rate for these tumors appeared to be steady[4]; however, for undetermined reasons, the yearly incidence of soft tissue sarcoma now appears to be steadily increasing in both men and women.[1, 5–7]

The above-mentioned numbers include all histologic types of sarcomas. Further, sarcomas arise in virtually all sites within the body, from the scalp to the toes, including the parenchymal organs. The most common sites are the lower and upper extremities (Table 24–1); within the lower extremity, the proximal thigh and buttock comprise the majority of the lesions. This broad spectrum of histologic subtypes and anatomic sites, combined with the overall rarity of soft tissue sarcomas, means that the knowledge base on the natural history and response of these tumors to different therapies is limited relative to that of more common cancers. Because these lesions occur at all body sites, their treatment is challenging and requires individualization for each patient. Therefore, it is important that patients with these tumors are treated at centers where there is a multidisciplinary team that is experienced in their management.

Etiology

Most soft tissue sarcomas occur sporadically. Their etiology is undefined, although, in rare cases, there is an association with familial disease syndromes:

TABLE 24–1. **Anatomic Distribution of Soft Tissue Sarcoma from Massachusetts General Hospital (1988–1995) in 738 Patients**

Site	%
Lower extremity	44
Upper extremity	21
Head and neck	12
Torso	10
Retroperitoneum	6
Other	7

- desmoid tumors among patients with *familial polyposis*[8, 9]
- sarcomas of soft tissue and bone in patients with *hereditary* or *bilateral retinoblastoma*[10]
- *neurofibromatosis type 1*, in which benign neurofibromas and malignant neurofibrosarcomas are seen[5, 11]
- bone and soft tissue sarcomas in patients with *Li-Fraumeni syndrome*[5, 12]

In addition to genetic causes, soft tissue sarcomas are occasionally associated with exposure to carcinogens. For example, radiation therapy has been linked to the development of bone and soft tissue sarcomas,[13] although this occurrence is uncommon and cohort studies of this phenomenon are rare.[14] The frequency of radiation-induced sarcoma is higher following treatment in children, particularly those with Ewing's sarcoma and retinoblastoma.[15, 16] In addition to radiation, exposure to chemicals, such as chemotherapeutic agents, phenoxyacetic acid, chlorophenols, and vinyl chloride, is similarly related to the development of sarcomas.[17–20]

An interesting feature of soft tissue sarcomas is that some of these tumors display stable chromosomal translocations; these translocations eventually may serve as diagnostic criteria. For example, a study in the Netherlands found patterns of structural and numeric imbalances in a series of malignant fibrous histiocytomas, the most common subtype of malignant soft tissue sarcomas. Through the use of comparative genomic hybridization and conventional cytogenetic and Southern blot analyses, researchers have found increases in 1q21-q22 (69%) and 20q (66%), and decreases in 9p21-pter (55%) and 11q23-qter (55%), along with loss of *TP53* and amplification of *MDM2* genes.[21]

Many of these chromosomal abnormalities have been characterized at the molecular level, and the chimeric genes that are associated with these cytogenetic changes have been cloned. Some of these developments are now providing clues to the molecular alterations that are fundamental to the development of soft tissue sarcomas:

- Myxoid liposarcomas display a t(12;16)(q13;p11) translocation.[22–24] The fusion gene, known as *TLS/FUS-CHOP*, fails to induce G_1/S arrest, whereas the nononcogenic form of *CHOP* induces a normal G_1/S arrest.[24]
- Synovial cell sarcomas are characterized by the translocation t(X;18)(p11.2;q11.2), which has been cloned and has led to the identification of two novel genes, *SYT* and *SSX*.[25]
- Alveolar rhabdomyosarcomas show a translocation at t(2;13)(q35;q14). This chimeric gene has also been cloned and has been termed *PAX3-FKHR*.[26] Molecular determination of minimal residual disease in alveolar rhabdomyosarcoma is possible with this gene, but the clinical significance of this finding is uncertain.[27]
- Clear cell sarcomas often exhibit a t(12;22)(q13-14;q12) translocation. This entity is sometimes referred to as malignant melanoma of soft parts, although it should be noted that the t(12;22)(q13-14;q12) translocation is not seen in cutaneous malignant melanoma.[28]
- Alterations of the retinoblastoma gene (*RB*) are a common finding in the sporadic development of soft tissue sarcomas. Loss of *RB* immunoreactivity[29] and *RB* loss of heterozygosity[30] have been correlated with a poorer outcome.
- Somatic alterations of the *TP53* gene are also common in soft tissue sarcomas.[31–34] It is now well recognized that the high cancer incidence in patients with Li-Fraumeni syndrome, in which soft tissue and bone sarcomas are prominent, is the consequence of germ line mutations on the *TP53* gene.[35, 36]
- The *MDM2* gene, located at 12q13-14, was observed to be frequently amplified in soft tissue sarcomas.[37–39] *SAS,* another gene located at 12q13-14, was similarly amplified in soft tissue sarcomas.[40, 41]

Molecular characterization of these chromosomal abnormalities now serves as diagnostic criteria for soft tissue sarcomas. It is expected that diagnoses will be made on the basis of histology, immunohistochemistry, cytogenetics, and molecular biology in the near future.[2, 42] Indeed, genetic evaluation already is proving to be a useful complement to histopathologic assessment.[43]

Detection and Diagnosis

Clinical Detection

Patients with a soft tissue sarcoma commonly present with a painless mass of a few months' duration. Occasionally, patients present with pain secondary to pressure effects or direct invasion of neural structures by the tumor. Frequently, patients recall a history of a traumatic incident, which suggests that the trauma brought the mass to the patient's attention.

Diagnostic Procedures

The diagnostic evaluation includes a complete history and physical examination to evaluate the involved anatomic part for evidence of involvement of skin, major vessels, nerves, or bone and regional lymph nodes.

- *Plain radiographs* are useful for indicating primary bone tumors with soft tissue masses, bone involvement by soft tissue tumors, calcification within the soft tissue mass (e.g., synovial sarcoma), and are of value in excluding some benign tumors, such as myositis ossificans.
- *Magnetic resonance imaging* (MRI) is the most useful method for imaging the extremities and the head and neck in order to detect lesions that require further work-up.[44]
- If plain films indicate either a periosteal reaction or other bone involvement, a *computed tomography (CT) scan* of the primary site with bone windows should be performed. Figure 24–1A and B demonstrates the merits of MRI relative to CT scan in the evaluation of soft tissue sarcoma of the thigh.
- *CT-guided core-needle biopsy* and *fine-needle cytologic aspirates* have all but replaced open or incisional biopsy except in the absence of adequate tissue.[45] These procedures are rapid, minimally invasive, and

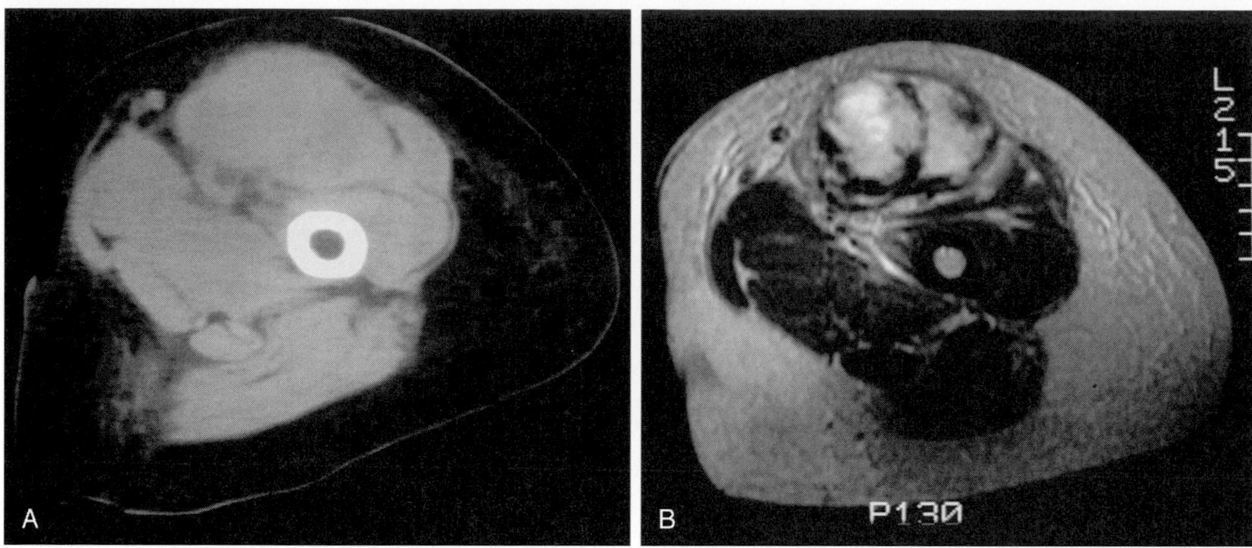

Figure 24–1. Axial sections of the thigh by (A) CT and (B) MRI demonstrating a soft tissue sarcoma. The margins are much more easily appreciated by MRI.

less costly, and they are well suited for deeply situated pelvic or retroperitoneal and extremity lesions. The needle biopsy should be performed by an experienced radiologist, and it should lie within tissue planes to be encompassed in the primary resection. If an incisional biopsy is necessary, it should be performed by the surgeon who will be performing the definitive surgery. The incision, made along the long axis of the limb, is short in length, with meticulous attention paid to hemostasis. Inappropriate biopsy with large areas of potential contamination as evidenced by ecchymosis may preclude limb salvage techniques.[46]

- A *chest CT scan* is recommended for sarcomas larger than 5 cm in diameter,[47] and it is used also for assessment of lung metastases in patients with grade 3 and 4 lesions.[44, 48] For patients with retroperitoneal sarcoma, evaluation of the liver is recommended, because the liver is often the first site of metastatic involvement. Patients with large, high-grade extremity liposarcomas should undergo abdominal CT scans, because these tumors can metastasize to the retroperitoneum and liver.

Classification and Staging

Histopathology

Accurate assignment of histopathologic grade is a central component in the accurate staging of the patient's sarcoma. Grade is generally assigned by a pathologist after review of nuclear and cellular morphology and pleomorphism, the number of mitoses per high-powered field, the presence of necrosis, and the degree of cellularity[49]; grade increases with the relative frequency of these features. Of note, the diagnosing and grading of sarcomas are facilitated by cytohistochemistry, immunohistochemistry, electron microscopy, flow cytometry, cytogenetics, and molecular genetics. Examination of hematoxylin and eosin–stained sections alone is no longer considered to be a sufficient pathologic study in a large proportion of cases.

The histopathologic subtype should be determined, because certain entities, for example, epithelioid sarcomas and liposarcomas, can have unique patterns of spread. Soft tissue sarcomas are subtyped according to the normal cell or tissue type that they resemble. For example, the cells of a liposarcoma resemble fat cells; those of leiomyosarcomas resemble smooth muscle cells; and those of fibrosarcomas resemble fibroblasts. For other sarcomas, the designation reflects the histologic pattern that the tumor mimics, such as alveolar sarcoma that resembles lung parenchyma. The two most common histopathologic subtypes are malignant fibrous histiocytoma and liposarcoma.[47] There seems to be less use of terms such as spindle cell sarcoma and fibrosarcoma, whereas the diagnosis of malignant fibrous histiocytoma now accounts for 40% of soft tissue sarcoma diagnoses (Table 24–2). The relationship between tumor type and histopathologic grade can be seen in Figure 24–2.

Sarcomas grow by local extension, infiltrate adjacent tissues, and extend along tissue planes. They rarely traverse

TABLE 24–2. **Histopathologic Subtypes from Massachusetts General Hospital (1988–1995) in 738 Patients**

Subtype	%
Malignant fibrous histiocytoma	40
Liposarcoma	14
Synovial sarcoma	13
Neurofibrosarcoma	12
Leiomyosarcoma	9
Clear cell sarcoma	3
Angiosarcoma	3
Alveolar soft part sarcoma	2
Fibrosarcoma	1
Epithelioid sarcoma	1
Spindle cell sarcoma	<1
Not specified	<1

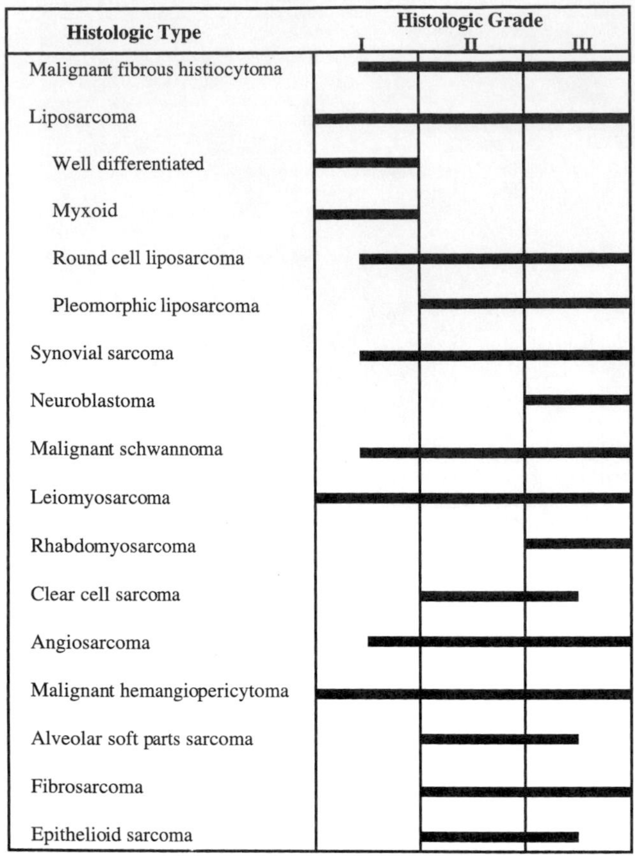

Histologic Type
Histologic Grade
I
II
III
Malignant fibrous histiocytoma
Liposarcoma
Well differentiated
Myxoid
Round cell liposarcoma
Pleomorphic liposarcoma
Synovial sarcoma
Neuroblastoma
Malignant schwannoma
Leiomyosarcoma
Rhabdomyosarcoma
Clear cell sarcoma
Angiosarcoma
Malignant hemangiopericytoma
Alveolar soft parts sarcoma
Fibrosarcoma
Epithelioid sarcoma

Figure 24–2. Estimated range of degree of malignancy based on histologic type and grade. (Modified from Enzinger FM, Weiss SW: Soft Tissue Tumors, 1st ed, p 9. St. Louis, C.V. Mosby Co., 1983, with permission.)

major fascial planes or bone. At diagnosis, more than 90% of sarcoma patients will have localized disease,[50] although eventual tumor spread to distant sites is the most common form of failure, especially for large and high-grade sarcomas.[51, 52] Among these patients, many (>50%) will develop disease in the lung as the first metastatic site.[53–55] Patients with liposarcoma are the exception to the above-mentioned observation, with 59% showing isolated extrapulmonary disease as the site of first metastasis.[56] Sarcomas infrequently spread to regional lymph nodes, with the exception of rhabdomyosarcoma, epithelioid sarcoma, and high-grade synovial sarcoma. The rate of metastasis to the regional lymph nodes at diagnosis or as the first metastasis is approximately 4%, and it increases as a function of grade: grade 1, 0 out of 63; grade 2, 2 out of 118; and grade 3, 17 out of 142.[57]

Staging

The staging of soft tissue sarcoma from the fourth edition of the American Joint Committee on Cancer's (AJCC) staging manual was based primarily on grade and secondarily on size[58]; however, the revised fifth edition includes significant changes to the staging system, incorporating both size and grade with equal weight (Table 24–3).[59] In addition, anatomic location is now incorporated, based on the finding that superficial tumors have a better prognosis.[60] The staging for soft tissue sarcomas is illustrated in Figure 24–3.

The designation of *low grade* is defined as 1 (well differentiated) or 2 (moderately differentiated), whereas *high grade* is designated as 3 (poorly differentiated) or 4 (undifferentiated). Tumors that are 5 cm are still designated as T1, and tumors larger than 5 cm are designated as T2. Superficial tumors, further designated as *a*, are superficial to the investing fascia. Deep tumors, further designated as *b*, are those lesions that are as deep as, or invade, the superficial fascia; all intraperitoneal visceral tumors or lesions with major vessel invasion, intrathoracic lesions, and the majority of head and neck tumors are considered to be deep.[59]

The new staging system was designed on the basis of treatment as well as prognosis: Stage I lesions are generally believed to be manageable by surgery alone; stage II tumors are managed by surgery and radiation therapy; and stage III tumors are often treated with chemotherapy. Retrospective and prospective studies will be needed to validate this system.

Principles of Treatment

Multidisciplinary Treatment Decisions

The preferred management of sarcoma patients is by a multidisciplinary and multispecialty sarcoma team composed of individuals who have a primary clinical and research interest in connective tissue oncology (Table 24–4). Team members should include bone and soft tissue diagnostic radiologists, sarcoma pathologists, orthopedic and general oncologic surgeons, medical and pediatric oncologists, radiation oncologists, nurses, physiotherapists, and data managers. In this manner, the diagnostic evalua-

TABLE 24–3. **Staging of Soft Tissue Sarcomas**

Stage	Grade	Grouping	Descriptor
IA	G1-2	T1a-1b N0 M0	T1a: Superficial tumor; T1b: Deep tumor G1: Well differentiated, low grade G2: Moderately differentiated, low grade N0: No regional lymph node metastasis M0: No distant metastasis
IB	G1-2	T2a N0 M0	T2a: Superficial tumor
IIA	G1-2	T2b N0 M0	T2b: Deep tumor
IIB	G3-4	T1a-1b N0 M0	G3: Poorly differentiated, high grade
IIC	G3-4	T2a N0 M0	G4: Undifferentiated, high grade
III	G3-4	T2b N0 M0	
IVA	Gany	Any T N1 M0	N1: Regional lymph node metastasis
IVB	Gany	Any T Any N M1	M1: Distant metastasis

T1 = tumor ≤5 cm in greatest dimension; T2 = tumor >5 cm in greatest dimension.

Used with the permission of the American Joint Committee on Cancer (AJCC®), Chicago, Illinois. The original source for this material is the AJCC® Cancer Staging Manual, 5th ed, 1997, published by Lippincott-Raven, Philadelphia, Pennsylvania.

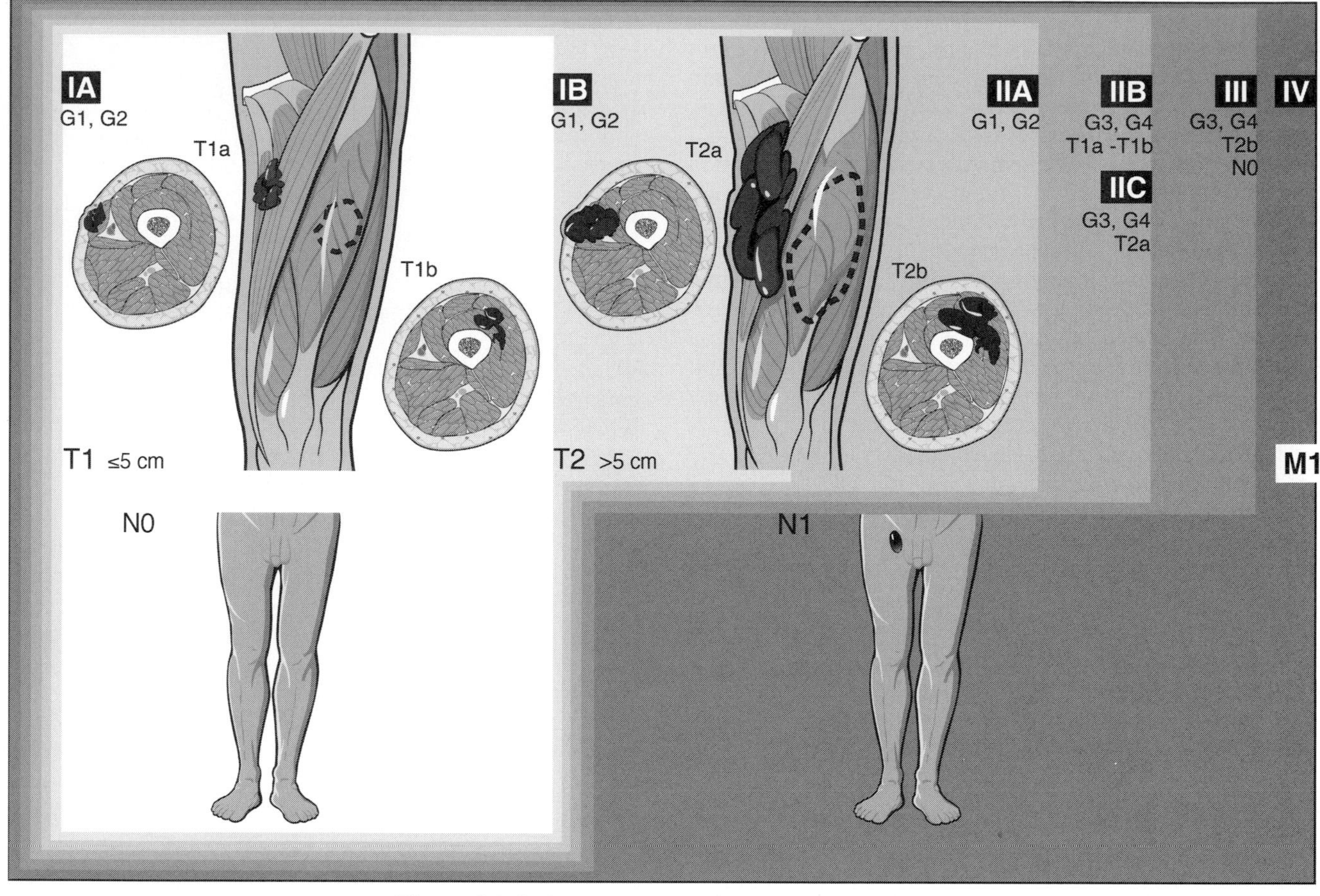

Figure 24–3. Anatomic staging for soft tissue sarcoma.

tion, treatment, and follow-up are performed by the team at a major cancer center, where these patients are seen in substantial numbers.

Surgery

Surgery is considered to be the primary treatment for soft tissue sarcomas. In the 1980s, there was a movement away from amputation, because although the removal of large volumes of grossly normal tissue reduced local failure rates to lower than 20%, it was at the expense of function and cosmesis. Nonetheless, historically, treatment with marginal surgery has been associated with local failure rates of 30% to 50%.[61, 62] In a randomized trial at Memorial Sloan-Kettering Cancer Center, patients undergoing limb-sparing surgery alone had a local failure rate of 33%, despite aggressive surgery by highly experienced oncologic surgeons.[63] In other series with surgery alone, local failure rates of 0% (for amputation) to 31% (for limb-sparing techniques) have been shown.[62, 64–66] In general, patients who have undergone an unplanned tumor resection or resection by a nononcologic surgeon will require additional surgery because of the higher frequency of close or positive margins.[67] In addition, a number of studies have indicated that 37% to 59% of such patients will have residual tumor in the subsequent resection specimen.[68, 69] For large tumors, total compartmental resection or amputation may be required.

TABLE 24–4. **Multidisciplinary Treatment Decisions for Soft Tissue Sarcomas**

Stage	Surgery		Radiation Therapy	Chemotherapy
IA, IB, IIA (G1, G2)	Conservative surgery		If microresiduum, ART: pre/postop 50–60 Gy	NR
IIB, IIC, III (G3, G4)	Conservative surgery		ART: pre/postop 50–60 Gy or BT 45 Gy	ACT: SAC/MAC/IC
IVA (Any G N1)	Conservative surgery		ART: pre/postop 50–60 Gy	ACT: SAC/MAC/IC
	Lymphadenectomy		ART: pre/postop 50–60 Gy	ACT: SAC/MAC/IC
IVB (Any G Any N M+)	Conservative surgery		ART or DRT: 75–80 Gy ± ACT	MAC/IC
	Resect pulmonary metastases		ART or DRT: 75–80 Gy ± ACT	MAC/IC
Recurrent or very advanced	Palliative amputation	or	PRT	SAC/MAC

ART = adjuvant radiation therapy; BT = brachytherapy; DRT = definitive radiation therapy; PRT = palliative radiation therapy; NR = not recommended; ACT = adjuvant chemotherapy; SAC = single-agent chemotherapy; MAC = multiagent chemotherapy; IC = investigational trials. Physicians Data Query recommendations: SAC = doxorubicin; MAC = MAID (mesna, driamycin, ifosfamide, decarbazine), other doxorubicin-based protocols.[47]

In general, wide or radical margins are mandated for high-grade lesions together with adjuvant radiation, whereas wide margins are adequate for low-grade and smaller, more localized lesions (Table 24–5).[70] However, with inadequate margins, even low-grade tumors should be considered for preoperative or postoperative radiation therapy.[71, 72] For patients receiving surgery alone, resection should be radical. A radical margin encompasses all structures within every compartment involved by the tumor, whereas a wide margin encompasses the tumor, its reactive zone or pseudocapsule, and at least 2 cm of normal (negative) tissue in all directions around the lesion,[73] although a fascial plane of minimal thickness also may constitute an adequate resection margin. The excision of the tumor must be *en bloc*, through normal tissues on all sides, with at least a 1-cm margin on all sides of the biopsy scar; any needle biopsy tract or drain tract used for previous biopsy should be included in the resection.

When adjuvant radiation therapy is to be used, the location of the scar should be oriented in anticipation. For an extremity sarcoma, the scar should be vertical along the limb and lateral if possible, because the lymphatic drainage medially is generally richer. When this has not been performed, subsequent attempts to resect are compromised if margins prove to be positive. An example is given in Figure 24–4A, which illustrates a forearm that had a transverse incision placed across the dorsum. Re-resection was deemed to be very difficult; therefore, the patient was treated with radiation. In this instance, the patient has progressed quite well and had an excellent cosmetic and functional outcome; however, the illustrated placement of the incision precluded our usual practice of sparing the medial aspect of the extremity to allow for adequate lymphatic drainage.

For radical surgery, the resected specimen should include the entire musculoaponeurotic structures with contiguous neurovascular tissues and, if possible, regional lymph nodes. Neurologic deficits resulting from resection of major nerves can often be managed effectively postoperatively with appropriate orthotic devices, braces, or tendon transfers. If major blood vessels traverse the tumor or reactive zone, in some cases they can be resected, and anastomotic grafts can be placed by a vascular surgeon. Further surgical details are beyond the scope of this chapter, but they may be found in surgical atlases.[74, 75]

To improve the functional outcome and cosmesis of patients who undergo radical surgery, radiation therapy has been combined with more conservative surgical procedures. The expectation is that moderate doses of radiation can inactivate microscopic deposits of tumor in grossly normal-appearing tissue beyond the surgical resection margin. The merit of this approach was demonstrated in a randomized

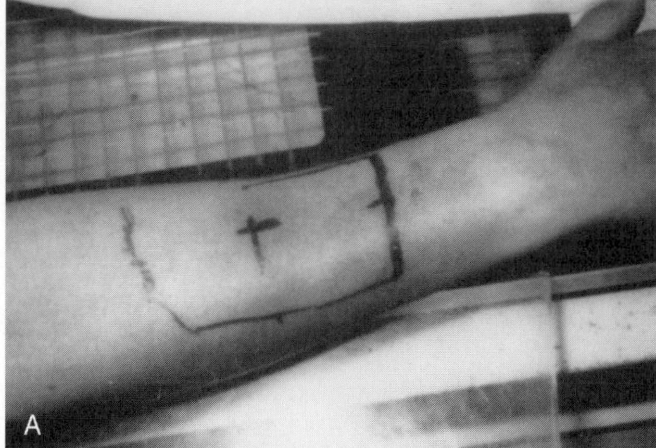

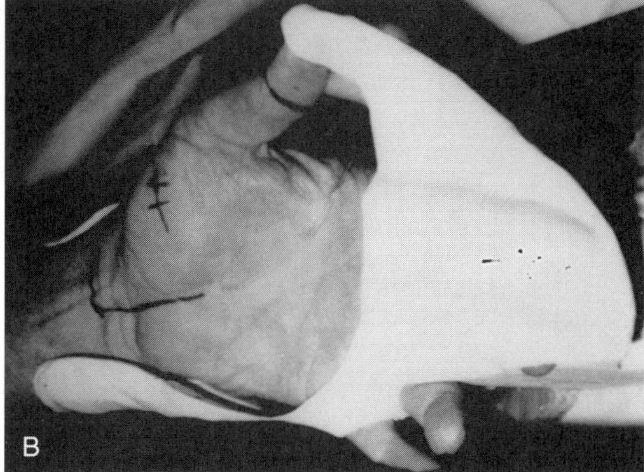

Figure 24–4. (A) The position of a transverse, small surgical excision scar on the dorsal aspect of the forearm. The scar is immediately adjacent to the center cross mark for the radiation field setup. Treatment was by means of opposed lateral fields; the volar or anterior margin of the fields extends just anterior to the interosseous membrane. (B) An immobilization device is shown for a patient who is receiving preoperative radiation for a sarcoma of the thenar eminence.

TABLE 24–5. **Margin Definitions for Surgical Procedures for Soft Tissue Sarcomas**

Margin	Limb Salvage	Amputation	Plane of Dissection	Microscopic Appearance
Intracapsular	Intracapsular piecemeal excision	Intracapsular amputation	Within lesion	Tumor at margin
Marginal	Marginal *en bloc* excision	Marginal amputation	Within reactive zone, extracapsular	Reactive tissue ± microsatellites
Wide	Wide *en bloc* excision	Wide amputation through bone	Beyond reactive zone, through normal tissue, within compartment	Normal tissue ± skips
Radical	Radical *en bloc* resection	Radical disarticulation	Normal tissue, extracompartmental	Normal tissue

From Enneking WF: Staging of musculoskeletal neoplasms. In: Uhthoff HK (ed): Current Concepts of Diagnosis and Treatment of Bone and Soft Tissue Tumors, p. 1. New York, Springer-Verlag, 1984, with permission.

trial at the National Cancer Institute.[76] Since that time, many clinical studies have demonstrated that local control rates with the combined-modality approach are equivalent to those seen with radical surgery alone.[2, 63, 64, 77–83] The success of this approach is reflected in the amputation rate for primary extremity sarcoma at most major centers falling to approximately 5%. Radiation, in combination with surgery, may be delivered pre-, post-, or intraoperatively (electron beam or brachytherapy techniques), allowing for limb preservation.

Radiation Therapy

When planning radiation therapy for a sarcoma patient, the goals are to define accurately the target volume and to estimate the distribution of reproductively intact tumor cells within that target. This estimate includes the probable relative number of clonogenic cells in the gross disease volume and the subclinical disease volume. MRI scanning and, more recently, dynamic MRI have greatly improved and simplified this task; these imaging techniques allow the radiation oncologist to discern the extent of tumor spread and edema in the tissues in which the tumor arises, as well as the likely involvement of adjacent tissues. Minimizing radiation dose to nontarget tissues is essential for improving cosmetic and functional outcome. The extent to which this is achieved increases the patient's tolerance of radiation. The consequence is a higher dose to the tumor and, hence, a better probability of tumor control. Further, the reduced dose to normal tissues means a lower frequency and severity of normal tissue complications.

In the planning of radiation treatment, the radiation oncologist has the same target volume as the surgeon. Treatment plans that incorporate two or more fields, wedges, compensators, and three-dimensional treatment planning can minimize normal tissue effects and generally improve homogeneity within the treatment volume. After defining the target, the anatomic part must be immobilized to minimize the margin allowed for set-up error. As an example, a cast or so-called alpha cradle for immobilizing the hand is presented in Figure 24–4B. If feasible, a sector of uninvolved tissue of the extremity should be spared from full radiation dose in order to preserve lymphatic drainage. Poorly vascularized skin, such as the pretibial, prepatellar, and preolecranon skin, should also be protected, because these areas tend to receive minor, but repeated trauma that may become significant if a full radiation dose has been delivered. Dose maximums in areas in which surgical wounds will be placed also should be avoided.

There is an ongoing debate regarding the relative effectiveness of preoperative versus postoperative radiation. Advocates for preoperative radiation list a number of advantages, but postoperative radiation is thought to have an advantage with regard to wound healing:

- Preoperative radiation allows treatment volumes to be limited to the clinically and radiographically evident disease and tissues judged to be microscopically involved. This is advantageous for radioresponsive tumors, such as liposarcomas, in which a significant reduction in tumor volume is an aid for a more limited resection.
- In contrast, the postoperative radiation portal has to include all of the tissues handled operatively, including drainage sites. A prospective study of portal sizes at Princess Margaret Hospital showed a 62% increase in field size for postoperative treatment versus preoperative.[84] Thus, it can be predicted that there would be a higher *late* morbidity frequency in patients irradiated postoperatively as a consequence of the larger treatment volumes.
- The risk of tumor autotransplantation (wound seeding) is virtually eliminated, as well as the establishment of distant metastases from cells exfoliated into vascular spaces during surgery.
- When surgery precedes radiation, wound complications can delay the start of radiation therapy, permitting residual tumor cells to proliferate during the waiting period. For that time, the viable cells in the surgical bed are exposed to an array of powerful cytokines for cell proliferation.
- In contrast, postoperative radiation is thought to produce fewer delays in wound healing.[85] In addition, the entire untreated pathologic specimen can be assessed for grade and histopathologic subtype when postoperative therapy is used.

The role of preoperative versus postoperative radiation in wound complications is being addressed in a phase III trial being conducted by the National Cancer Institute of Canada.

The local control rates for combined surgery and radiation therapy for a number of institutions are shown in Table 24–6.[77, 78, 86–99] Of note, results from Massachusetts General Hospital indicate that there is a local control advantage for preoperative radiation in the treatment of large lesions, especially those 10 cm or larger in maximum diameter (Table 24–7).

TABLE 24–6. **Local Control Results in Patients Treated with Surgery and Radiation**

Investigators	No. of Patients	% Local Control
Preoperative RT		
Barkley et al[86]	110	90
Suit et al[87]	181	90
Brant et al[77]	58	91
Wilson et al[88]	39	97
Postoperative RT		
Lindberg et al[89]	300	78
Abbatucci et al[90]	89	86
Karakousis et al[91]	53	86
Potter et al[92]	128	90
Keus et al[93]	64	92
Pao et al[78]	35	86
Suit et al[87]	176	86
Wilson et al[88]	23	91
Fein et al[94]	67	87
Mundt et al[95]	50	76
Brachytherapy		
Schray et al[96]	63	92
Alekhteyar et al[97]	87	82
IA/IV Doxorubicin + RT		
Eilber et al[98]	371	~90
Wanebo et al[99]	55	98

RT = radiation therapy; IA/IV = intra-arterial/intravenous.

TABLE 24–7. **5-Year Actuarial Local Control Results from Massachusetts General Hospital According to Size of Primary Soft Tissue Sarcoma**

	Preoperative RT		Postoperative RT	
Size (mm)	***No. of Patients***	***% Local Control***	***No. of Patients***	***% Local Control***
<25	11	80	20	100
26–49	16	100	45	95
50–100	63	93	64	83
101–150	34	100	12	91
151–200	25	79	6	50
>200	11	100	3	67
TOTAL	**160**	**92**	**150**	**87**

DEFINITIVE RADIATION

Radiation alone is a treatment option for the small number of patients whose cancer is medically small or technically inoperable, those who refuse an operation, and for some with radiosensitive subtypes of sarcoma, for example, embryonal rhabdomyosarcomas.[100] Even for T1 tumors, doses of 75 Gy are required if tumor control probabilities of 90% are anticipated. In a randomized trial of radiotherapy versus radiotherapy plus razoxane (a radiosensitizer), the nonsurgical, gross disease arm showed 7-year local control rates of 30% for radiotherapy alone using doses of 56 to 58 Gy, which improved to 64% for radiotherapy plus razoxane.[101] For larger tumors, 5-year control rates of 33% have been reported.[102]

PREOPERATIVE RADIATION THERAPY

Preoperative radiation therapy is planned using current MRI or CT imaging information. Biopsy incisions and needle tracks are included within the treatment volume. Generally, 50 Gy is delivered in 25 to 28 fractions over 5 to 5.5 weeks followed by a 3-week rest period before surgery. Occasionally, a daily dose per fraction of 1.8 Gy is employed if

- the treatment volume is large (linear dimension >30 cm)
- the tumor encompasses visceral organs
- the patient is of advanced age or has comorbid disease

At Massachusetts General Hospital, a few patients have been treated on a twice-per-day (b.i.d.) schedule to a dose of 46.4 Gy, using a daily dose per fraction of 1.6 Gy b.i.d. without additional wound healing morbidity. This schedule has been used mainly to accelerate the treatment as a convenience to the patient, but it also has been used for patients with rapidly growing tumors. At 2.0 Gy b.i.d., we have experienced difficulty in wound healing.

For patients with microscopically positive surgical margins (i.e., tumor is present at a resection edge), a postoperative boost of 16 Gy is delivered at 2.5 to 3 weeks after surgery or when the wound is adequately healed. This boost is intended to cover only the tumor bed with a small margin, not the entire surgical bed. It is advantageous if the surgeon identifies the tumor bed with clips and areas of suspected margin involvement. For patients with greater than a microscopic residual, reoperation to obtain negative margins should be considered. If reoperation is not feasible, then a boost of 26 Gy is given to a small volume of tissue, where the margins are known to be positive.

Obese, elderly patients with large tumors of the proximal medial thigh are at a significant risk of delayed healing. This setting presents a problem for surgery alone, but two of the most critical aspects of the resection of tumor in the patient who has received radiation therapy are closure of the wound without tension and elimination of dead space. Therefore, these patients often require the use of a skin graft or a vascularized myocutaneous flap. In our experience, there have been very few wound healing difficulties in patients who have had grafting, thus avoiding tension in closure after resection over selected sites.

POSTOPERATIVE RADIATION THERAPY

Postoperative radiation therapy generally starts 3 weeks after surgery to allow for adequate wound healing. Additional time may be needed if a seroma develops. The initial treatment volume includes all tissues handled at the time of surgery, including drainage sites, and is carried to a dose of 50 Gy. For the situation in which all gross disease has been removed, a total dose of 60 to 66 Gy is usually delivered through two subsequent field reductions. If gross residual disease remains and cannot be resected, then the dose is carried to 72 to 76 Gy with appropriate field reductions. The planning of postoperative radiation therapy following resection of a large tumor requires an understanding of how normal tissue planes may be altered or shifted in the postoperative state and is the basis for the total dose in patients treated postoperatively being 10 to 15 Gy higher than for preoperative treatment.

INTRAOPERATIVE RADIATION

Intraoperative techniques can be used for boost if the margin status is known at the time of surgery or if it is otherwise indicated, and it is particularly advantageous for retroperitoneal sarcomas in which external beam doses are limited by the small bowel and liver. Boost doses in the range of 15 Gy are used. In a study at Memorial Sloan-Kettering Cancer Center, patients with retroperitoneal sarcomas (associated with very poor prognosis) were treated with surgery, high-dose-rate intraoperative radiation, and postsurgical external beam radiation.[103] The overall 5-year actuarial local control rate was 62%, and the 5-year disease-free survival rate was 55%.

BRACHYTHERAPY

Brachytherapy involves placement of catheters in the long axis of the extremity; catheters are spaced at 1-cm intervals in a single plane. The implant volume is intended to cover the tumor bed plus margin, but it is not intended to cover the entire surgical bed or drain sites. As practiced at Memorial Sloan-Kettering Cancer Center, catheters are loaded on postoperative day 5, and a dose of 45 Gy is administered to a distance of 1 cm from the implant plane. Catheters can be safely placed over neurovascular structures and adjacent to pedicle and free flaps. This technique has the advantage that treatment is complete approximately 10 days postsurgery.

The Massachusetts General Hospital experience is to use brachytherapy as a boost modality at doses of 16 to 30 Gy (prescribed at 0.5 cm). However, these investigators recommend that brachytherapy not be used for low-grade lesions, and it should constitute only a fraction of the treatment for patients with positive surgical margins. Nonetheless, the technique appears to be well suited for smaller high-grade sarcomas. Brachytherapy also may be indicated in patients who have previously received radiation treatment, thus limiting the dose of external beam irradiation that can be delivered.

Chemotherapy

Chemotherapy alone does appear to have some activity in the treatment of soft tissue sarcomas. However, there is no consensus regarding the benefit of the use of postoperative adjuvant chemotherapy. Some researchers argue that no clear survival benefit has been established, designating small nonrandomized trials as inconclusive and calling for adjuvant chemotherapy to be regarded as experimental or investigational.[104–107] Others support the use of chemotherapy, even high-dose chemotherapy, as a valuable tool in the treatment of initially inoperable tumors and metastases.[47, 55, 106, 108] Of note, as with other disease sites, the extent of necrosis can be assessed in patients receiving preoperative chemotherapy, which may be a useful indicator of the response of any metastatic disease.

Distant metastases are the principal sites of relapse in patients with soft tissue sarcomas treated with surgery and radiation. This fact led to a number of trials with adjuvant chemotherapy to include a systemic therapy, and, in general, comparisons of disease-free survival with historic controls frequently have shown some benefit with chemotherapy. For example, results of the EORTC experience with adjuvant cyclophosphamide, vincristine, doxorubicin, and dacarbazine (CyVADIC) chemotherapy has shown that the relapse-free survival rate was 56% in the chemotherapy group versus 43% in control patients.[109] However, this difference was largely due to a decrease in local failure in the chemotherapy group (17% versus 31%) and, in fact, freedom from distant metastasis was identical in both groups.

Results and Prognosis

Results

Surgery

Since the mid- to late 1980s, there has been a general move toward more conservative surgery in an attempt to improve function and cosmesis. However, the use of limb-sparing techniques highlighted the need for adequate surgical margins.[110] Analysis from a number of early trials identified a preference for wide excisions over marginal excisions, particularly for high-grade tumors,[111, 112] and a more recent study of 90 patients supports this approach.[113] Other investigators have attempted to define further the margins required. One group, looking at 88 pediatric non-rhabdomyosarcomas, suggested that pathologic margins of greater than 1 cm reduced local recurrence in both low-grade and high-grade sarcomas,[114] although an earlier study, albeit in adult soft tissue sarcomas, had shown that the extent of the negative margin was not a significant factor.[115] Further, an analysis of 95 patients from the University of Texas M. D. Anderson Cancer Center has suggested that although the achievement of negative margins impacts local control, it has no effect on overall survival.[116] The effect of negative versus positive margins on local control in a number of studies is shown in Table 24–8.[60, 115–118]

Data regarding the functional outcome of patients undergoing limb-salvage procedures alone are limited. Long-term treatment complications were analyzed in patients with sarcoma undergoing limb-sparing therapy at the National Cancer Institute[119]; all of the patients received surgery and radiation therapy. Bone fracture was observed in 6%, contracture in 20%, edema greater than 2+ in 19%, a moderate to severe decrease in strength in 20%, and induration in 57% of the patients. However, the percentage of patients ambulating without assistive devices with mild or no pain was 84%. In another study, in a group of patients with lower limb sarcomas, it was concluded that adjuvant radiation therapy was associated with reduced muscle power and range of motion compared with patients treated with surgery alone.[120] However, overall, most patients retained good to excellent limb function and quality of life with excellent local control. Of note, these authors noted that large doses per fraction were associated with increased fibrosis and poorer outcome. In a series from Toronto of 88 patients treated with either preoperative or postoperative radiation therapy, 68 patients had acceptable functional results, and 61 of these patients returned to work.[118] In this series, large tumors, neural sacrifice, proximal thigh tumors, and postoperative complications were associated with a poor outcome. The authors suggested that limiting complications of wound healing would impact favorably on functional outcome.

Surgery alone can result in significant problems of wound healing, with rates reported to be as high as 40%.[121] This rate, although not the severity, is comparable to results obtained with preoperative radiation therapy (see next sec-

TABLE 24–8. **Surgical Margins and Local Control**

	Local Control %	
Investigators	***M−***	***M+***
Sadoski et al[115]	97	81
Tanabe et al[116]	91	62
Herbert et al[117]	100	55
LeVay et al[118]	87	76
Pisters et al[60]	80	60

tion). Higher rates of wound complication are reported for patients treated with radiation preoperatively as compared with postoperatively.

Based on current results and the experience of others as described in the literature, we suggest strategies that may lead to reduced wound morbidity:

- Increase gentle handling of tissue during surgery.
- Pay meticulous attention to achieving hemostasis before wound closure.
- Avoid closure under tension.
- Eliminate all dead space in the wound. If rotation of a flap is needed to fill the space, then it should be used.
- Drain the wound and leave the tubes in place until the drainage is less than 35 mL per day.
- Make use of a compression dressing; it is advantageous in many situations.
- Immobilize the affected part for at least 7 days.
- Use plastic surgical soft tissue coverage procedures aggressively, such as free tissue transfer, either primarily or secondarily, if signs of healing difficulties or necrosis become evident.

Overall, treatment for soft tissue sarcomas with limb-sparing techniques can now achieve excellent local control rates when they are combined with adjuvant radiation therapy (≥90%), but the 25%-to-50% distant failure rate requires the use of a systemic therapy.[88] In addition, it has been suggested by a small number of reports that there are subsets of patients that do not require adjuvant radiation[81, 114, 122]; this suggestion requires further investigation.

Radiation Therapy

Despite the hypothesis that late complications should be reduced with the use of preoperative radiation due to smaller treatment volumes,[84] there is evidence that acute wound complications are higher with preoperative versus postoperative therapy.[123] Wound healing was assessed in 202 consecutive patients treated at Massachusetts General Hospital with preoperative radiation therapy.[124] The overall wound complication rate was 37%. In 16.5% of the patients, secondary surgery was necessary, including 6 (3%) patients who required amputation. Multivariate analyses of the data showed that the following factors were significantly associated with wound morbidity:

- tumor in the lower extremity ($p < .001$)
- increasing age ($p = .004$)
- postoperative boost with interstitial implant ($p = .016$)

Wound healing among 180 patients treated with conservative surgery and radiation has been reported by a Canadian group.[125] In this study, the significant factors associated with increased risk of wound healing delay were size of the specimen, width of the skin incision, use of preoperative radiation, a history of smoking, and vascular disease.

One multi-institutional study has reported the results of the use of preoperative radiation in conjunction with doxorubicin used as a radiation sensitizer.[99] This trial resulted in excellent local control rates of 98.5%; however, the 5-year disease-free survival rate was 49%, and distant metastases were identified as a major problem.

BRACHYTHERAPY

Both intraoperative and postoperative adjuvant brachytherapy have been used to improve local control rates. A prospective randomized trial has been performed at Memorial Sloan-Kettering Cancer Center to study the use of adjuvant intraoperative brachytherapy.[63, 126, 127] Patients were randomized to receive either adjuvant brachytherapy (42 to 45 Gy over 4 to 6 days) or no further treatment. There was a significant improvement in local control rates with brachytherapy compared with no further treatment (89% versus 66%, respectively).[127] However, this result was not seen with the low-grade tumors,[126] and it was not associated with improvements in either distant failure rates or disease-specific survival.[127]

A French study has reported a 5-year actuarial local control rate of 89% that resulted from intraoperative brachytherapy combined with external radiation.[128] This rate supports the earlier findings from the Memorial Sloan-Kettering group of the advantages seen with the use of a brachytherapy boost, particularly with tumors with positive margins.[97] However, some investigators have reported a higher rate of complication that results from intraoperative brachytherapy, although it has been shown that this could be minimized by delaying the brachytherapy delivery until 5 days postsurgery.[105, 129]

For patients with retroperitoneal sarcoma, treatment is usually pre- or postoperative external beam radiation with either intraoperative radiation or brachytherapy. At Massachusetts General Hospital, the combination of preoperative radiation, grossly complete resection, and an intraoperative boost dose of 12 to 15 Gy has shown an 80% local control rate.[129a] This result was supported by a phase III NCI trial in which there was an 80% local control rate for external beam radiation combined with intraoperative radiation compared to a 20% local control rate for external beam radiation alone.[129b]

Chemotherapy

As noted repeatedly earlier, despite the ready achievement of good local control, 50% of soft tissue sarcoma patients will die from distant metastasis.[130] To this end, multiple investigators have explored the use of adjuvant systemic chemotherapy for high-grade tumors, with early trials centering around the use of doxorubicin (Table 24–9).[109, 131–139] A randomized trial from the Scandinavian Sarcoma Group administered doxorubicin as a single agent postoperatively (both with and without adjuvant radiation), but it failed to show any significant clinical benefit.[133] However, in multiagent protocols, doxorubicin-based regimens have appeared to provide a survival advantage[137]; this advantage has been supported by a 1997 meta-analysis.[140] Investigators from the University of Texas M. D. Anderson Cancer Center have demonstrated a similar benefit from preoperative doxorubicin-based chemotherapy.[141]

An early phase II trial demonstrated a substantial response as a result of the addition of ifosfamide to doxorubicin-based chemotherapy (the MAID chemotherapy regimen).[142] This combination produced a flurry of activity that produced higher response rates in advanced disease, although with indications of increased toxicity from myelo-

TABLE 24–9. **Randomized Adjuvant Chemotherapy Trials with Soft Tissue Sarcomas**

Investigators	Institution	No. of Patients*	DFS (%)	OS (%)
Doxorubicin alone				
Wilson et al[131]	Boston/ECOG	38 controls	62	68
		37 A	74	68
Antman et al[132]	Intergroup (USA)	32 controls	67	89
		32 A	67	82
Alvegard et al[133]	SSG†	77 controls	56	70
		77 A	62	75
	SSG‡	11 controls	64	73
		16 A	62	69
Eilber et al[134]	UCLA	62 controls	54	80
		57 A	58	84
Doxorubicin combination				
Benjamin et al[135]	MDAH	23 controls	35	57
		20 VAC-VAdC	55	65
Edmonson et al[136]	Mayo Clinic	31 controls	68	82
		30 VADIC/VAdC	88	82
Chang et al[137]	NCI	28 controls	54	60
		39 AC-Mtx	75	83
Bramwell et al[109]	EORTC	172 controls	43	56
		145 CyVADIC	56	63

DFS = disease-free survival; OS = overall survival; A = doxorubicin alone; VAC = vincristine, doxorubicin, cyclophosphamide; VAdC = vincristine, actinomycin D, cyclophosphamide; VADIC = vincristine, doxorubicin, dacarbazine; AC-Mtx = doxorubicin, cyclophosphamide, high-dose methotrexate; CyVADIC = cyclophosphamide, vincristine, doxorubicin, dacarbazine.

*All patients received localized treatment in the form of surgery ± radiation therapy.

†Patients received radical resection.

‡Patients received marginal resection.

Adapted from Mertens WC, Bramwell VHC: Adjuvant chemotherapy in the treatment of soft-tissue sarcoma. Clin Orthop Rel Res 1993; 289:81, and Benjamin RS: Evidence for using adjuvant chemotherapy as standard treatment of soft tissue sarcoma. Semin Radiat Oncol 1999; 9:349.

suppression.[143, 144] Some efforts in Europe have attempted to reduce these toxic effects through the use of granulocyte–colony-stimulating factor support.[145–147] Other frequently used protocols include the use of vincristine and cyclophosphamide: VAdC (vincristine, actinomycin D, and cyclophosphamide),[148] VACA (vincristine, cyclophosphamide, actinomycin D, and doxorubicin),[149] and other combinations. However, in an EORTC trial, it was demonstrated that patients receiving doxorubicin alone did as well as those receiving either doxorubicin plus ifosfamide or CyVADIC.[150]

A meta-analysis was performed that combined the results of 15 published randomized trials.[151] These data suggested an improvement in survival at 5 years, although the authors believed that the data needed to be viewed with caution. More recently, these data were reanalyzed, using individual data from 1568 patients treated on 14 trials.[140] Analysis of these data showed a statistically significant improvement in disease-free survival for doxorubicin-based chemotherapy. There was a trend toward improved overall survival, although this result was not statistically significant. There was a 30% reduction in the risk of metastasis, which translated into an absolute benefit of 10%, with an increase in distant relapse-free interval from 60% to 70%. At present in the United States, many high-risk patients are being offered adjuvant multiagent chemotherapy as the so-called standard of care.

Prognosis

Site

The location of the primary tumor affects both the 5- and 10-year survival rates, with extremities yielding better outcomes than either retroperitoneal or visceral sites.[152]

Surgical Margins

In a number of studies, positive surgical margins have been predictive of local failure in soft tissue sarcomas (see Table 24–8). Of interest, for patients treated with preoperative radiation, local control was the same for patients with close (e.g., <1 mm) but negative margins versus those with no tumor in the resection specimen.[115] The completeness of surgical resection may also determine the survival pattern, especially in retroperitoneal sarcomas (Fig. 24–5).[153]

Tumor Size

Several investigators have identified tumor size as an independent tumor-related predictor of outcome.[82, 118, 154] Two review articles have cited 5 cm as the threshold value for poor prognosis,[155, 156] whereas others have used 10 cm as the threshold.[88]

Histologic Grade

Histologic grade has been identified as a prognostic factor in a retrospective review of 1041 patients who presented with localized extremity soft tissue sarcoma.[60] However, comparing results from clinical trials requires caution, because many different grading systems are used.[157–159]

Metastatic Disease

Of the 20% of patients that go on to develop metastases, the majority will have pulmonary metastases only.[153] Importantly, a series from Memorial Sloan-Kettering Cancer Center demonstrated that of the patients that undergo thoracotomy, complete resection results in a 3-year survival rate

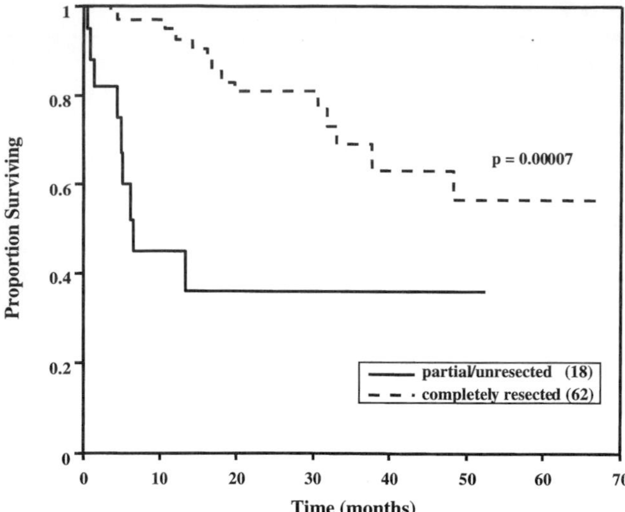

Figure 24–5. Complete surgical resection is the primary factor in outcome of retroperitoneal sarcoma. (From Brennan MF, Casper ES, Harrison LB: Soft tissue sarcoma. In: De Vita VT Jr, Hellman S, Rosenberg SA [eds]: Cancer: Principles & Practice of Oncology, 5th ed, p 1738. Philadelphia, Lippincott-Raven, 1997, with permission.)

of 23% compared with *no* survivors if resection is not performed.[160]

Specific Soft Tissue Sarcomas

Locally Aggressive Benign Soft Tissue Tumors

Desmoid tumors are uncommon and locally aggressive, but nonmalignant lesions with significant local recurrence rates following surgical extirpation.[161] Recurrence can occur both proximally or distally to the primary site and, even more rarely, in the contralateral limb. Treatment of primary lesions is surgical if grossly negative margins can be obtained. Patients with microscopically positive margins after primary surgery can be followed with observation alone *if* they will comply with follow-up, because 25% to 50% of patients will not experience local regrowth despite the positive margins.[162] Patients with primary tumors with grossly positive margins or recurrent tumors with microscopically positive margins are recommended to receive postoperative radiation therapy with doses of 56 to 60 Gy.[163, 164] In addition, definitive external beam radiation therapy can control gross disease in either recurrent or primary disease.[162, 163, 165, 166] Chemotherapy in the form of methotrexate, with or without a second agent, also has been reported to be useful.[167]

Dermatofibrosarcoma protuberans are low-grade tumors of the dermis, managed by surgery with wide margins (2 cm). Of three patients managed at Massachusetts General Hospital by radiation therapy alone, all are demonstrating local control at 9 years.[168]

Malignant Fibrous Histiocytoma

Since the introduction of the term *malignant fibrous histiocytoma* in the 1960s, this class of tumor has become the most commonly diagnosed extremity sarcoma.[153] These tumors have a fibrous histiocytic appearance, and the subtypes consist of the following:

- storiform-pleomorphic fibrous histiocytoma
- myxoid fibrous histiocytoma
- giant cell fibrous histiocytoma (malignant giant cell of soft parts)
- xanthomatous (inflammatory type) fibrous histiocytoma

This lesion characteristically appears in late adulthood, although it can occur in younger patients, originating from a primitive mesenchymal cell or fibroblast.[169] The principles of treatment described in the main body of this chapter should be applied to this sarcoma.

Liposarcoma

Liposarcomas are the second most frequent histologic type of the soft tissue tumors.[170] They can occur almost anywhere that fat is present, and they are usually malignant at inception; only rarely do they arise from lipomas.[170] They appear at all ages, but they are most common in patients between 40 and 60 years of age. Grossly, the tumors are frequently large with multiple convolutions, and they may attain tremendous proportions. In 1859, Delamater reported a liposarcoma weighing 180 pounds; this tumor grew to about 250 pounds at the time of the patient's death.[171] Liposarcomas may be yellowish and resemble fat, or they may have a more myxoid appearance. Of note, the myxoid liposarcoma is often classified as an intermediate-grade tumor with a large metastatic potential.[172] Because histologic subtype is a significant prognostic indicator, pathologic determination is important.[173]

The treatment of choice is resection with a wide surgical margin.[174–176] For high-grade lesions, such as pleomorphic liposarcoma, management is as discussed earlier for all types of high-grade tumor; a complete (extended) resection is particularly critical in younger patients or patients with retroperitoneal tumors.[177–179] Liposarcoma is among the most radioresponsive of the soft tissue sarcomas. Therefore, adjuvant radiation therapy can be given, either preoperatively or postoperatively, and its role is a function of margin status.[99, 173, 180]

There is a predilection for extrapulmonary metastases. Patients with M1 disease should be treated aggressively with systemic chemotherapy as well as appropriate local therapy. The myxoid variant of liposarcoma also shows a higher incidence of regional nodal metastases; therefore, any regional nodes that appear to be suspicious either at physical examination or on MRI or CT scanning should be removed surgically, although routine lymph node dissections are not recommended. However, complete responses that may be sustained for greater than 1 year are not uncommon following the initial aggressive treatment.

The role of adjuvant chemotherapy in the liposarcoma is not yet clearly defined, and it has not been routinely used. Nonetheless, a group from the University of Texas M. D. Anderson Cancer Center has reported some success with doxorubicin-based and dacarbazine-based regimens with the myxoid subtype.[172]

Rhabdomyosarcoma

These tumors are discussed in Chapter 19, Pediatric Solid Tumors. The rhabdomyosarcomas are tumors of the striated muscle, with several types being recognized, for example, *embryonal* and *alveolar*, occurring primarily in children and young adults (less often in adults) and *adult pleomorphic* rhabdomyosarcoma.

- The botryoid type of embryonal rhabdomyosarcoma (sarcoma botryoides) is named after its polypoid, grapelike appearance, and it frequently originates in mucosa-lined organs. It is, therefore, found most commonly in the genitourinary tract, orbit, and nasopharynx.
- Alveolar rhabdomyosarcoma is found chiefly in the extremities. The patient typically complains of severe intermittent or persistent pain in the area, sometimes months before a tumor mass becomes apparent. The tumor is often grayish white and almost cartilaginous, and it has cystic areas. Although there is a pseudocapsule, adjacent tissues are almost always infiltrated.
- The adult pleomorphic rhabdomyosarcoma is the most common form of rhabdomyosarcoma, and it arises most frequently in the extremities, with a special predilection for certain muscle groups: quadriceps, adductors, semimembranous muscles, biceps, and brachialis. They occur most frequently in the fourth to seventh decades, and the typical patient tends to experience repeated local recurrences with ultimate metastases. A few, however, demonstrate explosive growth and early hematogenous and lymphatic spread. The tumor in these cases is hemorrhagic, cystic, and necrotic, with little apparent viable tumor. Overall, this lesion is treated much like other high-grade adult sarcomas.

Treatment of the rhabdomyosarcomas has, like the majority of soft tissue sarcomas, evolved from radical surgery to a more multimodal approach. For example, a number of studies have demonstrated the benefit of adding chemotherapy to the treatment of embryonal rhabdomyosarcoma, both with and without adjuvant radiation.[181, 182] An investigation by Callender and associates showed that combining chemotherapy and irradiation, with or without surgery, produced 5-year survival rates of 60% in patients with head and neck rhabdomyosarcoma compared with survival rates of only 19% in those patients receiving only single modality or surgery with either chemotherapy or radiation alone.[183] Nonetheless, surgery still plays a major role in the treatment of these lesions. Blakely and colleagues have demonstrated that although a combined-modality approach produces good results, debulking significantly improves survival rates,[184] whereas other groups continue to mandate surgery alone when possible, thereby reducing the late effects associated with alternative therapies.[185]

Of note, the prognosis for alveolar rhabdomyosarcomas is worse than for embryonal rhabdomyosarcomas.[184] However, in general, age is the most important prognostic factor, with survival time decreasing in older patients.[186]

Angiosarcoma

Angiosarcomas are extremely rare and are most commonly high-grade tumors derived from vascular endothelial cells.[187] The etiology of vascular sarcomas, like that of other sarcoma types, is unknown; the cutaneous form of angiosarcoma shows a predilection for exposed areas of skin, particularly of the head and neck, raising sun exposure as a possible etiologic agent. In addition, angiosarcomas frequently have been associated with previous irradiation sites, although the mechanism for the radiation induction is unknown.[188] Vascular sarcomas generally present with a mass that may be asymptomatic. With high-grade lesions, warmth, distended venous patterns in overlying skin, and occasionally, a pulsatile nature of the mass may be present. The cutaneous form of angiosarcoma presents with one or more small reddish or purplish nodules that grow gradually.

These tumors are so rare that accurate statistical data are not readily available, but in general, the prognosis of angiosarcoma is poor, depending on size and histologic grade[189]; high-grade angiosarcoma has a dismal prognosis, with its progression frequently described as being relentless.[188, 190] The so-called standard treatment approach involves surgical resection according to the principles elaborated previously for other high-grade soft tissue sarcomas. These tumors are managed in a fashion similar to that of other sarcomas with adjuvant radiation.[191–193] There have been a few reports of limited success with chemotherapy,[188] most recently with paclitaxel,[194] but unfortunately, to date, the outlook for patients with angiosarcoma remains bleak.

REFERENCES

1. Greenlee RT, Murray T, Bolden S, et al: Cancer statistics, 2000. CA Cancer J Clin 2000; 50:7.
2. Suit H: Regaud Lecture, Granada 1994. Tumors of the connective and supporting tissues. Radiother Oncol 1995; 34:93.
3. Enzinger FM, Weiss SW: Soft Tissue Tumors, 1st ed, p 1. St. Louis, C.V. Mosby Co., 1983.
4. Ross JA, Severson RK, Davis S, et al: Trends in the incidence of soft tissue sarcomas in the United States from 1973 through 1987. Cancer 1993; 72:486.
5. Zahm SH, Fraumeni JF Jr: The epidemiology of soft tissue sarcoma. Semin Oncol 1997; 24:504.
6. Landis SH, Murray T, Bolden S, et al: Cancer statistics, 1998. CA Cancer J Clin 1998; 48:6.
7. Landis SH, Murray T, Bolden S, et al: Cancer statistics, 1999. CA Cancer J Clin 1999; 49:8.
8. Lambroza A, Tighe MK, DeCosse JJ, et al: Disorders of the rectus abdominis muscle and sheath: a 22-year experience. Am J Gastroenterol 1995; 90:1313.
9. Sagar PM, Moslein G, Dozois RR: Management of desmoid tumors in patients after ileal-anal anastomosis for familial adenomatous polyposis. Dis Colon Rectum 1998; 41:1350.
10. Moll AC, Imhof SM, Bouter LM, et al: Second primary tumors in patients with retinoblastoma. A review of the literature. Ophthalmic Genet 1997; 18:27.
11. Roos KL, Muckway M: Neurofibromatosis. Dermatol Clin 1995; 13:105.
12. Carnevale A, Lieberman E, Cardenas R: Li-Fraumeni syndrome in pediatric patients with soft tissue sarcoma or osteosarcoma. Arch Med Res 1997; 28:383.
13. Brady MS, Gaynor JJ, Brennan MF: Radiation-induced sarcoma of the bone and soft tissue. Arch Surg 1992; 127:1379.
14. Taghian A, DeVathaire F, Terrier M, et al: Long-term risk of sarcoma following radiation treatment for breast cancer. Int J Radiat Oncol Biol Phys 1991; 21:361.
15. Eng C, Li FP, Abramson DH, et al: Mortality from second tumors among long-term survivors of retinoblastoma. J Natl Cancer Inst 1993; 85:1121.
16. Hawkins MM, Wilson LM, Burton HS, et al: Radiotherapy, alkylat-

ing agents, and risk of bone cancer after childhood cancer. J Natl Cancer Inst 1996; 88:270.
17. Wingren G, Fredrikson M, Brage N, et al: Soft tissue sarcoma and occupational exposures. Cancer 1990; 66:806.
18. Vineis P, Faggiano F, Tedeschi M, et al: Incidence rates of lymphomas and soft tissue sarcomas and environmental measurements of phenoxy herbicides. J Natl Cancer Inst 1991; 83:362.
19. Kogevinas M, Becher H, Benn T, et al: Cancer mortality in workers exposed to phenoxy herbicides, chlorophenols, and dioxins. An expanded and updated cohort study. Am J Epidemiol 1997; 145:1061.
20. Hoppin JA, Tolbert PE, Flanders WD, et al: Occupational risk factors for sarcoma subtypes. Epidemiology 1999; 10:300.
21. Simons A, Schepens M, Jeuken J, et al: Frequent loss of 9p21 (p16(INK4A)) and other genomic imbalances in human malignant fibrous histiocytoma. Cancer Genet Cytogenet 2000; 118:89.
22. Crozat A, Aman P, Mandahl N, et al: Fusion of CHOP to a novel RNA-binding protein in human myxoid liposarcoma. Nature 1993; 363:640.
23. Rabbitts TH, Forster A, Larson R, et al: Fusion of the dominant negative transcription regulator CHOP with a novel gene FUS by translocation t(12;16) in malignant liposarcoma. Nat Genet 1993; 4:175.
24. Barone MV, Crozat A, Tabaee A, et al: CHOP (GADD153) and its oncogenic variant, TLS-CHOP, have opposing effects on the induction of G_1/S arrest. Genes Dev 1994; 8:453.
25. Clark J, Rocques PJ, Crew AJ, et al: Identification of novel genes, SYT and SSX, involved in the t(X;18)(p11.2;q11.2) translocation found in human synovial sarcoma. Nat Genet 1994; 7:502.
26. Barr FG, Galli N, Hollick J, et al: Rearrangement of the PAX3 in the solid tumour alveolar rhabdomyosarcoma. Nat Genet 1993; 3:113.
27. Kelly KM, Womer RB, Barr FG: Minimal disease detection in patients with alveolar rhabdomyosarcoma using a reverse transcriptase-polymerase chain reaction method. Cancer 1996; 78:1320.
28. Fletcher JA: Translocation (12;22)(q13-14;q12) is a non-random aberration in soft tissue clear cell sarcoma. Genes Chromosomes Cancer 1992; 5:184.
29. Cance WG, Brennan MF, Dudas ME, et al: Altered expression of the retinoblastoma gene product in human sarcomas. N Engl J Med 1990; 323:1457.
30. Feugeas O, Guriec N, Babin-Boilletot A, et al: Loss of heterozygosity of the RB gene is a poor prognostic factor in patients with osteosarcoma. J Clin Oncol 1996; 14:467.
31. Stratton MR, Moss S, Warren W, et al: Mutation of the p53 gene in human soft tissue sarcomas: association with abnormalities of the RB1 gene. Oncogene 1990; 5:1297.
32. Wadayama F, Toguchida J, Yamaguchi T, et al: p53 expression and its relationship to DNA alterations in bone and soft tissue sarcomas. Br J Cancer 1993; 68:1134.
33. Andreassen A, Oyjord T, Hovig E, et al: p53 abnormalities in different subtypes of human sarcomas. Cancer Res 1993; 53:468.
34. Patterson H, Gill S, Fisher C, et al: Abnormalities of the p53 MDM2 and DCC genes in human leiomyosarcomas. Br J Cancer 1994; 69:1052.
35. Malkin D: p53 and the Li-Fraumeni syndrome. Cancer Genet Cytogenet 1993; 66:83.
36. McIntyre JF, Smith-Sorensen B, Friend SH, et al: Germline mutations of the p53 tumor suppressor gene in children with osteosarcoma. J Clin Oncol 1994; 12:925.
37. Cordon-Cardo C, Latres E, Drobnjak M, et al: Molecular abnormalities of mdm2 and p53 genes in adult soft tissue sarcomas. Cancer Res 1994; 54:794.
38. Florenes VA, Maelandsmo GM, Forus A, et al: MDM2 gene amplification and transcript levels in human sarcomas: relationship to TP53 gene status. J Natl Cancer Inst 1994; 86:1297.
39. Nilbert M, Rydholm A, Willén H, et al: MDM2 gene amplificant correlates with ring chromosomes in soft tissue tumors. Genes Chromosomes Cancer 1994; 9:261.
40. Forus A, Florenes VA, Maelandsmo GM, et al: Mapping of amplification units in the q13-14 region of chromosome 12 in human sarcomas: some amplica do not include MDM2. Cell Growth Differ 1993; 4:1065.
41. Pedeutour F, Suijkerbuijk RF, Forus A, et al: Complex composition and co-amplification of SAS and MDM2 in ring and giant rod marker chromosomes in well-differentiated liposarcoma. Genes Chromosomes Cancer 1994; 10:85.
42. Barr FG, Chatten J, D'Crus CM, et al: Molecular assays for chromosomal translocations in the diagnosis of pediatric soft tissue sarcomas. JAMA 1995; 273:553.
43. Graadt van Roggen JF, Bovee JV, Morreau J, et al: Diagnostic and prognostic implications of the unfolding molecular biology of bone and soft tissue tumours. J Clin Pathol 1999; 52:481.
44. De Schepper AM, De Beuckeleer L, Vandevenne J, et al: Magnetic resonance imaging of soft tissue tumors. Eur Radiol 2000; 10:213.
45. Heslin MJ, Lewis JJ, Woodruff JM, et al: Core needle biopsy for diagnosis of extremity soft tissue sarcoma. Ann Surg Oncol 1997; 4:425.
46. Singer S, Antman K, Corson JM, et al: Long-term salvageability for patients with locally recurrent soft-tissue sarcoma. Arch Surg 1992; 127:548.
47. Physicians Data Query: Adult soft tissue sarcoma. Bethesda, National Cancer Institute, 1999.
48. Sauter ER, Hoffman JP, Eisenberg BL: Diagnosis and surgical management of locally recurrent soft-tissue sarcomas of the extremity. Semin Oncol 1993; 20:451.
49. Gaynor JJ, Tan CC, Casper ES, et al: Refinement of the clinicopathologic staging for localized soft tissue sarcoma of the extremity: a study of 423 adults. J Clin Oncol 1992; 10:1317.
50. Rydholm A, Berg NO, Gullberg B, et al: Epidemiology of soft-tissue sarcoma in the locomotor system. Acta Pathol Microbiol Immunol Scand 1984; 92:363.
51. Guillou L, Coindre JM, Bonichon F, et al: Comparative study of the National Cancer Institute and French Federation of Cancer Centers Sarcoma Group grading systems in a population of 410 adult patients with soft tissue sarcoma. J Clin Oncol 1997; 15:350.
52. Hayes AJ, Thomas JM: Soft tissue tumours. Postgrad Med J 1997; 73:705.
53. Lewis JJ, Brennan MF: Soft tissue sarcomas. Curr Prob Surg 1996; 33:817.
54. Billingsley KG, Burt ME, Jara E, et al: Pulmonary metastases from soft tissue sarcoma: analysis of patterns of diseases and postmetastasis survival. Ann Surg 1999; 229:602.
55. Sawyer M, Bramwell V: The treatment of distant metastases in soft tissue sarcoma. Semin Radiat Oncol 1999; 9:389.
56. Cheng EY, Springfield DS, Mankin HJ: Frequent incidence of extrapulmonary sites of initial metastasis in patients with liposarcoma. Cancer 1995; 75:1120.
57. Mazeron JJ, Suit HD: Lymph nodes as sites of metastases from sarcomas of soft tissue. Cancer 1987; 60:1800.
58. American Joint Committee on Cancer: Manual for Staging of Cancer, 4th ed. Philadelphia, Lippincott, 1992.
59. American Joint Committee on Cancer: AJCC Cancer Staging Manual, 5th ed. Philadelphia, Lippincott-Raven, 1997.
60. Pisters PW, Leung DH, Woodruff J, et al: Analysis of prognostic factors in 1041 patients with localized soft tissue sarcomas of the extremities. J Clin Oncol 1996; 14:1679.
61. Berlin O, Stener B, Angervall L, et al: Surgery for soft tissue sarcoma in the extremities. A multivariate analysis of the 6-26-year prognosis in 1337 patients. Acta Orthop Scand 1990; 61:475.
62. Azzarelli A: Surgery in the soft tissue sarcoma. Eur J Cancer 1993; 29A:618.
63. Harrison LB, Franzese F, Gaynor JJ, et al: Long-term results of a prospective randomized trial of adjuvant brachytherapy in the management of completely resected soft tissue sarcomas of the extremity and superficial trunk. Int J Radiat Oncol Biol Phys 1993; 27:259.
64. Keus RB, Rutgers EJ, Ho GH, et al: Limb-sparing therapy of extremity soft tissue sarcomas: treatment outcome and long-term functional results. Eur J Cancer 1994; 30:1459.
65. Midis GP, Pollock RE, Chen NP, et al: Locally recurrent soft tissue sarcoma of the extremities. Surgery 1998; 123:666.
66. Gustafson P, Arner M: Soft tissue sarcoma of the upper extremity: descriptive data and outcome in a population-based series of 108 adult patients. J Hand Surg (Am) 1999; 24:668.
67. Siebenrock KA, Hertel R, Ganz R: Unexpected resection of soft-tissue sarcoma. More mutilating surgery, higher local recurrent rates, and obscure prognosis as consequences of improper surgery. Arch Orthop Trauma Surg 2000; 120:65.
68. Zornig C, Peiper M, Schroder S: Re-excision of soft tissue sarcoma after inadequate initial operation. Br J Surg 1995; 82:278.
69. Noria S, Davis A, Kandel R, et al: Residual disease following

unplanned excision of a soft-tissue sarcoma of an extremity. J Bone Joint Surg Am 1996; 78A:650.
70. Enneking WF: Staging of musculoskeletal neoplasms. In: Uhthoff HK (ed): Current Concepts of Diagnosis and Treatment of Bone and Soft Tissue Tumors, p 1. New York, Springer-Verlag, 1984.
71. Suit HD, Spiro IJ, Spear M: Benign and low-grade tumors of the soft tissues: role for radiation therapy. Cancer Treat Res 1997; 91:95.
72. Lindner NJ, Scarborough MT, Powell GJ, et al: Revision surgery in dermatofibrosarcoma protuberans of the trunk and extremities. Eur J Surg Oncol 1999; 25:392.
73. Pisters PWT, Brennan MF: Sarcomas of soft tissue. In: Abeloff MD, Armitage JO, Lichter AS, et al (eds): Clinical Oncology, 2nd ed, p 2273. New York, Churchill Livingstone, 2000.
74. Levine BA: Current Practice of Breast, Skin, and Soft Tissue Surgery. New York, Churchill Livingstone, 1994.
75. Karakousis CP: Surgery for soft tissue sarcomas. In: Bland KI, Karakousis CP, Copeland EM (eds): Atlas of Surgical Oncology, p 283. Philadelphia, W.B. Saunders, 1995.
76. Rosenberg SA, Tepper J, Glatstein E, et al: The treatment of soft tissue sarcoma of the extremities. Ann Surg 1982; 196:305.
77. Brant TA, Parson JT, Marcus RB, et al: Preoperative irradiation for soft tissue sarcomas of the trunk and extremities in adults. Int J Radiat Oncol Biol Phys 1990; 19:899.
78. Pao WJ, Pilepich MV: Postoperative radiotherapy in the treatment of extremity soft tissue sarcomas. Int J Radiat Oncol Biol Phys 1990; 19:907.
79. Shiu MH, Hilaris BS, Harrison L, et al: Brachytherapy and function-saving resection of soft tissue sarcoma arising in the limb. Int J Radiat Oncol Biol Phys 1991; 21:1485.
80. Valle AA, Kraybill WG: Management of soft tissue sarcomas of the extremity in adults. J Surg Oncol 1996; 63:271.
81. Yang JC, Chang AE, Baker AR, et al: Randomized prospective study of the benefit of adjuvant radiation therapy in the treatment of soft tissue sarcomas of the extremity. J Clin Oncol 1998; 16:197.
82. Wilson RB, Crowe PJ, Fisher R, et al: Extremity soft tissue sarcoma: factors predictive of local recurrence and survival. Austral NZ J Surg 1999; 69:344.
83. Wylie JP, O'Sullivan B, Catton C, et al: Contemporary radiotherapy for soft tissue sarcoma. Semin Surg Oncol 1999; 17:33.
84. Nielsen OS, Cummings B, O'Sullivan B, et al: Preoperative and postoperative irradiation of soft tissue sarcomas: effect of radiation field size. Int J Radiat Oncol Biol Phys 1991; 21:1595.
85. Cheng EY, Dusenbery KE, Winters MR, et al: Soft tissue sarcoma: pre-operative versus postoperative radiotherapy. J Surg Oncol 1996; 61:90.
86. Barkley HT, Martin RG, Romsdahl MM, et al: Treatment of soft tissue sarcomas by preoperative irradiation and conservative surgical resection. Int J Radiat Oncol Biol Phys 1988; 14:693.
87. Suit HD, Rosenberg AE, Harmon DC, et al: Soft tissue sarcomas. In: Halnan K, Sikora K (eds): Treatment of Cancer, 2nd ed, p 657. London, Chapman and Hall, 1990.
88. Wilson AN, Davis A, Bell RS, et al: Local control of soft tissue sarcoma of the extremity: the experience of a multidisciplinary sarcoma group with definitive surgery and radiotherapy. Eur J Cancer 1994; 30A:746.
89. Lindberg RD, Martin RG, Romsdahl MM, et al: Conservative surgery and postoperative radiotherapy in 300 adults with soft-tissue sarcomas. Cancer 1981; 47:2391.
90. Abbatucci JS, Boulier N, de Ranieri J, et al: Local control and survival in soft tissue sarcomas of the limbs, trunk walls and head and neck: a study of 113 cases. Int J Radiat Oncol Biol Phys 1986; 12:579.
91. Karakousis CP, Emrich LJ, Rao U, et al: Feasibility of limb salvage and survival in soft tissue sarcomas. Cancer 1986; 57:484.
92. Potter DA, Kinsella T, Glatstein E, et al: High-grade soft tissue sarcomas of the extremities. Cancer 1986; 58:190.
93. Keus RB, Bartelink H: The role of radiotherapy in the treatment of desmoid tumours. Radiother Oncol 1986; 7:1.
94. Fein DA, Lee WR, Lanciano RM, et al: Management of extremity soft tissue sarcomas with limb-sparing surgery and postoperative irradiation: do total dose, overall treatment time, and the surgery-radiotherapy interval impact on local control? Int J Radiat Oncol Biol Phys 1995; 32:969.
95. Mundt AJ, Awan A, Sibley GS, et al: Conservative surgery and adjuvant radiation therapy in the management of adult soft tissue sarcoma of the extremities: clinical and radiobiological results. Int J Radiat Oncol Biol Phys 1995; 32:977.
96. Schray MF, Gunderson LL, Sim FH, et al: Soft tissue sarcomas. Integration of brachytherapy, resection, and external irradiation. Cancer 1990; 66:451.
97. Alekhteyar KM, Leung DH, Brennan MF, et al: The effect of combined external beam radiotherapy and brachytherapy on local control and wound complications in patients with high-grade soft tissue sarcomas of the extremity with positive microscopic margin. Int J Radiat Oncol Biol Phys 1996; 36:321.
98. Eilber FR, Eckardt JJ, Rosen G, et al: Neoadjuvant chemotherapy and radiotherapy in the multidisciplinary management of soft tissue sarcomas of the extremity. Surg Oncol Clin North Am 1993; 2:611.
99. Wanebo HJ, Temple WJ, Popp MB, et al: Preoperative regional therapy for extremity sarcoma. A tricenter update. Cancer 1995; 75:2299.
100. O'Sullivan B, Wylie J, Catton C, et al: The local management of soft tissue sarcoma. Semin Radiat Oncol 1999; 9:328.
101. Rhomberg W, Hassenstein EO, Gefeller D: Radiotherapy vs. radiotherapy and razoxane in the treatment of soft tissue sarcomas: final results of a randomized study. Int J Radiat Oncol Biol Phys 1996; 36:1077.
102. Tepper JE, Suit HD: Radiation therapy alone for sarcoma of soft tissue. Cancer 1985; 56:475.
103. Alektiar KM, Hu K, Anderson L, et al: High-dose-rate intraoperative radiation therapy (HDR-IORT) for retroperitoneal sarcomas. Int J Radiat Oncol Biol Phys 2000; 47:157.
104. Umeda T, Ishii T, Hatakeyama K, et al: Chemotherapy for soft tissue sarcoma—current concepts and review. Gan To Kagaku Ryoho 1993; 20:1937.
105. McGrath PC, Sloan DA, Kenady DE: Adjuvant therapy of soft-tissue sarcomas. Clin Plast Surg 1995; 22:21.
106. Elias AD: High-dose therapy for adult soft tissue sarcoma: dose response and survival. Semin Oncol 1998; 25 (suppl):19.
107. Verweij J, Seynaeve C: The reason for confining the use of adjuvant chemotherapy in soft tissue sarcoma to the investigational setting. Semin Radiat Oncol 1999; 9:352.
108. Levy E, Thirion P, Piedbois P: Adjuvant chemotherapy of soft tissue sarcoma. Cancer Radiother 1997; 1:462.
109. Bramwell V, Rouesse J, Steward W, et al: Adjuvant CYVADIC chemotherapy for adult soft tissue sarcoma—reduced local recurrence but no improvement in survival: a study of the European Organization for Research and Treatment of Cancer Soft Tissue and Bone Sarcoma Group. J Clin Oncol 1994; 12:1137.
110. Collin C, Hajdu SI, Godbold J, et al: Localized operable soft tissue sarcoma of the upper extremity. Presentation, management, and factors affecting local recurrence in 108 patients. Ann Surg 1987; 205:331.
111. Alho A, Alvegard TA, Berlin O, et al: Surgical margin in soft tissue sarcoma. The Scandinavian Sarcoma Group experience. Acta Orthop Scand 1989; 60:687.
112. Antognoni P, Cerizza L, Vavassori V, et al: Postoperative radiation therapy for adult soft tissue sarcomas: a retrospective study. Ann Oncol 1992; 3 (suppl):S103.
113. Flugstad DL, Wilke CP, McNutt MA, et al: Importance of surgical resection in the successful management of soft tissue sarcoma. Arch Surg 1999; 134:856.
114. Blakely ML, Spurbeck WW, Pappo AS, et al: The impact of margin of resection on outcome in pediatric nonrhabdomyosarcoma soft tissue sarcoma. J Pediatr Surg 1999; 34:672.
115. Sadoski C, Suit HD, Rosenberg A, et al: Preoperative radiation, surgical margins, and local control of extremity sarcomas of soft tissue. J Surg Oncol 1993; 52:223.
116. Tanabe KK, Pollock RE, Ellis LM, et al: Influence of surgical margins on outcome in patients with preoperatively irradiated extremity soft tissue sarcomas. Cancer 1994; 73:1652.
117. Herbert SH, Corn BW, Solin LJ, et al: Limb-preserving treatment for soft tissue sarcomas of the extremities. Cancer 1993; 72:1230.
118. LeVay J, O'Sullivan B, Catton C, et al: Outcome and prognostic factors in soft tissue sarcoma in the adult. Int J Radiat Oncol Biol Phys 1993; 27:1091.
119. Stinson SF, Delaney TF, Greenberg J, et al: Acute and long-term effects on limb function of combined modality limb sparing therapy for extremity soft tissue sarcoma. Int J Radiat Oncol Biol Phys 1991; 21:1493.

120. Robinson MH, Spruce L, Eeles R, et al: Limb function following conservation treatment of adult soft tissue sarcoma. Eur J Cancer 1991; 27:1567.
121. Saddegh MK, Bauer HC: Wound complication in surgery of soft tissue sarcoma. Analysis of 103 consecutive patients managed with adjuvant therapy. Clin Orthop Rel Res 1993; 289:247.
122. Baldini EH, Goldberg J, Jenner C, et al: Long-term outcomes after function-sparing surgery without radiotherapy for soft tissue sarcoma of the extremities and trunk. J Clin Oncol 1999; 17:3252.
123. Frezza G, Barbieri E, Ammendolia I, et al: Surgery and radiation therapy in the treatment of soft tissue sarcomas of extremities. Ann Oncol 1992; 3 (suppl):S93.
124. Bujko K, Suit HD, Springfield DS, et al: Wound healing after preoperative radiation for sarcoma of soft tissues. Surgery, Gynecology, and Obstetrics 1992; 176:124.
125. Peat BG, Bell RS, Davis A, et al: Wound-healing complications after soft-tissue sarcoma surgery. Plast Reconstr Surg 1994; 93:980.
126. Pisters PW, Harrison LB, Woodruff JM, et al: A prospective randomized trial of adjuvant brachytherapy in the management of low-grade soft tissue sarcomas of the extremity and superficial trunk. J Clin Oncol 1994; 12:1150.
127. Pisters PW, Harrison LB, Leung DH, et al: Long-term results of a prospective randomized trial of adjuvant brachytherapy in soft tissue sarcoma. J Clin Oncol 1996; 14:859.
128. Delannes M, Thomas L, Martel P, et al: Low-dose-rate intraoperative brachytherapy combined with external beam irradiation in the conservative treatment of soft tissue sarcoma. Int J Radiat Oncol Biol Phys 2000; 47:165.
129. Ormsby MV, Hilaris BS, Nori D, et al: Wound complications of adjuvant radiation therapy in patients with soft-tissue sarcoma. Ann Surg 1989; 210:93.
129a. Willett CG, Suit HD, Tepper JE, et al: Intraoperative electron beam therapy for retroperitoneal soft tissue sarcoma. Cancer 1991; 68:278.
129b. Sindelar WF, Kinsella TJ, Chen PW, et al: Intraoperative radiotherapy in retroperitoneal sarcomas. Final results of a prospective randomized clinical trial. Arch Surg 1993; 128:402.
130. Delaney TF, Yang JC, Glatstein E: Adjuvant therapy for adult patients with soft tissue sarcomas. Oncology 1991; 5:105.
131. Wilson RE, Wood WC, Lerner HL, et al: Doxorubicin chemotherapy in the treatment of soft-tissue sarcoma. Combined results of two randomized trials. Arch Surg 1986; 121:1354.
132. Antman K, Suit H, Amato D, et al: Preliminary results of a randomized trial of adjuvant doxorubicin for sarcomas: lack of apparent difference between treatment groups. J Clin Oncol 1984; 2:601.
133. Alvegard TA, Sigurdsson H, Mouridsen H, et al: Adjuvant chemotherapy with doxorubicin in high-grade soft tissue sarcoma: a randomized trial of the Scandinavian Sarcoma Group. J Clin Oncol 1989; 7:1504.
134. Eilber FR, Giuliano AE, Huth JF, et al: A randomized prospective trial using postoperative adjuvant chemotherapy (adriamycin) in high-grade extremity soft-tissue sarcoma. Am J Clin Oncol 1988; 11:39.
135. Benjamin R, Terjanian T, Fenoglio C, et al: The importance of combination chemotherapy for adjuvant treatment of high risk patients with soft-tissue sarcomas of the extremities. In: Salmon S (ed): Adjuvant Therapy of Cancer V, p 735. Orlando, Grune & Stratton, 1987.
136. Edmonson JH, Fleming TR, Ivins JC, et al: Randomized study of systemic chemotherapy following complete excision of nonosseous sarcomas. J Clin Oncol 1984; 2:1390.
137. Chang AE, Kinsella T, Glatstein E, et al: Adjuvant chemotherapy for patients with high-grade soft-tissue sarcomas of the extremity. J Clin Oncol 1988; 6:1491.
138. Mertens WC, Bramwell VHC: Adjuvant chemotherapy in the treatment of soft-tissue sarcoma. Clin Orthop Rel Res 1993; 289:81.
139. Benjamin RS: Evidence for using adjuvant chemotherapy as standard treatment of soft tissue sarcoma. Semin Radiat Oncol 1999; 9:349.
140. Sarcoma Meta-Analysis Collaboration: Adjuvant chemotherapy for localised resectable soft-tissue sarcoma of adults: meta-analysis of individual data. Lancet 1997; 350:1647.
141. Pisters PW, Patel SR, Varma DG, et al: Preoperative chemotherapy for stage IIIB extremity soft tissue sarcoma: long-term results from a single institution. J Clin Oncol 1997; 15:3481.
142. Elias A, Ryan L, Sulkes A, et al: Response to mesna, doxorubicin, ifosfamide, and dacarbazine in 108 patients with metastatic or unresectable sarcoma and no prior chemotherapy. J Clin Oncol 1989; 7:1208.
143. Edmonson JH, Ryan LM, Blum RH, et al: Randomized comparison of doxorubicin alone versus ifosfamide plus doxorubicin or mitomycin, doxorubicin, and cisplatin against advanced soft tissue sarcomas. J Clin Oncol 1993; 11:1269.
144. Antman K, Crowley J, Balcerzak SP, et al: An intergroup phase III randomized study of doxorubicin and dacarbazine with or without ifosfamide and mesna in advanced sarcomas. J Clin Oncol 1993; 11:1276.
145. Bui BN, Chevallier B, Chevreau C, et al: Efficacy of lenograstim on hematologic tolerance to MAID chemotherapy in patients with advanced soft tissue sarcoma and consequences on treatment dose-intensity. J Clin Oncol 1995; 13:2629.
146. Erkisi M, Erkurt E, Ozbarlas S, et al: The use of recombinant human granulocyte colony-stimulating factor in combination with single or fractionated doses of ifosfamide and doxorubicin in patients with advanced soft tissue sarcoma. J Chemother 1996; 8:224.
147. Reichardt P, Tilgner J, Hohenberger P, et al: Dose-intensive chemotherapy with ifosfamide, epirubicin, and filgrastim for adult patients with metastatic or locally advanced soft tissue sarcoma: a phase II study. J Clin Oncol 1998; 16:1438.
148. Ruymann FB, Vietti T, Gehan E, et al: Cyclophosphamide dose escalation in combination with vincristine and actinomycin-D (VAC) in gross residual sarcoma. A pilot study without hematopoietic growth factor support evaluating toxicity and response. J Pediatr Hematol Oncol 1995; 17:331.
149. Pratt CB, Maurer HM, Gieser P, et al: Treatment of unresectable or metastatic pediatric soft tissue sarcomas with surgery, irradiation, and chemotherapy: a Pediatric Oncology Group study. Med Pediatr Oncol 1998; 30:201.
150. Santoro A, Tursz T, Mouridsen H, et al: Doxorubicin versus CY-VADIC versus doxorubicin plus ifosfamide in first-line treatment of advanced soft tissue sarcomas: a randomized study of the European Organization for Research and Treatment of Cancer Soft Tissue and Bone Sarcoma Group. J Clin Oncol 1995; 13:1537.
151. Tierney JF, Mosseri V, Stewart LA, et al: Adjuvant chemotherapy for soft-tissue sarcoma: review and meta-analysis of the published results of randomised clinical trials. Br J Cancer 1995; 72:469.
152. Linehan DC, Lewis JJ, Leung D, et al: Influence of biologic factors and anatomic site in completely resected liposarcoma. J Clin Oncol 2000; 18:1637.
153. Brennan MF, Casper ES, Harrison LB: Soft tissue sarcoma. In: DeVita VT Jr, Hellman S, Rosenberg SA (eds): Cancer. Principles & Practice of Oncology, 5th ed, p 1738. Philadelphia, Lippincott-Raven, 1997.
154. Vraa S, Keller J, Nielsen OS, et al: Prognostic factors in soft tissue sarcomas: the Aarhus experience. Eur J Cancer 1998; 34:1876.
155. Zagars GK, Mullen JR, Pollack A: Malignant fibrous histiocytoma: outcome and prognostic factors following conservation surgery and radiotherapy. Int J Radiat Oncol Biol Phys 1996; 34:983.
156. Gibbs CP, Peabody TD, Mundt AJ, et al: Oncologic outcomes of operative treatment of subcutaneous soft-tissue sarcomas of the extremities. J Bone Joint Surg (Am) 1997; 79:888.
157. Borders AC, Hargrave R, Meyerding HW: Pathologic features of soft tissue sarcoma with special reference to the grading of its malignancy. Surg Gynecol Obstet 1939; 69:267.
158. Trojani M, Contesso G, Coindre JM, et al: Soft tissue sarcoma of adults: study of pathologic prognostic variables and definition of a histologic grading system. Cancer 1984; 33:37.
159. Alvegard TA, Berg NO: Histopathology peer review of high-grade soft tissue sarcoma: The Scandinavian Sarcoma Group experience. J Clin Oncol 1989; 7:845.
160. Gadd MA, Casper ES, Woodruff J, et al: Development and treatment of pulmonary metastases in adult patients with extremity soft tissue sarcoma. Ann Surg 1993; 218:705.
161. Nuyttens JJ, Rust PF, Thomas Jr CR, et al: Surgery versus radiation therapy for patients with aggressive fibromatosis or desmoid tumors: a comparative review of 22 articles. Cancer 2000; 88:1517.
162. Spear MA, Jennings LC, Mankin HJ, et al: Individualizing management of aggressive fibromatoses. Int J Radiat Oncol Biol Phys 1997; 40:637.
163. Kamath SS, Parsons JT, Marcus RB, et al: Radiotherapy for local control of aggressive fibromatosis. Int J Radiat Oncol Biol Phys 1996; 36:325.

164. Ballo MT, Zagars GK, Pollack A: Radiation therapy in the management of desmoid tumors. Int J Radiat Oncol Biol Phys 1998; 42:1007.
165. Acker JC, Bossen EH, Halperin EC: The management of desmoid tumors. Int J Radiat Oncol Biol Phys 1993; 26:851.
166. Ballo MT, Zagars GK, Pollack A, et al: Desmoid tumor: prognostic factors and outcome after surgery, radiation therapy, or combined surgery and radiation therapy. J Clin Oncol 1999; 17:158.
167. Skapek SX, Hawk BJ, Hoffer FA, et al: Combination chemotherapy using vinblastine and methotrexate for the treatment of progessive desmoid tumor in children. J Clin Oncol 1998; 16:3021.
168. Suit HD, Spiro IJ, Mankin HJ, et al: Radiation in management of patients with dermatofibrosarcoma protuberans. J Clin Oncol 1996; 14:2365.
169. Schneider P, Busch U, Meister H, et al: Malignant fibrous histiocytoma (MFH). A comparison of MFH in man and animals. A critical review. Histol Histopathol 1999; 14:845.
170. Springfield D: Liposarcoma. Clin Orthop Rel Res 1993; 289:50.
171. Delamater J: Mammoth tumor. Cleveland Med J 1859; 1:31.
172. Patel SR, Burgess MA, Plager C, et al: Myxoid liposarcoma. Experience with chemotherapy. Cancer 1994; 74:1265.
173. Zagars GK, Goswitz MS, Pollack A: Liposarcoma: outcome and prognostic factors following conservation surgery and radiation therapy. Int J Radiat Oncol Biol Phys 1996; 36:311.
174. Witz M, Shapira Y, Dinbar A: Diagnosis and treatment of primary and recurrent retroperitoneal liposarcoma. J Surg Oncol 1991; 47:41.
175. Lucas DR, Nascimento AG, Sanjay BK, et al: Well-differentiated liposarcoma. The Mayo Clinic experience with 58 cases. Am J Clin Pathol 1994; 102:677.
176. Zahir KS, Quin JA, Brown W, et al: Trends in the incidence of upper extremity soft tissue malignancies: a 40-year review of the Connecticut State Tumor Registry. Conn Med 1998; 62:9.
177. La Quaglia MP, Spiro SA, Ghavimi F, et al: Liposarcoma in patients younger than or equal to 22 years of age. Cancer 1993; 72:3114.
178. van Doorn RC, Gallee MP, Hart AA, et al: Resectable retroperitoneal soft tissue sarcomas. The effect of extent of resection and postoperative radiation therapy on local tumor control. Cancer 1994; 73:637.
179. Ferrari A, Casanova M, Spreafico F, et al: Childhood liposarcoma: a single-institutional twenty-year experience. Pediatr Hematol Oncol 1999; 16:415.
180. Pollack A, Zagars GK, Goswitz MS, et al: Preoperative vs. postoperative radiotherapy in the treatment of soft tissue sarcomas: a matter of presentation. Int J Radiat Oncol Biol Phys 1998; 42:563.
181. Balat O, Balat A, Verschraegen C, et al: Sarcoma botryoides of the uterine endocervix: long-term results of conservative surgery. Eur J Gynaecol Oncol 1996; 17:335.
182. Hahlin M, Jaworski RC, Wain GV, et al: Integrated multimodal therapy for embryonal rhabdomyosarcoma of the lower genital tract in postpubertal females. Gynecol Oncol 1998; 70:141.
183. Callender TA, Weber RS, Janjan N, et al: Rhabdomyosarcoma of the nose and paranasal sinuses in adults and children. Otolaryngol Head Neck Surg 1995; 112:252.
184. Blakely ML, Lobe TE, Anderson JR, et al: Does debulking improve survival rates in advanced-stage retroperitoneal embryonal rhabdomyosarcomas? J Pediatr Surg 1999; 34:736.
185. Daya H, Chan HS, Sirkin W, et al: Pediatric rhabdomyosarcoma of the head and neck: is there a place for surgical management? Arch Otolaryngol Head Neck Surg 2000; 126:468.
186. La Quaglia MP, Heller G, Ghavini F, et al: The effect of age at diagnosis on outcome in rhabdomyosarcomas. Cancer 1994; 73:109.
187. Enzinger FM, Weiss SW: Soft Tissue Tumors, 3rd ed. St. Louis, Mosby, 1995.
188. Lydiatt WM, Shaha AR, Shah JP: Angiosarcoma of the head and neck. Am J Surg 1994; 168:451.
189. Naka N, Ohsawa M, Tomita Y, et al: Prognostic factors in angiosarcoma: a multivariate analysis of 55 cases. J Surg Oncol 1996; 61:170.
190. Haustein UF: Angiosarcoma of the face and scalp. Int J Dermatol 1991; 30:851.
191. Morrison WH, Byers RM, Garden AS, et al: Cutaneous angiosarcoma of the head and neck. A therapeutic dilemma. Cancer 1995; 76:319.
192. Mark RJ, Poen JC, Tran LM, et al: Angiosarcoma. A report of 67 patients and a review of the literature. Cancer 1996; 77:2400.
193. Aust MR, Olsen KD, Lewis JE, et al: Angiosarcomas of the head and neck: clinical and pathologic characteristics. Ann Otol Rhinol Laryngol 1997; 106:943.
194. Fata F, O'Reilly E, Ilson D, et al: Paclitaxel in the treatment of patients with angiosarcoma of the scalp or face. Cancer 1999; 86:2034.

25 *Bone Tumors*

RANDY N. ROSIER, MD, PhD, Orthopedic Oncology
REGIS J. O'KEEFE, MD, PhD, Orthopedic Oncology
DEEPAK M. SAHASRABUDHE, MD, Medical Oncology

Is this the poultice for my aching bones?

WILLIAM SHAKESPEARE,
Romeo and Juliet

Perspective

Primary malignant bone tumors are relatively rare compared with other types of cancer, but nowhere else is the value of the multidisciplinary approach to cancer management better exemplified than in the area of bone tumors. Diagnosis often depends on input from the orthopedist, pathologist, and radiologist. Improvements in multidisciplinary management, multiagent chemotherapy, and diagnostic techniques have led to an increase in survival time of patients with these traditionally devastating neoplasms. For example, the 5-year survival rate for the management of primary tumors of the bone in children younger than age 15 has risen from 20% in 1963 to 67% for the period of 1989 to 1995.[10]

Both the diagnosis and the treatment decisions are based on the multidisciplinary process. Chemotherapy has contributed substantially to the management of bone tumors and the control of metastases, and aggressive drug combinations have been developed, particularly in the pediatric and young adult age groups.[11–13] Immunotherapy is still experimental, but it has shown some promise.[14] However, surgery remains the mainstay of treatment of the primary tumor, and limb-salvage procedures are firmly established as viable therapeutic methods for maintaining function and cosmesis.[15, 16] Previous data raised the possibility that the improvement in therapy results was due to changes in the natural history of certain tumors. However, subsequent studies have indicated that improvements in survival time of patients with these tumors are more likely related to better staging technology and adjuvant therapy.[17]

Epidemiology and Etiology

Epidemiology

Approximately 2500 new tumors of the bone and joint are expected to arise in the United States in the year 2000,[10] with the highest incidence occurring during adolescence at the age of 15 years, which coincides with adolescent growth spurts.[18] The incidence rate is the same in both sexes until about the age of 13, at which point cases in the male population become more common.[19] In spite of the high incidence in this age group, bone tumors comprise only 5% to 6% of childhood malignancies.[20] The incidence falls to 0.5 per 100,000 at ages 30 to 44 years and, thereafter, rises slowly until, at 75 to 79 years, the incidence is 2 per 100,000.[21]

Etiology

- The observation of a high incidence in children supports the assumption that skeletal neoplasms arise in areas of rapid growth, that is, that growing or modeling bone is susceptible to neoplastic transformation.[4] In addition, the most common location of primary bone sarcomas is the metaphyseal region, that is, near the growth plate. This area is the region in the bone with the most intense cellular proliferation and remodeling activity during long bone growth. The highest incidences of primary bone tumors occur in the distal femur and proximal tibia, the two areas with the most active growth plates. Figure 25–1 indicates the relative anatomic origins of the common bone tumors.[22]
- Prolonged growth or overstimulated metabolism may blend imperceptibly with neoplasia. This situation can be recognized in neoplasms arising in adult tissues affected by metabolic stimulation from longstanding conditions, for example, Paget's disease (giant cell tumors or osteosarcomas),[23] hyperparathyroidism (brown tumors),[24] chronic osteomyelitis (squamous cell carcinomas and osteosarcomas),[25] and old bone infarctions (malignant fibrous histiocytoma).[26]
- External beam irradiation, as well as internal bone-seeking radioisotopes from occupational and medicinal use, has been linked to the formation of osteogenic sarcomas, chondrosarcomas, and fibrosarcomas.[27, 28]
- Certain developmental anomalies and benign tumors are prone to malignant transformation. Chromosomal translocations (e.g., those induced by radiation) have been identified in a large number of sarcomas (Table 25–1).[29] As described in earlier chapters, chromosomal translocations can allow for the activation of oncogenes or the inactivation of tumor suppressor genes. For instance, in 95% of Ewing's sarcoma cases, there is a translocation between chromosomes 11 and 22 that has been postulated as being responsible for the

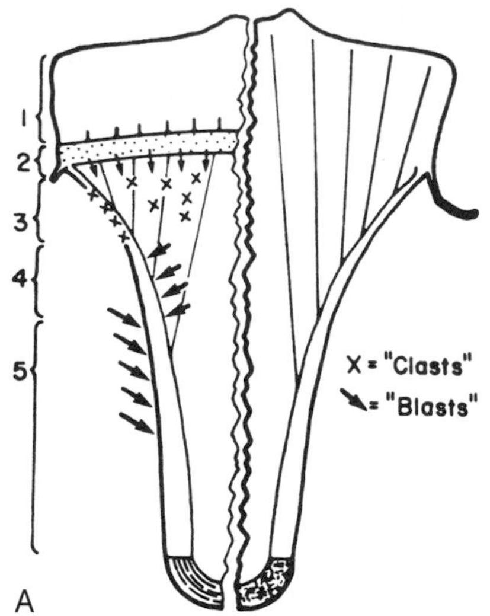

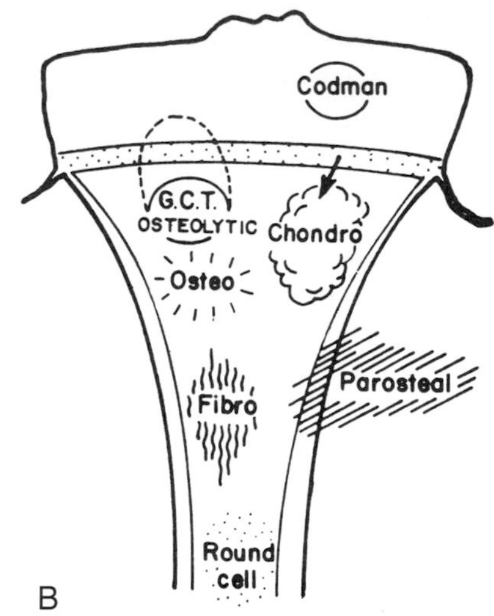

Figure 25–1. The relationship of modeling processes to bone tumors. (A) Cross section of growing long bone illustrates the geographic distribution of osteoclasts and osteoblasts. Five zones of endochondral growth: epiphysis, growth plate, subadjacent half of metaphysis, diaphyseal half of metaphysis, diaphysis. (B) Corresponding bone tumors in different sites to illustrate possible modeling aberrations (G.C.T. = giant cell tumor; Codman = chondroblastoma). (From Johnson LC: A general theory of bone tumors. Bull NY Acad Med 1953; 29:164, with permission).

development of the sarcoma.[30] This translocation results in the formation of a fusion protein between the *EWS* and *Fli1* genes, and related small round cell tumors have been shown to share this site, including peripheral primitive neuroectodermal tumor (PNET), Ewing's sarcoma, and Askin's tumor.[31–33] This fusion creates an abnormal transcription factor (EWS-Fli1), which binds to DNA and stimulates target genes. Because of variations in this chromosomal breakpoint, different EWS-Fli1 fusion proteins exist; the most common are type 1 (60%) and type 2 (25%), with tumors that exhibit type 2 having a better prognosis.[34]

- One gene worth noting is the focal adhesion kinase (*FAK*) gene that codes for pp125^{FAK} tyrosine kinase. This kinase is involved in cell adhesion, motility, and anchorage-independent growth,[35, 36] and it has been demonstrated in increased amounts in 13 different sarcomas relative to normal tissue,[37] which suggests that pp125^{FAK} may be involved in invasion and metastasis.[38]
- As described in earlier chapters, the two most well-studied tumor suppressor genes are the retinoblastoma (*RB*) and *TP53* genes. Patients with hereditary retinoblastoma are at risk for other neoplasms, with approximately 30% to 50% of the additional tumors that develop in these patients being osteosarcomas.[39, 40] In addition, analysis of a series of osteosarcomas from patients who had no known evidence of retinoblastoma revealed that 15% to 35% of the tumors had *RB* mutations.[41] It also has been shown that 28% to 65% of osteosarcomas have *TP53* mutations.[41–43] However, only a few patients appear to have a germline mutation, that is, a mutation that affects all of the cells of the individual.[44, 45]
- The murine double minute–2 (*MDM2*) gene has been shown in soft tissue sarcomas to bind to wild-type p53 protein, inhibiting p53-DNA binding and normal p53-regulated growth.[41, 46] Overexpression of this gene leads to p53 inactivation, which has been found to occur in 10% of osteosarcomas and 13% of Ewing's sarcomas,[47, 48] although not in chondrosarcomas. However, it also must be noted that alterations in the *MDM2* and *TP53* pathways appear to occur independently of each other.[41]

The roles played by both tumor suppressor genes and oncogenes in sarcoma progression are under intensive investigation, and some identified chromosomal aberrations are listed in Table 25–1. As specific genetic targets are identified, there is the increasing probability of the formulation of therapeutic approaches, including specific tumor vaccines.[49]

Detection and Diagnosis

Clinical Detection

Patients generally present with pain in the area of the lesion. The pain tends *not* to be activity related, as with many other types of musculoskeletal problems, and commonly, it may be worse at night. In more advanced lesions, patients may note a mass or swelling (but, generally, only if there is significant periosteal reaction or the tumor has eroded through the bony cortex), and he or she may occa-

TABLE 25–1. **Characteristic Cytogenetic Aberrations in Malignant Bone**

Histology	Characteristic Cytogenetic Event	Frequency (%)	Comments
Ewing's sarcoma	T(11;22)(g24;q11.2-12)	95%	Fusion protein EWS-Fli1, which is a transcription factor
Synovial sarcoma	T(X;18)	95%	Fusion of *SSX* with *SYT*
Malignant fibrous histiocytoma	Complex	90%	
Myxoid chondrosarcoma	T(9;22)	50%	
Multiple hereditary exostosis	8q24.1, 11p13, 19q		Mutations in *EXT1, 2,* or *3*

Modified from Fletcher JA: Cytogenetics and experimental models of sarcomas. Curr Opin Oncol 1994; 6:367, with permission.

sionally present with a pathologic fracture. If the lesion is near a joint, a sympathetic effusion or stiffness of the joint may be seen. Occasionally, symptoms distant from the primary site may occur, either through pain referral patterns (such as a hip lesion that presents with pain referred to the knee) or by nerve compression that causes distal neurologic symptoms. Systemic or constitutional symptoms, such as weight loss, fevers, malaise, or night sweats, are quite uncommon with most bone sarcomas, but they occur more commonly with Ewing's sarcoma, or in cases with multiple metastases at the time of presentation.

A complete patient history is extremely important for a number of reasons:

- A past history of carcinoma may suggest a metastatic etiology of a new bone lesion; previous radiation treatment to an area may suggest a radiation-induced sarcoma.
- A long history (months to years) of symptoms from a bone lesion may indicate a benign nature, such as an osteoid osteoma, whereas symptoms that rapidly progress over weeks or a few months would signify a higher likelihood of a malignant process.
- In patients with known cartilaginous lesions, for example, enchondroma or osteochondroma, occurrence of further growth in adulthood or pain may be an early indication of malignant transformation.

Consideration of demographics is essential for the differential diagnosis. For example, a lytic bone tumor with a permeative appearance in the distal femur would likely be

- an osteosarcoma or Ewing's sarcoma in a 15-year-old patient
- a lymphoma in a 45-year-old patient
- a myeloma in a 55-year-old patient
- metastases in a 70-year-old patient

Location is also an important consideration. Both giant cell tumors of bone and chondroblastomas typically occur in the epiphysis of the bone, adjacent to the joint surface. Thus, a lytic lesion with a geographic appearance in the epiphysis would likely be

- a chondroblastoma in a 15-year-old patient
- a giant cell tumor in a 30-year-old patient

Early detection of primary bone tumors is extremely difficult because of their rarity, and in general, it is the presence of pain that leads to evaluation for a bone tumor. As most of these tumors progress rapidly, incidental discovery of these lesions is rare.

Diagnostic Procedures

Conventional radiographs of the involved bone are mandatory, and together with the patient's age (see earlier), they are most important in developing a differential diagnosis before biopsy. Oblique or magnification views may occasionally be needed. *Magnetic resonance imaging* (MRI) and *computed tomography* (CT) scanning are required to rule out a malignancy or in preoperative planning.

A number of radiographic features should be considered in the evaluation of a bone lesion as they influence the differential diagnosis:

- Lesions may be lytic (destroying bone) or blastic (either forming bone or inducing reactive bone formation).
- Osteosarcoma is an example of a blastic, bone-forming tumor. However, osteosarcomas also can be completely lytic, and there is great overlap in the appearance of many tumors.

With regard to the lytic areas, a bone tumor may demonstrate several different patterns of bone destruction:

- Geographic lesions are well circumscribed, and they frequently have a well-defined, sclerotic border. There is typically no extension of the tumor beyond the radiographically evident lesion border, implying a slow growth rate. This, typically, is seen in benign tumors, such as osteoblastomas, giant cell tumors, or nonossifying fibromas. This pattern also can be observed in low-grade malignant lesions, such as a low-grade chondrosarcoma.
- A so-called moth-eaten pattern suggests an aggressive tumor, with multiple lytic areas and, frequently, cortical destruction. The tumor extends within the bone beyond the radiographically evident lytic areas and suggests an intermediate rate of growth.
- A permeative pattern implies extremely rapid and infiltrative growth, with diffuse areas of lytic destruction invading the bone. Permeative lesions are often associated with cortical disruption and extraosseous soft tissue mass, and they are characteristic of high-grade lesions. However, acute infection also can have this appearance, as well as, occasionally, benign tumors, such as eosinophilic granulomas. This overlap underscores the necessity for accurate diagnostic biopsy.
- Periosteal reactions can be of several types. A so-called sunburst periosteal reaction implies very proliferative malignant bone formation, and it is characteristic of an aggressive tumor, such as osteosarcoma or Ewing's sarcoma. Codman's triangle refers to the raised, normal periosteum at the margin of a bone tumor associated with reactive periosteal new bone formation; it can be seen with a variety of malignant bone tumors. A lamellar periosteal reaction (onion skin) implies rapid cyclic tumor growth, and it is most classically associated with Ewing's sarcoma, although it is not specific for this tumor. Spiculated periosteal reactions also occur in aggressive, rapidly growing tumors such as Ewing's sarcoma, and they represent reactive periosteal bone being deposited along periosteal vessels as the expanding tumor stretches the periosteum.

MRI has replaced CT in many circumstances.[50] MRI scans precisely delineate soft tissue components and their relationship to other anatomic structures. They also demonstrate clearly the reactive zone of the tissue, and edema in the marrow or soft tissues are also evident.[51] In the case of highly malignant bone tumors with cortical destruction and a soft tissue mass, MRI shows the relationship between normal tissues, neurovascular structures, and the tumor tissue—which is essential when planning a biopsy or treatment. Subtle marrow changes, indicative of skip metastases, can be readily visualized; however, soft tissue involvement can be overestimated because of hematoma, reactive edema, and inflammatory response.

Gadolinium has proved to be useful in further delineating differences between normal and neoplastic tissue, for example, distinguishing enchondroma from chondrosarcoma,[52] and clarifying intra- and periarticular extension. In addition, *gadolinium-enhanced MRI scans* can be used to assess histologic response to chemotherapy by comparing pretherapy and post-therapy scans; this information can be useful to both the medical oncologist and the surgeon. The medical oncologist may alter ongoing drug regimens, and the tumor response helps in surgical planning; a poor response requires wider surgical margins. Nonetheless, gadolinium contrast should be ordered selectively.

MRI is considered to be the so-called gold standard by most practitioners; however, *radionuclide bone scintigraphy,* particularly using technetium-99m, is useful for evaluating the extent of the lesion within the bone of origin, as well as for ruling out skip metastases or distant bony metastases.[53] Although bone scans lack specificity for neoplasms, the studies are extremely sensitive, and they can detect tumor foci in bone that is not visualized on standard radiographs. Bone scan results are frequently negative in multiple myeloma; therefore, if multiple myeloma is suspected, a skeletal survey of standard radiographs is indicated,[54] although this is the only malignant bone lesion in which the skeletal survey is routinely useful.

CT scanning also demonstrates soft tissue extension of the lesion and is important in staging. In particular, a CT scan is excellent for determining if there is any disruption of the bony cortex. However, assessment of extension into soft tissue planes or near major neurovascular structures is better accomplished with MRI. Although CT scan remains the standard for detecting occult metastases in the chest, it has been largely replaced by MRI for three-dimensional evaluation of the local tumor.

A number of laboratory studies have proved to be useful in bone sarcoma evaluation. These include blood cell count and sedimentation rate, alkaline phosphatase, serum calcium, and lactic dehydrogenase:

- The white blood cell count, differential, and sedimentation rate may be useful to exclude osteomyelitis, which can frequently mimic a primary bone tumor.[55] The sedimentation rate may also be elevated in myeloma, Ewing's sarcoma, eosinophilic granuloma, and bone lymphomas, but generally not to the high levels seen in osteomyelitis.[56] Of note, anemia is found in over 90% of patients with myeloma.
- Alkaline phosphatase concentration may be elevated, particularly in osteosarcoma, and it is at extremely high levels in the secondary osteosarcoma of Paget's disease.[57, 58] The levels of elevation of both alkaline phosphatase and L-lactate dehydrogenase have been shown to correlate with survival time in Ewing's sarcoma and osteosarcoma, respectively.[59, 60]
- Metastatic prostatic carcinoma can be excluded by the lack of elevated levels of acid phosphatase or absence of prostate-specific antigen.[61, 62]
- Hypercalcemia may suggest myeloma or metastatic disease, but it can also be present in brown tumors of hyperparathyroidism; although, with this latter lesion, there is associated hypophosphatemia.[63]
- Multiple myeloma can be diagnosed by serum protein electrophoresis if a significant level of abnormal immunoglobulin is present; serum immunoelectrophoresis is a more sensitive test to detect a monoclonal gammopathy, and presence of light chains in the urine by Bence Jones testing, or immunoelectrophoresis also can be helpful.[64]

Biopsy

Biopsy is essential in the diagnosis of any primary bone neoplasm. Nonetheless, accurate localization of the lesion before biopsy facilitates selection of an appropriate biopsy site that will not interfere with resection of the tumor and will minimize compartmental contamination:

- In general, biopsy sites should be placed so that major neurovascular structures and blood vessels are not encountered during the procedure, because contamination may hinder subsequent limb salvage.
- Any incision on the extremities should be longitudinal so that the biopsy tract or incision, along with at least 1 cm of skin and subcutaneous tissue on all sides, can be excised *en bloc* with the specimen during subsequent definitive surgery.
- Biopsy should not involve dissection of any structures. It should be performed *through* muscle that is expected to contain tumor spillage from the biopsy and can be resected with the specimen. Biopsy *between* muscles can result in significant contamination.
- If a bony defect exists in the cortex, biopsy should be performed at this site rather than making any additional surgical defect in the bone that could weaken and predispose it to pathologic fracture. Presence of a pathologic fracture in the extremities leads to contamination of multiple compartments and usually precludes limb-salvage procedures.
- Meticulous hemostasis must be maintained after biopsy to prevent seeding additional tissue planes. Use of a drain tract that is placed in line with and near the biopsy incision in order to facilitate its subsequent excision at the time of resection may also minimize hematoma formation.
- Another useful technique is packing of the biopsy defect in the bone with methyl-methacrylate cement, bone cement, or thrombin-soaked gel foam, which is performed to stop any bleeding from the bone.

The area of the tumor chosen for biopsy is also critical:

- Biopsy of the tumor should be performed through the compartment in which the tumor has risen to prevent contamination to other structures.
- The periphery of the lesion, where the interface between the tumor and normal tissues can be examined, generally provides the best assessment, because osteosarcomas and other bone sarcomas tend to demonstrate fewer differentiated characteristics peripherally, whereas central areas may contain more differentiated bone formation or necrosis.
- This approach is also helpful in differentiating myositis ossificans from an osteosarcoma, which it can resemble radiographically. In myositis, the lesion tends

to be most mature and differentiated at the periphery and more cellular and proliferative centrally.[65, 66]

- Finally, a frozen section always should be obtained to be sure that there is adequate tissue for definitive diagnosis; however, in general, permanent sections are needed for final diagnosis on which to base definitive therapy. A preoperative discussion with the pathologist is useful. Tissue also should be sent for aerobic, anaerobic, fungal, and tuberculosis cultures, because some lesions can prove to be infections and, in rare cases, tumor and infection coexist.

Because of the reaction of normal bone and periosteal elements to the lesion, sampling error is a potential problem and can make diagnosis difficult. For this reason, incisional biopsy is preferred by many, although needle biopsies are effective and can achieve a diagnostic accuracy of 70% to 90% at institutions with experience with this technique.[67–69] Even cytogenetic analysis can be performed on fine-needle aspirations of Ewing's sarcoma.[70]

In 1992, a repeat study was performed by the Musculoskeletal Tumor Society (MSTS) to determine the rates of complication, as well as other issues, from biopsies.[71] The study confirmed previous results that showed an increase in complications performed in referring institutions compared with treatment centers, supporting the view that biopsy should be performed by the surgeon who is going to provide the definitive treatment.

TABLE 25–2. **General Classification of Bone Tumors**

Histologic Type	(%)
Sarcoma	
Fibrosarcoma	5.7
Malignant fibrous histiocytoma	3.0
Other	2.7
Osteosarcoma	35.1
Osteosarcoma	29.4
Specified osteosarcoma	5.7
Osteosarcoma in Paget's disease	0.9
Juxtacortical osteosarcoma	1.6
Other	3.2
Chondrosarcoma	25.8
Ewing's sarcoma	16.0
Adamantinoma of long bones	0.2
Hemangiosarcoma	1.4
Chordoma	8.4
Other	6.2
Unspecified	1.2

Modified from Dorfman HD, Czerniak B: Bone cancers. Cancer 1995; 75:203.

Classification and Staging

Histopathology

A primary bone cancer is any neoplasm that arises from the tissues or cells present within bone and has the capability of producing metastases. Because many types of cells are present within the medullary space of bone and adjacent to the bone surface, a number of histologic tumor types are possible, including tumors derived from osteoblasts, cartilage cells, fat, fibrous tissue, vascular elements, and hematopoietic and neural tissues. These tumor types are all referred to as *sarcomas*, a term that signifies a common derivation from mesenchymal tissues.

Bone sarcomas are named in relation to the predominant differentiated tissue type, although obviously multiple cellular elements may be present in any given tumor. Bone-forming tumors are referred to as *osteosarcomas*, cartilage tumors as *chondrosarcomas*, fibroblastic tumors as *fibrosarcomas* or *malignant fibrous histiocytomas*, fat-forming tumors as *liposarcomas*, and tumors derived from vascular elements as *angiosarcomas*. Table 25–2 gives the classification and incidence of various benign and malignant bone tumors derived from SEER data for the period of 1973 to 1987.

- *Osteosarcoma* is the most common of the primary malignant bone sarcomas,[4, 72] and it is defined as a tumor in which osteoid is synthesized by malignant cells. In general, it is a tumor of adolescents and young adults between the ages of 10 and 30, and it commonly occurs around the knee. A second peak of incidence occurs in the elderly, frequently as a complication of Paget's disease[73, 74] or in pre-existing lesions,[75] and it may also be secondary to radiation therapy for other tumors.[27, 76] The commonest form of osteosarcoma (85%) occurs in the metaphysis of the long bones and is a high-grade intramedullary variant. Others of the eight recognized variants of osteosarcoma include both high- (e.g., high-grade surface, periosteal) and low-grade (e.g., parosteal, intraosseous well-differentiated) variants.[77]
- The second most common type of bone tumor is the *chondrosarcoma*, which makes up approximately 25% of malignant bone sarcomas.[21] Unlike the majority of other primary bone tumors, the incidence of chondrosarcomas increases with age, and the tumors frequently involve the axial skeleton. Chondrosarcomas may be primary, but they frequently occur as secondary malignancies that develop in pre-existing benign lesions, such as the enchondroma or osteochondroma.[78, 79] In multiple forms of these lesions, such as enchondromatosis (Ollier's disease) or hereditary multiple exostoses, the incidence of malignant transformation of one or more lesions can be as high as 25%.[80, 81]

  Whereas secondary chondrosarcomas rarely occur in patients younger than 50 years of age, those arising in conditions with multiple lesions, such as Ollier's disease or multiple hereditary osteochondromatosis, frequently occur early in adulthood. Biologic behavior also is dependent on the location of the lesion: more centrally located tumors have a worse prognosis and an increased risk of metastasis. Thus, cartilage tumors in the hands are rarely considered to be malignant, even though their histologic feature may appear more aggressive than more centrally located lesions.
- *Fibrosarcoma* is relatively rare as a primary sarcoma in bone, and it is seen more commonly either as a soft tissue sarcoma or as a complication of other conditions, such as Paget's disease[82]; the diagnosis of fibrosarcoma has largely been replaced by *malignant fibrous histiocytoma.* Although less frequent, the tumor can occur as a primary lesion and may be associated

with pre-existing or predisposing conditions, such as bone infarctions, fibrous dysplasia, or previous therapeutic irradiation to bone.[26] Malignant fibrous histiocytomas occur over a wide age range (6 to 81 years), although over 50% of the cases occur in patients older than 40 years of age; the most common site of malignant fibrous histiocytoma is the femur.

- *Round cell tumors,* which include primary lymphomas of bone, Ewing's sarcoma, and metastatic neuroblastoma, are discussed in other chapters. Ewing's sarcoma, the second most common primary bone tumor of childhood, comprises about 10% to 15% of all primary malignant bone tumors,[4, 83] and, similar to osteosarcoma, occurs in individuals between the ages of 10 and 30.
- Most malignant lesions in bone are of *metastatic* origin. In men, the most common metastatic tumors found in bone are from the lung and prostate, whereas in women the most common is from the breast. Metastatic carcinoma is encountered most frequently in the spine, proximal femur, proximal humerus, and pelvis; it becomes less frequent as the anatomic site moves further from the trunk. Metastatic bone lesions distal to the elbow or the knee are extremely rare, but the primary tumor associated most frequently with these distal or acrometastases is lung carcinoma.[84] Other primary tumor sites commonly associated with bony metastases are the kidney and thyroid.

Staging

An anatomic staging system using the tumor, node, metastasis (TNM) parameters has been formalized by the American Joint Committee on Cancer (AJCC). Table 25–3 shows the suggested AJCC guidelines for staging; see also Figure 25–2.[9] In addition, the MSTS has developed a surgical staging system for malignant bone tumors, which uses the same variables as the AJCC, but with different weighting. This system correlates well with prognosis, and it is widely used by orthopedic oncologists (Table 25–4); the system also stages benign bone tumors.

TABLE 25–3. **AJCC's TNM Staging System of Bone Cancer**

Stage	Grouping	Grade	Descriptor
IA	T1,N0,M0	G1, 2	T1: Tumor confined within cortex
IB	T2,N0,M0	G1, 2	T2: Tumor invades beyond the cortex G1: Well differentiated—low grade G2: Moderately differentiated—low grade N0: No regional lymph node metastasis M0: No distant metastasis
IIA	T1,N0,M0	G3, 4	G3: Poorly differentiated—high grade
IIB	T2,N0,M0	G3, 4	G4: Undifferentiated—high grade
III			Not defined
IVA	Any T,N1,M0	Any G	N1: Regional lymph node metastasis
IVB	Any T,Any N,M1	Any G	M1: Distant metastasis

Used with the permission of the American Joint Committee on Cancer (AJCC®), Chicago, Illinois. The original source for this material is the AJCC® Cancer Staging Manual, 5th edition (1997), published by Lippincott-Raven Publishers, Philadelphia, Pennsylvania.

TABLE 25–4. **MSTS Staging System for Bone Sarcomas**

Stage	Grouping	Grade	Descriptor
IA	T1,M0	G1	T1: Intracompartmental
IB	T2,M0	G1	T2: Extracompartmental G1: Low grade M0: No distant metastasis
IIA	T1,M0	G2	G2: High grade
IIB	T2,M0	G2	
III	T1-2,M1	G1-2	M1: Regional or distant metastasis

Modified from Enneking WF: A system of staging musculoskeletal neoplasms. Clin Orthop Rel Res 1986; 204:9.

The MSTS staging system is based on the concept of compartmental localization of the tumor. Compartments are composed of bone, musculofascial envelopes (such as the muscular compartments of the extremities), joints, skin, and subcutaneous tissues.[85] Neurovascular sheaths, although not technically separate compartments, are like fascial boundaries in providing a relative barrier to tumor penetration, and this consideration may influence surgical decisions regarding limb-salvage procedures.

Involvement of more than one compartment leads to placement in a higher surgical stage and correlates with poorer prognosis. Thus, the anatomic *T* parameter is similar in both staging systems: T1 is within the bone (intracompartmental); T2 indicates extension beyond the cortex of the bone. Spread of bone tumors to lymph nodes is rare; the usual pattern is hematogenous spread to pulmonary and other sites. In addition, distant metastases carry a similar poor prognosis, whether the metastasis is to regional nodes or to the lung. Therefore, the MSTS staging system does not differentiate N1 or M1, and nodal or other metastases place the patient in stage III; in this regard, the two staging systems differ. Finally, tumor grade is limited to G1 and G2 (low grade or high grade) in the MSTS system, as opposed to G1 to G4 in the AJCC system, owing to frequent disagreement among pathologists on specific grading of tumors, particularly with intermediate-grade lesions.

Principles of Treatment

Malignant tumors are managed best by a combination of surgery, chemotherapy, and radiation therapy, although the exact treatment is strongly dependent on the tumor type (Table 25–5).[86–88] Lower grade sarcomas (MSTS stage I) are almost always treated with definitive surgery alone, with results often depending on the adequacy of the resection margins.[89, 90] Such tumors include secondary chondrosarcomas, arising in enchondromas or osteochondromas, and parosteal osteosarcomas. Even higher grade chondrosarcomas are generally treated primarily with surgery, because all cartilage tumors are relatively resistant to chemo-

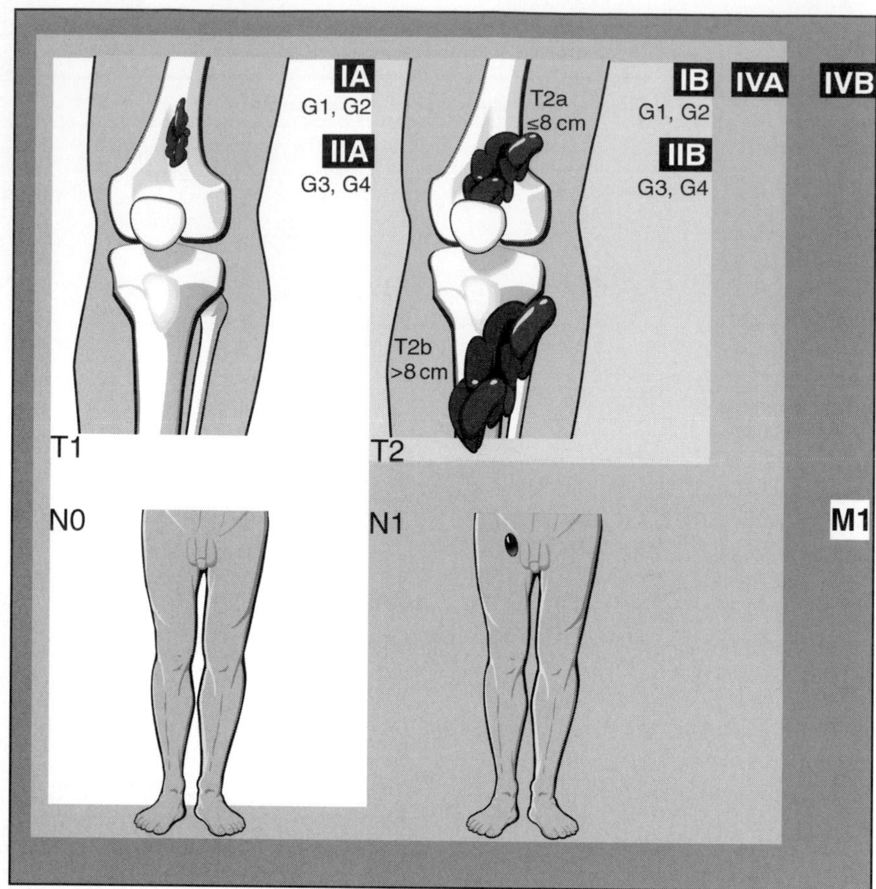

Figure 25–2. Anatomic staging for bone tumors.

therapy and radiation. Central, high-grade osteosarcomas and Ewing's sarcomas are treated with surgery and adjuvant chemotherapy; however, Ewing's sarcoma is radiosensitive, so supplemental radiation is occasionally used, depending on the surgical margins. This use is particularly true for pelvic Ewing's sarcomas, in which a combination of radiation and surgery has decreased local recurrence rates in some cases. In those tumors for which more limited data are available, the role of local radiation therapy and adjuvant chemotherapy is still controversial. A concise tabulation of multidisciplinary decisions in managing osteogenic sarcomas, Ewing's sarcoma, and other tumors of the bone is seen in Table 25–5.

Surgery

Nonmalignant tumors are best removed surgically by the most direct route possible. Large defects in the bone are filled with suitable bone grafts, and occasionally, protective internal fixation may be needed to prevent fracture or to stabilize a pathologic fracture. Intralesional resection (generally curettage) or, occasionally, marginal resection is generally adequate for treatment of these lesions. Marginal resection is sometimes used for more aggressive benign tumors, such as chondromyxoid fibroma, juxtacortical chondroma, and giant cell tumor, although curettage supplemented with an adjuvant, such as the chemical agent phenol or methyl methacrylate cement, also gives acceptable local control.[91] This approach also has been used successfully with low-grade chondrosarcomas.

There has been a shift away from radical surgical amputation of a limb, which often included the joint above the tumor as well as the entire bone, to more conservative surgery, and it is now performed in only 10% to 15% of patients. Limb-salvage surgery can allow for better function

TABLE 25–5. **Multidisciplinary Treatment Decisions for Bone Tumors**

Tumor	Surgery	Radiation Therapy	Chemotherapy
Osteosarcoma			
Low grade	Intralesional or marginal resection	NR	NCT*
High grade	Wide or radical resection	NR	NCT* + Postop CT*
Ewing's sarcoma	Amputation or limb salvage	RT 50–60 Gy	NCT: VAC ± IE
Chondrosarcoma	Amputation or limb salvage	NR	NR
Solitary plasmacytoma	NR	Definitive RT 50 Gy	NR

NR = not recommended; RT = curative radiation therapy; NCT = neoadjuvant chemotherapy; Postop CT = postoperative chemotherapy; VAC ± IE = vincristine, doxorubicin, cyclophosphamide ± etoposide, ifosfamide.

*Chemotherapy protocols consist of combinations of high-dose methotrexate, cisplatin, doxorubicin, cyclophosphamide, etoposide ± ifosfamide.

and cosmesis without compromise of local control or survival.[15, 16, 92] Improvements in imaging methods have allowed for better preoperative assessment of disease extent, facilitating assessment of patient suitability for limb-sparing surgery. In addition, development of new techniques of limb reconstruction, such as custom prosthetic implants, and use of allografts have made limb salvage an increasingly available treatment option.

Surgical Definitions. For consistency in evaluation of the surgical aspects of tumor treatment, some definitions have been proposed by MSTS.[6, 85] These definitions pertain to the anatomic extent and types of surgical procedures that are performed, and they provide a common ground for judging the efficacy of a given surgical treatment. Tumor resection margins are named similarly to the corresponding surgical procedure[93]:

- An *intralesional margin* or surgical procedure means gross macroscopic tumor is left behind. This procedure would generally be associated with incisional biopsy for diagnosis of a malignant lesion, or curettage of a known benign lesion.
- A *marginal resection* or *marginal margin* indicates that the resection plane goes through the reactive zone of the tumor, allowing for the possibility of residual microscopic disease within this zone.
- A *wide resection* or *margin* refers to removal of a tumor *en bloc*, with normal tissue surrounding the reactive zone in all planes. The amount of normal tissue considered to constitute a wide margin varies greatly, depending on the location and tissue type. For instance, a resection through bone is generally considered to be wide if the resection level is 3 to 5 cm above the reactive zone of the lesion, whereas a layer of fascia from a muscular compartment might constitute a wide margin because of its efficacy as an anatomic barrier, even though the tissue may be only a few millimeters thick.
- Finally, a *radical* surgical procedure (or *curative margin*) refers to a situation in which all structures in every compartment involved by the tumor are removed in their entirety. For a bone tumor, at a minimum, this means removal of the entire bone involved; any compartments with soft tissue extension would also have to be removed.

Amputation nomenclature is identical; therefore, an amputation may be intralesional, marginal, wide, or radical, depending on the level with regard to the above-mentioned definitions. Figure 25–3 illustrates this scheme diagrammatically.

Local control can be achieved in 90% of patients with primary malignant bone tumors treated with wide resection, limb salvage, and chemotherapy.[94, 95] A wide resection is generally considered to be acceptable if careful preoperative evaluation discloses no evidence of skip metastases and if the tumor responds well to chemotherapy.[96, 97] Bone scans should be used to detect skip areas; a margin of at least 3 to 5 cm above the proximal extension of tumor is recommended. In addition, MRI may show subtle marrow abnormalities indicative of skip lesions, and it should be included for preoperative assessment of the intraosseous extent of disease.[98]

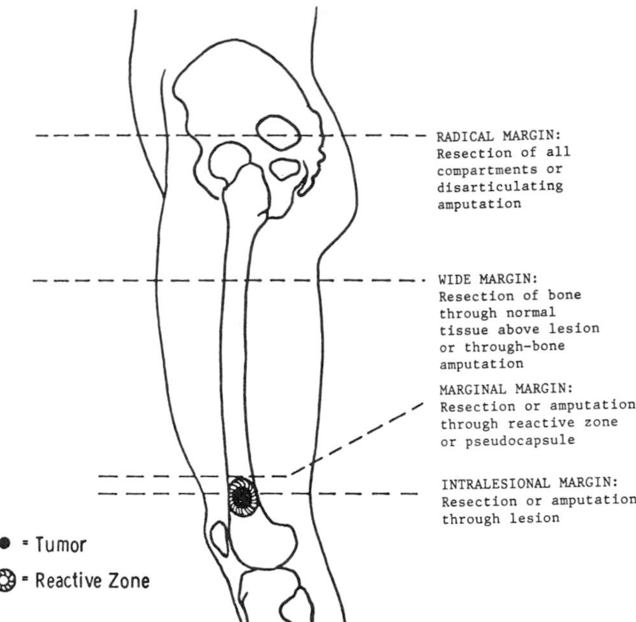

Figure 25–3. Surgical procedures and terminology in the treatment of osteosarcoma: limb preservation.

Limb-Salvage Surgery

At present, limb-salvage surgery is the treatment of choice for patients with extremity sarcomas, and the rate of local recurrence with high-grade bone sarcomas is approximately 10%.[99, 100] Although this rate is slightly higher than that observed with amputation,[101] there is no difference in long-term survival. In addition, a cost analysis has shown that, overall, limb salvage costs less than amputation and prostheses.[102]

In the application of limb salvage, the principles of oncologic surgery must be applied (see Fig. 25–3). First, the level of function after surgical and adjuvant treatment must be considered, and the patient should be considered to be a candidate for limb salvage only if function of the extremity is expected to equal or exceed function with a prosthetic limb after ablative surgery. Preservation of major nerves and blood vessels must be feasible, and three-dimensional imaging is critical for surgical planning; a wide margin (normal tissues or tissue planes removed in contiguity with the lesion in all directions) must be achievable. The extent of preoperative necrosis, surgical margins, and tumor volume are important prognostic factors.[103] Finally, a relative factor is the availability of an effective adjuvant therapy (chemotherapy, radiation therapy, or both) for a given tumor type. For example, the risk of local recurrence is reduced in patients with osteosarcoma who show an excellent response to chemotherapy (>95% necrosis).[94]

Preoperative systemic chemotherapy leads to a high degree of tumor sterilization with some tumor types, such as osteosarcoma, and it may be predictive of final outcome.[104, 105] This sterilization also may facilitate conservative surgery by shrinking a tumor mass away from major neurovascular structures. Together with MRI, chemotherapy allows for evaluation of the responsiveness of the tumor to the chemotherapeutic regimen before surgery and may, therefore, alter the subsequent protocol. Intra-arterial perfusion of chemotherapeutic agents, for example, doxorubicin, can also facilitate limb-sparing surgery,[106–108] but it is not widely used.

Reconstructive Techniques

Reconstructive techniques may allow replacement of large skeletal defects by any of several methods, although all are associated with high complication and failure rates.

1. *Resection arthrodesis* is infrequently used, but it is a choice for juxta-articular tumors of the knee, which may be accomplished using allograft, sliding local bone, or distant autogenous grafts with internal fixation devices.[109, 110] However, the large defects usually require allograft replacement. Similar procedures can be performed for tumors about the hip, shoulder girdle, and other locations.
2. *Bone* or *osteochondral allografts* are available in many centers and can be used to replace all or part of a bone or joint, avoiding the possibility of aseptic loosening.[111, 112] These allografts are stored fresh-frozen in licensed tissue banks after being obtained from carefully selected donors. Tissue typing is not performed owing to minimal antigenicity, and grafts are used on the basis of size availability. However, in children and adolescents, limb length discrepancies of greater than 2 cm have been recorded in one third or more of patients with the use of allografts, owing to a lack of functional growth plates in these transplants.[109, 113] Nonetheless, satisfactory results have been reported in many patients receiving allografts,[114, 115] although there is a high complication rate associated with allografts:
   - The rate of infection is 10% in the first year.
   - Allograft fractures occur at rates of 10% to 60%,[116, 117] and they appear between 2 and 3 years postsurgery.
   - Nonunion of the allograft-host junction appears in 8% to 30% of patients and appears more frequently in patients receiving adjuvant treatment.[118, 119]
3. Prosthetic bone and joint replacement with computer-designed, custom or modular metallic implants of titanium or stainless steel alloys provides another method of limb reconstruction. With the advent of porous ingrowth fixation systems, there may be a decreased risk of long-term prosthetic loosening and failure. Consequently, these devices are being used increasingly in orthopedic oncology.[120–122] In addition, modular and expandable prostheses have been developed for use in growing children, allowing sequential limb lengthening to simulate growth,[123–125] although these require multiple procedures.

Contraindications to limb salvage include invasion of major regional nerves or blood vessels or pathologic fractures in which the resulting hematoma contaminates many tissue planes and compartments.[126, 127] Of note, internal hemipelvectomy offers a method of resecting all or part of the hemipelvis while retaining a limb with some level of function, and it may be applicable to many pelvic sarcomas. A number of reconstructive techniques can be used to enhance the function of the remaining extremity, including fusion of the femur to the remaining portion of the pelvis or sacrum, creation of a pseudarthrosis, or reconstruction with allografts, prosthetic devices, or both.[128–130]

Radiation Therapy

Historically, radiation therapy has not been the primary treatment modality in the treatment of most bone tumors. Whereas radiation therapy is used almost exclusively for plasma cell tumors, metastatic tumors, and histiocytic lymphomas, tumors such as osteosarcoma, fibrosarcoma, and chondrosarcoma are relatively radioresistant. As early as 1969, Phillips and Sheline showed that doses in the order of 100 Gy are required for complete eradication of osteogenic sarcoma cells in pathologic specimens.[131] Later investigators, such as Gaitan-Yanguas,[132] demonstrated that sterilization of pathologic specimens occurred when moderate doses of radiation were given over a short period of time, but it required higher doses if the fractionation course was prolonged longer than 40 days. Therefore, when radiation therapy is used, the amount of radiation and the size of the treatment portal necessary for treatment of bone tumors are dictated primarily by the histology of the tumor. Doses in the range of 10 to 40 Gy are required for adequate local control and palliation of tumors such as lymphomas, multiple myeloma, metastatic carcinomas, and leukemias, whereas osteogenic sarcomas, chondrosarcomas, Ewing's sarcoma, fibrosarcomas, and solitary plasmacytoma and histiocytic lymphomas require higher doses (50 to 70 Gy) with prolonged fractionated treatment schedules.

Radiation treatment for benign tumors may eradicate the lesion, but it also may cause secondary cancers, both in the lesional tissue and in the normal surrounding bone.[133, 134] In children, irradiation of the bones can lead to scoliosis, epiphyseal slippage, and avascular necrosis, whereas in adults, osteoporosis, medullary fibrosis, and cytotoxicity may result in fracture or necrosis.[135] For this reason, radiation therapy to benign lesions in bone is limited to surgically inaccessible tumors or lesions that are responsive to very low doses of radiation, such as aneurysmal bone cysts in difficult surgical locations and eosinophilic granuloma.[136, 137]

Because of improved surgical techniques and the availability of radiosensitizing chemotherapeutic agents, radiation is beginning to be used, preoperatively and postoperatively, as part of multimodality treatments. Limb preservation is an important aspect of radiation treatment. Important points of limb preservation include sparing a strip of soft tissue to better preserve lymphatic drainage, if possible, making an accurate delineation of the tumor volume with MRI or CT scans, and using shrinking-field techniques to limit the high-dose treatment volume to as small a volume as possible.

Preoperative Radiation

Surgical management along with chemotherapy has been the treatment of choice for osteosarcomas, with radiation therapy given only to patients who are unable to undergo definitive surgical resection because of medical contraindications to surgery or the location of the primary. One multi-institutional study examined the use of preoperative radiation using an intra-arterial infusion of doxorubicin as a sensitizer.[138] The investigators demonstrated good local control (98.5%) with adequate resection margins, although metastases continued to be a problem.

Ewing's Sarcoma

Radiation therapy has a role in the treatment of Ewing's sarcoma, particularly when surgery is not possible or when adequate surgical margins cannot be obtained. Volume considerations are essential for radiation treatment planning for Ewing's sarcoma, and through the use of MRI and CT scan, excellent three-dimensional volumetric definition of bone and the large soft tissue component is possible, with careful field shaping and so-called beam's eye view. Although generous margins are used, sparing of medial skin and lymphatic strips is important to maintain lymphatic flow, and some institutions have made use of high-dose-rate brachytherapy to limit treatment volume and the resultant late effects.[139]

The standard dose range employed is 40 to 45 Gy to the medullary cavity, with boost to the 55- to 60-Gy level.[140, 141] Dose modification depends on the role of surgery or the inaccessibility of the tumor. There has been some limited success with low-dose irradiation (median dose 30 Gy) when used in conjunction with targeted resection.[142] However, consideration also must be given to the documented risk of secondary malignant tumors in patients with Ewing's sarcoma. Radiation alone, at doses higher than 60 Gy, and particularly in combination with alkylating agents, has been found to significantly increase the risk of secondary neoplasms.[143, 144]

Chemotherapy

Since the early 1970s, several important developments in the treatment of osteosarcoma and Ewing's sarcoma have led to improved chemotherapy regimens. Acting in conjunction with other techniques, such as limb-salvage therapy, chemotherapy has been successful in improving local control. Another major impact of chemotherapy has been in the treatment of micrometastases.[145] In addition, in both osteosarcoma and Ewing's sarcoma, the extent of tumor necrosis following chemotherapy is a measure of tumor responsiveness and is an important prognostic marker. At present, many protocols use multidrug, combination chemotherapy regimens to allow for synergistic effects between complementary agents. Table 25–6 lists the common agents, their drug classification, and mechanisms of action.[146]

Osteosarcoma

In the early 1970s, high-dose methotrexate and doxorubicin (Adriamycin) were the first agents to demonstrate a significant tumor regression in patients.[147, 148] Since that time, combination regimens with cisplatin[149, 150] and, more recently, with ifosfamide have been used.[151, 152]

Neoadjuvant Chemotherapy. Neoadjuvant therapy avoids any delay in systemic therapy, which would otherwise be necessitated by a postoperative recovery period. Rosen and associates[153] were the original advocates for preoperative adjuvant chemotherapy. They treated primary osteogenic sarcoma with high-dose methotrexate and leucovorin calcium rescue, doxorubicin, and BCD (bleomycin, cyclophosphamide, and dactinomycin) for 4 to 16 weeks before definitive surgery. The effect of the preoperative chemotherapy was assessed according to the percentage of tumor necrosis in the resected specimen. Postoperatively, the patients with greater than 90% necrosis were continued on the same chemotherapy program. The results from this study suggest that those patients who had chemoresponsive tumors had the better prognosis. This finding has been subsequently supported by larger studies.[154–156]

The agents most commonly used are high-dose metho-

TABLE 25–6. **Common Chemotherapeutic Agents Used for Bone Sarcomas**

Drug	Mechanism of Action	Complication/Side Effect
Alkylating Agent		
Cyclophosphamide	Reactive intermediates cause DNA cross-links	Myelosuppression, hemorrhagic cystitis, infertility
Ifosfamide		
Agent with Alkylating Activity		
Cisplatin		Nephrotoxicity, ototoxicity, myelosuppression
Antitumor Antibiotic		Myelosuppression
Doxorubicin	DNA intercalation impairs DNA/RNA synthesis, leads to strand breaks	Cumulative cardiotoxicity
Actinomycin D		
Bleomycin		Pneumonitis, pulmonary fibrosis
Plant Alkyloid		
Vincristine	Binds to tubulin, inhibits microtubules with metaphase arrest	Neurotoxicity
Etoposide	Type II topoisomerase inhibitor	Myelosuppression, transient hypotension
Antimetabolite		
Methotrexate	Dihydrofolate inhibitor	Myelosuppression

Modified from O'Keefe RJ, Terek RM: Musculoskeletal oncology. In: Beaty JH (ed): Orthopaedic Knowledge Update 6, p 167. Rosemont, American Academy of Orthopaedic Surgeons, 1999, with permission.

trexate, doxorubicin, cisplatin, cyclophosphamide, vincristine, ifosfamide, and etoposide.[87] Of note, one randomized trial found that despite the widespread use of polychemotherapy protocols, the two-drug regimen of doxorubicin and cisplatin produced the same survival rate as multidrug regimens and was better tolerated.[155] Indeed, in general, preoperative chemotherapy has permitted limb-salvage surgery for some patients who would have had an amputation if surgery had been performed first. Chemotherapy can shrink the tumor away from vital neurovascular structures, facilitating limb salvage. However, as suggested by Rosen's work, patients who are nonresponsive or poorly responsive to preoperative chemotherapy are poor candidates for limb-sparing surgery unless wide surgical margins can be achieved.[157] Therefore, the tumor response to chemotherapy frequently influences the subsequent treatment and also the prognosis of the patient.[94, 103]

Intra-Arterial Versus Intravenous Administration. In an attempt to improve survival time by creating a higher local concentration of chemotherapeutic agents, particularly with cisplatin, some investigators have used an intra-arterial infusion approach. However, to date, no additive benefit has been achieved through the use of this route.[154, 158, 159]

Immunotherapy

The role of immunotherapy in the treatment of bone tumors remains controversial. There exists the potential for great promise, but the clinical application of knowledge about the immune response has been disappointingly inconclusive.

Interferon

Strander and coworkers reported on a study that compared 33 osteosarcoma patients treated with a daily dose of human leukocyte interferon (IFN)—administered intramuscularly for 1 month, followed by the same dose three times a week for 17 months—with 30 contemporary patients who did not receive adjuvant therapy. The investigators reported a 5-year survival rate of 58% in the study group.[160, 161] An update from the group with a more intensive IFN treatment (3 mU given subcutaneously daily for 3 to 5 years) produced a 5-year disease-free survival rate of 63%.[162] However, apart from case studies that have demonstrated the successful use of interferon-alfa in the decrease of pulmonary metastasis and stabilization of disease in patients with giant cell tumors,[163, 164] little progress has been reported in this field.

Special Considerations of Treatment

Chondrosarcoma of Bone

Wide surgical excision of chondrosarcomas is the treatment of choice, with 5-year survival rates of 65% to 80% being reported following resection alone[165–167]; prognostic factors include tumor grade and adequate surgical margins. Part of the reasoning behind the use of surgery has been reports of chondrosarcomas of bone being relatively chemoresistant tumors.[168] Nonetheless, the poor prognosis with increasing tumor grade has led some investigators to include systemic therapy for high-grade lesions, but it has had mixed results.[165, 169, 170]

Fibrosarcoma and Malignant Fibrous Histiocytoma of Bone

In general, fibrosarcomas and malignant fibrous histiocytomas are treated according to osteosarcoma protocols; therefore, combined-modality regimens with chemotherapy is the treatment of choice for these tumors. Despite having an apparent lower chemosensitivity than osteosarcoma, malignant fibrous histiocytomas have similar prognoses and survival rates.[156, 171, 172]

Solitary Plasmacytoma

Plasmacytomas are rarely solitary lesions, so diagnosis and careful staging is required to exclude the presence of multiple myeloma. Careful delineation of the tumor volume, including CT scans of the affected area, is required to encompass any soft tissue component of the disease. The treatment of choice is radiation therapy, with doses of 45 to 50 Gy required for local control. However, despite successful local control, approximately 50% of patients develop other foci (multiple myeloma), with a median time to progression of 2 years.[173, 174]

A number of investigators have analyzed results from small groups of patients with solitary plasmacytoma of the bone.[173–175] The most frequent pattern of failure was the development of multiple myeloma. Although the presence of serum myeloma protein has been reported as not influencing prognosis,[173] at least one group has suggested that the disappearance of the protein following radiation treatment indicates a higher likelihood of cure.[174] Of note, one group has reported a small trial that has shown a benefit to the inclusion of adjuvant chemotherapy postradiation in the treatment of this lesion.[176]

Aneurysmal Bone Cysts

Aneurysmal bone cysts occur in all the bones of the body. Surgery is the treatment of choice using curettage and bone graft.[177–179] Aneurysmal cysts can arise as a secondary lesion in other tumors as well, most commonly with giant cell tumors.

Metastatic Bone Disease

Metastatic tumors of bone constitute the majority of bone tumors. Their treatment is discussed in detail in Chapter 31, Metastases and Disseminated Disease.

Results and Prognosis

The prognosis for patients with malignant bone tumors has improved on account of aggressive treatment. Because most studies are small in patient number (fewer than 100), statistical percentages are unreliable and can be misleading. Each series of reported cases can include multiple tumor types or variants, and a comparison of case reports is sometimes difficult. Each patient must be treated as a separate entity based on a full study of the specific lesion.

Surgery

A number of studies have been performed to analyze the use of limb-sparing techniques. One review has shown no difference in outcome between ablative and limb-sparing surgeries,[97] and in general, most reports support the use of limb salvage in cases in which adequate surgical margins are obtainable and the tumor has been shown to respond to preoperative chemotherapy.[96, 99, 100] However, a multicenter study from Sweden has suggested that limb sparing is associated with a higher rate of local recurrence.[101]

Radiation Therapy

As stated earlier, radiation therapy maintains a role in the treatment of Ewing's sarcoma. In an updated analysis of the CESS 86 study, 177 patients with Ewing's sarcoma were treated between 1986 and 1991.[140] All patients received systemic therapy in the form of either VACA (vincristine, actinomycin D, cyclophosphamide, and doxorubicin) or VAIA (vincristine, actinomycin D, ifosfamide, and doxorubicin) for low-risk and high-risk tumors, respectively. Local therapy was in the form of surgery alone, definitive radiation therapy, or a combination of surgery and radiation therapy. There was an apparent improvement in local control following radical surgery compared with radiation alone or in combination (100%, 86%, and 95%, respectively). However, this trend was not reflected in improvements in either relapse-free or overall survival because of an increase in the frequency of distant metastases following surgery alone (29%, 26%, and 16%, respectively). In this study, therefore, it was believed that radiation yielded equivalent survival results to radical surgery.

A final report from a Pediatric Oncology Group (POG) study, POG 8346, investigated the effects of involved field irradiation compared with standard whole bone irradiation on tumor response and survival rates in Ewing's sarcoma.[141] The group concluded that field size was not a prognostic factor unless inadequate doses were administered or an inappropriate volume was irradiated. Overall, the major determinant of relapse-free survival was shown to be the effectiveness of the systemic chemotherapy.

Chemotherapy

In the late 1980s, investigators reported an improvement in relapse-free survival rate for patients with bone tumors from 40% to 60% with the aggressive use of chemotherapy.[180] However, since that time, despite dose intensification schedules and the introduction of promising agents, only a limited improvement has been seen in these numbers.

A series of studies by the Cooperative Osteosarcoma Study Group (COSS) have examined the effect of both adjuvant and neoadjuvant chemotherapy, the addition of ifosfamide to a multidrug regimen, and the scheduling of doxorubicin or cisplatin for patients with osteosarcoma.[154, 159, 181, 182] This group initially reported, from COSS-80, a 4-year metastasis-free survival rate of 84% in patients histologically classified as good responders compared with 52% for those identified as poor responders, that is, those with resistant disease.[183] In an overview of a number of their subsequent completed studies, encompassing 20 years of caring for patients, they reported 5- and 10-year actuarial and relapse-free survival rates of 72.5% and 66.3%, and 62.1% and 59.4%, respectively.[182] Despite the associated toxicity, aggressive multiagent neoadjuvant chemotherapy was believed to be more effective than less aggressive protocols, although variations in the dose scheduling of both doxorubicin and cisplatin had no effect on outcome. Tumor size, tumor site, and the initial histologic response to the preoperative drug regimen were identified as prognostic factors.

Ewing's Sarcoma

Ewing's sarcoma used to have a very poor prognosis, but chemotherapy has improved survival rates. Clinical trials in the late 1980s suggested that the prognosis for Ewing's sarcoma may be improved by addition of surgical resection as an adjunct to radiation therapy and chemotherapy.[184] Overall 5-year survival rates were 52%, with 92% in the surgically treated group versus 37% in the nonsurgically treated group. The authors suggested that this result was due to an increase in local control.

Since that time, the majority of studies have reported similar survival rates. A number of groups have tried to improve these numbers through the addition of more aggressive agents, notably ifosfamide. Although one early, small study indicated some benefit of administering ifosfamide before the standard induction therapy,[185] a number of nonrandomized trials have shown no improvement in outcome with its use.[186–188]

Prognostic Factors

Tumor Response

Since the early 1980s, it has been recognized that the initial histologic response of the tumor to preoperative chemotherapy is a major prognostic factor.[60, 100, 189] This has led to the practice of tailoring the postoperative treatment to the preoperative tumor response.

Tumor Site

The site of a tumor greatly affects the patient's survival. A tumor of the pelvis is generally of a higher order of malignancy than one of the same type occurring in the hand. Both tumors may show similar histology, but the more centrally located tumors metastasize earlier and more extensively. Two separate randomized trials, one for osteosarcoma and the other for Ewing's sarcoma,[189, 190] have identified the pelvis and proximal femur as sites associated with a worse prognosis.

Tumor Size

An easily measurable factor that may affect prognosis, that is, the risk of metastasis, is tumor volume or size.[191–193] However, the reported threshold for the cutoff point attributable to the poor response has been reported between 150 and 200 cm^3.[191, 193]

Summary

For optimal management, patients with bone tumors must have a multidisciplinary approach to their disease. In addition, every attempt should be made to enter each of these patients into randomized studies to further clarify and advance the role of chemotherapy. Of note, especially in light of the previously reported poor survival rates with this disease, all patients with Ewing's sarcoma should have the benefit of chemotherapy, because complete responses are now possible in advanced disease.

Recommended Reading

Atlas of Bone Pathology from Marcove and associates,[1] *Tumors of the Bones and Joints* from the Armed Forces Institute of Pathology,[2] and *Tumors and Tumorous Conditions of the Bones and Joints* by Jaffe[3] are good starting places for an understanding of bone tumor pathology and pathogenesis. *Pathology of Bone and Joint Disorders* by McCarthy and Frassica[4] provides an up-to-date and comprehensive review of the clinicopathologic features of bone tumors, and the section on musculoskeletal tumors in *Surgery of the Musculoskeletal System*[5] has a very thorough description of clinical features and treatment of bone tumors. *Musculoskeletal Tumor Surgery* by Enneking[6] gives excellent detail on musculoskeletal tumor surgery and the rationale for surgical staging, and it can be complemented by *Musculoskeletal Tumors and Diseases* from the American Academy of Orthopaedic Surgeons,[7] together with the latest edition of *Musculoskeletal Cancer Surgery: Principles and Practice*, edited by Malawer and Sugarbaker.[8] Finally, the *AJCC Cancer Staging Manual* contains detailed information on sarcoma staging classifications and procedures.[9]

REFERENCES

General

1. Marcove RC, Jaffe HL, Arlen M: Atlas of Bone Pathology. With Clinical and Radiographic Correlations. Based on Henry L. Jaffe's Course. Philadelphia, Lippincott, 1992.
2. Fechner RE, Mills SE: Tumors of the Bones and Joints. Washington, DC, Armed Forces Institute of Pathology, 1993.
3. Jaffe HL: Tumors and Tumorous Conditions of the Bones and Joints. Philadelphia, Lea & Febiger, 1958.
4. McCarthy EF, Frassica FJ: Pathology of Bone and Joint Disorders with Clinical and Radiographic Correlation. Philadelphia, W.B. Saunders Co., 1998.
5. McCollister Evarts C: Surgery of the Musculoskeletal System, 2nd ed. New York, Churchill Livingstone, 1990.
6. Enneking WF: Musculoskeletal Tumor Surgery. New York, Churchill Livingstone, 1983.
7. Johnston JO: Musculoskeletal Tumors and Diseases. Rosemont, American Academy of Orthopaedic Surgeons, 1993.
8. Malawer MM, Sugarbaker PH: Musculoskeletal Cancer Surgery. Boston, Kluwer Academic Publishers, 2000.
9. American Joint Committee on Cancer: AJCC Cancer Staging Manual, 5th ed. Philadelphia, Lippincott-Raven Publishers, 1997.

Specific

10. Greenlee RT, Murray T, Bolden S, et al: Cancer statistics, 2000. CA Cancer J Clin 2000; 50:7.
11. Velez-Yanguas MC, Warrier RP: The evolution of chemotherapeutic agents for the treatment of pediatric musculoskeletal malignancies. Orthop Clin North Am 1996; 27:545.
12. Hahn M, Dormans JP: Primary bone malignancies in children. Curr Opin Pediatr 1996; 8:71.
13. Philip T, Blay JY, Brunat-Mentigny M, et al: Standards, options and recommendations (SOR) for diagnosis, treatment and follow-up of osteosarcoma. Groupe de travail SOR. Bull Cancer 1999; 86:159.
14. Fan Q, Ma B, Guo A, et al: Surgical treatment of bone tumors in conjunction with microwave-induced hypothermia and adjuvant immunotherapy. A preliminary report. Chin Med J (Engl) 1996; 109:425.
15. McDonald DJ: Limb-salvage surgery for treatment of sarcomas of the extremities. Am J Roentgenol 1994; 163:509.
16. Choong PF, Sim FH: Limb-sparing surgery for bone tumors: new developments. Semin Surg Oncol 1997; 13:64.
17. Wolf RE: Sarcoma and metastatic carcinoma. J Surg Oncol 2000; 73:39.
18. Gurney JG, Swensen AR, Bulterys M: Malignant bone tumors. In: Ries LAG, Smith MA, Gurney JG, et al (eds): Cancer Incidence and Survival among Children and Adolescents. United States SEER Program 1975–1995. NIH Pub. No 99-4649, p 111. Bethesda, National Cancer Institute, 1999.
19. Marina NM, Bowman LC, Pui C, et al: Pediatric solid tumors. In: Murphy GP, Lawrence WL, Lenhard RE Jr (eds): American Cancer Society Textbook of Clinical Oncology, p 524. Atlanta, American Cancer Society, 1995.
20. American Cancer Society: 2000 Facts and Figures. Atlanta, American Cancer Society, 2000.
21. Dorfman HD, Czerniak B: Bone cancers. Cancer 1995; 75:203.
22. Johnson LC: A general theory of bone tumors. Bull NY Acad Med 1953; 29:164.
23. Hadjipavlou A, Lander P, Srolovitz H, et al: Malignant transformation in Paget disease of bone. Cancer 1992; 70:2802.
24. Parisien M, Silverberg SJ, Shane E, et al: Bone disease in primary hyperparathyroidism. Endocrinol Metabol Clin North Am, 1990; 19:19.
25. McGrory JE, Pritchard DJ, Unni KK, et al: Malignant lesions arising in chronic osteomyelitis. Clin Orthop Rel Res 1999; 362:181.
26. Kenan S, Abdelwahab IF, Hermann G, et al: Malignant fibrous histiocytoma associated with a bone infarct in a patient with hereditary bone dysplasia. Skeletal Radiol 1998; 27:463.
27. Nekolla EA, Kreisheimer M, Kellerer AM, et al: Induction of malignant bone tumors in radium-224 patients: risk estimates based on the improved dosimetry. Radiat Res 2000; 153:93.
28. Leis AA, Fratkin J: Chondrosarcoma of the spine and thyroid carcinoma following radiation therapy for Hodgkin's lymphoma. Neurology 1997; 48:1710.
29. Fletcher JA: Cytogenetics and experimental models of sarcomas. Curr Opin Oncol 1994; 6:367.
30. Kovar H, Aryee D, Zoubek A: The Ewing family of tumors and the search for the Achilles' heel. Curr Opin Oncol 1999; 11:275.
31. Winters JL, Geil JD, O'Connor WN: Immunohistology, cytogenetics, and molecular studies of small round cell tumors of childhood. A review. Ann Clin Lab Sci 1995; 25:66.
32. Clark J, Benjamin H, Gill S, et al: Fusion of the EWS gene to CHN, a member of the steroid/thyroid receptor gene superfamily, in a human myxoid chondrosarcoma. Oncogene 1996; 12:229.
33. Labelle Y, Bussieres J, Courjal F, et al: The EWS/TEC fusion protein encoded by the t(9;22) chromosomal translocation in human chondrosarcomas is a highly potent transcriptional activator. Oncogene 1999; 18:3303.
34. Lin PP, Brady RI, Hamelin AC, et al: Differential transactivation of alternative EWS-FLI-1 fusion proteins correlates with clinical heterogeneity in Ewing's sarcoma. Cancer Res 1999; 59:1428.
35. Friedl P, Brocker EB, Zanker KS: Integrins, cell matrix interactions and cell migration strategies: fundamental differences in leukocytes and tumor cells. Cell Adhes Commun 1998; 6:225.
36. Ridyard MS, Sanders EJ: Potential roles for focal adhesion kinase in development. Anat Embryol 1999; 199:1.
37. Kornberg LJ: Focal adhesion kinase and its potential involvement in tumor invasion and metastasis. Head Neck 1998; 20:745.

38. Schlaepfer DD, Hauck CR, Sieg DJ: Signaling through focal adhesion kinase. Prog Biophys Mol Biol 1999; 71:435.
39. Moll AC, Imhof SM, Bouter LM, et al: Second primary tumors in patients with retinoblastoma. A review of the literature. Ophthal Genet 1997; 18:27.
40. Allison JW, James CA, Figarola MS: Pediatric case of the day. Osteogenic sarcoma as a second malignancy with bilateral hereditary retinoblastoma. Radiographics 1999; 19:830.
41. Miller CW, Aslo A, Won A, et al: Alterations of the p53, Rb and MDM2 genes in osteosarcoma. J Cancer Res Clin Oncol 1996; 122:559.
42. Radig K, Schneider-Stock R, Haeckel C, et al: p53 gene mutations in osteosarcomas of low-grade malignancy. Hum Pathol 1998; 29:1310.
43. Yokoyama R, Schneider-Stock R, Radig K, et al: Clinicopathologic implications of MDM2, p53 and K-ras gene alterations in osteosarcomas: MDM2 amplification and p53 mutations found in progressive tumors. Pathol Res Pract 1998; 194:615.
44. McIntyre JF, Smith-Sorensen B, Friend SH, et al: Germline mutation of the p53 suppressor gene in children with osteosarcoma. J Clin Oncol 1994; 12:925.
45. Panizo C, Patino A, Calasanz MJ, et al: Emergence of secondary acute leukemia in a patient treated for osteosarcoma: implications of germline TP53 mutations. Med Pediatr Oncol 1998; 30:165.
46. Hung J, Anderson R: p53: functions, mutations and sarcomas. Acta Orthop Scand 1997; 273 (suppl):68.
47. Radig K, Schneider-Stock R, Rose I, et al: p53 and ras mutations in Ewing's sarcoma. Pathol Res Pract 1998; 194:157.
48. Ragazzini P, Gamberi G, Benassi MS, et al: Analysis of SAS gene and CDK4 and MDM2 proteins in low-grade osteosarcomas. Cancer Detect Prev 1999; 23:129.
49. Himelstein BP, Dormans JP: Malignant bone tumors of childhood. Pediatr Clin North Am 1996; 43:967.
50. Bader TR, Imhof I, Dominkus M, et al: Pitfalls in MRI diagnosis of primary malignant bone tumors. Radiologe 1998; 38:530.
51. Janzen L, Logan PM, O'Connell JX, et al: Intramedullary chondroid tumors of the bone: Correlation of abnormal peritumoral marrow and soft-tissue MRI signal with tumor type. Skeletal Radiol 1997; 26:100.
52. De Beuckeleer LH, De Schepper AM, Ramon F, et al: Magnetic resonance imaging of cartilaginous tumors: a retrospective study of 79 patients. Eur J Radiol 1995; 21:34.
53. Soderlund V: Radiological diagnosis of skeletal metastases. Eur Radiol 1996; 6:587.
54. Lecouvet FE, Malghem J, Michaux L, et al: Skeletal survey in advanced multiple myeloma: radiographic versus MR imaging survey. Br J Haematol 1999; 106:35.
55. Juhn A, Healey JH, Ghelman B, et al: Subacute osteomyelitis presenting as bone tumors. Orthopedics 1989; 12:245.
56. Hannisdal E, Solheim OP, Theodorsen L, et al: Alterations of blood analyses at relapse of osteosarcoma and Ewing's sarcoma. Acta Oncol 1990; 29:585.
57. Schwartz MK: Bone tumors. Immunol Ser 1990; 53:423.
58. Davie MW, Worsfold M, Sharp CA: Differential response of serum alkaline phosphatase and serum osteocalcin in Paget's osteosarcoma. Ann Clin Biochem 1991; 28:194.
59. Pochanugool L, Subhadharaphandou T, Dhanachai M, et al: Prognostic factors among 130 patients with osteosarcoma. Clin Orthop Rel Res 1997; 345:206.
60. Tomer G, Cohen IJ, Kidron D, et al: Prognostic factors in nonmetastatic limb osteosarcoma: a 20-year experience of one center. Int J Oncol 1999; 15:179.
61. Romas NA, Kwan DJ: Prostatic acid phosphatase. Biomolecular features and assays for serum determination. Urol Clin North Am 1993; 20:581.
62. Gao X, Porter AT, Grignon DJ, et al: Diagnostic and prognostic markers for human prostate cancer. Prostate 1997; 31:264.
63. Schweitzer VG, Thompson NW, McClatchey KD: Sphenoid sinus brown tumor, hypercalcemia, and blindness: an unusual presentation of primary hyperparathyroidism. Head Neck Surg 1986; 8:379.
64. Ganeval D, Lacour B, Chopin N, et al: Proteinuria in multiple myeloma and related diseases. Am J Nephrol 1990; 10 (suppl 1):58.
65. Wakely PE Jr, Almeida M, Frable WJ: Fine-needle aspiration biopsy cytology of myositis ossificans. Mod Pathol 1994; 7:23.
66. Wybier M, Quillard A, Parlier C, et al: Myositis ossificans circumscripta and its variants. Ann Radiol 1997; 40:201.
67. Ayala AG, Ro JY, Fanning CV, et al: Core needle biopsy and fine-needle aspiration in the diagnosis of bone and soft-tissue lesions. Hematol Oncol Clin North Am 1995; 9:633.
68. Arca MJ, Biermann JS, Johnson TM, et al: Biopsy techniques for skin, soft-tissue, and bone neoplasms. Surg Clin North Am 1995; 4:157.
69. Elsheikh TM, Herzberg AJ, Silverman JF: Fine-needle aspiration cytology of metastatic malignancies involving unusual sites. Am J Clin Pathol 1997; 108:S12.
70. Bakhos R, Andrey J, Bhoopalam N, et al: Fine-needle aspiration cytology of extraskeletal Ewing's sarcoma. Diagn Cytopathol 1998; 18:137.
71. Mankin HJ, Mankin CJ, Simon MA: The hazards of the biopsy, revisited. Members of the Musculoskeletal Tumor Society. J Bone Joint Surg Am 1996; 78:656.
72. Bridge JA, Schwartz HS, Neff JR: Bone sarcomas. In: Abeloff MD, Armitage JO, Lichter AS, et al (eds): Clinical Oncology, p 1715. New York, Churchill Livingstone, 1995.
73. Harrington KD: Surgical management of neoplastic complications of Paget's disease. J Bone Miner Res 1999; 14 (suppl 2):45.
74. Jattiot F, Goupille P, Azais I, et al: Fourteen cases of sarcomatous degeneration in Paget's disease. J Rheumatol 1999; 26:150.
75. Yabut SM Jr, Kenan S, Sissons HA, et al: Malignant transformation of fibrous dysplasia. A case report and review of the literature. Clin Orthop Rel Res 1988; 228:281.
76. Logan PM, Munk PL, O'Connell JX, et al: Post-radiation osteosarcoma of the scapula. Skeletal Radiol 1996; 25:596.
77. Vander Griend RA: Osteosarcoma and its variants. Orthop Clin North Am 1996; 27:575.
78. Wuisman PI, Jutte PC, Ozaki T: Secondary chondrosarcoma in osteochondromas. Medullary extension in 15 of 45 cases. Acta Orthop Scand 1997; 68:396.
79. Peiper M, Zornig C: Chondrosarcoma of the thumb arising from a solitary enchondroma. Arch Orthop Trauma Surg 1997; 116:246.
80. Schwartz HS, Zimmerman NB, Simon MA, et al: The malignant potential of enchondromatosis. J Bone Joint Surg Am 1987; 69:269.
81. Lopes A, Morini S, Vieira LJ, et al: Chondrosarcoma secondary to hereditary multiple exostosis treated by extended internal hemipelvectomy. Rev Paul Med 1997; 115:1440.
82. Cossetto D, Nade S, Blackwell J: Malignant fibrous histiocytoma in Paget's disease of the bone. A report of seven cases. Aust NZ J Surg 1992; 62:52.
83. Vlasak R, Sim FH: Ewing's sarcoma. Orthop Clin North Am 1996; 27:591.
84. De Maeseneer M, Machiels F, Naegels S, et al: Hand and foot acrometastases in a patient with bronchial carcinoma. J Belge Radiol 1995; 78:274.
85. Enneking WF: A system of staging musculoskeletal neoplasms. Clin Orthop Rel Res 1986; 204:9.
86. Zehr RJ: Treatment options for orthopaedic entities. Instruct Course Lect 1999; 48:591.
87. Physicians Data Query: Osteosarcoma. Bethesda, National Cancer Institute, 1999.
88. Physicians Data Query: Ewing's sarcoma/primitive neuroectodermal tumor (PNET). Bethesda, National Cancer Institute, 1999.
89. Schreuder HW, Pruszczynski M, Veth RP, et al: Treatment of benign and low-grade malignant intramedullary chondroid tumours with curettage and cryosurgery. Eur J Surg Oncol 1998; 24:120.
90. Wirbel RJ, Remberger K: Conservative surgery for chondrosarcoma of the first metacarpal bone. Acta Orthop Belg 1999; 65:226.
91. Vander Griend RA, Funderburk CH: The treatment of giant-cell tumors of the distal part of the radius. J Bone Joint Surg 1993; 75:899.
92. Yasko AW, Johnson ME: Surgical management of primary bone sarcomas. Hematol Oncol Clin North Am 1995; 9:719.
93. Kawaguchi N, Matumato S, Manabe J: New method of evaluating the surgical margin and safety margin for musculoskeletal sarcoma, analyzed on the basis of 457 surgical cases. J Cancer Res Clin Oncol 1995; 121:555.
94. Picci P, Sangiorgi L, Rougraff BT, et al: Relationship of chemotherapy-induced necrosis and surgical margins to local recurrence in osteosarcoma. J Clin Oncol 1994; 12:2699.
95. Szendroi M, Papai Z, Koos R, et al: Limb-saving surgery, survival, and prognostic factors for osteosarcoma: the Hungarian experience. J Surg Oncol 2000; 73:87.

96. Sluga M, Windhager R, Lang S, et al: Local and systemic control after ablative and limb sparing surgery in patients with osteosarcoma. Clin Orthop Rel Res 1999; 358:120.
97. Weis LD: The success of limb-salvage surgery in the adolescent patient with osteogenic sarcoma. Adolesc Med 1999; 10:451.
98. McKenzie AF: The role of magnetic resonance imaging. When to use it and what to look for. Acta Orthop Scand 1997; 273 (suppl):21.
99. Tsuchiya H, Tomita K: Prognosis of osteosarcoma treated by limb-salvage surgery: the ten-year intergroup study in Japan. Jpn J Clin Oncol 1992; 22:347.
100. Bacci G, Ferrari S, Mercuri M, et al: Predictive factors for local recurrence in osteosarcoma: 540 patients with extremity tumors followed for a minimum 2.5 years after neoadjuvant chemotherapy. Acta Orthop Scand 1998; 69:230.
101. Brosjo O: Surgical procedure and local recurrence in 223 patients treated 1982–1997 according to two osteosarcoma chemotherapy protocols. The Scandinavian Sarcoma Group experience. Acta Orthop Scand 1999; 285 (suppl):58.
102. Bruns J, Luessenhop S, Behrens P: Cost analysis of three different surgical procedures for treatment of a pelvic tumour. Langenbecks Arch Surg 1998; 383:359.
103. Lindner NJ, Ramm O, Hillmann A, et al: Limb salvage and outcome of osteosarcoma. The University of Muenster experience. Clin Orthop Rel Res 1999; 358:83.
104. Lindner NJ, Scarborough MT, Spanier SS, et al: Local host response in osteosarcoma after chemotherapy referred to radiographs, CT, tumour necrosis and patient survival. J Cancer Res Clin Oncol 1998; 124:575.
105. Fujii J, Ozaki T, Kawai A, et al: Angiography for assessment of preoperative chemotherapy in musculoskeletal sarcomas. Clin Orthop Rel Res 1999; 360:197.
106. Kashdan BJ, Sullivan KL, Lackman RD, et al: Extremity osteosarcomas: intraarterial chemotherapy and limb-sparing resection with 2-year follow-up. Radiology 1990; 177:95.
107. Malawer M, Buch R, Reaman G, et al: Impact of two cycles of preoperative chemotherapy with intraarterial cisplatin and intravenous doxorubicin on the choice of surgical procedure for high-grade bone sarcomas of the extremities. Clin Orthop Rel Res 1991; 270:214.
108. Rha SY, Chung HC, Gong SJ, et al: Combined pre-operative chemotherapy with intra-arterial cisplatin and continuous intravenous adriamycin for high grade osteosarcoma. Oncol Rep 1999; 6:631.
109. Alman BA, De Bari A, Krajbich JI: Massive allografts in the treatment of osteosarcoma and Ewing sarcoma in children and adolescents. J Bone Joint Surg Am 1995; 77:54.
110. Salai M, Nerubay J, Caspi I, et al: Resection arthrodesis of the knee in the treatment of tumours--a long-term follow-up. Int Orthop 1997; 21:101.
111. Tomford WW, Springfield DS, Mankin HJ: Fresh and frozen articular cartilage allografts. Orthopedics 1992; 15:1183.
112. Springfield DS: Allograft reconstructions. Semin Surg Oncol 1997; 13:11.
113. Finn HA, Simon MA: Limb-salvage surgery in the treatment of osteosarcoma in skeletally immature individuals. Clin Orthop Rel Res 1991; 262:108.
114. Shelton WR, Treacy SH, Dukes AD, et al: Use of allografts in knee reconstruction: II. Surgical considerations. J Am Acad Orthop Surg 1998; 6:169.
115. Manfrini M, Gasbarrini A, Malguti C, et al: Intraepiphyseal resection of the proximal tibia and its impact on lower limb growth. Clin Orthop Rel Res 1999; 358:111.
116. San-Julian M, Canadell J: Fractures of allografts used in limb preserving operations. Int Orthop 1998; 22:32.
117. Thompson RC Jr, Garg A, Clohisy DR, et al: Fractures in large-segment allografts. Clin Orthop Rel Res 2000; 370:227.
118. Ortiz-Cruz E, Gebhardt MC, Jennings LC, et al: The results of transplantation of intercalary allografts after resection of tumors. A long-term follow-up study. J Bone Joint Surg Am 1997; 79:97.
119. Roebuck DJ, Griffith JF, Kumta SM, et al: Imaging following allograft reconstruction in children with malignant bone tumours. Pediatr Radiol 1999; 29:785.
120. Sim FH, Frassica FJ, Chao EY: Orthopaedic management using new devices and prostheses. Clin Orthop Rel Res 1995; 312:160.
121. Damron TA: Endoprosthetic replacement following limb-sparing resection for bone sarcoma. Semin Surg Oncol 1997; 13:3.
122. Cannon SR: Massive prostheses for malignant bone tumours of the limbs. J Bone Joint Surg Br 1997; 79:497.
123. Kenan S, DeSimone DP, Lewis MM: Limb sparing for skeletally immature patients with osteosarcoma: the expandable prosthesis. Cancer Treat Res 1993; 62:205.
124. Eckardt JJ, Safran MR, Eilber FR, et al: Expandable endoprosthetic reconstruction of the skeletally immature after malignant bone tumor resection. Clin Orthop Rel Res 1993; 297:188.
125. Ward WG, Yang RS, Eckardt JJ: Endoprosthetic bone reconstruction following malignant tumor resection in skeletally immature patients. Orthop Clin North Am 1996; 27:493.
126. Shih LY, Chen TS, Lo WH: Limb salvage surgery for locally aggressive and malignant bone tumors. J Surg Oncol 1993; 53:154.
127. Scully SP, Temple HT, O'Keefe RJ, et al: The surgical treatment of patients with osteosarcoma who sustain a pathologic fracture. Clin Orthop Rel Res 1996; 324:227.
128. O'Connor MI, Sim FH: Salvage of the limb in the treatment of malignant pelvic tumors. J Bone Joint Surg Am 1989; 71:481.
129. Harrington KD: The use of hemipelvic allografts or autoclaved grafts for reconstruction after wide resections of malignant tumors of the pelvis. J Bone Joint Surg Am 1992; 74:331.
130. Bruns J, Luessenhop SL, Dahmen G: Internal hemipelvectomy and endoprosthetic pelvic replacement: long-term follow-up results. Arch Orthop Trauma Surg 1997; 116:27.
131. Phillips TL, Sheline GE: Radiation therapy of malignant bone tumors. Radiology 1969; 92:1537.
132. Gaitan-Yanguas M: A study of the response of osteogenic sarcoma and adjacent normal tissues to radiation. Int J Radiat Oncol Biol Phys 1981; 7:593.
133. Habrand JL, Bondiau PY, Dupuis O, et al: Late effects of radiotherapy in children. Cancer Radiother 1997; 1:810.
134. Mosher RB, McCarthy BJ: Late effects in survivors of bone tumors. J Pediatr Oncol Nurs 1998; 15:72.
135. Ramuz O, Bourhis J, Mornex F: Late effects of radiations on mature and growing bone. Cancer Radiother 1997; 1:801.
136. Jereb B, Smith J: Giant aneurysmal bone cyst of the innominate bone treated with irradiation. Br J Radiol 1980; 53:489.
137. Chowdhury AD, Nagappan R, Benjamin CS: Eosinophilic granuloma of mandible in an adult (a case report). Australas Radiol 1989; 33:406.
138. Wanebo HJ, Temple WJ, Popp MB, et al: Preoperative regional therapy for extremity sarcoma. A tricenter update. Cancer 1995; 75:2299.
139. Potter R, Knocke TH, Kovacs G, et al: Brachytherapy in the combined modality treatment of pediatric malignancies. Principles and preliminary experience with treatment of soft tissue sarcoma (recurrence) and Ewing's sarcoma. Klin Padiatr 1995; 207:164.
140. Dunst J, Jurgens H, Sauer R, et al: Radiation therapy in Ewing's sarcoma: an update of the CESS 86 trial. Int J Radiat Oncol Biol Phys 1995; 32:919.
141. Donaldson SS, Torrey M, Link MP, et al: A multidisciplinary study investigating radiotherapy in Ewing's sarcoma: end results of POG# 8346. Pediatric Oncology Group. Int J Radiat Oncol Biol Phys 1998; 42:125.
142. Merchant TE, Kushner BH, Sheldon JM, et al: Effect of low-dose radiation therapy when combined with surgical resection for Ewing sarcoma. Med Pediatr Oncol 1999; 33:65.
143. Kuttesch JF Jr, Wexler LH, Marcus RB, et al: Second malignancies after Ewing's sarcoma: radiation dose-dependency of secondary sarcomas. J Clin Oncol 1996; 14:2818.
144. Hawkins MM, Wilson LM, Burton HS, et al: Radiotherapy, alkylating agents, and risk of bone cancer after childhood cancer. J Natl Cancer Inst 1996; 88:270.
145. Braun S, Pantel K: Micrometastic bone marrow involvement: detection and prognostic significance. Med Oncol 1999; 16:154.
146. O'Keefe RJ, Terek RM: Musculoskeletal oncology. In: Beaty JH (ed): Orthopaedic Knowledge Update 6, p 167. Rosemont, American Academy of Orthopaedic Surgeons, 1999.
147. Cortes EP, Holland JF, Wang JJ, et al: Doxorubicin in disseminated osteosarcoma. JAMA 1972; 221:1132.
148. Jaffe N: Recent advances in the chemotherapy of metastatic osteogenic sarcoma. Cancer 1972; 30:1627.
149. Leung S, Marshall GM, al Mahr M, et al: Prognostic significance of chemotherapy dosage characteristics in children with osteogenic sarcoma. Med Pediatr Oncol 1997; 28:179.

150. Bacci G, Ferrari S, Delepine N, et al: Predictive factors of histologic response to primary chemotherapy in osteosarcoma of the extremity: study of 272 patients preoperatively treated with high-dose methotrexate, doxorubicin, and cisplatin. J Clin Oncol 1998; 16:658.
151. Harris MB, Gieser P, Goorin AM, et al: Treatment of metastatic osteosarcoma at diagnosis: a Pediatric Oncology Group Study. J Clin Oncol 1998; 16:3641.
152. Bacci G, Briccoli A, Ferrari S, et al: Neoadjuvant chemotherapy for osteosarcoma of the extremities with synchronous lung metastases: treatment with cisplatin, adriamycin and high dose methotrexate and ifosfamide. Oncol Rep 2000; 7:339.
153. Rosen G, Marcove RC, Caparros B, et al: Primary osteogenic sarcoma: the rationale for preoperative chemotherapy and delayed surgery. Cancer 1979; 43:2163.
154. Winkler K, Bielack SS, Delling G, et al: Treatment of osteosarcoma: experience of the Cooperative Osteosarcoma Study Group (COSS). Cancer Treat Res 1993; 62:269.
155. Souhami RL, Craft AW, Van der Eijken JW, et al: Randomised trial of two regimens of chemotherapy in operable osteosarcoma: a study of the European Osteosarcoma Intergroup. Lancet 1997; 350:911.
156. Bramwell VH, Steward WP, Nooij M, et al: Neoadjuvant chemotherapy with doxorubicin and cisplatin in malignant fibrous histiocytoma of bone: a European Osteosarcoma Intergroup study. J Clin Oncol 1999; 17:3260.
157. Schulte M, Brecht-Krauss D, Werner M, et al: Evaluation of neoadjuvant therapy response of osteogenic sarcoma using FDG PET. J Nucl Med 1999; 40:1637.
158. Bacci G, Ferrari S, Forni C, et al: The effect of intra-arterial versus intravenous cisplatinum in the neoadjuvant treatment of osteosarcoma of the limbs: the experience of the Rizzoli Institute. Chir Organi Mov 1996; 81:369.
159. Fuchs N, Bielack SS, Epler D, et al: Long-term results of the cooperative German-Austrian-Swiss osteosarcoma study group's protocol COSS-86 of intensive multidrug chemotherapy and surgery for osteosarcoma of the limbs. Ann Oncol 1998; 9:893.
160. Nilsonne U: Treatment of osteosarcoma by interferon and differentiated surgery. Semaine de Hopitaux 1982; 58:1764.
161. Strander H, Adamson U, Aparisi T, et al: Adjuvant interferon treatment of human osteosarcoma: recent results. Cancer Res 1979; 68:40.
162. Strander H, Bauer HC, Brosjo O, et al: Long-term adjuvant interferon treatment of human osteosarcoma. A pilot study. Acta Oncol 1995; 34:877.
163. Kaiser U, Neumann K, Havemann K: Generalised giant-cell tumour of bone: successful treatment of pulmonary metastases with interferon alpha, a case report. J Cancer Res Clin Oncol 1993; 119:301.
164. Kaban LB, Mulliken JB, Ezekowitz RA, et al: Antiangiogenesis therapy of a recurrent giant cell tumor of the mandible with interferon-alfa-2a. Pediatrics 1999; 103:1145.
165. Mark RJ, Tran LM, Sercarz J, et al: Chondrosarcoma of the head and neck. The UCLA experience. Am J Clin Oncol 1993; 16:232.
166. Martini N, Huvos AG, Burt ME, et al: Predictors of survival in malignant tumors of the sternum. J Thorac Cardiovasc Surg 1996; 111:96.
167. Kawai A, Healey JH, Boland PJ, et al: Prognostic factors for patients with sarcomas of the pelvic bones. Cancer 1998; 82:851.
168. Terek RM, Schwartz GK, Devaney K, et al: Chemotherapy and P-glycoprotein expression in chondrosarcoma. J Orthop Res 1998; 16:585.
169. Hoekstra HJ, Szabo BG: Internal hemipelvectomy with intraoperative and external beam radiotherapy in the limb-sparing treatment of a pelvic girdle chondrosarcoma. Arch Orthop Trauma Surg 1998; 117:408.
170. Lee FY, Mankin HJ, Fondren G, et al: Chondrosarcoma of bone: an assessment of outcome. J Bone Joint Surg Am 1999; 81:326.
171. Picci P, Bacci G, Ferrari S, et al: Neoadjuvant chemotherapy in malignant fibrous histiocytoma of bone and in osteosarcoma located in the extremities: analogies and differences between the two tumors. Ann Oncol 1997; 8:1107.
172. Bielack SS, Schroeders A, Fuchs N, et al: Malignant fibrous histiocytoma of bone: a retrospective EMSOS study of 125 cases. European Musculo-Skeletal Oncology Society. Acta Orthop Scand 1999; 70:353.
173. Jyothirmayi R, Gangadharan VP, Nair MK, et al: Radiotherapy in the treatment of solitary plasmacytoma. Br J Radiol 1997; 70:511.
174. Liebross RH, Ha CS, Cox JD, et al: Solitary bone plasmacytoma: outcome and prognostic factors following radiotherapy. Int J Radiat Oncol Biol Phys 1998; 41:1063.
175. Bolek TW, Marcus RB, Mendenhall NP: Solitary plasmacytoma of bone and soft tissue. Int J Radiat Oncol Biol Phys 1996; 36:329.
176. Aviles A, Huerta-Guzman J, Delgado S, et al: Improved outcome in solitary bone plasmacytoma with combined therapy. Hematol Oncol 1996; 14:111.
177. Bollini G, Jouve JL, Cottalorda J, et al: Aneurysmal bone cyst in children: analysis of twenty-seven patients. J Pediatr Orthop 1998; 7:274.
178. Gibbs CP Jr, Hefele MC, Peabody TD, et al: Aneurysmal bone cyst of the extremities. Factors related to local recurrence after curettage with a high-speed burr. J Bone Joint Surg Am 1999; 81:1671.
179. Hemmadi SS, Cole WG: Treatment of aneurysmal bone cysts with saucerization and bone marrow injection in children. J Pediatr Orthop 1999; 19:540.
180. Rosier RR, Konski A, Boros L: Bone tumors. In: Rubin P (ed): Clinical Oncology: a Multidisciplinary Approach for Physicians and Students, 7th ed, p 509. Philadelphia, W.B. Saunders Co., 1993.
181. Winkler K, Bieling P, Bielack S, et al: Local control and survival from the Cooperative Osteosarcoma Study Group studies of the German Society of Pediatric Oncology and the Vienna Bone Tumor Registry. Clin Orthop Rel Res 1991; 270:79.
182. Bielack S, Kempf-Bielack B, Schwenzer D, et al: Neoadjuvant therapy for localized osteosarcoma of extremities. Results from the Cooperative Osteosarcoma Study Group COSS of 925 patients. Klin Padiatr 1999; 211:260.
183. Winkler K, Beron G, Delling G, et al: Neoadjuvant chemotherapy of osteosarcoma: results of a randomized cooperative trial (COSS-82) with salvage chemotherapy based on histological tumor response. J Clin Oncol 1988; 6:329.
184. Sailer SL, Harmon DC, Mankin HJ, et al: Ewing's sarcoma: surgical resection as a prognostic factor. Int J Radiat Oncol Biol Phys 1988; 15:43.
185. Meyer WH, Kun L, Marina N, et al: Ifosfamide plus etoposide in newly diagnosed Ewing's sarcoma of bone. J Clin Oncol 1992; 10:1737.
186. Oberlin O, Habrand JL, Zucker JM, et al: No benefit of ifosfamide in Ewing's sarcoma: a nonrandomized study of the French Society of Pediatric Oncology. J Clin Oncol 1992; 10:1407.
187. Antman K, Crowley J, Balcerzak SP, et al: A Southwest Oncology Group and Cancer and Leukemia Group B phase II study of doxorubicin, dacarbazine, ifosfamide, and mesna in adults with advanced osteosarcoma, Ewing's sarcoma, and rhabdomyosarcoma. Cancer 1998; 82:1288.
188. Bacci G, Picci P, Ferrari S, et al: Neoadjuvant chemotherapy for Ewing's sarcoma of bone: no benefit observed after adding ifosfamide and etoposide to vincristine, actinomycin, cyclophosphamide, and doxorubicin in the maintenance phase—results of two sequential studies. Cancer 1998; 82:1174.
189. Provisor AJ, Ettinger LJ, Nachman JB, et al: Treatment of nonmetastatic osteosarcoma of the extremity with preoperative and postoperative chemotherapy: a report from the Children's Cancer Group. J Clin Oncol 1997; 15:76.
190. Hense HW, Ahrens S, Paulussen M, et al: Factors associated with tumor volume and primary metastases in Ewing's tumors: results from the (EI)CESS studies. Ann Oncol 1999; 10:1073.
191. Bieling P, Rehan N, Winkler P, et al: Tumor size and prognosis in aggressively treated osteosarcoma. J Clin Oncol 1996; 14:848.
192. Werner M, Fuchs N, Salzer-Kuntschik M, et al: Therapy-induced changes in osteosarcoma after neoadjuvant chemotherapy (COSS 86 Therapy Study). Correlation between morphologic findings and clinical follow-up. Pathologe 1996; 17:35.
193. Ahrens S, Hoffmann C, Jabar S, et al: Evaluation of prognostic factors in a tumor volume-adapted treatment strategy for localized Ewing sarcoma of bone: the CESS 86 experience. Cooperative Ewing Sarcoma Study. Med Pediatr Oncol 1999; 32:186.

26 *Cancer of the Endocrine Glands*

MARTIN SCHLUMBERGER, MD, Oncology
MAURICE TUBIANA, MD, Oncology
PHILIPPE CHANSON, MD, Endocrinology
GILBERT SCHAISON, MD, Endocrinology

Thyroid Cancer

In all thy humours, whether grave or mellow,
Thou'rt such a touchy, testy, pleasant fellow.

JOSEPH ADDISON

Perspective

Most differentiated thyroid cancers are characterized by an indolent course with low morbidity and mortality. Although they account for less than 1% of all cancer deaths, they command our attention because they most often present as a thyroid nodule; therefore, they must be identified from among the many other more common causes of thyroid nodules seen in 4% to 7% of the population.[1, 2] Furthermore, although the clinical course of most thyroid cancers is among the most prolonged of all human cancers, thyroid cancers do cause death in sufficient number to justify early diagnosis and treatment. For these reasons, controversy continues over the proper diagnosis and treatment of thyroid cancer[3]; fine-needle biopsy has improved our diagnostic acumen, and surgery and radioactive iodine therapy have been the touchstones of therapy for papillary and follicular thyroid cancers.[4]

General Definitions

- *Goiter* is any enlargement of the thyroid, either diffuse or nodular.
- *Thyroid nodule* is a lump in the gland. A clinical thyroid nodule is usually located on or near the anterior surface of the gland and measures larger than 1 cm in diameter.

Thyroid nodules have been classified according to thyroid scan, with either technetium-99m or radioiodine, as hyperfunctioning or hot (and usually benign) or hypofunctioning or cold (10% being malignant). According to ultrasonography, they are classified as cystic (and usually benign), solid, or mixed. Most thyroid carcinomas are observed among nodules that are cold on thyroid scan and solid or mixed at thyroid ultrasonography. At the present time, the preoperative diagnosis of thyroid cancer relies on fine-needle biopsy.[1, 2, 4]

Epidemiology and Etiology

Epidemiology

Magnitude of the Problem

The annual incidence of thyroid carcinoma per 10^5 population ranges from 1.2 to 2.6 in men and from 2.0 to 3.8 in women. Mortality rate per 10^5 population ranges from 0.2 to 1.2 in men and from 0.4 to 2.8 in women. Annually in the United States, there are an estimated 14,000 new cases of thyroid cancer and approximately 1100 thyroid cancer–related deaths. A total of 500,000 people receive follow-up for thyroid carcinoma. The disparity between the incidence and mortality in thyroid carcinoma is a reflection of the low morbidity associated with thyroid cancer.[5]

Surgical Evidence

Before needle biopsy, a screened population had a 9% incidence rate of cancer in nodular goiters (24% in solitary nodules). There is a 0.5% incidence rate of cancer reported in toxic nodular goiters. With the routine use of fine-needle biopsy, less than 5% of thyroid nodules are malignant.[1]

The autopsy incidence rate in clinically normal thyroid glands ranges from 0% to more than 30%. Data vary with the care and number of sections studied. These cancers are predominantly occult papillary thyroid carcinomas. They are rare in children, whereas in adults, prevalence is similar in all age groups and in both sexes, which suggests that they appear in young adults and that the majority will remain occult.

Epidemiologic Characteristics

- Thyroid cancers are two to four times more frequent in women than in men.[5, 6]
- Thyroid carcinoma is rare in children younger than 16 years of age, with an annual incidence ranging from 0.02 to 0.3 per 10^5 children. It is exceptional before the age of 10 years.
- In adults, the incidence of thyroid carcinoma increases with the age of the patient. The median incidence age is between 45 and 50 years.
- The histologic type depends on the iodine intake. In countries in which iodine intake is normal, papillary and follicular histologic types account for more than 80% of thyroid carcinomas, with papillary cancers being the most frequent and accounting for 60% to 80% of cases. In countries in which iodine intake is low, follicular and anaplastic carcinomas represent a much higher proportion of thyroid carcinomas, but the global incidence of thyroid carcinomas is not significantly increased in such countries.

There has been a rising incidence of papillary and follicular thyroid cancer during the 1980s and 1990s in industrialized countries.[5, 6] This increase is probably a result of earlier and more efficient detection of thyroid cancers.

Etiology

External irradiation to the thyroid during childhood is the only well-established causative factor for thyroid carcinoma (mainly papillary).[7–10] Latency period between exposure and diagnosis is at least 5 years. The risk is maximal at about 20 years, and then decreases gradually but remains high for a further 20 years. The excess risk is important, being estimated at 7.7 for 1 Gy delivered to the thyroid gland during childhood. The risk is significant for radiation doses as low as 9 cGy during early childhood and increases linearly for higher doses up to 15 Gy. At doses higher than 15 Gy, the risk per gray decreases, probably because of cell killing, but the overall risk remains high. Young age at the time of exposure is the main risk factor; after 15 to 20 years of age, the risk is not significant.

The risk of thyroid carcinoma is not increased in patients given iodine-131 for diagnostic or therapeutic purposes.[10] However, it must be noted that iodine-131 given for the treatment of hyperthyroidism induces cell killing. Furthermore, the number of studied patients exposed to iodine-131 for medical reasons during childhood is too small to rule out a carcinogenic effect at a young age. The increased incidence of papillary thyroid carcinomas in children in the Marshall Islands after atomic bomb testing and, more recently, in Belarus and Ukraine after the Chernobyl nuclear accident, suggests that radioactive isotopes of iodine, both iodine-131 and short-lived isotopes, have a direct tumorigenic effect on the thyroid. In Belarus and Ukraine, the incidence of thyroid cancer started to increase as early as 4 years after the accident.[10, 11] To date, more than 1200 cases have been reported, mostly in children who were younger than 10 years of age at the time of the accident, which corresponds to an incidence 100 times that in nonirradiated children in some highly contaminated regions.

Other Factors

As already reported, the proportion of papillary carcinomas varies with iodine intake. Factors such as diet, body weight, and number of pregnancies may modify the risk of thyroid carcinoma.[6] A high incidence of papillary carcinomas has been reported in patients with adenomatous polyposis and Cowden disease (the multiple hamartoma syndrome). About 3% of cases of papillary carcinoma are familial.[12]

Undifferentiated (Anaplastic) Carcinoma

Undifferentiated thyroid cancer composes less than 10% of all thyroid carcinomas. It occurs in elderly patients and is thought to represent a dedifferentiation of a differentiated thyroid tumor. It is found most frequently in iodine-deficient areas.[13–16]

Medullary Thyroid Carcinoma

Medullary thyroid carcinoma (MTC) accounts for about 10% of all thyroid cancers. It is familial in 20% to 30% of cases, being transmitted as an autosomal dominant trait with a high penetrance.[17, 18] Hereditary MTC may be transmitted on its own (familial MTC) or be part of multiple endocrine neoplasia type 2 (MEN 2). There are two MEN 2 syndromes: MEN 2a, the more frequent, is characterized by the association of MTC in nearly all patients, pheochromocytoma in half, and less frequently, hyperparathyroidism; MEN 2b is characterized by the occurrence of an aggressive MTC, pheochromocytoma, marfanoid body habitus, ganglioneuromatosis, and skeletal abnormalities.[18]

Hereditary MTCs are due to germline point mutations of the *RET* gene. A germline mutation can be evidenced in almost all patients with MEN 2a (mainly in codon 634, exon 11) and MEN 2b (mainly in codon 918, exon 16) and in over 80% of patients with familial MTC (in exons 10, 13, 14, and 15).[17–19] The direct search for these mutations in index cases allows the identification of hereditary cases. If found, the mutation is then sought in all first-degree relatives younger than 6 years of age, which will identify gene carriers who should be submitted to prophylactic surgery.

Detection and Diagnosis

Diagnostic Procedures

Most papillary and follicular thyroid carcinomas present as asymptomatic thyroid nodules, but the first sign of the disease is occasionally lymph node metastases or, in rare cases, lung and bone metastases. Hoarseness, dysphagia, cough, and dyspnea suggest advanced disease.

On *physical examination,* the carcinoma, which is usually single, is firm, moves freely during swallowing, and is not distinguishable from a benign nodule. Among patients with thyroid nodules, the nodule is more likely to be a carcinoma in children, adolescents, patients older than 60 years, and men who are 20 to 60 years old. Carcinoma should be suspected if a hard, irregular thyroid nodule is found, ipsilateral lymph nodes are enlarged or compressive

TABLE 26–1. **Imaging Modalities for Evaluating Thyroid Tumors***

Method	Diagnosis and Staging Capability
Primary tumor and regional nodes	
Fine-needle aspiration	Distinguish between benign and malignant thyroid nodules
CT and MRI	Only in patients with large tumors, or suspicion of involvement of the esophagotracheal tract or mediastinum
Ultrasonography	Assess size and liquid or solid patterns, detect other nodules, and guide fine-needle biopsy
Radionuclide thyroid scan	Show hyperfunctioning or hypofunctioning solitary thyroid nodule
Metastatic evaluation	
Radionuclide total body ^{131}I scan	Detect functioning metastases after thyroid ablation

CT = computed tomography; MRI = magnetic resonance imaging.
*Depending on histologic type and clinical or surgical estimate of extent of lesion.

symptoms are present, and if there is a history of a progressive increase in the size of the nodule.[1, 2, 4]

Whatever the presentation, *fine-needle aspiration cytology* is the best test for distinguishing between benign and malignant thyroid nodules. Among large series, 15% to 20% of specimens are considered inadequate, 70% benign, 4% malignant, and 10% indeterminate or suspicious.[1, 2] False-negative results, usually from sampling or interpretive errors, and false-positive results are rare. Only about 20% of patients with indeterminate findings have malignant nodules, reflecting the difficulty of differentiating between benign follicular adenomas and their malignant counterparts. The routine use of fine-needle aspiration permits a reduction by two thirds of the number of patients referred to surgery.

Thyroid ultrasonography is useful for assessing the size and the liquid or solid patterns of the nodule, detecting other nodules, and guiding fine-needle biopsy in the case of a nodule that is small or difficult to palpate. It may also show echographic patterns of autoimmune thyroiditis.

Thyroid scan may show a hyperfunctioning nodule that is rarely malignant or a hypofunctioning nodule that is malignant (about 10% of cases). Optimal work-up of thyroid nodules is still controversial. Fine-needle biopsy is the key procedure for all investigators. Whether other procedures should be routinely performed, such as ultrasonography; thyroid scintigraphy; blood measurements of thyrotropin, antithyroid antibodies, and calcitonin, remains controversial. In fact, these procedures have not been shown to be beneficial.[1, 2, 4] CT scan and MRI are indicated only in patients with large tumors or with suspicion of involvement of the esophagotracheal tract or of the mediastinum.

Anaplastic thyroid carcinoma and thyroid lymphoma usually present as a rapidly enlarging thyroid mass. Fine-needle biopsy may be indicative of a tumor, but surgical biopsy is necessary for diagnosis.[13–16, 20–22]

MTC may be suspected if the thyroid nodule, located at the upper third of the thyroid lobe, is painful, if flushes or diarrhea are present, or in patients with a familial history of MTC or pheochromocytoma. Fine-needle biopsy and plasma calcitonin measurement will establish the diagnosis in patients with a clinical tumor (Table 26–1).

Classification and Staging

Histopathology

Thyroid cancers of follicular origin are classified as differentiated (papillary and follicular) or undifferentiated (anaplastic) (Table 26–2). Differentiated thyroid carcinomas retain some functional characteristics of the normal follicular cell, including the production of thyroglobulin in almost all cases, which can be evidenced by immunohistochemistry, and iodine trapping ability in two thirds of cases. However, undifferentiated thyroid carcinomas lack totally any functional property of the normal follicular cell.

The medullary thyroid carcinoma arises from parafollicular thyroid cells (C-cells). A number of rare tumors have been described to arise in the thyroid gland, including lymphomas.[15, 16, 21, 22]

Papillary Carcinoma

Papillary carcinoma, the most common type in countries in which iodine intake is normal, constitutes more than 50% of all adult thyroid cancers and more than 80% of all childhood thyroid cancers.[6, 21–23] The typical appearance of papillary thyroid carcinoma is that of an uncapsulated tumor with papillary and follicular structures and characteristic nuclear changes (70% of the total). The papillae have a fibrovascular core covered by a single layer of neoplastic cells. Psammoma bodies, present in 40% to 50% of cases, consist of degenerative calcified changes within the papillae and are almost pathognomonic of papillary thyroid carcinoma. The typical nuclear features include large-sized, overlapping nuclei that have a ground glass appearance and longitudinal grooves, with invaginations of cytoplasm into the nuclei. The tumor is multicentric in 20% to 80% of patients (with the wide range attributable to variations in the care used to examine the thyroid) and bilateral in about one third.[24] It spreads through the lymphatics within the thyroid to the regional lymph nodes and, less frequently, to the lungs.

The histologic variants include the encapsulated, follicular (without papillae), columnar-cell, tall-cell, clear-cell, and diffuse sclerosing carcinomas; they are classified as

TABLE 26–2. **Histologic Classification of Thyroid Tumors**

Tumor Type	Incidence (%)
Differentiated carcinoma	
Follicular carcinoma	10–15
Papillary carcinoma	65–75
Medullary carcinoma	5–9
Undifferentiated (anaplastic) carcinoma	2–15

papillary carcinomas because of their characteristic nuclear features. Papillary oxyphilic carcinoma is devoid of the typical nuclear features.

Follicular Carcinoma

Follicular carcinoma is characterized by follicular differentiation but without the nuclear changes characteristic of papillary carcinoma. Follicular carcinomas are encapsulated, and invasion of the capsule and vessels is the key feature distinguishing follicular carcinomas from adenomas. Two forms are recognized according to the pattern of invasion: minimally invasive and widely invasive carcinomas. The growth pattern may also vary, ranging from a well-differentiated pattern with macrofollicular structures to a poorly differentiated pattern with areas of solid, trabecular growth, and a high degree of atypia.[25]

Hürthle cell tumors are defined as solitary masses in the thyroid composed of Hürthle cells exclusively, or at least over 50% are Hürthle cells, and confined by a capsule. Hürthle cell carcinomas are classified as an oxyphilic or oncocytic variant of follicular carcinoma, and they account for 3% to 10% of all thyroid carcinomas. When compared with differentiated follicular cancers, they are usually more aggressive, metastasize more frequently (including in lymph nodes), and are less prone to take up radioiodine. Insular carcinoma is a rare and aggressive variant of poorly differentiated thyroid carcinoma.

Multicentricity and lymph node involvement are less frequent than in papillary carcinoma, and metastases to the lungs and bones stem from hematologic spread.

Anaplastic Carcinoma

Anaplastic carcinoma of the thyroid is one of the most aggressive cancers encountered in humans. In most cases, it represents the terminal stage in the dedifferentiation of a follicular or papillary carcinoma. In fact, anaplastic cells do not produce thyroglobulin, they are not able to transport iodine, and thyrotropin receptors are not found in their plasma cell membrane.[15, 16]

The tumor is typically composed of varying proportions of spindle, polygonal, and giant cells, often including squamous cells and sarcomatoid foci. Keratin is the most useful epithelial marker and is present in 40% to 100% of tumors.[20] Many anaplastic carcinomas have a well-differentiated component. Conversely, differentiated carcinomas with small undifferentiated foci should be considered to be anaplastic. Immunohistochemical studies indicate that most tumors previously called small cell undifferentiated carcinomas were in fact primary malignant lymphomas (positive for leukocyte common antigen) or, less often, medullary thyroid carcinoma (positive for calcitonin and carcinoembryonic antigen), poorly differentiated follicular carcinoma (positive for thyroglobulin), or a thyroid metastasis from another primary tumor. Some tumors do not react with any antibody; they are considered anaplastic carcinomas and have the same prognosis.

Anaplastic carcinomas have a rapidly progressing course. At the time of diagnosis, many patients have metastases in lymph nodes and invasion of adjacent organs (trachea, esophagus, vessels, muscles, and skin). Distant metastases ultimately occur in many patients, most commonly in the lungs, followed by bones, liver, and brain.

Medullary Thyroid Carcinoma

MTC is a tumor of the C-cells. C-cells physiologically produce calcitonin and are located at the junction between the upper third and the lower two thirds of thyroid lobes.[18] MTC presents as a white-red, hard lesion. At microscopy, it presents as sheets of spindle or round cells, typical of neuroendocrine tumors. Nuclei are usually uniform with rare mitosis. Deposits of amyloid are frequently found. Immunohistochemistry with anti-CT antibodies will establish the diagnosis; in familial MTC, it will show C-cell hyperplasia, which is seldom found in sporadic cases. Metastatic spread to regional lymph nodes is frequent and occurs early. Distant metastases, usually slow growing, are frequent. The sites most frequently affected are the liver, lungs, and bones.[18, 26]

Staging

While there are many staging systems for thyroid carcinomas (Table 26–3), the tumor, node, metastasis (TNM) system is the most widely used (Table 26–4).[27, 28]

TABLE 26–3. **Staging of Differentiated Thyroid Carcinoma: Components of Staging Systems**

	TNM	EORTC	IGR	AMES	AGES	MACIS	CHICAGO	OHIO
Age	+	+	+	+	+	+		
Cell type	+	+	+					
Histologic grade					+			
Tumor size	+			+	+	+	+	+
Extension beyond thyroid	+	+		+	+	+	+	+
Lymph node metastases	+						+	+
Distant metastases	+	+		+	+	+	+	+
Incomplete resection						+		

TNM = tumor, node, metastases; EORTC = European Organization for Research on Treatment of Cancer; IGR = Institut Gustave-Roussy; AMES = *a*ge, distant *m*etastases, *e*xtent and *s*ize of the primary tumor; AGES = *a*ge, *g*rade (according to Broder's classification), tumor *e*xtent and *s*ize of the tumor; MACIS = *m*etastases, *a*ge, *c*ompleteness of surgery, *i*nvasion of extrathyroidal tissues, and *s*ize; CHICAGO = University of Chicago; OHIO = Ohio State University.

Adapted from Schlumberger M, Pacini F: Thyroid Tumors, p 320. Paris, Editions Nucleon, 1999.

TABLE 26–4. **Staging of Thyroid Gland Carcinomas**

	Papillary or Follicular			
Stage	***<45 Years***	***>45 Years***	**Medullary**	**Descriptor**
I	Any T,Any N,M0	T1,N0,M0	T1,N0,M0	T1: ≤1 cm in greatest dimension; limited to thyroid N0: No regional lymph node metastasis M0: No distant metastasis
II	Any T,Any N,M1	T2–3,N0,M0	T2–4,N0,M0	T2: Tumor >1 cm but <4 cm in greatest dimension; limited to thyroid T3: Tumor >4 cm in greatest dimension; limited to thyroid T4: Tumor any size extending beyond thyroid capsule M1: Distant metastasis
III		T4,N0,M0 Any T,N1,M0	Any T,N1,M0	N1: Regional lymph node metastasis*
IV†		Any T,Any N,M1	Any T,Any N,M1	

*N1a: Metastasis in ipsilateral cervical lymph nodes; N1b: Metastasis in bilateral, midline, or contralateral cervical or mediastinal lymph nodes.
†All anaplastic carcinomas are stage IV.
Used with the permission of the American Joint Committee on Cancer (AJCC®), Chicago, Illinois. The original source for this material is the AJCC® Cancer Staging Manual, 5th edition (1997), published by Lippincott-Raven Publishers, Philadelphia, Pennsylvania.

Principles of Treatment

Papillary and Follicular Carcinoma

Surgery

Surgery is the first therapeutic procedure in patients with papillary and follicular thyroid carcinoma, with the aim of removing all tumor tissue in the neck. Therefore, the thyroid gland and affected cervical lymph nodes should be resected. The surgical strategy used at Institut Gustave-Roussy is given in Figure 26–1.

Although there is still some controversy about the extent of thyroid surgery, there are strong arguments in favor of a total or near-total thyroidectomy (leaving no more than 2 to 3 g of thyroid tissue at an upper pole) in all patients. Total or near-total thyroidectomy results in a lower recurrence rate than more limited thyroidectomy because many papillary carcinomas are multifocal and bilateral.[2, 4, 29–36] Furthermore, removal of most, if not all, of the thyroid gland facilitates total ablation with iodine-131. The argument against total thyroidectomy is that it increases the risk of surgical complications such as recurrent nerve injuries and hypoparathyroidism. Even with total thyroidectomy, often some thyroid tissue remains, as detected by postoperative scanning with iodine-131.

In patients who are at low risk for recurrence (those with papillary carcinoma smaller than 1.0 to 1.5 cm in diameter, if unifocal and intralobar), a lobectomy may be appropriate. If the microcarcinoma is discovered during surgery, a near-total thyroidectomy is advisable, because this will facilitate

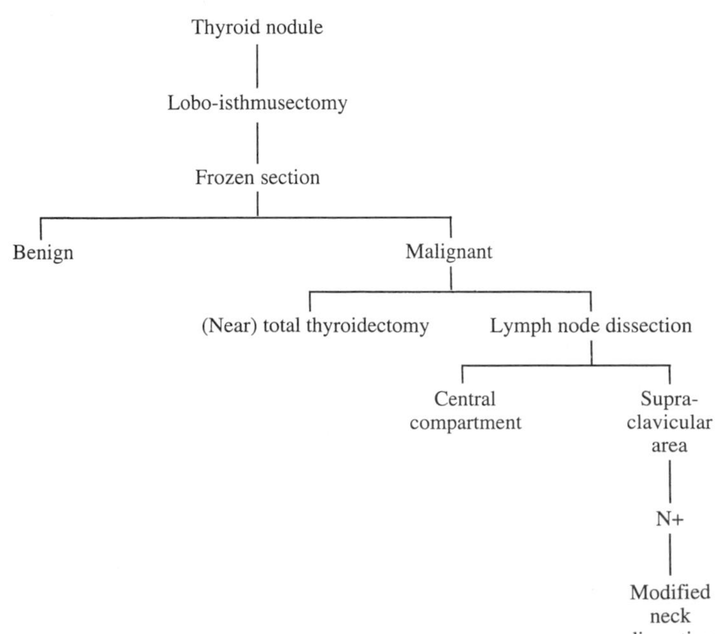

Figure 26–1. Surgical strategy at Institut Gustave-Roussy, Villejuif.

the long-term follow-up. If the microcarcinoma is discovered at the final histologic examination, the decision of complete thyroidectomy should take into account the low relapse rate (less than 3%) and the virtual absence of mortality of these tumors after lobectomy only.[37, 38]

In patients with papillary carcinoma, lymph nodes in the central compartment (paratracheal and esophagotracheal areas) are dissected. This may be extended to the ipsilateral supraclavicular area and lower third of the jugulocarotid chain. A modified neck dissection is performed if the supraclavicular area is involved or if there are palpable lymph node metastases in the jugulocarotid chain, sparing the jugular vein, the sternocleidomastoid muscle, and the spinal nerve. Dissection of lymph nodes is preferable to sampling. Although this type of lymph node dissection has not been shown to improve recurrence and survival rates, its routine use in patients with papillary carcinomas is warranted for several reasons. About two thirds of patients have lymph node metastases, and in more than 80% of patients with lymph node metastases, the central compartment is involved.[39] In addition, metastases are difficult to detect in lymph nodes located behind the vessels or in the paratracheal groove; neck lymph nodes are frequently found via ultrasonography, and the knowledge of initial tumor extent helps the interpretation of follow-up data. Finally, iodine-131 therapy is generally not effective on large tumor deposits (>1 cm in diameter).

Among patients with follicular carcinoma, a smaller proportion (about 35%) have lymph node metastases.[39] In these patients, a lymph node dissection is performed only if the diagnosis of follicular carcinoma is established during surgery or lymph nodes are palpable at surgery.

Iodine-131 Therapy

Iodine-131 therapy is given postoperatively for three reasons:

1. It destroys any remaining normal thyroid tissue, thereby increasing the sensitivity of subsequent iodine-131 total body scanning and the specificity of measurements of serum thyroglobulin for the detection of persistent or recurrent disease.
2. Iodine-131 therapy may destroy occult microscopic carcinoma, thereby decreasing the long-term risk of recurrent disease.
3. The use of a large amount of iodine-131 for therapy permits postablative total body scanning, a sensitive test for detecting persistent carcinoma.[4]

Postoperative iodine-131 therapy should be used selectively.[40] In patients who are at low risk, the long-term prognosis after surgery alone is so favorable that iodine-131 ablation is usually not recommended. In fact, ablation therapy is clearly not beneficial in patients with small intrathyroid tumors (smaller than 1.0 to 1.5 cm in diameter), and it does not influence recurrence rates in patients with lymph node–positive papillary thyroid microcarcinomas.[37, 38]

In patients with larger tumors, multifocality, and tumor extension beyond the thyroid capsule or lymph node metastases, the beneficial effects of radioactive iodine ablation continue to be controversial. This protocol was suggested in studies of Ohio State University[32, 33]; however, in patients treated at the Mayo Clinic with similar stages of disease and using an identical statistical analysis, no benefits were found.[29] The main difference between these two studies was the much higher rate of recurrences in nonablated patients in the study from Ohio State University than in the other groups of patients. These data strongly suggest that completeness of surgical excision is a major prognostic factor for recurrence. This belief is in accordance with previous studies in which the recurrence and survival rates were improved by iodine-131 ablation therapy only in patients for whom surgery was incomplete.[41, 42]

Therefore, only patients who are at high risk for recurrent disease should be treated with iodine-131, because it will decrease both recurrence and death rates. Furthermore, it permits postablative iodine-131 total body scanning to be performed, a sensitive procedure for controlling the completeness of surgery.[43–45] Uptake foci outside the thyroid bed may then warrant further therapeutic procedures and, in particular, surgical excision when they are located in the neck or in the mediastinum.

Iodine-131 ablation therapy is performed 4 to 6 weeks after surgery, with no thyroid treatment given in the interim. A total body scan is obtained 4 to 7 days after the dose,[43–45] and thyroxine therapy is initiated. Total ablation is routinely verified by performing iodine-131 total body scanning 6 to 12 months later using 2 mCi. In case of uptake outside the thyroid bed on postablation scan, another large amount of iodine-131 (3.7 GBq) is given 4 to 6 months after initial treatment. Total ablation (no visible uptake) is achieved after the administration of either 100 mCi (3.7 GBq) or 30 mCi (1.1 GBq) in more than 90% of patients who have undergone a total or a near-total thyroidectomy. After less extensive surgery, ablation with 30 mCi of iodine-131 is achieved in only two thirds of patients. Therefore, total or near-total thyroidectomy should be performed in all patients who are to be treated with iodine-131. Total ablation requires that a radiation dose of at least 300 Gy be delivered to the thyroid remnant; a dosimetric study may allow a more precise estimate of the dose of iodine-131 to be given.[46, 47]

External Radiotherapy

External radiotherapy to the neck and mediastinum (50 Gy in 25 fractions over 5 weeks) is indicated only in older patients (older than 45 years) in whom total surgical excision is impossible and the tumor tissue does not take up iodine-131 or when no tumor regression is observed following iodine-131 treatments (Table 26–5).[41, 48]

Anaplastic Thyroid Carcinoma

Only combined treatment may improve the survival rate of patients with anaplastic thyroid carcinoma. Combined treatment includes surgical excision of tumor masses present in the neck followed by a combination of systemic chemotherapy and external radiotherapy to the neck and mediastinum.

A chemotherapy regimen consists of either fractionated doses of doxorubicin (10 mg/m^2 per week)[49] or a combination of doxorubicin (60 mg/m^2) and cisplatinum (90 mg/m^2)

TABLE 26–5. **Multidisciplinary Treatment Decision for Well-Differentiated Thyroid Cancer**

Patient Age	Size of Lesion	Extrathyroidal Disease	Recommended Therapy
Any	≤2 cm	Absent	Thyroid lobectomy or NTT with suppression
<45	2–4 cm	Absent	NTT/TT with suppression
≥45	2–4 cm	Absent	NTT/TT with suppression and ^{131}I ablation
Any	>4 cm	Present with direct invasion	NTT/TT with suppression and ^{131}I ablation*
Any	Any	Distant metastases (bone or lung)	NTT/TT with suppression and ^{131}I ablation

NTT/TT = Near-total/total thyroidectomy; suppression = thyroxine to decrease thyroid-stimulating hormone levels; ^{131}I = treatment with iodine-131.
*One may consider additional local radiation therapy.

every 3 to 4 weeks.[50] External radiotherapy may be hyperfractionated and consists of fractions of 1.25 Gy, given twice a day for 5 days per week to a total dose of 40 Gy. It is given either in combination with fractionated doxorubicin or between the second and third courses of the combination of doxorubicin and cisplatinum.[49–52]

Severe toxicity is observed in one third of patients. Complete local control is obtained in 60% to 80% of patients, thus avoiding death from local invasion and suffocation. Long-term survival is obtained in 20% to 30% of patients who have undergone surgery and who had no initial distant metastases. The absence of response in distant metastases underlines the need to treat these patients rapidly.

Medullary Thyroid Carcinoma

Surgery is the main procedure in patients with MTC. It is performed after having ruled out the presence of a pheochromocytoma.[18, 53] In patients with clinical MTC, surgery includes a total thyroidectomy, with a dissection of the central compartment of the neck, and a bilateral modified neck dissection. Even after extensive lymph node dissection, the biochemical cure rate, as shown by undetectable calcitonin levels 5 days after surgery, is only 20% to 30% of clinical MTCs. In those patients with residual detectable calcitonin level, a complete work-up should be performed to search for regional and distant metastases. The complete work-up includes a CT scan of the neck, chest, and abdomen, ultrasonography of the liver and bone scintigraphy. If these procedures show a normal result, the venous sampling catheterization with selective measurements of the calcitonin level is the most precise tool for localizing persistent disease.[54, 55] If a calcitonin gradient is found only in the neck or in the mediastinum, further surgery may be indicated. This further surgery will find neoplastic tissue in most cases, but it will rarely permit a biochemical cure. Therefore, if the calcitonin level remains elevated after further surgery, external radiotherapy to the neck and mediastinum is indicated, which decreases the risk of local recurrence by a factor of 3 to 4.[48, 56]

In patients without clinical disease in whom surgery is undertaken on the basis of genetic testing, a total thyroidectomy with dissection of the central compartment of the neck is performed. The biochemical response rate is over 90%, and it is higher in surgical patients whose preoperative pentagastrin-stimulated calcitonin level is either normal or only weakly positive, and who also have no lymph node metastases.[17, 18, 53]

Thyroxine Treatment

Papillary and Follicular Thyroid Carcinoma

The aims of L-thyroxine (LT4) treatment are to restore euthyroidism and to suppress thyroid-stimulating hormone (TSH) secretion. The initial treatment dose is 2.5 μg/kg body weight in adults, being higher in children (3.0 μg/kg) and lower in the elderly. The serum TSH level is measured 3 months after initiation of therapy and should be below 0.1 μU/mL. When the TSH level is undetectable, the free triiodothyronine (T_3) level should be maintained within the normal range in order to avoid any overdose of LT4. When the TSH level is above 0.1 μU/mL, the daily dose of LT4 is increased by 25 μg and the TSH level is measured again 3 months later. Once the serum TSH level is below 0.1μU/mL, LT4 dosage is maintained, and the TSH level is measured once a year.[57, 58]

Other Thyroid Malignancies

The aim of LT4 treatment is to restore euthyroidism after thyroidectomy. A daily dose of 1.8 μg/kg body weight is given with the aim of obtaining a TSH level within the normal range.

Follow-Up

Papillary and Follicular Carcinoma

The goals of follow-up after initial therapy are to maintain adequate thyroxine therapy and to detect persistent or recurrent thyroid carcinoma. Recurrences are usually detected during the early years of follow-up, but they may occur later. Therefore, follow-up is necessary throughout the patient's life.[4, 32, 33, 42] The early discovery of recurrence has a paramount prognostic significance on both cure rate and survival rate after recurrence.[59, 60] This is made possible by the combined use of serum thyroglobulin measurement and iodine-131 total body scanning.[4, 10]

Routine Methods

- Palpation of the thyroid bed and lymph node areas is performed routinely.
- Ultrasonography is performed in patients at high risk for recurrent disease and in any patient with suspicious clinical findings. Lymph nodes that are small, thin, or oval, or those that are reduced in size after an interval of 3 months, are considered benign. Serum thyroglobulin concentrations are undetectable in 20% of patients

receiving thyroxine treatment who have isolated lymph node metastases; therefore, undetectable values do not rule out metastatic lymph node disease. The knowledge of initial lymph node status, which is determined by lymph node dissection at initial surgery, helps to interpret any lymph node abnormality. If there is a question of metastasis, a lymph node fine-needle biopsy may be performed, with cytology and thyroglobulin measurement in liquid aspirate[61]; genetic analysis of thyroid-specific transcripts (thyroglobulin, TSH-receptor mRNA) in liquid aspirate permits the early diagnosis in small lymph node metastases.[62]

- Chest radiography is no longer routinely performed in patients with undetectable thyroglobulin concentrations. The reason is that virtually all patients with abnormal radiographs have detectable serum thyroglobulin concentrations.[4, 60, 63]

Serum Thyroglobulin Measurement

Thyroglobulin (Tg) is a glycoprotein that is produced only by normal or neoplastic thyroid follicular cells. It should not be detectable in patients who have undergone total thyroid ablation, and its detection in such patients signifies the presence of persistent or recurrent disease.[63–68]

METHODS

Modern Tg assays can detect concentrations as low as 1 ng/mL or even lower. The results, however, can be artifactually altered by the presence of serum Tg antibodies, which are found in 15% to 25% of patients with thyroid carcinoma. Tests for these antibodies should always be performed when serum Tg is measured, but the extent to which the presence of antibodies alters the results of serum Tg assays depends on whether a radioimmunoassay (RIA) or an immunoradiometric assay (IRMA) is performed.[69–71]

At the present time, all European researchers advocate the use of IRMA methods. In these assays, interferences only lead to underestimated or falsely negative values. Serum should be screened for Tg antibodies with a sensitive Tg-antibody immunoassay before Tg measurement is undertaken. As an alternative, a recovery test has been advocated in parallel with each Tg determination. It consists of adding a known amount of Tg to the serum sample and measuring the recovery; it distinguishes between sera with interference (recovery less than 70% to 80%) and those without interference (recovery greater than 70% to 80%). Some of the modern IRMAs, using monoclonal antibodies with high-binding constants and incubation steps of more than a few hours, often allow extraction from weakly bound endogenous Tg-Tg antibody complexes to occur. In these IRMAs, interference is found in approximately 1% of sera from thyroid cancer patients and causes a small underestimate. Therefore, in the presence of interference, any detectable Tg level indicates the presence of thyroid tissue; however, when Tg is undetectable, a degree of caution is advisable in the presence of Tg antibodies, even if the recovery test is normal.

From a clinical point of view, Tg antibodies are sought at the first Tg determination, preferably using an RIA method. In the absence of Tg antibodies a recovery test is performed on each subsequent determination. The recovery test is necessary to detect falsely low Tg values as a result of the high-dose hook effect, which, unfortunately, occurs rather early in some assays. Furthermore, it is helpful to disclose nonspecific effects such as human antimouse antibody interference. If such interference is present, Tg antibodies should be sought at each subsequent Tg determination. In patients in complete remission after total thyroid ablation, serum Tg antibodies decline to low or undetectable values on or before the second postoperative year; their persistence or their reappearance during follow-up should be considered to be indicative of recurrent disease.[71] Despite the reported high frequency of Tg antibodies, false-negative Tg measurements are extremely rare.

RESULTS

The production of thyroglobulin by both normal and neoplastic thyroid tissue is, in part, dependent on thyrotropin.[72, 73] Thus, when interpreting the serum thyroglobulin value, serum thyrotropin value should be taken into account, as well as the presence or absence of thyroid remnants. If the serum thyroglobulin concentration is detectable during thyroxine treatment, then it will increase after the treatment has been withdrawn.

In patients receiving thyroxine treatment after total thyroid ablation, serum thyroglobulin is undetectable in 98% of patients considered to be in complete remission; it is detectable in almost all patients with large distant metastases and is often at a high level. However, in this situation, about 20% of patients with isolated lymph node metastases and 5% of those with small lung metastases, which are not visible on a standard chest x-ray film, have undetectable Tg value.[4, 63] In these patients with neoplastic disease, Tg concentration will increase following withdrawal of thyroid hormone treatment and frequently will reach high levels. In contrast, Tg level will remain undetectable in most patients considered to be in complete remission. Therefore, TSH stimulation obtained by withdrawing thyroid hormone treatment or by intramuscular injections of recombinant human TSH[74, 75] increases the sensitivity of Tg measurement.

In patients receiving thyroid hormone treatment after total thyroidectomy, Tg level is undetectable in 93% of cases. Following withdrawal of thyroid hormone treatment, it remains undetectable in 80% of cases. Therefore, Tg measurement can be used during patient follow-up after total thyroidectomy, even if an ablation dose of iodine-131 has not been given. The few patients with detectable Tg levels may then be treated with iodine-131, in particular, when Tg levels increase at two consecutive measurements.[63]

In patients receiving thyroid hormone treatment after lobectomy, Tg level is detectable in about half of cases. Ultrasonography has shown thyroid abnormalities (micronodules) in a high number of these patients with detectable Tg levels. Because of their small size, fine-needle biopsy may be impossible, and in the case of progression, surgery may be warranted. These data favor a near-total thyroidectomy in all patients with differentiated thyroid carcinoma. Following thyroid hormone withdrawal, the Tg level is poorly informative in these patients because it can be produced both by normal and by neoplastic thyroid tissue.[63]

Serum thyroglobulin concentration is an excellent prognostic indicator. Patients with undetectable serum thyroglobulin concentrations after thyroxine has been withdrawn have been free of relapse after more than 15 years of follow-up. Conversely, 60% to 80% of patients with serum Tg concentrations above 10 ng/mL after withdrawal of treatment, and with no other evidence of disease, have detectable foci of iodine-131 uptake in the neck or at distant sites after the administration of a large amount (3.7 GBq) of iodine-131.[43, 44, 76–78]

Iodine-131 Total Body Scanning

The results of iodine-131 total body scanning (TBS) depend on the ability of thyroid cancer tissue to take up iodine-131 in the presence of high serum TSH concentrations, which are achieved by withdrawing thyroxine for 4 to 6 weeks.[79] However, the resulting hypothyroidism is poorly tolerated by some patients.[80] This problem can be attenuated by substituting the more rapidly metabolized triiodothyronine for thyroxine for 3 weeks and withdrawing it for 2 weeks,[79] or by simply reducing the dose of thyroxine by about half.[72] The serum TSH concentration should be higher than some arbitrary level (e.g., 30 μU/mL) in patients treated in this way, and if necessary, the administration of iodine-131 should be delayed for 1 or 2 weeks until the value has exceeded that level. This is the case in some patients treated with totally suppressive doses of thyroxine or in the elderly.[72] Intramuscular injections of recombinant human TSH (0.9 mg each day for 2 days, with iodine-131 administration on the third day) is a promising alternative, because thyroxine treatment does not need to be discontinued and the side effects are minimal. The results of iodine-131 TBS performed after the administration of recombinant human TSH and after the withdrawal of thyroxine are similar in most patients.[74]

Even in the presence of high-serum TSH concentration, only two thirds of patients with metastatic disease exhibit some iodine-131 uptake. This is more frequently observed in young patients who have small metastases and a differentiated thyroid tumor.[46, 59, 60]

When iodine-131 TBS is planned, patients should be instructed to avoid iodine-containing medications and iodine-rich foods, and urinary iodine should be measured in doubtful cases.[81] In women of childbearing age, pregnancy must be ruled out. For routine diagnostic iodine-131 TBS, 2 to 5 mCi (74 to 185 MBq) of iodine-131 is given; higher doses may reduce the uptake of a subsequent therapeutic dose of iodine-131.[82] Scanning is performed and uptake, if any, is measured 3 days after the dose has been administered, with the use of a double-head gamma camera equipped with high-energy collimators.

Assuming equivalent fractional uptake after the administration of a diagnostic or high dose of iodine-131, an uptake too low to be detected with 2 to 5 mCi may be detectable after the administration of 100 mCi. This is the rationale for administering 100 mCi (or more) of iodine-131 in patients with a high likelihood of persistent or recurrent thyroid carcinoma. When this dose is administered, a TBS should be performed 4 to 7 days later.[43]

False-positive results are infrequent. They may be related to skin contamination, axillary perspiration, to thymus hypertrophy, or to various conditions such as pleuropericardial cysts, hiatal hernia, abnormal esophagus, and inflammatory processes. They are often easily diagnosed.[8, 47, 83–85]

Other Diagnostic Procedures

Other procedures can be useful in patients with a high likelihood of persistent or recurrent thyroid carcinoma in whom a TBS performed with a high iodine-131 dose (100 mCi or more) has not shown any foci of uptake. They may consist of a CT scan or MRI of the chest and neck, bone scintigraphy,[86] nonspecific isotopic scan, and a positron emission tomography scan.

CT scan and MRI may localize tumor deposits in the neck, chest, and bones. However, interpretation of data in an area already submitted to surgery may be difficult. These procedures are mostly useful to visualize abnormalities already seen on isotopic scans.

Nonspecific isotopic markers include thallium-201, technetium-99m tetrofosmin, technetium-99m MIBI (technetium-99m methoxyisobutryl isonitrile), and indium-111 pentetreotide.[87–90] They can be used to perform TBS while the patient is on thyroxine treatment. In some reports, the sensitivity of these techniques appeared to be high, but they cannot substitute for iodine-131 TBS in patients with suspected disease. Therefore, none of the nonspecific isotopic markers is routinely recommended.

Use of positron emission tomography (PET) is proving to be promising because enhanced glucose metabolism is a nonspecific feature of tumor cells. The use of PET scans, using (^{18}F) fluorodeoxyglucose (FDG), has been investigated in patients with differentiated thyroid carcinoma. It can be performed while the patient is taking thyroxine treatment; however, FDG uptake was higher when LT4 treatment was withdrawn. FDG uptake was detected more frequently in patients with poorly differentiated thyroid carcinoma, in whom no detectable iodine-131 uptake could be demonstrated. In addition, uptake was detected in neck lymph nodes, even in those smaller than 1 cm in diameter, thus confirming the high sensitivity of PET scan. PET scan did not, however, detect small lung metastases that could be evidenced by a spiral CT scan. Therefore, PET scan with FDG cannot substitute for iodine-131 TBS, but it should be performed in patients with a high likelihood of persistent or recurrent disease and in those in whom a high-dose iodine-131 TBS result is negative.[91–95]

Strategy of Follow-Up

If the iodine-131 TBS obtained after the administration of iodine-131 to destroy the thyroid remnants does not show any uptake outside the thyroid bed, then serum TSH and Tg concentrations are measured during thyroxine treatment 3 months later (Fig. 26–2).

Diagnostic iodine-131 TBS with 2 to 5 mCi is obtained after thyroxine withdrawal 6 to 12 months after iodine-131 treatment.[4, 10] This procedure is advocated by most clinicians in order to check that ablation is total and to search for foci of uptake outside the thyroid bed. If any uptake is detected, then 100 mCi of iodine-131 is given. If no uptake

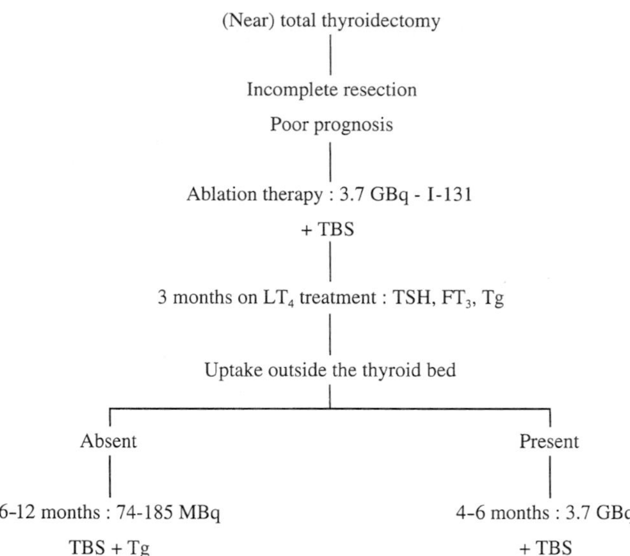

Figure 26–2. Initial treatment and follow-up in patients with papillary or follicular thyroid carcinoma.

is detected, subsequent follow-up is based on prognostic factors and on serum Tg concentration. However, the yield of routine control iodine-131 TBS is very low: ablation is achieved in more than 90% of patients after total thyroidectomy, and the discovery of foci of uptake not shown on postablation iodine-131 TBS is extremely rare.[10, 40] Furthermore, nearly all patients with foci of uptake outside the thyroid bed have detectable Tg concentrations after thyroid hormone withdrawal or recombinant human TSH stimulation. In the near future, the use of recombinant human TSH will probably permit the selection of patients in whom scanning should be performed, namely those with detectable Tg level after stimulation.[74]

In patients at low risk for recurrence and considered to be cured (i.e., with undetectable serum Tg concentration after thyroid hormone treatment withdrawal and negative results on iodine-131 TBS), the dose of thyroxine is decreased to maintain a low but detectable serum TSH concentration (0.1 to 0.5 μU/mL). The risk of recurrence is, in fact, so low in these patients that any overdose of thyroxine is unjustified. Patients at low risk represent the great majority (more than 80%) of patients.

In patients at high risk for recurrence, even those considered to be cured, higher doses of thyroxine are continued, with the objective of attaining serum TSH concentration of 0.1 μU/mL or less; the free triiodothyronine concentration should be maintained within the normal range to avoid any overdose.[57] Clinical and biochemical evaluations are performed annually; any other testing is unnecessary as long as the serum Tg concentration is undetectable.

If the serum Tg concentration becomes detectable in a patient receiving thyroxine, then the thyroxine should be withdrawn, iodine-131 TBS should be performed, and a serum Tg should be measured. If any uptake is detected, then 100 mCi of iodine-131 should be given. In patients with no uptake on iodine-131 diagnostic TBS, any detectable Tg concentration indicates the presence of thyroid tissue; in patients with a Tg level above some arbitrary limit (>10 ng/mL), the administration of a large dose (100 mCi) of iodine-131 has been advocated by several researchers in order to obtain highly sensitive iodine-131 TBS.[43, 44, 76–78] This procedure may also be warranted in those patients with a Tg concentration below 10 ng/mL, depending on the clinical context. This highly sensitive iodine-131 TBS has permitted the discovery of foci of uptake in 60% to 80% of such patients. Besides its diagnostic interest, it also permitted the cure of a significant proportion of them.[43, 77, 78] However, much controversy persists with regard to this procedure, mainly because of the indolent course of this disease and the absence of a controlled trial.[96, 97] In the absence of iodine-131 uptake, any other administration of iodine-131 is unnecessary. In these patients, CT scan or MRI of the neck and lungs and bone scintigraphy may be useful. PET scan also is a promising tool, because it more frequently shows a positive result in patients without iodine-131 uptake and even in small lesions (<1 cm in diameter), when localized in the neck or mediastinum.

The interest of diagnostic iodine-131 TBS should be questioned, because whatever the results, patients with a Tg concentration above 10 ng/mL will be given a large amount of iodine-131. Again, the availability of recombinant human TSH in the near future will allow patients with a stimulated Tg level attaining an arbitrary limit to be selected for treatment with a high dose of iodine-131, without undergoing diagnostic iodine-131 TBS.[74]

In patients at low risk for recurrence who have undergone a total thyroidectomy but have not been given iodine-131 postoperatively, iodine-131 TBS is performed 6 to 12 months after surgery. The follow-up protocol previously described is then applied on the basis of serum Tg concentration.

In patients at low risk for recurrence who have undergone a lobectomy, follow-up consists of a yearly neck examination and serum Tg measurement during thyroxine treatment. In most patients with detectable Tg concentrations, ultrasonography will show abnormalities in the remaining lobe. If the lesions are small, fine-needle biopsy may be impossible, and surgery is frequently the only option.

Medullary Thyroid Carcinoma

- Follow-up of patients with medullary thyroid carcinoma is designed to detect recurrences and associated lesions in familial cases.
- Recurrent disease is diagnosed by measurement of blood tumor markers (calcitonin and carcinoembryonic antigen) and by imaging procedures, including ultrasonography of the neck and the abdomen (liver and adrenal glands), bone scintigraphy, and CT scan of the neck, chest, and abdomen.[10, 18]
- Patients with an undetectable basal calcitonin level should undergo a pentagastrin test at 3 months, and again at 1 year after initial treatment. The absence of an increase in calcitonin following pentagastrin stimulation at two intervals signifies a cure. These patients are then followed at a yearly interval with basal calcitonin and carcinoembryonic antigen measurements.
- Patients with a detectable calcitonin level should be followed every 6 months. Notably, calcitonin levels

may vary by 20% to 30% at short intervals of time.[98] Venous sampling catheterization with calcitonin measurements is the most sensitive tool for localizing persistent or recurrent MTC.[54, 55]

- Patients with known, distant metastases also may be followed at regular intervals in case of an apparently stable disease; progression of the disease may warrant systemic chemotherapy.
- In familial cases, pheochromocytoma should be sought annually, with 24-hour urinary measurement of metanephrines and adrenal ultrasonography. Hyperparathyroidism is diagnosed with serum calcium and PTH 1–84 measurements.[10, 18]

Special Considerations

Papillary and Follicular Carcinoma

Complications of Disease

- Local or regional recurrences occur in 5% to 20% of patients with differentiated thyroid carcinoma. Some are related to incomplete initial treatment (recurrent disease in a thyroid remnant or lymph nodes). Others indicate the presence of an aggressive tumor (in the thyroid bed after total thyroidectomy or in soft tissues), and they are often associated with distant metastases.[29, 31, 36, 39]
- Distant metastases, usually in the lungs and bones, occur in 10% to 15% of patients with differentiated thyroid carcinoma.[99] Lung metastases are most frequent in young patients with papillary carcinomas, and the lungs are almost the only site of distant spread in children. Bone metastases are more common in older patients and those with follicular carcinomas. Other less common sites of metastases are the brain, liver, and skin. Symptoms associated with lung metastases are uncommon. In contrast, pain, swelling, or fracture occurs in more than 80% of patients with bone metastases.[23, 59, 60, 100–102]

Complications of Treatment

SURGERY

- Recurrent nerve paralysis is rare (for patients with experienced surgeons) and is mostly transient.
- Hypoparathyroidism is a difficult problem to manage medically. Its incidence is decreased by performing a near-total thyroidectomy and by using methylene blue staining and autotransplantation of the parathyroid glands.

IODINE-131 TREATMENT

Acute Side Effects. Acute side effects (nausea and sialadenitis) are common after treatment with large doses of iodine-131, but they are usually mild and resolve rapidly. Radiation-associated thyroiditis is usually minimal, but if the thyroid remnant is large, patients may have enough pain and swelling to warrant glucocorticoid therapy for a few days.[46] Tumors in certain locations (the brain, spinal cord, or paratracheal region) may swell in response to thyrotropin stimulation. If high doses of iodine-131 (>150 mCi) are administered at short intervals (<3 months),[103] radiation fibrosis may develop and eventually prove fatal in patients with diffuse lung metastases.

Genetic Defects and Infertility. Particular care must be taken to ensure that iodine-131 is not given to pregnant women.

After iodine-131 treatment, men may have a transient reduction in spermatogenesis, and women may have transient ovarian failure.[104, 105] Genetic damage induced by exposure to iodine-131 before conception has been a major concern. However, the only abnormality reported to date is an increased frequency of miscarriages in women treated with iodine-131 during the year preceding conception.[106, 107] Therefore, it is recommended that conception be postponed for 1 year after treatment with iodine-131. There is no evidence that pregnancy affects tumor growth in women receiving adequate thyroxine therapy.

Carcinogenesis and Leukemogenesis

Mild pancytopenia may occur after repeated iodine-131 therapy, especially in patients with bone metastases who have also been given external radiotherapy. The overall relative risk of secondary carcinoma or leukemia is increased only in patients given a large cumulative dose of iodine-131 (>500 mCi), as well as those given external radiotherapy.[106, 108, 109]

Medullary Thyroid Carcinoma

- In practical terms, a surgical cure of MTC is defined as a normal postoperative calcitonin stimulation test result at 3 months and again at 1 year after treatment.[10, 18]
- Overall, the rate of persistent hypercalcitoninemia is nearly 80% for patients presenting a palpable MTC. This high frequency of persistent disease is often a result of early metastases to regional lymph nodes. Patients with persistent hypercalcitoninemia but no other evidence of disease have an excellent long-term prognosis (86% overall survival at 10 years).[98]
- A surgical cure is achieved in more than 90% of patients undergoing operation on the basis of genetic testing. Surgery is advocated in gene carriers before the age of 6 years, or as soon as a pentagastrin test becomes positive.[10, 18, 110]

Results and Prognosis

Papillary and Follicular Carcinoma

Survival and Prognosis

The overall survival rate at 10 years for middle-aged adults with thyroid carcinomas is about 80% to 95%. Five percent to 20% of patients have local or regional recurrences, and 10% to 15% of patients have distant metastases.

The prognostic indicators of recurrent disease and death are the patient's age at diagnosis and the histologic subtype and extent of the tumor. The risk of death increases with age at diagnosis in patients with widely invasive or poorly differentiated thyroid carcinoma, as well as in those with a large extent of the tumor, that is, large tumor size, extension of the tumor beyond the thyroid capsule, and distant metastases.*

There are many staging systems for thyroid carcinoma, but the TNM system is the most widely used[27, 28] (see Tables 26–3 and 26–4). On the basis of these systems, 80% to 85% of patients are classified as being at low risk (<2% at 20 years of death from thyroid carcinoma).

Some patients have a higher risk of recurrence, even if their risk of death is low. This group includes younger (<16 years old) and older patients (>45 years), those with certain histologic subtypes (some papillary carcinomas: the tall-cell, columnar-cell, and diffuse sclerosing variants; some follicular carcinomas: the widely invasive and poorly differentiated subtypes and Hürthle-cell carcinomas), and those with large tumors, extension of the tumor beyond the thyroid capsule, or large and bilateral lymph node metastases. Older patients (>45 years) have the most aggressive thyroid cancers. The extent of initial treatment and follow-up should be determined according to these prognostic indicators.

Treatment of Recurrences

LOCAL AND REGIONAL RECURRENCES

A local or regional recurrence of the tumor that is palpable or easily visualized with ultrasonography or CT scanning should be excised. Our protocol includes the administration of 100 mCi with TBS 4 to 7 days later that may identify additional tissue that should be excised. Surgery is performed one day after scanning, with the use of an intraoperative probe. The completeness of resection is verified 1 to 2 days after surgery by obtaining another scan. This strategy allows for the resection of all foci of uptake in 92% of patients (Table 26–6).[115]

External radiotherapy to the neck is indicated in patients with soft tissue recurrences that cannot be completely excised and do not take up iodine-131.[42, 48]

DISTANT METASTASES

- Palliative surgery is required for bone metastases when there are neurologic or orthopedic complications or a high risk of such complications. Surgery may also be useful to debulk large tumor masses. In patients with a single bone metastasis, it is aimed to completely resect the metastasis, and this procedure has provided remarkable results in some patients.[102, 116]
- Patients with metastases that take up iodine-131 are treated with 100 to 150 mCi (3700 to 5500 MBq) every 4 to 6 months. The effective radiation dose, which depends on the ratio of total uptake to the mass of thyroid tissue, is correlated to the outcome of iodine-131 therapy.[10, 46, 117] For this reason, higher doses (200 mCi or more) have been recommended in patients with bone metastases, but their effectiveness remains to be demonstrated. Lower doses (1 mCi [37 MBq] per kg body weight) are given to children. There is no limit to the cumulative dose of iodine-131 that can be given to patients with distant metastases, although the risk of leukemia rises slightly when the cumulative dose is higher than 500 mCi (18,500 MBq); furthermore, higher cumulative doses have little benefit.[60, 109] External radiotherapy is given to patients who have bone metastases visible on radiographs or CT scans.[48, 60] Chemotherapy is not effective and should be considered only in patients with progressive metastases that do not take up iodine-131, or within the frame of controlled trials.[60, 118, 119]

*See references 4, 10, 29–31, 35–38, 41, 42, 111–114.

TABLE 26–6. **Treatment of Locoregional Recurrences**

Day 0	Administration of 100 mCi (3.7 GBq) ^{131}I
Day 4	TBS
Day 5	Surgery (intraoperative probe)
Day 6 or 7	TBS

TBS = total body scanning.

Complete responses to treatment have been observed in 45% of patients with distant metastases that take up iodine-131, with a higher frequency of complete responses in young patients and those with small metastases. Few relapses have been observed in patients with complete remission despite detectable serum Tg concentrations in some patients.[59, 60, 100]

The overall survival rate 10 years after the discovery of distant metastases is about 40%. Young patients with well-differentiated thyroid carcinomas that take up iodine-131 and those with metastases that are small when discovered have the most favorable outcome.[59, 60] When the size is considered, the location of the metastases (lungs or bone) has no independent prognostic influence. The poor prognosis of patients with bone metastases is linked to the bulkiness of the lesions.[60] The prognostic importance of the size of metastases at the time of their discovery has led to the administration of 100 mCi of iodine-131 in patients with elevated serum Tg concentrations and no other evidence of disease.[43]

Medullary Thyroid Carcinoma

Survival and Prognosis

- The overall prognosis of MTC is intermediate between well-differentiated papillary and follicular carcinoma and poorly differentiated carcinoma. Patients with normal postoperative calcitonin levels have a potentially normal life expectancy.[18, 56, 120]
- For patients with residual disease, several factors have been reported to have prognostic value: genetic background, age at initial treatment, extent of the disease, and histopathologic features.

Patients with MEN 2b have the most aggressive forms of MTC[10, 18]; those with MEN 2a or a sporadic form of the disease have the same long-term prognosis when the tumor extent is taken into account; some patients with familial MTC have an indolent course. Prognosis worsens with increasing age at diagnosis.

The extent of the disease has a paramount prognostic

significance: large tumor size, extension of the tumor beyond the thyroid capsule, lymph node metastases, or distant metastases are correlated with a poor outcome. Calcitonin immunostaining is also a strong prognostic factor, and loss of this endocrine differentiation correlates with tumor growth and metastases. A rapid increase in the carcinoembryonic antigen level, particularly in the setting of a stable calcitonin level, is indicative of tumor progression.

Treatment of Recurrences

- A locoregional relapse should be surgically treated when this is feasible. External radiotherapy to the neck and mediastinum may then be indicated.[48, 56]
- Distant metastases may be stable for years. In most patients, they are very slowly progressing. They are often multiple and involve the liver,[10, 18, 98] lungs, and bones.

In cases of progression only, systemic chemotherapy may be considered using a combination of several drugs, such as dacarbazine and 5-fluorouracil or dacarbazine, cyclophosphamide, and vincristine. Response rate is about 30%, all responses being partial, without any evidence of prolonged survival.[121–123] Biologic response modifiers, such as somatostatin analogues or interferon are ineffective. Diarrhea and flushing should be managed medically. Loperamide and diphenoxylate can be useful for diarrhea. Histamine-receptor blockers can be useful for flushing.

Pituitary Tumors

Epidemiology and Etiology

Epidemiology

Pituitary tumors are frequently occurring neoplasms of adenohypophyseal cells, and they represent approximately 15% of all intracranial tumors.[124, 125] Prevalence and incidence of clinically recognizable pituitary adenomas are about 200 cases per million and 15 new cases per million per year.[126] At autopsy, asymptomatic adenomas (mostly microadenomas) are found in 6% to 20% (mean, 11%) of presumably normal pituitary glands.[127, 128] In addition, in the general population, images compatible with the presence of a pituitary adenoma are found in 10% of systematic MRI studies of the pituitary gland.[129] The female-to-male ratio for a given adenoma type varies greatly with age; age ranges vary depending on the clinical syndrome.[130]

Etiology

Most tumors arise from epithelial cells of the anterior pituitary. Understanding of subcellular mechanisms for the pathogenesis and progression of pituitary adenomas is incomplete, but data have accumulated in recent years on the role of intrinsic pituitary genetic alterations, disordered transcription factors and growth factors, and signaling proteins in pituitary tumorigenesis.[131, 132] The potential role of the hypothalamus in causing tumor development in the pituitary (by means of hypersecretion or abnormal elaboration of releasing factors by the hypothalamus) has been challenged by the demonstration of the clonal origin of most pituitary adenomas.[133, 134] In fact, both events (spontaneous development of the tumor in a clone of cells within the pituitary and stimulation by hypothalamic hormones) may participate. Hypothalamic hormones or other local growth factors may promote the growth of already transformed pituitary cell clones and the expansion of small adenomas into large or invasive tumors. A large variety of molecular abnormalities has been explored in pituitary adenomas. With the exception of the *GSP* oncogene (heterozygous, activating, somatic point mutations in the α-subunit of the stimulatory G_s protein identified in up to 40% of growth hormone–secreting pituitary adenomas,[135, 136] there are only isolated instances of activating mutations in known oncogenes. Although loss-of-heterozygosity studies have identified changes associated with pituitary tumor initiation and progression, the search for mutations (the second hit) in the retained allele of known tumor suppressor genes has, to date, failed to reveal inactivating mutations.

Pituitary adenomas are usually benign, localized, and incapable of metastasis. Although the component cells are clearly transformed, cellular restraining factors (one of the candidates being an unidentified protein that is distinct from the Rb protein, but coded by chromosome 13q and adjacent to the *Rb* locus) prevent the expression of a true malignancy.[131] Alternatively, *HRAS* mutations may also play a role in aggressive tumors and in the very rare pituitary metastasis formation and growth.[131, 132] The combined data reported so far have allowed, albeit tentatively, some of the changes to be put into place along this multistep pathway (Fig. 26–3).

Malignant pituitary tumors are very rare (0.1% to 0.5% of pituitary tumors).[137, 138] Current opinion suggests that pituitary carcinomas arise after transformation of an initially benign pituitary adenoma.[131, 132, 138] Their malignant nature is not usually obvious in terms of their microscopic appearance, and several authors have advocated that the necessary criterion for the diagnosis of malignancy is the presence of metastasis to remote areas of the cerebrospinal subarachnoid space, the brain tissue, or extra–central nervous system sites.

Detection and Diagnosis

Clinical Detection

Pituitary tumors cause symptoms by secreting hormones or depressing the secretion of hormones or by mass-related

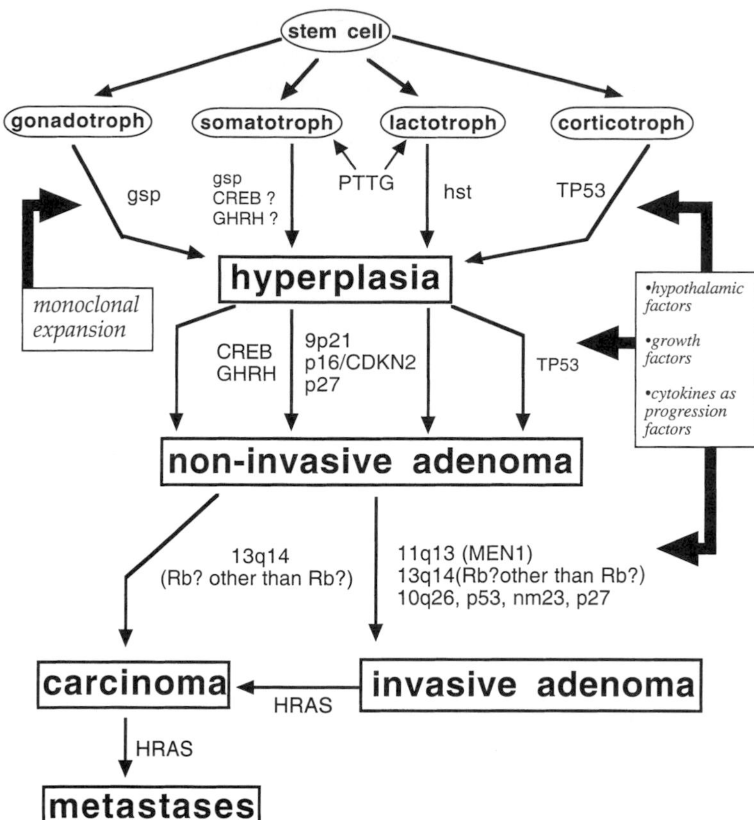

Figure 26–3. Schematic representation of molecular and biochemical events in pituitary tumor progression (gsp = mutated form of Gs protein; CREB = cAMP response element binding factor; GHRH = growth hormone-releasing hormone; PTTG = pituitary-tumor transforming gene; hst = heparin-binding secretory transforming gene; CDK = cyclin-dependent kinase; Rb = retinoblastoma susceptibility gene). (Adapted from Shimon I, Melmed S: Genetic basis of endocrine disease: pituitary tumor pathogenesis. J Clin Endocrinol Metab 1997; 82:1675–1681 and Farrell WE, Clayton RN: Molecular genetics of pituitary tumours. Trends Endocrinol Metab 1998; 9:20–26.)

effects. The variety of functions (Table 26–7) regulated by pituitary hormones accounts for the variety of syndromes caused by these tumors:

- *Acromegaly.* Characteristic clinical presentations for excess growth hormone include coarsened facial features (primarily of the brow and jaw), exaggerated growth of hands and feet, and soft tissue hypertrophy. Weight gain, hyperhidrosis, paresthesia, and fatigue are additional features.[139–142]
- *Cushing's syndrome.* Sustained hypercortisolism causes central obesity, hypertension, hirsutism, glucose intolerance, easy bruising, striae, osteoporosis, weakness, and psychological changes.[143, 144]
- *Nelson's syndrome.* This may follow bilateral adrenalectomy for Cushing's disease with development of hyperpigmentation.[143]
- *Prolactin-hypersecretion syndromes.* Women present with galactorrhea, amenorrhea, oligomenorrhea, or infertility. Men complain of decreased libido or impotence. Galactorrhea may also occur in men in the presence of gynecomastia.[145, 146]
- *Hyperthyroidism.* Rare TSH-secreting adenomas may stimulate the thyroid gland and produce thyrotoxicosis

TABLE 26–7. **Cellular Origin and Main Biologic Actions of Anterior Pituitary Hormones**

Hormone	Pituitary Cells	Hormone Structure (amino acids [aa] number)	Main Biologic Actions
Growth hormone	Somatotrophs	Peptide (191 aa)	Growth of bone, cartilage, muscle, connective tissues, viscera; increases glycemia; lipolytic
Prolactin	Lactotrophs	Peptide (199 aa)	Promotes lactation
Follicle-stimulating hormone (FSH)	Gonadotrophs	Dimeric glycoprotein α-subunit (92 aa) FSH-β (112 aa)	Female: promotes maturation and development of ovarian follicles and synthesis of estradiol; Male: promotes spermatogenesis
Luteinizing hormone (LH)	Gonadotrophs	Dimeric glycoprotein α-subunit (92 aa) LH-β (121 aa)	Female: triggers ovulation, stimulates corpus luteum; Male: stimulates testosterone formation by Leydig cells of testis
Thyroid-stimulating hormone (TSH)	Thyrotrophs	Dimeric glycoprotein α-subunit (92 aa) TSH-β (121 aa)	Increases thyroid growth and synthesis of thyroid hormones
Adrenocorticotropic hormone	Corticotrophs	Peptide (39 aa)	Promotes adrenocortical growth and steroidogenesis

and goiter simulating Graves' disease, with the difference that TSH is not suppressed in the presence of high plasma thyroid hormone levels (syndrome of inappropriate secretion of TSH).[147]
- *Gonadal hyperstimulation.* Macro-orchidism in men and ovarian hyperstimulation syndrome in premenopausal women may rarely be observed in patients with follicle-stimulating hormone secreting tumors.[148, 149]

Mass-related symptoms are also manifold because of the many critical structures in the vicinity of the pituitary gland[146, 150, 151]:

- *Optic nerve compression* with bilateral visual field loss that often begins in the superior temporal quadrants is the most common mass effect. Loss of visual acuity with optic disc atrophy may occur.
- *Cranial nerves III, IV* and *VI* may be compressed by lateral tumor extension. Abnormalities in extraocular muscle function result. Cranial nerve V is rarely affected.
- The *hypothalamus* is rarely involved by tumor extension superiorly through the diaphragm sellae. Increased appetite or changes in anterior pituitary hormone secretion may occur. Along with defects in pituitary hormone secretion, pituitary stalk compression may produce hyperprolactinemia by disinhibition of the dopaminergic tone normally acting at the level of the pituitary lactotrophs. By contrast, diabetes insipidus never occurs in pituitary adenomas: its presence rules out this diagnosis.
- Headache, increased intracranial pressure, seizures, or cerebrospinal fluid rhinorrhea may all occur. Pituitary apoplexy may be the presenting clinical picture with severe headaches of sudden onset, meningismus, variably depressed sensorium, and visual disturbances.
- *Hypopituitarism* may be caused by anterior pituitary compression, pituitary stalk interruption, or hypothalamic involvement. Sequential loss of hormone secretion usually begins with loss of growth hormone or the gonadotropins (luteinizing hormone [LH] and FSH). Decrease in TSH and adrenocorticotropic hormone (ACTH) secretion may follow.

Although hormonally active tumors are usually detected before the occurrence of mass effects, exceptions can be expected (e.g., prolactin-secreting tumors in men or in postmenopausal women or so-called clinically nonfunctioning pituitary adenomas [NFPA], which are generally gonadotropin-secreting adenomas without specific hyperstimulation symptoms). In addition, an increasing proportion of pituitary incidental (up to 15% of clinically NFPAs) are detected by chance on brain imaging by CT or MRI that is performed for independent reasons.

Diagnostic Procedures

All patients with suspected or documented pituitary tumors should be evaluated for gonadal, thyroid, and adrenal function, as well as prolactin and growth hormone secretion:

- gonadal: LH, FSH, free uncombined α-subunit, plasma estradiol in women, plasma testosterone in men
- thyroid: free T_4, free T_3, TSH
- adrenal: basal plasma cortisol at 8:00 A.M. The ability of the pituitary-adrenal axis to respond to stress, trauma, or surgery should be assessed by testing cortisol and ACTH response to insulin-induced hypoglycemia or corticotropin-releasing hormone, or by measuring 11-deoxycortisol (and eventually ACTH) increase after metyrapone. Hypersecretion of ACTH and cortisol are best assessed by measuring plasma cortisol and ACTH at 8:00 or 11:00 P.M. and 24-hour urinary free cortisol.
- prolactin secretion: Presence of hyperprolactinemia does not necessarily imply the presence of a prolactinoma (prolactin-secreting adenoma). It may also be observed when nonlactotroph tumors (whether adenomatous or nonadenomatous) compress the hypothalamus or pituitary stalk and impair normal inhibition by dopamine of normal pituitary lactotroph cells.
- growth hormone secretion: In normal adults, basal growth hormone is generally undetectable except during 3 to 5 spontaneous burst episodes occurring randomly over 24 hours. Assessment of growth hormone hypersecretion may thus be done by measuring growth hormone plasma levels sequentially (e.g., hourly) during 4 to 8 hours, in order to demonstrate the presence of sustained increased levels.

Specific stimulation and suppression tests for pituitary hormones (Table 26–8) are performed in selected situations for detecting the type of hypersecretion or the response to treatment.

Imaging procedures determine the presence, size, and extent of the lesion[152, 153] (Table 26–9):

- *Plain radiographs* can demonstrate gross enlargement of the sella turcica with a rounded, ballooned configuration or concavity of the anterior sellar wall, or a double-floor image.
- *Sellar polytomography, pneumoencephalography, and angiography* are now of no use. CT and MRI have totally replaced the need for these risky and uncomfortable procedures.
- *CT* provides substantial three-dimensional information on tumor size and extension.
- *MRI* has improved the quality of definition of the tumor (its extension and invasiveness are provided by CT) and increased the capability of delineating intraglandular pathology as well as (or even better than) CT. Furthermore, there is no ionizing radiation exposure, and MRI may be performed in any plane and does not require extension of the neck to obtain the very important direct coronal plane.
- *Visual perimetry and other neuro-ophthalmologic testing* is carefully performed.
- *Inferior petrosal sinus catheterization with simultaneous bilateral sampling of corticotropin* is a procedure that may be useful, in difficult cases, to confirm a pituitary source of corticotropin secretion and to establish the site of the adenoma.[144, 154]

Classification and Staging

Histopathology

The traditional classification of pituitary tumors is based on the tinctorial staining properties of the cell cytoplasm

TABLE 26–8. **Stimulation and Suppression Tests for Pituitary Hormones**

Hormone	Diagnosis Agent	Normal Response	Response with Tumor
PRL	TRH (or MCP)	Increase	Usually no change in case of prolactinoma and increase in secretion when hyperprolactinemia is related to hypothalamic deconnection
Growth hormone	Insulin hypoglycemia (also arginine, ornithine, L-dopa, GHRH)	Increase	No change in case of somatotropic failure
	Oral glucose tolerance test	Decrease	No decrease in case of acromegaly
	TRH	No change	Paradoxical increase in 25% of acromegalic patients
	Somatostatin analogue	Decrease	Variable response in acromegalic patients (predicts treatment response)
LH, FSH, free α-subunit	LHRH	Increase	Increase (in the presence or not of gonadotropic failure)
	TRH	No change	Paradoxical increase in 30–60% of gonadotropin-secreting adenomas
TSH	TRH	Increase	Increase (in the presence or not of thyrotropic failure); sometimes amplified and/or delayed response in case of thyrotropic failure of hypothalamic origin
ACTH	Metyrapone	Increase (together with 11-deoxycortisol)	No change in case of corticotropic failure; exaggerated response in Cushing's disease
	CRH (or insulin-induced hypoglycemia)	Increase	No change in case of corticotropic failure; exaggerated response in Cushing's disease
	Dexamethasone	Decrease	Low dose: no change in Cushing's disease; high-dose: decrease (incomplete) in Cushing's disease

PRL = prolactin; TRH = thyrotropin-releasing hormone; MCP = metoclopramide; GHRH = growth hormone–releasing hormone; LHRH = luteinizing hormone–releasing hormone; ACTH = adrenocorticotropic hormone; CRH = corticotropin-releasing hormone.

viewed by light microscopy. The four commonly recognized types include chromophobe adenomas, assumed to be endocrinologically inactive; acidophilic (eosinophilic) adenomas, primarily associated with acromegaly; basophilic adenomas, associated with Cushing's disease; and mixed types.

The use of electron microscopy and specific immunohistochemical techniques reveal the limitations of conventional histopathology.[124, 125, 155] Essentially all pituitary cells (except the follicular cells) have identifiable granules, including those considered to be chromophobic by classic techniques. Cells with a paucity of granules may, in fact, be secreting hormones so rapidly that accumulation is not observed, or alternatively, may be cells in a relative resting state. The classic types of adenomas and hormones produced are summarized in Table 26–10. The demonstration of hormone-specific granules in tumor cells may not correlate to a clinical endocrinologic syndrome (such adenomas are called silent adenomas of the somatotropic, corticotropic, or gonadotropic types according to their immunocytochemical characteristics). Thus, the classification most commonly used is based on the secretory characteristics of the cells. Such a classification with associated tumor prevalence in over 3000 surgically resected pituitary tumors studied by Kovacs and Horvath's group appears in Table 26–10.

TABLE 26–9. **Imaging Modalities for Evaluating Pituitary Tumors**

Method	Diagnosis and Staging Capability
CT	Provides substantial three-dimensional information on tumor size and extension
MRI	Indicates tumor definition while increasing the capability of delineating intraglandular pathology
Radiograph	Demonstrate gross enlargement of the sella turcica with a rounded, ballooned configuration or concavity of the anterior sellar wall
Inferior petrosal sinus catheterization with simultaneous bilateral sampling of corticotropin	Useful, in difficult cases, to confirm pituitary source of corticotropin secretion and establish site of adenoma

Staging

Because of the correlation of tumor growth characteristics and size with outcome, anatomic staging systems are also used in conjunction with the endocrinologic classifications. Pituitary tumors are defined as invasive on the basis of sphenoid sinus invasion on CT or cavernous sinus invasion on MRI, and they can be graded using criteria modified from Hardy's classification (initially based on the extent of expansion and erosion of the sella on plain radiographs and sellar polytomograms).[156] In this modified classification (Table 26–11), grade 2 tumors are macroadenomas ($\geq$10 mm) with or without suprasellar extension and grade 1 tumors are microadenomas ($<$10 mm). Grades 3 and 4 are considered invasive. Patients with tumors with extrasellar extension are further subclassified.

Staging Work-Up

Light microscopy shows small cells with large, round nuclei and scant cytoplasm lacking fibrils. Useful stains in-

TABLE 26–10. **Functional Classification of Pituitary Tumors by Means of Immunocytochemistry and Electron Microscope**

Type	Secretory Granules	Respective Prevalence (%)
Growth hormone (GH) adenomas		
Densely granulated GH adenomas	Dense 400–500 nm	8
Sparsely granulated GH adenomas	Dense 100–250 nm	9
Prolactin (PRL) adenomas		
Densely granulated PRL adenomas	Dense 200–1200 nm	0.5
Sparsely granulated PRL adenomas	Dense 150–300 nm	30
GH and PRL adenomas		
Mixed GH-PRL adenomas		4.5
Acidophil stem cell adenomas	Dense 150–200 nm	3.5
Mammosomatotroph adenomas	Dense 400–1200 nm	1.5
Corticotroph adenomas		
Densely granulated ACTH adenomas	Dense 150–450 nm	8
Sparsely granulated ACTH adenomas	Scanty 200–250 nm	<0.5
Silent corticotroph adenomas (3 subtypes)		6
Glycoprotein hormone–producing adenomas		
Gonadotroph adenomas	Dense 150–200 nm	2.5
TSH adenomas	Dense 150–250 nm	<1.0
Other		
Null cell adenomas	(halo) 150–250 nm	17
Oncocytomas	150–250 nm	6
Unclassified plurihormonal adenomas		2.5

Adapted from Singer PA, Cooper DS, Daniels GH, et al: Treatment guidelines for patients with thyroid nodules and well-differentiated thyroid cancer. Arch Intern Med 1996; 156:2165 and Mazzaferri EL, Jhiang SM: Long-term impact of initial surgical and medical therapy on papillary and follicular thyroid cancer. Am J Med 1994; 97:418.

clude Herlant's tetrachrome and periodic acid–Schiff–orange G. Electron microscopy demonstrates angulated polyhedral cells with granules that can be quantified by size. Fluorescent-labeled antibodies to the peptide hormones are used in the identification of endocrinologic types (see Table 26–10).

Clinical Classification

From a practical point of view, and for simplifying the therapeutic indications, a clinical classification based on the presence or absence of a clinical syndrome in relation to hypersecretion is employed. Generally, this clinical classification overlaps the histopathologic classification:

- *Growth hormone (GH)–secreting adenomas* are responsible for acromegaly. They may be purely GH-secreting adenomas or mixed adenomas (GH-PRL, GH-α-subunit) at the immunocytochemical level.
- *Prolactin (PRL)-secreting adenomas* are responsible for hyperprolactinemia. Immunocytochemically, they can be composed of pure PRL-secreting adenomatous cells or mixed (PRL-GH, PRL-α-subunit) cells.
- *Corticotropin-secreting adenomas* are associated with Cushing's syndrome (when Cushing's syndrome is the result of a pituitary microadenoma, the condition is called Cushing's disease). In immunocytochemistry, adenomatous cells stain for ACTH either alone or in association with other peptides.
- *TSH-secreting pituitary adenomas* are responsible for thyrotoxicosis and inappropriate secretion of TSH. TSH immunostaining may be isolated or associated with α-subunit GH, and PRL.
- *Clinically nonfunctioning pituitary adenoma* (NFPA) is the preferred term for designating all the pituitary adenomas that are not hormonally active (that is, not associated with one of the above-stated clinical syndromes).

Patients with NFPA have no acromegaly, no hyperprolactinemic syndrome, no Cushing's syndrome, and no hyperthyroidism, and their tumors are generally revealed by tumor mass effect or are discovered incidentally. The term *clinically NFPA* is preferred to that of *chromophobic* adenoma (proposed in the past, before the routine use of immunocytochemical staining) or *nonsecreting adenomas*, because immunocytochemistry demonstrates that the ma-

TABLE 26–11. **Classification of Pituitary Tumors According to Size, Expansion, and Invasiveness**

Grade 0	Normal
Grade I	Sella of normal size but asymmetry of the floor (tumor < 10 mm in diameter)
Grade II	Enlarged sella but with an intact floor (tumor ≥ 10 mm)
Grade III	Localized erosion or destruction of the sellar floor
Grade IV	Diffusely eroded floor
Grade V	Tumor spread via the cerebrospinal fluid or blood
Suprasellar extension	
O	None
A	Tumor occupies the chiasmatic cistern
B	Tumor obliterates recesses of the third ventricle
C	Tumor grossly displaces the third ventricle
Parasellar extension	
D	Intracranial (intradural) extension: anterior fossa = 1; middle fossa = 2; posterior fossa = 3
E	Extension into or beneath the cavernous sinus (extradural)

Modified classification of Hardy J: Transsphenoidal surgery of hypersecreting pituitary tumors. In: Kohler PO, Ross GT (eds): Diagnosis and Treatment of Pituitary Tumors, pp 179–194. Amsterdam, Excerpta Medica, 1973.

jority of these tumors are, in fact, able to secrete at least one of the pituitary hormones but either are not associated with increased plasma levels of the hormone (silent adenoma) or are associated with increased levels of a hormone (e.g., FSH, LH, or free uncombined α-subunit) that does not produce a recognizable clinical hypersecretion syndrome. Whatever the results of immunocytochemical studies of the removed clinically NFPA, the therapeutic management will be, grossly, the same.

Principles of Treatment

Management

Management begins with careful definition of the tumor extent and endocrinologic abnormalities. The principles of therapy are based on these factors and their clinical sequelae.[157–159] Any direct effect of the mass (e.g., visual) must be addressed, and endocrinologic dysfunction must be corrected. Certain deficiencies, particularly corticosteroid, should immediately be corrected. Complications of therapy (most prominently hypopituitarism) and tumor recurrence can be manifested many years (up to 30 years) after therapy, and they must be carefully and continuously considered:

- need for immediate relief of mass effect or endocrinologic abnormalities
- potential for obtaining long-term control
- character and frequency of possible morbidities

Table 26–12 presents a concise summary of recommended therapeutic procedures using a multidisciplinary approach.

Surgery

The role of surgery in the management of pituitary adenomas includes histologic confirmation of the diagnosis; cyst evacuation; decompression of a hemorrhagic tumor, the optic chiasm, or cranial nerves; reduction of obstructive hydrocephalus; complete excision of microadenomas and macroadenomas; and reduction of the tumor bulk of invasive adenomas. Either a subfrontal transcranial or transsphenoidal approach is used (Fig. 26–4 and Table 26–13).[160–167]

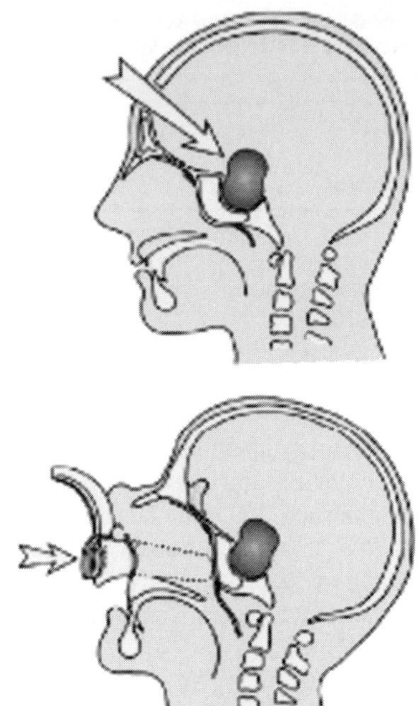

Figure 26–4. Schematic representation of the two surgical approaches used for excision of pituitary adenomas: transfrontal, intracranial route (*top*); transsphenoidal route (*bottom*).

Subfrontal Approach

The subfrontal approach via craniotomy provides added visualization of the tumor and surrounding structures. Indications include suprasellar or lateral tumor extension, dumbbell-shaped lesions, involvement of the chiasm or

TABLE 26–12. **Multidisciplinary Treatment Decisions Based on Tumor Type in Pituitary Adenoma**

Type	Surgery		Chemotherapy		Radiation Therapy
PRL-secreting adenomas					
Microadenoma	TSS	or	DA agonists*		NR
Macroadenoma	**		DA agonists		**
GH-secreting adenomas					
Microadenoma	TSS				
Macroadenoma	TSS	and/or	Somatostatin analogues†	and/or	ART†
ACTH-secreting adenomas					
Microadenoma	TSS		Mitotane‡	and/or	ART‡
Macroadenoma	TSS	and	Mitotane	and	ART
Clinically NFPA					
Microadenoma	TSS				
Macroadenoma	TSS			and	ART§

TSS = transsphenoidal surgery; DA = dopamine; NR = not recommended; ART = adjuvant radiotherapy.
*DA agonists either as first-line therapy or in case of persistent hyperprolactinemia after surgery.
**TSS not recommended as first-line treatment, may be proposed in case of resistance to DA agonists, eventually completed with radiation therapy.
†Somatostatin analogues and/or radiation therapy are proposed when surgery has failed to cure GH hypersecretion.
‡Mitotane alone or in combination with radiation therapy is proposed when surgery has failed to cure Cushing's disease.
§ART is proposed in case of invasive tumoral postoperative remnant.

TABLE 26–13. **Respective Place of Transfrontal and Transsphenoidal Approaches in the Surgical Treatment of Pituitary Adenomas Operated for the First Time According to Large Series**

Authors	Number of Interventions	Transsphenoidal Approach (%)	Transfrontal Approach (%)
Laws and Thapar[161]	2372	2254 (95)	18 (5)
Giovanelli et al[162]	932	882 (95)	48 (5)
Fahlbusch et al[164]	498	479 (96)	19 (4)
Wilson[166]	1010	1000 (99)	10 (1)

cranial nerves by tumor, and invasion of the surrounding vascular structures or pituitary apoplexy. Disadvantages of the subfrontal approach include the high morbidity (seizures, memory loss, increased duration of hospitalization) and mortality that result from damage to vital structures, the substantial incidence of postoperative hypopituitarism, and diabetes insipidus.

Transsphenoidal Technique

The transsphenoidal technique via a sublabial incision involves entry into the facial portion of the sphenoid sinus, thereby gaining access to the pituitary fossa. The binocular surgical microscope is coupled with fluoroscopic monitoring for direct visualization of the surgical field. The transsphenoidal approach offers the capability for tumor destruction by freezing, coagulation, or resection. Indications include removal of tumor confined to the sella turcica, tumors associated with cerebrospinal fluid (CSF) rhinorrhea, pituitary apoplexy, tumors with sphenoidal extension, and tumors with only modest suprasellar extension, or those whose fluid characteristics will allow the suprasellar part of the adenoma to flow down by gravity in the sellar cavity. Contraindications to this approach include dumbbell-shaped tumors with constriction at the diaphragm sellae, massive suprasellar tumors, lateral suprasellar extension, and incompletely pneumatized sphenoids. Morbidities include transient diabetes insipidus and, rarely, meningitis or persistent CSF rhinorrhea (Table 26–14). When selective resection of an adenoma is possible, hypopituitarism is uncommon.

TABLE 26–14. **Mortality and Morbidity of Transsphenoidal Surgery for Pituitary Adenomas**

Complication	Rate (%)
Mortality	0.6
Major complications	2.6
CSF leaks	1–8
Early postoperative hemorrhage	1
Meningitis	<1
Permanent diabetes insipidus	<1
Transient diabetes insipidus	10
New defect in at least one pituitary hormone	20

Adapted from Wartofsky L, Sherman SI, Gopal J, et al: The use of radioactive iodine in patients with papillary and follicular thyroid cancer. J Clin Endocrinol Metab 1998; 83:4195–4203 and Tenenbaum F, Corone C, Schlumberger M, et al: Thyroglobulin measurement and postablative ^{131}I total body scan after total thyroidectomy for differentiated thyroid carcinoma in patients with no evidence of disease. Eur J Cancer 1996; 32A:1262.

Combined Transsphenoidal and Subfrontal Approaches

Because there is a lesser risk of side effects with the transsphenoidal operation compared with the subfrontal approach, transsphenoidal surgery is generally used as a primary operation, and the removal of the tumoral remnant is performed, if necessary, in a second procedure.

Radiation Therapy

Radiation therapy has been proposed extensively in the treatment of pituitary adenomas before the era of transsphenoidal surgery.[168–179] External megavoltage photon therapy is generally used, although proton beams, cobalt gamma-knife radiosurgery, and linear accelerator focal stereotactic technology are all potentially applicable to pituitary adenomas.[178, 180, 181] Implantation of pellets containing radioactive isotopes (e.g., yttrium-90, gold-198) has been completely abandoned.

Indications include:

- primary treatment of intrasellar adenomas (very rarely)
- adjunct to the surgical treatment of tumors with suprasellar extension or of large tumors presenting with mass effects
- adjunct to medical or surgical management of hormone-secreting adenomas in patients with a suboptimal response, or an inability to tolerate medical therapy
- primary therapy in patients whose tumors are inoperable, or for invasive adenomas when surgical excision carries high risks
- primary therapy for selected patients with tumors having limited suprasellar extension

Treatment techniques vary, with the treatment volume tailored to the tumor volume and a minimum dose delivered to adjacent structures. Optimal techniques include bilateral coaxial wedge fields plus a vertex field, moving arc fields, and 360-degree rotational field.[169, 178, 182] The use of bilateral opposed fields is occasionally necessary for large, asymmetric tumors, but it is to be discouraged because of the increased dose delivered to the temporal lobes. Modern radiotherapy simulator facilities, together with current generation CT (or MRI) scanning, allow the fields to be accurately molded around the tumor volume (*conformational* irradiation). The day-to-day reproducibility of the field setup should be within 2.0 mm. Optimum doses are based on evidence that doses under 40 Gy provide a lower probability of tumor control, and doses above 50 Gy, or fractions above 2 Gy per day, are associated with higher complication rates, including injury to the optic nerves or chiasm and hypopituitarism. A dose of 50 Gy plus or minus 5 Gy is recommended. If the adenoma is completely removed with microresiduum and the patient is young, 45 to 50 Gy is advisable, but if there is recurrent tumor, macroresiduum postresection, or suprasellar extension, then a higher dose, 50 to 55 Gy (depending on tumor bulk), is recommended.[169, 178, 182]

Quantitatively, the major problem following pituitary irradiation (particularly when proposed in adjunct to surgery) is the development of partial or panhypopituitarism. Panhypopituitarism develops in about half of patients.[172] Figures are variably quoted for ACTH deficiency (30% to 45%), gonadotropin deficiency (40% to 50%), and TSH deficiency (5% to 20%).[168, 169, 172] The prevalence of deficiencies increases with the duration of follow-up (e.g. 100%, 96%, 84%, and 49% of patients being growth hormone–deficient, gonadotropin-deficient, ACTH-deficient, and TSH-deficient, respectively, after a mean follow-up of 8 years[173]). Hypothalamopituitary dysfunction may take up to 20 years to develop.[177] The exquisite sensitivity of hypothalamus and pituitary to the effects of radiation is better illustrated by the very frequent dysfunction observed in patients irradiated for nasopharyngeal, extracranial or primary brain tumors, even though these tumors are anatomically distinct from the hypothalamic pituitary region.[176] Prolonged and repeated assessment of pituitary functions is thus mandatory after radiation therapy: This assessment allows a precise detection of pituitary deficiencies and adequate replacement therapy. However, it must be emphasized that these side effects of radiation therapy, when precociously diagnosed, are not clinically problematic and are easily medically manageable.

Other disadvantages of this method of treatment include the delay in therapeutic benefit for patients with hormonally active tumors, radiation-induced optic neuropathy or cortical scarring, and the rare occurrence of radiation-induced malignancies (meningiomas, astrocytomas).[174, 183]

Chemotherapy

Increased understanding of the hypothalamic control of pituitary function has led to the development of drugs to modulate pituitary hormone secretion.[145, 184–186]

Dopaminergic Agonists

Bromocriptine effectively reduces elevated serum prolactin levels in most patients with prolactin-secreting pituitary adenomas.[145, 186, 187] Bromocriptine therapy may thus be indicated as primary treatment for microadenomas. Macroadenomas have also been successfully medically managed[145, 157, 188, 189]: bromocriptine not only decreases prolactin levels but is also able to produce a dramatic reduction in tumoral volume. The antitumoral effect of bromocriptine may be very rapid. In the presence of chiasmal compression by the tumor, visual improvement often manifests within the first hours following the initiation of the treatment. Ovulatory and menstrual cycles may resume in 75% to 80% of patients.[145, 157] Patients with macroadenomas who become pregnant are at risk for complications related to tumor growth. For these patients, pregnancy should either be prevented by contraceptive methods or definitive ablative therapy should be performed before pregnancy.[145, 157] Patients with intrasellar microadenomas (or macroadenomas less than 12 mm) are at a risk of greater than 6% for substantial tumor growth and associated complications.[190–192] Bromocriptine should be discontinued when pregnancy is confirmed, although concerns regarding the teratogenicity of bromocriptine have not, to date, been substantiated.[145]

Quinagolide and *cabergoline* are two other dopamine agonists more recently available in the United States and Europe. Quinagolide is not an ergot derivative and is able to bind specifically to dopamine type 2 receptors. It is at least as efficient as bromocriptine[193] and may be useful in rare cases of bromocriptine resistance[194–196] or intolerance.[196] It offers the advantage of being taken once daily. Cabergoline is characterized by its very long duration of action (half-life is approximately 70 hours), allowing a once- or twice-weekly oral administration.[197] Efficacy is at least equal to and tolerance better than that of bromocriptine.[197, 198] In patients with macroprolactinomas, cabergoline also seems effective in reducing prolactin levels and in producing tumoral shrinkage.[199–201] In addition, cabergoline seems able to normalize PRL levels in a significant number of patients resistant to bromocriptine or quinagolide.[200] Bromocriptine and other dopamine agonists are able to improve symptoms of acromegaly in few patients and to decrease GH secretion.[202]

Whereas a number of case reports of *cyproheptadine*-induced remission in Cushing's disease have been described, in the vast majority of patients, no beneficial effect or only a moderate improvement was observed.[203] Because cyproheptadine causes increased appetite, weight gain, and tiredness, it has been largely abandoned in the treatment of Cushing's disease. Thus, chemotherapy in Cushing's disease is limited to the use of compounds directed to the adrenal gland, able to inhibit steroidogenesis, such as mitotane, ketoconazole, metyrapone, etomidate, trilostane, or aminoglutethimide.[143, 203]

Somatostatin (the Hypothalamic GH Release Inhibitory Factor) and Its Analogues

SMS 201–995 (octreotide) and *BIM 23014 (lanreotide)* are able to reduce GH secretion. The native peptide had too short a half-life to be administered easily. Octreotide, given subcutaneously three times daily has been proven to control GH hypersecretion and to decrease tumoral volume in a significant proportion of acromegalic patients, with a few side effects (e.g., cholelithiasis, digestive symptoms).[184, 185, 204–208] The availability of a long-acting form of octreotide allows once-monthly intramuscular injections with the same efficiency.[209] Another somatostatin analogue, lanreotide, also encapsulated in microspheres and allowing a prolonged release, has proven to be effective in lowering GH and insulin-like growth factor I (IGF-I) levels and decreasing tumoral mass of acromegalic patients, in a manner comparable to octreotide[210–213]:

- Octreotide and lanreotide are very effective in reducing TSH levels in patients with TSH-secreting adenomas, thus allowing a high proportion of patients to normalize their plasma thyroid hormone levels.[214, 215]
- Octreotide and lanreotide have no established place in the treatment of Cushing's disease, although a minority of patients may respond with a decrease in ACTH secretion.[203]
- In clinically NFPAs, octreotide has proven to be useful in improving visual defects owing to chiasmal compression in some patients.[216, 217]

Scintigraphy with labeled octreotide (somatostatin receptor scintigraphy) allows visualization of pituitary tumors.[218] The detected images are thought to reflect the importance of somatostatin receptor present at the surface of the tumoral cells. However, scintigraphic results are poor predictors of long-term results of treatment with somatostatin analogues, whatever the type of pituitary adenoma.[219]

Side effects of somatostatin analogues are benign. Digestive problems are minor and most often transitory (abdominal cramps, diarrhea, flatulence). Cholelithiasis occurred in 10% to 55% of patients and varied according to the country where the study was performed, the duration of the study, and the type of analysis.[204, 205, 207, 208] Generally, cholelithiasis is asymptomatic and must be treated conservatively. Despite reduction in insulin secretion due to somatostatin analogues, glucose tolerance alterations are of minor significance.

Treatment Recommendations

(see Table 26–12)

Clinically Nonfunctioning Pituitary Adenomas

- Transsphenoidal surgery with or without postoperative radiation therapy (50 Gy) is performed for almost all patients with a clinically NFPA whether or not they have visual consequences of their tumor.
- Selected patients with small, incidentally discovered microadenomas may be carefully followed without immediate therapy.

GH-Secreting Adenomas

- Transsphenoidal surgery is the first-line therapy except when the macroadenoma is giant or if surgery is contraindicated.
- Postoperative radiation therapy (50 to 55 Gy) is performed for partially resected tumors or when GH levels remain elevated.
- Somatostatin analogues are proposed when surgery is contraindicated or has failed to normalize GH levels, or while waiting for the delayed effects of radiation therapy.

Prolactin-Secreting Adenomas

Selected patients with microadenomas may be carefully followed without treatment if hyperprolactinemia does not have consequences on gonadal function (if regular ovulatory cycles persist).

Patients with microadenomas may be treated surgically with a transsphenoidal operation or medically with dopamine agonists. If a surgical option is chosen, then dopamine agonists may be useful when prolactin levels remain elevated postoperatively. Alternatively, when medical therapy with dopamine agonists is the primary treatment, secondary surgery may be proposed in the case of resistance or intolerance to dopamine agonists. During this time, pregnancy is acceptable, but dopamine agonists are generally interrupted as soon as a pregnancy is confirmed.

In patients with macroadenomas, even in the presence of chiasmatic syndrome, dopamine agonists are now proposed as primary treatment. Indeed, effects on visual disturbances are often very rapid (within a few hours or days), and tumoral shrinkage is usually very significant. Thus, the results provided by dopamine agonists are generally much better than those obtained with surgery, even when performed by a skilled surgeon. However, in the case of visual disturbances, if dopamine agonists are not rapidly effective, surgery is recommended. Postoperatively, if PRL levels remain increased (which is likely the case for macroadenomas, particularly when they are large), dopamine agonists are given.

When pregnancy is planned in patients with macroprolactinomas, one might propose to pursue dopamine agonists during the entire pregnancy. Alternatively, surgery may be decided on before pregnancy for removal of the pituitary adenoma. Thereafter, dopamine agonists are given in case of remaining hyperprolactinemia until the onset of pregnancy; at that time, they are interrupted.

Radiotherapy is now a very rare therapeutic option. It must be limited to rare cases of patients with large, incompletely resected tumors who keep high PRL levels resistant to dopamine agonists.

Corticotropin-Secreting Adenomas

- Primary therapy for children and adults is generally transsphenoidal surgery.
- Radiotherapy (50 Gy) is reserved for patients who are subtotally resected or remain hypersecretory after surgery.
- In waiting for the effects of radiotherapy, adrenal steroidogenesis inhibitors (mitotane) may be indicated.

TSH-Secreting Adenomas

- Primary therapy is transsphenoidal surgery, whatever the size of the tumor.
- Radiation therapy (40 to 50 Gy) is generally proposed when resection is incomplete, particularly when the remnant is invasive.
- Somatostatin analogues are indicated in cases of persistent postoperative hyperthyroidism, while awaiting for the effects of radiotherapy.

Results and Prognosis

Results

Clinically Nonfunctioning Pituitary Adenomas

The strategy of observation only for patients with clinically evident but apparently inactive pituitary adenomas is inap-

TABLE 26–15. **Recurrence Rate According to Therapy in NFPAs**

	Surgical Therapy Alone		Surgery and Radiation Therapy	
Authors	***Total Number***	***Recurrences***	***Total Number***	***Recurrences***
Chun et al[171]	60	9 (15%)	54	4 (7%)
Sheline et al[182]	29	20 (69%)	80	9 (11%)
Ebersold et al[220]	42	5 (12%)	50	9 (18%)
Hayes et al[224]	29	13 (45%)	42	9 (21%)
Ciric et al[225]	32	9 (28%)	67	4 (6%)
Vlahovitch et al[226]	89	14 (16%)	46	4 (8%)
Jaffrain-Rea et al[227]	33	9 (27%)	24	2 (8.8%)
Gittoes et al[229]	63	20 (66%)	63	4 (7%)
Total	**377**	**99 (26%)**	**426**	**45 (11%)**

propriate. Transsphenoidal surgery allows improvement in visual disturbances owing to chiasmal syndrome in 44% to 70% of patients with a clinically NFPA.[149, 220–223]

When NFPAs are gonadotropin-secreting adenomas associated with supranormal levels of gonadotropins or free subunits, surgery reduces supranormal plasma FSH and α-subunit levels and normalizes them in the vast majority of cases.[149] When an NFPA is responsible for pituitary failure, surgery is able to improve pituitary function in 15% to 50% of cases. Alternatively, surgery may aggravate preoperative pituitary deficiency.

After surgery alone, nearly 30% (between 10% and 69%) of patients relapse within 5 to 10 years.[149, 171, 182, 220, 222, 224–229] These variable figures reflect, in part, not only differences in neurosurgical expertise but also progress in imaging techniques used postoperatively to assess the quality of tumoral excision (Table 26–15).

Radiotherapy is proposed either as a systematic adjunct or only if a significant remnant persists. Systematic radiation therapy is supported by the low relapse rate observed (mean, 11%; range, 6% to 21%) when radiation therapy is systematically associated with surgery (see Table 26–15).[149, 171, 177, 182, 220, 224–229] However, irradiation is most always followed by hypopituitarism, and several epidemiologic studies have demonstrated that postradiation hypopituitarism might be associated with a reduction in life expectancy, despite appropriate replacement therapy (see "Prognosis").[230–232]

Somatostatin analogues are able to improve visual problems in 20% to 40% of cases, but reduction in tumoral volume is anecdotal.[216, 217]

GH-Secreting Tumors

Results of the various types of treatment must be analyzed according to stringent criteria that have been reassessed. At the present time, a so-called cure (*good control* is the preferred term) of acromegaly is defined by mean GH levels of less than 2 or 2.5 μg/L and normal insulin-like growth factor I (IGF-I).[141, 233] Indeed, when this goal is achieved, life expectancy of patients with acromegaly seems comparable to that of the general population.[234, 235]

According to stringent criteria as stated above, 42% to 62% of patients can be considered to be cured by transsphenoidal surgery alone (Table 26–16).[141, 163, 236–240] Results depend on the size of the tumor. Surgery is able to cure 60% to 75% and 23% to 48% of patients with microadenomas and macroadenomas, respectively. When the macroadenoma is giant or in the presence of parasellar or sphenoid sinus invasion, the cure rate decreases to 17%

TABLE 26–16. **Results of Transsphenoidal Surgery in Patients with Acromegaly, According to Stringent Criteria of Cure**

Authors	**Type of Adenoma**	**Number**	**GH <2.5 μg/L**	**GH <2.5 μg/L and normal IGF-I**
Derome et al*	Microadenoma	44		38 (86%)
	Macroadenoma	96		44 (46%)
	Total	140		82 (59%)
Fahlbusch et al[163]	Microadenoma	74	53 (72%)	
	Macroadenoma	170	73 (43%)	
	Total	224	126 (56%)	
Roelfsema et al[236]	Microadenoma	9	6 (66%)	
	Macroadenoma	51	31 (60%)	
	Total	60	37 (62%)	
Sheaves et al[237]	Microadenomas	44	27 (61%)	
	Macroadenomas	56	15 (26%)	
	Total	100	42 (42%)	
Yamada et al[238]	Total	61		34 (56%)
Colao et al[239, 240]	Total	86		37 (62%)

IGF-I = insulin-like growth factor I.
*Personal communication.

TABLE 26–17. **Success Rate of Radiation Therapy in Acromegaly, Using Different Criteria of Cure**

Authors	Number	GH <10 μg/L	GH <5 μg/L	GH <2.5 μg/L and normal IGF-I
Lamberg et al (1976)[243]	31		50%	
Feek et al (1984)[244]	48	62%	42%	
Kliman et al (1986)[245]	435	78%	44%	
Speirs et al (1990)[246]	17		46%	
Eastman et al (1992)[175]	87	92%	80%	
Barkan et al (1997)[179]	38		65%	5%
Chanson (1997)[247]	34		71%	38%

IGF-I = insulin-like growth factor I.

and 40%, respectively.[163] The success rate of surgery in patients with acromegaly also varies according to preoperative GH levels: about 70%, 43% to 55%, and 18% to 40% when GH levels are less than 10, between 10 and 50, and above 50 μg/L, respectively.[163, 237] Relapse rate after surgical cure (using stringent criteria, i.e., GH levels less than 2 or 2.5 μg/L) is less than 3%.[236, 237, 241, 242]

Radiation therapy is able to decrease GH levels in a large proportion of patients. A mean plasma GH level less than 5 μg/L is obtained in about 50% of patients (40% to 80%, according to the length of follow-up of each study),[175, 179, 243–247] and when more stringent criteria for a cure are applied, radiation therapy leads to a cure of the disease in 5% to 38% of the cases after a median follow-up of about 7 years (Table 26–17).[179, 247] However, the irradiation is almost always followed by hypopituitarism, and its effects on GH hypersecretion are delayed for many years.

Bromocriptine or other dopaminergic agonists produce improvement in clinical symptoms of acromegaly in 50% of patients and substantially decrease GH levels in some patients, but they rarely normalize GH and IGF-I levels (less than 10% of cases).[202]

Treatment with somatostatin analogue has now gained wide acceptance in the treatment of acromegaly. GH levels are decreased in 50% to 80% of patients treated with octreotide subcutaneously three times daily.[141, 204–208, 248] Up to 50% of patients with acromegaly may be considered to be cured (GH plasma levels less than 2 μg/L [20% to 30%] or normal IGF-I level [20% to 60%]) with this treatment (Table 26–18). Similar results are obtained with 30 mg of lanreotide administered intramuscularly every 10 or 14 days (GH plasma levels less than 2 μg/L [30% to 70%] or normal IGF-I level [40% to 70%]),[210–213] or with octreotide long-acting release (LAR), which may be administered every month at the dose of 20 to 30 mg (GH plasma levels less than 2 μg/L [50% to 60%] or normal IGF-I level [60% to 90%] (see Table 26–18).[209, 249–251] Such variation in the figures obtained from one study to another is probably explained by the variation in the method of IGF-I assay

TABLE 26–18. **Effects of Various Somatostatin Analogues (Octreotide and Lanreotide) with Various Modes of Preparation and Administration in Large Series of Patients with Acromegaly, Treated Long-Term According to Different Criteria of Cure**

Authors	Number	Type of Treatment (Dosage)	% of Patients with GH <5 μg/L	% of Patients with GH <2.5 μg/L and/or Normal IGF-I	% of Patients with More Than 20% Reduction in Tumoral Volume
Sassolas et al (1990)[204]	58	octreotide SC (300–1500 μg/d)	43	29 (GH)	47
Vance and Harris (1991)[205]	189	octreotide SC (50–500 μg/d)	45	46 (IGF-I)	44
Ezzat et al (1992)[206]	115	octreotide SC (300–750 μg/d)	51	18 (GH) 61 (IGF-I)	28
Arosio et al (1995)[248]	68	octreotide SC (300–600 μg/d)		20 (IGF-I)	27
Morange et al (1994)[211]	19	lanreotide PR IM (30 mg q10–14 days)	89	68 (IGF-I)	
Giusti et al (1996)[212]	57	lanreotide PR IM (30 mg q10–14 days)	85	76 (GH) 38 (IGF-I)	17
Caron et al (1997)[213]	22	lanreotide PR IM (30 mg q10–14 days)	68	27 (GH) 63 (IGF-I)	13
Stewart et al (1995)[249]	8	octreotide LAR IM (20–40 mg q28–42 days)	100	63 (GH) 88 (IGF-I)	43
Lancranjan et al (1996)[250]	101	octreotide LAR IM (20–40 mg q28 days)	94	54 (GH) 65 (IGF-I)	72
Fløgstad et al (1997)[251]	14	octreotide LAR IM (20–40 mg q28 days)	86	64 (GH) 64 (IGF-I)	29

q = every; IM = intramuscularly; SC = subcutaneously; PR = prolonged release; LAR = long-acting release.

and by the differences in the inclusion criteria for each study. Indeed, in some of the studies assessing the efficiency of the long-acting forms of somatostatin analogue, patients were included if they were previously demonstrated to be responsive to subcutaneous octreotide, whereas in others, patients were entered blindly, without knowing whether they were responsive to octreotide.

A small reduction in tumor volume (in general at the level of the suprasellar expansion) may be observed in 15% to 70% of patients with acromegaly (see Table 26–18).[141, 204–209, 211–213, 248–251]

PRL-Secreting Adenomas

Transsphenoidal resection of microprolactinomas allows normalization of PRL levels in 71.2% of patients, according to a compilation of various studies on a total of 1224 patients performed by Mollitch.[145] Cure rates vary according to preoperative PRL level. When the PRL level is above 200 μg/L, the cure rate decreases to 13%. Up to 88% of women desiring conception conceived within 1 year.[145, 252] The recurrence rate after surgical success was initially thought to be as high as 50%; in fact, more recent series give a recurrence rate ranging between 5% and 18% after a 10-year follow-up.[145, 252, 253] However, even if hyperprolactinemia relapses, it remains generally mild, without any clinical consequences. Finally, 10 years after surgery, 55% to 73% of patients have normal PRL levels and 75% have normal menstrual cycles.[252–254]

The success rate of transsphenoidal surgery in macroprolactinomas is much lower. According to a compilation of various reported series concerning 1256 patients, the mean cure rate is 31.8%.[145] Moreover, after initial cure, 18% of patients relapse. Surgical results are proportional to the preoperative size of the tumor and to the level of PRL. When the adenoma is larger than 20 mm and PRL levels are higher than 200 μg/L, the cure rate is lower than 15%.[145]

Dopamine agonists are able to decrease PRL levels in 73% to 95% of patients and produce a decrease in tumor volume in 77% of patients with a macroprolactinoma.[145, 188, 189, 193, 199, 201] This tumoral shrinkage may be dramatic (more than 50% of initial volume in half of the patients) (Fig. 26–5). Treatment with dopamine agonists may need to be prolonged. Indeed, after treatment withdrawal, a tumor generally returns to its original size, often within days to weeks, and PRL levels increase.

In patients resistant to bromocriptine, other dopamine agonists, such as quinagolide or cabergoline, may be an interesting alternative because they allow normalization of PRL levels in 16% to 20% and in 80% of cases, respectively.[194–196, 200] In the case of intolerance to bromocriptine, PRL may be normalized by quinagolide in 58% of patients.[196] Tolerance of cabergoline also proved to be better than that of bromocriptine, thus allowing a larger dose to be used in case of incomplete response.[197–201]

Radiation therapy, which is only indicated in rare cases of surgical failure associated with dopamine agonists, intolerance, or resistance, requires time to be effective.[145, 169, 255, 256] Three to 4 years after radiation therapy, 20% to 30% of patients have normalized PRL levels, and after 8 years, the normalization rate climbs to only half of patients.[257]

TSH-Secreting Adenomas

Forty percent of patients with TSH-secreting adenomas are not cured by surgery, and they maintain increased thyroid hormone levels responsible for thyrotoxicosis.[147]

Octreotide, the somatostatin analogue, is able to reduce TSH and free α-subunit levels in 91% of patients, and it allows normalization of thyroid hormone levels in 73% of patients.[214] Reduction in tumoral volume is similar to that obtained in patients with acromegaly who are treated with octreotide. Lanreotide has very similar effects.[215]

Cushing's Disease

When surgery is performed by skilled neurosurgeons, the cure rate of transsphenoidal surgery is 70% to 80%[144, 203, 258–268] in the case of microadenomas. The criteria for a cure should be an undetectable plasma cortisol concentration in the morning and a plasma ACTH concentration of less than 5 pg/mL 4 to 7 days after surgery.[144] Less strict criteria result in higher rates of apparent cure but higher rates of recurrence as well (Table 26–19). The recurrence rate of the disease is more frequent than was previously thought,

TABLE 26–19. **Results of Transsphenoidal Surgery for Cushing's Disease, According to Studies Published 1988 to 1995**

Authors	Success Rate	Recurrences	Mean Follow-Up (mos)
Guilhaume et al (1988)[258]	42/61 (69%)	6/42 (14.3%)	24
Mampalam et al (1988)[259]	171/216 (79%)	9/171 (5.3%)	46
Arnott et al (1990)[260]	24/28 (85%)	3/24 (12.5%)	22
Burke et al (1990)[261]	44/54 (81%)	2/44 (4.5%)	56
Post and Habas (1990)[262]	29/37 (78%)	1/29 (3.4%)	NA
Tindall et al (1990)[263]	46/53 (86%)	1/46 (2.1%)	57
Robert and Hardy (1991)[264]	60/78 (77%)	5/60 (8.3%)	77
Tahir and Sheeler (1992)[265]	34/45 (75%)	7/34 (20.6%)	69
Trainer et al (1993)[266]	39/48 (81%)	3/39 (7.7%)	NA
Ram et al (1994)[267]	205/222 (92%)	NA	NA
Bochicchio et al (1995)[268]	510/668 (76%)	65/510 (12.7%)	46

NA = not available.

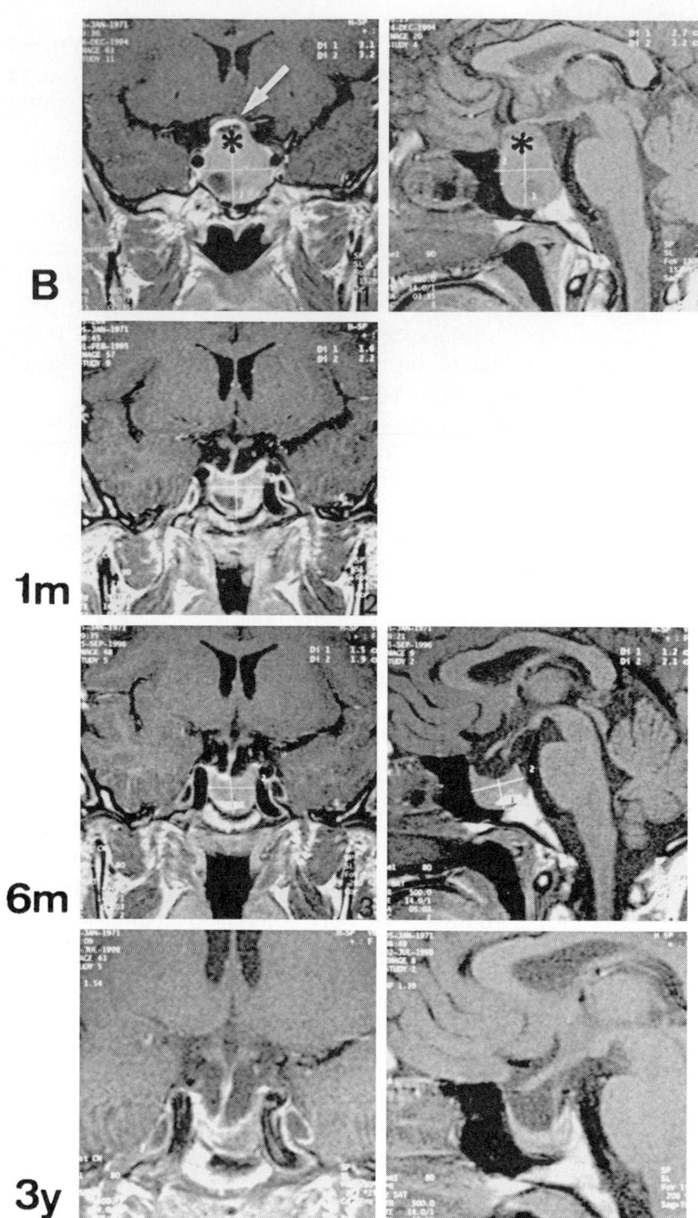

Figure 26–5. Dramatic shrinkage of a macroprolactinoma with suprasellar extension (*) compressing the optic chiasm (*white arrow*) in a young male patient treated with the new dopamine agonist, cabergoline (B = before treatment; 1m = after 1 month of treatment; 6m = after 6 months; 3y = after 3 years). Coronal (*left panels*) and sagittal (*right panels*) views on MRI.

and it shows a progressive upward trend with time.[258] In a series of studies from 1988 to 1995, the recurrence rate is approximately 10% to 20% (see Table 26–19). Only 50% of patients with macroadenomas achieve remission after initial pituitary microsurgery.

In children, the rate of cure following transsphenoidal surgery is 70% to 86%,[241, 259, 269–271] even reaching 97% for one team.[272] However, as in adults, owing to extended follow-up and more stringent criteria used, figures will probably be less optimistic, approaching 50% to 75%.[270, 271]

Pituitary irradiation, in the case of surgical failure, is seen to produce remission in 56%[273] to 83%[274] of patients with Cushing's disease after a median follow-up of about 3 years. Primary radiotherapy in Cushing's disease is effective in 50% to 60% of adults, and 85% of children.[143, 167, 178, 203] During the months or years required to achieve maximal benefits from irradiation, hypercortisolism is easily controlled with adrenal enzyme inhibitors (mitotane).[143]

Prognosis

Prognosis depends on the type of tumor and a combination of other factors, including:

- severity of the endocrinologic disturbance or mass-related symptoms and signs (the size and the extent of the tumor [as reflected in the staging systems] are also correlated to the outcome [see "Results"])
- success of therapy in reversing these abnormalities
- morbidities due to therapy
- permanency of the therapeutic response

Although pituitary tumors are generally benign, the failure to provide adequate therapy can lead to severe func-

TABLE 26–20. **Epidemiologic Studies Demonstrating an Increased Mortality in Patients with Hypopituitarism**

Authors	Number	SMR (95% confidence interval)			SMR from Total Cardiac and Vascular Causes			SMR from Cerebrovascular Causes			SMR from Malignancy
		Total	***Male***	***Female***	***Total***	***Male***	***Female***	***Total***	***Male***	***Female***	***Total***
Rosen et al (1990)[230]	333	1.81*	1.46	2.82	1.94*	1.70	2.70				0.49*
Bates et al (1996)[231]	172	1.73 (1.28–2.28)*	1.50 (1.02–2.13)*	2.29 (1.37–3.58)*	1.35 (0.84–2.07) ns	1.32 (0.94–2.17) ns	1.46 (0.50–3.20) ns				1.41 (0.73–2.47) ns
Bülow et al (1997)[232]	344	2.17 (1.88–2.51)*	1.91 (1.59–2.28)*	2.93 (2.28–3.75)*	1.75 (1.40–2.19)*	1.54 (1.16–2.03)*	2.39 (1.60–3.52)*	3.39 (2.27–4.99)*	2.64 (1.44–4.42)*	4.91 (2.62–8.40)*	1.71 (1.21–2.37)*

SMR = standardized mortality ratio, calculated by dividing observed mortality by expected mortality in an age- and sex-matched control population; when available, 95% confidence interval is given; ns = not statistically significant; * = statistically significant.

tional deficits and death. Optimal therapy can vastly improve quality and duration of life. When untreated, patients with acromegaly have a 10-year life expectancy reduction, particularly because of cardiovascular and respiratory problems and the increased risk of neoplasms. Standardized mortality ratio (SMR) (observed-to-expected mortality in a sex- and age-matched control population) is 2.63 (95% confidence interval [CI], 1.8 to 3.9) in a 1993 series.[234] The most important predictive factor of mortality is the so-called final post-therapeutic GH level.[234, 235] When the final GH level is less than 2.5 μg/L, the SMR is 1.42 (95% CI, 0.46 to 3.31), which is not significantly different from that of the general population. However, if the final GH level is between 2.5 and 5 μg/L, then the SMR is 2.01 (95% CI, 0.9 to 3.8), which is statistically different from the general population. This indicates that the more stringent criteria applied to define cure or successful outcome in acromegaly at present (GH levels less than 2.5 μg/L) are probably associated with better survival than those used in the past.

Incidence of mortality in patients with Cushing's disease is higher than that expected for the control population (SMR 3.8; 95% CI, 2.5 to 17.9). The first cause of death is vascular disease. Higher age, persistence of hypertension, and abnormalities in glucose metabolism after treatment are independent predictors of mortality.[275]

Hypopituitarism, particularly following surgery or radiation therapy for pituitary adenomas, is also associated with an increase in mortality (SMR, 1.70 to 2.10), according to concordant results of three studies,[230–232] and is mainly because of an increase in cardiovascular deaths for some studies[230, 232] but not for others (Table 26–20).[231] GH deficiency is cited as a potential cause of the increased incidence of mortality in these patients because they were supposed to be adequately replaced by other pituitary hormones, but they did not receive GH replacement therapy. However, this assertion remains highly questionable because the presence of a GH deficiency was not assessed in all the patients of these studies and there was evidence of long-term lack or inadequacy of substitution for other pituitary hormones in many of the patients. It is presently unknown if a substitutive therapy with GH, as recommended by some investigators,[276] would improve the prognosis of hypopituitary adults.

One might re-emphasize the importance of assessing regularly, during many years (up to 30 years after radiation therapy), the pituitary function of patients treated for pituitary adenomas, in order to provide an adequate replacement therapy, as soon as possible, in hypopituitary patients.

Summary

The management of pituitary adenomas is presently well defined.[277] Diagnostic challenges are rare, except in the case of Cushing's disease, in which occult ectopic ACTH-secreting tumors (often bronchial carcinoids) may mimic Cushing's disease resulting from a nonvisible, corticotropic microadenoma. It is unlikely that improvement in imaging techniques will allow better definition of microadenomas in this setting. Bilateral inferior petrosal sinus catheterization generally solves the issue. Early recognition of pathologies such as acromegaly, which is responsible for important morbidity and cosmetic consequences, also needs to be improved. Progress in imaging techniques has greatly ameliorated the quality of diagnosis, but the improvement in technique also has led to an increasing frequency of incidental images. The management of such pituitary incidentalomas, in terms of cost and benefits, needs to be determined more precisely.

Surgical resection by transsphenoidal route has very low morbidity and mortality rates. In skilled hands, it allows a complete cure of the disease in many cases. Surgical progress thus may apply to invasive tumors in order to obtain a better removal. It is presently unknown if endoscopic techniques, the use of intraoperative MRI, or intraoperative computer-assisted neuronavigation with robots would improve the outcome.

Histopathologic techniques (and particularly immunocytochemistry) have greatly ameliorated the classification of nonfunctioning pituitary adenomas, demonstrating that the majority of them were gonadotropin-secreting adenomas. Markers of invasiveness and aggressiveness, routinely applicable on tumor specimens removed at surgery, are lacking. Prospective studies of molecular genetic alterations demonstrated on pituitary adenomas will determine whether these markers are truly predictive of subsequent behavior and can be used to aid clinical management in a manner not possible when current histologic criteria are used. This may help, in particular, to decide which patients need systematic, postoperative radiation therapy.

Although our understanding of the molecular and biochemical changes associated with pituitary tumor initiation and progression has significantly increased in recent years, the pathogenesis of pituitary adenomas remains largely unknown. Progress is thus expected in this field in order to improve the understanding of the pathogenesis of these very peculiar benign tumors, which become malignant in exceedingly rare cases.

Adrenocortical Carcinoma

Epidemiology and Etiology

Epidemiology

Adrenocortical carcinoma (ACC) is a rare tumor with a poor prognosis. Its annual incidence is 0.6 to 1.67 cases per 10^6 population.[278] It occurs at all ages and is more frequent in those older than the age of 45. Tumors producing clinical syndromes are more frequent in women, the most usual presentation being Cushing's or virilizing syndromes, seen either singly or in association. Conversely, non–syndrome-producing tumors occur more frequently in men.[279–294] In recent years, incidental findings of ACC have increased with the more frequent use of ultrasound, CT scan, or MRI of the abdomen. This may change both the clinical picture and the epidemiology of this tumor. Bilaterality has been reported in 2% to 10% of cases.

Etiology

No etiologic factors have been elicited for ACCs. In children, ACC is uncommon and often manifested by a virilizing syndrome, although it occasionally occurs in the context of a tumor-predisposing syndrome such as Beckwith-Wiedemann or Li-Fraumeni.[285, 286] Also, adrenal tumors have been reported to occur with an increased frequency in patients with Carney's complex or multiple endocrine neoplasia type 1. Reports from Europe and throughout the United States do not suggest any particular geographic, racial, or climatic distribution. Carcinoma development in longstanding suppressible adrenal hyperplasia has been reported. Some tumors may be sensitive to endogenous corticotropin and, therefore, are analogous to TSH-sensitive thyroid cancer.

Detection and Diagnosis

Clinical Detection

Clinical Presentation

Frequently, local extension causes pain, hemorrhage, distention, and a large, palpable abdominal mass. Weight loss, fatigue, anorexia, fever, and sweating are common, as in any advanced malignancy. ACC tends to invade the veins locally, producing thrombosis and occlusion. Embolic complications are common.

Metastatic lesions can erupt in any organ, causing symptoms. Metastases to both deep and superficial lymph nodes can appear as silent lymphadenopathy on a chest film or be detected during a physical examination. Lungs and liver are the most common sites of distant spread, and they occur in the course of most patients affected. Bone metastases are less frequent and can be lytic or blastic.[279–285, 287, 288]

Hormonal Pattern

ACCs can produce large amounts of steroid hormones; approximately half of all ACCs produce mainly hormonal precursors with low bioactivity,[280] and they may be nonfunctioning. The following terminology may help to classify ACCs according to their hormonal pattern:

- *Nonfunctioning:* Steroid production is normal and emanates from normal adrenal residue.
- *Functioning:* Steroid production is increased but no clinical syndrome is produced. These ACCs produce mainly hormonal precursors with low bioactivity.
- *Syndrome producing:* Steroid production is increased and there is a clinical endocrine syndrome. Cushing's syndrome is the most frequently associated endocrine syndrome in adults, and is observed in half of ACC patients. It is either isolated or appears in association with virilizing features. Virilization is frequent in women and children; pure feminization in men and hyperaldosteronism are rare. One particular pattern often predominates, but mixed syndromes are common.

Inappropriate production of polypeptide hormones has been reported in rare cases, for example, IGF and calcitonin.

Adrenal Incidentaloma

Commonly, small adrenocortical tumors are discovered in the context of an imaging procedure, such as ultrasound, CT scan, or MRI, which happens to be performed for an unrelated reason. Studies show that 0.4% to 4.4% of abdominal CT scans performed for other indications will incidentally identify an adrenal mass. The frequency of adrenal masses increases with the age of the patient, and the discovery of adrenal incidentalomas is likely to increase as imaging technology is able to resolve smaller masses (the prevalence of these masses at autopsy is 1.4% to 8.9%[288–291]).

Over 80% of incidentally discovered adrenal masses are nonsecreting adenomas. Hormone-secreting cortical adenomas (mainly producing aldosterone) and pheochromocytomas each have a calculated frequency of 7.0%; ACC is found in less than 1% of these tumors.

The evaluation of adrenal incidentalomas, by taking into account their sizes and patterns of hormonal production, allows selection of the minority of patients for operations. Diabetes, obesity, and hypertension are sought. The minimal laboratory work-up should include:

- *serum electrolytes* during normal salt diet
- *serum cortisol* (A.M. and P.M.) with a 1-mg, overnight dexamethasone suppression test
- 24-hour urinary excretion of *free cortisol*
- 24-hour urinary excretion of *metanephrines*

Other diagnostic testing should be performed as indicated clinically. An accurate measurement of tumor size should be obtained from CT scan or MRI. Hormone-secreting adrenal tumors and hormonally silent adrenal masses with a diameter of 5 cm or more, or smaller masses with a suspicious imaging appearance should be excised. Nonoperated tumors should be followed at regular intervals with ultrasound, CT scan, or MRI: 3 months later, then every 6 months for 2 years, and then annually. An increase in the size of the tumor dictates surgery.

Diagnostic Procedures

Imaging Procedures

The diagnosis of adrenal neoplasms depends on the identification of an adrenal mass on CT scan, MRI, or both. The presence of a large unilateral adrenal mass with irregular borders is virtually diagnostic of adrenal cancer.

- A *CT scan* provides information about size, homogeneity, presence of calcifications, areas of necrosis, and extent of local invasion, thus aiding in decision making about the resectability of the lesion. A Hounsfield attenuation of 10 or less with a uniform distribution throughout the mass on an unenhanced CT represents an adrenal adenoma in virtually all cases.[290, 291]

- *MRI* can distinguish, with a fair degree of accuracy, various adrenal tumors by comparing the ratio of signal intensity on T2-weighted images of each adrenal mass with that of liver: nonfunctional adenomas have a low signal intensity; ACCs have an intermediate to high signal intensity; and pheochromocytomas have an extremely high signal intensity.[290, 291]
- Other imaging modalities are rarely indicated: iodocholesterol scanning usually gives a negative result in malignant ACCs and a positive result in steroid-secreting adenomas.[292] Inferior vena cava venography may be indicated if CT or MRI findings suggest the presence of a tumor thrombus.

Laboratory Studies

Several laboratory studies are useful in the establishment or confirmation of excessive steroid secretion and the monitoring of patients with adrenocortical neoplasms. These include:

- *glucocorticosteroids:* A.M. and P.M. serum cortisol with a 1-mg, overnight dexamethasone suppression test and precursors 17-hydroxyprogesterone and 11-deoxycortisol. Hypercorticolism is best established by measuring 24-hour urinary excretion of free cortisol; more subtle evidence of cortisol excess, as detected by loss of diurnal variation in cortisol production, lack of suppression with an overnight dexamethasone suppression test, and low levels of ACTH, can be recognized.
- *androgens:* testosterone that can be produced by ACC, dehydroepiandrosterone sulfate, and 4-androstenedione
- *estrogens:* estradiol that can be produced by ACC
- *mineralocorticosteroids:* aldosterone, 11-deoxycorticosterone, corticosterone, and renin
- *minimal steroid determinations:* Preoperatively, assessment should be made of autonomous cortisol production that could lead to suppression of the contralateral adrenal gland. Patients with cortisol overproduction should receive cortisol substitution postoperatively to avoid adrenal insufficiency. Other measurements are guided by the clinical presentation.

Classification and Staging

Histopathology

Grossly, ACCs are characteristically large, bulky tumors whose cut surfaces are yellow, frequently hemorrhagic, cystic, and necrotic. They are partly encapsulated. Pleomorphism, multinucleated and nucleoli cells, and spindle shapes compose the usual picture.

The diagnosis of malignancy can be difficult among primary adrenal tumors. A number of histologic characteristics and hormonal tests have been used to differentiate adenomas from carcinomas. In the absence of distant metastasis or regional spread, no single finding can absolutely resolve this issue, but several features may be useful:

- the large size of malignant tumors, with a tumor weight above 100 g being usually indicative of malignancy
- the combination of histologic features such as high mitotic rate, atypical mitoses, high nuclear grade, low percentage of clear cells, necrosis, diffuse architecture of the tumor, and capsular or vascular invasion [293, 294]; among them, mitotic rate is strongly associated with patient outcome
- the increased production of steroid precursors or androgens
- a dysfunction of the aldosterone pathway with hypoaldosteronism, and normal or increased levels of aldosterone precursors
- the absence of expression of the class II major histocompatibility complex antigens
- the evaluation of molecular abnormalities of the 11p15 region (paternal isodisomy and IGF-II overexpression)[295, 296]

In the case of a nonfunctioning tumor, diagnosis may be difficult with either a primary neuroendocrine tumor of the adrenal or an adrenal metastasis, because some ACCs may express neuroendocrine features.[297, 298]

In the case of a nonfunctioning tumor with involvement of both the adrenal and other sites, such as the lungs, the question of the primary tumor may arise. In fact, metastases to the adrenals are frequent, being observed in 9% of all malignant tumors, particularly in patients with breast and bronchial carcinoma, whereas nonfunctioning metastatic ACCs are rare. In these patients, a complete work-up is mandatory before any invasive procedure or treatment. Immunohistochemistry may help to differentiate ACC from an adrenal metastasis or a renal carcinoma.[297]

In the majority of patients with a history of nonadrenal cancer, masses that are 3 cm in size or larger represent metastases. If the presence of cancer in the adrenal gland would alter the patient's oncologic management, a fine-needle aspiration should be considered: cytology can provide a diagnosis in most cases regarding metastatic cancer, but it is less helpful in differentiating a nodule containing an adenoma from a localized adrenal carcinoma.

Staging

Patients are staged according to MacFarlane's classification, modified by Icard and colleagues[281, 299]: a stage I tumor is smaller than 5 cm in diameter, whereas a stage II tumor is larger than 5 cm. Neither has nodes, local invasion, or metastases, and these two stages define a local cancer. A stage III tumor has nodes, local invasion without distant metastases, or both, and it defines a locoregional cancer. A stage IV tumor has distant metastases (Table 26–21).

Principles of Treatment

Surgery

A complete adrenalectomy is the minimal surgical procedure for local cancer. Systematic nephrectomy does not improve survival time in patients with local cancer. An associated regional cellular lymphadenectomy is performed

TABLE 26–21. **Clinical Staging System for Carcinoma of the Adrenal Cortex**

Stage	Grouping	Descriptor
I	T1, M0, R0, D1	T1: Tumor <5 cm and confined to adrenal gland M0: No demonstrable metastases R0: Tumor completely excised D1: Differentiated, no capsular or vascular invasion
II	T2, M0, R1, D2	T2: Tumor >5 cm but <10 cm, or adherence to kidney R1: Tumor entered at operation D2: Moderately undifferentiated, either capsular or vascular invasion
III	T3, M1, R1, D2	T3: >10 cm, or invasion of surrounding structures including renal vein M1: Metastases-regional lymphatics
IV	T3, M2, R2, D3	M2: Distant metastases (e.g., liver, lung, bone) R2: Tumor tissue remaining after resection D3: Differentiation anaplastic, both capsular and vascular invasion

for locoregional cancer. Resection of tumor thrombus from the vena cava may be performed. Few benefits have been obtained from the primary resection of distant metastases.[281]

Radiation Theapy

Preoperative and postoperative radiation therapy has been used in an attempt to eradicate local extension. However, no beneficial effect has been found. Radiation therapy can be useful in palliation of bone pain from metastasis.

Chemotherapy

Mitotane (o,p′-DDD or 1,1-(o,p′-dichlorodiphenyl)-2,2-dichloroethane) controls endocrine hypersecretion in 60% to 75% of patients with ACC. It provides an objective tumor response rate of 14% to 38% (mean, 23%). A high percentage of tumor responses has been partial and transient, but some complete responses, lasting a few years, have been reported. Tumor responses are rarely observed before 8 weeks of continuous therapy.[282, 300–303]

The response rate is not related to age, gender, tumor burden, hormonal production, or histologic characteristics. The prognostic value of genetic abnormalities of the 11p15 region (paternal isodisomy and *IGF-II* gene overexpression) is still under study.[296] In a retrospective study, the only significant prognostic factor for tumor response to mitotane was its serum level: tumor response rate was 59% in patients whose serum mitotane level could be maintained above 14 mg/L and 0% in the patients whose serum mitotane level remained below that. Furthermore, a multivariate analysis showed that a serum mitotane level above 14 mg/L was associated with a significantly longer survival ($p < .01$). Clinical side effects may be avoided by maintaining a serum mitotane level below 20 mg/L.[303] The serum mitotane level cannot be predicted from the daily dose or the morphotype of the patient. Therefore, it has to be measured at a monthly interval initially, then every 2 to 3 months.

Mitotane is given by mouth as tablets at a daily dose of 2.3 g or as capsules containing 0.5 g of micronized mitotane mixed with cellulose acetate phthalate at a daily dose of 10 g for 2 months; it is then adapted according to its serum level. In most patients, mitotane dosage can be decreased progressively to 3 to 6 g per day, given in three divided doses. To offset adrenal insufficiency induced by mitotane, 30 to 60 mg oral hydrocortisone and 50 μg oral fludrocortisone are administered daily, with the salt diet being normal. Education of the patient is mandatory to avoid adrenal insufficiency.[304]

Drugs that block the synthesis of steroids (metyrapone, aminoglutethimide, ketoconazole), or that block the action of steroids in their target tissues (mifepristone), may control the clinical manifestations induced by hypersecretory tumors, but they do not inhibit tumor growth.[203]

In cytotoxic chemotherapy, the most tested drug is cisplatin. When used alone, the tumor response rate was 27%. Efficacy seems to be dose dependent.[305–307] However, in some patients with isolated or prominent liver metastases, chemoembolization with cisplatin has provided remarkable responses. Combinations of mitotane with cisplatin have not seemed to be synergic in terms of tumor response rate.[308] Similarly, the combination of cisplatin and doxorubicin did not provide a higher response rate than cisplatin alone.[309, 310] Presently, the combination of cisplatin and VP-16 is considered to be the reference combination. It provides tumor response rates of 35% to 40%, with most responses being transient and partial.[311–313] It appears that there is no cross-resistance between mitotane and cisplatin.

Other drugs have been used only in isolated cases, and none have proved to be efficient.[285, 305] Combinations of doxorubicin and mitotane did not provide higher response rates than mitotane alone.[314] Clearly, there is a need for trials using other combinations.

Suramin sodium may prove useful against ACC. Responses to suramin sodium have been reported in a few patients with metastatic ACC, some of whom have received previous chemotherapy with mitotane or other agents. However, its high toxicity limits its use.[315, 316]

Complications of Disease and Treatment

In functioning cancers, there can be severe and complete contralateral atrophy, requiring hormonal substitutive therapy starting postoperatively. Local recurrences encroach on bowel and retroperitoneal structures. Mitotane drug toxicity is usually dose-related and is reversible when therapy is discontinued or when its daily dose is decreased. It may be avoided by maintaining a serum mitotane level below 20 mg/L. The observed toxicities include:

- neurotoxicity (weakness, somnolence, lethargy, vertigo, headache, ataxia, dysarthria)
- gastrointestinal side effects (anorexia, nausea, vomiting, diarrhea)

- hepatotoxicity that should be monitored regularly by biochemical testing
- skin rashes, toxic retinopathy with papilledema, interstitial cystitis, ovary cysts, gynecomastia (all less frequently)
- hypercholesterolemia, hypouricemia, prolongation of bleeding time

In addition, steroid replacement therapy is required during mitotane treatment and should be maintained after its withdrawal.

Results and Prognosis

Surgery

Total ablation of functioning cancer is accompanied by a gradual regression of the clinical syndrome. Recurrence is common and it is often heralded by a recurring increase in steroid production. The 5-year survival rate is 34%, being higher after curative resection (42%) than after incomplete resection (34%) ($p < .02$). The 5-year survival rate is 53% in local disease and 24% in locoregional disease. The 1-year survival rate is 9% in patients with metastases.[283] The 5-year survival rate after local recurrence is 16%. After reoperation, the 5-year survival rate is 28% in the curative reoperated group and 8% in the noncurative reoperated group. The high recurrence rate, even after apparently curative resection, and the poor prognosis after recurrence, either at local or distant sites, emphasizes the interest in adjuvant treatment.

Adjuvant Treatment

External radiotherapy has not proved to be useful. Mitotane or chemotherapy with a cisplatin-based regimen has been advocated by several researchers. Owing to the absence of a randomized study, benefits of either treatment modalities in terms of disease-free interval or global survival have yet to be shown.

Treatment of Persistent or Recurrent Disease

After incomplete surgery and in patients with metastatic disease, therapy has two aims: control of hormonal overproduction and control of tumor growth. The first-line treatment is oral mitotane. In the absence of disease progression, a continuous treatment with mitotane should be given for at least 3 months before concluding it to be inefficient. In patients with disease progression during mitotane treatment, a chemotherapy with a cisplatin-based regimen is given.

In patients who achieve a partial response during mitotane treatment or chemotherapy, excision of residual tumors is performed, when it is feasible. In fact, disease control has been obtained in some of those metastatic patients with extensive and repeated surgical procedures. In contrast, surgery as a first-line treatment for metastatic disease provides poor results.[281, 287] In patients with local recurrence, surgery is also performed, when it is feasible.

Recommended Reading

An overview of pituitary adenomas with particular attention to endocrinologic evaluation is given in Thorner and associates' chapter entitled "The Anterior Pituitary" in the 9th edition of *Williams Textbook of Endocrinology.*[186] Comprehensive discussions on diagnosis (description of syndromes and physical, endocrinologic, and neuroradiographic examination), pathology, and therapy (surgical, radiation, and chemical) are presented in Melmed's *The Pituitary.*[277] Additional details on pathology are available in Horvath and Kovacs,[125] on surgery in Laws,[160, 161] Wilson,[165, 166] and Fahlbusch,[163] and on radiation therapy in Plowman.[178] A recent article by Klibanski and Zervas[157] gives information on advances in diagnostic techniques and therapeutic indications. An excellent overview of the different diagnostic and therapeutic problems addressed by Cushing's syndrome is provided by Orth.[144] A brief summary of the recent developments in the molecular genetics of pituitary adenomas is given in Shimon and Melmed[131] and in Farrell and Clayton.[132]

REFERENCES

1. Mazzaferri EL: Management of a solitary thyroid nodule. N Engl J Med 1993; 328:553.
2. Singer PA, Cooper DS, Daniels GH, et al: Treatment guidelines for patients with thyroid nodules and well-differentiated thyroid cancer. Arch Intern Med 1996; 156:2165.
3. Vanderpump MPJ, Alexander L, Scarpello JHB, et al: An audit of the management of thyroid cancer in a district general hospital. Clin Endocrinol 1998; 48:419–424.
4. Schlumberger MJ: Papillary and follicular thyroid carcinoma. N Engl J Med 1998; 338:297.
5. Parkin DM, Muir CS, Whelan SL, et al: Cancer Incidence in Five Continents, vol 6, IARC Scientific Publication 120. Lyon, France, International Agency for Research on Cancer, 1992.
6. Franceschi S, Boyle P, Maisonneuve P, et al: The epidemiology of thyroid carcinoma. Crit Rev Oncog 1993; 4:25.
7. Shore RE: Issues and epidemiological evidence regarding radiation-induced thyroid cancer. Radiat Res 1992; 131:98.
8. Ron E, Lubin JH, Shore RE, et al: Thyroid cancer after exposure to external radiation: a pooled analysis of seven studies. Radiat Res 1995; 141:259–277.
9. Schneider AB, Ron E: Carcinoma of follicular epithelium: pathogenesis. In: Braverman LE, Utiger RD (eds): Werner and Ingbar's The Thyroid. A Fundamental and Clinical Text, 7th ed, p 902. Philadelphia, Lippincott-Raven, 1996.
10. Schlumberger M, Pacini F: Thyroid Tumors, p 320. Paris, Editions Nucleon, 1999.
11. Kazakov VS, Demidchik EP, Astakhova LN: Thyroid cancer after Chernobyl. Nature 1992; 359:21.
12. Goldgar DE, Easton DF, Cannon-Albright LA, et al: Systematic population-based assessment of cancer risk in first-degree relatives of cancer probands. J Natl Cancer Inst 1994; 86:1600.
13. Nel CJC, Van Heerden JA, Goellner JR, et al: Anaplastic carcinoma of the thyroid: a clinicopathologic study of 82 cases. Mayo Clin Proc 1985; 60:51.
14. Venkatech YSS, Ordonez NG, Schultz PN, et al: Anaplastic carcinoma of the thyroid. A clinicopathologic study of 121 cases. Cancer 1990; 66:321.
15. Schlumberger M, Caillou B: Miscellaneous tumors of the thyroid. In: Braverman LE, Utiger RD (eds): Werner and Ingbar's The Thyroid. A Fundamental and Clinical Text, 7th ed, p 961. Philadelphia, Lippincott-Raven, 1996.
16. Ain KB: Anaplastic thyroid carcinoma: behavior, biology, and therapeutic approaches. Thyroid 1998; 8:715.
17. Eng C, Clayton D, Schuffenecker I, et al: The relationship between specific RET proto-oncogene mutation and disease phenotype in multiple endocrine neoplasia type 2: International RET Mutation Consortium Analysis. JAMA 1996; 276:1575.

18. Ball DW, Baylin SB, de Bustros A: Medullary thyroid carcinoma. In: Braverman LE, Utiger RD (eds): Werner and Ingbar's The Thyroid. A Fundamental and Clinical Text, 7th ed, p 946. Philadelphia, Lippincott-Raven, 1996.
19. Pasini B, Ceccherini I, Romeo G: Ret mutations in human disease. Trends Genet 1996; 12:138.
20. Livolsi VA, Brooks JJ, Arendash-Durand B: Anaplastic thyroid tumors: immunohistology. Am J Clin Pathol 1987; 87:434.
21. Hedinger C, Williams ED, Sobin LH: Histological typing of thyroid tumours. In: World Health Organization: International Histological Classification of Tumours, vol 11, 2nd ed. Berlin, Springer-Verlag, 1988.
22. Rosai J, Carcangiu ML, De Lellis RA: Tumors of the thyroid gland. In: AFIP Atlas of Tumor Pathology, vol 5. Washington, DC, Armed Forces Institute of Pathology, 1992.
23. Schlumberger M, De Vathaire F, Travagli JP, et al: Differentiated thyroid carcinoma in childhood: long term follow-up of 72 patients. J Clin Endocrinol Metab 1987; 65:1088.
24. Russel WO, Ibanez ML, Clark RL, et al: Thyroid carcinoma. Classification, intraglandular dissemination, and clinicopathological study based upon whole organ sections of 80 glands. Cancer 1963; 16:1425.
25. Sakamoto A, Kasai N, Sugano H: Poorly differentiated carcinoma of the thyroid. A clinico-pathologic entity for a high-risk group of papillary and follicular carcinomas. Cancer 1983; 52:1849.
26. Gautvik KM, Talle K, Hafer B, et al: Early liver metastases in patients with medullary carcinoma of the thyroid gland. Cancer 1989; 63:175.
27. Brierley JD, Panzarella T, Tsang RW, et al: A comparison of different staging systems predictability of patient outcome. Thyroid carcinoma as an example. Cancer 1997; 79:2414.
28. Hermanek P, Sobin LH: Thyroid gland (ICD-OC73). In: Hermanek P, Sobin LH (eds): TNM Classification of Malignant Tumors, vol 35, 4th ed. Berlin, Springer-Verlag, 1992:35.
29. Hay ID, Grant CS, Taylor WF, et al: Ipsilateral lobectomy versus bilateral lobar resection in papillary thyroid carcinoma: a retrospective analysis of surgical outcome using a novel prognostic scoring system. Surgery 1987; 102:1088.
30. De Groot LJ, Kaplan EL, McCormick M, et al: Natural history, treatment, and course of papillary thyroid carcinoma. J Clin Endocrinol Metab 1990; 71:414.
31. Demeure MJ, Clark OH: Surgery in the treatment of thyroid cancer. Endocrinol Metab Clin North Am 1990; 19:663.
32. Mazzaferri EL, Jhiang SM: Long-term impact of initial surgical and medical therapy on papillary and follicular thyroid cancer. Am J Med 1994; 97:418.
33. Mazzaferri EL: Carcinoma of follicular epithelium: radioiodine and other treatment outcomes. In: Braverman LE, Utiger RD (eds): Werner and Ingbar's The Thyroid: a Fundamental and Clinical Text, 7th ed, p 922. Philadelphia, Lippincott Raven, 1996.
34. Solomon BL, Wartofsky L, Burman KD: Current trends in the management of well differentiated papillary thyroid carcinoma. J Clin Endocrinol Metab 1996; 81:333.
35. Grebe SKG, Hay ID: Follicular cell-derived thyroid carcinomas. In: Arnold A (ed): Endocrine Neoplasms, p 91. Boston, Kluwer Academic Publishers; 1997.
36. Hay ID, Feld S, Garcia M, the Thyroid Cancer Task Force: AACE clinical practice guidelines for the management of thyroid carcinoma. Endocrine Practice 1997; 3:60.
37. Hay ID, Grant CS, Van Heerden JA, et al: Papillary thyroid microcarcinoma: a study of 535 cases observed in a 50-year period. Surgery 1992; 112:1139.
38. Baudin E, Travagli JP, Ropers J, et al: Microcarcinoma of the thyroid gland: the Gustave-Roussy Institute experience. Cancer 1998; 83:553.
39. Grebe SKG, Hay ID: Thyroid cancer nodal metastases: biologic significance and therapeutic considerations. Surg Oncol Clin North Am 1996; 5:43.
40. Wartofsky L, Sherman SI, Gopal J, et al: The use of radioactive iodine in patients with papillary and follicular thyroid cancer. J Clin Endocrinol Metab 1998; 83:4195–4203.
41. Tubiana M, Schlumberger M, Rougier P, et al: Long-term results and prognostic factors in patients with differentiated thyroid carcinoma. Cancer 1985; 55:794.
42. Simpson WJ, Panzarella T, Carruthers JS, et al: Papillary and follicular thyroid cancer: impact of treatment in 1578 patients. Int J Radiat Oncol Biol Phys 1988; 14:1063.
43. Sherman SI, Tielens ET, Sostre S, et al: Clinical utility of posttreatment radioiodine scans in the management of patients with thyroid carcinoma. J Clin Endocrinol Metab 1994; 78:629.
44. Tenenbaum F, Corone C, Schlumberger M, et al: Thyroglobulin measurement and postablative ^{131}I total body scan after total thyroidectomy for differentiated thyroid carcinoma in patients with no evidence of disease [Abstract]. Eur J Cancer 1996; 32A:1262.
45. Schlumberger M, Mancusi F, Baudin E, et al: ^{131}I therapy for elevated thyroglobulin levels. Thyroid 1997; 7:273.
46. Maxon HR, Smith HS: Radioiodine-131 in the diagnosis and treatment of metastatic well differentiated thyroid cancer. Endocrinol Metab Clin North Am 1990; 19:685.
47. Maxon HR, Englaro EE, Thomas SR, et al: Radioiodine-131 therapy for well-differentiated thyroid cancer. A quantitative radiation dosimetric approach: outcome and validation in 85 patients. J Nucl Med 1992; 33:1132.
48. Tubiana M, Haddad E, Schlumberger M, et al: External radiotherapy in thyroid cancers. Cancer 1985; 55:2062.
49. Kim JH, Leeper RD: Treatment of locally advanced thyroid carcinoma with combination doxorubicin and radiation therapy. Cancer 1987; 60:2372.
50. Schlumberger M, Parmentier C, Delisle MJ, et al: Combination therapy for anaplastic giant cell thyroid carcinoma. Cancer 1991; 67:564.
51. Tallroth E, Walling G, Lundell G, et al: Multimodality treatment in anaplastic giant cell carcinoma. Cancer 1987; 60:1428.
52. Tennvall J, Lundell G, Hallquist A, et al: Combined doxorubicin, hyperfractionated radiotherapy, and surgery in anaplastic thyroid carcinoma. Swedish Anaplastic Thyroid Cancer Group. Cancer 1994; 74:1348.
53. Wahl RA, Roher AD: Surgery of C-cell carcinoma of the thyroid. Progress in Surgery 1988; 19:100.
54. Frank-Raue K, Raue F, Buhr HJ, et al: Localization of occult persisting medullary thyroid carcinoma before microsurgical reoperation: high sensitivity of selective venous catheterization. Thyroid 1992; 2:113.
55. Abdelmoumene N, Schlumberger M, Gardet P, et al: Selective venous sampling catheterisation for localisation of persisting medullary thyroid carcinoma. Br J Cancer 1994; 69:1141.
56. Brierley JD, Tsang R, Simpson WJ, et al: Medullary thyroid cancer: analysis of survival and prognostic factors and the role of radiation therapy in local control. Thyroid 1996; 6:305.
57. Bartalena L, Martino E, Pacchiarotti A, et al: Factors affecting suppression of endogenous thyrotropin secretion by thyroxine treatment: retrospective analysis in athyreotic and goitrous patients. J Clin Endocrinol Metab 1987; 64:849.
58. Marcocci C, Golia F, Bruno-Bossio G, et al: Carefully monitored levothyroxine suppressive therapy is not associated with bone loss in premenopausal women. J Clin Endocrinol Metab 1994; 78:818.
59. Casara D, Rubello D, Saladini G, et al: Different features of pulmonary metastases in differentiated thyroid cancer: natural history and multivariate statistical analysis of prognostic variables. J Nucl Med 1993; 34:1626.
60. Schlumberger M, Challeton C, DeVathaire F, et al: Radioactive iodine treatment and external radiotherapy for lung and bone metastases from thyroid carcinoma. J Nucl Med 1996; 37:598.
61. Pacini F, Fugazzola L, Lippi F, et al: Detection of thyroglobulin in fine needle aspirates of nonthyroidal neck masses: a clue to the diagnosis of metastatic differentiated thyroid cancer. J Clin Endocrinol Metab 1992; 74:1401.
62. Arturi F, Russo D, Giuffrida D, et al: Early diagnosis by genetic analysis of differentiated thyroid cancer metastases in small lymph nodes. J Clin Endocrinol Metab 1997; 82:1638.
63. Schlumberger M, Baudin E: Serum thyroglobulin determination in the follow-up of patients with differentiated thyroid carcinoma. Eur J Endocrinol 1998; 138:249.
64. Ashcraft MW, VanHerle AJ: The comparative value of serum thyroglobulin measurements and ^{131}I total body scans in the follow-up study of patients with treated differentiated thyroid cancer. Am J Med 1981; 71:806.
65. Pacini F, Lari R, Mazzeo S, et al: Diagnostic value of a single serum thyroglobulin determination on and off thyroid suppressive therapy in the follow-up of patients with differentiated thyroid cancer. Clin Endocrinol (Oxf) 1985; 23:405.

66. Ozata M, Suzuki S, Miyamoto T, et al: Serum thyroglobulin in the follow-up of patients with treated differentiated thyroid cancer. J Clin Endocrinol Metab 1994; 79:98.
67. Roelants V, DeNayer P, Bouckaert A, et al: The predictive value of serum thyroglobulin in the follow-up of differentiated thyroid cancer. Eur J Nucl Med 1997; 24:722.
68. Utiger RD: Follow-up of patients with thyroid carcinoma. N Engl J Med 1997; 337:928.
69. Van Herle AJ, Uller RP, Matthews NL, et al: Radioimmunoassay for measurement of thyroglobulin in human serum. J Clin Invest 1973; 52:1320.
70. Mariotti S, Barbesino G, Caturegli P, et al: Assay of thyroglobulin in serum with thyroglobulin autoantibodies: an unobtainable goal? J Clin Endocrinol Metab 1995; 80:468.
71. Spencer CA, Takeuchi M, Kazarosyan M, et al: Serum thyroglobulin autoantibodies: prevalence, influence on serum thyroglobulin measurement, and prognostic significance in patients with differentiated thyroid carcinoma. J Clin Endocrinol Metab 1998; 83:1121.
72. Schlumberger M, Charbord P, Fragu P, et al: Circulating thyroglobulin and thyroid hormones in patients with metastases of differentiated thyroid carcinoma: relationship to serum thyrotropin levels. J Clin Endocrinol Metab 1980; 51:513.
73. Schneider AB, Line BR, Goldman JM, et al: Sequential serum thyroglobulin determinations, ^{131}I scans, and ^{131}I uptakes after triiodothyronine withdrawal in patients with thyroid cancer. J Clin Endocrinol Metab 1981; 53:1199.
74. Ladenson PW, Braverman LE, Mazzaferri EL, et al: Comparison of administration of recombinant human thyrotropin with withdrawal of thyroid hormone for radioactive iodine scanning in patients with thyroid carcinoma. N Engl J Med 1997; 337:888.
75. Rudavsky AZ, Freeman LM: Clinical case seminar: Treatment of scan-negative, thyroglobulin-positive metastatic thyroid cancer using radioiodine ^{131}I and recombinant human thyroid stimulating hormone. J Clin Endocrinol Metab 1997; 82:11.
76. Pacini F, Lippi F, Formica N, et al: Therapeutic doses of ^{131}I reveal undiagnosed metastases in thyroid cancer patients with detectable serum thyroglobulin levels. J Nucl Med 1987; 28:1888.
77. Schlumberger M, Arcangioli O, Piekarski JD, et al: Detection and treatment of lung metastases of differentiated thyroid carcinoma in patients with normal chest x-rays. J Nucl Med 1988; 29:1790.
78. Pineda JD, Lee T, Ain K, et al: ^{131}I therapy for thyroid cancer patients with elevated thyroglobulin and negative diagnostic scan. J Clin Endocrinol Metab 1995; 80:1488.
79. Goldman JM, Line BR, Aamodt RL, et al: Influence of triiodothyronine withdrawal time on ^{131}I uptake postthyroidectomy for thyroid cancer. J Clin Endocrinol Metab 1980; 50:734.
80. Guimaraes V, DeGroot LJ: Moderate hypothyroidism in preparation for whole body ^{131}I scintiscans and thyroglobulin testing. Thyroid 1996; 6:69.
81. Regalbuto C, Gullo D, Vigneri R, et al: Measurement of iodine before ^{131}I in thyroid cancer. Lancet 1994; 344:1501–1502.
82. Park HM, Perkins OW, Edmondson JW, et al: Influence of diagnostic radioiodines on the uptake of ablative dose of ^{131}I. Thyroid 1994; 4:49–54.
83. Vermiglio F, Baudin E, Travagli JP, et al: Iodine concentration by the thymus in thyroid carcinoma. J Nucl Med 1996; 37:1830–1831.
84. Veronikis IE, Simkin P, Braverman LE: Thymic uptake of ^{131}I in the anterior mediastinum. J Nucl Med 1996; 37:991–992.
85. Salvatori M, Saletnich I, Rufini V, et al: Unusual false-positive radioiodine whole-body scans in patients with differentiated thyroid carcinoma. Clin Nucl Med 1997; 22:380–384.
86. Tenenbaum F, Schlumberger M, Bonnin F, et al: Usefulness of technetium-99 m hydroxymethylene diphosphonate scans in localizing bone metastases of differentiated thyroid carcinoma. Eur J Nucl Med 1993; 20:1168–1174.
87. Baudin E, Schlumberger M, Lumbroso J, et al: Octreotide scintigraphy in patients with differentiated thyroid carcinoma: contribution for patients with negative radioiodine scan. J Clin Endocrinol Metab 1996; 81:2541–2544.
88. Hoefnagel CA, Delprat CC, Marcuse HR, et al: Role of Thallium-201 total body scintigraphy in follow-up of thyroid carcinoma. J Nucl Med 1986; 27:1854–1857.
89. Lind P, Gallowitsch HJ, Langsteger W, et al: Technetium 99m-Tetrofosmin whole-body scintigraphy in the follow-up of differentiated thyroid carcinoma. J Nucl Med 1997; 38:348–352.
90. Miyamoto S, Kasagi K, Misaki T, et al: Evaluation of Technetium-99m-MIBI scintigraphy in metastatic differentiated thyroid carcinoma. J Nucl Med 1997; 38:352–356.
91. Dietlein M, Scheidhauer K, Voth E, et al: Fluorine-18 fluorodeoxyglucose positron emission tomography and ^{131}I whole-body scintigraphy in the follow-up of differentiated thyroid cancer. Eur J Nucl Med 1997; 24:1342–1348.
92. Feine U, Lietzenmayer R, Hanke JP, et al: Fluorine-18-FDG and ^{131}I uptake in thyroid cancer. J Nucl Med 1996; 37:1468–1472.
93. Grünwald F, Menzel C, Bender H, et al: Comparison of 18FDG-PET with ^{131}I and 99mTc-Sestamibi scintigraphy in differentiated thyroid cancer. Thyroid 1997; 7:327–335.
94. Grünwald F, Schomburg A, Bender H, et al: Fluorine-18 fluorodeoxyglucose positron emission tomography in the follow-up of differentiated thyroid cancer. Eur J Nucl Med 1996; 23:312–319.
95. Sisson JC, Ackermann RJ, Meyer MA, et al: Uptake of 18-fluoro-2-deoxy-D-glucose by thyroid cancer: implications for diagnosis and therapy. J Clin Endocrinol Metab 1993; 77:1090–1094.
96. Mazzaferri EL: Treating high thyroglobulin with radioiodine. A magic bullet or a shot in the dark? J Clin Endocrinol Metab 1995; 80:1485–1487.
97. McDougall IR: ^{131}I treatment of ^{131}I negative whole body scan, and positive thyroglobulin in differentiated thyroid carcinoma: what is being treated? Thyroid 1997; 7:669–672.
98. Van Heerden JA, Grant CS, Gharib H, et al: Long-term course of patients with persistent hypercalcitoninemia after apparent curative primary surgery for medullary thyroid carcinoma. Ann Surg 1990; 212:395–401.
99. Hoie J, Stenwig AE, Kullmann G, et al: Distant metastases in papillary thyroid cancer. A review of 91 patients. Cancer 1988; 61:1–6.
100. Dinneen SF, Valimaki MJ, Bergstralh EJ, et al: Distant metastases in papillary thyroid carcinoma: 100 cases observed at one institution during 5 decades. J Clin Endocrinol Metab 1995; 80:2041–2045.
101. Vassilopoulou-Sellin R, Klein MJ, Smith TH, et al: Pulmonary metastases in children and young adults with differentiated thyroid cancer. Cancer 1993; 71:1348–1352.
102. Marcocci C, Pacini F, Elisei R, et al: Clinical and biologic behavior of bone metastases from differentiated thyroid carcinoma. Surgery 1989; 106:960–966.
103. Rall JE, Alpers JB, Lewallen CG, et al: Radiation pneumonitis and fibrosis: a complication of radioiodine treatment of pulmonary metastases from cancer of the thyroid. J Clin Endocrinol Metab 1957; 17:1263–1276.
104. Pacini F, Gasperi M, Fugazzola L, et al: Testicular function in patients with differentiated thyroid carcinoma treated with radioiodine. J Nucl Med 1994; 35:1418–1422.
105. Raymond JP, Izembart M, Marliac V, et al: Temporary ovarian failure in thyroid cancer patients after thyroid remnant ablation with radioactive iodine. J Clin Endocrinol Metab 1989; 69:186–190.
106. Dottorini ME, Lomuscio G, Mazzucchelli L, et al: Assessment of female fertility and carcinogenesis after ^{131}I therapy for differentiated thyroid carcinoma. J Nucl Med 1995; 36:21–27.
107. Schlumberger M, De Vathaire F, Ceccarelli C, et al: Exposure to radioactive ^{131}I for scintigraphy or therapy does not preclude pregnancy in thyroid cancer patients. J Nucl Med 1996; 37:606–612.
108. Hall P, Holm LE, Lundell G, et al: Cancer risks in thyroid cancer patients. Br J Cancer 1991; 64:159–163.
109. De Vathaire F, Schlumberger M, Delisle MJ, et al: Leukaemias and cancers following ^{131}I administration for thyroid cancer. Br J Cancer 1997; 75:734–759.
110. Gagel RF, Tashjian AH, Cummings T, et al: The clinical outcome of prospective screening for multiple endocrine neoplasia type 2a. An 18-years experience. N Engl J Med 1988; 318:478–484.
111. Byar DP, Green SB, Dor P, et al: A prognostic index for thyroid carcinoma. A study of the EORTC thyroid cancer cooperative group. Eur J Cancer 1979; 15:1033–1041.
112. Cady B, Rossi R: An expanded view of risk-group definition in differentiated thyroid carcinoma. Surgery 1988; 104:947–953.
113. Samaan NA, Schultz PN, Hickey RC, et al: The results of various modalities of treatment of well differentiated thyroid carcinoma: a retrospective review of 1599 patients. J Clin Endocrinol Metab 1992; 75:714–720.
114. Hay ID, Bergstralh EJ, Goellner JR, et al: Predicting outcome in papillary thyroid carcinoma: development of a reliable prognostic

scoring system in a cohort of 1779 patients surgically treated at one institution during 1940 through 1989. Surgery 1993; 114:1050–1058.

115. Travagli JP, Cailleux AF, Ricard M, et al: Combination of radioiodine (^{131}I) and probe-guided surgery for persistent or recurrent thyroid carcinoma. J Clin Endocrinol Metab 1998; 83:2675–2680.
116. Niederle B, Roka R, Schemper M, et al: Surgical treatment of distant metastases in differentiated thyroid cancer: indication and results. Surgery 1986; 100:1088–1097.
117. Maxon HR, Thomas SR, Hertzberg VS, et al: Relation between effective radiation dose and outcome of radioiodine therapy for thyroid cancer. N Engl J Med 1983; 309:937–941.
118. Shimaoka K, Schoenfeld DA, Dewys WD, et al: A randomized trial of Doxorubicin versus Doxorubicin plus Cisplatin in patients with advanced thyroid carcinoma. Cancer 1985; 56:2155–2160.
119. Williams SD, Birch R, Einhorn LH: Phase II evaluation of Doxorubicin plus Cisplatin in advanced thyroid cancer: a Southeastern Cancer Study Group Trial. Cancer Treat Rep 1986; 70:405–407.
120. Modigliani E, Cohen R, Campos JM, et al: Prognostic factors for survival and for biochemical cure in medullary thyroid carcinoma: results in 899 patients. Clin Endocrinol (Oxf) 1998; 48:265–273.
121. Orlandi F, Caraci P, Berruti A, et al: Chemotherapy with dacarbazine and 5-fluorouracil in advanced medullary thyroid cancer. Ann Oncol 1994; 5:763–765.
122. Wu LT, Averbuch SD, Ball DW, et al: Treatment of advanced medullary thyroid carcinoma with a combination of cyclophosphamide, vincristine, and dacarbazine. Cancer 1994; 73:432–436.
123. Schlumberger M, Abdelmoumene N, Delisle MJ, et al: Treatment of advanced medullary thyroid cancer with an alternative combination of 5FU-Streptozotocin and 5FU-Dacarbazine. Br J Cancer 1995; 71:363–365.
124. Kovacs K, Horvath E: Tumors of the pituitary gland. In: Hartman WH (ed): Atlas of Tumor Pathology, pp 1–264. Washington, DC, Armed Forces Institute of Pathology, 1986.
125. Horvath E, Kovacs K: The adenohypophysis. In: Kovacs K, Asa L, (eds): Functional Endocrine Pathology, pp 247–281. Boston, Blackwell Science, 1998.
126. Ambrosi B, Faglia G: Epidemiology of pituitary tumors. In: Faglia G, Beck-Peccoz P, Ambrosi B, et al (eds): Pituitary Adenomas: New Trends in Basic and Clinical Research, pp 159–169. Amsterdam, Excerpta Medica, 1991.
127. Molitch ME, Russell EJ: The pituitary "incidentaloma." Ann Intern Med 1990; 112:925–931.
128. Teramoto A, Hirakawa K, Sanno N, et al: Incidental pituitary lesions in 1000 unselected autopsy specimens. Radiology 1994; 193:161–164.
129. Hall WA, Luciano MG, Doppman JL, et al: Pituitary magnetic resonance imaging in normal human volunteers: occult adenomas in the general population. Ann Intern Med 1994; 120:817–820.
130. Mindermann T, Wilson CB: Age-related and gender-related occurrence of pituitary adenomas. Clin Endocrinol (Oxf) 1994; 41:359–364.
131. Shimon I, Melmed S: Genetic basis of endocrine disease: pituitary tumor pathogenesis. J Clin Endocrinol Metab 1997; 82:1675–1681.
132. Farrell WE, Clayton RN: Molecular genetics of pituitary tumours. Trends in Endocrinology and Metabolism 1998; 9:20–26.
133. Alexander JM, Biller BM, Bikkai H, et al: Clinically nonfunctioning pituitary tumors are monoclonal in origin. J Clin Invest 1990; 86:336–340.
134. Herman V, Fagin J, Gonski R, et al: Clonal origin of pituitary adenomas. J Clin Endocrinol Metab 1990; 71:1427–1430.
135. Spada A, Arosio M, Bochicchio D, et al: Clinical, biochemical, and morphological correlates in patients bearing growth hormone–secreting pituitary tumors with or without constitutively active adenylate cyclase. J Clin Endocrinol Metab 1990; 71:1421–1426.
136. Landis CA, Harsh G, Lyons S, et al: Clinical characteristics of acromegalic patients whose pituitary tumors contain mutant Gs protein. J Clin Endocrinol Metab 1990; 71:1416–1420.
137. Pernicone PJ, Scheithauer BW, Sebo TJ, et al: Pituitary carcinoma: a clinicopathologic study of 15 cases. Cancer 1997; 79:804–812.
138. Kaltsas GA, Grossman AB: Malignant pituitary tumours. Pituitary 1998; 1:69–81.
139. Melmed S: Acromegaly. N Engl J Med 1990; 322:966–977.
140. Ezzat S, Forster MJ, Berchtold P, et al: Acromegaly. Clinical and biochemical features in 500 patients. Medicine (Baltimore) 1994; 73:233–240.
141. Melmed S, Ho K, Klibanski A, et al: Clinical review 75: Recent advances in pathogenesis, diagnosis, and management of acromegaly. J Clin Endocrinol Metab 1995; 80:3395–3402.
142. Melmed S: Acromegaly. In: Melmed S (ed): The Pituitary, pp 413–442. Boston, Blackwell Science, 1995.
143. Bertagna X, Raux-Demay MC, Guilhaume B, et al: Cushing's disease. In: Melmed S (ed): The Pituitary, pp 478–545. Boston, Blackwell Science, 1995.
144. Orth DN: Cushing's syndrome. N Engl J Med 1995; 332:791–803.
145. Molitch M: Prolactinoma. In: Melmed S (ed): The Pituitary, pp 443–477. Boston, Blackwell Science, 1995.
146. Molitch ME: Evaluation and treatment of the patient with a pituitary incidentaloma. J Clin Endocrinol Metab 1995; 80:3–6.
147. Beck-Peccoz P, Brucker-Davis F, Persani L, et al: Thyrotropin-secreting pituitary adenomas. Endocr Rev 1996; 17:610–638.
148. Samuels MH, Ridgway EC; Glycoprotein-secreting pituitary adenomas. Baillieres Clin Endocrinol Metab 1995; 9:337–358.
149. Chanson P, Petrossians P: Les adénomes hypophysaires cliniquement nonfonctionnels. Paris-Montrouge, John-Libbey-Eurotext, 1998.
150. Arnold AC: Neuroophthalmologic evaluation of pituitary disorders. In: Melmed S (ed): The Pituitary, pp 687–707. Boston, Blackwell Science, 1995.
151. Abboud CF: Anterior pituitary failure. In: Melmed S (ed): The Pituitary, pp 341–410. Boston, Blackwell Science, 1995.
152. Wolpert SM: The radiology of pituitary adenomas. Endocrinol Metab Clin North Am 1987; 16:553–584.
153. Pressman BD: Pituitary imaging. In: Melmed S (ed): The Pituitary, pp 663–686. Boston, Blackwell Science, 1995.
154. Oldfield EH, Chrousos GP, Schulte HM, et al: Preoperative lateralization of ACTH-secreting pituitary microadenomas by bilateral and simultaneous inferior petrosal venous sinus sampling. N Engl J Med 1985; 312:100–103.
155. Thapar K, Kovacs K, Laws ER, et al: Pituitary adenomas: current concepts in classification, histopathology, and molecular biology. The Endocrinologist 1993; 3:39–56.
156. Hardy J: Transsphenoidal surgery of hypersecreting pitutary tumors. In: Kohler PO, Ross GT (eds): Diagnosis and Treatment of Pituitary Tumors, pp 179–194. Amsterdam, Excerpta Medica, 1973.
157. Klibanski A, Zervas NT: Diagnosis and management of hormone-secreting pituitary adenomas. N Engl J Med 1991; 324:822–831.
158. Molitch ME: Pituitary adenomas. Ann Intern Med 1995; 122:476.
159. Molitch ME, Thorner MO, Wilson C: Management of prolactinomas. J Clin Endocrinol Metab 1997; 82:996–1000.
160. Laws ER Jr: Pituitary surgery. Endocrinol Metab Clin North Am 1987; 16:647–665.
161. Laws ER Jr, Thapar K: Surgical management of pituitary adenomas. Baillieres Clin Endocrinol Metab 1995; 9:391–405.
162. Giovanelli M, Losa M, Mortini P: Surgical therapy of pituitary adenomas. Metabolism 1996; 45:115–116.
163. Fahlbusch R, Honegger J, Buchfelder M: Surgical management of acromegaly. Endocrinol Metab Clin North Am 1992; 21:669–692.
164. Fahlbusch R, Honegger J, Buchfelder M: Acromegaly—the place of the neurosurgeon. Metabolism 1996; 45:65–66.
165. Wilson CB: Extensive clinical experience: surgical management of pituitary tumors. J Clin Endocrinol Metab 1997; 82:2381–2385.
166. Wilson CB: A decade of pituitary microsurgery. J Neurosurg 1984; 61:814–833.
167. Tyrrell JB, Wilson CB: Cushing's disease. Therapy of pituitary adenomas. Endocrinol Metab Clin North Am 1994; 23:925–938.
168. Snyder PJ, Fowble BF, Schatz NJ, et al: Hypopituitarism following radiation therapy of pituitary adenomas. Am J Med 1986; 81:457–462.
169. Sheline G, Tyrrell J: Pituitary tumors. In: Perez C, Brady L (eds): Principles and Practice of Radiation Oncology, pp 1108–1125. Philadelphia, J.B. Lippincott Co., 1987.
170. Grigsby PW, Stokes S, Marks JE, et al: Prognostic factors and results of radiotherapy alone in the management of pituitary adenomas. Int J Radiat Oncol Biol Phys 1988; 15:1103–1110.
171. Chun M, Masko GB, Hetelekidis S: Radiotherapy in the treatment of pituitary adenomas. Int J Radiat Oncol Biol Phys 1988; 15:305–309.
172. Nelson PB, Goodman ML, Flickinger JC, et al: Endocrine function in patients with large pituitary tumors treated with operative decompression and radiation therapy. Neurosurgery 1989; 24:398–400.
173. Littley MD, Shalet SM, Beardwell CG, et al: Hypopituitarism following external radiotherapy for pituitary tumours in adults. Q J Med 1989; 262:145–160.

174. Brada M, Ford D, Ashley S, et al: Risk of second brain tumour after conservative surgery and radiotherapy for pituitary adenoma. Br Med J 1992; 304:1343–1346.
175. Eastman RC, Gorden P, Glatstein E, et al: Radiation therapy of acromegaly. Endocrinol Metab Clin North Am 1992; 21:693–712.
176. Constine LS, Woolf PD, Cann D, et al: Hypothalamic-pituitary dysfunction after radiation for brain tumors. N Engl J Med 1993; 328:87–94.
177. Brada M, Rajan B, Traish D, et al: The long-term efficacy of conservative surgery and radiotherapy in the control of pituitary adenomas. Clin Endocrinol (Oxf) 1993; 38:571–578.
178. Plowman PN: Radiotherapy for pituitary tumours. Baillieres Clin Endocrinol Metab 1995; 9:407–420.
179. Barkan AL, Halasz I, Dornfeld KJ, et al: Pituitary irradiation is ineffective in normalizing plasma insulin-like growth factor I in patients with acromegaly. J Clin Endocrinol Metab 1997; 82:3187–3191.
180. Thorén M, Rähn T, Guo WY, et al: Stereotactic radiosurgery with the cobalt-60 gamma unit in the treatment of growth hormone-producing pituitary tumors. Neurosurgery 1991; 29:663–668.
181. Pollock BE, Kondziolka D, Lunsford LD, et al: Stereotactic radiosurgery for pituitary adenomas: imaging, visual, and endocrine results. Acta Neurochir Suppl (Wien) 1994; 62:33–38.
182. Sheline GE: Proceedings: treatment of nonfunctioning chromophobe adenomas of the pituitary. Am J Roentgenol Radium Ther Nucl Med 1974; 120:553–561.
183. Tsang RW, Laperriere NJ, Simpson WJ, et al: Glioma arising after radiation therapy for pituitary adenoma. A report of four patients and estimation of risk. Cancer 1993; 72:2227–2233.
184. Lamberts SW, Hofland LJ, de Herder WW, et al: Octreotide and related somatostatin analogs in the diagnosis and treatment of pituitary disease and somatostatin receptor scintigraphy. Front Neuroendocrinol 1993; 14:27–55.
185. Lamberts SW, van der Lely AJ, de Herder WW, et al: Octreotide. N Engl J Med 1996; 334:246–254.
186. Thorner M, Vance ML, Laws ER Jr, et al: The anterior pituitary. In: Wilson JD, Foster DW, Kronenberg HM, Larsen PR (eds): Williams Textbook of Endocrinology, pp 249–340. Philadelphia, W.B. Saunders, 1998.
187. Vance ML, Evans WS, Thorner MO: Drugs five years later. Bromocriptine. Ann Intern Med 1984; 100:78–91.
188. Liuzzi A, Dallabonzana D, Oppizzi G, et al: Low doses of dopamine agonists in the long-term treatment of macroprolactinomas. N Engl J Med 1985; 313:656–659.
189. Bevan JS, Webster J, Burke CW, et al: Dopamine agonists and pituitary tumor shrinkage. Endocr Rev 1992; 13:220–240.
190. Gemzell C, Wang CF: Outcome of pregnancy in women with pituitary adenoma. Fertil Steril 1979; 31:363–372.
191. Molitch ME: Pregnancy and the hyperprolactinemic woman. N Engl J Med 1985; 312:1364–1370.
192. Kupersmith MJ, Rosenberg C, Kleinberg D: Visual loss in pregnant women with pituitary adenomas. Ann Intern Med 1994; 121:473–477.
193. van't Verlaat JW, Croughs RJ, Brownell J: Treatment of macroprolactinomas with a new non-ergot, long-acting dopaminergic drug, CV 205-502. Clin Endocrinol (Oxf) 1990; 33:619–624.
194. Duranteau L, Chanson P, Lavoinne A, et al: Effect of the new dopaminergic agonist CV 205–502 on plasma prolactin levels and tumour size in bromocriptine-resistant prolactinomas. Clin Endocrinol (Oxf) 1991; 34:25–29.
195. Brue T, Pellegrini I, Gunz G, et al: Effects of the dopamine agonist CV 205–502 in human prolactinomas resistant to bromocriptine. J Clin Endocrinol Metab 1992; 74:577–584.
196. Vilar L, Burke CW: Quinagolide efficacy and tolerability in hyperprolactinaemic patients who are resistant to or intolerant of bromocriptine. Clin Endocrinol (Oxf) 1994; 41:821–826.
197. Rains CP, Bryson HM, Fitton A: Cabergoline: a review of its pharmacological properties and therapeutic potential in the treatment of hyperprolactinaemia and inhibition of lactation. Drugs 1995; 49:255–279.
198. Webster J, Piscitelli G, Polli A, et al: A comparison of cabergoline and bromocriptine in the treatment of hyperprolactinemic amenorrhea. Cabergoline Comparative Study Group. N Engl J Med 1994; 331:904–909.
199. Biller BM, Molitch ME, Vance ML, et al: Treatment of prolactin-secreting macroadenomas with the once-weekly dopamine agonist cabergoline. J Clin Endocrinol Metab 1996; 81:2338–2343.
200. Colao A, Di Sarno A, Sarnacchiaro F, et al: Prolactinomas resistant to standard dopamine agonists respond to chronic cabergoline treatment. J Clin Endocrinol Metab 1997; 82:876–883.
201. Colao A, Di Sarno A, Landi ML, et al: Long-term and low-dose treatment with cabergoline induces macroprolactinoma shrinkage. J Clin Endocrinol Metab 1997; 82:3574–3579.
202. Jaffe CA, Barkan AL: Treatment of acromegaly with dopamine agonists. Endocrinol Metab Clin North Am 1992; 21:713–735.
203. Miller JW, Crapo L: The medical treatment of Cushing's syndrome. Endocr Rev 1993; 14:443–458.
204. Sassolas G, Harris AG, James-Deidier A: Long term effect of incremental doses of the somatostatin analog SMS 201-995 in 58 acromegalic patients. French SMS 201-995 Acromegaly Study Group. J Clin Endocrinol Metab 1990; 71:391–397.
205. Vance ML, Harris AG: Long-term treatment of 189 acromegalic patients with the somatostatin analog octreotide. Results of the International Multicenter Acromegaly Study Group. Arch Intern Med 1991; 151:1573–1578.
206. Ezzat S, Snyder PJ, Young WF, et al: Octreotide treatment of acromegaly. A randomized, multicenter study. Ann Intern Med 1992; 117:711–718.
207. Chanson P, Timsit J, Harris AG: Clinical pharmacokinetics of octreotide. Therapeutic applications in patients with pituitary tumours. Clin Pharmacokinet 1993; 25:375–391.
208. Newman CB, Melmed S, Snyder PJ, et al: Safety and efficacy of long-term octreotide therapy of acromegaly: results of a multicenter trial in 103 patients—a clinical research center study. J Clin Endocrinol Metab 1995; 80:2768–2775.
209. Gillis JC, Noble S, Goa KL: Octreotide long-acting release (LAR). A review of its pharmacological properties and therapeutic use in the management of acromegaly. Drugs 1997; 53:681–699.
210. Heron I, Thomas F, Dero M, et al: Pharmacokinetics and efficacy of a long-acting formulation of the new somatostatin analog BIM 23014 in patients with acromegaly. J Clin Endocrinol Metab 1993; 76:721–727.
211. Morange I, De Boisvilliers F, Chanson P, et al: Slow release lanreotide treatment in acromegalic patients previously normalized by octreotide. J Clin Endocrinol Metab 1994; 79:145–151.
212. Giusti M, Gussoni G, Cuttica CM, et al: Effectiveness and tolerability of slow release lanreotide treatment in active acromegaly: six-month report on an Italian multicenter study. Italian Multicenter Slow Release Lanreotide Study Group. J Clin Endocrinol Metab 1996; 81:2089–2097.
213. Caron P, Morange-Ramos I, Cogne M, et al: Three year follow-up of acromegalic patients treated with intramuscular slow-release lanreotide. J Clin Endocrinol Metab 1997; 82:18–22.
214. Chanson P, Weintraub BD, Harris AG: Octreotide therapy for thyroid-stimulating hormone-secreting pituitary adenomas. A follow-up of 52 patients. Ann Intern Med 1993; 119:236–240.
215. Gancel A, Vuillermet P, Legrand A, et al: Effects of a slow-release formulation of the new somatostatin analogue lanreotide in TSH-secreting pituitary adenomas. Clin Endocrinol (Oxf) 1994; 40:421–428.
216. Warnet A, Timsit J, Chanson P, et al: The effect of somatostatin analogue on chiasmal dysfunction from pituitary macroadenomas. J Neurosurg 1989; 71:687–690.
217. Warnet A, Harris AG, Renard E, et al: A prospective multicenter trial of octreotide in 24 patients with visual defects caused by nonfunctioning and gonadotropin-secreting pituitary adenomas. Neurosurgery 1997; 41:786–797.
218. Krenning EP, Kwekkeboom DJ, Bakker WH, et al: Somatostatin receptor scintigraphy with [^{111}In-DTPA-D-Phe1]-and [^{123}I-Tyr3]-octreotide: the Rotterdam experience with more than 1000 patients. Eur J Nucl Med 1993; 20:716–731.
219. Chanson P: Predicting the effects of long-term medical treatment in acromegaly. At what cost? For what benefits? Eur J Endocrinol 1997; 136:359–361.
220. Ebersold MJ, Quast LM, Laws ER Jr, et al: Long-term results in transsphenoidal removal of nonfunctioning pituitary adenomas. J Neurosurg 1986; 64:713–719.
221. Harris PE, Afshar F, Coates P, et al: The effects of transsphenoidal surgery on endocrine function and visual fields in patients with functionless pituitary tumours. Q J Med 1989; 71:417–427.

222. Comtois R, Beauregard H, Somma M, et al: The clinical and endocrine outcome to transsphenoidal microsurgery of non secreting pituitary adenomas. Cancer 1991; 68:860–866.
223. Sassolas G, Trouillas J, Treluyer C, et al: Management of non-functioning pituitary adenomas. Acta Endocrinol 1993; 129 (suppl 1):21–26.
224. Hayes TP, Davis RA, Raventos A: The treatment of pituitary chromophobe adenomas. Radiology 1971; 98:149–153.
225. Ciric I, Mikhael M, Stafford T, et al: Transsphenoidal microsurgery of pituitary macroadenomas with long-term follow-up results. J Neurosurg 1983; 59:395–401.
226. Vlahovitch B, Reynaud C, Rhiati J, et al: Treatment and recurrences in 135 pituitary adenomas. Acta Neurochir (Wien) 1988; 42 (suppl):120–123.
227. Jaffrain-Rea ML, Derome P, Bataini JP, et al: Influence of radiotherapy on long-term relapse in clinically non-secreting pituitary adenomas. A retrospective study (1970–1988). Eur J Med 1993; 2:398–403.
228. Bradley KM, Adams CBT, Potter CPS, et al: An audit of selected patients with non-functioning pituitary adenoma treated by transsphenoidal surgery without irradiation. Clin Endocrinol 1994; 41:655–659.
229. Gittoes NJL, Bates AS, Tse W, et al: Radiotherapy for non-functioning pituitary tumours. Clin Endocrinol 1998; 48:331–337.
230. Rosen T, Bengtsson A-G: Premature mortality due to cardiovascular disease in hypopituitarism. Lancet 1990; 336:285–288.
231. Bates AS, Van't Hoff W, Jones PJ, et al: The effects of hypopituitarism on life expectancy. J Clin Endocrinol Metab 1996; 81:1169–1172.
232. Bülow B, Hagmar L, Mikoczy Z, et al: Increased cerebrovascular mortality in patients with hypopituitarism. Clin Endocrinol 1997; 46:75–81.
233. Frohman LA: Acromegaly: what constitutes optimal therapy? J Clin Endocrinol Metab 1996; 81:443–445.
234. Bates AS, Van't Hoff W, Jones JM, et al: An audit of outcome of treatment in acromegaly. Q J Med 1993; 86:293–299.
235. Rajasoorya C, Holdaway IM, Wrightson P, et al: Determinants of clinical outcome and survival in acromegaly. Clin Endocrinol (Oxf) 1994; 41:95–102.
236. Roelfsema F, van Dulken H, Frolich M: Long-term results of transsphenoidal pituitary microsurgery in 60 acromegalic patients. Clin Endocrinol (Oxf) 1985; 23:555–565.
237. Sheaves R, Jenkins P, Blackburn P, et al: Outcome of transsphenoidal surgery for acromegaly using strict criteria for surgical cure. Clin Endocrinol (Oxf) 1996; 45:407–413.
238. Yamada S, Aiba T, Takada K, et al: Retrospective analysis of long-term surgical results in acromegaly: preoperative and postoperative factors predicting outcome. Clin Endocrinol (Oxf) 1996; 45:291–298.
239. Colao A, Ferone D, Cappabianca P, et al: Effect of octreotide pretreatment on surgical outcome in acromegaly. J Clin Endocrinol Metab 1997; 82:3308–3314.
240. Colao A, Merola B, Ferone D, et al: J Clin Endocrinol Metab 1997; 82:2777–2781.
241. Buchfelder M, Fahlbusch R: Neurosurgical treatment of Cushing's disease in children and adolescents. Acta Neurochir Suppl (Wien) 1985; 35:101–105.
242. Losa M, Oeckler R, Schopohl J, et al: Evaluation of selective transsphenoidal adenomectomy by endocrinological testing and somatomedin-C measurement in acromegaly. J Neurosurg 1989; 70:561–567.
243. Lamberg BA, Kivikangas V, Vartianen J, et al: Conventional pituitary irradiation in acromegaly. Effect on growth hormone and TSH secretion. Acta Endocrinol (Copenh) 1976; 82:267–281.
244. Feek CM, McLelland J, Seth J, et al: How effective is external pituitary irradiation for growth hormone–secreting pituitary tumors? Clin Endocrinol (Oxf) 1984; 20:401–408.
245. Kliman B, Kjellberg RN, Swisher B, et al: Long-term effects of proton-beam therapy for acromegaly. In: Robbins RJ, Melmed S (eds): Acromegaly, pp 221–228. New York, Plenum Press, 1986.
246. Speirs CJ, Reed PI, Morrison R, et al: The effectiveness of external beam radiotherapy for acromegaly is not affected by previous pituitary ablative treatments. Acta Endocrinol (Copenh) 1990; 122:559–565.
247. Chanson P, Grellier-Fouqueray P, Young J, et al: Comment et avec quelle efficacité traite-t-on l'acromégalie en 1997? Enquête transversale sur une population de 74 acromégales [Abstract]. Ann Endocrinol (Paris) 1997; 58 (suppl 2):2S69.
248. Arosio M, Macchelli S, Rossi CM, et al: Effects of treatment with octreotide in acromegalic patients—a multicenter Italian study. Italian Multicenter Octreotide Study Group. Eur J Endocrinol 1995; 133:430–439.
249. Stewart PM, Kane KF, Stewart SE, et al: Depot long-acting somatostatin analog (Sandostatin-LAR) is an effective treatment for acromegaly. J Clin Endocrinol Metab 1995; 80:3267–3272.
250. Lancranjan I, Bruns C, Grass P, et al: Sandostatin LAR: a promising therapeutic tool in the management of acromegalic patients. Metabolism 1996; 45:67–71.
251. Fløgstad AK, Halse J, Bakke S, et al: Sandostatin LAR in acromegalic patients: long-term treatment. J Clin Endocrinol Metab 1997; 82:23–28.
252. Feigenbaum SL, Downey DE, Wilson CB, et al: Transsphenoidal pituitary resection for preoperative diagnosis of prolactin-secreting pituitary adenoma in women: long term follow-up. J Clin Endocrinol Metab 1996; 81:1711–1719.
253. Thomson JA, Davies DL, McLaren EH, et al: Ten year follow up of microprolactinoma treated by transsphenoidal surgery. Br Med J 1994; 309:1409–1410.
254. Serri O, Hardy J, Massoud F: Relapse of hyperprolactinemia revisited. N Engl J Med 1993; 329:1357.
255. Nabarro JD: Pituitary prolactinomas. Clin Endocrinol (Oxf) 1982; 17:129–155.
256. Grossman A, Cohen BL, Charlesworth M, et al: Treatment of prolactinomas with megavoltage radiotherapy. Br Med J (Clin Res Ed) 1984; 288:1105–1109.
257. Tsagarakis S, Grossman A, Plowman PN, et al: Megavoltage pituitary irradiation in the management of prolactinomas: long-term follow-up. Clin Endocrinol (Oxf) 1991; 34:399–406.
258. Guilhaume B, Bertagna X, Thomsen M, et al: Transsphenoidal pituitary surgery for the treatment of Cushing's disease: results in 64 patients and long term follow-up studies. J Clin Endocrinol Metab 1988; 66:1056–1064.
259. Mampalam TJ, Tyrrell JB, Wilson CB: Transsphenoidal microsurgery for Cushing disease. A report of 216 cases. Ann Intern Med 1988; 109:487–493.
260. Arnott RD, Pestell RG, McKelvie PA, et al: A critical evaluation of transsphenoidal surgery in the treatment of Cushing's disease: prediction of outcome. Acta Endocrinol (Copenh) 1990; 123:423–430.
261. Burke CW, Adams CB, Esiri MM, et al: Transsphenoidal surgery for Cushing's disease: does what is removed determine the endocrine outcome? Clin Endocrinol (Oxf) 1990; 33:525–537.
262. Post KD, Habas JE: Comparison of long term results between prolactin secreting adenomas and ACTH secreting adenomas. Can J Neurol Sci 1990; 17:74–77.
263. Tindall GT, Herring CJ, Clark RV, et al: Cushing's disease: results of transsphenoidal microsurgery with emphasis on surgical failures. J Neurosurg 1990; 72:363–369.
264. Robert F, Hardy J: Cushing's disease: a correlation of radiological, surgical, and pathological findings with therapeutic results. Pathol Res Pract 1991; 187:617–621.
265. Tahir AH, Sheeler LR: Recurrent Cushing's disease after transsphenoidal surgery. Arch Intern Med 1992; 152:977–981.
266. Trainer PJ, Lawrie HS, Verhelst J, et al: Transsphenoidal resection in Cushing's disease: undetectable serum cortisol as the definition of successful treatment. Clin Endocrinol (Oxf) 1993; 38:73–78.
267. Ram Z, Nieman LK, Cutler GB Jr, et al: Early repeat surgery for persistent Cushing's disease. J Neurosurg 1994; 80:37–45.
268. Bochicchio D, Losa M, Buchfelder M: Factors influencing the immediate and late outcome of Cushing's disease treated by transsphenoidal surgery: a retrospective study by the European Cushing's Disease Survey Group. J Clin Endocrinol Metab 1995; 80:3114–3120.
269. Styne DM, Grumbach MM, Kaplan SL, et al: Treatment of Cushing's disease in childhood and adolescence by transsphenoidal microadenomectomy. N Engl J Med 1984; 310:889–893.
270. Dyer EH, Civit T, Visot A, et al: Transsphenoidal surgery for pituitary adenomas in children. Neurosurgery 1994; 34:207–212.
271. Leinung MC, Kane LA, Scheithauer BW, et al: Long term follow-up of transsphenoidal surgery for the treatment of Cushing's disease in childhood. J Clin Endocrinol Metab 1995; 80:2475–2479.

272. Magiakou MA, Mastorakos G, Oldfield EH, et al: Cushing's syndrome in children and adolescents. Presentation, diagnosis, and therapy. N Engl J Med 1994; 331:629–636.
273. Howlett TA, Plowman PN, Wass JA, et al: Megavoltage pituitary irradiation in the management of Cushing's disease and Nelson's syndrome: long-term follow-up. Clin Endocrinol (Oxf) 1989; 31:309–323.
274. Estrada J, Boronat M, Mielgo M, et al: The long-term outcome of pituitary irradiation after unsuccessful transsphenoidal surgery in Cushing's disease. N Engl J Med 1997; 336:172–177.
275. Etxabe J, Vazquez JA: Morbidity and mortality in Cushing's disease: an epidemiological approach. Clin Endocrinol (Oxf) 1994; 40:479–484.
276. De Boer H, Blok GJ, van der Veen EA: Clinical aspects of growth hormone in adults. Endocrine Rev 1995; 16:63–86.
277. Melmed S: The Pituitary. Boston, Blackwell Science, 1995.
278. Cutler SJ, Young JL (eds): Third national cancer survey: incidence data. National Cancer Institute, Monograph 41. NLM 7512783 (DHEW publication no. NIH 75–787). Washington D.C., Government Printing Office, 1975.
279. Gicquel C, Baudin E, Lebouc Y, et al: Adrenocortical carcinoma. Ann Oncol 1997; 8:423–427.
280. Luton JP, Cerdas S, Billaud L, et al: Clinical features of adrenocortical carcinoma, prognostic factors, and the effect of mitotane therapy. N Engl J Med 1990; 322:1195–1201.
281. Icard P, Chapuis Y, Andreassian B, et al: Adrenocortical carcinoma in surgically treated patients: a retrospective study on 156 cases by the French Association of Endocrine Surgery. Surgery 1992; 112:972–980.
282. Pommier RF, Brennan MF: An eleven-year experience with adrenocortical carcinoma. Surgery 1992; 112:963–971.
283. Sabagga C, Avilla S, Schulz C, et al: Adrenocortical carcinoma in children: clinical aspects and prognosis. J Pediatr Surg 1993; 28:841–843.
284. Mendonca BB, Lucon AM, Menezes CAV, et al: Clinical, hormonal, and pathological findings in a comparative study of adrenal cortical neoplasms in childhood and adulthood. J Urol 1995; 154:2004–2009.
285. Venkatesh S, Hickey RC, Sellin RV, et al: Adrenal cortical carcinoma. Cancer 1989; 64:765–769.
286. Teinturier C, Brugieres L, Lemerle J, et al: Corticosurrénalomes de l'enfant: analyse rétrospective de 54 cas. Arch Pediatr 1996; 3:235–240.
287. Jensen JC, Pass HI, Sindelar WF, et al: Recurrent or metastatic disease in selected patients with adrenocortical carcinoma. Arch Surg 1991; 126:457–461.
288. Latronico AC, Chrousos GP: Adrenocortical tumors. J Clin Endocrinol Metab 1997; 82:1317–1324.
289. Ross NS, Aron DC: Hormonal evaluation of the patient with an incidentally discovered adrenal mass. N Engl J Med 1990; 323:1401–1405.
290. Kloos RT, Gross RT, Francis IR, et al: Incidentally discovered adrenal masses. Endocr Rev 1995; 16:460–484.
291. Peppercorn PD, Grossman AB, Reznek RH: Imaging of incidentally discovered adrenal masses. Clin Endocrinol (Oxf) 1998; 48:379–388.
292. Shapiro B, Fig LM, Gross MD, et al: Contributions of nuclear endocrinology to the diagnosis of adrenal tumors. Recent Results Cancer Res 1990; 118:113–138.
293. Weiss LM: Comparative histologic study of 43 metastasizing and non-metastasizing adrenocortical tumors. Am J Surg Pathol 1984; 8:163–169.
294. Weiss LM, Medeiros J, Vickey A: Pathologic features of prognostic significance in adrenocortical carcinomas. Am J Surg Pathol 1989; 13:202–206.
295. Gicquel C, Bertagna X, Schneid H, et al: Rearrangements at the 11p15 locus and overexpression of insulin-like growth factor–II gene in sporadic adrenocortical tumors. J Clin Endocrinol Metab 1994; 78:1444–1453.
296. Gicquel C, Bertagna X, Le Bouc Y: Recent advances in the pathogenesis of adrenocortical tumours. Eur J Endocrinol 1995; 133:133–144.
297. Tartour E, Caillou B, Tenenbaum F, et al: Immunohistochemical study of adrenocortical carcinoma. Predictive value of the D11 monoclonal antibody. Cancer 1993; 72:3296–3303.
298. Haak HR, Fleuren GJ: Neuroendocrine differentiation of adrenocortical tumors. Cancer 1995; 75:860–864.
299. MacFarlane DA: Cancer of the adrenal cortex: the natural history, prognosis, and treatment in a study of fifty-five cases. Ann R Coll Surg Engl 1958; 23:155–186.
300. Boven E, Vermorken JB, Van Slooten H, et al: Complete response of metastasized adrenal cortical carcinoma with Op′DDD. Cancer 1984; 53:26–29.
301. Van Slooten H, Moolenaar AJ, Van Seters AP, et al: The treatment of adrenocortical carcinoma with Op′DDD: prognostic implications of serum level monitoring. Eur J Cancer 1984; 20:47–53.
302. Epelman S, Gorender EF, Lopes LF, et al: The role of Op′DDD in childhood adrenal carcinoma [Abstract]. Proceedings of the American Society of Clinical Oncology 1990; 9:296.
303. Haak HR, Hermans J, Van de Velde CJH, et al: Optimal treatment of adrenocortical carcinoma with mitotane: results in a consecutive series of 96 patients. Br J Cancer 1994; 69:947–951.
304. Robinson BG, Hales IB, Henniker AJ, et al: The effect of Op′DDD on adrenal steroid replacement therapy requirements. Clin Endocrinol 1987; 27:437–444.
305. Haq MH, Legha SS, Samaan NA, et al. Cytotoxic chemotherapy in adrenal cortical carcinoma. Cancer Treat Rep 1980; 64:909–913.
306. Chun HG, Yogoda A, Kemeny N: Cisplatinum for adrenal cortical carcinoma. Cancer Treat Rep 1983; 76:513–514.
307. Hesketh PJ, McCaffrey RP, Finkel HE, et al: Cisplatin-based treatment of adrenocortical carcinoma. Cancer Treat Rep 1987; 71:222–224.
308. Bukowski RM, Wolfe M, Levine HS, et al: Phase II trial of mitotane and cisplatin in patients with adrenal carcinoma: a Southwest Oncology Group Study. J Clin Oncol 1993; 11:161–165.
309. Van Slooten H, Van Oosterom AT: CAP (Cyclophosphamide, Doxorubicin, and Cisplatinum) regimen in adrenal cortical carcinoma. Cancer Treat Rep 1983; 67:377–379.
310. Schlumberger M, Brugieres L, Gicquel C, et al: 5 Fluorouracil, Doxorubicin, and Cisplatin as treatment for adrenal cortical carcinoma. Cancer 1991; 67:2997–3000.
311. Johnson DH, Greco FA: Treatment of metastatic adrenal cortical carcinoma with cisplatin and etoposide (VP16). Cancer 1986; 58:2198–2202.
312. Burgess MA, Legha SS, Sellin RV: Chemotherapy with cisplatinum and etoposide (VP16) for patients with advanced adrenal cortical carcinoma (ACC) [Abstract]. Proceedings of the American Society of Clinical Oncology 1993; 12:188.
313. Bonacci R, Gigliotti A, Baudin E, et al: Cytotoxic therapy with etoposide and cisplatin in advanced adrenocortical carcinoma. Br J Cancer 1998; 78:546–549.
314. Decker RA, Elson P, Hogan TF, et al, for the Eastern Cooperative Oncology Group: Eastern Cooperative Oncology Group Study 1879. Mitotane and adriamycin in patients with advanced adrenocortical carcinoma. Surgery 1991; 110:1006–1013.
315. La Rocca RV, Stein CA, Danesi R, et al: Suramin in adrenal cancer: modulation of steroid hormone production, cytotoxicity in vitro, and clinical antitumor effect. J Clin Endocrinol Metab 1990; 71:497–504.
316. Dorfinger K, Niederle B, Vierhapper H, et al: Suramin and the human adrenocortex: results of experimental and clinical studies. Surgery 1991; 100:1100–1105.

27 *Alimentary Cancer*

LEONARD L. GUNDERSON, MD, Radiation Oncology
MICHAEL G. HADDOCK, MD, Radiation Oncology
RICHARD GOLDBERG, MD, Medical Oncology
PATRICK BURCH, MD, Medical Oncology
VICTOR TRASTEK, MD, Thoracic Surgery
JOHN DONOHUE, MD, General Surgery
HEIDI NELSON, MD, Colorectal Surgery

I hav finally kum to the konklusion that a good reliable sett ov bowels iz wurthmore tu a man than enny quantity ov brains.

HENRY WHEELER SHAW[1]

Perspective

Cancer of the alimentary tract continues to be a common health problem. Approximately 226,600 new cases of gastrointestinal (GI) malignancy were estimated to occur in the United States in 2000. Although colorectal tumors account for more than 50% of the relative incidence, cancer of the esophagus and stomach continue to occur with calculated regularity and high mortality. Hereditary factors play some role in the etiology of GI cancer, and increasing evidence implicates environmental toxins as causative agents.

A problem with some alimentary tract cancers relates to delay in clinical presentation. Signs that give early warning for other types of cancer (i.e., pain or palpation of a mass) do not occur early. Instead, patients often present with symptoms of obstruction or gross hemorrhage, which are usually associated with large primary tumors, high risk of metastasis, and a lower chance of cure. Physicians must search for earlier signs of GI cancer, and educate their patients to be aware of certain symptoms in order to make earlier diagnoses. In general, the early warning signs include vague abdominal discomfort, unexplained weight loss, change in bowel habits, or new onset of anemia. Routine sigmoidoscopy and stool testing for occult blood are recommended screening procedures. Other tests such as routine contrast radiography, upper endoscopy, or cytology analysis have yet to demonstrate cost effectiveness. Eventually, these screening procedures may apply to high-risk populations.

Although surgery remains the primary mode of treatment for cure of gastric and large bowel cancers, combined chemoradiation has become the primary treatment for anal cancer and offers an equivalent option to surgery alone for esophageal cancers. Surgery alone, however, has been unable to change survival rates over the last decade for gastric, esophageal, and large bowel cancers. Adjuvant and neoadjuvant utilization of radiation and chemotherapy offer the best prospect of improving cure rates.

A large number of investigational studies are being or have been performed with regard to the above strategies. With unresected esophageal cancers, combined chemoradiation has improved disease control and 5-year survival over irradiation alone in phase III randomized trials. For resected high-risk rectal and gastric cancers, postoperative chemoradiation has improved disease control and disease-free and overall survival when compared with surgery alone (both rectal and gastric) or adjuvant irradiation (rectal alone) control arms. Preoperative irradiation has also demonstrated improved local control and survival when compared with surgery alone for resectable rectal cancer in a large randomized trial from Sweden. For resected node-positive colon cancers, adjuvant chemotherapy with 12 months of 5-fluorouracil (5-FU) and levamisole or 6 months of 5-FU and leucovorin has produced improvements in disease-free and overall survival when compared with surgery-alone control arms. Finally, chemoradiation with its preservation of sphincter function has replaced surgical resection as the primary mode of treatment for most anal carcinomas, with surgical resection being reserved for salvage therapy. Although all of these positive trials are exciting and encouraging, refinements in multimodality therapy will necessitate continued enrollment of patients in clinical trials to help develop the most effective combined-modality treatment strategies for the future.

Esophagus

Perspective

The standard of care for limited esophageal cancer is surgery alone or external beam irradiation (EBRT) plus concomitant and maintenance 5-FU plus cis-diamminedichloroplatinum (cisplatin, CDDP). The finding that EBRT plus chemotherapy is better than EBRT alone represents the first major therapeutic advance with a documented impact on survival since the development of esophagectomy nearly 80 years ago.[11, 12] As with nearly all other significant advances in the treatment of malignant disease, this advance occurred as a result of a prospective randomized clinical trial.

Despite the aforementioned advance, long-term results for esophageal cancers remain poor regardless of method of treatment. The best hope for continued improvement remains a commitment by all physicians to entry of patients into well-designed clinical trials.

Epidemiology and Etiology

Epidemiology

Esophageal cancer accounts for approximately 5% of all GI malignancies.[2, 3] An estimated 12,300 new cases were expected to occur in the United States in 2000, with a male-to-female ratio of 3:1. The incidence is higher among blacks (3.5:1). Worldwide, China and southern Africa have the highest incidence, and other areas of relatively high risk are eastern Africa, South America, and southern Asia.[3] Esophageal cancer was the eighth most common cancer worldwide, with 316,000 new cases in 1990.[3] The estimated death rate for esophageal cancer was 12,100 in the United States in 2000. Worldwide it was the sixth most common cause of cancer deaths in 1990 at 286,000. Esophageal cancer is most common in elderly males over age 60, yet it may appear at a younger age in association with achalasia or hiatal hernia, although cancer is not associated frequently with either of these entities.

Etiology

Direct causative factors for esophageal cancer have not been established. However, numerous associated conditions have been identified as risk factors.[2, 3, 13, 14]

- *Environmental carcinogens* believed to be responsible or associated seem to show important geographic differences.[2, 15]
    - *Heavy alcohol* and *tobacco* use are independent risk factors for developing esophageal cancer and are associated with 80% to 90% of all cases of squamous cell cancers of the esophagus in North America and western Europe.[3] A combination of these two factors multiplies the risk even more.
    - Chronic consumption of *hot or heavily seasoned foods and liquids* has been associated with this disease, especially in regions of eastern and southern Africa; in South America, hot beverages, particularly hot maté (herbal infusion), are believed to be suspect.[3]
    - The extraordinarily high incidences of human esophageal cancer in humans and domestic chickens in northern China are believed to be related to *nitrosamines* in the food or water.[16] Similarly, it is thought that nutritional deficiencies, in addition to exogenous carcinogens, lead to high rates in China and central Asia.[3]
- Patients with *Plummer-Vinson syndrome* (sideropenic anemia, glossitis, esophagitis) have a 10% incidence of esophageal cancer, particularly common in Sweden.
- *Esophageal strictures* resulting from lye injuries put patients at risk for development of carcinoma.[17]
- Long-standing *achalasia* is associated with a 5% incidence of esophageal cancer. Performing a myotomy to relieve achalasia does not decrease this risk.
- *Barrett's esophagus,* a condition of gastric columnar epithelium extending more than 3 cm into the distal esophagus, is commonly associated with the occurrence of adenocarcinoma.[18–20] Although most adenocarcinomas of the distal esophagus arise from Barrett's esophagus, the incidence of this cancer developing in patients monitored with Barrett's epithelium is approximately 1 in 175 to 441 patient years. Antireflux therapy, medical or surgical, does not reduce this risk, which is almost 30 times the normal risk of developing carcinoma of the esophagus.
- The only hereditary transmission of esophageal cancer is among patients with *tylosis,* an autosomal dominant disorder characterized by hyperkeratosis of the palms and soles. Thirty-seven percent of these patients will develop squamous cell carcinoma of the esophagus.[21]

Detection and Diagnosis

Clinical Detection

Dysphagia and *weight loss* are the most common symptoms at presentation, occurring in 90% of patients. Other symptoms that may portend early disease include chest pain or *odynophagia* (pain with swallowing), but these are usually not severe enough to result in medical attention. Although screening procedures, such as endoscopy and cytology brushings, are common in Asia, they have not been cost effective in the United States.

Late signs due to invasion of adjacent organs include hoarseness (recurrent laryngeal nerve), superior vena cava syndrome, cough related to tracheal-esophageal or bronchial-esophageal fistula, Horner's syndrome (sympathetic nerves), paralyzed diaphragm (phrenic nerve), malignant pleural effusion, or massive hematemesis related to aorta-esophageal fistula, which is ominous.

Diagnostic Procedures

The basic work-up of a patient with esophageal cancer should consist of history, physical examination, barium esophagram, basic laboratory studies including complete blood count (CBC) and liver function tests, and esophagoscopy with ultrasound (Table 27–1).[4, 22–25] Patients with lesions of the middle or upper third of the esophagus should also have bronchoscopy. Computed tomography (CT) scan of the chest and upper abdomen is a useful adjunct to treatment planning and helps to exclude lung, liver and adrenal metastases.

- *Fluoroscopy* and *barium swallow*: Barium swallow is used to determine the length of the lesion, the extent of circumferential involvement, and the degree of obstruction. Characteristic findings of carcinoma include irregular filling defects, ulcerative strictures, and deviation or angulation of the barium column. Double contrast with air and barium may be used to find smaller lesions.
- *Esophagoscopy*: Flexible endoscopy with biopsy and cytology capabilities have improved the diagnosis of esophageal cancer. The combination of cytology brushings and biopsies of a mass will make the diagnosis of cancer with 90% accuracy.
- *Ultrasound*: Ultrasound with endoscopy, although a relatively new mode of assessment, is felt to be the most accurate diagnostic tool for determining depth of penetration through the esophageal wall and into surrounding structures,[26, 27] and it may also demonstrate enlarged nodes.
- *CT scans* of the chest and abdomen evaluate the presence of enlarged nodes, invasion of adjacent structures, as well as metastatic spread to lung, liver, or adrenal glands.[28]
- *Bronchoscopy* is especially important for lesions in the middle third of the esophagus to rule out invasion of the left main stem bronchus. Vocal cord function can also be assessed with this procedure.[28]
- *Exploratory laparotomy* with *biopsy* of celiac lymph nodes or sites of distant spread, or of both, is an important maneuver for clinical staging, which if positive may contraindicate radical surgery. For lower third lesions, celiac nodes are regional in nature, and microscopic involvement should not preclude resection, even though the current staging system classifies such involvement as M1a disease.

Classification and Staging

Histopathology

Although many esophageal cancers are still squamous histopathology (50% to 60%), the incidence of adenocarcinomas has increased in recent years, especially in the distal thoracic esophagus (40% to 50%).[12, 29, 30] It has been questioned whether these are true esophageal cancers or gastric cancers that have invaded the esophagus. The most convincing pathologic differences between these adenocarcinomas and gastric adenocarcinomas is the presence of Barrett's epithelium in the esophageal site.[29] Other unusual malignancies of the esophagus include adenosquamous variants, oat cell carcinoma, carcinosarcomas, and melanoma (usual incidence of 1% or less for each).

Anatomy and Pathways of Spread

The various divisions of the esophagus are as follows:

1. Cervical—from the bottom of the cricoid cartilage (C6) to the suprasternal notch, which spans 15 to 18 cm from the incisors; areas of potential direct extension—larynx, trachea, prevertebral fascia
2. Upper thoracic—from the suprasternal notch to the carina (T4 or T5), 18 to 24 cm from incisors; areas of direct extension—aorta, trachea, prevertebral fascia
3. Midthoracic—from tracheal bifurcation to esophagogastric junction, 24 to 32 cm; areas of possible direct extension—aorta, pericardium, left main stem bronchus, prevertebral fascia

TABLE 27–1. **Diagnostic and Imaging Procedures for Esophageal Cancer**

Method	Diagnosis and Staging Capability	Recommended for Routine Use
Primary Tumor and Regional Nodes		
Esophagogram	Useful to detect and define primary lesion, occasionally to demonstrate second tumor	Yes
Upper endoscopy	Detects and defines primary lesion; for lower 1/3 lesions, can determine extension into stomach	Yes
Endoscopy with ultrasound	Most accurate method of determining degree of extension within and beyond esophagus wall	Yes
CT—chest, abdomen	Most useful of all modalities for determining local invasion, regional node status, and metastasis	Yes
Percutaneous CT-guided biopsy	Used in neck and abdomen, rarely in chest	No (select cases only)
Metastatic Tumors		
Chest films	Good for detecting metastases and second primary	Yes
Ultrasound	CT as good or better than ultrasound in evaluating clinically suspected abdominal metastases	No
RN scans—liver, brain, bone	CT better than RN scans for liver, brain; bone scans used to define extent of metastases	No

CT = computed tomography; RN = radionuclide.

4. Lower thoracic—approximately 8 cm in length, which includes the abdominal esophagus, 32 to 40 cm from the incisors; areas of direct extension—aorta, pericardium, diaphragm, prevertebral fascia

The esophagus lies in close proximity to a number of vital structures in the neck and mediastinum, as noted in the preceding section on divisions of the esophagus. Once extension beyond the esophageal wall occurs, it is difficult to achieve good radial resection margins. Even with lesions limited to the esophageal wall, total removal of tumor may be difficult in view of tumor spread longitudinally (along mucosal layers, intermuscular spaces, and submucosal lymphatics), multicentric lesions, and skip metastases. The longitudinal growth pattern accounts for the 10% to 15% incidence of positive margins in esophagectomy specimens and for the predisposition of this tumor to relapse at the margins of surgical resection or irradiation fields.

The esophagus is permeated by an extensive submucosal lymphatic plexus, which results in the risk for skip metastases and frequent nodal involvement. Lymph node involvement is found in 50% to 70% of patients with carcinoma of the esophagus.[31–33] The main nodal areas at risk include the cervical, supraclavicular, mediastinal, and subdiaphragmatic areas (celiac axis, perigastric), although distribution of nodal involvement varies with the site of origin.[34] Nodal mapping data indicate that supraclavicular nodes are involved in 20% to 30% of patients and are usually nonpalpable.[31, 32] Neck or abdominal nodal involvement is not uncommon with an esophageal primary at any site.

Staging

Clinical staging (cTNM; Table 27–2) is based on the extent of the primary tumor as determined by pretreatment studies (Fig. 27–1).[5] These studies include physical examination, laboratory findings, radiologic imaging and esophagoscopy, and possibly endoscopy. Most cancers occur in the middle or distal third of the esophagus. Fifteen percent occur in the upper third of the esophagus and, by their critical location, are associated with a different mode of treatment.

Pathologic staging is based on data acquired clinically, along with the findings of surgical exploration and histologic examination of the pathologic specimen and regional lymph nodes (Fig. 27–2). A single staging classification serves both clinical and pathologic staging and all regions of the esophagus. Although celiac lymph node involvement constitutes metastatic disease (M1a) currently in the American Joint Committee on Cancer (AJCC) staging system, for distal third thoracic lesions it amounts to regional node disease. In the AJCC system, supraclavicular lymph node involvement is considered as regional nodal disease for patients with cervical lesions, but as distant metastasis in patients with thoracic esophageal cancer. For upper thoracic lesions, supraclavicular nodes can be considered as regional disease for the purposes of treatment planning and philosophy.

TABLE 27–2. **TNM Classification for Esophageal Cancer**

Stage	Grouping	TNM Descriptor
Stage 0	Tis, N0, M0	Tis: Carcinoma *in situ* (into mucosa only) N0: No regional node metastases M0: No distant metastasis
Stage I	T1, N0, M0	T1: Tumor invades lamina propria or submucosa
Stage IIA	T2–3, N0, M0	T2: Invades muscularis propria T3: Invades adventitia
Stage IIB	T1–2, N1, M0	N1: Regional lymph node metastasis
Stage III	T3, N1, M0 T4, Any N, M0	T4: Invades adjacent structures (or adherent to)
Stage IV	Any T, Any N, M1	M1: Distant metastasis*

T = tumor; N = node; M = metastases.

*Lower thoracic tumors: M1a—celiac nodes, M1b—other distant metastases; upper thoracic tumors: M1a—cervical nodes, M1b—other distant metastases; midthoracic—only M1b applicable.

Used with permission of the American Joint Committee on Cancer (AJCC®), Chicago, Illinois. The original source for this material is the AJCC® Cancer Staging Manual, 5th ed, 1997, published by Lippincott-Raven Publishers, Philadelphia, Pennsylvania.

Principles of Treatment

Esophageal cancer is a disease that is rarely localized at diagnosis, and it is characterized by a high incidence of local-regional and distant spread at death. Any successful treatment strategy must address these issues. Frequent sites of local disease outside the esophagus at autopsy include trachea (54%), mediastinum (13%), lung (16%), pleura (7%), aorta (6%), and heart (5%).[35] Patterns of failure at autopsy include 83% with local plus regional plus distant spread, 53% liver, 35% lung, 11% bone, 8% adrenals, and 4% brain.[36] For patients who present without distant metastases, a multidisciplinary approach is essential to achieve desirable outcomes and is presented in Table 27–3.

Surgery

Surgery is the standard treatment of choice for patients with early stage cancers of the esophagus (stage 0, I, or IIa) who are capable of withstanding a major operation. Operative mortality ranges from 3% to 10% depending on patient selection and the experience and expertise of the individual surgeon.[33] Following esophagectomy, the 5-year survival for curative resections is as high as 22%, but for all patients resected, 5-year survival is less than 10%.[21, 23, 33, 37] Despite low overall survival rates, surgical resection offers good palliation of dysphagia. In one study, over 50% of patients had no recurrence of dysphagia after esophagectomy, and most patients with recurrent dysphagia were eating satisfactorily.[33]

The principles of surgical treatment for esophageal cancer include extended longitudinal resection because of the tendency for submucosal spread. More than 40% of patients will have involvement of the submucosa 5 cm beyond the gross extent of the tumor.[38] Attempts at maximal radial resection margins are also optimal, although difficult to obtain. Many surgeons, including those at the Mayo Clinic, recommend near total thoracic esophagectomy as minimal treatment. The most widely used approach is a midline laparotomy to mobilize the stomach and rule out metastatic disease. This is followed by a right thoracotomy

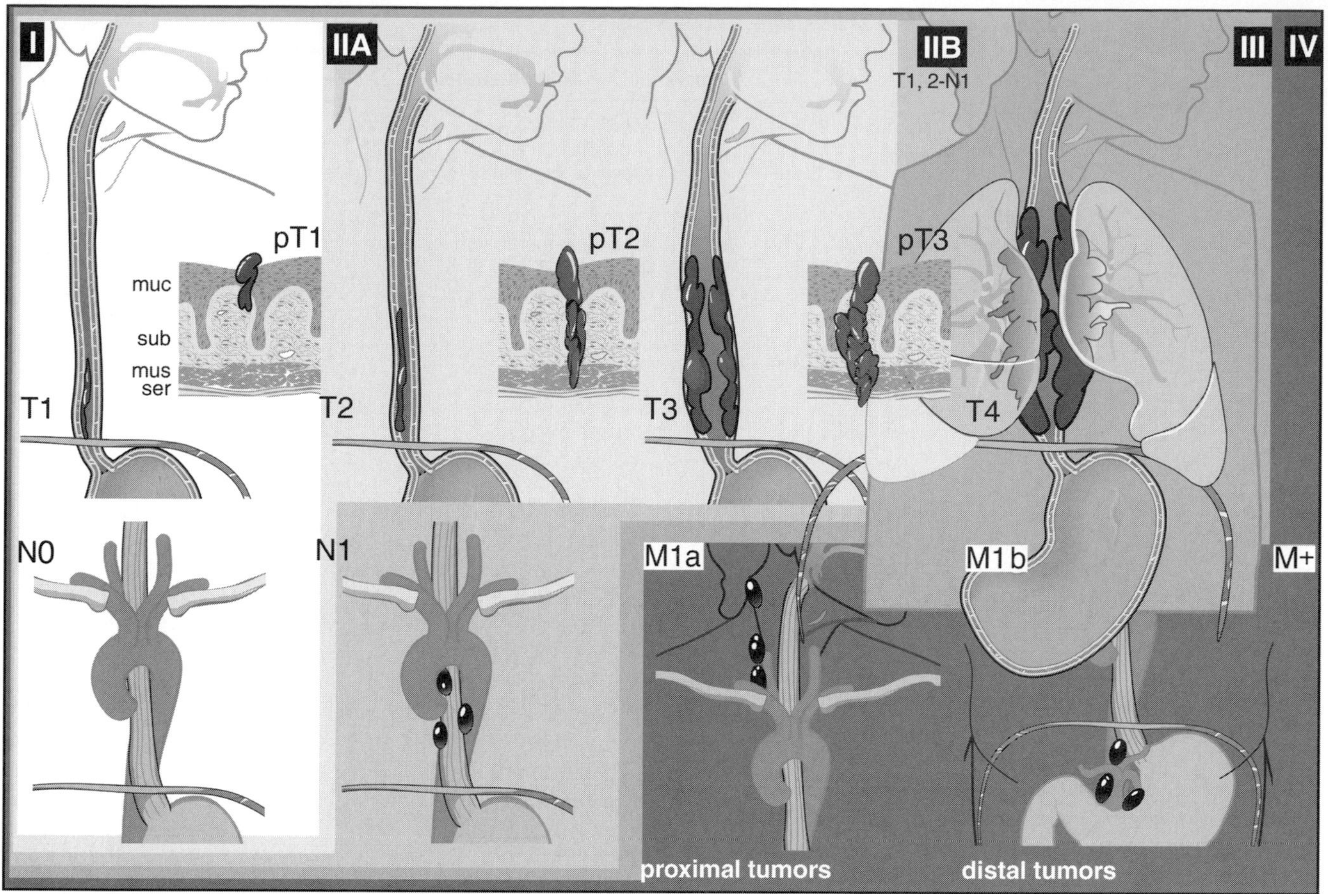

Figure 27–1. Anatomic staging for cancer of the esophagus.

for esophagogastrectomy and subsequent anastomosis (the Ivor-Lewis approach).

Reconstruction is usually accomplished by esophagogastrostomy in the posterior mediastinum with the stomach brought through the resection bed. Depending on the location of the primary tumor, anastomosis may be at the level of the apex of the chest or in the neck through a separate cervical incision. Other alternatives include interposition with colon or jejunal segments.[39] Following preoperative irradiation or chemoradiation, the anastomosis is preferably placed in the neck because the risk of anastomotic leak may be increased. An anastomotic leak in the neck is more easily controlled and less morbid than are those that occur in the thorax.

Some surgeons have converted to esophagectomy without thoracotomy (transhiatal esophagectomy). The esophagogastric anastomosis is performed in the neck. The abdominal exploration and mobilization of the stomach is the same as for the Ivor-Lewis approach. Comparative studies have shown reduced respiratory morbidity with this procedure and no differences in tumor relapse.[40]

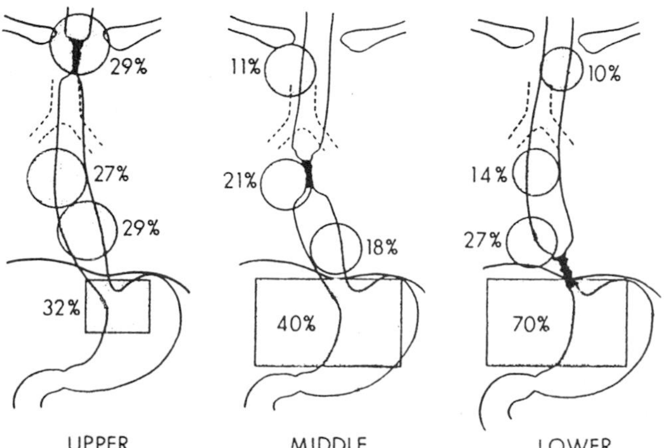

Figure 27–2. Percentage of positive nodes found at surgery for esophageal carcinoma in the upper, middle, and lower esophagus.

Radiation Therapy

Esophageal epidermoid carcinomas are radioresponsive[6, 7, 11, 12, 41–44] and local tumor eradication is attainable with irradiation alone; however, both disease control and survival are better with irradiation plus concurrent and maintenance chemotherapy (standard of treatment for nonsurgical disease). Combined chemoradiation is favored over surgery for lesions above the aortic arch because surgical mortality rates rise for upper thoracic esophageal lesions without improvement in surgical outcome.[45]

Irradiation alone, or in conjunction with chemotherapy, has also been successful in palliating pain and improving dysphagia in 65% to 80% of cases. In 1.8- to 2.0-Gy fractions, the palliation dose is close to the definitive dose

TABLE 27–3. **Multidisciplinary Treatment Decisions: Esophagus**

	Stage	Surgery	Irradiation + Chemotherapy		Chemotherapy
I	T1, N0, M0	Esophagectomy and anastomosis	DCCRT 50–60 Gy for lesions above aortic arch	and	5-FU + cisplatin, concurrent with RT and maintenance
II	T1–2, N1, M0 and T3, N0	If good response to RT, then resection attempted	ACCRT preop or postop 45–50 Gy	and	Same chemo
III	T3, N1, M0 and T4, N0–1	Bypass procedure if obstruction is severe	DCCRT 50–70 Gy or preop ACCRT 45–50 Gy then attempt resection	and	Same chemo
IV	Any T, Any N, M+	Bypass procedure if obstruction is severe	NR or PCCRT 50 Gy		Same or IC II

5-FU = 5-fluorouracil; RT = irradiation; DCCRT = definitive concurrent chemotherapy and irradiation; ACCRT = adjuvant concurrent chemotherapy and irradiation; PCCRT = palliative concurrent chemotherapy and irradiation; NR = not recommended; IC II = investigational chemotherapy, phase I/II clinical trials.

Adapted from Physicians' Data Query. Esophageal cancer. Bethesda, National Cancer Institute, June 1999.

at 50 to 60 Gy. Another potentially palliative schedule is 50 Gy in 20 fractions of 2.5 Gy over 4 weeks.[29, 46, 47]

Technical Considerations—Irradiation

Technical considerations in the radiotherapeutic management of esophageal cancer can be divided into field size considerations, treatment planning considerations, and total dose.

The only paper to address the issue of field size comes from Princess Margaret Hospital in the era before combined chemoradiation. No relationship between field size and long-term survival was found.[43] A 5-cm margin or preferably greater is traditionally recommended both proximal and distal to the primary lesion, and this margin is reasonable in view of the propensity for submucosal spread of this disease. Although Pearson initially suggested margins of 5 cm or greater,[41, 42] others have demonstrated a marginal failure rate of 15% to 25% with 5-cm margins.[48, 49] On the basis of this information, Wayne State investigators have recommended inclusion of the entire thoracic esophagus in the initial target volume.[49] The field should be large enough to include major nodal areas at risk, as long as this does not result in a major increase in morbidity. Most treatment plans that adequately cover the primary lesion will also treat the immediate lymph nodes at risk. Treatment of supraclavicular nodes is optional for patients with thoracic esophagus lesions, but it is probably worthwhile in upper and middle third thoracic lesions, assuming fields can be designed to result in no appreciable increase in morbidity. Major increase in field size to cover the celiac axis is of uncertain benefit, but those nodal groups should definitely be included for lower thoracic lesions or those that extend into the stomach.

In treatment planning, three-point setup and isocentric technique with the patient supine are basic techniques used in the treatment of esophageal cancer at the Mayo Clinic. When setting up treatment for a patient with a middle or upper third lesion, the lateral setup marks will invariably fall on the shoulders, arms, or axilla. Such a three-point setup is certain to be unreliable because slight movements of the arms will result in significant deviation of the lateral setup marks. Therefore, a second set of points lower on the thorax should be used to position the patient. After the patient has been positioned in the actual treatment position, the anteroposterior (AP) setup distance should be carefully checked. If it is not the same on a day-to-day basis, the patient is probably not being consistently set up in the same way each day. Anteroposterior-posteroanterior (AP-PA) fields are generally the most reproducible.

Generally, up to 40 Gy can usually be delivered safely by AP-PA fields. The remainder of the dose can be given via obliques or laterals to keep the spinal cord dose at 45 Gy or less. After a dose of 45 Gy, field length is usually reduced to tumor plus 2 to 2.5 cm, and boost fields receive an additional 5.4 to 25 Gy (total dose of 50 Gy or greater for chemoradiation and 60 to 70 Gy for irradiation alone in patients who cannot tolerate concomitant chemotherapy). Lateral fields are easier to verify on port films than obliques, but they have the disadvantage of treating more lung; the dose via lateral fields should therefore be limited to 18 Gy or less. An axis of rotation isocentric technique should be used to set up lateral and oblique fields. For bulky lower esophageal lesions, lateral fields have an advantage over oblique fields in sparing the heart. Use of lateral fields for transcervical-thoracic lesions generally requires some form of compensation technique, such as tissue equivalent wax bolus material.[50] As an alternative to the use of laterals, obliques can be highly reproducible if extreme care is used in patient setup.

Although doses of 60 to 70 Gy were typically recommended in the treatment of esophageal cancer prior to the routine use of combined-modality therapy, there are very few data on which to base this recommendation. In an Eastern Cooperative Oncology Group (ECOG) study, for example, no difference in survival was seen between patients receiving greater or less than 55 Gy (with or without bleomycin). At Massachusetts General Hospital, local failure rates were consistently about 50% over a range of doses from 50 to 69 Gy.[51] At the University of Florida, 3 of 5 patients were locally controlled with greater than 67 Gy and 1 of 9 was controlled with less than 67 Gy.[50] At Rush Presbyterian St. Luke's, complete symptom relief was seen in 77% of patients treated with a time-dose fractionation (TDF) of less than 100 (TDF of 100 is approximately equal to 60 Gy at 2.0 Gy/day).[48]

Radiation Tolerance of Esophagus and Surrounding Structures

The esophagus is quite tolerant to irradiation alone in the 60- to 70-Gy range. In order to treat to this high dose, it is necessary to avoid exceeding tolerance to the spinal cord, heart, and lungs, as discussed previously. Acute side effects of irradiation are mainly dysphagia, which has its onset after 20 to 30 Gy and regresses within 1 to 2 weeks of completion. Because of the marginal nutritional status of many of these patients, alimentation in the form of percutaneous gastric tubes, percutaneous endoscopic gastrostomy tubes, or a feeding jejunostomy may be necessary. Although irradiation has been implicated as a cause of esophageal strictures, the stricture is often related to persistent or recurrent disease or may also be related to fibrous tissue replacement of a circumferential cancer that has completely regressed after chemoradiation. Myelitis as a complication should be rare given the knowledge of spinal cord tolerance, CT treatment planning, and off cord oblique or lateral fields. Pericarditis or significant radiation pneumonitis should be rare with the use of careful irradiation fields as discussed previously. There is further discussion in Chapter 34, Late Effects of Cancer Treatment.

Chemotherapy

There have been a number of phase II studies with traditional chemotherapy agents for locally advanced or metastatic esophageal cancer. Cytotoxic drugs with objective response rates greater than 10% include bleomycin, cisplatin, 5-FU, mitomycin C, doxorubicin, methotrexate, lomustine, and vindesine.[52–54] In addition, 2 newer drugs, paclitaxel and vinorelbine, have demonstrated single-agent activity.[55, 56]

Several phase II studies of multiagent chemotherapy have been performed for locally advanced or metastatic esophageal cancer or both (Table 27–4). Caution needs to be employed in interpreting results especially when comparing studies. Problems include mixtures of regional and metastatic cases, evaluable and measurable disease, and variable amounts of squamous versus adenocarcinoma histologies. In addition, some studies used local treatment modalities after chemotherapy. Table 27–4 includes results of a number of phase II studies, almost all of which are based on combination regimens that include cisplatin. An effort has been made to identify the breakdown of local-regional compared with metastatic disease. Reports where a significant percentage of patients subsequently received surgery or irradiation were excluded. Generally, response rates are in the range of 30% to 50% and median survival is 6 to 8 months. Some of the newer paclitaxel-containing regimens have looked more promising; however, randomized trials have not been performed. These responses have generated enthusiasm for a number of current studies looking at neoadjuvant regimens that include chemotherapy and irradiation.

Combined-Modality Therapy

Attempts to improve response rates, disease control, and survival in this disease have resulted in combined-modality chemoradiation used in combination with surgical resection or as definitive therapy (see Table 27–3).

- *Preoperative irradiation* alone or in combination with chemotherapy has theoretical advantages, such as reduction of tumor bulk to improve surgical resectability, reduction in transplantable tumor cells by the surgery, curative effect on disease in the paraesophageal region, and sterilization of occult foci in lymph nodes. A variety of studies for preoperative irradiation alone have been reported; most have shown no improvement in survival but rather an increase in complications.[78–83] Initial trials evaluating preoperative irradiation plus

TABLE 27–4. **Combination Chemotherapy in Esophageal Cancer**

Treatment	No.	Met/Loc	Resp (%)	Med Surv (Mos)	Reference
CDDP/Bleo	29	14/15	52	7.0	Marcuello[57]
CDDP/Bleo	18	18/0	17	4.0	Coonley[58]*
CDDP/Vind	31	NR/NR	19	NR	Iizuka[59]
CDDP/Bleo/Mtx	34	16/18	26	5.0	DeBesi[60]
CDDP/Bleo/Mtx	10	9/1	50	7.5	Vogl[61]
CDDP/Vind/Bleo	68	26/0	33	NR	Kelsen[62]*
CDDP/Vind/Bleo	27	20/7	29	3.5	Dinwoodie[63]
CDDP/MMC/Ifos	20	7/13	20	NS	Allen[64]
CDDP/VP-16	73	70/3	48	8.5	Kok[65]
CDDP/5-FU	39	NR/NR	36	NR	Iizuka[66]
CDDP/5-FU	40	19/21	35	NR	DeBesi[67]
CDDP/5-FU/Dox	21	15/6	33	8.0	Gisselbrecht[68]
CDDP/5-FU/Epi	107	NR/NR	55	NR	Bamias[69]†
5-FU/IFL	40	30/10	27	6.4	Kelsen[70]
5-FU/IFL	21	11/10	25	NR	Wadler[71]
CDDP/5-FU/IFL	27	23/4	50	7.6	Ilson[72]
CDDP/5-FU/IFL	23	13/10	65	8.6	Wadler[73]
CDDP/5-FU/IFL	22	22/0	73	6.0	Pai[74]
CDDP/5-FU/Tax	19	7/12	69	13.0	Garcia-Alfonso[75]
CDDP/5-FU/Tax	61	47/14	48	10.8	Ilson[76]
CDDP/CPT-11	21	20/1	53	NR	Enzinger[77]

CDDP = cisplatin; Bleo = bleomycin; Vind = vindesine; Mtx = methotrexate; MMC = mitomycin C; Ifos = ifosfamide; VP-16 = etoposide; 5-FU = 5-fluorouracil; Dox = doxorubicin; Epi = epirubicin; IFL = interferon; Tax = paclitaxel; CPT-11 = irinotecan; NR = not reported; Met = metastatic disease; Loc = local-regional; Resp = response; Med Surv = median survival; Mos = months.

*Metastatic patients only.

†Esophagus and esophagogastric junction patients only.

chemotherapy also suggested no improvement in survival.[84, 85] More recently, studies utilizing preoperative irradiation plus concomitant chemotherapy have, however, shown improvement in both disease control and survival.[86–93]

- *Postoperative irradiation* should ideally allow one to select the most suitable patients for adjuvant therapy. However, survival has not been improved with postoperative irradiation as a single adjuvant in most reports.[94–96] Pilot studies are ongoing in our institution to evaluate adjuvant postoperative chemoradiation.

Primary Chemoradiation

Investigators at Wayne State were the first to report on a combined-modality approach for squamous cell carcinoma of the esophagus using preoperative chemoradiation. Surgical specimens were pathologically free of disease in 5 of 15 patients (33%).[85] In a larger, nonrandomized study performed by Southwest Oncology Group (SWOG), 71 of 106 evaluable patients had surgery; pathology specimens were free of disease in 18 of 71 (25%) and complete responders had a longer survival.[97] The Radiation Therapy Oncology Group (RTOG) reported on a similar trial with similar results[98]; however, toxicity was significant and surgical mortality was increased.

Because the role of surgery came into question from the preoperative chemoradiation trials, various investigators decided to proceed with chemoradiation alone.[44, 49, 99–104] Both nonrandomized and randomized trials show improvement over historical controls of irradiation alone (nonrandom Wayne State[49] and Princess Margaret Hospital[44]) or randomized controls.[11, 12, 44, 49, 99–106] Results have been improved with regard to disease control and survival at 2 years (30% to 40%) and at 5 years (15% to 30%). Accordingly, combined chemoradiation has become the treatment of choice for nonsurgical candidates.

Treatment According To Clinical Stage

Stages I and II

Surgical resection with reconstruction is the primary mode of treatment. Preoperative chemoradiation can be used to decrease local relapse but has not been demonstrated in randomized studies to alter overall survival. Postoperative adjuvant chemoradiation pilot studies may be applicable depending on the pathologic stage (ongoing at the Mayo Clinic).

Stage III

Chemoradiation alone can achieve significant palliation, if not cure, of these patients. Selected patients may be candidates for an attempt at resection after preoperative chemoradiation, depending on the performance status of the patient and location of the primary tumor. Many of these patients may require parenteral or enteral hyperalimentation during treatment. Smaller (boost) irradiation fields should be used to deliver the higher doses of irradiation that are being evaluated to determine the impact of higher dose on local control and survival.

Stage IV

Radical surgery or irradiation is contraindicated in this group of patients with disseminated disease. Effective palliation without major morbidity and mortality is difficult. Silastic tubes can be used to bypass obstructive lesions. Laser therapy offers hope for better palliation of this group.

Special Considerations of Treatment

Treatment Complications

Esophagectomy and *reconstruction* is an extensive surgical endeavor that may result in considerable morbidity and significant mortality. Early complications include anastomotic leak and respiratory failure. Later complications may include anastomotic strictures, reflux esophagitis, and motility disorders.[107, 108]

The *intolerance* to *irradiation* or *chemoradiation* depends upon normal tissue tolerance and varies with type of tissue, volume irradiated, total dosage, and rate of administration. The type of complication depends upon the structure involved:

- *Esophagus*: During therapy, soreness with swallowing is common; perforation or hemorrhage due to rapid tumor dissolution is rare. A late effect is stricture.
- *Lung*: Radiation pneumonitis may occur during the early post-treatment period, and late effects include radiation fibrosis. This is fortunately an infrequent complication that usually occurs in a small volume of lung.
- Other structures, such as heart and spinal cord, are rarely involved with serious intolerance. Transverse myelitis should be avoidable with modern multiple field design shielding techniques.

There is a wide range of *chemotherapy toxicities* that depend upon which drugs are given. Using chemotherapeutic agents requires careful consideration because of their limited palliative gains.

Palliation

Local invasion of vital structures, presence of distant metastases, or severe debilitation renders 60% of patients with esophageal cancer unresectable. The alternatives for palliative care include:

- *Substernal gastric bypass*: Substernal gastric bypass leaves the esophagus in place and creates a bypass conduit using the stomach placed through the anterior mediastinum. This procedure has become less desirable with reports of significant morbidity and mortality (26%), and survival no greater than 5 months.[109, 110]
- *Irradiation*: External irradiation is 50% to 60% successful for palliation of dysphagia. Intracavitary supplementation with radioactive iridium may improve this figure,[111, 112] but an increase in the occurrence of treatment-related fistulas has also been reported in at least one pilot study.[113]
- *Dilatation* and *intubation*: Placement of prosthetic tubes to stent malignant obstructions of the esophagus

has been used for many years. These devices are probably no more successful at palliation than dilation alone with Bougie or Maloney dilators. Morbidity from aspiration pneumonia and migration of the prosthetic tubes is high.[114, 115]

- *Laser therapy*: Endoscopic Nd:YAG and argon laser treatments, with or without photodynamic dyes, are recent advances in palliation of the unresectable carcinoma. Generally, three to five sessions of laser therapy are required in conjunction with dilation to establish patency in most obstructing tumors. Bleeding, perforation, and fistula formation have been reported, but symptoms are improved in 80% to 90% of patients.[116, 117]
- *Gastrostomy* and *cervical esophagostomy*: These procedures rarely provide good palliation and are discouraged except for the rare situations in which a debilitated patient is receiving neoadjuvant treatment with the hope of undergoing subsequent resection. Feeding jejunostomy would be preferable in these cases to preserve later use of the stomach for reconstruction.

Results and Prognosis

Single-Modality Treatment

Surgical Results

Surgery remains the primary strategy in patients with stage I and IIa disease. Surgical results will be discussed as a reference point for comparing results with irradiation alone or various forms of combined-modality treatment.

In a survey of 122 reports describing results in 83,783 patients, 58% underwent surgical resection.[37] Of this group of approximately 48,594 patients, 22% died as a result of surgery. The 5-year survival of patients undergoing surgery was 7%. It is critical to recognize that these results reflect a broad overview of the world's literature.

In centers where a large volume of surgery for esophageal carcinoma is performed, results are often much better. For example, in a survey of 748 patients treated at the Mayo Clinic between 1956 and 1965, the 3-year and 5-year survival rates were 23% and 15% and the hospital death rate was 12%.[118] A later report of 100 patients treated at the Mayo Clinic disclosed a 5-year survival of 22% and a 3% hospital mortality rate.[33] For early stage patients (T1–2,N0), 5-year survival was 86% (7 patients T1,N0) or 34% (11 patients T2,N0) versus 15% for the remaining 82 patients with positive nodes or higher T stage. Immediate palliation of dysphagia was satisfactory in 97% of patients. Although 40 patients developed late dysphagia, the dysphagia was satisfactorily palliated with dilation in the 35 cases in which the etiology was benign. Results from other centers also suggest that when surgeons have extensive experience in the treatment of esophageal cancer, mortality can be kept to a minimum.

Radiation Alone

Results of irradiation alone for esophageal cancer are extremely poor. Pearson has reported 5-year survival in the range of 17% to 20%.[41, 42] These numbers are the best figures in the literature, and other reports have not come close to these results. This finding is probably related to case selection. In the original 1969 paper,[41] the 20% survival figure was quoted for patients "treated radically." In that paper, no indication was provided regarding factors that led to selection of a patient for "radical treatment." It is worth noting, however, that only 39% of patients treated by irradiation were treated "radically." In a 1977 paper, it was stated that "The main reason for not attempting radical treatment was extensive tumor; for instance, a primary tumor demonstrably more than 10 cm long (or less for particularly frail, old patients), tumor infiltrating the trachea or bronchi, remote lymphatic metastases, or demonstrable liver or lung or other blood borne metastasis."[42] In general, most reports indicate a 2-year survival rate of 11% or 12%.[44, 51] Three-year to 5-year survival rates run in the range of less than 1% to 7%.

Patterns of Relapse

Local-regional relapse (or persistence) and distant metastases are both extremely frequent after any treatment ap-

TABLE 27–5. **Clinical Relapse Patterns in Esophageal Carcinoma**

Treatment Modality	Series Analyzed, n	Total Patients, n	Site of Relapse, %		
			Primary	*Mediastinum/neck*	*DM*
Irradiation (EBRT)	6	1382	56–85	10–43	36–50
Surgery	5	729	8–50	40–50	17–69
Surgery ± EBRT*	3		Locoregional		DM
1. Surgery		189	30; 67; 52		46; 50
2. Pre- or postop EBRT		156	15; 46; 48		52; 50
EBRT ± Chemo	2				
1. EBRT		93	62; 84		40; 23
2. EBRT + Chemo		89	44; 61		23; 32

DM = distant metastases; EBRT = external beam irradiation; n = number; Chemo = chemotherapy.

*Randomized trials only; each randomized group is paired by a vertical line.

Adapted from Gunderson LL, Martenson JA, Smalley SR, et al: Upper gastrointestinal cancers: rationale, results, and techniques of treatment. Front Radiat Ther Oncol 1994; 28:121–139.

proach (Table 27–5). Autopsy series in untreated patients reveal nodal involvement in 80% to 85% and cancer restricted to the local-regional area in about one third. Autopsy series[119] demonstrate the problem with distant metastases (chiefly lung and pleura, liver, and bone) as well as local-regional recurrence, which occurs as the only failure in 25% to 40% of patients.

In irradiation-only series, local-regional disease is the dominant clinical problem and site of relapse (see Table 27–5).[42, 120, 121] Although Pearson's results with irradiation alone surpass other published results, 80% of the radically irradiated patients failed to survive 5 years, and approximately half died from local relapse.[42]

Evaluations of failure patterns after surgical resection and adjuvant treatment also reveal a high incidence of local-regional failure (see Table 27–5).[121] This failure results from tumor bed or anastomotic relapse and progression in dissected or undissected nodal regions.

Combined-Modality Treatment

In an effort to improve the dismal results with irradiation alone or surgery alone in the treatment of esophageal cancer, various combinations of irradiation, surgery, and chemotherapy have been applied (Table 27–6). Combined-modality therapy (CMT) in any form subjects patients to the toxicity of more than one modality of treatment. Trials showing superior results for irradiation plus chemotherapy compared with irradiation alone will be described.

Preoperative External Beam Irradiation

Preoperative external beam irradiation (EBRT) has been employed in an attempt to improve on the results of conventional therapy. Some retrospective comparisons of EBRT plus surgery versus surgery alone do suggest improvement in survival with CMT. In Akakura's report from Keio University, 5-year survival among patients receiving EBRT plus surgery was 25% versus 14% among patients treated with surgery alone.[78] However, fatal complications were higher among patients receiving CMT at 21% versus 13%. Other retrospective studies suggest a worse survival with EBRT plus surgery in comparison to surgery alone.[122, 123]

Five prospective randomized studies of surgery versus preoperative EBRT plus surgery have been performed in patients with esophageal cancer. Three of these studies have not shown any difference in survival.[79, 81–83] Guo-Jun and associates have reported a randomized prospective study in which patients treated with preoperative EBRT plus surgery had a 5-year survival of 45% in comparison to only 25% among those patients treated with surgery alone.[80] No details regarding the time-dose fractionation scheme for the preoperative EBRT are provided in the brief report. Moreover, no information is provided regarding whether the difference in survival is statistically significant. Clearly, although this report is intriguing, full-length detailed publication of results will be needed before any consideration can be given regarding this study as evidence favoring combined-modality preoperative EBRT plus surgery. A study from Scandinavia comparing results in patients randomized to 35 Gy preoperative EBRT (with or without chemotherapy) followed by surgery versus surgery (with or without preoperative chemotherapy) without preoperative EBRT suggested a survival benefit for patients who received preoperative EBRT.[90] An imbalance in prognostic factors favored the preoperatively irradiated patients (there were nearly twice as many T1 patients who received EBRT).

Preoperative Chemotherapy

Preoperative chemotherapy as a single adjuvant has been tested in single-institutions[124–126] and randomized trials.[90, 127–129] Neither the three small randomized trials[90, 127, 128] nor

TABLE 27–6. **Nonsurgical Treatment of Locoregional Esophageal Cancer**

Reference	Treatment Plan	No. of Patients	Survival			
			Median (mo)	*1-Year (%)*	*2-Year (%)*	*5-Year (%)*
Randomized						
Herskovic[11]	Cisplatin 75 mg/m² + 5-FU 1000 mg/m²/d × 96 h weeks 1, 5, 8, 11 + RT 50 Gy (2-Gy Fx) vs.	61	12.5*	52*	36*	27
Al-Saraf[12]	RT 64 Gy (2-Gy fx)	60	8.9	34	10	0
Pilot Studies						
Leichman[85]	Cisplatin 100 mg/m² + 5-FU 1000 mg/m² × 96 h × 2 cycles + RT 30 Gy, mitomycin + bleomycin + RT 20 Gy	20	22	—	—	
Coia[105]	Mitomycin 10 mg/m² day 1 + 57; 5-FU 1000 mg/m²/d × 96 h days 2 + 29 + RT 60 Gy	57	18	—	—	
Lokich[101]	5-FU 300 mg/m² CI weeks 1–6; 5-FU + RT weeks 6–10	13	16	—	—	

RT = irradiation; CI = continuous infusion; Gy = gray; Fx = fractions.
*Survival at 1, 2 and 5 yr.
Difference statistically significant; p = 0.0001 in randomized Radiation Therapy Oncology Group trial (chemotherapy concurrent with irradiation weeks 1 and 5 and as maintenance weeks 8 and 11).
Updated from Al-Saraf M, Martz K, Herkovic A, et al: Progress report of combined chemo-radiotherapy vs radiotherapy alone in patients with esophageal cancer: an intergroup study. J Clin Oncol 1997; 15:277–284.

the larger intergroup phase III trial[129] demonstrated a survival benefit for preoperative chemotherapy.

Preoperative External Beam Irradiation Plus Chemotherapy

Combined preoperative treatment with chemotherapy and EBRT is another method that has been employed in an attempt to improve upon the dismal results of single-modality therapy[86–93, 130] (Table 27–7). At Wayne State University, a combination of EBRT, 30 Gy in 3 weeks, with 5-FU and mitomycin C was used preoperatively.[84] Surgery followed 4 to 6 weeks after completion of EBRT-chemotherapy. Patients with residual tumor following surgery had additional EBRT and chemotherapy. Among 30 patients initially entered into the protocol, 23 subsequently underwent surgery. The hospital mortality rate among this group of patients was 30%. Six patients had no residual cancer at the time of their operation and four of these patients were 5-year survivors. Seventeen patients had residual cancer and all died. One of 6 patients who did not have surgery was alive at 4 years. The overall results with this regimen were not better than that which might have been expected with single-modality therapy alone. A second regimen, similar to the first Wayne State program, substituted cisplatin for mitomycin C. Similar poor results were achieved in terms of survival and hospital mortality in patients who underwent surgery.[85]

The most important study of preoperative chemotherapy and radiation therapy was published in 1996 by Walsh and colleagues[86] (Fig. 27–3). Patients with adenocarcinoma of the esophagus were randomized to receive preoperative EBRT (40 Gy in 15 fractions), 5-FU (15 mg/kg per day continuous infusion [*approximately* equivalent to 600 mg/m^2] per day for 5 days, weeks 1 and 6) and cisplatin (75 mg/m^2 on the first day of each 5-FU infusion), followed by surgical resection 8 weeks after completion of radiation therapy *or* immediate surgery. A highly significant difference in survival was observed with CMT (intent to treat—median survival 16 vs. 11 months, 3-year survival 32% vs. 6%, p = 0.01; actual treatment—median survival 32 vs. 11 months—p = 0.001, 3-year survival 37% versus 7%—p = 0.006).

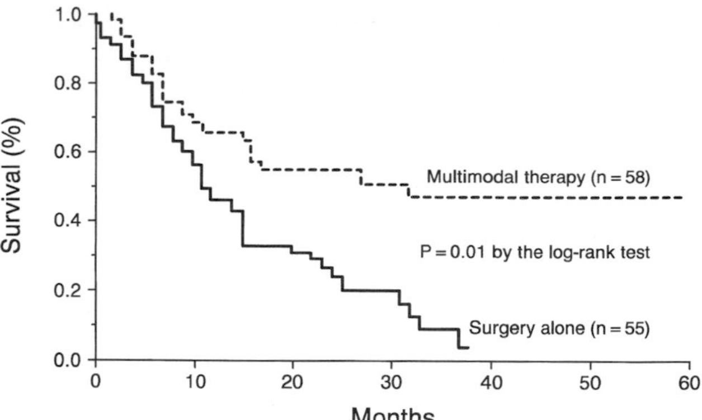

Figure 27–3. Dublin phase III trial of preoperative combined-modality therapy versus surgery alone for adenocarcinoma of the esophagus. Survival analysis by intent to treat favors the multimodal therapy (p = 0.01). (From Walsh TN, Noonan N, Hollywood D, et al: A comparison of multimodal therapy and surgery for esophageal adenocarcinoma. N Engl J Med 1996; 335:462–467.)

Urba and colleagues, from the University of Michigan, have also found a survival advantage for patients treated with preoperative chemoradiation versus surgery alone.[87–89] Preoperative treatment involved 5-FU, cisplatin, and vinblastine given concurrently with irradiation. Patients with either squamous or adenocarcinomas were eligible, but a

TABLE 27–7. **Preoperative Chemoradiotherapy for Eosophageal Cancer—Phase II–III Trials**

Reference	No. of Patients	Preoperative Treatment	Pathologic CR Rate (%)	Survival: *Median (mo)*	*3 yr OS*	*p*
Pilot Studies						
Leichman[85]	21	EBRT 30 Gy/5-FU–CDDP	5/19 (26)	18	—	—
Forastiere[87]	43	EBRT 37–45 Gy/5-FU–CDDP–VBL	10/41 (24)	29	—	—
Poplin[97]	113	EBRT 30 Gy/5-FU–CDDP	18/71 (25)	12	—	—
Seydel[98]	41	EBRT 30 Gy/5-FU–CDDP	8/27 (29)	13*	—	—
Randomized						
Walsh (Dublin Trial)[86]	55	a) Surgery alone vs.	—	11	6%	
	58	b) EBRT 40 Gy in 15 Fx; 5-FU–CDDP	13/52 (25)	16 †	32%	0.01
Urba (U Michigan)[87–89]	50	a) Surgery alone vs.	—	18	15	
	50	b) EBRT 45 Gy/1.5 Gy b.i.d.; 5-FU–CDDP–VBL	14/50 (28)	18	32	0.04‡
Nygaard (Scandinavian)[90]	91	a) Surgery ± CDDP/Bleo vs.	—	7.2§	6	
	95	b) EBRT 35 Gy in 20 Fx ± CDDP Bleo	—	9.2§	19	0.009
Bosset (French/ EORTC)[91]	139	a) Surgery alone vs.	—	18.6	28 (DFS)	
	143	b) EBRT 37 Gy in 10 Fx; CDDP 0–2 d before EBRT	29/112 (26)	18.6	40 (DFS)	0.003

CR = complete response; EBRT = external beam irradiation; 5-FU = 5-fluorouracil; CDDP = cisplatin; VBL = vinblastine; Bleo = bleomycin; Fx = fractions; OS = overall survival; DFS = disease-free survival.
*Mean survival.
†Actual treatment—median survival: 11 vs. 32 mo [p = 0.001] and 3-yr survival: 7% vs. 37% [p = 0.006].
‡p value = 0.07 (log-rank) or 0.04 (Cox regression).
§Data taken from published figure.

majority of the 100 randomized patients had adenocarcinoma. Survival differences favoring trimodality treatment did not appear until several years of follow-up with 3-year survival of 15% for surgery alone and 32% for multimodality treatment (p = 0.04 Cox regression, 0.07 log-rank). A confirmatory intergroup trial was initiated in North America in an attempt to validate the positive results found in the small trials by Walsh and associates[86] and Urba and coworkers.[87–89]

In a trial conducted by the French Foundation of Digestive Cancer and the European Organization for Research and Treatment of Cancer (EORTC) (Fig. 27–4), 297 patients were randomized to surgery alone versus preoperative chemoradiation.[91] Of the 282 eligible patients, 139 were assigned to surgery alone and 143 to preoperative adjuvant treatment. Those randomized to receive preoperative treatment had longer disease-free survival at 3 years (p = 0.003), improved local control (p = 0.01), a lower rate of cancer-related deaths (p = 0.002), and a higher rate of curative resection (p = 0.017). There was also a higher rate of postoperative death in the preoperative chemoradiation group (p = 0.012), which along with the lack of maintenance chemotherapy likely contributed to a lack of difference in both median and long-term survival.

Postoperative External Beam Irradiation or Chemotherapy

Postoperative EBRT has been advocated as yet another method of improving on the dismal results of single-modality therapy. Such treatment has been advocated for patients with adverse prognostic factors such as positive mediastinal lymph nodes, invasion of tumor through the entire esophageal wall, or close surgical margins. Published data on this topic, however, show lack of benefit for postoperative EBRT as a single adjuvant in patients with surgical-pathologic stage III esophageal cancer. Kasai and associates, for example, found the 5-year survival to be 18% in node-positive patients with surgery alone versus only 11% in patients with postoperative EBRT.[94] Although results in node-negative patients were more optimistic (surgery alone—17%, postoperative EBRT—85%), such results have not been evaluated in detail in other series. Two randomized trials have either shown no benefit for postoperative EBRT[93] or have indicated that postoperative EBRT may result in decreased survival.[92] Available evidence indicates, then, that postoperative EBRT, as a single adjuvant, subjects patients to the additional toxicity and expense of EBRT without any benefit.

In summary, it is our feeling that neither postoperative adjuvant EBRT nor adjuvant chemotherapy should be used as a single adjuvant. At the Mayo Clinic, we are evaluating combined-modality postoperative EBRT in conjunction with interrupted infusion 5-FU plus CDDP in a controlled phase I–II clinical trial.

External Beam Irradiation Plus Chemotherapy

For unresected lesions, the combined chemoradiotherapy approach appeared to improve both local control and survival in nonrandomized trials,[44, 49, 98–104, 131] and it has definitely demonstrated such in randomized trials.[12, 104, 106, 111, 132]

Although two early prospective randomized trials failed to establish a role for EBRT plus chemotherapy,[133, 134] several nonrandomized single-institution reports of EBRT plus infusion 5-FU combinations were encouraging.[44, 49, 99–104, 131] A report from Princess Margaret Hospital was particularly interesting.[44] Patients treated with infusion 5-FU and mitomycin C plus EBRT to doses of 40 to 50 Gy in 20 fractions were compared with patients treated with EBRT alone. Although the study was nonrandomized, patients were matched for major prognostic factors. Both survival and local control were better in the combined-modality group. Although this study cannot substitute for a randomized prospective trial, the findings of the Princess Margaret Group were encouraging.

ECOG completed a phase III trial comparing (1) EBRT, 5-FU, and mitomycin C plus surgery with (2) EBRT with or without surgery.[104, 106] The decision for patients to receive surgery in the ECOG trial was not randomized but was based on clinical choice following randomization. Median survival was 9 months for EBRT with or without surgery versus 14.9 months for EBRT, 5-FU, mitomycin C with or without surgery (p = 0.03), and overall survival at 2 years was 12% versus 27%.

The landmark study in esophagus cancer was the phase III trial by the RTOG, which compared EBRT alone (64 Gy) with EBRT (50 Gy) plus concomitant and maintenance 5-FU and CDDP.[11, 12] A marked survival benefit and disease control were noted among the combined-modality patients[11] (Table 27–8; Fig. 27–5). Actuarial 2-year survival was 42% versus 10% (p = 0.0009) and actuarial local control at 2 years was 53% versus 30% (p = 0.01) favoring chemoradiation. The final results of this study have been reported.[12]

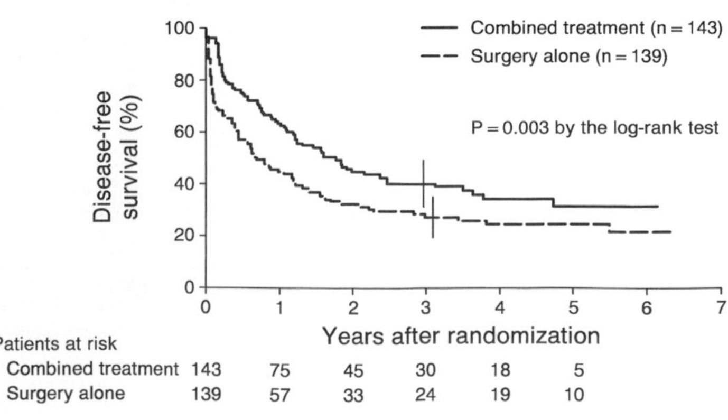

Figure 27–4. French/EORTC phase III trial of surgery ± preoperative chemoradiation. Disease-free survival rate is better with the combined-modality treatment (p = 0.003). (From Bosset JF, Gignoux M, Triboulet JP, et al: Chemoradiotherapy followed by surgery compared with surgery alone in squamous cell cancer of the esophagus. N Engl J Med 1997; 337:165.)

TABLE 27–8. **Primary Irradiation Without or with Chemotherapy for Esophageal Cancer—RTOG 85–01 Phase III Trial**

Survival Estimates (Kaplan-Meier)						
			EBRT-CT			
	EBRT Only (Randomized)		***Randomized***		***Nonrandomized***	
Years	*At Risk (No.)*	*Alive (%)*	*At Risk (No.)*	*Alive (%)*	*At Risk (No.)*	*Alive (%)*
0	62	100	61	100	69	100
1	21	34	32	52	42	63
2	6	10	22	36	23	35
3	0	0	18	30	13	26
4	0	0	15	30	3	—
5	0	0	10	27	0	—
Dead/Total	62/62		45/61		50/69	
Median (mo.)	9.3		14.1		17.2	

RTOG = Radiation Therapy Oncology Group; EBRT = external beam irradiation; CT = chemotherapy.
Randomized comparison: Log-rank $p < 0.0001$; Cox $p < 0.0001$.
Modified from Al-Saraf M, Martz K, Herkovic A, et al: Progress report of combined chemo-radiotherapy vs radiotherapy alone in patients with esophageal cancer: an intergroup study. J Clin Oncol 1997; 15:277–284.

With a minimum follow-up of 5 years, the 5-year survival is 27% in the patients treated by CMT and 0% in the patients treated by EBRT alone ($p < 0.0001$). Results in the CMT arm of the study are comparable to some of the best single-institution results found in the surgical literature. The RTOG trial establishes combined EBRT plus 5-FU and CDDP as the standard of care for the nonsurgical management of esophageal cancer.

Clinical Investigations

Screening

Screening of high-risk populations with endoscopy and cytology brushings is an important area of investigation. Asian investigators have shown that earlier detection of carcinoma of the esophagus should lead to higher cure rates. For patients in the United States, however, it is difficult to define a group of patients at high enough risk to justify routine screening.

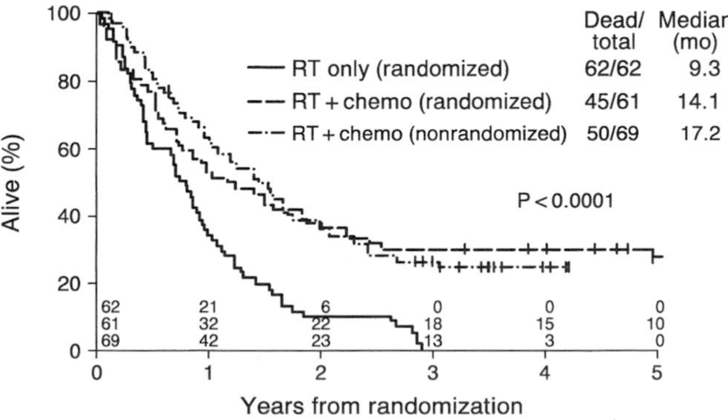

Figure 27–5. RTOG trial 85-01 of primary irradiation ± chemotherapy, with survival rate advantage to chemoradiation ($p < 0.0001$). (From Al-Saraf M, Martz K, Herkoric A, et al: Progress report of combined chemo-radiotherapy vs radiotherapy alone in patients with esophageal cancer: An intergroup study. J Clin Oncol 1997; 15:283.)

Combined-Modality Treatment

For patients with resectable early cancers who are suitable candidates for surgery (Tis–T2, N0), surgery alone remains the standard of treatment in the United States. For patients with a high risk factor of extension beyond the muscularis propria (T3 or T4) or nodal involvement (N1 or M1a), results from the Walsh study for adenocarcinoma of the esophagus and gastric cardia and from the University of Michigan for squamous cell and adenocarcinomas of the esophagus suggest that trimodality therapy may be preferable if it can be given safely. In the United States, a GI intergroup study was initiated to serve as a confirmatory study to both the Walsh and University of Michigan trials, in that patients with either squamous cell cancer or adenocarcinomas were eligible. The control arm was surgery alone and the study arm was preoperative chemoradiation (50.4 Gy in 28 fractions over 5½ weeks plus concurrent and maintenance 5-FU plus cisplatin). However, the study was closed early due to poor accrual.

In patients who are not suitable candidates for or who do not desire surgery, the current standard of care is combined-modality chemoradiation with external irradiation plus concurrent and maintenance 5-FU plus cisplatin. Since approximately 50% of patients in the positive RTOG trial had local relapse or persistence of disease at the dose of 50 Gy plus 5-FU plus cisplatin and approximately 25% developed distant metastases, a replacement intergroup phase III trial was designed to test an increase in EBRT dose intensity but was closed when no advantage was seen with the higher dose of 64.4 Gy versus 50 Gy. An alternate approach to irradiation dose intensification would be utilization of a brachytherapy supplement to EBRT (50 Gy) plus chemotherapy. A single-institution pilot study of 95 patients was presented at the American Radium Society meeting in 1999[135] (personal communication). In this study, patients received 45 to 55.8 Gy per EBRT (1.8 Gy per fraction) plus concomitant 5-FU plus cisplatin, followed by high-dose rate (HDR) brachytherapy (63 of the 95 received 10 Gy in 2 fractions with a 2-week break after EBRT and between fractions). There were no treatment-related deaths or fistulas.

For patients with T4,N0–1 lesions who are potential candidates for resection, acceptable treatment options would include either definitive chemoradiation or well-controlled phase II trials testing preoperative chemoradiation and resection. Supplemental intraoperative irradiation with electrons or HDR brachytherapy could be given in institutions with those options available. Maintenance chemotherapy should also be considered. Randomized trials could compare definitive chemoradiation with trimodality treatment or definitive chemoradiation with 5-FU plus cisplatin versus taxol-containing chemoradiation regimens.

Systemic Therapy

The current focus of systemic therapy revolves around two major areas: advanced disease and preoperatively with or without irradiation. As previously discussed, single adjuvant preoperative chemotherapy has not improved survival in three small trials and one large randomized trial.[90, 127–129] Intergroup efforts have been conducted to evaluate preoperative chemoradiation in a confirmatory large study to follow up on the positive smaller trials by Walsh and colleagues[86] and Urba and coworkers[87–90] for preoperative chemoradiation versus surgery alone.

Given reports of activity both as a single agent and in combination with cisplatin and 5-FU, paclitaxel is being evaluated in a number of pilot regimens for locally advanced and potentially resectable disease.[136] Ongoing trials are also in progress evaluating new agents such as irinotecan, vinorelbine and gemcitabine in combination with cisplatin for patients with advanced disease.

Irradiation Field Design

In the positive RTOG trial for chemoradiation versus irradiation as primary treatment,[11, 12] the initial irradiation field extended from the supraclavicular fossa to the esophagogastric junction except in lower third lesions where inclusion of the supraclavicular region was optional. Nodal groups were included to 50 Gy in the irradiation-alone patients (plus 14-Gy primary boost) versus 30 Gy with combined irradiation plus chemotherapy (plus 20-Gy primary boost).

The current intergroup phase III chemoradiation trials are using fields that encompass the primary tumor plus initial esophageal margins of at least 5 cm. After a dose of 45 to 50 Gy, fields are reduced to tumor plus 2 cm, and the boost field dose is carried to 50 to 64.4 Gy. Because more extended fields were used in the positive RTOG trial, results in the two studies will need to be compared to determine potential differences in local control or survival between extended versus more restrictive irradiation fields.

At present, a high percentage of patients still have persistence or relapse of the primary lesion. Until better local control can be achieved, it will be hard to determine the relevance of extended-field lymphatic irradiation, dose levels necessary for nodal regions, and so forth. This information may be more easily collected in an adjuvant setting where the addition of surgery should improve the ability to control the primary lesion.

Stomach

Perspective

The standard of care for resectable gastric cancer in patients who can tolerate a surgical procedure is surgical resection. However, many patients with gross total resection of their malignancy are not cured by surgery alone. Because both local and systemic relapses are common after resection of high-risk gastric cancers (beyond wall, nodes positive, or both), trimodality treatment is indicated for these patients. Results of a phase III trimodality trial that confirmed a benefit for trimodality treatment versus surgery alone will be presented in this section, and future trial designs will be discussed.

For patients with locally advanced disease that appears unresectable for cure, several treatment options appear to favorably impact disease control and survival. These include primary EBRT plus concomitant chemotherapy, maximal resection plus intraoperative irradiation (IORT) and preoperative chemotherapy or chemoradiation prior to resection. Results of these approaches and future trial design will be presented.

In the setting of metastatic disease, there are many active chemotherapy agents that can produce meaningful response alone or in combination with other agents, but the duration of response is often limited. Trials now exist that demonstrate both a survival and quality of life benefit for multidrug chemotherapy versus best supportive care for patients with metastatic cancers. Results of these trials will be discussed.

Epidemiology and Etiology

Epidemiology

Gastric carcinoma is expected to be the tenth leading cause of cancer death in the United States in 2000 with 13,000 deaths.[2] However, for unknown reasons, the frequency of gastric cancer has been steadily decreasing over the past 50 years; the death rate from this disease was five times greater in the 1930s. The estimated new cases for 2000 in the United States are 21,500; 13,400 will be male and approximately 8100 will be female.

Although the incidence of gastric cancer has decreased

significantly in the United States, on a worldwide scale, gastric cancer has a very high incidence and is still a leading cause of cancer death.[3, 137] In 1999, the expected world incidence was 798,000 (the third most common malignancy, exceeded only by lung and breast cancers) with an expected 628,000 deaths (exceeded only by lung at 921,000).[3] Gastric cancer is especially common in Japan (78 per 100,000 males, 33.3 per 100,000 females), other eastern Asia countries, China, eastern Europe, and South American countries.

Etiology

Gastric cancer is associated with dietary and environmental causes, as well as other factors.[138]

- *Diet*: Diets high in poorly preserved, highly salted, and smoked foods are associated with an increased risk of gastric cancer,[139, 140] whereas diets rich in fruits and vegetables are associated with a reduced risk.[141] Nitrosamines and nitrosamides are known gastric carcinogens. Some evidence suggests that food containing ascorbic acid antagonizes these mutagenic chemicals.
- *Environment*: Potential occupational risks for developing gastric cancer are the following: coal mining, nickel refining, rubber working, and asbestos exposure.
- The *transformation* of a benign gastric ulcer into a cancer is rare. However, gastric carcinomas are frequently ulcerative and misdiagnosed as benign ulcers. A gastric ulcer that fails to heal is always suspect for malignancy.
- *Gastric polyps* are not precancerous unless villous changes are found on histopathology; villous adenomas of the stomach have a definite association with malignancy. In general, biopsies should be performed on all gastric polyps, and all polyps greater than 2 cm in size should be excised.
- The risk of developing gastric carcinoma is 2.4 times greater in individuals who have previously had *resection for ulcer disease.* These cancers occur anywhere from 15 to 40 years after the initial resection.
- *Helicobacter pylori* infection is associated with increased risk of gastric cancer.[142–144] The precise role of this bacterium in the etiology of gastric cancer, however, remains unknown.[143, 144] Only a minority of infected patients develop gastric cancer, and data do not yet exist on the effect of treatment of the *H. pylori* infection on subsequent malignancy.

Detection and Diagnosis

Clinical Detection

Vague epigastric discomfort is the most frequent symptom associated with gastric cancer, and other common presenting symptoms or signs include loss of appetite, weight loss, weakness (due to anemia), nausea, and vomiting and melena. None of the symptoms or signs are usually manifestations of early disease. Duration of symptoms is less than 3 months in about 40% of patients and longer than 1 year in only 20%.[145, 146]

- *Physical findings*: Positive findings on physical examination for gastric cancer are invariably related to metastatic or locally unresectable disease. One third of patients will have signs of metastatic or locally advanced primary disease, that is, palpable abdominal or epigastric mass (primary tumor, liver or ovarian metastasis), ascites, jaundice, left supraclavicular adenopathy (Virchow's node), left axillary adenopathy (Irish's node), rectal shelf (peritoneal seeding), or generalized cachexia on initial presentation.
- *Laboratory findings* indicate that about 85% of patients have anemia and 50% have guaiac-positive stools. Hypoalbuminemia is also common.

Diagnostic Procedures

Diagnostic procedures for gastric cancer are described in Table 27–9.[4, 145]

- *Stool examination* for occult blood.
- *Upper GI series* is an accurate (and the most common) method of detecting malignant gastric lesions, but approximately 10% of malignant gastric lesions may be missed unless a double-contrast technique is used. Lesions with smooth, sharply defined borders and rugal folds that radiate from the ulcer are usually benign. Malignant lesions generally have elevated irregular margins and rugal folds that do not radiate from the ulcer. Duodenal invasion carries a poor prognosis. The UGI contrast study usually underestimates the extent of disease.
- *Endoscopy*: Flexible gastroscopy allows visualization and biopsy of most gastric lesions and yields diagnosis in approximately 90% of cases. Generous biopsies of all gastric ulcers should be performed. Infiltrative lesions are least likely to be biopsied accurately. *Ultrasound* performed at the time of endoscopy has become the most accurate method of defining degree of extension of the primary lesion.
- *CT scan* of the abdomen and pelvis is a valuable technique for detecting evidence of metastatic spread to liver or ovaries and the degree of extragastric local extension. CT scanning adds information for presurgical staging of the primary lesion.[147] In addition, extragastric extension posteriorly, relative to the celiac vessels or pancreas, may be visualized on CT as well as the presence of enlarged nodes. Obliterations of the lesser sac might indicate unresectability of the primary tumor. CT has not been successful in the determination of local invasion into the gastric wall and is even less sensitive for gastric lymph node involvement, although helical CT studies may be more sensitive than standard CT for evaluation of nodes.[148]
- *Staging or diagnostic laparoscopy* should be considered in patients with more than early cancer who have no obstruction, bleeding, or other cause for surgical palliation. This technique has proven to be very sensitive and specific for disease in both the Memorial Sloan Kettering and M.D. Anderson experiences.[149, 150] This technique will spare patients nontherapeutic and nonpalliative laparotomies.
- At present, *laparotomy* remains the final and most accurate procedure for staging and assessment of resectability. Studies have shown that using laparotomy

TABLE 27–9. **Diagnostic and Imaging Procedures for Gastric Cancer**

Method	Diagnosis and Staging Capability	Recommended for Use
Primary Tumor and Regional Nodes		
Single-contrast upper GI studies	Useful in detecting and defining primary lesions in stomach	Yes
Double-contrast upper GI studies	Very useful in detecting early gastric cancers	Yes—should be performed along with single-contrast
Gastroscopy	Very accurate modality to detect and define primary lesions: ~90% confirmation rate	Yes—use to confirm lesion detected in UGI series and to screen high-risk patients
CT—abdomen ± chest	Most valuable of all modalities for determining degree of extragastric extension and distant metastases	Yes
Endoscopic ultrasound	Most accurate method of determining extension within and beyond gastric wall	Yes—if plan preoperative chemoirradiation
Metastatic Tumors		
Chest films	Good for detecting metastases	Yes
Laparoscopy	May allow visualization of small serosal implants or liver metastases	Yes—if plan preoperative chemotherapy or chemoradiation
Bone film	Useful only for confirming metastases	No—unless patient has bone pain
Radionuclide scans—liver, brain, bone	Useful in evaluation of clinically suspected metastases; CT is better than nuclide scans for liver and brain	No—unless suspected bone metastases

GI = gastrointestinal; UGI = upper gastrointestinal; CT = computed tomography.

for staging does not increase mortality rates and provides the best information for effecting cure or palliation.[151] However, in view of increased experience with laparoscopy, this procedure may replace laparotomy as the tool for assessing abdominal dissemination of malignancy in institutions that are evaluating preoperative chemotherapy or chemoirradiation prior to resection.

- *Exfoliative cytology* using abrasive balloon or chymotrypsin lavage is highly accurate when positive. However, it is time consuming and requires skilled personnel.[152]

Classification and Staging

Histopathology

Adenocarcinoma is the most common malignant tumor of the stomach, comprising 90% to 95% of these lesions.[153] Other histologies include lymphoma, leiomyosarcoma, carcinoid, and squamous cell carcinomas.[153] Histologic subtypes of adenocarcinomas include intestinal (because it resembles intestinal mucosa), signet ring cells, and anaplastic. The gross appearance of gastric adenocarcinomas is characterized by four different types of presentation, which are important for their varied prognosis:

1. Ulcerative carcinoma is the most common and is the reason to perform biopsies on all gastric ulcers.
2. Polypoid cancers or fungating are also common, and all polypoid lesions should be surgically excised.
3. Diffusely infiltrating or scirrhous carcinoma has the worst prognosis. These lesions infiltrate the gastric wall producing a thickened, nodular, foreshortened stomach that is referred to as *linitis plastica.*
4. Superficial gastric cancer is an uncommon variety that is characterized by sheet-like collections of cancer cells replacing the normal mucosa.

Staging

Clinical staging: The current TNM (tumor, lymph nodes, metastasis) staging system[5, 153, 154] is depicted in Table 27–10[5] and Figure 27–6. Portions of this system are compared in Table 27–11 with a modification of the Astler-Coller rectal system suitable for all alimentary tract carcinomas.[154] The modified Astler-Coller system is more inclusive with respect to degree of extension beyond the wall, but the TNM system has a better description of nodal involvement and level of gastric invasion for lesions confined to the gastric wall.

Stage grouping (see Tables 27–10 and 27–11): Stage classification depends on anatomic extent of the disease that is most reliably assessed at the time of surgical exploration. Some clinical studies such as CT scanning, gastroscopy with or without endoscopic ultrasound, and laparoscopy are helpful for identifying patients with advanced local disease or metastases, which may obviate the need for surgical exploration.

Principles of Treatment

All methods of treating gastric cancer suffer from the predominance of advanced stage disease at the time of presentation; stage of disease is the most important predictor of outcome for any treatment modality. Most patients who present with gastric cancer have disease outside the stomach at diagnosis, but this may not be known without surgical staging with laparoscopy or laparotomy. Generally about 20% to 30% of patients will be considered inoperable at diagnosis because of metastatic disease or medical contraindications. The remaining patients will undergo surgery, which at this time is the main treatment modality that influences survival for patients in whom complete resection with negative margins can be attained. Of the 75% of patients who undergo surgical exploration, 20% will be

TABLE 27–10. **TNM Staging for Carcinoma of the Stomach**

Stage	Grouping	TNM Descriptor
Stage 0	Tis, N0, M0	Tis: Carcinoma *in situ*; intraepithelial tumor without invasion of the lamina propria N0: No regional lymph node metastasis M0: No distant metastasis
Stage IA	T1, N0, M0	T1: Tumor invades lamina propria or submucosa
Stage IB	T1, N1, M0	N1: Metastasis in 1–6 regional nodes
	T2, N0, M0	T2: Tumor invades the muscularis propria or the subserosa
Stage II	T1, N2, M0	N2: Metastasis in 7–15 regional nodes
	T2, N1, M0	
	T3, N0, M0	T3: Tumor penetrates the serosa (visceral peritoneum) without invasion of adjacent structures
Stage IIIA	T2, N2, M0	
	T3, N1, M0	
	T4, N0, M0	T4: Tumor invades adjacent structures
Stage IIIB	T3, N2, M0	
	T4, N1, M0	
Stage IV	T1, N3, M0	N3: Metastasis in more than 15 regional nodes
	T2, N3, M0	
	T3, N3, M0	
	T4, N1–3, M0	
	Any T, Any N, M1	M1: Distant metastasis present

Metastasis to other intra-abdominal lymph nodes such as hepatoduodenal, retropancreatic, portal, mesenteric, or para-aortic are considered distant metastasis within this system, but are N3 or N4 in the Japanese Research Society Classification.[153]

Used with permission of the American Joint Committee on Cancer (AJCC®), Chicago, Illinois. The original source for this material is the AJCC® Cancer Staging Manual, 5th ed, 1997, published by Lippincott-Raven Publishers, Philadelphia, Pennsylvania.

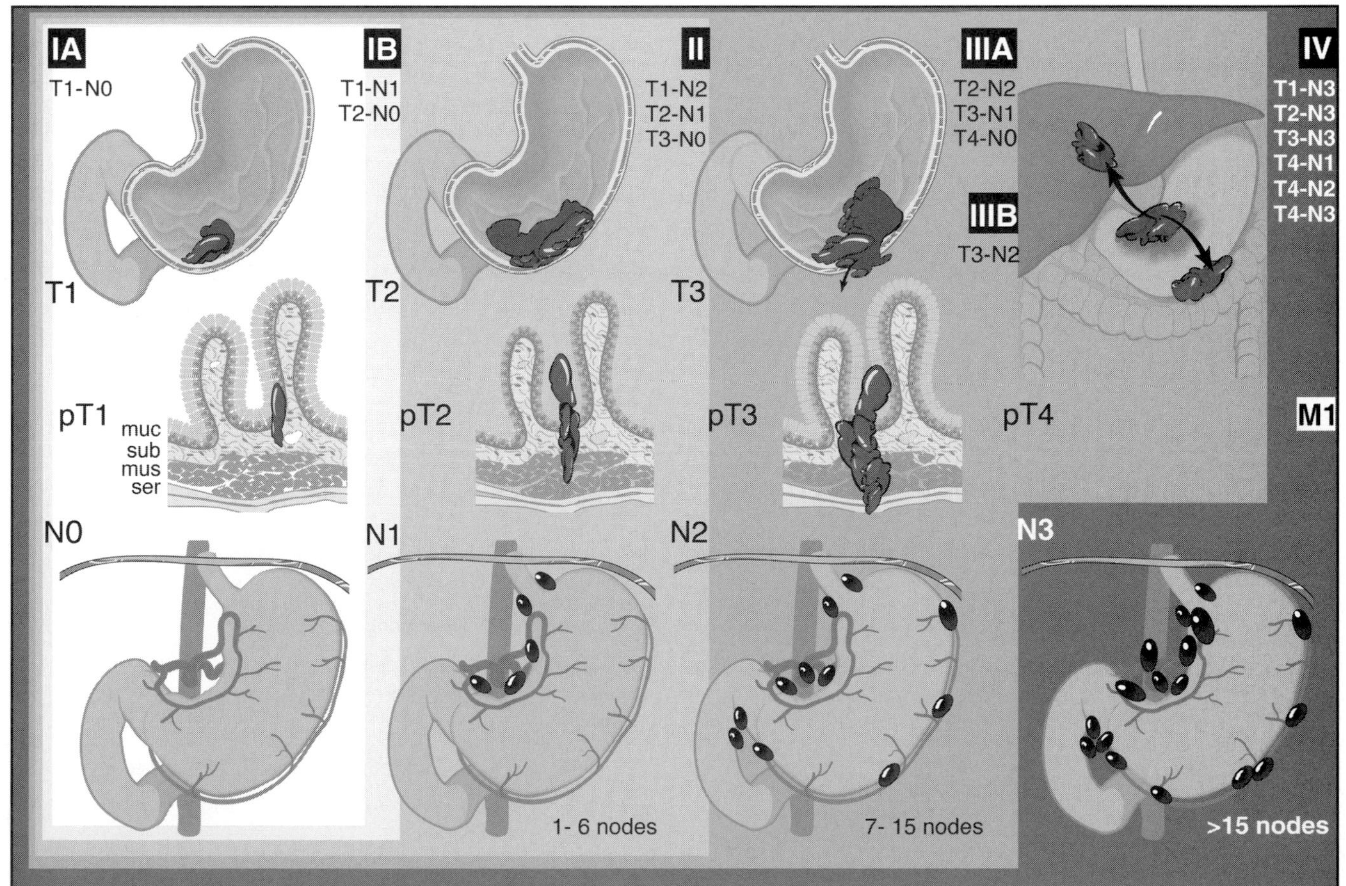

Figure 27–6. Anatomic staging for cancer of the stomach.

TABLE 27–11. **Staging Systems for Gastric Carcinoma: Comparison of TNM System[5] with a Modification of the Astler-Coller Rectal System by Gunderson and Sosin[154]**

Staging System		
Modified Astler-Coller	***TNM***	**Characteristics**
A	Tis, N0	Nodes negative; lesion limited to mucosa
B1	T1–2, N0	Nodes negative; extension of lesion beyond mucosa but still within gastric wall
B2	T3, N0	Nodes negative; extension beyond the entire wall (including serosa if present)
B3	T4, N0	Nodes negative, beyond wall with adherence to or invasion of surrounding organs or structures
C1	Tis–T2, N1–3	Nodes positive; lesion limited to gastric wall
C2	T3, N1–3	Nodes positive; extension of lesion through the entire wall (including serosa)
C3	T4, N1–3	Nodes positive; beyond wall with adherence to or invasion of surrounding organs or structures

found to be unresectable, 25% have noncurative resections (palliative), and 30% will have "curative" resections (approximately 45% of those explored); these figures will undoubtedly vary among institutions by 5% to 15%. Local-regional relapse, liver metastases, and peritoneal seeding, however, will be common patterns of failure in most surgical series. A multidisciplinary approach is essential to managing gastric cancers, and a concise summary is offered in Table 27–12.

Surgery

Surgical excision of the gastric primary and nodal components of disease remains the primary therapy of potentially resectable gastric cancers and is the only single modality capable of curing gastric cancer. Results with surgery alone, however, continue to be poor except for T1–2,N0 lesions. The goals of surgery are to provide safe removal of all tumor, palliate symptoms such as bleeding and obstruction, and produce the least mortality and morbidity.

The extent of gastric resection is governed by the location of the primary tumor. Total gastrectomy should be reserved for removal of lesions of the proximal stomach. Radical distal subtotal gastrectomy is the most common operation. This entails removal of approximately 80% of the stomach along with the first portion of the duodenum, greater and lesser omenta, and, occasionally, splenectomy and distal pancreatectomy. Direct expansion into contiguous organs, such as liver and transverse colon, is treated by *en bloc*-extended resection of involved areas, if feasible. Reconstruction is generally accomplished with a gastrojejunostomy. Cancer of the cardia can be resected with a more limited esophagogastrectomy and reconstruction with an esophagogastrectomy in the chest.[155–158]

The optimal required extent of lymph node dissection is controversial. Although Japanese surgeons advocate as standard an extended regional node dissection as a means to improve both local control and survival, these benefits have been demonstrated only in nonrandomized series.[159, 160] Separate randomized trials from Britain[161, 162] and the Netherlands[163–166] have not demonstrated any survival benefit for extended lymphadenectomy to date but have demonstrated increased morbidity from the more aggressive approach of a D2 versus D1 node dissection. These findings are not unexpected in view of patterns of relapse data generated in the University of Minnesota reoperative analysis for patients with gastric cancer that included patients with extensive node dissections.[154] When wide lymph node dissection is preferred by the surgeon, nodal regions dissected should include greater curvature, lesser curvature, splenic, celiac, and hepatic lymph nodes. Splenectomy and distal pancreatectomy may be indicated to facilitate a wide lymphadenectomy,[159, 160] but this results in increased morbidity.[166]

For patients with locally advanced primary tumors that appear unresectable for cure or for patients with distant

TABLE 27–12. **Multidisciplinary Treatment Decisions: Stomach**

Stage	Surgery	Radiation Therapy	Chemotherapy
IA T1, N0	Radical subtotal and regional nodes	NR	NR
IB T1, N1	Radical subtotal and regional nodes	NR routinely; ART postop 45–50 Gy or postop EBRT-CT in T1, N1	MACT in T1, N1
T2, N0		Observe in T2, N0	
II T1, N2; T2, N1	Radical subtotal and regional nodes	ART postop 45–50 Gy or postop EBRT-CT all subsets	MACT
T3, N0		Evaluate preop EBRT-CT in T3, N0	
III T2, N2; T3, N1–2	Radical subtotal and regional nodes; T4—resect involved organs *en bloc*	ART preop or postop 45–50 Gy or postop EBRT-CT	MACT
T3, N1–2; T4, N0–1		Evaluate preop EBRT-CT	
IV T4, N3, M0–1	Radical subtotal and regional nodes; T4—resect involved organs *en bloc*	ART 45–50 Gy preop. Evaluate preop EBRT-CT, resection, IORT	MACT
V Local relapse; metastases	Palliative if feasible	PRT if indicated	MACT, ICT I or II

ART = adjuvant irradiation; EBRT-CT = external beam irradiation + chemotherapy; IORT = intraoperative irradiation; postop = postoperative; preop = preoperative; PRT = palliative; NR = not recommended; MACT = multiagent chemotherapy; ICT I/II = investigational chemotherapy, phase I/II clinical trials.
Recommended chemotherapy for MACT = FAMTx = 5-fluorouracil, doxorubicin, and methotrexate; also FAP, FAB, EAP, ELF, ECF (see Table 27–16). From Physicians Data Query: Gastric cancer. Bethesda, National Cancer Institute, October 1999.

metastases, palliation is best accomplished by resection, but the extent of resection must be tempered by the knowledge that cure is improbable. Patients with symptomatic obstruction, hemorrhage, and ulceration, and some with perforation, can be successfully relieved of symptoms by even limited gastric resection. Radical subtotal or total gastrectomy may be indicated in some patients whose lesions cannot be completely resected with negative pathologic margins in order to achieve symptomatic palliation. Results with total gastrectomy in advanced gastric cancer showed good quality of life when this procedure was indicated for bulky or proximal tumors, but symptom relief was less likely for patients with linitis plastica.[167] Although adjacent organ resection should be undertaken if all gross tumor can be removed, it is rarely justified if gross residual tumor (visible or palpable) would remain.

Adjuvant Chemoradiation—Rationale and Principles

Although neither irradiation alone (postoperative) nor chemotherapy alone (preoperative or postoperative) has significant benefit as adjuvant therapy for gastric cancer, there is excellent rationale for pursuing combined irradiation and chemotherapy adjuvant approaches. This rationale is based on five principles:

1. Surgical resection has anatomic limitations with regard to achieving wide tumor-free margins when there is tumor extension either within or beyond the gastric wall. It is also difficult to accomplish a complete regional node dissection. Although gastric cancers are localized and surgically resectable in approximately 50% of patients at the time of diagnosis, nodal metastases or direct invasion of surrounding organs or structures is frequently encountered and precludes cure by surgery alone in many patients[154, 168] (Table 27–13).
   - *Pathways of tumor spread—direct extension or lymphatic:* Both direct tumor extension and lymphatic spread can present difficulties for the surgeon with regard to achieving complete resection of gastric cancers with tumor-free margins. The stomach is surrounded by a number of organs and structures that can be involved once a lesion has extended beyond the gastric wall. Abundant lymphatic channels are present within the submucosal and subserosal layers of the gastric wall; microscopic or subclinical spread beyond the visible gross lesion (intramural spread) occurs via these lymphatic channels. Accordingly, frozen sections of the gastric resection margins should be obtained intraoperatively to assure that margins of resection are uninvolved microscopically. The submucosal lymphatic plexus is also prominent in the esophagus and the subserosal plexus in the duodenum, allowing both proximal and distal intramural tumor spread.
   - Although initial lymphatic drainage is usually to lymph nodes along the lesser and greater curvatures (perigastric or N1 nodes [Japan]),[153] primary node drainage includes nodes along all three branches of the celiac axis (common hepatic, splenic, left gastric) and the celiac itself (Japan N2 nodes). Node groups, which are more distal, include hepatoduodenal, peripancreatic, root of mesentery (Japan N3), periaortic, and middle colic (Japan N4). When proximal gastric lesions extend into the distal esophagus, that nodal system becomes at risk.
2. *Relapse patterns after "curative resection"*: Local relapse or failures in the tumor bed and regional lymph nodes or distant failures via hematogenous or peritoneal routes are all common mechanisms of relapse after curative resection in clinical,[169, 170] reoperative,[154] and autopsy series.[171–175] For lesions of the esophagogastric junction, both the liver and lungs are common sites of distant failure via hematogenous routes. With gastric lesions that do not extend to the esophagus, the initial site of distant failure is usually the liver, and many relapses could be prevented if an effective abdominal or systemic therapy could be combined with treatment of the primary tumor and regional lymph nodes.
   - Local-regional failures occur commonly within the region of the gastric bed and nearby lymph nodes (Table 27–14). Tumor relapse in anastomoses, the gastric remnant, or the duodenal stump is also frequent. In a University of Minnesota reoperative analysis,[154] local-regional failure occurred as the only evidence of relapse in 29% of the 86 patients with relapse (23% of the 105 evaluable patients at risk) and as any component of relapse in 88%. More extensive operative procedures including routine splenectomy, omentectomy, and radical lymph node dissection neither improved survival[176] nor decreased the incidence of local-regional failure in the reoperative analysis.[154] Subsequent relapse within the scope of the initial node dissection occurred in a high percentage of patients even when radical node dissections were performed (D1 + D2 or D3 resection) (Table 27–15). This finding indicates the difficulty of obtaining a complete lymph node dissection in this anatomic location.
   - Patterns of relapse by stage were analyzed in detail in a series of 130 patients who underwent resection with curative intent at the Massachusetts General

TABLE 27–13. **Surgery: Five-Year Survival and Initial Stage of Gastric Cancer**

Extent of Disease	5-Year Survival Clinical Series (%)[168]	5-Year Survival (%) U Minn[154]
Lymph nodes (−)		
Mucosa only	85	—
Mucosa and gastric wall	52	—
Through gastric wall	47	—
Lymph nodes (+)		
Extent of lymph node involvement		19
Regional only	17	—
Other areas	5	—
Extent of primary		
Confined to wall (T1–2)	—	
Beyond wall (T3–4)	—	40

U Minn = University of Minnesota Reoperative Data.

TABLE 27–14. **Gastric Cancer—Patterns of Local-Regional Relapse in Clinical, Reoperation, and Autopsy Series**

	Incidence—Any Component of Local or Regional Relapse			
	MGH (Clinical)[170] (n = 130)	*U. Minn (Reoperation)[154] (n = 105)*	*McNeer (Autopsy)[174] (n = 92)*	*Thomson and Robins (Autopsy)[172] (n = 28)*
Failure Area	*No. (%)*	*No. (%)*	*No. (%)*	*No. (%)*
Gastric bed	27 (21)	58 (55)	48 (52)	19 (68)
Anastomosis or stumps	33 (25)	28 (27)	55 (60)	15 (54)
Abdominal or stab wound	—	5 (5)	—	—
Lymph node(s)	11 (8)	45 (43)	48 (52)	—

Hospital.[170] Local-regional failure occurred as any component of relapse in 49 patients (38%) and as the sole relapse in 21 (16% of 130 patients at risk and 24% of the 88 patients with disease progression). The incidence of local-regional failure by stage was in excess of 35% for modified Astler Coller stages B2 (T3,N0), B3 (T4,N0), C2 (T3,N1–3), and C3 (T4,N1–3). The sites at highest risk for local-regional failure included the gastric bed (27 of 130 patients, 21%) and the anastomosis or gastric remnant (33 of 130 patients, 25%). The true incidence of gastric bed, regional lymph node, and peritoneal relapse may be higher because this series was neither a reoperative nor an autopsy series (see comparative findings in Table 27–14). Additional information exists on patterns of relapse by stage in both the University of Minnesota reoperation analysis[154] and the University of Washington autopsy analysis.[175] Although patterns of relapse data are more accurate in such analyses, patient selection is biased.

- All these data suggest that the development of an effective therapy for local-regional disease as an adjuvant to surgery could potentially benefit at least 20% of patients. However, effective systemic therapy is also essential to improve the outcome for resected high-risk gastric cancer patients in view of the high incidence of distant metastases.

3. Patients with locally advanced gastric cancer who have an incomplete resection have achieved a 10% to 20% 5-year survival following treatment with a combination of external irradiation and chemotherapy or intraoperative electron irradiation (IOERT) alone[6, 7] (see subsequent section on "Results and Prognosis"). Because the combination of irradiation and chemotherapy is capable of sterilizing known residual disease, adjuvant irradiation of the local-regional area (plus simultaneous chemotherapy) following complete resection can be assumed capable of sterilizing subclinical disease present in many patients who have either involved nodes or T3–4 primary gastric cancers. Improved local control with the addition of irradiation (plus simultaneous chemotherapy) is especially important for those patients destined to fail local-regionally but will impact survival in only the approximately 20% of patients with local-regional failure alone. Therefore, the integration of systemic treatment is also necessary.
4. Most positive phase III trials in GI cancer (improvements in survival alone or plus disease control) have been due to combinations of irradiation and chemotherapy (plus resection when feasible).[6–8] These have

TABLE 27–15. **Operative Method Versus Patterns of Relapse—Reoperation Series***

		Patterns of Relapse‡					
		Local-Regional		*Peritoneal Seeding*		*Distant Metastasis*	
Operative Procedure†	**# of Relapses/ Total at Risk**	*Alone No. (%)*	*Component No. (%)*	*Alone No. (%)*	*Component No. (%)*	*Alone No. (%)*	*Component No. (%)*
Method 1 (pre-1950)	25/36	9 (25)	23 (64)	1 (3)	12 (33)	0	7 (19)
Method 2 (1950–1954)	29/32	6 (19)	24 (75)	1 (9)	17 (53)	3 (9)	9 (28)
Method 3 (1954 on)	26/37	8 (22)	23 (62)	1 (3)	15 (41)	2 (5)	7 (19)
Totals	80/105	23 (22)	70 (67)	3 (3)	44 (42)	5 (5)	23 (22)

*86 patients with relapse, 80 evaluable by all parameters.

†Method 1 (pre-1950): subtotal or total gastrectomy, greater omentectomy, regional node dissection.

Method 2 (1950–1954): method 1 plus splenectomy, total omentectomy, additional node dissection regarding splenic, suprapancreatic, and central celiac axis.

Method 3 (1954 on): methods 1 and 2 plus extension of node dissection to porta hepatis and pancreaticoduodenal (intent: total lymph node dissection of all primary node areas equivalent to D2 or D3 dissection).

‡Data represent number of patients with relapse; data in parentheses represent percent total group at risk who had complete follow-up.

From MacDonald JS, Steele G, Gunderson LL: Carcinoma of the stomach. In: DeVita V, Hellman S, Rosenberg SA (eds): Principles and Practice of Oncology, 3rd ed, pp 765–799. Philadelphia, J.B. Lippincott, 1989.

involved the simultaneous use of both modalities. The most significant trials have attempted to deliver one to two cycles of chemotherapy during irradiation and at least two additional cycles of systemic chemotherapy. The Mayo North Central Cancer Treatment Group (NCCTG) adjuvant rectal[8] and RTOG esophagus phase III trials[11, 12] both demonstrated improvements in local control, distant control, disease-free and overall survival with such treatment arms. Additional phase III trials with positive combined-modality arms include the Gastrointestinal Tumor Study Group (GITSG) adjuvant rectal and pancreas protocols,[6–8] Mayo Clinic and GITSG unresectable pancreas[6, 7] and locally advanced gastric cancer trials[6, 7, 177–180] (unresectable or residual), and a Mayo Clinic locally unresectable or residual colorectal study.[8]

5. Finally, positive results from several gastric adjuvant phase II trials and a number of prospectively randomized phase III adjuvant studies using irradiation with or without chemotherapy for adenocarcinoma of the stomach, esophagus, or esophagogastric junction suggest that further definitive trials are warranted[86, 181–186] (see subsequent section on "Results and Prognosis"). Combined-modality treatment is reasonably well tolerated,[9, 10, 181, 182] decreases local-regional failure,[6–8, 181–186] and improves survival.[182–186] A large U.S. intergroup protocol has been completed in which approximately 600 completely resected high-risk patients were randomized to a surgery-alone control arm versus postoperative EBRT (45 Gy in 25 fractions over 5 weeks) plus chemotherapy (5-FU plus low-dose leucovorin before, during, and after irradiation). Results confirmed both disease-free and overall survival benefit from adjuvant EBRT plus chemotherapy.[186a, 186b]

Locally Advanced Disease (Unresectable for Cure)—Treatment Principles

The term *locally advanced disease* has different interpretations depending on the author and institution. At the Mayo Clinic, and for the purpose of this presentation, the term refers to cancers that the surgeon would not expect to resect with negative pathologic margins, that is, unresectable for cure as determined at surgical exploration or as defined preoperatively with CT, endoscopic ultrasound, laparoscopy, or other studies. For other authors, the category of *locally advanced disease* is also used to include lesions that are completely resected but have high risk factors for local recurrence or distant metastasis (nodal involvement, extension beyond the gastric wall, or both).

Surgical Aspects

The extent of the surgical procedure for patients with locally advanced cancers must be tempered by the knowledge that cure is, at best, improbable. As described earlier, some patients can be relieved of symptoms by limited gastric resection. In other patients whose lesions cannot be completely resected, radical subtotal or total gastrectomies may be indicated to achieve symptomatic palliation. Sites of residual disease should be judiciously marked with clips to aid the delivery of postoperative irradiation plus chemotherapy.

Irradiation and Chemotherapy

Although some patients without resection have long-term survival with irradiation alone or with chemotherapy, irradiation is not a preferable alternative to surgical resection plus adjuvant therapy as indicated because the initial bulk of disease and the limited tolerance of the stomach and surrounding organs prevents a suitable therapeutic ratio between cure and complications. Radiation is preferably used in combination with chemotherapy (concomitant and maintenance) plus resection of all gross primary and lymph node disease.

Metastatic Disease—Treatment Principles

Chemotherapy

For patients with metastatic disease, a number of chemotherapy agents can produce meaningful chemotherapy response alone or combined with other agents, but the duration of response is often short. A number of multiple-drug chemotherapy regimens have response rates of 30% to 50%, but most regimens do not affect long-term survival (Table 27–16). Phase III trials have been conducted that demonstrate both response rate and survival benefit for FAMTx (5-FU plus doxorubicin plus methotrexate) versus FAM (5-FU plus doxorubicin plus mitomycin C) (EORTC) and better tolerance for FAMTx versus EAP (etoposide plus doxorubicin plus cisplatin) (Memorial Sloan-Kettering Cancer Center [MSKCC]). Successor trials by the EORTC suggest that FAMTx is equivalent to ELF (etoposide plus leucovorin plus 5-FU) or 5-FU plus cisplatin with regard

TABLE 27–16. **Combination Chemotherapy for Gastric Cancer**

Drug Combination	% Response (Range)	Median Survival (mos)
5-FU, mitomycin C	24 (14–32)	4–6
5-FU, BCNU	26 (11–41)	3–8
FAM (original)	33 (17–55)	6–8
Intensified	32	7–9
Variants	26	6–9
FAB	43	6–8
FAP	36	6–13
FAMTx	43	8
EAP	56	9–18
ELF	52	11
ECF	45	9

F = 5-FU; BCNU = bis-chloroethyl-nitrosourea; A = doxorubicin; M = mitomycin C; B = carmustine; P = cisplatin; MTx = methotrexate; E = etoposide; L = leucovorin; ECF = epirubicin, cisplatin, infusion 5-FU.

Modified from MacDonald JS, Steele G, Gunderson LL: Carcinoma of the stomach. In: De Vita V, Hellman S, Rosenberg SA (eds): Principles and Practice of Oncology, 3rd ed, pp 765–799. Philadelphia, J.B. Lippincott, 1989, and Wilke H, Preusser P, Fink U, et al: New developments in the treatment of gastric carcinoma. Semin Oncol 1990; 17:(1 suppl 2):61–70.

to response rates and survival. Furthermore, a United Kingdom trial suggests that ECP (epirubicin plus cisplatin plus 5-FU) results for response rates, survival, and quality of life exceed those for FAMTx and should now be considered the standard treatments for advanced esophagogastric cancers. Results of these trials will be presented in the "Results and Prognosis" section.

Randomized trials have also demonstrated both a quality of life and survival benefit for multidrug chemotherapy versus best supportive care for patients with metastatic gastric cancer. Results of these trials will be discussed in the section entitled "Results and Prognosis."

Treatment According to Clinical Stage

Stages I and II

Total surgical resection of adenocarcinoma with a radical subtotal gastrectomy (see "Surgery" for details) and reconstruction with gastrojejunostomy is recommended as standard treatment. Neither chemotherapy nor radiotherapy is routinely recommended as a single-modality adjuvant. In the clinical trial setting, combined-modality postoperative chemoradiation has been tested against a surgery-alone control arm for T2,N1 and T3,N0 lesions (also for resectable stage III) in a phase III U.S. intergroup trial. Results have demonstrated a benefit in both disease-free and overall survival, confirming the role of adjuvant chemoradiation as a component of the standard treatment.

Stage III

For resectable stage III lesions, complete resection with or without *en bloc* resection of adjacent organs is recommended. Postoperative chemoradiation has been tested in randomized fashion and has shown benefits in completely resected T2,N2, T3,N1–2, or T4,N0–1 lesions. Preoperative chemoradiation is being tested in phase II multi-institution studies.

In locally unresectable stage III gastric cancers, preoperative or primary chemoradiation or multiple drug chemotherapy can be utilized, preferably in the setting of controlled prospective clinical trials.

Stage IV

For locally unresectable stage IV gastric cancers (T4,N0–3,M0), preoperative chemoradiation followed by resection with or without IOERT should be further evaluated in controlled trials. For metastatic cancers, multidrug chemotherapy combinations are applicable[187, 188] and patients should be placed on randomized trials when available (see Table 27–16 with regard to response rates and median survival with multidrug chemotherapy for advanced or metastatic disease). Radiation therapy can be used for painful metastatic lesions but is otherwise not indicated.

Results and Prognosis

Overall Survival

Despite decreasing incidence and overall mortality of this disease, success with treatment has improved only slightly in the past 30 years. Overall 5-year survival in the United States is 21%, compared with 15% from 1974 to 1976 ($p < 0.05$) and 10% in 1960.[2] Survival for early gastric cancer (node negative, confined to wall) is reported as high as 50% to 90% dependent on the depth of penetration; with metastatic disease, 0% to 5% 5-year survival is expected.

- Only 10% to 20% of patients who present with gastric cancer will have disease capable of curative resection. For this subgroup, however, survival rates of 30% to 50% over 5 years are commonly reported. Five-year survival rates adjusted for stage were presented in Table 27–13 for surgery alone.
- Prognostic factors: As with other alimentary tract cancers, the two most important prognostic features are depth of invasion and lymph nodc involvement. In Table 27–13, the 5-year survival is shown by depth of invasion or T stage (47% to 85% 5-year survival when N0) and nodal involvement, which may reduce survival (overall survival with node involvement <20%) especially when found in conjunction with T3 or T4 primaries. If the primary lesion is confined to the gastric wall (T1 or T2) when nodes are involved, the prognosis at 5 years (40% survival) is similar to that of patients with T2,N0 or T3,N0 lesions (approximately 50% 5-year survival).

Adjuvant Chemotherapy

WESTERN TRIALS

The results of surgery alone for resectable gastric cancer justify the evaluation of adjuvant chemotherapy with regard to systemic risks and survival. However, adjuvant chemotherapy programs to date are of potential rather than therapeutic benefit. Although many active single agents exist and a number of drug combinations are purported to have response rates of 40%,[187, 189] randomized western trials have generally failed to yield positive findings for adjuvant chemotherapy. Results of western randomized trials with a surgery-alone control arm versus multidrug chemotherapy arms are seen in Table 27–17.[190–205]

The GITSG surgical adjuvant chemotherapy trial using 5-FU and methyl CCNU (MeCCNU, semustine) is the only U.S. study that showed a survival benefit (50% vs. 31% survival at 5 years).[190] Two other U.S. trials using the same drug combination (Veterans Administration Surgical Oncology Group, ECOG) did not show a survival benefit.[191, 192] A report from the Italian Gastrointestinal Tumor Study Group did not support the positive results of the GITSG study using 5-FU and MeCCNU either alone or combined with levamisole in the adjuvant setting.[193] Finally, the addition of Adriamycin (doxorubicin) to either 5-FU alone or with 5-FU and MeCCNU produced the same negative results.[194, 195]

Following the reports of high response rates to FAM in advanced gastric cancer, several studies were initiated to test the role of this promising regimen in the adjuvant setting. The International Collaborative Cancer Group could not detect a survival advantage for adjuvant FAM chemotherapy in the overall study population; however, some suggestive benefit was seen in patients with T3 and T4 disease in a retrospective subset analysis.[196] Studies

TABLE 27–17. **Adjuvant Multidrug or Single-Drug Chemotherapy for Gastric Cancer: Western Studies**

			Survival		
Author	**Regimen**	**Patients**	***Interval***	**%**	***p Value***
GITSG[190]	5-FU/MeCCNU	71	5 yr	50	p <0.03
	Control	71		31	
Higgins[191] (VASOG)	5-FU/MeCCNU	66	3.5 yr	37.8	p = 0.88
	Control	68		38.9	
Engstrom[192] (ECOG)	5-FU/MeCCNU	91	2 yr	57	p = 0.73
	Control	89		57	
IGITSG[193]	5-FU/MeCCNU	75	5 yr	~50	p = 0.9
	5-FU/MeCCNU/levamisole	69		~50	
	Control	69		~50	
Krook[194] (NCCTG)	5-FU/adria	61	5 yr	32	p = 0.88
	Control	64		33	
Estrada[195]	5-FU/adria/MeCCNU	31	5 yr	29	p = 0.31
	Control	35		37	
Coombes[196] (ICCG)	5-FU/adria/mito C	133	5 yr	45.7	p = 0.21
	Control	148		35.4	
MacDonald[197] (SWOG)	5-FU/adria/mito C	93	5 yr	37	p = 0.59
	Control	100		32	
Hallissey[198] (BSCG)	5-FU/adria/mito C	138	5 yr	19	p = 0.69
	Control	145		20	
Lise[199] (EORTC)	5-FU/adria/mito C	159	Med	42 mo	p = 0.295
	Control	155	Surv	36 mo	
Tsavaris[200]	5-FU/epirubicin/mito C	42	Med	42 mo	p = 0.248
	Control	42	Surv	39 mo	
Huguier[201]	5-FU/vinblastine/cycloph	27	5 yr	18	p = NS
	Control	26		16	
Rake[202]	5-FU/cycloph/vinc/MTx + mito C	17	Med	10 mo	p = 0.034
	Control	17	Surv	6 mo	
Jakesz[203]	5-FU/Ara-C/mito C ± OK−432	53	5 yr	45	p = NS
	Control	34		29	
Estape[204]	Mito C	68	5 yr	41	p <0.03
	Control	66		26	
Neri[205]	Epirubicin/5-FU/leucovorin	48	3 yr	25	p <0.01
	Control	55		13	

NS = not significant; mo = months; yr = year; Med = median; Surv = survival; 5-FU = 5-fluorouracil; MeCCNU = semustine; adria = doxorubicin; mito C = mitomycin C; cycloph = cyclophosphamide; vinc = vincristine; MTx = methotrexate; Ara-C = cytosine arabinoside.

both by the SWOG and British Stomach Cancer Group (BSCG) did not show an advantage for the postoperative use of FAM.[197, 198] An intensified FAM (FAM2) was used for surgical adjuvant therapy by the EORTC.[199] Although time to progression was superior for FAM2 (p = 0.02), survival was not improved (p = 0.295). A group from Greece studied 5-FU, epirubicin, and mitomycin (FEM) compared with surgical controls.[200] Although a trend toward improved survival in patients with histologic grade III tumor was observed (p = 0.085), no statistically significant survival benefit for the entire study group was detected.

Other 5-FU–based multidrug chemotherapy regimens have been tested in the adjuvant setting as shown in Table 27–17. None have demonstrated a survival benefit for the total group of patients at risk except for a small trial of 34 patients reported by Rake and coworkers who were randomized to receive an induction course of 5-FU, cyclophosphamide, vincristine, and methotrexate followed by 6 weekly courses of 5-FU and mitomycin C.[202] Median survival was improved from 6 months in the surgical controls to 10 months for adjuvant-treated patients (p = 0.034). When the BSCG looked at a similar combination of 5-FU and mitomycin C alone or following an induction course of 5-FU, cyclophosphamide, vincristine, and methotrexate in more than 400 patients, no survival benefit was derived from treatment with either chemotherapy regimen in the subset of patients who underwent complete resection.[206] A large number of patients (80%) in this study, however, had residual disease following surgery.

Positive results for adjuvant systemic treatment have been reported in two other western trials, although the numbers of patients in both studies are small. A study from Spain involving 70 patients suggested a significant survival benefit for single-agent mitomycin C at 5 and 10 years.[204] This trial has been extended to 134 patients with a median follow-up of 8.75 years and still shows a survival advantage for postoperative mitomycin C (p = 0.025).[207] Interestingly, an adjuvant trial from Spain comparing mitomycin C and tegafur plus uracil showed no benefit for the treated patients versus surgical controls.[208] Neri and colleagues randomized surgically resected node-positive patients to receive or not receive adjuvant epirubicin, 5-FU, and leucovorin.[205] An improvement in 3-year survival from 13% to 25% (p <0.01) was noted for patients receiving adjuvant systemic treatment.

JAPANESE TRIALS

Stomach cancer is a common disease in Japan, and a number of adjuvant studies have been performed using postoperative chemotherapy and chemoimmunotherapy following resection. Most Japanese trials include patients with stages I to IV disease (Japanese Research Society for Gastric Cancer),[153] whereas adjuvant trials in the United States would exclude patients with early (stage I) and advanced cancers (stage IV). Because some Japanese studies do not include surgical controls, are not prospectively randomized, or are not available in the English language, only those randomized trials that are published in English and include surgically treated controls are summarized in Table 27–18.[209–213]

Imanaga and Nakazato reviewed the early Japanese cooperative group experience with adjuvant systemic treatment in four studies involving over 2,500 patients.[209] Treatment included mitomycin C, either alone or combined with other agents, utilizing different routes and schedules. In the first study, mitomycin C was given intravenously twice a week for 5 weeks, with the first dose given on the day of surgery. Survival favored treated patients at 5 years (68% vs. 54%). Subset analysis of this study showed particular benefit for treatment in stage II patients. In subsequent studies, no survival advantage for the treated group was seen.

Nakajima and colleagues performed a series of three adjuvant studies with mitomycin C plus other drugs for resected gastric cancer.[210–212] In the initial study, mitomycin C was given on a twice-a-week schedule for 5 weeks. Although no survival benefit was seen for the whole cohort of patients, a striking benefit was seen for patients with involved serosa or advanced lymph node metastasis.[210] A three-arm adjuvant study was subsequently performed in which patients were randomized to surgery alone, mitomycin C alone, or the combination of MFC (mitomycin C, 5-FU, and ara-C).[211] A survival benefit for MFC-treated patients was seen at 5 years when compared with surgical controls, but no significant benefit was seen for the mitomycin C arm alone. These same investigators then studied the regimen of MFC followed by either long-term oral 5-FU or ftorafur compared with surgical controls.[212] A significant survival benefit was seen for patients with stages I to III disease treated with MFC and oral 5-FU.

Finally, Ochiai and colleagues conducted a trial that randomized patients to surgery alone, MFC chemotherapy or MFC plus bacille Calmette-Guérin cell wall skeleton.[213] A survival benefit was demonstrated for the patients treated with chemoimmunotherapy.

The above data form the basis for the routine use of postoperative systemic therapy following the resection of gastric cancer in Japan. Currently, a common adjuvant regimen includes intravenous mitomycin C, 5-FU, and ara-C, followed by the prolonged use of tegafur. Most current studies are examining issues of adding new drugs, intensifying the mitomycin dose, and the use of immunostimulants in addition to chemotherapy.[214–219]

SUMMARY—ADJUVANT CHEMOTHERAPY

In attempting to resolve the differences between the results of western and Japanese adjuvant chemotherapy studies, Nakajima and associates and others have pointed out some features of the Japanese trials that may contribute to a positive experience for postoperative chemotherapy.[220, 221] These include the initiation of systemic therapy in the immediate perioperative period, less postoperative tumor burden, and the use of mitomycin C. Some of the shortcomings of these same studies include high exclusion rates, the frequent use of subset analysis, and the lack of surgical

TABLE 27–18. **Adjuvant Therapy of Gastric Cancer: Japanese Studies***

			Survival		
Author	**Regimen**	**Patients**	***Interval***	**%**	***Stat. Result***
Imanaga[209]	Mitomycin C (5 wk)	242	5 yr	67.8	Pos
	Control	283		54.3	
	Mitomycin C (2 days)	265	5 yr	60.3	Neg
	Control	255		59.9	
	Mitomycin C IA/cycloph	146	5 yr	70.8/29.4†	Neg
	Mitomycin C IA	135		68.4/36.0	
	Control	152		73.4/40.9	
	Mitomycin C	197	3 yr	73.5	Neg
	Mitomycin C/5-FU/Ara-C	208		68.9	
	Control	217		68.5	
Nakajima[210]	Mitomycin C	207	5 yr	52.2	Neg
	Control	223		43.5	
Nakajima[211]	Mitomycin C	42	5 yr	64.3	Pos
	Mitomycin C/5-FU/Ara-C	40		66.9	
	Control	38		50.0	
Nakajima[212]	Mitomycin C/5-FU/Ara-C/5-FU (oral)	73	5 yr	64.3	Pos‡
	Mitomycin C/ftorafur/Ara-C/5-FU (oral)	76		65.5	
	Control	74		53.1	
Ochiai[213]	Mitomycin C/5-FU/Ara-C	49		NR	Pos
	Mitomycin C/5-FU/Ara-C/BCG	49			
	Control	40			

Neg = negative; Pos = positive; NR = not reported; cycloph = cyclophosphamide; 5-FU = 5-fluorouracil; Ara-C = cytosine arabinoside; BCG = bacille Calmette-Guérin.

*Includes stages I–IV.

†Survival stage II/stage III.

‡Positive for curative resections.

controls. It is noteworthy that only two small western surgical adjuvant studies have ever shown a positive result using a mitomycin C–containing regimen.[202, 207]

Currently, large cooperative group studies are still evaluating the role of adjuvant therapy after resection of gastric carcinoma. The EORTC is testing sequential 5-FU/methotrexate and Adriamycin (FAMTx) in a randomized study. A combined intraperitoneal and systemic chemotherapy approach, compared with surgery alone, has been under investigation as an adjuvant approach in Japan. The recently completed U.S. intergroup study of approximately 600 patients tested the role of combined-modality postoperative adjuvant treatment with irradiation plus concomitant and maintenance chemotherapy with 5-FU and leucovorin based on the patterns of failure following surgery and demonstrated a survival benefit for adjuvant chemoradiation.

Adjuvant Irradiation

POSTOPERATIVE IRRADIATION

Irradiation has only been minimally evaluated as the sole adjuvant treatment following complete surgical resection in randomized phase III trials. Adjuvant EBRT reduced local-regional failures when compared with the surgery-alone control arm in a British adjuvant trial, but no survival benefits were found.[184] Although phase III trials from Japan[222, 223] and China[224] suggest some survival benefit for IORT versus a surgery-alone control arm, the advantage was found only in subset analyses. At the National Cancer Institute (NCI), Sindelar and associates performed a small randomized trial of IORT versus EBRT following complete surgical resection; this trial demonstrated improved local control with IORT but no survival benefit.[225] A surgery-alone control arm did not exist in the NCI trial. Phase II studies combining EBRT and IORT have been conducted in Pamplona (Spain) and the United States (by RTOG) and are still under way in Lyon (France).

The BSCG's prospectively randomized trial compared surgery alone with adjuvant postoperative FAM or EBRT (45 Gy in 25 fractions with or without 5-Gy boost).[184] A total of 436 patients were randomized and followed for a minimum of 12 months. Although no survival differences by treatment arm were found (median: 15 months), local-regional failure was documented in only 15 of 153 patients (10%) in the irradiation arm versus 39 of 145 (27%) in the surgery-alone arm, and 26 of 138 (19%) in the FAM group. Interpretation of the BSCG results is complicated by the inclusion of 93 patients who would not be candidates for gastric surgical adjuvant trials in the United States. In addition, nearly one third of patients randomized to receive adjuvant treatment did not receive the assigned therapy; of 153 patients randomized to the irradiation arm, only 104 (68%) received a dose of 40.5 Gy or more, and 36 (24%) received none.

Abe and Takahashi[222, 223] reported results from a Japanese trial in which 211 patients were randomized on the basis of day of hospital admission to either surgery only or surgery plus IORT (28 to 35 Gy). Five-year survival rates for Japanese stages II to IV improved approximately 15% to 25% in the IORT versus surgery-alone patients (stage II, 84% vs. 62%; stage III, 62% vs. 37%; stage IV, 15% vs. 0%). This magnitude of survival improvement correlates nicely with the approximately 20% of patients who fail local-regionally after complete surgical resection. Although the data are intriguing, this method of randomization is susceptible to bias in treatment selection, and the trial failed to stratify for important prognostic factors.

In an analysis from Beijing, patients with stage III (serosal involvement or node-positive tumors) or stage IV (unresectable metastasis or adjacent organ involvement) disease were randomized to surgery alone or IORT (single dose, 25 to 40 Gy).[224] In a report of 200 patients, a survival advantage with IORT was demonstrated for stage III patients (5-year survival: 65% versus 30%; 8-year survival: 52% versus 22%; $p < 0.01$).

PREOPERATIVE IRRADIATION

Randomized trials testing preoperative irradiation have been performed in both Russia and China. All have reported a positive survival benefit when compared with surgery-alone control arms. Three prospective randomized Russian trials evaluated preoperative irradiation for patients with potentially resectable gastric cancer.[226–228] The first trial assigned 293 patients to receive either surgery alone, surgery after preoperative EBRT (20 Gy in four fractions), or surgery after the same EBRT plus daily hyperthermia. The survival rates at 3 and 5 years were improved in both irradiation arms compared with surgery alone, and the improvement with combined EBRT and hyperthermia was statistically significant at both 3 and 5 years.[228] The second trial compared preoperative EBRT (20 Gy) versus surgery alone in 279 patients. Three-year and 5-year survival rates were improved with EBRT, and no increase in operative morbidity was observed.[226] The third trial compared surgery alone versus preoperative EBRT plus oxygen inhalation (32 Gy with concomitant inhalation of 8% oxygen).[227] A survival advantage was observed with preoperative treatment, and the resection rate was increased by 17%.

A randomized double-blind trial from Beijing compared a surgery-alone control arm ($n = 199$) with preoperative EBRT plus surgery ($n = 171$) for patients with adenocarcinoma of the gastric cardia.[229] Irradiation was given with 8 MeV photons or cobalt 60 with AP-PA fields to a dose of 40 Gy in 20 fractions of 2 Gy over 4 weeks. Surgery was performed 3 to 8 weeks after completion of irradiation. Downstaging of disease and improvements in radical resection rates were found with the addition of preoperative EBRT (radical resection rates of 80% vs. 62% with preoperative EBRT vs. surgery alone). Survival and local-regional disease control were improved for patients assigned to the preoperative EBRT arm. Five-year and 10-year survival rates were 30% versus 20% and 20% versus 13%, respectively (Fig. 27–7, $p = 0.009$ log rank). Local-regional disease control was also improved with preoperative EBRT, with local relapse rates of 39% versus 52% ($p < 0.025$) and regional node relapse rates of 39% versus 54% ($p < 0.005$). The rate of distant metastases was the same, at 24% versus 25%. Improvements in survival and disease control (local-regional) were accomplished with no apparent increase in treatment-related morbidity or mortality (operative mortality 0.6% vs. 2.5% with or without

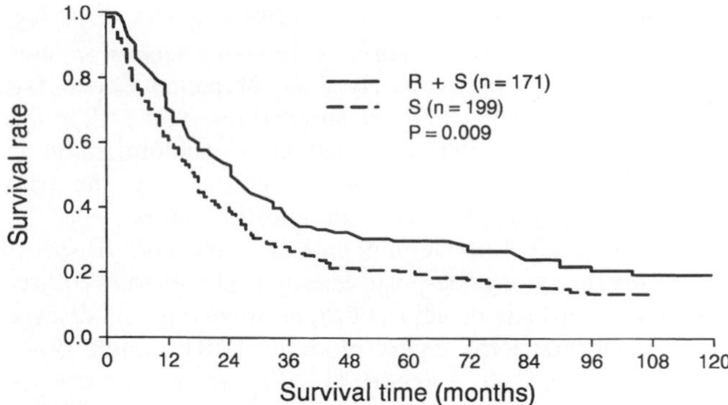

Figure 27–7. Overall survival in Beijing phase III trial comparing surgery alone with preoperative EBRT for adenocarcinoma of the gastric cardia (40 Gy/20 fractions/4 wks), with advantage to preoperative EBRT (p = 0.009 log rank). (From Zhang ZX, Gu XZ, Yin WB, et al: Randomized clinical trial combination on the preoperative irradiation and surgery in the treatment of adenocarcinoma of the gastric cardia [AGC]—report on 370 patients. Int J Radiat Oncol Biol Phys 1998; 42:931.)

preoperative EBRT; intrathoracic leak rates of 1.8% and 4.2%, respectively).

In view of the survival advantage (alone or plus disease control) and radical resection rates demonstrated for preoperative EBRT in the four published trials,[226–229] such approaches need to be evaluated further in U.S. and European study groups. As suggested by the authors from the Beijing trial, factors to be evaluated include radiation dose escalation to 45 to 50 Gy (1.8- to 2.0-Gy fractions) and the addition of chemotherapy (concomitant with EBRT and maintenance).

Adjuvant Chemoradiation

Although adjuvant therapy following complete surgical resection of gastric cancers is indicated on the basis of failure patterns and survival results with surgery alone (high incidence of local-regional relapse and distant metastases), single-modality adjuvant therapy has not had a meaningful impact on outcome (disease control or survival). Most western chemotherapy trials are negative for both single and multiple drugs. As an adjuvant, irradiation alone reduces local-regional relapse, but it does not alter survival unless given preoperatively. Data from single-institution phase II and small phase III trials suggest that combined-modality adjuvant therapy (irradiation plus chemotherapy) may have a positive outcome on both disease control and survival. A large confirmatory U.S. intergroup trial was therefore performed to evaluate disease control and survival benefit trends for combined-modality postoperative irradiation plus chemotherapy that were found in a small Mayo Clinic randomized study.

POSTOPERATIVE EBRT PLUS CHEMOTHERAPY

Phase II single-institution gastric cancer trials that show promise for combination postoperative adjuvant therapy have been reported from Massachusetts General Hospital (MGH),[181] Israel (Hadassah),[183] Thomas Jefferson University Hospital (TJUH),[186] and the University of Pennsylvania.[185] Gunderson and associates from the MGH reported a median survival of 24 months and 4-year survival of 43% in 14 patients who had complete resection of tumors with extension beyond the wall, nodal involvement, or both.[181] Patients received postoperative EBRT (45 to 52 Gy, 1.8 Gy/d) plus concomitant 5-FU–based chemotherapy. Subsequent local-regional relapse was documented in only 2 of the 14 patients (14%) in contrast to a 42% incidence in a similar high-risk group of 110 patients treated with surgery alone at MGH.[170] Hadassah University investigators reported on 25 patients with gross tumor resection but at high risk for relapse who were treated with EBRT (50 Gy over 7 weeks, 2 to 2.5 Gy/fraction with a 2-week split) and 5-FU on days 1 to 3 of each EBRT cycle plus 1 year of maintenance 5-FU.[183] Median survival was 33 months, and the 5-year actuarial survival was 40% (of the 13 survivors, 12 were disease free). Local failure was documented in only two patients (8%). In the series from TJUH, 120 patients had surgical resection but were at high risk for relapse because of extension beyond the gastric wall, nodal metastases, or positive margins of resection.[186] Seventy patients had surgery alone and 50 received adjuvant therapy. Apparent improvements in local control as well as median and 5-year survival were noted with additional therapy. In patients with negative resection margins, 2-year local control with surgery alone was 55% versus 93% with adjuvant EBRT with or without chemotherapy ($p = 0.03$). For patients with T3–4 tumors and lymph node involvement, median survival was 9 months versus 13 months (surgery with or without adjuvant treatment), and 5-year survival was 4% versus 22% ($p = 0.03$). In a University of Pennsylvania analysis, the incidence of local failure with surgery alone was 75% (31 of 40) versus 24% with adjuvant EBRT (4 of 17) and 15% with adjuvant EBRT plus chemotherapy (4 of 27).[185]

A prospective randomized trial conducted at the Mayo Clinic included 62 patients with poor-prognosis completely resected gastric cancers who were randomized to either surgery alone or surgery followed by EBRT (37.5 Gy in 24 fractions over 4 to 5 weeks) plus concomitant 5-FU (15 mg/kg/d for 3 days week one of EBRT by IV bolus).[182] A nonstratified, prerandomization scheme was used with a 2:3 ratio favoring treatment. Informed consent was requested only of the 39 patients randomized to treatment; 10 of the 39 refused further therapy and were observed. When analyzed by intent to treat, the adjuvant arm had statistically significant improvement in both relapse-free and overall survival (overall 5-year survival 23% vs. 4%; $p < 0.05$). When patient outcome was compared by actual treatment received (29 adjuvant treatment, 33 surgery alone), 5-year survival still favored the adjuvant group (20% vs. 12%), but the differences were not statistically significant in view of small patient numbers. When analyzed by treatment delivered, local-regional relapse was decreased with adjuvant treatment (54% incidence with surgery alone vs. 39% with irradiation plus 5-FU). As seen in Table 27–19, the 10 patients who refused assignment to adjuvant treatment had more favorable prognostic findings than the other two groups of patients. When the two groups with equally poor prognostic factors were compared, the 5-year overall survival was 20% versus 4%, with an advantage to those receiving adjuvant treatment. The survival data with adjuvant chemoradiation parallel the high-risk

TABLE 27–19. **Randomized Gastric Adjuvant Trial at the Mayo Clinic***

	Adjuvant EBRT + 5-FU (%) (n = 29)	Surgery Control (%) (n = 23)	Refused Adjuvant (%) (n = 10)
Pathologic Characteristics			
Cardia	55	56	30
Ulcerative	72	70	50
Grade 2	7	9	30
Grade 3, 4	93	91	70

	Adjuvant EBRT + 5-FU (%)	Surgery Alone (%)
Five-Year Survival		
Treatment intent (39 vs 23 patients)	23	4 ($p < 0.05$)
Treatment delivered (29 vs 33 patients)		
Overall	20	12
Disease free	17	9
Local Failure (treatment delivered)	39	54

EBRT = external beam irradiation; 5-FU = 5-fluorouracil.
*Surgery ± Irradiation + 5-FU
Modified from Moertel CG, Childs DS, O'Fallon JR, et al: Combined 5-fluorouracil and radiation therapy as a surgical adjuvant for poor prognosis gastric carcinoma. J Clin Oncol 1984; 2:1249–1254.

TJUH gastric data with adjuvant chemoradiation discussed in the prior paragraph[186] and the GITSG adjuvant pancreas phase III trial that resulted in 19% versus 5% 5-year survival for adjuvant irradiation plus 5-FU versus surgery alone ($p < 0.05$).[6, 7]

In a recent retrospective Mayo analysis, 63 patients received postoperative EBRT plus 5-FU after resection of carcinoma of the stomach or gastroesophageal junction.[230] Twenty-five of the 63 patients had complete resection with no residual disease but had high-risk factors for disease relapse (extension beyond gastric wall—92% of patients; involved nodes—92%; both high-risk factors—84%). Concomitant 5-FU plus leucovorin was given with EBRT in 84% of the 25 adjuvantly treated patients, but maintenance chemotherapy was given in only 20%. Local-regional control was achieved in 20 of the 25 (80%) with median survival of 19 months. Four-year survival was 31% in spite of the very poor prognostic factors in these 25 patients.

PREOPERATIVE EBRT PLUS CHEMOTHERAPY

Although no randomized trials testing preoperative EBRT plus chemotherapy for gastric cancer alone have yet been published, the Walsh and colleagues trial for adenocarcinoma of the esophagus and gastric cardia certainly has relevance.[86] A highly significant difference in survival was observed with CMT over surgery alone (intent to treat—median survival 16 vs. 11 months, 3-year survival 32% vs. 6%, p = 0.01; actual treatment—median survival 32 vs. 11 months—p = 0.001, 3-year survival 37% vs. 7%—p = 0.006). A confirmatory (North America) intergroup trial was attempted for either esophagus or esophagogastric junction cancers (squamous or adenocarcinoma), but it was discontinued in 2000 because of inadequate patient accrual.

SUMMARY—ADJUVANT CHEMORADIATION

In summary, although neither irradiation nor chemotherapy alone has significant benefit as adjuvant therapy for gastric cancer, there is an excellent rationale for pursuing combined irradiation and chemotherapy approaches either postoperatively or preoperatively (Table 27–20). This rationale is based on the five principles previously discussed.

1. Anatomic limitations of surgical resection exist with regard to achieving wide tumor-free margins with tumor extension within and beyond the gastric wall; in addition, it is more difficult to perform a complete regional node dissection.
2. Patterns of relapse data following surgical resection demonstrate a significant incidence of local-regional failure in the tumor bed, regional nodes, gastric remnant, or anastomosis following potentially curative surgery and a high rate of distant metastases (see "Surgery," earlier, and Tables 27–14 and 27–15). In the reoperative series, approximately 20% of all evaluable patients undergoing resection and 30% of those with relapse failed only in local-regional sites.
3. Patients with locally advanced gastric cancer have a 10% to 20% 5-year survival following treatment with chemoradiation or IORT alone (see subsequent section on "Locally Advanced Disease").
4. Most positive phase III trials in GI cancer (improvements in survival, disease control, or both) have been due to combinations of irradiation and chemotherapy (plus resection where feasible). These trials have involved the simultaneous use of both modalities. The most significant trials have attempted to deliver either one to two cycles of bolus 5-FU–based chemotherapy or protracted venous infusion (PVI) 5-FU during EBRT and two to four additional cycles of systemic or maintenance chemotherapy.
5. Finally, positive results from gastric adjuvant phase II trials and a number of prospectively randomized phase III adjuvant studies using irradiation, with or without chemotherapy, for adenocarcinoma of the stomach, esophagus, or esophagogastric junction suggest that further definitive trials are warranted.

The methodologic flaws in the Japanese IOERT,[222, 223] Russian preoperative EBRT,[226–228] and Mayo postoperative EBRT plus 5-FU trials[182] and the negative results of the

TABLE 27–20. **Surgery ± Adjuvant Therapy for Resected Gastric Cancer (or Esophageal-Gastric Junction)**

		Survival			Local Regional Relapse			
	Patient No.	***Median (mo)***	***Long-Term* (%)***	***P Value***	***No.***	***(%)***	***P Value***	**Ref. No.**
Phase III Studies								
1. British Stomach Group		15	(3 yr)					184
Surgery alone	145	—	20	—	39	27	—	—
Postop chemo	138	—	19	—	26	19	—	—
Postop EBRT	153	—	12	—	15	10	—	—
2. Japan—Surgery ± IOERT†	S IOERT		S IOERT					222, 223
	110 101							
Stage I	43 24	—	93 vs. 87%	—	—	—	—	—
Stage II	11 20	—	62 vs. 84%	—	—	—	—	—
Stage III	38 30	—	37 vs. 62%	—	—	—	—	—
Stage IV	18 27	—	0 vs. 15%	—	—	—	—	—
3. China—Surgery ± IOERT†	100 100							224
Stage III (5 yr)	— —	—	30 vs. 65%	<0.01	—	—	—	—
Stage III (8 yr)	— —	—	22 vs. 52%		—	—	—	—
4. Mayo Clinic‡								182
Surgery alone	23	15	4	—	—	54	—	—
Postop EBRT + 5-FU	39	24	23	0.05	—	39	—	—
5. China-Beijing								
Surgery alone	199	—	20		—	52		229
Postop EBRT + 5-FU	171	—	30	0.009	—	39	<0.025	
6. USGI Intergroup△	603	—	(3 yr)	—	—	—	—	186a, 186b
Surgery alone	—	—	41	—	—	—	—	
Postop IORT + 5-FU	—	—	52	0.03	—	—	—	
Phase II Trials								
1. MGH (gastric)								
Surgery alone	110	—	38 (B2, B3) 15 (C1–3)	—	46	42	—	170
Postop EBRT + chemo	14	24	43 (4 yr)	—	2	14	—	181
2. TJUH (gastric)								
Total group T3, T4, or N+	120							186
Surgery alone	70	12	13		17/38	45	—	—
Postop chemo, EBRT, or both	50	19	17	<0.05	13/36	36	—	—
Postop EBRT + chemo	20 of 50	19	21		3/16	19	—	—
T3/T4, N1/N2 (Surg ± adj)	44, 30	9 vs. 13	4 vs. 22	0.04	—	—	—	—
3. U Penn (gastric or EG)§			(2 yr)					
Surgery alone	40	16	31	—	31	75	—	185
Postop EBRT	17	15	50	—	4	24	—	—
Postop EBRT + chemo	27	21	55	—	4	15	—	—
4. TJUH (EG junction)‖	S EBRT		S EBRT					189
Surgery ± EBRT + chemo	37 18	12 vs. 20		—	—	74 vs. 36	0.0014	—
T3, T4	— —	—	11 14	—	—	87 vs. 47	0.0016	—
LN (−)	— —	—	42 100	—	—	—	—	—
LN (+)	— —	—	0 15	0.001	—	97 vs. 14	0.0001	—
5. Mayo Clinic (gastric, EG)			(4 yr)					
Postop EBRT ± chemo T3, T4 or N+	25	19	31	—	5	20	—	230

postop = postoperative; chemo = chemotherapy; EBRT = external beam irradiation; IOERT = intraoperative electron irradiation; S = surgery; 5-FU = 5-fluorouracil; IORT = intraoperative irradiation; MGH = Massachusetts General Hospital; TJUH = Thomas Jefferson University Hospital; adj = adjuvant treatment; EG = esophagogastric; LN = lymph nodes.

*Long-term survival = 5-year data unless otherwise specified.

†Advantage to IOERT in subset analyses—Japan Stage II–IV, China Stage III (37% of patients).

‡Survival data based on intent to treat, relapse data on actual treatment.

△ = disease-free survival at 3 yrs: 32% versus 49% favoring chemoradiation (p = 0.001).

§Long-term data—2-year survival, negative margins.

‖Mehta and Mohuidden[189]

BSCG trial preclude definitive judgments regarding the value of preoperative EBRT alone or postoperative irradiation (EBRT or IORT) with or without chemotherapy. However, the added positive data from the Beijing trial for preoperative EBRT[229] and from the Walsh and colleagues trial for preoperative EBRT plus chemotherapy[86] adds credibility in questioning whether surgery alone is an appropriate control arm in future phase III studies. Combined-modality treatment is reasonably well tolerated,[9, 10, 181, 182] decreases local-regional failure,[6–8, 181–186] and may improve survival.[182–186] A large U.S. intergroup protocol has been completed in which approximately 550 completely resected high-risk patients were randomized to a surgical-alone control arm versus postoperative EBRT plus chemotherapy.

Results presented at national meetings confirmed the benefit from adjuvant chemoradiation.[186a, 186b]

Locally Advanced Disease

As described above, although some patients in whom resection is not performed have long-term survival using irradiation with or without chemotherapy, this treatment is not a viable alternative to surgical resection plus adjuvant therapy. When locally advanced disease that appears unresectable for cure is diagnosed before surgical exploration, preoperative EBRT would preferably be used in combination with chemotherapy (concomitant during EBRT and maintenance), followed by restaging and an attempted resection of all gross primary and lymph node disease alone or with IORT.

Irradiation Alone

The available literature suggests that adenocarcinoma of the stomach is radioresponsive. Wieland and Hymmen used 60 Gy when feasible (1.5–2.0 Gy daily) with 11% (9 of 82) 3-year and 7% (5 of 72) 5-year survival.[231] Takahashi compared historical controls with patients who were unresectable or who had palliative procedures and received postoperative radiation (unknown if chemotherapy also used).[232] The average survival for the irradiated patients was 9 to 10 months longer, with 74% 1-year (32 of 43) and 27% 2.5-year survival (12 of 43). Abe and Takahashi reported 15% 5-year survival with a single dose of IORT (28–35 Gy) in a group of 27 patients with stage IV disease.[222, 223] Three of the four long-term survivors had proven residual disease after resection. In the same study, 18 stage IV patients were randomized to a surgery-alone control arm with 5-year survival of 0%.

Irradiation plus Chemotherapy

Most reports of combined irradiation and chemotherapy for gastric cancer involve patients with unresectable or residual primary disease, and the majority of phase III trials in this setting show an advantage for combined-modality treatment over single-modality treatment (Table 27–21).

In a Mayo Clinic NCCTG dose escalation pilot study, EBRT was combined with 5-FU plus low-dose leucovorin (400 mg/m^2 and 20 mg/m^2, respectively, for 3 to 4 days, weeks 1 or 1 plus 5 of irradiation).[236] Two of six patients with locally advanced gastric cancer were alive and disease-free beyond 3 years. In the most recent Mayo Clinic analyses of irradiation plus chemotherapy for gastric or esophagogastric cancers by Henning and coworkers,[237] an improvement in survival was suggested for patients with gross total resection but microscopic residual disease when compared with higher risk subsets of patients. In these analyses, the results of irradiation or chemoradiation were evaluated in 87 patients with either locally advanced primary or locally recurrent adenocarcinoma of the stomach or esophagogastric junction treated from July 1980 to January 1996 at the Mayo Clinic. Chemotherapy with 5-FU (plus leucovorin) was given during or following EBRT in 75% of the patients with microscopic residual disease and 92% of the other subgroups (concomitant with EBRT in 84%). An IOERT supplement to EBRT was given in 13 patients. Median survival in primary cancer patients with microscopic residual disease was 16.7 months versus 9.2 months in patients with subtotal resection and gross resid-

TABLE 27–21. **Unresectable or Residual Gastric Cancer: Treatment Results**

Group or Institution	Treatment Arms	EBRT Dose/ Schedule (Gy)	Chemotherapy	No. of Patients	Results (Failure Patterns and Survival)
Randomized					
Mayo Clinic[177, 178]	EBRT ± 5-FU	35–40/9–12 Gy/wk	5-FU 15 mg/kg, d 1–3, wk 1 EBRT	48	Increased SR for EBRT + 5-FU with mean SR 13 vs. 5.9 mo and 3/25 (12%) vs. 0/23 5-yr SR
GITSG[179, 180]	CT ± EBRT	50/8 wk—2 wk split after 25/3 wk	5-FU 500 mg/m^2, d 1–3, wk 1 + 6 EBRT; 5-FU + MeCCNU maintenance vs. 5-FU + MeCCNU	90	Advantage in long-term SR with EBRT + CT at 18% vs. 7% ($p < 0.05$)
Japan[222, 223]	Operation ± IORT*	IORT, 28–40	None	110 operation 101 IORT	Increased 5-yr SR for 27 patients with IORT + operation for stage IV disease vs. 18 patients with operation alone (15% vs. 0%)
Nonrandomized					
MGH[181]	EBRT ± CT	45–55/5–6½ wk	5-FU 500 mg/m^2, 3 d wk 1 EBRT ± maintenance FAM or 5-FU MeCCNU	32†	Median SR res(m) 24 mo, res(g) 15 mo, unresectable 14 mo; survival ≥30 mo, unresected 0%, residual after resection ~10%.
Mayo Clinic[230, 237]	EBRT ± CT ± IOERT	45–54/5–6½ wk; IOERT boost 13 patients	5-FU 500 mg/m^2 3 d wk 1, 5 or 5-FU 400 mg/m^2 leucovorin 20 mg/m^2	87	Median SR res(m)—17 mo, res(g)—9 mo, unresectable—12 mo, locally recurrent—10 mo; 4-year SR ≤9% res(m) and res(g), 18% unresectable or locally recurrent

EBRT, external beam irradiation; SR, survival rate; GITSG, Gastrointestinal Tumor Study Group; CT, chemotherapy; IORT, intraoperative irradiation; MGH, Massachusetts General Hospital; res(m), microscopic residual; res(g), gross residual; IOERT = intraoperative electron irradiation. For chemotherapy abbreviations, see footnotes to Tables 27–16 and 27–22.

*Treatment method based on date of hospitalization.

†An additional 14 had "curative resection" with high-risk LF: 43% 4-yr actuarial SR with EBRT + CT.

ual disease or 12 months in those with unresectable disease. Patients who presented with local or regional relapse had a median survival of 10 months.

Prognostic factor analyses showed that long-term survival appeared slightly poorer in patients who had resection before irradiation or chemoradiation in this latest Mayo Clinic analysis.[237] Actuarial 4-year survival was 0% versus 9% in patients with gross residual disease after partial resection (1 of 11 patients alive with no evidence of disease 2 years after treatment), 9% in those with microscopic residual disease after gross total resection, and 18% in patients with unresectable primary or locally recurrent cancers. The survival trends may be a reflection of both treatment sequence and higher irradiation dose inasmuch as 12 of 13 patients with EBRT plus IOERT had unresectable primary or locally recurrent cancers. In the 21 patients with locally or regionally recurrent cancers, irradiation dose greater than 54 Gy had a trend for improved survival (median survival 25.6 vs. 5.5 months, $p = 0.06$). If patients with microscopic residual disease are excluded, an increase in the number of cycles of chemotherapy appeared to correlate with an improvement in median survival (<2 cycles—median 5.2 months vs. 11.5 months with 2 or 3 cycles and 14.5 months with 4 or more cycles, $p = 0.014$). Because maintenance chemotherapy is not routinely given to gastric cancer patients at the Mayo Clinic, the trend for improved survival with an increased number of cycles of chemotherapy is not a function of which patients were doing well enough to tolerate multiple cycles.

Preoperative Chemotherapy Alone or Plus Irradiation

As a result of the inability of adjuvant (postoperative) systemic therapy to prolong survival in surgically managed gastric cancer, several investigators have pursued the neoadjuvant (preoperative) chemotherapy approach in an attempt to increase resectability and improve survival.[238–251] These studies involve a mix of patients including either those determined as unresectable for cure either surgically or clinically, locally advanced (as defined by the study authors), or clinically operable patients. Some patients were staged clinically by a variety of methods, making it difficult to know which patients were truly resectable prior to neoadjuvant treatment. Table 27–22 summarizes the results of these reports. All but one of these studies are phase II protocols.

UNRESECTABLE DISEASE

One of the earliest reports of neoadjuvant systemic therapy came from Wilke and associates, who examined the role of etoposide, doxorubicin (Adriamycin), and cisplatin (EAP) in a group of 34 patients with laparotomy-determined unresectable stomach cancer.[238] This study was prompted by their promising results with EAP in advanced disease patients (21% complete remission and 64% overall response rate). Following exploratory laparotomy, patients were begun on EAP. Twenty patients (59%) who achieved a clinical response went on to a second-look operation followed by two additional courses of chemotherapy. Fifteen of the original 34 patients (44%) could be resected. Five patients were pathologic complete responders (15% of the original 34). Median survival was 18 months for the entire study group. In an update of this data at an international GI cancer symposium in Germany, results were reported in a series of 21 patients who had total resection after EAP chemotherapy for locally unresectable disease.[239] Fourteen of 21 patients had relapsed, and 11 of 14 had a local-regional component of disease (79% of relapses, 52% of group at risk).

High rates of local-regional relapse after preoperative chemotherapy and resection have also been reported by Verschueren and colleagues, who evaluated 17 patients with unresectable gastric cancer.[240] Fifteen of the patients had undergone laparotomy whereas two patients were deemed unresectable on the basis of CT. After receiving

TABLE 27–22. **Neoadjuvant Chemotherapy for Gastric Cancer**

Author (ref.)	No. Pts.	Regimen	Explored (%)	Resected (%)	Overall Response Rate (%)	Pathologic CR (%)	Survival Med (mo)
Unresectable							
Wilke[238]	34	EAP	59	44	68	15	18
Verschueren[240]	17	5-FU/MTx	76	41	NS	NS	14
Locally Advanced							
Rougier[241]	30	5-FU/CDDP	93	77	50	0	16
Fink[242]	30	EAP	90	80	57	0	17
Alexander[243]	22	5-FU/LV/IFN	91	70	36	NS	18
Kang[244]	53	EFP	89	70	NS	7	43
	54	Control	100	61	—	—	30
Resectable							
Ajani[245]	25	EFP	100	72	24	0	15
Ajani[246]	48	EAP	85	77	31	0	15.5
Kelsen[247]	56	FAMTx preop; ip 5-FU/ CDDP postop 5-FU	89	61	51	0	15.3
Crookes[248]	56	5-FU/CF/CDDP preop, ip FUDR/CDDP postop	95	68	54	9	52

EAP = etoposide, Adriamycin, cisplatin; 5-FU = 5-fluorouracil; MTx = methotrexate; CDDP = cisplatin; FAMTx = 5-FU, Adriamycin, high-dose methotrexate; LV = leucovorin; IFN = interferon; EFP = etoposide, 5-FU, cisplatin; ip = intraperitoneal; ci = continuous infusion; med (mo) = median (months); NS = not stated.

up to four courses of sequential 5-FU and high-dose methotrexate, 13 patients (76%) underwent attempted resection. Although seven patients were found to be resectable (41%), local-regional relapse subsequently occurred in five of seven. No postoperative systemic therapy was administered. The median survival for the entire group was 14 months.

Additional trials in patients with unresectable disease have demonstrated that preoperative chemotherapy was feasible and resulted in clinical response rates of 30% to 68%, as well as curative resections in 8% to 73% of patients. This wide range of resectability likely reflects patient selection rather than superiority of any one regimen. Unfortunately, pathologic complete responses (CRs) were uncommon except for the Wilke study.[238]

BORDERLINE RESECTABLE/LOCALLY ADVANCED DISEASE

A number of phase II studies have tested the use of preoperative systemic treatment in patients defined by the study authors as having locally advanced stomach cancer. Presumably this category represents a mix of clinically resectable and unresectable or borderline resectable patients. In a trial by Rougier and coworkers, patients received two to three cycles of cisplatin and 5-FU before surgery.[241] In the 23 resected patients, no pathologic CRs were seen and the overall median survival was 16 months. EAP was studied in 30 patients by Fink and colleagues.[242] In resected patients, no pathologic CRs were seen and median survival was 17 months. Alexander and associates used 5-FU, leucovorin, and interferon both preoperatively and postoperatively in 22 patients.[243] No pathologic CRs were reported and median survival was 17 months.

Kang and associates presented an updated report of the only phase III trial of neoadjuvant chemotherapy in locally advanced or borderline resectable gastric cancer in 107 patients randomized to receive two to three cycles of etoposide, 5-FU, and cisplatin (EFP) followed by surgery versus surgery alone.[244] Of the 53 patients randomized to preoperative treatment, 47 (89%) were explored, and 37 (70%) were resected for cure. A 7% pathologic CR rate was noted. In the control group of 54 patients, 100% were explored and 61% curatively resected. Median survival was 43 months versus 30 months in favor of neoadjuvant treatment, but this difference did not reach statistical significance ($p = 0.114$).

RESECTABLE DISEASE

Several investigators have examined the role of neoadjuvant chemotherapy in patients with clinically resectable disease (see Table 27–22). Ajani and colleagues have performed two phase II studies of preoperative chemotherapy in this setting. In the first study, 25 patients were treated with two preoperative cycles of etoposide, 5-FU, and cisplatin (EFP).[245] In the 25 patients who underwent surgery, 72% were resected for cure; no pathologic CRs were seen, and median survival was 15 months overall. Following Wilke and associates' report of a 15% pathologic CR to EAP chemotherapy,[238] Ajani and colleagues treated 48 potentially curable patients with three cycles of preoperative EAP and two cycles following surgery if a response to preoperative treatment was observed.[246] Of the 48 patients, 85% underwent exploration, and 77% were resectable; no pathologic CRs were seen in resected patients. The overall median survival was 15.5 months. Unfortunately, in this group of resectable patients with potentially smaller tumor burdens, the impressive results obtained with neoadjuvant EAP in Wilke and associates' study could not be reproduced.

In the late 1990s, other investigators examined the utility of combining preoperative chemotherapy and postoperative treatment with intraperitoneal chemotherapy in view of the high peritoneal failure rate following resection of gastric cancer. Kelsen and coworkers studied 56 patients with high-risk (clinical T3 or T4) gastric cancer who received three cycles of neoadjuvant FAMTx, surgery, and postoperative intraperitoneal 5-FU and cisplatin along with infusional 5-FU for three cycles.[247] Although 51% of patients were downstaged as determined by comparing the initial endoscopic ultrasonography and the final pathologic staging, no pathologic CRs were observed and the median survival was 15.3 months. Crookes and colleagues had somewhat similar trial design, treating 59 potentially resectable patients with two cycles of 5-FU, leucovorin, and cisplatin preoperatively, and two cycles of intraperitoneal 5-FUDR and cisplatin postoperatively in resected patients.[248] The pathologic CR rate in resected patients was only 9%, although the estimated median survival was an impressive 52 months.

SUMMARY—PREOPERATIVE CHEMOTHERAPY ALONE OR PLUS IRRADIATION

Advantages to preoperative systemic treatment include the potential of reducing tumor bulk, increasing surgical resectability, and affecting micrometastatic disease. In addition, some investigators point to experimental models where surgical resection may serve as a stimulus for increased growth of residual disease.[249] Theoretically, the stimulus to proliferate may lead to more spontaneous mutations and enhanced chemotherapy resistance. In addition, the altered vascular supply to tumor cells caused by surgery, which may compromise drug delivery, would be circumvented by a neoadjuvant approach.[250] Potential negatives to preoperative treatment include toxicity, delay in definitive therapy, and potential increased surgical morbidity and mortality.[249, 250] The high response rates achieved with neoadjuvant chemotherapy are of interest, and this form of treatment will undoubtedly be the subject of further investigation over the next several years.

Because no survival advantage has been demonstrated in phase III trials, neoadjuvant chemotherapy should be considered investigational. Although resectability rates in neoadjuvantly treated patients seem higher than the median rate of 40% from several surgical studies, the patients in these studies are highly selected. Except for the trials in which some patients were unresectable on the basis of prior exploration, the successful operations in these reports may not have been influenced by neoadjuvant chemotherapy. In general, pathologic CR rates are low (<15%), and no proof exists that clinically staged patients are made more resectable by such treatment. The impact of preoperative systemic treatment on survival is even less clear. The one reported randomized trial shows a nonsignificant improvement in survival for neoadjuvant treatment in borderline resectable/locally advanced disease.[244] Newer technologies such as endoscopic ultrasonography [EUS] may identify patients who will do poorly with standard therapy alone and would be reasonable candidates for future neoadjuvant studies.[247] The reports of combined systemic and intraperitoneal approaches are provocative and may warrant future phase III trials because only through such studies will any impact on survival be determined.

In view of the high incidence of local-regional relapse noted in several series of patients resected after neoadjuvant chemotherapy for initially unresectable lesions, irradiation has been incorporated into the study design of recent trials for patients with high-risk factors. The positive results of the esophagus and gastric cardia trial by Walsh and colleagues[86] and high pathologic CR rates in similar pilot studies with gastric-only cancers[251] have led to larger confirmatory trials of neoadjuvant CMT in carcinoma of the esophagus and gastroesophageal junction and potentially a separate trial for gastric cancers.

Metastatic Cancers—Results

Comparison of Single-Drug or Multidrug Chemotherapy Regimens

The combination of 5-FU and a nitrosourea (MeCCNU or BCNU) represents one of the earliest combined drug regimens evaluated for advanced gastric cancer. Although early response rates were encouraging, survival was no better than single-agent 5-FU.[252] In the early 1980s, the combination of 5-FU, doxorubicin (Adriamycin), and mitomycin C (FAM) became widely used. This was based on a report from MacDonald and associates, who demonstrated a 42% response rate in 62 patients with advanced measurable gastric cancer.[187, 253] Although the overall median survival was a modest 5.5 months, the median survival for responding patients was 12.5 months. Subsequent randomized trials, however, could not demonstrate a survival advantage for FAM versus 5-FU alone.[254] The addition of cisplatin to 5-FU and Adriamycin (FAP) yielded response rates of 53% in a phase II Mayo Clinic study. A phase III Mayo/NCCTG study, however, did not show an advantage for FAP over 5-FU alone.[255]

In 1989, Wilke and colleagues reported interesting results for the combination of etoposide, doxorubicin, and cisplatin (EAP) in 67 patients with advanced gastric cancer; the overall response rate was 64%, and the CR rate was 21%.[188] Follow-up phase II studies revealed response rates of 13% to 73%, but some authors reported worrisome toxicity. Interestingly, Presseur and colleagues developed a less toxic regimen for patients medically unfit for EAP using a combination of etoposide, leucovorin, and 5-FU (ELF). ELF produced a response rate of 53% and median survival of 11 months.[256]

Sequential methotrexate and 5-FU followed by doxorubicin (Adriamycin) (FAMTx) has also been widely studied based on a large phase II trial, which revealed a response rate of 58% and median survival of 9 months. When compared with FAM in a randomized study by the EORTC, FAMTx showed both superior response rates (41% vs. 9%, $p < 0.0001$) and survival (median 42 versus 29 weeks, $p = 0.004$).[257] FAMTx also has been shown to be less toxic than EAP in a randomized trial of 60 patients from MSKCC by Kelsen and coworkers.[258] Finally, FAMTx has been compared with ELF and 5-FU/cisplatin in a preliminary report of an EORTC study. No apparent differences in response rates or survival have been demonstrated at present.[259]

Investigators from Great Britain studied the regimen of epirubicin, cisplatin, and infusional 5-FU (ECF) and demonstrated a 71% response rate in 139 patients. A subsequent phase III study from Great Britain showed superiority for ECF over FAMTx for both overall response rate (45% vs. 21%) and median survival (8.9 months vs. 5.7 months).[260]

Supportive Care Versus Chemotherapy

In 1993, Murad and coworkers published results of a randomized trial in which a modified FAMTx regimen was compared with best supportive care.[261] The trial was interrupted after entry of 22 patients because the treated patients were enjoying a significantly better outcome. The next 18 patients were assigned directly to treatment. Median survival for all the treated patients was 10 months versus 3 months for the untreated controls ($p = 0.001$).

Pyrhonen and associates reported the results of 41 patients randomized to 5-FU, epirubicin, and methotrexate (FEMTx) plus vitamins A and E versus the same vitamins and best supportive care.[262] In FEMTx patients, 29% had an objective response and 33% had stable disease for greater than 2 months. In control patients, 20% had stable disease. Median time to progression (5.4 vs. 1.7 months) and median survival (12.3 vs. 3.1 months) both favored treatment with FEMTx ($p = 0.0013$ and $p = 0.0006$, respectively).

Glimelius and colleagues studied, in a group of 61 patients with inoperable gastric cancer, the cost-effectiveness of palliative therapy by randomly assigning patients to primary chemotherapy with ELF or 5-FU plus leucovorin versus best supportive care.[263] Improved or prolonged high quality of life was documented in patients receiving chemotherapy versus supportive care alone. Chemotherapy patients had a significantly longer median survival at 8 months versus 5 months (adjusted p value $= 0.003$) and quality-of-life analysis also favored the treated patients ($p < 0.05$).

Survival by Stage

Stage 0

Experience in Japan, where stage 0 is diagnosed frequently, indicates that 85% to 90% of patients treated by radical subtotal gastrectomy with lymphadenectomy will survive beyond 5 years.

Stage I, II, and Resectable Stage III

Total surgical resection of the cancer with a radical subtotal gastrectomy and reconstruction with gastrojejunostomy is recommended. The expected 5-year survival rate with surgery alone for stage I is 50% to 85% and for stage II, 20% to 50%. IORT of gastric cancer has shown a modest improvement in results by Japanese investigators[222, 223] for stage II and for stage III and by Chinese investigators for stage III disease.[224]

Neither chemotherapy nor radiation therapy nor both in combination were previously recommended except in prospective controlled trials (see Table 27–12). However, for patients with high-risk factors for local relapse, adjuvant irradiation or chemoradiation has been shown to reduce local relapse rates and increase survival in single-institution and small randomized trials. Confirmatory postoperative chemoradiation trials have been completed, and adjuvant chemoradiation has demonstrated a survival benefit for high-risk patients at 3 years.[186a, 186b] Compared with patients treated with surgery alone, the patients treated with chemoradiation had an overall survival rate of 52% versus 41% ($p = 0.03$) and a disease-free survival rate of 49% versus 32% ($p = 0.001$).

Stage III

For resectable stage III disease, see the preceding two paragraphs. In locally unresectable or resected but residual gastric cancer, combined-modality chemoradiation or combination chemotherapy can be utilized. Expected 5-year survival is 10% to 20%.

Stage IV

For patients with locally unresectable or resected but residual stage IV malignancies with no evidence of metastases, 5-year survival rates of 10% to 20% have been achieved with IORT or EBRT plus chemotherapy. In metastatic cancer, combined drug chemotherapy is appropriate and improves both quality and duration of life when compared with best supportive care. Radiation can be used for painful local metastatic lesions. With metastatic cancer, it would be rare to have any survivors at 5 years.

Special Considerations and Treatment

Malignant Lymphoma

The GI tract is the most common extranodal site for non-Hodgkin's lymphoma, with the highest incidence of primary disease in the western world arising in the stomach. The Ann Arbor staging system is utilized to stage these patients; however, the degree of gastric wall penetration and histology do have prognostic significance. The standard approach to gastric lymphoma in the past was surgical resection, which was both therapeutic and served to pathologically stage the disease, but combined chemoradiation is an appropriate if not preferable option in many patients.[264] Better diagnostic (endoscopy and biopsy) and staging tests (CT, lymphangiography, laparoscopy) obviate the need for surgical staging. Although concern exists that chemotherapy and radiation could lead to rapid tumor lysis with gastric hemorrhage and perforation, this concept has been challenged by authors including Maor and coworkers, who treated a group of patients primarily with combined chemotherapy and radiation and obtained favorable results without increased morbidity.[264] The optimal staging-treatment strategy of surgery, radiation, and chemotherapy is still in a state of debate for patients with stage IE and IIE disease.

Gastric Leiomyosarcoma

Resection is effective for GI stromal sarcomas (including prior histologic subtype of leiomyosarcoma) and may be less radical than with carcinoma. These lesions rarely metastasize to lymph nodes and do not require *en bloc* node removal. If lesions extend beyond the wall and marginal resection relative to other structures occurs, local relapse rates of 70% to 90% would be likely based on retroperitoneal sarcoma literature. Adjuvant preoperative irradiation plus chemotherapy and IOERT may be indicated in such cases.

Clinical Investigations

Screening

Screening tests (i.e., brush cytology) for high-risk subgroups are being developed. These populations might include patients with pernicious anemia, chronic atrophic gastritis, and previous gastrectomy for ulcer disease. Earlier diagnosis is essential to improving cure rates.

Completely Resected Lesions

Many patients with gross complete resection of their gastric cancer are not cured with surgery alone. If patients with early gastric cancer are excluded (lesions confined to the mucosa or submucosa without nodal involvement), the remaining patients benefit from adjuvant local-regional and systemic treatment. Because both local and systemic relapses are common following complete resection of gastric cancers, combinations of chemotherapy and irradiation have been evaluated in a confirmatory intergroup trial in the United States, which tested combined-modality postoperative EBRT plus chemotherapy (before, during, and after EBRT) versus a surgery-alone control arm in approximately 600 patients. Because survival benefit has been shown with adjuvant chemoradiation, trimodality therapy will serve as the new standard of treatment for resected high-risk patients. Successive trials will test issues of treatment intensification with alternate chemotherapy regimens or treatment sequencing.

On the basis of encouraging results with preoperative chemotherapy or chemoradiation for locally advanced disease, future phase III intergroup studies are being considered to evaluate preoperative chemoradiation in combination with resection plus IORT and postoperative chemotherapy for patients with potentially resectable lesions. Because some of the newer drug combinations have CR rates of approximately 20%, the hope is that these regimens will alter systemic failure rates more than previous combinations. This response has not yet been demonstrated in phase III trials.

Locally Advanced Disease

For patients with locally advanced disease, it seems reasonable to build on positive segments of treatment data (EBRT plus chemotherapy, IOERT, preoperative chemotherapy, preoperative EBRT, and preoperative chemoradiation) plus patterns of failure information. EBRT plus chemotherapy or IOERT alone or with EBRT has improved local control of disease and produced long-term survival in 10% to 20% of patients in most single-institution analyses and randomized trials in patients with locally unresectable cancers or residual disease after resection. Preoperative chemotherapy for locally advanced disease has resulted in subsequent total resection of disease in approximately 40% of patients in several European trials with EAP or other regimens. However, the incidence of subsequent local-regional relapse is significant, even after total resection.

The evaluation of high-dose preoperative irradiation plus simultaneous chemotherapy is reasonable if laparoscopy or laparotomy have ruled out peritoneal spread and diagnostic imaging has been used to define extragastric extent of disease (endoscopic ultrasound, CT, etc.). In patients with subtotal resection and residual disease after neoadjuvant chemotherapy or resection but high-risk factors for relapse (beyond the gastric wall, nodes positive, or both), IORT should be evaluated in conjunction with maintenance chemotherapy.

For patients whose malignancy is unresectable but still localized after preoperative chemotherapy alone (no EBRT) on the basis of preoperative staging, including laparoscopy or exploratory laparotomy, preoperative EBRT plus infusion chemotherapy should be considered before resection is attempted. Decisions regarding attempts at later resection alone or with IORT and maintenance chemotherapy could be individualized by institution.

Metastatic Disease

Innovative combination chemotherapy and intraperitoneal chemotherapy trials are under way, and new drugs being tested include the topoisomerase I inhibitors and taxanes. Alternative approaches that should be evaluated include biologicals, gene therapy, and angiogenesis and metastasis inhibitors. Response rates must be correlated to survival as these new treatment programs are evaluated. Only durable responses are clinically meaningful.

Small Intestine

Epidemiology and Etiology

Although 90% of the mucosal surface of the alimentary tract is small bowel, less than 5% of GI tumors or carcinomas occur in this organ.[265] The estimated incidence of small bowel cancers in the United States for 2000 is 4700, split proportionally between men and women. The estimated number of deaths in the United States for 2000 is 1200 patients.[2]

The most common benign tumors of this organ are leiomyomas and adenomatous polyps.[266] The most common malignant tumor is adenocarcinoma in the proximal small bowel and carcinoid in the distal bowel. Lymphomas and sarcomas are less frequent malignancies. A typical distribution of small bowel tumors is outlined in Table 27–23.

Several factors contribute to the low rate of mutagenesis in the small bowel[266, 267]:

1. Neutralization of acids by pancreatic and small bowel secretions protects against carcinogenic effects of nitrosamines, which usually require the presence of acid for activity.[267, 268]
2. Rapid peristalsis decreases exposure of mucosal surfaces to intraluminal carcinogens.
3. High concentrations of IgA and abundant lymphoid tissue are immunologic factors that probably help protect the small bowel from the development of cancer.
4. There may be competitive inhibition of malignant cells as a result of the rapid proliferation rates seen in the normal mucosa.

One of the most important causes of small bowel cancer is inherited disorders. These disorders include familial adenomatous polyposis (FAP), Gardner's syndrome, Peutz-Jeghers syndrome, and Crohn's disease.

Detection and Diagnosis

Clinical Detection

Clinical detection of small bowel tumors can be very difficult and requires special attention to various signs and

TABLE 27–23. **Distribution of Malignant Neoplasms in the Small Intestine**

Type of Neoplasm	Number and Percentage by Region			
	Duodenum	*Jejunum*	*Ileum*	*Total*
Adenocarcinoma	427 (40%)	408 (38%)	241 (22%)	1076 (46%)
Sarcoma	46 (10%)	162 (36%)	239 (54%)	447 (19%)
Lymphoma	4 (16%)	9 (36%)	12 (48%)	25 (1%)
Carcinoid	48 (6%)	78 (10%)	682 (84%)	808 (34%)
Total	525 (22%)	660 (28%)	1171 (50%)	2356 (100%)

From Sindelar WF: Cancer of the small intestine. In: De Vita VT Jr, Hellman S, Rosenberg SA (eds): Cancer, Principles and Practice of Oncology, 3rd ed, pp 875–894. Philadelphia, J.B. Lippincott Co., 1989, with permission.

symptoms. Frequently, the symptoms of these lesions are insidious and nonspecific. Over one third of patients have symptoms for 6 to 12 months before diagnosis is made.

Symptoms

- *Abdominal pain* is usually cramping in nature and related to obstruction. A benign small bowel tumor is the most common cause of intussusception in adults.[267] Carcinomas are more likely to cause a napkin ring obstruction. Lymphomas generally obstruct by extrinsic compression and dysmotility through nerve invasion.
- *Hemorrhage* is usually slow and chronic. Hemangiomas, on the other hand, are the exception that can bleed massively. Carcinoid tumors rarely bleed.
- *Weight loss* occurs in 50% of patients and is especially associated with lymphoma.

Signs and Syndromes

- An *abdominal mass* is palpable in nearly 25% of patients and is usually moveable.
- *Jaundice* is a particular finding in duodenal tumors that involve the ampulla.
- *Occult or gross blood* per rectum can be an early sign of a small bowel neoplasm.

Syndromes that are associated with small bowel tumors[268] help the clinician diagnose small bowel cancers that might otherwise be silent. Examples include the following:

1. *Carcinoid syndrome*: Carcinoid tumors have the capacity to produce serotonin, histamine, and bradykinin. These compounds cause a clinical syndrome manifested by attacks of watery diarrhea, cutaneous flushing, and asthmatic-type respiratory distress. Lesions of tricuspid and pulmonic valves also occur. This syndrome does not occur in all instances of carcinoid tumor. The syndrome is most frequently associated with carcinoids of the ileum or extensive hepatic metastases. Carcinoids most commonly occur on the appendix, but rarely produce carcinoid syndrome from this site.[269]
2. *Peutz-Jeghers syndrome* is a genetically determined syndrome transmitted in a dominant sex-linked pattern of inheritance. Hamartomas appear along the small bowel, with malignant transformation being rare. The syndrome includes pigmented lesions of the skin and mucous membranes at an early age.[268]
3. *Gardner's syndrome* is a familial syndrome of small and large intestinal polyps; these polyps are true adenomas. Associated anomalies are desmoid tumors, osteomas, and abnormalities of the teeth. Periampullary carcinomas are increased in these patients.

Diagnostic Procedures

- The small bowel is difficult to evaluate by radiographic methods. An *upper GI series* extended with a *small bowel follow-through* can characterize some lesions, although the redundancy of the small bowel frequently obscures the ability of this examination to detect small lesions.
- The small bowel *enema* or *enteroclysis* is a more sensitive method of examining the small bowel by passing a nasoenteral tube and instilling contrast with pressure in the region of the ligament of Treitz in order to delineate smaller lesions in the intestine. A *barium enema* can be used to visualize the terminal ileum if reflux is obtained through the ileocecal valve.
- Other radiographic methods for evaluating small bowel cancers include *angiography* through the superior mesenteric artery. This test is helpful for cases of acute hemorrhage. Also, *CT scan* may be helpful to evaluate metastatic disease. Magnetic resonance imaging is of no value because of bowel motion.
- *Flexible endoscopy* allows for a direct visualization of the luminal aspect of many tumors and also offers the opportunity for biopsy or polypectomy.
- Pertinent *laboratory studies* in patients who are thought to have small bowel tumors include a CBC (to detect anemia) and liver function tests, with particular interest in bilirubin and amylase. In cases of carcinoid tumors, a 5-hydroxyindole acetic acid level is indicated.
- *Abdominal exploration* is frequently the best diagnostic test and is usually required when a specific diagnosis or site of bleeding cannot be determined. Unfortunately, explorations for small bowel tumors are usually unproductive when preoperative x-rays are negative and the patient does not have acute obstruction or hemorrhage.

Classification and Staging

Classification of small bowel tumors correlates to their histopathologic type (see Table 27–23). The current TNM staging classification is depicted in Table 27–24.

Principles of Treatment

Surgery

Surgery remains the therapeutic mainstay for all intestinal malignancies. A wide mesenteric margin is indicated in curative procedures for carcinoma. Palliative resections are indicated for advanced stage tumors that present with GI obstruction, bleeding, or perforation. Periampullary invasive malignancies require a pancreaticoduodenectomy, whereas a segmental duodenal resection may be sufficient for cancers elsewhere in the duodenum. Bowel lymphomas are still managed initially with surgical resection, but postoperative therapy is required for the curative management of these patients.

Small bowel carcinoids most commonly occur in the distal ileum, necessitating a right hemicolectomy to achieve clearance of metastatic nodal tissue. Patients with carcinoid syndrome in whom more than 90% to 95% of the hepatic tumor mass can be resected benefit from tumor debulking.

Irradiation or Chemoradiation

The rationale for and method of irradiation for small bowel cancers is related both to the histology and location of the

TABLE 27–24. **TNM Staging for Small Intestine**

Stage	Grouping	TNM Descriptor
Stage 0	Tis, N0, M0	Tis: Carcinoma *in situ* N0: No regional lymph node metastasis M0: No distant metastasis
Stage I	T1, N0, M0 T2, N0, M0	T1: Tumor invades lamina propria or submucosa T2: Tumor invades the muscularis propria
Stage II	T3, N0, M0	T3: Tumor invades through the muscularis propria into the subserosa or into the nonperitonealized perimuscular tissue with extension of ≤2 cm
	T4, N0, M0	T4: Tumor perforates visceral peritoneum or directly invades other organs or structures
Stage III	Any T, N1, M0	N1: Regional lymph node metastasis
Stage IV	Any T, Any N, M1	M1: Distant metastasis present

Used with permission of the American Joint Committee on Cancer (AJCC®), Chicago, Illinois. The original source for this material is the AJCC® Cancer Staging Manual, 5th ed, 1997, published by Lippincott-Raven Publishers, Philadelphia, Pennsylvania.

primary cancer and what the surgeon can accomplish with regard to degree of surgical resection. Whole abdominal irradiation is used in some institutions for patients with lymphoma or carcinoid lesions that are surgically unresectable or are partially resected but with residual disease because the entire abdominal cavity may be at risk. Adjuvant irradiation to the tumor bed alone, or plus nodal areas at risk, can be considered following complete resection of most histologic types of small bowel cancers, but is dependent on the following:

- the location of the primary lesion (anatomically mobile vs. immobile component of the small bowel)
- presence or absence of high-risk factors with regard to local relapse (primary tumor extension beyond the muscularis propria [rctropcritoncal small bowel] or serosa [intraperitoneal small bowel]), with adherence to or adjacency to an unresected structure
- presence or absence of nodal involvement

The indications for adjuvant irradiation, alone or in combination with concomitant and maintenance chemotherapy, at the Mayo Clinic are based on tumor extent as determined on preoperative imaging or surgical-pathologic findings, or both:

1. If *preoperative CT imaging* suggests the likelihood of unresectability as a result of tumor fixation or a *marginal gross total resection* with narrow or microscopically involved margins, histologic diagnosis is usually achieved with CT-guided biopsy. Consultations are then obtained with both the surgeon and the radiation oncologist and also, in preference, with the medical oncologist to determine if preoperative adjuvant irradiation (alone or with concomitant chemotherapy) is indicated. If the histology is adenocarcinoma or carcinoid, 5-FU–based chemotherapy is combined with the preoperative irradiation; if the biopsy reveals sarcoma, cisplatin-based chemotherapy may be combined with the irradiation. If the lesion is found to be a lymphoma, multiple-drug chemotherapy precedes any consideration of resection or preoperative irradiation. Patients with carcinoma, carcinoid, or sarcoma histology are scheduled for restaging, resection, and IOERT 3 to 5 weeks following completion of the preoperative adjuvant treatment (see "Colon and Rectum" section of this chapter for a discussion of indications and results with IOERT as a component of treatment).
2. If preoperative imaging or surgical exploration suggests that *total resection* can be accomplished *with acceptable margins*, the surgical resection is performed. Postoperative adjuvant treatment is considered for patients with high-risk lesions in the anatomically immobile segments of small bowel (duodenum, proximal jejunum, occasionally distal ileum) or for lesions at any site in which there is tumor adherence to an adjacent organ or structure that cannot be resected with wide margins. For patients with resected carcinoma, carcinoid, or lymphoma in an anatomically immobile segment of small bowel, it would be reasonable to offer postoperative adjuvant treatment with the pathologic finding of tumor extension beyond the bowel wall, nodal involvement, or both. This treatment is currently done for rectal cancers, an anatomically similar situation with regard to the potential for compromised surgical margins of resection. Because it would be rare to have nodal involvement with small bowel sarcomas, adjuvant treatment is indicated primarily for lesions in an anatomically immobile site with extension beyond the wall and narrow margins of resection. In all instances, surgical clip placement to mark the tumor and nodal areas at risk along with surgical reconstruction, if feasible, would improve the accuracy of irradiation fields and potentially decrease the risk of treatment-related morbidity.

The potential indications for, and results of, adjuvant irradiation alone or with chemotherapy are demonstrated in an MGH series of resected ampullary carcinomas analyzed by Willett and associates.[270] Survival and patterns of relapse were determined in a series of 41 patients. For 12 patients with low-risk pathologic features (limited to the ampulla or duodenum, well or moderately differentiated, uninvolved margins and nodes), the 5-year actuarial local control and survival rates were 100% and 80% respectively, after surgery alone. In 17 high-risk patients treated with surgery alone, those rates were 50% and 38% respectively ($p < 0.05$); high risk was defined as tumor invasion of the pancreas, poorly differentiated lesions, and involved nodes or margins. An additional 12 patients with high-risk cancers received postoperative irradiation alone or with 5-FU. Although the adjuvant treatment appeared to improve 5-year local control and survival rates, with values of 83% versus 50% and 51% versus 38% respectively, these differences were not statistically significant in view of small patient numbers and distant relapse (liver, peritoneum, pleura).

Chemotherapy

Indications for concomitant chemoradiation are discussed in the prior section on principles of irradiation, and indications for primary chemotherapy for metastatic disease will be mentioned only briefly here. For adenocarcinomas, the combination of 5-FU and leucovorin is used most commonly on the basis of positive results with large bowel carcinomas. Lymphomas have shown response to common chemotherapeutic programs. Streptozotocin and 5-FU are standard systemic agents for unresectable carcinoid tumors. Carcinoid syndrome is treated with antiserotonin agents and somatostatin analogue.

Results and Prognosis

Overall Survival

The 5-year survival results vary by site in the small intestine and by tumor histology, with a 5-year survival range of 20% to 70%.

Survival by Tumor Type

1. *Adenocarcinoma* most frequently occurs in the duodenum, and 5-year survival rates following resection are 20% to 30%.[268]
2. *Sarcomas* have an overall better prognosis with a 5-year survival rate of 20% to 50%.[268]
3. Resectable *lymphomas* have a 40% to 70% survival rate if radiation is added.[268] Unresectable lymphomas have a prognosis of 25% survival.
4. Survival of *carcinoid* tumor also depends on resectability. Generally, however, these tumors are slow growing and have relatively longer survival rates. Even metastatic carcinoid disease has a 60% to 70% 5-year survival if the metastatic tumors can be resected. A 40% 5-year survival rate is reported in those instances where the carcinoid tumors are unresectable.

Clinical Investigations

In view of the small number of cases of primary small bowel cancers each year, meaningful phase III clinical trials are unlikely to be performed in a single country, even at an intergroup level. Institutions are encouraged to conduct single-or multi-institution prospective phase II studies in which patients are treated in standardized fashion to test clinical hypotheses in patients with locally unresectable or resected high-risk lesions, as previously defined. Until results from expanded phase II studies are available, we can only theorize with regard to the rationale for multimodality treatment in specific circumstances.

Prospective phase II studies that would be of interest include the following:

1. To evaluate resected ampullary cancer patients to determine if the data from MGH,[270] discussed in the section on "Irradiation and Chemoradiation," is accurate with regard to high-risk factors for local relapse and survival following resection, and whether the use of adjuvant irradiation alone or with 5-FU can improve disease control and survival. Both postoperative and preoperative sequencing of adjuvant treatment need to be evaluated.
2. To evaluate preoperative irradiation plus concomitant infusion 5-FU in the treatment of duodenal adenocarcinomas (or other anatomically immobile small bowel sites). This investigation is based on the high rates of pathologic CR following preoperative irradiation plus infusion 5-FU for patients with primary duodenal cancers treated at the Fox Chase Cancer Center that contrasted with a nonexistent rate of CR in patients treated in similar fashion for primary adenocarcinoma of the pancreas.[271]

Colon and Rectum

Perspective

Combined-modality chemoradiation is commonly used as a component of treatment, in combination with maximum resection, for both high-risk resectable and locally advanced primary or recurrent rectal cancers. With surgically resected but high-risk rectal cancers, postoperative chemoradiation has been shown to improve both disease control (local and distant) and survival (disease-free and overall) and was recommended as standard adjuvant treatment at the 1990 National Institutes of Health (NIH) Consensus Conference on adjuvant treatment for patients with rectal and colon cancers. In a large Swedish trial, preoperative irradiation achieved similar improvements in local control and survival when compared with a surgery-alone control arm for resectable primary rectal cancers. Subsequently, trials are being conducted in high-risk primary rectal cancers to help define optimal combinations of postoperative chemoradiation (United States Intergroup), to test sequencing issues of preoperative versus postoperative chemoradiation (National Surgical Adjuvant Breast and Bowel Program [NSABP]) and to define if concomitant and maintenance 5-FU plus leucovorin add to the benefits found with preoperative irradiation (EORTC).

With locally unresectable primary or recurrent colorectal cancers, standard therapy with surgery, EBRT, and concomitant chemotherapy is often unsuccessful. When IOERT is added to standard treatment, local control and survival appear to be improved when compared with historical controls in separate analyses from the Mayo Clinic and the MGH. However, maintenance systemic therapy is also needed as a component of treatment, in view of high rates of systemic failure.

For patients with resected node-positive colon cancers, the addition of postoperative chemotherapy improves disease-free and overall survival. Six months of bolus 5-FU plus leucovorin is equivalent to 12 months of 5-FU plus levamisole, and the shorter regimen has become the standard adjuvant treatment in the United States. The addition of irradiation to surgical resection and chemotherapy was tested in a randomized phase III United States Intergroup trial for patients at high risk for local relapse.

Epidemiology and Etiology

Epidemiology

Colorectal cancer was projected to afflict 130,200 Americans in 2000 (colon—93,800, rectum—36,400).[2] The incidence is equal among men and women. Overall, 56,300 deaths due to colorectal cancer were anticipated in 2000: 47,700 from cancer of the colon and 8600 from rectal cancers.[2] These results are second only to lung cancer in terms of nationwide mortality. Most patients are over 50 years of age, with a median age of approximately 60 years. Subgroups of patients, including those with familial polyposis or ulcerative colitis, can develop colorectal cancer at a much earlier age. Rectal carcinoma is uncommon below 20 years of age.

Several series have reported an increasing incidence of cancer in the right side of the large bowel, as opposed to more distal lesions.[272, 273] Wider use of screening sigmoidoscopy and polypectomy may have decreased the relative incidence of rectal cancers. Approximately 50% of colorectal cancers are now found to originate beyond the range of the rigid sigmoidoscope. A typical distribution of cancers in the large bowel is as follows: ascending, 24%; transverse, 16%; descending, 7%; sigmoid, 38%; rectum, 15%.[273]

Etiology

Environmental Factors

The prevalence of colorectal cancer in the western world is attributed to a diet high in animal fat and low in fiber. Supportive data are derived from studies of Japanese immigrants to the United States who develop colorectal cancer with a frequency 2.5 times greater than Japanese people who still live in Japan. In rural Africa, where fiber and cellulose comprise a high percentage of the daily diet, colon cancer is rare. An NCI review article noted an inverse relationship between dietary fiber intake and large bowel cancer in most studies.[274] Armstrong and Doll reported a strong association between total fat consumption and mortality rates for large bowel cancers.[275]

Dietary fat stimulates the production of bile acids that influence proliferation of gut epithelium. Fiber increases fecal bulk, lowers transit time, and decreases fecal pH; all of these are factors that potentially reduce the impact of intraluminal carcinogens.

Genetic Causes

Genetic conditions that increase the risk of developing a large bowel cancer include familial adenomatous polyposis syndrome (FAP) and its variants and hereditary nonpolyposis colorectal cancer. FAP is a hereditary disease with an autosomal dominant transmission pattern characterized by pancolonic adenomatous polyps. If not treated by surgical removal of the large bowel, most patients die of colorectal cancer before age 60.[276] Gardner's syndrome includes desmoid tumors, osteomas, and fibromas in addition to colorectal adenomas. The risk for developing adenocarcinoma is similar to those patients with FAP. Peutz-Jeghers syndrome and juvenile polyposis are also associated with an increased risk of developing large bowel or other GI cancers.

Inherited familial cancer syndromes also have been described in which affected members have fewer polyps than are seen with FAP. The genetic condition is inherited in an autosomal dominant pattern and includes Lynch syndromes I and II. Patients are typically young, have multiple large bowel lesions, and have a higher incidence of other intraabdominal malignancies.[277]

Polyps—Progression to Cancer

Polyps are mucosal tumors that may be pedunculated on a stalk or sessile; they have variable degrees of malignant potential. Hyperplastic polyps are most common but do not progress to adenomas or carcinomas. Adenomatous polyps have a higher likelihood of progressive malignant evolution. Histologically they may be tubular or villous. Risk factors for malignancy include size greater than 2 cm, villous features, and degree of dysplasia. One of the most exciting research discoveries was the uncovering of the multistep gene mutations that accompany progression in colonic neoplasia.[277a]

Inflammatory Bowel Disease

The risk of large bowel cancer increases markedly in patients with inflammatory bowel disease, particularly chronic ulcerative colitis. The risk correlates with the duration of ulcerative colitis and the degree of large bowel involvement. At any time during the process of ulcerative colitis, the finding of dysplasia in the mucosa confers a 50% chance of developing carcinoma[278]; after 30 years, the incidence of cancer reaches 35%.

Crohn's Disease

Crohn's disease results in a slight increased risk in large bowel cancer. This risk, however, is less than is noted in patients with ulcerative colitis.

Diverticulosis

Diverticulosis and cancer may be found together, but there is no evidence that the presence of diverticula predisposes to the development of cancer.

Detection and Diagnosis

Clinical Detection

History and Physical Examination

History and physical examination can alert the physician to colorectal cancer. A change in bowel function (constipation or diarrhea) is often the first symptom of this disease. Other symptoms are related to the location of the primary in the large bowel.

- *Right colon*: Microcytic anemia, occult blood in stool, diarrhea, or palpable mass in right lower quadrant.
- *Left colon*: Hematochezia (usually red blood mixed with stool), decreased stool caliber, or obstructive symptoms.
- *Rectum*: Rectal lesions often present with rectal bleeding (65% to 90%), change in bowel habits (45% to 80%), and diminished stool caliber. Pain and tenesmus may occur as later symptoms. Rectal bleeding is often initially ascribed to hemorrhoids and the lesions may go uninvestigated for long periods of time, especially in patients 40 years of age or younger. Most rectal cancers can be detected and their mobility defined by a digital rectal examination (65% to 80%). Proctosigmoidoscopy should then be performed with appropriate biopsies to establish the diagnosis.[279]
- *Metastatic disease*: Hepatomegaly or right upper quadrant pain (liver), cough or chest pain (lungs), bone or soft tissue masses may indicate the presence of metastatic disease.

Laboratory Studies

- *Liver function studies*: Alkaline phosphatase or lactate dehydrogenase elevations may be the first indication of liver metastases; serum glutamate oxaloacetate transaminase and bilirubin values are needed if chemotherapy is indicated.
- *Renal function:* An elevated creatinine value suggests ureteral obstruction in the pelvis or para-aortic region.
- *Serum carcinoembryonic antigen (CEA)* is an oncofetal antigen that may be expressed by colorectal tumors. CEA should be obtained preferably after the diagnosis of adenocarcinoma has been made and before treatment is initiated (an elevated value before treatment suggests that subsequent CEA may be a useful component of studies used to monitor for relapse). CEA is not useful as a screening test as a result of numerous benign conditions that may also elevate CEA levels.[280] If the CEA is 100 or above, liver metastases should be suspected.

Screening

Screening recommendations for colorectal cancer are individualized depending on risk factors.[281] Mass screening of the average risk population with fecal occult blood testing will produce between 2% and 6% positive findings. One third of these positive tests will be benign adenomas; 5% to 10% will be carcinoma.[282]

- *Average risk population*: Digital rectal examination and occult blood testing should be performed annually after age 50. Screening sigmoidoscopy can be offered every 5 years, colonoscopy every 10 years, or double-contrast barium enema every 5 to 10 years.[281]
- *Population with positive family history* for colorectal cancer should have the same screening as in the average risk group except to begin at age 40.
- *Ulcerative colitis* patients with pancolitis for more than 10 years' duration should, at a minimum, have an annual colonoscopy with biopsies for dysplasia. Although the efficacy of dysplasia evaluation has not been fully and properly evaluated, it is preferred at present over prophylactic colectomy.
- *Patients with familial polyposis* should have an elective proctocolectomy, preferably with a restorative procedure of ileal pouch–anal anastomosis. In selected young individuals with fewer than 20 rectal polyps, a rectal sparing resection with ileorectal anastomosis is reasonable. Such patients should have endoscopic follow-up twice per year with conversion to an ileal pouch–anal anastomosis reserved until after their family is established.

Diagnostic Procedures

Similar diagnostic procedures are used for both the colon and the rectum (Table 27–25).[4]

- *Rectal digital examination* should be a part of every physical examination on patients older than age 40 regardless of symptoms or physical condition. If a lesion is found, the inferior extent should be noted (relative to anal verge and coccyx) as well as location (anterior, posterior, left, right), degree of circumference involved and degree of mobility (mobile, tethered, fixed).
- *Sigmoidoscopy* is indicated for screening and should be performed on any patient with lower GI symptoms or a positive occult blood test. Flexible sigmoidoscopy (60–65 cm) provides the best yield for the cost and discomfort involved.
- *Colonoscopy* has not been tested as a screening device, but can be offered as a screening approach every 10 years. Colonoscopy is the procedure of choice for evaluation of the patient with GI bleeding or follow-up of high-risk patients.
- *Barium enema* is indicated for unexplained iron deficiency anemia. The contrast technique may assist in detection of mucosal polyps.[283, 284] A barium enema is especially important for patients who have suboptimal colonoscopy.
- *Endorectal ultrasound* and *coil magnetic resonance imaging* studies are both techniques for determining the degree of local spread into and beyond the rectal wall and occasionally perirectal node detection.[285]
- *CT of pelvis and abdomen* is the most useful procedure to define extrarectal or extracolonic spread of the pri-

TABLE 27–25. **Diagnostic and Imaging Procedures for Colorectal Cancer**

Method	Diagnosis and Staging Capability	Recommended for Use
Primary Tumor ± Regional Nodes		
Barium enema (BE)	Very useful in detecting and defining primary lesions in the colon. Single-contrast study may be less sensitive than double-contrast in detecting polyps.	Yes
Endoscopy	Very accurate modality for detecting and defining primary lesions in rectum, sigmoid (flex sig), or remaining colon (colonoscopy).	Yes, if used to confirm lesion detected on BE or to screen high-risk patients
Endorectal ultrasound or coil MRI	Useful in defining depth of penetration of the primary lesion.	Yes, if preoperative chemoRT is considered
CT	Most valuable of all modalities for determining extrarectal or extracolonic local invasion and nodal metastases.	Yes
Metastases		
Chest film ± CT	Chest film—best for metastasis screening; CT chest—rules out multiple metastases.	Yes
CT abdomen	Most useful study to define para-aortic node enlargement or liver metastases.	Yes
Liver ultrasound	Can differentiate between cystic and solid lesions.	Yes

MRI = magnetic resonance imaging; CT = computed tomography; chemoRT = chemoradiation.

mary lesion and whether negative radial or circumferential surgical margins may be compromised (i.e., lack of free space relative to pelvic side wall or presacrum with rectal or sigmoid cancer). The abdominal component of the CT can also evaluate para-aortic nodes and the liver to rule out metastatic disease.

- *Liver ultrasound*—can be used to differentiate between cystic and solid lesions when seen on the abdomen CT.
- *Virtual colonoscopy,* a potentially important advance that combines CT imaging and air or barium enema contrast, may be competetive with endoscopic studies.[4]

Classification and Staging

Histopathology

The vast majority of cancers are adenocarcinoma (>90%).[5] Other histologic types encountered include carcinoid tumors, leiomyosarcomas, lymphoma, and squamous cell cancers. [5] The grading system used for adenocarcinomas refers to the degree of differentiation and anaplasticity. Some institutions use a 3-grade system (well, moderate, poor) and others use a 4-grade system.

Staging

Staging classifications for large bowel cancers depend on the degree of primary tumor invasion both within and beyond the bowel wall, and the presence or absence of nodal or distant metastasis (Table 27–26; Fig. 27–8).[5] Differences in or incorrect interpretations of staging systems may create difficulties when comparing treatment results by series.[287] Although both the original Dukes' system and the current TNM system are useful in predicting survival outcome after surgical resection, categories of patients within each stage have markedly different outcomes. A modification of the Astler-Coller rectal staging system (MAC) by Gunderson and Sosin[286] subdivided Astler-Coller B2 and C2 stages on the basis of degree of extrarectal or extracolonic tumor extension and operative or pathologic adherence to or invasion of surrounding organs or structures (B3 or C3; T4b,N0, T4b,N1–2). When the MAC system was used to analyze survival and patterns of release after potentially curative resection of either rectal or colon cancers, survival and local relapse rates differed in subsets of patients within both Dukes' B and C stages, and the rate of systemic metastasis differed within Dukes' C stage.

In the 1990 NIH Consensus Conference statement, it was noted that the MAC staging system was commonly used within the United States, but a plea was made for more standard use of the TNM system. The TNM system applies to both clinical and pathologic staging, has a more precise definition of the degree of primary tumor extension for lesions confined to the bowel wall, and node involvement is defined by the number of nodes involved (N1—≤3, N2—≥4). The TNM system is confusing, however, with regard to the correct T stage for lesions with primary tumor adherence to other organs or structures because adherence is not defined within the TNM system. Although adherent lesions are preferably substaged as T4b, the most important factor in presentations and publications is a clear definition of disease extent with regard to both the primary lesion and nodes. If stage is defined only by TNM stages I to IV or Dukes' A to C, much valuable prognostic information is lost or ignored. Differential survival and local relapse risks are found within both TNM stages II and III (Dukes' B and C) and differential systemic risks within stage III (Dukes' C).

Metastatic Spread

Spread to regional lymph nodes generally correlates with the depth of invasion by the primary tumor and the grade of differentiation. Nodal spread occurs in 10% to 20% of tumors confined to the bowel wall. Overall, low-grade tumors have a 30% chance of nodal spread, whereas high-grade lesions have an 80% probability.

TABLE 27–26. **Comparison of Staging Systems for Colorectal Adenocarcinoma**

Dukes' Stage	TNM Stage	TNM Grouping	Modified Astler-Coller (MAC)*	TNM Classification
	0	Tis, NO, MO	A	Tis: carcinoma *in situ* NO: no regional lymph node metastases MO: no distant metastasis
A	I	T1, NO, MO T2, NO, MO	B1	T1: tumor invades submucosa T2: tumor invades muscularis propria
B	II	T3–4a, NO, MO	B2	T3: tumor invades through the muscularis propria into the subserosa or into nonperitonealized pericolic or perirectal tissues T4a: tumor perforates the visceral peritoneum
		T4b, NO, MO	B3	T4b: tumor (is adherent to) directly invades other organs or structures (surgical or pathologic definition)
C	III	T1–2, N1–2, MO T3–4a, N1–2, MO T4b, N1–2, MO	C1 C2 C3	N1: metastasis in 1 to 3 pericolic or perirectal lymph nodes N2: metastasis in ≥4 pericolic or perirectal lymph nodes
D	IV	Any T, Any N, M1	D	M1†: distant metastasis

*From Gunderson LL, Martenson JA: Postoperative adjuvant irradiation with or without chemotherapy for rectal cancer. Semin Radiat Oncol 1993; 1:55–63 and Gunderson LL: Indications for and results of combined modality treatment of colorectal cancer. Acta Oncol 1999; 38:7–21.

†Lymph nodes beyond those encompassed by standard resection of the primary tumor and regional lymphatics (e.g., retroperitoneal nodes) are considered distant metastases.

Used with permission of the American Joint Committee on Cancer (AJCC®), Chicago, Illinois. The original source for this material is the AJCC® Cancer Staging Manual, 5th ed, 1997, published by Lippincott-Raven Publishers, Philadelphia, Pennsylvania.

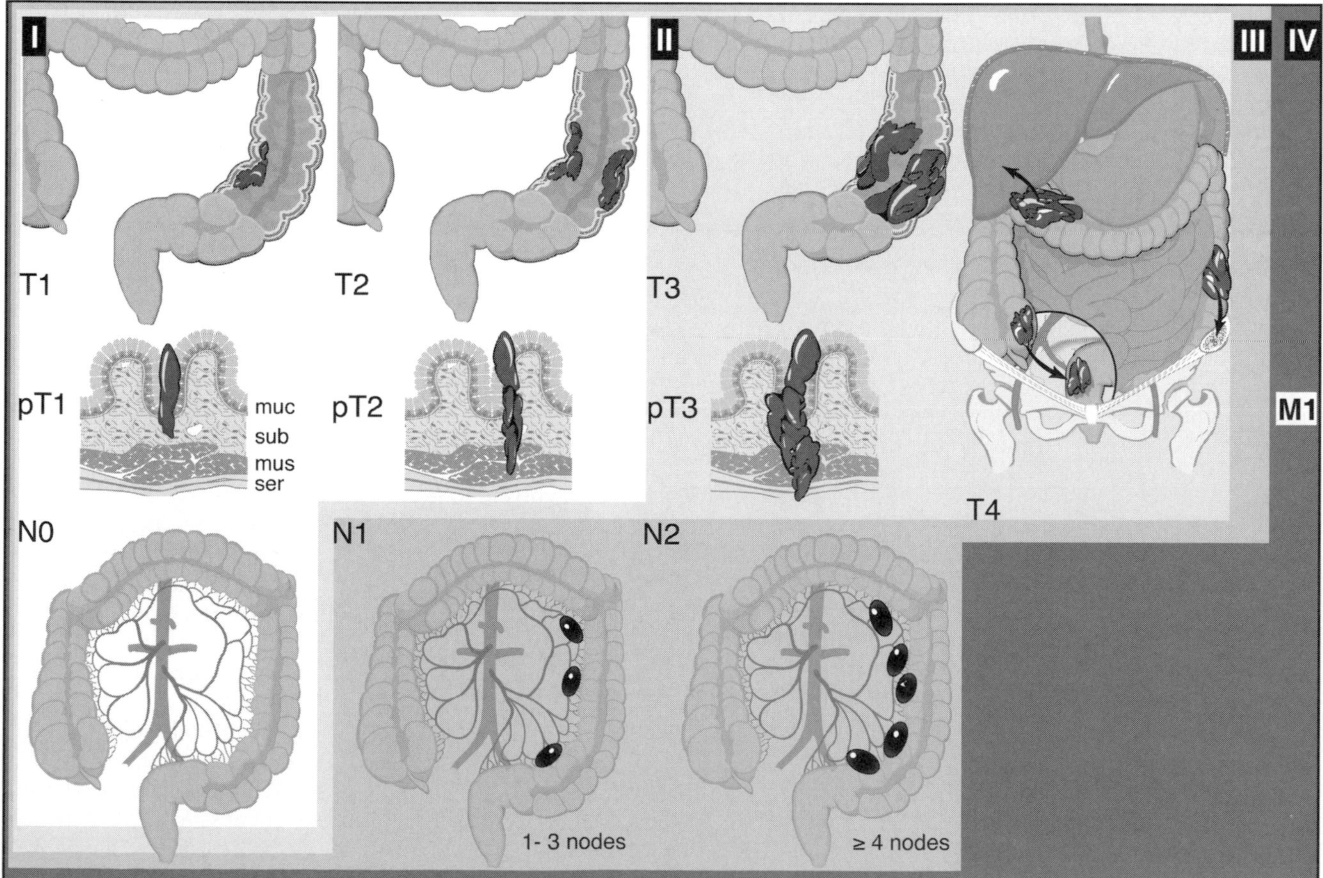

Figure 27–8. Anatomic staging of the colon and rectum.

Hematogenous spread of colon cancers is usually to the liver via the portal venous drainage, but for rectal cancers, the lung and liver are at nearly equal risk. The upper rectum has venous drainage via the superior hemorrhoidal into the inferior mesenteric system (to the portal system and liver), and the midrectum and lower rectum can, in addition, drain via the internal iliac system (to the vena cava and lung).

Staging Work-Up

The colon and rectum should be evaluated to determine intraluminal and extraluminal extension. The recommended procedures for evaluating local extent include digital rectal examination; barium enema (in the absence of obstructing symptoms) plus flexible sigmoidoscopy or colonoscopy, or both; transrectal ultrasound or coil magnetic resonance imaging (regarding depth of penetration for rectal primaries); and pelvic or abdominal CT (degree of extraluminal involvement). If lack of free space exists between the bladder and a primary tumor of the rectum or sigmoid, cystoscopy can be performed to determine whether there is invasion of the mucosal surface. For the purpose of defining metastatic disease, studies include serum for CEA, liver function tests, and renal function, chest film (with or without CT) and abdomen CT (liver, para-aortic nodes).

Principles of Treatment

The large bowel measures approximately 1.5 meters (about 5 feet) and is comprised of the distal rectum and proximal colon (sigmoid, descending, transverse, ascending, cecum). Because different treatment strategies are used for the rectum and "proximal" colon, principles of treatment[288, 289] will be discussed separately following a discussion of general surgical principles.

Surgery—General Principles

Surgical Methods—Interaction with Irradiation

The objective of surgery is to remove the tumor and primary nodal drainage with as wide a margin around both as is technically feasible and safe. If adjacent organs are involved, they should be removed *en bloc* with the specimen, assuming associated morbidity would be minimal. If a primary lesion is adherent to prostate or base of bladder, it may be preferable to use preoperative EBRT plus concurrent chemotherapy, followed by gross total resection and supplemental IOERT or high-dose-rate brachytherapy. This multimodality approach may allow preservation of the involved organ if favorable downstaging occurs. Small clips should be placed around areas of adherence or presumed microscopic residual disease for the purpose of boost-field EBRT if IORT options do not exist, and to mark the tumor bed for follow-up evaluation with serial CT studies. With rectal lesions, the pelvic floor should be reconstructed after resection to minimize the amount of small bowel within the true pelvis, and primary or partial closure of the perineum should be performed after abdominoperineal resection to hasten healing and decrease the interval to initiation of postoperative adjuvant treatment.

When deciding whether sphincter-preserving procedures are suitable for rectal lesions, the surgeon and pathologist commonly refer to the distal bowel margin (amount of resected normal bowel below the primary lesion). When lesions extend beyond the entire rectal wall, however, the narrowest transected or dissected surgical margin is often the lateral or anteroposterior margin. Therefore, attention should always be placed on obtaining adequate radial and mesorectal margins.

An anterior resection with reanastomosis can safely be performed following moderate-dose preoperative irradiation (45 to 50 Gy in 1.8 to 2 Gy fractions). An unirradiated limb of large bowel should be used for the proximal limb of the anastomosis, with temporary diverting stomas done only on the basis of operative indications (typically for ultra-low anterior resection, coloanal anastomoses, or tension on the anastomosis). Published data confirm that this approach results in an acceptably low risk of anastomotic leak.[290]

In some colonic sites, gross posterior or lateral tumor extension may result in narrow or compromised operative margins as more commonly occurs with rectal cancers. If colonic lesions are adherent to surrounding organs or structures, *en bloc* resection of the involved site should be performed.

Patterns and Rates of Relapse After Curative Resection of Large Bowel Cancers

Patterns of relapse after curative resection of primary rectal cancer have been defined in clinical, reoperative (Fig. 27–9), and autopsy series.[286, 287, 291] Pelvic relapse is a function of both tumor bed and nodal relapse that occurs because of direct tumor extension or lymphatic spread. Distant metastases with low or mid rectal cancers can occur in either the lungs or liver (see Fig. 27–8); with proximal rectal cancers, the liver is primarily at risk.

The rate of local relapse after curative resection of primary rectal cancers is related both to tumor extension beyond the rectal wall and to nodal spread.[286, 287, 291] For patients with a single high-risk factor of either direct tumor extension beyond the rectal wall, nodes negative (T3 or T4,N0; MAC B2 or B3), or involved nodes but primary tumor confined to the rectal wall (T1–2,N1–2; MAC C1), local relapse varies from 20% to 40%. For patients with both involved nodes and extension beyond the wall (T3 or T4,N1–2; MAC C2 or C3), the risk of local relapse is nearly additive (40% to 65% in clinical series and 70% in the reoperative series). When lesions extend beyond the rectal wall, the amount of uninvolved tissue on microscopic review (circumferential or radial margin) may be as, or more, important than the degree of extrarectal extension in determining the risk of local relapse.[292]

The rate of systemic metastases, in both adjuvant rectal and colon analyses, appears to be significantly higher in patients with both high-risk pathologic factors (extension beyond bowel wall and positive nodes; MAC C2 and C3) as opposed to those with only a single risk factor (MAC B2, B3, C1). In published data from adjuvant rectal cancer patients irradiated at either MGH or the Mayo Clinic, the

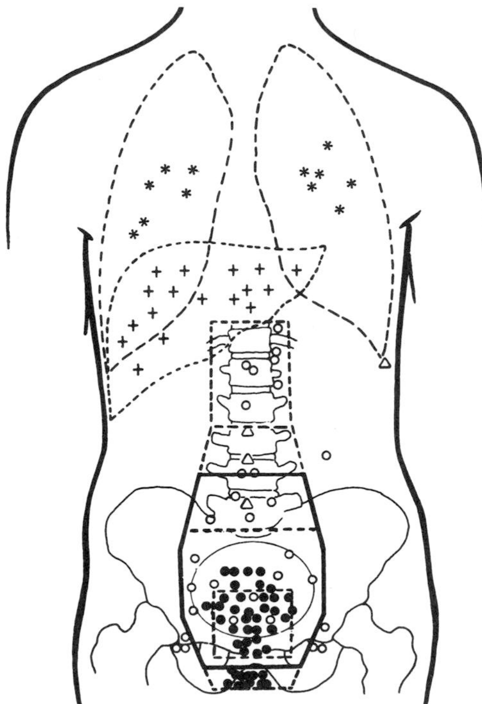

Figure 27–9. Patterns of relapse in University of Minnesota rectal reoperation series, with superimposed irradiation fields to pelvis alone or with perineum. * = lung metastasis; + = liver metastasis; △ = wound implant; ● = local failure in pelvic or perineal tissues; ○ = lymph node involvement. (From Gunderson LL, Sosin H: Adenocarcinoma of the rectum: areas of failure found at reoperation [second or symptomatic look] following curative surgery for adenocarcinoma of the rectum. Clinicopathologic correlation and implications for adjuvant therapy. Cancer 1974; 34:1278–1292, with permission.)

incidence of subsequent systemic relapse was approximately 20% with B2, B3, and C1 lesions versus 40% to 60% with C2 with or without C3 lesions.[293, 294] Similar differences are seen in adjuvant colon data from MGH in patients treated with either surgery alone[295] or surgery plus adjuvant irradiation.[296, 297]

Chemotherapy—Principles and Rationale

Metastatic Colorectal Cancer

Colorectal cancer is traditionally regarded as a relatively chemotherapy resistant disease. When chemotherapy is administered to patients with advanced colorectal cancer, it is, at best, a palliative modality. Despite phase II studies in many patients with colorectal cancer in which dozens of drugs were evaluated, relatively few agents produce tumor shrinkage. Of the active drugs, the most widely studied has been 5-FU, an agent that has been in clinical use for 40 years. Used alone, it results in partial or, rarely, complete tumor shrinkage in 10% to 20% of patients with advanced disease.[298] Until recently, among the multitude of drugs tested in phase II trials, only two other agents, mitomycin C and the nitrosourea MeCCNU, have produced responses in more than 10% of treated patients.

There is a burgeoning literature of clinical investigations in which 5-FU is administered by bolus, infusion, bolus loading dose followed by infusion, intraperitoneal, and hepatic intra-arterial approaches. Although the precise mechanism of action of 5-FU is debated, it appears that 5-FU cytotoxicity arises from interference with both DNA and RNA replication. Bolus administration of 5-FU is felt to inhibit *de novo* pyrimidine synthesis, resulting in the lethal incorporation of this fraudulent base into RNA during replication.[299, 300] The bolus administration of 5-FU in the clinic is efficient and commonplace.

The half-life of 5-FU after bolus injection in humans is 6 to 20 minutes.[299] Because relatively few cells cycle during the brief period of exposure of cells to cytotoxic drug levels when 5-FU is administered as a bolus injection, continuous infusion of 5-FU was attempted as a strategy to sustain meaningful drug levels. A number of clinical trials documented favorable response rates and reduced toxicity for 5-FU infusion over 5-FU bolus administration. The discovery that 5-FU also inhibits thymidylate synthase, thus interfering with DNA synthesis, and that this mechanism of action appears to be more important in cell death with continuous drug infusion than with bolus administration, led to widespread use of infusion schedules. The difference in mechanism of action led to the prediction that patients resistant to bolus 5-FU might respond to infusion of the drug.[299] Intraperitoneal administration of 5-FU has been shown to result in the presence of tumoricidal doses in the peritoneal cavity as well as high portal vein drug levels, leading to its use in clinical trials for both advanced and adjuvant therapy of colorectal cancer.[301, 302]

In vitro studies in which folinic acid (leucovorin) was mixed with 5-FU found that sequential administration of the two drugs in combination potentiated the binding of 5-FU to thymidylate synthase and led to increased cell kill in colon cancer cell cultures.[303, 304] In patients, this combination increases the incidence and severity of side effects, including diarrhea and stomatitis, as compared with that seen with 5-FU alone, suggesting that this biochemical modulation occurs in normal as well as tumor cells.

Intrahepatic chemotherapy with floxuridine (FUDR) has been investigated in patients with metastatic disease limited to the liver. The approach takes advantage of the dual blood supply to the liver and the fact that most macroscopic metastatic lesions draw upon the hepatic artery for blood supply. In contrast, most hepatocytes are nourished by portal venous blood flow.[305] Although hepatic artery catheters can be placed in most patients, in 10% to 15% of patients, anomalous circulation precludes establishing uniform liver perfusion. Initial reports indicated a high level of activity with response rates of as high as 80% noted.[306] Later reports indicated response rates that exceed those seen for systemic therapy, and are in the 40% to 50% range.

Irinotecan (CPT-11) is a topoisomerase I inhibitor that interferes with the uncoiling of helical DNA necessary for replication and thus leads to double-strand DNA breaks and apoptosis rather than cell division.[307] It is one of several agents tested in the past decade and is now commonly used in clinical practice. As a single agent in previously untreated patients with metastatic colorectal cancer, response rates of 23% to 27% have been reported.[308–310]

Oxaliplatin is a platinum analogue with a diaminocyclohexane carrier ligand that forms intrastrand links between DNA nucleotides, preventing strand separation and replication.[311] Oxaliplatin shows activity in a number of cell lines resistant to cisplatin and carboplatin.[312]

Principles and Rationale of Treatment—Rectal Cancer

Anatomy and Pathways of Spread

The rectum comprises the distal 12 to 15 cm of the large bowel, and the anus is the terminal 3 to 4 cm of the alimentary tract. It is important to separate rectal lesions from colon lesions for purposes of discussion and data presentation because the rates of local failure and treatment strategies differ.

The rectum begins in the upper to middle presacrum as a continuation of the sigmoid colon. Although the sigmoid colon has a complete peritoneal covering (serosa) and mesentery, the upper rectum is covered by peritoneum only anteriorly and laterally (the rectum begins where mesosigmoid ends). The lower one half to two thirds of the rectum is infraperitoneal and is surrounded by fibro-fatty tissue as well as organs and structures that can be involved by direct tumor extension (bladder, prostate, seminal vesicles, ureters, vagina, uterus, sacrum, nerves, and vessels).

The venous drainage of the upper rectum via the superior hemorrhoidal veins is to the inferior mesenteric vein and then to the portal system, whereas the lower rectum can also drain to the internal iliac veins and inferior vena cava. Therefore, either liver or pulmonary metastases or both can occur with rectal lesions.

Lymphatic drainage follows the inferior mesenteric vein in the upper rectum, whereas the middle and lower third rectal lymphatics drain to internal iliac and presacral nodes. Lesions that extend beyond the rectal wall spread through the lymphatic system of the invaded tissue or organ (bladder, prostate or cervix to external iliac). Inguinal lymph nodes are not at risk for metastases unless the lesion extends to the dentate line and anus or invades the distal vagina.

There has always been an emphasis on adequate proximal and distal surgical margins in alimentary tract cancers, but circumferential or radial margins are also important as a potential cause of local failure.[292] Adequate radial margins may be difficult for the surgeon to obtain within the anatomic confines of the pelvis. The pathologist should identify the amount of tumor extension beyond the muscularis propria and the amount of uninvolved fat. Local relapse in the pelvis after surgical resection alone occurs in 25% to 40% of MAC B2, B3, C1 cases and 40% to 65% of C2, C3 lesions.[286, 287, 291, 313] Local relapse is important not only because it portends an almost uniformly poor outcome but also because of the local pain symptoms,[314] bladder dysfunction, and sepsis; hence the emphasis on adjuvant therapy.

Surgery

Surgery remains the mainstay of curative treatment for all T1–4,N1–2,M0 (Dukes' A, B, C; MAC A, B2–3, C1–3) lesions; other modalities are adjunctive. The principles of surgical therapy are as follows:

1. laparotomy for staging
2. wide *en bloc* resection of the primary tumor
3. lymphadenectomy for staging as well as possible therapeutic benefit

The proper application of surgical techniques is as critical as the accuracy of the staging component of the procedure. Although numerous aspects of surgery for rectal cancer have been scrutinized, it is increasingly evident that local failures typically occur as a result of the inability to provide complete local clearance of the tumor, either along the distal bowel margin, radial tumor margin, or mesorectal tissues. Furthermore, it has been demonstrated in at least one study that inadvertent perforation of the rectum at surgery has a significant and adverse impact on the risk of local failure and death from recurrence. Increasing attention is being focused on the role of proper surgery for primary rectal cancer, emphasizing the importance and curative role of surgery.

The traditional operations for rectal cancers have been either an abdominoperineal resection (APR), which implies a permanent colostomy, or a low anterior resection (LAR) or rectal resection with coloanal anastomosis, in which bowel continuity is restored after resection of the involved segment of bowel. The abdominoperineal resection, also called the Miles procedure, involves a separate abdominal and perineal incision in order to radically excise the entire rectum, most of the sigmoid colon and mesocolon with its regional lymphatic drainage, anal sphincter and canal, the levator ani muscles and ischiorectal fat. Lesions within 5 to 6 cm of the anal verge usually require APR, whereas more proximal lesions are treated with LAR or rectal resection with coloanal anastomosis.[315, 316] Operative mortality for APR is, on average, 3% but varies between 1% to 8% depending on the surgical series. Complications related to surgery in this site include fistulas (vesicovaginal, vesicoperineal, ureteroperineal), abscess, hemorrhage, stomal problems, and small bowel obstruction.[317]

New techniques are emerging for preservation of the anal sphincter and GI continuity and are being tested to determine if adequate tumor control is obtained.[318] These operations include combined abdominal transsacral resection, transsacral resection (Kraske procedure), abdominal transsphincteric resection, and various pull-through procedures.[316] The circular, intraluminal stapling device has offered great technical advantages.

Conservative local therapies that have been used on rare occasions for early rectal cancer and as palliation to avoid obstruction include electrocoagulation, local excision (with or without adjuvant irradiation or chemotherapy), cryosurgery, laser vaporization, and contact radiation therapy, all of which have their proponents.[316] Colostomy, without some form of local therapy, is rarely palliative for incurable rectal lesions. The procedure may be done, however, in preparation for preoperative irradiation plus concomitant chemotherapy to be followed by APR or other multimodal treatment.

With the trend toward adjuvant postoperative irradiation plus concomitant chemotherapy (Table 27–27),[289] there has been emphasis on pelvic reconstruction to decrease the amount of small intestine in the irradiation field. This reconstruction may take the form of reperitonealization of

TABLE 27–27. **Multidisciplinary Treatment Decisions: Rectum**

Stage TNM/MAC		Surgery	Radiation Therapy	Chemotherapy
I	(A, B1)	Abdominoperineal or low anterior resection and regional nodes; local excision	Contact therapy for selected cases 30 Gy × 3–4 surface dose	NR
II	(B2)	Abdominoperineal or anterior resection and regional nodes	ART postop 50–54 Gy	CCR*
	(B3)	Resect after preop CCR	ART preop 50–54 Gy	CCR
III	(C1, C2)	Resect before or after CCR	ART preop or postop 50–54 Gy	CCR
	(C3)	Resect after preop CCR	ART preop 50–54 Gy	CCR
IV	(D)	If unresectable, colostomy	PRT or CCR 50–60 Gy	IC II

RT = irradiation; ART = adjuvant irradiation; PRT = palliative irradiation; NR = not recommended; CCR = concurrent chemotherapy and irradiation; IC II = investigational chemotherapy, phase I/II clinical trials; preop = preoperative; postop = postoperative.
*CCR = 5-fluorouracil + ART 50 Gy. From Physicians' Data Query. Rectal cancer. Bethesda, National Cancer Institute, January 1998.

the pelvic floor, use of omental slings or pedicle flaps, or less commonly the application of absorbable polyglycolic acid mesh[319] or temporary pelvic prosthetic devices. For patients with locally recurrent rectal cancer following adjuvant EBRT alone or with chemotherapy, pelvic reconstruction with a vascularized muscle flap (rectus abdominis, other) may be preferable to other maneuvers.[320]

Irradiation

The role of irradiation alone or usually in conjunction with concurrent and maintenance chemotherapy for rectal cancers is as follows:

1. Primary treatment if the patient is considered medically inoperable.
2. Primary treatment in some early, T1–2 lesions (exophytic, ≤3 × 5 cm in size, well to moderately well differentiated histology) using contact irradiation (Papillon technique), depending on the experience and expertise of the radiation oncologist.[321, 322]
3. Palliative treatment for pain or bleeding in patients with metastatic disease.
4. Treatment for locally recurrent disease.
5. Adjuvant therapy after primary resection (T3–4,N0–2, any T,N1–2; MAC B2–3, C1–3) for patients with completely resected lesions at high risk for local relapse.
6. Combined-modality treatment for those with microscopic or macroscopic disease remaining after maximal resection.

Primary radiation treatment is not recommended for rectal carcinoma, except for patients who refuse surgery or are medically inoperable[323–325] or have select early lesions appropriate for endocavitary irradiation.[321, 322]

The rationale for using combinations of irradiation and chemotherapy as a component of adjuvant treatment in rectal cancer is based on the risks of relapse after surgery alone and evidence of radioresponsiveness in both preoperative and primary irradiation series for rectal cancers. Cummings and associates presented a series from Princess Margaret Hospital (PMH)[324, 325] in which primary irradiation was given to patients with tumor fixation (n = 77), partial fixation (n = 37), or clinically mobile lesions (n = 97). The clinically mobile lesions were either medically inoperable or the patients refused abdominoperineal resection. The most common irradiation dose was 45 to 50 Gy in 20 fractions over 4 weeks. In the 97 patients with mobile lesions, complete clinical regression was achieved in 48 patients (50%), but 18 relapsed locally for an ultimate local control rate of 31% (30 of 97). Five-year actuarial survival for those with mobile lesions was 48%. Surgical salvage was attempted in 25 patients with initially mobile lesions that persisted or relapsed and was successful in 18. Although the PMH results are not as good as those reported with the use of combined-modality treatment that includes resection, they support the curative potential of irradiation as a single modality.

When both surgery and radiation are indicated in an adjuvant setting, differences of opinion exist regarding the preferred sequence of each modality. Potential advantages of preoperative irradiation (with or without concomitant and maintenance chemotherapy) include the damaging effect on cells that may be spread locally or distantly at the time of resection, as well as downstaging of lesions in an attempt to improve the rate of sphincter preservation. The major advantage of postoperative irradiation (with or without concomitant and maintenance chemotherapy) is that the only patients irradiated are those without metastases and at high risk for local recurrence on the basis of operative and pathologic findings.

Irradiation Fields

Most tumor bed relapses are in the posterior one half to two thirds of the true pelvis, and the internal iliac and presacral nodes have a posterior location relative to external iliac nodes. Lateral treatment fields can logically be combined with AP/PA fields to reduce the dose to anteriorly located normal structures, including small bowel.[8, 326]

Field arrangements can be individualized[8, 326] depending on the location of the primary tumor, presence or absence of adjacent organ involvement, and area and number of nodes involved, but some generalizations can be made. The width of AP/PA ports should cover the pelvic inlet with margin around the desired iliac nodes (Fig. 27–10A). Lateral margins extending 1 to 2 cm beyond the widest point of the bony pelvis usually are sufficient, depending on treatment energy and penumbrum. The superior margin should usually be at least 1.5 cm above the level of the sacral promontory (occasionally mid-L5 to L4, depending on the superior extent of the lesion; infrequently, periaortic coverage to T12 or T11). This margin may depend on the extent of inferior mesenteric or iliac nodal involvement,

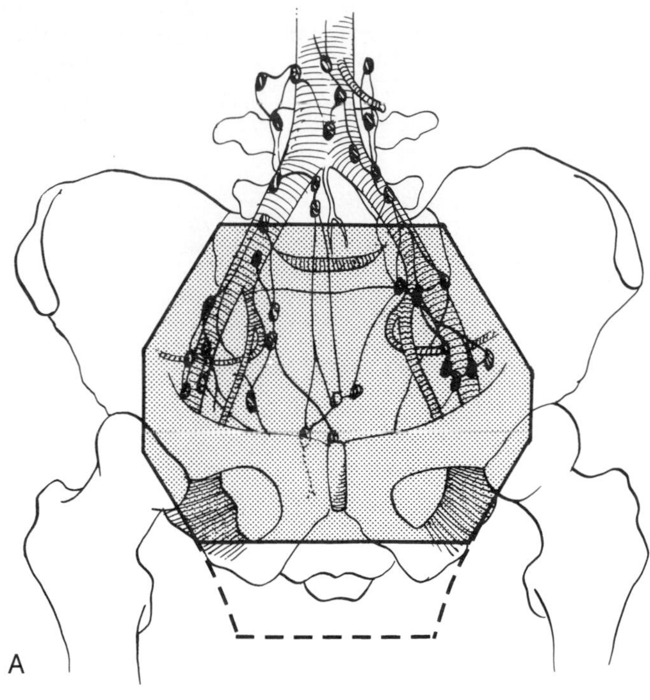

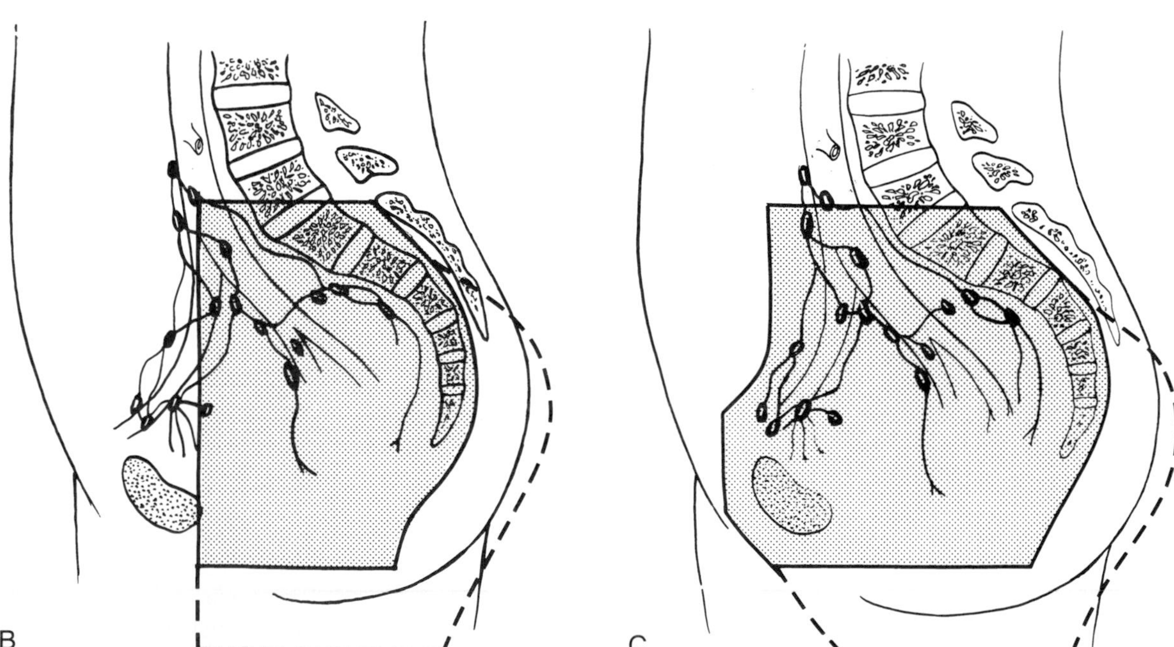

Figure 27–10. Idealized EBRT fields, rectal cancer preceding or following resection. (A) Posteroanterior/anteroposterior (PA-AP). (B, C) Lateral fields (B = internal iliac and presacral nodes at risk; C = external iliac nodes at risk). Copyright © Mayo Foundation.

which usually is not known preoperatively. The inferior field extent is also somewhat variable. For both preoperative and postoperative radiation, the minimal extent should usually be 3 to 5 cm below the gross tumor (preoperative) or below the most inferior extent of dissection or mobilization of the distal limb (postoperative). Ideally, this level should be marked with surgical clips (approximately bottom of obturator foramen). The perineum should be included after abdominoperineal resection.

When using lateral fields (Figs. 27–10B and C), treatment in the prone position allows visualization of the sacrum and a more positional shift in the small bowel. The posterior field margin is vital, because the rectum and perirectal tissues (tumor plus target volume) lie just anterior to the sacrum and coccyx. Accordingly, the posterior field margin should be a minimum of 1.5 to 2 cm behind the anterior bony sacral margin to allow for some daily patient movement. Individually shaped blocks can be used to spare posterior muscle and soft tissues. The anterior margin can be shaped to reduce the amount of irradiation to the femoral head and bladder inferiorly or when external iliac lymph nodes need to be included in order to decrease the amount of small bowel superiorly and anteriorly. Anteriorly, the lower one third of the rectum abuts the posterior vaginal wall and prostate, and these structures should be included. In female patients, inclusion of the vagina can be verified at stimulation if a contrast-soaked gauze pad or tampon is placed therein during treatment planning.

Irradiation Dose

The dose to the extended tumor bed nodal field should be 45 to 50 Gy in 5 to 6 weeks (usually two or more fields per day, 1.8- to 2.0-Gy fractions 5 days per week). Strong consideration should be given to the use of a boost field to the primary tumor bed and possibly the immediately adjacent nodes, if the large field dose is in the 45-Gy range. Our usual total dose in the boost field with both preoperative and postoperative irradiation of rectal cancer is 50.4 to 54 Gy in 6 to 6½ weeks. Boost fields are defined by imaging studies or surgical clip placement, and usually are 10 × 10 cm or 12 × 12 cm to ensure adequate coverage to at least the 50 Gy level. When doses greater than 50 Gy are contemplated, small bowel films should be used to help define both dose limits and field shaping.[8–10, 326] Doses greater than 50 Gy in 1.8-Gy fractions, 5 days per week, are rarely administered unless small bowel mobility is good or the amount of small bowel within the field is minimal.

For patients with subtotal resection but residual disease, locally recurrent cancer, or fixed pelvic lesions in posterior or lateral locations, a major difference in treatment technique is the necessity of including the sacral canal as target volume for the initial 45 to 50 Gy. Definition of this area as target volume is indicated because of the increased risk of tumor spread along nerve roots in such cases. Failure to do so may result in a marginal recurrence in the sacral canal.

Boost pelvic fields usually are treated with 3-field (PA and lateral) or 4-field techniques (lateral and paired posterior obliques). Field shaping of the lateral boost portals is often helpful in deleting additional small intestine anteriorly and superiorly. Bladder distention alone or in conjunction with an anterior compression device may be extremely useful in displacing small bowel loops superiorly and anteriorly out of both large and boost fields.

Small bowel films can help to identify those patients in whom immobile loops remain in an area at high risk for relapse. In such instances, the radiation oncologist must limit the dose to conform to small bowel tolerance, or the surgeon must re-explore the patient and reconstruct the pelvis or allow the delivery of an intraoperative component of irradiation with electrons or high-dose-rate brachytherapy while the small bowel is displaced.

Chemotherapy

The role of chemotherapy in rectal cancer has been studied in both the adjuvant setting and for metastatic disease. Chemotherapy alone as a surgical adjuvant does not reduce the risk of local relapse and has not consistently demonstrated any survival advantage over surgery alone.[326] An NSABP study did demonstrate an improved survival in the chemotherapy adjuvant arm (MeCCNU, vincristine, 5-FU) as compared with surgery alone, but only in subset analysis for men younger than 65 years.[327] When used concurrently with EBRT, PVI 5-FU (225 mg/m²/24 hrs 7 days/wk or until intolerance) improved disease control and survival when compared with concurrent bolus 5-FU (500 mg/m² for 3 days weeks 1 and 5 of EBRT) in a U.S. Intergroup trial.[328] Based upon the recommendations of an NCI-sponsored consensus conference in 1990, such CMT is considered standard in stages II and III rectal cancer (MAC B2, B3, C1, C2, C3).

Single agents or combinations of drugs used for the systemic treatment of rectal cancers are similar to those for colon cancer because there is no evidence to suggest that large bowel cancers originating in the rectum differ in chemotherapy response when compared with cancers originating in the colon. 5-FU has long been the standard of systemic treatment but produces only a 20% response rate for metastatic disease. Various drug combinations (5-FU + MeCCNU, 5FU + MeCCNU + VCR, 5-FU + leucovorin, 5-FU + levamisole, etc.) have been used, but none have been better than 5-FU alone. Recently, there has been enthusiasm for the combination of 5-FU and leucovorin in metastatic colorectal cancers. CPT-11 can also achieve response in patients who progress on 5-FU–containing regimens and recently has been shown to increase survival and improve quality of life in 5-FU–refractory patients as compared with best supportive care alone.

Combined-Modality Therapy

The search for improved disease control and survival for resectable but high-risk rectal cancer has led to studies that combine all three modalities. There have now been three randomized studies that have demonstrated improved overall survival and better local control for patients treated with postoperative irradiation and chemotherapy, when compared with surgery alone or surgery plus irradiation control arms (two U.S. trials—GITSG and Mayo/NCCTG; Norway trial). A large preoperative EBRT trial from Sweden also demonstrated local control and survival advantages when compared with a surgery-alone control arm.

The now classic study performed by the GITSG randomized patients with postoperative Dukes' Stages B or C lesions to one of four arms: (1) observation alone, (2) pelvic irradiation to a dose of 40–48 Gy, (3) chemotherapy with bolus 5-FU and MeCCNU, or (4) irradiation and chemotherapy (concomitant with EBRT and maintenance). Both disease-free and overall survival in the adjunctive radiation-chemotherapy arm were statistically better than in the surgery-alone control arm.[329, 330]

In a study by the Mayo Clinic and the NCCTG,[331] patients with Dukes' B and C disease were randomized between postoperative EBRT alone (50 Gy) or postoperative EBRT plus concomitant bolus 5-FU and maintenance chemotherapy with bolus 5-FU and MeCCNU. Improved disease-free and overall survival were found with combined-modality treatment, as well as reduced rates of local relapse and distant metastases.

In the most recent trial from Norway, combined-modality postoperative chemoradiation was compared with a surgery-alone control arm for Dukes' B and C patients.[332] Statistically significant improvements in local control and survival were again found with the chemoradiation adjuvant.

At this time, combined-modality postoperative chemoradiation appears to be the most rational treatment approach for patients with resected but high-risk lesions. The concomitant administration of 5-FU and irradiation takes advantage of the radiosensitizing effects of the 5-FU. Recently completed studies tested EBRT plus 5-FU alone, 5-FU plus levamisole, 5-FU plus low-dose leucovorin, and 5-FU plus levamisole plus leucovorin. Preoperative CMT is also being investigated for both resectable as well as locally unresectable or locally recurrent cancers. Although most preoperative EBRT trials demonstrate reductions in local relapse with the addition of preoperative EBRT to resection, only the recent large Swedish trial in approximately 1100 patients demonstrated a survival improvement.[333]

Principles and Rationale of Treatment—Colon Cancer

Anatomy and Pathways of Spread

The ascending and descending colon, as well as splenic and hepatic flexures, are anatomically somewhat similar to the rectum. They are relatively immobile structures that lack a true mesentery and usually do not have a peritoneal covering (serosa) on the posterior and lateral surfaces. Lesions that extend through the entire bowel wall in these locations may have narrow transected or dissected operative radial margins, especially with moderate posterior to lateral extension. Lesions on the anterior wall or medial wall have closer access to a free peritoneal surface.

The sigmoid and transverse colon are intraperitoneal organs with a complete mesentery and serosa. Each is freely mobile except for their proximal and distal segments, in which moderate extracolonic extension may result in narrow surgical margins. When lesions are in the mid-transverse or midsigmoid colon, operative margins usually are excellent. An exception occurs when the tumor is adherent to or is invading adjacent organs or structures (i.e., sigmoid cancer involving the bladder or lateral pelvic sidewall; transverse colon malignancy invading the greater curvature of the stomach or adherent to the anterior abdominal wall). The cecum has a variable mesentery and some mobility. When lesions extend posteriorly, radial surgical margins may be narrow because of the iliac wing and associated musculature and vessels.

Lymphatic and venous drainage of the colon is by the mesenteric system (inferior mesenteric for the left colon and superior mesenteric for the right) unless adjacent organs or structures are involved. If lesions in the sigmoid, cecal, proximal ascending, or distal descending colon involve organs or structures in the true or false pelvis, the iliac nodes may be at risk. When extrapelvic lesions involve the posterior abdominal wall, direct spread to periaortic lymph nodes can occur. If the anterior abdominal wall is involved at or below the level of the umbilicus, inguinal nodes are also at risk.

Surgery

Polyps larger than 3 to 5 mm should be completely removed endoscopically and histologically examined, if technically possible. Recurrent or persistent polyps that are not amenable to endoscopic removal or that are of concern for malignancy should be removed surgically. The finding of invasive cancer within a sessile polyp requires laparotomy and resection of the involved segment. Pedunculated polyps with invasion into only the head, neck, or stalk with established clean margins and favorable histologic features (well differentiated and without lymphatic or venous invasion) can be treated with observation, without resection.

Surgery is the primary mode of therapy for colon cancers. The principles of surgical therapy are as previously discussed:

1. Laparotomy for staging (hepatic, peritoneal, retroperitoneal and local tumor assessment)
2. Wide *en bloc* resection of the primary tumor with anastomotic reconstruction
3. Lymphadenectomy for staging as well as possible therapeutic benefit[334]

For anatomic reasons, it is rarely difficult to accomplish wide bowel margins for colon cancers; hence, anastomotic recurrences are not common. However, there is some evidence that margins of 5 cm for stage II disease and 10 cm for stage III disease provide advantage. Little evidence exists to suggest that implantation of tumor cells onto the suture line during resection contributes significantly to local relapse. Although randomized trials of the "no touch" technique have failed to confirm a significant difference in survival, reasonable efforts should be made intraoperatively to prevent intraluminal and intraperitoneal spread of tumor cells.[335]

Synchronous metastatic disease to the ovaries is reported in almost 8% of colorectal cancers. Although a slight survival benefit has been suggested for prophylactic oophorectomy in some analyses,[336] benefits have not been established in randomized trials, and routine oophorectomy is not recommended.

Resection of metastases can prolong survival in patients with metastasis to a single organ (liver or lung). Five-year survival rates of 20% to 40% have been seen in selected series following such resections. Patients who appear to benefit most from salvage surgical resection of metastases are those with single lesions limited to a single organ and a long disease-free interval between primary disease and discovery of metastasis.[337]

Patterns of Relapse

After complete resection of adjuvant colon cancers, most relapses appear within 2 years (about 70%) and almost all (90%) within 5 years.[295, 338, 339] Local relapse is related to stage, with a 10% or lower risk in patients with MAC stages A, B1, B2, C1, and 30% or greater for MAC stages B3, C2, C3.[295] Adherence to or invasion of the primary tumor to local structures (T4b) and perforation of the bowel (T4a) are factors associated with significantly earlier tumor relapse.[340] The liver is the prime organ for metastatic disease (65%); extra-abdominal metastases in lung (25%), and bone and brain (10%) are much less common.

A multidisciplinary approach is essential for node-positive and selected high-risk node-negative colon cancers and is summarized in Table 27–28.[288]

TABLE 27–28. **Multidisciplinary Treatment Decisions: Colon**

Stage	TNM/MAC	Surgery	Radiation Therapy	Chemotherapy
I	(A, B1)	Wide segmental resection and regional nodes in mesentery; primary anastomosis	NR	NR
II	(B2, B3)	Wide segmental resection and regional nodes in mesentery; primary anastomoses	IRCT (T4b,N0; B3)	IC III
III	(C1, C2)	Wide surgical resection if feasible; primary anastomoses	NR routinely; IRCT (T3,4a or proximal nodes)	MDC
	(C3)	Restage and resect after preop IRCT	IRCT	MDC ± ART
IV	(D)	Bypass colostomy or palliative resection	NR routinely	MDC ± PRT

IRCT = investigational radiochemotherapy; NR = not recommended; IC III = investigational chemotherapy, phase III clinical trials; MDC = multidrug chemotherapy; ART = adjuvant irradiation; PRT = palliative irradiation; 5-FU = 5-fluorouracil.

*MDC = 5-FU + leucovorin for 6 months. From Physicians' Data Query. Colon cancer. Bethesda, National Cancer Institute, January 1998.

Adjuvant Chemotherapy

In the 1970s, an empiric attempt to use the antihelminthic agent levamisole as an "immunostimulant" indicated a possible benefit result when a treated cohort exhibited decreased relapse rates when compared with control patients with resected colon cancer.[341] A trial, initiated in 1979, led to the combination of 5-FU with levamisole in this setting.[342] Subsequent laboratory investigation suggested that levamisole may be a cytotoxic agent by virtue of its inhibition of tyrosine kinase.[343] The increased response rates seen for metastatic disease when 5-FU and leucovorin were combined led to testing of that regimen in the adjuvant setting.[344] As a consequence, it is now felt that chemotherapy with 5-FU and levamisole or 5-FU and leucovorin reduces the risk of relapse in patients with stage III colon cancer (positive nodes, confined to or beyond colonic wall—MAC C1, C2, C3).

At this time, the standard adjuvant therapy for stage III colon cancer in the United States is a 6-month combination of 5-FU plus leucovorin, with the leucovorin given either as a high-dose weekly program or as a low-dose program for 5 consecutive days each month. The Mayo/NCCTG program is leucovorin 20 mg/m^2 daily with 5-FU 425 mg/m^2 as a low-dose program.[345] The NSABP regimen is leucovorin 500 mg/m^2 before 5-FU 500 mg/m^2 weekly for 6 of every 8 weeks.[346] The principal differences between these two regimens are the higher incidence of stomatitis and leukopenia associated with the Mayo/NCCTG regimen and the higher incidence of grade 4 diarrhea as well as additional drug-related expense as a result of the use of high-dose leucovorin noted with the NSABP regimen. The results of a large trial that examined 5-FU plus levamisole, the NSABP high-dose leucovorin plus 5-FU regimen, the NCCTG low-dose leucovorin plus 5-FU regimens, and 5-FU plus leucovorin plus levamisole have been reported in preliminary fashion.[347] This trial indicates that both the NCCTG and NSABP regimens given for 6 months are equivalently effective. The NSABP trial of 5-FU plus leucovorin with or without interferon alfa showed additional toxicity but no added benefit to the regimen containing immunotherapy.[348]

The potential value of adjuvant therapy in patients with stage II disease (node negative, beyond colonic wall—MAC B2 or B3) remains controversial. Although the major adjuvant therapy trials have included such patients, the trials had different eligibility requirements. In the Mayo NCCTG trials, only patients judged to be at high risk of relapse, based on the presence of colonic perforation or obstruction, tumor cell aneuploidy, or adherence to or invasion of surrounding structures (T4b,N0 or MAC B3), were enrolled; in the NSABP trials, any stages II patient was eligible. Often the results of stages II and III patients are pooled in the available reports. The NSABP has reported in preliminary fashion on the experiences of stage II patients enrolled in their serial trials.[349] Their conclusion was that the magnitude of the reduction in the rate of relapse and death related to colon cancer seen in stage II patients was similar to that seen in stage III patients. However, the relatively good prognosis seen with stage II disease means that more patients are cured by surgery alone and therefore fewer have the potential to benefit from adjuvant therapy. A meta-analysis of five adjuvant trials in which stage II patients were randomly assigned to a control group or a 5-FU plus leucovorin regimen noted a 2% difference in 5-year survival (80% versus 82%) for treated over untreated patients.[350]

Immunotherapy has been the subject of a number of adjuvant trials. A murine monoclonal antibody known as 17-1A, which recognizes a 34-kDa glycoprotein on the cell membrane of epithelial cells, has been studied in a group of 189 patients.[351] The treatment provided an equivalent improvement in disease-free and overall survival for stage III patients, as has been reported for 5-FU plus leucovorin or levamisole when compared with a surgery-only control group. Trials of the antibody alone in stage II patients or antibody plus chemotherapy in stage III patients are ongoing in the United States.

Another novel approach to adjuvant chemotherapy for colon cancer has been infusion of 5-FU into the portal vein in the perioperative period. This approach is based on the knowledge that the liver is the most frequent site of metastatic disease, that early metastases derive their blood supply from the portal vein, and that 5-FU has very little toxicity when administered in this manner because of hepatic drug degradation. Although some trials have shown efficacy of this approach, others have not.[352, 353] A meta-analysis demonstrated only a modest benefit to this therapy.[354] The approach has been largely superseded by the more effective systemic therapy discussed earlier.

Irradiation (and Chemotherapy)

There is no defined role for irradiation either as primary treatment in colon cancer or as an adjuvant therapy. The basis for consideration of either adjuvant irradiation alone or in conjunction with chemotherapy is the high incidence of local relapse in certain stages of disease (≥30% rate for MAC stages B3, C2, C3). These data have been accumulated by a number of institutions from second-look surgery in asymptomatic and symptomatic patients as well as in clinical or autopsy series.[295, 338, 339, 355, 356]

Irradiation Fields

Radiation oncologists have investigated the role of both postoperative radiation using tumor bed plus nodal fields or even whole abdominal fields for resected high-risk patients (MAC stages B3, C2, C3; TNM: T4b,N0, T3–4,N1–2, T4b,N1–2).[296, 297, 357, 358] These studies have been nonrandomized and selected and usually are from single institutions.

The target volume should include the tumor bed as well as areas of potential or proven nodal involvement.[8, 296, 297, 359] Wherever feasible, the initial margin beyond tumor bed should be 5 cm (minimum 3 cm; tumor bed is defined as the affected segment of the large bowel, and when present, the adjacent organ or structure to which it was adherent or invading). Node groups are included routinely if nodes were involved at the level of the proximal surgical vascular ligature or an area of tumor adherence places a group of nodes at risk (para-aortic with posterior abdominal wall adherence; external iliac with iliac fossa or pelvic side wall adherence). When such tumor adherence occurs, the acceptable superior-inferior extent of nodal coverage is the same as tumor bed plus margin. If the adjacent organ was totally resected (ovary, uterus, or kidney), no alteration is necessary in the initial volume. If the tumor was adherent to an organ (bladder, stomach, other) that has been only partially resected, it is desirable to include a majority of that organ in the field that receives 45 Gy. If adherence was to structures such as pelvic side wall, diaphragm, or muscle, a 3- to 5-cm margin beyond the area of adherence is used.

An excretory urogram should be done at, or before, the start of treatment to define renal function if more than one third of one kidney may be in the field, because at least two thirds of the other kidney needs to be excluded from the high-dose fields. With cephalad right colon lesions, it is common to include 50% or more of the right kidney, and therefore the left kidney must be spared. For proximal left colon lesions, one may have to include 50% or more of the left kidney, emphasizing the need to spare the right kidney.

Multifield techniques are useful with primary lesions of the sigmoid colon. For such lesions in other parts of the colon, parallel opposed AP-PA fields are used for the major portion of treatment unless pretreatment CT studies or surgical clip placement suggests that multifield techniques can spare normal tissues. For extrapelvic right or left colon locations, the patient should be in a decubitus position for a portion of treatment if small bowel films reveal a good shift of small intestine and this position can be reproduced reliably (largest benefit may be achieved if done on the days the patient receives concomitant chemotherapy).

Treatment Tolerance for Surgery plus Irradiation—Colorectal Cancers

An optimal therapeutic ratio between local control and complications is achieved only with close interaction between the surgeon and the radiation oncologist.[9, 10, 326, 359] Major surgical considerations include use of clips to mark areas at high risk as well as the use of reconstruction techniques to displace small bowel (indicated especially with rectal primary lesions). The radiation oncologist should consider certain things as well. For both rectal and colonic primary lesions, shrinking or boost field techniques should be used after a dose of 45 to 50 Gy. With rectal and sigmoid primary lesions, lateral fields should be used for a portion of treatment to avoid as much small bowel as possible while still including the area at risk, and treatment with bladder distention should be considered unless the tumor is adherent to the bladder. With extrapelvic primary lesions, the volume of small bowel within the field often can be reduced by treating the patient in the decubitus position for a portion of treatment.

In postoperative rectal series, the incidence of small bowel obstruction requiring reoperation appears to vary by treatment technique. When parallel-opposed techniques were used in an M.D. Anderson series, the incidence was 17.5%, in comparison with 5% with surgery alone. When the superior extent of the field was shifted from the L2–3 region to L5, the incidence of operative intervention decreased to about 12%.[360] In an MGH series in which multifield techniques and bladder distention were used, the incidence of small bowel obstruction requiring operative intervention in the group receiving irradiation was 6%, which was essentially equal to that in the group undergoing operation alone at 5%.[293] In an MGH adjuvant colon irradiation series, the incidence of small bowel obstruction requiring reoperation was less than 5%.[296, 297]

When multifield irradiation techniques are used in combination with chemotherapy in the adjuvant treatment of rectal cancer, no apparent increase occurs in the risk of small bowel complications. In a 1989 analysis of the Mayo/NCCTG randomized trial (minimum 3 years' follow-up),[331] the incidence of severe small bowel complications was less than 5% with either irradiation alone or irradiation plus chemotherapy.

Follow-Up After Treatment—Colorectal Cancer

The detection and treatment of asymptomatic cancer relapse may have an impact on survival and quality of life. Detection requires a plan of regular follow-up and specific diagnosis tests.

- Patients should be examined every 3 to 4 months for the first 2 to 3 years after initial treatment. Rectal examination with or without occult blood tests should be done on each visit. Colonoscopy or colon radiograph and flexible sigmoidoscopy should be done yearly for 3 years, then at 2- to 3-year intervals. Chest x-ray should be done at 6-month intervals for 2 to 3 years and then yearly.
- CEA levels can detect disease relapse by a rising serum titer. Two thirds of colorectal cancer relapses

have been heralded by a rising CEA as the first indication in those institutions that perform serial CEA studies. In patients with an elevated CEA prior to their initial resection, this test is justifiably performed every 2 to 3 months after surgery. Although several studies justify re-exploration based on a rising CEA as the only sign of disease relapse,[361, 362] in our institution a suspicious or positive imaging study must also exist.

- The use of abdominal pelvic CT as a component of routine follow-up is the only way to screen the tumor bed, regional nodes (para-aortic), and liver with a single imaging study. Although recommended in some guidelines as a component of follow-up, it is not a routine study in other guidelines on the basis of cost-benefit issues. If obtained, a 3-month baseline CT after resection is useful, followed by scans at 6-month intervals for 2 to 3 years, then yearly to year 5 or 8. If screening of the liver only is desired, ultrasound is cheaper. Alternating liver ultrasound and abdominal pelvic CT scan is another option.

Special Considerations of Treatment—Colorectal Cancer

Surgical Issues

Familial Polyposis

Patients with familial polyposis syndromes should have total proctocolectomy once the diagnosis is established. If the rectum is preserved, a 7% to 20% incidence of carcinoma is reported; patients should, therefore, either have proctoscopy every 6 months or undergo rectal mucosectomy with ileal pouch–anal anastomosis.

Polyps (Not Polyposis)

Most polyps can be removed by colonoscopic polypectomy. The finding of carcinoma in a polyp does not necessarily mandate colon resection. The following conditions in a polyp would mitigate in favor of resection versus observation following endoscopic polypectomy: poorly differentiated histology, positive margins, venous or lymphatic invasion, sessile lesion, or invasion of base of pedunculated polyp.

Locally Advanced Lesions

Aggressive surgical resection of advanced local disease without metastasis is warranted. This approach may require *en bloc* removal of adjacent organs or, in the case of rectal cancer, total pelvic exenteration. Such heroic measures have been associated with improved survival in select series.[363]

A persistent or recurrent sinus in the perineum after abdominal perineal resection suggests residual or recurrent tumor in the pelvis. Likewise, persistent pelvic or perineal pain is most often a sign of pelvic recurrence and deserves careful and thorough diagnostic evaluation.

Circumferential carcinoma of the descending and sigmoid colon may present with obstruction or perforation. This situation requires a two-stage surgical approach with formation of a diverting colostomy. More proximal lesions can be treated safely with a one-step procedure in spite of these complications.

Laparoscopic Colon Resection

The role of minimally invasive (laparoscopic) surgery in the curative treatment of colon cancer has not been definitively established. Current data suggest that the same extent of resection and nodal staging can be accomplished. However, concern has been raised, and not yet resolved, regarding the possibility of altered patterns of relapse, specifically wound tumor implants, rates of which range from 0% to 21%. Clinical trials are under way and should be completed within the next few years.

Endoscopic Laser Therapy

Patients who are medically inoperable may have obstruction palliated by laser therapy.

Endocavitary Irradiation

Select early rectal cancers may be appropriately treated with endocavitary irradiation.[321, 322] Selection criteria include the following: exophytic lesion—maximum size 3 × 5 cm, well or moderately well differentiated, superficial (mucosa, submucosa, or inner muscularis propria), location with superior extent 12 cm or less above anal verge and inferior extent 1 to 2 cm or more above top of anal canal.

Results and Prognosis—Colorectal Cancer

Results will be presented as a function of disease presentation (local, regional, systemic) and whether complete surgical resection is feasible for primary lesions. For completely resected but high-risk primary rectal and colon cancers, results in adjuvant trials will be discussed (rectal—single vs. combined modality; colon—chemotherapy with or without irradiation). For locally advanced primary or recurrent colorectal cancers, results of aggressive trimodality approaches will be presented that include the addition of intraoperative irradiation to maximal resection, external irradiation, and concurrent plus maintenance chemotherapy. With metastatic lesions, chemotherapy results will be discussed.

Prognostic Factors—Colorectal Cancer

Survival and disease relapse after surgery with or without adjuvant treatment for colon and rectal cancer are a function of both degree of bowel wall penetration of the primary lesion and nodal status.[8, 286, 291, 295, 338] It is pertinent to understand that nodal involvement *per se* is not the most important pathologic factor that determines survival and relapse. Therein lies the weakness of the current TNM stage I, II, III and Dukes' A, B, C. Patients with the best survival are those with the primary lesion confined to the bowel wall and uninvolved nodes (T1–2,N0,M0, TNM stage I, MAC A or B1, Dukes' A) with an expected 5-year survival of approximately 90% for such patients. For such patients, local recurrence rates are 5% or less and distant relapse rates are approximately 10%.

Intermediate, but still excellent, results are found in patients with one high-risk feature—either primary tumor extension beyond the bowel wall (T3 or T4,N0, MAC B2 or B3, TNM II, Dukes' B) or confined to the wall but with positive nodes (T1–2,N1–2, MAC C1, TNM III, Dukes' C). Five-year survival rates can range from 70% to 90%. The higher survival expectation is for the MAC B2 patients (T3–4a,N0) and MAC C1 patients with 1 to 3 nodes (T1–2,N1) who are treated with surgery plus adjuvant therapy (surgery plus chemotherapy for colon cancers; surgery plus chemoradiation for rectal cancers). For such patients, local relapse risks are 10% to 20% or lower and distant metastasis risks are 20% to 25%. The lower survival component of the intermediate-risk group includes the node-negative patients with adherence to or invasion of surrounding organs or structures (T4b,N0, MAC B3) or C1 patients with a higher number of involved nodes (T1–2,N2). Five-year survival expectancy of these patients would be 60% to 80%. Overall relapse rates are similar for both groups of patients, but patterns of relapse differ. For B3 patients, tumor bed relapse rates with surgery alone are 30% or greater with distant metastasis rates of 20% to 25% (same as B2). For T1–2,N2 patients, systemic risks are higher than for T1–2,N1 patients, and the risk of regional node relapse is higher. For patients in the intermediate-risk group, factors of ploidy and percentage of cells in S phase are felt to have independent prognostic significance.

The poorest survival and highest relapse rates are found in patients with both high-risk factors of nodal involvement and tumor extension beyond the colonic or rectal wall with or without adherence to or invasion of surrounding structures (T3–4b,N1–2, MAC C2 or C3, TNM III, Dukes' C). Five-year survival of these patients after resection plus adjuvant therapy is 30% to 50% with variability by virtue of the presence or absence of primary tumor adherence, number and location of nodes involved, ploidy, and other factors. The rate of local relapse after surgery alone is approximately 35% with MAC C2 lesions versus approximately 50% with MAC C3. The risk of distant metastasis for patients with C2, C3 lesions is 40% to 60%, which is approximately double that of patients with a single risk factor (MAC B2, B3, C1).

Many clinical and other histopathologic factors also have potential influence on the prognosis of colorectal cancers[356, 364, 365]:

- *Gender*: Women tend to have a higher survival rate than men.
- *Symptoms*: Asymptomatic patients have a better prognosis. Those patients with a very short duration of symptoms tend to have worse prognosis.[366, 367]
- *Obstruction* or *perforation*: These complications increase operative mortality and may result in decreased overall survival.[368]
- *Transfusion*: Multivariate analysis has shown conflicting results, but in a number of series, perioperative blood transfusion is inversely related to survival. Whether this relationship is related to the need for transfusions in higher stage disease or to the effects of blood elements is not entirely known.[125, 369, 370]
- *Blood vessel invasion*: This histopathologic finding is associated with a threefold increase in the incidence of liver metastasis.[371]

Adjuvant Results—Rectal Cancer

Scientific End Points

Trial design and results of pertinent randomized studies will be presented with a focus on three independent scientific end points, identified at the 1990 NIH Colorectal Consensus Conference (disease-free survival, overall survival, and local control).[372] A point that must be made is that therapeutic gains achieved with combination adjuvant treatment programs may be offset by an unnecessary increase in complications unless physicians select patients that have definite indications for treatment and work closely to optimize delivery of the combined modalities.

Preoperative Irradiation

Low-dose preoperative irradiation (≤20 Gy in 1.8- to 2.0-Gy fractions) has had no significant impact on either tumor control (local or distant) or survival (disease-free, overall). This was demonstrated most definitively in the MRC trial that compared a surgery-alone control arm with treatment arms of 5 Gy in 1 fraction and 20 Gy in 10 fractions.[366]

Although moderate-dose preoperative irradiation has demonstrated improved local control in two randomized European trials, improved survival was demonstrated only in subset analyses (Table 27–29). In both series, the dose delivered was 34.5 Gy in 15 fractions of 2.3 Gy over 19 days (equivalent to 39.6 to 44 Gy in standard fractionation). Subset analyses suggested a survival advantage in irradiated T3 and T4 patients in the Rotterdam series ($p = 0.001$) and for patients with curative resection in the EORTC trial (5-year survival of 70% vs. 60%, $p = 0.08$). In the EORTC trial, no difference in distant metastasis rates was identified.

A large Swedish trial has been published that demonstrated that a significant improvement in local control also could translate into improved survival (Fig. 27–11; see Table 27–29).[333] Patients were randomized to a surgery-alone control arm ($n = 557$) or to short-course high-dose-per-fraction preoperative irradiation (25 Gy in 5 fractions) followed by resection in 1 week ($n = 553$). After a follow-up interval of 5 years, the rate of local relapse was 27% with surgery alone versus 11% with preoperative irradiation ($p < 0.001$). The 5-year overall survival rate was 48% versus 58% respectively ($p = 0.004$). There was no impact by adjuvant irradiation on distant metastases, with rates of 24% and 23%.

Preoperative Versus Postoperative Irradiation

A Swedish trial compared single adjuvant, high-dose-per-fraction preoperative irradiation (25.5 Gy in 5 fractions over 1 week) to postoperative irradiation (60 Gy in 30 fractions over 8 weeks with planned 2-week split).[376, 377] The local relapse rate in patients with curative resection was less in the preoperative irradiation patients at 13% versus 22% ($p = 0.02$).[377] No significant difference was seen in survival or distant metastasis rates.[375]

TABLE 27–29. **Adjuvant Rectal–Preoperative ± Postoperative Irradiation, Impact on Survival and Disease Control***

Trial		Advantage Seen	Actuarial Survival: *Disease-free %, (p value)*	Actuarial Survival: *Overall %, (p value)*	Incidence Local Recurrence (%): *Surg*	Incidence Local Recurrence (%): *EBRT*	Incidence Local Recurrence (%): *p*	Incidence Distant Metastasis (%): *Surg*	Incidence Distant Metastasis (%): *EBRT*	Incidence Distant Metastasis (%): *p*
Preop (All Stages)										
EORTC[374]	Curative	Preop EBRT vs. surg alone	Not given	69 vs. 59 (.08)	30	15	.003	25	25	.87
	Total	None	56 vs. 51 (.54)	52 vs. 49 (.69)	35	20	.02	—	—	—
Rotterdam[375]	T3, T4	Preop EBRT vs. surg alone	Not given	50 vs. 18 (.001)	36	14	.08	45	32	NS
	T2	None	Not given	62 vs. 70 (NS)	18	0	NS	26	45	NS
Swedish[333]	Total	Preop EBRT vs. surg alone	—	58 vs. 48 (.004)	27	11	<.001	—	—	—
	Curative	Preop EBRT	—	—	33	9	<.001	24	23	NS
Preop vs. Postop (all stages)										
Swedish[376, 377]		Preop vs. postop	Not given for total group	43 vs. 37 (.43)	—	13 vs. 22	.02	—	28 vs. 37	.30

Preop = preoperative; Postop = postoperative; EBRT = external beam irradiation; Surg = surgery; NS = not significant.
*All data are from controlled multi-institution randomized trials.

Postoperative Irradiation and Chemotherapy

A summary of results in six published randomized adjuvant trials for resected high-risk rectal cancers is shown in Table 27–30. Results are reported as a function of treatment impact on patterns of relapse (local, distant) and survival (disease-free, overall). Positive survival results were reported in five of the trials.

UNITED STATES TRIALS

The NSABP three-arm trial (NSABP R01) compared surgery alone with postoperative irradiation and postoperative chemotherapy as single adjuvants.[328] An advantage in disease-free survival was demonstrated with adjuvant chemotherapy versus surgery alone ($p = 0.006$), but neither local relapse nor distant metastasis was significantly altered with the addition of chemotherapy. In patients randomized to receive irradiation, there was a significant decrease in local relapse from 25% to 16% when compared with surgery alone ($p = 0.06$), but overall survival was equal (14% of patients randomized to the irradiation arm did not receive such).

Two randomized postoperative trials from the United States, GITSG 7175 and Mayo/NCCTG 79-47-51,[329–331] and a trial from Norway[332] documented a decrease in local relapse and improvement in both disease-free and overall survival with combined postoperative chemoradiation for resected high-risk patients (Dukes' B or C lesions; TNM stages II, III; MAC B2, B3, C1, C2, C3). In the GITSG 7175 trial, patients were randomized to a surgery-alone control arm and adjuvant arms of postoperative irradiation, postoperative chemotherapy, or a combination thereof.[329, 330] Statistically significant advantages in disease-free and overall survival with the chemoradiation arm were achieved in

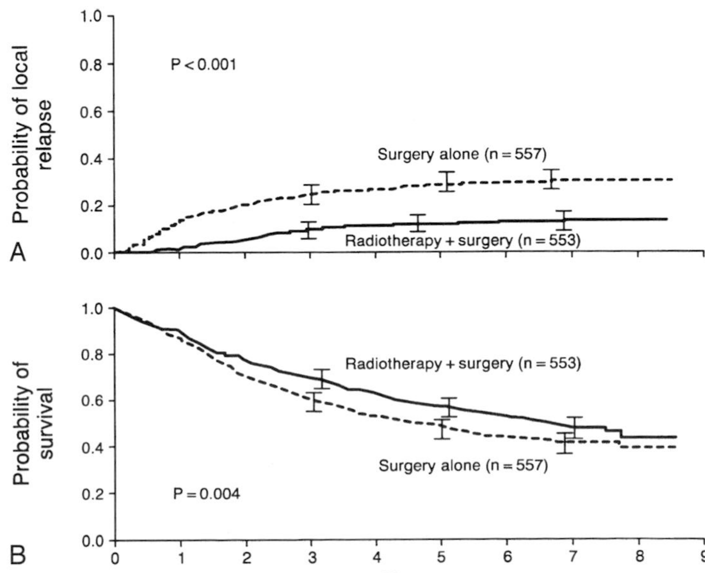

Figure 27–11. Swedish adjuvant rectal phase III trial comparing surgery ± short course, high-dose-per-fraction preoperative irradiation. (A) Local control. (B) Overall survival. (From Swedish Rectal Cancer Trial: Improved survival with preoperative radiotherapy in resectable rectal cancer. N Engl J Med 1997; 336:980–987, with permission.)

TABLE 27–30. **Adjuvant Rectal Postoperative Irradiation ± Chemotherapy—Impact On Survival and Disease Control***

		Actuarial Survival		Incidence of Local Recurrence (%)					Incidence of Distant Metastases (%)				
Sequence EBRT/Surg	**Advantage Seen**	**Disease-Free % (p value)**	**Overall % (p value)**	**Surg**	**CT**	**EBRT**	**EBRT/ CT**	**p**	**Surg**	**CT**	**EBRT**	**EBRT/CT**	**p**
Postop[a] (5-yr actuarial data and 2-tail p values unless specified)													
GITSG 7175[329, 330]	EBRT CT vs. Surg	70 vs. 46 (.009)	58 vs. 45 (.005, 1 tail)	24	27	20	11	.08§	34	27†	30	26†	—
NSABP R01[328]	CT vs. Surg	41 vs. 30 (.006)	53 vs. 43 (.05)	25	21	16	—	.06	26	24	31	—	NS
NCCTG/Mayo 794751[331]	EBRT CT vs. EBRT	59 vs. 37 (.002)	58 vs. 48 (.025)‡	—	—	25	13.5	.04	—	—	46	29	.01
Norwegian[332]	EBRT 5-FU vs. Surg	64 vs. 46 (.01)	64 vs. 50 (.05)	30	—	—	12	.01	39	—	—	33	—
GITSG 7180 (3-yr data)[378]	EBRT 5-FU ± MeCCNU	68 vs. 54 (.20)	75 vs. 66 (.58)	—	—	—	17 vs. 16	NS	—	—	—	26 vs. 40	.05
NCCTG 864751 (4-yr data)[379]	EBRT PVI 5-FU vs EBRT bolus 5-FU	63 vs. 53 (.01)	70 vs. 60 (.005)	—	—	—	8 vs. 12	.11‖	—	—	—	31 vs. 40 (p = .03)	.03‖
Preop vs. Postop (all stages)													
Swedish[376, 377]	Preop vs. postop	Not given for total group	43 vs. 37 (.43)	—	—	13 vs. 22	—	.02	—	—	28 vs. 37	—	.30

EBRT = external beam irradiation; Surg = operation; CT = chemotherapy; PVI 5-FU = protracted venous infusion 5-fluorouracil; MeCCNU = methyl-chloroethyl-cyclo-hexyl-nitrosourea; SR = survival.

[a]MAC stages B2, B3, C1, C2, C3 (TNM stages: II, III, or T3–4,N0; Tis–4,N1–2).

*All data are from controlled multi-institution randomized trials.

†GITSG—advantage to chemotherapy vs. no chemotherapy at 20% vs. 30% (distant metastases only), 27% vs. 32% (any distant metastases).

‡Mayo alone series: 5-yr overall SR 70% vs. 57% postop EBRT CT vs EBRT (p = 0.01) and distant metastasis rate of 33% vs 52%. From Schild SE, Martenson JA, Gunderson LL, et al: Postoperative adjuvant therapy of rectal cancer. Int J Radiat Oncol Biol Phys 1989; 17:55–62.

§EBRT vs. no EBRT.

‖Advantage to EBRT PVI 5-FU vs. EBRT bolus 5-FU.

a comparison with the surgery-alone control arm (p = 0.009 and 0.005, respectively). The best local control was achieved with combined chemoradiation (local relapse rate of 11% versus 20% with irradiation alone). No impact on local control was seen with chemotherapy as a single adjuvant. Although rates of distant metastasis were lower in the two arms that contained chemotherapy when compared with the two arms without chemotherapy, no single arm had a significant impact on the rate of distant metastases (see Table 27–30). The survival advantage achieved with combined chemoradiation appeared to relate primarily to the marked reduction in local relapse.

In the initial Mayo/NCCTG trial (79-47-51),[331] the minimum irradiation dose within the boost field in both the irradiation and radiochemotherapy arms was higher than in the GITSG 7175 trial (50.4 Gy versus 40 to 48 Gy). The chemoradiation arm achieved statistically improved results with regard to both disease control and survival. Local relapse, as an initial pattern of failure, was reduced from 25% to 13.5% (p = 0.04), and distant metastases were decreased from 46% to 29% (p = 0.01). Both disease-free survival (DFS) and overall survival (OS) were also statistically improved. This study was the first randomized trial in which a course of full-dose chemotherapy was given before as well as after combined chemoradiation in an attempt to decrease the incidence of distant metastases (one dose of MeCCNU, two cycles of 5-FU in both the pre- and post-chemoradiation arms). This study was also the first trial in which both local relapse and distant metastases were reduced significantly in the experimental treatment arm.

Two subsequent randomized postoperative trials, GITSG 7180[378] and the intergroup 86-47-51 trial coordinated by NCCTG,[379] demonstrated that MeCCNU did not produce an incremental benefit when added to irradiation plus 5-FU. The intergroup trial NCCTG 86-47-51 also tested the best method of giving 5-FU concomitant with irradiation in a 2 × 2 randomization design in 664 patients.[379] A planned interim analysis of disease control (initial patterns of relapse) and time to relapse indicated a significant advantage for patients who received PVI 5-FU during irradiation. The analysis also revealed a significant improvement in overall survival (Fig. 27–12).

As a result of the lack of additive benefit from MeCCNU, the control arm in the subsequent U.S. Intergroup rectal adjuvant study (INT 0114) was postoperative irradiation plus bolus 5-FU.[380] INT 0114 tested four different systemic regimens before and after irradiation plus bolus 5-FU with or without leucovorin: 5-FU alone; 5-FU and levamisole; 5-FU plus low-dose leucovorin; and all three drugs. Accrual to INT 0114 was initiated in 1990 and completed in late 1992 before results from 86-47-51 were available concerning the advantage of infusion 5-FU over bolus 5-FU when given as a single drug during irradiation. An initial analysis showed no statistical benefit for any treatment arm versus another with regard to either disease control or survival.[380]

NORWAY TRIAL

The trial conducted by the Norwegian Adjuvant Rectal Cancer Project Group[332] was initiated in 1986–87 when only the GITSG 7175 trial had demonstrated both a local

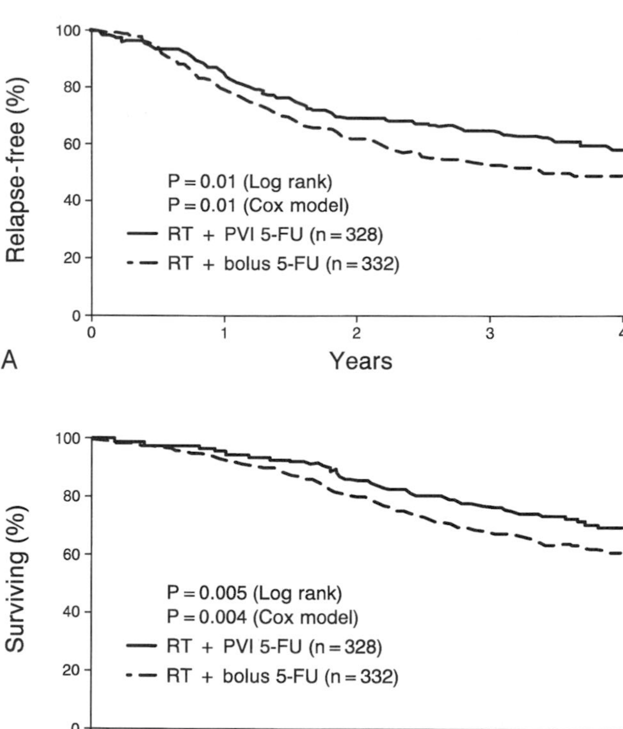

Figure 27–12. Mayo/NCCTG 86-47-51 relapse-free (A) and overall survival (B) curves, showing advantage of PVI versus bolus 5-FU during irradiation in resected high-risk rectal cancer. (From O'Connell MJ, Martenson JA, Wieand HS, et al: Improving adjuvant therapy for rectal cancer by combining protracted infusion fluorouracil with radiation therapy after curative surgery. N Engl J Med 1994; 331:502–507, with permission.)

control and a survival benefit for combined postoperative chemoradiation. Therefore, the investigators chose to conduct a two-arm trial of surgery alone (n = 70 patients) with or without postoperative chemoradiation (n = 66 patients). The combined adjuvant arm differed from the GITSG 7175 and subsequent trials in that the adjuvant 5-FU was given only concomitantly with adjuvant EBRT (46 Gy in 2-Gy fractions over 4½ to 5 weeks) and no maintenance chemotherapy was given. With minimum follow-up of 4 years, an improvement in local control was demonstrated in the chemoradiation arm. Local relapse rates were 30% with surgery alone versus 12% with adjuvant chemoradiation. No significant impact on distant metastases was achieved; however, the improvement in local control translated into improvements in both 5-year DFS and OS (Fig. 27–13).

Complications and Therapeutic Ratio

An optimal therapeutic ratio between local control and complications is achieved only with close interaction between the surgeon and the radiation oncologist and the use of sophisticated radiation techniques.[9, 10, 326, 359] In the MGH postoperative rectal adjuvant series, which used shaped multifield irradiation techniques, bladder distention, and the like, the incidence of small bowel obstruction requiring operative intervention was the same in patients receiving

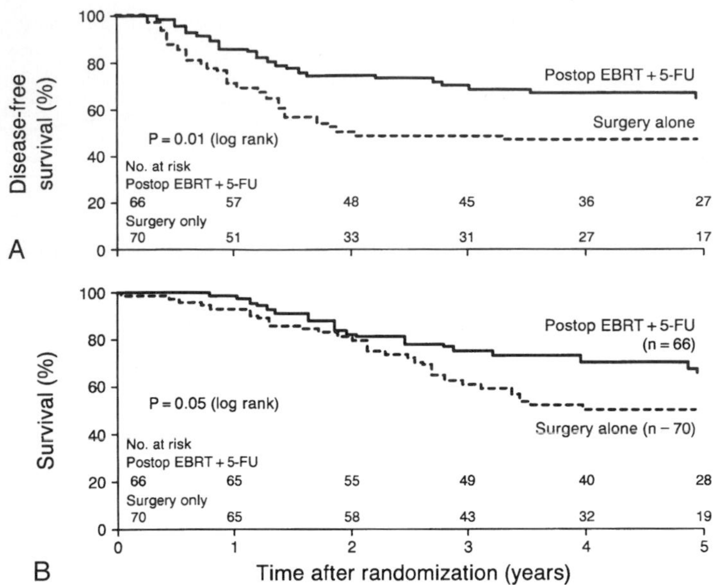

Figure 27–13. Norwegian phase III rectal adjuvant trial comparing surgery ± postoperative irradiation plus concomitant 5-FU. (A) Disease-free survival rate. (B) Overall survival. (From Tveit KM, Guldvog I, Hagen S, et al: Randomized controlled trial of postoperative radiotherapy and short-term time-scheduled 5-fluorouracil against surgery alone in the treatment of Dukes B and C rectal cancer. Norwegian Adjuvant Rectal Cancer Project Group. Am J Surg 1997; 84:1130–1135, with permission.)

adjuvant postoperative irradiation (with or without chemotherapy) as in those with surgery alone at 6% versus 5%, respectively.[293, 381] In the Mayo/NCCTG 79-47-51 adjuvant rectal trial using multifield irradiation techniques, the incidence of acute enteritis was higher in the patients with irradiation plus 5-FU versus irradiation alone at 20% versus 5%.[331] This finding did not translate into increased chronic intolerance; the incidence of severe small bowel problems was 6% or less with either adjuvant irradiation alone or adjuvant radiochemotherapy. In the subsequent NCCTG 86-47-51 trial, acute GI intolerance was higher with PVI 5-FU than with bolus 5-FU during irradiation. Severe diarrhea occurred in 24% versus 14% of patients ($p < 0.01$).[379] Severe hematologic intolerance was lower with PVI 5-FU versus bolus 5-FU, with the white blood cell count below 2000 in 2% versus 11% of patients ($p < 0.01$).

In a single-institution retrospective analysis of rectal function following adjuvant treatment, Kollmorgen and associates[382] suggested that rectal function was unfavorably altered by postoperative irradiation with or without chemotherapy for high-risk lesions when compared with surgery alone for low-risk lesions. This finding was manifested primarily as increased frequency of bowel movements, occasional stool incontinence, and the need for periodic anti-diarrheal agents. Flaws in the analysis included the nonrandom selection of treatment, the presence of early-stage versus late-stage disease in the surgery-alone versus adjuvant treatment groups, the retrospective nature of the analysis, and nonblinding of the interviewer with regard to treatment method. Nonetheless, it is not surprising that postoperative irradiation with or without chemotherapy may reduce compliance of the reconstructed stool reservoir and result in some dysfunction. Such dysfunction can usually be ameliorated by the use of antidiarrheal agents. The incidence of severe treatment-related dysfunction was judged to be low, and this risk must be placed in proper perspective by considering the severe morbidity and dysfunction of pelvic relapse. Prospective quality-of-life studies need to be performed to determine both the actual level of dysfunction with preoperative versus postoperative adjuvant chemoradiation and whether treatment-related effects can be modified or prevented with agents such as somatostatin and sucralfate.

Summary and Future Directions for Adjuvant Therapy

The impact of preoperative and postoperative irradiation with or without chemotherapy on both disease control and survival in major randomized adjuvant rectal cancer trials is summarized in Tables 27–28 and 27–29.

Single-Modality Rectal Adjuvants

Neither irradiation nor chemotherapy as single-adjuvant modalities achieves all suggested criteria of efficacy. Adjuvant irradiation reduces the rate of local relapse in both prospective nonrandomized and randomized preoperative and postoperative trials, but in most series, this reduction has not translated into an improvement in OS because of a lack of impact on distant metastases. The only published trial in which single-modality adjuvant treatment improved both local control and survival was the large Swedish trial of over 1100 patients testing surgery with or without preoperative irradiation.[333] The adjuvant irradiation did not reduce distant metastases. In a Swedish trial that compared high-dose-per-fraction preoperative irradiation to postoperative irradiation as single adjuvants, the local relapse rate in patients with curative resection was lower in the patients treated with preoperative irradiation at 13% versus 22%.[376, 377] No significant difference was seen between the treatment approaches in survival or distant metastasis rates.

Adjuvant chemotherapy produced a significant improvement in DFS and marginal improvement in overall survival in the NSABP R-01 trial.[328] However, no significant improvement in local control has been seen with single-modality adjuvant chemotherapy in any randomized study (incidence of 21% in NSABP R-01 and 27% in GITSG 7175 as initial patterns of relapse).

Combined-Modality Rectal Adjuvants

Only combined-modality postoperative adjuvant treatment has consistently demonstrated efficacy in all scientific end points, as noted in two prospectively randomized U.S. trials (GITSG 7175[329,330] and Mayo/NCCTG 79-47-51[331]) and a third trial from Norway.[332] In both of the U.S. studies, bolus 5-FU was administered during irradiation, and patients received additional chemotherapy either after irradiation plus 5-FU (GITSG) or both before and after (Mayo/NCCTG) the combined-modality segment of treatment. In the Norwegian study, patients received 5-FU only during irradiation. Subsequent randomized trials by the same two U.S. study groups have determined that MeCCNU does not provide additional benefit over bolus 5-FU as the systemic component of treatment in adjuvant rectal combined-modality regimens.[378, 379] However, in the NCCTG intergroup trial, the use of PVI 5-FU during irradiation produced a reduction in both local relapse and distant metastases and improvements in both DFS and OS.[379]

Despite the advantages noted with combined-modality treatment, there is a need to further improve both local control and systemic control of disease. Although the reported NCCTG intergroup trial suggested a decrease in local relapse with the use of PVI versus bolus 5-FU during irradiation (8% vs. 12% as initial relapse), the true incidence of local relapse as a component of failure at any time in follow-up is probably 10% to 12.5%, even with combinations of irradiation and PVI 5-FU chemotherapy (possibly higher for the highest risk C2 and C3 patients; T3–4b,N1–2). This inference is based on the single-institution analysis by Schild and colleagues that demonstrated that use of initial failure data to predict local relapse risks underestimates the total risk of local relapse by approximately 33%.[294] To accomplish further improvements in local control, it may be necessary to investigate administration of the best local and systemic adjuvants simultaneously instead of delaying postoperative irradiation for two cycles of chemotherapy. Alternatively, preoperative chemoradiation may be more effective than postoperative chemoradiation.

Systemic metastases as an initial pattern of relapse occurred in 26% to 29% of patients in spite of combined chemoradiation in both GITSG 7175 and NCCTG 79-47-51. In the NCCTG intergroup study, distant metastases were decreased with PVI 5-FU versus bolus 5-FU from 40% to 31%, but the magnitude of the problem is still significant. There is a need to evaluate the delivery of the most effective systemic therapy during as well as before and after irradiation to avoid delays of 2.5 to 3 months between sequences of the most effective systemic therapy. As systemic control of disease is optimized, drug combinations may need to be tailored based upon the relative risk of systemic metastasis.

Adjuvant Results—Colon Cancer

Adjuvant Chemotherapy

5-FU PLUS LEVAMISOLE

The initial dramatic studies that began the advances in adjuvant colon treatment were two controlled clinical trials using 5-FU plus levamisole for Dukes' stage C colon cancer (Mayo/NCCTG 784852; confirmatory intergroup 0035). In the initial study by Mayo/NCCTG,[342] DFS was improved by 15% to 20% at 5 years when compared with a surgery-alone control arm ($p < 0.003$), and OS was also increased at 52% versus 42% (from published figures; $p = 0.03$). The original report of intergroup trial 0035 noted the experience of 1247 patients with stages II and III colon cancer who were randomized after resection to 5-FU plus levamisole, levamisole alone, or to no postoperative adjuvant therapy (surgery-alone control group).[383] After a median follow-up of 3.5 years, there was a 41% reduction in odds of relapse ($p < 0.001$) and a 33% reduction in the overall death rate ($p = 0.006$) when the cohort treated with 5-FU plus levamisole was compared with the untreated surgery-alone control group. A later report, which focused on the subset of patients with stage III disease after a median follow-up of 6.5 years, noted a reduction in the rate of relapse by 40% and the death rate by 33% ($p = 0.0007$).[384] With confirmation of the Mayo/NCCTG trial (784852)[342] by the Intergroup trials (0035) (Fig. 27–14), the conclusions seem firm for patients with positive nodes.

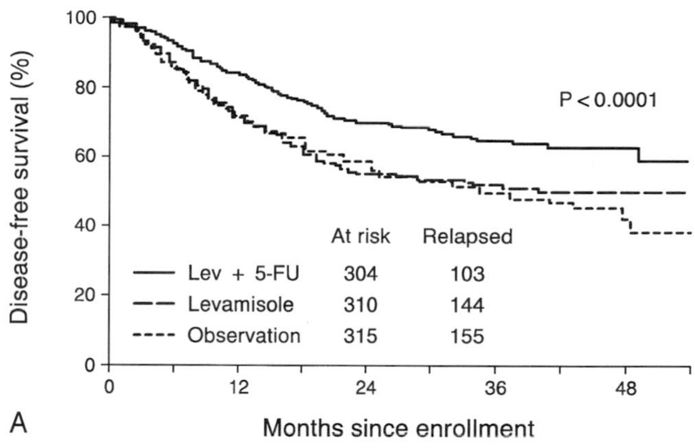

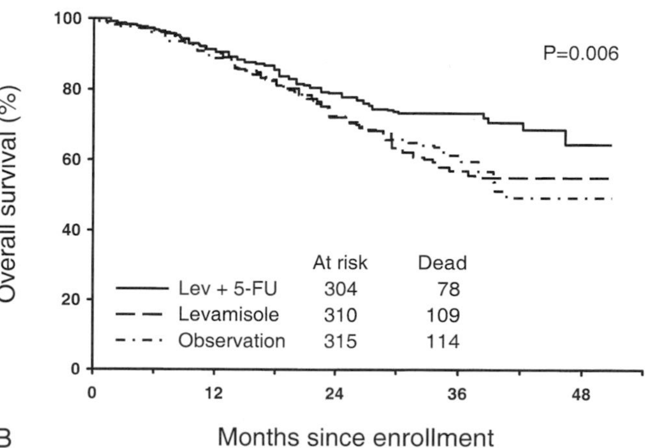

Figure 27–14. Colon adjuvant chemotherapy with 12 months of 5-FU–levamisole versus surgery alone for node-positive patients in the confirmatory U.S. intergroup trial: (A) Disease-free survival rate. (B) Overall survival. (From Moertel CG, Fleming TR, McDonald JS, et al: Fluorouracil plus levamisole as an effective adjuvant therapy after resection of stage II colon cancer: a final report. Ann Intern Med 1995; 122:321–326, with permission.)

In Dukes' stage B colon cancer, the results with 5-FU plus levamisole were less conclusive. Because nearly 80% of patients are alive at 5 years with surgery alone, it becomes more difficult to alter outcome. Larger numbers of patients will be necessary to show differences in disease control and survival, and only the highest risk patients should probably be considered for adjuvant therapy (T4 disease, aneuploid, high S phase).

5-FU PLUS LEUCOVORIN

5-FU plus leucovorin was noted to be effective in a study of 309 patients who were randomized to 5-FU plus leucovorin or a control group of surgery alone after complete resection.[345] This trial indicated that the relapse-free rate with therapy (77%) was statistically better than was seen with no postoperative therapy (64%) at 3.5 years of median follow-up time (p = 0.004, Fig. 27–15). In a subsequent trial, stage III and high-risk stage II patients were randomly assigned to 5-FU plus levamisole or 5-FU plus leucovorin and levamisole for either 6 months or 12 months. This trial showed that the 5-FU plus leucovorin regimen administered for 6 months was equivalent to the 5-FU plus levamisole regimen given for 12 months.[385]

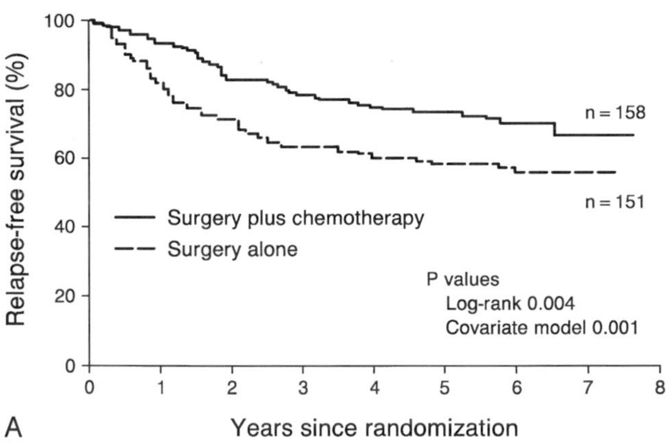

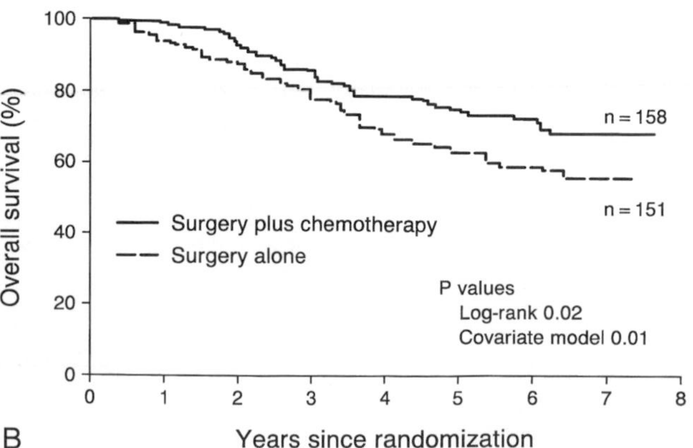

Figure 27–15. Colon adjuvant chemotherapy with 6 months of 5-FU–low-dose leucovorin versus surgery alone for node-positive patients in the Mayo/NCCTG trial: (A) Disease-free survival rate. (B) Overall survival. (From O'Connell MJ, Mailliard JA, Kahn MJ: Controlled trial of fluorouracil and low dose leucovorin given for six months as postoperative adjuvant therapy for colon cancer. J Clin Oncol 1997; 15:246–250, with permission.)

In a trial by the NSABP of 5-FU plus high-dose leucovorin compared with a regimen of MeCCNU, vincristine, and 5-FU (MOF), the experience in 1091 patients favored the 5-FU plus leucovorin regimen.[346] The overall survival was 84% for 5-FU plus leucovorin and 77% for MOF-treated cohorts after a median of 48 months of follow-up (p = 0.003).

17 1-A ANTIBODY

Immunotherapy has been the subject of a number of adjuvant trials. In a group of 189 patients,[351] 17-1A antibody treatment was reported to provide an equivalent relative improvement in DFS and OS for a group of stage III patients, as has been reported for 5-FU plus leucovorin or levamisole, when compared with the control group in that trial. Trials of the antibody alone in stage II patients and of the antibody plus chemotherapy in stage III patients are ongoing in the United States.

The aforementioned results are summarized in Table 27–31.

Adjuvant Postoperative Irradiation and Chemotherapy

Significant data have been accumulated in autopsy, clinical, and reoperative series to indicate that local-regional relapse in the tumor bed or regional nodes is a significant risk after resection of selected stages of colonic as well as rectal lesions.[295, 338, 339] The risk of local regional relapse is felt to be 30% or greater with surgery alone for MAC stages B3, C3, and C2 (TNM: T4b,N0, T4b,N1–3, T3–4a,N1–3).

PHASE II—SINGLE-INSTITUTION OR GROUP STUDIES

Results from a large MGH pilot study using adjuvant tumor bed–nodal irradiation for patients with high-risk colon cancers were compared with those achieved by surgery alone.[296, 297] Patients defined as at high risk for local relapse included those with a MAC B3 or C3 lesion or C2 lesions except for midtransverse or midsigmoid. Patients with B2 lesions were included only if the surgeon felt the radial margins (usually posterior) were narrow. EBRT doses of 45 to 50 Gy in 1.8-Gy fractions were given to tumor bed plus 3- to 5-cm margins with or without regional nodes. In a 1993 publication of 169 adjuvant colon patients irradiated at MGH (52 with simultaneous 5-FU with EBRT), 5-year actuarial local control and survival appeared to be better in irradiated B3 and C3 patients.[297] Those differences may have been due in part to patient selection because this was not a controlled randomized trial. Simultaneous 5-FU during EBRT produced a trend for improved local control and DFS, as found in randomized rectal adjuvant studies.

Estes, Giri, and Fabian compared patterns of relapse for MAC C2 patients on SWOG 8591[386] (arms of surgery alone or surgery plus 5-FU plus levamisole), SWOG 8572[387] (whole abdomen irradiation plus tumor bed EBRT and infusion 5-FU), and the surgery-alone arm from the MGH analysis.[297] In SWOG 8591, although lung relapse was decreased from 34% to 21% with the addition of 5-FU plus levamisole to surgical resection, the chemotherapy adjuvant had no impact on the rate of local-regional relapse (surgery alone—20%; 5-FU plus levamisole—27%). This incidence was equivalent to the 32% incidence with surgery alone in the MGH analysis. Patients who received chemora-

TABLE 27–31. **Colon Cancer Adjuvant Chemotherapy Trials**

Study	Chemotherapy	Immunotherapy	Results	Ref. #
NCCTG	5-FU	Levamisole	5-FU + levamisole results in increased relapse-free and overall survival in Dukes' C	342
Confirmatory Intergroup	5-FU	Levamisole	Increased relapse-free and overall survival in Dukes' C over surgery alone	383, 384
NCCTG	5-FU + leucovorin (low dose)	—	Increased relapse-free and overall survival in Dukes' C over surgery alone	345
NSABP	5-FU + leucovorin (high dose)	—	Increased relapse-free and overall survival in Dukes' C over surgery alone	346
ECOG	5-FU	Levamisole		347
	5-FU + leucovorin (low dose)	—		
	5-FU + leucovorin (high dose)	—		
	5-FU + leucovorin + levamisole	—	5-FU + leucovorin arms equivalent	
NSABP	5-FU + leucovorin	Interferon-α	No benefit to interferon	348
Reithmuller	—	17-1A monoclonal Ab	Increased relapse-free survival in Dukes' C over surgery alone	351

5-FU = 5-fluorouracil; Ab = antibody.

diation on SWOG 8592 had only a 12% tumor bed nodal relapse rate along with a reduction in liver and peritoneal relapse rates (liver relapse rate of 22% with chemoradiation vs. 54% and 57% in the two arms of SWOG 8591; peritoneal relapse rates of 15% in SWOG 8572 vs. 37% and 40% in SWOG 8591).

Results–Locally Advanced Colorectal Cancer

External Irradiation (and Resection and Chemotherapy)

EBRT has been combined with surgical resection, chemotherapy, or immunotherapy for locally advanced cancers.[291, 388] In separate series from the PMH[324] and Mayo Clinic using EBRT alone or with immunotherapy,[389] local persistence or relapse was 90% or greater in evaluable patients. As seen in Table 27–32, attempts to control locally recurrent disease with EBRT with or without resection are primarily palliative. An Australian publication by Guiney and coworkers discussed results in 135 patients with pelvic relapse of rectal cancer who had no evidence of extrapelvic metastases.[391] A select group of 39 patients were treated with radical intent—re-resection in 54% and EBRT doses of 50 to 60 Gy in all 39. Median survival in the radically treated group was 18 months and 5-year survival was 9% or lower.

Local relapse has been reduced in patients with locally advanced primary lesions by combining irradiation with surgical resection with or without chemotherapy.[291, 388] External irradiation has been given either after subtotal resection of locally advanced lesions (45 to 70 Gy in 1.8- to 2.0-Gy fractions) or before an attempt at resection for disease that is initially unresectable for cure (45 to 60 Gy in 5 to 6.5 weeks preoperatively, followed by resection in

TABLE 27–32. **Locally Recurrent or Primary Colorectal Cancer Survival and Disease Relapse with EBRT, Various Series**

		Overall Survival (%)				Disease Relapse Actuarial 3-yr (%)	
Disease Category and Treatment	**No. Pts.**	***Median (mo)***	***2 yr***	***3 yr***	***5 yr***	***Local No. (%)***	***Distant No. (%)***
Recurrent + Primary—EBRT							
Mayo Clinic—Moertel[177]	65						
EBRT alone	—	10.5	24	9	—	—	—
EBRT + 5-FU	—	16	38	19	5	—	—
Recurrent—EBRT							
Netherlands—Lybeert[390]	76	14	25	13	5	43/63 (68)	26/63 (41)
EBRT <50 Gy	—	12	20	6	0	—	—
EBRT ≥50 Gy	—	20	40	18	10	—	—
Australian—EBRT[391]	135	15	—	—	—	—	—
Low-dose palliative	16	9	13	6	—	—/(94)	—
High-dose palliative*	80	15	26	12	4	—/(94)	—/(38)†
Radical (50–60 Gy/2 Gy Fx)	39	18	31	28	≤9	—/(82)	—/(49)†

EBRT = external beam irradiation; 5-FU = 5-fluorouracil; Fx = fractions.
*High-dose palliative patients had 45 Gy/3 Gy Fx with 1 week treatment break after 30 Gy in 10 Fx.
†Incidence of metastasis underestimated because patients were investigated as warranted by symptoms.

3 to 5 weeks). Long-term local control and survival can be obtained in a minority of patients, but the risk of local recurrence is still too high at 30% to 70%.

Intraoperative Electron Irradiation and External Irradiation

PRIMARY LESIONS

When IOERT is combined with conventional treatment for locally advanced primary colorectal cancers, separate analyses from the MGH and the Mayo Clinic suggest an improvement in both local control and survival.[392–396] In an early MGH series of patients with locally advanced rectal cancer, disease relapse within irradiation fields was 43% versus 0% for 17 non-IOERT versus 16 IOERT patients, and 1- and 2-year survival were statistically better with IOERT. An updated MGH analysis by Willett and colleagues reports actuarial 5-year survival of 43% in 42 IOERT patients.[395] In the MGH analysis, patients with gross total resection before IOERT did better with regard to local control and survival than those with gross residual disease.

In a Mayo Clinic comparison of 17 non-IOERT[394] and 56 IOERT plus EBRT patients with locally advanced primary rectal or colon cancers,[396] local control was 24% versus 87%, median survival was 18 versus 40 months, and the 3-year survival was 24% versus 55% (Table 27–33). Prognostic factors that had a statistically positive impact on disease control and survival in IOERT patients included EBRT plus 5-FU versus EBRT alone, treatment sequence of preoperative EBRT plus 5-FU versus postoperative EBRT plus 5-FU, microscopic or no residual disease after maximal resection, and colon versus rectal primary.

A separate Mayo Clinic analysis was performed regarding the use of EBRT (with or without chemotherapy) with or without IOERT as a supplement to maximal resection for 103 patients with locally advanced colon cancers.[398] The 5-year actuarial local relapse rate was 10% for patients with no residual disease, 54% for patients with microscopic residual disease, and 79% for patients with gross residual disease ($p < 0.0001$). For patients with residual disease, local relapse occurred in 11% of patients receiving IOERT compared with 82% of patients receiving only EBRT ($p = 0.02$). The 5-year actuarial survival rate was 66% for patients with no residual disease, 47% for patients with microscopic residual and 23% for patients with gross residual disease ($p = 0.0009$). The 5-year survival rate in patients with residual disease was 76% for patients receiving IOERT and 26% for patients receiving EBRT alone ($p = 0.04$).

LOCALLY RECURRENT CANCERS

For locally recurrent colorectal cancers, standard treatment with EBRT, with or without chemotherapy, results in excellent short-term palliation (usually less than 1 year), median survival of 10 to 18 months, but rare long-term survival (0% to 7% at 5 years).[291, 399] With the addition of IOERT supplements to standard treatment, 5-year survivals of approximately 20% have been achieved in series from both MGH and the Mayo Clinic.[395, 397, 399, 400]

In a Mayo Clinic analysis of 106 locally recurrent rectal cancer patients who had a palliative resection and no extrapelvic disease, 42 received IOERT.[397] Overall survival was significantly better with IOERT versus no IOERT ($p = 0.0006$) (see Table 27–33). The 3-year survival differences favoring IOERT also persisted when subset analyses were done that evaluated results in patients who presented with pain or had gross residual disease remaining after maximal resection (overall 3-year survival: 43% vs. 19% and 44% vs. 15%, respectively; DFS: 25% vs. 8% and 29% vs. 6%, respectively).

In an updated Mayo Clinic analysis, 123 previously unirradiated patients with local-regional relapse of colorectal cancer received IOERT as a component of treatment.[400] Disease control and survival were similar to that reported by Suzuki (see Table 27–33). The only prognostic factor that showed a trend for improved OS and DFS was EBRT plus 5-FU versus EBRT alone.

Sequencing of Modalities

The preferred sequencing of modalities in IOERT-containing regimens is usually preoperative external irradiation

TABLE 27–33. **Locally Advanced Primary and Recurrent Colorectal—EBRT ± IOERT, Mayo Clinic**

		Overall Survival (%)				**Disease Relapse Actuarial 3-yr (%)**	
Treatment	**Patients at Risk**	***Median (mo)***	***2 yr***	***3 yr***	***5 yr***	***Local (%)***	***Distant (%)***
Primary Disease							
External (EBRT)*[394]	17	18	35	24	24	76	59
EBRT + IOERT[396]	56	40	70	55	46	16	49
Localized Recurrence							
Suzuki[397]							
No IOERT	64	17	26	18	7	93	54
IOERT ± EBRT	42	30	62	43	19	40	60
IOERT ± EBRT							
No prior EBRT[395]	123	28	62	39	20	25	64
Prior EBRT[399]	51	23	48	28	12	55	71

EBRT = external beam irradiation; IOERT = intraoperative electron irradiation.
*All deaths within 30 mo. Local failure range 3–15 mo. Distant failure range 3–17 mo.

plus chemotherapy followed by maximal resection and IOERT. Several analyses, including those of MGH, have shown the advantage of achieving a gross total resection, whenever such is safe and feasible, for patients with both primary and recurrent lesions even when IOERT is a component of treatment.[395, 401–403] In recent Mayo Clinic IOERT analyses, the advantage of gross total resection with regard to local control and survival was demonstrated in the 56 IOERT patients who presented with locally advanced primary lesions[396] (see Table 27–33). In the 123 IOERT patients who presented at the time of local relapse without prior EBRT,[395] however, the 5-year survival in the 65 patients with gross residual was equivalent to the patients with no residual or microresidual disease at 18% versus 24%.

The risk of systemic failure is 50% or greater in patients with locally advanced colorectal cancers, which provides rationale for the routine addition of maintenance chemotherapy to concomitant radiochemotherapy and resection. Pilot trials have demonstrated that either the two-drug bolus combination of 5-FU plus leucovorin[236] or PVI 5-FU[379] can be combined with external irradiation with acceptable tolerance, thus starting effective local and systemic treatment simultaneously. Therefore, it is reasonable to have patients receive both concomitant and maintenance 5-FU–based chemotherapy.

Metastatic Colorectal Disease

Chemotherapy Results

Combinations of 5-FU and MeCCNU, with or without vincristine, were initially reported to produce response rates of 32% to 43%.[404–406] In subsequent larger trials, lower responses rates were noted: 5-FU plus MeCCNU plus vincristine gave a 27% response rate in 137 patients; and 5-FU plus MeCCNU gave a 16% response rate in 61 patients.[298] The finding that these multidrug combinations provided no response or survival advantage over treatment with 5-FU alone was reported in a series of 1314 patients in ECOG trials.[407] Consequently, MeCCNU is seldom prescribed today for therapy of advanced colorectal cancer. Indeed, MeCCNU was never approved by the Food and Drug Administration and was only available to patients in the United States through enrollment in a clinical trial. Many drugs with broad spectrums of activity among a multitude of tumor types, such as the anthracyclines, taxanes, and platinum-based agents, have failed to provide clinical benefit in colorectal cancer.

Selected patients who are resistant to bolus 5-FU may respond to infusion 5-FU.[408] In one large randomized phase II trial that investigated a variety of methods of 5-FU administration, the activity of the various regimens was similar.[409] The favorable toxicity profile of 5-FU by continuous infusion and the fact that, in a meta-analysis, response rates to 5-FU by infusion (22%) were higher than response rates to 5-FU bolus (14%) have led some investigators to advocate routine use of this administration method.[410]

A meta-analysis of 10 randomized trials of 5-FU alone compared with 5-FU plus leucovorin indicated an improvement in response rate from 10% to 23% but did not demonstrate a survival advantage for patients treated with leucovorin-modulated 5-FU.[344] The median survivals of groups of patients treated with a variety of 5-FU plus leucovorin chemotherapy regimens have been remarkably consistent at approximately 12 months. A few individual trials have suggested that groups of patients treated with leucovorin-modulated 5-FU may have a survival advantage over those treated with 5-FU alone.[411, 412]

The optimal method of administering these two drugs in combination has been the aim of numerous trials. In the United States, the use of bolus schedules predominates. In Europe, infusion of 5-FU over 24 to 48 hours is common practice.[413, 414] In one common regimen, named after its originator Aimery de Gramont, leucovorin is followed by bolus and then 22-hour infusion of 5-FU, repeated on each of 2 consecutive days every 2 weeks. When the de Gramont regimen was compared with the Mayo/NCCTG low-dose leucovorin (20 mg/m^2 daily days 1–5) plus 5-FU (425 mg/m^2 daily days 1–5) regimen, no survival differences were noted. However, there was a difference in the response rate of 33% for the de Gramont regimen and 14% for the Mayo/NCCTG regimen. A review of trials in progress worldwide suggests that the most common regimen still employed as the control regimen for phase III trials in advanced colorectal cancers is the Mayo/NCCTG regimen.

The high response rates of 40% to 80% for intrahepatic chemotherapy with floxuridine have failed to translate into a statistically significant survival advantage in randomized trials where systemic has been compared with intrahepatic chemotherapy administration.[415] Additionally, toxicity including biliary tract sclerosis, gastric ulceration, and arterial thrombosis has been reported. Because floxuridine is broken down in the liver and systemic levels are subtherapeutic, patients receiving and responding to intra-arterial chemotherapy may progress in extrahepatic sites. The concomitant use of dexamethasone with floxuridine has been reported to decrease toxicity.[416]

Two randomized trials have recently been reported that have identified a survival and quality-of-life advantage for CPT-11 over supportive care alone or retreatment with an additional 5-FU–based regimen in patients with colorectal cancer that is refractory to 5-FU.[417, 418] In one trial, 189 patients were randomized to receive CPT-11, 350 mg/m^2 every 3 weeks, plus supportive care or best supportive care alone.[418] At 1-year, 36% of those who received CPT-11 were alive compared with 14% in the supportive care group. In the other trial, 133 patients were randomized to CPT-11 and 134 to one of several 5-FU plus leucovorin regimens.[417] At 1-year the survival was 45% in the CPT-11 group, and 32% in the 5-FU plus leucovorin groups.

In trials of oxaliplatin for patients with colorectal cancer, response rates of 18% have been reported for previously untreated and 10% for previously treated patients.[419, 420] Oxaliplatin is commonly administered with 5-FU and leucovorin because of preclinical indications of synergy and reports of enhanced clinical activity when the drugs are administered in combination.[421–423] Response rates exceeding 50% have been reported in phase II studies.[422]

Clinical Investigations

Adjuvant—Rectal Cancer

Future trials need to continue to define optimal combinations of chemoradiation (what drugs, route and timing of delivery, sequencing of irradiation and chemotherapy, etc.) and to determine whether some patients can be spared the most aggressive treatment combinations (i.e., limited T3,N0 and T1–2,N1 lesions). There is a need to evaluate which drug(s) and what method of administration should be used during irradiation in order to enhance its effect, and which drugs are necessary to alter systemic patterns of relapse.

The current U.S. intergroup rectal adjuvant study, coordinated by SWOG (INT 0144), was developed to further pursue optimal combinations of postoperative irradiation and chemotherapy. One of the study arms will determine whether the systemic benefit of PVI 5-FU can be enhanced with irradiation. In addition, full-dose preoperative chemoradiation was compared with postoperative chemoradiation for potentially resectable T3 and tethered T4 rectal cancers by NSABP. This trial was designed to test quality-of-life issues in addition to disease control and survival. The NSABP study randomly tested some of the conclusions raised about rectal function in the retrospective Mayo Clinic analysis by Kollmorgen and associates.[382]

Adjuvant—Colon Cancer

Chemotherapy Trials

A number of randomized trials testing alternative chemotherapy for high-risk patients have completed accrual. The final results of the four-arm INT 0089 trial where 3759 patients were randomized to low-dose leucovorin plus 5-FU (Mayo Clinic regimen), high-dose leucovorin plus 5-FU (NSABP regimen), levamisole plus 5-FU, and low-dose leucovorin plus levamisole plus 5-FU are not yet available. Preliminary results were noted in a 1999 review article that indicated 5-year survival rates for patients treated on study ranged from 63% to 67% for the four regimens.[424] Preliminary results have not been made public for the completed NSAPB study CO-5 in which patients were randomized to intravenous 5-FU plus leucovorin or oral UFT (tegafur plus uracil); analysis is expected shortly. The trial of high-dose versus standard-dose levamisole with 5-FU and leucovorin performed by the NCCTG and National Cancer Institute of Canada clinical trials group has completed accrual and will be analyzed in 2001.

Additional adjuvant therapy trials are in progress in the United States, both in the NCI-funded cooperative groups and through industry-sponsored consortia. SWOG is coordinating a trial of 5-FU administered by infusion compared with 5-FU plus leucovorin and levamisole as bolus therapy. The Cancer and Acute Leukemia Group B has a trial in progress of monoclonal antibody 17-1A versus no therapy for stage II patients. In addition, a consortium is randomizing patients to 5-FU and levamisole, with or without monoclonal antibody 17-1A in stage III disease. In Europe, trials are under way using the low-dose leucovorin plus 5-FU Mayo Clinic regimen compared with the de Gramont infusion regimen and, in a separate trial, the German high-dose 5-FU infusion regimen. In the near future, trials of CPT-11 plus 5-FU and leucovorin and oxaliplatin plus 5-FU and leucovorin will be initiated to explore the potential value of those regimens in the adjuvant setting.

Chemoradiation

PHASE III INTERGROUP TRIAL

In view of the high local relapse risks in selected subsets of colon cancer patients,[295, 338, 339] encouraging pilot study results with postoperative irradiation with or without 5-FU for such patients at MGH,[296, 297] and the positive results of 5-FU and levamisole in high-risk adjuvant colon cancer,[342, 383] a U.S. Intergroup randomized trial was conducted comparing 5-FU and levamisole with 5-FU and levamisole plus irradiation (tumor bed with or without regional nodes).[425] Eligible patients felt to be at high risk for local relapse following surgical resection included MAC stage B3, C3 and retroperitoneal C2 lesions (TNM: T4b,N0, T4b,N1–2, T3–4a,N1–2). This protocol did not reach revised accrual objectives of 400 patients (initial accrual goal—700 patients) because 6 months of adjuvant 5-FU plus leucovorin has become the standard of adjuvant chemotherapy for resected high-risk colon cancer patients.[345, 346] Of the 222 randomized patients, 34 were ineligible, leaving 188 eligible for disease control, survival, and tolerance analyses. Initial results showed no difference in either DFS or OS for either arm. This trial should be regarded as inconclusive, rather than definitive, in view of premature closure as a result of inadequate accrual and study limitations. These limitations included the lack of reliable information about the radial surgical margins, surgical clip placement to guide EBRT fields in only 19% of patients, and lack of both clip placement and preoperative imaging in 18% of cases.

FUTURE TRIALS

An alternate treatment approach for patients with adherence to or invasion of other organs or structures (T4b,N0–2; MAC B3 or C3) is preoperative irradiation plus chemotherapy followed by resection (with or without IORT) and maintenance chemotherapy. When imaging studies are not performed preoperatively to select out such patients, the surgeon should be willing to identify them at laparotomy and defer resection. Clips should be placed to identify the extent of disease, a diverting colostomy performed if indicated, and the patient referred for preresection chemoradiation. Randomized trials could test the intensity of the chemoradiation components of treatment or types of chemotherapy.

Locally Advanced Colorectal Cancer

When IOERT-containing trials are compared with standard treatment approaches in separate analyses from MGH and Mayo Clinic, encouraging trends are seen with regard to improvement in local control and possibly survival of patients with locally advanced primary and recurrent colorectal lesions. However, the incidence of systemic failure is 50% or greater, and local failures within the IOERT and EBRT fields still occur, especially when a gross total resection is not surgically feasible. In an attempt to improve local control, it seems reasonable to consistently add PVI 5-FU or bolus 5-FU plus leucovorin or other enhancing or additive agents during EBRT and to evaluate the use of dose modifiers in conjunction with IOERT (sensitizers, hyperthermia, etc.). In view of the high systemic failure rates, clinical trials should evaluate the use of more aggressive chemotherapy during and after external irradiation. Because survival advantages with 5-FU plus leucovorin versus 5-FU alone have been demonstrated in some randomized trials for metastatic disease, this regimen is currently being employed as the maintenance systemic component of treatment. PVI 5-FU as systemic treatment and during EBRT is also a reasonable strategy to evaluate in locally advanced primary or recurrent disease in view of results in the adjuvant setting.

Although it would be of scientific interest to randomly compare standard treatment with or without an IORT electron or brachytherapy boost, such trials were attempted in the United States and could not be completed. Many patients are referred to institutions with IORT or brachytherapy expertise with the expectation of receiving the specialized boost technique and will not consent to randomization. Trials that will be easier to complete in the United States are those in which surgical, external beam, and intraoperative irradiation options with electrons or brachytherapy are standard and the randomization tests optimal chemotherapy during as well as after external irradiation. These trials would allow for testing the presence or absence of radiation sensitizers or dose modifiers during IORT.

Metastatic Colorectal Cancer

Two large intergroup trials investigating a number of therapies for previously untreated patients with metastatic colorectal cancer are just getting under way. ECOG and SWOG are randomizing patients to 5-FU infusion plus leucovorin or to oral 5-FU given with the oral dihydropyrimidine dehydrogenase (DPD) inhibitor 776C85 (5-ethynyluracil, 5-EU). 5-EU irreversibly inhibits DPD and causes oral absorption to be less variable and prolongs the half-life of 5-FU to approximately 4 hours.[426] The NCCTG, Cancer and Acute Leukemia Group B, and National Cancer Institute of Canada are randomizing patients to one of six treatments. The trial has a low-dose leucovorin plus 5-FU Mayo Clinic regimen control arm, two regimens of 5-FU plus leucovorin plus CPT-11, two regimens of 5-FU plus leucovorin plus oxaliplatin, and a regimen of CPT-11 plus oxaliplatin. Phase II trials of a variety of CPT-11 and oxaliplatin plus 5-FU and leucovorin regimens have shown promising activity for these multidrug regimens.[421, 427–429] The combination of CPT-11 plus oxaliplatin has also shown encouraging activity in preliminary trials.[430]

Other oral 5-FU–related agents are in clinical trials. The 5-FU prodrug capecitabine is activated by the enzyme thymidine phosphorylase, which is present in higher concentrations in tumor than in normal cells.[431] This condition leads to the potential to cause selective cytotoxicity in tumor cells. UFT plus oral leucovorin and S-1 are two combinations of tegafur with other agents that have shown activity in colorectal cancer and remain under investigation.[432, 433] Tomudex, a specific thymidylate synthase inhibitor, has been extensively investigated in phase II trials and appears to have little advantage to offer over 5-FU although it is approved for treatment of colorectal cancer in the United Kingdom and Canada.[434] LY 231514, a multitargeted antifol, also has produced tumor shrinkage in patients with colorectal cancer and is undergoing further evaluation in this setting.[435]

Clinical trials looking at noncytotoxic therapy, such as matrix metalloproteinase inhibitors, antiangiogenesis factors, monoclonal antibodies to tumor-related extracellular matrix components, farnesyl transferase inhibitors, and other agents that inhibit tumor unique signaling pathways, are also under investigation.

Anal Carcinoma

Perspective

Organ preservation with radiochemotherapy has become standard treatment for most patients with anal cancer, but questions still exist with regard to treatment optimization. Irradiation, with or without local excision,[436, 437] and irradiation plus chemotherapy[438, 439] have resulted in excellent local control and survival. Further improvements in current standard treatment have the potential to maximize local control and colostomy-free survival and, it is hoped, to improve overall survival. Although surgery is now used infrequently as the primary treatment modality for anal cancer, an understanding of anatomy, pathways of tumor spread, and patterns of relapse after surgery alone are useful in designing and optimizing radiochemotherapy.

Epidemiology and Etiology

Anal carcinomas are relatively rare in comparison with other alimentary tract malignancies. An estimated 3400 cases were expected in the United States in 2000 (1400 male, 2000 female), with an estimated 500 deaths.[2] In most series, the incidence in females exceeds that in males, but male-female ratios in different series vary from 1:1.5 to 1:6. Exact statistics for anal carcinomas are altered because they are frequently included with rectal cancers, and the anatomic nomenclature used varies by series (e.g., definition of anal margin cancers). The average age for most series is between 60 and 65 years, with a broad range of ages between 30 to 85 years.[440]

The exact cause of anal carcinoma is uncertain. It has been associated with a variety of chronic anorectal conditions, such as condylomata (human papillomavirus), fistulas, fissures, leucoplakia, and Bowen's disease. An association with certain genital infections and cigarette smoking also exists. The incidence of anal cancer is higher in homosexual versus heterosexual males, irrespective of human immunodeficiency virus status.[441] Anal cancer is also much more common in both men and women with acquired immunodeficiency syndrome, with an absolute risk of 1:1000. Human papillomavirus (HPV) is a suspected sexually transmitted agent in anal cancer; the average age of patients with HPV-associated anal cancer is 10 years younger than HPV-negative patients. Although the exact role of HPV in anal carcinogenesis is unknown, HPV E6 and E7 proteins have been implicated in laboratory evaluations. The incidence of anal cancer is also high in transplant patients with chronic immunosuppression; this finding suggests that immunodeficiency may play a role.[442]

Detection and Diagnosis

Clinical Detection

The symptoms that usually lead to the detection of anal carcinoma include GI bleeding (50%), rectal pain (20% to 40%), or a palpable mass (25%). Other potential symptoms include pressure sensation, change in bowel habits, rectal discharge or tenesmus.[442, 443]

Diagnostic Procedures

- *Physical examination* with digital anorectal examination and bimanual vaginal examination in females will confirm the presence of an anal margin or anal canal cancer and whether rectal or vaginal involvement is suspected. The presence of hepatomegaly or enlarged inguinal nodes is a sign of metastatic disease.
- *Proctoscopic examination* and *biopsy* will confirm the diagnosis, clinically stage the extent of local disease and exclude a second proximal lesion.
- *Barium enema* or *colonoscopy* should be performed to rule out another cause of lower GI bleeding.
- *Transluminal ultrasound* is felt by some to be of minimal value with lesions below the dentate line, but others note that by using a hard plastic applicator, depth of anal invasion can be discerned.[444] For lesions extending into the rectum, transrectal ultrasound can help determine depth of penetration of the rectal wall.
- *Laboratory evaluation* should include CBC, creatinine, and liver function studies (suspicion for liver metastasis).
- *CT scan* of the *pelvis* and *abdomen* provides evidence for or against local extension into prostate, bladder, uterus, or vagina. It also helps to define nodal status (inguinal, iliac, para-aortic) and to rule out liver metastases.
- *Chest film* is used to rule out lung metastases.

Classification and Staging

Histopathology

The two predominant histologic types of anal carcinomas are both variants of squamous cell carcinoma: squamous cell (epidermoid), and basaloid (cloacogenic, transitional). Less common histologic types include mucoepidermoid, adenocarcinoma, small cell, and undifferentiated carcinoma. The squamous histology predominates in most series (≥70%) with the basaloid type comprising nearly 30%. Malignant lymphoma, melanoma, and sarcoma may also occur as rare primary malignancies of the anus. Perianal tumors other than the squamous variety include extramammary Paget's, Bowen's disease, and basal cell carcinoma.[445]

Anatomy and Pathways of Spread

For evaluation of both tumor spread and ultimate prognosis, anal cancers are commonly divided into those of the anal canal (extending from rectum to perianal skin) versus the perineal aspect of the anus (also known as anal margin). Anal margin lesions (distal to the anal verge where the hair-bearing skin begins) should be staged and treated as skin cancers. Anal canal lesions more frequently exhibit local invasion of adjacent perianal tissues and can also involve the sphincter muscles or adjacent organs.

Lymphatics of the anal canal drain either to the superficial inguinal nodes or to nodes of the low rectum (perirectal, internal iliac, and inferior mesenteric). Lesions on the anal margin drain primarily to the superficial inguinal nodes. Perirectal or inferior mesenteric node involvement at the time of initial resection has varied from 28% to 64% and inguinal node involvement from 13% to 25%. In a Mayo Clinic analysis by Boman and coworkers,[445] the incidence of nodal involvement at diagnosis was 30% or greater with lesion size larger than 2 cm independent of histology, and with grades 3 or 4 nonkeratinizing basaloid tumors of any size.

Staging

T stage for T1–3 lesions is based on size (≤2 cm, >2 cm but ≤5 cm, >5 cm), but T4 lesions are those that invade adjacent organs, independent of size (Table 27–34; Fig.

TABLE 27–34. **TNM Classification—Anal Canal**

Stage	Grouping	TNM Descriptor
0	Tis, N0, M0	Tis: Carcinoma *in situ* N0: No regional lymph node metastasis M0: No distant metastasis
I	T1, N0, M0	T1: Tumor ≤2 cm in greatest dimension
II	T2, N0, M0	T2: Tumor >2 cm, but ≤5 cm in greatest dimension
	T3, N0, M0	T3: Tumor >5 cm
IIIA	T1–3, N1, M0	N1: Metastasis in perirectal lymph node(s)
	T4, N0, M0	T4: Tumor of any size invades adjacent organ(s)*
IIIB	T4, N1, M0; Any T, N2–3, M0	N2: Metastasis in unilateral internal iliac and/or inguinal lymph node(s) N3: Metastasis in perirectal and inguinal lymph nodes and/or bilateral internal iliac and/or inguinal lymph nodes
IV	Any T, Any N, M1	M1: Distant metastasis present

T = tumor; N = node; M = metastases.

*Adjacent organs include vagina, urethra, bladder; involvement of the sphincter muscle(s) is not classified as T4.

Used with permission of the American Joint Committee on Cancer (AJCC®), Chicago, Illinois. The original source for this material is the AJCC® Cancer Staging Manual, 5th ed, 1997, published by Lippincott-Raven Publishers, Philadelphia, Pennsylvania.

27–16).[5] The staging system applies to all anal canal carcinomas but not melanoma or sarcoma.

The usual staging work-up is accomplished with a thorough history and physical examination (anorectal examination and nodal palpation) complemented by laboratory and imaging studies:

- Careful *anorectal/vaginal examination* and *proctosigmoidoscopy* with appropriate biopsies.
- *Inguinal nodes*—if palpable, perform a fine-needle aspirate and a biopsy only if aspirate is negative.
- *Blood tests*: CBC, creatinine, and liver function studies (bilirubin, alkaline phosphatase, lactate dehydrogenase, serum glutamate oxaloacetate transaminase).
- *Chest x-ray.*
- *CT scan* of abdomen and pelvis searching for metastatic inguinal, pelvic, or para-aortic nodes or liver metastases.

Principles of Treatment

Surgery

For most patients with anal cancer, surgical removal with APR has been replaced by chemoradiation as the standard of care (Table 27–35). APR is usually reserved for salvage of the 15% to 20% of lesions that fail to respond completely to chemoradiation or those with incontinence due to sphincter invasion. In the rare patient where irradiation with or without chemotherapy may be contraindicated (pelvic irradiation for prior pelvic malignancy), APR would be excellent primary treatment. Local excision alone also is an excellent treatment option for anal margin cancers and selected early cancers of the anal canal that are limited to the mucosa or submucosa. The main technical issue with local excision is to maintain sphincter preservation, thus avoiding fecal incontinence.

Patterns of Relapse—Surgery Alone

Although APR has been replaced with irradiation plus chemotherapy as the standard of care for most anal cancers, some excellent data exist on patterns of relapse after surgery alone. In a Mayo analysis by Boman and coworkers,[445] local-regional relapse was shown to be the predominant relapse pattern in 106 evaluable patients with APR. Of the 38 evaluable patients who relapsed, 84% had a local-regional component of failure, and 29% had a distant component. The risk of local relapse was related to the degree of local invasion and nodal involvement. Fifteen of 38 patients (39%) with relapse had an inguinal node component. In seven patients who had inguinal node dissection for clinically apparent involvement at the time of abdominoperineal resection, the 5-year relapse-free survival was 71% (5 of 7).

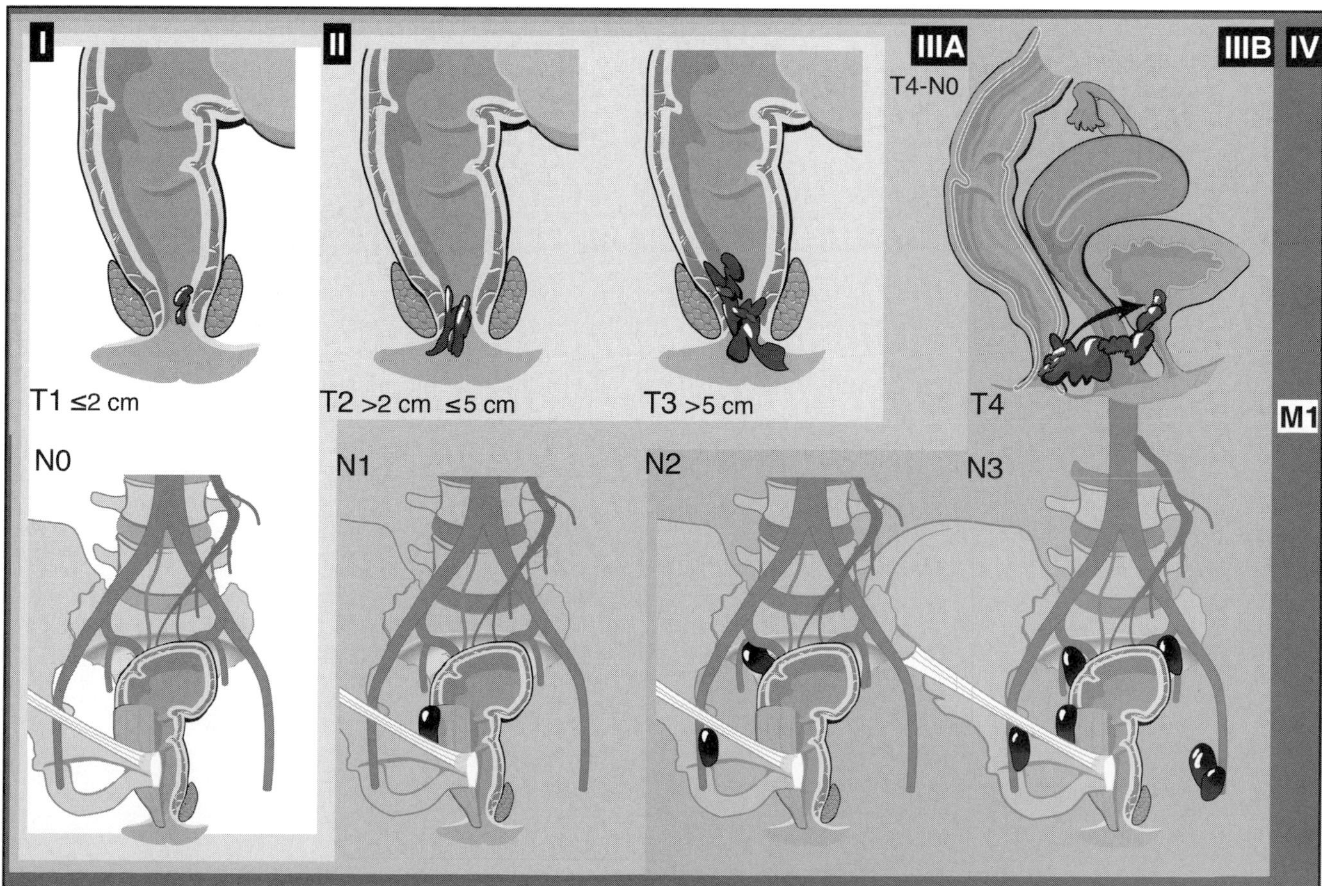

Figure 27–16. Anatomic staging for cancer of the anus.

TABLE 27–35. **Multidisciplinary Treatment Decisions: Anus**

Stage	Radiation		Chemotherapy	Surgery
I–III	RT-C† 50–60 Gy	plus	CCRT	NR*
IV	RT-P 50 Gy		CCRT	NR

RT-C = curative irradiation; RT-P = palliative irradiation; NR = not recommended; CCRT = concurrent chemotherapy and irradiation.
*NR, not recommended unless chemoradiation response is less than complete response or with limited Stage I lesion (amenable to local excision).
†RT-C plus CCR-5-fluorouracil + mitomycin C. From Physicians' Data Query. Anal cancer. Bethesda, National Cancer Institute, July 1999.

Irradiation Versus Chemoradiation

Anal carcinomas are radioresponsive, and local tumor eradication can be achieved with irradiation alone (Table 27–36). However, both local tumor control and colostomy-free survival are better with concurrent chemoradiation (Table 27–37).[457, 458] Definitive irradiation for anal cancers was initially rejected as an alternative to APR because the perianal skin and mucocutaneous juncture were sensitive to irradiation. Severe reactions commonly occurred in the orthovoltage era.

Most combined-modality treatment schedules used in practice today were derived from the Wayne State regimen combining EBRT with 5-FU plus mitomycin C.[459] In the initial series, patients received 30 Gy in 15 fractions over 3 weeks as planned preoperative treatment before combined abdominoperineal resection. In view of unexpected pathologic CRs in an initial group of 12 patients, 16 subsequent patients had local excisions or biopsy only after similar doses of EBRT plus 5-FU and mitomycin C.

Local Control Versus Irradiation Dose, Field Design, and Fractionation

Separate analyses by investigators from PMH,[438, 446] RTOG,[439] University of Kansas,[460] M.D. Anderson,[461] and MGH[462] support the need to evaluate both irradiation dose as well as type and duration of chemotherapy in an attempt to improve both local control and systemic control of disease. The pelvic failure rates (anal primary or pelvic and inguinal nodes, or both) in the preceding series range from 20% to 30% at dose levels of approximately 40 to 50 Gy plus chemotherapy (1.8- to 2.0-Gy fractions in the U.S. analyses and 2.0–2.5 Gy in the PMH trial). In the PMH analysis, the most optimal combination of irradiation plus 5-FU plus mitomycin C still resulted in a 19% pelvic failure rate (13 of 69 patients) and 17% systemic relapse rate (12 of 69) (Table 27–38). A nodal component of failure was found in 5 of 69 patients (7%), a percentage that may be falsely low because intrapelvic node relapse is difficult to diagnose without reoperation or autopsy. In the RTOG trial 83-14, in which irradiation to 40.8 Gy was combined with 5-FU plus mitomycin C, the 3-year colostomy-free survival was 63%.[439] Pelvic recurrence occurred in 24 of 77 patients (5-year actuarial rate of 32%) and systemic relapse in 12 of 77 patients (5-year actuarial rate of 19%).

Primary tumor control may increase as a function of irradiation dose level. In pooled data on 57 patients from five Kansas City institutions, 77% of patients received chemotherapy with irradiation—5-FU.[451] Local control was achieved in 81%; all local failures occurred within 1.5 years of treatment and salvage was achieved in 8 of 11 for an eventual local control rate of 95%. The local control rate by irradiation dose level was as follows: 45 Gy or less, 64%; 45 to 55 Gy, 72%, and greater than 55 Gy, 92% ($p = 0.05$). On the basis of Cox multivariate analysis, the EBRT dose of greater than 55 Gy was the only variable associated with improved local control. In a separate analysis from MGH, both local control and survival appeared to increase as a function of irradiation dose of 54 Gy or greater versus less than 54 Gy.[462] Doses of 54 Gy or greater were associated with improved local control and 5-year OS and DFS. In a multivariate analysis, dose independently affected all three parameters ($p = 0.02, 0.01, 0.02$).

As higher doses of irradiation are used in aggressive concurrent radiochemotherapy regimens, a clinical issue that arises is whether to utilize a planned treatment interruption at a particular EBRT dose level versus as clinically indicated. In the sequential regimens used at PMH, investigators initially combined EBRT with 5-FU and mitomycin C without a planned break, but found an excessive incidence of acute and chronic perineal reactions.[438, 446] In their

TABLE 27–36. **Local Control and Survival with Radiation Alone—Anal Canal**

Study	N	Tumor Size	5-Year Overall Survival Rate (%)	Local Control (%)	Radiation Dose (Gy)
Doggett[436]	35	1.3–4.5 cm	92	77	45–76
Martenson and Gunderson[437]	18	T1–2 in 17 of 18	94 (5 yr)	100% (5 yr)	47–67
			86 (7 yr)	90% (7 yr)	
Cummings[438, 446]	25	—	75	56	45–60
Eschwege[447]	33	T1–2	72	91	60–65
	31	T3–4	35	71	
Dobrowsky[448]	23	—	65	83	45–70
Newman[449]	72	—	78	—	50 Gy/20 Fx
Svensson[450]	78	—	74	70	66–68
Schlienger[440]	193	—	70	76	60–65

N = number of patients; Fx = fraction.

TABLE 27–37. **Local Control and Survival—EBRT plus 5-FU plus Mitomycin C—Anal Canal**

Reference	N	Tumor Size	Total Dose (Gy)	Local Control (%)	Survival (%)
Sischy[439]	79	<3 cm	41	84	85 (3 yr)
		>3 cm		62	68 (3 yr)
Leichman[451]	45	—	30	84	76 (50 mo median)
Flam[452]	30	—	41–50	97	58 (6–90 mo)
Tveit[453]	24*	—	50	83	58 (40–70 mo)
Flam[454, 455] (RTOG Phase III)	146	—	45–50	71†	78‡ (4 yr)
	145		45–50	59†	71‡ (4 yr)
Martenson[456]	50	—	50–53	80	58 (7 yr)

N = number.
*Includes 3 patients with distant metastasis before treatment began.
†Colostomy-free survival was statistically different between the two groups with an advantage to external beam irradiation (EBRT) plus 5-fluorouracil (5-FU) and mitomycin C vs. those with EBRT and 5-FU.
‡Not statistically significant.

subsequent EBRT plus 5-FU—mitomycin C regimen, a 4- to 6-week break was utilized. Although primary tumor control was equivalent at 87% versus 85%, nodal relapse was 0% versus 9% and total pelvic relapse rates were 13% (non–split-course irradiation) versus 21% (split-course irradiation). Some additional data on the potential of increased local relapse with planned split-course irradiation is found in the section on "Clinical Investigations."

Irradiation field design has a probable impact on nodal control. In early trials by Papillon and associates, no attempt was made to include pelvic nodes, and the incidence of documented nodal relapse was 24%.[463] This incidence was reduced to 3.6% after fields were appropriately altered to include pelvic nodes. Elective inguinal irradiation appears to decrease the risk of subsequent inguinal failure (risk of 11% to 24% without irradiation versus 0% to 5% with irradiation). In the PMH analysis by Cummings and coworkers,[446] the risk was 18% without versus 3% with elective inguinal EBRT, and in Papillon's series was 13% versus 0%.

Irradiation Field Design

Currently most single-institution and group studies design irradiation fields to include the primary lesion as well as major nodal groups (inguinal and pelvic). The initial large field is carried to 30 to 36 Gy in 1.8- to 2.0-Gy fractions when irradiation is combined with concomitant chemotherapy, or 45 Gy in 25 fractions for schemas employing irradiation alone. A majority of investigators utilize parallel-opposed fields to those dose levels, with the superior field extent varying by series from the level of the sacral promontory to the bottom of the sacroiliac joint (Fig. 27–17). If the superior field extent is at the sacral promontory level and a nodal dose of 45 Gy is planned, lateral fields could be considered as a component of treatment in order to reduce dose to the small bowel. When the superior field extent is at the bottom of the sacroiliac joint, lateral fields would be of little value except for boost field irradiation to the primary lesion.

In patients with uninvolved nodes who are treated with irradiation plus 5-FU plus mitomycin C, the nodal groups are excluded above a dose of 30 to 36 Gy (Fig. 27–18; see Fig. 27–17). The primary lesion plus a 2- to 2.5-cm margin is then carried to a higher dose with multifield techniques, including lateral fields. Lymphangiograms (LAGs) can be useful in designing the nodal portion of shaped fields for both AP-PA and lateral fields (see Fig. 27–18). In order to decrease dose to the femoral head and neck, inguinal nodes can be excluded from the PA field and an anterior electron boost can be used to supplement the dose delivered to those nodes with the anterior photon field. As shown in Figure 27–18C–E, use is made of a LAG-altered field design in a particular patient. The decision was made to

TABLE 27–38. **Cancer of the Anus: Survival and Patterns of Relapse with Irradiation ± Chemotherapy (PMH)**

Treatment	Primary *n*	Primary %	Nodal *n*	Nodal %	Distant *n*	Distant %	Total *n*	Total %	5-Year Survival, % (Cause-Specific)	
Continuous EBRT										
EBRT	25	44	11	19	10	18	28/57	49	68	} p = 0.14
EBRT, 5-FU, mito-C	2	13	0	—	1	6	3/16	19	} 76	
Split-Course EBRT										
EBRT, 5-FU, mito-C	8*	15	5*	9	11	21	17/53	32		} p = 0.02
EBRT, 5-FU	26	40	5	8	8	12	31/65	48	64	

EBRT = External beam irradiation; 5-FU = 5-fluorouracil; mito-C = mitomycin C; n = number; PMH = Princess Margaret Hospital.
*11/53 or 21% had pelvic failure (primary or nodal).
Modified from Cummings BJ, Keane TJ, O'Sullivan MB, et al: Epidermoid anal cancer: Treatment by radiation alone or by radiation and 5-fluorouracil with and without mitomycin C. Int J Radiat Oncol Biol Phys 1991; 21:1115–1125.

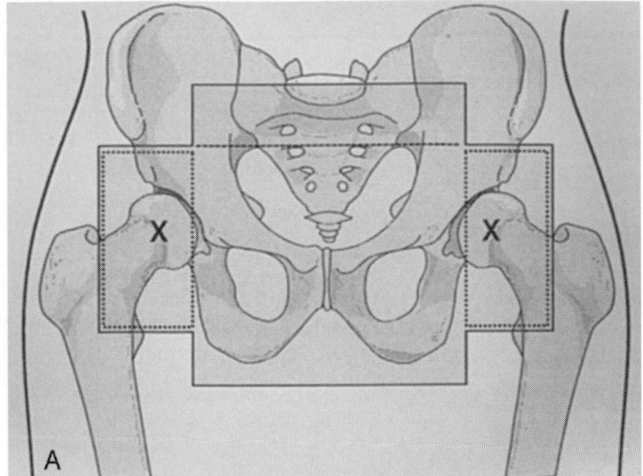

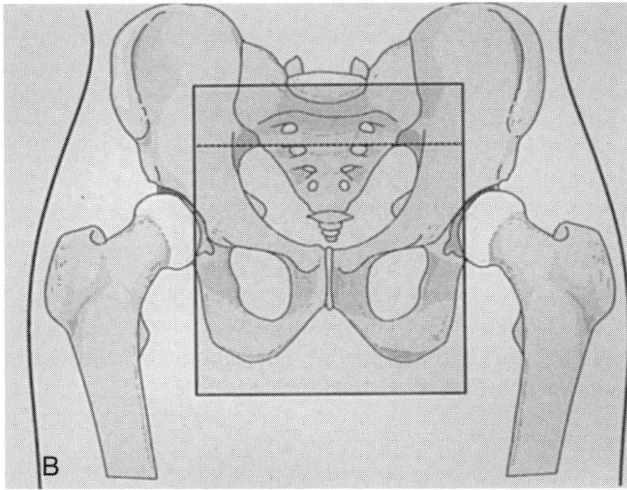

Figure 27–17. Idealized AP-PA irradiation fields for primary anal cancer. (A) Anteroposterior (AP) field includes primary tumor plus pelvic and inguinal nodes. Lateral inguinal nodes are brought to prescribed dose with the aid of electron boost fields *(interrupted lines)*. (B) Posteroanterior (PA) field includes primary tumor plus pelvic nodes and medial inguinal nodes. Copyright © Mayo Foundation.

minimally alter the PA field to include all inguinal nodes instead of using an anterior electron boost. The LAG also demonstrated an involved right common iliac node that altered boost field design and may have altered initial field design in some institutions.

Chemotherapy

As a general rule, distant metastases occur less frequently with anal carcinomas when compared with other GI carcinomas. An exception is the subset of patients with small cell cancers. The most active multidrug regimens for squamous variants include 5-FU plus cisplatin[463–465] and 5-FU plus mitomycin C.

Special Considerations of Treatment

Surgery as Salvage Treatment or for Incontinence

APR with colostomy is utilized after chemoradiation in patients with persistent fecal incontinence, persistent tumor, or local relapse. Fecal incontinence is often not a result of the chemoradiation; it is usually preexistent in patients with massive tumors that have sphincter invasion with resultant destruction or anal sphincter weakness. Even if lesions resolve nicely with chemoradiation, the sphincter may remain incompetent.

Surgery is more commonly used as salvage treatment in patients in whom complete regression does not occur with chemoradiation or in whom local relapse occurs after complete regression.[466] This finding exists in 15% to 25% of all patients treated with chemoradiation and up to 30% to 40% of those with T3 to T4 lesions. Therefore, patients should be followed closely during years 1 and 2 after chemoradiation so that local relapse is diagnosed early, whereas APR still has curative potential.

A common evaluation routine after treatment has been completed is to follow the patient monthly until a complete clinical regression has occurred, at 3-month intervals for 2 years, every 6 months to 5 years, then annually to year 8 or 10. The most important components of evaluation are anorectal examination (digital and scope) and inguinal node examination complemented with periodic chest film, labs, and pelvis plus abdomen CT scan. Multidisciplinary follow-up with a high degree of continuity is key to the early recognition of persistent or recurrent disease especially as it pertains to differentiating it from treatment related changes (induration, fibrosis).

Results and Prognosis

Surgery Alone

The general survival for anal cancers of all stages treated surgically with an APR and colostomy has been in the range of 50% to 70% at 5 years. For select early lesions of the anal canal, local excision can yield local control and 5-year survival in 90% or greater of patients.[445]

Radiation Alone

Treatment with irradiation alone to doses of 45 to 76 Gy in 4.5 to 8 weeks (usually >60 Gy) yielded excellent local control and survival in a series reported by Doggett and associates.[436] In 35 patients with lesion size of 1.3 to 4.5 cm, 5-year survival was 92% and a local control rate of 77% was reported. In a select series of 18 patients reported by Martenson and Gunderson from Mayo Clinic, similar results were achieved.[437] With a minimum follow-up of 2.5 years, 5-year actuarial local control and survival were 100% and 94%, respectively.

Local control and survival with irradiation alone were less optimal in a series from PMH reported by Cummings and coworkers in which larger as well as smaller lesions were treated[438, 446] (see Tables 27–35 and 27–37). In the 57 patients treated with irradiation alone, relapse at the primary site occurred in 25 patients (44%), with nodal relapse in 11 (19%). Five-year cause-specific survival was 68%.

In the largest published series using irradiation alone (60–65 Gy), Schlienger and associates reported results in 193 patients.[440] Local control was achieved in 76% of patients and 5-year overall survival was 70%.

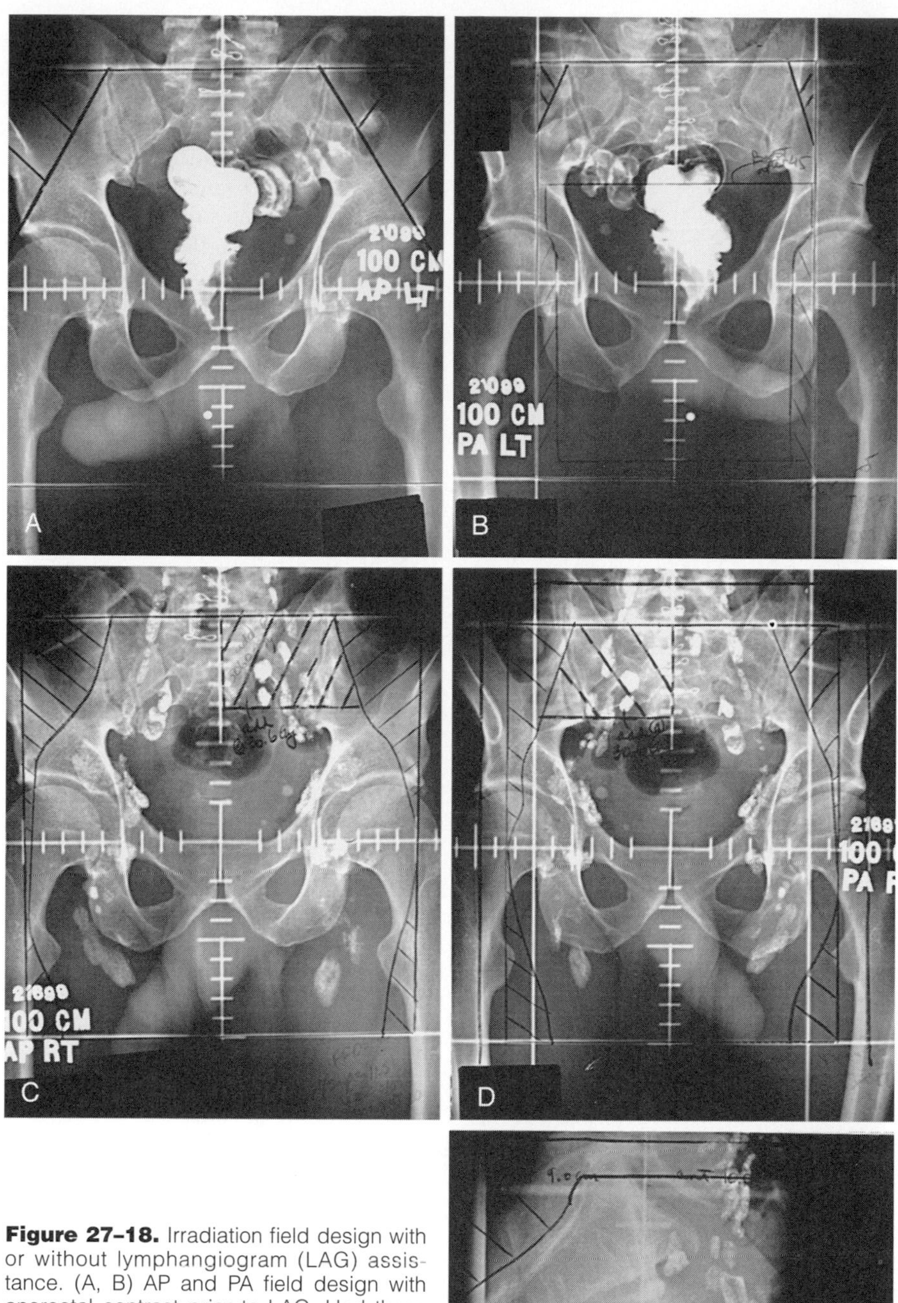

Figure 27-18. Irradiation field design with or without lymphangiogram (LAG) assistance. (A, B) AP and PA field design with anorectal contrast prior to LAG. Had these fields been maintained, an AP electron field would have been designed to supplement lateral inguinal dose (see Fig. 27-17A). (C-E) Modification of AP and PA fields and development of lateral field after LAG to demonstrate actual location of nodes. Note filling defect approximately 1.0 cm in diameter in right common iliac node at the inferior level of the sacroiliac (SI) joint (would have bisected involved node in institutions that design fields with superior field extent at the bottom of the SI joint). The involved node was kept within boost field #1 to the level of 45 Gy in 25 fractions (block added to left common iliac region after 30.6 Gy).

Chemoradiation

Chemoradiation has been used with increasing frequency and success since being introduced by Nigro.[459] Generally, the combination of 5-FU and mitomycin C or the combination of 5-FU plus cisplatin has been used concurrently with irradiation. The irradiation dose has been increased from the 30-Gy level used in the initial Nigro studies to doses of 45 to 50 Gy or greater. A pilot study was carried out by RTOG using an EBRT dose of 40.8 Gy in 24 fractions plus 5-FU plus mitomycin C (RTOG 83-14). In a preliminary report of 79 patients by Sischy and associates,[439] local control appeared to be better with lesion sizes of less than 3 cm versus 3 cm or greater (local relapse in 4 of 26 patients with lesion sizes <3 cm versus 18 of 50 with lesions ≥3 cm). Three-year actuarial survival trends were also better in smaller lesions at 85% versus 68%.

EBRT plus or minus 5-FU or 5-FU–Mitomycin

In a 1984 PMH report by Cummings and coworkers,[438] the colostomy-free survival rates with EBRT plus 5-FU–mitomycin appeared to be superior to those achieved with EBRT alone, but overall 3- to 5-year survival rates were similar. In a 1991 update,[446] the combination of EBRT plus 5-FU and mitomycin C appeared to achieve improved local control when compared with results achieved with EBRT alone or EBRT plus 5-FU (see Table 27–38). Cause-specific survival at 5 years also favored the EBRT plus 5-FU–mitomycin C combination. In view of the nonrandomized nature of the PMH series, differences in local control and survival could have been a reflection of patient selection and disease factors rather than a result of treatment regimens.

The relative efficacy of EBRT alone versus EBRT plus 5-FU–mitomycin C has been addressed in separate randomized trials performed by both EORTC[458] and British investigators.[457] The EORTC reported an increased CR rate of 80% versus 54%, which resulted in an advantage in local control ($p = 0.02$) and colostomy-free survival ($p = 0.002$) for the radiochemotherapy arm.[458] Overall survival was similar in the two treatment arms. In the British trial of 585 patients,[457] the radiochemotherapy arm was also superior to irradiation alone with regard to 3-year local control ($p < 0.0001$) and cause-specific survival ($p = 0.02$). Absolute rates of local failure were 36% versus 59%. Overall survival was not statistically better in the radiochemotherapy patients, although suggestive trends exist (3-year survival of 65% vs. 58%).

A randomized trial coordinated by RTOG (RTOG 87-04) addressed the question of EBRT plus 5-FU versus EBRT plus 5-FU–mitomycin C (see Tables 27–34 and 27–36). Interim results were reported at the American Society of Clinical Oncology in 1993[454] and updated in 1995[455] and 1998.[467] The 5-FU–mitomycin C radiochemotherapy arm had statistically significant advantages over EBRT plus 5-FU with regard to local control, rate of colostomy, and DFS (Table 27–39). Overall 5-year survival rates were equivalent at 67% versus 65% (univariate value of $p = 0.41$).

Differences in DFS do not necessarily translate into improved overall survival in the treatment of anal cancers. As discussed previously, local relapse can be potentially salvaged with combined APR if diagnosed early as a function of close follow-up evaluation.

Clinical Investigations

An intergroup U.S. study was initially designed to test in a 2 × 2 fashion the separate questions of irradiation dose (45 vs. 59.4 Gy) and type of concurrent chemotherapy (5-FU plus mitomycin C versus 5-FU plus cisplatin). The rationale for testing 5-FU plus cisplatin is based on excellent response rates achieved in patients with locally recurrent or metastatic anal cancer.

The tolerance of the higher EBRT doses of 59.4 Gy plus concurrent two-drug chemotherapy was tested in separate phase II studies conducted by RTOG (EBRT plus 5-FU and mitomycin C, RTOG 9208) and ECOG (EBRT plus 5-FU and cisplatin) in a planned, coordinated fashion.[456, 467] A planned 2-week treatment interruption after 36 Gy and one cycle of chemotherapy was used in the initial component of both pilot studies in an attempt to improve tolerance at the higher EBRT dose (use of a planned interruption was based on the prior experience of PMH[438, 446] and the need for periodic treatment interruptions in the earlier RTOG 87-04 study).[455] Although satisfactory tolerance was achieved in both pilot studies, the incidence of colostomy in the RTOG 92-08 pilot exceeded that seen in the earlier RTOG 87-04 phase III trial using doses of 45 to 50.4 Gy plus 5-FU plus mitomycin C.[455, 467] Although this difference

TABLE 27–39. **Anal Cancer: Disease Control and Survival with EBRT plus 5-FU Versus EBRT plus 5-FU and Mitomycin C—RTOG 87-04 Phase III Trial**

	Estimated 5-Yr Rates (%)		P Value	
End Point	***5-FU***	***5-FU + MMC***	***Univariate***	***Multivariate***
Positive postinduction biopsy	15	8	.062	.13
Local regional failure	36	17	.0005	.0014
Colostomy	22	11	.009	.019
Colostomy-free survival	58	64	.092	.17
NED survival	50	67	.0025	.006
Overall survival	65	67	.41	.7

EBRT = External beam irradiation; 5-FU = 5-fluorouracil; MMC = mitomycin C; RTOG = Radiation Therapy Oncology Group; NED = no evidence of disease.

Data from Flam et al.[454, 455, 467]

may have been due to patient selection factors (i.e., physicians may place only higher risk patients on a higher dose pilot study), both the RTOG and ECOG pilots were reopened for additional patient accrual. The automatic 2-week treatment interruption was deleted and an optional interruption was inserted. Accrual was completed in both pilot studies, which demonstrated that high-dose radiochemotherapy can be completed with an optional rather than planned interruption.[468]

Of note, in view of the large patient numbers required for a 2 × 2 design, the U.S. intergroup study was redesigned as a two-arm study testing the method of chemotherapy only. This study was opened for accrual in 1998.

REFERENCES

General

1. Strauss MB: Familiar Medical Quotations. Boston, Little, Brown and Co., 1968.
2. Greenlee RT, Murray T, Bolden S, et al: Cancer statistics, 2000. CA Cancer J Clin 2000; 50:7–33.
3. Parkin DM, Pisani P, Ferlay J: Global cancer statistics. CA Cancer J Clin 1999; 48:33–64.
4. Bragg DG, Rubin P, Hricak H (eds): Oncologic Imaging, 2nd ed. Philadelphia, W.B. Saunders Co., 2001.
5. Fleming ID, Cooper JS, Henson DE, et al: AJCC Staging Manual, 5th ed. Philadelphia, J.B. Lippincott-Raven, 1997.
6. Gunderson LL, Martenson JA, Smalley SR, et al: Upper gastrointestinal cancers: rationale, results, and techniques of treatment. Front Radiat Ther Oncol 1994; 28:121–139.
7. Gunderson LL, Haddock MG, Foo M: Role of radiation therapy in the management of upper gastrointestinal cancers. Curr Radiat Oncol 1997; 3:177–202.
8. Gunderson LL, Martenson JA, Smalley SR, et al: Lower gastrointestinal cancers: rationale, results, and techniques of treatment. Front Radiat Ther Oncol 1994; 28:140–154.
9. Gunderson LL, Martenson JA: Gastrointestinal tract radiation tolerance. Front Radiat Ther Oncol 1989; 23:277–298.
10. Gunderson LL, Martenson JA, Smalley SR: Gastrointestinal tract tolerance with irradiation ± chemotherapy. In: John M, Flam M, Legha S, Phillips T (eds): Chemoradiation: An Integrated Approach to Cancer Treatment, pp 430–444. Philadelphia, Lea & Febiger, 1993.

Specific

Esophagus

11. Herskovic A, Martz K, Al-Saraf M, et al: Combined chemotherapy and radiotherapy compared with radiotherapy alone in patients with cancer of the esophagus. N Engl J Med 1992; 326:1593–1598.
12. Al-Saraf M, Martz K, Herkovic A, et al: Progress report of combined chemo-radiotherapy vs radiotherapy alone in patients with esophageal cancer: an intergroup study. J Clin Oncol 1997; 15:277–284.
13. Broitman SA, Vitale JJ, Gottlief LS: Ethanolic beverage consumption, cigarette smoking, nutritional status and digestive tract cancers. Semin Oncol 1983; 10:322–329.
14. Schottenfeld D: Epidemiology of cancer of the esophagus. Semin Oncol 1984; 11:92–100.
15. Munoz N, Day N: Esophageal cancer. In: Schottenfeld D, Frammeni JF (eds): Cancer Epidemiology and Prevention, 2nd ed. New York, Oxford University Press, 1996.
16. Rubio CA, Fu-Sheng L: Spontaneous squamous carcinoma of the esophagus in chickens. Cancer 1989; 64:2511–2514.
17. Appelquist P, Salmo M: Lye corrosion carcinoma of the esophagus. Cancer 1980; 45:2655–2658.
18. Camerson AJ, Oh BJ, Payne WS: The incidence of adenocarcinoma in columnar-lined (Barrett's) esophagus. N Engl J Med 1985; 313:857–859.
19. Kuster GG, Foroozan P: Early diagnosis of adenocarcinoma developing in Barrett's esophagus. Arch Surg 1989; 124:925–927.
20. Sjogren RW, Johnson LF: Barrett's esophagus: a review. Am J Med 1983; 74:313–321.
21. DeMeester TR, Barlow AP: Surgery and current management for cancer of the esophagus and cardia. Curr Prob Cancer 1988; 12:243–327.
22. Lightdale DJ, Winawe SJ: Screening diagnosis and staging of esophageal cancer. Semin Oncol 1984; 11:101–112.
23. McFarlane SD, Ilver R: Carcinoma of the esophagus. In: Hill L, Kozarek R, McCallum R, et al (eds): The Esophagus, Medical and Surgical Management, pp 237–256. Philadelphia, W.B. Saunders Co., 1988.
24. McLean AM, Reznek RH: Radiologic diagnosis and assessment. In: Hurt RL (ed): Management of Oesophageal Carcinoma, pp 69–101. London, Springer-Verlag, 1989.
25. Thompson WM: Esophageal cancer. In: Bragg DG, Rubin P, Youker JE (eds): Oncologic Imaging, pp 207–242. Elmsford, NY, Pergamon Press, 1985.
26. Murata Y, Muroi M, Yoshida M, et al: Endoscopic ultrasound in the diagnosis of esophageal carcinoma. Surg Endosc 1986; 1:11.
27. Tio TL, Cohen P, Coene PP, et al: Endosonography and computed tomography of esophageal carcinoma: preoperative classification compared to new (1987) TNM system. Gastroenterology 1989; 96:1478–1486.
28. Inculet TI, Keller SM, Dwyer A, et al: Evaluation of noninvasive tests for the preoperative staging of carcinoma of the esophagus: a preoperative study. Ann Thorac Surg 1985; 40:561–565.
29. Hesketh PJ, Clapp RW, Doos WG, et al: The increasing frequency of adenocarcinoma of the esophagus. Cancer 1989; 64:526–530.
30. Blot WJ, Devera SS, Kneller RW, et al: Rising incidence of adenocarcinoma of the esophagus and gastric cardia. JAMA 1991; 265:1287–1289.
31. Guernsey JM, Knudsen DF, Mark JB: Abdominal exploration in the evaluation of patients with carcinoma of the thoracic esophagus. J Thorac Cardiovasc Surg 1970; 59:62–66.
32. Akiyama H, Tsurumara M, Kawamura T, et al: Principles of surgical treatment for carcinoma of the esophagus. Ann Surg 1981; 194:438–446.
33. King RM, Pairolero PC, Trastek VF, et al: Ivor-Lewis esophagogastrectomy for carcinoma of the esophagus: early and late functional results. Ann Thorac Surg 1987; 44:119–122.
34. Quint LE, Glazer GM, Orringer MB: Esophageal imaging by MR and CT: Study of normal anatomy and neoplasms. Radiology 1985; 156:727–731.
35. Demeester TR, Lafontaine ER: Surgical therapy. In: Demeester TR, Levin B (eds): Cancer of the Esophagus, pp 141–197. New York, Grune and Stratton, 1985.
36. Flores AD, Nelems B, Evans K, et al: Impact of new radiotherapy modalities on the surgical management of cancer of the esophagus and cardia. Int J Radiat Oncol Biol Phys 1986; 17:482–487.
37. Earlam R, Cunha-Melo JR: Oesophageal squamous cell carcinoma: I. A critical review of surgery. Br J Surg 1980; 67:381–390.
38. Maillet P, Baulieux J, Boulez J, et al: Carcinoma of the thoracic esophagus: Results of one-stage surgery (271 cases). Am J Surg 1982; 143:629–634.
39. DeMeester TR: Carcinoma of the esophagus (Part I & II). Curr Prob Surg 1988; 25:477–605.
40. Orringer MB: Surgical therapy for esophageal carcinoma. In: Sawyers JL, Williams LF (eds): Difficult Problems in General Surgery, pp 21–42. Chicago, Year Book Medical Publishers Inc., 1989.
41. Pearson JG: The value of radiotherapy in the management of esophageal cancer. Am J Roentgenol 1969; 105:500–513.
42. Pearson JG: The present status and future potential of radiotherapy in the management of esophageal cancer. Cancer 1977; 39:882–890.
43. Beatty JD, DeBoer G, Rider WD: Carcinoma of the esophagus—pretreatment assessment, correlation of radiation treatment parameters with survival and identification and management of radiation treatment failure. Cancer 1979; 43:2254–2267.
44. Keane TJ, Harwood AR, Rider WD, et al: Concomitant radiation and chemotherapy for squamous cell carcinoma of esophagus [abstract]. Int J Radiat Oncol Biol Phys 1984; 10:89.
45. Mendenhall WM: Carcinoma of the cervical esophagus. In: Million RR, Cassisi NJ (eds): Management of Head and Neck Cancer, A Multidisciplinary Approach, pp 393–405. Philadelphia, J.B. Lippincott Co., 1984.
46. Rider WD, Diaz Mendoza R: Some opinions on the treatment of cancer of the esophagus. Am J Roentgenol 1969; 105:514–517.
47. Pringle R, Winsey HS: The palliation of esophageal carcinoma. J R Coll Surg Edinb 1973; 18:188–190.

48. Elkon D, Lee MS, Hendrickson FR: Carcinoma of the esophagus: sites of recurrence and palliative benefits after definitive radiotherapy. Int J Radiat Oncol Biol Phys 1978; 4:615–620.
49. Herskovic A, Leichman L, Lattin P, et al: Chemo/radiation with and without surgery in the thoracic esophagus: the Wayne State experience. Int J Radiat Oncol Biol Phys 1988; 15:655–662.
50. Mendenhall WM, Million RR, Bova FJ: Carcinoma of the cervical esophagus treated with radiation therapy using a four-field box technique. Int J Radiat Oncol Biol Phys 1982; 8:1435–1439.
51. Langer M, Choi NC, Orlow E, et al: Radiation therapy alone or in combination with surgery in the treatment of carcinoma of the esophagus. Cancer 1986; 58:1208–1213.
52. Kelsen DP: The role of chemotherapy in the treatment of esophageal cancer. Chest Surg Clin North Am 1994; 4:173–184.
53. Heitmiller RF, Forastiere AA, Kleinberg LR: Esophagus. In: Abeloff MD, Armitage JO, Lichter AS, et al (eds): Clinical Oncology, 2nd ed, pp 1517–1544. New York, Churchill-Livingstone, 2000.
54. Roth JA, Putnam JB Jr, Rich TA, et al: Cancer of the esophagus. In: De Vita VT, Hellman S, Rosenberg SA (eds): Cancer Principles and Practice of Oncology. Philadelphia, Lippincott-Raven, 1997.
55. Ajani JA, Ilson DH, Daugherty K, et al: Activity of taxol in patients with squamous cell carcinoma and adenocarcinoma of the esophagus. J Natl Cancer Inst 1994; 86:1086–1091.
56. Conroy T, Etienne PL, Adenis A, et al: Phase II trial of vinorelbine in metastatic squamous cell esophageal carcinoma. European Organization for Research and Treatment of Cancer, Gastrointestinal Tract Cancer Cooperative Group. J Clin Oncol 1996; 14:164–170.
57. Marcuello E, Alba E, Gomez de Segura G, et al: Cisplatin and intravenous continuous infusion of bleomycin in advanced and metastatic esophageal cancer. Eur J Cancer Clin Oncol 1988; 24:633–635.
58. Coonley CJ, Bains M, Hilaris B, et al: Cisplatin and bleomycin in the treatment of esophageal carcinoma. A final report. Cancer 1984; 54:2351–2355.
59. Iizuka T, Kakegawa T, Ida H, et al: Phase II evaluation of combined cisplatin and vindesine in advanced squamous cell carcinoma of the esophagus: Japanese Esophageal Oncology Group trial. Jpn J Clin Oncol 1991; 21:176–179.
60. DeBesi P, Salvagno L, Endrizzi L, et al: Cisplatin, bleomycin and methotrexate in the treatment of advanced oesophageal cancer. Eur J Cancer Clin Oncol 1984; 20:743–747.
61. Vogl SE, Greenwald E, Kaplan BH: Effective chemotherapy for esophageal cancer with methotrexate, bleomycin, and cis-diaminedichloroplatinum II. Cancer 1981; 48:2555–2558.
62. Kelsen D, Hilaris B, Coonley C, et al: Cisplatin, vindesine, and bleomycin chemotherapy of local-regional and advanced esophageal carcinoma. Am J Med 1983; 75:645–652.
63. Dinwoodie WR, Bartolucci AA, Lyman GH, et al: Phase II evaluation of cisplatin, bleomycin, and vindesine in advanced squamous cell carcinoma of the esophagus: a Southeastern Cancer Study Group trial. Cancer Treat Rep 1986; 70:267–270.
64. Allen SM, Duffy JP, Walker SJ, et al: A phase II study of mitomycin, ifosfamide and cisplatin in operable and inoperable squamous cell carcinoma of the oesophagus. J Clin Oncol 1994; 6:91–95.
65. Kok TC, Van der Gasst A, Dees J, et al: Cisplatin and etoposide in oesophageal cancer: a phase II study. Rotterdam Oesophageal Tumour Study Group. Br J Cancer 1996; 74:980–984.
66. Iizuka T, Kakegawa T, Ide H, et al: Phase II evaluation of cisplatin and 5-fluorouracil in advanced squamous cell carcinoma of the esophagus: A Japanese Esophageal Oncology Group trial. Jpn J Clin Oncol 1992; 22:172–176.
67. DeBesi P, Sileni VC, Salvagno L, et al: Phase II study of cisplatin, 5-FU, and allopurinol in advanced esophageal cancer. Cancer Treat Rep 1986; 70:909–910.
68. Gisselbrecht C, Calvo F, Mignot L, et al: Fluorouracil, adriamycin, and cisplatin (FAP): combination chemotherapy of advanced esophageal carcinoma. Cancer 1983; 52:974–977.
69. Bamias A, Hill ME, Cunningham D, et al: Epirubicin, cisplatin, and protracted venous infusion of 5-fluorouracil for esophagogastric adenocarcinoma. Cancer 1996; 77:1978–1985.
70. Kelsen D, Lovett D, Wong J, et al: Interferon alfa-2a and fluorouracil in the treatment of patients with advanced esophageal cancer. J Clin Oncol 1992; 10:269–274.
71. Wadler S, Fell S, Haynes J, et al: Treatment of carcinoma of the esophagus with 5-fluorouracil and recombinant alfa-2a-interferon. Cancer 1993; 71:1726–1730.
72. Ilson DH, Sirott M, Saltz L, et al: A phase II trial of interferon alpha-2a, 5-fluorouracil, and cisplatin in patients with advanced esophageal carcinoma. Cancer 1995; 75:2197–2202.
73. Wadler S, Haynes H, Beitler JJ, et al: Phase II clinical trial with 5-fluorouracil, recombinant interferon-alpha-2b, and cisplatin for patients with metastatic or regionally advanced carcinoma of the esophagus. Cancer 1996; 78:30–34.
74. Pai C, Bazarbashi S, Rahal M, et al: Phase II study of cis-platinum, 5-fluorouracil and interferon-a-2b in advanced/metastatic epidermoid esophageal carcinoma [Abstract]. Proceedings of the American Society of Clinical Oncology 1998; 17:1158A.
75. Garcia-Alfonso P, Guevara S, Lopez P, et al: Taxol and cisplatin + 5-fluorouracil sequential in advanced esophageal cancer [Abstract]. Proceedings of the American Society of Clinical Oncology 1998; 17: 998A.
76. Ilson DH, Ajani J, Bhalla K, et al: Phase II trial of paclitaxel, fluorouracil, and cisplatin in patients with advanced carcinoma of the esophagus. J Clin Oncol 1998; 16:1826–1834.
77. Enzinger PC, Ilson DH, Saltz LB, et al: A phase II trial of cisplatin and irinotecan in patients with advanced esophageal cancer [abstract]. Proceedings of the American Society of Clinical Oncology 1998; 17:1085A.
78. Akakura I, Nakamura Y, Kakegawa T, et al: Surgery of carcinoma of the esophagus with preoperative radiation. Chest 1970; 57:47.
79. Launois B, Delarue D, Campion JP, et al: Preoperative radiotherapy for carcinoma of the esophagus. Surg Gynecol Obstet 1981; 153:690.
80. Guo-Jun H, Xiang-Zhi G: Experience with combined preoperative irradiation and surgery for squamous cell carcinoma of the esophagus. In: Wagner G, Zhang Y-H (eds): Cancer of the Liver, Esophagus, and Nasopharynx. Berlin, Springer-Verlag, 1987.
81. Gignoux M, Roussel A, Pallot B, et al: The value of preoperative radiotherapy in esophageal cancer: results of a study of the EORTC. World J Surg 1987; 11:426–432.
82. Gignoux M, Roussel A, Paillot B, et al: The value of preoperative radiotherapy in esophageal cancer: results of a study by the EORTC. Recent Results Cancer Res 1988; 110:1–13.
83. Mei W, Xian-Zhi G, Weibo Y, et al: Randomized clinical trial on the combination of preoperative irradiation and surgery in the treatment of esophageal carcinoma: report of 206 patients. Int J Radiat Oncol Biol Phys 1989; 16:325–327.
84. Franklin R, Steiger Z, Vaishampayan G, et al: Combined modality therapy for esophageal squamous cell carcinoma. Cancer 1983; 51:1062–1071.
85. Leichman L, Steiger Z, Seydel HG, et al: Combined preoperative chemotherapy and radiation therapy for cancer of the esophagus: the Wayne State University, Southwest Oncology Group and Radiation Therapy Oncology Group experience. Semin Oncol 1984; 11:178–185.
86. Walsh TN, Noonan N, Hollywood D, et al: A comparison of multimodal therapy and surgery for esophageal adenocarcinoma. N Engl J Med 1996; 335:462–467.
87. Forastiere AA, Orringer MB, Perez-Tamayo C, et al: Concurrent chemotherapy and radiation therapy followed by transhiatal esophagectomy for local-regional cancer of the esophagus. J Clin Oncol 1990; 8:119–127.
88. Forastiere AA, Urba SG: Combined modality therapy for cancer of the esophagus. PPO Updates. Principles and Practice of Oncology 1996; 10:1–15.
89. Urba S, Orringer M, Turrisi A, et al: A randomized trial comparing surgery to preoperative concomitant chemoirradiation plus surgery in patients with resectable esophageal cancer: updated analysis [abstract]. Proceedings of the American Society of Clinical Oncology 1997; 16:277A.
90. Nygaard K, Hagen S, Hansen HS, et al: Pre-operative radiotherapy prolongs survival in operable esophageal carcinoma: A randomized, multicenter study of preoperative radiotherapy and chemotherapy. The second Scandinavian trial in esophageal cancer. World J Surg 1992; 16:1104–1110.
91. Bosset JF, Gignoux M, Triboulet JP, et al: Chemoradiotherapy followed by surgery compared with surgery alone in squamous cell cancer of the esophagus. N Engl J Med 1997; 337:161–167.
92. Kok TC: Chemotherapy in esophageal cancer. Cancer Treat Rev 1997; 23:65–85.
93. Vokes EE, Mauer AM: Multimodality therapy for esophageal cancer: an emerging role. Cancer J Sci Am 1998; 4:226–229.

94. Kasai M, Mori S, Watanabe T: Follow-up results after resection of thoracic esophageal carcinoma. World J Surg 1978; 2:543–551.
95. Teniere P, Hay J, Fingerhut A, et al: Postoperative RT does not increase survival after curative resection for squamous cell carcinoma of the middle and lower esophagus. Surg Gynecol Obstet 1991; 173:123–130.
96. Fok M, Cheng SWK, Wong J: Endosonography in patient selection for surgical treatment of esophageal carcinoma. World J Surg 1992; 16:1098–1103.
97. Poplin E, Fleming T, Leichman L, et al: Combined therapies for squamous-cell carcinoma of the esophagus: A Southwest Oncology Group Study (SWOG-8037). J Clin Oncol 1987; 5:622–628.
98. Seydel HG, Leichman L, Byhardt R, et al: Preoperative radiation and chemotherapy for localized squamous cell carcinoma of the esophagus: a RTOG study. Int J Radiat Oncol Biol Phys 1988; 14:33–35.
99. Byfield JE, Barone R, Mendelsohn J, et al: Infusional 5-fluorouracil and x-ray therapy for non-resectable esophageal cancer. Cancer 1980; 45:703–708.
100. Coia LR, Engstrom PF, Paul A: Nonsurgical management of esophageal cancer: report of a study of combined radiotherapy and chemotherapy. J Clin Oncol 1987; 5:1783–1790.
101. Lokich JJ, Shea M, Chaffey J: Sequential infusional 5-fluorouracil followed by concomitant radiation for tumors of the esophagus and gastroesophageal junction. Cancer 1987; 60:275–279.
102. Coia LR, Paul AR, Engstrom PF: Combined radiation and chemotherapy as primary management of adenocarcinoma of the esophagus and gastroesophageal junction. Cancer 1988; 61:643–649.
103. Coia LR: Esophageal cancer. Is esophagectomy necessary? Oncology 1989; 3:101–110.
104. Sischy B, Ryan L, Heller D, et al: Interim report of EST 1282 phase III protocol for the evaluation of combined modalities in the treatment of patients with carcinoma of the esophagus, stage I and II [Abstract]. Proceedings of the American Society of Clinical Oncology 1990; 9:105.
105. Coia LR, Engstrom PF, Paul AR, et al: Long-term results of infusional 5-FU, mitomycin-C, and radiation as primary management of esophageal carcinoma. Int J Radiat Oncol Biol Phys 1991; 20:29–36.
106. Smith TJ, Ryan LM, Douglas HO Jr, et al: Combined chemotherapy vs radiotherapy alone for early stage squamous cell carcinoma of the esophagus: a study of the Eastern Cooperative Oncology Group. Int J Radiat Oncol Biol Phys 1998; 42:269–276.
107. Skinner DB: Surgical treatment for esophageal carcinoma. Semin Oncol 1984; 11:136–143.
108. Abe S, Tachibana M, Shimokawa T, et al: Surgical treatment of advanced carcinoma of the esophagus. Surg Gynecol Obstet 1989; 168:115–120.
109. Orringer MB: Substernal gastric bypass of the excluded esophagus—results of an ill-advised operation. Surgery 1984; 96:467–470.
110. Mannell A, Becker PJ, Nissenbaum M: Bypass surgery for unresectable esophageal cancer: early and late results in 124 cases. Br J Surg 1988; 75:283–286.
111. Pagliero KM: Brachytherapy (intracavitary irradiation). In: Hurt RL (ed): Management of Oesophageal Carcinoma, pp 243–250. London, Springer-Verlag, 1989.
112. Hishikawa Y, Kurisu K, Taniguchi M, et al: High-dose rate intraluminal brachytherapy (HDRIBT) for esophageal cancer. Int J Radiat Oncol Biol Phys 1991; 21:1133–1136.
113. Gaspar LE, Quian C, Kocha WI, et al: A phase I/II study of external beam radiation, brachytherapy, and concurrent chemotherapy in localized cancer of the esophagus (RTOG 92–07): preliminary toxicity report. Int J Radiat Oncol Biol Phys 1997; 37:593–599.
114. Boyce HW: Palliation of advanced esophageal cancer. Semin Oncol 1984; 11:186–195.
115. Watson A: Palliative therapy. In: Hurt RL (ed): Management of Oesophageal Carcinoma, pp 211–222. London, Springer-Verlag, 1989.
116. Manyak MH, Russo A, Smith PD, et al: Photodynamic therapy. J Clin Oncol 1988; 6:380–391.
117. Murray FE, Bowers GJ, Birkett DH, et al: Palliative laser therapy for advanced esophageal carcinoma: an alternative perspective. Am J Gastroenterol 1988; 83:816–819.
118. Gunnlaugsson GH, Wychulis AR, Roland C, et al: Analysis of the records of 1,657 patients with carcinoma of the esophagus and cardia of the stomach. Surg Gynecol Obstet 1970; 130:997–1005.
119. Mandard AM, Chasle J, Marnay J, et al: Autopsy findings in 111 cases of esophageal cancer. Cancer 1981; 48:329–335.
120. Cox JD: Failure analysis of inoperable carcinoma of the lung of all histopathologic types and squamous cell carcinoma of the esophagus. Cancer Treat Symp 1983; 2:77–86.
121. Aisner J, Forastiere A, Aroney R: Patterns of recurrence for cancer of the lung and esophagus. Cancer Treat Symp 1983; 2:87–105.
122. Sugimachi K, Matsufuji H, Kai H, et al: Preoperative irradiation for carcinoma of the esophagus. Surg Gynecol Obstet 1986; 162:174–176.
123. Sugimachi K, Matsuoka H, Matsufuji H, et al: Survival rates of women with carcinoma of the esophagus exceed those of men. Surg Gynecol Obstet 1987; 164:541–544.
124. Kelsen DP, Ahuja R, Hopfan S, et al: Combined modality therapy of esophageal carcinoma. Cancer 1981; 48:31–37.
125. Kelsen D: Neoadjuvant therapy of esophageal cancer. Can J Surg 1989; 32:410–414.
126. Kelsen DP, Bains M, Burt M: Neoadjuvant chemotherapy and surgery of cancer of the esophagus. Semin Surg Oncol 1990; 6:268–273.
127. Roth JA, Pass HU, Flanagan MM, et al: Randomized clinical trial of preoperative and postoperative chemotherapy with cisplatin, vindesine, and bleomycin for carcinoma of the esophagus. J Thorac Cardiovasc Surg 1988; 96:242–248.
128. Schlag PM: Randomized trial of preoperative chemotherapy for squamous cell cancer of the esophagus. Arch Surg 1992; 127:1446–1450.
129. Kelsen DP, Ginsberg R, Pajak TF, et al: Chemotherapy followed by surgery compared with surgery versus operation alone for localized esophageal cancers. N Engl J Med 1998; 339:1979–1984.
130. MacFarlane SD, Hill LD, Jolly PC, et al: Improved results of surgical treatment for esophageal and gastroesophageal junction carcinomas after preoperative combined chemotherapy and radiation. J Thorac Cardiovasc Surg 1988; 95:415–422.
131. Richmond J, Seydel HG, Bae Y, et al: Comparison of three treatment strategies for esophageal cancer within a single institution. Int J Radiat Oncol Biol Phys 1987; 13:1617–1620.
132. Araujo CMM, Souhami L, Gil RA, et al: A randomized trial comparing radiation therapy versus concomitant radiation therapy and chemotherapy in carcinoma of the thoracic esophagus. Cancer 1991; 67:2258–2261.
133. Earle JD, Gelber RD, Moertel CG, et al: A controlled evaluation of combined radiation and bleomycin therapy for squamous cell carcinoma of the esophagus. Int J Radiat Oncol Biol Phys 1980; 6:821–826.
134. Andersen AP, Berdal P, Edsmyr T, et al: Irradiation, chemotherapy, and surgery in esophageal cancer: a randomized clinical study. Radiother Oncol 1984; 2:179–188.
135. Mantravadi RVP, Hayes J, Gates JO, et al: External radiotherapy, high dose rate brachytherapy combined with chemotherapy in the treatment of carcinoma of the esophagus. Proceedings of the American Radium Society. Hawaii, April 1999.
136. Bhalla KN, Kumar GN, Walle UK, et al: Phase I and pharmacologic study of a 3-hour infusion of paclitaxel followed by cisplatin and 5-fluorouracil in patients with advanced solid tumors. Clin Cancer Res 1999; 5:1723–1730.

Stomach

137. Franceschi S, Levi F, LaVecchia C: Epidemiology of gastric cancer in Europe. Eur J Cancer Prev 1994; 3:5–10.
138. Correa P: Clinical implications of recent developments in gastric cancer pathology and epidemiology. Semin Oncol 1985; 12:2–10.
139. Wadström T: An update on *Helicobacter pylori.* Curr Opin Gastroenterol 1995; 11:69–75.
140. Nomura A: Stomach cancer. In: Schottenfeld D, Fraumeni JF Jr (eds): Cancer Epidemiology and Prevention, pp 707–724. Oxford, Oxford University Press, 1996.
141. Neugut AI, Hayeh M, Howe G: Epidemiology of gastric cancer. Semin Oncol 1996; 23:281–291.
142. Parsonnet J, Friedman GD, Vandersteen DP, et al: Helicobacter pylori infection and the risk of gastric carcinoma. N Engl J Med 1991; 325:1127–1136.
143. The Eurogast Study Group: An international association between H. pylori infection and gastric cancer. Lancet 1993; 341:1359–1362.
144. Nomura A, Stemmerman GN, Chyon PH, et al: Helicobacter pylori

infection and gastric carcinoma among Japanese Americans in Hawaii. N Engl J Med 1995; 325:1132–1136.
145. Kurtz RC, Sherlock P: The diagnosis of gastric cancer. Semin Oncol 1985; 12:11–18.
146. Hendricks JC: Malignant tumors of the stomach. Surg Clin North Am 1986; 66:683–693.
147. Moss AA, Schnyder P, Marks W, et al: Gastric adenocarcinoma: a comparison of the accuracy and economics of staging by computed tomography and surgery. Gastroenterology 1981; 80:45–90.
148. Fukuya T, Honda H, Hayashi T, et al: Lymph-node metastases: efficacy of the detection with helical CT in patients with gastric cancer. Radiology 1995; 197:705–711.
149. Lowy AM, Mansfield PF, Leach SD, Ajana J: Laparoscopic staging for gastric cancer. Surgery 1996; 119:611–614.
150. Burke EC, Karpeh MS, Conlon KC, et al: Laparoscopy in the management of gastric adenocarcinoma. Ann Surg 1997; 225:262–267.
151. Gupta JP, Jain AL, Agrawal BK, et al: Gastroscopic cytology and biopsies in diagnosis of gastric malignancies. J Surg Oncol 1983; 22:62–64.
152. Douglass HO, Nava HR: Gastric adenocarcinoma—management of the primary disease. Semin Oncol 1985; 12:32–45.
153. Japanese Research Society for Gastric Cancer. The general rules for the gastric cancer study in surgery and pathology. Part I. Clinical Classification. Jpn J Surg 1981; 11:127–139.
154. Gunderson LL, Sosin H: Adenocarcinoma of the stomach: areas of failure in a reoperation series (second or symptomatic looks): clinicopathologic correlation and implications for adjuvant therapy. Int J Radiat Oncol Biol Phys 1982; 8:1–11.
155. ReMine WH: Preoperative assessment and palliative surgery. In: Fielding JWL, Newman CE, Ford CHJ, et al (eds): Gastric Cancer: Advances in the Biosciences, volume 32, pp 123–138. Oxford, Pergamon Press, 1981.
156. Shiu MH, Moore E, Sanders M, et al: Influence of the extent of resection on survival of the curative treatment of gastric carcinoma. Arch Surg 1987; 122:1347–1351.
157. Salo JA, Saario I, Kimilankao EO, et al: Near total gastrectomy for gastric cancer. Am J Surg 1988; 155:486–489.
158. Gouzi JL, Huguier M, Gagniez PL, et al: Total versus subtotal gastrectomy for adenocarcinoma of the gastric antrum. A French prospective controlled study. Ann Surg 1989; 209:162–166.
159. Okamura T, Tsujitan S, Korenaga O, et al: Lymphadenectomy for cure in patients with early gastric cancer and lymph node metastasis. Am J Surg 1988; 155:476–480.
160. Baker T, Nakane Y, Okusa T, et al: Strategy for lymphadenectomy of gastric cancer. Surgery 1989; 105:585–592.
161. Cuschieri A, Fayers P, Fielding J, et al: Postoperative morbidity and mortality after D_1 and D_2 resections for gastric cancer: preliminary results of the MRC randomized controlled surgical trial. Lancet 1996; 347:995–999.
162. Cuschieri A, Weeden S, Fielding J, et al: Patient survival after D_1 and D_2 resections for gastric cancer: long-term results of the MRC randomized surgical trial. Br J Cancer 1999; 79:1522–1530.
163. Sasako M, Maruyama K, Kinoshita T: Quality control of surgical technique in a multicenter, prospective, randomized, controlled study on the surgical treatment of gastric cancer. Jpn J Clin Oncol 1992; 22:41–48.
164. Bonnenkamp JJ, Songum I, Hermans J, et al: Randomized comparison of morbidity after D1 and D2 dissection for gastric cancer in 996 Dutch patients. Lancet 1995; 345:745–748.
165. Sasako M: Risk factors for surgical treatment in the Dutch gastric cancer trial. Br J Surg 1997; 84:1567–1571.
166. Bonnenkamp JJ, Hermans J, Sasako M, et al: Extended lymph node dissection for gastric cancer. Dutch Gastric Cancer Group. N Engl J Med 1999; 340:908–914.
167. Monson JRT, Donohue JH, McIlrath DC, et al: Total gastrectomy for advanced cancer. A worthwhile palliative procedure. Cancer 1991; 68:1863–1873.
168. Kennedy BJ: TNM classification for stomach cancer. Cancer 1970; 26:971–983.
169. Papachristou DN, Fortner JG: Local recurrence of gastric adenocarcinomas after gastrectomy. J Surg Oncol 1981; 18:47–53.
170. Landry J, Tepper J, Wood W, et al: Analysis of survival and local control following surgery for gastric cancer. Int J Radiat Oncol Biol Phys 1990; 19:1357–1362.
171. Stout AP: Pathology of carcinoma of the stomach. Arch Surg 1943; 46:807–822.
172. Thomson FB, Robins RE: Local recurrence following subtotal resection for gastric carcinoma. Surg Gynecol Obstet 1952; 95:341–344.
173. Horn RC: Carcinoma of the stomach. Autopsy findings in untreated cases. Gastroenterology 1955; 29:515–525.
174. McNeer G, Vandenberg H, Donn FY, Bowden LA: A critical evaluation of subtotal gastrectomy for the cure of cancer of the stomach. Ann Surg 1957; 134:2–7.
175. Wisbeck WM, Becher EM, Russell AH: Adenocarcinoma of the stomach: autopsy observations with therapeutic implications for the radiation oncologist. Radiother Oncol 1986; 7:13–18.
176. Gilbertson VA: Results of treatment of stomach cancer: an appraisal of efforts for more extensive surgery and a report of 1,938 cases. Cancer 1969; 23:1305–1308.
177. Moertel CG, Childs DS Jr, Reitemeier RJ, et al: Combined 5-fluorouracil and supervoltage radiation therapy of locally unresectable gastrointestinal cancer. Lancet 1969; 2:865–867.
178. Holbrook MA: Current concepts in cancer—radiation therapy for gastric cancer: treatment principles. JAMA 1974; 228:1289–1290.
179. Schein PS, Novak J: Combined modality therapy (XRT-chemo) versus chemotherapy alone for locally unresectable gastric cancer. GITSG. Cancer 1982; 49:1771–1777.
180. Chevalier TL, Smith FP, Harter WK, et al: Chemotherapy and combined-modality therapy for locally advanced and metastatic gastric carcinoma. Semin Oncol 1985; 12:46–53.
181. Gunderson LL, Hoskins B, Cohen AM, et al: Combined modality treatment of gastric cancer. Int J Radiat Oncol Biol Phys 1983; 9:965–975.
182. Moertel CG, Childs DS, O'Fallon JR, et al: Combined 5-fluorouracil and radiation therapy as a surgical adjuvant for poor prognosis gastric carcinoma. J Clin Oncol 1984; 2:1249–1254.
183. Gez E, Sulkes A, Yablonsky-Peretz T, et al: Combined 5-fluorouracil (5-FU) and radiation therapy following resection of locally advanced gastric carcinoma. J Surg Oncol 1986; 31:139–142.
184. Allum WH, Hallissey MT, Ward LC, et al for the British Stomach Cancer Group: A controlled, prospective, and randomized trial of adjuvant chemotherapy or radiotherapy in resectable gastric cancer: Interim report. Br J Cancer 1989; 60:739–744.
185. Whittington R, Coia L, Haller DG, et al: Adenocarcinoma of the esophagus and esophagogastric junction: the effects of single and combined modalities on the survival and patterns of failure following treatment. Int J Radiat Oncol Biol Phys 1990; 19:593–603.
186. Regine WF, Mohuidden M: Impact of adjuvant therapy on locally advanced adenocarcinoma of the stomach. Int J Radiat Oncol Biol Phys 1992; 24:921–927.
186a. MacDonald JS, Smalley S, Benedetti J, et al: Postoperative combined radiation and chemotherapy improves disease free survival (DFS) and overall survival (OS) in resected adenocarcinoma of the stomach and gastroesophageal junction [Abstract]. J Clin Oncol 2000; 19:1a.
186b. Smalley S, Benedetti J, Gunderson L, et al: Intergroup 0116–phase III trial of postoperative adjuvant radiochemotherapy for high risk gastric and gastroesophageal junction adenocarcinoma: evaluation of efficacy and radiotherapy treatment [Abstract]. Int J Radiat Oncol Biol Phys 2000; 47(suppl):111.
187. MacDonald JS, Steele G, Gunderson LL: Carcinoma of the stomach. In: DeVita VT, Hellman S, Rosenberg SA (eds): Principles and Practice of Oncology, 3rd ed, pp 765–799. Philadelphia, J.B. Lippincott, 1989.
188. Wilke H, Preusser P, Fink U, et al: New developments in the treatment of gastric carcinoma. Semin Oncol 1990; 17(1 suppl 2):61–70.
189. Mehta K, Mohuidden M: Improved local control with adjunctive therapy for cancers of the gastroesophageal junction [Abstract]. Int J Radiat Oncol Biol Phys 1994; 30(suppl):272.
190. The Gastrointestinal Tumor Study Group: Controlled trial of adjuvant chemotherapy following resection for gastric cancer. Cancer 1982; 49:1116–1122.
191. Higgins GA, Amadeo JH, Smith DE, et al: Efficacy of prolonged intermittent therapy with combined 5-FU and methyl CCNU following resection for gastric carcinoma: Veterans Administration Surgical Oncology Group report. Cancer 1983; 52:1105–1112.
192. Engstrom PF, Lavin PT, Douglass HO, et al: Postoperative adjuvant 5-FU plus methyl CCNU therapy for gastric cancer patients: Eastern Cooperative Oncology Study Group 3275. Cancer 1985; 55:1868–1873.
193. Italian Gastrointestinal Tumor Study Group: Adjuvant treatments

following curative resection for gastric cancer. Br J Surg 1988; 75:1100–1104.

194. Krook JE, O'Connell MJ, Wieand HS, et al: A prospective, randomized evaluation of intensive-course 5-fluorouracil plus doxorubicin as surgical adjuvant chemotherapy for resected gastric cancer. Cancer 1991; 67:2454–2458.
195. Estrada E, Lacave AJ, Valle M, et al: Methyl-CCNU, 5-fluorouracil and Adriamycin (MeFA) as adjuvant chemotherapy in gastric cancer [Abstract]. Proceedings of the American Society of Clinical Oncology 1988; 7:358.
196. Coombes RC, Schein PS, Chilvers CE, et al: A randomized trial comparing adjuvant fluorouracil, doxorubicin, and mitomycin with no treatment in operable gastric cancer. J Clin Oncol 1990; 8:1362–1369.
197. MacDonald JS, Fleming TR, Peterson RF, et al: Adjuvant chemotherapy with 5-FU, adriamycin, and mitomycin-C (FAM) versus surgery alone for patients with locally advanced gastric adenocarcinoma: a Southwest Oncology Group study. Ann Surg Oncol 1995; 2:488–494.
198. Hallissey MT, Dunn JA, Ward LC, et al: The second British Stomach Cancer Group trial of adjuvant radiotherapy or chemotherapy in resectable gastric cancer: five-year follow-up. Lancet 1994; 343:1309–1312.
199. Lise M, Nitti D, Marchet A, et al: Final results of a phase III clinical trial of adjuvant chemotherapy with the modified fluorouracil, doxorubicin, and mitomycin regimen in resectable gastric cancer. J Clin Oncol 1995; 13:2757–2763.
200. Tsavaris N, Tentas K, Dosmidis P, et al: A randomized trial comparing adjuvant fluorouracil, epirubicin, and mitomycin with no treatment in operable gastric cancer. Chemotherapy 1996; 42:220–226.
201. Huguier M, Destroyes JP, Baschet C, et al: Gastric carcinoma treated by chemotherapy after resection. A controlled study. Am J Surg 1980; 139:197–199.
202. Rake MO, Mallinson CN, Cocking JB, et al: Assessment of the value of cytotoxic therapy in the treatment of carcinoma of the stomach. Gut 1976; 17:832.
203. Jakesz R, Dittrich C, Funovics J, et al: The effect of adjuvant chemotherapy in gastric carcinoma is dependent on tumor histology: 5-year results of a prospective randomized trial. Recent Results Cancer Res 1988; 110:44–51.
204. Estape J, Grau JJ, Lcobendas F, et al: Mitomycin C as an adjuvant treatment to resected gastric cancer. A 10-year follow-up. Ann Surg 1991; 213:219–221.
205. Neri B, de Leonardis V, Romano S, et al: Adjuvant chemotherapy after gastric resection in node-positive cancer patients: a multicentre randomized study. Br J Cancer 1996; 73:549–552.
206. Allum WH, Hallissey MT, Kelly KA: Adjuvant chemotherapy in operable gastric cancer. Five-year follow-up of first British Stomach Cancer Group trial. Lancet 1989; 1:571–574.
207. Grau JJ, Estape J, Alcobendas F, et al: Positive results of adjuvant mitomycin-C in resected gastric cancer: a randomized trial on 134 patients. Eur J Cancer 1993; 29A:340–342.
208. Carrato A, Diaz-Rubio E, Medrano J, et al: Phase III trial of surgery versus adjuvant chemotherapy with mitomycin C and tegafur plus uracil, starting within the first week after surgery for gastric adenocarcinoma [Abstract]. Proceedings of the American Society of Clinical Oncology 1995; 14:198.
209. Imanaga H, Nakazato H: Results of surgery for gastric cancer and effect of adjuvant mitomycin-C on cancer recurrence. World J Surg 1977; 2:213–221.
210. Nakajima T, Fukami A, Ohashi I, et al: Long-term follow-up study of gastric cancer patients treated with surgery and adjuvant chemotherapy with mitomycin C. Int J Clin Pharmacol Biopharm 1978; 16:209–216.
211. Nakajima T, Fukami A, Takagi K, et al: Adjuvant chemotherapy with mitomycin C, and with a multi-drug combination of mitomycin C, 5-fluorouracil and cytosine arabinoside after curative resection of gastric cancer. Jpn J Clin Oncol 1980; 10:187.
212. Nakajima T, Takahashi T, Takagi K, et al: Comparison of 5-fluorouracil with ftorafur in adjuvant chemotherapies with combined inductive and maintenance therapies for gastric cancer. J Clin Oncol 1984; 2:1366–1371.
213. Ochiai T, Sato H, Hayashi R, et al: Postoperative adjuvant immunotherapy of gastric cancer with BCG-cell wall skeleton. Three- to six-year follow-up of a randomized clinical trial. Cancer Immunol Immunother 1983; 14:167–171.
214. Hattori T, Niimoto M, Toge T, et al: Effects of levamisole in adjuvant immunochemotherapy for gastric cancer: a prospective randomized controlled study. Jpn J Surg 1983; 13:480–485.
215. Ochiai T, Sato H, Sato H, et al: Randomly controlled study of chemotherapy versus chemoimmunotherapy in postoperative gastric cancer patients. Cancer Res 1983; 43:3001–3007.
216. Niimoto M, Hattori T, Tamada R, et al: Postoperative adjuvant immunochemotherapy with mitomycin-C, futraful and PSK for gastric cancer. An analysis of data on 579 patients followed for five years. Jpn J Surg 1988; 18:681–686.
217. Niimoto M, Saeki T, Toi M, et al: Prospective randomized controlled study on bestatin in resectable gastric cancer. Third report. Jpn J Surg 1990; 20:186–191.
218. Hattori T, Nakajima T, Nakazato H, et al: Postoperative adjuvant immunochemotherapy with mitomycin C, tegafur, PSK and/or OK-432 for gastric cancer, with special reference to the change in stimulation index after gastrectomy. Jpn J Surg 1990; 20:127–136.
219. Fukushima M: Adjuvant therapy of gastric carcinoma: the Japanese experience. Semin Oncol 1996; 23:369–378.
220. Nakajima T: Adjuvant chemotherapy for gastric cancer in Japan: present status and suggestions for rational clinical trials. Jpn J Clin Oncol 1990; 20:30–42.
221. Bleiberg H, Gerard B, Deguiral P: Adjuvant therapy in resectable gastric cancer. Br J Cancer 1992; 66:987–991.
222. Abe M, Takahashi M: Intraoperative radiotherapy: the Japanese experience. Int J Radiat Oncol Biol Phys 1981; 5:863–868.
223. Takahashi M, Abe M: Intraoperative radiotherapy for carcinoma of the stomach. Eur J Surg Oncol 1986; 12:247–250.
224. Chen G, Song S: Evaluation of intraoperative radiotherapy for gastric carcinoma analysis of 247 patients. In: Abe M, Takahashi M (eds): Proceedings of Third International IORT Symposium, Kyoto, Japan, pp 190–191. New York, Pergamon Press, 1991.
225. Sindelar WF, Kinsella TJ, Tepper JE, et al: Randomized trial of intraoperative radiotherapy in carcinoma of the stomach. Am J Surg 1993; 165:178–187.
226. Talaev MI, Starinskii VV, Kovalev BN, et al: Results of combined treatment of cancer of the gastric antrum and gastric body. Vopr Onkol 1990; 36:1485–1488.
227. Kosse VA: Combined treatment of gastric cancer using hypoxic radiotherapy. Vopr Onkol 1990; 36:1349–1353.
228. Shchepotin IB, Evans SRT, Chorny V, et al: Intensive preoperative radiotherapy with local hyperthermia for the treatment of gastric carcinoma. Surg Oncol 1994; 3:37–44.
229. Zhang ZX, Gu XZ, Yin WB, et al: Randomized clinical trial combination on the preoperative irradiation and surgery in the treatment of adenocarcinoma of the gastric cardia (AGC)—report on 370 patients. Int J Radiat Oncol Biol Phys 1998; 42:929–934.
230. Henning GT, Schild SF, Stafford SL, et al: Results of irradiation or chemoirradiation following resection of gastric adenocarcinoma. Int J Radiat Oncol Biol Phys 2000; 46:589–598.
231. Wieland C, Hymmen U: Mega–volt therapy for malignant stomach tumors. Strahlenther 1970; 40:20–26.
232. Takahashi T: Studies on preoperative and postoperative telecobalt therapy in gastric cancer. Nippon Acta Radiol 1964; 24:129–132.
233. The Gastrointestinal Tumor Study Group: The concept of locally advanced gastric cancer. Cancer 1990; 66:2324–2330.
234. Bleiberg H, Goffin JC, Dalesie O, et al: Adjuvant radiotherapy and chemotherapy in resectable gastric cancer. Eur J Surg Oncol 1989; 15:535–543.
235. O'Connell MJ, Gunderson LL, Moertel CG, et al: A pilot study of intensive combined therapy for locally unresectable gastric cancer. Int J Radiat Oncol Biol Phys 1985; 11:1827–1831.
236. Moertel CG, Gunderson LL, Malliard JA, et al: Early evaluation of combined fluorouracil and leucovorin as a radiation enhancer for locally unresectable, residual, or recurrent gastrointestinal carcinoma. The North Central Cancer Treatment Group. J Clin Oncol 1994; 12:21–27.
237. Henning GT, Schild SF, Stafford SL, et al: Results of irradiation or chemoirradiation for primary unresectable, locally recurrent, or grossly incomplete resection of gastric adenocarcinomas. Int J Radiat Oncol Biol Phys 2000; 46:109–118.
238. Wilke H, Preusser P, Fink U, et al: Preoperative chemotherapy in locally advanced and nonresectable gastric cancer: a phase II study with etoposide, doxorubicin, and cisplatin. J Clin Oncol 1989; 7:1318–1326.
239. Wilke H, Preusser P, Fink U, et al: Neoadjuvant chemotherapy of primarily unresectable gastric cancer. International Conference on

Biology and Treatment of Gastrointestinal Malignancies. Frankfurt, Germany, 1992.
240. Verschueren R, Willemse P, Sleijfer D, et al: Combined chemotherapeutic-surgical approach of locally advanced gastric cancer [Abstract]. Proceedings of the American Society of Clinical Oncology 1988; 7:355.
241. Rougier P, Mahjoubi M, Lasser P, et al: Neoadjuvant chemotherapy in locally advanced gastric carcinoma—a phase II trial with combined continuous intravenous 5-fluorouracil and bolus cisplatinum [Abstract]. Eur J Cancer 1994; 30A:1269.
242. Fink U, Schuhmacher C, Stein HJ, et al: Preoperative chemotherapy for stage III–IV gastric carcinoma: feasibility, response and outcome after complete resection. Br J Surg 1995; 82:1248–1252.
243. Alexander HR, Grem JL, Hamilton JM, et al: Thymidylate synthase protein expression. Association with response to neoadjuvant chemotherapy and resection for locally advanced gastric and gastroesophageal adenocarcinoma. Cancer J Sci Am 1995; 1:49.
244. Kang YK, Choi DW, Im YH, et al: A phase III randomized comparison of neoadjuvant chemotherapy followed by surgery versus surgery for locally advanced stomach cancer [Abstract]. Proceedings of the American Society of Clinical Oncology 1996; 15:215.
245. Ajani JA, Ota DM, Jessup JM, et al: Resectable gastric carcinoma. An evaluation of preoperative and postoperative chemotherapy. Cancer 1991; 68:1501.
246. Ajani JA, Mayer RJ, Ota DM, et al: Preoperative and postoperative combination chemotherapy for potentially resectable gastric carcinoma. J Natl Cancer Inst 1993; 85:1839–1844.
247. Kelsen D, Karpeh M, Schwartz G, et al: Neoadjuvant therapy of high-risk gastric cancer: a phase II trial of preoperative FAMTX and postoperative intraperitoneal fluorouracil-cisplatin plus intravenous fluorouracil. J Clin Oncol 1996; 14:1818–1828.
248. Crookes P, Leichman CG, Leichman L, et al: Systemic chemotherapy for gastric carcinoma followed by postoperative intraperitoneal therapy: a final report. Cancer 1997; 79:1767–1775.
249. Fink U, Stein HJ, Schuhmacher C, et al: Neoadjuvant chemotherapy for gastric cancer: update. World J Surg 1995; 19:509–516.
250. Kelsen DP: Adjuvant and neoadjuvant therapy for gastric cancer. Semin Oncol 1996; 23:379–389.
251. Ajani JA, Mansfield PF, Janjan N, et al: Preoperative chemoirradiation therapy in patients with potentially resectable gastric carcinoma: a multi-institution pilot [Abstract]. Proceedings of the American Society of Clinical Oncology 1998; 17:283A.
252. Moertel CG, Engstrom P, Lavin PT, et al: Chemotherapy of gastric and pancreatic carcinoma: a controlled evaluation of combinations of 5-fluorouracil with nitrosoureas and "lactones." Surgery 1979; 85:509–513.
253. MacDonald JS, Schein PS, Woolley PV, et al: 5-Fluorouracil, doxorubicin, and mitomycin (FAM) combination chemotherapy for advanced gastric cancer. Ann Intern Med 1980; 93:533–536.
254. Cullinan SA, Moertel CG, Fleming TR, et al: A comparison of three chemotherapeutic regimens in the treatment of advanced pancreatic and gastric carcinoma. Fluorouracil vs fluorouracil and doxorubicin vs fluorouracil, doxorubicin, and mitomycin. JAMA 1985; 253:2061–2067.
255. Cullinan SA, Moertel CG, Wieand HS, et al: Controlled evaluation of three drug combination regimens versus fluorouracil alone for the therapy of advanced gastric cancer. North Central Cancer Treatment Group. J Clin Oncol 1994; 12:412–416.
256. Stahl M, Wilke H, Preusser P, et al: Etoposide, leucovorin, and 5-fluorouracil (ELF) in advanced gastric carcinoma—final results of a phase II study in elderly patients or patients with cardiac risk [Abstract]. Onkologie 1991; 14:314.
257. Wils JA, Klein HO, Wagner DJT, et al: Sequential high-dose methotrexate and fluorouracil combined with doxorubicin—a step ahead in the treatment of advanced gastric cancer: a trial of the European Organization for Research and Treatment of Cancer Gastrointestinal Tract Cooperative Group. J Clin Oncol 1991; 9:827–831.
258. Kelsen D, Atiq OT, Saltz L, et al: FAMTx versus etoposide, doxorubicin, and cisplatin: a random assignment trial in gastric cancer. J Clin Oncol 1992; 10:541–548.
259. Wilke H, Wils J, Rougier P, et al: Preliminary analysis of a randomized phase III trial of FAMTx versus ELF versus cisplatin/FU in advanced gastric cancer. A trial of the EORTC Gastrointestinal Tract Cancer Cooperative Group and the AIO (Arbeitsge-Meinschaft Internistische Onkologie) [Abstract]. Proceedings of the American Society of Clinical Oncology 1995; 14:206.
260. Webb A, Cunningham D, Scarffe JH, et al: Randomized trial comparing epirubicin, cisplatin, and fluorouracil versus fluorouracil, doxorubicin, and methotrexate in advanced esophagogastric cancer. J Clin Oncol 1997; 15:261–267.
261. Murad AM, Santiago FF, Petroianu A, et al: Modified therapy with 5-fluorouracil, doxorubicin and methotrexate in advanced gastric cancer. Cancer 1993; 72:37–41.
262. Pyrhonen S, Kuitunen T, Nyandoto P, et al: Randomised comparison of fluorouracil, epidoxorubicin and methotrexate (FEMTx) plus supportive care with supportive care alone in patients with non-resectable gastric cancer. Br J Cancer 1995; 71:587–591.
263. Glimelius B, Ekstrom K, Hoffman K, et al: Randomized comparison between chemotherapy plus best supportive care with best supportive care in advanced gastric cancer. Ann Oncol 1997; 8:163–168.
264. Maor MH, Velasquez WS, Fuller LM, et al: Stomach conservation in stage IE and IIE gastric non-Hodgkin's lymphoma. J Clin Oncol 1990; 8:266–271.

Small Intestine

265. Garvin PJ, Herrman V, Kaminski DL, et al: Benign and malignant tumors of the small intestine. Curr Publ Cancer 1979; 3:1–46.
266. Sindelar WF: Cancer of the small intestine. In: DeVita VT Jr, Hellman S, Rosenberg SA (eds): Cancer, Principles and Practice of Oncology, 3rd ed, pp 875–894. Philadelphia, J.B. Lippincott Co., 1989.
267. Ashley SW, Wills SA Jr: Tumors of the small intestine. Semin Oncol 1989; 15:116–128.
268. Coit DG: Cancer of the small intestine. In: DeVita VT Jr, Hellman S, Rosenberg SA (eds): Cancer, Principles and Practice of Oncology, 4th ed, pp 1128–1143. Philadelphia, Lippincott-Raven, 1997.
269. Marks C: Carcinoid Tumors. A Clinicopathologic Study, pp 1–154. Boston, G.K. Hall, 1979.
270. Willett C, Warshaw AL, Convery K, et al: Patterns of failure after pancreatoduodenectomy for ampullary carcinoma. Surg Gynecol 1993; 176:33–38.
271. Coia L, Hoffman J, Scher R, et al: Preoperative chemoradiation for adenocarcinoma of the pancreas and duodenum. Int J Radiat Oncol Biol Phys 1994; 30:161–167.

Colon and Rectum

272. Welch CE, Giddings WP: Carcinoma of colon and rectum. Observations on Massachusetts General Hospital cases. N Engl J Med 1951; 244:859–867.
273. Morgenstern L, Lee SE: Spatial distribution of colonic carcinoma. Arch Surg 1978; 113:1142–1143.
274. Greenwald P, Lanza E, Eddy GA: Dietary fiber in the reduction of colon cancer risk. J Am Diet Assoc 1987; 87:1178–1188.
275. Armstrong B, Doll R: Environmental factors and cancer incidence and mortality in different countries, with special reference to dietary practices. Int J Cancer 1975; 15:617–631.
276. Bussey HJR: Familial Polyposis Coli. Family Studies, Histopathology, Differential Diagnosis, and Results of Treatment. Baltimore, Johns Hopkins University Press, 1975.
277. Cannon-Albright LA, Skolnick MH, Bishop DT, et al: Common inheritance of susceptibility to colonic adenomatous polyps and associated colorectal cancers. N Engl J Med 1988; 319:533–537.
277a. Feinberg AP, Vogelstein B: Alterations in DNA methylation in human neoplasia. Semin Surg Oncol 1987; 3:149–151.
278. Fenoglio-Preiser CM, Hutter RVP: Colorectal polyps: Pathologic diagnosis and clinical significance. Cancer 1985; 35:322–344.
279. McDermott FT: Carcinoma of the colon. In: Hughes E, Cuthbertson AM, Killingback MK (eds): Colorectal Surgery, pp 382–412. New York, Churchill-Livingstone, 1983.
280. Sugarbaker PH: Role of carcinoembryonic antigen assay in the management of cancer. Adv Immunol Cancer Ther 1985; 1:167–193.
281. Winawer ST, Fletcher RH, Miller L, et al: Colorectal cancer screening: clinical guidelines and rationale. Gastroenterology 1997; 112:594–642.
282. Fleischer DE, Goldberg SB, Browning TH, et al: Detection and surveillance of colorectal cancer. JAMA 1989; 261:580–586.
283. Kelvin GM: Radiologic approach to the detection of colorectal neoplasia. Radiol Clin North Am 1982; 20:743–759.
284. Dent TL, Kukora JS, Buinewicz BR: Endoscopic screening and surveillance for gastrointestinal malignancy. Surg Clin North Am 1989; 69:1205–1225.
285. Beynon J: An evaluation of the role of rectal endosonography in rectal cancer. Ann Royal Coll Surg (Engl) 1989; 71:131–139.
286. Gunderson LL, Sosin H: Adenocarcinoma of the rectum: areas of

failure found at reoperation (second or symptomatic look) following curative surgery for adenocarcinoma of the rectum. Clinicopathologic correlation and implications for adjuvant therapy. Cancer 1974; 34:1278–1292.

287. Gunderson LL, Martenson JA: Postoperative adjuvant irradiation with or without chemotherapy for rectal cancer. Semin Radiat Oncol 1993; 1:55–63.
288. Physicians' Data Query. Colon cancer. Bethesda, National Cancer Institute, January 1998.
289. Physicians' Data Query. Rectal cancer. Bethesda, National Cancer Institute, January 1998.
290. Kerman HD, Roberson SH, Bloom TS, et al: Rectal carcinoma. Long-term experience with moderately high-dose preoperative radiation and low anterior resection. Cancer 1992; 69:2813–2819.
291. Gunderson LL: Indications for and results of combined modality treatment of colorectal cancer. Acta Oncol 1999; 38:7–21.
292. Chan KW, Boey J, Wong SKC: A method of reporting radial invasion and surgical clearance of rectal carcinoma. Histopathology 1983; 9:1319–1327.
293. Hoskins RB, Gunderson LL, Dosoretz DE, et al: Adjuvant postoperative radiotherapy in carcinoma of the rectum and rectosigmoid. Cancer 1985; 55:61–71.
294. Schild SE, Martenson JA, Gunderson LL, et al: Postoperative adjuvant therapy of rectal cancer. Int J Radiat Oncol Biol Phys 1989; 17:55–62.
295. Willett CG, Tepper JE, Cohen AM, et al: Failure patterns following curative resection of colonic carcinoma. Ann Surg 1984; 200:685–690.
296. Duttenhaver JR, Hoskins RB, Gunderson LL, et al: Adjuvant postoperative radiation therapy in the management of adenocarcinoma of the colon. Cancer 1986; 57:955–963.
297. Willett CG, Fung CY, Kaufman DS, et al: Postoperative radiation therapy for high-risk colonic carcinoma. J Clin Oncol 1993; 11:1112–1117.
298. Moertel CG: Chemotherapy of gastrointestinal cancer. N Engl J Med 1978; 299:1049–1059.
299. Parker WB, Cheng YC: Metabolism and mechanism of action of 5-fluorouracil. Pharmacol Ther 1990; 48:381–395.
300. Sobrero AF, Aschele C, Bertino JR: Fluorouracil in colorectal cancer—a tale of two drugs: implications for biochemical modulation. J Clin Oncol 1997; 15:368–381.
301. Cunliffe WJ, Sugarbaker PH: Gastrointestinal malignancy: rationale for adjuvant therapy using early postoperative intraperitoneal chemotherapy. Br J Surg 1985; 76:1082–1090.
302. Sugarbaker PH, Gianola FJ, Speyer JC, et al: Prospective randomized trial of intravenous versus intraperitoneal 5-fluorouracil in patients with advanced primary colon or rectal cancer. Surgery 1985; 98:414–421.
303. Houghton JA, Maroda SJ, Phillips JO, et al: Biochemical determination of responsiveness to 5-fluorouracil and its derivatives in xenographs of human colorectal adenocarcinoma in mice. Cancer Res 1981; 41:144–149.
304. Keyomarsi K, Moran RG: Folinic acid augmentation of the effects of fluoropyrimidines on murine and human leukemic cells. Cancer Res 1986; 46:5229–5235.
305. Ensminger WD, Gyves JW: Clinical pharmacology of hepatic arterial chemotherapy. Semin Oncol 1983; 10:176–182.
306. Niederhuber JE, Ensminger W, Gyves J, et al: Regional chemotherapy of colorectal cancer metastatic to the liver. Cancer 1984; 53:1336–1344.
307. Hsian YH, Hertzberg R, Hecht S, et al: Camptothecin induces protein-linked DNA breaks via mammalian DNA topoisomerase I. J Biol Chem 1985; 260:14873–14878.
308. Shimada Y, Yoshino M, Wakui A, et al: Phase II study of CPT-11, a new camptothecin derivative, in metastatic colorectal cancer. J Clin Oncol 1993; 11:909–913.
309. Conti JA, Kemeny N, Saltz L, et al: Irinotecan is an active agent in untreated patients with metastatic colorectal cancer. J Clin Oncol 1996; 14:709–715.
310. Pitot HC, Wender DB, O'Connell MJ, et al: A phase II trial of irinotecan (CPT-11) in patients with metastatic colorectal carcinoma. J Clin Oncol 1997; 15:2910–2919.
311. Woynarowski JM, Chapman WG, Napier C, et al: Sequence- and region-specificity of oxaliplatin adducts in naked and cellular DNA. Mol Pharmacol 1998; 54:770–777.
312. Petersen LN, Mamonta EL, Stevajsner T, et al: Increased gene specific repair of cisplatin induced crosslinks in cisplatin resistant cell lines and studies on carrier liquid specificity. Carcinogenesis 1996; 17:2597–2602.
313. Williams NS: Changing patterns in the treatment of rectal cancer. Br J Surg 1989; 76:5–6.
314. Gilbert SG: Symptomatic local tumor failure following abdominoperineal resection. Int J Radiat Oncol Biol Phys 1978; 4:801–807.
315. Rothenberger DA, Wong WD: Rectal cancer—adequacy of surgical management. Surg Ann 1985; 17:309–331.
316. Curley SA, Roh MS, Rich TA: Surgical therapy of early rectal carcinoma. Hematol Oncol Clin North Am 1989; 3:87–102.
317. Rosen L, Veidenheimer MC, Coller JA, et al: Mortality, morbidity and patterns of recurrence after abdominoperineal resection for cancer of the rectum. Dis Colon Rectum 1982; 25:202–208.
318. Mohiuddin M, Marks G: High dose preoperative irradiation for cancer of the rectum, 1976–1988. Int J Radiat Oncol Biol Phys 1991; 20:37–43.
319. Devereux DF, Eisenstat T, Zinkin L: The safe and effective use of postoperative radiation therapy in modified Astler Coller stage C3 rectal cancer. Cancer 1989; 63:2393–2396.
320. Radice E, Nelson H, Merrill S, et al: Primary myocutaneous flap closure following resection of locally advanced pelvic malignancies. Br J Surg 1999; 86:349–354.
321. Lavery IC, Jones IT, Weakley FL, et al: Definitive management of rectal cancer by contact (endocavitary) irradiation. Dis Colon Rectum 1987; 30:835–838.
322. Gerard JP, Ayzac L, Coquard R, et al: Endocavitary irradiation for early rectal carcinomas T1 (T2). A series of 101 patients treated with the Papillon's technique. Int J Radiat Oncol Biol Phys 1996; 34:775–783.
323. Leaming R: Radiation therapy in the clinical management of neoplasm of the colon, rectum and anus. In: Stearns MW (ed): Neoplasms of the Colon, Rectum and Anus, pp 143–153. New York, John Wiley and Sons, 1980.
324. Cummings BJ: Radiation therapy and rectal carcinoma: The Princess Margaret Hospital experience. Br J Surg 1985; 72(suppl):64–65.
325. Brierly JD, Cummings BJ, Wong CS, et al: Adenocarcinoma of the rectum treated by radical external radiation therapy. Int J Radiat Oncol Biol Phys 1995; 31:255–259.
326. Gunderson LL, Russell AH, Llewellyn HJ, et al: Treatment planning for colorectal cancer: radiation and surgical techniques and value of small-bowel films. Int J Radiat Oncol Biol Phys 1985; 11:1379–1393.
327. O'Connell MJ, Gunderson LL, Fleming TR: Surgical adjuvant therapy of rectal cancer. Semin Oncol 1988; 15:138–145.
328. Fisher B, Wolmark N, Rockette H, et al: Postoperative adjuvant chemotherapy or radiation therapy for rectal cancer: Results from NSABP protocol R-01. J Natl Cancer Inst 1988; 80:21–29.
329. Gastrointestinal Tumor Study Group: Prolongation of the disease-free interval in surgically treated rectal carcinoma. N Engl J Med 1985; 312:1465–1472.
330. Gastrointestinal Tumor Study Group: Survival after postoperative combination treatment for rectal cancer. N Engl J Med 1986; 314:1294–1295.
331. Krook J, Moertel C, Gunderson LL, et al: Effective surgical adjuvant therapy for high-risk rectal carcinoma. N Engl J Med 1991; 324:709–715.
332. Tveit KM, Guldvog I, Hagen S, et al: Randomized controlled trial of postoperative radiotherapy and short-term time-scheduled 5-fluorouracil against surgery alone in the treatment of Dukes B and C rectal cancer. Norwegian Adjuvant Rectal Cancer Project Group. Am J Surg 1997; 84:1130–1135.
333. Swedish Rectal Cancer Trial: Improved survival with preoperative radiotherapy in resectable rectal cancer. N Engl J Med 1997; 336:980–987.
334. Enker WE, Laffer VT, Block GE: Enhanced survival of patients with colon and rectal cancer is based upon wide anatomic resection. Ann Surg 1979; 190:350–360.
335. Umpleby HC, Williamson RCW: Anastomotic recurrence in large bowel cancer. Br J Surg 1987; 74:873–878.
336. Cotait R, Lesser MC, Enker WE: Prophylactic oophorectomy in surgery for large bowel cancer. Dis Colon Rectum 1983; 26:6–11.
337. Goldberg RM, Fleming TR, Tangen CM, et al: Surgery for recurrent colon cancer: strategies for identifying resectable recurrence and success rates after resection. Eastern Cooperative Oncology Group, the North Central Cancer Treatment Group, and the Southwest Oncology Group. Ann Intern Med 1998; 129:27–35.
338. Gunderson LL, Sosin H, Levitt S: Extrapelvic colon—areas of

failure in a reoperation series: Implications for adjuvant therapy. Int J Radiat Oncol Biol Phys 1985; 11:731–741.
339. Russell AH, Pelton J, Reheis CE, et al: Adenocarcinoma of the colon: an autopsy study with implications for new therapeutic strategies. Cancer 1985; 56:1446–1451.
340. Galandiuk S, Wieand HS, Moertel CG, et al: Patterns of recurrence after curative resection of carcinoma of the colon and rectum. Surg Gynecol Obstet 1992; 174:27–32.
341. Verhaegen H, DeCree J, DeCock W, et al: Levamisole therapy in patients with colorectal cancer. In: Terry WD, Rosenberg SA (eds): Immunotherapy of Human Cancer, pp 225–229. New York, Excerpta Medica, Elsevier North Holland, 1982.
342. Laurie JA, Moertel CG, Fleming TR, et al: Surgical adjuvant therapy of large-bowel carcinoma: an evaluation of levamisole and fluorouracil: the North Central Cancer Treatment Group and Mayo Clinic. J Clin Oncol 1989; 7:1447–1456.
343. Kovach JS, Svingen PA, Schaid DJ: Levamisole potentiation of fluorouracil antiproliferative activity mimicked by orthovanadate, an inhibitor of tyrosine phosphatase. J Natl Cancer Inst 1992; 84:515–519.
344. Einhorn LH: Improvement in fluorouracil chemotherapy. J Clin Oncol 1989; 7:1377–1379.
345. O'Connell MJ, Mailliard JA, Kahn MJ: Controlled trial of fluorouracil and low dose leucovorin given for six months as postoperative adjuvant therapy for colon cancer. J Clin Oncol 1997; 15:246–250.
346. Wolmark N, Rockette H, Fisher B, et al: The benefit of leucovorin-modulated fluorouracil as postoperative adjuvant therapy for primary colon cancer: Results from National Surgical Adjuvant Breast and Bowel Project protocol C-03. J Clin Oncol 1993; 11:1879–1887.
347. Haller DG, Catalano P, Macdonald JS, et al: Fluorouracil (FU), leucovorin (LV), and levamisole (LEV) adjuvant therapy for colon cancer: four-year results of INT-0089 [Abstract]. Proceedings of the American Society of Clinical Oncology 1997; 16:265a.
348. Wolmark N, Bryant J, Smith R, et al: Adjuvant 5-fluorouracil and leucovorin with or without interferon alfa-2a in colon carcinoma: National Surgical Adjuvant Breast and Bowel Project protocol C-05. J Natl Cancer Inst 1998; 90:1810–1816.
349. Mamounas EP, Rockette H, Jones J, et al: Comparative efficacy of adjuvant chemotherapy in patients with Dukes' B vs Dukes' C colon cancer. Results from four NSABP adjuvant studies (C-01, C-02, C-03, C-04) [Abstract]. Proceedings of the American Society of Clinical Oncology 1996; 15:205.
350. Erlichman C, Marsoni S, Seitz JF, et al: Event-free and overall survival is increased by FUFA in resected B colon cancer: a pooled analysis of five randomized trials [Abstract]. Proceedings of the American Society of Clinical Oncology 1997; 16:280.
351. Reithmuller G, Holz E, Schlimok G, et al: Monoclonal antibody therapy for resected Dukes' C colorectal cancer: seven-year outcome of a multicenter randomized trial. J Clin Oncol 1998; 16:1788–1794.
352. Taylor I, Machin D, Mullee M, et al: Randomized controlled trial of adjuvant portal vein cytotoxic perfusion in colorectal cancer. Br J Surg 1985; 72:359–363.
353. Rougier P, Sahmoud T, Nitti D, et al: Adjuvant portal-vein infusion of fluorouracil and heparin in colorectal cancer: a randomized trial. Lancet 1998; 351:1677–1681.
354. Liver Infusion Meta-Analysis Group: Portal vein infusion of cytotoxic drugs after colorectal cancer surgery: a meta-analysis of 10 randomized studies involving 4000 patients. J Natl Cancer Inst 1997; 89:497–505.
355. Russell AH, Tong D, Dawson LE, et al: Adenocarcinoma of the proximal colon. Sites of initial dissemination and patterns of recurrence following surgery alone. Cancer 1984; 53:360–367.
356. Minsky BD, Mies C, Rich TA, et al: Potentially curative surgery of colon cancer: Patterns of failure and survival. J Clin Oncol 1988; 6:106–118.
357. Turner SS, Vieira EF, Ager PJ, et al: Elective postoperative radiotherapy for locally advanced colorectal cancer. A preliminary report. Cancer 1977; 40:105–108.
358. Shehata WM, Meyer RL, Jazy FK, et al: Regional adjuvant irradiation for adenocarcinoma of the cecum. Int J Radiat Oncol Biol Phys 1987; 13:843–846.
359. Gunderson LL, Martenson JA: Cancers of the colon and rectum. In: Levitt S, Kahn F, Potish R (eds): Technological Basis of Radiation Therapy, 2nd ed, pp 342–350. Philadelphia, Lea & Febiger, 1991.
360. Withers R, Cuasay L, Mason K, et al: Elective radiation therapy in the curative treatment of cancer of the rectum and rectosigmoid. In: Strocklin JR, Romsdahl MM (eds): Gastrointestinal Cancer, pp 351–362. New York, Raven Press, 1981.
361. Atliych FF, Stearns MW: Second-look laparotomy based on CEA elevation in colorectal cancer. Cancer 1981; 47:2119–2125.
362. Martin EW, Minton JP, Carey LC: CEA-directed second-look surgery in the asymptomatic patient after primary resection of colorectal carcinoma. Ann Surg 1985; 202:310–317.
363. Williams LF, Huddleston CB, Sawyers JL, et al: Is total pelvic exenteration reasonable primary treatment for rectal carcinoma? Ann Surg 1988; 207:670–678.
364. Minsky BD, Mies C, Rich TA, et al: Colloid carcinoma of the colon and rectum. Cancer 1987; 60:3103–3112.
365. Minsky BD, Mies C, Rich TA, et al: Potentially curative surgery of colon cancer: The influence of blood vessel invasion. J Clin Oncol 1988; 6:119–127.
366. McDermott FT, Hughes ESR, Paihl E, et al: Prognosis in relation to symptom duration in colon cancer. Br J Surg 1981; 68:846–849.
367. Rosemungy AS, Block GE, Shihab F: Surgical treatment of carcinoma of the abdominal colon. Surg Gynecol Obstet 1988; 167:399–405.
368. Saadia R, Schain M: Local treatment of carcinoma of the rectum. Surg Gynecol Obstet 1988; 166:481–486.
369. Blumberg N, Heal JM, Murphy P, et al: Association between transfusion of whole blood and recurrence of cancer. Br J Med 1986; 293:530–533.
370. Donohue JH, Williams S, Cha S, et al: Perioperative blood transfusions do not affect disease recurrence of patients undergoing curative resection of colorectal carcinoma: a Mayo/North Central Cancer Treatment Group study. J Clin Oncol 1995; 13:1671–1678.
371. Krasna MJ, Glancbaum L, Cody RP, et al: Vascular and neural invasion in colorectal carcinoma. Incidence and prognostic significance. Cancer 1988; 61:1018–1023.
372. NIH Consensus Conference: Adjuvant therapy for patients with colon and rectal cancer. JAMA 1990; 264:1444–1450.
373. MRC Working Party: The evaluation of low dose preoperative x-ray therapy in the management of operable rectal cancer: results of a randomly controlled trial. Br J Surg 1984; 71:21–25.
374. Gerard A, Buyse M, Nordlinger B, et al: Preoperative radiotherapy as adjuvant treatment in rectal cancer: final results of a randomized study (EORTC). Ann Surg 1988; 208:606–614.
375. Wassif SB, Langenhorst BL, Hop CJ: The contribution of preoperative radiotherapy in the management of borderline operability rectal cancer. In: Salmon SE, Jones SE (eds): Adjuvant Therapy of Cancer, pp 612–626. New York, Grune & Stratton, 1974.
376. Pahlman L, Glimelius B: Pre- or postoperative radiotherapy in rectal and rectosigmoid carcinoma. Ann Surg 1990; 211:187–195.
377. Frykholm GJ, Glimelius B, Pahlman L: Preoperative or postoperative irradiation in adenocarcinoma of the rectum: final treatment results of a randomized trial and an evaluation of late secondary effects. Dis Colon Rectum 1993; 36:564–572.
378. Gastrointestinal Tumor Study Group: Radiation therapy and fluorouracil with or without semustine for the treatment of patients with surgical adjuvant adenocarcinoma of the rectum. J Clin Oncol 1992; 10:549–557.
379. O'Connell MJ, Martenson JA, Wieand HS, et al: Improving adjuvant therapy for rectal cancer by combining protracted infusion fluorouracil with radiation therapy after curative surgery. N Engl J Med 1994; 331:502–507.
380. Tepper JE, O'Connell MJ, Petroni G, et al: Adjuvant postoperative 5-FU-modulated chemotherapy combined with pelvic radiation therapy for rectal cancer. J Clin Oncol 1997; 15:2030–2039.
381. Willett CG, Kaufman DS, Shellito PC, et al: Adjuvant postoperative radiation therapy of rectal adenocarcinoma. Am J Clin Oncol 1992; 15:371–375.
382. Kollmorgen CF, Meagher AP, Wolff BG, et al: The long-term effect of adjuvant postoperative chemoradiotherapy for rectal carcinoma on bowel function. Ann Surg 1994; 220:676–682.
383. Moertel CG, Fleming TR, MacDonald JS, et al: Levamisole and fluorouracil for adjuvant therapy of resected colon carcinoma. N Engl J Med 1990; 322:352–358.
384. Moertel CG, Fleming TR, McDonald JS, et al: Fluorouracil plus levamisole as an effective adjuvant therapy after resection of stage II colon cancer: a final report. Ann Intern Med 1995; 122:321–326.
385. O'Connell MJ, Laurie JA, Kahn MJ, et al: Prospectively randomized trial of postoperative adjuvant chemotherapy in patients with high-risk colon cancer. J Clin Oncol 1998; 16:295–300.
386. Fabian C, Giri S, Estes N, et al: Adjuvant continuous infusion 5-

FU, whole abdominal radiation and tumor bed boost in high risk stage III colon carcinoma: A Southwest Oncology Group Pilot Study. Int J Radiat Oncol Biol Phys 1995; 32:457–464.
387. Estes NC, Giri S, Fabian C: Patterns of recurrence for advanced colon cancer modified by whole abdominal radiation and chemotherapy. Am J Surg 1996; 62:546–550.
388. Gunderson LL, Dozois RR: Intraoperative irradiation for locally advanced colorectal carcinomas. Perspectives in Colon and Rectal Surgery 1992; 5:1–23.
389. O'Connell MJ, Childs DS, Moertel CG, et al: A prospective controlled evaluation of combined pelvic radiotherapy and methanol extraction residue of BCG (MER) for locally unresectable or recurrent rectal carcinoma. Int J Radiat Oncol Biol Phys 1982; 8:1115–1119.
390. Lybeert ML, Martijn H, de Neve W, et al: Radiotherapy for locoregional relapses of rectal carcinoma after initial radical surgery: definite but limited influence of relapse free survival and survival. Int J Radiat Oncol Biol Phys 1992; 24:241–246.
391. Guiney MJ, Smith JG, Worotniuk V, et al: Radiotherapy treatment for isolated loco-regional recurrence of rectosigmoid cancer following definitive surgery: Peter MacCullum Cancer Institute experience, 1981–1990. Int J Radiat Oncol Biol Phys 1997; 38:1019–1025.
392. Gunderson LL, Cohen AM, Dosoretz DE, et al: Residual, unresectable or recurrent colorectal cancer: external beam irradiation and intraoperative electron beam boost ± resection. Int J Radiat Oncol Biol Phys 1983; 9:1597–1606.
393. Gunderson LL, Martin JK, Beart RW, et al: External beam and intraoperative electron irradiation for locally advanced colorectal cancer. Ann Surg 1988; 207:52–60.
394. Schild SE, Martenson JA, Gunderson LL, et al: Long-term survival and patterns of failure after postoperative radiation therapy for subtotally resected rectal adenocarcinoma. Int J Radiat Oncol Biol Phys 1989; 16:459–463.
395. Willett CG, Shellito PC, Tepper JE, et al: Intraoperative electron beam radiation therapy for primary locally advanced rectal and rectosigmoid carcinoma. J Clin Oncol 1991; 9:843–849.
396. Gunderson LL, Nelson H, Martenson J, et al: Locally advanced primary colorectal cancer: Intraoperative electron and external beam irradiation ± 5FU. Int J Radiat Oncol Biol Phys 1997; 37:601–614.
397. Suzuki K, Gunderson LL, Devine RM, et al: Intraoperative irradiation after palliative surgery for locally recurrent rectal cancer. Cancer 1995; 75:939–952.
398. Schild SE, Gunderson LL, Haddock MG, et al: The treatment of locally advanced colon cancer. Int J Radiat Oncol Biol Phys 1997; 37:51–58.
399. Gunderson LL, Willett CG, Haddock M, et al: Recurrent colorectal-EBRT with or without IOERT or HDR-IORT. In: Gunderson LL, Willett CG, Harrison LB (eds): Intraoperative Irradiation: Techniques and Results, pp 273–306. Totowa, NJ, Humana Press, 1999.
400. Gunderson LL, Nelson H, Martenson J, et al: Intraoperative electron and external beam irradiation with or without 5FU and maximal surgical resection for previously unirradiated locally recurrent colorectal cancer. Dis Colon Rectum 1996; 39:1380–1396.
401. Kramer T, Share R, Kiel K, et al: Intraoperative radiation therapy of colorectal cancer. In: Abe M (ed): Intraoperative Radiation Therapy, pp 308–310. New York, Pergamon Press Inc., 1991.
402. Lanciano R, Calkins A, Wolkov H, et al: A phase I, II study of intraoperative radiotherapy in advanced unresectable or recurrent carcinoma of the rectum: an RTOG study. In: Abe M (ed): Intraoperative Radiation Therapy, pp 311–313. New York, Pergamon Press Inc., 1991.
403. Abuchaibe O, Calvo FA, Azinovic I, et al: Intraoperative radiotherapy in locally advanced recurrent colorectal cancer. Int J Radiat Oncol Biol Phys 1993; 26:859–867.
404. Moertel CG, Schutt AJ, Hahn RG, et al: Therapy of advanced colorectal cancer with a combination of 5-FU, Methyl-CCNU, and Vincristine. J Natl Cancer Inst 1975; 54:69–71.
405. Falkson G, Falkson HC: Fluorouracil, methyl-CCNU, and vincristine in cancer of the colon. Cancer 1976; 38:1468–1470.
406. Posey LE, Morgan LR: Methyl-CCNU vs. Methyl-CCNU and 5-FU in carcinoma of the large bowel. Cancer Treat Rep 1977; 61:1453–1458.
407. Lavin P, Mittelman A, Douglas H, et al: Survival and response to chemotherapy for advanced colorectal carcinoma. An Eastern Cooperative Oncology Group report. Cancer 1980; 46:1536–1543.
408. Lokich J, Fine N, Perri J, et al: Protracted ambulatory venous infusion of 5-fluorouracil. Am J Clin Oncol 1983; 6:103–107.
409. Leichman CG, Fleming TR, Muggia F, et al: Phase II study of fluorouracil and its modulation in advanced colorectal cancer: A Southwest Oncology Group study. J Clin Oncol 1995; 13:1303–1322.
410. Rougier P, Buyse M, Ryan L, et al: Meta-analysis of all trials comparing intravenous bolus administration compared to continuous infusion of 5-fluorouracil in patients with advanced colorectal cancer [Abstract]. Proceedings of the American Society of Clinical Oncology 1997; 16:267a.
411. Gastrointestinal Tumor Study Group: The modulation of 5-fluorouracil with folinic acid (Leucovorin) in metastatic colorectal carcinoma: a prospective randomized phase III trial. J Clin Oncol 1989; 7:1419–1426.
412. Poon MA, O'Connell MJ, Moertel CG, et al: Biochemical modulation of fluorouracil: Evidence of significant improvement of survival and quality of life in advanced colorectal carcinoma. J Clin Oncol 1989; 7:1407–1418.
413. de Gramont A, Bosset JF, Milan C, et al: Randomized trial comparing monthly low-dose leucovorin and fluorouracil bolus with bimonthly high-dose leucovorin and fluorouracil bolus plus continuous infusion for advanced colorectal cancer. J Clin Oncol 1997; 15:808–815.
414. Kohne CH, Schoffski P, Wilke H, et al: Effective biomodulation by leucovorin of high-dose infusion fluorouracil given as a weekly 24-hour infusion: results of a randomized trial in patients with advanced colorectal cancer. J Clin Oncol 1998; 16:418–426.
415. Meta-Analysis Group in Cancer: Reappraisal of hepatic arterial infusion in the treatment of nonresectable liver metastases from colorectal cancer. J Natl Cancer Inst 1996; 88:252–258.
416. Kemeny N, Conti JA, Cohen A, et al: Phase II study of hepatic arterial floxuridine, leucovorin, and dexamethasone for unresectable liver metastases from colorectal carcinoma. J Clin Oncol 1994; 12:2288–2295.
417. Rougier P, Van Cutsem E, Bajetta E, et al: Randomized trial of irinotecan versus fluorouracil by continuous infusion after fluorouracil failure in patients with metastatic colorectal cancer. Lancet 1998; 352:1407–1412.
418. Cunningham D, Pyrrhohen S, James RD, et al: Randomized trial of irinotecan plus supportive care versus supportive care alone after fluorouracil failure for patients with metastatic colorectal cancer. Lancet 1998; 352:1413–1418.
419. Machover D, Diaz-Rubio E, de Gramont A, et al: Two consecutive phase II studies of oxaliplatin (L-OHP) for treatment of patients with advanced colorectal carcinoma resistant to previous treatment with fluoropyrimidines. Ann Oncol 1996; 7:95–98.
420. Diaz-Rubio E, Sastre J, Zaniboni A, et al: Oxaliplatin as a single agent in previously untreated colorectal carcinoma patients: a multicentric study. Ann Oncol 1998; 9:105–108.
421. Levi FA, Zidani R, Vannetzel JM, et al: Chronomodulated versus fixed-infusion-rate delivery of ambulatory chemotherapy with oxaliplatin, fluorouracil, and folinic acid (leucovorin) in patients with colorectal cancer metastases. A randomized multi-institutional trial. J Natl Cancer Inst 1994; 86:1608–1617.
422. Bertheault-Cvitkovic F, Jami A, Ithzaki M, et al: Biweekly intensified ambulatory chronomodulated chemotherapy with oxaliplatin, fluorouracil, and leucovorin in patients with metastatic colorectal cancer. J Clin Oncol 1996; 14:2950–2958.
423. Raymond E, Buquet-Fagot F, Djelloul C, et al: Antitumor activity of oxaliplatin in combination with 5-fluorouracil and the thymidylate synthase inhibitor AG337 in human colon, breast, and ovarian cancers. Anticancer Drugs 1997; 8:876–885.
424. Peeters M, Haller DG: Therapy for early-stage colorectal cancer. Oncology 1999; 13:307–315.
425. Martenson J, Willett C, Sargent D, et al: A phase III study of adjuvant radiation therapy (RT), 5-Fluorouracil (5-FU), and levamisole (Lev) vs 5-FU and Lev in selected patients with resected high risk colon cancer: initial results of INT O130 [Abstract]. Proceedings of the American Society of Clinical Oncology 1999; 18:235a.
426. Adjei AA, Doucette M, Spector T, et al: 5-Ethynyluracil (776C85), an inhibitor of dihydropyrimidine dehydrogenase, permits reliable oral dosing of 5-fluorouracil and prolongs its half-life [Abstract]. Proceedings of the American Society of Clinical Oncology 1995; 14:459.
427. Saltz LB, Kanowitz J, Kemeny NE, et al: Phase I clinical and pharmacokinetic study of irinotecan, fluorouracil, and leucovorin in patients with advanced solid tumors. J Clin Oncol 1996; 14:2959–2967.

428. Fonseca R, Goldberg RM, Erlichman C, et al: Phase I study of CPT-11/5-FU/leucovorin [Abstract]. Proc Am Assoc Canc Res 1997; 38:76.
429. Vanhoefer U, Hastrick A, Kohne CH, et al: Phase I study of a weekly schedule of irinotecan, high-dose leucovorin, and infusional fluorouracil as first-line chemotherapy in patients with advanced colorectal cancer. J Clin Oncol 1999; 17:907–913.
430. Scheithauer W, Kornek GV, Rudere M, et al: Combined irinotecan and oxaliplatin plus granulocyte colony stimulating factor in patients with advanced fluoropyrimidine/leucovorin pretreated colorectal cancer. J Clin Oncol 1999; 17:902–906.
431. Ishikawa T, Sekiguchi F, Fukase Y, et al: Positive correlation between efficacy of capecitabine and doxifluridine and the ratio of thymidine phosphorylase to dihyropyrimidine dehydrogenase activities in tumors in human cancer xenografts. Cancer Res 1998; 58:685–690.
432. Pazdur R, Lassere Y, Rhodes V, et al: Phase II trial of uracil plus tegafur plus oral leucovorin in the treatment of metastatic colorectal carcinoma. J Clin Oncol 1994; 12:2296–2300.
433. Baba H, Ohtsu A, Sakata Y, et al: Late phase II study of S-1 patients with advanced colorectal cancer in Japan [Abstract]. Proceedings of the American Society of Clinical Oncology 1998; 17:277a.
434. Cunningham D: Mature results from three large controlled studies with raltitrexed ('Tomudex'). Br J Cancer 1998; 77(suppl 2):15–21.
435. John W, Clark J, Burris H, et al: Phase II trial of LY 231514 in patients with metastatic colorectal cancer [Abstract]. Proceedings of the American Society of Clinical Oncology 1997; 16:292a.

Anal Carcinoma

436. Doggett SW, Green JP, Cantril ST: Efficacy of radiation therapy alone for limited squamous cell carcinoma of the anal canal. Int J Radiat Oncol Biol Phys 1988; 15:1069–1072.
437. Martenson JA, Gunderson LL: Radiation therapy without chemotherapy in the management of cancer of the anal canal. Cancer 1993; 71:1736–1740.
438. Cummings B, Keane T, Thomas G, et al: Results and toxicity of the treatment of anal canal carcinoma by radiation therapy or radiation therapy and chemotherapy. Cancer 1984; 54:2062–2068.
439. Sischy B, Doggett RLS, Krall JM, et al: Definitive irradiation and chemotherapy for radiosensitization in management of anal carcinoma: interim report on RTOG 83-14. J Natl Cancer Inst 1989; 81:850–856.
440. Schlienger M, Krzisch D, Pene F, et al: Epidermoid carcinoma of the anal canal: Treatment results and prognostic variables in a series of 242 cases. Int J Radiat Oncol Biol Phys 1989; 17:1141–1151.
441. Daling JR, Weiss NS, Hislop TG, et al: Sexual practices, sexually transmitted diseases and the incidence of anal cancer. N Engl J Med 1987; 317:973–977.
442. Mitchell EP: Carcinoma of the anal region. Semin Oncol 1988; 15:146–153.
443. Beahrs OH: Management of cancer of the anus. Am J Roentgenol 1979; 133:791–795.
444. Herzog U, Boss M, Spichtin HP: Endoanal ultrasonography in the follow-up of anal carcinoma. Surg Endosc 1994; 8:1186–1189.
445. Boman BM, Moertel CG, O'Connell MJ, et al: Carcinoma of the anal canal. A clinical and pathologic study of 188 cases. Cancer 1984; 54:114–125.
446. Cummings BJ, Keane TJ, O'Sullivan MB, et al: Epidermoid anal cancer: Treatment by radiation alone or by radiation and 5-fluorouracil with and without mitomycin C. Int J Radiat Oncol Biol Phys 1991; 21:1115–1125.
447. Eschwege F, Lasser P, Chavy A, et al: Squamous cell carcinoma of the anal canal: Treatment by external beam irradiation. Radiother Oncol 1985; 3:145–150.
448. Dobrowsky W: Radiotherapy of epidermoid and anal cancer. Br J Radiol 1989; 62:53–58.
449. Newman G, Calverley DC, Acker BD, et al: The management of carcinoma of the anal canal by external beam radiotherapy, experience in Vancouver 1971–1988. Radiother Oncol 1992; 25:196–202.
450. Svensson C, Goldman S, Friberg B: Radiation treatment of epidermoid cancer of the anus. Int J Radiat Oncol Biol Phys 1993; 27:67–73.
451. Leichman L, Nigro N, Vaitkevicius VK, et al: Cancer of the anal canal: model for preoperative adjuvant combined modality therapy. Am J Med 1985; 78:211–215.
452. Flam MS, John MJ, Mowry PA, et al: Definitive combined modality therapy of carcinoma of the anus: a report of 30 cases including results of salvage therapy in patients with residual disease. Dis Colon Rectum 1987; 30:495–502.
453. Tveit KM, Karlsen KO, Fossa SD, et al: Primary treatment of carcinoma of the anus by combined radiotherapy and chemotherapy. Scand J Gastroenterol 1989; 24:1243–1247.
454. Flam MS, John MJ, Peters T, et al: Radiation and 5-fluorouracil (5-FU) vs radiation, 5-FU, mitomycin C in the treatment of anal canal carcinoma: preliminary results of a phase III randomized RTOG/ECOG intergroup trial [Abstract]. Proceedings of the American Society of Clinical Oncology 1993; 12:192.
455. Flam MS, John M, Pajak T, et al: Radiation (RT) and 5-fluorouracil (5-FU) vs radiation, 5-FU, mitomycin-C (MMC) in the treatment of anal carcinoma: results of a phase III randomized RTOG/ECOG intergroup trial. J Clin Oncol 1996; 14:2527–2539.
456. Martenson JA, Lipsitz S, Wagner H, et al: Phase II trial of radiation therapy, 5-fluorouracil and cisplatin in patients with anal cancer [Abstract]. Int J Radiat Oncol Biol Phys 1995; 32(suppl):158.
457. UK CCCR Anal Cancer Trial Working Party: Epidermoid anal cancer: results from the UK CCCR randomized trial of radiotherapy alone versus radiotherapy, 5-fluorouracil and mitomycin. Lancet 1996; 348:1049–1054.
458. Bartelink H, Roelefson F, Bosset JF, et al: Concomitant radiotherapy and chemotherapy is superior to radiotherapy alone in the treatment of locally advanced anal cancer. Results of a phase III randomized trial of the EORTC radiotherapy and gastrointestinal cooperative groups. J Clin Oncol 1997; 15:2040–2049.
459. Nigro ND, Vaitkevicius VK, Considine B Jr: Combined therapy for cancer of the anal canal a preliminary report. Dis Colon Rectum 1974; 17:354–356.
460. Nigh SS, Smalley SR, Elman AT, et al: Conservative therapy for anal carcinoma: an analysis of prognostic factors [Abstract]. Int J Radiat Oncol Biol Phys 1991; 21(suppl):224.
461. Hughes LL, Rich TA, Delclos L, et al: Radiotherapy for anal cancer: experience from 1979–1987. Int J Radiat Oncol Biol Phys 1989; 17:1153–1160.
462. Constantinou EC, Daly W, Fung CY, et al: Time-dose considerations in the treatment of anal cancer. Int J Radiat Oncol Biol Phys 1997; 39:651–657.
463. Papillon J, Mayer M, Montbarbon JF, et al: A new approach to the management of epidermoid carcinoma of the anal canal. Cancer 1983; 51:1830–1837.
464. Mahjoubi M, Sadek H, Francois E, et al: Epidermoid and carcinoma (EACC): activity of cisplatin (P) and continuous 5-fluorouracil (5-fluorouracil) in metastatic (M) and/or local recurrent (LR) disease [Abstract]. Proceedings of the American Society of Clinical Oncology 1990; 9:114.
465. Brunet R, Sadek H, Vignoud J, et al: Cisplatin (P) and 5-fluorouracil (5-FU) for the neoadjuvant treatment of epidermoid anal canal carcinoma (EACC) [Abstract]. Proceedings of the American Society of Clinical Oncology 1990; 9:104.
466. Ellenhorn JD, Enker WE, Quan SH: Salvage abdominoperineal resection following combined chemotherapy and radiotherapy for epidermoid carcinoma of the anus. Ann Surg Oncol 1994; 1:105–110.
467. John M, Flam M, Berkey B, et al: Five-year results and analyses of a Phase 3 randomized RTOG/ECOG chemoradiation protocol for anal cancer [Abstract]. Proceedings of the American Society of Clinical Oncology 1998; 17:989.
468. John M, Pajak T, Flam M, et al: Dose escalation in chemoirradiation for anal cancer: preliminary results of RTOG 92-08. Cancer J Sci Am 1996; 2:205–211.

28 Cancer of the Major Digestive Glands: Pancreas, Liver, Bile Ducts, Gallbladder

AJAY SANDHU, MD, Radiation Oncology
JAMES L. PEACOCK, MD, Surgical Oncology
JULIA L. SMITH, MD, Medical Oncology

Now good digestion wait on appetite, and health on both!
WILLIAM SHAKESPEARE, *Macbeth*

Perspective

Cancer of the pancreas is the most common cancer of the major digestive glands in the United States; the other sites are affected much less frequently. However, all cancers of the major digestive glands have in common a propensity for advanced stage at presentation. Our ability to image these tumors has been refined and improved over the past two decades, as has the technique for histopathologic diagnosis using fine-needle aspirates. Epidemiologic studies have not been clinically useful in identifying high-risk groups for close surveillance, except in hepatic cancer, and new markers for these cancers have not been found. Recent treatment strategies have included combined-modality therapy, but in most cases a significant survival advantage has not been realized. Nonetheless, numerous innovations, including bone marrow and liver transplantation, now offer a considerable chance for cure in hepatocellular cancer.

Pancreatic Cancer

Epidemiology

In the United States, 28,300 new cases of pancreatic carcinoma were diagnosed in 2000, with an almost equal sex distribution.[6] This incidence rate reflects a slight decline, observed principally among white men, in which the incidence has fallen from 12.8 cases per 100,000 in 1973 to 9.6 cases per 100,000 in 1997.[7] In 2000, there were approximately 28,200 deaths[6]; the incidence-to-death ratio is virtually equal and reflects the almost universally fatal outcome for this lesion. Therefore, despite the decline in incidence, pancreatic cancer remains the fourth leading cause of cancer deaths in this country.[6] Pancreatic cancer is rare before the age of 40, and the majority of cases occur between ages of 60 and 80 years.[7, 8]

Since the 1970s, long-term survival has shown some improvement as a result of better surgical management and improving combined-modality therapies.[9–12] Unfortunately, this improved rate is mostly composed of those patients with localized resectable cancers, negative nodes, and little or no invasion. These patients have a 5-year survival rate of greater than 20% compared with a 7% 5-year survival rate for the remaining cases in most large series.[13]

Etiology

Direct causes of pancreatic cancer have not been identified; however, certain associations and contributing risk factors have been established:

- *Cigarette smoking* is a well-established risk factor, although the incidence does not approach that of lung cancer. The relative risk of pancreatic cancer in smokers is approximately 1.5 times that of the nonsmoking population, and this rate rises with the amount and duration of smoking activity.[14, 15]
- Studies of *dietary relationships* to pancreatic cancer indicate a high fat intake or high meat consumption, or both, are positive risk factors for pancreatic cancer.[16, 17] *Coffee and alcohol consumption* also have been extensively studied.[18, 19] However, although coffee consumption has previously been identified as a risk factor, a comprehensive review by Gordis indicated no such association.[20]
- *Diabetes mellitus* has long been known to be associated with pancreatic cancer, and a meta-analysis showed an increased frequency of pancreatic cancer in

patients with diabetes mellitus.[21] However, despite the association, it is unlikely that diabetes mellitus is a cause-and-effect mechanism.

- Previous *peptic ulcer surgery* has been related not only to a higher risk of gastric cancer but also to greater incidence rates of pancreatic cancer.[22] Similarly, the occurrence of *chronic pancreatitis* often correlates with the incidence of pancreatic cancer, but the extent to which this is a causal relationship remains under investigation.[23–25]
- *Genetic predisposition* may be present in nearly 5% of the cases of pancreatic cancer.[26] The associated syndromes include multiple endocrine neoplasia type I,[27, 28] von Hippel–Lindau syndrome,[29] and hereditary pancreatitis.[30–32]
- The genetics of cancer of the pancreas has been under investigation, particularly with regard to the tumor suppressor genes related to chromosome karyotyping abnormalities (Table 28–1).[33]

Detection and Diagnosis

Clinical Detection

Unfortunately, because of the lack of specific symptoms or signs, pancreatic cancer is invariably diagnosed when it is advanced. The insidious onset of abdominal or back pain, anorexia, early satiety, weight loss, dyspepsia, weakness, fatigue, bloating, nausea, and vomiting are the most common symptoms. These symptoms are typically very vague and, frequently, are overlooked for many months before diagnosis is made. New-onset hyperglycemia without a family history of diabetes mellitus could be a clue. Back pain that characteristically worsens when lying flat or stretching the back occurs in about 25% of cases and is related to the retroperitoneal location of the gland; this pain occurs more with lesions in the body of the gland. If the cancer is located in the head of the pancreas, signs of obstructive jaundice predominate.[34] If the periampullary region or duodenum is involved, gastrointestinal (GI) bleeding may be noted. Lesions in the body or tail of the gland often go undiagnosed until there are advanced locoregional extensions or distant metastases. Less common presentations include psychiatric disturbances (e.g., depression) and migratory thrombophlebitis or thromboembolic phenomenon.

Physical signs of pancreatic cancer may include weight loss, jaundice, abdominal mass, epigastric tenderness, palpable gallbladder, and hepatomegaly; however, at least half of the patients have no physical findings. Metastatic signs include supraclavicular adenopathy (Virchow's nodule), umbilical nodule (Sister Joseph's node), or peritoneal shelf on rectal examination (Blumer's shelf).

Diagnostic Procedures

Diagnosis requires a biopsy of the pancreas or peripancreatic area demonstrating a carcinoma of ductal origin. Frequently, however, the diagnosis is made indirectly by a biopsy of a metastatic site that reveals a histology compatible with pancreatic origin, along with a constellation of other findings that include (1) appropriate presentation for pancreatic carcinoma; (2) a mass in the pancreas detected on ultrasound, computed tomography (CT), magnetic resonance imaging (MRI), or endoscopic retrograde cholangiopancreatography (ERCP) (Table 28–2); and (3) absence of another primary. Tissue or cells for cytology for diagnosis may be obtained from duodenal drainage, ERCP or fine-needle aspirates under ultrasound or CT guidance. It is of interest that, in some series, from 1% to 57% of cases do not have histologic proof of cancer.[35]

Once pancreatic carcinoma is highly suspected, it is usually the surgeon's preference whether percutaneous confirmation is needed before exploration. If the tumor is considered to be operable and the patient is medically fit for major surgery, a biopsy is generally not performed. Percutaneous biopsies tend to have poor sensitivity and, therefore, negative results are unreliable. Angiograms are rarely necessary now that techniques in CT have improved sufficiently to visualize relationships and anatomy of surrounding vessels.

A variety of procedures are being used to diagnose pancreatic cancers:

- *Physical examination* is essential, with emphasis on sites of metastases or local extension: abdominal mass, hepatomegaly, palpable gallbladder, supraclavicular adenopathy, rectal shelf, and umbilical nodule.

TABLE 28–1. **Genes Associated with Pancreatic Cancer**

Chromosome	Gene	Function	Associated Syndrome
Allelic Loss			
3p	Tumor suppressor gene locus		MEN-1, VHL
8p	Multiple genes	Transcription regulation	
9p	p16	Cell cycle	
17p	p53	Cell cycle, apoptosis	
18q	*DPC4*	TGFβ signaling	MEN-1
13q	*BRCA2*	DNA repair?	MEN-1
Chromosome Gain			
8q	Multiple genes	Transcription regulation	
11q	*BCL1*	Cell cycle	MEN-1
20q	*TP53TG5*	Cell cycle, apoptosis	

MEN-1 = multiple endocrine neoplasia type I; VHL = von Hippel–Lindau syndrome; TGFβ = transforming growth factor, type beta.
Modified from Abrams RA: Primary malignancies of the pancreas, periampullary region and hepatobiliary tract—considerations for the radiation oncologist. 41st Annual Scientific Meeting of the American Society for Therapeutic Radiology and Oncology, San Antonio, Texas, October 31 to November 4, 1999.

TABLE 28–2. **Imaging Modalities for Evaluating Carcinoma of the Pancreas**

Method	Diagnosis and Staging Capability	Recommended for Use
Abdominal ultrasound	Helpful in defining primary tumor and evaluating dilated bile ducts and ascites. Useful for evaluating suspected abdominal metastases, especially hepatic.	Yes
Computed tomography (CT)	Most useful of all imaging modalities in determining local invasion and distant metastases.	Yes
Endoscopic retrograde cholangiopancreatography/ percutaneous transhepatic cholangiography (ERCP/PTC)	Very accurate in defining deformity of bile and pancreatic duct and localizing site of obstruction. Useful in the jaundiced patient.	No
Magnetic resonance imaging (MRI)	Morphologic imaging of pancreas and peripancreatic duct for local and distant metastases.	No

- *Ultrasound*: This test is almost invariably used for the initial screening of anyone presenting with jaundice, because of its low cost and ready availability. It has a 95% accuracy in diagnosing obstructive jaundice, and is sensitive in detecting both intrahepatic and extrahepatic bile duct dilatation. Ultrasound has a reported sensitivity and specificity of 80% to 90% in tumor detection[36]; however, the presence of abdominal gas limits its accuracy, as does residual barium in the bowel, obesity, ascites, and hemoclips. Liver metastases can be detected with this modality.
- *Endoscopic ultrasonography*: Recently, endoscopic ultrasonography has been added to the diagnostic armamentarium. This is a relatively new, but highly sensitive, tool that shows much promise in detecting the extent, invasiveness,[37] staging,[38] and resectability of a pancreatic tumor.[39] This technique provides information not available with conventional studies, particularly for small sized tumors.[39] In addition, endoscopic ultrasound–guided fine-needle aspirate biopsies have provided a significant improvement in histologic confirmation.[40]
- *Laparoscopy*: This procedure allows direct visualization of the peritoneal cavity; laparoscopic ultrasonography has a significantly high predictive value for assessing tumor resectability.[41] Nearly one third of patients deemed operable during their routine work-up are found to have small metastases with a laparoscopy. Laparoscopic ultrasound can help identify hepatic and peritoneal metastases and enlarged lymph nodes, and some studies have shown improved staging accuracy over spiral CT.[42, 43]
- *Computed tomography*: Helical CT is the current test of choice for pancreatic carcinoma, and the initial test for suspected carcinoma of the body or tail of the pancreas. It is more reliable than ultrasound in determining and localizing the position and level of bile duct obstruction, and it is also helpful in determining local and nodal extension and liver metastases. It has a diagnostic accuracy rate of over 95% and is close to 100% in staging unresectable tumors.[44]

Although ultrasound is widely used, it is limited by variations inherent to the expertise of the evaluator and the body's physical parameters. Therefore, at present, helical CT scan remains the gold standard, providing an accurate definition of tumor extent. The addition of dynamic CT enhances the physician's ability to predict tumor resectability.

- *Endoscopic retrograde cholangiopancreatography*: If the patient is jaundiced and the site of obstruction is not defined, then ERCP is extremely helpful. It allows visualization (and biopsy) of the duodenum and Vater's ampulla, as well as visualization (and cytology) of both the pancreatic and bile duct, which could be important for resection. ERCP also allows direct visualization and biopsy of ampullary and duodenal cancers. The diagnostic yield is increased by cytologic examinations of pancreatic juice obtained during this procedure. Preoperative stent placement for relief of jaundice is unnecessary in patients with localized cancers who are of good operative risk, and it has been shown to cause a higher risk of perioperative infections.[45] ERCP stent placement is valuable for unresectable tumors and those patients who participate in neoadjuvant treatment protocols.
- *Magnetic resonance imaging*: MRI of the biliary and pancreatic systems has improved significantly with magnetic resonance cholangiopancreatography. Contrast-enhanced MRI with a heavily T2-weighted sequence can illuminate ductal structures with a quality comparable to ERCP or percutaneous cholangiography. However, conventional MRI adds little to the diagnostic evaluation, and it is currently held that there is no definitive advantage in the use of MRI over CT scanning.[46]
- *Positron emission tomography*: Although its use is still experimental, positron emission tomography can be employed to differentiate pancreatic cancer from chronic pancreatitis, and it may be developed as a noninvasive modality to detect and stage pancreatic cancer in the future.[47]
- *Laboratory tests* must include complete blood cell counts, with differential and platelet count, liver enzyme tests, creatinine and blood urea nitrogen, glucose, coagulation tests, and calcium and electrolytes measurements. These tests determine if the patient has any medical contraindications for surgery and evaluate for paraneoplastic manifestation.

A wide variety of serologic markers have been investigated for their usefulness in the diagnosis of pancreatic cancer: serum levels of carbohydrate antigens (CA19-9,

TABLE 28–3. **Histologic Classification of Pancreatic Cancer**

Histologic Type	% Incidence
Carcinoma, all	98
Adenocarcinoma	82
Adenocarcinoma, NOS	69
Papillary adenocarcinoma	0.8
Mucinous	2
Mucin producing	3
Infiltrating duct	4
Other adenocarcinoma*	2
Other carcinoma†	3
Squamous cell carcinoma	0.4
Carcinoma, NOS	13
Sarcoma	0.1
Other and unspecified	1

NOS = not otherwise specified
*Includes adenosquamous, cystadenocarcinoma, acinar cell and others.
†Includes islet cell carcinomas and others.
Modified from Carriaga MT, Henson DE: Liver, gallbladder, extrahepatic, bile ducts, and pancreas. Cancer 1995; 75(suppl):171.

CA50, CA125, CA195, and CA242), and carcinoembryonic antigen (CEA). CA19-9 remains the most useful and extensively studied tumor marker in this disease as a result of its high sensitivity (up to 85% in some studies),[48] but is limited by its low specificity. Nonetheless, it has proved useful in prognosis and follow-up because CA19-9 levels have been shown to predict for tumor volume, survival time after tumor resection,[48] and the success of radiation therapy.[49] Studies also have indicated that using tumor markers in combination can increase the rate of accurate diagnosis. For example, CEA alone is useful in differentiating between cancer and pancreatitis,[50] but it does not have the same level of sensitivity as CA19-9 and CA50. However, when CEA is used in conjunction with CA19-9 and CA125, or CA195 alone, both sensitivity and specificity rates improve.[51, 52]

Classification and Staging

Histopathology

The most common pancreatic carcinoma is the solid adenocarcinoma that arises from the ductal epithelial cells.[53] Other exocrine varieties are rare and include acinar cell carcinomas, cystadenocarcinomas, anaplastic, and squamous cell carcinomas. Cancers of the pancreas may also arise from islet cell components of the gland (Table 28–3).[54]

In approximately 50% to 60% of cases, the tumor is situated in the head of the gland, and in the remaining cases, the cancer is distributed evenly in the body and tail, or some combination of sites. Lesions of the head of the gland tend to be smaller at diagnosis than tail and body lesions; tumor size is a significant prognosis factor, with 2 to 3 cm being the cutoff point.[55, 56] In addition, more than 70% of cases are found to have extension outside the gland at diagnosis[57]; extension affects prognosis, particularly of ampullary carcinomas.[58] Direct extension to the duodenum, stomach, retroperitoneum (especially body and tail), and portal vein is common, as is local lymph node and para-aortic nodal metastases. Liver metastases are frequent and distant metastases to lung, brain, bone, and other sites also occur; indeed there are few distant sites where it has not been described.

Staging

The present staging classification for exocrine pancreatic cancer is shown in Table 28–4[59] and illustrated in Figure 28–1.

Principles of Treatment

A multidisciplinary approach is essential because the median survival time for untreated pancreatic cancer is approximately 6 months.[60] Table 28–5 summarizes the treatment options.

Surgery

Surgery is the only known curative modality, but, even with surgery, cure is infrequent. The percentage of cases deemed resectable is about 5% to 25%, depending on the experience and enthusiasm of the surgeon.[61] The reporting of a large retrospective analysis of approximately 13,560 patients from Britain found only 60 5-year actuarial survivors.[62, 63] The majority of patients had not received resective surgery; however, the largest percentage of survivors came from that group. Indeed, this group was the only one that demonstrated an improvement in outcome over

TABLE 28–4. **TNM Classification of Exocrine Pancreatic Cancer**

Stage	Grouping	Descriptor
I	T1, N0, M0 T2, N0, M0	T1: Primary tumor limited to pancreas; ≤2 cm in greatest dimension T2: Primary tumor limited to pancreas; >2 cm in greatest dimension N0: No regional lymph node metastasis M0: No distant metastases
II	T3, N0, M0	T3: Tumor extends directly to duodenum, common bile duct, or peripancreatic tissues
III	T1–3, N1, M0	N1*: Regional lymph node metastasis
IVA	T4, Any N, M0	T4: Tumor extends directly to stomach, spleen, colon, or adjacent large blood vessels
IVB	Any T, Any N, M1	M1: Distant metastasis

TNM = tumor, nodes, metastases.
*pN1a = metastasis in single regional lymph node; pN1b = metastasis in multiple lymph nodes.
Used with the permission of the American Joint Committee on Cancer (AJCC®), Chicago, Illinois. The original source for this material is the AJCC® Cancer Staging Manual, 5th edition (1997), published by Lippincott-Raven Publishers, Philadelphia, Pennsylvania.

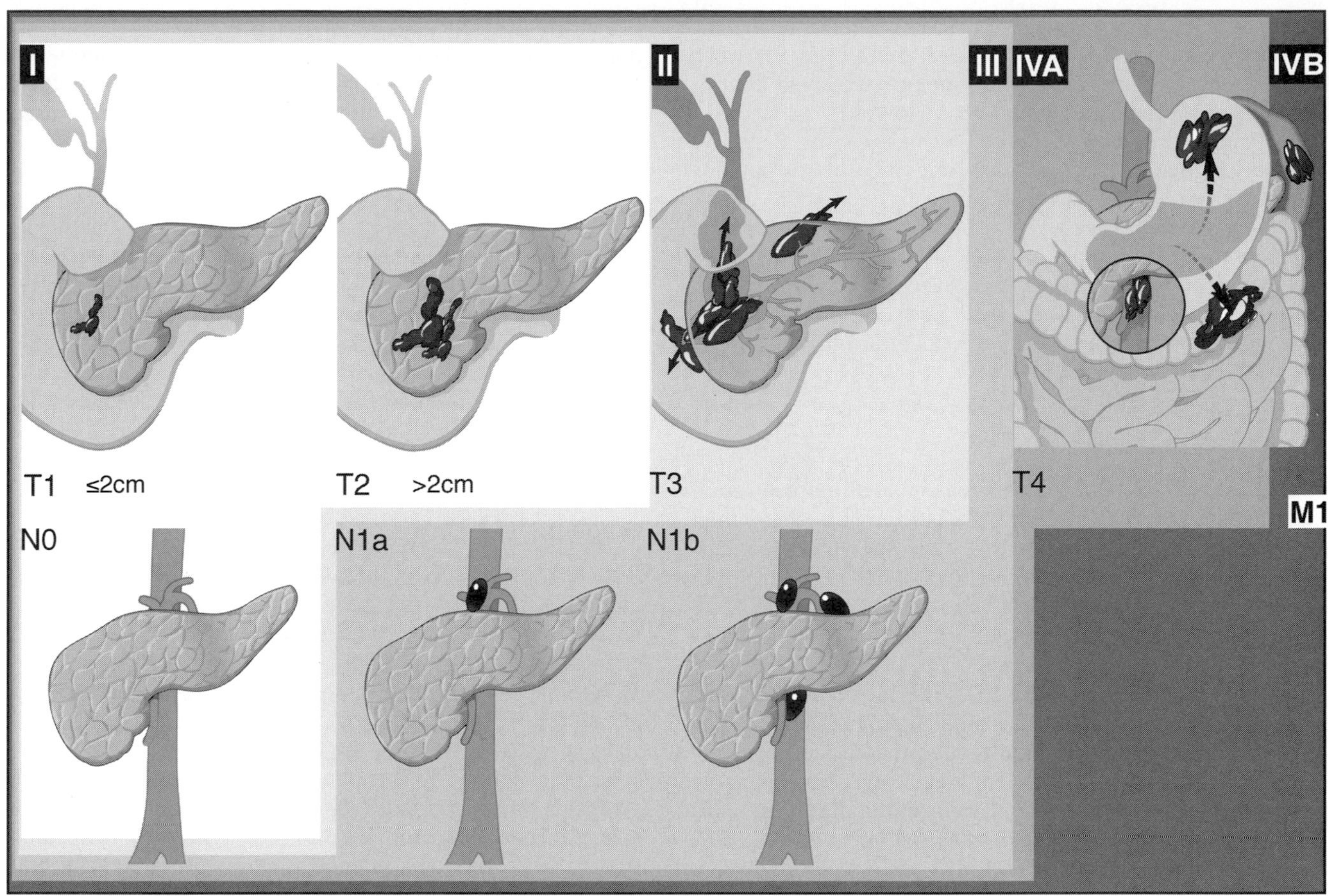

Figure 28–1. Anatomic staging for cancer of the pancreas.

sequential time periods. In general, 20% of patients are deemed operable at presentation, and another 15% have a laparotomy with biopsy only. Approximately 35% are explored and undergo some type of palliative bypass procedure, but only 15% to 20% are eligible for a total resection.

The standard operation for lesions of the tail and body of the gland is a distal or total pancreatectomy.[64] For lesions in the head of the pancreas, a pancreaticoduodenectomy, or Whipple procedure, is standard. This operation consists of *en bloc* removal of the duodenum, head of the pancreas, distal portion of the common duct and, occasionally, the distal stomach with the pylorus. The gastric pouch is reanastomosed to the jejunum, and the common duct and pancreatic duct are joined to the jejunum proximal to the gastrojejunostomy. Complications of surgery include GI bleeding, sepsis, and anastomotic leaks; recent reports document improvements in morbidity and survival, and, in general, perioperative mortality has fallen to about 1% at present.[65] Some surgeons prefer a total pancreatectomy for a lesion anywhere in the gland because it avoids pancreaticojejunal anastomotic problems; however total pancreatectomy is not a widely accepted technique.[66, 67]

In recent years, duodenopancreatectomy has gained acceptance because it leaves the pylorus intact and avoids the effects of a partial gastrectomy.[64] Pyloric sparing, where possible, avoids a vagotomy and gastric resection, reduces operating time, and avoids some nutritional problems. Clips can also be placed around the tumor area for identification, if postoperative radiation therapy is planned.[35]

Radiation Therapy

Potentially, radiation therapy could be used in several postoperative settings: (1) when there is no residual disease, but

TABLE 28–5. **Multidisciplinary Treatment Decisions: Pancreas**

Stage	Surgery		Radiation Therapy	Chemotherapy
Localized T1, T2, N1: head	Whipple procedure ± pyloric sparing		± Postop RT	± Postop CT
tail	Distal pancreatectomy	or		
	Radical pancreatic resection		+ Postop RT	+ Postop CT
Advanced T3, T4, N1	Palliative bypass		Chemoradiation	
Any T, Any N, M1	NR		Palliative RT	IC

RT = radiation therapy; CT = chemotherapy; IC = investigational clinical trials; NR = not recommended.

still a high incidence of recurrence; (2) when microscopic or macroscopic disease has been left behind; or (3) when the disease is considered locally unresectable, and there is no evidence of distant metastases. However, as in other cancers that originate in the abdominal cavity, definitive radiation is made difficult by the tolerance of surrounding structures, such as spinal cord, stomach, liver, small bowel, and kidney. Some investigators have suggested the use of postoperative irradiation for patients with a high risk of residual microscopic disease; however, the few small trials that were performed, both with and without additional chemotherapy, have demonstrated no improvement in survival or local control.[61, 65]

Chemotherapy

For adenocarcinoma of the pancreas, a small percentage of patients may have temporary palliation with chemotherapy.[69] Single-agent regimens that have shown some measurable activity include 5-fluorouracil (5-FU) (28% response),[70] mitomycin C (27%),[71] and gemcitabine (11%).[72, 73] In general, the combination regimens that have been investigated have been based on 5-FU, and newer clinical trials include combinations of 5-FU, cisplatin, or gemcitabine.[74, 75] However, the nucleoside analogue gemcitabine alone has been shown to be effective in advanced pancreatic cancer. In one randomized trial, comparing gemcitabine with 5-FU, gemcitabine demonstrated significant survival and symptomatic benefits over 5-FU.[76]

Combined-Modality Therapy

Gastrointestinal Tumor Study Group (GITSG) trials established the role of postoperative chemoradiotherapy in resected tumors by demonstrating improvements in patient survival.[77, 78] These are old studies, however, and have been criticized for small patient size and suboptimal radiation therapy, which involved a split course of delivery. A subsequent prospective, single-institution study has reported results of adjuvant therapy based on the GITSG studies.[79] Standard dose schedule and intensity with modern techniques was employed for the delivery of the radiation therapy. Although this study was nonrandomized, there was, nonetheless, a favorable effect on survival with the use of adjuvant therapy by both univariate and multivariate analysis. However, another study comparing neoadjuvant and postoperative chemoradiotherapy for resectable pancreatic carcinoma found no significant differences in patterns of disease recurrence between the two modalities, and the median survival times were identical.[80] The use of rapid fractionated radiation with gemcitabine has been under study; however, treatment-related toxicity keeps this protocol investigational at present.[81]

Palliation

At the time of surgery, palliation procedures, which include biliary-enteric bypass to relieve the jaundice and gastroenteric bypass if duodenal obstruction exists, are often performed.[82] Endoscopically placed biliary stents can also palliate obstructive jaundice. In addition, celiac axis blocks may be used for pain relief.[83, 84] These blocks have been shown to provide pain relief in 10% to 25% of patients until death, and they are effective in 80% of cases when used in combination with other treatments.[85] Radiation therapy has also helped to relieve pain and is frequently used for symptomatic metastatic disease.[86, 87]

Results

Overall, despite the general improvement in techniques and increased understanding of the molecular biology underlying the disease, the survival of patients with pancreatic adenocarcinoma is poor. For example, in one study, the median survival of all patients who underwent resection but received no adjuvant therapy is 1 year, but even with a combined-modality approach, the 2-year survival rate is only 30% (Fig. 28–2).[9]

Surgery

With the improvement in morbidity and mortality, especially at high-volume hospitals, 5-year survival rates greater than 30% have been reported for resectable pancreatic cancer, an improvement from comparative reports of 10% in the 1970s.[9] Results from the 1990s following Whipple resection have shown a significant increase in some subgroups, with as high as 40% 5-year survivors in one series for node-negative patients.[9] In a review from the same institution of a large series of 650 patients undergoing pancreaticoduodenectomies during the 1990s, the median survival for pancreatic adenocarcinoma and for distal bile duct and ampullary cancers was reported as 18, 20, and 42

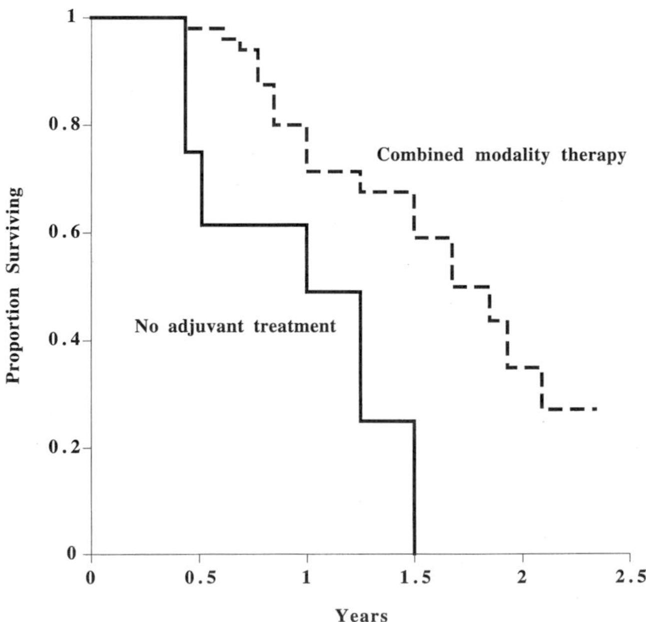

Figure 28–2. The actuarial survival curves for patients undergoing pancreaticoduodenectomy for pancreatic carcinoma from 1991 to 1994. Shown is the comparison of patients receiving combined-modality therapy (n = 56) compared with those receiving no adjuvant therapy (n = 22). Survival time is significantly better for patients receiving adjuvant therapy (p = .001). (From Yeo CJ, Cameron JL, Lillemoe KD, et al: Pancreaticoduodenectomy for cancer of the head of the pancreas. 201 patients. Ann Surg 1995; 221:721, with permission.)

months, respectively.[88] The prognostic factors for a favorable survival rate have been identified as patients with a tumor diameter smaller than 3 cm, negative resection margins, an absence of lymph node metastases, well-differentiated histology, and no reoperation.[89, 90]

A prospective randomized trial has evaluated the role of prophylactic gastrojejunostomy for unresectable periampullary carcinoma. There was a significant decrease in the incidence of late gastric outlet obstruction, thereby supporting the routine use of this procedure for palliation.[91]

Radiation Therapy

Many investigators have attempted to use novel radiotherapeutic techniques in order to improve outcome; these have included intraoperative radiation therapy (IORT) and brachytherapy.[92, 93] Zerbi and colleagues demonstrated improvement in local control after adjuvant IORT following resection of pancreatic cancer.[92] However, this was based on a retrospective study, and results were compared with surgery alone, instead of standard adjuvant therapy. A Japanese study comparing external beam radiotherapy with or without IORT found a significant survival advantage for nonmetastatic patients using either radiation modality over no adjuvant therapy.[94] There was a modest advantage to including IORT in the regimen. A feasibility study assessing the role of interstitial brachytherapy as the primary therapy for unresectable pancreatic carcinoma showed no promise.[95]

Chemoradiation

Chemoradiation produces its best results when used adjuvantly.[96] Investigators continue to explore its use, using both preoperative and postoperative protocols.[80, 88, 97, 98] However, despite the early Eastern Cooperative Oncology Group study that demonstrated no advantage to chemoradiation over 5-FU alone in unresectable patients[99] because of the continued poor prospects for these patients, investigations continue into the use of chemoradiation, with the latest efforts using altered fractionation in the radiation therapy, continuous infusion of chemotherapeutic agents, and including the use of radiosensitizers.[69]

Prognostic Factors

A number of postresection prognostic factors have been identified, including tumor size, lymph node metastases, histologic differentiation, DNA ploidy, intraoperative blood transfusions, positive margins of resection, decade of resection, and adjuvant therapy.[9, 100] However, a 1999 study evaluating these prognostic factors found during multivariate analysis that negative resection margins and an absence of intraoperative blood transfusion were the only significant independent factors improving survival.[101]

Clinical Trials

Clinical trials in pancreatic cancer are mostly directed at attempts to downstage locally advanced disease. Paclitaxel and gemcitabine are currently being tested because of their radiation sensitizing capabilities.[102] Other strategies involve targeted immunotherapy. The *KRAS* oncogene is activated in over 90% of pancreatic cancers, and the protein products of this oncogene are processed onto the plasma membrane; these membrane-bound products make an attractive target for cytotoxic T cells.

Islet Cell or Neuroendocrine Tumors

Other tumors of the pancreas include the infrequent islet cell or neuroendocrine tumors. In general, these tumors have been recognized by their autonomous secretion of various hormones that originate in the pancreas. However, 15% to 25% are nonfunctioning or have as yet no detectable hormone abnormality.[103] Fifty percent to 70% of these tumors are considered malignant, based not on their histologic features but on metastases outside the pancreas (especially abdominal lymph nodes and liver).[104, 105] Many are associated with an inherited disorder, multiple endocrine neoplasia type 1 (MEN-1), for which the responsible gene was cloned in 1997.[106, 107] The hereditary aspects of this syndrome are associated with both hyperplasia and neoplasia in an endocrine tissue, for example, parathyroid and pituitary.[108] In addition to neuroendocrine tumors, mutations in the *MEN1* gene are associated with parathyroid adenomas (>20%), gastrinomas (>30%), insulinoma (15% to 20%) and bronchial carcinoids (36%).[104, 108]

The neuroendocrine tumors can be divided into functioning and nonfunctioning types, with the functioning tumors producing a variety of substances (e.g., peptides or serotonin). The functioning tumors are classified according to their dominant clinical syndrome, for example, insulinomas, gastrinomas (Zollinger-Ellison syndrome), glucagonomas, and VIPomas (neuroendocrine tumors secreting vasoactive intestinal peptide).[105, 109–111] There is no staging system for these lesions and the treatment is frequently symptomatic, usually surgical, with chemotherapy for symptomatic, metastatic disease.[112, 113]

Principles of Treatment

In 1989, the Food and Drug Administration approved the drug octreotide, an analogue of somatostatin, which is effective in controlling some of the symptoms of the hormonal excess (e.g., hypoglycemia, diarrhea, and nausea).[114, 115] By extension, the analogues of octreotide are now finding increasing use in both imaging and as a primary treatment, particularly through radiolabeling with indium or yttrium.[116, 117] The chemotherapy agents used in the treatment of this disease include steptozotocin, doxorubicin, cisplatin, cyclophosphamide, dacarbazine, etoposide, and 5-FU[112, 118–121]; interferon has also been used.[122] These agents are mainly used in some combination and often include concomitant somatostatin analogue treatment.

The treatment of liver metastases, the most common site, commonly employs embolization or chemoembolization[121, 123]; some institutions have performed total hepatectomies followed by liver transplantation with some success.[124, 125] A more detailed discussion of the individual pathophysiology, diagnosis, and treatment of the different tumor types and their hormonal derivatives is beyond the scope of this chapter, and interested readers are referred to the above-mentioned references.

Results

The role of surgery in patients with Zollinger-Ellison syndrome has been controversial. A 1999 prospective study evaluated the efficacy of surgery, including duodenotomy, in this group.[126] Among those patients with sporadic gastrinomas, who comprised more than 81% of patients, 34% were disease-free at 10 years, compared with none of the patients with MEN-1. The overall 10-year survival rate was 94%.

Primary Liver (Hepatocellular) Cancer

Epidemiology and Etiology

Epidemiology

In the United States, although only approximately 15,300 new cases of hepatocellular cancer (HCC) are expected to be diagnosed in the year 2000,[6] nonetheless, HCC is one of the most common malignancies worldwide.[127] Most cases occur in individuals older than 40 years of age; it is uncommon before age 20 in the United States, but not in the areas with a higher incidence. Indeed, a number of studies have suggested that the incidence rates of HCC are increasing worldwide, with a shift toward a younger age group.[128–131] Various reasons suggested for this change are the increasing incidence of hepatitis C virus and the changing age structure in the populations.

Men are more likely to contract this disease than are women; the excess of HCC among men is worldwide, with recorded male-to-female sex ratios of 1.5 to 3.0.[132] There also is an overall geographic variability in the risk rates: countries of highest risk are in eastern Asia, with risks varying from 27.6 to 36.6 per 100,000 men; the risk varies across Africa, with rates of 20.8 to 38.1 in middle Africa, rising to 30 to 48 in west Africa; the countries of lowest risk are northern Europe, Australia and New Zealand, and the white populations in both Latin and North America.[132]

Etiology

- There is extensive evidence that chronic infection with *hepatitis B* and *hepatitis C* virus plays a role in the etiology of HCC.[131–134] The risk is higher in the presence of concurrent infections of both hepatitis B and C viruses.[135] Infection leads sequentially through chronic hepatitis, cirrhosis, to hepatocellular carcinoma. Both viruses can be used for screening: hepatitis B can be identified as a serum surface antigen, occurring in 60% to 80% of Asian patients, and hepatitis C as a serum antibody, and is found to be positive in 20% to 40% of Asians and up to 30% in whites.[136, 137] Efforts to decrease the levels of hepatitis B in hyperendemic areas through vaccination programs have led to decreasing levels of HCC incidence.[134]
- *Cirrhosis* itself is a risk factor for HCC, irrespective of etiology. Almost 80% of HCCs occur in cirrhotic livers.[138, 139] This association has led many to look at the influence of alcohol on HCC etiology, and alcohol consumption, particularly when combined with smoking, shows a strong influence on HCC incidence.[128, 132, 140]
- Other etiologic factors include *aflatoxins,* which are derived from the fungus *Aspergillus flavus* in poorly stored grain crops.[141, 142] This factor has been shown to act synergistically with hepatitis B virus.
- A radiocontrast agent, *Thorotrast,* is associated with hepatocellular carcinoma.[143, 144] Other therapies associated with HCC include anabolic steroids and oral contraceptives.[145, 146]

Detection and Diagnosis

Screening

There have been no randomized trials testing the usefulness of screening for HCC. The most commonly used screening tests use serum alpha-fetoprotein (AFP) and ultrasonography. Patients with cirrhosis who have persistently elevated serum levels of AFP are at a higher risk of developing HCC; however, it has been shown that no advantage was gained with respect to resectability when asymptomatic tumors diagnosed at the start of a surveillance program are compared with those detected during the course of continued surveillance.[147] The screening issue becomes even more questionable if cost-effectiveness is taken into account.[148]

Clinical Detection

The presenting symptoms relate to the effects of hepatomegaly and ascites and include pain, anorexia, weight loss, malaise, occasionally abdominal mass, and, rarely, jaundice. Patients with cirrhosis may have unexplained changes in liver enzymes, clinical deterioration, pain, or fever. On physical examination, there is usually hepatomegaly, right upper quadrant tenderness, occasionally an audible bruit, ascites, and portal hypertension with associated esophageal varices and splenomegaly. Associated paraneoplastic syndromes include hypoglycemia, hypertension, erythrocytosis from an erythropoietin-like substance secreted by the tumor, hypercalcemia, and hypercholesterolemia.[149–151]

Diagnostic Procedures

At diagnosis, the majority of patients have advanced disease. Imaging studies with ultrasound are highly sensitive for detecting the disease and directing percutaneous fine-needle aspirate biopsies. These tumors are hypervascular and biopsy can be associated with bleeding, even with normal coagulation studies. In addition, liver biopsy has a small, but finite, risk of tumor seeding along the needle tract.[152, 153]

IMAGING

- *Helical CT*: Helical CT eliminates problems of respiratory misregistration and enables subcentimeter lesions to be detected. This technique allows both hepatic arterial and portal venous phases to be imaged separately. Hypervascular tumors such as HCC are en-

TABLE 28–6. **Histologic Classification of Malignant Tumors in the Liver**

Type of Tumor	% Incidence
Hepatocellular carcinoma (liver cell carcinoma)	85–95
Cholangiocarcinoma (intrahepatic bile duct carcinoma)	5–15
Mixed hepatocellular cholangiocarcinoma	<1
Undifferentiated	<1

hanced dramatically during the hepatic arterial phase of contrast enhancement as a result of their blood supply pattern, thereby resulting in a higher yield of tumor detection.

- *Angiographically assisted CT*: CT arterial portography and CT hepatic angiography are employed to determine the resectability of tumors by improving characterization of lesions.[154]
- Dynamic multiphase *gadolinium-enhanced MRI* may be superior to a spiral CT scan in the early detection of HCC. It also is useful in the characterization of diffuse liver entities. So far, MRI remains a problem-solving technique for additional information not available with other modalities.[155]
- *Sonography*: The sensitivity of sonography for the detection of HCC in end-stage cirrhotic liver is only 50%, and it is mostly seen as hyperechoic as a result of the homogeneous structure of lesions smaller than 3 cm. Larger lesions are typically hyperechoic as a result of heterogeneous echogenicity. Duplex and color Doppler sonography are useful in detecting vascular invasion.[156]

Laboratory tests include abnormal hepatic enzymes.

- *AFP*, a carcinoembryonic antigen, is present in approximately 75% of symptomatic cases of HCC.[157] Levels higher than 400 ng/mL are 95% predictive for HCC.[158] However, AFP levels alone cannot distinguish between benign and malignant disease at levels lower than 1000 ng/mL.[159, 160]

Once the diagnosis is suspected, further diagnostic work-up is necessary to determine resectability. CT, MRI, and arteriography may be used. Comparative studies show that MRI, with T2-weighted spin echo, is the single best test.[161] The addition of Lipiodol as a contrast agent is very helpful during angiography or CT, or both.[162] Laparoscopic ultrasound is a new technique that assists in staging and operative planning.

Classification and Staging

Histopathology

Cancers of the liver may arise in the parenchymal cells (HCCs) or from the intrahepatic bile ducts (cholangiocarcinomas). The bulk of these cancers (85% to 95%) originate in the liver cells (Table 28–6), and eight histologic varieties have been described: childhood, spindle cell, carcinosarcoma, clear cell, sclerosing, giant cell, fibrolamellar, and mixed; the fibrolamellar variant is more frequent in young women.[163] The remaining cancers (5% to 15%), generally arising from the bile duct, are adenocarcinomas and they differ from HCCs in that the sex incidence is equal, patients are usually older than those with HCC, cirrhosis is much less common, and AFP is usually normal.[164] Malignant hemangioendothelioma (angiosarcoma or Kupffer cell sarcoma) is a rare liver malignancy, but is an important variant because of its strong association with Thorotrast, arsenic, and vinyl chloride.

Metastatic spread of these tumors occurs by direct extension within the liver and to adjacent organs. It can also spread by lymphatic and vascular invasion, principally to bone and lungs.[165]

Staging

This classification system applies to primary hepatocellular and intrahepatic bile duct carcinomas of the liver (Table 28–7; Fig. 28–3).[59]

Principles of Treatment

The treatment modality for HCC is dictated by the potential resectability of the tumor. The presence of unifocal or

TABLE 28–7. **TNM Classification of Liver and Intrahepatic Bile Ducts**

Stage	Grouping	Descriptor
I	T1, N0, M0	T1: Solitary tumor, ≤2 cm in greatest dimension, without vascular invasion N0: No regional lymph node metastasis M0: No distant metastasis
II	T2, N0, M0	T2: Solitary tumor, ≤2 cm in greatest dimension, with vascular invasion, or multiple tumors limited to one lobe, none more than 2 cm in greatest dimension, without vascular invasion, or solitary tumor >2 cm in greatest dimension, without vascular invasion
IIIA	T3, N0, M0	T3: Solitary tumor >2 cm in greatest dimension, with vascular invasion, or multiple tumors limited to one lobe, none more than 2 cm in greatest dimension, with vascular invasion, or multiple tumors limited to one lobe, some more than 2 cm in greatest dimension, ± vascular invasion
IIIB	T1–3, N1, M0	N1: Regional lymph node metastasis
IVA	T4, Any N, M0	T4: Multiple tumors in more than 1 lobe, or tumor(s) involve(s) a major branch of the portal or hepatic vein(s), or invasion of adjacent organs other than gallbladder or perforation of the visceral peritoneum
	Any T, Any N, M1	M1: Distant metastasis

Used with the permission of the American Joint Committee on Cancer (AJCC®), Chicago, Illinois. The original source for this material is the AJCC® Cancer Staging Manual, 5th edition (1997), published by Lippincott-Raven Publishers, Philadelphia, Pennsylvania.

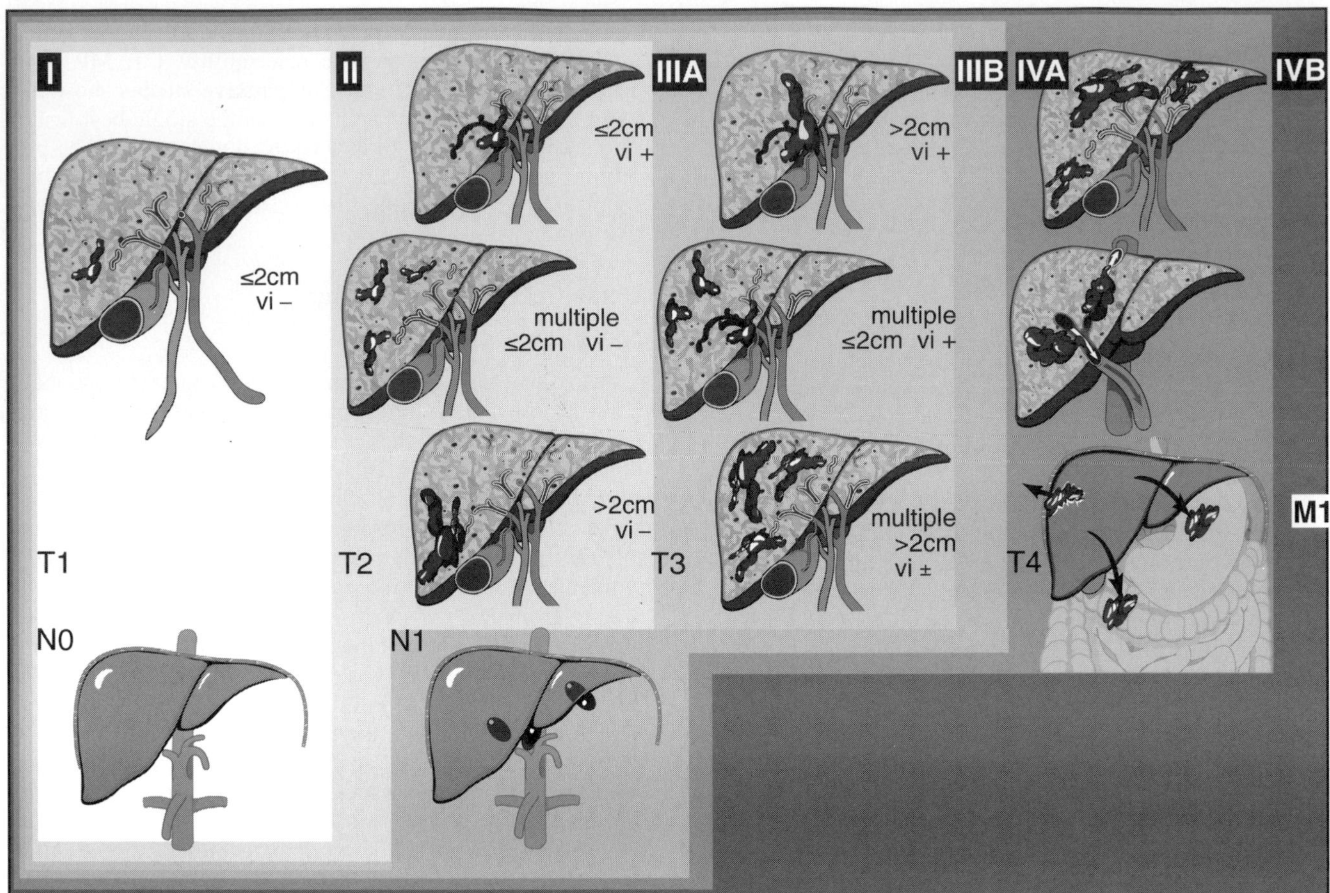

Figure 28–3. Anatomic staging for cancer of the liver.

multifocal disease, the extent of cirrhosis and functional reserve of liver, the degree of portal hypertension, patient age, and so forth all aid in the classification of the tumor with respect to its resectability. If the tumor is deemed unresectable, a number of alternative treatments are available; therefore, a multidisciplinary approach is necessary to explore all potential therapeutic options.[166] Generalized treatment options are summarized in Table 28–8.

Surgery

Subtotal hepatectomy is the treatment of choice for most patients[124, 167, 168]; the selection of patients for resection depends on the stage of disease and the functional hepatic reserve of the non–tumor-bearing liver. Cirrhosis increases the morbidity and mortality[169] but does not necessarily preclude limited resections unless there is increased portal pressure.[170] More important in treatment choice is the assessment of liver function rather than presence or absence of cirrhosis. Variables indicating liver reserve include total bilirubin and serum albumin levels, as well as protime, presence of ascites, encephalopathy, or muscular wasting. In general, patients should be free of jaundice and ascites, and the lesion should be solitary or localized to a single lobe.

TABLE 28–8. **Multidisciplinary Treatment Decisions: Liver**

Stage	Surgery	Radiation Therapy	Chemotherapy
T1–3, N0	Resection	RT for +/close margins	NR
T4, Any N	Unresectable	External RT	Regional: hepatic arterial infusion IC

NR = not recommended; RT = radiation therapy; IC = investigational clinical trials.

Resection can be total or partial, with partial varying according to sector or segment. Segmental resection is usually restricted to patients with solitary HCC without evidence of vascular or extrahepatic spread. In general, it is a safe and effective approach, with operative mortality rates as low as 2% being reported[171]; the overall estimated 5-year survival rate is 30% following segmental resection.[171–173] For cirrhotic patients, patients with poor hepatic reserve, and for locally extensive tumors, total hepatectomy and orthotopic liver transplantation (OLT) is an alternative strategy.[174, 175] Success also has been achieved through the use of liver transplantation for small tumors, although there have been no randomized trials to accurately assess the impact of this treatment modality.[176, 177]

OLT has the advantage of treating not only HCC but also any underlying cirrhosis. This technique leads to a relatively low rate of recurrence because (1) the unresected liver is the most frequent site of metastatic nodules; and (2) cirrhosis is a premalignant condition.[178] Some impressive results have been reported with this technique (Table 28–9); for example, the University of Pittsburgh reported an overall 5-year survival rate of 49% in patients undergoing OLT for HCC; a select group of patients with negative margins, negative nodes, and no vascular invasion or metastases had a 5-year survival rate of 62%.[190]

Hepatic ligation for palliation is no longer recommended. However, cryosurgery may become a useful modality for ablating liver tumors in the near future.[191, 192] Cryoablation, using radiofrequencies, also is under investigation.[193]

INTERSTITIAL LASER COAGULATION

Interstitial laser coagulation, a technique first presented in 1983, is a procedure for the treatment of unresectable hepatic tumors using local light delivery to thermally coagulate solid tumors. According to some studies, the effective tumor size for this procedure is 5 cm or less,[194] although this figure is currently under debate.[195] Some limitations of this procedure are (1) the absence of a means for real-time monitoring of heat buildup and charring effects[194, 195]; (2) the ineffectiveness of this procedure on high fibrous tumors[195]; and (3) the lack of any evidence of actual patient survival benefit.[194]

Radiation Therapy

The liver does not tolerate so-called definitive doses of external irradiation. The generally accepted tolerance dose of the whole liver is 30 to 35 Gy, delivered in 1.8- to 2.0-Gy fractions[196]; at higher fractions, the chance of significant radiation hepatitis increases. The radiation injury site is the hepatic venules, producing a clinical picture that resembles obstruction of the suprahepatic vein, that is, similar to Budd-Chiari syndrome. Hepatic tolerance may be further reduced when chemotherapy also is used.[197, 198] Thus external irradiation, alone or with chemotherapy, plays little role in this disease.

Greater success has been achieved when radiation is used in combined-modality treatments:

- Order and colleagues at Johns Hopkins developed protocols combining external radiation, chemotherapy (5-FU and doxorubicin), and iodine-labeled ferritin antibodies that were subsequently taken to clinical trial.[199] Iodine-131 radiolabeling of Lipiodol also has been used, with tolerable side effects.[200, 201]
- Durable response rates and encouraging median survival durations have been reported through the use of conformal radiation therapy with regional chemotherapy.[202]
- Combined transcatheter arterial chemoembolization (TACE) and local radiation therapy have yielded a high response rate,[203] and combined TACE, percutaneous ethanol injection, and radiation therapy have been shown to effectively control large HCCs (≤8 cm) with little toxicity.[204]

Chemotherapy

Systemic administration of conventional chemotherapeutic agents, single agent or in combination, has been unable to produce significant tumor responses in most cases.[165] Doxorubicin, etoposide, cisplatin, and 5-FU have been used, but have demonstrated no measurable benefit, either as single agents or in combination. Therefore, because of poor response rates, toxicity, and a restricted applicable patient population, this modality is limited in its usefulness for the treatment of HCC.[205] Nonetheless, randomized clinical trials that compare systemic chemotherapy with other therapies currently used to treat HCC are necessary.

NEOADJUVANT CHEMOTHERAPY

Neoadjuvant chemotherapy has produced some encouraging results. Most trials have used bolus infusions of a

TABLE 28–9. **Results of Liver Transplantation in Patients with Hepatocellular Carcinoma**

Investigator	No.	Patient Characteristics	Treatment	Survival Rate (%) 1–3 yrs	Survival Rate (%) 5 yrs	Prognosis Factors
Romani et al[179]	27	HCC, + cirrhosis, ≤5 cm	OLT	82–71		HBV/HCV reinfection
McPeake et al[180]	56	HCC, + cirrhosis	OLT		57.1	Lesions >4 cm
	31	HCC, − cirrhosis	OLT		44.4	
Bismuth et al[181]	60	HCC, + cirrhosis	OLT	47		Diffuse form, >2 nodules >3-cm
	60	HCC, + cirrhosis	R	50		Uninodular
Iwatsuki et al[182]	220	HCC	OLT	68–46	37	Multiple tumors, metastasis, + margins, >2 lobes involved
Ojogho et al[183]	26	HCC ± HBV/HCV	OLT	73–65.4		Multiple tumors
Michel et al[184]	113	HCC, + cirrhosis	OLT		32	Multiple tumors, tumor size
	102	HCC, + cirrhosis	R		31	
Gugenheim et al[185]	30	HCC, + cirrhosis	OLT		32.6	Multiple nodules, nodule size
	34	HCC, + cirrhosis	R		13	
Klintmalm et al[186]	410	HCC, ± HBV/HCV	OLT	72.2–63.4	44.4	Tumor size (>5 cm), + nodes, vascular invasion, tumor grade
Bechstein et al[187]	52	HCC	OLT	88	71	Bilobar, Stage IVA, multiple nodes
Colella et al[188]	55	HCC ± cirrhosis	OLT	72	68	Tumor variables, liver disease
	41	HCC ± cirrhosis	R	64	44	
Closset et al[189]	16	HCC ± cirrhosis	OLT	62–54	54	
	40	HCC ± cirrhosis	R	67–34	18	Extension to both lobes

HCC = hepatocellular carcinoma; HBV = hepatitis B virus; HCV = hepatitis C virus; OLT = orthotopic liver transplant; R = resection.

chemotherapeutic agent, for example, doxorubicin, cisplatin, or mitomycin C, and included some form of embolization, such as Lipiodol, Gelfoam, or microspheres, with partial response rates in the 40% to 60% range.[206–208] Postoperative treatment for the prevention of recurrence after hepatic resection, in the form of chemotherapy and chemoembolization, has had mixed results. A 1997 study by Ono and associates evaluated the usefulness of postoperative adjuvant chemotherapy with epirubicin or 1-hexylcarbamoyl-5-fluorouracil, and found neither course to be effective.[209] However, in a 1999 study, Asahara's group reported promising results from their clinical study on the effectiveness of postoperative adjuvant hepatic arterial infusion chemotherapy, such as improved overall survival rates as well as higher disease-free survival rates.[210]

TRANSCATHETER ARTERIAL CHEMOEMBOLIZATION

TACE delays tumor growth by inducing tumor necrosis; however, it also may promote tumor dissemination. Nonetheless, this modality is effective for treatment of unresectable HCC, particularly in elderly patients[211] and in cases involving multiple HCC nodules.[212]

PERCUTANEOUS ETHANOL INJECTION

Percutaneous ethanol injection is a widely accepted and useful procedure of tumor ablation because it has high antitumor activity, and it is simple and inexpensive. It has been used with some success in Europe and Asia for poor-risk patients but is generally limited to small tumors ($\leq$3 cm) because of the number of treatments required.[213, 214] It becomes more effective in larger lesions if used in conjunction with TACE.[215]

HORMONE THERAPY

Despite its success in other gastric tumors, hormone therapy has not been promising in the treatment of HCC. Results from tamoxifen clinical trials have been varied, but a 1998 article by the Cancer of the Liver Italian Programme, detailing a large-scale randomized trial involving nearly 500 patients from 30 institutions, concluded that tamoxifen had no effect on survival time in patients with HCC.[216]

Results and Prognosis

Proliferation in hepatocellular carcinoma is closely related to tumor differentiation,[217] so that at sizes of 1 to 1.5 cm or smaller, the nodules are well differentiated, and resection offers a high rate of cure, with 5-year survival rates of greater than 90%.[218] However, once the lesions exceed this size, the nodules become increasingly undifferentiated, and the prognosis worsens. Liver transplantation offers the potential for a cure rate of approximately 50%[187] or, at the least, prolonged palliation (see Table 28–9)[219]; however, the donor shortage means that this option is not always available.

Prognostic factors vary between modalities; general factors include the lack of cirrhosis, female sex, and resectability. Specific factors associated with recurrence following resection are tumor size (>2 cm),[175, 185] and solitary versus multiple tumors.[175] Liver transplantation has produced better outcomes with patients with cirrhosis,[175] but nonetheless recurrence is increased with macroscopic vascular invasion,[175, 182] as well as tumor size (>3–5 cm),[180–182] and number.[185]

Clinical Investigations

Gene therapy for the treatment of HCC is in its infancy. However, there have been some encouraging results at the laboratory level with the HSV-TK (herpes simplex virus-thymidine kinase) gene under the control of a radioinducible promoter.[220] In addition, researchers have observed that T-cell–mediated immune responses elicited by suicide gene/prodrug systems CD5-FC (cytosine deaminase 5-fluorocytosine) and HSV-TK/GCV (herpes simplex virus thymidine kinase/ganciclovir) have a significant role in antitumor effects *in vivo*.[221]

Extrahepatic Bile Duct Cancer

Epidemiology and Etiology

Epidemiology

Bile duct cancers, or cholangiocarcinomas, are uncommon cancers and the least common of those categorized as liver and biliary passage cancers. The annual incidence in the United States is approximately 2500 cases, and the mortality rate approaches the incidence.[222] The incidence of cholangiocarcinoma increases with age, there are fewer incidences in the younger age groups than with HCC and, unlike HCC, there is a more even distribution between men and women.[54] As with HCC, there is a geographic variability in incidence, with a higher incidence rate seen among American Indians, as well as such countries as Israel and Japan.[223]

Etiology

- Patients with inflammatory bowel disease (especially ulcerative colitis and, to a lesser degree, Crohn's disease) may have associated sclerosing cholangitis and, with this, there is an increased incidence of cholangiocarcinoma.[224, 225] The neoplastic progression in some of these patients has been associated with *KRAS* mutations and *TP53* dysfunction.[226]
- Although gallstones are found in 30% of cholangiocarcinoma cases, this finding is not unexpected in the elderly population at risk.[223]
- Biliary passage parasites also have been associated with this cancer in a higher than expected ratio, especially in areas endemic with the liver fluke, *Opisthorchis viverrini*.[227, 228]
- There is an increased incidence in patients with choledochal cysts.[229]

Detection and Diagnosis

Clinical Detection

The majority of patients present with cholestatic (obstructive) jaundice, defined as jaundice (mostly direct hyperbilirubinemia) associated with an aspartate aminotransferase level of less than 300 U/L and a serum alkaline phosphatase level more than three times the upper limit of normal. In addition, the majority of patients have an elevated serum bilirubin level[223]; of note, total serum bilirubin levels of 10 mg/dL or higher are prognostic of a worse outcome.[230] However, this presentation is not specific for this type of cancer and can be found in a number of other conditions causing bile duct obstruction, for example, cholecystitis, sclerosing cholangitis, primary biliary cirrhosis, cholestatic hepatitis (frequently drug related), intrahepatic cholestasis, and alcoholic hepatitis.

Symptoms of obstructive jaundice include nausea, vomiting, epigastric pain, weight loss (frequently secondary to malabsorption), and pruritus. The pruritus itself can be severely debilitating. Dark urine, light-colored stools, steatorrhea, and hepatomegaly are common. The gallbladder is palpable in about one third of cases (Courvoisier's sign). A palpable gallbladder is tantamount to bile duct obstruction; bile calculi rarely lead to a palpable gallbladder. Signs of liver failure are a late manifestation. Laboratory tests invariably demonstrate the liver pattern mentioned earlier but also elevated prothrombin time (corrected by administration of vitamin K) and frequently anemia. Serum tumor markers CA19-9 and CA50 are commonly elevated, although levels may fall when biliary obstruction is relieved and, in general, these markers are considered to be unreliable.[231]

Diagnostic Procedures

The best tests for patients with obstructive jaundice, if no clues are forthcoming from the history and physical examination, are among ultrasound, CT scan, and cholangiography (Table 28–10). The major questions asked of these tests include: (1) site and possible cause of the obstruction; (2) extent of disease locally; and (3) evidence of metastatic disease. Diagnostic and therapeutic interventional procedures have shown recent progression with the refinement of imaging techniques.[232]

- *Ultrasound*: This test is performed early because it is associated with few complications, is readily available, and is cost effective. Ultrasound is 90% to 100% accurate in detecting bile duct dilatation, but its accuracy in detecting the tumor is less (80% to 90%).[233] Ultrasound also helps to detect nodal enlargement and hepatic metastases.
- *CT scan* is 90% to 95% accurate in detecting dilated bile ducts and is better than ultrasound in determining the level of obstruction (88%) and the cause (70%). CT scan is also used to determine local extent of disease and liver metastases. This test is undoubtedly our best single noninvasive test. Spiral CT can be used to further delineate tumor extent.[223]
- *Cholangiography*: Direct cholangiography may be performed either from above (percutaneous transhepatic cholangiography) or below (ERCP). Percutaneous transhepatic cholangiography is preferred for proximal lesions, whereas ERCP is beneficial for more distal lesions. These tests are associated with more complications; therefore, they usually are performed after ultrasound or CT scans. Complications include sepsis, bile duct leakage, hemorrhage, perforation, and pancreatitis.
- Tissue diagnosis can be performed using exfoliative cytology from brush biopsies or with fine-needle aspiration biopsy.[222] However, if surgery is contemplated, a preoperative tissue diagnosis is not necessary.[223]

Tumor markers have included CEA, CA19-9, glycoprotein, BCA-2257, MUC1 and MUC2 mucin antigens,[234] and hepatocarcinoma-intestine-pancreas/pancreatic associated protein.[235] The first two markers of the list have been commonly used for diagnosis, although, as noted earlier, their low specificity has limited their accuracy.[231]

Classification and Staging

Histopathology

The majority of cholangiocarcinomas are perihilar, accounting for 50% to 70% of cases,[222] whereas the remainder are distal or, rarely, intrahepatic. Almost all of these lesions are adenocarcinomas (Table 28–11).[54] They are frequently considered multicentric, and significant submucosal spread is not unusual.

Anatomically, these cancers have been divided into three locations. The upper third is the area from the main right and left hepatic ducts to the confluence with the common hepatic duct at the level of the cystic duct. The middle third encompasses from the entrance of the cystic duct down to the intrapancreatic part of the common bile duct. The lower third is that portion of the common duct that runs through the pancreas and wall of the duodenum. Over

TABLE 28–10. **Imaging Modalities for Biliary Tree Tumors**

Method	Capability	Recommended for Use
Computed tomography (CT)	Minimally invasive with IV contrast. Most useful for determining local invasion, extent of tumor, defining site of biliary ductal obstruction and evaluating for distant metastases.	Yes
Ultrasound	Excellent for evaluating metastatic disease and for evaluating the biliary tract. Even when the primary tumor is not seen, the bile ducts may be visualized.	Yes
Endoscopic retrograde cholangiopancreatography/ percutaneous transhepatic cholangiography (ERCP/PTC)	Defines biliary anatomy. PTC is preferred for proximal lesions, ERCP for distal.	Yes
Angiography	To determine surgical resection for pancreatic cancers.	Yes

TABLE 28–11. **Histologic Classification of Extrahepatic Bile Duct Cancers**

Histologic Type	% Incidence
Carcinoma	99
Adenocarcinoma	91
Adenocarcinoma, NOS	72
Papillary adenocarcinoma	9
Mucinous and mucin producing	5
Other adenocarcinoma	6
Squamous cell carcinoma	0.2
Carcinoma, NOS	7
Other specific carcinomas	0.5
Sarcoma	0.2
Other and unspecified	0.4

NOS = not otherwise specified.
Modified from Carriaga MT, Henson DE: Liver, gallbladder, extrahepatic bile ducts, and pancreas. Cancer 1995; 75(suppl):171.

half the cases of bile duct cancers are found in the upper one third of the duct. Those found at the bifurcation of the hepatic duct within the porta hepatis have been called Klatskin tumors, after the clinician who stressed their small size, their tendency to remain localized, and the need for cholangiography to establish the site of obstruction.[236] About one fourth of tumors are found in the middle third and the other fourth in the distal third. Direct extension to liver, portal vein, or pancreas occurs in 70% to 80% of patients, and local node metastases (choledochal, pancreaticoduodenal, hepatic artery) are found in 50%. However, peritoneal seeding and distant metastases are rare: Most patients die from hepatic failure or infections.

Staging

Staging for these tumors is given in Table 28–12. In the past, surgical exploration in the form of laparotomy was required for diagnosis. However, currently, diagnosis and extent of disease can be established using ultrasound or CT, as with HCC, with additional information from cholangiography and angiography; refinements in spiral CT and MRI are leading to less use of angiography.[223]

Principles of Treatment

Surgery

Surgery is the only known curative modality. Its aim is resection of the tumor and reanastomosis of bile drainage to the bowel. Unfortunately, only 20% to 50% of cases are available for curative resection, and locoregional recurrences are the norm (60% to 85%). The type of surgery performed is related to the location of the carcinomatous obstruction, status of the common bile duct, and the extent of disease.

Resectable disease in the *distal duct* is best managed with a pancreaticoduodenal resection (Whipple procedure), both with and without pylorus preservation; no difference in long-term survival or recurrence has been seen between the two procedures.[237] Approximately 40% of cancers in this area are resectable. Those that involve the Vater's ampulla have a more favorable prognosis than patients with cancer of the head of the pancreas because these lesions are more frequently localized.

Resectable lesions in the *mid common bile duct* are rare because of the probable involvement of the portal vein and hepatic artery, and are usually treated with block resection of the gallbladder, common hepatic and common bile ducts, and surrounding lymph nodes. The hepatic ducts are then anastomosed to a defunctionalized portion of the jejunum (Roux-Y-hepaticojejunostomy) to reduce the incidence of cholangitis. Many surgeons prefer to perform a Whipple procedure.

Until recently, lesions in the *common hepatic duct* or *right* or *left hepatic ducts* were frequently considered to be unresectable (50% to 70%).[238] When resection is undertaken, in addition to the structures removed for mid duct lesions, the confluence of ducts and partial hepatectomy is added with Roux-Y-intrahepatic cholangiojejunostomy. Recently, a more radical approach has been taken by some institutions that includes hepatectomy with the tumor resection; 5-year survival rates of 25% to 45% have been reported.[239–241]

Bile duct resection, with or without partial hepatectomy, is the procedure of choice for anatomically resectable *hilar* and *peripheral* cholangiocarcinoma, with 3-year survival rates of 25% to 35%.[242, 243] However, total hepatectomy

TABLE 28–12. **Staging Classification of Extrahepatic Bile Duct Carcinomas**

Stage	Grouping	Descriptor
I	T1, N0, M0	T1*: Tumor invades subepithelial connective tissue or fibromuscular layer N0: No regional lymph node metastasis M0: No distant metastasis
II	T2, N0, M0	T2: Tumor invades perifibromuscular connective tissue
III	T1, N1,2, M0	N1: Metastasis in cystic duct, pericholedochal and/or hilar lymph nodes (i.e., in the hepatoduodenal ligament)
	T2, N1,2, M0	N2: Metastasis in peripancreatic (head only), periduodenal, periportal, celiac, and/or superior mesenteric and/or posterior pancreaticoduodenal lymph nodes
IVA	T3, Any N, M0	T3: Tumor invades adjacent structures: liver, pancreas, duodenum, gallbladder, colon, stomach
IVB	Any T, Any N, M1	M1: Distant metastasis

*T1a: Tumor invades subepithelial connective tissue; T1b: Tumor invades fibromuscular layer.
Used with the permission of the American Joint Committee on Cancer (AJCC®), Chicago, Illinois. The original source for this material is the AJCC® Cancer Staging Manual, 5th edition (1997), published by Lippincott-Raven Publishers, Philadelphia, Pennsylvania.

with liver transplantation is required for patients with underlying cirrhosis, sclerosing cholangitis, or when tumor extension prevents resection, although recurrence rates remain a problem.[243, 244]

For situations in which resection is not possible, palliative procedures include biliary enteric bypass, transtumoral or paratumoral bypass, and stenting.[245]

Radiation Therapy

The techniques available to the radiation oncologist for treatment include (1) external irradiation with high-energy machines, with field size reduction for boost; (2) intraoperative irradiation using orthovoltage equipment or electrons; and (3) intracavitary irradiation using a ^{192}Ir ribbon in a cholangiogram decompression tube, primarily used for boost to the tumor field. As in other areas of the abdomen, normal surrounding structures (liver, kidney, small bowel, and spinal cord) limit the external dose, hence the rationale for intracavitary or intraoperative irradiation.[246]

In general, the use of external irradiation alone, as adjuvant therapy for gross or microscopic residual disease after palliative resection, or as definitive treatment in cases of unresectable disease, has provided reasonable (>80%) palliation (relief of jaundice, pruritus, and pain) in small series from single institutions. However, the benefits due to its use are unclear because of the reporting of both positive[247–249] and negative results.[250, 251] Conformal irradiation, which is coplanar/noncoplanar high-dose external beam irradiation delivered with the assistance of three-dimensional planning, is being investigated.[252] In addition, in order to obtain higher doses while avoiding exceeding tolerance to normal tissue, brachytherapy and intraoperative techniques have come into use.

Intraluminal brachytherapy has been used by a few institutions for palliation, both with and without external beam, with some degree of success.[253–255] In addition, encouraging results have been reported with the use of brachytherapy as part of a combined-modality approach with external beam radiation therapy and chemotherapy.[256]

Chemotherapy

Because of the rarity of this type of cancer, there have been no large studies of chemotherapy. Occasional reports are made of responses seen with 5-FU alone,[257] but the focus of investigations in the 1990s has been on the use of 5-FU–based combinations, such as FAM (5-FU, doxorubicin, and mitomycin-C), in patients with advanced disease.[258–260] Overall response rates of 30% to 50% of cases have been seen, with durations from 8.5 to 18 months. However, because of these generally low response rates, the use of chemotherapy has remained primarily palliative. At present, there is no evidence that chemotherapy affects survival rate; however, a patient's quality of life can be improved.[261]

Palliation

Biliary-enteric bypass may be accomplished surgically or with stents placed through or around the tumor at the time of surgery.[262] Catheters also can be placed, either percutaneously or endoscopically, for external or internal decompression; their use is based on many individual factors, including the medical condition of the patient, his or her performance status, prospect for curative resection, and patient preferences. Biliary drainage is another percutaneous palliative procedure for patients with inoperable tumors.[263]

Results

Surgery

Survival for patients with distal lesions where radical pancreaticoduodenectomy is possible ranges from 15% to 56% at 5 years, dependent on the ability to perform curative resection.[237, 264–266] Mid duct cancer, for the most part, is much less common and generally unresectable; 5-year survival is less than 5%. Carcinomas of the proximal ducts are resectable in only 30% to 40% of cases, however recent employment of a more radical approach has increased 5-year survival rates to 30% to 45%.[240, 241]

Radiation Therapy

At the end of the 1980s, Fields and Emami[267] and Hayes and associates[268] retrospectively reviewed their experience of the radiation therapy treatment of 17 and 24 patients, respectively. Many of these patients were treated with combined external and transcatheter brachytherapy irradiation. Side effects, including infections and GI bleeding, were not insignificant; however, it was not always clear how much these complications were related to the long-term presence of percutaneous catheters.

Since that time, the use of intraluminal brachytherapy has continued to be explored. In at least two studies, it has appeared that its use, both with and without external beam irradiation, has improved survival rate and local control.[254, 269]

Combined-Modality Therapy

As a result of the relatively few resectable tumors and the low responses with alternative therapy, investigators are looking increasingly at multimodality treatments. In two recent studies employing chemoradiation, median survivals of 20 months were reported, with 5-year survival rates of 15% to 25%.[270, 271] In the one study in which resection was possible, with complete resection and negative margins the 5-year actuarial survival was reported at 53.5%.[270]

Prognosis

The prognosis for patients with this disease is generally poor. The absence of metastases, both nodal and distant, has been identified as a positive prognostic factor (Fig. 28–4).[237, 272, 273] However, surgeons should be aware that, regardless of the biologic characteristics of the tumor, most patients die of local recurrence if curative resection is not performed.[274] Further study is required to better define the roles of radiation and chemotherapy in the treatment of this disease.

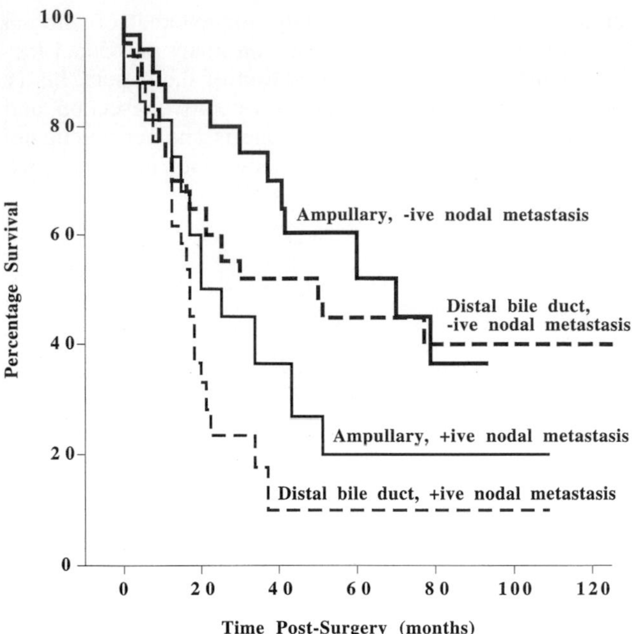

Figure 28–4. Comparison of actuarial survival curves of patients with ampullary or distal bile duct cancer who were node negative (n = 32 and 37, respectively) or node positive (n = 17 and 27, respectively). Five-year survival rates between patients who were node negative (60% and 43%) and those who were node positive (19% and 12%), respectively, showed significant differences ($p < .05$). (From Takao S, Aikou T, Shinchi H, et al: Comparison of relapse and long-term survival between pylorus-preserving and Whipple pancreaticoduodenectomy in periampullary cancer. Am J Surg 1998; 176:467, with permission from Excerpta Medica.)

Gallbladder Carcinoma

Epidemiology and Etiology

Epidemiology

Cancer of the gallbladder is a relatively rare form of cancer, but, nonetheless, is the fifth most common GI cancer.[223] Approximately 7000 cases are diagnosed in the United States each year, and the estimated mortality rate in 2000 was 3400.[6] The incidence in the United States is about 2.5 per 100,000 persons.[223] Although rare among most Caucasian populations, it has an increased risk in the native populations of both North and South America and New Zealand, and in Israel.[275] It also is increasing in incidence in India, although there is a geographic split between the northern and southern rates.[276]

It is rarely seen in patients younger than 50 years old, and the peak incidence occurs between 75 and 79 years of age.[54] The female-to-male ratio is approximately 3:1, which is similar to the incidence of cholelithiasis.

Etiology

The direct cause of this disease is unknown, although several associations have been noted:

- Most patients with gallbladder cancer have associated gallstones (45% to 100%),[277] but there is no conclusive evidence that this is a cause-and-effect relationship.[278] American Indians from the Southwest, who have a high rate of gallstones, also have a high rate of gallbladder cancer at an early age.[223] Although a study from the National Cancer Institute on the Danish National Registry of Patients identified an increased risk for gallbladder cancer of 2.7 in gallstone patients who had not undergone a cholecystectomy,[279] prophylactic cholecystectomy cannot be recommended for patients with gallstones.
- Women, especially postmenopausal women who were multiparous and smokers, are at a higher risk for gallbladder carcinoma.[280]
- There is some evidence to suggest that an anomalous pancreaticobiliary union with associated reflux of pancreatic secretion may be an etiologic relationship. In those patients with an anomalous union, as judged by a cholangiopancreatography, gallbladder cancer was found to be significantly increased.[281, 282]
- Gallbladder polyps are a risk factor for cancer.[283] Polyps larger than 1 cm are most likely to become malignant and are an indication for cholecystectomy.[223]

Detection and Diagnosis

Clinical Detection

The most common symptoms reported by patients with this disease include pain (75%); jaundice (45%); and nausea, vomiting, anorexia, and weight loss (40%). The symptoms of right upper quadrant pain, nausea, and vomiting are similar to those seen in patients with cholelithiasis and cholecystitis. Jaundice implies tumor extension, producing common duct obstruction, or, less frequently, metastases to the liver. Malaise, anorexia, fever, and weight loss all suggest advanced disease. Hepatomegaly suggests liver metastases, as does elevated alkaline phosphatase with hyperbilirubinemia; the gallbladder may be palpably enlarged. Nearly 20% of gallbladder cancers are not detected until pathologic examination of a gallbladder removed for symptomatic cholelithiasis.[223]

Diagnostic Procedures

Because fewer than 5% of patients are diagnosed preoperatively, the surgeon or pathologist makes the diagnosis in the majority of cases.

- *Ultrasound*: This procedure is capable of diagnosing the disease by detecting polypoid, solid masses, even if the patient is seen early.[284] Although there are many shortcomings to this test, bile duct obstruction, gallstones, regionally enlarged nodes, and hepatic metastases can be detected with this procedure. Nonetheless, diagnosis is established in less than 50% of patients.[285] The use of *endoscopic ultrasonography* has significantly improved the specificity of diagnosing gallbladder cancer.[286]
- *CT scan*: This modality is capable of detecting wall thickness, masses, and liver, nodal, and duodenal extension, and complements ultrasound. *Spiral CT* can identify liver invasion.
- *MRI*: Improvements in magnetic resonance technology now allow for assessment of the tumor before therapeutic intervention.[287, 288]

TABLE 28–13. **Histologic Classification of Gallbladder Cancers**

Histologic Type	% Incidence
Carcinoma	96
Adenocarcinoma	86
Adenocarcinoma, NOS	71
Papillary adenocarcinoma	6
Mucinous and mucin producing	5
Other adenocarcinoma	4
Squamous cell carcinoma	0.2
Carcinoma, NOS	7
Other specific carcinomas	0.5
Sarcoma	0.2
Other and unspecified	0.8

NOS = not otherwise specified.
Modified from Carriaga MT, Henson DE: Liver, gallbladder, extrahepatic bile ducts, and pancreas. Cancer 1995; 75(suppl):171.

- *Magnetic resonance cholangiography and angiography*: Cholangiography with vascular enhancement can identify extension of tumor into the hepatoduodenal ligament, and angiography can identify encasement of the portal vein.[289] However, MRI and spiral CT may provide the same information.[223]

In summary, to improve the survival rate of patients with gallbladder carcinoma, early detection and diagnosis is crucial. The primary imaging modalities used include CT, ultrasonography, endosonography,[290] and cholangiography. A combination of these methods has improved the accuracy of diagnosis. In addition, cytology and the analysis of *TP53* expression are useful for intraoperative diagnosis.[291]

Classification and Staging

Histopathology

Adenocarcinomas comprise 86% of these cancers, with similar types and incidences as seen with the extrahepatic cancers (Table 28–13).[54] From a prognostic viewpoint, the papillary adenocarcinomas are generally low grade and have a better survival than all of the others. Tumor type has an influence on survival, as does grade.[54]

TABLE 28–15. **Multidisciplinary Treatment Decisions: Gallbladder**

Stage	Surgery	Radiation Therapy	Chemotherapy
T1–2, N0	Resection	NR	NR
T3, N0	Palliative resection	DRT Intraluminal BRT	IC
T4, Any N	Unresectable	DRT Intraluminal BRT	IC

NR = not recommended; DRT = definitive radiation therapy; BRT = brachytherapy; IC = investigational clinical trials.

As with most intra-abdominal cancers, the pattern of spread may be hematogenous, lymphatic, by direct extension, or peritoneal seeding; the last is uncommon. The predominant pattern of spread, as determined from surgery and postmortem examination, is by direct extension: (1) gallbladder fossa of the liver, 60% to 83%; (2) extrahepatic bile ducts, 57%; (3) duodenum or transverse colon, 40%; (4) portal vein or hepatic artery, 15%; and (5) pancreas, 23%. Positive regional cystic, choledochal, or pancreaticoduodenal nodes occur in 42% to 70% of patients, and para-aortic nodes in 25%. Frequent sites of hematogenous spread include the liver (64%), lung (24%), and bone (12%).

Staging

Staging for the gallbladder is shown in Table 28–14.

Principles of Treatment

Multidisciplinary decisions are essential for optimal outcomes (Table 28–15).

Surgery

Surgery is the only known curative modality. The patients who do best are those in which the disease is found incidentally and early; however, this cancer is rarely detected

TABLE 28–14. **Staging Classification of the Gallbladder**

Stage	Grouping	Descriptor
I	T1, N0, M0	T1*: Tumor invades lamina propria or muscle layer N0: No regional lymph node metastasis M0: No distant metastasis
II	T2, N0, M0	T2: Tumor invades perimuscular connective tissue; no extension beyond serosa or into liver
III	T1–2, N1, M0	N1: Metastasis in cystic duct, pericholedochal and/or hilar lymph nodes (i.e., in the hepatoduodenal ligament)
	T3, N0,1, M0	T3: Tumor perforates the serosa (visceral peritoneum) or directly invades one adjacent organ, or both (extension of ≤2 cm into liver)
IVA	T4, N0,1, M0	T4: Tumor extends >2 cm into liver, and/or into ≥2 adjacent organs (stomach, duodenum, colon, pancreas, omentum, extrahepatic bile ducts, any involvement of liver)
IVB	Any T, N2, M0	N2: Metastasis in peripancreatic (head only), periduodenal, periportal, celiac, and/or superior mesenteric lymph nodes
	Any T, Any N, M1	M1: Distant metastasis

*T1a: Tumor invades lamina propria; T1b: Tumor invades muscle layer.
Used with the permission of the American Joint Committee on Cancer (AJCC®), Chicago, Illinois. The original source for this material is the AJCC® Cancer Staging Manual, 5th edition (1997), published by Lippincott-Raven Publishers, Philadelphia, Pennsylvania.

early. Indeed, only about 10% of cases have disease confined to the gallbladder, and another 10% to 20% involve associated local spread that is resectable. Nonetheless, if found early, small cancers confined to the gallbladder wall (tumor stage T1 or T2) have an 80% curability rate.[292] Unfortunately, the remaining 75% are inoperable for cure, but bypass for obstruction is frequently performed.

The standard surgery for patients with stage I and II disease is a cholecystectomy. More radical procedures, including resection of the gallbladder fossa of the liver, regional nodes, and the gallbladder, are recommended for stage III disease, with a survival advantage of approximately 30%.[293–295] However, there is no clear agreement on the use of radical resection in cases of gallbladder carcinoma. In a study by Bartlett and associates, in which resection was performed on 23 patients, 51% experienced a 5-year disease-free survival.[296] In a larger study that included 135 patients who had gallbladder resection, the 5-year overall survival rate was only 36%[297]; however, this percentage may be skewed by the large number of stage IV patients (96) who underwent resection.

For patients with resectable locally advanced gallbladder cancer, combined pancreaticoduodenectomy and hepatectomy is effective, even with the presence of peripancreatic lymph node disease.[298] If simple cholecystectomy reveals cancer, the extraction of residual disease by re-resection is recommended for stage T2 and T3 tumors because this procedure can affect long-term survival.[296] Both gross and microscopic residual disease, left untreated, are associated with a poor prognosis.[299]

Radiation Therapy

It was often stated in the past that this tumor was radioresistant; however, relief of jaundice and osseous pain using radiation suggest that it may not be radioresistant. Again, the limiting feature of irradiation is the tolerance of surrounding structures. Numerous small series have been reported, but none have demonstrated improvement in survival. The usual doses recommended are 45 to 50 Gy to include the tumor bed and regional lymphatic drainage. Some investigators have suggested postoperative irradiation for patients with high risk of residual microscopic disease, for example, transmural penetration or regional nodes, or both. Data, however, are too sparse to recommend this routinely.

Chemotherapy

Currently, chemotherapy for this disease is investigational. A number of agents have been tried, including 5-FU, mitomycin C, streptozotocin, and lomustine, either alone or in combination. However, for patients with advanced gallbladder carcinoma, survival and response rates have not been very promising. In a study by Gebbia and colleagues, 5-FU in modulation with levofolinic acid and hydroxyurea achieved only a 30% response rate,[300] and Jones and associates concluded that it is improbable that paclitaxel is effective in treating unresectable adenocarcinomas of the gallbladder.[301] However, de Aretxabala and coworkers have reported encouraging results with preoperative chemoradiotherapy.[302]

Palliation

Biliary-enteric bypass is reasonable if biliary obstruction is present. The decision for operative, percutaneous catheter decompression or use of an endoprosthesis is often debated, but final decisions are often individualized, based on risk of surgery, extent of disease, clinical status of the patient, and patient preference.[303] Radiation therapy also can be used to palliate symptomatic metastatic disease.

Prognosis

Although nodal status is the strongest factor for prognosis, tumor type and grade, presence of distant metastases, jaundice, cancer stage, and residual tumor level are also important predictors of the success of surgical resection.[296, 297] Curative resection is not recommended in cases involving nodal metastases beyond pericholedochal nodes.[296]

Recommended Reading

There are rich sources of multiauthored references on all aspects of cancer of the major digestive glands. Recent texts on hepatobiliary disease have included *Liver Cancer*, edited by Steven Curley,[1] as well as comprehensive sections in *Diseases of the Liver and Bile Ducts: A Practical Guide to Diagnosis and Treatment*, edited by Wu and Israel.[2] An insight into the underlying molecular mechanisms of pancreatic disease can be found in *Pancreatic Cancer: Molecular and Clinical Advances*, edited by Neoptolemos and Lemoine.[3] For those interested in the histologic aspects of these diseases, a series on the international histologic classification of tumors includes *Histological Typing of Tumours in the Liver*, edited by Ishak, Anthony, and Sobine,[4] and *Histological Typing of Endocrine Tumours*, edited by Solcia, Klöppel, and Sobine.[5]

REFERENCES

General

1. Curley SA (ed): Liver Cancer. New York, Springer, 1998.
2. Wu GY, Israel J (eds): Diseases of the Liver and Bile Ducts: A Practical Guide to Diagnosis and Treatment. Totowa, NJ, Humana Press, 1998.
3. Neoptolemos J, Lemoine NR (eds): Pancreatic Cancer: Molecular and Clinical Advances. Oxford, Blackwell Science, 1996.
4. Ishak KG, Anthony PP, Sobine LH, et al (eds): Histological Typing of Tumours in the Liver, 2nd ed. New York, Springer-Verlag, 1994.
5. Solcia E, Klöppel G, Sobine LH, et al (eds): Histological Typing of Endocrine Tumours, 2nd ed. New York, Springer-Verlag, 2000.

Specific

6. Greenlee RT, Murray T, Bolden S: Cancer Statistics, 2000. CA Cancer J Clin 200; 50:7.
7. Ries LAG, Kosary CL, Hankey BF, et al (eds): SEER Cancer Statistics Review, 1973–1997, National Cancer Institute. Bethesda, National Cancer Institute, 2000.
8. Falk, R: Pancreas. In: Harras A, Edwards BK, Blot WJ (eds): Cancer Rates and Risks, 4th ed, p 182. Bethesda, National Cancer Institute, 1996.
9. Yeo CJ, Cameron JL, Lillemoe MD, et al: Pancreaticoduodenectomy for cancer of the head of the pancreas. 201 patients. Ann Surg 1995; 221:721.
10. Mohiuddin M, Rosato F, Barbot D, et al: Long-term results of combined modality treatment with I-125 implantation for carcinoma of the pancreas. Int J Radiat Oncol Biol Phys 1992; 23:305.

11. Jessup JM, Posner M, Huberman M: Influence of multimodality therapy on the management of pancreas carcinoma. Semin Surg Oncol 1993; 9:27.
12. Schuricht AL, Spitz F, Barbot D, et al: Intraoperative radiotherapy in the combined-modality management of pancreatic cancer. Am Surg 1998; 64:1043.
13. Nitecki SS, Sarr MG, Colby TV, et al: Long-term survival after resection for ductal adenocarcinoma of the pancreas: is it really improving? Ann Surg 1995; 221:59.
14. Farrow DC, Davis S: Risk of pancreatic cancer in relation to medical history and the use of tobacco, alcohol and coffee. Int J Cancer 1990; 45:816.
15. Howe GR, Jain M, Burch JD, et al: Cigarette smoking and cancer of the pancreas: evidence from a population-based case-control study in Toronto, Canada. Int J Cancer 1991:47:323.
16. Farrow DC, Davis S: Diet and the risk of pancreatic cancer in men. Am J Epidemiol 1990; 132:423.
17. Lyon JL, Slattery ML, Mahoney AW, et al: Dietary intake as a risk factor for cancer of the exocrine pancreas. Cancer Epidemiol Biomarkers Prev 1993; 2:513.
18. Clavel R, Benhamou E, Auquier A, et al: Coffee, alcohol, smoking and cancer of the pancreas: a case-control study. Int J Cancer 1989; 43:17.
19. Harnack LJ, Anderson KE, Zheng W, et al: Smoking, alcohol, coffee, and tea intake and incidence of cancer of the exocrine pancreas: the Iowa Women's Health Study. Cancer Epidemiol Biomarkers Prev 1997; 6:1081.
20. Gordis L: Consumption of methylxanthine-containing beverages and risk of pancreatic cancer. Cancer Lett 1990; 52:1.
21. Everhart J, Wright D: Diabetes mellitus as a risk factor for pancreatic cancer. A meta-analysis. JAMA 1995; 273:1605.
22. Offerhaus GJ, Tersmette AC, Tersmette KW, et al: Gastric, pancreatic, and colorectal carcinogenesis following remote peptic ulcer surgery. Review of the literature with the emphasis on risk assessment and underlying mechanism. Mod Pathol 1988; 1:352.
23. Ekbom A, McLaughlin JK, Karlsson BM, et al: Pancreatitis and pancreatic cancer: a population-based study. J Natl Cancer Inst 1994; 86:625.
24. Schlosser W, Schoenberg MH, Rhein E, et al: Pancreatic carcinoma in chronic pancreatitis with inflammatory tumor of the head of the pancreas. Z Gastroenterol 1996; 34:3.
25. Talamini G, Falconi M, Bassi C, et al: Incidence of cancer in the course of chronic pancreatitis. Am J Gastroenterol 1999; 94:1253.
26. Lynch HT, Smyrk T, Kern SE, et al: Familial pancreatic cancer: a review. Semin Oncol 1996; 23:251.
27. Wang EH, Ebrahimi SA, Wu AY, et al: Mutation of the MENIN gene in sporadic pancreatic endocrine tumors. Cancer Res 1998; 58:4417.
28. Hessman O, Lindberg D, Einarsson A, et al: Genetic alterations on 3p, 11q13, and 18q in nonfamilial and MEN 1-associated pancreatic endocrine tumors. Genes Chromosomes Cancer 1999; 26:258.
29. Kogire M, Hosotani R, Kondo M, et al: Pancreatic lesions in von Hippel-Lindau syndrome: the coexistence of metastatic tumors from renal cell carcinoma and multiple cysts. Surg Today 2000; 30:380.
30. Lowenfels AB, Maisonneuve P, DiMagno EP, et al: Hereditary pancreatitis and the risk of pancreatic cancer. International Hereditary Pancreatitis Study Group. J Natl Cancer Inst 1997; 89:442.
31. Gates LK Jr, Ulrich CD Jr, Whitcomb DC: Hereditary pancreatitis. Gene defects and their implications. Surg Clin North Am 1999; 79:711.
32. Whitcomb DC, Applebaum S, Martin SP: Hereditary pancreatitis and pancreatic carcinoma. Ann N Y Acad Sci 1999; 880:201.
33. Abrams RA: Primary malignancies of the pancreas, periampullary region and hepatobiliary tract—considerations for the radiation oncologist. Refresher course lectures presented at American Society for Therapeutic Radiology and Oncology, November 1, 1999, San Antonio, TX.
34. Bastidas JA, Poen JC, Niederhuber JE: Pancreas. In: Abeloff MD, Armitage JO, Lichter AS, et al (eds): Clinical Oncology, 2nd ed, p 1749. New York, Churchill Livingstone, 2000.
35. Gudjonsson B: Cancer of the pancreas: 50 years of surgery. Cancer 1987; 60:2284.
36. Taylor KJ, Buchin PJ, Viscomi GN, et al: Ultrasonographic scanning of the pancreas: prospective study of clinical results. Radiology 1981; 138:211.
37. Stevens PD, Lightdale CJ: The role of endosonography in the diagnosis and management of pancreatic cancer. Surg Oncol Clin North Am 1998; 7:125.
38. Bhutani MS: Endoscopic ultrasound in pancreatic diseases. Indications, limitations, and the future. Gastroenterol Clin North Am 1999; 28:747.
39. Buscail L, Pagés P, Berthélemy P, et al: Role of EUS in the management of pancreatic and ampullary carcinoma: a prospective study assessing resectability and prognosis. Gastrointest Endosc 1999; 50:34.
40. Hawes RH, Xiong Q, Waxman I, et al: A multispecialty approach to the diagnosis and management of pancreatic cancer. Am J Gastroenterol 2000; 95:17.
41. John TG, Wright A, Allan PL, et al: Laparoscopy with laparoscopic ultrasonography in the TNM staging of pancreatic carcinoma. World J Surg 1999; 23:870.
42. Callery MP, Strasberg SM, Doherty GM, et al: Staging laparoscopy with laparoscopic ultrasonography: optimizing resectability in hepatobiliary and pancreatic malignancy. J Am Coll Surg 1997; 185:33.
43. Minnard EA, Conlon KC, Hoos A, et al: Laparoscopic ultrasound enhances standard laparoscopy in the staging of pancreatic cancer. Ann Surg 1998; 228:182.
44. Freeny PC: Computed tomography in the diagnosis and staging of cholangiocarcinoma and pancreatic carcinoma. Ann Oncol 1999; 10(suppl):12.
45. Heslin MJ, Brooks AR, Hochwald SN, et al: A preoperative biliary stent is associated with increased complications after pancreaticoduodenectomy. Arch Surg 1998; 133:149.
46. Thoeni RF, Blankenberg F: Pancreatic imaging. Computed tomography and magnetic resonance imaging. Radiol Clin North Am 1993; 31:1085.
47. Berberat P, Friess H, Kashiwagi M, et al: Diagnosis and staging of pancreatic cancer by positron emission tomography. World J Surg 1999; 23:882.
48. Safi F, Schlosser W, Falkenreck S, et al: Prognostic value of CA 19-9 serum course in pancreatic cancer. Hepatogastroenterology 1998; 45:253.
49. Okusaka T, Okada S, Sato T, et al: Tumor markers in evaluating the response to radiotherapy in unresectable pancreatic cancer. Hepatogastroenterology 1998; 45:867.
50. Nakaizumi A, Uehara H, Takenaka A, et al: Diagnosis of pancreatic cancer by cytology and measurement of oncogene and tumor markers in pure pancreatic juice aspirated by endoscopy. Hepatogastroenterology 1999; 46:31.
51. Cappelli G, Paladini S, D'Agata A: Tumor markers in the diagnosis of pancreatic cancer. Tumori 1999; 85(suppl 1):S19.
52. Andicoechea A, Vizoso F, Alexandre E, et al: Comparative study of carbohydrate antigen 195 and carcinoembryonic antigen for the diagnosis of pancreatic carcinoma. World J Surg 1999; 23:227.
53. Wilentz RE, Hruban RH: Pathology of cancer of the pancreas. Surg Oncol Clin North Am 1998; 7:43.
54. Carriaga MT, Henson DE: Liver, gallbladder, extrahepatic bile ducts, and pancreas. Cancer 1995; 75(suppl):171.
55. Benassai G, Mastrorilli M, Quarto G, et al: Factors influencing survival after resection for ductal adenocarcinoma of the head of the pancreas. J Surg Oncol 2000; 73:212.
56. Wenger FA, Peter F, Zieren J, et al: Prognosis factors in carcinoma of the head of the pancreas. Digest Surg 2000; 17:29.
57. Ohta T, Nagakawa T, Ueno K, et al: The mode of lymphatic and local spread of pancreatic carcinomas less than 4.0 cm in size. Int Surg 1993; 78:208.
58. Bakkevold KE, Kambestad B: Staging of carcinoma of the pancreas and ampulla of Vater. Tumor (T), lymph node (N), and distant metastasis (M) as prognostic factors. Int J Pancreatol 1995; 17:249.
59. American Joint Committee for Cancer: Manual for Staging Cancer, 5th ed. Philadelphia, Lippincott-Raven, 1997.
60. Kalser MH, Barkin J, MacIntyre JM: Pancreatic cancer. Assessment of prognosis by clinical presentation. Cancer 1985; 56:397.
61. Foo ML, Gunderson LL: Adjuvant postoperative radiation therapy ± 5-FU in resected carcinoma of the pancreas. Hepatogastroenterology 1998; 45:613.
62. Bramhall SR, Allum WH, Jones AG, et al: Treatment and survival in 13,560 patients with pancreatic cancer, and incidence of the disease, in the West Midlands: an epidemiological study. Br J Surg 1995; 82:111.
63. Gudjonsson B: Treatment and survival in 13,560 patients with pan-

creatic cancer, and incidence of the disease, in the West Midlands: an epidemiological study [letter]. Br J Surg 1996; 83:874.
64. Wagner M, Dikopoulos N, Kulli C, et al: Standard surgical treatment in pancreatic cancer. Ann Oncol 1999; 10(suppl 4):247.
65. Rios G, Conrad A, Cole D, et al: Trends in indications and outcomes in the Whipple procedure over a 40-year period. Am Surg 1999; 65:889.
66. Albertson DA: Pancreaticoduodenectomy with reconstruction by Roux-en-Y pancreaticojejunostomy: no operative mortality in a series of 25 cases. South Med J 1994; 87:197.
67. Ihse I, Anderson H, Andren-Sandberg A: Total pancreatectomy for cancer of the pancreas: is it appropriate? World J Surg 1996; 20:288.
68. Willett CG, Lewandrowski K, Warshaw AL, et al: Resection margins in carcinoma of the head of the pancreas. Implications for radiation therapy. Ann Surg 1993; 217:144.
69. Evans DB, Abbruzzese JL, Rich TA: Cancer of the pancreas. In: DeVita VT Jr, Hellman S, Rosenberg SA (eds): Cancer Principles & Practice of Oncology, 5th ed, p 1054. Philadelphia, Lippincott-Raven, 1997.
70. Carter SK, Comis RL: The integration of chemotherapy into a combined modality approach for cancer treatment. IV. Pancreatic adenocarcinoma. Cancer Treat Rev 1975; 2:193.
71. Haller DG: Chemotherapy in gastrointestinal malignancies. Semin Oncol 1988; 15(suppl 4):50.
72. Casper ES, Green MR, Kelsen DP, et al: Phase II trial of gemcitabine (2,2′-difluorodeoxycytidine) in patients with adenocarcinoma of the pancreas. Invest New Drugs 1994; 12:29.
73. Rothenberg ML, Moore MJ, Cripps MC, et al: A phase II trial of gemcitabine in patients with 5-FU-refractory pancreas cancer. Ann Oncol 1996; 7:347.
74. Sporn JR, Buzaid AC, Slater D, et al: Treatment of advanced pancreatic adenocarcinoma with 5-FU, leucovorin, interferon-alpha-2b, and cisplatin. Am J Clin Oncol 1997; 20:81.
75. Cascinu S, Silva RR, Barni S, et al: A combination of gemcitabine and 5-fluorouracil in advanced pancreatic cancer, a report from the Italian Group for the Study of Digestive Tract Cancer (GISCAD). Br J Cancer 1999; 80:1595.
76. Burris HA III, Moore MJ, Andersen J, et al: Improvements in survival and clinical benefit with gemcitabine as first-line therapy for patients with advanced pancreas cancer: a randomized trial. J Clin Oncol 1997; 15:2403.
77. Gastrointestinal Tumor Study Group: Treatment of locally unresectable carcinoma of the pancreas: comparison of combined-modality therapy (chemotherapy plus radiotherapy) to chemotherapy alone. J Natl Cancer Inst 1988; 80:751.
78. Seydel HG, Stablein DM, Leichman LP, et al: Hyperfractionated radiation and chemotherapy for unresectable localized adenocarcinoma of the pancreas. The Gastrointestinal Tumor Study Group experience. Cancer 1990; 65:1478.
79. Yeo CJ, Abrams RA, Grochow LB, et al: Pancreaticoduodenectomy for pancreatic adenocarcinoma: postoperative adjuvant chemoradiation improves survival. A prospective, single-institution experience. Ann Surg 1997; 225:621.
80. Spitz FR, Abbruzzese JL, Lee JE, et al: Preoperative and postoperative chemoradiation strategies in patients treated with pancreaticoduodenectomy for adenocarcinoma of the pancreas. J Clin Oncol 1997; 15:928.
81. Wolff R, Janjan N, Lenzi R, et al: Treatment related toxicities with rapid-fractionation external beam radiation therapy and concomitant gemcitabine for locally advanced nonmetastatic adenocarcinoma of the pancreas. Int J Radiat Oncol Biol Phys 1998; 42(suppl 1):201.
82. van den Bosch RP, van der Schelling GP, Klinkenbijl JH, et al: Guidelines for the application of surgery and endoprostheses in the palliation of obstructive jaundice in advanced cancer of the pancreas. Ann Surg 1994; 219:18.
83. Polati E, Finco G, Gottin L, et al: Prospective randomized double-blind trial of neurolytic coeliac plexus block in patients with pancreatic cancer. Br J Surg 1998; 85:199.
84. Sohn TA, Lillemoe KD, Cameron JL, et al: Surgical palliation of unresectable periampullary adenocarcinoma in the 1990s. J Am Coll Surg 1999; 188:658.
85. Ischia S, Ischia A, Polati E, et al: Three posterior percutaneous celiac plexus block techniques. A prospective, randomized study in 61 patients with pancreatic cancer pain. Anesthesiology 1992; 76:534.
86. Tisdale BA, Paris KJ, Lindberg RD, et al: Radiation therapy for pancreatic cancer: a retrospective study of the University of Louisville experience. South Med J 1995; 88:741.
87. Kamthan AG, Morris JC, Dalton J, et al: Combined modality therapy for stage II and stage III pancreatic carcinoma. J Clin Oncol 1997; 15:2920.
88. Yeo CJ, Cameron JL, Sohn TA, et al: Six hundred and fifty consecutive pancreaticoduodenectomies in the 1990s: pathology, complications, and outcomes. Ann Surg 1997; 226:248.
89. Fernandez-del Castillo C, Rattner DW, Warshaw AL, et al: Standards for pancreatic resection in the 1990s. Arch Surg 1995; 130:295.
90. Yeo CJ, Cameron JL: Improving results of pancreaticoduodenectomy for pancreatic cancer. World J Surg 1999; 23:907.
91. Lillemoe KD, Cameron JL, Hardacre JM, et al: Is prophylactic gastrojejunostomy indicated for unresectable periampullary cancer? A prospective randomized trial. Ann Surg 1999; 230:322.
92. Zerbi A, Fossati V, Parolini D, et al: Intraoperative radiation therapy adjuvant to resection in the treatment of pancreatic cancer. Cancer 1994; 73:2930.
93. Willett CG, Warshaw AL: Intraoperative electron beam irradiation in pancreatic cancer. Front Biosci 1998; 3:E207.
94. Nishimura Y, Hosotani R, Shibamoto Y, et al: External and intraoperative radiotherapy for resectable and unresectable pancreatic cancer: analysis of survival rates and complications. Int J Radiat Oncol Biol Phys 1997; 39:39.
95. Raben A, Mychalczak B, Brennan MF, et al: Feasibility study of the treatment of primary unresectable carcinoma of the pancreas with ^{103}Pd brachytherapy. Int J Radiat Oncol Biol Phys 1996; 35:351.
96. Carr JA, Ajlouni M, Wollner I, et al: Adenocarcinoma of the head of the pancreas: effects of surgical and nonsurgical therapy on survival—a ten-year experience. Am Surg 1999; 65:1143.
97. Hoffman JP, Weese JL, Solin LJ, et al: A pilot study of preoperative chemoradiation for patients with localized adenocarcinoma of the pancreas. Am J Surg 1995; 169:71.
98. Miller AR, Pisters PW, Lee JF, et al: Preoperative chemoradiation and pancreaticoduodenectomy for adenocarcinoma of the pancreas. Hepatogastroenterology 1998; 45:624.
99. Klaassen DJ, MacIntyre JM, Catton GE, et al: Treatment of locally unresectable cancer of the stomach and pancreas: a randomized comparison of 5-fluorouracil alone with radiation plus concurrent and maintenance 5-fluorouracil: an Eastern Cooperative Oncology Group study. J Clin Oncol 1985; 3:373.
100. Geer RJ, Brennan MF: Prognostic indicators for survival after resection of pancreatic adenocarcinoma. Am J Surg 1993; 165:68.
101. Millikan KW, Deziel DJ, Silverstein JC, et al: Prognostic factors associated with resectable adenocarcinoma of the head of the pancreas. Am Surg 1999; 65:618.
102. Pisters PW, Hudec WA, Lee JE, et al: Preoperative chemoradiation for patients with pancreatic cancer: toxicity of endobiliary stents. J Clin Oncol 2000; 18:860.
103. Oberg K, Janson ET, Eriksson B: Tumour markers in neuroendocrine tumours. Ital J Gastroenterol Hepatol 1999; 31(suppl 2):S160.
104. Fajans SS, Vinik AI: Insulin-producing islet cell tumors. Endocrinol Metab Clin North Am 1989; 18:45.
105. Phan GQ, Yeo CJ, Hruban RH, et al: Surgical experience with pancreatic and peripancreatic neuroendocrine tumors: review of 125 patients. J Gastrointest Surg 1998; 2:472.
106. Komminoth P: Review: multiple endocrine neoplasia type 1, sporadic neuroendocrine tumors, and MENIN. Diagn Mol Pathol 1999; 8:107.
107. Pape UF, Hocker M, Seuss U, et al: New molecular aspects in the diagnosis and therapy of neuroendocrine tumors of the gastroentero-pancreatic system. Recent Results Cancer Res 2000; 153:45.
108. Marx SJ, Agarwal SK, Kester MB, et al: Multiple endocrine neoplasia type 1: clinical and genetic features of the hereditary endocrine neoplasias. Recent Prog Horm Res 1999; 54:397.
109. Meriney DK: Pathophysiology and management of VIPoma: a case study. Oncol Nurs Forum 1996; 23:941.
110. Soga J, Yakuwa Y: Glucagonomas/diabetico-dermatogenic syndrome (DDS): a statistical evaluation of 407 reported cases. J Hepatobiliary Pancreat Surg 1998; 5:312.
111. Cadiot G, Jais P, Mignon M: Diagnosis of Zollinger-Ellison syndrome. From symptoms to biological evidence. Ital J Gastroenterol Hepatol 1999; 31(suppl 2):S147.
112. Faiss S, Scherubl H, Riecken EO, et al: Drug therapy in metastatic

neuroendocrine tumors of the gastroenteropancreatic system. Recent Results Cancer Res 1996; 142:193.
113. Goldstone AP, Scott-Coombes DM, Lynn JA: Surgical management of gastrointestinal endocrine tumours. Baillieres Clin Gastroenterol 1996; 10:707.
114. de Herder WW, van der Lely AJ, Lamberts SW: Somatostatin analogue treatment of neuroendocrine tumours. Postgrad Med J 1996; 72:403.
115. Degen L, Beglinger C: The role of octreotide in the treatment of gastroenteropancreatic endocrine tumors. Digestion 1999; 60(suppl 2):9.
116. De Jong M, Breeman WA, Bernard HF, et al: Therapy of neuroendocrine tumors with radiolabeled somatostatin-analogues. Q J Nucl Med 1999; 43:356.
117. Tiensuu Janson E, Eriksson B, Oberg K, et al: Treatment with high dose [(111)In-DTPA-D-PHE1]-octreotide in patients with neuroendocrine tumors—evaluation of therapeutic and toxic effects. Acta Oncol 1999; 38:373.
118. Hatton MQ, Reed NS: Chemotherapy for neuroendocrine tumors: the Beatson Oncology Centre experience. Clin Oncol 1997; 9:385.
119. Bajetta E, Rimassa L, Carnaghi C, et al: 5-Fluorouracil, dacarbazine, and epirubicin in the treatment of patients with neuroendocrine tumors. Cancer 1998; 83:372.
120. Oberg K: Neuroendocrine gastrointestinal tumors—a condensed overview of diagnosis and treatment. Ann Oncol 1999; 10(suppl 2):S3.
121. Kirchhoff T, Chavan A, Galanski M: Chemoembolization of hepatic metastases from intestinal neuroendocrine tumours. Eur J Gastroenterol Hepatol 2000; 12:141.
122. Frank M, Klose KJ, Wied M, et al: Combination therapy with octreotide and alpha-interferon: effect on tumor growth in metastatic endocrine gastroenteropancreatic tumors. Am J Gastroenterol 1999; 94:1381.
123. Venook AP: Embolization and chemoembolization therapy for neuroendocrine tumors. Curr Opin Oncol 1999; 11:38.
124. DeMatteo RP, Fong Y, Blumgart LH: Surgical treatment of malignant liver tumours. Best Pract Res Clin Gastroenterol 1999; 13:557.
125. Lang H, Schlitt HJ, Schmidt H, et al: Total hepatectomy and liver transplantation for metastatic neuroendocrine tumors of the pancreas—a single center experience with ten patients. Langenbecks Arch Surg 1999; 384:370.
126. Norton JA, Fraker DL, Alexander HR, et al: Surgery to cure the Zollinger-Ellison syndrome. N Engl J Med 1999; 341:635.
127. Okuda K: Hepatocellular carcinoma: recent progress. Hepatology 1992; 15:948.
128. Benhamiche AM, Faivre C, Minello A, et al: Time trends and age-period-cohort effects on the incidence of primary liver cancer in a well-defined French population: 1976–1995. J Hepatol 1998; 29:802.
129. El-Serag HB, Mason AC: Rising incidence of hepatocellular carcinoma in the United States. N Engl J Med 1999; 340:745.
130. Kaczynski J, Oden A: The rising incidence of hepatocellular carcinoma. N Engl J Med 1999; 341:451.
131. Okuda K: Hepatocellular carcinoma. J Hepatol 2000; 32(suppl 1):225.
132. Bosch FX, Ribes J, Borras J: Epidemiology of primary liver cancer. Semin Liver Dis 1999; 19:271.
133. Colombo M: Hepatitis C virus and hepatocellular carcinoma. Best Pract Res Clin Gastroenterol 1999; 13:519.
134. Chang MH, Chen DS: Prospects for hepatitis B virus eradication and control of hepatocellular carcinoma. Best Pract Res Clin Gastroenterol 1999; 13:511.
135. Benvegnu L, Fattovich G, Noventa F, et al: Concurrent hepatitis B and C virus infection and risk of hepatocellular carcinoma in cirrhosis. A prospective study. Cancer 1994; 74:2442.
136. Kew MC: Hepatitis C virus and hepatocellular carcinoma. FEMS Microbiol Rev 1994; 14:211.
137. Hwang SJ, Tong MJ, Lai PP, et al: Evaluation of hepatitis B and C viral markers: clinical significance in Asian and Caucasian patients with hepatocellular carcinoma in the United States of America. J Gastroenterol Hepatol 1996; 11:949.
138. Kato Y, Nakata K, Omagari K, et al: Risk of hepatocellular carcinoma in patients with cirrhosis in Japan. Analysis of infectious hepatitis viruses. Cancer 1994; 74:2234.
139. Ikeda K, Saitoh S, Koida I, et al: A multivariate analysis of risk factors for hepatocellular carcinoma: a prospective observation of 795 patients with viral and alcoholic cirrhosis. Hepatology 1993; 18:47.
140. Kuper H, Tzonou A, Kaklamani E, et al: Tobacco smoking, alcohol consumption and their interaction in the causation of hepatocellular carcinoma. Int J Cancer 2000; 85:498.
141. Sylla A, Diallo MS, Castegnaro J, et al: Interactions between hepatitis B virus infection and exposure to aflatoxins in the development of hepatocellular carcinoma: a molecular epidemiological approach. Mutat Res 1999; 428:187.
142. Jackson PE, Groopman JD: Aflatoxin and liver cancer. Best Pract Res Clin Gastroenterol 1999; 13:545.
143. dos Santos Silva I, Jones M, Malveiro F, et al: Mortality in the Portuguese thorotrast study. Radiat Res 1999; 152(suppl 6):S88.
144. Mori T, Fukutomi K, Kato Y, et al: 1998 results of the first series of follow-up studies on Japanese thorotrast patients and their relationships to an autopsy series. Radiat Res 1999; 152(suppl 6):S72.
145. Kosaka A, Takahashi H, Yajima Y, et al: Hepatocellular carcinoma associated with anabolic steroid therapy: report of a case and review of the Japanese literature. J Gastroenterol 1996; 31:450.
146. Stuver SO: Towards global control of liver cancer? Semin Cancer Biol 1998; 8:299.
147. Colombo M, de Franchis R, Del Ninno E, et al: Hepatocellular carcinoma in Italian patients with cirrhosis. N Engl J Med 1991; 325:675.
148. Collier J, Sherman M: Screening for hepatocellular carcinoma. Hepatology 1998; 27:273.
149. Nizam R, Ahmed F: Hyperthyroxinemia and elevated lipids as paraneoplastic phenomena in hepatocellular carcinoma. A case report. J Clin Gastroenterol 1995; 21:246.
150. Chu CW, Hwang SJ, Luo JC, et al: Manifestations of hypercholesterolaemia, hypoglycaemia, erythrocytosis and hypercalcaemia in patients with hepatocellular carcinoma: report of two cases. J Gastroenterol Hepatol 1999; 14:807.
151. Arai H, Saitoh S, Matsumoto T, et al: Hypertension as a paraneoplastic syndrome in hepatocellular carcinoma. J Gastroenterol 1999; 34:530.
152. John TG, Garden OJ: Needle track seeding of primary and secondary liver carcinoma after percutaneous liver biopsy. HPB Surg 1993; 6:199.
153. Chapoutot C, Perney P, Fabre D, et al: Needle-tract seeding after ultrasound-guided puncture of hepatocellular carcinoma. A study of 150 patients. Gastroenterol Clin Biol 1999; 23:552.
154. Kemmerer SR, Mortele KJ, Ros PR: CT scan of the liver. Radiol Clin North Am 1998; 36:247.
155. Krinsky GA, Lee VS, Theise ND: Focal lesions in the cirrhotic liver: high resolution ex vivo MRI with pathologic correlation. J Comput Assist Tomogr 2000; 24:189.
156. Fernandez MP, Redvanly RD: Primary hepatic malignant neoplasms. Radiol Clin North Am 1998; 36:333.
157. Johnson PJ: Role of alpha-fetoprotein in the diagnosis and management of hepatocellular carcinoma. J Gastroenterol Hepatol 1999; 14 (suppl): S32.
158. Jones DB, Koorey DJ: Screening studies and markers. Gastroenterol Clin North Am 1987; 16:563.
159. Aoyagi Y: Carbohydrate-based measurements on alpha-fetoprotein in the early diagnosis of hepatocellular carcinoma. Glycoconj J 1995; 12:194.
160. Ogawa A, Kanda T, Sugihara S, et al: Correlation between serum level of, and tissue positivity for, alpha-fetoprotein in hepatocellular carcinoma. J Med 1996; 27:33.
161. Tabor E, DiBisceglie AM, Purcell RH (eds): Etiology, Pathology and Treatment of Hepatocellular Carcinoma in North America, p 255. Woodlands, TX, Portfolio Publishing, 1991.
162. Torzilli G, Minagawa M, Takayama T, et al: Accurate preoperative evaluation of liver mass lesions without fine-needle biopsy. Hepatology 1999; 30:889.
163. Physicians' Data Query. National Cancer Institute; 1984–2000, updated monthly. Adult primary liver cancer. Updated March 2000. Available from the National Cancer Institute, Bethesda, MD.
164. Parkin DM, Ohshima H, Srivatanakul P, et al: Cholangiocarcinoma: epidemiology, mechanisms of carcinogenesis and prevention. Cancer Epidemiol Biomarkers Prev 1993; 2:537.
165. Carr BI, Flickinger JC, Lotze MT: Hepatobiliary cancers. In: DeVita VT Jr, Hellman S, Rosenberg SA (eds): Cancer Principles & Practice of Oncology, 5th ed, p 1087. Philadelphia, Lippincott-Raven, 1997.

166. Ellis LM, Demers ML, Roh MS: Current strategies for the treatment of hepatocellular carcinoma. Curr Opin Oncol 1992; 4:741.
167. Nagasue N: Liver resection for hepatocellular carcinoma: indications, techniques, complications, and prognostic factors. J Hepatobiliary Pancreat Surg 1998; 5:7.
168. Hemming AW, Greig PD, Langer B: Current surgical management of primary hepatocellular carcinoma. Adv Surg 1999; 32:169.
169. Moser MA, Kneteman NM, Minuk GY: Research toward safer resection of the cirrhotic liver. HPB Surg 2000; 11:285.
170. Bruix J, Castells A, Bosch J, et al: Surgical resection of hepatocellular carcinoma in cirrhotic patients: prognostic value of preoperative portal pressure. Gastroenterology 1996; 111:1018.
171. Billingsley KG, Jarnagin WR, Fong Y, et al: Segment-oriented hepatic resection in the management of malignant neoplasms of the liver. J Am Coll Surg 1998; 187:471.
172. Nagorney DM, Gigot JF: Primary epithelial hepatic malignancies: etiology, epidemiology, and outcome after subtotal and total hepatic resection. Surg Oncol Clin North Am 1996; 5:283.
173. Taschieri AM, Elli M, Cristaldi M, et al: Hepatocarcinoma: considerations on surgical treatment in a personal series of 23 patients. Hepatogastroenterology 2000; 46:2500.
174. Mazzaferro V, Regalia E, Doci R, et al: Liver transplantation for the treatment of small hepatocellular carcinomas in patients with cirrhosis. N Engl J Med 1996; 334:693.
175. Figueras J, Jaurrieta E, Valls C, et al: Resection or transplantation for hepatocellular carcinoma in cirrhotic patients: outcomes based on indicated treatment strategy. J Am Coll Surg 2000; 190:580.
176. Llovet JM, Fuster J, Bruix J: Intention-to-treat analysis of surgical treatment for early hepatocellular carcinoma: resection versus transplantation. Hepatology 1999; 30:1434.
177. Olthoff KM: Surgical options for hepatocellular carcinoma: resection and transplantation. Liver Transpl Surg 1998; 4(suppl 1):S98.
178. Regalia E, Fassati LR, Valente U, et al: Pattern and management of recurrent hepatocellular carcinoma after liver transplantation. J Hepatobiliary Pancreat Surg 1998; 5:29.
179. Romani F, Belli LS, Rondinara GF, et al: The role of transplantation in small hepatocellular carcinoma complicating cirrhosis of the liver. J Am Coll Surg 1994; 178:379.
180. McPeake JR, O'Grady JG, Zaman S, et al: Liver transplantation for primary hepatocellular carcinoma: tumor size and number determine outcome. J Hepatol 1993; 18:226.
181. Bismuth H, Chiche L, Adam R, et al: Liver resection versus transplantation for hepatocellular carcinoma in cirrhotic patients. Ann Surg 1993; 218:145.
182. Iwatsuki S, Marsh JW, Starzl TE: Survival after liver transplantation in patients with hepatocellular carcinoma. Princess Takamatsu Symp 1995; 25:271.
183. Ojogho ON, So SK, Keeffe EB, et al: Orthotopic liver transplantation for hepatocellular carcinoma. Factors affecting long-term patient survival. Arch Surg 1996; 131:935.
184. Michel J, Suc B, Montpeyroux F, et al: Liver resection or transplantation for hepatocellular carcinoma? Retrospective analysis of 215 patients with cirrhosis. J Hepatol 1997; 26:1274.
185. Gugenheim J, Baldini E, Casaccia M, et al: Hepatic resection and transplantation for hepatocellular carcinoma in patients with cirrhosis. Gastroenterol Clin Biol 1997; 21:590.
186. Klintmalm GB: Liver transplantation for hepatocellular carcinoma: a registry report of the impact of tumor characteristics on outcome. Ann Surg 1998; 228:479.
187. Bechstein WO, Guckelberger O, Kling N, et al: Recurrence-free survival after liver transplantation for small hepatocellular carcinoma. Transpl Int 1998; 11(suppl 1):S189.
188. Colella G, Bottelli R, De Carlis L, et al: Hepatocellular carcinoma: comparison between liver transplantation, resective surgery, ethanol injection, and chemoembolization. Transpl Int 1998; 11(suppl 1):S193.
189. Closset J, Van de Stadt J, Delhaye M, et al: Hepatocellular carcinoma: surgical treatment and prognostic variables in 56 patients. Hepatogastroenterology 1999; 46:2914.
190. Molmenti, EP, Marsh W, Dvorchik I, et al: Hepatobiliary malignancies: primary hepatic malignant neoplasms. Surg Clin North Am 1999; 79:43.
191. Feifel G, Schuder G, Pistorius G: Cryosurgery—renaissance or real progress? Chirurg 1999; 70:154.
192. Kemeny NE, Atiq OT: Non-surgical treatment for liver metastases. Best Pract Res Clin Gastroenterol 1999; 13:593.
193. Pearson AS, Izzo F, Fleming RY, et al: Intraoperative radiofrequency ablation or cryoablation for hepatic malignancies. Am J Surg 1999; 178:592.
194. Heisterkamp J, van Hillegersberg R, Ijzermans JN: Interstitial laser coagulation for hepatic tumours. Br J Surg 1999; 86:293.
195. Jiao LR, Habib NA: Interstitial laser coagulation for hepatic tumours. Br J Surg 1999; 86:1224.
196. Lawrence TS, Robertson JM, Anscher MS, et al: Hepatic toxicity resulting from cancer treatment. Int J Radiat Oncol Biol Phys 1995; 31:1237.
197. Finley RS: Drug interactions in the oncology patient. Semin Oncol Nurs 1992; 8:95.
198. Flentje M, Weirich A, Potter R, et al: Hepatotoxicity in irradiated nephroblastoma patients during postoperative treatment according to SIOP9/GPOH. Radiother Oncol 1994; 31:222.
199. Order S, Pajak T, Leibel S, et al: A randomized prospective trial comparing full dose chemotherapy to 131I antiferritin: an RTOG study. Int J Radiat Oncol Biol Phys 1991; 20:953.
200. Ho S, Lau WY, Leung TW, et al: Internal radiation therapy for patients with primary or metastatic hepatic cancer: a review. Cancer 1998; 83:1894.
201. Risse JH, Grunwald F, Kersjes W, et al: Intraarterial HCC therapy with I-131-Lipiodol. Cancer Biother Radiopharm 2000; 15:65.
202. Robertson JM, Lawrence TS, Dworzanin LM, et al: Treatment of primary hepatobiliary cancers with conformal radiation therapy and regional chemotherapy. J Clin Oncol 1993; 11:1286.
203. Seong J, Keum KC, Han KH, et al: Combined transcatheter arterial chemoembolization and local radiotherapy of unresectable hepatocellular carcinoma. Int J Radiat Oncol Biol Phys 1999; 43:393.
204. Yasuda S, Ito H, Yoshikawa M, et al: Radiotherapy for large hepatocellular carcinoma combined with transcatheter arterial embolization and percutaneous ethanol injection therapy. Int J Oncol 1999; 15:467.
205. Okada S: Chemotherapy in hepatocellular carcinoma. Hepatogastroenterology 1998; 45:1259.
206. Carr BI, Zajko A, Bron K, et al: Phase II study of Spherex (degradable starch microspheres) injected into the hepatic artery in conjunction with doxorubicin and cisplatin in the treatment of advanced-stage hepatocellular carcinoma: interim analysis. Semin Oncol 1997; 24(suppl 6):S6.
207. Schmassmann A: Nonsurgical therapies for hepatocellular and cholangiocellular carcinoma. Swiss Surg 1999; 5:116.
208. Caturelli E, Siena DA, Fusilli S, et al: Transcatheter arterial chemoembolization for hepatocellular carcinoma in patients with cirrhosis: evaluation of damage to nontumorous liver tissue—long-term prospective study. Radiology 2000; 215:123.
209. Ono T, Nagasue N, Kohno H, et al: Adjuvant chemotherapy with epirubicin and carmofur after radical resection of hepatocellular carcinoma: a prospective randomized study. Semin Oncol 1997; 24(suppl 6):S6.
210. Asahara T, Itamoto T, Katayama K, et al: Adjuvant hepatic arterial infusion chemotherapy after radical hepatectomy for hepatocellular carcinoma—results of long-term follow-up. Hepatogastroenterology 1999; 46:1042.
211. Poon RT, Fan ST, Lo CM, et al: Hepatocellular carcinoma in the elderly: results of surgical and nonsurgical management. Am J Gastroenterol 1999; 94:2460.
212. Acunas B, Rozanes I: Hepatocellular carcinoma: treatment with transcatheter arterial chemoembolization. Eur J Radiol 1999; 32:86.
213. Belli G, Iannelli A, Romano G, et al: Hepatic resection and percutaneous ethanol injection for the treatment of selected patients with more than one hepatocellular carcinoma. Eur J Surg 1999; 165:647.
214. Khan KN, Yatsuhashi H, Yamasaki K, et al: Prospective analysis of risk factors for early intrahepatic recurrence of hepatocellular carcinoma following ethanol injection. J Hepatol 2000; 32:269.
215. Kirchhoff T, Chavan A, Galanski M: Transarterial chemoembolization and percutaneous ethanol injection therapy in patients with hepatocellular carcinoma. Eur J Gastroenterol Hepatol 1998; 10:907.
216. Cancer of the Liver Italian Programme: Tamoxifen in treatment of hepatocellular carcinoma: a randomized controlled trial. CLIP Group. Lancet 1998; 352:17.
217. Kojiro M, Nakashima O: Histopathologic evaluation of hepatocellular carcinoma with special reference to small early stage tumors. Semin Liver Dis 1999; 19:287.
218. Takayama T, Makuuchi M, Hirohashi S, et al: Early hepatocellular

carcinoma as an entity with a high rate of surgical cure. Hepatology 1998; 28:1241.
219. Heneghan MA, O'Grady JG: Liver transplantation for malignant disease. Best Pract Res Clin Gastroenterol 1999; 13:575.
220. Kawashita Y, Ohtsuru A, Kaneda Y, et al: Regression of hepatocellular carcinoma in vitro and in vivo by radiosensitizing suicide gene therapy under the inducible and spatial control of radiation. Hum Gene Ther 1999; 10:1509.
221. Kuriyama S, Mitoro A, Yamazaki M, et al: Comparison of gene therapy with the herpes simplex virus thymidine kinase gene and the bacterial cytosine deaminase gene for the treatment of hepatocellular carcinoma. Scand J Gastroenterol 1999; 34:1033.
222. Pitt HA, Dooley WC, Yeo CJ, et al: Malignancies of the biliary tree. Curr Prob Surg 1995; 32:1.
223. Pitt HA, Grochow LB, Abrams RA: Cancer of the biliary tree. In: DeVita VT Jr, Hellman S, Rosenberg SA (eds): Cancer Principles & Practice of Oncology, 5th ed, p 1114. Philadelphia, Lippincott-Raven, 1997.
224. Broome U, Lofberg R, Veress B, et al: Primary sclerosing cholangitis and ulcerative colitis: evidence for increased neoplastic potential. Hepatology 1995; 22:1404.
225. van Leeuwen DJ, Reeders JW: Primary sclerosing cholangitis and cholangiocarcinoma as a diagnostic and therapeutic dilemma. Ann Oncol 1999; 10(suppl 4):89.
226. Boberg KM, Schrumpf E, Bergquist A, et al: Cholangiocarcinoma in primary sclerosing cholangitis: K-ras mutations and Tp53 dysfunction are implicated in the neoplastic development. J Hepatol 2000; 32:374.
227. Okuda K, Kojiro M, Okuda H: Neoplasms of the liver. In: Schiff L, Schiff ER (eds): Diseases of the Liver, 7th ed, p 1242. Philadelphia, J.B. Lippincott, 1993.
228. Watanapa P: Cholangiocarcinoma in patients with opisthorchiasis. Br J Surg 1996; 83:1062.
229. Nakeeb A, Lipsett PA, Lillemoe KD, et al: Biliary carcinoembryonic antigen levels are a marker for cholangiocarcinoma. Am J Surg 1996; 171:147.
230. Su CH, Tsay SH, Wu CC, et al: Factors influencing postoperative morbidity, mortality, and survival after resection for hilar cholangiocarcinoma. Ann Surg 1996; 223:384.
231. Bjornsson E, Kilander A, Olsson R: CA 19-9 and CEA are unreliable markers for cholangiocarcinoma in patients with primary sclerosing cholangitis. Liver 1999; 19:501.
232. Dondelinger RF: Advances in abdominal interventional radiology. Lancet 1999; 353:15.
233. Looser C, Stain SC, Baer HU, et al: Staging of hilar cholangiocarcinoma by ultrasound and duplex sonography: a comparison with angiography and operative findings. Br J Radiol 1992; 65:871.
234. Higashi M, Yonezawa S, Ho JJ, et al: Expression of MUC1 and MUC2 mucin antigens in intrahepatic bile duct tumors: its relationship with a new morphological classification of cholangiocarcinoma. Hepatology 1999; 30:1347.
235. Christa L, Simon MT, Brezault-Bonnet C, et al: Hepatocarcinoma-intestine-pancreas/pancreatic associated protein (HIP/PAP) is expressed and secreted by proliferating ductules as well as by hepatocarcinoma and cholangiocarcinoma cells. Am J Pathol 1999; 155:1525.
236. Klatskin G: Adenocarcinoma of the hepatic duct at its bifurcation within the porta hepatis. An unusual tumor with distinctive clinical and pathologic features. Am J Med 1965; 38:241.
237. Takao S, Aikou T, Shinchi H, et al: Comparison of relapse and long-term survival between pylorus-preserving and Whipple pancreaticoduodenectomy in periampullary cancer. Am J Surg 1998; 176:467.
238. Mena FJ, Velicia R, Valbuena MC, et al: Carcinoma of the extrahepatic biliary tree: analysis of 15 cases. Rev Esp Enferm Dig 1999; 91:297.
239. Miyazaki M, Ito H, Nakagawa K, et al: Aggressive surgical approaches to hilar cholangiocarcinoma: hepatic or local resection? Surgery 1998; 123:131.
240. Kusano T, Tamai O, Miyazato H, et al: Surgical treatment for proximal bile duct carcinoma. Int Surg 1998; 83:119.
241. Launois B, Terblanche J, Lakehal M, et al: Proximal bile duct cancer: high resectability rate and 5-year survival. Ann Surg 1999; 230:266.
242. Bismuth H, Nakache R, Diamond T: Management strategies in resection for hilar cholangiocarcinoma. Ann Surg 1992; 215:31.
243. Iwatsuki S, Todo S, Marsh JW, et al: Treatment of hilar cholangiocarcinoma (Klatskin tumors) with hepatic resection or transplantation. J Am Coll Surg 1998; 187:358.
244. Burke EC, Jarnagin WR, Hochwald SN, et al: Hilar cholangiocarcinoma. Ann Surg 1998; 228:385.
245. Finch MD, Butler JA: Palliation for nonpancreatic malignant obstruction of the biliary tract. Surg Gynecol Obstet 1990; 170:437.
246. Rich TA, Evans DB, Curley SA, et al: Adjuvant radiotherapy and chemotherapy for biliary and pancreatic cancer. Ann Oncol 1994; 5(suppl 3):75.
247. Grove MK, Hermann RE, Vogt DP, et al: Role of radiation after operative palliation in cancer of the proximal bile ducts. Am J Surg 1991; 161:454.
248. Mahe M, Romestaing P, Talon B, et al: Radiation therapy in extrahepatic bile duct carcinoma. Radiother Oncol 1991; 21:121.
249. Zlotecki RA, Jung LA, Vauthey JN, et al: Carcinoma of the extrahepatic biliary tract: surgery and radiotherapy for curative and palliative intent. Radiat Oncol Investig 1998; 6:240.
250. Langer JC, Langer B, Taylor BR, et al: Carcinoma of the extrahepatic bile ducts: results of an aggressive surgical approach. Surgery 1985; 98:752.
251. Pitt HA, Nakeeb A, Abrams RA, et al: Perihilar cholangiocarcinoma. Postoperative radiotherapy does not improve survival. Ann Surg 1995; 221:788.
252. Gunderson LL, Haddock MG, Foo ML, et al: Conformal irradiation for hepatobiliary malignancies. Ann Oncol 1999; 10(suppl 4):221.
253. Righi D, Maass J, Zanon E, et al: Percutaneous treatment of hilar cholangiocarcinoma completed by high-dose rate brachytherapy. Experience in the first 5 cases. Radiol Med 1994; 88:79.
254. Montemaggi P, Morganti AG, Dobelbower RR Jr, et al: Role of intraluminal brachytherapy in extrahepatic bile duct and pancreatic cancers: is it just for palliation? Radiology 1996; 199:861.
255. Leung J, Guiney M, Das R: Intraluminal brachytherapy in bile duct carcinomas. Aust N Z J Surg 1996; 66:74.
256. Alden ME, Mohiuddin M: The impact of radiation dose in combined external beam and intraluminal Ir-192 brachytherapy for bile duct cancer. Int J Radiat Oncol Biol Phys 1994; 28:945.
257. Kitagawa K, Taniguchi H, Koh T, et al: A case of successful management of nonresectable advanced cholangiocellular carcinoma by intermittent hepatic arterial infusion at home. Gan To Kagaku Ryoho 2000; 27:605.
258. Kajanti M, Pyrhonen S: Epirubicin-sequential methotrexate-5-fluorouracil-leucovorin treatment in advanced cancer of the extrahepatic biliary system. A phase II study. Am J Clin Oncol 1994; 17:223.
259. Todoroki T: Chemotherapy for primary bile duct cancer. Nippon Geka Gakkai Zasshi 1997; 98:479.
260. Takada T, Nimura Y, Katoh H, et al: Prospective randomized trial of 5-fluorouracil, doxorubicin, and mitomycin C for non-resectable pancreatic and biliary carcinoma: multicenter randomized trial. Hepatogastroenterology 1998; 45:2020.
261. Furue H: Cancer of the liver, pancreas, gallbladder, and bile duct. Gan To Kagaku Ryoho 1999; 26(suppl 1):139.
262. Marcos-Alvarez A, Jenkins RL: Cholangiocarcinoma. Surg Oncol Clin North Am 1996; 5:301.
263. Pichlmayr R, Weimann A, Klempnauer J, et al: Surgical treatment in proximal bile duct cancer. A single-center experience. Ann Surg 1996; 224:628.
264. Yoshikawa T, Hirano H, Araida T, et al: The study for the surgical treatment on distal bile duct carcinoma. Nippon Geka Gakkai Zasshi 1997; 98:501.
265. Zerbi A, Balzano G, Leone BE, et al: Clinical presentation, diagnosis and survival of resected distal bile duct cancer. Dig Surg 1998; 15:410.
266. Sohn TA, Lillemoe KD, Cameron JL, et al: Reexploration for periampullary carcinoma: resectability, perioperative results, pathology, and long-term outcome. Ann Surg 1999; 229:393.
267. Fields JN, Emami B: Carcinoma of the extrahepatic biliary system results of primary and adjuvant radiotherapy. Int J Radiat Oncol Biol Phys 1987; 13:331.
268. Hayes JK, Sapozink D, Miller FJ: Definitive radiation therapy in bile duct carcinoma. Int J Radiat Oncol Biol Phys 1988; 15:735.
269. Foo ML, Gunderson LL, Bender CE, et al: External radiation therapy and transcatheter iridium in the treatment of extrahepatic bile duct carcinoma. Int J Radiat Oncol Biol Phys 1997; 39:929.
270. Urego M, Flickinger JC, Carr BI: Radiotherapy and multimodality

management of cholangiocarcinoma. Int J Radiat Oncol Biol Phys 1999; 44:121.

271. Morganti AG, Trodella L, Valentini V, et al: Combined modality treatment in unresectable extrahepatic biliary carcinoma. Int J Radiat Oncol Biol Phys 2000; 46:913.
272. Flickinger JC, Epstein AH, Iwatsuki S, et al: Radiation therapy for primary carcinoma of the extrahepatic biliary system. An analysis of 63 cases. Cancer 1991; 68:289.
273. Kurosaki I, Tsukada K, Watanabe H, et al: Prognostic determinants in extrahepatic bile duct cancer. Hepatogastroenterology 1998; 45:905.
274. Ishiyama S, Fuse A, Kuzu H, et al: Results of surgical treatments and prognostic factors for hepatic hilar bile duct cancer. J Hepatobiliary Pancreat Surg 1998; 5:429.
275. Lowenfels AB, Maisonneuve P, Boyle P, et al: Epidemiology of gallbladder cancer. Hepatogastroenterology 1999; 46:1529.
276. Dhir V, Mohandas KM: Epidemiology of digestive tract cancers in India IV. Gall bladder and pancreas. Indian J Gastroenterol 1999; 18:24.
277. Paraskevopoulos JA, Dennison AR, Johnson AG: Primary carcinoma of the gallbladder. HPB Surg 1991; 4:277.
278. Pastor FA, Duran I, Montalban S, et al: Cholelithiasis and cancer: a study using precursor changes in a population with low incidence of cholelithiasis. Rev Esp Enferm Dig 1992; 81:403.
279. Chow WH, Johansen C, Gridley G, et al: Gallstones, cholecystectomy and risk of cancers of the liver, biliary tract and pancreas. Br J Cancer 1999; 79:640.
280. Khan ZR, Neugut AL, Ahsan H, et al: Risk factors for biliary tract cancers. Am J Gastroenterol 1999; 94:149.
281. Kato O, Hattori K, Suzuki T, et al: Clinical significance of anomalous pancreaticobiliary union. Gastrointest Endosc 1983; 29:94.
282. Kimura K, Ohto M, Saisho H, et al: Association of gallbladder carcinoma and anomalous pancreaticobiliary ductal union. Gastroenterology 1985; 89:582.
283. Okamoto M, Okamoto H, Kitahara F, et al: Ultrasonographic evidence of association of polyps and stones with gallbladder cancer. Am J Gastroenterol 1999; 94:446.
284. Elvin A, Erwald R, Muren C, et al: Gallbladder carcinoma. Diagnostic procedures with emphasis on ultrasound diagnosis. Ann Radiol (Paris) 1989; 32:282.
285. Tsuchiya Y: Early carcinoma of the gallbladder: macroscopic features and US findings. Radiology 1991; 179:171.
286. Mizuguchi M, Kudo S, Fukahori T, et al: Endoscopic ultrasonography for demonstrating loss of multiple-layer pattern of the thickened gallbladder wall in the preoperative diagnosis of gallbladder cancer. Eur Radiol 1997; 7:1323.
287. Brink JA, Borrello JA: MR imaging of the biliary system. Magn Reson Imaging Clin N Am 1995; 3:143.
288. Wagreich JM, Shapiro RS, Glajchen N, et al: MRI findings in adenosquamous carcinoma of the gallbladder. Clin Imaging 1998; 22:130.
289. Vahldiek G, Broemel T, Klapdor R: MR-cholangiopancreaticography (MRCP) and MR-angiography: morphologic changes with magnetic resonance imaging. Anticancer Res 1999; 19:2451.
290. Inui K, Nakazawa S: Diagnosis of depth of invasion of gallbladder carcinoma with endosonography. Nippon Geka Gakkai Zasshi 1998; 99:696.
291. Onoyama H, Yamamoto M, Takada M, et al: Diagnostic imaging of early gallbladder cancer: retrospective study of 53 cases. World J Surg 1999; 23:708.
292. Tsukada K, Kurosaki I, Uchida K, et al: Lymph node spread from carcinoma of the gallbladder. Cancer 1997; 80:661.
293. Gall FP, Kockerling F, Scheele J, et al: Radical operations for carcinoma of the gallbladder; present status in Germany. World J Surg 1991; 15:328.
294. Eckhauser FE, Rayes SE, Mulholland MW, et al: Carcinoma of the gallbladder. In: Niederhuber JE (ed): Current Therapy In Oncology, p 402. St. Louis, Mosby-Year Book, 1993.
295. Schoenthaler R, Phillips TL, Castro J, et al: Carcinoma of the extrahepatic bile ducts: the University of California at San Francisco experience. Ann Surg 1994; 219:267.
296. Bartlett DL, Fong Y, Fortner JG, et al: Long-term results after resection for gallbladder cancer. Ann Surg 1996; 224:639.
297. Todoroki T, Kawamoto T, Takahashi H, et al: Treatment of gallbladder cancer by radical resection. Br J Surg 1999; 86:622.
298. Shirai Y, Ohtani T, Tsukada K, et al: Combined pancreaticoduodenectomy and hepatectomy for patients with locally advanced gallbladder carcinoma: long term results. Cancer 1997; 80:1904.
299. North JH Jr, Pack MS, Hong C, et al: Prognostic factors for adenocarcinoma of the gallbladder: an analysis of 162 cases. Am Surg 1998; 64:437.
300. Gebbia V, Majello E, Testa A, et al: Treatment of advanced adenocarcinomas of the exocrine pancreas and the gallbladder with 5-fluorouracil, high dose levofolinic acid and oral hydroxyurea on a weekly schedule. Results of a multicenter study of the Southern Italy Oncology Group (G.O.I.M.). Cancer 1996; 78:1300.
301. Jones DV Jr, Lozano R, Hoque A, et al: Phase II study of paclitaxel therapy for unresectable biliary tree carcinomas. J Clin Oncol 1996; 14:2306.
302. de Aretxabala X, Roa I, Burgos L, et al: Preoperative chemoradiotherapy in the treatment of gallbladder cancer. Am Surg 1999; 65:241.
303. Hall RI, Denyer ME, Chapman AH: Percutaneous-endoscopic placement of endoprostheses for relief of jaundice caused by inoperable bile duct strictures. Surgery 1990; 107:224.

29 Central Nervous System Tumors

DIANA F. NELSON, MD, Radiation Oncology
ROBERT B. JENKINS, MD, PhD, Cytogenetics
BERND W. SCHEITHAUER, MD, Neuropathology
COREY RAFFEL, MD, Surgical Oncology
ROBERT DINAPOLI, MD, Neuro-Oncology
STEVEN E. SCHILD, MD, Radiation Oncology
RALPH A. BRASACCHIO, MD, Radiation Oncology
DAVID N. KORONES, MD, Medical Oncology

Whenever God prepares evil for a man, He first damages his mind.

SCHOLIAST on Sophocles, *Antigone*

Perspective

Any malignancy is devastating, but none are more so than tumors of the central nervous system (CNS). A brain tumor poses the same threat that any tumor poses, that is, uncontrolled growth and dissemination; however, it wreaks additional havoc by virtue of its location. Even a so-called benign tumor within the cranial vault can rob a person of his or her ability to walk, talk, feel, communicate, remember, and think. CNS tumors can cause symptoms by compressing the brain against the rigid bony calvarium or by obstructing the ventricular system, which creates hydrocephalus, thereby producing symptoms associated with increased intracranial pressure. Without therapy to remove or eradicate it, even a benign tumor in the brain or upper cervical spinal cord can ultimately lead to death.

Low-grade benign tumors tend to grow slowly and some may be cured by surgery or radiation therapy, or a combination of the two. However, inevitably, many of the benign tumors progress to become malignant and fatal. The malignant or high-grade tumors grow more rapidly and are associated with a shorter survival. In addition, even though brain tumors are far less likely to metastasize outside the CNS without surgical intervention, some disseminate within the CNS. These tumors include medulloblastoma and other primitive neuroectodermal tumors (PNET), ependymoma, germinoma, primary central nervous system lymphoma (PCNSL), 5% of glioblastoma multiforme tumors, and, albeit very rarely, lower grade tumors located within the ventricles or periventricular space.

Survival is dependent upon histopathology, grade, and, in most tumors, performance status and, in particular, age.[8] In numerous clinical trials, particularly in malignant gliomas, these prognostic factors have had a greater influence on survival than the type or extent of the therapy being evaluated. Unfortunately, one of the most common adult brain tumors, glioblastoma multiforme (GBM), is one of the most lethal, and despite decades of basic and clinical research to improve the prognosis of patients with this disease (and other similar malignant brain tumors), progress has been slow and disappointing. However, with the advent of newer and innovative therapies, along with a willingness of physicians and patients to enter clinical trials, it is hoped that the outcome for these unfortunate patients will improve.

Epidemiology and Etiology

Epidemiology

Based on population data from the United States Bureau of the Census and cancer incidence rates from the National Cancer Institute Surveillance, Epidemiology, and End Results program, the American Cancer Society estimated that, in the year 2000, there were 16,500 new cases of primary CNS tumors (or 1.3% of all new cancers) and 13,000 deaths from primary CNS tumors (or 2.3% of all cancer deaths).[9] There is an early peak in CNS tumor incidence between age 0 and 4 years, and these neoplasms are the most prevalent tumors of childhood.[10] Indeed, CNS primary tumors are the second leading cause of cancer-related deaths in young children, and for ages 15 to 35, primary

CNS tumors are the third most common cause of death in men and the fourth in women. The incidence rates of primary CNS tumors are, in general, higher in whites than in nonwhites, and differences in incidence between ethnic groups in the United States suggest that there is a substantial contribution to tumor frequencies from genetic predisposition.[11]

The incidence of primary brain tumors has been increasing for a number of years, particularly in the elderly.[12, 13] A number of factors may be responsible for this increase:

- an increase in life span of the population
- the increasing availability and usage of computed tomography (CT) and magnetic resonance imaging (MRI), resulting in an increased detection of underlying tumors
- an increased interest in geriatrics and an overall improvement in health care of the elderly

Etiology

Hereditary Aspects

Twenty percent to 30% of patients with primary CNS tumors have a positive family history of cancer, although only 5% or less of primary CNS tumors are hereditary. Most hereditary CNS tumors identified to date are associated with the following predisposing genetic syndromes; all but Turcot syndrome demonstrate an autosomal dominant pattern of inheritance.[14]

- Germline mutations of *TP53* on the 17p chromosome have been described in patients with *Li-Fraumeni syndrome*, as well as in association with sporadic breast cancers and some soft tissue sarcomas.[14, 15] Although *TP53* mutation is a common lesion in many human tumors, a specific role for *TP53* has been proposed in the initiation and progression of gliomas.[16]
- *Von Recklinghausen's disease*, or type 1 neurofibromatosis (NF1), is associated with pilocytic astrocytoma of the optic pathways (optic gliomas) or cerebellum, and high-grade gliomas. *NF1* is a tumor suppressor gene located on chromosome 17q12–17q22[17]; mutation of this gene has proved to be rare in most sporadic gliomas, with the exception of some sporadic pilocytic astrocytomas.[18, 19]
- *Type 2 neurofibromatosis* (NF2) is associated with schwannomas of the cranial and spinal nerve roots (particularly acoustic schwannoma), as well as meningioma, ependymoma, and astrocytoma. *NF2* is a tumor suppressor gene located on chromosome 22q.[14,20]
- *Von Hippel–Lindau disease* is associated with hemangioblastoma, renal carcinoma, and pheochromocytoma; hemangioblastomas occur most frequently in the cerebellum. This syndrome has been associated with tumor suppressor genes on chromosome 3p13–14.3 and 3p25–26.[14,20]
- *Cowden's disease*, an autosomal inherited disorder characterized by multiple hamartomas in skin, brain, thyroid, and breast, is associated with an increased risk of malignancies in these organs, especially in the breast and thyroid.[21] Germline mutations in *PTEN*, a phosphatase gene, have been found in the majority of patients with both sporadic and familial Cowden's syndrome.[21–23]
- In *Turcot's syndrome*, patients have an association between primary neuroepithelial tumors (typically, medulloblastoma and glioblastoma) and gastrointestinal polyposis. Affected family members with medulloblastoma have germline mutations in the *APC* gene.[24] Those Turcot's syndrome patients with glioblastoma have germline mutations in the region of the *hPMS2* mismatch repair complex, and frequently display chromosomal instability.[25,26]

Environmental, Chemical, and Viral Causes

Environmental factors frequently have been implicated as a cause of increasing incidence. A recurring subject for investigation has been childhood exposure to electromagnetic fields; however, despite many studies, the findings are still inconclusive.[27, 28] Other environmental and occupational factors studied are exposure to pesticides,[29–31] petrochemicals,[29, 32] and lead,[33] but, to date, no significant associations have been proved.

There have been a number of reports of organ transplant patients demonstrating an increased risk of developing primary CNS malignancies, notably lymphomas,[34–36] with suggested risks of 1% to 2% for renal transplant recipients and 2% to 7% for cardiac, lung, and liver transplant recipients.[37] Acquired immunodeficiency syndrome (AIDS) patients also have an increased incidence of primary non-Hodgkin's lymphoma of the brain[37,38]; whether immunodeficiency is a cause or effect remains to be determined.

Radiation Treatment

Ionizing radiation may induce tumors many years after treatment. Meningiomas, schwannomas, lymphomas, and gliomas have all been associated with childhood irradiation for tinea capitis,[39, 40] and gliomas have developed in patients receiving cranial irradiation for leukemia, especially when administered in conjunction with antimetabolites.[41]

Molecular Biology: Cytogenetics

Intracranial neoplasms arise from a highly complex, and incompletely understood, series of events. A wide variety of chromosomal and genetic changes have been demonstrated using cytogenetic and molecular techniques on human brain tumor samples obtained at surgery. Some abnormalities identified in various brain tumors may ultimately provide further clues to more specific molecular mechanisms underlying tumor development and progression. Because the specific brain tumor, the astrocytoma, typically progresses through three histologically defined stages (low-grade astrocytoma, anaplastic astrocytoma and GBM),[42, 43] genetic variations in these subtypes have been carefully scrutinized. Nonetheless, although there may be an underlying genetic basis for gliomas (and other brain tumors), most tumors have acquired somatic mutations in genes responsible for control of cell growth, and these mutations are not thought to be inherited. The characteristic molecular alterations associated with glioma evolution are illustrated in Figure 29–1.

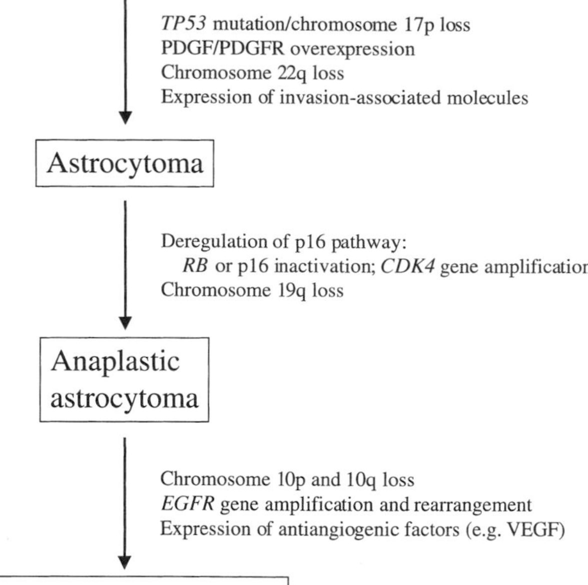

Figure 29–1. Molecular alterations characteristic of different stages of astrocytoma progression. PDGF = platelet-derived growth factor; R = receptor; VEGF = vascular endothelial growth factor. (From Louis DN, Cavenee WK: Molecular biology of central nervous system neoplasms. In: DeVita VT Jr, Hellman S, Rosenberg SA [eds]: Cancer. Principles & Practice of Oncology, 5th ed, p 2013. Philadelphia, Lippincott-Raven, 1997, with permission.)

Low-Grade Astrocytomas

Low-grade astrocytomas have cytogenetic abnormalities that include deletions of chromosome 10[44, 45] and alterations of the p arm of chromosome 17 where the tumor suppressor gene, *TP53*, resides.[43, 45] *TP53* has an integral role in a number of cellular processes, and loss of this gene is, therefore, presumed to be involved in the initial stages of tumor transformation.[46] However, one group from New York University Medical Center has observed significant accumulations of p53 protein in gliomas without detectable *TP53* gene mutation,[47] and have proposed alternative pathways for glioma progression independent of *TP53* alterations.[48] Indeed, studies correlating p53 expression with prognosis in astrocytic tumors have shown that *TP53* status has little relevance to progression in high-grade tumors, although it may be predictive of recurrence.[49,50] Although there appeared to be prognostic significance for p53 overexpression with grade II astrocytomas, this did not reach significance. Other investigators have identified a downregulation of human β2-chimaerin, associated with chromosome 7p, suggesting that this chromosome also may be a feature of progression in gliomas.[51]

High-Grade Astrocytomas

There are a number of hypothesized pathways of glioma progression to a grade IV astrocytoma (GBM): one primary pathway and two or more secondary pathways[46, 48, 52]:

- Primary GBM tumors, or grade IV astrocytomas, arise *de novo*. They usually occur in older adults and have a very short history of symptoms.
- Secondary gliomas arise following progression from a previous low-grade glioma and have a relatively long clinical course. Patients with secondary gliomas are generally younger adults.
- There are at least two types of secondary GBM: those that progress through the astrocytic lineage (see Fig. 29–1); those that progress through the oligodendroglial lineage.

Specific genetic anomalies have been associated with the primary and each of these secondary pathways.[46]

Of the many studies on the genetic alterations associated with anaplastic astrocytomas, there has been a focus on genes that are identified with a critical cell cycle regulatory complex that controls cell proliferation; this complex includes p16, cyclin-dependent kinase 4 (CDK4), and retinoblastoma (Rb) proteins. The $p16^{INK4a}$ protein inhibits the CDKs that control the phosphorylation of the Rb protein.[53] The $p16^{INK4a}$ gene is on chromosome 9p, and its loss has been correlated with increasing grade in astrocytomas.[54] In addition, the *INK4a-ARF* locus encodes for $p14^{ARF}$, whose product can complex with and sequester the MDM2 protein, thus modulating *TP53* activity.[53] In addition, a number of other genetic and biologic patterns are seen in anaplastic astrocytoma: an atypical accretion of the protein p53,[55, 56] gains of 1q, 11q, Xq, and chromosome 7, as well as loss of 9p, 10q, and 13q.[57]

There is an increasing frequency in total or partial chromosome 10 deletion with astrocytic glioma progression.[45] Primary GBMs have a high incidence of this alteration (~90%), suggesting that loss of this chromosome results in rapid development of the tumor. Recently, a strong candidate for one of the critical chromosome 10 genes has been cloned, the *PTEN-MMAC1-TEP1* gene; alterations in this gene have been demonstrated in about 20% of fresh glioma specimens and 30% of glioma cell lines, and they are limited to high-grade gliomas.[58–61]

Gene amplification is rare in gliomas, although amplification of the *ERBB* oncogene, encoding for epidermal growth factor receptor (EGFR), occurs in approximately 30% to 40% of GBMs, primarily in older patients with a more rapid clinical course.[43, 62] Amplification of *EGFR* results in overexpression of the EGFR; receptor binding leads to activation of a transmembrane tyrosine kinase. The tyrosine kinase phosphorylates a number of substrates, activating pathways that ultimately lead to cell growth, DNA synthesis and expression of oncogenes (e.g., *fos* and *jun*).[63] *EGFR* amplification almost never occurs in the absence of chromosome 10 loss,[64] and, in general, *EGFR* amplification is associated with *de novo* glioblastomas. This compares with *TP53* mutation, which appears to be associated with the progressive glioma subtype.[48, 65]

Oligodendroglioma

In more than 80% of oligodendrogliomas, loss of heterozygosity is observed for 19q[66]; approximately 75% of these tumors also show loss of heterozygosity on 1p.[66–68] Of interest, some mixed oligoastrocytomas have been shown to demonstrate 1p and 19q deletions, whereas others demonstrate *TP53* mutations (chromosome 17). Allelic loss of chromosomes 1p and 19q has been found to be inversely correlated with *TP53* mutation, suggesting that there are two subtypes of oligoastrocytomas, one genetically related to oligodendrogliomas and the other to astrocytomas.[69]

One result of genetic typing has been a potential for a prognostic correlation with outcome. It is hoped that, in the future, a more accurate system of identification and classification, in addition to histopathology, can be defined, inasmuch as mixed oligoastrocytomas are notoriously difficult to classify morphologically.[70] Such a system of identification leads to more individualized treatment planning.

Detection and Diagnosis

Clinical Detection

Brain tumors can cause generalized symptoms and signs due to increased pressure within the skull. They can also cause localized symptoms and signs through direct compression, invasion, or irritation of the brain. The diagnosis of a brain tumor depends on the recognition of clinical symptoms and signs of brain dysfunction. These, in turn, are determined by the location of the lesion, its size, and its rate of growth. In general, patients present with a subacute progressive course over weeks, months, or, occasionally, years.

Increased intracranial pressure may be produced by the increasing bulk of the tumor itself, by associated peritumoral edema, by obstruction of cerebrospinal fluid pathways, by venous obstruction, or by increased production or decreased absorption, of cerebrospinal fluid (CSF). In most cases, it is due to a combination of these factors. Symptoms and signs of increased intracranial pressure include headache, vomiting with or without nausea, papilledema, cognitive and behavioral changes, and alterations in consciousness.

- *Headache* associated with increased intracranial pressure is usually intermittent, generalized, and exacerbated by activities that normally increase intracranial pressure (e.g., coughing or straining). Typically, it is more pronounced in the morning, presumably as a result of recumbency during sleep. In patients without increased intracranial pressure, headaches are more often localized and may provide some clue as to the location of the tumor. Traction on pain-sensitive structures, such as arteries, veins, meninges, and cranial nerves containing branches of the trigeminal system, can produce orbital, frontal, and temporal-parietal headaches. Posterior fossa structures, supplied by the ninth and tenth cranial nerves and upper cervical nerves, produce mastoid, occipital, and nuchal headaches.

  Headaches occur in approximately 50% of patients with brain tumors, but are almost always associated with other symptoms. In general, the headaches gradually worsen in frequency, severity, or both over time.
- *Vomiting*, with or without nausea, usually indicates increased intracranial pressure.
- *Papilledema* may develop early with deep subcortical or intraventricular lesions that obstruct CSF pathways and produce hydrocephalus. Large tumors eventually produce papilledema by virtue of their size.
- *Cognitive* and *behavioral changes* include decreased spontaneity, slowness, and inattention, with patients becoming increasingly fatigued and drowsy. They may fall asleep easily during the day, or at inappropriate times.
- *Seizures* associated with gliomas may be generalized or partial. Seizures constitute one of the more dramatic and obvious presenting symptoms, usually prompting neurologic evaluation. In some series, seizures have been associated with a more favorable prognosis.[71] In patients older than the age of 30 with new-onset seizures, 10% to 15% have some type of brain tumor. Seizures generally are associated with tumors affecting sensorimotor cortex.

Attention to focal symptoms and signs may lead to earlier diagnosis and, it is hoped, a more prolonged survival or improved quality of survival. The following regional brain syndromes emphasize early localizing symptoms and signs:

- *Frontal lobe*: Anterior involvement is characterized by behavioral and cognitive decline. Apathy, jocularity, and socially inappropriate behavior occur in unilateral or bilateral involvement. Posterior and premotor involvement may produce forced grasping, whereas motor involvement produces a contralateral paresis of face, arm, or leg. Lateral dominant hemispheric tumors result in language dysfunction, with motor aphasia or apraxia. Partial motor seizures are sometimes associated with eye and head turning.
- *Temporal lobe*: Nondominant, anterior lesions may reach a large size before producing memory or visual field defects (superior homonymous quadrantanopsia). Midtemporal dominant hemisphere lesions result in aphasia, primarily receptive aphasia. Posterior lesions involving inferior parietal and lateral occipital regions produce more extensive language deficits and a variety of apraxias. An expanding temporal lobe mass may eventually produce contralateral hemiparesis. Medial inferior involvement may reach the tentorial incisura, compressing the third cranial nerve and eventually the midbrain, producing early uncal herniation. Simple partial seizures or more complex seizures with impairment of consciousness can also occur.
- *Parietal lobe*: Anterior parietal lobe tumors produce partial, usually sensory, seizures by involvement of the postcentral gyrus. Motor phenomena may also occur by contiguous spread to the precentral gyrus. Posterior and superior lobe tumors produce a variety of complex cortical symptoms: inattention, tendency to neglect contralateral limbs, and vague heaviness or weakness of the limbs. Examination shows astereognosis, tactile inattention, and loss of topesthesia. Nondominant involvement may produce more complex body image disturbances, such as neglect, denial of deficits, and spatial neglect. Dominant parietal lesions are manifested by receptive dysphasia, dysgraphia, dyslexia, and dyscalculia. Deeper lesions may affect optic radiations and produce visual field defects.
- *Occipital lobe*: Patients with occipital lobe lesions present with complaints of blurred or loss of vision, or a history suggestive of visual field loss, such as bumping into door frames or having an automobile

accident. There may be unformed visual hallucinations, such as bright flashes or flickerings, with or without partial or secondarily generalized seizures.

- *Thalamic/basal ganglia*: Deep subcortical tumors in these regions usually produce contralateral sensory or motor symptoms and signs of increased intracranial pressure secondary to trapping of the lateral horn of a ventricle.
- *Brain stem*: Tumors involving the brain stem are unusual in adults, but relatively common in infants and children. A combination of cranial nerve deficits and contralateral sensory and motor pathway deficits are seen. Midbrain lesions that compress the aqueduct of Sylvius present with hydrocephalus combined with Parinaud's syndrome (vertical gaze palsy, pupillary abnormalities and oculomotor nerve pareses). Pontine lesions produce gaze palsies, nystagmus, and facial numbness, or weakness, or a combination of these symptoms. Patients with these tumors tend to develop increased intracranial pressure later in their course. Medullary tumors produce dysphagia, dysarthria, nausea, vomiting, and weight loss.
- *Cerebellum*: Hemispheric lesions produce homolateral incoordination of limbs, intention tremor, and ataxia of gait. Midline or vermis lesions produce gait ataxia and symptoms of obstructive hydrocephalus (headache, nausea, and vomiting). Alteration of gait is a common symptom in all of these patients. Examination may only show a mild ataxia of station and gait, but may show dysdiadochokinesia or nystagmus on lateral gaze, or both.

Diagnostic Procedures

Diagnosis may be accomplished by use of physical and neurologic examinations, funduscopic examination, visual field examination, CT, MRI, cerebral angiography, positron emission tomography (PET), single photon emission computed tomography (SPECT), lumbar puncture, and stereotactic biopsy (Table 29–1).

- *Physical* and *neurologic examinations* are indicated with new onset of seizures, cognitive changes (including inappropriate behavior, somnolence, lethargy, disorientation, subtle degrees of aphasia or apraxia), behavioral or personality changes, or unexplained focal neurologic deficits. A neurologic history should include a careful evaluation of the chronologic history of the illness from the patient and also from an observer, such as spouse, family member, or companion. Focal signs and deficits should be meticulously elicited in the course of a thorough neurologic examination. A clinical diagnosis including location and histologic type should be proposed, accompanied by an appropriate differential diagnosis depending on the age of the patient.
- *Funduscopic examination* should be routine, primarily to look for papilledema. If the room is darkened, this usually can be performed without mydriatics. These drugs should be avoided, if possible, because they can interfere with the subsequent neurologic evaluation.
- *Visual field examination* can give precise information about the location of a tumor and may be abnormal in sellar, parasellar, occipital, and some parietal and temporal lobe lesions. For lesions in these locations that do not need urgent surgery, pretreatment visual field examination is recommended.
- *CT* is almost universally available and, with contrast enhancement, is a reliable screening and diagnostic method in many cases. CT is usually performed in the axial plane and, in some cases, multiple planar images are desirable, particularly for surgical planning. CT is less accurate than MRI for the detection of meningeal involvement and for tumors near the skull, including the posterior fossa, because of bone hardening artifacts. However, CT is better than MRI in detecting intracranial calcifications and differentiating them from acute hemorrhage.
- *MRI* is a noninvasive, safe, painless, highly sensitive, and efficient technique. MRI of the brain has become the screening procedure of choice for diagnosing and localizing tumors in the brain stem, posterior fossa, and spinal cord, and for defining the extent of low-grade gliomas. MRI is now more frequently used in patients with malignant brain tumors, and it has shown advantages over CT in some studies.[72, 73]

In high-grade tumors, MRI, including T1- and T2-weighting and T1-weighting with gadolinium (Gd), more reliably defines the extent of tumor (T1 with Gd) and peritumoral edema (T2-weighting). The multiplanar capacity of MRI is also an advantage for surgery or radiation therapy treatment planning. Other advantages of MRI include the lack of radiation exposure, as well as the elimination of iodine-containing contrast agents with the risk of potentially serious allergic reactions. MRI can be used to differentiate between

TABLE 29–1. **Imaging Modalities for Evaluating Brain and Spinal Cord**

Method	Diagnosis and Staging Capability
CT	Most economical screening and diagnostic method in many cases. If nondiagnostic, then order MRI. Can confirm presence of calcifications and hemorrhage.
MRI	Best procedure for low-grade gliomas, posterior fossa tumors, tumors of cerebellopontine angle, meningeal carcinomatosis, and brain stem & spinal cord evaluation. Has replaced myelogram as an initial procedure for evaluating spinal cord tumors & discs. Better than CT in differentiating stroke & ischemic changes from low-grade glioma. Presence of classic multiple sclerosis (MS) plaques may suggest an apparent tumor is really an MS lesion. Better than CT in identifying multiple brain metastases.
Angiography	Aids in differentiating tumors from AV malformation. Aids in planning surgical approach. Used to follow AV malformations after radiosurgery.
Myelography	Best test for small epidural and nerve root lesions, whether primary or secondary, when MRI is negative or indeterminate.

CT = computed tomography; MRI = magnetic resonance imaging; AV = arteriovenous.

intrinsic and extrinsic spinal cord problems, and metastatic disease versus disc problems. MRI of the spine is routinely performed for staging purposes in medulloblastoma, ependymoblastoma, ependymoma of the posterior fossa, pineoblastoma, PNET, and primary CNS lymphoma. In childhood tumors, when meningeal spread is suspected, gadolinium enhancement provides confirmation.

- *Cerebral angiography* is used by surgeons who desire information about the intrinsic vasculature of the tumor and its relationship to adjacent blood vessels—of importance when planning surgery. However, increasingly, special MRI techniques (magnetic resonance angiography or venography) and spiral CT scans with contrast are being used to define cerebral vasculature.[74, 75]
- *PET, SPECT,* or MRI SPECT may provide additional useful information in certain settings, particularly in differentiating active tumor from necrosis, or low-grade gliomas from nontumoral lesions, based on evaluating metabolic patterns.[76, 77] For example, PET uses a positron-emitting radioisotope-labeled tracer to provide metabolic data about tissue. Actively metabolizing (higher grade) tumors incorporate the fluorinated glucose analogue (^{18}F-2-fluoro-2-deoxyglucose [^{18}FDG]) at a greater rate than necrotic or normal tissue or low-grade tumors. SPECT utilizes thallium-201, which is similarly preferentially taken up by active tumors.
- *Lumbar puncture* is avoided when there is obvious evidence of increased intracranial pressure because there is definite risk of herniation when this procedure is used under such circumstances. When CSF is withdrawn, or when CSF continues to leak through the hole made by the puncture in the leptomeninges, there can be a shift in the intracranial contents; this can aggravate, or even cause, an impending transtentorial herniation. Nonetheless, *CSF examination* is most helpful in staging primary CNS lymphoma, medulloblastoma, pineoblastoma, and PNET to rule out microscopic seeding of the craniospinal axis. However, a positive cytology obtained within 7 to 10 days of surgery can be falsely positive, and should be repeated 2 weeks after surgery.

CSF examination or MRI of the spine, or both, should be considered in low-grade tumors when there is tumor in the intraventricular or periventricular locations, or in both locations. CSF cytology is usually positive in meningeal carcinomatosis and with tumors that involve the meninges or are situated in a subependymal location. CSF examination is also helpful in differentiating patients with meningitis or subarachnoid hemorrhage from those with suspected tumors, although unenhanced MRI or CT scans should demonstrate hemorrhage. Overall, CSF examination is valuable because CSF protein is elevated in approximately one third of patients in the presence of intracranial tumor, and almost always in the presence of a spinal cord tumor. CSF glucose may be low in the presence of highly malignant tumors or metastatic meningeal deposits.

Stereotactic Biopsy

Stereotactic biopsy, performed with CT or MRI, provides tissue for diagnosis, with an accuracy of greater than 95% in experienced hands.[78, 79] Error is most often the result of insufficient tissue, resulting in an underestimation of the grade of the neoplasm. Nowadays, it is almost mandatory that a stereotactic biopsy be performed and a tissue diagnosis made before external beam irradiation or radiosurgery is given. Exceptions to this rule are highly vascular lesions (e.g., arteriovenous malformations) or inaccessible tumors in the brain stem, pons, and the like, because of a potential disastrous outcome.

Classification and Staging

Histopathology

Reliance on a pathologic classification of brain tumors is a requisite for treatment. Indeed, histopathology is more important than anatomic staging in determining the clinical behavior and prognosis of these tumors. Tissue diagnosis should be obtained in all patients with a brain tumor; the few exceptions include patients with diffuse intrinsic brain stem gliomas and optic nerve gliomas.

Central nervous system tumors are generally classified as follows: (1) gliomas, (2) neuronal/glioneuronal neoplasms, (3) embryonal neoplasms, (4) meningeal neoplasms, and (5) miscellaneous nonglial neoplasms (Table 29–2). *Tumor classification is based on histologic evidence of differentiation;* however, expression of histologic features may vary widely within tumors of a given type, particularly diffuse gliomas. This regional heterogeneity makes interpretation of small biopsy samples difficult; this is especially true of astrocytomas. Unfortunately, these difficulties can have significant implications on the diagnosis and grading of these tumors.

Gliomas

The majority of primary brain tumors are "diffuse" gliomas, which include:

- astrocytoma, anaplastic astrocytoma, and GBM
- low- and high-grade oligodendrogliomas, and mixed oligoastrocytomas[80]

As a rule, the diffuse gliomas are associated with a relatively unfavorable outcome because of a tendency for widespread parenchymal invasion and "anaplastic transformation." The more circumscribed astrocytomas, such as the pilocytic astrocytoma, pleomorphic xanthoastrocytoma, and subependymal giant cell astrocytomas, have distinctive pathologic features, a low-to-negligible frequency of transformation, and a more favorable prognosis. Low- and high-grade ependymomas are also circumscribed gliomas.

Attempts to provide prognostically significant diagnostic categories for gliomas have resulted in the use of several histologic grading systems. As a rule, these schemes have divided the continuum of malignancy into grades based upon the presence or absence of key histologic features: nuclear atypia, mitoses, endothelial proliferation, and necrosis, with or without peripheral palisading of nuclei

TABLE 29–2. **Histopathology of Brain Tumors**

Major Classification	Variants	WHO Grades
Glioma		
Astrocytic: circumscribed	Pilocytic astrocytoma	I
	Subependymal giant cell astrocytoma (SEGA)	I
	Pleomorphic xanthoastrocytoma (PXA)	II
Astrocytic: diffuse	Astrocytoma	II
	Anaplastic astrocytoma	III
	Glioblastoma multiforme	IV
Oligodendroglial	Oligodendroglioma	II
	Anaplastic oligodendroglioma	III
Mixed gliomas	Oligoastrocytoma	II
	Anaplastic oligoastrocytoma	III
Ependymal	Subependymoma	I
	Myxopapillary ependymoma	I
	Ependymoma	II
	Anaplastic ependymoma*	III
Choroid plexus	Choroid plexus papilloma	I
	Choroid plexus carcinoma*	III
Cranial & Peripheral Nerve Tumors	Schwannoma	I
Neuronal & Glioneuronal Tumors	Gangliocytoma/ganglioglioma	I–III
	Desmoplastic infantile ganglioma (DIG)	I
	Dysplastic cerebellar gangliocytoma	I
	Central neurocytoma	I
	Dysembryoplastic neuroepithelial tumor	I
	Paraganglioma	I
Pineal Parenchymal Tumors (PPT)	Pineocytoma	II
	PPT with intermediate differentiation	III
	Pineoblastoma	IV
Embryonal Tumors	Medulloepithelioma*	IV
	Primitive neuroectodermal tumor (PNET),*	IV
	including medulloblastoma and variants*	IV
	Atypical teratoid/rhabdoid tumor (AT/RT)	IV
	Cerebral neuroblastoma/ganglioneuroblastoma	IV
	Ependymoblastoma*	IV
	Olfactory neuroblastoma (esthesioneuroblastoma)	IV
Meningeal Tumors	Meningioma	I
	Atypical meningioma	II
	Anaplastic (malignant) meningioma	III
Germ Cell Tumors	Hemangiopericytoma†	II–III
	Germinoma	NA
	Mature teratoma	NA
	Nongerminomatous germ cell tumors	NA
Tumors of the Sellar Region	Craniopharyngioma: adamantinomatous	I
	Craniopharyngioma: papillary	I
Hemopoietic Neoplasms	Primary CNS lymphoma (PCNSL)	NA
	Secondary lymphoma/leukemia	NA
	Histiocytic tumors and histiocytoses	NA
Secondary Tumors/Metastases	Carcinomas and sarcomas	NA

WHO = World Health Organization; NA = not applicable.
*Indicates those tumors with a tendency to disseminate throughout the CNS.
†Origin of hemangiopericytoma is uncertain.

(pseudopalisading). Of the numerous grading schemes that have been applied to diffuse astrocytomas, four systems are best known: the Kernohan,[81] the Ringertz/Burger,[82] the St. Anne–Mayo,[83] and the 2000 World Health Organization (WHO) classification and grading system[84] (Table 29–3).

The grading scheme most commonly used today is the 2000 WHO classification.[84] As applied to diffuse gliomas, the WHO classification employs a three-tier grading system based on the same four basic histologic criteria described earlier, and is a simplification of the St. Anne–Mayo system[83]:

- Grade II tumors show atypia.
- Grade III lesions acquire mitotic activity.
- Grade IV tumors show either endothelial proliferation or necrosis, or both.

The WHO classification system designates astrocytomas, anaplastic astrocytomas, and GBM as grades II, III, and IV, respectively. Grade II astrocytomas are sometimes referred to as low or intermediate grade; grades III and IV are high grade. In the WHO classification, the designation *grade I* is reserved for a variety of glial and glioneuronal tumors, such as pilocytic astrocytoma, subependymal giant cell astrocytoma, and ganglioglioma; all carry favorable prognoses and are not diffusely infiltrative neoplasms.[84] Although the WHO and the St. Anne–Mayo methods provide comparable results, this situation is not true of other

TABLE 29–3. **Classification Schemes for Gliomas**

Kernohan	Ringertz-Burger	St. Anne–Mayo	WHO
Grade 1 Mild cellularity, normal appearing astrocytes, no anaplasia, no mitoses		Grade I No features present	Grade 1 Pilocytic astrocytoma
Grade 2 Mild cellularity, mild anaplasia, no mitoses	Astrocytoma: mild pleomorphism, hypercellularity, mitoses rare	Grade 2 One feature present (pleomorphism)	Grade II Diffuse growth of well-differentiated astrocytes, nuclear atypia only, no mitoses
Grade 3 Increased cellularity, moderate anaplasia, mitoses present; vascular proliferation & necrosis may be seen	Anaplastic astrocytoma: moderate pleomorphism, hypercellularity, increased mitoses	Grade 3 Two features present (usually pleomorphism and mitoses)	Grade III Nuclear atypia, increased mitoses, pleomorphism, some vascular proliferation
Grade 4 Marked cellularity, numerous mitoses, extensive anaplasia, necrosis & vascular proliferation present	Glioblastoma multiforme: Features of anaplastic astrocytoma plus necrosis	Grade 4 3 or 4 features present (pleomorphism, mitoses, necrosis and/or endothelial proliferation)	Grade IV Necrosis or endothelial proliferation, mitoses, undifferentiated or primitive appearing cells

WHO = World Health Organization.
Modified from Coons SW, Johnson PC: Pathology of primary intracranial malignant neoplasms. In: Morantz RA, Walsh JW (eds): Brain Tumors: A Comprehensive Text, p 45. New York, Marcel Dekker, 1994.

classification and grading schemes. Thus, it is important for the pathologist to specify which system is being used.

ASTROCYTOMAS (WHO GRADES I–IV)

Because of their infiltrative nature and lack of encapsulation, all astrocytomas can be regarded as malignant lesions and are classified as diffuse versus circumscribed. The circumscribed astrocytomas have a favorable prognosis and are readily cured by surgical excision. Based upon histologic appearance, the diffuse astrocytomas are infiltrative and are sometimes further classified as fibrillary, gemistocytic, giant cell, small cell, or disease extent, as in gliomatosis cerebri. With the exception of gliomatosis cerebri, the diffuse astrocytomas display a continuum of malignancy from low to high grade (grade II to grade IV). The characteristic feature of anaplastic astrocytoma is mitotic activity; other features include a moderate degree of hypercellularity, cellular pleomorphism, and nuclear atypia. An astrocytoma of lower grade has fewer or none of these features.

Glioblastoma Multiforme (WHO grade IV). GBM is the most common adult CNS malignancy and the deadliest.[8] The incidence gradually increases from childhood into adulthood, peaking in the sixth and seventh decades. Approximately 40% of all CNS malignancies in adults are glioblastoma.[86] The disease is more common in men than in women. Histologically, the hallmark of GBM is the presence of necrosis with pseudopalisading of neoplastic nuclei; necrosis distinguishes GBM from astrocytomas of lesser grade.[87]

Pilocytic Astrocytoma (WHO grade I). Pilocytic astrocytoma is the most frequent brain tumor in children and young adults, and is found in the cerebellum, hypothalamus, third ventricle, optic nerve, cerebral hemisphere, and spinal cord.[88] Histologically, pilocytic astrocytomas are composed of bipolar or piloid cells with dense fibrillation. Rosenthal fibers (elongated eosinophilic club-shaped structures) and eosinophilic granular bodies are characteristic of this tumor, and glial fibrillary acidic protein immunoreactivity is always present, although to varying degrees. A biphasic compact and loose microcystic pattern may predominate. Pilocytic astrocytomas rarely undergo malignant transformation, although the presence of cytologic atypia and rare mitoses are not uncommon.[89] In general, these tumors have a favorable prognosis and the 10- and 20-year survival rates are 95% and 85%, respectively.[90, 91]

Subependymal Giant Cell Astrocytoma (WHO grade I). Subependymal giant cell astrocytomas present as large, sharply demarcated, solid, and often calcified, intraventricular tumors near the foramen of Monro.[92] There is no infiltration into the surrounding tissue. Histologically, these neoplasms have a mixed architecture with spindle, epithelioid, and occasional giant cells with primarily glial features, but occasionally neuronal-like giant cells; true giant cells are uncommon.[93] The prognosis of this tumor is excellent.

Pleomorphic Xanthoastrocytoma (WHO grade II). Pleomorphic xanthoastrocytoma is an unusual, often seizure-associated, cystic tumor with nodular enhancement presenting in children and young adults. It occurs in the temporal lobes more frequently than in the parietal lobes, and is superficial in location, often involving the leptomeninges.[92, 94] Pleomorphic xanthoastrocytoma lesions feature cellular pleomorphism, xanthomatous cells that vary in number, bizarre nuclei often having cytoplasmic pseudoinclusions, and eosinophilic granular bodies.[95] Anaplastic transformation is infrequent (10% to 20%), so the prognosis is favorable. Despite nuclear abnormalities, cellular pleomorphism and focal necrosis, such tumors should not be mistaken for GBMs.

OLIGODENDROGLIOMAS (WHO GRADE II/III)

Oligodendrogliomas (WHO grade II) arise from oligodendrocytes or from precursor cells committed to oligodendroglial differentiation.[80] Oligodendrogliomas are comprised of uniform cells with round uniform nuclei, surrounded either by a rim of clear cytoplasm, resulting in the classic "fried egg" appearance, or by a scant, slightly eccentric rim of pink cytoplasm, and a few processes. The "fried egg" appearance results as an artifact of delayed fixation. In addition to these distinctive rounded cells, oligodendrogliomas may contain "transitional" cells; these range from gliofibrillary oligodendrocytes to miniature gemistocytic cells; their finding does not indicate a mixed tumor.[96] Oligodendrogliomas have a tendency to infiltrate overlying cortex and exhibit perineuronal satellitosis. Typically, a dense network of thin-walled, branching capillaries gives a "chicken-wire" appearance. Spherical microcalcifications are often present.

Anaplastic oligodendrogliomas (WHO grade III), as distinct from anaplastic astrocytomas, have proved to be responsive to multiagent chemotherapy and, therefore, the two lesions need to be distinguished. Glial fibrillary acidic protein fragments can provide the distinction; these fragments may be identified using such techniques as one- or two-dimensional electrophoresis.[97]

Mixed oligodendroglioma–astrocytomas are not rare. The diagnosis requires finding an obvious population of fibrillary or gemistocytic astrocytes, or both. The relative proportion of oligodendroglial and astrocytic elements affects the prognosis.

EPENDYMAL TUMORS (WHO GRADES I–III)

Ependymal tumors arise from ependymal or subependymal cells lining the cerebral ventricles and the central canal of the spinal cord.

Ependymoma (WHO grade II). Ependymomas most commonly develop in the posterior fossa, lateral ventricles, and spinal cord. Intracranial ependymomas primarily affect children, whereas spinal ependymomas are more common in adults.[98] The cells form typical perivascular pseudorosettes and, infrequently, true rosettes.[99] Uniform round nuclei are present in a fibrillary background and nucleoli are distinct. Histologic variants include cellular, papillary, clear cell, and tanycytic. Histologically, these lesions are sharply demarcated, like metastases.

Anaplastic Ependymoma (WHO grade III). Anaplastic ependymomas are less common and constitute about one quarter of the intracranial ependymomas. They have significant mitotic activity, nuclear polymorphism, high cell density, necrosis, and microvascular endothelial proliferation. They have a greater propensity to invade adjacent brain tissue and disseminate through the cerebrospinal axis.

Myxopapillary Ependymoma (WHO grade I). Myxopapillary ependymomas primarily occur in the filum terminale and, rarely, in the pre- or postsacral soft tissues. Despite its grade I histology, myxopapillary ependymoma can metastasize to the lung,[100] although it is uncommon. Myxopapillary ependymoma has a characteristic feature of abundant intercellular and perivascular mucin.

Subependymoma (WHO grade I). Subependymomas are slow-growing, distinctive nodular tumors of the ventricular surface that are sharply circumscribed like an ependymoma; most occur in the lateral or 4th ventricle. These tumors are hypocellular and characterized by nests of benign cell bodies in a high fibrillar background. Nonetheless, subependymomas are benign, and simple resection is curative.

Neuronal and Glioneuronal Neoplasms

These neoplasms include ganglion cell tumors (WHO grade I–III), central neurocytomas (WHO grade II), dysembryoplastic neuroepithelial tumors (WHO grade I), and paragangliomas (WHO grade II). With the possible exception of anaplastic gangliogliomas (WHO grade III) and central neurocytomas (WHO grade II), these tumors need only to be treated surgically.

PINEAL PARENCHYMAL TUMORS (PINEOCYTOMA/PINEOBLASTOMA)

Pineocytomas occur primarily in middle and late adulthood and, on CT and MRI, appear as discrete, contrast-enhancing lesions in the pineal region that are often globular; calcification may be seen.[101] Histologically, the cells possess round nuclei with "salt and pepper" and chromatin form pineocytic rosettes (large, exaggerated Homer Wright rosettes) filled with argyrophilic processes having club-shaped endings. Bizarre nuclei may be seen, but mitoses are lacking.

Pineoblastomas, in contrast, occur primarily in children and are rare and highly malignant.[101] Frequently, there is CSF seeding with drop metastases or leptomeningeal enhancement, or both, on MRI. Histologically, these are classified as small "blue cell tumors" (primitive neuroectodermal tumors or PNETs). There are no pineocytomatous rosettes, but Homer Wright rosettes are often present. Pineal parenchymal tumors with intermediate differentiation are also seen; the range of reported incidences of the various pineal parenchymal tumors reflects difficulties in their classification.[102]

EMBRYONAL TUMORS

Embryonal tumors include medulloepithelioma, medulloblastoma and its variants, PNET (a medulloblastoma-like tumor outside the cerebellum), atypical teratoid/rhabdoid tumor, central neuroblastoma/ganglioneuroblastoma, ependymoblastoma, olfactory neuroblastoma, and retinoblastoma.

Medulloblastoma/PNET. The medulloblastoma is a prototypical PNET that occurs predominantly in children.[103] Histologically, the lesions feature small cells with round or "carrot shaped" nuclei, inapparent nucleoli, and scant cytoplasm; however, the cell of origin is still uncertain.[103, 104] The classic medulloblastoma variant is infiltrative, and usually involves the cerebellar vermis. The desmoplastic form occurs primarily in the lateral cerebellar hemispheres of adults, and exhibits both reticulin rich and "germinal center"–like nodules in which glioneuronal differentiation may be seen. Medullomyoblastoma is characterized by rhabdomyoblastic differentiation, and melanotic medulloblastoma by melanosome-associated melanin production. Medulloblastomas are aggressive tumors; this is particularly true of extracerebellar PNETs.

Atypical Teratoid/Rhabdoid Tumor (AT/RT). The AT/RT is a recently described tumor that has long been included with medulloblastoma/PNET.[84] Most of these tumors present before the age of 2 years and arise in either the cerebrum or cerebellum. Fully one third are disseminated at initial diagnosis. They are characterized by varying combinations of rhabdoid or large "pale" cells with open chromatin and prominent nucleoli and mesenchyme or epithelial cells. Their immunophenotype is therefore far more complex than that of medulloblastoma/PNET. Despite the term "teratoid," the AT/RT is not a germ cell tumor because it lacks the serum markers of the latter and has a much worse prognosis. Resistance to treatment and death by 6 months is the rule.

Olfactory Neuroblastoma. The olfactory neuroblastoma, also known as esthesioneuroblastoma, involves the vault of the nose and cribriform plate region; intracranial extension may be seen. Histologically, these tumors form a morphologic spectrum from paraganglioma to neuroblastomas, but typically with a closer resemblance to paraganglioma.[105] Aggressive behavior is associated with histologic malignancy; a high MIB-1, and a neuroblastic predominance.

Meningeal Neoplasms and Pseudotumors

Meningeal neoplasms include meningioma, hemangiopericytoma, and other primary mesenchymal neoplasms, both benign (chondroma, fibrous histiocytoma, hemangioma, solitary fibrous tumor) and malignant (hemangiopericytoma, malignant fibrous histiocytoma/fibrosarcoma, osteosarcoma, chondrosarcoma) and melanocytic tumors. Secondary neoplasms also are found in the meninges, the majority originating from lung or breast carcinomas. Primary brain tumors occasionally show meningeal attachment, for example, GBM, desmoplastic infantile astrocytoma, ganglioglioma, and the like. There are also inflammatory pseudotumors, dural based masses of unknown etiology, such as rheumatoid nodules, Rosai-Dorfman disease, Erdheim-Chester disease, and various granulomatous disorders. Clinically and radiologically, these processes can mimic meningioma.

MENINGIOMAS

The histology of meningiomas is highly variable. Meningothelial in derivation, they consist of cells ranging from epithelioid to elongated, often feature nuclear pseudo-inclusions, whorls, psammoma bodies, and hyalinized vessels, and the tumors vary in terms of the amount of stromal collagen present.

In the past, the definition of *atypical meningioma* has been debated; however, atypical meningiomas are now well characterized and considered to be WHO grade II.[106] The most important histologic characteristic of an atypical meningioma is frequent mitoses, at least four mitoses per 10 high power fields. In the absence of this level of mitotic activity, the Mayo Clinic definition of atypical meningioma also includes at least three of the five following features:

- a sheeting pattern of growth with loss of whorls and fascicles
- small cells (lymphocyte-like nests with high nucleus-to-cytoplasm ratios)
- hypercellularity
- macronucleoli
- necrosis, often with pseudopalisading

Malignant meningiomas are considered WHO grade III. Diagnosis requires that any one of the following criteria be met:

- greater than 15 mitoses per 10 high power fields
- histology resembling that of carcinoma, sarcoma, or melanoma

Brain invasion alone is equated with "atypical meningioma," not malignancy.[106] Differentiation between intermediate and higher grades is suggested by loss of alkaline phosphatase activity, which correlates with loss of the distal part of chromosome 1p.[107]

HEMANGIOPERICYTOMA

Once termed *angioblastic meningiomas*, hemangiopericytomas are now considered to be true meningeal sarcomas.[108] Histologically, there is dense cellularity, "staghorn vessels," pale zones, variable mitotic activity and, often, a rich intercellular pattern of reticulin staining.

Other Nonglial Neoplasms

LYMPHOMA/LEUKEMIA

Primary CNS Lymphoma. Primary CNS lymphoma is increasing in frequency and occurs primarily in elderly and immunosuppressed patients.[37, 109] Favorite sites include the basal ganglia, subependymal zone, and temporal lobes where they appear contrast enhanced on CT and MRI. Central necrosis may be seen, particularly in the setting of AIDS. The tumor tends to be multifocal in nature; however, the tumor only occasionally involves the brain stem or spinal cord. Greater than 95% of CNS lymphomas are composed of large B-cell lymphocytes. In addition, small, reactive CD3+ T-cells are often present in varying numbers.

It is of note that the lesions can completely disappear with steroid therapy, a frustration to pathologists who see only chronic inflammation, a picture resembling demyelination, or no significant abnormality. This problem for clinicians and patients, as well as pathologists, can be avoided, if primary CNS lymphoma is suspected on imaging studies, by withholding steroid therapy until after a biopsy or diagnosis has been obtained.

Secondary (Systemic) Lymphoma/Leukemia. Unlike primary CNS lymphoma, which is a parenchymal disease, secondary lymphoma/leukemia involves the dura, leptomeninges, and epidural space. When seen, parenchymal involvement is secondary. Cranial nerve or spinal nerve root involvement, or both, is commonly seen. Intravascular lymphoma, a rare condition, may present with multifocal infarcts as a result of plugging of blood vessels by lymphoma cells. Despite initial responsiveness to steroid therapy, survival is short.

SECONDARY TUMORS (METASTASES)

Secondary CNS involvement by carcinoma occurs as a result of:

- hematogenous metastases from lung, breast, gastrointestinal and skin melanomas
- direct perineural extension from head and neck primaries

Although the majority of metastases are intraparenchymal and involve the gray-white matter junction, meningeal metastases also occur, primarily from breast, gastrointestinal, and prostate primaries. Melanoma, renal cell carcinoma, and choriocarcinoma produce hemorrhagic metastases. Involvement by sarcomas is rare, but is present in proportion to their frequency of occurrence.

Staging

The purpose of staging is to determine treatment, estimate prognosis, and compare treatment results between centers and between techniques. An earlier attempt by the American Joint Committee on Cancer (AJCC) to formulate a tumor-node-metastasis (TNM) staging system was based on tumor grade, tumor size (≤5 cm or >5 cm), tumor location (ipsilateral versus contralateral infiltration), and the presence or absence of distant metastasis.[110] However, this system had many faults; for example, primary brain tumors do not typically disseminate outside the central nervous system. Therefore, this cumbersome system was not found to have prognostic value and, subsequently, has been abandoned by the AJCC.[111] Tumor histology and grade and, in many instances, patient age and patient performance status are considered far more significant determinants of outcome than the TNM stage. Of note, neither the brain nor spinal cord have lymphatic drainage, and hematogenic metastases are extremely rare.

Principles of Treatment

Multidisciplinary Decisions

Because many CNS tumors are not cured by surgical resection, a multidisciplinary approach is essential for both diagnostic evaluation and for correct therapeutic decision making (Table 29–4). The goal of therapy is to maintain a good quality of life, with the least neurologic symptoms from either the tumor or the treatment, for as long as is possible. At diagnosis, progressive neurologic deterioration can usually be stabilized or reversed, or both, by corticosteroid therapy, allowing time for consultation by all disciplines. The poor results for aggressive malignancies require careful consideration for new combined-modality approaches in investigative clinical trials. Optimal management has been summarized by treatment category and histopathologic type in the appropriate following sections.

Surgery

The advent of CT scanning in 1974 and MRI scanning in 1983 has resulted in significant improvement in the preoperative delineation of tumor. The use of microsurgical techniques, stereotactic equipment, cortical mapping, intraoperative imaging, and image-guided surgery has decreased both the morbidity and mortality of neurosurgery. In addition, anesthesia safety has improved. The purpose of surgery is both diagnostic and therapeutic. Whenever possible, following biopsy and histologic confirmation of malignancy, resection should be attempted immediately.

Complete Surgical Resection

Obviously, the ideal treatment for benign and malignant tumors is complete surgical resection of tumor without causing significant permanent neurologic deficit.[112] New sophisticated technical adjuncts that aid in maximizing the amount of tumor removed safely include image-guided techniques, both frame based and frameless, and the use of intraoperative MRI.[113–116] Unfortunately, for most CNS malignancies, the ideal treatment of complete resection of the tumor is seldom possible because of the infiltrative nature of so many brain tumors. Thus, the surgical goal is reduced to maximal resection, leaving some microscopic or macroscopic disease.

TABLE 29–4. **Multidisciplinary Treatment Decisions for Various Brain Tumors**

Tumor Type	Surgery	Radiation Therapy	Chemotherapy
Astrocytoma (low-grade)	Gross total resection* followed by observation	At tumor progression, postop RT 50–55 Gy	NR
	Gross total resection*	Postop RT 50–55 Gy	NR
Astrocytoma, mixed astrocytoma (high grade)	Gross total resection*	Postop RT 60–70 Gy ± 50–60 Gy BT/RS	BCNU (patients <60 years of age)
Oligodendroglioma	Gross total resection*	Postop RT 60–70 Gy ± 50–60 Gy BT/RS	NR
Anaplastic oligodendroglioma	Gross total resection*	Postop RT 60–70 Gy	PCV
Meningioma	Subtotal resection	Postop RT 50–55 Gy	NR
	Gross total resection	NR	
Malignant meningioma	Gross total resection*	Postop RT 60 Gy	
Ependymoma	Subtotal resection	Postop RT 54–59 Gy	
	Gross total resection	Postop RT 54 Gy ± RS boost	
Medulloblastoma, anaplastic ependymoma	Gross total resection*	Postop RT 30–36 Gy to entire brain and spine; 20–25 Gy tumor boost	
Spinal cord tumors	Biopsy vs. resection	Postop RT 50 Gy	BCNU
CNS lymphoma	Biopsy	WBI 40–45 Gy	MTX or MAC

Postop RT = immediate postoperative radiation therapy (unless otherwise stated); BT = brachytherapy; RS = radiosurgery; WBI = whole brain irradiation; NR = not recommended; BCNU = carmustine; PCV = procarbazine, lomustine (CCNU), and vincristine; MTX = methotrexate; MAC = multiagent chemotherapy; CNS = central nervous system.

*Gross total resection where possible; also includes subtotal resection or biopsy.

TABLE 29–5. **Brain Tumors Treated with Surgery Alone (Complete Resection)**

Grade	Tumor Type
WHO grade I	Pilocytic astrocytoma, subependymal giant cell astrocytoma (SEGA), myxopapillary ependymoma (if totally resected without violation of capsule), subependymoma, choroid plexus papilloma, ganglioglioma/gangliocytoma, desmoplastic infantile ganglioglioma (DIG), dysplastic cerebellar gangliocytoma, pineocytoma, dysembryoplastic neuroepithelial tumor (DNT), paraganglioma, meningioma,* mature teratoma
WHO grade II	Pleomorphic xanthoastrocytoma (PXA), atypical meningioma, mature teratoma, olfactory neuroblastoma

*Excluding skull-based meningiomas, parasellar meningiomas, and meningiomas involving the cavernous sinus where surgical resection would produce significant neurologic deficit(s). In such instances, conformal external beam radiation therapy or radiosurgery should be considered.

The appropriate management following total resection of benign WHO grade I and some WHO grade II tumors is observation only. A list of tumors treated adequately with surgery alone is given in Table 29–5. Other tumors that have higher recurrence rates following surgery alone, listed in Table 29–6, are among those lesions best treated with surgery and adjuvant radiation therapy. There is some controversy as to whether there is a role for radiation therapy in ependymoma that is completely resected without being peeled off the remaining brain tissue, hence its inclusion in both tables.

In patients with malignant gliomas, although the goal of complete resection is rarely, if ever, realized, operative resection reduces the mass effect and pressure on the functional normal brain surrounding the tumor and provides adequate tissue for diagnosis. However, even with new sophisticated techniques, including intraoperative MRI, survival of patients with malignant gliomas treated with surgery alone is dismal, with a median survival of 14 weeks and a 1-year survival of 3%. These results suggest that total resection of all neoplastic cells does not occur and, indeed, tumor cells are present beyond the area of contrast enhancement seen on CT and MRI. Even for WHO grade I astrocytomas, meningiomas, ependymomas, medulloblastomas, and solitary brain metastases, survival is best when gross total resection has been achieved. Nonetheless, when total resection is not feasible, for many of the tumor types, for example, meningioma, subtotal resection followed by localized radiation therapy delivered with precise treatment planning techniques and adjuvant radiation therapy can achieve results comparable to those of total resection (Table 29–7).

TABLE 29–6. **Brain Tumors Appropriate for Treatment with Surgery plus Radiation Therapy**

Tumor Type	Defining Condition
Astrocytoma	Low grade (grade II); ?RT at diagnosis vs. at relapse Anaplastic astrocytoma (grade III) Glioblastoma multiforme (grade IV)
Ependymoma	Treatment with postoperative RT S/P MRI is controversial, but is standard following subtotal resection
Embryonal tumors	WHO grade IV
Medulloepithelioma	
Primitive neuroectodermal tumor (PNET)	Including: medulloblastoma; pineoblastoma; ependymoblastoma; retinoblastoma; central neuroblastoma/ ganglioneuroblastoma
Pineal parenchymal tumors	Malignant
Mixed pineocytoma/ pineoblastoma	WHO grade III
PPT with intermediate differentiation	WHO grade III
Meningioma	Atypical (WHO grade II); malignant (WHO grade III)
Hemangiopericytoma	WHO grades II–III
Craniopharyngioma	Adamantinomatous; papillary
Germ cell tumors	Germinoma
Nongerminomatous germ cell tumors	Immature teratoma
Incompletely excised tumors	With the exception of pilocytic astrocytomas
Recurrent tumors	S/P surgery, or RT

PPT = pineal parenchymal tumor; RT = radiation therapy; S/P = status post; MRI = magnetic resonance imaging; WHO = World Health Organization.

Partial Resection

If critical structures are involved by the tumor, partial resection may be all that is possible. According to Dr. Robert Ojemann: "The first priority is to try and preserve or improve neurologic function. For patients in whom total removal carries significant risk of morbidity, it may be better judgment to leave some tumor and plan to follow the patient or treat the residual tumor with radiation therapy,"[112] depending upon the histology, grade, and age.

Subsequent treatment following subtotal resection of some benign or WHO grade I tumors, such as a cerebellar pilocytic astrocytoma, is observation only; for most other partially resected tumors, postoperative radiation therapy is recommended (see Table 29–6). For subtotally resected

TABLE 29–7. **Results of Various Treatments of Meningioma**

Technique	5-Year Recurrence Rate (%)
Total resection	5–10
Subtotal resection	20–50
Subtotal resection + XRT	10–30
Subtotal resection + MRI/CT-based XRT*	2
Radiosurgery	<5

XRT = radiation therapy; MRI/CT = magnetic resonance imaging/computed tomography.

*Data from Goldsmith BJ, Wara WM, Wilson CB, et al: Postoperative irradiation for subtotally resected meningiomas. A retrospective analysis of 140 patients treated from 1967 to 1990. J Neurosurg 1994; 80:195.

From Larson DA: Adult brain tumors. Presented at the 41st Annual Scientific Meeting of the American Society for Therapeutic Radiology and Oncology, San Antonio, Texas, November 2, 1999.

WHO grade II astrocytomas or oligodendrogliomas, it is not yet known whether it is better to administer irradiation (with or without chemotherapy) immediately after surgery or at the time of tumor progression. The 5-year survival data from the European Organization for Research and Treatment of Cancer/Medical Research Council (EORTC/MRC) randomized trial addressing this question indicated that there was no difference in survival between those who received prompt treatment after surgery versus those who were treated at the time of progression.[119] However, because the median survival of similar patients on the North Central Cancer Treatment Group low-grade glioma trial is 9.6 years,[120] 10- and 15-year follow-up data on the EORTC/MRC trial is needed before we can definitely conclude this supposition to be true. Nonetheless, because most ependymomas cannot be completely excised because of their growth pattern or location, or both, and because radiation improves both local control and survival, postoperative radiation therapy is considered standard with these lesions if subtotally resected or peeled off the floor of the 4th ventricle.

Stereotactic Biopsy

When tumors involve functionally important brain parenchyma or deep, midline structures, stereotactic biopsy replaces the conventional open operation in order to prevent postoperative neurologic deficits. This procedure is described further in "Diagnostic Procedures."

Reoperation

Reoperation in patients with recurrent low-grade tumors may provide additional years of improved neurologic function. However, in order to try to prevent additional recurrences, the addition of postoperative radiation therapy should be considered. Alternatively, if the lesion is small and the risk of conversion to a higher grade or malignant tumor is low, gamma knife– or linear accelerator–based stereotactic radiosurgery can be considered.

Reoperation is appropriately considered in young patients with good performance status and recurrences amenable to resections that do not involve functionally important brain areas, such as those tumors located in the frontal, temporal, or occipital poles, or posterior parietal region. If such patients are treated with brachytherapy or radiosurgery, or both, at the time of reoperation, occasionally there can be gratifying results.[121–123] Nonetheless, reoperation in patients with recurrent malignant tumors, such as malignant gliomas, is controversial. No randomized, prospective trials have been performed, and no retrospective trial has convincingly demonstrated prolongation of survival from the date of tumor recurrence. One difficulty is that confounding variables can make differences in survival difficult to ascribe to surgical intervention alone. For example, the patients chosen for reoperation are, often, of a cohort that is younger and has a better performance status.[124] Survivor selection bias, in which patients that have already survived longer than average are given additional therapy, is another form of bias in these studies.[125] In a randomized study addressing the efficacy of reoperation for malignant glioma, the authors concluded that reoperation may prolong survival by 8 weeks.[124]

Reoperation can be palliative by gaining some additional time with absent or decreased symptoms, and may allow a patient to live long enough to undergo chemotherapy. Reoperation is also the only definitive way to establish the diagnosis of radiation necrosis, and is the most effective way to treat symptomatic radiation necrosis.

Radiation Therapy

At present, radiation therapy is the most important post-surgery treatment modality for malignant gliomas, embryonal tumors, malignant meningiomas, hemangiopericytomas, hemangioblastomas, craniopharyngiomas, and primitive neuroectodermal tumors, and it also plays a role in the treatment of so-called benign tumors, such as low-grade gliomas and meningiomas (see Table 29–6). Radiation therapy produces cures in certain tumors and prolonged survival in others, and it also can allay symptoms when tumors are unresectable or recur. With the possible exception of PCNSL, radiation therapy is more effective than chemotherapy alone, or any other systemic agent, in producing long-term tumor control in brain tumors.

When considering treatment for more "benign" tumors, one must consider:

- the natural course of the disease
- the risks from possible late radiation effects on cognitive function
- the possible benefits of improved symptoms, potential increased survival, or delayed tumor recurrence

In general, radiation therapy is indicated when the tumor is

- *malignant*, such as anaplastic oligodendroglioma, anaplastic oligoastrocytoma, anaplastic astrocytoma, GBM, gliosarcoma, meningiosarcoma, medulloblastoma, ependymoblastoma, pineoblastoma
- *low grade and incompletely excised*, especially if it is producing symptoms, such as low-grade astrocytoma or oligodendroglioma, ependymoma, meningioma, pinealoma, oligoastrocytoma
- *centrally located and involves critical structures*, so that surgical intervention is not possible without a great deal of morbidity or mortality, such as parasellar meningiomas, base of skull meningiomas, brain stem gliomas, and tumors involving midbrain or third ventricle, or both. It may not even be possible to safely perform a biopsy on some of these tumors.
- *a symptomatic lesion*, even a low-grade "benign" lesion, that is unresectable because of location or tumor extent
- *a metastatic lesion*; although clinically only one lesion may be suspected, MRI scan reveals that more than 50% of patients have multiple metastases, which are, in general, not amenable to surgical resection
- *a pituitary tumor* (see Chapter 26, Cancer of the Endocrine Glands)

The normal tissue tolerance, patient age, tumor histologic type and radioresponsiveness, and anatomic site determine the radiation treatment dose. However, the anatomic extent of the tumor, tumor biology, and the potential areas of spread determine the treatment fields. Because of the infiltrative pattern of growth of many CNS neoplasms into surrounding normal tissue, it is often necessary to irradiate significant areas of normal CNS tissue within the treatment volume. In addition, elective irradiation of the spinal cord is advocated for neoplasms with a high potential for meningeal seeding, such as medulloblastomas, high-grade ependymomas, pineoblastomas, and malignant gliomas of the posterior fossa with positive CSF cytology.

Normal Tissue Tolerance–Related Dose Considerations. The total radiation dose that can be administered to the CNS is limited by normal tissue tolerance. Tolerance depends on radiation factors, such as the dose per fraction, the total time of treatment, and the volume treated, and host factors, such as patient age, the presence of diabetes mellitus or hypertension, and adjunctive therapies. When normal tissue tolerance is exceeded in the brain, the classical late effect, radiation necrosis, develops.[126, 127] The risk of brain necrosis, balanced against the risk of tumor progression, determines the dose that can be given. In adults with malignant tumors, such as GBM where survival is usually measured in months, the risk of rapid tumor recurrence is high enough that a higher risk of necrosis is accepted, and doses of 60 Gy in 30 to 35 fractions are routinely used. The risk of injury increases with larger daily doses or at total doses of greater than 60 Gy.[127, 128] For adults with low-grade astrocytomas or meningiomas, whose survival is measured in years, an incidence rate of 5% or less for necrosis is, in general, acceptable. Therefore, doses of approximately 50 to 55 Gy, delivered in 1.8-Gy fractions, are frequently used, especially because the benefit of higher doses has not been established.[120] In patients with pituitary adenomas, survival is long and there is a potential risk of blindness from injury to the optic chiasm or nerves, which have a slightly lower tolerance to radiation than the brain in general. Thus, the total dose is usually restricted to 45 to 50 Gy in 25 to 28 fractions in these patients.

In general, the dose for whole brain irradiation is limited to 35 to 40 Gy, and spinal axis irradiation is given to total doses of 25 to 40 Gy, the lower doses being used for potential microscopic disease. Whole brain irradiation to 30 Gy in 10 fractions is the most commonly used schedule. This schedule produces a median survival time of 4.5 months.[128a] Of note, a number of investigators now advocate a movement away from whole brain irradiation in the treatment of brain metastases, except in small patient subsets (>65 years of age, Karnofsky performance status [KPS] of >70), in favor of more aggressive local treatment in the form of radiosurgery.[129]

Age-Related Dose Considerations. In children with malignant tumors, further dose modification is required depending upon the age of the child, as the developing brain is more sensitive to radiation therapy. Treatment in children younger than 4 years is avoided, if possible; very young children (<4 years of age) are given chemotherapy or are simply followed after surgical resection, until either tumor progression requires the use of radiation therapy or until the patient reaches 4 years of age, at which time brain growth and development is nearly complete. The young brain is more sensitive to irradiation, and postradiation learning and behavioral difficulties become a particularly severe problem for ages up to 6 years; therefore, doses in this patient age range are usually modified.[130, 131]

When a substantial portion of the brain is irradiated, patients may develop short-term memory loss and difficulty with concentration.[132, 133] In addition, radiation may cause hypothalamic pituitary axis dysfunction, which can lead, in children, to growth hormone deficiency; this dysfunction can occur at doses as low as 18 Gy, and is seen in nearly all children at doses above 35 Gy.[134] In addition, deficiencies of gonadotrophin, thyroid-stimulating hormone, and adrenocorticotrophins may be seen with doses of greater than 30 Gy.[135] More discussion can be found in Chapter 34, Late Effects of Cancer Treatment.

Postoperative Radiation Therapy

Postoperative radiation therapy is recommended for the following tumors:

1. *Symptomatic low-grade gliomas*, except pilocytic astrocytoma, and including optic glioma: Postoperative radiation appears to prolong the survival of patients, even with incompletely resected low-grade astrocytomas.[136, 137] However, a 2000 study has suggested that conventional adjuvant radiation therapy is associated with high rates of local progression in both grade II and incompletely resected grade I low-grade gliomas.[138] Nonetheless, in general, patients who are older than 35 to 40 years old, symptomatic, or have intractable seizurcs receive postoperative treatment: the usual dose is 55 Gy.
2. *Ependymoma*: Radiation therapy improves tumor control and survival and is standard treatment following partial (and total) resection.[139, 140] A local radiation field (i.e., tumor plus a margin of approximately 1–2.5 cm) based on operative and radiographic findings, to a dose of approximately 55 Gy, is usually recommended. As local control is a problem, an additional tumor boost to 59 Gy may be given.
3. *Meningioma*: Radiation therapy is effective in controlling the growth of subtotally resected and recurrent meningiomas.[117, 141] Long-term control can be achieved with a dose of 52 to 55 Gy; of note, higher doses may place the optic nerve and chiasm at risk when treating optic sheath or parasellar meningiomas.
4. *Chordoma*: Postoperative radiation improves disease-free survival in these patients[142, 143]; in addition, charged particle radiation appears to be superior to conventional radiation.[144]
5. *Neurilemoma*: Radiation therapy, delivered by stereotactic external beam technique, has efficacy for eighth cranial nerve neurilemomas or schwannoma. Radiosurgery also may be used, with hearing preservation using lower doses than previously recommended.
6. *Oligodendroglioma*: The use of postoperative radiation in this tumor is controversial, although most series report better survival with its addition, particularly apparent in patients whose tumors were subtotally resected.[145–147] It is difficult to determine the benefit with certainty because of the retrospective nature of many of the series.[145–148]

7. *High-grade astrocytomas or glioblastoma multiforme*: Following two prospective clinical trials supporting the use of radiation therapy in the treatment of malignant gliomas,[149, 150] institutions continue to use adjuvant radiation as standard, either with or without the addition of chemotherapy, in the treatment of these difficult lesions.[151–153]

Special Treatment Considerations and Techniques

LOCAL RECURRENCE

Hochberg and Pruitt reported on 35 patients who had CT scans within 2 months of autopsy, and found gross and microscopic tumor within 2 cm of the contrast-enhancing lesion identified on CT scan in 29 of 35 patients.[154] An additional two patients, who had multifocal disease identified on a previous CT scan, had additional nodules identified on postmortem examination that had not been previously identified. Similarly, Wallner and colleagues reported that 78% of 32 patients with unifocal tumors had recurrence within 2 cm of the presurgical initial tumor margin, as defined on the enhancing edge of the tumor by CT scan.[155]

Therefore, inasmuch as local control is the challenge with malignant gliomas, various means of dose escalation have been used in an attempt to increase survival. Among the techniques that have been studied are the use of neutrons, heavy particle therapy, a brachytherapy boost, radiosurgery boost, and dose escalation with three-dimensional conformal therapy. With the exception of neutrons, all of the aforementioned are currently being evaluated in clinical trials. Radiosensitizers also have been used in an attempt to increase the effectiveness of radiation, as described earlier, and radiation has been combined with chemotherapy for an additive effect.

STEREOTACTIC IMPLANTS

The use of interstitial brachytherapy, in combination with CT or MRI, allows for the delivery of much higher doses to the primary tumor while sparing much of the surrounding normal tissue; this effect is secondary to the rapid dose fall-off. The ability to deliver higher doses of radiation to the primary raised the hopes that the local control rate could be increased with this technique, especially since the use of stereotactic CT and MRI techniques allows for a more precise placement of afterloading catheters.

In general, patients are selected for stereotactic implants if they have a good performance status (KPS >70), and a single, peripheral, well-circumscribed lesion measuring less than 5 cm in size. Patients with more central lesions, or lesions involving the corpus callosum, optic chiasm, or brain stem are excluded from receiving implants.[153] Several authors have evaluated the role of stereotactic implants in the management of malignant glioma patients and have demonstrated good tolerance and improved survival rates.[156–158] Of interest, the use of stereotactic brachytherapy also may change the pattern of failure for GBM patients. Loeffler and associates noted a predominance of failures after brachytherapy occurred either at the margin of the tumor or at distant sites.[159] This result was attributed to improved control of the primary site, resulting in patients living long enough to develop metastases elsewhere.

The limiting toxicity of stereotactic implants is tumor or brain necrosis or persistent peritumoral edema. The severity of these toxicities depends on multiple factors, including the total dose, the implanted tumor volume, and the dose rate. The resultant late effects may require long-term steroid use or additional surgery for resection of the necrotic tissue. Surgery may stop or reverse the progressive neurologic deterioration and relieve the steroid dependency caused by mass effect and edema associated with irritation from necrotic tissue.

STEREOTACTIC RADIOSURGERY

Stereotactic radiosurgery is an external radiation technique in which multiple narrow radiation beams are precisely aimed at a target in order to deliver a high radiation dose to a small volume, while sparing the tissue surrounding the target. The dose is delivered using high energy x-rays created by a linear accelerator, or by γ-rays produced by an array of cobalt sources; this latter device is known as the *gamma knife*.

Stereotactic radiosurgery has been shown to produce prolonged survival when used as a boost in patients with appropriate lesions. For example, Loeffler and associates have reported a median survival rate of 26 months for 69 patients with malignant glioma (GBM) treated with radiosurgery boost.[160] However, this and similar results have raised the question of whether the improved survival was related solely to patient selection or to treatment effect.[161] The Radiation Therapy Oncology Group (RTOG) has an ongoing phase III clinical trial answering this question.

Because of the important influence of prognostic factors on survival, no conclusions can be drawn from small radiosurgery studies, unless, perhaps, recursive partitioning analysis (RPA) is performed to determine survival for each RPA class of patients. RPA was carried out by Sarkaria and his associates, who demonstrated that radiosurgery did indeed prolong survival in GBM patients, although the patients' prognosis could not be defined.[162]

RADIOSENSITIZERS

Several radiosensitizers, including IUdR, BUdR, misonidazole, and terazapine, have been used in conjunction with radiation therapy in the treatment of malignant gliomas. Misonidazole, a hypoxic cell radiosensitizer, was one of the first agents to be tested in clinical trials. The enhancement ratio for misonidazole was in the range of 1.3 to 1.7, meaning that for a given dose of radiation, there would be a 30% to 70% increase in its effectiveness with the use of misonidazole.[163] The first randomized trial looking at postoperative radiation therapy with or without misonidazole (metronidazole) showed an initial gain in overall survival with the addition of misonidazole.[164] However, this benefit of survival was short lived, and prognosis and survival beyond 12 months was not altered. Subsequent studies, by the RTOG,[165] the Cambridge glioblastoma study,[166] and the Brain Tumor Cooperative Group (BTCG),[167] have revealed no added benefit to the use of misonidazole with concurrent radiation therapy in the treatment of malignant gliomas. In fact, both the RTOG and

BTCG observed a worse survival in patients with anaplastic astrocytoma who received misonidazole.

The ability of halogenated pyrimidines to alter the radiation responsiveness of tumor cells has made them an intriguing mode of adjuvant therapy. Both IUdR and BUdR have been used in this setting.[168–170] However, none of these studies has demonstrated a clear improvement in overall survival with the use of halogenated pyrimidines.

OLDER PATIENTS WITH POOR KARNOFSKY PERFORMANCE STATUS

Consideration should be given to using an abbreviated course of irradiation when treating older patients with poor performance status because, historically, they have had a very poor prognosis.[171–173] When their survival is measured in weeks to months, treating them with a 6-week course of radiation therapy may negatively impact the quality of their short survival because they are spending precious time that might better be spent with family and friends. Of note, Bauman and associates reported on 29 patients who were older than 65 years of age or had a KPS of below 50, or both, who were treated to only 30 Gy in 10 fractions over 2 weeks.[174] When compared with historical controls who had received 60 Gy in 30 fractions, for patients with KPS below 50, there was no difference in length of survival. Similar results have been observed with short-course hypofractionated regimens in poor KPS patients.[175]

ALTERED FRACTIONATION

The poor results in patients with GBM treated with conventional doses and the potential for an increase in complications with increased total doses using standard fractionation led to hyperfractionation and accelerated hyperfractionation trials. In the accelerated hyperfractionation trials, smaller fraction doses were delivered two to three times a day, to total doses of up to 82 Gy.[167, 176, 177] The RTOG, in a randomized dose searching phase I/II trial, identified 72 Gy as having the best median survival.[176,177] However, when tested in a phase III randomized trial, RTOG 90–06, there was no significant difference in median survival between 72 Gy, in 60 fractions of 1.2 Gy delivered b.i.d., and 60 Gy in 30 fractions, given once daily.[178] Indeed, those patients with better prognostic factors, based on either age younger than 50 years or anaplastic astrocytoma histology, had a worse outcome, suggesting that brain tolerance had been exceeded.

Other fractionation regimens that have been evaluated in the treatment of malignant gliomas include hypofractionation,[172] split course,[179] and other accelerated hyperfractionated regimens.[180–183] Although none of these studies demonstrated an increase in the severe toxicity rate, none has demonstrated improvement in overall survival or median survival when compared with standard fractionation.

TOXICITY

The higher toxicity seen in patients with anaplastic astrocytoma on RTOG trial 90–06 confirms previous experience that these patients have a worse survival when treated with more aggressive therapy. This was observed in neutron trials,[184, 185] in the BTCG and RTOG misonidazole trials,[165, 167] and in the BTCG intra-arterial carmustine (BCNU) versus intravenous BCNU trial, BTCG 83–01.[186] One explanation for this phenomenon is that because patients with anaplastic astrocytoma survive longer than patients with GBM, they live long enough to manifest toxicity that can be life shortening. This possibility needs to be considered when designing clinical trials, and it has resulted in conducting trials for anaplastic astrocytoma histology that are separate from trials for GBM.

Chemotherapy

Although the role of surgery and radiation in treating brain tumors in adults is firmly established, the role of chemotherapy is on less firm footing. Indeed, many brain tumors are not sensitive to the agents currently available,[187] and the blood-brain barrier presents a formidable obstacle to many cytotoxic drugs. These factors, coupled with the toxicity of chemotherapy, have conspired to result in only a modest benefit of this modality in prolonging the lives of patients with brain tumors.

Recently, there has been an explosive growth and interest in the development of new chemotherapeutic agents and innovative approaches for treating brain tumors. Although many of these agents are still under active investigation, for the first time in decades there is great hope for dramatic improvements in the treatment of these diseases. The challenges of using chemotherapy for treating brain tumors and the novel approaches now being investigated are discussed in the following sections.

The Blood-Brain Barrier

Brain tumors are unique among malignancies because access to them by chemotherapy is impeded by the blood-brain barrier. The anatomic basis of this barrier appears to be tight interendothelial junctions unique to brain capillaries.[188] As a result, only substances that are lipid soluble, nonionized, nonprotein bound, and of low molecular weight can penetrate these capillaries.[189] In addition, recent studies of P-glycoproteins have revealed that there is a functionally defensive component to the blood-brain barrier, known as the P-glycoprotein pump.[190] The P-glycoprotein pump is ATP dependent, and is located on cell surfaces, pumping a broad range of compounds out of cells into the interstitium.[8] The presence of P-glycoprotein in brain and brain tumor capillaries suggests that it may play a role in actively extruding toxic compounds back into the intravascular space.[191, 192]

Brain tumor capillaries differ from normal brain capillaries. They are thicker walled, fenestrated, contain numerous pinocytotic vesicles, and have open endothelial gaps.[193] Hence, the blood-tumor barrier may not have the same integrity as the blood-brain barrier. However, the vessels at the edge of the tumor, closer to normal brain, resemble normal brain vessels and, like normal brain vessels, are less permeable to water-soluble compounds.[194]

The strategies for chemotherapy over the past few decades have been centered on overcoming both the blood-brain (and blood-tumor) barrier, and tumor chemoresistance. These strategies include using lipophilic agents, high-dose chemotherapy, local therapy (e.g., intratumoral or intrathecal drug delivery), and blood-brain barrier disruption. Other more biologic approaches include gene therapy, immunotherapy, differentiation therapy, and antiangiogenic therapy; the principles of these approaches are discussed in the following sections. Because the most common adult malignancy is GBM, most experience with chemotherapy is in the setting of this disease and, thus, much of the discussion refers to this disease.

Drug Delivery Strategies

CONVENTIONAL CHEMOTHERAPY

The vast majority of experience with chemotherapy for treatment of brain tumors is in the use of conventional chemotherapy, that is, modest doses of chemotherapy that cause modest toxicity. The nitrosoureas (BCNU, lomustine [CCNU]) are the most commonly used agents. They are lipophilic, have excellent penetration of the blood-brain barrier, show *in vitro* activity against a variety of CNS tumors, and have proven efficacy in patients with a broad spectrum of CNS malignancies.[10] Other commonly used agents have included procarbazine, vincristine, carboplatin, and cisplatin.[195–198] Temozolomide is a new oral alkylating agent that shows great promise in treating malignant gliomas and anaplastic astrocytoma,[199–201] and irinotecan (CPT-11) is a new topoisomerase inhibitor that also has shown activity against malignant gliomas.[202] It is likely that these and other new agents will eventually replace the more established agents, such as the nitrosoureas, because their efficacy is comparable, if not better, and there are fewer toxicities. A series of response rates for a number of single and multiagent chemotherapeutic regimens are shown in Table 29–8.

REGIONAL CHEMOTHERAPY

Regional chemotherapy employs the strategy of delivering high doses of chemotherapy to the tumor site while sparing the rest of the body from systemic toxicity. One approach is carmustine (BCNU)-impregnated polymers. Such polymers are surgically implanted in the tumor cavity at the time of initial tumor resection or at recurrence. Preliminary studies in patients with recurrent glioblastoma suggest increased efficacy with this approach.[224] Current studies are examining the role of higher concentrations of BCNU or other agents in the polymers.

Other regional approaches include intra-arterial therapy. Although this approach may result in higher "first-pass" exposure of tumor to chemotherapy, it also is associated with a higher risk of blindness and focal neurologic deficits.[225, 226] Intrathecal chemotherapy may prove to be a

TABLE 29–8. **Response Rates for Single-Agent and Multiagent Therapy in Brain Tumors**

Investigators (ref. no)	Tumor Type	No. Patients	Drug(s)	Other Therapy	Response Rate (%)
Single Agent					
Yung et al[203]	Recurrent glioma	29	Carboplatin (IV)	PRT	48
Fujiwara et al[204]	Malignant glioma	6	ACNU (IA)—high dose	—	50
		6	ACNU (IA)—low dose	—	17
Eyre et al[205]	Low-grade glioma	54	CCNU	RT	54
				RT	79
Watanabe et al[206]	Malignant glioma	19	MCNU (IA)	RT	43
		7	MCNU (IA)		33
Chauveinc et al[207]	Malignant glioma	10	ACNU (IA)	RT	30
	Anaplastic astrocytoma	17	ACNU (IA)	RT	65
Prados et al[208]	Recurrent glioma	41	Paclitaxel	PRT ± PCT	35
Fujiwara et al[209]	Malignant glioma	20	Carboplatin (IA)	—	12.5
		22	ACNU (IA)	—	45
Forsyth et al[210]	Recurrent glioma	18	Docetaxel	—	0
Newlands et al[211]	Malignant glioma	27	Temozolomide	RT	30
	Recurrent glioma	48	Temozolomide	PRT	25
Cloughesy et al[212]	Recurrent glioma	19	Carboplatin (IA)	—	70
Phuphanich et al[213]	Recurrent glioma	25	All-*trans*-retinoic acid	PRT	12
Kuratsu et al[214]	Recurrent glioma	37	MX2 (IV)	—	11
Clarke et al[215]	Recurrent glioma	49	MX2 (IV)	—	43
Multiagent					
Coyle et al[216]	Recurrent glioma	27	MOP	PRT ± PCT	52
Watne et al[217]	Recurrent glioma	79	PCV	—	60
Galanis et al[218]	Recurrent low grade glioma	61	PCV	± PCT	19
	Recurrent anaplastic astrocytoma			± PCT	11
	Recurrent oligodendrogliomas			± PCT	25
	Recurrent glioblastoma			± PCT	4.3
Soffietti et al[219]	Recurrent oligodendrogliomas	26	PCV	± PRT	62
Hildebrand et al[220]	Recurrent glioblastoma	26	PCD	—	12
	Recurrent anaplastic astrocytoma	11	PCD	—	55
van den Bent et al[221]	Recurrent glioma	16	Cisplatin + etoposide	RT	31
Brandes et al[222]	Recurrent glioma	51	Procarbazine + tamoxifen	PCT	30
Dazzi et al[223]	Malignant glioma	18	BCNU + cisplatin	RT	54

IV = intravenous; IA = intra-arterial; ACNU = nimustine; CCNU = lomustine; MCNU = ranimustine; BCNU = carmustine; MX2 = KRN8602 (novel morpholino-anthracycline); MOP = mechlorethamine + vincristine + procarbazine; PCV = carmustine + vincristine + procarbazine; PCD = dibromodulcitol + carmustine + procarbazine; RT = radiation therapy; PRT = previous radiation therapy; PCT = previous chemotherapy.

useful adjunct, but, to date, it has no proven efficacy in treating brain tumors.

BLOOD-BRAIN BARRIER DISRUPTION

Although the blood-brain barrier is significantly altered and made more penetrable by brain neoplasms, nonetheless, it is still a major obstacle to penetration of chemotherapy into brain tumors. One approach taken by many researchers has been to administer chemotherapy in conjunction with agents that increase the permeability of brain tumor vessels. One of the first attempts included the use of intra-arterial mannitol along with methotrexate, cyclophosphamide and procarbazine[227]; although responses were seen, there was considerable toxicity.

More recently, investigators have focused on RMP-7, a bradykinin analogue, that renders the brain and tumor capillaries more porous. Preliminary studies of this agent, in conjunction with carboplatin, have demonstrated responses in patients with recurrent, high-grade glioma, but the impact on overall survival is not known.[228] Other studies are focused on functional disruption of the blood-brain barrier; for example, there is an ongoing, multicenter trial in which cyclosporine is administered with vincristine and oral etoposide in children with brain stem gliomas. Cyclosporine is an inhibitor of the endothelial P-glycoprotein pump and may allow greater access of the vincristine and etoposide to the tumor, although this approach previously has been shown to induce increased systemic toxicity.[229] Another approach used recently by French scientists has attached doxorubicin to peptides, which are "acceptable" to P-glycoproteins, in order to deliver the antineoplastic agent, thus bypassing the blood-brain barrier.[230]

HIGH-DOSE CHEMOTHERAPY WITH STEM CELL RESCUE (AUTOLOGOUS BONE MARROW TRANSPLANTATION)

The rationale for high-dose chemotherapy in the treatment of brain tumors is that higher doses of chemotherapy may result in a higher proportion of the drug penetrating the blood-brain barrier, resulting in greater tumor kill, shrinkage of the tumor volume, or hindrance of tumor relapse, or a combination of these results.[201] Furthermore, there may be greater efficacy in those tumors that respond to chemotherapy in a dose-responsive fashion. Unfortunately, results of studies employing this approach in adults with newly diagnosed or recurrent high-grade gliomas have been disappointing. Tumor control has not improved over conventional therapy, and patients have suffered from major nonhematologic toxicities.[231, 232] Indeed, a retrospective study by Kramer and colleagues noted that 54% of patients at participating institutions who were treated with high-dose chemotherapy and autologous bone marrow rescue suffered acute neurologic complications.[233]

STRATEGIES TO OVERCOME TUMOR RESISTANCE

Although penetrating the blood-brain barrier is a major obstacle to the effectiveness of chemotherapy, overcoming intrinsic chemoresistance of the tumor is critical. In order to address this major problem, there is a push to develop drugs that overcome tumor chemoresistance. For example, one approach now under active investigation is the use of O^6-benzylguanine (O^6BG) to prevent resistance to the nitrosoureas and temozolomide. These agents render their cytotoxic effect by methylating the oxygen moiety at the sixth position of the DNA base guanine; however, some brain tumors have an enzyme, alkylguanine transferase (AGT), that can reverse this cytotoxic effect by cleaving the methyl group at the O^6 position of guanine and transferring it to the AGT enzyme itself. A substantial number of patients with malignant gliomas have high tumor AGT content; these patients appear to have a worse outcome than those with low tumor AGT content and are less likely to respond to temozolomide.[234, 235] Friedman and colleagues have reported that a dose of 100 mg/m^2 of O^6BG can lower AGT levels to below 10 fmol/mg for 18 hours.[236] Therefore, when O^6BG is given along with temozolomide or BCNU, the O^6BG binds to and inactivates tumor AGT and clears the route for chemotherapeutic methylation. Currently, phase I and II trials of BCNU or temozolomide plus O^6BG are under way to determine whether the two agents can be given safely together, and whether this combination results in increased tumor response and prolonged survival.

Biologic Therapy

The modest benefit of chemotherapy, coupled with the lack of progress over the past 30 years in improving the dismal prognosis of patients with high-grade gliomas, is a potent stimulus for clinician-investigators to look beyond traditional approaches to these humbling diseases. In the past decade, innovative approaches ranging from gene therapy to antiangiogenesis inhibitors have come to clinical trial and may provide a fertile ground for major breakthroughs in the coming decade.

ANTIANGIOGENIC THERAPY

The most aggressive CNS malignancies, such as glioblastoma, anaplastic astrocytoma, and anaplastic oligodendroglioma, are highly vascular and are characterized by intense endothelial proliferation. It follows that agents that can inhibit vascular proliferation might reduce blood flow to the tumor and, thereby, inhibit tumor cell growth. Thalidomide is the most developed of the antiangiogenic agents, and trials of this drug alone[237] and in combination with carboplatin[238] have established the potential for antiangiogenic agents in controlling brain tumors. Antiangiogenic agents targeting endothelial growth factor receptors, endothelial growth factors themselves, metalloproteinases, cell adhesion molecules, and protein inhibitors of angiogenesis (angiostatin and endostatin) are under development and should come to clinical trial in the near future.[239]

GENE THERAPY

There have been several clinical trials involving inoculation of retroviral vectors into the surgical cavity of resected tumors.[240, 241] Vectors introduced into the central nervous system can be designed to selectively infect replicating cells, thus sparing the normal, quiescent brain cells. The most widely used vector has been the herpes simplex thymidine kinase; this vector selectively infects replicating tumor cells and renders them susceptible to subsequent treatment with ganciclovir. Preliminary trials have suggested some tumoricidal effect, but progression at the tumor margin also has indicated problems delivering the vector to all sites of active tumor.[240, 241] Another vector in development is an adenovirus that selectively infects and kills *TP53*-deficient cells.[242]

IMMUNOTHERAPY

The observation that white blood cells are seen in and around brain tumors has raised the possibility of using the immune system to combat these tumors; however, to date, immunotherapy has not had an impact on the survival of patients with brain tumors. Clinical trials using interferon and preliminary studies of interleukin-2 plus lymphocyte-activated killer cells show some promise. Injection of a radiolabeled monoclonal antibody (^{131}I-conjugated antitenascin antibody) into the tumor cavity of patients with recurrent glioblastoma resulted in improved survival and suggests there may be a role for antitumor monoclonal antibody immunotoxins.[243] Interleukin-4 receptor, found in 60% to 80% of high-grade gliomas but not normally expressed in normal brain tissue, is being examined as a possible delivery site for pseudomonas exotoxin A.[187]

OTHER BIOLOGIC APPROACHES

A number of other approaches targeting specific intracellular biochemical pathways are in development or early clinical trials. Tamoxifen, a protein kinase C inhibitor, has shown activity against glioblastoma in several small clinical trials. The farnesyl transferase inhibitors, agents that inhibit the *RAS*-signaling pathway, an important pathway in tumor growth, may prove beneficial in treating patients with brain tumors. The differentiating agents phenylacetate and *cis*-retinoic acid, compounds that cause tumor cells to mature and stop dividing, are now in clinical trial.[244]

Toxicity

The toxicity of chemotherapy is highly variable, depending on the agents used and the condition of the patient. Side effects common to most drugs include nausea and vomiting, hematotoxicity, and fatigue. For most of the standard and newer agents used, the toxicity is mild to moderate and manageable:

- Nausea and vomiting are easily controlled with the 5-hydroxytryptamine 3 receptor blockers ondansetron or granisetron.[245]
- Hematotoxicity includes anemia, thrombocytopenia, and neutropenia. Although hematotoxicity is initially mild, cumulative doses of chemotherapy, especially with the nitrosoureas and procarbazine, often result in a heightened risk of infection and the need for transfusions.
- Fatigue is particularly problematic with procarbazine, but it also can occur with any chemotherapy regimen.

In addition to these toxicities, most agents have other, more specific toxicities. For example, cumulative doses of nitrosoureas may cause pulmonary fibrosis, and cisplatin can cause renal damage and hearing loss.[246, 247]

Results and Prognosis

There is a vast array of CNS lesions, particularly when tumor types, variants, and grades are taken into account; this array leads to hundreds of tumor categories, each with a different survival rate highly dependent on patient age and anatomic location. To maintain a perspective, the vast majority of primary CNS tumors (>60%) are related to either gliomas or meningiomas. Although great strides have been made over the past decade in using combined modalities, together with the introduction of conformal surgery, three-dimensional stereotactic radiosurgery, and brachytherapy, any significant improvement in patient survival that is measured in years remains a work in progress.

In general, the approach to treating all brain tumors has been similar, that is, surgery followed by consideration of radiation or chemotherapy, or both; nonetheless, specific therapy must be based on the precise histology of the tumor. The treatment results for some of the more common brain tumors are discussed in the following sections.

Glioblastoma Multiforme

Despite various combinations of therapy including surgery, radiation, and chemotherapy, the prognosis is dismal for these patients, with almost all succumbing to their disease within 2 years of diagnosis. The standard of care for glioblastoma remains gross total resection of the tumor, when it can be safely performed, followed by approximately 60 Gy of radiation therapy to the tumor plus 2.5 cm, given in 1.8- to 2-Gy daily fractions. The initial field is generally defined as the tumor plus edema plus 2 cm, with a total dose of 45 to 50 Gy and the boost fields treat the tumor plus 2.5 cm. Adjuvant chemotherapy with BCNU is reserved for younger, more functional patients. Every effort should be made to enroll these patients on institutional or multicenter trials exploring new approaches in surgery, radiation therapy, chemotherapy, and biologic approaches.

Surgery

The best results have been achieved when patients were treated with surgery (gross total resection) followed by radiation, with or without chemotherapy. However, because patients who are the most amenable to undergoing complete resection of their tumor are those with positive prognostic variables, that is, younger age, good KPS, or small tumors that are not adjacent to critical structures, the effect of gross total resection is difficult to assess. Nonetheless, Keles and colleagues found that patients with total resection had a significantly higher postoperative KPS score, a longer median survival rate, and a longer median time to tumor progression.[248] In addition, several studies have suggested that gross total resection or subtotal resection results in better survival than biopsy alone. The combined analysis of three RTOG trials has suggested that patients undergoing biopsy alone had a significantly worse outcome than those patients undergoing gross total resection (median survival 6.6 months vs. 11.3 months).[153, 249] These results confirmed a randomized trial by the Princess Margaret Hospital in which patients who had a biopsy only fared significantly worse than patients who underwent more extensive resection (median survival 252 days vs. 354 days).[250]

In a Brain Tumor Cooperative Group Study, it was found

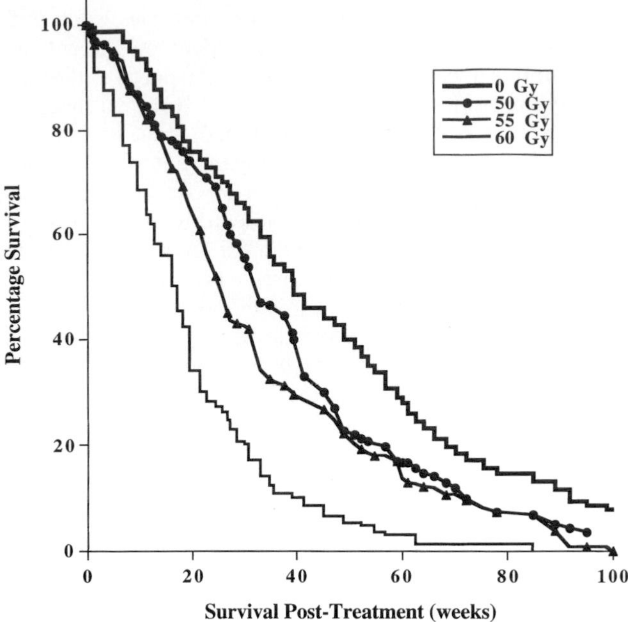

Figure 29–2. Survival curves for patients with malignant glioma who showed an increase in survival as the postoperative radiation dose increased from 0 to 60 Gy. (Modified from Walker MD, Strike TA, Sheline GE: An analysis of dose-effect relationship in radiotherapy of malignant gliomas. Int J Radiat Oncol Biol Phys 1979; 5:1725, with permission from Elsevier Science.)

that the preoperative size of the brain tumor on CT scan did not correlate with outcome, but the postoperative volume of tumor did (those with minimal residual disease fared best).[251] Indeed, in a compelling study aimed at improving a patient's chance of total resection, Knauth and colleagues measured the usefulness of intraoperative MRI.[115] Intraoperative MRI was performed when the neurosurgeon believed that all tumor had been removed; in 53.7% of the cases (n = 38), residual tumor was detected and surgery was continued.

Radiation Therapy

Postoperative radiation therapy clearly prolongs survival in patients with GBM.[252] Walker and colleagues first demonstrated this result in a large, multicenter, randomized clinical trial in which the median survival of patients who received surgery alone was 14 weeks versus 36 weeks for the patients who received surgery followed by 50 Gy of whole brain radiation.[149] In addition, by pooling data from three Brain Tumor Cooperative Group Study randomized protocols, Walker and associates retrospectively evaluated survival as a function of dose, and found that survival increased with an increase in radiation dose from 50 to 60 Gy (Fig. 29–2). Nonetheless, it has been possible to reduce radiation fields without compromising survival; Shapiro and colleagues demonstrated that patients with glioblastoma who received a lower whole brain radiation dose, but with a full dose to the coned down region of the tumor, fared as well as patients who received full-dose whole brain radiation therapy (WBRT).[254] However, studies of hyperfractionated radiation with total doses reaching as high as 81.6 Gy have not offered any survival advantage with doses greater than 60 Gy[180–183]; neither have studies using radiation with radiosensitizers.[164–167]

Brachytherapy and stereotactic radiosurgery have shown some promise in preliminary studies. Loeffler's group reported a median survival of 18 months and a 34% 2-year survival in 56 patients who received limited field external beam radiation followed by a 50-Gy boost using an implant.[255] A group from the Netherlands recently compared two brachytherapy strategies in patients with primary GBM[256]; in one arm (A) (n = 45), following biopsy, the patients were implanted with temporary or permanent ^{125}I seeds followed by 10- to 30-Gy external beam radiation therapy (EBRT), whereas patients in the other arm (B) (n = 21) underwent cytoreductive surgery, then received 60 Gy EBRT before the implantation of temporary ^{192}Ir wires. The median survival for both arms was 16 months; however, reoperations were performed in 9% of patients in arm A and 33% of patients in arm B. In addition, only patients in arm B experienced complications or late effects (n = 4). Koot and colleagues observed that despite the significant differences in radiation dose rates between the two isotopes, the median survival was the same for both arms, concluding that dose rate did not play a role in long-term survival.

Loeffler's group also has reported encouraging results using stereotactic radiosurgery; they treated 78 glioblastoma patients with EBRT followed by a radiosurgery boost.[152] The median survival was 20 months and the 2-year survival was 36%. Although the therapy was well tolerated, half of the patients required a second surgery, many because of radionecrosis. It should be noted that patients eligible for brachytherapy or stereotactic radiosurgery protocols, or both, are generally healthier, younger, and have smaller tumors and, thus, are not representative of the full spectrum of patients with this disease. Indeed, the University of California at San Francisco group analyzed survival following the use of brachytherapy or radiosurgery, and identified five selection variables: lower pathologic grade, younger age, increased KPS, smaller tumor volume, and unifocal tumor. By applying these variables, they were able to show improved survival in patients chosen for radiosurgical treatment (Table 29–9).[287] Nonetheless, some radiation oncologists advise a stereotactic radio-

TABLE 29–9. **Survival in Glioma Patients Following Radiosurgery or Brachytherapy**

		Survival (%)	
Initial Pathology	**Treatment**	***1-Year***	***2-Year***
Glioblastoma	RS	60	30
	B	50	20
Anaplastic astrocytoma	RS	70	60
	B	50	30
Astrocytoma	RS	80	70
	B	60	50

RS = radiosurgery; B = brachytherapy.

Data from Sneed PK (unpublished data), and from Larson DA, Gutin PH, McDermott M, et al: Gamma knife for glioma: selection factors and survival. Int J Radiat Oncol Biol Phys 1996; 36:1045.

From Larson DA: Adult brain tumors. Presented at the 41st Annual Scientific Meeting of the American Society for Therapeutic Radiology and Oncology, San Antonio, Texas, November 2, 1999.

surgery boost only if the area of postoperative residual enhancing tumor is less than 3 cm in diameter.

Chemotherapy

The role of chemotherapy in treating patients with glioblastoma is debatable. In two large, multicenter, randomized clinical trials conducted in the 1970s, Walker and coworkers showed that patients with glioblastoma treated with radiation plus BCNU had improved survival at 18 months (19% to 27%) compared with those patients treated with radiation alone (4% to 15%).[149, 258] However, there was no difference in the median survival or survival at 1 or 2 years. In these studies, the major prognostic factors for improved survival were age (<45 years) and KPS of 90 or higher. Fine and colleagues performed a meta-analysis of 16 trials of radiation, with or without adjuvant chemotherapy, for patients with high-grade gliomas.[259] Although there were design flaws in many of the studies, they concluded from this meta-analysis that adjuvant chemotherapy provided a modest survival benefit.

Because of their activity against glioblastoma, their penetration of the blood-brain barrier, and their mild toxicity, the nitrosoureas are the most extensively used agents for glioblastoma. Numerous other agents have been studied as adjuvant chemotherapy or in the setting of recurrent disease. Although many demonstrate activity, none have, as yet, proved superior to the nitrosoureas.

New Approaches

There is much excitement over newer agents currently under study for the treatment of glioblastoma:

- Temozolomide is an oral alkylating agent that is well absorbed, well tolerated, and has excellent CNS penetration. Friedman and associates demonstrated a 50% response rate in 33 patients with glioblastoma treated with four cycles of temozolomide before radiation therapy.[235]
- Irinotecan (CPT-11) is a topoisomerase inhibitor and another well-tolerated agent with activity against glioblastoma.[202] In patients with recurrent disease, 15% responded and 55% had stable disease. Activity of the drug is hampered by increased clearance of its active metabolite, SN-38, in patients on anticonvulsants. Studies are currently under way to assess its true activity in patients who are not on anticonvulsants.

There is a great deal of interest in investigating other, more biologic, approaches in the treatment of this disease:

- Brem and colleagues demonstrated a survival advantage in patients with recurrent glioblastoma who received locally implanted BCNU-impregnated wafers.[224]
- Gene therapy with direct inoculation of a herpes simplex thymidine kinase vector into the resection bed of patients with recurrent glioblastoma has proved to be technically feasible and has resulted in some responses.[240, 241]
- A trial of the antiangiogenic agent thalidomide for patients with recurrent glioblastoma did show a few responses.[199]

None of these approaches have proved to be any more beneficial than chemotherapy or even observation. However, the significance of these studies is that they demonstrate that the new technologies are feasible and the biologic rationale underpinning them is plausible. It is hoped that these pioneering studies will provide a foundation upon which to develop more effective therapies—polymers impregnated with multiagent chemotherapy, more effective gene therapies, targeted biologic approaches, and more potent antiangiogenic agents.

Anaplastic Astrocytoma

Anaplastic astrocytoma is a high-grade glioma that corresponds to a WHO or St. Anne–Mayo grade III astrocytoma. Efforts to characterize the impact of therapy on the outcome of patients with this disease have been hampered by their small numbers and that they are "lumped in" with the patients with glioblastoma in most studies. Nonetheless, their less malignant histology coupled with their more favorable prognosis merit their consideration as a separate disease entity. Patients with this disease are generally younger than patients with glioblastoma (median age at diagnosis 40 to 45 years vs. 55 years for glioblastoma) and their overall survival is better: 50% at 2 to 3 years.

The approach to treatment of anaplastic astrocytoma has been similar to that of glioblastoma and gross total resection is recommended if possible. Approximately 60 Gy radiation is delivered to the tumor with a 2- to 3-cm margin. There appears to be a survival benefit with adjuvant chemotherapy. A phase III study by Levin and colleagues compared BCNU with the regimen PCV (procarbazine, CCNU, and vincristine) when both were administered in combination with 60 Gy radiation and oral hydroxyurea.[196] In the treatment of anaplastic gliomas, excluding GBM, the CCNU arm achieved a median overall survival of 157.1 weeks, whereas the BCNU arm attained 82.1 weeks. The Levin study established PCV as the standard adjuvant treatment of anaplastic astrocytoma following radiation. However, in 1999, Prados and associates retrospectively reviewed the outcome of 432 patients with anaplastic astrocytoma treated with BCNU or PCV on four different RTOG protocols, and found no difference in outcome in patients treated with BCNU versus PCV.[260] Improved survival was correlated with younger age, higher KPS, and complete resection. There have been no specific studies of anaplastic astrocytoma in which patients were treated with radiation alone versus radiation plus adjuvant chemotherapy.

As with glioblastoma, many other agents have been studied in patients with newly diagnosed or recurrent anaplastic astrocytoma. Temozolomide holds great promise for this disease. For example, Yung and associates demonstrated an objective response rate of 35% in patients with recurrent anaplastic astrocytoma, and a median overall survival of 13.6 months from the time of recurrence.[261]

Low-Grade Astrocytoma

Low-grade astrocytomas fall into two categories: the WHO grade I tumors, which are associated with a very favorable outcome, and the WHO grade II tumors, which carry a much worse prognosis. Unfortunately, the WHO grade II tumors are the more common of the two tumor types and constitute approximately 5% to 10% of all adult brain tumors. Although the median duration of symptoms is 6 months, symptoms may precede diagnosis by years.[262] The tumors are almost always supratentorial, are often ill defined on CT and MRI studies, and seldom enhance.

The WHO grade I tumors are rare in adults. They are typically well circumscribed and amenable to subtotal or gross total resection, with the major histologic type being pilocytic. Laws and coworkers reported an 85% 5-year survival and 79% 10-year survival for 41 patients with pilocytic astrocytoma.[263] For the 10 patients who had gross total or radical subtotal resection, the 5- and 10-year survival rates were both 100% compared with 95% and 84%, respectively, for the 22 patients who underwent subtotal resection. The 10-year survival rate was only 44% for the 9 patients who had a biopsy only. The addition of postoperative radiation only improves survival for those patients who had subtotal resection or biopsy of the tumor.

There are many unresolved issues in the treatment of patients with this complex and variable disease. Most oncologists recommend biopsy of newly diagnosed patients with astrocytoma, and gross total resection if possible. Patients younger than 40 years of age with gross total resection are followed, and patients older than 40 generally receive radiation therapy, regardless of extent of resection. Chemotherapy is usually withheld until the time of recurrence.

Surgery

The treatment of patients with low-grade astrocytomas is controversial. Some clinicians would argue that patients who are otherwise well, and who present with CT or MRI findings consistent with a low-grade astrocytoma, may be observed without biopsy. Recht and associates reported on 26 patients followed in this fashion and compared their outcome with that of 20 patients who had prompt surgery (with or without radiation therapy).[264] There was no difference in outcome between the two groups. In symptomatic patients, there is a different story. Afra and colleagues, focusing on patients presenting with seizure, reported a notable difference in the survival times of patients treated aggressively soon after diagnosis, as compared with patients in the "delayed" surgery group: 67.5 months versus 57.5 months, respectively.[265] Indeed, in two studies of patients who presented with supratentorial nonenhancing masses on CT or MRI (typical for a low-grade astrocytoma), 30% of patients had an anaplastic astrocytoma.[266, 267]

It appears that gross total resection of low-grade astrocytoma improves outcome in these patients. This result is best illustrated in a review of 221 patients in whom extent of resection was based on postoperative CT or MRI.[268] Patients were categorized as having a gross total resection, near gross total resection ($\leq$10 cm^3 of residual tumor) or subtotal resection ($>$10 cm^3 of residual tumor). The disease-free survival of patients with gross total resection, near gross total resection, and subtotal resection was 100% and 85% at 4.5 years, and 54% at 2.5 years, respectively. Other studies have relied more upon anecdotal reports of extent of resection. Some of these reports have shown a survival benefit for patients with gross total resection,[269, 270] whereas others have not.[271, 272]

Radiation Therapy

There is considerable controversy regarding the role of radiation therapy in the treatment of patients with low-grade astrocytoma. Most of the studies cited in the literature are retrospective reviews, and the groups of patients who are or are not treated with radiation therapy are not comparable. For example, Leighton and colleagues noted an improved survival in patients who received surgery versus surgery plus radiation therapy; however, there were more patients with a gross total resection in the surgery-only arm.[273] In one of the few studies showing a dose-response benefit of radiation therapy, Shaw's group reported 5- and 10-year survivals of 68% and 39% for patients who received 53 or more Gy radiation therapy, 49% and 20% for patients who had less than 53 Gy, and 32% and 11%, respectively, for those who had surgery alone.[136] Others similarly have reported a benefit from radiation therapy,[271] but several other studies have suggested no survival benefit for patients receiving radiation.[274]

In general, most retrospective studies suggest a benefit to postoperative radiation therapy following incomplete resection, especially if the patients are symptomatic or older than 35 to 40 years of age. However, following complete resection, the benefit of radiation is more controversial and may be reserved until recurrence.

Chemotherapy

There is no proven benefit of chemotherapy in the treatment of low-grade astrocytoma. Eyre and associates conducted a randomized clinical trial of radiation, with or without CCNU, for patients with incompletely resected low-grade astrocytoma, and found no difference in median survival between the two groups.[205] Lote and coworkers also demonstrated that adjuvant chemotherapy with vincristine, procarbazine, and intra-arterial BCNU or with PCV did not improve outcome.[262] Currently, an RTOG study in progress is designed to answer some of the unresolved issues regarding treatment of patients with low-grade astrocytoma. Patients younger than 40 years of age with gross total resection are observed; patients 40 years old or older or with subtotal resection are randomized to receive radiation therapy alone versus radiation therapy plus PCV.

Oligodendroglioma

Because oligodendroglioma is a rare lesion, constituting 4% of CNS tumors, there are no prospective comparative trials of surgery, radiation, or chemotherapy. Thus the role of radiation therapy and chemotherapy is not precisely defined and is controversial. Of note, Smith and colleagues observed that patients whose tumors had loss of chromosome fragment 1p coupled with the loss of 19q could be linked to extended survival after therapy.[70]

Surgery

Surgery is the mainstay of therapy and the goal of surgery is gross total resection. Because the tumors are generally well circumscribed, gross total resection often is feasible, and these patients appear to have a better outcome than patients with subtotal resection. Shaw and associates reported median, 5-year, and 10-year survivals of 12.6 years, 74%, and 59%, respectively, for 19 patients who had gross total resection of oligodendroglioma[145]; these results compared to 2 years, 25%, and 25%, respectively, for the 8 patients who had a subtotal resection and no further therapy. Other studies corroborate the poor outcome of subtotally resected patients who do not receive radiation therapy.[146, 275]

Radiation Therapy

Most studies examining the impact of radiation on the outcome of patients with oligodendroglioma consist of retrospective reviews of small series of patients seen at single institutions over several decades. The variability of techniques over time in diagnostic imaging, surgery, neuropathology, and delivery of radiation therapy, as well as institutional biases in the approach to treatment, have made it difficult to assess the impact of radiation on survival of these patients. Nonetheless, there is some consensus on treatment that can be distilled from the aggregate of these studies. Wallner and associates reported a 56% 10-year survival in irradiated patients, compared with 18% in nonirradiated patients.[275] Gannet and colleagues showed 5- and 10-year survivals of 83% and 46% for patients treated with radiation, compared with only 51% and 36% for patients who had surgery alone.[146] In a meta-analysis of studies of oligodendroglioma, Shimuzu and associates reported a 14% improvement in 5-year survival in irradiated patients[276]; this result was supported by Shaw and colleagues, who noted an increased 5-year survival in subtotally resected, irradiated versus nonirradiated patients, although there was no difference in survival between the two groups at 10 years.[145] Indeed, in the aggregate, studies have shown an improvement in survival at 5 years in irradiated patients, but less of an effect at 10 years.

Based on these and other studies, the usual approach to patients with oligodendroglioma is to withhold radiation therapy in those patients who have had a gross total resection, particularly if they are young.[277] For those patients with large, unresectable, symptomatic tumors, radiation is generally given following surgery. Patients who have had subtotal resection, who are asymptomatic, and have only small residual disease, can be followed or treated with radiation therapy.

Chemotherapy

The long-term impact of adjuvant chemotherapy in the treatment of oligodendroglioma is unknown. Based on growing numbers of small reports, it appears that this tumor is remarkably sensitive to PCV.[8] Most studies of PCV therapy have been in patients with recurrent disease or anaplastic oligodendroglioma.[278–282] However, one group has reported a 100% disease-free survival at a median follow-up of 125 months in 6 patients with newly diagnosed oligodendroglioma who received radiation therapy and adjuvant PCV chemotherapy.[147] Nonetheless, at this time, there are not enough data to support the routine use of adjuvant PCV chemotherapy in newly diagnosed patients with oligodendroglioma. An RTOG study is currently under way to examine this approach.

Anaplastic Oligodendroglioma or Oligoastrocytoma

Patients with anaplastic oligodendroglioma or mixed anaplastic oligoastrocytoma do not fare as well as patients with pure oligodendroglioma. These patients are treated with radiation in a similar fashion to high-grade astrocytomas, even when the tumor is completely resected. In addition, these tumors are also very sensitive to PCV chemotherapy; hence, most patients are treated with PCV following radiation. Cairncross and coworkers have reported responses in 18 of 24 patients with newly diagnosed or recurrent anaplastic oligodendroglioma or mixed anaplastic oligoastrocytoma.[282] They further showed that patients whose tumors had loss of chromosome fragment 1p were more likely to respond to PCV and had a better outcome.[283] Of note, Paleologos and colleagues reported a response rate of 70% in patients treated for anaplastic oligodendrogliomas with neoadjuvant chemotherapy (PCV); the remaining 30% required preoperative radiation as a result of chemoresistance or unacceptable chemotoxicity.[284]

Nonetheless, overall survival and disease-free survival for this more aggressive variant of oligodendroglioma remains poor with 5- and 10-year survivals of 41% and 20%, respectively.[145] These rates are improving through the use of adjuvant chemotherapy; Cairncross reported a 5-year survival of 66% in 39 patients with anaplastic oligodendroglioma who received radiation and PCV chemotherapy.[282] In a phase II study, 23 patients underwent tumor resection followed by postoperative irradiation (total 60 Gy), and postradiation chemotherapy with "modified" PCV (procarbazine 60 mg/m^2, days 1–14; CCNU, 100 mg/m^2, day 1; vincristine, 1.4 mg/m^2, days 1 and 8) administered every 6 weeks for up to 6 cycles.[285] With this regimen, both the 2-year overall and progression-free survival rates were 100%, and both the 5-year overall and progression-free survival rates were 52%.

Meningioma

Meningiomas are often considered benign because they grow so slowly and can be cured by complete surgical resection alone. However, the vascularity of these tumors and their precarious location deep within the cranial cavity often precludes complete resection and any guarantee of a cure. The extra-axial location of meningiomas is evident on MRI scan, where a "dural tail" sign is often seen, that is, enhancement beyond the tumor that may be neoplastic or granulation tissue in composition.[286] Occasionally, meningiomas are aggressive, as evidenced by rapid growth and local invasiveness.[8] Signs and symptoms depend on the location of the tumor. There may be hyperostosis of overlying skull, thus a "lump on the skull" may be the presenting symptom; other symptoms include altered mentation, headaches, seizures, and in sphenoid ridge tumors, unilateral exophthalmos and vision loss.

Surgery

Meningiomas usually can be removed completely, and survival is best when gross total resection has been achieved. Generally, this goal can be accomplished when the tumor overlies the convexity of the brain or is attached to the falx cerebri or tentorium. Totally excised, benign meningiomas require no additional therapy, but where there is malignancy, adjuvant radiation therapy reduces the risk of recurrence.[287] If the tumor is highly vascular, preoperative embolization should be considered. Partial resection of meningiomas provides symptomatic relief. Because meningiomas can grow slowly, recurrent symptoms may not be a problem for years.

Meningiomas can be multiple and more than one craniotomy may be necessary for excision of all the tumors. Sometimes, there are so many tumors that some, particularly if they are indolent and not causing symptoms, are allowed to remain and are followed with serial scans at intervals of 6 to 12 months. In the same way, small, asymptomatic meningiomas may be found incidentally on scans, usually in older patients. When the tumors are not symptomatic, again they may be followed with serial scans. If they appear to be enlarging, they should be irradiated or excised.[287]

Meningiomas often occur in areas that preclude gross total resection:

- Along the superior sagittal sinus. In its posterior two thirds, this structure cannot be ligated unless it is already occluded by tumor, and this procedure also may require leaving some tumor along its wall at the time of surgery.
- Meningiomas of the clivus can almost never be removed completely.

Olfactory groove tumors, which formerly were treated only with partial resection, now can be fully resected by a unilateral frontal craniotomy with orbital osteotomy.[288] Meningiomas arising from the base of the skull may be difficult to remove completely because of their involvement with the internal carotid arteries, the nerves entering the cavernous sinus, or the optic nerves. Often the bulk of the tumor can be excised, but a small portion meshing these vital structures must be allowed to remain rather than destroy their function. Any residual tumor in these critical regions is best irradiated postoperatively while the tumor is small.

Radiation Therapy

Numerous studies support the use of radiation therapy to treat patients with subtotally resected meningiomas. Although there has been some controversy as to the timing in this setting, most studies support immediate radiation therapy, rather than waiting until the time of progression.

Recurrence rates after total excision of meningiomas are low, varying between 0% and 25%, and have been shown to be predicated on the degree of peritumoral edema.[289, 290] Hence radiation is not recommended for these patients. Recurrence rates after partial surgical excision are considerably higher, ranging from 39% at 5 years to 60% at 10 years.[289, 291] When postoperative radiation therapy has been added to subtotal resection, the recurrence rates have been low and comparable to nonirradiated patients who had gross total resections.[117, 141] The Royal Marsden Hospital has reported a 77% 10-year actuarial survival after partial removal of the tumor followed by postoperative radiation therapy; inoperable patients treated with radiation alone had a survival rate of 46%.[292] In patients with base of skull meningiomas, the same institution has demonstrated 5- and 10-year progression-free survival rates of 92% and 83%, respectively, with surgery and postoperative radiation.[293] In a 1994 series, Goldsmith reported 5- and 10-year survivals of 89% and 77% in a large cohort of patients who received radiation therapy after subtotal resection[117]; 20-year survival was 90% for patients who received 52 or more Gy. This result indicates that radiation therapy is effective in this subset of patients. Deferring the use of radiation therapy until the time of recurrence, as opposed to postoperatively, has been associated with a much higher subsequent recurrence rate. In one series of patients with subtotally resected tumors, 54 patients who had immediate radiation therapy had a median survival of 10.4 years compared with 5.5 years for 30 similar patients in whom treatment was deferred until the time of progression.[294] However, stereotactic radiosurgery and interstitial brachytherapy have a role in some refractory or recurrent meningiomas.[295, 296]

Chemotherapy

There is no role for chemotherapy in the treatment of meningioma. Although some agents, such as cyclophosphamide, doxorubicin, and ifosfamide, have been used in patients with malignant meningioma or recurrent meningioma refractory to other, more standard approaches, results have been disappointing.[10] Treatment with mifepristone (RU-486), an antiprogesterone, has been moderately effective. Several investigators report that a third of patients with refractory disease responded to this approach.[297, 298]

Malignant Meningioma

Malignant meningiomas, which constitute 10% to 15% of all meningiomas, require more aggressive therapy. Adjuvant radiation therapy is recommended for all patients with malignant meningioma, even in those whose tumors are completely resected.[10] In general, the postoperative radiation doses used are 54 Gy in 1.8- to 2-Gy fractions for benign meningiomas, and 60 Gy for malignant tumors. In some centers, stereotactic radiosurgery is now being used for patients with small residual tumors, and results appear comparable to standard EBRT.[299] However, patients with malignant meningioma do not fare as well. The recurrence rate after complete resection is 33%, after complete resection plus radiation 12%, after subtotal resection plus radiation 55%, and 100% following subtotal resection alone.[300] However, a small study of 14 patients with primary malignant meningiomas who received combined-modality therapy, including CAV (cyclophosphamide, doxorubicin, and vincristine), had a median survival of 5.3 years, with a median time to progression of 4.6 years.[301]

Ependymoma

Ependymomas are derived from the ependymal lining of the ventricles, the obliterated central canal of the spinal cord, or ependymal rests within supratentorial white matter. Ependymoma is one of the more common brain tumors of childhood, but is unusual in adults.[8] Approximately two thirds of these tumors in adults are supratentorial, and one third infratentorial (including the spinal cord).[277] There are three pathologic subtypes: ependymoma, anaplastic ependymoma, and myxopapillary ependymoma; the last is an indolent tumor, commonly found in spinal cord lesions. These tumors can disseminate throughout the craniospinal axis, so once the diagnosis is established, patients should have imaging of the entire neuraxis to assess for dissemination of tumor.

Surgery is the initial treatment for intracranial ependymoma and outcome is significantly improved with gross total resection[302]; even patients with nonanaplastic ependymoma who have subtotal resections have a poor prognosis. Most clinicians recommend radiation therapy following surgery; however, there is debate over the radiation fields. Because ependymoma can disseminate, some oncologists recommend craniospinal radiation up to 36 Gy, with a boost to 54 Gy at the primary site. However, the primary site of recurrence is, in general, local. Furthermore, there appears to be as high a rate of disseminated recurrences in patients who receive craniospinal radiation as in those who receive local therapy alone.[303] Thus, most patients with local disease are treated with radiation therapy to the primary tumor alone. The impact of chemotherapy has been disappointing. Most studies of chemotherapy involve children, and although ependymomas respond to chemotherapy, this response seldom translates into increased survival. The most active agents are cisplatin and nitrosourea-based regimens.[10, 304]

Spinal cord ependymomas should be considered separately. Most are well circumscribed, the lesions are usually myxopapillary, and many are located near the cauda equina. When gross total resection is achieved, radiation is not necessary. However, when the tumor is subtotally resected or removed piecemeal, radiation is recommended.[139] In a 1999 study, 5- and 10-year survival rates of 93.8% and 67.5%, respectively, were achieved with total or partial resection and external beam radiation.[305] The authors of the study noted that the presence of cysts within or around the tumor was a positive prognostic indicator.

Neurilemoma (Schwannoma)

Neurilemoma is chiefly a tumor of adults. Surgery by the translabyrinthine or suboccipital approach is often successful, with large clinics reporting total tumor removal achieved in 95% of cases.[306] Stereotactic radiosurgery is a viable alternative, aimed at preserving hearing. Flickinger and colleagues reported preservation of useful hearing in 46% of patients treated with radiosurgery, but they also reported a negative tumor size–hearing loss relationship.[307]

Chordoma

Chordoma is an uncommon tumor that arises at the base of the skull just behind the sella turcica. Surgical resection can be performed, but does not lead to a cure, even though it may palliate symptoms; local irradiation and brachytherapy are also used. Irradiation with heavy particles has produced encouraging results, with some prolonged cures and 5-year local control rates as high as 55%.[308]

Spinal Cord Tumors

Spinal cord tumors account for approximately 10% to 20% of CNS tumors in adults.[309] The tumors are either intramedullary (arising from within the spinal cord), such as astrocytoma or ependymoma, or extramedullary (arising from structures adjacent to the cord and compressing it), such as meningioma, neurilemomas, or metastases. Management of specific tumor types is similar to management of their intracranial counterparts, and is discussed in previous sections; however, total radiation doses delivered to spinal cord tumors are usually modified to account for the lower tolerance of spinal cord to radiation.

Primary CNS Lymphoma

Although primary CNS lymphoma is a rare malignancy, the incidence appears to be on the rise. Immunocompromised patients are at increased risk of CNS lymphoma; thus, with the AIDS epidemic, CNS lymphoma has become more common.[310] In addition, for reasons that are unknown at present, there also has been a significant increase in the incidence of CNS lymphomas within the immunocompetent patient population.[311]

Immunocompetent Host

CNS lymphoma can occur at any age, but it is most common between the ages of 50 and 70. The tumor grows rapidly; thus, the time from first symptoms to presentation is short, often measured in only weeks. Thirty percent of patients have multiple lesions, 20% have ocular involvement, and, in 42% of patients, there is evidence of leptomeningeal dissemination.[311]

Because CNS lymphoma is sensitive to both radiation therapy and chemotherapy, aggressive resection is not necessary and does not improve survival.[312, 313] Until recently, radiation has been the principal therapy for CNS lymphoma[314]; whole brain or spinal radiation of 40 Gy has been shown to improve the median survival from 4 months to 10 to 18 months.[311, 314] However, unlike the response of non-CNS diffuse lymphomas, radiation oncologists have shown that WBRT with a further boost to the tumor does not improve survival[315, 316]; use of craniospinal radiation also does not appear to improve survival consistently.[317, 318] The addition of high-dose methotrexate to the treatment regimen for CNS lymphoma, however, has significantly increased survival. DeAngelis and associates treated 31 patients with intravenous high-dose methotrexate and intrathecal methotrexate followed by WBRT; the median survival was 41 months.[319]

Although there have been no comparative studies of intrathecal methotrexate with high-dose methotrexate versus the high-dose methotrexate alone, most investigators recommend the addition of intrathecal therapy given the propensity of this tumor for leptomeningeal dissemination. One group from Japan has studied methotrexate infusion schedules by comparing rapid versus regular infusion of high-dose methotrexate.[320] All 28 patients in the study received 100 mg/kg of methotrexate, on a rapid (n = 16) or regular (n = 12) schedule, followed by irradiation. The rapid infusion arm had a 93.8% partial (PR) or complete response (CR) rate, and a median survival of 60 months, compared with a 58.3% PR/CR in the regular infusion arm, with a median survival of 20 months. Notably, after the first course of therapy, the rapid infusion arm showed an overall tumor volume reduction of 66%, a figure significantly greater than that of the regular infusion arm (46%).

Neurotoxicity is a major problem for patients treated with radiation therapy for CNS lymphoma, particularly for those 60 years of age or older. For example, Abrey and colleagues have noted that almost all of their patients older than 60 years, treated with high dose methotrexate, high dose Ara-C, and whole brain irradiation, developed late neurologic sequelae, including dementia, ataxia, and incontinence.[321] For this reason, some clinicians have investigated treating older patients with chemotherapy alone. Freilich and associates treated 13 patients older than 50 years of age with high-dose methotrexate-based multiagent chemotherapy regimens[322]; their median survival was 30.5 months, and neurotoxicity was observed in only one patient.

Immunocompromised Host

The majority of immunocompromised patients who develop CNS lymphoma have AIDS. It is typically a late complication of the disease, occurring when the CD4 count is below 100/mm^3. Unlike normal hosts, CNS lymphoma in AIDS patients is caused by Epstein-Barr virus infection.[310] Its appearance on MRI is different than in normal hosts: It is often a ring-enhancing cavitary lesion resembling CNS toxoplasmosis. This appearance frequently presents a dilemma for clinicians; that is, whether the patient has lymphoma or toxoplasmosis. There are two useful tests to distinguish these disparate diseases: A PET scan shows increased uptake with lymphoma and decreased uptake with infection; Epstein-Barr virus DNA is usually detected in the cerebrospinal fluid of HIV patients with CNS lymphoma, but not in those with toxoplasmosis. Empiric treatment for toxoplasmosis and follow-up scans to assess response is not recommended if CNS lymphoma is a strong possibility.

The treatment for AIDS patients is similar to the treatment for normal immunocompetent hosts; however, WBRT results in a median survival of only 2 to 5 months in these patients.[312] The addition of high-dose methotrexate-based treatment improves survival in some AIDS patients[323]; interestingly, the newer, more effective antiretroviral therapy also has resulted in increased responses and survival.[324] Nonetheless, in general, the treatment of AIDS patients with CNS lymphoma remains largely undefined. Many regimen combinations have been used, but small patient populations and the varied dosages and drug combinations have meant that no single regimen has been adequately studied. One of the more successful, albeit inconclusive, studies treated 38 patients with the oral combination chemotherapy regimen of CCNU, etoposide, cyclophosphamide, and procarbazine.[325] This regimen has had an overall response rate of 66% and a median survival of 7 months, with a 33% overall survival at 1 year and 11% at 2 years.

Central Nervous System Metastases

Metastases to the brain are the most frequently seen CNS tumors, whereas metastases to the spinal cord are rare (see Chapter 31, Metastases and Disseminated Diseases). The most common sources are the lung, breast, and gut, but metastases may come from any malignant tumor within the body. Any patient with cancer should be evaluated with a contrasted CT scan or MRI scan if he or she develops CNS symptoms, including unexplained nausea. Metastases are usually associated with a large amount of edema; thus, if brain metastases are confirmed, the patient should be started on dexamethasone.

If the metastasis is solitary and is in a favorable location, such as the anterior frontal region, surgical excision usually is advisable. WBRT in addition to surgery may improve survival[326, 327]; however, its role is now in question. Recently, the use of stereotactic radiosurgery for patients with single (or few) lesions, with or without WBRT, has offered promise for local control of metastatic disease.[328, 329] Indeed, even in cases with multiple metastases, radiosurgery is playing a significant role. A recent study comparing WBRT alone versus WBRT plus radiosurgery showed that the group receiving WBRT alone had a median time to local failure of 6 months and a median survival of 7.5 months, compared with 36 months and 11 months, respectively, with WBRT plus radiosurgery.[330] Use of brachytherapy with ^{125}I implants[331, 332] and chemotherapy[333, 334] also has resulted in good control rates.

Prognosis

Statisticians in the RTOG have performed one of the best meta-analyses of prognostic factors for GBM and anaplastic astrocytoma. They used a database that encompassed several trials and more than 1000 patients and identified a number of broad categories, shown in Table 29–10.[335] The results from this analysis are shown in Figure 29–3, which illustrates the number of patients in each prognostic group, together with the 2-year survival rate. The approach of recursive partitioning analysis (RPA) allows for the examination of the interaction between prognostic variables and can be used to refine stratification and design of clinical trials.

AGE

In all of the histologic variants of CNS tumors, age is one of the strongest factors associated with survival. In patients with meningiomas, the 5-year survival rate has been shown to be 81% in patients aged 21 to 64 years, but drops to 56% for patients 65 years of age or older.[336] Survival is significantly better in younger patients with low-grade astrocytomas (age <40 years) and those who undergo gross total resection. In a multivariate analysis of predictors of outcome in 379 patients with low-grade astrocytoma, Lote and coworkers noted a 60% 10-year survival in patients younger than 50 years, WHO performance score of 0 to 1, normal mental status and neurologic examination, and no enhancement on CT scan.[262] Patients who did not meet any two of these criteria had only a 16% 10-year survival. In high-grade gliomas, age is again one of the most important factors for survival, although there is uncertainty as to the defining age threshold.[335, 337, 338]

TABLE 29–10. **RTOG Recursive Partitioning Analysis for Malignant Glioma Prognostic Groups**

Class	Age	KPS	Histology	Other
I	<50	—	AAF	Normal mental status
II	≥50	70–100	AAF	Symptoms for >3 months
III	<50	—	AAF	Abnormal mental status
	<50	90–100	GBM	—
IV	<50	<90	GBM	—
	≥50	70–100	AAF	Symptoms for ≤3 months
	≥50	70–100	GBM	Partial/total resection, able to work
V	≥50	70–100	GBM	Partial/total resection, unable to work
	≥50	70–100	GBM	Biopsy, RT >54.4 Gy
	≥50	<70	—	Normal mental status
VI	≥50	70–100	GBM	Biopsy, RT ≤54.4 Gy
	≥50	≤70	—	Abnormal mental status

RTOG = Radiation Therapy Oncology Group; KPS = Karnofsky performance status; AAF = astrocytoma with anaplastic or atypical foci; GBM = glioblastoma multiforme; RT = radiation therapy.

Modified from Curran WJ Jr, Scott CB, Horton J, et al: Recursive partitioning analysis of prognostic factors in three Radiation Therapy Oncology Group malignant glioma trials. J Natl Cancer Inst 1993; 85:704.

Age is also strongly linked with the adjuvant treatment; in both low- and high-grade gliomas, it has been shown that younger patients (<35 to 40 years) benefit from more radical surgery, whereas in the older patients, benefit is seen from surgery with adjuvant radiation,[339, 340] although in the elderly (≥70 years), it is suggested that reduced doses of limited field radiation therapy should be used.[341]

KARNOFSKY PERFORMANCE STATUS

In numerous clinical trials using univariate and multivariate analyses, a high (80–100) preoperative or postoperative KPS has been shown to be a favorable prognostic factor.[172, 338, 342] Through the use of RPA, a significant split has been shown to occur in survival prognosis at KPS below 70.[343]

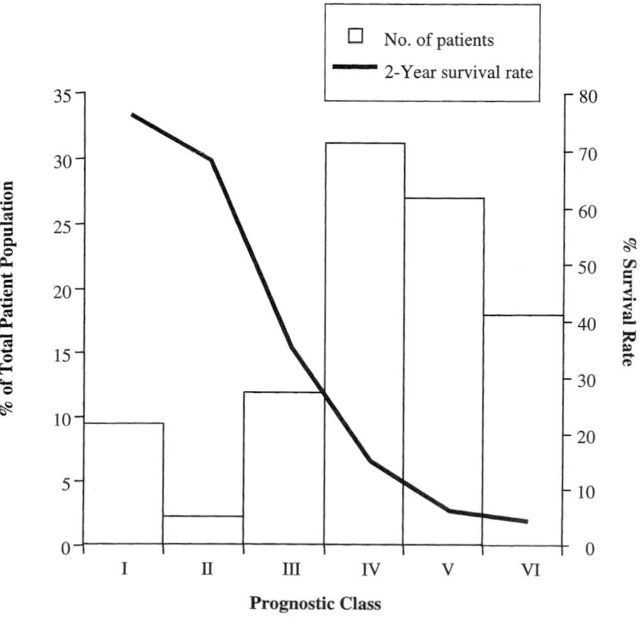

Figure 29–3. Combined data from three RTOG malignant glioma trials showing the percentage of patients found in each prognostic class (see Table 29–11) and the 2-year survival rate for each class. Data from Curran and associates.[335]

TUMOR SIZE

Many studies of low-grade CNS tumors and some high-grade gliomas have shown that tumor size (3 to 5 cm) is an important factor as an indicator of an individual's survival.[318, 320, 325] Indeed, the EORTC in a study of 399 patients showed that tumor size, that is, the T parameter, was a highly important factor.[345]

TUMOR MARKERS

The DNA labeling index may predict outcome in gliomas using an immunohistochemical stain (designed to detect the nuclear proliferating antigen Ki-67) to detect the proportion of tumor cells actively replicating. In several small studies, investigators have demonstrated an overall survival of 80% in patients with a labeling index of less than 5%, but a 0% overall survival in patients with a labeling index of above 5%.[346, 347] In an immunohistochemical study by Dehghani and colleagues, they revealed that oligodendrogliomas overexpressing vimentin or a high MIB-1 (Ki-67) nuclear labeling index, or both, corresponded to significantly lower 5-year survival rates in patients.[348]

The overexpression of oncogenes also has been looked at as a predictor of survival. One group in Germany showed that overexpression of the mdm2 protein in malignant glioma patients was a statistically significant negative prognostic indicator.[349] However, a 1998 study from the Mayo Clinic examined a large series of known oncogenes and markers (*EGFR,* CDK4, *MYC,* and others) and showed no apparent correlation between gene amplification and patient survival, suggesting that many of the genes are parts of much larger signaling pathways.[350]

Recommended Reading

The following literature is highly recommended: *Brain Tumors* by Greenberg, Chandler, and Sandler[1]; *Cancer Principles and Practice of Oncology*, 5th edition, edited by DeVita, Hellman, and Rosenberg[2]; *Clinical Oncology*, 2nd edition, edited by Abeloff, Armitage, Lichter, and Niederhuber[3]; *Principles and Practice of Radiation Oncology*, 3rd edition, edited by Perez and Brady,[4] *Textbook of Radiation Oncology*, edited by Leibel and Phillips,[5] and *Clinical Radiation Oncology*, edited by Gunderson and Tepper.[5a] For a more defined look at radiosurgery, readers are referred to *Gamma Knife Brain Surgery*, edited by Lunsford, Kondziolka, and Flickinger,[6] as well as a 1999 review article by Sims and colleagues.[7]

REFERENCES

General

1. Greenberg H, Chandler WF, Sandler HM: Brain Tumors. New York, Oxford University Press, 1999.
2. DeVita VT Jr, Hellman S, Rosenberg SA (eds): Cancer Principles and Practice of Oncology, 5th ed. Philadelphia, Lippincott-Raven, 1997.
3. Abeloff MD, Armitage JO, Lichter AS, et al (eds): Clinical Oncology, 2nd edition. New York, Churchill Livingstone, 2000.
4. Perez CA, Brady LW (eds): Principles and Practice of Radiation Oncology, 3rd ed. Philadelphia, Lippincott-Raven, 1997.
5. Leibel SA, Phillips TL (eds): Textbook of Radiation Oncology. Philadelphia, W.B. Saunders Co., 1998.

5a. Gunderson LL, Tepper JE (eds): Clinical Radiation Oncology. New York, Churchill Livingstone, 2000.

6. Lunsford LD, Kondziolka D, Flickinger JC (eds): Gamma Knife Brain Surgery. New York, Karger, 1998.
7. Sims E, Doughty D, Macaulay E, et al: Stereotactically delivered cranial radiation therapy: a ten-year experience of linac-based radiosurgery. Clin Oncol Royal Coll Radiol 1999; 11:303.

Specific

8. Shapiro WR, Shapiro JR, Walker RW: Central nervous system. In: Abeloff MD, Armitage JO, Lichter AS, et al (eds): Clinical Oncology, 2nd ed, p 1103. New York, Churchill Livingstone, 2000.
9. Greenlee RT, Murray T, Bolden S, et al: Cancer statistics, 2000. CA Cancer J Clin 2000; 50:7.
10. Levin VA, Leibel SA, Gutin PH: Neoplasms of the central nervous system. In: DeVita VT Jr, Hellman S, Rosenberg SA (eds): Cancer Principles and Practice of Oncology, 5th ed, p 2022. Philadelphia, Lippincott-Raven, 1997.
11. Stiller CA, Nectoux J: International incidence of childhood brain and spinal tumours. Int J Epidemiol 1994; 23:458.
12. Grieg NH, Ries LG, Yancik R, et al: Increasing annual incidence of primary malignant brain tumors in the elderly. J Natl Cancer Inst 1990; 82:1621.
13. Riggs JE: Longitudinal Gompertzian analysis of primary malignant brain tumor mortality in the U.S., 1962–1987: rising mortality in the elderly is the natural consequence of competitive deterministic dynamics. Mech Ageing Dev 1991; 60:225.
14. Bondy M, Wiencke J, Wrensch M, et al: Genetics of primary brain tumors: a review. J Neurooncol 1994; 18:69.
15. Kyritsis AP, Bondy ML, Xiao M, et al: Germline p53 mutation in subsets of glioma patients. J Natl Cancer Inst 1994; 86:344.
16. Bogler O, Huang HJ, Kleihues P, et al: The p53 gene and its role in human brain tumors. Glia 1995; 15:308.
17. Li Y, Bollag G, Clark R, et al: Somatic mutations in the neurofibromatosis 1 gene in human tumors. Cell 1992; 69:275.
18. von Deimling A, Louis DN, Menon AG, et al: Deletions on the long arm of chromosome 17 in pilocytic astrocytoma. Acta Neuropathol 1993; 86:81.
19. Platten M, Giordano MJ, Dirven CMF, et al: Up-regulation of specific NF1 gene transcripts in sporadic pilocytic astrocytomas. Am J Pathol 1996; 149:621.
20. Kleihues P, Cavenee WK (eds): Pathology and Genetics of Tumours of the Nervous System. Lyon, International Agency for Research on Cancer, 1998.
21. Celebi JT, Ping XL, Zhang H, et al: Germline mutations in three families with Cowden syndrome. Exp Dermatol 2000; 9:152.
22. Liaw D, Marsh DJ, Li J, et al: Germline mutations of the PTEN gene in Cowden disease, an inherited breast and thyroid cancer syndrome. Nat Genet 1997; 16:64.
23. Eng C: The role of PTEN, a phosphatase gene, in inherited and sporadic nonmeduallary thyroid tumors. Recent Prog Horm Res 1999; 54:441.
24. Hamilton SR, Liu B, Parsons RE, et al: The molecular basis of Turcot's syndrome. N Engl J Med 1995; 332:839.
25. McLaughlin MR, Gollin SM, Lese CM, et al: Medulloblastoma and glioblastoma multiforme in a patient with Turcot syndrome: a case report. Surg Neurol 1998; 49:295.
26. Taylor MD, Perry J, Zlatescu MC, et al: The hPMS2 exon 5 mutation and malignant glioma. Case report. J Neurosurg 1999; 90:946.
27. Dockerty JD, Elwood JM, Skegg DC, et al: Electromagnetic field exposures and childhood cancers in New Zealand. Cancer Causes Control 1998; 9:299.
28. UK Childhood Cancer Study: Exposure to power-frequency magnetic fields and the risk of childhood cancer. Lancet 1999; 354:1925.
29. Brownson RC, Reif JS, Chang JC, et al: An analysis of occupational risks for brain cancer. Am J Public Health 1990; 80:169.
30. Smith-Rooker JL, Garrett A, Hodges LC, et al: Prevalence of glioblastoma multiforme subjects with prior herbicide exposure. J Neurosci Nurs 1992; 24:260.
31. Bohnen NI, Kurland LT: Brain tumor and exposure to pesticides in humans: a review of the epidemiologic data. J Neurol Sci 1995; 132:110.
32. Pan BJ, Hong YJ, Chang GC, et al: Excess cancer mortality among children and adolescents in residential districts polluted by petrochemical manufacturing plants in Taiwan. J Toxicol Environ Health 1994; 43:117.
33. Cocco P, Dosemeci M, Heineman EF: Brain cancer and occupational exposure to lead. J Occup Environ Med 1998; 40:937.
34. Colquhoun SD, Robert ME, Shaked A, et al: Transmission of CNS malignancy by organ transplantation. Transplantation 1994; 57:970.
35. Jonas S, Bechstein WO, Lemmens HP, et al: Liver graft-transmitted glioblastoma multiforme. A case report and experience with 13 multiorgan donors suffering from primary cerebral neoplasia. Transplant Int 1996; 9:426.
36. Bustillo M, Perez MC, Otero GA, et al: High grade lymphoma in a post-renal transplant patient. Description of a case and literature review. Nephron 2000; 84:189.
37. Schaber M: Epidemiology of primary CNS lymphoma. J Neurooncol 1999; 43:199.
38. Franceschi S, Dal Maso L, La Vecchia C: Advances in the epidemiology of HIV-associated non-Hodgkin's lymphoma and other lymphoid neoplasms. Int J Cancer 1999; 83:481.
39. Stein M, Haim N, Kuten A, et al: Primary brain lymphoma after X-ray irradiation to the scalp for tinea capitis in childhood. J Surg Oncol 1992; 50:270.
40. Marconi F, Parenti G: Radiation-induced cerebral meningiomas. Case reports. J Neurosurg Sci 1997; 41:413.
41. Relling MV, Rubnitz JE, Rivera GK, et al: High incidence of secondary brain tumours after radiotherapy and antimetabolites. Lancet 1999; 354:34.
42. Fults D, Brockmeyer D, Tullous MW, et al: p53 mutation and loss of heterozygosity on chromosomes 17 and 10 during human astrocytoma progression. Cancer Res 1992; 52:674.
43. Kleihues P, Lubbe J, Watanabe K, et al: Genetic alterations associated with glioma progression. Verhand Deutsch Gesell Pathol 1994; 78:43.
44. Ng HK, Lam PY: The molecular genetics of central nervous system tumors. Pathology 1998; 30:196.
45. Ichimura K, Schmidt EE, Miyakawa A, et al: Distinct patterns of deletion on 10p and 10q suggest involvement of multiple tumor suppressor genes in the development of astrocytic gliomas of different malignancy grades. Genes Chromosomes Cancer 1998; 22:9.
46. Louis DN, Cavenee WK: Molecular biology of central nervous system neoplasms. In: DeVita VT Jr, Hellman S, Rosenberg SA (eds): Cancer Principles and Practice of Oncology, 5th ed, p 2013. Philadelphia, Lippincott-Raven, 1997.
47. Newcomb EW, Madonia WJ, Pisharody S, et al: A correlative study of p53 protein alteration and p53 mutation in glioblastoma multiforme. Brain Pathol 1993; 3:229.
48. Lang FF, Miller DC, Koslow M, et al: Pathways leading to glioblastoma multiforme: a molecular analysis of genetic alterations in 65 astrocytic tumors. J Neurosurg 1994; 81:427.
49. Chozick BS, Pezzullo JC, Epstein MH, et al: Prognostic implications of p53 overexpression in supratentorial astrocytic tumors. Neurosurgery 1994; 35:831.
50. Watanabe K, Sato K, Biernat W, et al: Incidence and timing of p53 mutations during astrocytoma progression in patients with multiple biopsies. Clin Cancer Res 1997; 3:523.
51. Yuan S, Miller DW, Barnett GH, et al: Identification and character-

ization of human beta 2-chimaerin: association with malignant transformation in astrocytomas. Cancer Res 1995; 55:3456.
52. Louis DN, Gusella JF: A tiger behind many doors: multiple genetic pathways to malignant glioma. Trends Genet 1995; 11:412.
53. Newcomb EW, Alonso M, Sung T, et al: Incidence of p14ARF gene deletion in high-grade adult and pediatric astrocytomas. Hum Pathol 2000; 31:115.
54. Shuangshoti S, Navalitloha Y, Kasantikul V, et al: Genetic heterogeneity and progression in different areas within high-grade diffuse astrocytoma. Oncol Rep 2000; 7:113.
55. Danks RA, Chopra G, Gonzales MF, et al: Aberrant p53 expression does not correlate with the prognosis in anaplastic astrocytoma. Neurosurgery 1995; 37:246.
56. Hwang SL, Hong YR, Sy WD, et al: Expression and mutation analysis of the p53 gene in astrocytoma. J Formos Med Assoc 1999; 98:31.
57. Nishizaki T, Ozaki S, Harada K, et al: Investigation of genetic alterations associated with the grade of astrocytic tumor by comparative genomic hybridization. Genes Chromosomes Cancer 1998; 21:340.
58. Li J, Yen C, Liaw D, et al: PTEN, a putative protein tyrosine phosphatase gene mutated in human brain, breast, and a prostate cancer. Science 1997; 275:1943.
59. Li D-M, Sun H: PTEN/MMAC1/TEP1 suppresses the tumorigenicity and induces G1 cell cycle arrest in human glioblastoma cells. Proc Natl Acad Sci U S A 1998; 95:15406.
60. Morimoto AM, Berson AE, Fujii GH, et al: Phenotypic analysis of human glioma cells expressing the MMAC1 tumor suppressor phosphatase. Oncogene 1999; 18:1261.
61. Rasheed BK, Stenzel TT, McLendon RE, et al: PTEN gene mutations are seen in high-grade but not in low-grade gliomas. Cancer Res 1997; 57:4187.
62. Hayashi Y, Ueki K, Waha A, et al: Association of EGFR gene amplification and CDKN2 (p16/MTS1) gene deletion in glioblastoma multiforme. Brain Pathol 1997; 7:871.
63. Voldborg BR, Damstrup L, Spang-Thomsen M, et al: Epidermal growth factor receptor (EGFR) and EGFR mutations, function and possible role in clinical trials. Ann Oncol 1997; 8:1197.
64. von Deimling A, Louis DN, von Ammon K, et al: Association of epidermal growth factor receptor gene amplification with loss of chromosome 10 in human glioblastoma multiforme. J Neurosurg 1992; 77:295.
65. Rasheed BK, Wiltshire RN, Bigner SH, et al: Molecular pathogenesis of malignant gliomas. Curr Opin Oncol 1999; 11:162.
66. Reifenberger J, Reifenberger G, Liu L, et al: Molecular genetic analysis of oligodendroglial tumors shows preferential allelic deletions on 19q and 1p. Am J Pathol 1994; 145:1175.
67. Bigner SH, Matthews MR, Rasheed BK, et al: Molecular genetic aspects of oligodendrogliomas including analysis by comparative genomic hybridization. Am J Pathol 1999; 155:375.
68. Smith JS, Alderete B, Minn Y, ct al: Localization of common deletion regions on 1p and 19q in human gliomas and their association with histological subtype. Oncogene 1999; 18:4144.
69. Maintz D, Fiedler K, Koopmann J, et al: Molecular genetic evidence for subtypes of oligoastrocytomas. J Neuropathol Exp Neurol 1997; 56:1098.
70. Smith JS, Perry A, Borell TJ, et al: Alterations of chromosome arms 1p and 19q as predictors of survival in oligodendrogliomas, astrocytomas, and mixed oligoastrocytomas. J Clin Oncol 2000; 18:636.
71. Shady JA, Black PM, Kupsky WJ, et al: Seizures in children with supratentorial astroglial neoplasms. Pediatr Neurosurg 1994; 21:23.
72. Valk J, de Slegte RG, Crezee FC, et al: Contrast enhanced magnetic resonance imaging of the brain using gadolinium-DTPA. Acta Radiol 1987; 28:659.
73. Stack JP, Antoun NM, Jenkins JP, et al: Gadolinium-DTPA as a contrast agent in magnetic resonance imaging of the brain. Neuroradiology 1988; 30:145.
74. Ohkawa M, Fujiwara N, Katoh T, et al: Detection of subependymal veins using high-resolution magnetic resonance venography. Acta Med Okayama 1997; 51:321.
75. Vieco PT: CT angiography of the intracranial circulation. Neuroimaging Clin N Am 1998; 8:577.
76. Herholz K, Holzer T, Bauer B, et al: ^{11}C-methionine PET for differential diagnosis of low-grade gliomas. Neurology 1998; 50:1316.
77. Mineura K, Shioya H, Kowada M, et al: Blood flow and metabolism of oligodendrogliomas: a positron emission tomography study with kinetic analysis of ^{18}F-fluorodeoxyglucose. J Neurooncol 1999; 43:49.
78. Krieger MD, Chandrasoma PT, Zee CS, et al: Role of stereotactic biopsy in the diagnosis and management of brain tumors. Semin Surg Oncol 1998; 14:13.
79. Kondziolka D, Lunsford LD: The role of stereotactic biopsy in the management of gliomas. J Neurooncol 1999; 42:205.
80. Burger PC, Scheithauer BW: Tumors of the Central Nervous System. Atlas of Tumor Pathology, Third Series, Fascicle 10. Washington, Armed Forces Institute of Pathology, 1994.
81. Kernohan JW, Mabon RF, Svien HJ, et al: A simplified classification of the gliomas. Proc Staff Meet Mayo Clin 1949; 24:71.
82. Ringertz N: Grading of gliomas. Acta Pathol Microbiol Scand 1950; 27:51.
83. Daumas-Duport C, Scheithauer B, O'Fallon J, et al: Grading of astrocytomas. A simple and reproducible method. Cancer 1988; 62:2152.
84. Kleihues P, Cavenee WK (eds): Pathology and Genetics of Tumours of the Nervous System. Lyon, France, International Agency for Research on Cancer, 2000.
85. Coons SW, Johnson PC: Pathology of primary intracranial malignant neoplasms. In: Morantz RA, Walsh JW (eds): Brain Tumors: A Comprehensive Text, p 45. New York, Marcel Dekker, 1994.
86. Polednak AP, Flannery JT: Brain, other CNS, and eye cancer. Cancer 1995; 75:330.
87. Leibel SA: Primary and metastatic brain tumors in adults. In: Leibel SA, Phillips TL (eds): Textbook of Radiation Oncology, p 293. Philadelphia, W.B. Saunders Co., 1998.
88. Kleihues P, Soylemezoglu F, Schauble B, et al: Histopathology, classification, and grading of gliomas. Glia 1995; 15:211.
89. Tomlinson FH, Scheithauer BW, Hayostek CJ, et al: The significance of atypia and histologic malignancy in pilocytic astrocytoma of the cerebellum: a clinicopathologic and flow cytometric study. J Child Neurol 1994; 9:301.
90. Pollack IF, Claassen D, al-Shboul O, et al: Low-grade gliomas of the cerebral hemispheres in children: an analysis of 71 cases. J Neurosurg 1995; 82:536.
91. Kayama T, Tominaga T, Yoshimoto T: Management of pilocytic astrocytoma. Neurosurg Rev 1996; 19:217.
92. Chen TC, Gonzalez-Gomez I, McComb JG: Uncommon glial tumors. In: Kaye AH, Laws ER Jr (eds): Brain Tumors, p 525. Edinburgh, Churchill Livingstone, 1995.
93. Lopes MB, Altermatt HJ, Scheithauer BW, et al: Immunohistochemical characterization of subependymal giant cell astrocytomas. Acta Neuropathol 1996; 91:368.
94. Kepes JJ: Pleomorphic xanthoastrocytoma: the birth of a diagnosis and a concept. Brain Pathol 1993; 3:269.
95. Giannini C, Scheithauer BW, Burger PC, et al: Pleomorphic xanthoastrocytoma: what do we really know about it? Cancer 1999; 85:2033.
96. Kros JM, Schouten WC, Janssen PJ, et al: Proliferation of gemistocytic cells and glial fibrillary acidic protein (GFAP)-positive oligodendroglial cells in gliomas: a MIB-1/GFAP double labeling study. Acta Neuropathol 1996; 91:99.
97. Luider TM, Kros JM, Sillevis Smitt PA, et al: Glial fibrillary acidic protein and its fragments discriminate astrocytoma from oligodendroglioma. Electrophoresis 1999; 20:1087.
98. Applegate GL, Marymont MH: Intracranial ependymomas: a review. Cancer Invest 1998; 16:588.
99. Liberski PP: The ultrastructure of ependymoma: personal experience and the review of the literature. Folia Neuropathol 1996; 34:212.
100. Rickert CH, Kedziora O, Gullotta F: Ependymoma of the cauda equina. Acta Neurochir 1999; 141:781.
101. Bruce JN, Connolly ES Jr, Stein BM: Pineal cell and germ cell tumors. In: Kaye AH, Laws ER Jr (eds): Brain Tumors, p 725. Edinburgh, Churchill Livingstone, 1995.
102. Jouvet A, Saint-Pierre G, Fauchon F, et al: Pineal parenchymal tumors: a correlation of histological features with prognosis in 66 cases. Brain Pathol 2000; 10:49.
103. Provias JP, Becker LE: Cellular and molecular pathology of medulloblastoma. J Neurooncol 1996; 29:35.
104. Katsetos CD, Burger PC: Medulloblastoma. Semin Diagn Pathol 1994; 11:85.
105. Hirose T, Scheithauer BW, Lopes MB, et al: Olfactory neuroblastoma. An immunohistochemical, ultrastructural, and flow cytometric study. Cancer 1995; 76:4.

106. Perry A, Stafford SL, Scheithauer BW, et al: Meningioma grading: an analysis of histologic parameters. Am J Surg Pathol 1997; 21:1455.
107. Neidermayer I, Feiden W, Henn W, et al: Loss of alkaline phosphatase activity in meningiomas: a rapid histochemical technique indicating progression-associated deletion of a putative tumor suppressor gene on the distal part of the short arm of chromosome 1. J Neuropathol Exp Neurol 1997; 56:879.
108. Perry A, Scheithauer BW, Nascimento AG: The immunophenotypic spectrum of meningeal hemangiopericytoma: a comparison with fibrous meningioma and solitary fibrous tumor of meninges. Am J Surg Pathol 1997; 21:1354.
109. Nuckols JD, Liu K, Burchette JL, et al: Primary central nervous system lymphomas: a 30-year experience at a single institution. Mod Pathol 1999; 12:1167.
110. American Joint Committee on Cancer: Manual for Staging of Cancer, 4th ed. Philadelphia, Lippincott, 1992.
111. American Joint Committee on Cancer: AJCC Cancer Staging Manual, 5th ed, p 281. Philadelphia, Lippincott-Raven, 1997.
112. Ojemann RG: Surgical principles in the management of brain tumors. In: Kaye AK, Laws ER Jr (eds): Brain Tumors, p 293. Edinburgh, Churchill Livingstone, 1995.
113. Kelly PJ: Computed tomography and histologic limits in glial neoplasms: tumor types and selection for volumetric resection. Surg Neurol 1993; 39:458.
114. Schwartz RB, Hsu L, Wong TZ, et al: Intraoperative MR imaging guidance for intracranial neurosurgery: experience with the first 200 cases. Radiology 1999; 211:477.
115. Knauth M, Wirtz CR, Tronnier VM, et al: Intraoperative MR imaging increases the extent of tumor resection in patients with high-grade gliomas. Am J Neuroradiol 1999; 20:1642.
116. Kelly PJ: Stereotactic surgery: what is past is prologue. Neurosurgery 2000; 46:16.
117. Goldsmith BJ, Wara WM, Wilson CB, et al: Postoperative irradiation for subtotally resected meningiomas. A retrospective analysis of 140 patients treated from 1967 to 1990. J Neurosurg 1994; 80:195.
118. Larson DA: Adult brain tumors. Presented at 41st Annual Scientific Meeting of the American Society for Therapeutic Radiology and Oncology, San Antonio, Texas, November 2, 1999.
119. Karim AB, Cornu P, Bleehen N, et al: Immediate postoperative radiotherapy in low grade glioma improves progression free survival, but not overall survival: preliminary results of an EORTC/MRC randomized phase III study [abstract]. Proc Am Soc Clin Oncol 1998; 17:400a.
120. Shaw EG, Arusell R, Scheithauer B, et al: A prospective randomized trial of low-versus-high-dose radiation therapy in adults with supratentorial low-grade glioma: initial report of NCCTG-RTOG-ECOG study [abstract]. Proc Am Soc Clin Oncol 1998; 17:401a.
121. Gutin PH, Leibel SA Wara WM, et al: Recurrent malignant gliomas: survival following interstitial brachytherapy with high-activity iodine-125 sources. J Neurosurg 1987; 67:864.
122. Hall WA, Djalilian HR, Sperduto PW, et al: Stereotactic radiosurgery for recurrent malignant gliomas. J Clin Oncol 1995; 13:1642.
123. Shrieve DC, Alexander E III, Wen PY, et al: Comparison of stereotactic radiosurgery and brachytherapy in the treatment of recurrent glioblastoma multiforme. Neurosurgery 1995; 36:275.
124. Barker FG II, Chang SM, Gutin PH, et al: Survival and functional status after resection of recurrent glioblastoma multiforme. Neurosurgery 1998; 42:709.
125. Florell RC, MacDonald DR, Irish WD, et al: Selection bias, survival, and brachytherapy for glioma. J Neurosurg 1992; 76:179.
126. Marks JE, Baglan RJ, Prassad SC, et al: Cerebral radionecrosis: incidence and risk in relation to dose, time, fractionation and volume. Int J Radiat Oncol Biol Phys 1981; 7:243.
127. Schultheiss TE, Kun LE, Ang KK, et al: Radiation response of the central nervous system. Int J Radiat Oncol Biol Phys 1995; 31:1093.
128. Leibel SA, Sheline GE: Tolerance of the brain and spinal cord to conventional irradiation. In: Gutin PH, Leibel SA, Sheline GE (eds): Radiation Injury to the Nervous System, p 239. New York, Raven Press, 1991.
128a. Murray KJ, Scott C, Greenberg HM, et al: A randomized phase III study of accelerated hyperfractionation versus standard in patients with unresected brain metastases: a report of the Radiation Therapy Oncology Group (RTOG) 9104. Int J Radiat Oncol Biol Phys 1997; 39:571.
129. Shaw EG: Radiotherapeutic management of multiple brain metastases: "3000 in 10" whole brain radiation is no longer a "no brainer." Int J Radiat Oncol Biol Phys 1999; 45:253.
130. Mulhern RK, Fairclough D, Ochs J: A prospective comparison of neuropsychologic performance of children surviving leukemia who received 18-Gy, 24-Gy, or no cranial irradiation. J Clin Oncol 1991; 9:1348.
131. Yang TF, Wong TT, Cheng LY, et al: Neuropsychological sequelae after treatment for medulloblastoma in childhood—the Taiwan experience. Childs Nerv Syst 1997; 13:77.
132. Maire JP, Coudin B, Guerin J, et al: Neuropsychologic impairment in adults with brain tumors. Am J Clin Oncol 1987; 10:156.
133. Armstrong C, Ruffer J, Corn B, et al: Biphasic patterns of memory deficits following moderate-dose partial-brain irradiation: neuropsychologic outcome and proposed mechanisms. J Clin Oncol 1995; 13:2263.
134. Clayton PE, Shalet SM: Dose dependency of time of onset of radiation-induced growth hormone deficiency. J Pediatr 1991; 118:226.
135. Sklar CA, Constine LS: Chronic neuroendocrinological sequelae of radiation therapy. Int J Radiat Oncol Biol Phys 1995; 31:1113.
136. Shaw EG, Daumas-Duport C, Scheithauer BW, et al: Radiation therapy in the management of low-grade supratentorial astrocytomas. J Neurosurg 1989; 70:853.
137. Trautmann TG, Shaw EG: Supratentorial low-grade glioma: is there a role for radiation therapy? Ann Acad Med Singapore 1996; 25:392.
138. Mansur DB, Hekmatpanah J, Wollman R, et al: Low grade gliomas treated with adjuvant radiation therapy in the modern imaging era. Am J Clin Oncol 2000; 23:222.
139. Wen BC, Hussey DH, Hitchon PW, et al: The role of radiation therapy in the management of ependymomas of the spinal cord. Int J Radiat Oncol Biol Phys 1991; 20:781.
140. Stuben G, Stuschke M, Kroll M, et al: Postoperative radiotherapy of spinal and intracranial ependymomas: analysis of prognostic factors. Radiother Oncol 1997; 45:3.
141. Peele KA, Kennerdell JS, Maroon JC, et al: The role of postoperative irradiation in the management of sphenoid wing meningiomas. A preliminary report. Ophthalmol 1996; 103:1761.
142. Forsyth PA, Cascino TL, Shaw EG, et al: Intracranial chordomas: a clinicopathological response and prognostic study of 51 cases. J Neurosurg 1993; 78:741.
143. York JE, Kaczaraj A, Abi-Said D, et al: Sacral chordoma: 40-year experience at a major cancer center. Neurosurgery 1999; 44:74.
144. Catton C, O'Sullivan B, Bell R, et al: Chordoma: long-term follow-up after radical photon irradiation. Radiother Oncol 1996; 41:67.
145. Shaw EG, Scheithauer BW, O'Fallon JR, et al: Oligodendrogliomas: the Mayo experience. J Neurosurg 1992; 76:428.
146. Gannett DE, Wisbeck WM, Silbergeld DL, et al: The role of postoperative irradiation in the treatment of oligodendroglioma. Int J Radiat Oncol Biol Phys 1994; 30:567.
147. Allison RR, Schulsinger A, Vongtama V, et al: Radiation and chemotherapy improve outcome in oligodendroglioma. Int J Radiat Oncol Biol Phys 1997; 37:399.
148. Allam A, Radwi A, El Weshi A, et al: Oligodendroglioma: an analysis of prognostic factors and treatment results. Am J Clin Oncol 2000; 23:170.
149. Walker MD, Alexander E, Hunt WE, et al: Evaluation of BCNU and/or radiotherapy in the treatment of anaplastic glioma. J Neurosurg 1978; 49:333.
150. Kristiansen K, Hagen S, Kollevold T, et al: Combined modality therapy of operated astrocytomas grade III and IV: confirmation of the value of postoperative irradiation and the lack of potentiation on survival time: a prospective multicentric trial of the Scandinavian Glioblastoma Study Group. Cancer 1981; 47:649.
151. Obwegeser A, Ortler M, Seiwals M, et al: Therapy of glioblastoma multiforme: a cumulative experience of 10 years. Acta Neurochir 1995; 137:29.
152. Shrieve DC, Alexander E III, Black PM, et al: Treatment of patients with primary glioblastoma multiforme with standard postoperative radiotherapy and radiosurgical boost: prognostic factors and long-term outcome. J Neurosurg 1999; 90:72.
153. Leibel SA, Pajak TF: The management of malignant gliomas with radiation therapy: therapeutic results and research strategies. Semin Radiat Oncol 1991; 1:32.
154. Hochberg FH, Pruitt A: Assumptions in the radiotherapy of glioblastoma. Neurology 1980; 30:907.
155. Wallner KE, Galicich JH, Krol G, et al: Patterns of failure following

treatment for glioblastoma multiforme and anaplastic astrocytoma. Int J Radiat Oncol Biol Phys 1989; 16:1405.
156. Ostertag CB, Kreth FW: Iodine-125 interstitial irradiation for cerebral gliomas. Acta Neurochir 1992; 119:53.
157. Scharfen CO, Sneed PK, Wara WM, et al: High activity iodine-125 interstitial implant for gliomas. Int J Radiat Oncol Biol Phys 1992; 24:583.
158. Gaspar LE, Zamarano LJ, Shamsa F, et al: Permanent ^{125}iodine implants for recurrent malignant gliomas. Int J Radiat Oncol Biol Phys 1999; 43:977.
159. Loeffler JS, Alexander E, Wen PY, et al: Results of stereotactic brachytherapy used in the initial management of patients with glioblastoma. J Natl Cancer Inst 1990; 82:1918.
160. Loeffler JS, Alexander E 3rd, Shea WM, et al: Radiosurgery as part of the initial management of patients with malignant gliomas. J Clin Oncol 1992; 10:1379.
161. Curran WJ Jr, Scott CB, Weinstein AS, et al: Survival comparison of radiosurgery-eligible and -ineligible malignant glioma patients treated with hyperfractionated radiation therapy and carmustine: a report of Radiation Therapy Oncology Group 83-02. J Clin Oncol 1993; 11:857.
162. Sarkaria JN, Mehta MP, Loeffler JS, et al: Radiosurgery in the initial management of malignant gliomas: survival comparison with the RTOG recursive partitioning analysis. Radiation Therapy Oncology Group. Int J Radiat Oncol Biol Phys 1995; 32:931.
163. Urtasun RC, Miller JDR, Frunchat V, et al: Radiotherapy pilot trials with sensitizers of hypoxic cells: metronidazole in supratentorial glioblastomas. Br J Radiol 1977; 50:602.
164. Urtasun R, Band P, Chapman JD, et al: Radiation and high dose metronidazole in supratentorial glioblastoma. N Engl J Med 1976; 294:1354.
165. Nelson DF, Diener-West M, Weinstein AS, et al: A randomized comparison of misonidazole sensitized radiotherapy plus BCNU and radiotherapy plus BCNU for treatment of malignant glioma after surgery: Final report of an RTOG study. Int J Radiat Oncol Biol Phys 1986; 12:1793.
166. Bleehan NM: The Cambridge glioma trial and radiation therapy with associated studies. Cancer Clin Trials 1980; 3:267.
167. Deutsch M, Green SB, Strike TA, et al: Results of a randomized trial comparing BCNU plus radiotherapy, streptozotocin plus radiotherapy, BCNU plus hyperfractionated radiotherapy, and BCNU following misonidazole plus radiotherapy in the postoperative treatment of malignant glioma. Int J Radiat Oncol Biol Phys 1989; 16:1389.
168. Phillips TL, Levin VA, Ahn DK, et al: Evaluation of bromodeoxyuridine in glioblastoma multiforme: a Northern California Cancer Center Phase II study. Int J Radiat Oncol Biol Phys 1990; 18:205.
169. Rodriguez R, Kinsella TJ: Halogenated pyrimidines as radiosensitizers for high grade glioma: revisited. Int J Radiat Oncol Biol Phys 1991; 21:859.
170. Phillips TL, Scott CB, Leibel SA, et al: Results of a randomized comparison of radiotherapy and bromodeoxyuridine with radiotherapy alone for brain metastases: report of RTOG trial 89-05. Int J Radiat Oncol Biol Phys 1995; 33:339.
171. Peschel RE, Wilson L, Haffty B, et al: The effect of advanced age on the efficacy of radiation therapy for early breast cancer, local prostate cancer and grade III–IV gliomas. Int J Radiat Oncol Biol Phys 1993; 26:539.
172. Slotman BJ, Kralendonk JH, van Alphen HA, et al: Hypofractionated radiation therapy in patients with glioblastoma multiforme: results of treatment and impact of prognostic factors. Int J Radiat Oncol Biol Phys 1996; 34:895.
173. Gaspar L, Scott C, Rotman M, et al: Recursive partitioning analysis (RPA) of prognostic factors in three Radiation Therapy Oncology Group (RTOG) brain metastases trials. Int J Radiat Oncol Biol Phys 1997; 37:745.
174. Bauman GS, Gaspar LE, Fisher BJ, et al: A prospective study of short-course radiotherapy in poor prognosis glioblastoma multiforme. Int J Radiat Oncol Biol Phys 1994; 29:835.
175. Hercbergs AA, Tadmor R, Findler G, et al: Hypofractionated radiation therapy and concurrent cisplatin in malignant cerebral gliomas. Rapid palliation in low performance status patients. Cancer 1989; 64:816.
176. Murray KJ, Nelson DF, Scott C, et al: Quality adjusted survival analysis of malignant glioma. Patients treated with twice-daily radiation (RT) and carmustine: a report of Radiation Therapy Oncology Group (RTOG) 83-02. Int J Radiat Oncol Biol Phys 1995; 31:453.
177. Werner-Wasik M, Scott CB, Nelson DF, et al: Final report of a phase I/II trial of hyperfractionated and accelerated hyperfractionated radiation therapy with carmustine for adults with supratentorial malignant gliomas. Radiation Therapy Oncology Group Study 83-02. Cancer 1996; 77:1535.
178. Scott C, Curran W, Yung W, et al: Long term results of RTOG 90-06: a randomized trial of hyperfractionated radiotherapy (RT) to 72.0 Gy and carmustine vs. standard RT and carmustine for malignant glioma patients with emphasis on anaplastic astrocytoma (AA) patients [abstract]. J Clin Oncol 1998; 16:384.
179. Marcial-Vega VA, Wharam MD, Leibel S, et al: Treatment of supratentorial high grade gliomas with split course high fractional dose postoperative radiotherapy. Int J Radiat Oncol Biol Phys 1989; 16:1419.
180. Shenouda G, Souhami L, Freeman CR, et al: Accelerated fractionation for high-grade cerebral astrocytomas. Preliminary treatment results. Cancer 1991; 67:2247.
181. Gonzalez DG, Menten J, Bosch DA, et al: Accelerated radiotherapy in glioblastoma multiforme: a dose searching prospective study. Radiother Oncol 1994; 32:98.
182. Levin VA, Maor MH, Thall PF, et al: Phase II study of accelerated fractionation radiation therapy with carboplatin followed by vincristine chemotherapy for the treatment of glioblastoma multiforme. Int J Radiat Oncol Biol Phys 1995; 33:357.
183. Buatti JM, Marcus RB, Mendenhall WM, et al: Accelerated hyperfractionated radiotherapy for malignant gliomas. Int J Radiat Oncol Biol Phys 1996; 34:785.
184. Griffin TW, Davis R, Laramore GE, et al: Fast neutron radiation therapy for glioblastoma multiforme—results of an RTOG study. Am J Clin Oncol 1983; 6:661.
185. Laramore GE, Martz KL, Nelson JS, et al: Radiation Therapy Oncology Group (RTOG) survival data on anaplastic astrocytomas of the brain: does a more aggressive form of treatment adversely impact survival? Int J Radiat Oncol Biol Phys 1989; 17:1351.
186. Shapiro WR, Green SB, Burger PC, et al: A randomized comparison of intra-arterial versus intravenous BCNU, with or without intravenous 5-fluorouracil, for newly diagnosed patients with malignant gliomas. J Neurosurg 1992; 76:772.
187. Galanis E, Buckner J: Chemotherapy for high-grade gliomas. Br J Cancer 2000; 82:1371.
188. Reese TS, Karnovsky MJ: Fine structural localization of a blood brain barrier to exogenous peroxidase. J Cell Biol 1967; 37:207.
189. Rall DP, Zubrod CG: Mechanisms of drug absorption and excretion: passage of drugs in and out of the central nervous system. Ann Rev Pharmacol 1962; 2:109.
190. Fromm MF: P-glycoprotein: a defense mechanism limiting oral bioavailability and CNS accumulation of drugs. Int J Clin Pharmacol Ther 2000; 38:69.
191. Cordon-Cardo C, O'Brien JP, Casals D, et al: Multidrug resistance gene (P-glycoprotein) is expressed by endothelial cells at blood-brain barrier sites [abstract]. Proc Natl Acad Sci U S A 1989; 86:695.
192. Schinkel AH, Smit JJM, Tellingen O, et al: Disruption of the mouse mdr1a P-glycoprotein gene leads to a deficiency in the blood-brain barrier and to increased sensitivity to drugs. Cell 1994; 77:491.
193. Blasberg RG, Groothuis DR: Chemotherapy of brain tumors: physiological and pharmacokinetic considerations. Semin Oncol 1986; 13:70.
194. Levin VA, Freeman-Dove M, Landahl HD: Permeability characteristics of brain adjacent to tumors in rats. Arch Neurol 1975; 32:785.
195. Sposto R, Ertel IJ, Jenkin RD, et al: The effectiveness of chemotherapy for treatment of high grade astrocytoma in children: results of a randomized trial. A report from the Children's Cancer Group. J Neurooncol 1989; 7:165.
196. Levin VA, Silver P, Hannigan J, et al: Superiority of post-radiotherapy adjuvant chemotherapy with CCNU, procarbazine, and vincristine (PCV) over BCNU for anaplastic gliomas: NCOG 6G61 final report. Int J Radiat Oncol Biol Phys 1990; 18:321.
197. Friedman HS, Krischer JP, Burger P, et al: Treatment of children with progressive or recurrent brain tumors with carboplatin or iroplatin: a Pediatric Oncology Group randomized phase II study. J Clin Oncol 1992; 10:249.
198. Shinoda J, Sakai N, Hara A, et al: Clinical trial of external beam-radiotherapy combined with daily administration of low-dose cisplatin for supratentorial glioblastoma multiforme—a pilot study. J Neurooncol 1997; 35:73.
199. Cokgar I, Friedman HS, Friedman AH: Chemotherapy for adults with malignant glioma. Cancer Invest 1999; 17:264.

200. Friedman HS: Temozolomide in early stages of newly diagnosed malignant glioma and neoplastic meningitis. Semin Oncol 2000; 27:35.
201. Prados MD: Future directions in the treatment of malignant gliomas with temozolomide. Semin Oncol 2000; 27:41.
202. Friedman HS, Petros WP, Friedman AH, et al: Irinotecan therapy in adults with recurrent or progressive malignant glioma. J Clin Oncol 1999; 17:1516.
203. Yung WK, Mechtler L, Gleason MJ: Intravenous carboplatin for recurrent malignant glioma. J Clin Oncol 1991; 9:860.
204. Fujiwara T, Matsumoto Y, Tsuchida T, et al: Intra-arterial chemotherapy with ACNU in the treatment of malignant gliomas. Gan To Kagaku Ryoho 1992; 19:489.
205. Eyre HJ, Crowley JJ, Townsend JJ, et al: A randomized trial of radiotherapy versus radiotherapy plus CCNU for incompletely resected low-grade gliomas: a Southwest Oncology Group study. J Neurosurg 1993; 78:909.
206. Watanabe M, Takeda N, Tanaka R: Effect of intra-arterial and local administration of MCNU on cerebral malignant gliomas. Gan To Kagaku Ryoho 1995; 22:811.
207. Chauveinc L, Soal-Martinez MT, Martin-Duverneuil M, et al: Intra arterial chemotherapy with ACNU and radiotherapy in inoperable malignant gliomas. J Neurooncol 1996; 27:141.
208. Prados MD, Schold SC, Spence AM, et al: Phase II study of paclitaxel in patients with recurrent malignant glioma. J Clin Oncol 1996; 14:16.
209. Fujiwara T, Matsumoto Y, Honma Y, et al: A comparison of intraarterial carboplatin and ACNU for the treatment of gliomas. Surg Neurol 1995; 44:145.
210. Forsyth P, Cairncross G, Stewart D, et al: Phase II trial of docetaxel in patients with recurrent malignant glioma: a study of the National Cancer Institute of Canada Clinical Trials Group. Invest New Drug 1996; 14:203.
211. Newlands ES, O'Reilly SM, Glaser MG, et al: The Charing Cross Hospital experience with temozolomide in patients with gliomas. Eur J Cancer 1996; 32A:2236.
212. Cloughesy TF, Gobin YP, Black KL, et al: Intra-arterial carboplatin chemotherapy for brain tumors: a dose escalation study based on cerebral blood flow. J Neurooncol 1997; 35:121.
213. Phuphanich S, Scott C, Fischbach AJ, et al: All-trans-retinoic acid: a phase II Radiation Therapy Oncology Group study (RTOG 91-13) in patients with recurrent malignant astrocytoma. J Neurooncol 1997; 34:193.
214. Kuratsu J, Arita N, Kurisu K, et al: A phase II study of KRN8602 (MX2), a novel morpholino-anthracycline derivative, in patients with recurrent malignant glioma. J Neurooncol 1999; 42:177.
215. Clarke K, Basser RL, Underhill C, et al: KRN8602 (MX2-hydrochloride): an active new agent for the treatment of recurrent high-grade glioma. J Clin Oncol 1999; 17:2579.
216. Coyle T, Baptista J, Winfield J, et al: Mechlorethamine, vincristine, and procarbazine chemotherapy for recurrent high-grade glioma in adults: a phase II study. J Clin Oncol 1990; 8:2014.
217. Watne K, Hannisdal E, Nome O, et al: Combined intra-arterial and systemic chemotherapy for recurrent malignant brain tumors. Neurosurgery 1992; 30:223.
218. Galanis E, Buckner JC, Burch PA, et al: Phase II trial of nitrogen mustard, vincristine, and procarbazine in patients with recurrent glioma: North Central Cancer Treatment Group results. J Clin Oncol 1998; 16:2953.
219. Soffietti R, Ruda R, Bradac GB, et al: PCV chemotherapy for recurrent oligodendrogliomas and oligoastrocytomas. Neurosurgery 1998; 43:1066.
220. Hildebrand J, De Witte O, Sahmoud T: Response of recurrent glioblastoma and anaplastic astrocytoma to dibromodulcitol, BCNU and procarbazine—a phase II study. J Neurooncol 1998; 37:155.
221. van den Bent MJ, Pronk L, Sillevis Smitt PA, et al: Phase II study of weekly dose-intensified cisplatin chemotherapy with oral etopside in recurrent glioma. J Neurooncol 1999; 44:59.
222. Brandes AA, Ermani M, Turazzi S, et al: Procarbazine and high-dose tamoxifen as a second-line regiment in recurrent high-grade gliomas: a phase II study. J Clin Oncol 1999; 17:645.
223. Dazzi C, Cariello A, Giannini M, et al: A sequential chemo-radiotherapeutic treatment for patients with malignant gliomas: a phase II pilot study. Anticancer Res 2000; 20:515.
224. Brem H, Piantadosi S, Burger PC, et al: Placebo-controlled trial of safety and efficacy of intraoperative controlled delivery by biodegradable polymers of chemotherapy for recurrent gliomas. Lancet 1995; 345:1008.
225. Stewart DJ, Grahovac Z, Benoit B, et al: Intracarotid chemotherapy with a combination of BCNU, cisplatin, and VM-26 in the treatment of primary and metastatic brain tumors. Neurosurgery 1984; 15:828.
226. Bobo H, Kapp JP, Vance R: Effect of intra-arterial cisplatin and 1,3-bis(2-chloroethyl)-1-nitrosourea (BCNU) dosage on radiographic response and regional toxicity in malignant glioma patients: proposal of a new method of intra-arterial dosage calculation. J Neurooncol 1992; 13:291.
227. Neuwelt EA, Howieson J, Frankel EP, et al: Therapeutic efficacy of multiagent chemotherapy with drug delivery enhancement by blood-brain barrier modification in glioblastoma. Neurosurgery 1986; 19:573.
228. Ford J, Osborn C, Barton T, et al: A phase I study of intravenous RMP-7 with carboplatin in patients with progression of malignant glioma. Eur J Cancer 1998; 34:1807.
229. Theis JG, Chan HS, Greenberg ML, et al: Increased systemic toxicity of sarcoma chemotherapy due to combination with the P-glycoprotein inhibitor cyclosporin. Int J Clin Pharmacol Ther 1998; 36:61.
230. Rousselle C, Clair P, Lefauconnier JM, et al: New advances in the transport of doxorubicin through the blood-brain barrier by a peptide vector-mediated strategy. Mol Pharmacol 2000; 57:679.
231. Mbidde EK, Selby PJ, Perren TJ, et al: High dose BCNU chemotherapy with autologous bone marrow transplantation and full dose radiotherapy for grade IV astrocytoma. Br J Cancer 1988; 58:779.
232. Abrey LE, Rosenblum MK, Papadopoulos E, et al: High dose chemotherapy with autologous stem cell rescue in adults with malignant primary brain tumors. J Neurooncol 1999; 44:147.
233. Kramer ED, Packer RJ, Ginsberg J, et al: Acute neurologic dysfunction associated with high-dose chemotherapy and autologous bone marrow rescue for primary malignant brain tumors. Pediatr Neurosurg 1997; 27:230.
234. Jaeckle KA, Eyre HJ, Townsend JJ, et al: Correlation of tumor O^6 methylguanine-DNA methyltransferase levels with survival of malignant astrocytoma patients treated with BCNU: a Southwest Oncology Group Study. J Clin Oncol 1998; 16:3310.
235. Friedman HS, McLendon RE, Kerby T, et al: DNA mismatch repair and O^6-alkylguanine-DNA alkyltransferase analysis and response to Temodal in newly diagnosed malignant glioma. J Clin Oncol 1998; 16:3851.
236. Friedman HS, Kokkinakis DM, Pluda J, et al: Phase I trial of O^6-benzylguanine for patients undergoing surgery for malignant glioma. J Clin Oncol 1998; 16:3570.
237. Fine HA, Figg WD, Jaeckle K, et al: Phase II trial of the antiangiogenic agent thalidomide in patients with recurrent high-grade gliomas. J Clin Oncol 2000; 18:708.
238. Gruber ML, Glass J: Phase I/II study of carboplatin and thalidomide in recurrent glioblastoma multiforme. Presented at the Chemotherapy Foundation Symposium XVII Innovative Cancer Therapy for Tomorrow, New York, 1999.
239. Jones PH, Harris AL: The current status of clinical trials in antiangiogenesis. PPO Updates 2000; 14:1.
240. Klatzmann D, Valery CA, Bensimon G, et al: A phase I/II study of herpes simplex virus type I thymidine kinase "suicide" gene therapy for recurrent glioblastoma. Hum Gene Ther 1998; 9:2595.
241. Shand N, Weber F, Mariani L, et al: A phase 1–2 clinical trial of gene therapy for recurrent glioblastoma multiforme by tumor transduction with the herpes simplex thymidine kinase gene followed by gancyclovir. Hum Gene Ther 1999; 10:2325.
242. Lang FF, Yung WK, Sawaya R, et al: Adenovirus-mediated p53 gene therapy for human gliomas. Neurosurgery 1999; 45:1093.
243. Bigner DD, Brown MT, Friedman AH, et al: Iodine-131-labeled antitenascin monoclonal antibody 81C6 treatment of patients with recurrent malignant gliomas: phase I trial results. J Clin Oncol 1998; 16:2202.
244. Avgeropoulos NG, Batchelor TT: New treatment strategies for malignant gliomas. Oncologist 1999; 4:209.
245. Oge A, Alkis N, Oge O, et al: Comparison of granisetron, ondansetron and tropisetron for control of vomiting and nausea induced by cisplatin. J Chemother 2000; 12:105.
246. Ikeda H, Nagashima K, Matsuyama S, et al: Multidisciplinary treatment of advanced neuroblastoma—experience in treatment with the protocol of a group study supported by a grant from Ministry of Health and Welfare. Gan No Rinsho 1988; 34:953.
247. Massin F, Coudert B, Foucher P, et al: Nitrosourea-induced lung diseases. Rev Mal Respir 1992; 9:575.

248. Keles GE, Anderson B, Berger MS: The effect of extent of resection on time to tumor progression and survival in patients with glioblastoma multiforme of the cerebral hemisphere. Surg Neurol 1999; 52:371.
249. Simpson JR, Horton J, Scott C, et al: Influence of location and extent of surgical resection on survival of patients with glioblastoma multiforme: results of 3 consecutive Radiation Therapy Oncology Group (RTOG) clinical trials. Int J Radiat Oncol Biol Phys 1993; 26:239.
250. Payne DA, Simpson WJ, Keen C, et al: Malignant astrocytoma: hyperfractionated and standard radiotherapy with chemotherapy in a randomized prospective trial. Cancer 1982; 50:2301.
251. Wood JR, Green SB, Shapiro WR: The prognostic importance of tumor size in malignant glioma: a CT scan study by the Brain Tumor Cooperative Group. J Clin Oncol 1988; 6:338.
252. Huhn SL, Mohapatra G, Bollen A, et al: Chromosomal abnormalities in glioblastoma multiforme by comparative genomic hybridization: correlation with radiation treatment outcome. Clin Cancer Res 1999; 5:1435.
253. Walker MD, Strike TA, Sheline GE: An analysis of dose-effect relationship in radiotherapy of malignant gliomas. Int J Radiat Oncol Biol Phys 1979; 5:1725.
254. Shapiro WR, Green SB, Burger PC, et al: Randomized trial of 3 chemotherapy regimens and 2 radiotherapy regimens in the postoperative treatment of malignant glioma. BTCGT 8001. J Neurosurg 1989; 71:1.
255. Wen PY, Alexander E III, Black PM, et al: Long term results of stereotactic brachytherapy used in the initial treatment of patients with glioblastomas. Cancer 1994; 73:3029.
256. Koot RW, Maarouf M, Hulshof MC, et al: Brachytherapy: results of two different therapy strategies for patients with primary glioblastoma multiforme. Cancer 2000; 88:2796.
257. Larson DA, Gutin PH, McDermott M, et al: Gamma knife for glioma: selection factors and survival. Int J Radiat Oncol Biol Phys 1996; 36:1045.
258. Walker MD, Green SB, Byar DP, et al: Randomized comparison of radiotherapy and nitrosoureas for the treatment of malignant glioma after surgery. N Engl J Med 1980; 303:1323.
259. Fine HA, Dear KBG, Loeffler JS, et al: Meta-analysis of radiation therapy with and without adjuvant chemotherapy for malignant gliomas in adults. Cancer 1993; 71:2585.
260. Prados MD, Scott C, Curran WJ Jr, et al: Procarbazine, lomustine, and vincristine (PCV) chemotherapy for anaplastic astrocytoma: a retrospective review of radiation therapy oncology group protocols comparing survival with carmustine or PCV adjuvant chemotherapy. J Clin Oncol 1999; 17:3389.
261. Yung WK, Prados MD, Yaya-Tur R, et al: Multicenter phase II trial of temozolomide in patients with anaplastic astrocytoma or anaplastic oligoastrocytoma at first relapse. J Clin Oncol 1999; 17:2762.
262. Lote K, Egeland T, Hager B, et al: Survival, prognostic factors, and therapeutic efficacy in low-grade glioma: a retrospective study in 379 patients. J Clin Oncol 1997; 15:3129.
263. Laws ER, Taylor WF, Clifton M, et al: Neurosurgical management of low-grade astrocytoma of the cerebral hemispheres. J Neurosurg 1984; 61:665.
264. Recht LIB, Lew R, Smith TW: Suspected low-grade glioma: is deferring treatment safe? Ann Neurol 1992; 31:431.
265. Afra D, Osztie E, Sipos L, et al: Preoperative history and postoperative survival of supratentorial low-grade astrocytomas. Br J Neurosurg 1999; 13:299.
266. Wilden JN, Kelly PJ: CT computerized stereotactic biopsy for low density CT lesions presenting with epilepsy. J Neurol Neurosurg Psychiatry 1987; 50:1302.
267. Kondziolka D, Lunsford LD, Martinez HA: Unreliability of contemporary neurodiagnostic imaging in evaluating suspected adult supratentorial (low-grade) astrocytoma. J Neurosurg 1993; 79:533.
268. Berger MS, Deliganis AV, Dobbins J, et al: The effect of extensive resection on recurrence in patients with low-grade cerebral hemisphere gliomas. Cancer 1994; 74:1784.
269. North CA, North RB, Epstein JA, et al: Low-grade cerebral astrocytomas: survival and quality of life after radiation therapy. Cancer 1990; 66:6.
270. Janny P, Cure H, Mohr M, et al: Low-grade supratentorial astrocytomas: management and prognostic factors. Cancer 1994; 73:1937.
271. Shibomoto Y, Kitikabu Y, Takahashi M, et al: Supratentorial low-grade astrocytoma: correlation of computed tomography findings with effective radiation therapy and prognostic variables. Cancer 1993; 72:190.
272. Shaw EG, Scheithauer B, O'Fallon J: Supratentorial gliomas: a comparative study by grade and histologic type. J Neurooncol 1997; 31:273.
273. Leighton C, Fisher B, Bauman G, et al: Supratentorial low-grade glioma in adults: an analysis of prognostic factors and timing of radiation. J Clin Oncol 1997; 15:1294.
274. Philippon JH, Clemenceau SH, Fauchon FH, et al: Supratentorial low-grade astrocytomas in adults. Neurosurgery 1993; 32:554.
275. Wallner KE, Gonzalez M, Sheline GE: Treatment of oligodendrogliomas with or without radiation. J Neurosurg 1988; 68:684.
276. Shimuzu KY, Tran LM, Mark RJ, et al: Management of oligodendrogliomas. Radiology 1993; 186:569.
277. NCCN adult and brain tumor practice guidelines. Oncology (Huntingt) 1997; 11:237.
278. McDonald DR, Gasper LE, Cairncross JG: Successful chemotherapy for newly diagnosed aggressive oligodendroglioma. Ann Neurol 1990; 27:573.
279. Cairncross JG, Macdonald DR: Chemotherapy for oligodendroglioma. Arch Neurol 1991; 48:225.
280. Glass J, Hochberg FH, Gruber ML, et al: The treatment of oligodendrogliomas and mixed oligodendroglioma-astrocytomas with PCV chemotherapy. J Neurosurg 1992; 76:741.
281. Kyritsis AP, Yung WKA, Bruner J, et al: The treatment of anaplastic oligodendrogliomas and mixed gliomas. Neurosurgery 1993; 32:365.
282. Cairncross JG, MacDonald D, Ludwin S, et al: Chemotherapy for anaplastic oligodendroglioma. J Clin Oncol 1994; 12:2013.
283. Cairncross JG, Veki K, Zlatescu MC, et al: Specific genetic predictors of chemotherapeutic response and survival in patients with anaplastic oligodendrogliomas. J Natl Cancer Inst 1998; 90:1473.
284. Paleologos NA, Macdonald DR, Vick NA, et al: Neoadjuvant procarbazine, CCNU, and vincristine for anaplastic and aggressive oligodendroglioma. Neurology 1999; 53:1141.
285. Jeremic B, Shibamoto Y, Gruijicic D, et al: Combined treatment modality for anaplastic oligodendroglioma: a phase II study. J Neurooncol 1999; 43:179.
286. Ferrante L, Acqui M, Lunardi P, et al: MRI in the diagnosis of cystic meningiomas: surgical implications. Acta Neurochir 1997; 139:8.
287. Maor MH: Radiotherapy for meningiomas. J Neurooncol 1996; 29:261.
288. Babu R, Barton A, Kasoff SS: Resection of olfactory groove meningiomas: technical note revisited. Surg Neurol 1995; 44:567.
289. Stafford SL, Perry A, Suman VJ, et al: Primarily resected meningiomas: outcome and prognostic factors in 581 Mayo Clinic patients, 1978 through 1988. Mayo Clin Proc 1998; 73:936.
290. Mantle RE, Lach B, Delgado MR, et al: Predicting the probability of meningioma recurrence based on the quantity of peritumoral brain edema on computerized tomography scanning. J Neurosurg 1999; 91:375.
291. Wara WM, Bauman GS, Sneed PK, et al: Brain, brain stem, and cerebellum. In: Perez CA, Brady LW (eds): Principles and Practice of Radiation Oncology, 3rd ed, p 777. Philadelphia, Lippincott-Raven, 1997.
292. Glaholm J, Bloom HJ, Crow JH: The role of radiotherapy in the management of intracranial meningiomas: the Royal Marsden Hospital experience with 186 patients. Int J Radiat Oncol Biol Phys 1990; 18:755.
293. Nutting C, Brada M, Brazil L, et al: Radiotherapy in the treatment of benign meningioma of the skull base. J Neurosurg 1999; 90:823.
294. Barbaro NM, Gutin PH, Wilson CD, et al: Radiation therapy in the treatment of partially resected meningiomas. Neurosurgery 1987; 20:525.
295. Black PM: Benign brain tumors. Meningiomas, pituitary tumors, and acoustic neuromas. Neurol Clin 1995; 13:927.
296. Akeyson EW, McCutcheon IE: Management of benign and aggressive intracranial meningiomas. Oncology (Huntingt) 1996; 10:747.
297. Granberg SM, Weiss MH, Spitz IM, et al: Treatment of unresectable meningiomas with the antiprogesterone agent mifepristone. J Neurosurg 1991; 74:861.
298. Lamberts SW, Tanghe HL, Avezaat CJ, et al: Mifepriston (RU 486) treatment of meningiomas. J Neurol Neurosurg Psychiatry 1992; 55:486.
299. Hakim R, Alexander E 3rd, Loeffler JS, et al: Results of linear accelerator-based radiosurgery for intracranial meningiomas. Neurosurgery 1998; 42:446.
300. Wilson CB: Meningiomas: genetics, malignancy, and the role of

radiation in induction and treatment. The Richard C. Schneider lecture. J Neurosurg 1994; 81:666.

301. Chamberlain MC: Adjuvant combined modality therapy for malignant meningiomas. J Neurosurg 1996; 84:733.
302. Healey EA, Barnes PD, Kupsky WJ, et al: The prognostic significance of postoperative residual tumor in ependymoma. Neurosurgery 1991; 28:666.
303. Vanuytsel LJ, Bessell EM, Ashley SE, et al: Intracranial ependymoma: long term results of a policy of surgery and radiotherapy. Int J Radiat Oncol Biol Phys 1992; 23:313.
304. Bertolone SJ, Baum ES, Krivit W, et al: A phase II study of cisplatinum therapy in recurrent childhood brain tumors. J Neurooncol 1989; 7:5.
305. Abdel-Wahab M, Corn B, Wolfson A, et al: Prognostic factors and survival in patients with spinal cord gliomas after radiation therapy. Am J Clin Oncol 1999; 22:344.
306. Briggs RJ, Luxford WM, Atkins JS Jr, et al: Translabyrinthine removal of large acoustic neuromas. Neurosurgery 1994; 34:785.
307. Flickinger JC, Lunsford LD, Coffey RJ, et al: Radiosurgery of acoustic neurinomas. Cancer 1991; 67:345.
308. Schoenthaler R, Castro JR, Petti PL, et al: Charged particle irradiation of sacral chordomas. Int J Radiat Oncol Biol Phys 1993; 26:291.
309. Connolly ES: Spinal cord tumors in adults. In: Youmans JR (ed): Youmans' Neurological Surgery, p 3196. Philadelphia, W.B. Saunders Co., 1982.
310. Lister TA, Armitage JO: Non-Hodgkin's lymphoma. In: Abeloff MD, Armitage JO, Lichter AS, et al (eds): Clinical Oncology, 2nd ed, p 2658. New York, Churchill Livingstone, 2000.
311. Nasir S, DeAngelis LM: Update on the management of primary central nervous system lymphoma. Oncology (Huntingt) 2000; 14:228.
312. DeAngelis LM: Current management of primary central nervous system lymphoma. Oncology (Huntingt) 1995; 9:63.
313. DeAngelis LM: Primary CNS lymphoma: treatment with combined chemotherapy and radiotherapy. J Neurooncol 1999; 43:249.
314. Maher EA, Fine HA: Primary CNS lymphoma. Semin Oncol 1999; 26:346.
315. Nelson DF, Martz KL, Bonner H, et al: Non-Hodgkin's lymphoma of the brain: can high dose, large volume radiation therapy improve survival? Report on a prospective trial by the Radiation Therapy Oncology Group (RTOG): RTOG 8315. Int J Radiat Oncol Biol Phys 1992; 23:9.
316. Nelson DF: Radiotherapy in the treatment of primary central nervous system lymphoma (PCNSL). J Neurooncol 1999; 43:241.
317. Loeffler JS, Ervin TJ, Mauch P, et al: Primary lymphomas of the central nervous system: patterns of failure and factors influencing survival. J Clin Oncol 1985; 3:490.
318. Brada M, Dearnaley D, Horwich A, et al: Management of primary cerebral lymphoma with initial chemotherapy: preliminary results and comparison with patients treated with radiotherapy alone. Int J Radiat Oncol Biol Phys 1990; 18:787.
319. DeAngelis LM, Yahalom J, Thaler HT, et al: Combined modality therapy for primary central nervous system lymphoma. J Clin Oncol 1992; 10:635.
320. Hiraga S, Arita N, Ohnishi T, et al: Rapid infusion of high-dose methotrexate resulting in enhanced penetration into cerebrospinal fluid and intensified tumor response in primary central nervous system lymphomas. J Neurosurg 1999; 91:221.
321. Abrey LE, DeAngelis LM, Yahalom J: Longterm survival in primary central nervous system lymphoma. J Clin Oncol 1998; 16:859.
322. Freilich RJ, Delattre JY, Monjour A, et al: Chemotherapy without radiotherapy as initial treatment for primary central nervous system lymphoma in older patients. Neurology 1996; 46:435.
323. Forsyth PA, Yahalom J, DeAngelis LM: Combined modality therapy in the treatment of primary central nervous system lymphoma in AIDS. Neurology 1994; 44:1473.
324. McGowan JP, Shah S: Longterm remission of AIDS-related primary central nervous system lymphoma associated with highly active antiretroviral treatment. AIDS 1998; 12:952.
325. Remick SC, Sedransk N, Haase R, et al: Oral combination chemotherapy in the management of AIDS-related lymphoproliferative malignancies. Drugs 1999; 58(suppl):99.
326. Vecht CJ: Clinical management of brain metastasis. J Neurol 1998; 245:127.
327. Vermeulen SS: Whole brain radiotherapy in the treatment of metastatic brain tumors. Semin Surg Oncol 1998; 14:64.
328. Pirkall A, Debus J, Lohr F, et al: Radiosurgery alone or in combination with whole-brain radiotherapy for brain metastases. J Clin Oncol 1998; 16:3563.
329. Boyd TS, Mehta MP: Stereotactic radiosurgery for brain metastases. Oncology (Huntingt) 1999; 13:1397.
330. Kondziolka D, Patel A, Lunsford LD, et al: Stereotactic radiosurgery plus whole brain radiotherapy versus radiotherapy alone for patients with multiple brain metastases. Int J Radiat Oncol Biol Phys 1999; 45:427.
331. McDermott MW, Cosgrove GR, Larson DA, et al: Interstitial brachytherapy for intracranial metastases. Neurosurg Clin North Am 1996; 7:485.
332. Bogart JA, Ungureanu C, Shihadeh E, et al: Resection and permanent I-125 brachytherapy without whole brain irradiation for solitary brain metastasis from non-small lung cell carcinoma. J Neurooncol 1999; 44:53.
333. Korfel A, Thiel E: Chemotherapy of brain metastases. Front Radiat Ther Oncol 1999; 33:343.
334. Franciosi V, Cocconi G, Michiara M, et al: Front-line chemotherapy with cisplatin and etoposide for patients with brain metastases from breast carcinoma, nonsmall cell lung carcinoma, or malignant melanoma: a prospective study. Cancer 1999; 85:1599.
335. Curran WJ Jr, Scott CB, Horton J, et al: Recursive partitioning analysis of prognostic factors in three Radiation Therapy Oncology Group malignant glioma trials. J Natl Cancer Inst 1993; 85:704.
336. McCarthy BJ, Davis FG, Freels S, et al: Factors associated with survival in patients with meningioma. J Neurosurg 1998; 88:831.
337. Wurschmidt F, Bunemann H, Heilmann HP: Prognostic factors in high-grade malignant glioma. A multivariate analysis of 76 cases with postoperative radiotherapy. Strahlenther Onkol 1995; 171:315.
338. Hosli P, Sappino AP, de Tribolet N, et al: Malignant glioma: should chemotherapy be overthrown by experimental treatments? Ann Oncol 1998; 9:589.
339. Curran WJ Jr, Scott CB, Horton J, et al: Does extent of surgery influence outcome for astrocytoma with atypical or anaplastic foci (AAF)? A report from three Radiation Therapy Oncology Group (RTOG) trials. J Neurooncol 1992; 12:219.
340. Vecht CJ: Effect of age on treatment decisions in low-grade glioma. J Neurol Neurosurg Psych 1993; 56:1259.
341. Pierga JY, Hoang-Xuan K, Feuvret L, et al: Treatment of malignant gliomas in the elderly. J Neurooncol 1999; 43:187.
342. Nakamura M, Konishi N, Tsunoda S, et al: Analysis of prognostic and survival factors related to treatment of low-grade astrocytomas in adults. Oncology 2000; 58:108.
343. Steltzer KJ, Sauve KI, Spence AM, et al: Corpus callosum involvement as a prognostic factor for patients with high-grade astrocytoma. Int J Radiat Oncol Biol Phys 1997; 38:27.
344. Blankenberg FG, Teplitz RL, Ellis W, et al: The influence of volumetric tumor doubling time, DNA ploidy, and histologic grade on the survival of patients with intracranial astrocytomas. Am J Neuroradiol 1995; 16:1001.
345. Karim AB, Maat B, Hatlevoll R, et al: A randomized trial on dose-response in radiation therapy of low-grade cerebral glioma: European Organization for Research and Treatment of Cancer (EORTC) Study 22844. Int J Radiat Oncol Biol Phys 1996; 36:549.
346. Franzini A, Leocata F, Cajola L, et al: Low-grade glial tumors in basal ganglia and thalamus: natural history and biological reappraisal. Neurosurgery 1994; 35:817.
347. Schiffer D, Cavalla P, Chio A, et al: Proliferative activity and prognosis of low-grade astrocytomas. J Neurooncol 1997; 34:31.
348. Dehghani F, Schachenmayr W, Laun A, et al: Prognostic implication of histopathological, immunohistochemical and clinical features of oligodendrogliomas: a study of 89 cases. Acta Neuropathol 1998; 95:493.
349. Rainov NG, Dobberstein KU, Bahn H, et al: Prognostic factors in malignant glioma: influence of the overexpression of oncogene and tumor-suppressor gene products on survival. J Neurooncol 1997; 35:13.
350. Galanis E, Buckner J, Kimmel D, et al: Gene amplification as a prognostic factor in primary and secondary high-grade malignant gliomas. Int J Oncol 1998; 13:717.

30 *Lung Cancer*

PAUL VAN HOUTTE, MD, Radiation Oncology
SANDRA McDONALD, MD, Radiation Oncology
ALEX YUANG-CHI CHANG, MD, Medical Oncology
OMAR M. SALAZAR, MD, FACR, FACRO, Radiation Oncology

A being breathing thoughtful breath;
A traveller betwixt life and death.

WILLIAM WORDSWORTH, *Simon Lee*

Perspective

Lung cancer accounts for 15% of all cancer types in men, compared with 13% in women.[10] It is responsible for 31% of cancer-related deaths in men and 25% in women. Furthermore, the overall 5-year survival rate is lower than 14%.[10] Only one third of patients are eligible for surgical resection with curative intent. Among those patients, less than one third will be living 5 years after surgery. Nevertheless, all disciplines involved in lung cancer management have advanced considerably, and as a result, some small but significant improvements in long-term survival have been noted.[10] From 1974 to 1976, the relative 5-year survival rates for whites and blacks were 13% and 11%, respectively, whereas from 1989 to 1994, the rates had improved in whites to 15% but remained stable in blacks at 11%.[10] Today, lung cancer is not considered to be a single disease entity, but, rather, it is believed to be composed of several diseases, conditioned by histopathologic types that determine patterns of spread, treatment, and prognosis. Furthermore, the modern management of lung cancer requires, more than ever, cooperation between all specialties involved in diagnosis and therapy.

Epidemiology and Etiology

Epidemiology

In 2000, it was estimated that there were 164,100 new cases of lung cancer per year in the United States and 156,900 deaths from the disease.[10] According to the International Agency for Research on Cancer, 1.037 million new cases of lung cancer are diagnosed annually worldwide.[11] Of note, it has been estimated that 86% of lung cancer deaths among men and 49% among women are attributed to smoking, with the average age for onset for lung cancer being about 60 years (less than 1% of cases occur to those younger than age 30). Most striking is the rising incidence among women during the 1990s. In the United States, lung cancer is becoming the most common cause of death from any cancer among women, overtaking breast cancer.[10] Approximately 2 million cases of lung cancer were estimated for the year 2000, with 58% of them occurring in developing countries.[11]

Cigarette smoking increases the risk of developing lung cancer, as well as dying from it. The death rate increases with an increase in exposure. For smokers of less than half of a pack, half to one pack, one to two packs, two, and more than two packs daily, the death rates are 46, 95, 108, 229, and 264 per 100,000, respectively.[12, 13] There has been an overall decline in cigarette smoking in the United States. In 1965, 50.2% of men and 31.9% of women smoked; by 1993, these figures had declined to 31.7% and 26.8%, respectively.[14, 15] Cigarette smoking is more common in blacks (34%) than in whites (28.8%), although whites smoke more cigarettes per day.[13, 15] However, the largest difference in smoking habits has been seen in educated groups. In 1966, 36.5% of people with some education but no high school diploma smoked, compared with 33.7% of college graduates. By 1993, these figures stood at 35% and 13%, respectively, representing a drop of more than 50% among college graduates. The Public Health Service's stated goal for smoking rates in the year 2000 was a decrease in the percentage of adult smokers to 15% of the population; however, smoking prevalence among people 18 years or older in 1997 was still 24.7%.[15]

Today, through legislative efforts, there are antitobacco health policies in effect in most western countries. There has also been sweeping antitobacco legislation in the United States. However, among American high school students, the rate of smoking has increased dramatically since the early 1990s,[14] even though each state has laws prohibiting the sale of tobacco products to minors. In the United States and some Scandinavian countries, the incidence of lung cancer among young men appears to be decreasing. However, similar to the trend in the United States, there has been an increase in cigarette smoking among the younger population of many countries. Any major difference in mortality will be seen during the next century.

The smoke inhaled by nonsmokers has a similar chemical composition to that inhaled by smokers, but it has higher *N*-nitrosamine levels and smaller particles that remain suspended in air and can easily penetrate the bronchial tree. About one third of cases of lung cancer in nonsmokers who live with smokers and one fourth of cases of nonsmokers in general appear to be related to passive exposure to cigarettes.[14]

Etiology

A variety of agents has proven to be carcinogenic in humans:

- *Tobacco smoke* is the dominant agent. It represents a complex mixture of physical and chemical carcinogens. There is a direct relationship between amount of tobacco exposure and risk for developing lung cancer. In addition to the increased risk for lung cancer, smoking is also associated with an increased risk of upper respiratory, genitourinary, and digestive tract cancer. The type of cigarettes seems also to influence risk; that is, a filter apparently decreases the risk of cancer. Stopping smoking is associated with a gradual decrease in risk, but an appreciable diminution of risk occurs only after a long period of time (more than 6 years). Interestingly, in Asians, the proportion of cases attributable to active smoking may not be as high. The rate of deaths from smoking-related lung cancer has been reported to be as low as 6% among Asian women[16]; however, an additional lung cancer risk unrelated to smoking has been observed among Chinese women.[17] Nonsmoking risk factors in these patients include inhalation of combustion byproducts from cooking, heating stoves, and oil furnaces.
- *Asbestos exposure* is associated with the development of mesothelioma and bronchogenic carcinoma. The risk from asbestos is particularly pronounced when it is combined with cigarette smoking.[18, 19]
- *Atmospheric pollution* has been implicated as a causative agent because of the higher incidence of lung cancer in urban areas than in rural areas.[20]
- *Metals*, mostly nickel and silver but also chromium, cadmium, beryllium, cobalt, selenium, and steel, have been proven to be carcinogenic in animals, and they are occupational hazards, particularly when they are combined with other factors.[21]
- *Chemical products*, such as chloromethyl ethers, have been associated with the development of lung cancer, especially small cell lung cancer (SCLC).[22]

Molecular and Cell Biology

Cytogenetic and molecular genetic studies have demonstrated that mutations in both proto-oncogenes and tumor suppressor genes (TSGs) are critical in the multistep development and progression of lung tumors; typical targets include activation of oncogenes, including the *KRAS* and *MYC* genes, and the inactivation of tumor suppressor genes, which include the *RB*, *TP53*, and *CDKN2* genes.[23, 24] Inactivation of TSGs is by far the most common mutational event documented during the development of lung cancer. For example, loss of function of the *RB* or *TP53* genes has been detected in both SCLC and non–small cell lung cancer (NSCLC). In addition, allelic loss analyses have implicated the existence of other tumor suppressor gene loci on 9p, as well as on 3p, 5q, 8p, 9q, 11q, and 17q.[25]

Identifying the specific genes undergoing such changes and understanding their role in lung cancer progression may be useful in the development of biomarkers for the early detection of cells destined to become malignant, as well as for the prognosis of treatment. *KRAS* oncogene activation is frequently used as a prognostic indicator for a number of different histologic lung cancers.[26, 27] Moreover, such genetic changes can become targets of newly designed drugs and gene-based therapy (Table 30–1). Other molecular and genetic properties inherent within lung cancer cells may have prognostic importance. Therefore, they are potentially useful in monitoring response to therapy or recurrence.

Cell lines have been established from a variety of organ sites, including the primary tumor, bone marrow aspirates, lymph node biopsies, malignant effusions, and other surgically resected sites. These allow detailed studies of the biologic properties of these tumor cells and permit clinical correlation with patients. Stability in culture is usually noted for these cell lines over prolonged periods.

SCLC cell lines are subclassified into classic (70%) and variant (30%) subgroups:

1. *Classic* cell lines (Table 30–2)[28] express elevated levels of levodopa decarboxylase, bombesin/gastrin-releasing peptide (BBS/GRP), neuron-specific enolase (NSE) and creatinine (CR) kinase, have a relatively long doubling time, have low cloning efficiency *in vitro*, and are radiosensitive.
2. *Variant* cell lines have low or undetectable levels of levodopa decarboxylase, the marker of neuroendocrine differentiation. They lack BBS/GRP, but unlike non–small cell lung lines, they express elevated levels of NSE and CR kinase-BBS. They have more rapid growth than classic lines, are radioresistant, and, morphologically, more closely resemble large cell undifferentiated carcinomas. They also have 4 to 60 times the DNA amplification of the *MYC* oncogene and show increased expression of it.

Detection and Diagnosis

Clinical Detection

Clinical manifestations are varied and mimic other pulmonary conditions. A change of pulmonary habits is the most significant sign of lung cancer. Cough, chest pain, rust-streaked or purulent sputum production, hemoptysis, and dyspnea are common symptoms of lung cancer. Local complications depend on the location of the tumor and include:

- superior vena cava obstruction
- shoulder or arm pain with brachial plexus involvement
- recurrent pleural effusions and pneumonitis, resulting from pulmonary vein or bronchial obstruction, respectively

TABLE 30–1. **Molecular and Genetic Abnormalities in Lung Cancer**

Genes	Mutations	Abnormal Expression Frequency	
		NSCLC (%)	***SCLC (%)***
Oncogenes			
KRAS	Point mutation (codon 12)	30	Not reported
MYC	DNA amplification overexpression	10	10–40
ERBB2	Increased expression	25	Not reported
BCL2	Expression of protein	25	Not reported
Tumor suppressor genes			
3p	Deletion	50	90
RB	Deletion, altered protein expression, and phosphorylation	15	>90
TP53	Deletion, point mutation, and overexpression	50	80
CDKN2	Expression of protein	60	Not reported

From Salgia R, Skarin AT: Molecular abnormalities in lung cancer. J Clin Oncol 1998; 16:1207–1217, with permission.

- cardiac failure or arrhythmia, resulting from cardiac involvement
- hoarseness secondary to recurrent laryngeal nerve paralysis

Paraneoplastic Syndromes

Extrapulmonary manifestations of lung cancer may be recognized before the lung cancer itself produces any symptoms. Approximately 2% of patients present with a paraneoplastic syndrome. These may be categorized as follows:

- *Metabolic*: Cushing's syndrome, hypercalcemia, excessive antidiuretic hormone, and carcinoid syndrome
- *Neuromuscular*: peripheral neuritis, cortical or cerebellar degenerations, and myopathy
- *Dermatologic*: acanthosis nigricans and dermatomyositis
- *Skeletal*: pulmonary hypertrophic osteoarthropathy, including clubbing of fingers
- *Vascular*: migratory thrombophlebitis and nonbacterial verrucous endocarditis
- *Hematologic*: anemia and disseminated intravascular coagulopathy

An initial metastatic presentation may be cerebral metastases. A chest film is mandatory in suspected brain tumor to rule out a primary tumor in the lung. Bone and liver metastases are also possible.

Radiographic screening procedures or cytologic studies performed annually generally do not aid in early detection, although serial sputum cytologies can detect occult lesions. If cytology results are positive and radiograph results are negative, then the patient requires fiberoptic bronchoscopy and guided bronchial wash-out studies for localization. Large-scale, randomized trials involving periodic applications of these two procedures to individuals who were at high risk failed to demonstrate any significant benefit in terms of survival, although suggestions of overdiagnosis have been disproved.[29–32] The Lung Imaging Fluorescence

TABLE 30–2. **Biologic Properties of Lung Cancer Cell Lines**

Characteristic	SCLC		NSCLC
	Classic	***Variant***	
Growth morphology	Suspension	Suspension	Attached
Cytology	SCLC	SCLC	NSCLC
Colony forming efficiency	2%	13%	6%
Doubling time	72 hrs	32 hrs	40 hrs
Dense core granules	+	−	−
DDC	+ +	−	−
BLI/GRP	+ +	−	−
NSE	+ +	+	−
CKBB	+ +	+ +	−
Neurotensin	+ +	−	−
Peptide hormone	+ +	+/−	−
BLI receptors	+	−	−
EGF receptors	−	−	+
Chromosome 3, deletion	+	+	−
CD57 antigen	+	+	−
Radiation sensitivity	Sensitive	Resistant	Resistant
MYC amplification	−	+	+/−

SCLC = small cell lung cancer; NSCLC = non–small cell lung cancer; DDC = L-dopa decarboxylase; BLI/GRP = bombesin/gastrin-releasing peptide; NSE = neuron specific enolase; CKBB = creatine kinase; EGF = epidermal growth factor.
Form Carney DN, De Leij L: Lung cancer biology. Semin Oncol 1988; 15:199–214, with permission.

Endoscopy (LIFE) system has been developed based on the observation that when the bronchial surface is illuminated by a blue light from a laser (krypton or helium-cadmium), there is a progressive reduction in the fluorescence intensity as the tissue becomes more abnormal, particularly in the cases of intraepithelial and invasive cancer.[33] This test is now under investigation for patients at very high risk (heavy smokers or those at follow-up of resected cancer to detect secondary tumors).

Diagnostic Procedures

The management of clinically suspected lung cancer requires pathologic confirmation of a tumor, definition of its histology, determination of tumor extent, research of prognostic factors, and evaluation of the host's physiologic function in regard to the proposed treatment. A careful history and physical examination are most important in establishing the diagnosis of pulmonary neoplasm, because many benign lesions have radiologic characteristics similar to malignant lesions.

Radiographic studies (Table 30–3)[34] (posteroanterior and lateral chest films) are the most valuable tools for establishing diagnosis when there is clinical suspicion of bronchogenic carcinoma. They may show a peripheral parenchymal tumor, the effects of bronchial obstruction (atelectasis), or regional metastases (hilar and mediastinal enlargement, rib erosion). Computed tomography (CT), magnetic resonance imaging (MRI), and even angiography may be used to define further the nature and extent of involvement. Although CT scans are used for defining the disease extent both locally or distally,[35, 36] there are limitations in its accuracy; differentiation between tumor contiguity and subtle invasion of the mediastinum or chest wall remain a problem.[37] MRI has similar limitations, although it may be superior when defining minimal chest wall or mediastinal invasion.

Fiberbronchoscopy yields positive histology if the bronchogenic carcinoma involves a bronchus. Brush biopsy performed under videoscopy may even be positive for peripheral lesions. It has been found to be most useful for visualization and biopsy of central lesions. CT bronchoscopy may also play a significant role in volumetric analysis in patients with mediastinal or hilar tumors.[38]

Cytologic studies include sputum examinations by Papanicolaou technique. In the hands of expert cytologists, positive results may be found in as many as 75% of cases of bronchogenic carcinoma after repeated examinations. Routine bronchial washings at the time of bronchoscopy yield results in only 44% of cases, which is not as good as the sputum examinations performed after bronchoscopy. Selective bronchiolar washout techniques with fiberoptic scopes can identify occult lesions.

Percutaneous needle biopsy under videoscopic and CT scan control has been introduced to diagnose peripheral lesions. There is a risk of seeding along the needle tract, pneumothorax, and hemorrhage, but the risk is low when the procedure is performed by an experienced surgeon or radiologist; there is a 20% to 30% risk of pneumothorax, but only 5% of such patients require tubal thoracotomy. This technique has a high degree of accuracy. Histologic confirmation of a diagnosis of bronchogenic carcinoma may be forthcoming only after exploration and direct biopsy of the tumor or its metastases.

Scalene lymph node biopsy may be performed, especially for an apical tumor. It should be recognized that the right scalene fat pad drains the right lung and left lower lobe. The left scalene fat pad drains the lingula and the left upper lobe. If metastatic scalene lymph nodes are found, then thoracotomy is contraindicated.

Mediastinoscopy is another test of operability. This method explores the mediastinal lymph nodes to the level of the carina and yields better results for the right side than the left side, where the exploration is limited by the aortic arch. If metastases to lymph nodes are found, then the indication for a thoracotomy should be re-examined in favor of a combined approach, either preoperatively or not.

Radioisotopic procedures include technetium (^{99m}Tc) (used for angiograms to detect superior vena cava obstruction) coupled with medronate to detect possible bone me-

TABLE 30–3. **Imaging Modalities for Detection and Diagnosis of Lung Cancer**

Method	Capability	Recommended
Primary tumor and regional nodes work-up		
Chest films	Baseline image	Yes
CT/spiral CT	Most useful of all modalities for determining characteristics of T and N in the thorax and M in the brain and liver	Yes
MRI	Not as good as CT	No
Percutaneous needle biopsy	Guided by fluoroscopy or CT, accurate in establishing cytologic diagnosis from T (particularly peripheral lung lesions); M (especially liver or bone); less experience with N	Yes
Mediastinoscopy/thoracoscopy	Confirmation of nodal involvement	Yes
Metastatic work-up for clinically suspected metastases		
CT/echography	For liver, adrenals	Yes
CT/MRI	For brain	Yes
Bone scan	For the bone	Yes
PET scan/MRI spectroscopy	Diagnosis of peripheral lesions, staging	Yes, if clinically indicated

CT = computed tomography; MRI = magnetic resonance imaging; PET = positron emission tomography; T = tumor; N = node; M = metastasis.
Modified from Bragg DG: Imaging in primary lung cancer: the roles of detection, staging and follow-up. Semin Ultrasound CT MR 1989; 10:453–466.

tastases. Routine lung scanning, with macroaggregate or radioactive gas such as xenon, yields information on lung perfusion or ventilation and is used to assess the pulmonary function. Gallium may be fixed by the tumor, and gallium scans are advocated by some investigators as preoperative screens for mediastinal nodes.

Positron emission tomography (PET) is based on imaging of biochemical process *in vivo*; the process makes use of the increased uptake of a glucose analogue ([^{18}F] fluorodeoxyglucose) in transformed cells and has a 95% sensitivity with an 85% specificity.[39] There is an increased accuracy in the evaluation of hilar and mediastinal lymph node status compared with CT, and whole body PET is used in the detection of metastatic disease.[40] In addition, both PET and single photon emission computed tomography can reveal the differentiation between benign and malignant lesions.[41]

A variety of tumor markers, including hormones, antigens, and proteins, have been identified in lung cancer. Their major role is the monitoring of tumor response or the detection of early relapses. The carcinoembryonic antigen (CEA) remains the gold standard for non–small cell lung cancers; its concentration correlates well with tumor extent: 50% to 60% of patients with metastatic disease have elevated CEA titers.[42] In addition to CEA, tissue polypeptide antigen and immunoreactive calcitonin are two other possible markers for NSCLC. Furthermore, cytokeratin markers are a family of proteins that are part of the cytoskeleton of epithelial cells. CYFRA 21-1 is a tumor marker, especially for squamous cell carcinoma: CYFRA levels may be correlated with the stage of the disease.[43] For SCLC, the best marker is certainly the neuron-specific enolase (NSE), an isoenzyme of enolase that is a good marker for all neuroendocrine tumors. Elevated NSE titers are observed in 60% to 70% of patients with limited SCLC, and in 80% to 95% of those with extensive SCLC. Furthermore, NSE is a good marker to monitor tumor response. CEA and calcitonin may complement NSE, especially in patients with a normal NSE value. Several biologic markers (*RAS*, *TP53*, Ki-67, *RB*, epidermal growth factor [EGF] family genes) have been identified for lung cancers, but they are not yet established as prognostic markers in contrast to the classic factors, such as performance status, weight loss, symptoms, and TNM staging.[44]

Recommended Procedures

Chest radiography remains a useful tool for detecting lung cancer, but CT is the most useful procedure for the staging of intrathoracic disease. The major question is whether the disease is confined to the lung or if pleura, mediastinum, or other structures are invaded. For the nodal compartment, it is difficult to determine mediastinal and scalene nodal involvement. Sixteen common radiographic presentations are shown in Figure 30–1, which demonstrates how lung cancers can masquerade as benign or infectious disease problems.[45]

Tomograms were helpful at one time in determining the extent of the primary tumor within major bronchi, but they are no longer used because of the availability of much more accurate procedures, such as the CT scan or MRI. CT is the most important and valuable radiologic procedure in the diagnosis, staging, and therapeutic planning of lung cancer.

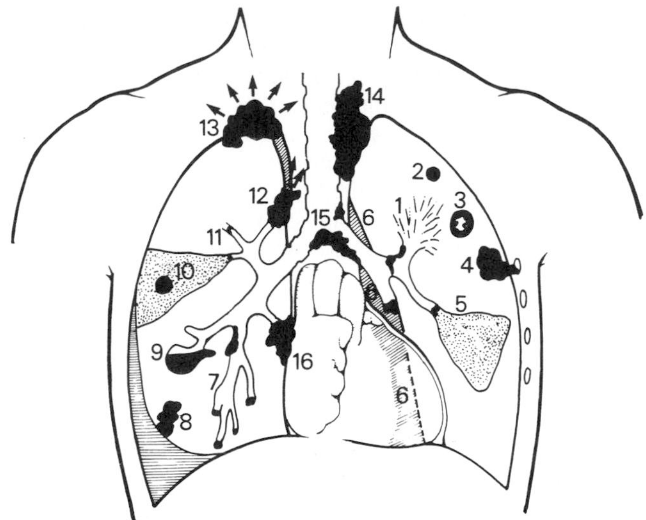

Figure 30–1. The most frequent manifestations of bronchial carcinoma (after Grunze): (1) hilar lung cancer with endobronchial growth (relatively early elicitation of the cough reflex); (2) typical round focus; (3) tumor cavern (note the thick irregular walls); (4) subpleural focus infiltrating the chest wall; (5) obstructive segmental discontinuation with retention in pneumonia, (10) already with abscess formation; (6) atelectasis, which is hidden behind the cardiac shadow (lateral radiograph); (7) secondary bronchiectasis due to partial stenosis; (8) focus near to the pleura, with effusion; (9) necrotizing tumor with draining bronchus (abscess symptom); (11) obstruction emphysema due to valve occlusion; (12, 13) outbreak of carcinoma into the mediastinum, for example, in the direction of the vena cava (upper inflow congestion) or as Pancoast's tumor; (14) lymph node involvement in the upper mediastinum and paratracheally, extending to the upper clavicular fossa. Detection by lymph node biopsy according to Daniels or by mediastinoscopy: (15) and (16) carcinoma spreading to the trachea and pericardium, respectively. Note, a bronchial carcinoma can be masked even in a normal radiograph. (From Bates M [ed]: Bronchial Carcinoma. An Integrated Approach to Diagnosis and Management. Berlin, Springer-Verlag, 1984, with permission.)

- Primary tumor staging with CT scan is preferred to MRI to delineate and diagnose most peripheral pulmonary nodules and central masses. However, primary staging is difficult with CT scan or MRI, because it is impossible to distinguish tumor from distal atelectasis or pneumonia. The disadvantage of chest film is the inability to determine chest wall, mediastinal, hilar, or subcarinal involvement. CT scan may provide more accurate information, but it is also insensitive. It is easier to find criteria to define the possible resectable cases than the unresectable tumors. MRI may improve specificity, but unless bone destruction is evident, it is limited to determining chest wall invasion; with vascular invasion, it can possibly define mediastinal extension. Its main advantage is to give better information for tumors located close to the heart or to the spinal cord.
- Nodal staging is well established by CT scan and relates to identifying enlarged nodes. Nodal enlargement is the only sign for nodal metastases. An enlargement may be a result of something other than metastasis: distal infection or coincidental occupational

granulomatous lung disorders. In a study by McLoud and coworkers, the rate of positive mediastinal lymph nodes rose from 13% for nodes measuring smaller than 1 cm to 62% for nodes that were 2 to 2.9 cm.[35] Such nodes may be sampled by mediastinoscopy, transbronchial needle aspiration, or limited thoracotomy. Gallium scans may be helpful.

- Metastases staging often is part of CT scan of the thorax, with liver and adrenal assessment. The adrenal is found to be abnormal in 10% to 40% of patients at autopsy, but 66% of adrenal masses identified on CT scan are found to be non-neoplastic and require needle biopsy.

CT scanning can determine if the tumor is limited to the lung or has involved the chest wall or mediastinum. It is also valuable to search for distant metastases (brain, liver, adrenals). Compared with CT, MRI offers two advantages: multiplanar images can be obtained easily and great vessels can be identified without contrast media. It has also proven to be as accurate as CT in evaluating the hilus and the mediastinum for enlarged lymph nodes. When making the decision for surgery, it must be remembered that an enlarged lymph node seen on a CT scan is not necessarily a metastatic deposit and, in general, histologic confirmation is recommended.

Mediastinoscopy assesses the status of mediastinal and scalene nodes. It is an important tool for diagnosis and tumor staging, especially if a surgery is planned.

To find occult metastases, *radioisotopic scans* are essential to determine the status of skeleton, but CT scan or MRI (or both) should be used to detect liver, adrenal, or brain metastases.

Video-assisted thoracic surgery provides surgeons with high-resolution images of the thorax and may be used for diagnosis and staging of thoracic disease. Indications may include the diagnosis of an indeterminate solitary pulmonary nodule, staging assistance for areas beyond the reach of cervical mediastinoscopy (left hilum, perioesophageal or inferior subcarinal lymph nodes).[46] Additional studies are required to show the safety and usefulness of this approach for the treatment of NSCLC.

If a *bone scan* has a positive finding, then a search for specific lesions should be made by detailed skeletal radiography, including CT scan or MRI, if necessary, rather than doing skeletal surveys with conventional radiographs.

Bone marrow aspiration and *biopsy* have been used in the staging of small cell carcinoma, but they should only be performed to detect a suspected bone marrow involvement.

Determination of the *immunologic status* of the patient may also be important to determine the outcome. CEA, CYFRA, or NSE, if elevated, can be used to monitor treatment responses.

Laboratory studies include the complete blood cell count and sonogram liver test. Abnormal laboratory values should be further defined, especially in the event of a paraneoplastic syndrome. In the case of surgery or even radiation, *pulmonary function tests* and a *cardiac evaluation* should be performed.

Classification and Staging

Histopathology

There are four major histologic types of invasive lung tumors: squamous cell carcinoma or epidermoid carcinoma (SCC); adenocarcinoma, including the bronchoalveolar type; large cell anaplastic carcinoma; and small cell anaplastic carcinoma, which includes the oat cell type. Other types encountered are sarcomas and other soft tissue tumors; these are rare.

There have been reports that the incidence of SCC, the most common form of lung cancer worldwide, has undergone an absolute and relative increase in the United States. However, based on Surveillance, Epidemiology, and End Results Program (SEER) data,[47] there has been a shift in the overall distribution of histologic types. The incidence of SCC was surpassed by adenocarcinoma during the period of 1983 to 1987 (Table 30–4).[48]

SCC arises from metaplastic bronchial epithelium; 50% to 60% of cases are proximal or involve the hilus. It tends to grow into the bronchial lumen and to produce obstruction early, with associated pneumonitis. Consequently, it is a form of lung cancer easy to diagnose through sputum cytology. It is also less likely to metastasize early.

Adenocarcinoma tends to be located more in the periphery of the lung, but it metastasizes widely and frequently to the other lung, liver, bone, kidney, and the central nervous system (CNS). *Bronchioalveolar carcinoma*, an unusual subtype of adenocarcinoma, appears to have a distinct presentation and biologic behavior.[49]

Small cell anaplastic carcinoma tends to be disseminated at the time of diagnosis. This is an aggressive and rapidly growing neoplasm. Disease is limited to the thorax at presentation in only 25% of patients. Metastases will be found in regional lymph nodes, lung, abdominal lymph nodes, liver, adrenal gland, bone, CNS, and bone marrow. A bone marrow biopsy may be positive in one third of patients at presentation. Histologic variants of small cell

TABLE 30–4. **Evolution of Histological Distribution Over the Years***

	1973–1977	1978–1982	1983–1987
Squamous cell carcinoma	13.4	15.1	15.3
Adenocarcinoma	10.5	14.2	16.7
Small cell carcinoma	5.9	8.2	9.4
Large cell carcinoma	N/A	3.9	4.9
Total carcinomas	39.5	46.8	51.4

*Expressed as incidence rates per 100,000 people per year

Adapted from Travis WD, Travis LB, DeVessa SS: Lung cancer. Cancer 1995; 75 (1 suppl):191–198. Reprinted by permission of Wiley-Liss, Inc., a subsidiary of John Wiley & Sons, Inc.

carcinoma have not proven to have different biologic behavior or chemotherapeutic response.[50] This form of lung cancer, like SCC, is mostly proximal (central) in location, but unlike SCC, it grows submucosally and distorts the bronchus by extrinsic (extraluminal) compression.

Large cell anaplastic carcinoma metastasizes in a pattern quite similar to adenocarcinoma, with a predilection for mediastinal lymph nodes, pleura, adrenals, CNS, and bone.

Staging

The definitions of tumor and node categories for carcinoma of the lung are shown in Table 30–5,[51] and they apply to NSCLC. For SCLC, the definition of limited disease (LD) versus extensive disease (ED) is the most widely used, with LD confined to the lung and regional nodes (mediastinum and scalene) and ED denoting metastatic disease outside the lung and regional nodes. For a staging diagram, see Figure 30–2.

Differences Between Staging Systems

Recent editions of the American Joint Committee on Cancer (AJCC) and International Union Against Cancer (IUAC) staging texts distinguish T3 from the T4 category. T3 is invasion of adjacent structures: pleura, pericardium, diaphragm, ribs, and chest wall. T4 denotes invasion of mediastinum, heart, great vessels, trachea, esophagus, vertebrae and pleural effusion (presence of malignant cells) (see Table 30–5). N2 and N3 categories distinguish between ipsilateral mediastinal and contralateral mediastinal nodes and supraclavicular nodes. The T1 or T2 equivalent to node involvement that indicates size is not an overriding factor. The new TNM (tumor, node, metastasis) classification varies from the old one, mainly in the stage grouping, by dividing stage I and II in two subgroups and by including T3,N0 within stage IIb.

Staging Work-Up

There are three types of staging work-up:

1. *Clinical and imaging evaluation* should be performed before thoracotomy is performed.
2. *Pathologic evaluation* (postsurgically) is performed after thoracotomy and includes both biopsies and the entire resected specimen of lungs and regional nodes.
3. *Recurrent staging* is done at the time of recurrence for a previously staged lung tumor.

Principles of Treatment

Multidisciplinary Approach

The strategy for control of bronchogenic carcinoma is based on an individual selection of the treatment modality or combinations of those that can offer the maximum benefit for the patient. Several important prognostic factors are considered: histology, tumor extent, and the patient's physical condition. Tables 30–6 and 30–7 are concise, multimodality treatment summaries of the role of surgery, radiation therapy, and chemotherapy according to disease stage. However, we should always remember that it is a patient that we must treat and not a cancer and that we must take into account the different prognostic factors (TNM staging, weight loss, performance status, histology), as well as the patient's status.

TABLE 30–5. **TNM Classification and Stage Grouping**

Stage	Grouping	Descriptor
IA	T1, N0, M0	T1: Tumor ≥3 cm in diameter, surrounded by lung or visceral pleura, with no bronchoscopic evidence of invasion more proximal than lobar bronchus.
IB	T2, N0, MO	T2: Tumor with any of the following features of size or extent: >3 cm in greatest dimension, involves main bronchus ≥2 cm distal to carina, invades visceral pleura, associated with atelectasis or obstructive pneumonitis extending to hilar region, but not involving entire lung.
		N0: No regional lymph node metastasis.
		M0: No distant metastasis.
IIA	T1, N1, M0	T3: Tumor of any size that directly invades any of the following: chest wall with or without superior sulcus tumors, diaphragm, mediastinal pleura, or parietal pericardium; *or* tumor in the main bronchus <2 cm distal to carina without carinal involvement; *or* tumor associated with atelectasis or obstructive pneumonitis of entire lung.
IIB	T2, N1, M0	N1: Metastasis to ipsilateral peribronchial and/or ipsilateral hilar lymph nodes, and intrapulmonary nodes involved by direct extension of primary tumor.
	T3, N0, M0	
IIIA	T3, N1, M0	T4: Tumor of any size that invades any of the following: mediastinum, heart, great vessels, trachea, esophagus, vertebral body, or carina; *or* tumor with malignant pleural or pericardial effusion; *or* tumor with satellite nodules within ipsilateral primary tumor lobe of lung.
	T1–3, N2, M0	N2: Metastasis to ipsilateral mediastinal and/or subcarinal nodes.
IIIB	Any T, N3, M0	N3: Metastasis to contralateral mediastinal, contralateral hilar, ipsilateral or contralateral scalene, or supraclavicular lymph nodes.
	T4, Any N, M0	
IV	Any T, Any N, M1	M1: Distant metastasis present.

Tumor (T) category includes above classifications plus the following: TX = primary tumor that cannot be assessed, or tumor proven by presence of malignant cell sputum or bronchial washing but not visualized by imaging or bronchoscopy; T0 = no evidence of primary tumor; Tis = carcinoma in situ; Node (N) category includes above classifications plus the following: NX = regional lymph nodes cannot be assessed; M = metastasis category.

Adapted from Mountain CF: Revisions in the international system for staging lung cancer. Chest 1997; 111:1710–1717.

From Strauss GM: NSCLC stage groupings; 1997 revisions to ISS. Paper presented at: Clinical Decision Making in NSCLC: Active Treatment vs Supportive Care Alone Meeting; October 25, 1997; New Orleans.

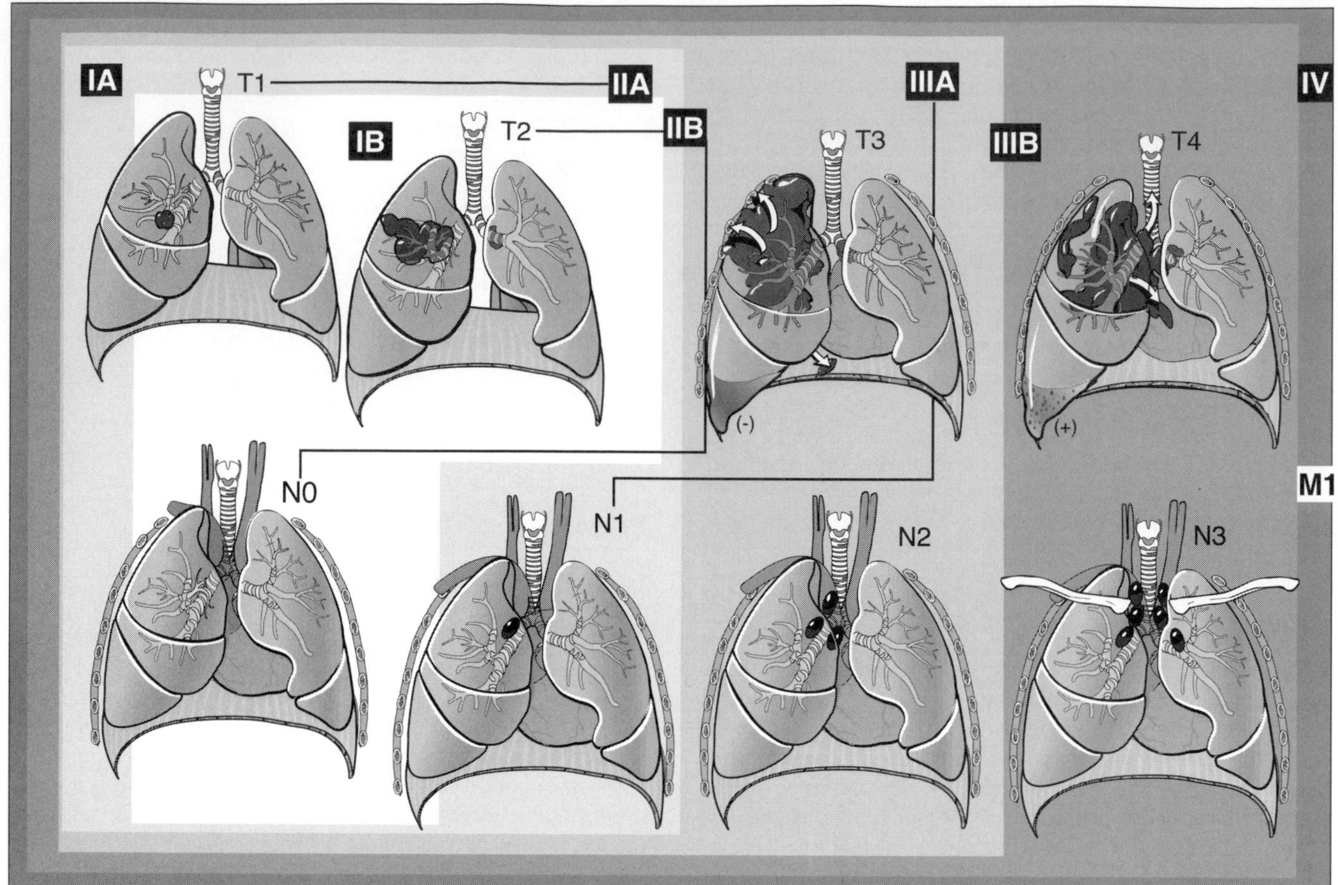

Figure 30–2. Anatomic stage grouping: lung.

Surgery

For localized non–small cell carcinomas (stages I and II), surgery is the treatment of choice,[52–56] because these lesions usually can be excised completely. The choice of surgical procedure—lobectomy, pneumonectomy, segmental or sleeve resection—depends on the extent of malignant disease and the patient's functional status. The procedure of choice is usually that which will encompass all existing disease and provide maximum conservation of normal lung

TABLE 30–6. **Multidisciplinary Treatment Decisions for Non–Small Cell Lung Cancer**

Stage	Surgery	Radiation Therapy		Chemotherapy
I				
T1-2, N0, M0	Lobectomy Pneumonectomy Sleeve resection, segmentectomy if necessary Plus hilar node resection	NR except for medically inoperable DRT 60–70 Gy		NR
II				
T1-2, N1, M0 T3, N0, M0	Lobectomy Pneumonectomy Plus hilar node resection	NR except for medically inoperable DRT 60–70 Gy		NR
III				
T3, N0–2, M0	Complete resection surgery	ART postoperatively 50–60 Gy/5–6 weeks		IC III
Any T, N3, M0	Usually unresectable	DRT if unresectable 60–70 Gy/6 weeks	and	YES
IV				
T4, N3, M0	NR	PRT 40–50 Gy/4–6 weeks	and/or	YES
Any T, Any N, M+	NR	PRT 5 Gy/wk for 10–12 wks, to 50–60 Gy/10–12 wks	and/or	YES

NR = not recommended; DRT = definitive radiation therapy; ART = adjuvant radiation therapy; PRT = palliative radiation therapy; IC III = investigational chemotherapy, phase II/III clinical trials.

TABLE 30–7. **Multidisciplinary Treatment Decisions for Small Cell Lung Cancer**

Stage	Surgery	Radiation Therapy		Chemotherapy
T1, T2, N0, M0	Lobectomy (selected cases)	ART 50 Gy after chemotherapy	and/or	MAC CCR
T3, T4, N1–3, M0	NR	RT 50 Gy CNS prophylaxis for CR 2 Gy × 12 (24 Gy)	and	CCR
Metastatic	NR	PRT selected sites—30 Gy HBI—6 Gy		MAC

NR = not recommended; ART = adjuvant radiation therapy; CR = complete remission; PRT = palliative radiation therapy; HBI = half-body irradiation; MAC = multiagent chemotherapy; CCR = concurrent chemotherapy and radiation.

tissue. Nevertheless, for T1,N0 tumor, a lobectomy is preferable to a segmentectomy whenever it is feasible; the overall survival after 2 years has proved superior in a randomized trial of the Lung Cancer Study Group (LCSG), owing to a significant reduction of local relapse.[57]

On occasion, stage III disease may present borderline cases for surgery. Localized chest wall or pericardium invasion, superior sulcus tumor, limited mediastinal nodal involvement, and phrenic nerve involvement are not absolute surgical contraindications. Each case must be carefully evaluated and individualized. The primary aim is to achieve complete tumor resection and to avoid an exploratory thoracotomy or an incomplete surgical resection. The presence of distant or extrathoracic metastases is indicative of inoperability, and a surgical procedure is an absolute contraindication, except for some very selected cases with single brain metastasis and an early lung cancer. Achieving palliation by resection in the presence of metastases is a myth, except for some very special and well-selected cases, such as one single brain metastasis from an early lung cancer without nodal involvement or other metastatic deposits. There is no proven place, to date, for debulking surgical procedures in lung cancer.

Immunotherapy

BCG (bacille Calmette-Guérin strain of *Mycobacterium bovis*), which is a living vaccine, levamisole, and *Corynebacterium parvum* have been used after surgery or radiotherapy; however, the early positive results of some studies[58, 59] were not confirmed by large-scale trials carried out by other groups.[60] Similar disappointing results have been encountered using different protocols with interferon. Nonetheless, the need for improved treatment options for lung cancer has spawned increased activity in this field using improved technologies and a greater understanding of the underlying biology.[61]

Radiation Therapy

Radiotherapy plays an important role in the multimodal management of lung cancer,[62–65] with the aim being to cure the patient or to palliate symptoms from primary tumors or metastases. At the time of diagnosis, at least one third of all patients are already considered to be inoperable because of locoregional extension (stage III disease) or compromised physiologic functions. Radiotherapy is often considered to be the treatment of choice, but it has been regarded to be more of a palliative than curative modality: the overall 5-year survival rates have varied between 4% and 9%.[7] Nevertheless, several factors related either to the tumor or to irradiation have been clearly identified as having an impact on local control and survival:

- Local control by radiotherapy has a direct influence on survival and is related to treatment parameters (dose, fractionation, volume, and the quality of the technique) (Fig. 30–3).[66]
- There is a clear dose-response relationship: for instance, Radiation Therapy Oncology Group (RTOG) trial 73-01 evaluated total radiation doses of 40, 50, and 60 Gy delivered with 2 Gy per fraction. The highest dose yielded a better 3-year survival rate: 15% after 60 Gy versus 6% after 40 Gy. The optimum doses with conventional treatment procedure appeared to be around 60 Gy.[66–68] Higher doses need to take into account the normal tissue tolerance and require special technical approaches.
- Thoracic irradiation is limited by the tolerance of vital

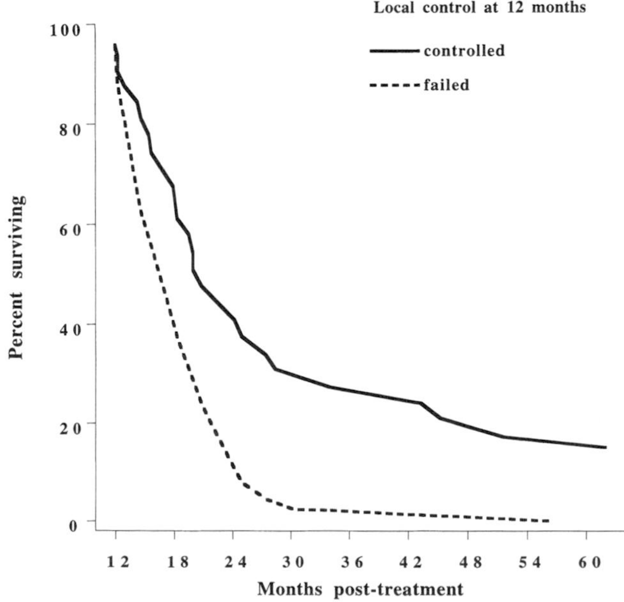

Figure 30–3. Correlation of survival from 12 months for patients with local tumor control or failure at 12 months for patients treated on protocol 73-02. (From Perez CA, Bauer M, Edelstein S, et al: Impact of tumor control on survival in carcinoma of the lung treated with irradiation. Int J Radiat Oncol Biol Phys 1986; 12:539–547, with permission from Elsevier Science.)

organs that lie within the treatment field. The main complications are pneumonopathy, myelopathy, and to some extent cardiomyopathy; they are all time-dose-volume–related events. Doses as low as 25 Gy to the whole lung can lead to severe radiation fibrosis, with or without effusion or pneumonitis. A dose higher than 45 Gy, delivered continuously to the spinal cord over 4 weeks, can also lead to a late, irreversible radiation myelopathy.

- The quality of the radiation procedure is an important factor, not only to avoid inducing severe late effects in normal tissues but also for local control and even survival. For example, prolongation of the radiation treatments by a few days or treatment interruptions of several weeks (such as the rest period in a split-course schedule) can lead to a decrease in tumor control or survival. In an analysis of three RTOG trials evaluating different hyperfractionated schedules, if the treatment was delayed for more than 5 days, then the 2-year survival rate dropped from 33% to 14%.[69]
- Even with the best classic radiation schedule, results remain disappointing and failures may be directly related both to local control and distant metastases. For example, in the French trial of Arriagada and colleagues, a precise pattern of failure analysis was performed, including repeated fiberoptic bronchoscopies: the local control at 1 year was only 17% for stage III tumor treated with 65 Gy, with or without induction chemotherapy.[70]
- Several approaches are under investigation to improve the treatment efficacy of radiation: increasing the biologic dose (radiosensitizers, concomitant chemotherapy, and modification of the fractionation), increasing the physical dose (conformal radiotherapy, brachytherapy, and intraoperative irradiation), and combined treatment modalities with surgery or chemotherapy.

Fractionation. Fractionation is aimed at taking advantage of the four radiobiologic principles. The classic radiation schedule is to deliver one fraction per day. Some of the newer schedules try to take advantage of more recent observations (e.g., the importance of fraction size) through the use of several small-dose fractions per day, with each fraction separated by several hours *(hyperfractionation).* This adjustment allows for an increase in the total dose without causing more late damage. In addition, the role played by tumor repopulation during a radiation course (see Chapter 5, Basic Principles of Radiobiology) leads to a reduction in the treatment duration to overcome this problem *(accelerated repopulation).*

The hyperfractionated schedule has been investigated by the RTOG. A 69.6-Gy hyperfractionated schedule was tested in a three-arm randomized trial, comparing the new experimental schedule (two fractions of 1.2 Gy per day separated by at least 4 hours) with 60 Gy in daily 2-Gy fractions and with an induction chemotherapy program followed by standard radiation therapy. The 1-, 2-, 3-, and 4-year survival rates were 46%, 20%, 9%, and 4%, respectively, after a standard radiation course and 51%, 24%, 14%, and 9%, respectively, after a hyperfractionated schedule.[71] These differences are not statistically significant but suggest a trend in favor of the hyperfractionated schedule.

Intraoperative Radiation. One way to increase the total dose delivered to the tumor without exposing normal surrounding structures is to implant radioactive sources or administer a single dose of external radiation at the time of surgery. Either one of these approaches requires close interaction and collaboration among surgeons and radiation oncologists. Calvo and colleagues[72] stressed that the real advantage for intraoperative radiation therapy (IORT) was in resected bronchogenic cancers, with a frequency-following response (local progression) of 44%. However, there was a high complication rate and only 10- to 15-Gy boost doses are recommended. Esophageal tolerance is one of the limiting factors for this boost dose. More recently, intraoperative radiation has been used in combination with external beam radiation and chemotherapy protocols.[73, 74]

Brachytherapy. The development of afterloading techniques, automatic source projectors, dosimetry facilities, and miniaturized sources have led to a renewed interest in endobronchial brachytherapy. This technique requires the insertion of a flexible catheter during a fibrobronchoscopy. If a high-dose rate unit is used, the treatment will take a few minutes and may be carried out in an outpatient setting. It requires several sessions to allow for normal tissue tolerance. The limits of this approach are directly related to the volume treated. Because of a rapid dose fall-off, the volume usually covered is a cylinder with a 2- to 3-cm diameter. Endobronchial brachytherapy may be used to relieve an endoluminal bronchial obstruction,[75] as a boost to a complete external course of radiation, or for the treatment of small endobronchial tumors.[76, 77] For the treatment of small endobronchial tumors, this approach has not yet been shown to be superior to surgery, but it is a potential alternative in selected patients who are not surgical candidates.

Three-Dimensional Conformal Radiotherapy. This approach results from advances in imaging techniques, computerized treatment planning techniques that allow a three-dimensional reconstruction of the radiation dose distribution, and inverse planning with intense dose modulation and in radiation delivery with the use of multileaf collimators. The goal of this approach is to define precisely and restrict the irradiated volume to the tumor (thus limiting the amount of normal tissue irradiated) and allow an increase in the total dose. The available data show the feasibility of this approach; the limiting factor remains the amount of normal lung volume irradiated.[63, 78, 79] Studies are ongoing for gating to correct for motion due to respiratory and cardiac movements.

Surgery and Radiotherapy

Preoperative irradiation is no longer generally advocated.[80, 81] Although radiation therapy can ablate gross tumors into microscopic deposits in 30% to 50% of instances and some tumors that initially were unresectable can be made operable, no improvements in survival have been noted. However, preoperative radiation therapy has been traditionally advocated for patients with a superior sulcus (Pancoast's) tumor,[82] who are considered to be good risk. More recently, triple therapy (chemoradiation, surgery, then further chemotherapy) has been explored.[82, 83]

Postoperative radiation has no role after complete resection of T1-T2, N0, or M0 NSCLC tumors.[84, 85] Randomized trials have failed to show any benefit from additional postoperative radiation, and the survival rate after surgery alone is approaching 60% at 5 years. In completely resected NSCLC with involvement of hilar or mediastinal nodes, postoperative irradiation decreases local relapses, but the possible gain in survival time is still not known and is likely to be very small: this group of patients has a high probability of subclinical metastases.[86]

Postoperative radiation represents a challenge: a dose able to control microscopic disease (at least 50 Gy in 5 weeks) must be delivered without inducing severe late effects to the heart or the lungs, which often already have compromised functions from either surgical resection or a long history of tobacco smoking. A precise technique using all modern facilities (CT-based treatment planning and linear accelerators) is highly recommended.

Pulmonary function tests have shown minimal impairment despite loss of some lung volume owing to irradiation, as shown by Choi and associates[87] in a convincing serial prospective study conducted for 10 to 12 years postoperatively. With adequate technique, postoperative radiation may be safely delivered even after pneumonectomy.[88]

In cases of incomplete resection, postoperative irradiation is always used. It is best to administer radiation doses immediately after surgery rather than wait for overt recurrences. When a local failure is detected after surgery, salvage therapy with irradiation has less efficacy because of increased tumor burden and disease spread.

Chemoradiotherapy Approaches

Distant metastases remain a common failure pattern in lung cancer. Consequently, a systemic treatment can be a key factor for improving survival.

Non–Small Cell Lung Cancer. For NSCLC, chemotherapy has been used for more than 40 years as an adjuvant treatment to either surgery or radiotherapy. Most of the early studies did not show a clear benefit from chemotherapy, owing to drug inadequacy rather than the concept itself. However, during the 1990s, positive results have been increasingly reported in well-conducted randomized trials, including a large meta-analysis; this analysis collected the data from 9387 patients included in 52 randomized trials.[89] From this analysis, it was shown that after surgery, long-term alkylating agents had a detrimental effect on survival, whereas regimens containing cisplatin yielded an absolute, although modest, benefit of 3% at 2 years, and 5% at 5 years. For locally advanced disease, a cisplatin-based chemotherapy program yielded an absolute benefit of 4% at 2 years and 2% at 5 years. This analysis suggests that chemotherapy may have an impact in the treatment of NSCLC, but further research is required to confirm this modest benefit and to define the best treatment approach.

When combining drugs with radiation or surgery, several aims may be pursued, depending on the type of drugs and the sequence used:

- Conventional cytostatic agents may achieve a spatial cooperation, controlling mainly subclinical metastatic spread.
- A sequential approach with chemotherapy may have to be temporally separated from radiation to reduce possible added toxicities.
- Alternatively, selected drugs may be given concurrently with radiation to achieve a radiosensitizing effect. However, timing becomes a critical factor that can lead to a possible increase in acute and late toxicities.

During the last decade, the concept of neoadjuvant chemotherapy or induction therapy has been introduced. It is defined as a cytoreductive therapy and is administered before a definitive locoregional treatment. It consists of two to three cycles of chemotherapy given before radiotherapy or surgery. This approach offers several theoretical advantages:

1. Any tumor shrinkage achieved with drugs may enhance reoxygenation of hypoxic cells, which increases radiosensitivity. This also may reduce the volume of normal tissue to be irradiated.
2. Chemotherapy given after radiation therapy seems to be less effective as a result of a subsequent impairment of blood supply.
3. Evaluation of tumor responses allows selection of patients for possible maintenance chemotherapy.

Disadvantages of neoadjuvant chemotherapy are as follows:

1. Tumor progression is more hypoxic and, therefore, has less effective radiosensitization.
2. There is a risk of recruiting tumor clonogens into active proliferation or inducing resistant clonogens to chemotherapy and, later, to radiation.
3. Acute toxicity is exacerbated, with its attendant need to reduce radiation doses or even interrupt a treatment.

Induction chemotherapy has been used before a definitive course of radiotherapy. Consecutive randomized trials have clearly demonstrated an improvement in long-term survival when a cisplatin-based chemotherapy was administered before 60 to 65 Gy (Table 30–8).[90]

A concurrent approach implies delivery of a drug or drugs in close association with radiation; the drug may be used as a radiosensitizer or as a cytoreductive modality. The former approach was well illustrated by an EORTC trial using daily doses of 6 mg/m^2 of cisplatin during split-course irradiation; this led to an improved 2-year survival rate because of better local control.[91] Another approach is to use a classic chemotherapy regimen with drugs known not to affect radiation-induced toxicity. This approach is usually associated with an increase in acute toxicity, including esophageal toxicity.[92] Preliminary data of phase II trials yield promising results with cisplatin-based chemotherapy. In a phase III trial, Furuse and coworkers observed better results after a concurrent approach than with an induction treatment using mitomycin, vindesine, and cisplatin followed by 56 Gy: the 5-year survival rates were 15.8% for the concurrent approach and 8.9% for the induction treatment, respectively.[93]

Preoperative chemotherapy has been used mainly in large series phase II trials and a few small phase II trials for stage III patients with NSCLC.[94] Two trials reported a

TABLE 30–8. **Intergroup Phase III Study: Preliminary Analysis of Survival Rate Based on 4-Year Follow-Up**

Regimen	1-Year	2-Year	3-Year	4-Year	Median Survival (mos)
Standard RT alone	46%	20%	9%	4%	11.4
Hyperfractionated RT	51%	24%	14%	9%	12.3
Chemotherapy followed by RT	60%	31%	13%	11%	13.6

RT = radiation therapy.
Adapted from Sause WT, Scott C, Taylor S, et al: Radiation Therapy Oncology Group (RTOG) 88-08 and Eastern Cooperative Oncology Group (ECOG) 4588: Preliminary results of a phase III trial in regionally advanced unresectable non–small-cell lung cancer. J Natl Cancer Inst 1994; 87:198–205; Sause WT, Scott C, Taylor S, et al: RTOG 88-08 ECOG 4588: Preliminary analysis of a phase III trial in regionally advanced unresectable non–small-cell lung cancer with minimum three-year follow-up [abstract]. Int J Radiat Oncol Biol Phys 1995; 32 (suppl):195; and Komaki R, Scott C, Sause WT, et al: Radiation Therapy Oncology Group (RTOG) 88-08 and Eastern Cooperative Oncology Group (ECOG) 4588: Induction cisplatin/vinblastine and irradiation vs. irradiation in unresectable squamous cell lung cancer. Int J Radiat Oncol Biol Phys 1997; 39 (3):533–535.

high response rate with a resectability rate above 75% and a better survival.[95, 96] Nevertheless, these two trials included only a limited number of patients, and additional studies are required to confirm the role of preoperative chemotherapy. Furthermore, a number of phase II trials have clearly shown that the only patients that have an advantage with this approach must have a complete resection without residual mediastinal lymph nodes.

Preoperative chemotherapy plus irradiation, given either concomitantly or sequentially, has been explored for regional disease. Most series show an increase in responses when the combined treatment is used, but there is additional toxicity. The optimal combination of these two modalities for regionally advanced NSCLC remains to be determined with respect to sequencing, dose, and duration of therapy, as well as the place of surgery. Preoperative chemotherapy used as an adjuvant has also shown some benefit.[89, 97]

Small Cell Lung Cancer. For SCLC, chemotherapy has been the main therapeutic modality for the last 15 years.[98, 99] The poor survival time after locoregional treatment, such as surgery and radiotherapy, underlines the fact that this is a systemic disease. Introducing active cytotoxic drugs has dramatically increased survival time.

In extensive disease, thoracic radiotherapy has a limited role to play except for palliation. For limited SCLC, controversies persist over how to sequence the standard modalities for the primary site. The case for using a local modality such as radiotherapy is based on the high rate of local relapse after chemotherapy alone; chest failures are observed in more than 80% of the patients.[100] Two meta-analyses that evaluate the role of radiotherapy in limited disease patients have been published. The results show that radiation improved 3-year survival rate by 5.4% and tumor control by 25.3%.[101, 102]

The continuing questions are (1) how to combine drugs and radiation, including the sequencing, the timing of radiation, total dose, fractionation, and (2) which drugs to use. No definitive answers are available, but the existing data offer suggestions:

- There is a dose response for SCLC; better local control and survival are observed with doses in excess of 45 Gy.[103]
- Concurrent approaches with cisplatin-based chemotherapy appear to give better long-term survival but added acute toxicity.
- Concerning the timing of radiotherapy, a meta-analysis carried out by Murray and coworkers suggests better results for concomitant administration compared with a true sequential approach, with radiation given after completion of the chemotherapy program (Fig. 30–4).[99, 104]
- The dose-response curve for SCLC with radiation presents almost no initial shoulder, making this tumor particularly appropriate for a hyperfractionated radiation schedule. A randomized trial that compared 45 Gy delivered with one daily fraction of 1.8 Gy to 45 Gy delivered with two daily fractions of 1.5 Gy showed a better survival rate after 2 years.[105]
- Using a concurrent approach, cisplatin-based chemotherapy is the current recommended choice; cisplatin does not enhance radiation effects on the lungs.
- Patients with superior vena cava syndrome should be treated according to their tumor extent. This clinical presentation has no negative impact on survival.[106]

Prophylactic (Elective) Cranial Irradiation

The CNS provides a tumor sanctuary from chemotherapy leading to a high rate of brain metastases. The actuarial probability of developing CNS metastases has been projected to reach 80% at 5 years.[107, 108] Prophylactic (elective) cranial irradiation (PCI) significantly decreases brain relapses in SCLC, but it may only have an impact on survival time in patients who achieve a complete response. In two large randomized trials, PCI decreased the risk of brain metastases with a trend toward better survival.[109, 110] This concept is being applied to both adenocarcinoma and large cell anaplastic carcinomas. However, because of fear of late damage and our current lack of knowledge with respect to normal brain tolerance under the impact of low daily doses, the optimal dose is yet to be defined. Indeed, late CNS damage has been reported, including neurologic deficits, deterioration in neuropsychological tests, and abnormalities detected by CT or MRI.[111] These problems have been observed after chemotherapy alone, but additional PCI increases the risk.[112]

Palliative Irradiation

One of the primary goals of radiation therapy is to relieve distressing symptoms of lung cancer. Some symptoms may

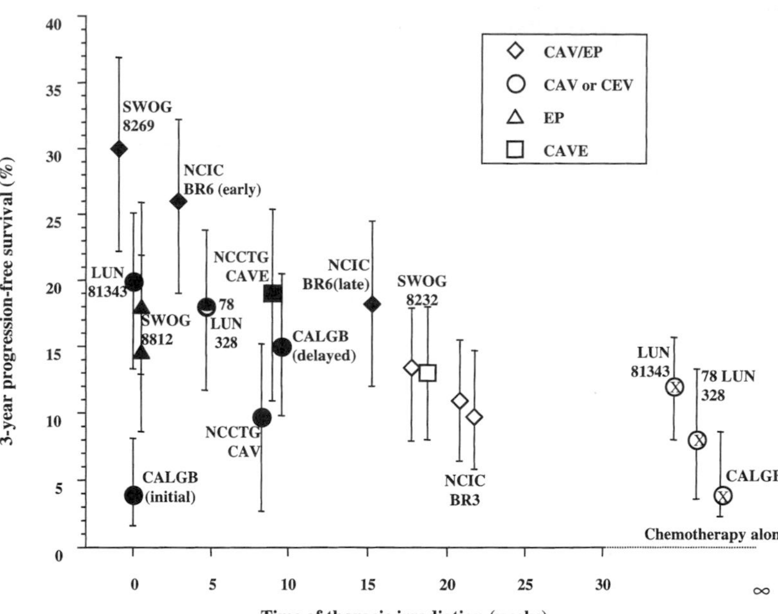

Figure 30–4. Limited-stage small cell lung cancer: 3-year progression-free survival versus time of thoracic irradiation relative to the beginning of chemotherapy. Solid symbols represent concurrent chemotherapy and thoracic irradiation. Open symbols represent sequential chemotherapy and thoracic irradiation. The half-solid symbol is alternating chemotherapy and split-course thoracic irradiation. Open symbols with an *X* indicate that thoracic irradiation was not given. Symbol shape indicates the type of chemotherapy: diamonds = CAV/EP (cyclophosphamide, doxorubicin, vincristine/etoposide, cisplatin); circles = CAV (cyclophosphamide, doxorubicin, vincristine) or CEV (cyclophosphamide, etoposide, vincristine); triangles = EP (etoposide, cisplatin); squares = CAVE (cyclophosphamide, doxorubicin, vincristine, etoposide). (From Murray N: Treatment of small cell lung cancer: the state of the art. Lung Cancer 1997; 17(suppl):S75–S89.)

be a result of the primary tumor (obstruction, hemoptysis, superior vena cava obstruction); others are from the advancement of local disease (chest pain, bone involvement, cord compression); and others are because of metastatic disease (brain, bone, liver, and abdomen). Radiation is very effective in relieving distressing symptoms, and this may be achieved through the use of quite moderate radiation doses.[113]

When facing true emergency situations, it is better to start with three large daily fractions (4 Gy each) on consecutive days, followed by normal fractions. Such an approach offers a rapid reversal of life-threatening signs and symptoms. More routine palliative situations are usually treated with 30 Gy in 2 weeks, with or without a boost. This treatment provides effective palliation in two thirds of all patients, without need for retreatment.

When metastatic disease is extensive, it is necessary to apply radiation fields to several areas. This carries an intrinsic danger of having to overlap radiation fields of previously treated areas. Such so-called chasing of disease can be obviated with the use of *large-field (hemibody) irradiation*. Irradiation of the upper, lower, or midsection of the body (half-body irradiation), with either single doses (6 Gy to upper and 8 Gy to middle or lower half) or fractionated doses of radiation (5 fractions of 3 Gy each), achieves rapid pain relief (70% to 80% within 24 to 48 hours). This strategy offers the advantage of consolidating large symptomatic areas within a single radiation field, which is particularly true for multiple symptomatic bone metastases.

A *hypofractionated* regimen of 5 Gy weekly for 10 to 12 fractions has offered excellent local palliation with reduced acute side effects. This schedule is convenient for patients with advanced lung cancer who are in poor general condition, as well as those who need to travel long distances or are difficult to transport.[114]

For relief of bronchial obstruction, one can use *high-dose-rate* or *low-dose-rate brachytherapy*, with a reported 84% and 67% relief of symptoms, respectively, with confirmed widening of bronchi upon bronchoscopy.[75, 76, 115] Some patients with intrinsic endobronchial obstructing lesions or extrinsic compression due to tumor have been palliated successfully with endobronchial laser or brachytherapy, or both (laser is used only if the lesion is endobronchial).

Chemotherapy

Because of the frequency of metastases on presentation (50%) and the inevitable development of metastases in the majority of patients (90%), chemotherapy is frequently used. Despite the widespread application of single-agent and multiagent chemotherapy, only small gains have been made in treating non–small cell bronchogenic carcinomas. Small cell anaplastic cancers, however, have proven to be highly responsive to combination chemotherapy. The majority of patients have partial response (30% to 50%) or complete response (10% to 40%) with prolongation of survival (Tables 30–9 and 30–10).

SQUAMOUS CELL CARCINOMA, ADENOCARCINOMA, LARGE CELL ANAPLASTIC CARCINOMA, AND NON–SMALL CELL LUNG CANCER

- At present, for NSCLC, chemotherapy is part of its management (see Table 30–9), not only for progressive (recurrent or metastatic) or advanced stage IV disease but also for the treatment of stage III disease with surgery or radiotherapy, or both. For advanced stage, chemotherapy may be accepted for palliation of inoperable symptoms in patients whose disease is beyond control by radiation therapy. It is superior to a best supportive approach, both in treatment efficacy and cost. Furthermore, a combined approach appears to be superior to surgery or radiotherapy alone for stage III disease.
- The overall response rate for most widely used single agents has not been higher than 25% (range varies from 0% to 35%). Active agents include cisplatin,

TABLE 30–9. **Response Rates of Different Classic Multiagent Chemotherapy in Non–Small Cell Lung Cancer**

Chemotherapy	Response Rate %
CAP: cyclophosphamide, doxorubicin, cisplatin	15–25
PV: cisplatin, vinblastine or vindesine	15–30
EP: etoposide, cisplatin	20–30
MVP: mitomycin, vinblastine, cisplatin	30–60
MIP: mitomycin, ifosfamide, cisplatin	35–50
ICE: ifosfamide, carboplatin, etoposide	25–40
Carboplatin and paclitaxel	12–63
Cisplatin and paclitaxel	35–47
Cisplatin and gemcitabine	30–58
Cisplatin and vinorelbine	25–30

Adapted from Shepherd FA: Treatment of advanced non–small cell lung cancer. Semin Oncol 1994; 21 (suppl):7–18. From Ramanathan RK, Belani CP: Chemotherapy for advanced non–small cell lung cancer: past, present, and future. Semin Oncol 1997; 24:440–454.

vinca alkaloid (vinblastine or vindesine), mitomycin C, ifosfamide, carboplatin, paclitaxel, docetaxel, vinorelbine, gemcitabine, and irinotecan.[116, 117] Most agents have a low-objective response rate with transient responses.

- With a few exceptions, combination chemotherapy has failed to increase long-term survival in patients with stage IV NSCLC, but it can increase 1-year survival rates and relieve symptoms. In general, 25% to 35% response rates can be expected. Higher response rates have been reported, but they are rarely substantiated. The majority of responding patients achieve palliation of symptoms. The response rates are higher for stage III than for stage IV disease, with figures as high as 70%.
- The use of new agents or new combination chemotherapy is under active investigation, including taxanes, gemcitabine, and vinorelbine; carboplatin and paclitaxel is the current, most accepted regimen. The number of agents available and the diversity of possible therapeutic schedules have generated a great number of combinations that may include from two to seven drugs. The general impression is that using any combination of two to four drugs produces an equal result as long as the associated drugs have proven effective when used alone.
- Although no regimen can be considered to be standard and none has been shown to be superior to any other, some regimens are commonly used and, in general, are well tolerated. They are listed in Table 30–9.
- The large variation in response rates to combination chemotherapy can be explained by factors such as patient selection, dose intensity, and tumor burden. In general, patients with good performance status, minimal tumor burden, and higher dose chemotherapy (at the expense of potentially having more complications) have a higher response possibility.
- Surgical *adjuvant chemotherapy* has not shown evidence of increased survival time over surgery alone in stage I or II operable cases. In 10 controlled trials that included more than 5000 patients, chemotherapy showed no advantage.[89] In two of those studies, there was evidence of adverse effects; this was particularly seen with alkylating agents that were given over a long period. Agents used included cyclophosphamide, methotrexate, 5-fluorouracil, and vinblastine, administered for short courses for months up to 2 years. The absence of effective chemotherapy with high response rates for NSCLC has limited its use as adjuvant therapy. However, the use of cisplatin-based chemotherapy has been shown to prolong disease-free survival and provide some survival benefit in patients with stage III disease, either completely or incompletely resected. Large phase III trials are ongoing worldwide.
- Chemotherapy can be used as a *radiosensitizer* to enhance local cell killing and could improve local tumor control. Investigators[91, 92] have produced evidence of radiosensitization using daily cisplatin plus radiation and demonstrated a significant improvement in overall survival compared with patients receiving irradiation alone. Radiosensitization is useful for the local control of the disease, but there is also a clear need for an effective systemic treatment because distant metastases are a common cause of failure.

TABLE 30–10. **Standard Chemotherapy Regimens for Small Cell Lung Cancer**

Chemotherapy	Regimen
CAV	
Cyclophosphamide	1000 mg/m² IV Day 1
Doxorubicin (Adriamycin)	45–50 mg/m² IV Day 1
Vincristine	1.4 mg/m² IV Day 1 (max. 2 mg)
	Repeat every 3 weeks
CAE	
Cyclophosphamide	1000 mg/m² IV Day 1
Doxorubicin (Adriamycin)	45 mg/m² IV Day 1
Etoposide	50 mg/m² IV Days 1–5
	Repeat every 3 weeks
PE	
Cisplatin	60–80 mg/m² IV Day 1
Etoposide	80–120 mg/m²/day IV Days 1–3
	Repeat every 3 weeks
CABCDA-E	
Carboplatin	100 mg/m²/day IV Days 1–3
Etoposide	120 mg/m²/day IV Days 1–3
	Repeat every 4 weeks
CAV alternating with PE	
CAV with	
Cisplatin	80 mg/m²/day IV Day 1
Etoposide	100 mg/m²/day IV Days 1–3
	Repeat every 3 weeks

IV = intravenously.
From Johnson DH, Eisert DR: Treatment of small cell lung cancer. In: Roth JA, Ruckdeschel JC, Weisenberger TH (eds): Thoracic Oncology, 2nd ed, pp 201–224. Philadelphia, W.B. Saunders, 1995, with permission. Modified from DeVore RF, Johnson DH: Lung cancer: chemotherapy. In: Brain MC, Carbone PP (eds): Current Therapy in Hematology-Oncology, 4th ed, pp 245–249. Philadelphia, B.C. Dekker, 1992.

SMALL CELL CARCINOMA

The most frequently used classification only makes distinctions between limited disease (e.g., confined to one hemithorax, including ipsilateral, positive, scalene lymph nodes) or extensive disease (all remaining cases). During the last decade, chemotherapy has become the primary treatment for this disease,[99, 118] but other modalities (e.g., radiation therapy and surgery) play an important role in obtaining locoregional disease control.

- Combination chemotherapy is now the accepted treatment for all stages (see Table 30–10),[119] particularly because this cancer tends to be widely disseminated in virtually all cases at the time of diagnosis. Surgery is rarely justified except in patients with small primary tumors without clinical evidence of mediastinal lymph node or distant metastases and those who have achieved a complete response to chemotherapy. In this case, chemotherapy followed by surgery may offer a better long-term, disease-free survival.[120]
- Virtually every combination of active agents has been used in the treatment of this disease. Regimens including three, four, or five drugs have been used without demonstrating clear superiority to any other regimens containing more than three drugs.
- Several effective agents have been identified: cyclophosphamide, doxorubicin, vincristine, nitrosoureas, etoposide, and cisplatin are the most commonly used, with individual response rates between 20% and 40%. Several combination regimens achieve a response rate of at least 80%. This response is usually achieved within the first 6 weeks of induction chemotherapy treatment and continues for four to six cycles. Maintenance chemotherapy for longer than 6 months does not appear to be beneficial to patients.
- Toxicity usually increases when the number of drugs is increased. The challenge is to achieve and maintain a complete response, because prolonged survivals are seen only in this group of patients. Although progress has been made in the management of this disease (better responses and increases in median survival), long-term survival (over 2 years) is still disappointingly low (up to 20% of patients with limited stage and 10% with extensive stage).
- For patients with limited-stage disease, a combined approach with systemic chemotherapy and radiotherapy for thoracic disease is likely to be better than chemotherapy alone. Radiation should be given early in the course of treatment. Failure within the chest is a common finding with chemotherapeutic regimens; therefore, the major contribution of thoracic radiotherapy has been to increase locoregional control.[102] The brain and leptomeninges continue to be sanctuary sites for chemotherapy. Prophylactic brain irradiation has reduced the incidence of metastasis by 50% (from 35% to 15%); however, this reduction has not led to any apparent survival benefit. This fact reflects the necessity for more effective systemic treatment to control the disease in other sites, rather than simply an indication of the failure of radiation as a local treatment.
- The evaluation of new drugs has many different strategies.[121, 122] One of the most controversial is testing new agents in untreated patients rather than in previously treated patients with recurrent or metastatic disease. The response rates can range from 80% in previously untreated patients to 10% for patients who received previous drug therapy.
- Controversy exists over the issue of whether increasing the dose rate intensity of commonly used front-line regimens above levels that produce modest toxicity will produce improved survival. Retrospective studies are plagued by methodologic difficulties and show inconsistency. The issue will be settled best through randomized clinical trials.[123, 124]
- Newer active agents include taxanes, gemcitabine, ifosfamide, topotecan, camptothecin-11, and vinorelbine. Some of these drugs in combination, including VIP (**V**P-16 [etoposide], **i**fosfamide, and cis**p**latin) and PPE (**p**aclitaxel, cis**p**latin, and **e**toposide), are showing response rates between 73% and 94%.[125, 126]

Results and Prognosis

Results: Non–Small Cell Cancers

The overall survival rate for all patients treated is 5% to 10%, with little impact made by current diagnostic screening procedures or newer multimodality approaches in the common adenocarcinomas and SCCs. With the rising incidence of all lung cancers, as noted earlier, the mortality rate for this malignancy is such that respiratory cancers represent the major cancers for which the burden of premature deaths has increased and accounts for 25% of all premature loss of life from any cancer.

Overall Survival

According to SEER data, the relative 5-year survival rate is 8% to 10%, and the 10-year survival rate is 5% to 7%.[127] For 5-year survivors, there is a small rate of attrition; however, 68% will still be alive at 10 years. The survival rate is somewhat better for females than for males—13% versus 10% at 5 years.[128] Some subsets of patients with metastatic disease live longer than others: good performance status, female gender, and age of 70 years or older appear to be associated with a modestly more favorable outcome.

BY STAGE

The AJCC has revised staging criteria, and there is an improvement in stage III—especially IIIa—patients, although this is from the creation of a new T4 and N3 category (Table 30–11 and Fig. 30–5).[26] This category is different from the previous classification, which included a very poor prognosis for patients in the T3 category.

BY HISTOPATHOLOGY

Patients with carcinoid tumors have the best prognosis for survival (5-year relative survival rate of 83.2%), whereas those with SCLC have the worst prognosis (5-year relative survival rate of 4.6%).[48] There is little difference in outcome for the common varieties of adenocarcinoma and SCC: 5-year survival rates range from 16% to 23% versus 15% to 21%, respectively (Table 30–12).

BY MODALITY

Surgical results: The survival results presented are largely from the successful resection of lung cancer.

Radiation therapy results—postoperative: The addition

TABLE 30–11. **Clinical and Pathologic Surgical Survival Results by Stage of Non–Small Cell Lung Cancer**

		Clinical		Surgical	
Stage	**TNM**	***1-Year Survival %***	***5-Year Survival %***	***1-Year Survival %***	***5-Year Survival %***
IA	T1, NO, MO	91	61	94	67
IB	T2, NO, MO	72	38	87	57
IIA	T1, N1, MO	79	34	89	55
IIB	T2, N1, MO	61	24	78	39
	T3, NO, MO	55	22	76	38
IIIA	T3, N1, MO	56	9	65	25
	T1-2-3, N2, MO	50	13	64	23
IIIB/IV	T4, NO-1-2, MO	37	7		
	Any T, N3, MO	32	3		
	Any T, Any N, M1	20	5		

T = tumor; N = node; M = metastasis.
Modified from Mountain CF: Revisions in the international system for staging lung cancer. Chest 1997; 111:1710–1717.

of irradiation postoperatively (Table 30–13) has failed to show any benefit in survival time in different randomized trials,[84, 86, 129] but there was better local control, especially for N2 disease. Whereas nonrandomized studies show a gain in 5-year survival, randomized studies do not.[81, 87, 130–132]

Radiation therapy—unresectable: Patients treated with definitive radiation have either an early stage tumor and are not surgical candidates (a result of compromised lung functions or other disease) or have locally advanced disease considered to be unresectable. Tables 30–8 and 30–14 summarize some of the results achieved with radiation alone, including the new fractionation schedules, or combinations with chemotherapy given either in a neoadjuvant or concomitant approach. It is important to remember that the patients were selected after an extensive work-up and often had good prognostic factors before treatment (good performance status, no weight loss, or no N3 disease).

Chemotherapy results: Although multiagent chemotherapy improves the response rate over single agents (see Table 30–9), the complete remission rate remains low (i.e., less than 10% to 15%) despite regressions that are observed in the majority of lung cancers (i.e., 53% to 87%). The median survival time for most advanced and metastatic disease patients (stages III and IV) treated with chemotherapy is usually less than 1 year.

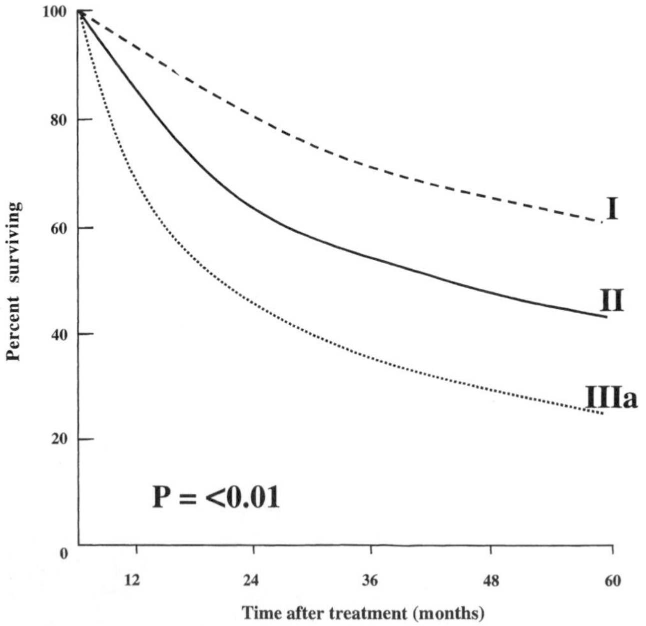

Figure 30–5. Cumulative proportion of patients surviving after complete resection for non–small cell lung cancer, according to surgical pathologic stage (deaths within 30 days excluded). Collected series: stage I, n = 865; stage II, n = 318; stage IIIa, n = 252. (From Mountain CF: New prognostic factors in lung cancer: biologic prophets of cancer cell aggression. Chest 1995; 108:246.)

Results: Small Cell Cancers

The expectation of increasing curability for SCLC in proportion to its response rates (80% to 100%) has not been realized in terms of survival. The median survival time at 1 year (10 to 16 months) in patients with limited-stage cancer in most randomized clinical trials using multiagent chemotherapy alone increased by 3 months with combined-modality approaches (13 to 17 months). Reports of 5-year survivors in some mature studies range from 2% to 19% for chemotherapy alone, but they increase to 14% to 36% with combined modality.[131–141]

With the incorporation of current chemotherapy regimens into treatment programs, however, survival is unequivocally prolonged, with at least a four- to five-fold improvement in median survival time compared with patients who are given no therapy.[142] Furthermore, about 10% of the total population of patients remains free of disease over 2 years from the start of therapy, a time period during which most relapses occur. However, even these patients are at risk of dying from lung cancer (both small and non–small cell types) at a later time.

Despite improved high response rates, the long-term 5-year survival rate, in general, is dismal, ranging from 1% to 12%, with most series being less than 5%, similar to non–small cell cancers.[143]

TABLE 30–12. **5-Year Relative Survival Rates for Non–Small Cell Lung Cancer by Histology**

Histologic Type	No. of Cases	5-Year Survival %			
		All Stages	*Local*	*Regional*	*Distant*
All carcinomas	87,128	13.9	39.6	14.4	1.5
Squamous cell carcinoma	26,407	15.4	34.3	14.9	1.5
Adenocarcinoma, NOS	20,991	16.6	49.9	16.1	1.5
Bronchoalveolar carcinoma	2382	42.1	65.1	31.8	4.2
Papillary adenocarcinoma	568	23.7	57.4*	25.8	5.4
Adenosquamous carcinoma	1056	21.6	49.6	19.1	2.2
Small cell carcinoma	15,656	4.6	12.3	7.5	1.4
Large cell carcinoma	7592	11.4	34.8	13.2	1.6

NOS = not otherwise specified.
*Standard error >5% and ≤10%.
Modified from Travis WD, Travis LB, DeVesa SS: Lung cancer. Cancer 1995; 75(1 suppl):191–198. Reprinted by permission of Wiley-Liss, Inc., a subsidiary of John Wiley & Sons, Inc.

TABLE 30–13. **5-Year Survival Rates Following Postoperative Radiation Therapy in Non–Small Cell Lung Cancer**

Studies	RT Dose	Histology	5-Year Survival (%)	
			RT	*Control*
Randomized				
Van Houtte et al[84]	60 Gy	All	24	43
Lung CSG[129]	50 Gy	Epidermoid (Epi)	38	38
Stephens et al[86]	40 Gy	Epi + Adenocarcinoma	36	21*
Nonrandomized				
Green et al[130]	50–60 Gy	Epidermoid	21	6
		Adenocarcinoma	50	14
Kirsh et al[131]	N/A	Epidermoid	34	0
		Adenocarcinoma	12	0
Choi et al[87]	40–60 Gy	Epidermoid	33	33
		Adenocarcinoma	43	8
Van Houtte et al[81]	55–60 Gy	Epidermoid	21	
		Adenocarcinoma	17	
Sawyer et al[132]	50 Gy	Epi + Adenocarcinoma	43	22†

RT = radiotherapy; N/A = not applicable.
*3-year survival rate for N2 disease.
†4-year survival rate.

TABLE 30–14. **Results of Radical Radiotherapy for Non–Small Cell Lung Cancer**

Authors	Stage	Radiation Dose (Gy)	No. of Patients	Survival Rate (%) at		
				2 Years	*3 Years*	*5 Years*
Zhang et al[133]	I	>50	44		55	32
Sandler et al[134]	I	>50	77		17	15
Krol et al[135]	I	>50	108		31	15
Morita et al[65]	I	>50	149		34	22
Perez et al[68]	I–III	40 S	101	18	7	4
		40 C	102	16	7	4
		50 C	90	10	12	4
		60 C	86	9	14	4
Sause et al[71]	I–III	60 C	149	19	6	
		60 H*	152	24	13	
Saunders et al[64]	I–III	60 C	225	20		
		54 H†	338	30		

C = continuous irradiation; S = split-course irradiation.
*Two fractions per day.
†Three fractions per day, treatment without interruption (CHART).

Clinical Investigations

Prevention

Prevention of lung cancer must be one of the primary aims of research. Reduction or elimination of the respiratory carcinogens conceptually are the simplest methods to improve the general outcome. Major efforts must be made to persuade patients to stop smoking, and the physician's role in tobacco control cannot be overemphasized. Self-help smoking cessation kits, counseling, and nicotine replacement are helpful to induce patients to quit smoking.[144, 145]

Lung cancer chemoprevention using retinoids was designed to reverse premalignant lesions, prevent an initial lung cancer in individuals who are at high risk for it, and prevent second primary tumors in patients previously treated for a lung cancer or another head and neck cancer. Retinoids act on normal bronchial epithelium by inducing mucins and blocking aberrant squamous cell differentiation.[146] However, some trials have failed to show any benefit in terms of survival time or in the number of cancers detected.[147] Recent studies using supplemental beta-carotene and retinol administered in high-risk groups have even suggested an adverse effect on the incidence of lung cancer; other trials are ongoing using either *N*-acetylcyseine or retinylpalmitate.[147–149]

Stages I and II Squamous Cell Carcinoma, Adenocarcinoma, and Large Cell Carcinoma

The failure of adjuvant radiation therapy, chemotherapy, and immunostimulation to increase overall survival time has shifted interest to specific immunostimulation, new drug combinations, or even chemoprevention of second cancers (a major challenge among long-term survivors). Furthermore, any adjuvant therapy trial must take into account the high proportion of patients with T1,N0,M0 tumors that are definitely cured by resection. The addition of an adjuvant treatment must always include an attempt to avoid an increase in morbidity or mortality.

Stage III Tumors

The major search is for an optimal combination of different modalities to improve the current results. Large phase III trials are ongoing to assess the impact of induction chemotherapy, the place of surgery after induction chemotherapy, and the role of adjuvant chemotherapy after a complete resection.

Stage IV Tumors

- For radiation therapy, different schedules testing hyperfractionation with higher total doses and additional boosting with intraluminal brachytherapy are being investigated. Studies to investigate the advantage of dose escalation and three-dimensional radiotherapy planning (applied in conformal therapy) are ongoing.
- Multiagent chemotherapy and new drugs are continuously being explored in an attempt to achieve higher response rates. This is the primary aim when using chemotherapy in combined approaches or as an adjuvant to surgery or irradiation; it is hoped that such uses will have a major impact on survival.
- Immunostimulation with chemotherapy or radiation therapy programs is also under study.
- Biologic response modifiers may prove to be promising. Other modes of therapy being investigated are gene therapy, for instance, inhalation gene transfer of manganese superoxide dismutase transgene[150]; anticytokine and antiadhesion molecule approaches; and targeting intracellular signal transduction pathways, including cyclic adenosine monophosphate metabolism, tyrosine kinases and mitogen-activated protein kinases.[151]

For SCLC, better drug combinations or new drugs and the best possible chemoradiation therapy schedule must be identified for limited disease.

Recommended Reading

During the 1990s, good reviews of the multidisciplinary approach in lung cancer have been published. These books are included in the General References section. We particularly recommend a *Seminars in Oncology* series,[1] the chapters on lung cancer in DeVita and colleagues' *Cancer Principles and Practice of Oncology*,[2, 3] as well as three books dedicated to lung cancer: Pass and coworkers' *Lung Cancer: Principles and Treatment*,[4] Roth and associates' *Thoracic Oncology*,[5] and Aisner and colleagues' *Comprehensive Textbook of Thoracic Oncology*.[6] A fine review also is found in the chapter in *Principles and Practice in Radiation Oncology*.[7] Staging for these cancers is defined in several publications.[8, 9]

REFERENCES

General

1. Johnson DH (ed): Lung cancer. Semin Oncol 1997; 24:387–499.
2. Ginsberg RJ, Vokes EE, Raben A: Non–small cell lung cancer. In: DeVita VT, Hellman S, Rosenberg SA (eds): Cancer. Principles & Practice of Oncology, 5th ed, pp 858–910. Philadelphia, Lippincott-Raven, 1997.
3. Ihde DC, Glatstein E, Pass HI: Small cell lung cancer. In: DeVita VT, Hellman S, Rosenberg SA (eds): Cancer. Principles & Practice of Oncology, 5th ed, pp 911–950. Philadelphia, Lippincott-Raven, 1997.
4. Pass HI, Mitchell JB, Johnson DH, et al (eds): Lung Cancer: Principles and Practice. Philadelphia, Lippincott-Raven, 1996.
5. Roth JA, Ruckdeschel JC, Weisenberger TH: Thoracic Oncology. Philadelphia, W.B. Saunders, 1995.
6. Aisner J, Arriagada R, Green MR, et al (eds): Comprehensive Textbook of Thoracic Oncology. Baltimore, Williams & Wilkins, 1996.
7. Emami B, Graham MV: Lung. In: Perez CA, Brady LW (eds): Principles and Practice of Radiation Oncology, pp 1181–1220. Philadelphia, Lippincott-Raven, 1997.
8. American Joint Committee on Cancer: AJCC Cancer Staging Manual, 5th ed. Philadelphia, Lippincott-Raven, 1997.
9. International Union Against Cancer (UICC): TNM Classification of Malignant Tumors, 5th ed. New York, Wiley-Liss, 1997.

Specific

10. Landis SH, Murray T, Bolden S, et al: Cancer statistics, 1999. CA Cancer J Clin 1999; 49:8–31.
11. Parkin DM, Pisani P, Ferlay J: Global cancer statistics. CA Cancer J Clin 1999; 49:33–64.

12. Hammond EC, Horn D: Smoking and death rates—report on forty-four months of follow-up of 187,783 men. Cancer 1988; 38:28–58.
13. Garfinkel L, Silverberg E: Lung cancer and smoking trends in the United States over the past 25 years. CA Cancer J Clin 1991; 41:137–145.
14. Redmond WH: Trends in adolescent cigarette use: the diffusion of daily smoking. J Behav Med 1999; 22:379–395.
15. Garfinkel L: Trends in cigarette smoking in the United States. Prev Med 1997; 26:447–450.
16. Koo LC, Ho JH: Worldwide epidemiological patterns of lung cancer in nonsmokers. Int J Epidemiol 1990; 19 (suppl):S14–S23.
17. Le Marchand L, Wilkens LR, Kolonel LN: Ethnic differences in the lung cancer risk associated with smoking. Cancer Epidemiol Biomarkers Prev 1992; 1:103–107.
18. Albin M, Magnani C, Krstev S, et al: Asbestos and cancer: an overview of current trends in Europe. Environ Health Perspect 1999; 107 (suppl):289–298.
19. Reif AE, Heeren T: Consensus on synergism between cigarette smoke and other environmental carcinogens in the causation of lung cancer. Adv Cancer Res 1999; 76:161–186.
20. Katsouyanni K, Perhagen G: Ambient air pollution exposure and cancer. Cancer Causes Control 1997; 8:284–291.
21. Waalkes MP, Coogan TP, Barter RA: Toxicological principles of metal carcinogenesis with special emphasis on cadmium. Crit Rev Toxicol 1992; 22:175–201.
22. Blair A, Kazerouni N: Reactive chemicals and cancer. Cancer Causes Control 1997; 8:473–490.
23. Spivack SD, Fasco MJ, Walker VE, et al: The molecular epidemiology of lung cancer. Crit Rev Toxicol 1997; 27:319–365.
24. Salgia R, Skarin AT: Molecular abnormalities in lung cancer. J Clin Oncol 1998; 16:1207–1217.
25. Testa JR, Liu Z, Feder M, et al: Advances in the analysis of chromosome alterations in human lung carcinomas. Cancer Genet Cytogenet 1997; 95:20–32.
26. Mountain CF: New prognostic factors in lung cancer: biologic prophets of cancer cell aggression. Chest 1995; 108:246–254.
27. Wiest JS, Franklin WA, Drabkin H, et al: Genetic markers for early detection of lung cancer and outcome measures for response to chemoprevention. J Cell Biochem 1997; 28–29 (suppl):64–73.
28. Carney DN, De Leij L: Lung cancer biology. Semin Oncol 1988; 15:199–214.
29. Frost JK, Ball WC Jr, Levin ML, et al: Early lung cancer detection: results of the initial (prevalence) radiologic and cytologic screening in the Johns Hopkins study. Am Rev Respir Dis 1984; 130:549–554.
30. Flehinger BJ, Melamed MR, Zaman MB, et al: Early lung cancer detection: results of the initial (prevalence) radiologic and cytologic screening in the Memorial Sloan-Kettering study. Am Rev Respir Dis 1984; 130:555–560.
31. Fontana RS, Sanderson DR, Woolner LB, et al: Screening for lung cancer. A critique of the Mayo Lung Project. Cancer 1991; 67 (suppl):1155–1164.
32. Strauss GM, Gleason RE, Sugarbaker DJ: Chest x-ray screening improves outcome in lung cancer. A reappraisal of randomized trials on lung cancer screening. Chest 1995; 107 (suppl):270S–279S.
33. Lam S, Becker HD: Future diagnostic procedures. Chest Surg Clin N Am 1996; 6:363–380.
34. Bragg DG: Imaging in primary lung cancer: the roles of detection, staging and follow-up. Semin Ultrasound CT MR 1989; 10:453–466.
35. McLoud TC, Bourgouin PM, Greenberg RW, et al: Bronchogenic carcinoma: analysis of staging in the mediastinum with CT by correlative lymph node mapping and sampling. Radiology 1992; 182:319–323.
36. Bragg DG: The diagnosis and staging of primary lung cancer. Radiol Clin N Am 1994; 32:1–14.
37. Bonomo L, Ciccotosto C, Guidotti A, et al: Lung cancer staging: the role of computed tomography and magnetic resonance imaging. Eur J Radiol 1996; 23:35–45.
38. Hopper KD: CT bronchoscopy. Semin Ultrasound CT MR 1999; 20:10–15.
39. Coleman RE: PET in lung cancer. J Nucl Med 1999; 40:814–820.
40. Schiepers C: Role of positron emission tomography in the staging of lung cancer. Lung Cancer 1997; 17 (suppl):S29–35.
41. Schiepers C, Hoh CK: Positron emission tomography as a diagnostic tool in oncology. Eur Radiol 1998; 8:1481–1494.
42. Concannon JP, Dalbow MH, Liebler GA, et al: The carcinoembryonic antigen assay in bronchogenic carcinoma. Cancer 1974; 34:184–192.
43. Bombardieri E, Seregni E, Bogni A, et al: Comparison of Cyfra 21-1, TPA and TPS in lung cancer, urinary bladder and benign diseases. Int J Biol Markers 1994; 9:89–95.
44. Graziano SL: Non-small cell lung cancer: clinical value of new biological predictors. Lung Cancer 1997; 17 (suppl):S37–S58.
45. Bates M (ed): Bronchial Carcinoma. An Integrated Approach to Diagnosis and Management. Berlin, Springer-Verlag, 1984.
46. Hau T, Forster F, Ganawidjaja L, et al: Thoracoscopic pulmonary surgery: indications and results. Eur J Surg 1996; 162:23–28.
47. Percy C: Introduction. Cancer 1995; 75:140–146.
48. Travis WD, Travis LB, DeVesa SS: Lung cancer. Cancer 1995; 75 (1 suppl):191–198.
49. Daly RC, Trastek VF, Pairolero PC, et al: Bronchoalveolar carcinoma: factors affecting survival. Ann Thorac Surg 1991; 51:368–376.
50. Aisner SC, Finkelstein DM, Ettinger DS, et al: The clinical significance of varient-morphology small-cell carcinoma of the lung. J Clin Oncol 1990; 8:402–408.
51. Mountain CF: Revisions in the international system for staging lung cancer. Chest 1997; 111:1710–1717.
52. Andreassian B: New techniques in thoracic surgery. I. Presse Med 1995; 24:1078–1083.
53. Johnston MR: The limits of surgical resection alone for non–small cell lung cancer. Lung Cancer 1997; 17 (suppl):S99–102.
54. Livingston RB: Combined modality therapy of lung cancer. Clin Cancer Res 1997; 3:2638–2647.
55. Martini N, McCormack PM: Evolution of the surgical management of pulmonary metastases. Chest Surg Clin N Am 1998; 8:13–27.
56. Lassen U, Hansen HH: Surgery in limited stage small cell lung cancer. Cancer Treat Rev 1999; 25:67–72.
57. Ginsberg RJ, Rubinstein LV: Randomized trial of lobectomy versus limited resection for T1 N0 non–small cell lung cancer. Lung Cancer Study Group. Ann Thorac Surg 1995; 60:615–622.
58. Amery WK: Adjuvant levamisole in the treatment of patients with resectable lung cancer. Ann Clin Res 1980; 12 (suppl):1–83.
59. McKneally MF, Maver C, Lininger L, et al: Four-year follow-up on the Albany experience with intrapleural BCG in lung cancer. J Thorac Cardiovasc Surg 1981; 81:485–492.
60. Shepherd FA: Alternatives to chemotherapy and radiotherapy as adjuvant treatment for lung cancer. Lung Cancer 1997; 17 (suppl):S121–S136.
61. Al-Moundhri M, O'Brien M, Souberbielle BE: Immunotherapy in lung cancer. Br J Cancer 1998; 78:282–288.
62. Dosoretz DE, Katin MJ, Blitzer PH, et al: Radiation therapy in the management of medically inoperable carcinoma of the lung: results and implications for future treatment strategies Int J Radiat Oncol Biol Phys 1992; 24:3–9.
63. Hazuka MB, Turrisi AT, Lutz ST, et al: Results of high-dose thoracic irradiation incorporating beam's eye view display in non–small cell lung cancer: a retrospective multivariate analysis. Int J Radiat Oncol Biol Phys 1993; 27:273–284.
64. Saunders MI, Dische S, Barrett A, et al: Randomised multicentre trials of CHART vs conventional radiotherapy in head and neck and non–small-cell lung cancer: an interim report Br J Cancer 1996; 73:1455–1462.
65. Morita K, Fuwa N, Suzuki Y, et al: Radical radiotherapy for medically inoperable non–small cell lung cancer in clinical stage I: a retrospective analysis of 149 patients. Radiother Oncol 1997; 42:31–36.
66. Perez CA, Bauer M, Edelstein S, et al: Impact of tumor control on survival in carcinoma of the lung treated with irradiation. Int J Radiat Oncol Biol Phys 1986; 12:539–547.
67. Perez CA, Stanley K, Grundy G, et al: Impact of irradiation technique and tumor extent in tumor control and survival of patients with unresectable non–oat cell carcinoma of the lung. Report by the Radiation Therapy Oncology Group. Cancer 1982; 50:1091–1099.
68. Perez CA, Pajak TF, Rubin P, et al: Long-term observations of the patterns of failure in patients with unresectable non–oat cell carcinoma of the lung treated with definitive radiotherapy. Report by the Radiation Therapy Oncology Group. Cancer 1987; 59:1874–1881.
69. Cox JD, Pajak TF, Asbell S, et al: Interruptions of high-dose radiation therapy decrease long-term survival of favorable patients with unresectable non-small cell carcinoma of the lung: analysis of 1244

cases from 3 Radiation Therapy Oncology Group (RTOG) trials. Int J Radiat Oncol Biol Phys 1993; 27:493–498.

70. Arriagada R, Le Chevalier T, Quoix E, et al: ASTRO plenary: effect of chemotherapy on locally advanced non–small lung carcinoma: a randomized study of 353 patients. GETCB, FNCLCC and the CEBI trialists. Int J Radiat Oncol Biol Phys 1991; 20:1183–1190.
71. Sause WT, Scott C, Taylor S, et al: Radiation Therapy Oncology Group (RTOG) 88-08 and Eastern Cooperative Oncology Group (ECOG) 4588: preliminary results of a phase III trial in regionally advanced unresectable non–small-cell lung cancer. J Natl Cancer Inst 1994; 87:198–205.
72. Calvo FA, Ortiz de Urbina D, Abuchaibe O, et al: Intraoperative radiotherapy during lung cancer surgery: technical description and early clinical results. Int J Radiat Oncol Biol Phys 1990; 19:103–111.
73. Smolle-Juettner FM, Geyer E, Kapp KS, et al: Evaluating intraoperative radiation therapy (IORT) and external beam radiation therapy (EBRT) in non–small cell lung cancer. Eur J Cardiothorac Surg 1994; 8:511–516.
74. Aristu J, Rebollo J, Martinez-Monge R, et al: Cisplatin, mitomycin, and vindesine followed by intraoperative and postoperative radiotherapy for stage III non–small cell lung cancer: final results of a phase II study. Am J Clin Oncol 1997; 20:276–281.
75. Cotter GW, Lariscy C, Ellingwood KL, et al: Inoperable endobronchial obstructing lung cancer treated with combined endobronchial and external beam irradiation: a dosimetric analysis. Int J Radiat Oncol Biol Phys 1993; 27:531–536.
76. Speiser B, Spratling L: Remote afterloading brachytherapy for the local control of endobronchial carcinoma. Int J Radiat Oncol Biol Phys 1993; 25:579–587.
77. Huber RM, Fischer R, Hautmann H, et al: Does additional brachytherapy improve the effect of external irradiation? A prospective randomized study in central lung tumors. Int J Radiat Oncol Biol Phys 1997; 38:533–540.
78. Hodapp N, Boesecke R, Schlegel W, et al: Three-dimensional treatment planning for conformation therapy of a bronchial carcinoma. Radiother Oncol 1991; 20:245–249.
79. Armstrong J, Raben A, Zelefsky M, et al: Promising survival with three-dimensional conformal radiation therapy for non-small cell lung cancer. Radiother Oncol 1997; 44:17–22.
80. Payne DG: Is preoperative or postoperative radiation therapy indicated in non–small cell cancer of the lung? Lung Cancer 1994; 10 (suppl):S205–S212.
81. Van Houtte P: Combined modality: non–small cell lung cancer: surgery and postoperative radiotherapy. In: Pass HI, Mitchell JB, Johnson DH, et al (eds): Lung Cancer: Principles and Practice, pp 851–862. Philadelphia, Lippincott-Raven, 1996.
82. Attar S, Krasna MJ, Sonett JR, et al: Superior sulcus (Pancoast) tumor: experience with 105 patients. Ann Thorac Surg 1998; 66:193–198.
83. Johnson DE, Goldberg M: Management of carcinoma of the superior pulmonary sulcus. Oncology 1997; 11:781–785.
84. Van Houtte P, Rocmans P, Smets P, et al: Postoperative radiation therapy in lung cancer: a controlled trial after resection of curative design. Int J Radiat Oncol Biol Phys 1980; 6:983–986.
85. Lafitte JJ, Ribet ME, Prevost BM, et al: Postresection irradiation for T2 NO MO non–small cell carcinoma: a prospective, randomized study. Ann Thorac Surg 1996; 62:830–834.
86. Stephens RJ, Girling DJ, Bleehen NM, et al: The role of postoperative radiotherapy in non–small-cell-lung cancer: a multicentre randomised trial in patients with pathologically staged T1-2, N1-2 M0 disease. Medical Research Council Lung Cancer Working Party. Br J Cancer 1996; 74:632–639.
87. Choi NC, Kanarek DJ, Grillo HC: Effect of postoperative radiotherapy on changes in pulmonary function in patients with stage II and IIIA lung carcinoma. Int J Radiat Oncol Biol Phys 1990; 18:95–101.
88. Phlips P, Rocmans P, Vanderhoeft P, et al: Postoperative radiotherapy after pneumonectomy: impact of modern treatment facilities. Int J Radiat Oncol Biol Phys 1993; 27:525–529.
89. Non–small Cell Lung Cancer Collaborative Group: Chemotherapy in non–small cell lung cancer: a meta-analysis using updated data on individual patients from 52 randomised clinical trials. BMJ 1995; 311:899–909.
90. Sause WT, Scott C, Taylor S, et al: RTOG 88-08 ECOG 4588, Preliminary analysis of a phase III trial in regionally advanced unresectable non–small-cell lung cancer with minimum three-year follow-up [Abstract]. Int J Radiat Oncol Biol Phys 1995; 32 (suppl):195.
91. Schaake-Koning C, van den Bogaert W, Dalesio O, et al: Effects of concomitant cisplatin and radiotherapy on inoperable non–small cell lung cancer. N Engl J Med 1992; 326:524–530.
92. Mirimanoff RO: Concurrent chemotherapy (CT) and radiotherapy (RT) in locally advanced non–small cell lung cancer (NSCLC): a review. Lung Cancer 1994; 11 (suppl):S79–S99.
93. Furuse K, Fukuoka M, Kawahara M, et al: Phase III study of concurrent versus sequential thoracic radiotherapy in combination with mitomycin, vindesine, and cisplatin in unresectable stage III non–small cell lung cancer. J Clin Oncol 1999; 17:2692–2699.
94. Ruckdeschel JC: Combined modality therapy for non–small cell lung cancer. Semin Oncol 1997; 24:429–439.
95. Rossell R, Gomez-Codina J, Camps C, et al: A randomized trial comparing preoperative chemotherapy plus surgery with surgery alone in patients with non–small cell lung cancer. N Engl J Med 1994; 330:153–158.
96. Roth JA, Fossella F, Komaki R, et al: A randomized trial comparing perioperative chemotherapy and surgery with surgery alone in resectable stage IIIA non–small cell lung cancer. J Natl Cancer Inst 1994; 86:673–680.
97. Niiranen A, Niitamo-Korhonen S, Kouri M, et al: Adjuvant chemotherapy after radical surgery for non–small-cell lung cancer: a randomized study. J Clin Oncol 1992; 10:1927–1932.
98. Comis RL: Chemotherapy of small cell lung cancer. In: Devita VT (ed): Updates in Cancer: Principles and Practice of Oncology, p 13. Philadelphia, Lippincott Co., 1987.
99. Murray N: Treatment of small cell lung cancer: the state of the art. Lung Cancer 1997; 17 (suppl):S75–S89.
100. Salazar OM: Combined modality treatment of small cell lung cancer. Chest 1989; 96 (suppl):74S–78S.
101. Warde P, Payne D: Does thoracic irradiation improve survival and local control in limited-stage small-cell carcinoma of the lung? A meta-analysis. J Clin Oncol 1992; 10:890–895.
102. Pignon JP, Arriagada R, Ihde DC, et al: A meta-analysis of thoracic radiotherapy for small-cell lung cancer. N Engl J Med 1992; 327:1618–1624.
103. Choi NC, Carey RW: Importance of radiation dose in achieving improved loco-regional tumor control in limited stage small-cell lung carcinoma: an update. Int J Radiat Oncol Biol Phys 1989; 17:307–311.
104. Murray N, Coy P, Pater JL, et al: Importance of timing for thoracic irradiation in the combined modality treatment of limited-stage small-cell lung cancer. The National Cancer Institute of Canada Clinical Trials Group. J Clin Oncol 1993; 11:336–344.
105. Wagner H Jr: Thoracic irradiation of limited small cell lung cancer: have we defined optimal dose, time, and fractionation? Lung Cancer 1997; 17 (suppl):S137–S148.
106. Wurschmidt F, Bunemann H, Heilmann HP: Small cell lung cancer with and without superior vena cava syndrome: a multivariate analysis of prognostic factors in 408 cases. Int J Radiat Oncol Biol Phys 1995; 33:77–82.
107. Turrisi AT: Brain irradiation and systemic chemotherapy for small-cell lung cancer: dangerous liaisons? J Clin Oncol 1990; 8:196–199.
108. Kristjansen PEG, Hansen HH: Prophylactic cranial irradiation in small cell lung cancer: an update. Lung Cancer 1995; 12 (suppl):S23–S40.
109. Arriagada R, Le Chevalier T, Borie F, et al: Prophylactic cranial irradiation for patients with small-cell lung cancer in complete remission. J Natl Cancer Inst 1995; 87:183–190.
110. Gregor A, Cull A, Stephens RJ, et al: Prophylactic cranial irradiation is indicated following complete response to induction therapy in small cell lung cancer: results of a multicentric randomised trial. United Kingdom Coordinating Committee for Cancer Research (UKCCR) and the European Organization for Research and Treatment of Cancer (EORTC). Eur J Cancer 1997; 33:1752–1758.
111. Lishner M, Feld R, Payne DG, et al: Late neurological complications after prophylactic cranial irradiation in patients with small-cell lung cancer: the Toronto experience. J Clin Oncol 1990; 8:215–221.
112. Komaki R, Meyers CA, Shin DM, et al: Evaluation of cognitive function in patients with limited small cell lung cancer prior to and shortly following prophylactic cranial irradiation. Int J Radiant Oncol Biol Phys 1995; 33:179–182.

113. Hoegler D: Radiotherapy for palliation of symptoms in incurable cancer. Curr Prob Cancer 1997; 21:129–183.
114. Salazar OM, Slawson RG, Poussin-Rosillo H, et al: A prospective randomized trial comparing once-a-week vs. daily radiation therapy for locally-advanced, non-metastatic, measurable lung cancer: a preliminary report. Int J Radiat Oncol Biol Phys 1986; 12:779–787.
115. Roach M 3d, Leidholdt EM, Tatera BS, et al: Endobronchial radiation therapy (EBRT) in the management of lung cancer. Int J Radiat Oncol Biol Phys 1990; 18:1449–1454.
116. Shepherd FA: Treatment of advanced non–small cell lung cancer. Semin Oncol 1994; 21 (suppl):7–18.
117. Ramanathan RK, Belani CP: Chemotherapy for advanced non–small cell lung cancer: past, present, and future. Semin Oncol 1997; 24:440–454.
118. Johnson DH, Eisert DR: Treatment of small cell lung cancer. In: Roth JA, Ruckdeschel JC, Weisenberger TH (eds): Thoracic Oncology, 2nd ed, pp 201–224. Philadelphia, W.B. Saunders, 1995.
119. DeVore RF, Johnson DH: Lung cancer: chemotherapy. In: Brain MC, Carbone PP (eds): Current Therapy in Hematology-Oncology, 4th ed, pp 245–249. Philadelphia, B.C. Dekker, 1992.
120. Deslauriers J: Surgery for small cell lung cancer. Lung Cancer 1997; 17 (suppl):S91–S98.
121. Ettinger DS: Evaluation of new drugs in untreated patients with small-cell lung cancer: its time has come. J Clin Oncol 1990; 8:374–377.
122. Ettinger DS: New drugs for treating small cell lung cancer. Lung Cancer 1995; 12 (suppl):S53–S61.
123. Klasa RJ, Murray N, Coldman AJ: Dose-intensity meta-analysis of chemotherapy regimens in small-cell carcinoma of the lung. J Clin Oncol 1991; 9:499–508.
124. Ihde DC, Mulshine JL, Kramer BS, et al: Prospective randomized comparison of high-dose and standard-dose etoposide and cisplatin chemotherapy in patients with extensive-stage small-cell lung cancer. J Clin Oncol 1994; 12:2022–2034.
125. Loehrer PJ Sr, Ansari R, Gonin R, et al: Cisplatin plus etoposide with and without ifosfamide in extensive small-cell lung cancer: a Hoosier Oncology Group study. J Clin Oncol 1995; 13:2594–2599.
126. Bunn PA Jr, Kelly K: A phase I study of cisplatin, etoposide, and paclitaxel in small cell lung cancer. Semin Oncol 1997; 24 (suppl):S144–S148.
127. SEER Cancer Statistics Review, 1973–1995. NIH Publication No. 98-2789. Bethesda, National Cancer Institute, 1998.
128. Myers MH, Gloeckler Ries LA: Cancer patient survival rates: SEER program results for 10 years of follow-up. CA Cancer J Clin 1989; 39:21–32.
129. The Lung Cancer Study Group: Effects of postoperative mediastinal radiation on completely resected stage II and III epidermoid cancer of the lung. N Engl J Med 1986; 315:1377–1381.
130. Green N, Kurohara SS, George FW 3rd, et al: Postresection irradiation for primary lung cancer. Radiology 1975; 116:405–407.
131. Kirsh MM, Rotman H, Argenta L, et al: Carcinoma of the lung: results of treatment over ten years. Ann Thorac Surg 1976; 21:371–377.
132. Sawyer TE, Bonner JA, Gould PM, et al: The impact of surgical adjuvant thoracic radiation therapy for patients with nonsmall cell lung carcinoma with ipsilateral mediastinal lymph node involvement. Cancer 1997; 80:1399–1408.
133. Zhang HX, Yin WB, Zhang LJ, et al: Curative radiotherapy of early operable non small cell lung cancer. Radiother Oncol 1989; 14:89–94.
134. Sandler HM, Curran WJ Jr, Turrisi AT 3rd: The influence of tumor size and pre-treatment staging on outcome following radiation therapy alone for non-small cell lung cancer. Int J Radiat Oncol Biol Phys 1990; 19:9–13.
135. Krol ADG, Aussems P, Noordijk EM, et al: Local irradiation alone for peripheral stage I lung cancer: could we omit the elective regional nodal irradiation? Int J Radiat Oncol Biol Phys 1996; 34:297–302.
136. Bunn PA, Carney DN: Overview of chemotherapy for small cell lung cancer. Semin Oncol 1997; 24 (suppl):S69–S74.
137. Johnson BE: Concurrent approaches to combined chemotherapy and chest radiography for the treatment of patients with limited stage small cell lung cancer. Lung Cancer 1994; 10 (suppl):S281–S287.
138. Sandler AB: Current management of small cell lung cancer. Semin Oncol 1997; 24:463–476.
139. Thiele KP: Prognostic factors and therapeutic strategies in small cell bronchial carcinoma. Schweiz Rundsch Med Prax 1997; 86:1660–1667.
140. Yokayama A: Multimodality therapy for small-cell lung cancer. Gan to Kagaku Ryoho 1997; 24 (suppl):405–411.
141. Ettinger DS: Concurrent paclitaxel-containing regimens and thoracic radiation therapy for limited-disease small cell lung cancer. Semin Radiat Oncol 1999; 9 (suppl):148–150.
142. Gregor A, Drings P, Burghouts J, et al: Randomized trial of alternating versus sequential radiotherapy/chemotherapy in limited-disease patients with small-cell lung cancer: a European Organization for Research and Treatment of Cancer Lung Cancer Cooperative Group Study. J Clin Oncol 1997; 15:2840–2849.
143. Johnson BE, Grayson J, Makuch RW, et al: Ten-year survival of patients with small-cell lung cancer treated with combination chemotherapy with or without irradiation. J Clin Oncol 1990; 8:396–402.
144. Tonnesen P, Fryd V, Hansen M, et al: Effect of nicotine chewing gum in combination with group counseling on the cessation of smoking. N Engl J Med 1988; 318:15–18.
145. Anda RF, Remington PL, Sienko DG, et al: Are physicians advising smokers to quit? The patient's perspective. JAMA 1987; 257:1916–1919.
146. Jetten AM, Nervi C, Vollberg TM: Control of squamous differentiation in tracheobronchial and epidermal epithelial cells: role of retinoids. J Natl Cancer Inst Monogr 1992; 13:93–100.
147. Omenn GS, Goodman G, Thornquist M, et al: Chemoprevention of lung cancer: the beta-Carotene and Retinol Efficacy Trial (CARET) in high-risk smokers and asbestos-exposed workers. IARC Sci Publ 1996; 136:67–85.
148. Alpha-Tocopherol Beta Carotene Cancer Prevention Study Group: The effect of vitamin E and beta carotene on the incidence of lung cancer and other cancers in male smokers. N Engl J Med 1994; 330:1029–1034.
149. Van Zandwijk N: N-Acetylcysteine for lung cancer prevention. Chest 1995; 107:1437–1441.
150. Greenberger JS, Bahri S, Jett J, et al: Considerations in optimizing radiation therapy for non–small cell lung cancer. Chest 1998; 113 (suppl):46S–52S.
151. Rogers DF, Laurent GJ: New ideas on the pathophysiology and treatment of lung disease. Thorax 1998; 53:200–203.

31 *Metastases and Disseminated Disease*

CHARLES W. SCARANTINO, MD, PHD, Radiation Oncology
ROBERT D. ORNITZ, MD, Radiation Oncology
SABRA A. WOODARD, MD, Radiology

Omnis cellula e cellula.

RUDOLPH VIRCHOW[5]

Perspective

The American Cancer Society estimates that there will be 1,220,100 new cases of invasive cancer diagnosed in 2000.[6] Approximately 30% of these patients will have detectable distant metastases at the time of first diagnosis (excluding skin cancer other than melanoma). Of the remaining patients, approximately 35% will be cured by local and regional therapy, whereas the remainder will develop metastatic disease. Therefore, 60% to 70% of patients with cancer will develop metastatic disease at some point before death.

Metastasis is the spread of malignant cells from the primary tumor to distant sites. In many respects, it represents the terminal event of a process that begins with the malignant transformation and proliferation of normal cells and signals the final phase in the natural history of malignant tumors. In general, current therapeutic maneuvers have been ineffective in eliminating overt disease.[7, 8] Therefore, an understanding of the process and mechanisms that result in a metastatic deposit should lead to an improved clinical outcome in the patient with metastatic disease.

The patient with metastatic disease poses one of the most challenging problems in oncology; effective treatment of the patient requires an understanding of the natural history of the primary tumor and the metastases. The therapeutic approach will vary according to the tumor burden, the presence or absence of clinical symptoms and diagnostic markers, performance status, the temporal development of progressive disease, and the psychosocial needs of the patient. Most patients require palliative and supportive care, because the relief of the symptoms caused by the presence of metastases becomes paramount to their well-being. Knowledge and understanding of available methods and techniques for the palliation of symptoms, supportive care, and interventions to improve the quality of life (QOL) are important, and they are required to effectively address the morbidity associated with the presence and treatment of malignant disease.

Several general references are included for a more in-depth perspective.[1–4]

Epidemiology and Etiology

Epidemiology

The four most favored sites of metastatic disease are bone, lung, brain, and liver. The most common malignancies responsible for metastases in the four major organs are summarized in Table 31–1.

The temporal identification of metastases differs significantly between time of diagnosis and autopsy (Table 31–2).[3] This may be related to either inadequate screening methods or an actual increase in metastatic deposits occurring over time.

- Bone metastases arise commonly from carcinoma of the breast, prostate, thyroid, and kidney. Given the

TABLE 31–1. **Primary Clinically Important Metastatic Patterns**

Primary Site	Bone	Lung	Liver	Brain
Head and Neck	+	+		
Neuroblastoma (age dependent)	+		+	
Thyroid	+	+		
Lung	+	+	+	+
Breast	+	+		+
Ovary		+	+	
Cervix	+	+		
Testis		+		+
Prostate	+	+		
Kidney	+	+		
Wilms'		+	+	+ (<15 yrs)
Bladder	+	+	+	
Stomach			+	
Pancreas			+	
Colorectal	+	+	+	+
Melanoma		+	+	+
Sarcoma		+		+ (<21 yrs)
Ewing's		+		+ (<15 yrs)

TABLE 31–2. **Incidence of Metastases at Diagnosis and Autopsy***

	Metastatic Site							
	% Bone		*% Lung*		*% Liver*		*% Brain*	
Primary Site	*Diagnosis*	*Autopsy*	*Diagnosis*	*Autopsy*	*Diagnosis*	*Autopsy*	*Diagnosis*	*Autopsy*
Lung	16 (38†)	20–36		21–60	17	25–48 (74†)	18–28 (8–14†)	18–37 (42†)
Breast	20–40	44–73		59–69		56–65	15	9–20
Prostate	20–40	50–70	5.0	15–53	1	5–13	<1	2
Kidney	6–10	24–50	5–30	50–75	13	27–40	4	7–8
Bladder	5	12–25	5–10	25–30	>5	30–50	<1	<1
Testis (germinal)	<1	20	2–12	70–80	<1	50–80	<1	<10
Colon-Rectum	<1	22	<5	25–40	20–24	60–71	4	8
Cervix	<1	8–20	<5	20–30	<1	20–35	<1	2–3
Ovary	<1	9	<5	5–10	<5	10–15	<1	<1
Uterus	<1	5–12	<1	30–40	<1	10–30	<1	<5

*Numbers represent estimates from several sources.
†Values for small cell carcinoma.

high prevalence of these cancers, more than 80% of cancer patients may show this dissemination pattern.[9]

- Lung metastases are the second most common site of metastases. They are seen most commonly in carcinoma of the breast and kidney (50% incidence), followed by melanomas, sarcomas, and probably the gastrointestinal (GI) tract.
- Liver metastases are most common in patients with carcinoma of the GI tract, particularly colorectal cancer, and less commonly in pancreas, lung, and breast.[10]
- Brain metastases may frequently present as solitary lesions, and they most commonly arise from the lung and breast.[11]

Etiology

During the last 10 years, our understanding of the metastatic process has increased, without a concomitant improvement in treatment outcome. Although the metastatic process is usually defined by its end points, that is, the identification of a deposit distant from its origin, the definition of the process itself has been more inferred than observed. However, it is generally agreed that the process is not the result of one gene product. Rather, it is due to a complex, coordinated cellular process that includes positive factors (activated oncogenes, growth factors, proteases, adhesion receptors, motility cytokines) and negative factors (tumor suppressor genes, growth inhibitors, metastasis suppressor genes, protease inhibitors).

Metastases result from an imbalance in the regulation of growth control, motility, and heterogeneity. The heterogeneity extends to karyotype, receptors, and growth properties, cell surface enzymes, morphology, and the ability to invade and produce metastases. The result of this heterogeneity, as suggested in the 1980s by Fidler and Hart,[12] is a subpopulation of cells within the neoplasm that was selected based on its propensity to invade and metastasize. This subpopulation exists and dominates the tumor early on in its growth, possibly in response to local cytokines[13]; this is important, because the measurement of a molecular marker in the primary tumor early in its growth could provide information on the metastatic potential of the tumor. In addition, the potential for metastases is thought to be related temporally to tumor vascularization, intrinsic aggressiveness, and histologic type but not to size.[14, 15]

The process of metastasis is not a random event but rather a series of linked and sequential steps that involve continued host-tumor interaction, resulting in the survival of a minor subpopulation of tumor cells. These interactions are summarized in the next section and have been reviewed by Liotta and Stetler-Stevenson.[16] In their review, they stated that "the process of metastasis is not random. Instead, it is a cascade of linked sequential steps that must be traversed by tumor cells if a metastasis is to develop. . . . Metastasis is the result of a highly selective competition favoring the survival of a minor subpopulation of metastatic cells that preexist within the primary neoplasm." Parenthetically, metastasis can be prevented by interruption at any one or more of these steps.

Suggested Steps in the Development of Metastases

1. *Premetastasis:* Genetic alterations in DNA result in oncogene activation and amplification, with production of autocrine growth factors and autonomy from the host microenvironment. The resultant cell population may manifest or exhibit many enzymatic, metabolic, and molecular perturbations,[17, 18] including critical membrane-associated changes that affect cellular adhesion and cell-cell contact.[19–21] The mechanism for conversion from a malignant to a metastatic phenotype is not known at present, but it probably involves a number of processes, including increased levels of proteinases, a decrease in proteinase inhibitors,[18, 22] and loss of tumor suppressor gene function.[23–25] More recently, important evidence has been presented[26] that supports the concept that cancer cells exhibit a mutator phenotype (i.e., mutate at a high rate), because the large number of mutations in tumor cells cannot be accounted for by the low mutation rates of normal somatic cells.[27]
2. *Metastasis:* The constant tumor-host interactions within the tumor microenvironment result in a break-

down of constraints inherent in normal tissue architecture and in the formation of malignant cells capable of surviving in a normal milieu.

a. *Angiogenesis:* This process involves the formation of a blood supply by a tumor through release of angiogenic factors.[28, 29] Both *in vitro* modeling and *in vivo* observation suggest an intimate relationship between angiogenesis and the production of a variety of growth factors and proteolytic enzymes, including metalloproteinases, tyrosine kinases, and some cytokines, for example, interleukin (IL)-8.[30–32]
b. *Invasion:* The tumor cells invade the host stroma, accompanied by lysis of host basement membrane and connective tissue through the release of proteolytic enzymes, such as cathepsin B, the plasminogen-activating system, and collagenases.[33, 34]
c. *Intravasation:* Tumor cells gain access to newly formed tumor vessels, as well as pre-established host vessels and lymphatics[4]; the lymphatics are significant, because the tumor lacks a well-defined lymphatic network per se. The cells entering the lymphatics are carried to regional nodes, arrest, and within 10 to 60 minutes, enter the afferent lymphatics. Experimental evidence indicates that 24 hours after gaining access to the circulation, less than 1% of all cells are viable and less than 0.1% of the cells will survive to form metastases.[35]

   A review by Chambers and Matrisian[8] examines the role of matrix metalloproteinases (MMPs), enzymes implicated in metastases, and reviews the results of a new technique—*in vivo* videomicroscopy—which permits direct visualization of the microcirculation.[36] The results of *in vivo* videomicroscopy suggest that the majority of tumor cells that undergo intravasation survive, arrest, and undergo extravasation; the metastatic inefficiency arises from a failure of cells to grow within the target organ.[37] There is no difference between the ability of highly or poorly differentiated cells to undergo extravasation[38]; however, the ability of cells to grow within the target organ reflects their growth potential.
d. *Arrest:* Tumor cells react with platelets while in the circulatory system and are influenced by both platelets and the coagulation system. The fate of tumor cells varies with the location and mechanism by which the cells are lodged. In the venules, the tumor emboli can induce a reaction in the endothelial cells,[39, 40] including dissolution of the basement membrane, and can frequently form pseudopodial projections in order to move into the tissue.[41] In the arterial tree, tumor cells proliferate, enlarge, and become covered by endothelial cells; eventually mechanic damage occurs and exposes the basement membrane. Tumor cells then invade the basement membrane to gain an extravascular position.
e. *Extravasation:* Escape or discharge of metastasized tumor cells from the systemic circulation occurs by mechanisms similar to those responsible for invasion (see Invasion, earlier). Tumor cells may recognize tissue-specific motility factors, respond to organ-specific factors, or produce their own growth factors (autocrine stimulation). The cells complete extravasation through destruction of the basement membrane, establish residence, and induce angiogenesis and proliferation.

Metastasis is clearly a multistep process (Fig. 31–1). The steps involved appear to be similar for all tumors, in contrast to our understanding of the genetic basis of tumorigenesis, which appears to vary greatly between different tumors. This concept is important because it provides a more general approach to antimetastases therapy.

Several antimetastases therapies are being tested, including antiangiogenic agents, for example, TNP-470, which inhibits proliferation of vascular endothelial cells,[42, 43] as well as inhibitors of MMPs (BB94, BB2516)[44, 45]:

- The results of preclinical testing of the antiangiogenic agents angiostatin and endostatin have shown that microscopic tumor dormancy can be achieved, that there is no induction of drug resistance, and that there is no toxicity with prolonged administration. However, although results suggest that these particular agents may not be used,[46, 47] similar angiogenesis inhibitors are proving successful as adjuncts to chemotherapy and radiotherapy, as well as maintenance therapy to prevent recurrence of metastases.[48]
- The MMPs are a family of zinc-binding enzymes involved in tissue remodeling and morphogenesis.[49, 50] They are capable of degrading all components of extracellular matrix, including collagen, elastin, and fibronectin, and play a role in wound healing.[8, 31] The activity of these enzymes has been found to be increased in a number of different solid tumors,[51] and good correlation has been noted between increased MMP activity and the aggressiveness of a variety of tumors.[52] Marimastat, the MMP inhibitor, has been tested clinically[53, 54]; marimastat is available orally and has been noted to significantly reduce the rise in cancer-specific antigen levels from several different tumor types.[55] It has now reached phase III clinical trial as an adjuvant therapy in pancreatic cancer.

Traditional cytotoxic therapies have and should continue to focus on the eradication of the malignant cell. However, as more is known about the process of metastasis and how normal cellular mechanisms are integrated to promote tumor invasion and vascularization, it will be important to incorporate these therapies into the multimodal approach to cancer.

Detection and Diagnosis

Clinical Detection

There is simply no substitute for the classic medical history and physical examination of a patient to provide initial narrative data and findings to focus a staging (metastatic) work-up. Often, one needs only the time to listen carefully to essentially allow a patient to self-diagnose. As John Milton observed that "he also serves who stands and

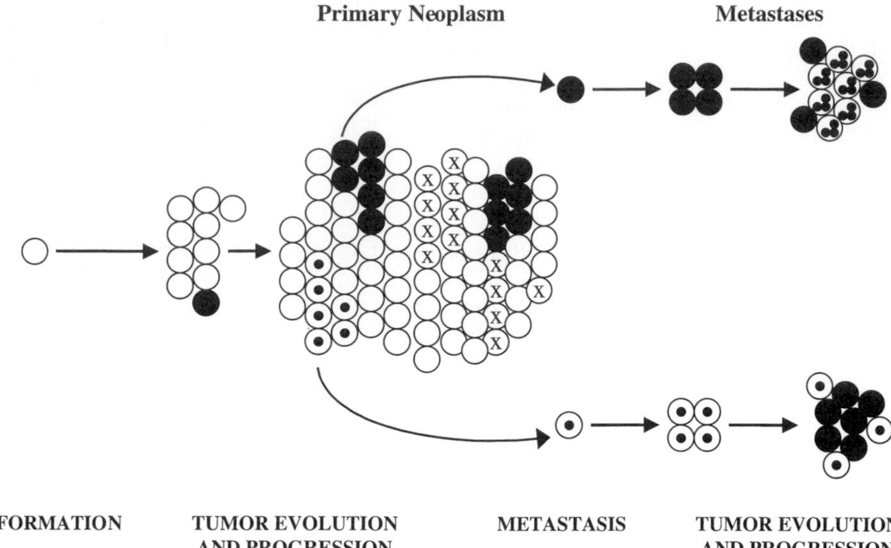

Figure 31–1. Biologic heterogeneity in tumors that are unicellular in origin is due to genetic and epigenetic instability (see Chapter 5, Basic Principles of Radiobiology). By the time of clinical diagnosis, most neoplasms consist of multiple subpopulations of cells with different properties. Metastases may have a clonal origin or can originate from different progenitor cells. Even in clonal metastases, biologic diversification gives rise to heterogeneous lesions. (From Fidler IJ: Molecular biology of cancer: invasion and metastasis. In: De Vita VT Jr, Hellman S, Rosenberg SA [eds]: Cancer. Principles & Practice of Oncology, 5th ed, pp 135–152. Philadelphia, Lippincott-Raven, 1997, with permission.)

waits," so the astute oncologist need only incorporate historic information from the patient or family member to chart an initial diagnostic course. This information, integrated with physical findings such as the presence of palpable lymphadenopathy, organomegaly, cutaneous exanthema, and localizing neurologic signs, can often lead almost immediately to either an initial diagnosis of malignancy or suspected pattern of metastatic dissemination.

The importance of the classic history and physical examination becomes even more relevant if one is to consider not only the classic description of tumor pathophysiology (e.g., lung cancer most commonly disseminates to bone, liver, central nervous system [CNS], or adrenal glands). In addition, with the advent of successful systemic therapy, it should be noted that as this behavior has been modified, patients are surviving long enough to express highly unusual patterns of metastatic involvement. Such examples, personally observed, have been colon cancer metastases to bone marrow as the first site of dissemination and biopsy-proven breast cancer to involve the bilateral pharyngeal tonsils and head of the pancreas. Whereas it cannot be argued that common dissemination patterns occur most frequently, it is probably equally true that the unusual is becoming more common.

The search for metastases is a principal goal of staging malignancies. Whereas careful history and physical examination are imperative, the use of laboratory and imaging tests is necessary for confirmation of clinical suspicions and for finding occult metastases. The detection of occult malignancies has tremendous impact on therapy and patient longevity. Detection of metastases is a balance between the sensitivity and specificity of a given test, the medical necessity of detection, and the cost-effectiveness of each test.

Diagnostic Procedures

Diagnostic imaging is an important component and first step in deciding the cause of symptoms and extent of disease. The symptoms that result from metastatic disease are often debilitating in varying degrees, thereby making it necessary to choose the most appropriate imaging modality as the initial diagnostic evaluation. The first section of this discussion deals with the imaging of oncologic emergencies, including brain metastases, spinal cord compression, carcinomatous meningitis, superior vena cava obstruction, neoplastic pericardial effusion, and obstructive uropathy. Next, the optimal radiologic evaluation of metastases to various organs is reviewed, consisting of metastases to the liver, lung, and bone. Finally, imaging of the lymphomas is discussed.

Brain Metastases (Breast, Lung, and Melanoma). Computed tomography (CT) and magnetic resonance imaging (MRI) are both useful in the detection of primary and metastatic brain tumors. CT is less expensive and more accessible than MRI; however, MRI is the modality of choice and can detect tumors in the early size range (less than 1 cm). MRI often detects more tumors than CT and allows for multiplanar imaging (axial, coronal, sagittal), which facilitates detection of metastatic disease and allows more accurate localization for stereotactic biopsy, surgical resection, or radiation therapy. In addition, certain patterns of brain metastases can be missed on CT scan (meningeal infiltration, invasion of skull base). Both CT and MRI are equally ineffective in differentiating tumor recurrence from radiation necrosis,[56–58] although it may be achieved through the use of positron emission tomography (PET).[59]

Spinal Cord Compression (Breast, Lung, and Prostate). Spine radiographs may show obvious vertebral body destruction, but they tend to underestimate the extent of disease; the majority of patients with cord compression from lymphoma or myeloma will have plain films with a normal result. MRI is the imaging modality of choice because it allows observation of the entire cord, in both the sagittal and axial planes, and can determine the exact location and extent of disease, as well as demonstrating other asymptomatic areas of involvement. This ability allows for appropriate surgical or radiation therapy intervention, with or without corticosteroids.[60] For patients who are unable to undergo MRI, that is, those with pacemakers or metal clips, diagnosis can be made using contrast myelography.

Carcinomatous Meningitis (Lymphoma, Leukemia, Breast, Lung, and Melanoma). This unusual form of metastatic disease is being seen with increasing frequency and is believed to be due to increased length of patient survival from more effective chemotherapy regimens. Sheets of tumor cells may cover the spinal cord, nerve roots, and lining membranes of the brain. This condition can be demonstrated by contrast-enhanced CT or contrast-enhanced MRI, with MRI being the more sensitive and specific. However, the diagnosis must be confirmed by cytologic evaluation of cerebrospinal fluid obtained from a lumbar puncture.[61]

Superior Vena Cava Obstruction (Lung, Lymphoma). The chest radiograph may show widening of the superior mediastinum, but a CT scan provides definitive diagnosis, also demonstrating the extent of disease, which may involve additional nodes in the mediastinum, hilar regions, and supraclavicular region. This definitive diagnosis allows for optimal radiation therapy planning, which may be combined with chemotherapy.[62] A select group of patients may undergo surgery.

Pericardial Effusion and Neoplastic Cardiac Tamponade (Lung, Breast, Leukemia, Lymphoma, Melanoma, GI, and Sarcoma). Tumor cells may spread to the pericardium and incite an inflammatory response, causing a rapid accumulation of fluid that can cause compression of the heart and interfere with its contractile function. The chest radiograph may show an enlarged heart with a classic so-called water-bottle silhouette; however, echocardiography of the chest is needed to make the definitive diagnosis.[63]

Obstructive Uropathy (Prostate, Cervix, Bladder, Rectum, Ovary, Sarcoma, and Lymphoma). Either the urethra or bladder neck may become obstructed by tumor. Renal ultrasound is readily available and noninvasive. It can document the presence of hydronephrosis, but it may not identify the level or cause of the obstruction. An intravenous (IV) pyelogram defines the site of obstruction in approximately 80% of patients with acute urinary obstruction. A retrograde pyelogram (contrast injected into the dilated renal pelvis under ultrasound or fluoroscopic guidance) can demonstrate the site of obstruction and allow percutaneous drainage of the kidney or placement of a ureteral stent to bypass the blockage. A CT scan may be necessary to show the location and extent of the tumor to allow for immediate radiation therapy to those tumors most likely to be radiosensitive.[64]

Hepatic Metastases (Colon, Breast, Lung, Pancreas, Melanoma, and Sarcoma). Helical (spiral) CT is the modality of choice. This technology allows rapid scanning with a single breath hold, which accounts for increased lesion detection from lack of respiratory motion and optimal IV contrast enhancement. Focal abnormalities within the liver can subsequently be categorized as either benign or malignant. This classification often requires a fine-needle aspiration (FNA) of the mass under CT guidance. If localized disease is demonstrated, the patient may be a candidate for a segmental hepatic resection. The threshold size for the detection of tumors using optimal IV contrast enhancement and breath hold appears to be about 1 cm.[65, 66]

With respect to metastases from the pancreas, frequent use is made of endoscopic retrograde cholangiopancreatography.[67] However, because of its invasive nature, this technique will, in all probability, be replaced in the future by less traumatic and more cost-effective procedures, such as MR pancreatography and endoscopic ultrasound.[68, 69]

Lung Metastases (Choriocarcinoma, Renal Cell, Testicular, Melanoma, Bone, and Soft Tissue Sarcomas). Although the routine chest x-ray film has been used to detect lung metastases in patients who are at low risk, its sensitivity in at least one study has been shown to be about 52%, significantly less than CT scan (82%), and is not cost-effective.[70] Helical CT scan is the modality of choice. This technology allows for minimal motion artifact and optimizes IV contrast enhancement of normal vascular structures, which improves the detection of pulmonary parenchymal nodules and nodal metastatic disease. CT scan will also show chest wall involvement.[71]

Bone Metastases (Breast, Prostate, and Lung). The radionuclide bone scan is the primary imaging modality for the detection of bony metastatic disease. The radioactive tracer will accumulate in the skeleton in areas of bone destruction and repair. False-positive scans are common because of the low specificity of the exam, with increased radionuclide uptake also occurring in multiple benign conditions, such as degenerative joint disease, trauma, and osteoporotic vertebral fractures. Plain radiographic correlation may be necessary to differentiate between metastatic disease and benign causes of increased uptake.

In myeloma patients, skeletal surveys with radiography have been used not only to assess metastases but also to evaluate bone response to chemotherapy[72]; bony involvement in multiple myeloma is usually not detected by bone scan; therefore, plain films and MRI are used instead.[73, 74] In addition, owing to the evolution of technology, MRI is being continuously refined; for example, use of echo-planar MRI is proving to be faster and simpler, and it improves staging.[75]

Lymphomas (Hodgkin's and Non-Hodgkin's). Whereas Hodgkin's disease (HD) spreads via contiguous nodal extension, the non-Hodgkin's lymphomas (NHL) disseminate widely by hematogenous routes; documenting the complete extent of disease before therapy (staging) greatly affects the outcome in both HD and NHL. CT scan of the chest, abdomen, and pelvis are considered to be essential to staging. The presence of enlarged nodes and solid or hollow organ involvement should be evaluated; as in all cases of anatomic imaging, enlarged lymph nodes are presumed to be involved with tumor (1 cm in the chest and 1.5 cm in the abdomen), whereas nonenlarged lymph nodes are assumed to be free of tumor. However, benign processes can cause nodal enlargement and normal-size nodes may contain microinvasion of the tumor. Therefore, in all tumors staged with CT scan or MRI, there will be false-positive and false-negative findings. Undoubtedly, this will have an impact on outcome.

Studies in the late 1990s compared PET with anatomic imaging (CT, MRI).[76, 77] Tumors are imaged through their uptake of (18F) fluorodeoxyglucose; the differential in uptake is caused by the accelerated metabolism of tumor cells compared with nontumor cells. Early evidence of PET compared with CT or MRI in lymphoma staging shows promising cost-effective data for better and more accurate staging and follow-up.[78] PET identifies more sites of disease and more accurately reflects response to therapy, thus avoiding unnecessary surgery and contributing to more accurate staging, which ultimately guides treatment strategies. Similar results have been found with PET versus anatomic imaging in the evaluation of non–small cell lung cancer, colorectal cancer, melanoma, and head and neck tumors. PET imaging also differentiates postsurgical and radiation changes from tumor recurrence.[79]

Gallium-67 scintigraphy is a widely used radiotracer technique that has been used in the management of lymphoma patients. Although its role in lymphoma staging has been questioned,[80, 81] gallium scintigraphy can play a role in defining prognosis and follow-up.[81, 82]

Biologic Markers

The generic definition of a tumor marker is any substance synthesized by a tumor and released into the general circulation or body fluids.[83, 84] Ideally, the marker should be detectable with tumor cell burdens below the threshold of common imaging technique and normalize with effective therapy. Clinical usefulness is enhanced when the marker is not ordinarily present in healthy controls, but it is found to be proportionally increased with an enlarging tumor compartment. Some tumor markers may not actually be produced by the malignant cell population per se, but they may represent the biomolecular response of the host to the tumor. Therefore, a critical aspect in the clinical usefulness of tumor markers involves an appreciation that very few markers used clinically today are truly tumor-specific but, rather, are tumor-associated.

Many tumor markers are entirely unsuitable as cancer screening tests, not because of poor sensitivity but because of a lack of specificity. Pragmatically, the clinical usefulness of a tumor marker rests with its return to normal following effective therapy. Markers are certainly becoming more heavily relied on to serve as bioindices to assess response to therapy earlier than is currently possible with imaging.

Applied Concepts of Oncomarkers

Some examples of tumor markers used in patients with metastatic disease are as follows:

1. *Carcinoembryonic antigen (CEA):*
   - *Colon:* Levels of CEA have been found to be stage specific.[85] There is a rising titer following resection, usually associated with recurrence and, in particular, metastasis, because only 19% to 30% of colon cancers recur locally.[86]
   - *Breast:* In a European study, CEA serum levels with erythrocyte sedimentation rate identified 84% of patients at diagnosis with metastasis.[87]
   - *Lung:* Rising levels of CEA may correlate with relapse. Use of newer methods of analysis, for example, reverse transcriptase–polymerase chain reaction, increases the sensitivity of this marker.[88]
2. *Human chorionic gonadotropin:* This serum tumor marker is a good predictor of outcome for a number of tumors, such as choriocarcinoma and embryonal cell carcinoma of the testes,[89] but it is less predictive of progression.[90]
3. *Prostate-specific antigen (PSA):* This marker is expressed independently of prostatic acid phosphatase, and elevated levels are found in 63% to 86% of patients with various stages of prostate cancer; it may be used to monitor recurrence.
4. *Acid phosphatase:* When combined with PSA, acid phosphatase is a good predictor of recurrence.[91]
5. *Free PSA (f-PSA):* The ratio of free PSA to total PSA (T-PSA) can distinguish between patients with benign prostatic hyperplasia or prostatic carcinoma. Patients with benign prostatic hyperplasia show a higher f-PSA–to–T-PSA ratio than patients with cancer. Criteria for f-PSA% cutoff are still under investigation.[92]
6. *Carbohydrate antigen (CA) 19-9:* CA 19-9 is detected by radioimmunoassay incorporating a monoclonal antibody raised against a human colorectal carcinoma line. Like CEA, CA 19-9 is stage specific,[85] and it has been found to correlate with metastasis.[93]
7. *CA 125:* CA 125 is a high-molecular-weight glycoprotein that has been found to be a useful marker for the detection of cervical, ovarian, and endometrial cancer.[94] CA 125 also has been found to correlate with disease progression and recurrence in some cancers,[94, 95] but not in others.[96, 97] CA 125 may predict for metastasis in gastric cancer patients.[98]
8. *CA 15-3:* CA 15-3 is showing increased usefulness in breast cancer patients. Although it is not reliable for the early detection of the cancer, an elevated serum level is a good indicator for both recurrent and metastatic disease.[87, 99, 100] In addition, a 1999 study has shown that breast cancer–associated glycoprotein CA 27.29 may prove more discriminatory in the early stages of the primary disease.[101]
9. *5-hydroxyindoleacetic acid (5-HIAA):* 5-HIAA, a biochemical end product of tryptophan metabolism, can be detected in the urine and may be useful in monitoring disease progression and response to therapy in malignant carcinoid tumors with liver metastases. The intermediate metabolite serotonin is responsible for the classic carcinoid syndrome.

The detection of metastases is not an academic exercise but the most important aspect of initial diagnosis and staging: it dictates appropriateness of care and identifies patient subsets that might be eligible for phase II or III clinical trials. Moreover, it may preclude any recommendation for locoregional therapy alone, which can carry significant morbidity and could not be justified unless it were administered with true curative intent. For example, a pneumonectomy could not be supported in the face of a malignant pleural effusion or a Whipple's resection for a pancreatic lesion associated with bulky celiac adenopathy and liver metastases. A patient with an endolaryngeal tumor associated with a fixed vocal cord and invasion of the preepiglottic space is certainly not a candidate for definitive external beam radiation. Conversely, the patient with non–small cell lung cancer associated with a solitary pulmonary nodule should not be precluded from potential resection unless a CT scan–directed FNA biopsy confirms metastases as opposed to an incidental granuloma. The holistic care of the cancer patient, including recruitment of paramedic support services, depends on the metastatic (M) status of the patient. The M0 or M1 condition is, indeed, the melody to which the therapeutic lyrics are cast.

Classification and Staging

The most commonly used system for staging metastases is that suggested by the American Joint Committee on Cancer (AJCC).[102] The M classification simply designates the presence or absence of metastases.

- MX: The presence of metastatic disease is not assessed.
- M0: There is no evidence of metastatic disease.
- M1: Distant metastases are present. Specific sites for metastatic disease should be individually noted.

A more detailed classification based on the criteria of number of metastases, number of organ systems involved, and the degree of functional impairment has been suggested by Rubin[103] (Table 31–3). Although cure is rare in patients with multiple metastases, it is being increasingly observed in patients with solitary metastasis, or metastases confined to one anatomic segment of an organ. As our understanding of the mechanisms of metastases improves and new therapeutic maneuvers become more effective, more patients with favorable prognoses will be identified and categorized accordingly.

Principles of Treatment

The concept of individualized therapy is never more apparent than in the treatment of a patient with metastatic disease. The presentations vary from a single asymptomatic focus of disease to multiple symptomatic sites affecting one or several organ systems. Therapeutic aggressiveness is tempered by numerous objective factors, including the temporal onset of the metastasis, site of the primary tumor, potential response of the tumor, organ system involved, age, and subjective findings. Subjective findings include degree of pain, presence of anorexia, cachexia, and nausea and vomiting, all of which affect the performance status and QOL of the patient. Formal QOL instruments will include the physical function part of performance scales, as well as role function, psychosocial function, and spiritual function. One of the most often used QOL instruments is the functional assessment of cancer treatment. All of these conditions are covered in detail in Chapter 32 (Cancer Pain Management), Chapter 33 (Palliative Care), and Chapter 14 (Principles of Psychosocial Oncology); therefore, they are mentioned only briefly here.

Symptoms Associated with Metastases

Pain

ETIOLOGY

The two broad categories of cancer pain are somatic/visceral and neuropathic.[104, 105]

1. Somatic/visceral pain arises from activation of nociceptors (receptors of noxious stimuli) in afferent nerves, caused by tumor infiltration of skin, soft tissue, or viscera. The visceral pain is poorly localized but can be described as a squeezing or pressure-like sensation. Somatic pain tends to be more localized, dull, or aching in nature. Common causes include bone metastases, capsular distention secondary to liver metastases, and ureteral or bowel obstruction.
2. Neuropathic pain arises from injury or chronic compression of peripheral nerves, tumor invasion of nerve, or spinal cord compression. It has been described as sharp, burning, or viselike, and it is often associated with dysesthesias or paresthesias.

TREATMENT

The approach to pain relief has become more complex and important because of the need for a compassionate assessment of the QOL of a cancer patient. A survey conducted by the Eastern Cooperative Oncology Group (ECOG) reported that although 67% of the patients experienced pain or had taken analgesics, as many as 42% con-

TABLE 31–3. **Proposed Classification Schema**

M Stage	Descriptor
M0	No evidence of metastases
M1a	Solitary, isolated metastasis confined to organ or one anatomic site
M1b	Multiple metastatic foci confined to one organ system or one anatomic site with no functional impairment
M1c	Multiple organs involved anatomically; no or minimal to moderate functional impairment of involved organs
M1d	Multiple organs involved anatomically; moderate to severe functional impairment of involved organs
Mx	No metastatic work-up done
M_*	Modified to show viscera involved by letter subscript: pulmonary (M_p), hepatic (M_h), osseous (M_o), skin (M_s), brain (M_b), and others
M+	Microscopic evidence of suspected metastases; confirmed by pathologic examination

sidered their treatment inadequate.[106] The World Health Organization (WHO)[107] and the Agency for Healthcare Policy and Research (AHCPR)[108] have published clinical guidelines for the management of cancer pain, and several reviews[109, 110] have reported effective analgesia in 70% to 95% of patients with their use. WHO has suggested a three-step ladder, indexed to a patient classification of pain intensity as mild, moderate, or severe; summaries of these guidelines are as follows:

1. *Mild pain* is treated with nonopioid analgesics with a potency similar to or greater than aspirin, and these are the drugs of choice. Failure to control pain has led to the more common use of combined narcotic and non-narcotic drugs.[111]
2. *Moderate pain* is treated with weak to moderate strength opioids, such as control-released codeine and oxycodone.[112, 113]
3. *Severe pain* is addressed with strong opioids, including morphine (prototype), hydromorphone, levorphanol, methadone, and oxymorphone; these opioids produce their effects by combining with the opiate receptors in the peripheral nervous system and CNS.

Response of neuropathic pain is usually poor, and it responds inconsistently to opioids and nonsteroidal anti-inflammatory agents. The additional use of anticonvulsant medications has proven effective in some cases. For example, phenytoin (Dilantin) was the first oral anticonvulsant shown to be effective against neuropathic pain; in addition, IV infusions have shown use for flare-ups in chronic situations.[114] Amitriptyline effectively reduces neuropathic pain[115]; however, its adverse side effects are leading to its replacement by the γ-aminobutyric acid analogue gabapentin.[116, 117]

Adequate treatment of the patient with pain requires a comprehensive evaluation for the cause of the pain, and the therapeutic approach, including choice of drug, must be individualized. Equianalgesic doses, which relate the amount of analgesic necessary to achieve a given level of pain control to the specific dose of morphine that would be required for the same result, are given in Table 31–4.

Cachexia

ETIOLOGY

Cancer cachexia is characterized by involuntary weight loss, anorexia, weakness, impaired immune function, lean body wasting, and poor performance status. The weight loss is characterized primarily by loss of skeletal muscle mass and adipose tissue compared with simple starvation, in which there is preservation of muscle mass. Therefore, although anorexia is common in cancer patients (35% to 80% on presentation),[118, 119] body composition changes suggest that anorexia alone is not responsible for the cachexia of cancer. The etiology of cancer cachexia is incompletely understood and is likely multifactorial. Three potential mechanisms have been hypothesized[120] to account for the changes noted in cancer cachexia, including maladaptive metabolism, decreased intake or anorexia, and mediators of cachexia (cytokines). Some of these factors may be related to the cause, whereas others may be a consequence of cachexia per se.

In general, the basal metabolic rate (BMR) or resting energy expenditure in cancer patients has been found to be elevated,[121, 122] and one study has reported an increase in the BMR before the onset of weight loss, suggesting that the increase in BMR may be a contributing factor to cachexia.[123] This situation could be explained by anaerobic metabolism of glucose being the main source of energy in most solid tumors. Because it is more inefficient than oxidative phosphorylation, it is usually accompanied by a decrease in glucose uptake by the host tissue and weight loss from overactivity of the glucose fatty acid cycle.[124] However, despite the weight loss, cancer patients also can experience a 40% increase in hepatic glucose production (gluconeogenesis).[125] In addition, alterations in fat and protein metabolism have also been observed in cancer cachexia.[126, 127]

Just as the alterations in the metabolic state in cachexia may be a component or consequence of cachexia, so have cytokines been postulated to play a role in the etiology of cancer cachexia. It has been suggested that cytokines, produced by host or tumor tissue, may induce anorexia and result in a decrease in the clearing enzyme lipoprotein lipase. The degree of lipoprotein lipase inhibition appears to be related to the effect of the cytokines. Some of the suggested important cytokines are tumor necrosis factor–α (TNFα), IL-1 and IL-6, and interferon-γ (γIFN).[119, 128]

- TNFα is a potent inhibitor of lipoprotein lipase,[129] which, following IV infusion, has been shown to cause an increase in plasma triglyceride, glycerol, and free

TABLE 31–4. **Equianalgesic Dose (ED) of Selected Opioids in Adults ≥ 50 Kg Who Are Opioid-Naïve**

	Approximate ED (mg)		Usual Starting Dose (mg) for Moderate to Severe Pain	
Drug	***Oral***	***Parenteral***	***Oral***	***Parenteral***
Morphine	30 q3–4 hrs	10 q3–4 hrs	30 q3–4 hrs	10 q3–4 hrs
Morphine, controlled-release	90–120 q12 hrs	N/A	90–120 q12 hrs	N/A
Hydromorphone (Dilaudid)	7.5 q3–4 hrs	1.5 q3–4 hrs	6 q3–4 hrs	1.5 q3–4 hrs
Meperidine (Demorol)	300 q2–3 hrs	100 q3 hrs	N/A	100 q3 hrs
Methadone (Dolophine)	20 q6–8 hrs	10 q6–8 hrs	20 q6–8 hrs	10 q6–8 hrs
Codeine (with ASA)	180–200 q3–4 hrs	130 q3–4 hrs	60 q3–4 hrs	60 q2 hrs IM/SC
Hydrocodone (Lorcet, Lortab)	30 q3–4 hrs	N/A	10 q3–4 hrs	N/A
Oxycodone (Percocet, Percodan, others)	30 q3–4 hrs	N/A	10 q3–4 hrs	N/A

q = every; IM = intramuscular; SC = subcutaneous.

fatty acid turnover.[124] However, several studies have failed to detect increased TNFα levels in patients with cachexia.[130, 131] In addition, pentoxifylline, a potent inhibitor of TNFα, has also failed to affect cachexia in patients.[132]

- The effects of IL-1 are similar to TNFα; however, the role of IL-1 in cancer cachexia is doubtful.[133]
- The role of IL-6 in cachexia has been supported in animal studies,[134] and, clinically, increased levels have been found in patients with non–small cell lung or colon cancers who are losing weight.[135]
- The properties of γIFN are similar to TNFα; however, although the levels were increased by 53% in one study of patients with myeloma,[136] no association was observed with the clinical parameters of the disease.

The lack of a specific relationship between any cytokines and cachexia suggests that other factors may be involved, such as catabolic substances or lipid- and protein-mobilizing factors, which act directly on host tissues.

TREATMENT

No single modality has been successful in reversing the cachexia of cancer. Of particular interest are those patients exhibiting more than 15% weight loss from, in large part, loss of total body protein, because physiologic function (e.g., respiratory muscle) can be impaired and may lead to death from cachexia without intervention.

The prevention of malnutrition in the cancer patient can lead to a reduction in morbidity and mortality.[137] However, attempts to replace lean body mass with total parenteral nutrition have not been successful. A number of studies on patients who received parenteral nutrition has not shown any significant advantage or even a decrease in survival time and, occasionally, a poorer tumor response.[138–140] Enteral nutrition is advised when possible.

The use of appetite stimulants has been more successful in terms of weight gain, which has been primarily adipose tissue, not lean body mass. Several pharmacologic agents have been evaluated in patients with cancer cachexia:

- *Corticosteroids* stimulate appetite and may or may not increase body weight.[141]
- *Dronabinol*, an orally active cannabinoid, has increased appetite in cancer patients without significant weight gain.[142]
- *Hydrazine sulfate*, an inhibitor of gluconeogenesis, and pentoxifylline have also been evaluated, but they have not been proven effective for weight gain or stabilization.[132, 143]
- *Ibuprofen* and *eicosapentaenoic acid* have been shown to reduce the resting energy expenditure, suggesting an effect on the catabolic process and stabilization of protein and fat stores.[144, 145]
- One of the most potent appetite stimulants is *megestrol acetate* (MA, Megace). At standard doses of 160 mg per day, MA produces weight gain in 25% to 30% of patients. Early phase I and II studies of MA, using doses up to 1600 mg per day, demonstrated an increase in weight regardless of tumor response or the presence of visceral disease.[146] Subsequently, randomized, double-blind, placebo-controlled trial of MA (800 mg per day) versus placebo reported an increase in appetite and substantial weight gain of up to 6.8 kg in the MA group. Patients in the MA group also reported significantly less nausea and emesis.[147, 148] Although MA stimulates weight gain in patients with cancer cachexia, the majority of the weight gained is adipose tissue rather than lean body mass.[149] However, as the intervention in the majority of studies is subsequent to the weight loss and initiation of treatment, an alternative approach would be to initiate treatment before the weight loss.

Whether the amelioration of cachexia will affect survival time directly is not known. However, in a subgroup of patients, reversal of the cachexia-anorexia syndrome could improve the ability of the patient to receive and tolerate cytotoxic therapy and, therefore, may indirectly affect survival time. In other patients with widely disseminated disease, the QOL becomes as important as the quantity of life and, therefore, an important consideration when evaluating the patient for anticachectic maneuvers.

Nausea and Vomiting

ETIOLOGY

Nausea in malignant disease is primarily associated with cytotoxic therapy (chemotherapy and radiotherapy) and, secondarily, as a consequence of disease. It is most prominent as a consequence of disease in patients with brain metastases, followed by those with cancer of the GI tract. Although the mechanisms underlying vomiting remain poorly understood, the vomiting center, located in the medulla oblongata, responds to stimuli from the chemoreceptor trigger zone and the GI tract (via the vagus nerve).

Studies indicate that radiation- and chemotherapy-induced emesis are mediated by the serum vasoconstrictor serotonin (5-hydroxytryptamine, 5HT)[150, 151] and, in particular, one of its receptors (5-HT3), which has been found in the brain, concentrated in the cortical and limbic areas.[152] Stimulation of the 5-HT3 receptors by serotonin release induces emesis, which can be antagonized by general agents, such as metoclopramide and dexamethasone,[153, 154] but it is better controlled through the use of selective antagonists of the 5-HT3 receptors, including ondansetron and tropisetron.[155, 156]

TREATMENT

There are several therapeutic options for the control of emesis and the choice should depend on the underlying cause and degree of emesis.

- *Metoclopramide (substituted benzamides):* Metoclopramide blocks dopamine receptors and is found to be 30% to 40% effective for cisplatin-induced emesis.[157] However, it is now being replaced by newer, more targeted treatments.[158]
- *Agents that block serotonin receptors: Hydroxytryptamines* have been identified in both the GI tract and CNS. A widely used agent for the treatment of nausea is *prochlorperazine;* however, the best-studied agent so far is *odansetron*, which has been found to be very effective for both chemotherapy- and radiation-induced emesis.[153, 154, 159, 160] In addition to having anti-

emetic properties, odansetron has been associated with fewer side effects than both metoclopramide and prochlorperazine.[160]
- *Corticosteroids:* The antiemetic mechanism of these remains unclear, but effectiveness has been established.[161]
- *Cannabinoids:* Dronabinol (delta 9-tetrahydrocannabinol) has been found to be better than placebo, but because of ongoing controversy, it is not recommended at present.[162]

The treatment and control of nausea requires knowledge of the agents available, clinical experience, and familiarity with the particular agents. The general opinion is that several agents may be necessary to ease the symptoms associated with the metastatic disease itself or the side effects of treatment.

Fatigue

Fatigue is one of the most common symptoms encountered by the cancer patient. Although there is no universal definition for fatigue, there are several agreed-on concepts:

- Fatigue is subjective and multidimensional.
- It is perceived as whole body tiredness, weakness, lethargy, and malaise.
- In a 1997 three-way assessment survey on the perceptions of cancer-related fatigue, 78% of patients reported experiencing fatigue during the course of their disease and 38% on a daily basis. Moreover, 61% of patients believed fatigue affected their daily lives more than cancer-related pain.[163]
- The cause of fatigue in the cancer patient is probably multifactorial and can be classified as physiologic, psychological, or situational. The most common physiologic causes are anemia and pain. Anemia can be addressed with transfusion or epoetin alfa[164] and pain with analgesics.
- The most common psychological causes include depression, anxiety, and nausea and vomiting (as discussed earlier).
- Finally, examples of situational factors include sleep disturbances and excessive inactivity. Patients usually complain of difficulty getting to sleep and staying asleep. Sleep aids may be helpful.

Several studies suggest that it may be a mistake to restrict the activities of cancer patients, because such activities may accelerate muscle wasting and decrease functional capacity. In a study of breast cancer patients receiving radiation, those assigned to a self-directed 15-minute aerobic walk had statistically significant improvement in physical and emotional functioning, including reduced fatigue.[165]

Therapeutic Management of Metastases

Because the majority of cancer patients will develop metastases at some point during the course of their disease, appropriate therapeutic management is extremely important. The improvement in QOL, owing to relief of symptoms from metastasis, can be a most rewarding experience to both the patient and physician. The performance status of the patient, type of symptoms, location of metastasis, histology, life expectancy, disease tempo, and patient wishes are factors to be considered when choosing appropriate palliative therapy.

Palliative treatment should relieve symptoms quickly and for as long as possible, with a minimum of side effects. For patients who are bedridden with widely disseminated metastatic disease and who have run the gamut of therapeutic programs, good supportive care at home or in a hospital can relieve suffering during the final days. Others with symptoms from a solitary metastasis to a vital organ may become symptom-free for several years with surgical treatment. It is the responsibility of the physician to evaluate all of the factors in the disease process and to develop an individualized program that will give the best palliation.

Surgery can be very effective for relieving symptoms quickly or preventing further loss of function, for example, with spinal cord compression. Prophylactic surgical stabilization of a metastasis to a weight-bearing bone can prevent fracture while receiving radiation therapy. Chemotherapy or hormonal therapy can sometimes relieve symptoms from widespread metastases. Radiation therapy can often relieve symptoms of pain, swelling, respiratory insufficiency, bleeding, or neurologic symptoms as a result of metastasis. The appropriate choice of pain medication, dose, and route of administration can control pain in the majority of patients. Often, a combination of therapies—cytotoxic, pharmacologic, and psychosocial—provides the best results.

Results and Prognosis

Brain Metastases

Surgery

The clinical status of the patient, solitary versus multiple foci, surgical accessibility of the tumor, histology of the primary cancer, and time interval between control of the primary tumor and appearance of metastases are the five most important factors when considering patients for surgical resection of metastases. The most important factor is the status of the primary cancer, with longer survivals expected in patients with absent, controlled, or limited primary disease. The most relevant histologic factor is the radiochemosensitivity of the primary. The more radiochemosensitive tumors (small cell lung, lymphoma) should be treated with irradiation and chemotherapy, whereas the more radioresistant tumors (melanoma and renal cell carcinoma) are best treated with surgery and metastases from non–small cell lung and breast cancers are best treated with surgery and radiation. Long-term survival of greater than 48 months has been demonstrated in 18% to 33% of patients in which the primary disease is controlled and no other metastases exist. Similarly, patients whose metastases appear later than 2 years after control of primary tumor will live longer than those whose metastases appear within 1 year.

Surgery, when possible, should be followed by whole brain irradiation to prevent the development of further brain metastases.[166] The results of two randomized studies have demonstrated that surgical resection followed by postoperative radiation was superior to radiation alone.[167, 168] The patients with a Karnofsky performance score (KPS) of 70, limited systemic disease, and a single metastasis had a longer median survival time (40 weeks versus 15 weeks; $p < .01$), significantly fewer recurrences at the initial metastatic site (52% versus 20%; $p < .02$), and improved QOL. However, the overall survival rate was less than 10% in both groups by week 90.

Surgery can be very effective at quickly relieving the symptoms associated with a solitary metastasis, or it may provide a tissue diagnosis in others. The symptoms of nausea, vomiting, and ataxia associated with a cerebellar metastasis will be relieved in nearly all patients after tumor resection, with very little risk of morbidity from surgery.

Radiation Therapy

Radiation therapy has been proven to be effective in relieving symptoms from solitary or multiple metastases in 60% to 80% of all patients.[169, 170] In an early Radiation Therapy Oncology Group study (RTOG 79-16), different treatment schedules of whole brain irradiation were compared—20 Gy x 4, 30 Gy x 10, and 40 Gy x 15 or 20—and the shorter schedules were found to be at least as effective as more protracted ones.[171] Improvement in functional neurologic performance was noted in 50% to 60% of patients, usually within 2 to 3 weeks, but sustained performance was brief in those responders surviving 6 months after therapy. A subsequent analysis identified four favorable prognostic factors, including a KPS of 70 to 100, absent or a controlled primary, patient age of younger than 60 years, and metastases limited to the brain. The probability of surviving 6 months was 52% in patients with all four factors, 33% with three of four factors, and only 8% if there were no favorable factors present.[172, 173] However, it must be noted that because patients receiving brain irradiation often have extensive disease elsewhere, median survival is generally only 4 to 6 months.

The literature provides some evidence for the need for reirradiation of brain metastases following the recurrence of tumor and symptoms. Some investigators have reported improvement in neurologic function; however, there is a median survival of only 3 to 4 weeks.[174, 175]

Stereotactic Radiosurgery

Stereotactic radiosurgery is a technique that was developed in the early 1950s by a Swedish neurosurgeon for the delivery of a very large fraction of ionizing radiation to a small intracranial target using stereotactically directed narrow beams.[176] The characteristics of brain metastases (smaller than 30 mm, nearly spherical, minimally invasive, and displacing normal brain parenchyma circumferentially beyond the target volume) often make them good radiosurgery targets. The local control rates using this technique vary from 85% to 95%,[177, 178] and the large dose per fraction obtained with this technique has proved to be more effective than conventional radiation therapy in more radioresistant tumors, such as renal cell carcinomas, sarcomas, and melanomas.[179, 180] In addition, the combination of radiosurgery and whole brain irradiation has been found to reduce the failure at both the radiosurgery site and elsewhere in the brain, and some survival time advantage has been noted.[181, 182]

Chemotherapy

The use of chemotherapy has, in general, been restricted to those select tumors of known chemosensitivity, for example, small cell carcinoma[183, 184] and breast cancer.[185] Some success has been found through the use of cisplatin in a number of combination regimens, for example, with etoposide, vinblastine, dacarbazine, and biologic agents such as the interferons.[185–187] Response rates of 15% to 60% have been reported with a median survival time of 6 to 11 months. Use of these regimens frequently results in severe, although not life-threatening hematologic toxicity. Corticosteroids (dexamethasone and prednisone) can quickly relieve symptoms from swelling.[188] New systemic protocols, including paclitaxel, are now in clinical trial.[189, 190]

Malignant Spinal Cord Compression

Malignant spinal cord compression (MSCC) is one of the most devastating consequences of metastatic cancer. The natural history of MSCC is one of relentless and progressive pain and, if untreated, paralysis, sensory loss, and sphincter incontinence. This clinical description, especially with unexplained back pain in a patient with a known malignancy, and minimal radiographic evidence of indentation of the theca or compression of the dural sac should alert the physician to the presence or possibility of cord compression. Surgery, radiotherapy, and steroids are accepted treatments for MSCC and some suggested guidelines exist; however, there is no consensus regarding the specific indications or sequence in which each modality should be employed.[191, 192]

Some general comments can be made regarding suggested approaches:

- Three distinct pretreatment categories—ambulatory, paretic, and paraplegic—have been identified and should be included when reporting the effectiveness of any modality.
- High-dose dexamethasone (96 mg per day) is effective,[193] although some older reports support a more moderate dose, using a 10 mg bolus followed by 16 mg per day (in divided doses four times a day), tapered over 2 weeks.
- The recommendations for surgical intervention include MSCC caused by so-called mechanical impingement, when the diagnosis of MSCC is in doubt, or in patients who have had previous radiation to the site. In a prospective study, when using these criteria, surgery preceded radiation in only 7% of the cases.[194, 195]
- Radiation therapy is the most commonly used modality for MSCC and it is usually combined with steroid treatment. The most commonly used schedule is 30 Gy in 10 fractions over 2 weeks, prescribed to a depth of 5 to 8 cm, using a single posterior field encompassing one uninvolved vertebra on either side of the compression and a width of 8 to 10 cm.
- Good prognostic factors are pretreatment motor func-

tion[196, 197] and neurologic status at the time of diagnosis.[198] In addition, the median duration of response and survival are tumor-type dependent.[199] Good responders are lymphoproliferative disorders and breast cancer, with a mean duration of response of 23 months and a mean survival time of 25 to 48 months.[198, 200] More resistant disorders, for example, myelomas and bronchogenic carcinomas, have a mean duration of 4.5 months and a survival time of 10 months.

Bone Metastases

Metastases to the skeletal system will develop in about 30% to 70% of all new cases of cancer at some point during the natural history of the disease, with the most common sites in decreasing incidence being the vertebra, pelvis, femur, skull, and upper extremity.[201] The principal symptom for initiating therapy is pain at the site of metastasis, and its relief is a measure of the effectiveness of therapy. The mechanisms of pain and recommendations for pharmacologic intervention were discussed earlier. The roles of surgery, radiation therapy, and chemotherapy are now discussed.

Surgery

Surgery should be considered for stabilization of a weight-bearing long bone if significant cortical destruction exists and the patient is ambulatory.[202] An intramedullary rod and cement often accomplish this, although a prosthesis may be necessary if the hip is involved. Removal of extradural bone fragments, debulking of tumor, and stabilization of vertebrae are effective in relieving pain from pathologic vertebral body compression if a patient otherwise is in good medical condition. Pathologic fractures requiring surgical intervention occur in approximately 9% of patients with metastatic bone disease.

Radiation Therapy

Radiation therapy has been very effective for relieving pain and improving function, either alone or following surgical stabilization of bone metastasis. A wide range of single and multifraction dose regimens have been used. The RTOG conducted an early randomized study that compared differing dose levels of radiation therapy.[203] Overall, 89% (547 out of 613) experienced at least minimal relief of pain, with 53% achieving complete relief and 30% partial relief. There was no significant difference in pain relief rates or promptness of minimal relief between the different schedules, although there was a significant difference in achieving complete relief. The data were reanalyzed by combining solitary and multiple metastasis groups.[204] The results suggested that the protracted course of treatment was associated with improved outcome and a greater degree of pain relief than short courses.

The most common schedule in use today is 30 Gy in 10 fractions over 2 weeks and has been reported to result in 50% good or complete relief of pain.[205] However, earlier reports from prospective trials have shown that a single fraction of 8 Gy is equally as effective as both 30 Gy in 10 fractions[206] and 24 Gy in 4 fractions,[207] so that the optimal dose of radiation required for pain relief is, as yet, undetermined. The RTOG is presently conducting a prospective randomized study (RTOG 97-14) that compares 30 Gy in 10 fractions to a single fraction of 8 Gy and, in order to address some of the questions and concerns noted earlier, is including QOL and patient assessment of pain.

Large Field and Systemic Radiotherapy

Some interest has centered on the ability of hemi body irradiation to affect occult or asymptomatic overt disease, thereby raising the idea of hemi body irradiation as a systemic agent.[208] However, a later study using fractionated hemi body irradiation demonstrated no additional improvement.[209] Systemically administered isotopes also have the ability to palliate pain caused by widespread osseous metastases.[210, 211] The rationale for their use lies in their ability to follow the metabolic pathways of calcium in bone. Several radiopharmaceuticals have been developed for systemic therapy of bone metastases (Table 31–5); the physical characteristic of each radiopharmaceutical varies, which determines how it is used. One of the most important factors is the nature of the emitting radiation following decay; for example, for beta emitters, the effective range is 80 to 100 mm, and for alpha emitters, it is 50 to 90 μm.

- *Phosphorus-32* has been used for relief of bone pain since its introduction in the 1950s. The results of clinical studies reported responses of 58% to ~100%, and the mean responses for breast and prostate metastases were 84% and 77%, respectively.[212] However, because it was found to have only a 2:1 ratio of uptake (tumor-to-bone), its use has become more limited.
- The use of *strontium-89* for treating painful bone metastases from prostate cancer has been reported.[213] The retention of strontium in bone varies with the degree of bone involvement, and the ratio of uptake in involved bone-to-marrow has been reported to be 10:1 with an average tumor dose of 20 to 24 Gy.[214] Response rates of 64% to 96% have been reported in patients with prostate cancer,[215, 216] and 47% to 62% in patients with breast cancer.[216, 217]
- More recently, radiopharmaceuticals have been developed that form metal complexes that localize in osteoblastic metastases when combined with chelating agents, which results in high target-to-nontarget ratios. *Samarium-153* has been reported to affect bone pain in 65% to 80% of patients up to 11 months after a single dose of 0.5 to 1.0 mCi/kg.[218] In a 1998 randomized study, pain relief was noted at 3 weeks in 62% to 72% of those treated and 40% of those in the placebo

TABLE 31–5. **Radionuclides Used for Bone Metastases**

Radionuclide	Half-Life (hrs)	Beta Energy (MeV)
Iodine-131	193	0.61
Samarium-153	46.7	0.81
Rhenium-186	90.6	1.07
Phosphorus-32	343	1.71
Strontium-89	1212	1.46

group. The pain relief persisted through 16 weeks in 43% of patients who received the drug. Bone marrow suppression was minimal.[219]

Chemotherapy

Bone is among the most common sites of metastatic disease of breast, prostate, and lung.[220] Indeed, a significant percentage of patients (50% to 70%) with metastatic breast cancer will demonstrate skeletal involvement, possibly owing to clonal selection mediated through parathyroid hormone–related proteins or other factors.[221] For patients with estrogen receptor–positive breast cancer or prostate cancer, hormonal treatment is among the treatments of choice. In patients with estrogen receptor–negative breast cancer who have failed hormonal therapy or who have liver metastases, systemic chemotherapy can be used, particularly in combination therapies.[222–224] However, complete responses of bone lesions to chemotherapy are rare, although partial responses and disease stabilization can lead to long-term patient benefit. Therefore, patients are in a favorable position to benefit from adjunctive supportive therapy, such as from bisphosphonates.

Bisphosphonates are potent inhibitors of bone resorption that were examined initially as a part of the pain management of bone metastases. Phase II studies, which were run until 1992, demonstrated bisphosphonate efficacy in reducing morbidity in terms of bone pain, fracture, and hypercalcemia.[225] At that time, randomized phase III trials began and, since then, bisphosphonates have begun to represent a valid therapy for bone metastases. Studies have been performed with pamidronate, given both orally and through IV, clodronate, and ibandronate,[226–228] and all have demonstrated a significant reduction in skeletal morbidity, although no increase has been shown in the duration of survival. Newer and more potent bisphosphonates, such as zoledronate, are presently under investigation.

Lung Metastases

Surgery

Surgery can remove a solitary lung metastasis for diagnostic or therapeutic purposes without significant morbidity. The techniques of pulmonary metastasectomy involve either median sternotomy or lateral thoracotomy. Surgical resection of pulmonary metastases can be considered if the primary cancer is controlled with an adequate disease-free interval, there are no other metastatic sites, and the metastases can be completely resected. This is especially relevant in renal cell, thyroid, colon, and osteogenic and soft tissue sarcomas, because long-term survival may be possible.

- Approximately 50% of all patients with renal cell cancer will present with or develop pulmonary metastases. In one series, the mean survival from metastasectomy was 43 months and included patients with multiple nodules and varying length of disease-free survival.[229] Survival was independent of the number of metastases resected if the patient was rendered disease-free at the time of resection.
- Only 1% of patients with colorectal cancer will present with isolated lung metastases. A report of a large series of patients demonstrated a 5-year survival rate of 31%, which was in agreement with several earlier, small series.[230] However, in comparison with other sites noted earlier, patients with multiple metastases or an elevated CEA level did less well.

Radiation Therapy

Radiation therapy can relieve or prevent symptoms of hemorrhage, obstruction, and pain associated with metastases. Often, small fields and abbreviated treatment courses may be used. Irradiation to the whole lung is limited by the sensitivity of normal lung tissue to relatively large doses (15 Gy). A more practical approach is the use of small boost fields to involved sites, to total doses of 30 to 50 Gy at 1.8 Gy per fraction, or even high single doses (6 Gy) can be used. In addition, symptoms that are related to recurrent obstructing endobronchial lung cancer might be resolved using debulking by laser treatment or endobronchial brachytherapy.

Chemotherapy

Chemotherapy can be curative in sensitive tumors such as germ cell tumors, choriocarcinoma, and Hodgkin's disease. Iodoantipyrine is effective in metastatic thyroid tumors that demonstrate uptake. Improvements in symptoms that are related to multiple pulmonary metastases from other cancers have occurred with chemotherapy and hormone therapy. Chest tube drainage and insertion of a sclerosing agent such as tetracycline or single-agent chemotherapy are effective in preventing recurrence of a malignant pleural effusion.

Superior Vena Cava Obstruction

Radiation Therapy

Superior vena cava obstruction (SVCO) is manifested by increasing shortness of breath; edema of the face, neck, and upper extremities; and a prominent venous pattern on the chest and upper abdomen. Death from the syndrome is unusual unless accompanied by severe complicating factors. Nevertheless, prompt administration of therapy will result in relief of shortness of breath in 60% of patients within 1 to 2 days and 86% within 3 to 4 days, whereas the edema usually lags and clearing is evident in 65% of patients within 7 days.[231] Although most patients with SVCO have lung cancer, it has been observed in lymphoma, small cell lung cancer, and occasionally in breast and germ cell cancers. Different schedules have been proposed, including large daily fractions (4 Gy $\times$ 3) followed by conventional doses. The total dose depends on the state of the individual and the disease, that is, whether the SVCO is the presenting symptom or one of many metastatic sites, and will range from a palliative (30 Gy) to a definitive (50 Gy) dose. In addition to instituting radiation therapy, diuretics and steroids should be considered and the head of the bed should be elevated; although, if there is unilateral extension of the obstruction, IV therapy should not be initiated on the affected side.

Chemotherapy

The focus of chemotherapy has been primarily on small cell lung cancer and lymphomas, because both tumors are chemosensitive.[232] Response rates of 81% have been reported in small cell cancer with chemotherapy alone.[233] However, the results from a meta-analysis suggest that the addition of thoracic radiation should be considered,[234] provided the patients have limited-stage disease, and a platinum-based approach, rather than a doxorubicin-based approach, is recommended.[235]

Liver Metastases

The prognosis for patients with extensive liver metastases is quite poor in most cases. The symptoms associated with liver metastases include anorexia, nausea, pyrexia, malaise, and a failure to thrive. Solitary metastases can be candidates for surgical resection or stereotactic radiosurgery (SRS).

Surgery

Surgery can remove a solitary metastasis, and some patients are cured without other metastatic disease. More extensive involvement of a single lobe can also be resected in certain cases with good palliation but with less chance of cure. Survival after resection of hepatic metastases in the absence of extrahepatic disease is related to a number of factors, including the following:

- *Number of metastases:* The 5-year survival rate in patients with fewer than four lesions is 37%; 23% with more than four lesions.
- *Disease-free interval (DFI):* The 5-year survival rate in patients with a DFI of less than 1 month is 27%; 42% with a DFI of more than 1 year.
- *CEA level before liver resection:* Patients with a CEA level lower than 5 ng/mL had a 5-year survival rate of 47%; patients with a CEA level higher than 30 ng/mL had a 5-year survival rate of 28%.

Radiation Therapy

Radiation therapy can relieve pain caused by a diffusely involved, massively enlarged liver with very little acute toxicity. The limiting factor in treating hepatic metastases is the tolerance of the normal liver, although the incidence of radiation hepatitis is low after doses less than 30 Gy. Dose schedules of 6 Gy × 1, 3 Gy × 7, 2.5 Gy × 10, and 2 Gy × 15 are all effective and well tolerated. An RTOG study compared radiation (21 Gy in 3 Gy fractions) with radiation plus misonidazole; there was an effective response rate of 80%, but no significant improvement in response was demonstrated with the addition of the radiation sensitizer.[236] Use of a hyperfractionated schedule has proved unsuccessful.[237] With SRS, single doses of 20 to 30 Gy can be delivered to well-targeted foci.

Chemotherapy

Hepatic arterial infusion is frequently used to achieve high drug levels in the intrahepatic tumor while maintaining low systemic levels, and it is presently under clinical study.[238] In the various combination protocols, the most commonly used drug is 5-fluorouracil, and response rates of 40% to 60% have been recorded.[239, 240] In addition, monoclonal antibodies have been successful in the treatment of primary hepatomas and may have a role in the treatment of metastatic disease.[241]

Clinical Investigations

The challenge for the health professional in caring for the patient with metastatic disease is to determine the best therapeutic plan for the patient after careful evaluation of all available subjective and objective findings. The information provided in this chapter should serve as a guide to formulating a therapeutic plan, because each patient, by definition, presents with his or her own set of complex variables. From the time-honored patient history and physical examination, using newer diagnostic procedures and careful subjective evaluation, one should begin to formulate a treatment plan that will lead to the use of an efficacious modality. Implicit in the management of the patient with metastatic disease is the concern for improving the QOL or minimizing the adverse effects of the disease or treatment.

Some of the key issues of the treatment of metastases were discussed at the First International Consensus Workshop on RT in the Treatment of Metastases, where Bates and coworkers[242] provided an overview of the management of bone metastases and its compression. However, it was evident from the consensus statement that treatment decisions are frequently based more on one's training and local custom than on clinical trials. In addition, in spite of broad agreement that the progress in metastatic management has been poor, there was disagreement as to whether or not treatment could be considered to be radical or palliative. To compare the benefits of different treatments, it is necessary, therefore, to consider the long-term control rates, life expectancy of patients, and the financial and human cost of treatment. Nonetheless, the ensuing years have witnessed a new paradigm in the attitude toward and, therefore, treatment of the patient with metastatic disease. The increasing manifestation of positive results has shifted the paradigm from a palliative to a more curative mode when evaluating the therapeutic algorithm for the patient with metastatic disease.

REFERENCES

General

1. Woodhouse EC, Chuaqui RF, Liotta LA: General mechanisms of metastases. Cancer 1997; 80 (suppl):1529–1537.
2. Groopman JE: Fatigue in cancer and HIV/AIDS. Oncology 1998; 12:335–344.
3. Hill RP: Metastasis. In: Tannock IF, Hill RP (eds): The Basic Science of Oncology, 2nd ed, pp 178–195. New York, McGraw-Hill Inc, 1992.
4. Fidler IJ: Molecular biology of cancer: invasion and metastasis. In: DeVita VT Jr, Hellman S, Rosenberg SA (eds): Cancer. Principles & Practice of Oncology, 5th ed, pp 135–152. Philadelphia, Lippincott-Raven, 1997.

Specific

5. Virchow R: Die Cellularpathologie in ihrer Begrundung auf Physiologische Gewebelebre. Berlin, Hirschwald, 1858.

6. Greenlee RT, Murray T, Bolden S, et al: Cancer Statistics, 2000. CA Cancer J Clin 2000; 50:7–33.
7. Effert PJ, Strohmeyer TG: Theories on the metastatic process and possible therapeutic options. Urol Res 1995; 23:11–19.
8. Chambers AF, Matrisian LM: Changing views of the role of matrix metalloproteinases in metastasis. J Natl Cancer Inst 1997; 89:1260–1270.
9. Rubens RD, Coleman RE: Bone metastases. In: Abeloff MD, Armitage JO, Lichter AS, et al. (eds): Clinical Oncology, pp 643–665. New York, Churchill Livingstone, 1995.
10. Kemeny NE, Kemeny M, Lawrence TS: Liver metastases. In Abeloff MD, Armitage JO, Lichter AS, et al. (eds): Clinical Oncology, pp 679–707. New York, Churchill Livingstone, 1995.
11. Patchell RA: Brain metastases and carcinomatous meningitis. In: Abeloff MD, Armitage JO, Lichter AS, et al. (eds): Clinical Oncology, pp 629–642. New York, Churchill Livingstone, 1995.
12. Fidler IJ, Hart IR: Biologic diversity in metastatic neoplasm—origins and implications. Science 1982; 217:998–1001.
13. Kerbel RS: Growth dominance of the metastatic cancer cell: cellular and molecular aspects. Adv Cancer Res 1990; 55:87–131.
14. Chu JS, Lee WJ, Chang TC, et al: Correlation between tumor angiogenesis and metastasis in breast cancer. J Formos Med Assoc 1995; 94:373–378.
15. Kumar R, Fidler IJ: Angiogenic molecules and cancer metastasis. In Vivo 1998; 12:27–34.
16. Liotta LA, Stetler-Stevenson WG: Principles of molecular cell biology of cancer: cancer metastasis. In: DeVita VT Jr, Hellman S, Rosenberg SA (eds): Cancer. Principles & Practice of Oncology, 4th ed, pp 134–149. Philadelphia, Lippincott, 1993.
17. Weinberg RA: Prospects for cancer genetics. Cancer Surv 1995; 25:3–12.
18. Weijzen S, Velders MP, Kast WM: Modulation of the immune response and tumor growth by activated Ras. Leukemia 1999; 13:502–513.
19. Tabata M, Sugihara K, Yonezawa S, et al: An immunohistochemical study of thrombomodulin in oral squamous cell carcinoma and its association with invasive and metastatic potential. J Oral Pathol Med 1997; 26:258–264.
20. Imai K, Itoh F, Hinoda Y: Regulation of integrin function in the metastasis of colorectal cancer. Nippon Geka Gakkai Zasshi 1998; 99:415–418.
21. Sneath RJ, Mangham DC: The normal structure and function of CD44 and its role in neoplasia. Mol Pathol 1998; 51:191–200.
22. Tuck AB, Wilson SM, Khokha R: Ras-responsive genes and tumor metastasis. Crit Rev Oncol 1991; 4:95–114.
23. MacDonald NJ, de la Rosa A, Steeg PS: The potential roles of nm23 in cancer metastasis and cellular differentiation. Eur J Cancer 1995; 31A:1096–1100.
24. Lee JH, Miele ME, Hicks DJ, et al: KiSS-1, a novel human malignant melanoma metastasis-suppressor gene. J Natl Cancer Inst 1996; 88:1731–1737.
25. Fidler IJ, Radinsky R: Search for genes that suppress cancer metastasis. J Natl Cancer Inst 1996; 88:1700–1703.
26. Richards B, Zhang H, Phear G: Conditional mutator phenotypes in $hMSH_2$-deficient tumor cell lines. Science 1997; 277:1523–1526.
27. Loeb LA: Mutator phenotype may be required for multistage carcinogenesis. Cancer Res 1991; 51:3075–3079.
28. Pluda JM: Tumor-associated angiogenesis: mechanisms, clinical implications, and therapeutic strategies. Semin Oncol 1997; 24:203–218.
29. Zetter BR: Angiogenesis and tumor metastasis. Ann Rev Med 1998; 49:407–424.
30. Rak JW, St Croix BD, Kerbel RS: Consequences of angiogenesis for tumor progression, metastasis and cancer therapy. Anti-Cancer Drugs 1995; 6:3–18.
31. Rabbani SA: Metalloproteases and urokinase in angiogenesis and tumor progression. In Vivo 1998; 12:135–142.
32. Bar-Eli M: Role of interleukin-8 in tumor growth and metastasis of human melanoma. Pathobiology 1999; 67:12–18.
33. Goldmann T, Suter L, Ribbert D, et al: The expression of proteolytic enzymes at the dermal invading front of primary cutaneous melanoma predicts metastasis. Pathol Res Pract 1999; 195:171–175.
34. Carroll VA, Binder BR: The role of plasminogen activation system in cancer. Semin Thromb Hemost 1999; 25:183–197.
35. Fidler IJ: Metastasis: quantitative analysis of distribution and fate of tumor emboli labeled with ^{125}I-iodo-2'deoxyuridine. J Natl Cancer Inst 1970; 45:773–782.
36. Chambers AF, MacDonald IC, Schmidt EE, et al.: Preclinical assessment of anti-cancer therapeutic strategies using in vivo videomicroscopy. Cancer Metastasis Rev 1998–1999; 17:263–269.
37. Koop S, MacDonald IC, Luzzi K, et al: Fate of melanoma cells entering the microcirculation: over 80% survive and extravasate. Cancer Res 1995; 55:2520–2523.
38. Morris VL, Koop S, MacDonald IC, et al: Mammary carcinoma cell lines of high and low metastatic potential differ not in extravasation but in subsequent migration and growth. Clin Exp Metastasis 1994; 12:357–367.
39. Lapis K, Paku S, Liotta LA: Endothelialization of embolized tumor cells during metastasis formation. Clin Exp Metastasis 1988; 6:73–76.
40. el-Sabban ME, Pauli BU: Adhesion-mediated gap junctional communication between lung-metastatic cancer cells and endothelium. Invasion Metastasis 1994–1995; 14:164–176.
41. Morris VL, Schmidt EE, MacDonald IC, et al: Sequential steps in hematogenous metastasis of cancer cells studied by in vivo videomicroscopy. Invasion Metastasis 1997; 17:281–296.
42. Folkman J: Clinical applications of research on angiogenesis. N Engl J Med 1995; 333:1757–1763.
43. Sheu JR, Fu CC, Tsai ML, et al: Effect of U-995, a potent shark cartilage-derived angiogenesis inhibitor, on anti-angiogenesis and anti-tumor activities. Anticancer Res 1998; 18:4435–4441.
44. Brown PD: Matrix metalloproteinase inhibitors. Breast Cancer Res Treat 1998; 52:125–136.
45. Brown PD: Clinical studies with matrix metalloproteinase inhibitors. APMIS 1999; 107:174–180.
46. Raymond E: Tumor angiogenesis inhibitors: media and scientific aspects. Presse Med 1998; 27:1221–1224.
47. Cao Y: Therapeutic potentials of angiostatin in the treatment of cancer. Haematologica 1999; 84:643–650.
48. Gasparini G: The rationale and future potential of angiogenesis inhibitors in neoplasia. Drugs 1999; 58:17–38.
49. Cockett MI, Murphy G, Birch ML, et al: Matrix metalloproteinases and metastatic cancer. Biochem Soc Symp 1998; 63:295–313.
50. Kahari VM, Saarialho-Kere U: Matrix metalloproteinases and their inhibitors in tumour growth and invasion. Ann Med 1999; 31:34–45.
51. Zeng ZS, Guillem JG: Distinct patterns of matrix metalloproteinase 9 and tissue inhibitor of metalloproteinase I in RNA expression in human colorectal and liver metastases. Br J Cancer 1995; 72:575–582.
52. Zeng ZS, Huang Y, Cohen AM, et al: Prediction of colorectal cancer relapse and survival via tissue RNA levels of matrix metalloproteinase 9. J Clin Oncol 1996; 14:3133–3140.
53. Steward WP: Marimastat (BB2516): current status of development. Cancer Chemother Pharmacol 1999; 43 (suppl):S56–S60.
54. Jones L, Ghaneh P, Humphreys M, et al: The matrix metalloproteinases and their inhibitors in the treatment of pancreatic cancer. Ann NY Acad Sci 1999; 880:288–307.
55. Millar A, Brain PB: 360 patient meta analysis of studies of marimastat: a novel matrix metalloproteinase inhibitor. Ann Oncol 1996; 7 (suppl):123–126.
56. Davis PC, Hudgins PA, Peterman SB, et al: Diagnosis of cerebral metastases: double dose delayed CT versus contrast enhanced MR imaging. AJNR Am J Neuroradiol 1991; 12:293–300.
57. Madison NT, Hall WA, Letchaw RE, et al: Radiological diagnosis, staging, and follow-up of adult central nervous system primary malignant glioma. Radiol Clin N Am 1994; 32:183–196.
58. Hendee WR, Manaster DJ, Harnsberger HR, et al: Oncologic imaging. In: Holleb AE, Fink OJ, Murphy GP (eds): American Cancer Society Textbook of Clinical Oncology, 4th ed, pp 519–520. Atlanta, American Cancer Society, 1994.
59. Ericson K, Kihlstrom L, Mogard J, et al: Positron emission tomography using ^{18}F-fluorodeoxyglucose in patients with stereotactically irradiated brain metastases. Stereotact Funct Neurosurg 1996; 66 (suppl):214–224.
60. Ruckdeschel JC: Spinal cord compression. In: Abeloff MD, Armitage JO, Lichter AS, et al. (eds): Clinical Oncology, pp 619–628. New York, Churchill Livingstone, 1995.
61. Glover B, Glick JM: Oncologic emergencies. In: Holleb AI, Fink OJ, Murphy GP (eds): American Cancer Society Textbook of Clinical Oncology, 4th ed, pp 519–524. Atlanta, American Cancer Society, 1994.

62. Murray MJ, Stewart JR, Johnson DH: Superior vena cava syndrome. In: Abeloff MD, Armitage JO, Lichter AS, et al. (eds): Clinical Oncology, pp 609–618. New York, Churchill Livingstone, 1995.
63. Pass HI: Malignant pleural and pericardial effusions. In: DeVita VT Jr, Hellman S, Rosenberg SA (eds): Cancer. Principles & Practice of Oncology, 5th ed, pp 2586–2606. Philadelphia, Lippincott-Raven, 1997.
64. Russo P: Urologic emergencies. In: DeVita VT Jr, Hellman S, Rosenberg SA (eds): Cancer. Principles & Practice of Oncology, 5th ed, pp 2512–2522. Philadelphia, Lippincott-Raven, 1997.
65. Blumke DA, Soyer P, Fishman EK: Medical (spiral) CT of the liver. Radiol Clin North Am 1995; 33:863–886.
66. Fishman EK: Imaging techniques in cancer management. In: DeVita VT Jr, Hellman S, Rosenberg SA (eds): Cancer. Principles & Practice of Clinical Oncology, 5th ed, pp 643–656. Philadelphia, Lippincott-Raven, 1997.
67. Barkin JS, Goldstein JA: Diagnostic approach to pancreatic cancer. Gastroenterol Clin North Am 1999; 28:709–722.
68. Takehara Y: MR pancreatography. Semin Ultrasound 1999; 20:324–339.
69. Bhutani MS: Endoscopic ultrasound in pancreatic diseases. Indications, limitations, and the future. Gastroenterol Clin North Am 1999; 28:747–770.
70. Lorenzen J, Beese M, Mester J, et al: Chest X ray: routine indication in the follow-up of differentiated thyroid cancer? Nuklearmedizin 1998; 37:208–212.
71. Touliopuolos P, Costello P: Helical (spiral) CT of the thorax. Radiol Clin North Am 1995; 33:843–861.
72. Sebes JI, Niell HB, Palmieri GM, Reidy TJ: Skeletal surveys in multiple myeloma. Radiologic-clinical correlation. Skeletal Radiol 1986; 15:354–359.
73. Krasnow AZ, Hellman RS, Timins ME, et al: Diagnostic bone scanning in oncology. Semin Nucl Med 1997; 27:107–141.
74. Larson SM: Imaging techniques in cancer management: radionuclide imaging. In: DeVita VT Jr, Hellman S, Rosenberg SA (eds): Cancer. Principles & Practice of Clinical Oncology, 5th ed, pp 663–669. Philadelphia, Lippincott-Raven, 1997.
75. Horvath LJ, Burtness BA, McCarthy S, et al: Total-body echo-planar MR imaging in the staging of breast cancer: comparison with conventional methods—early experience. Radiology 1999; 211:119–128.
76. Anzai Y, Carroll WR, Quint DJ, et al: Recurrence of head and neck cancer after surgery or irradiation: prospective comparison of 2-deoxy-2-[F-18]fluoro-D-glucose PET and MR imaging diagnosis. Radiology 1996; 200:135–141.
77. Bury T, Dowlati A, Paulus P, et al: Whole-body ^{18}FDG positron emission tomography in the staging of non–small cell lung cancer. Eur Respir J 1997; 10:2529–2534.
78. Newman JJ, Francis IN, Kaminski MS, et al: Imaging of lymphoma with PET with 2-[^{18}F]-fluoro-2-deoxyglucose: correlation with CT. Radiology 1994; 190:111–116.
79. Valk PE, Pounds TR, Ruth DT, et al: Cost effectiveness of PET imaging in clinical oncology. Nucl Med Biol 1996; 23:737–743.
80. Larcos G, Farlow DC, Antico VF, et al: The role of high dose 67-gallium scintigraphy in staging untreated patients with lymphoma. Aust N Z J Med 1994; 24:5–8.
81. Gallamini A, Biggi A, Fruttero A, et al: Revisiting the prognostic role of gallium scintigraphy in low-grade non-Hodgkin's lymphoma. Eur J Nucl Med 1997; 24:1499–1506.
82. Draisma A, Maffioli L, Gasparini M, et al: Gallium-67 as a tumor-seeking agent in lymphomas—a review. Tumori 1998; 84:434–441.
83. Bates SE, Longo DL: Use of serum tumor markers in cancer diagnoses and management. Semin Oncol 1987; 14:102–138.
84. Jacobs EL, Haskell CM: Clinical use of tumor markers in oncology. Curr Prob Cancer 1991; 15:299–360.
85. Sato T, Nishimura G, Nonomura A, et al: Serological studies on CEA, CA 19-9, STn and SLX in colorectal cancer. Hepato-Gastroenterol 1999; 46:914–919.
86. Hine KR, Dykes PW: Serum CEA testing in postoperative surveillance of colorectal carcinoma. Br J Cancer 1984; 49:689–693.
87. Robertson JF, Jaeger W, Syzmendera JJ, et al: The objective measurement of remission and progression in metastatic breast cancer by use of serum tumour markers. European Group for Serum Tumour Markers in Breast Cancer. Eur J Cancer 1999; 35:47–53.
88. Fujita J, Bandoh S, Namihara H, et al: A case of leptomeningeal metastasis from lung adenocarcinoma diagnosed by reverse transcriptase-polymerase chain reaction for carcinoembryonic antigen. Lung Cancer 1998; 22:153–156.
89. Bajorin DF, Mazumdar M, Meyers M, et al: Metastatic germ cell tumors: modeling for response to chemotherapy. J Clin Oncol 1998; 16:707–715.
90. Otto T, Virchow S, Fuhrmann C, et al: Detection of vital germ cell tumor cells in short-term cell cultures of primary tumors and of retroperitoneal metastasis—clinical implications. Urol Res 1997; 25:121–124.
91. Moul JW, Connelly RR, Perahia B, et al: The contemporary value of pretreatment prostatic acid phosphatase to predict pathological stage and recurrence in radical prostatectomy cases. J Urol 1998; 159:935–940.
92. Lein M, Stephan C, Jung K, et al: Relation of free PSA/total PSA in serum for differentiating between patients with prostatic cancer and benign hyperplasia of the prostate: which cutoff should be used? Cancer Invest 1998; 16:45–49.
93. Asano F, Matsushita T, Shinoda T, et al: Lung cancer with small intestine metastasis characterized by exceptionally high levels of serum CA 19-9. Nihon Kokyuki Gakkai Zasshi 1999; 37:577–582.
94. Borras G, Molina R, Xercavins J, et al: Tumor antigens CA 19.9, CA 125, and CEA in carcinoma of the uterine cervix. Gynecol Oncol 1995; 57:205–211.
95. Diez M, Gomez A, Hernando F, et al: Serum CEA, CA 125, and SCC antigens and tumor recurrence in resectable non–small cell lung cancer. Int J Biol Markers 1995; 10:5–10.
96. Price FV, Chambers SK, Carcangiu ML, et al: CA 125 may not reflect disease status in patients with uterine serous carcinoma. Cancer 1998; 82:1720–1725.
97. Krimmel M, Hoffmann J, Krimmel C, et al: Relevance of SCC-Ag, CEA, CA 19.9 and CA 125 for diagnosis and follow-up in oral cancer. J Craniomaxillofac Surg 1998; 26:243–248.
98. Nakata B, Hirakawa-YS, Chung K, et al: Serum CA 125 level as a predictor of peritoneal dissemination in patients with gastric carcinoma. Cancer 1998; 83:2488–2492.
99. Mangkharak J, Patanachak C, Podhisuwan K, et al: The evaluation of combined scintimammography and tumor markers in breast cancer patients. Anticancer Res 1997; 17:1611–1614.
100. Rubach M, Szymendera JJ, Kaminska J, et al: Serum CA 15.3, CEA and ESR patterns in breast cancer. Int J Biol Markers 1997; 12:168–173.
101. Gion M, Mione R, Leon AE, et al: Comparison of the diagnostic accuracy of CA27.29 and CA15.3 in primary breast cancer. Clin Chem 1999; 45:630–637.
102. American Joint Committee on Cancer: AJCC Cancer Staging Manual, 5th ed. Philadelphia, Lippincott-Raven, 1997.
103. Rubin P: A unified classification of tumor: an oncotaxonomy with symbols. Cancer 1973; 31:963–982.
104. Kelly J, Payne R: Cancer pain syndromes. Neurol Clin North Am 1991; 9:937–953.
105. Foley KM: Management of cancer pain. In: DeVita VT Jr, Hellman S, Rosenberg S (eds): Cancer. Principles & Practice of Oncology, 5th ed, pp 2807–2841. Philadelphia, Lippincott-Raven, 1997.
106. Cleeland CS, Gonin R, Hatfield AK, et al: Pain and its treatment in outpatients with metastatic cancer. N Engl J Med 1994; 330:592–596.
107. World Health Organization: Cancer Pain Relief. Geneva, World Health Organization, 1986.
108. Jacox A, Carr DB, Payne R: New clinical-practice guidelines for the management of pain in patients with cancer. N Engl J Med 1994; 330:651–655.
109. Hanks GW, Justins DM: Cancer pain: management. Lancet 1992; 339:1031–1036.
110. Cleeland CS: Strategies for improving cancer pain management. J Pain Symptom Manage 1993; 8:361–364.
111. Weinstein SM: New pharmacological strategies in the management of cancer pain. Cancer Invest 1998; 16:94–101.
112. Dhaliwal HS, Sloan P, Arkinstall WW, et al: Randomized evaluation of controlled-release codeine and placebo in chronic cancer pain. J Pain Symptom Manage 1995; 10:612–623.
113. Bruera E, Belzile M, Pituskin E, et al: Randomized, double-blind, cross-over trial comparing safety and efficacy of oral controlled-release oxycodone with controlled-release morphine in patients with cancer pain. J Clin Oncol 1998; 16:3222–3229.

114. McCleane GJ: Intravenous infusion of phenytoin relieves neuropathic pain: a randomized double-blinded, placebo-controlled, crossover study. Anesth Analg 1999; 89:985–988.
115. Eija K, Tiina T, Pertti NJ: Amitriptyline effectively relieves neuropathic pain following treatment of breast cancer. Pain 1996; 64:293–302.
116. Beydoun A: Postherpetic neuralgia: role of gabapentin and other treatment modalities. Epilepsia 1999; 40 (suppl):S51–S56.
117. Morello CM, Leckband SG, Stoner CP, et al: Randomized double-blind study comparing the efficacy of gabapentin with amitriptyline on diabetic peripheral neuropathy pain. Arch Intern Med 1999; 159:1931–1937.
118. Souba WW: Nutritional support. In: DeVita VT Jr, Hellman S, Rosenberg S (eds): Cancer. Principles & Practice of Oncology, 5th ed, pp 2807–2841. Philadelphia, Lippincott-Raven, 1997.
119. Tisdale MJ: Biology of cachexia. J Natl Cancer Inst 1997; 89:1763–1773.
120. Puccio M, Nathanson L: The cancer cachexia syndrome. Semin Oncol 1997; 24:277–287.
121. Dickerson RN, White KG, Curcillo PG II, et al: Resting energy expenditure of patients with gynecologic malignancies. J Am Coll Nutr 1995; 14:448–454.
122. Jatoi A, Daly BD, Hughes V, et al: The prognostic effect of increased resting energy expenditure prior to treatment for lung cancer. Lung Cancer 1999; 23:153–158.
123. Hyltander A, Drott C, Korner U, et al: Elevated energy expenditure in cancer patients with solid tumors. Eur J Cancer 1991; 27:9–15.
124. Gambardella A, Tortoriello R, Tagliamonte MR, et al: Metabolic changes in elderly cancer patients after glucose ingestion. The role of tumor necrosis factor-α. Cancer 1997; 79:177–184.
125. Tayek JA: A review of cancer cachexia and abnormal glucose metabolism in humans with cancer. J Am Coll Nutr 1992; 11:445–456.
126. Hyltander A, Korner U, Lundholm KG: Evaluation of mechanisms behind elevated energy expenditure in cancer patients with solid tumours. Eur J Clin Invest 1993; 23:46–52.
127. McMillan DC, Preston T, Fearon KC, et al: Protein synthesis in cancer patients with inflammatory response: investigations with [^{15}N]glycine. Nutrition 1994; 10:232–240.
128. Mantovani G, Maccio A, Lai P, et al: Cytokine activity in cancer-related anorexia/cachexia: role of megestrol acetate and medroxyprogesterone acetate. Semin Oncol 1998; 25:45–52.
129. Berg M, Fraker DL, Alexander HR: Characterization of differentiation factor/leukemia inhibitory factor effect on lipoprotein lipase activity and mRNA in 3T3-LI adipocytes. Cytokine 1994; 6:425–432.
130. Socher SH, Martinez D, Craig JB, et al: Tumor necrosis factor not detectable in patients with clinical cancer cachexia. J Natl Cancer Inst 1988; 50:595–598.
131. Maltoni M, Fabbri L, Nanni O, et al: Serum levels of tumor necrosis factor alpha and other cytokines do not correlate with weight loss and anorexia in cancer patients. Support Care Cancer 1997; 5:130–135.
132. Goldberg RM, Loprinzi CL, Malliard JA, et al: Pentoxifylline for treatment of cancer anorexia and cachexia? A randomized, double-blind, placebo-controlled trial. J Clin Oncol 1995; 13:2856–2859.
133. Gelin J, Moldawer LL, Lonnroth C, et al: Role of endogenous tumor necrosis factor and interleukin 1 for experimental tumor growth and the development of cancer cachexia. Cancer Res 1991; 51:415–421.
134. Strassmann G, Fong M, Kenny JS, et al: Evidence for the involvement of interleukin 6 in experimental cancer cachexia. J Clin Invest 1992; 89:1681–1684.
135. Scott HR, McMillan DC, Crilly A, et al: The relationship between weight loss and interleukin 6 in non–small cell lung cancer. Br J Cancer 1996; 73:1560–1562.
136. Pisa P, Stenke L, Bernell P, et al: Tumor necrosis factor and interferon γ in serum of multiple myeloma patients. Anticancer Res 1990; 10:817–820.
137. Pille S, Bohmer D: Options for artificial nutrition of cancer patients. Strahlenther Onkol 1998; 174 (suppl):52–55.
138. McGeer AJ, Detsky AS, O'Rourke K: Parenteral nutrition in cancer patients undergoing chemotherapy: a meta-analysis. Nutrition 1990; 6:233–240.
139. Mercadante S: Parenteral versus enteral nutrition in cancer patients: indications and practice. Support Care Cancer 1998; 6:85–93.
140. Body JJ: Metabolic sequelae of cancers (excluding bone marrow transplantation). Curr Opin Clin Nutr Metabol Care 1999; 2:339–344.
141. Tchekkmedyian NS, Heber D: Cancer and AIDS cachexia: mechanisms and approaches to therapy. Oncology 1993; 7:55–59.
142. Beal JE, Olson R, Laubenstein L, et al: Dronabinol as a treatment for anorexia associated with weight loss in patients with AIDS. J Pain Symptom Manage 1995; 10:89–97.
143. Loprinzi CL, Kuross SA, O'Fallon JR, et al: Randomized placebo controlled evaluation of hydrazine sulfate in patients with advanced colorectal cancer. J Clin Oncol 1994; 12:1126–1129.
144. Wigmore SJ, Falconer JS, Plester CE, et al: Ibuprofen reduces energy expenditure and acute-phase protein production compared with placebo in pancreatic cancer patients. Br J Cancer 1995; 72:185–188.
145. Wigmore SJ, Ross JA, Falconer JS, et al: The effect of polyunsaturated fatty acids on the progress of cachexia in patients with pancreatic cancer. Nutrition 1996; 12:S27–S30.
146. Tchekkmedyian NS, Tait N, Moody M, et al: High dose megestrol acetate: a possible treatment for cachexia. JAMA 1987; 9:1195–1198.
147. Loprinzi CL, Ellison NM, Schaid DJ, et al: Controlled trial of megestrol acetate for the treatment of cancer anorexia and cachexia. J Natl Cancer Inst 1990; 82:1127–1132.
148. Gebbia V, Testa A, Gebbia N: Prospective randomized trial of two dose levels of megestrol acetate in the management of anorexia cachexia syndrome in patients with metastatic cancer. Br J Cancer 1996; 73:1576–1580.
149. Loprinzi CL, Schaid DJ, Dose AM, et al: Body composition changes in patients who gain weight while receiving megestrol acetate. J Clin Oncol 1993; 11:52–154.
150. Scarantino CW, Ornitz RD, Hoffman LG, et al: On the mechanism of radiation-induced emesis: the role of serotonin. Int J Radiat Oncol Biol Phys 1994; 30:825–830.
151. Warr D: Standard treatment of chemotherapy-induced emesis. Support Care Cancer 1997; 5:12–16.
152. Kilpatrick GJ, Jones BJ, Tyers MB: Binding of the 5-HT3 ligands, [^{3}H]GR65630, to rat area postrema, vagus nerve and the brains of several species. Eur J Pharmacol 1989; 159:157–164.
153. Tavorath R, Hesketh PJ: Drug treatment of chemotherapy-induced delayed emesis. Drugs 1996; 52:639–648.
154. The Italian Group for Antiemetic Research in Radiotherapy: Radiation-induced emesis: a prospective observational multicenter Italian trial. Int J Radiat Oncol Biol Phys 1999; 44:619–625.
155. Drescheler S, Bruntsch U, Eggert J, et al: Comparison of three tropisetron-containing antiemetic regimens in the prophylaxis of acute and delayed chemotherapy-induced emesis and nausea. Support Care Cancer 1997; 5:387–395.
156. Yalcin S, Tekuzman G, Baltali E, et al: Serotonin receptor antagonism in prophylaxis of acute and delayed emesis induced by moderately emetogenic, single-day chemotherapy: a randomized study. Am J Clin Oncol 1999; 22:94–96.
157. Chang TC, Hsieh F, Lai CH, et al. Comparison of the efficacy of tropisetron versus a metoclopramide cocktail based on the intensity of cisplatin-induced emesis. Cancer Chemother Pharmacol 1996; 37:279–285.
158. Cunningham D, Dicato M, Verweij J, et al: Optimum anti-emetic therapy for cisplatin induced emesis over repeat courses: ondansetron plus dexamethasone compared with metoclopramide, dexamethasone plus lorazepam. Ann Oncol 1996; 7:277–282.
159. Maisano R, Pergolizzi S, Settineri N: Escalating dose of oral ondansetron in the prevention of radiation induced emesis. Anticancer Res 1998; 18:2011–2013.
160. Koseoglu V, Kurekci AE, Sarici U, et al: Comparison of the efficacy and side-effects of ondansetron and metoclopramide-diphenhydramine administered to control nausea and vomiting in children treated with antineoplastic chemotherapy: a prospective randomized study. Eur J Pediatr 1998; 157:806–810.
161. Fauser AA, Fellhauer M, Hoffmann M, et al: Guidelines for antiemetic therapy: acute emesis. Eur J Cancer 1999; 35:361–370.
162. Schwartz RH, Voth EA, Sheridan MJ: Marijuana to prevent nausea and vomiting in cancer patients: a survey in clinical oncologists. South Med J 1997; 90:167–172.
163. Vogelzang NJ, Breitbart W, Cella D, et al: Patient, caregiver, and oncologist perceptions of cancer-related fatigue: results of a tripart assessment survey. Semin Hematol 1997; 34 (suppl):4–12.

164. Thatcher N, De Campos ES, Bell DR, et al: Epoetin alpha prevents anaemia and reduces transfusion requirements in patients undergoing primarily platinum-based chemotherapy for small cell lung cancer. Br J Cancer 1999; 80:396–402.
165. Mock V, Dow KH, Meares CJ: et al: Effects of exercise on fatigue, physical functioning and emotional distress during radiation therapy for breast cancer. Oncol Nurs Forum 1997; 24:991–1000.
166. Ueoka H: Treatment for brain metastases of lung cancer. Gan To Kagaku Ryoho 1997; 24 (suppl):426–431.
167. Patchell RA, Tibbs PA, Walsh JW, et al: A randomized trial of surgery in the treatment of single metastases to the brain. N Engl J Med 1990; 322:494–500.
168. Vecht CJ, Haaxim-Reiche H, Noordijk EM, et al: Treatment of single brain metastasis: radiotherapy alone or in combination with neurosurgery? Ann Neurol 1993; 33:583–590.
169. Sundstrom JT, Minn H, Lertola KK, et al: Prognosis of patients treated for intracranial metastases with whole-brain irradiation. Ann Med 1998; 30:296–299.
170. Baumert B, Steinauer K, Lutolf UM: Therapy of CNS metastases. Ther Umsch 1999; 56:338–341.
171. Borgelt B, Gelber R: The palliation of brain metastases: final results of the first two studies by the RTOG. Int J Radiat Oncol Biol Phys 1980; 6:1–8.
172. Deiner-West M, Dobbins TW, Phillips TL, et al: Identification of an optimal subgroup for treatment evaluation of patients with brain metastases using RTOG study 79-16. Int J Radiat Oncol Biol Phys 1991; 16:669–673.
173. Coia LR: The role of radiation therapy in the treatment of brain metastases. Int J Radiat Oncol Biol Phys 1992; 23:229–238.
174. Wong WW, Schild SE, Sawyer TE, et al: Analysis of outcome in patients reirradiated for brain metastases. Int J Radiat Oncol Biol Phys 1996; 34:585–590.
175. Abdel-Wahab MM, Wolfson AH, Raub W, et al: The role of hyperfractionated re-irradiation in metastatic brain disease: a single institutional trial. Am J Clin Oncol 1997; 20:158–160.
176. Leksell L: The stereotactic method and radiosurgery of the brain. Acta Chirurgica Scandinavica 1951; 103:316–319.
177. Cho KH, Hall WA, Gerbi BJ, et al: Patient selection criteria for the treatment of brain metastases with stereotactic radiosurgery. J Neurooncol 1998; 40:73–86.
178. Becker G, Duffner F, Kortmann R, et al: Radiosurgery for the treatment of brain metastases in renal cell carcinoma. Anticancer Res 1999; 19:1611–1617.
179. Schoggl A, Kitz K, Ertl A, et al: Gamma-knife radiosurgery for brain metastases of renal cell carcinoma: results in 23 patients. Acta Neurochir (Wien) 1998; 140:549–555.
180. Seung SK, Sneed PK, McDermott MW, et al: Gamma knife radiosurgery for malignant melanoma brain metastases. Cancer J Sci Am 1998; 4:103–109.
181. Pirzkall A, Debus J, Lohr F, et al: Radiosurgery alone or in combination with whole-brain radiotherapy for brain metastases. J Clin Oncol 1998; 16:3563–3569.
182. Kondziolka D, Patel A, Lunsford LD, et al: Stereotactic radiosurgery plus whole brain radiotherapy versus radiotherapy alone for patients with multiple brain metastases. Int J Radiat Oncol Biol Phys 1999; 45:427–434.
183. Malacarne P, Santini A, Maestri A: Response of brain metastases from lung cancer to systemic chemotherapy with carboplatin and etoposide. Oncology 1996; 53:210–213.
184. Tummarello D, Lippe P, Bracci R, et al: First line chemotherapy in patients with brain metastases from non–small and small cell lung cancer. Oncol Rep 1998; 5:897–900.
185. Franciosi V, Cocconi G, Michiara M, et al: Front-line chemotherapy with cisplatin and etoposide for patients with brain metastases from breast carcinoma, nonsmall cell lung carcinoma, or malignant melanoma: a prospective study. Cancer 1999; 85:1599–1605.
186. Vinolas N, Graus F, Mellado B, et al: Phase II trial of cisplatinum and etoposide in brain metastases of solid tumors. J Neurooncol 1997; 35:145–148.
187. Legha SS, Ring S, Eton O, et al: Development of a biochemotherapy regimen with concurrent administration of cisplatin, vinblastine, dacarbazine, interferon alfa, and interleukin-2 for patients with metastatic melanoma. J Clin Oncol 1998; 16:1752–1759.
188. Oneschuk D, Bruera E: Palliative management of brain metastases. Support Care Cancer 1998; 6:365–372.
189. Hainsworth JD, Stroup SL, Greco FA: Paclitaxel, carboplatin, and extended schedule etoposide in the treatment of small cell lung cancer. Cancer 1996; 77:2458–2463.
190. Lee JS, Pisters KM, Komaki R, et al: Paclitaxel/carboplatin chemotherapy as primary treatment of brain metastases in non–small cell lung cancer: a preliminary report. Semin Oncol 1997; 24 (suppl):S52–S55.
191. Byrne TN: Spinal cord compression from epidermal metastases. N Engl J Med 1992; 327:614–619.
192. Scarantino CW: Metastatic spinal cord compression: criteria for effective treatment—regarding Maranzano et al, IJROBP 32:957–967; 1995. Int J Radiat Oncol Biol Phys 1995; 32:1259–1260.
193. Loblaw DA, Laperriere NJ: Emergency treatment of malignant extradural spinal cord compression: an evidence-based guideline. J Clin Oncol 1998; 16:1613–1624.
194. Maranzano E, Latini P, Beneventi S, et al: Radiation therapy in metastatic spinal cord compression. A prospective analysis of 105 consecutive patients. Ann Neurol 1991; 3:40–51.
195. Maranzano E, Latini P: Effectiveness of radiation therapy without surgery in metastatic spinal cord compression: final results from a prospective trial. Int J Radiat Oncol Biol Phys 1995; 32:959–967.
196. Kim RY, Spencer SA, Meredith RF, et al: Extradural spinal cord compression: Analysis of factors determining functional prognosis—prospective study. Radiology 1990; 176:279–282.
197. Solberg A, Bremnes RM: Metastatic spinal cord decompression: diagnostic delay, treatment, and outcome. Anticancer Res 1999; 19:677–684.
198. Wallington M, Mendis S, Premawardhana U, et al: Local control and survival in spinal cord compression from lymphoma and myeloma. Radiother Oncol 1997; 42:43–47.
199. Leviov M, Dale J, Stein M, et al: The management of metastatic spinal cord compression: a radiotherapeutic success ceiling. Int J Radiat Oncol Biol Phys 1993; 27:231–234.
200. Wagner W, Prott FJ, Rube C, et al: Radiotherapy of epidural metastases with spinal cord compression. Strahlenther Onkol 1996; 172:604–609.
201. Clain A: Secondary malignant disease of bone. Br J Cancer 1965; 19:15.
202. Harrington K: Orthopedic surgical management of skeletal complications of malignancy. Cancer 1997; 80:1614–1627.
203. Tong D, Gillich L, Henderson FR: The palliation of symptomatic osseous metastases: final results of the study by the radiation therapy oncology group. Cancer 1982; 50:893–899.
204. Blitzer P: Reanalysis of the RTOG study of the palliation of symptomatic osseous metastasis. Cancer 1985; 55:1468–1472.
205. Rasmusson B, Vejborg I, Jensen AB, et al: Irradiation of bone metastases in breast cancer patients: a randomized study with 1 year follow-up. Radiother Oncol 1995; 34:179–184.
206. Price P, Hoskin PJ, Easton D, et al: Prospective randomized trial of single and multifraction radiotherapy schedules in the treatment of painful bony metastases. Radiother Oncol 1986; 6:247–255.
207. Cole DJ: A randomized trial of a single treatment versus conventional fractionation in the palliative radiotherapy of painful bone metastases. Clin Oncol 1989; 1:59–62.
208. Poulter CA, Cosmatos D, Rubin P, et al: A report of RTOG 8206: a phase III study of whether the addition of single dose hemibody irradiation to standard fractionated local field irradiation is more effective than local field irradiation alone in the treatment of symptomatic osseous metastases. Int J Radiat Oncol Biol Phys 1992; 23:207–214.
209. Scarantino CW, Caplan R, Rotman M, et al: A phase I/II study to evaluate the effect of fractionated hemibody irradiation in the treatment of osseous metastases—RTOG 88-22. Int J Radiat Oncol Biol Phys 1996; 36:37–48.
210. Ben-Josef E, Porter AT: Radioisotopes in the treatment of bone metastasis. Ann Med 1997; 29:31–35.
211. Mertens WC, Filipczak LA, Ben-Josef E, et al: Systemic bone-seeking radionuclides for palliation of painful osseous metastases: current concepts. CA Cancer J Clin 1998; 48:361–374.
212. Silberstein EB, Elgazzar AH, Kapilivsky A: Phosphorus-32 radiopharmaceuticals for the treatment of painful osseous metastases. Semin Nucl Med 1992; 22:17–27.
213. Baumrucker S: Palliation of painful bone metastases: strontium 89. Am J Hospice Palliat Care 1998; 15:113–115.
214. Blake GM, Zivanovic MA, Blaquiere RM, et al: Strontium-89 ther-

apy: measurement of absorbed dose to skeletal metastases. J Nucl Med 1988; 29:549–557.

215. Dearnaley DP, Bayly RJ, A'Hern RP, et al: Palliation of bone metastases in prostate cancer. Hemibody irradiation or strontium-89? Clin Oncol (R Coll Radiol) 1992; 4:101–107.
216. Pons F, Herranz R, Garcia A, et al: Strontium-89 for palliation of pain from bone metastases in patients with prostate cancer. Eur J Nucl Med 1997; 24:1210–1214.
217. Berna L, Carrio I, Alonso C, et al: Bone pain palliation with strontium-89 in breast cancer patients with bone metastases and refractory bone pain. Eur J Nucl Med 1995; 22:1101–1104.
218. Resche I, Chatal JF, Pecking A, et al: A dose-controlled study of ^{153}Sm-ethylenediaminetetramethylenephosphonate (EDTMP) in the treatment of patients with painful bone metastases. Eur J Cancer 1997; 33:1583–1591.
219. Serafini AN, Houston SJ, Resche I, et al: Palliation of pain associated with metastatic bone cancer using samarium-153 lexidronum: a double-blind placebo-controlled clinical trial. J Clin Oncol 1998; 16:1574–1581.
220. Reichardt P: Systemic hormone- and chemotherapy in the management of skeletal metastases. Orthopade 1998; 27:240–244.
221. Harvey HA: Issues concerning the role of chemotherapy and hormonal therapy of bone metastases from breast carcinoma. Cancer 1997; 80 (suppl):1646–1651.
222. Louvet C, de Gramont A, Demuynck B, et al: Folinic acid, 5-fluorouracil bolus and infusion and mitoxantrone with or without cyclophosphamide in metastatic breast cancer. Eur J Cancer 1993; 29A:1835–1838.
223. Nomura Y, Tominga T, Adachi I, et al: Clinical evaluation of cyclophosphamide, methotrexate and 5-fluorouracil (CMF) on advanced and recurrent breast cancer. Clinical study group of CMF for breast cancer in Japan. Gan To Gakaku Ryoho 1994; 21:1949–1956.
224. Ardvanis A, Extra JM, Espie M, et al: Phase II trial of a combination of vinorelbine, cyclophosphamide and 5-fluorouracil in the treatment of advanced breast cancer. In Vivo 1998; 12:559–562.
225. Lortholary A, Jadaud E, Berthaud P: Bisphosphonates and bone metastases. Bull Cancer 1999; 86:732–738.
226. Theriault RL, Lipton A, Hortobagyi GN, et al: Pamidronate reduces skeletal morbidity in women with advanced breast cancer and lytic bone lesions: a randomized, placebo-controlled trial. Protocol 18 Aredia Breast Cancer Study Group. J Clin Oncol 1999; 17:846–854.
227. Kristensen B, Ejlertsen B, Groenvold M, et al: Oral clodronate in breast cancer patients with bone metastases: a randomized study. J Intern Med 1999; 246:67–74.
228. Coleman RE, Purohit OP, Black V, et al: Double-blind, randomised, placebo-controlled study of oral ibandronate in patients with metastatic bone disease. Ann Oncol 1999; 10:311–316.
229. Pogrebniak HW, Hass G, Linehan WM, et al: Renal cell carcinomas: resection of solitary and multiple metastases. Ann Thorac Surg 1992; 54:33–38.
230. McAfee MK, Allen MS, Trastek VF, et al: Colorectal lung metastases: results of surgical excision. Ann Thorac Surg 1992; 53:780–786.
231. Scarantino CW, Salazar OM, Rubin P, et al: The optimum schedule in treatment of superior vena canal obstruction: importance of ^{99m}Tc scintiangiograms. Int J Radiat Oncol Biol Phys 1979; 5:1987–1995.
232. Mehta MP, Kinsella TJ: Superior vena cava syndrome. In: Roth JA, Ruckdeschel JC, Weisenburger TH (eds): Thoracic Oncology, pp 239–258. Philadelphia, W.B. Saunders, 1995.
233. Urban T, LeBeau B, Chastang C, et al: Superior vena cava syndrome in small-cell lung cancer. Arch Intern Med 1993; 153:384–387.
234. Pignon JP, Arriagada R, Ihde DC, et al: A meta-analysis of thoracic radiotherapy for small-cell lung cancer. N Engl J Med 1992; 327:1618–1624.
235. Murray N, Coy P, Pater J, et al: Importance of timing for thoracic irradiation in the combined modality treatment of limited stage small cell lung cancer. J Clin Oncol 1993; 11:336–344.
236. Leibel SA, Pajak TF, Massullo V, et al: A comparison of misonidazole sensitized radiation therapy to radiation therapy alone for palliation of hepatic metastases: results of a Radiation Therapy Oncology Group randomized prospective trial. Int J Radiat Oncol Biol Phys 1987; 13:1057–1064.
237. Russell AH, Clyde C, Wasserman TH, et al: Accelerated hyperfractionated hepatic irradiation in the management of patients with liver metastases: results of the RTOG dose escalating protocol. Int J Radiat Oncol Biol Phys 1993; 27:117–123.
238. Kemeny NE, Ron IG: Hepatic arterial chemotherapy in metastatic colorectal patients. Semin Oncol 1999; 26:524–535.
239. Link KH, Pillasch J, Formentini A, et al. Downstaging by regional chemotherapy of non-resectable isolated colorectal liver metastases. Eur J Surg Oncol 1999; 25:381–388.
240. Giacchetti S, Itzhaki M, Gruia G, et al: Long-term survival of patients with unresectable colorectal cancer liver metastases following infusional chemotherapy with 5-fluorouracil, leucovorin, oxaliplatin and surgery. Ann Oncol 1999; 10:663–669.
241. Howell JD, Warren HW, Anderson JH, et al: Intra-arterial 5-fluorouracil and intravenous folinic acid in the treatment of live metastases from colorectal cancer. Eur J Surg 1999; 165:652–658.
242. Bates T, Yarold JR, Blitzer P, et al: Bone metastasis consensus statement. Int J Radiat Oncol Biol Phys 1992; 23:215–216.

32 Cancer Pain Management: An Essential Component of Comprehensive Cancer Care

RICHARD B. PATT, MD, Anesthesiology

We must all die. But that I can save him from days of torture, that is what I feel is my great and ever new privilege. Pain is a more terrible lord of mankind than even death himself.

ALBERT SCHWEITZER

Perspective

Until recently, curative and even palliative treatments for patients with neoplastic disease have focused on survival, whereas supportive care was more likely to be regarded as a secondary consideration, pertaining uniquely to the end of life.[1, 2] Initiatives in the 1990s, emphasizing the concept of comprehensive cancer care, mandated that attention to symptom control and psychosocial concerns be applied in an integrated fashion throughout the course of a cancer diagnosis.[3, 4] Contemporary approaches to managing pain and other symptoms emphasize earlier and more liberal use of opioids, recognizing their low addiction potential and overall favorable risk-benefit ratio.[5–7] A second important concept, which has only recently become well established, relates to the use of the less traditional adjuvant analgesics (e.g., antidepressants, anticonvulsants) for specific types of pain. The role of invasive pain therapies, though critical, remains less well defined.[8–10] Although the principles of contemporary pain management more than ever constitute a fundamental area of knowledge for providers of cancer care, unfortunately they are underused.

The prospect of suffering from unrelieved pain is one of the most feared aspects of a cancer diagnosis for most patients and their families. Optimal management parallels that of cancer treatment and involves careful assessment, individualization of therapy, close follow-up, and a proactive approach. Adequate control of pain can be achieved in the vast majority of patients with the rigorous and aggressive application of measures that are ultimately quite straightforward. Patients are reassured and symptoms are easier to control when it is communicated that pain is treatable, and that symptom control is one of the treatment team's priorities. Optimal control of pain and related symptoms facilitates cancer treatment and promotes an enhanced quality of life, improved functioning, better compliance, and a means for patients to focus on those things that give meaning to life.

Epidemiology and Undertreatment

Pain is among the most common symptoms associated with cancer, affecting about two thirds of patients overall.[11–13] A considerable proportion of patients (15% to 25%) experience significant pain in association with early, localized, even curable disease. If pain is poorly controlled in this setting, its effects may reduce the patient's compliance with plans for demanding cytotoxic therapies and, by influencing performance status, may exclude patients from entering protocols for investigational therapies. With the development of metastases, the incidence of pain increases to 40% to 60% of patients, and in far advanced disease, 60% to 90% of patients report significant pain. As curative options become exhausted, the focus of care shifts, and symptom control assumes paramount importance.

Despite vast improvements in our understanding of pain and its management over the last decade, it is curious and, indeed, tragic that despite the availability of straightforward, cost-effective therapies, cancer pain remains undertreated even in developed nations.[11, 14, 15] The factors contributing to undertreatment are complex but well documented. Undertreatment is usually conceived of as relating to knowledge deficits, beliefs, and attitudes maintained by (1) health care providers, (2) patients and family members, and (3) regulators and health care delivery systems.[16] Representative barriers are listed in Table 32–1. The most prevalent underlying issues relate to an inadequate understanding of the pharmacology of the opioid drugs, and exaggerated fears of addiction. Thus, workable solutions relate less to developing new drugs or technology, and

TABLE 32–1. **Barriers to Effective Cancer Pain Management**

A. Health Care Provider–Related Barrier

1. Lack of education and knowledge regarding:
   a. assessment and management of pain, e.g., pharmacology of chronically administered opioids, management of opioid-mediated side effects
   b. assessment and management of refractory pain, especially use of alternative treatments, e.g., adjuvant analgesics (antidepressants, anticonvulsants, etc.), parenteral routes, other treatment modalities
   c. risks of analgesic therapy, e.g., addiction vs. physical dependence vs. tolerance, respiratory depression
2. Outdated beliefs:
   a. Pain is an unmanageable and inevitable feature of advanced cancer.
   b. Use of opioids at effective doses is equivalent to euthanasia.
   c. Opioids should be reserved for the dying patient.
   d. Patient reports of pain are unreliable.
3. Reluctance to use triplicate prescriptions:
   a. added cost and effort
   b. fear of reprisal from regulatory agencies
   c. restrictions due to limits on quantities prescribed and telephone refills
4. Practice management:
   a. lack of time, energy, motivation to make the frequent changes necessary to maintain pain control
   b. inability to recognize patients' reluctance to discuss pain

B. Cultural or Health Care System–Related Barrier

1. War on drugs:
   a. failure to distinguish between illicit and medicinal use
   b. restrictive limits on prescribing
   c. failure of pharmacies to stock strong opioids
2. Medical education:
   a. Medical school curricula and residency training programs do not provide information or adequate reference material on management of chronic pain.
   b. They do not recognize pain management or palliative care as legitimate subspecialty.
   c. Texts fail to distinguish between acute and chronic pain.
3. Health care:
   a. Acute disease-oriented health care model leads to lack of accountability for control of chronic symptoms, failure to coordinate as patient moves between care settings (e.g., hospital, home, nursing home).
   b. There are inadequate resources for procedurally based pain management.
   c. There is fragmentation of care due to multiple specialists.
   d. There is resultant failure of some insurers to provide hospice care or to consider reimbursement for treatment aimed at comfort.

C. Patient and Family-Related Barriers

1. Beliefs:
   a. Pain inevitably accompanies cancer and is unmanageable.
   b. Painkillers must be withheld until late in the disease process or they will not be effective.
   c. Opioids have serious side effects, making people incoherent and high, and leading to addiction.
   d. Opioids are associated with serious illness; they may hasten death or signify the disease is incurable.
2. War on drugs:
   a. pressure (family, media, government) **never** to take opioids under any circumstances
3. Reluctance to discuss pain with health care provider:
   a. desire to be seen as a "good" patient
   b. complaints may be regarded as weak character or an insult to the providers
   c. reluctance to "use up" doctor's time
   d. fear of an acknowledgement that the cancer has returned or is progressing

instead involve improving the utilization of currently available techniques.

Assessment

Assessment is the cornerstone for developing a diagnosis and an effective treatment plan, and should be explicitly performed in all cancer patients (Tables 32–2 to 32–4). The experience of pain varies according to many factors, including the meaning it imparts to the patient, and, as a result, the initial encounter should be broad-based. In addition to focusing the inquiry on the pain syndrome *per se* (Table 32–5), the process should encompass evaluation of the person, his or her feelings and attitudes about pain and disease, and family concerns.

Published guidelines recommend that pain be assessed initially and then reassessed at regular intervals, at each new report of pain, and at suitable times following new interventions (e.g., 15–30 minutes after parenteral therapy and 1 hour after oral therapy) (see Table 32–3).

The assessment process may also serve an educational purpose. The prognosis for pain control is usually good, and orienting patients, family, and referring physicians to what realistically can be accomplished should be reassuring. A compassionate but objective approach to assessment establishes a therapeutic alliance and serves to instill confidence in the patient and family that will be of value throughout treatment (see Table 32–4).

Physiology of Nociception

Classically, pain is understood to be initiated by injury to peripheral tissue that results in the activation of deep and

TABLE 32–2. **General Principles of Pain Management in the Cancer Patient: Assessment**

- Assess the patient carefully prior to initiating treatment. A careful history and directed physical examination (especially of the painful region and neurologic and musculoskeletal systems) are essential.
- Assess pain in a global context. Elicit past medical history, oncologic and social history, and presence of other distressing symptoms. Seek history of alcohol or drug abuse.
- Listen to and believe the patient's reports of pain and other symptoms, as well as the observations of the patient's relations.
- Ask explicitly about the presence and nature of pain and other symptoms. Pertinent information is often not otherwise volunteered.
- Seek the presence of multiple complaints of pain. When multiple complaints exist, they should each be evaluated as discrete, independent entities, as well as in their wider context. When appropriate, prioritize complaints based on how distressing they are, as well as their treatability.
- Assess the characteristics of each pain complaint: chronicity, location and referral or radiation, severity (best, worst, average, current), quality, temporal features, associated symptoms, aggravating and relieving factors.
- Assess pain complaints globally: In addition to pertinent physical aspects, assessment and ultimately management should address emotional, psychological, environmental, and spiritual factors that influence pain and well-being.
- Determine beneficial and adverse effects for each analgesic in current use, as well as those taken in the past. Determine to what degree trials of other agents have been adequate and thorough.
- Determine to what degree pain and other symptoms are distressing and interfere with activities that are important to the patient.
- Consider the use of a simple, validated, written instrument that can be rapidly completed to document self-report (e.g., Brief Pain Inventory or Memorial Pain Assessment Card).
- Teach and encourage the consistent use of a simple verbal tool to monitor pain intensity (e.g., 0–10, none–slight–moderate–severe).
- Develop a problem list based on data obtained during assessment.
- Based on the initial evaluation, develop a provisional diagnosis for the cause and type of each pain.
- Formulate a treatment plan that includes primary recommendations for each targeted symptom, with contingencies for titration or alternate interventions.
- Obtain and personally review needed diagnostic tests.
- Document findings and recommendations in the medical record, and communicate with the patient and family and the referring and other treating physicians.

cutaneous pain receptors (nociceptors) by a variety of stimuli that involve both mechanical trauma and the release of biochemical mediators such as prostaglandins, serotonin, norepinephrine, substance P, and bradykinin.[17] Stimuli are relayed along sensory afferent pathways to the dorsal root ganglia. Neurons synapse in the dorsal root, where the first level of processing occurs. Incoming electrical impulses are modified by the integration of additional excitatory and inhibitory information from adjacent afferent neurons, and from descending pathways originating in the brain via the thalamus and other structures. From the dorsal root, the afferent signal crosses and ascends the spinothalamic tract. The spinothalamic tracts radiate branches to the medulla, pons, midbrain, and especially the thalamus, where further processing occurs. Finally, the neospinothalamic tract enters the cortex and terminates in the postcentral gyrus, producing an awareness of the initial stimulus, which is only then finally interpreted as pain.

TABLE 32–3. **General Principles of Pain Management in the Cancer Patient: Reassessment**

- Reassess at appropriate, individualized intervals: Gauge response to interventions; monitor for disease progression, development of new symptoms.
- Reassess at frequent intervals after initial evaluation/commencing new drugs/performing an intervention (e.g., nerve block).
- Use pre-established verbal tools to assess pain intensity longitudinally (e.g., 0–10, none–slight–moderate–severe).
- When reassessing, ask about efficacy and side effects of current treatment regimen.
- When reassessing, routinely inquire about bowel habit, nausea, and alertness.
- Be alert to findings consistent with epidural spinal cord compression and other neurologic syndromes. Pertinent information is often not otherwise volunteered.
- Review problem list and progress made in treating each distressing symptom.
- Encourage patients to focus on whether symptoms have improved, rather than whether they have been entirely eliminated.
- Determine overall satisfaction with treatment.
- Document findings and recommendations in medical record, and communicate changes in condition and modifications in treatment regimen with referring and other treating physicians.

Modulation occurs by descending signals that originate from the periaqueductal gray nuclei of the midbrain (a major locus for opioid receptors), synapse in the medulla, and then travel to the dorsal horn nuclei via the medial descending pathways, decreasing the intensity of incoming painful stimuli. Serotonin, substance P, dopamine, norepinephrine, and other neurotransmitters are all important modulators of the afferent and efferent limbs of pain sensation. These neurotransmitters, as well as the endogenous opioid peptides enkephalin, beta endorphin, and dynorphin, interact at a synaptic level within the spinal cord and brain to accentuate or diminish the sensation of pain. Synapses within the ascending and descending pathways also contain opioid receptors, which are the target sites for opioid analgesics. Research is under way to localize these receptors more accurately, and thus to allow more specific analgesia with potentially fewer side effects.

Physiology of Pain

Even a detailed account of tissue injury and nociception does not sufficiently characterize the end result of these events—the phenomenon of pain. Pain, as defined by the International Association for the Study of Pain, is "an unpleasant sensory and emotional experience associated with actual or potential tissue damage or described in terms

TABLE 32–4. **General Principles of Pain Management in the Cancer Patient: Management**

- Develop and apply an algorithmic approach to each pain problem, always being prepared to modify care plans based on individual features of a patient's presentation and response.
- When feasible, treat pain by attempting to modify its cause, usually with antineoplastic therapy. Institute concurrent symptomatic treatment with analgesics while awaiting therapeutic response, which may be delayed.
- Select specific drugs for specific reasons.
- Keep the treatment regimen simple whenever possible. Avoid polypharmacy unless indicated for specific reasons. Review drug regimen regularly and consider discontinuing agents that are of questionable value. They can always be restarted.
- Maintain exquisite familiarity with a core group of drugs that are frequently used. Ensure ready access to reliable information on less frequently prescribed drugs.
- Be knowledgeable about the range of side effects associated with prescribed drugs. When considering drugs with similar primary effects, be aware of the opportunity to exploit "side effects" (secondary effects) that may be beneficial in a given patient (e.g., nighttime use of a sedating antidepressant for neuropathic pain in a patient with concomitant insomnia).
- Start new drugs in low doses and be prepared to titrate dose upwards rapidly once a therapeutic response and the presence or absence of side effects have been established.
- Avoid starting multiple drugs simultaneously, both to minimize the risk of drug interactions and to avoid uncertainty about which agent is responsible for changes.
- Always express a generic willingness to help the patient and family. Ask explicitly what they want or need. Be aware that it may not be a prescription, but advice or just an empathetic listener. Never say or imply "nothing more can be done."
- Consider nonpharmacologic therapies, both invasive (antineoplastic, anesthetic, neurosurgical, orthopedic) and noninvasive (behavioral, counseling, physiatric), when appropriate.
- Discuss treatment decisions with patient and family members. When appropriate, present options in the context of their alternatives and relative risk and benefit. Always try to provide clear recommendations based on your knowledge of the patient and the merits of each treatment option.
- Provide education to the patient and family or significant others regarding all aspects of treatment. When appropriate, involve the family in establishing realistic goals. Seek their help in maintaining compliance with treatment recommendations. Interact with family members in a supportive manner that communicates concern about their well-being and a willingness to ease their distress.
- Encourage patients to understand their illness and the treatments they are receiving and to maintain and carry with them a list of medications they take. When appropriate, provide instructions on the use of pain diaries.
- Discuss advanced directives when appropriate.

of such."[18] This widely accepted concept of pain as a multiply determined personal experience recognizes that pain cannot be simply equated with tissue damage, even if the extent of such injury could be accurately determined. Pain is better understood as a process that is the product of the influence of multiple factors, both biochemical-physiologic (tumor site and size, associated inflammation, etc.), and psychological-spiritual (previous experiences, meaning or significance of pain, attendant suffering).[19–21] As such, patients with identical x-ray films may present with dramatically different symptoms and may respond to analgesics in widely disparate ways. This broader view of the experience of pain requires that a carefully individualized approach be applied to the patient, based on the clinician's willingness to believe the patient's self-report.[22]

TABLE 32–5. **Elements of a Comprehensive Pain History**

Premorbid chronic pain
Premorbid drug or alcohol use
Pain catalogue (number and locations)
For each pain:

- Onset and evolution
- Site and radiation
- Pattern (constant, intermittent, predictable, etc.)
- Intensity (best, worst, average, current): 0–10 scale
- Quality
- Exacerbating factors
- Relieving factors
- How the pain interferes
- Neurologic and motor abnormalities
- Vasomotor changes
- Other associated factors
- Current analgesics (use, efficacy, side effects)
- Prior analgesics (use, efficacy, side effects)

PAIN CHARACTERISTICS

Various schemata for classifying cancer pain have been suggested that, especially when applied together, have potential utility to aid in diagnosis and management (Table 32–6).[23] Although efforts at classification help guide treatment, pain in the cancer patient is ultimately an individual phenomenon, and optimal treatment requires careful assessment and management tailored to meet the unique needs of the individual patient.

Etiology and Pathophysiology

Given the variety of clinically relevant methods for classifying cancer pain, classification is best approached by considering a general schema first. Foremost in this context is a broad etiologic classification that distinguishes among the general causes of pain in patients with cancer (Table 32–7). Tumor invasion accounts for two thirds to three quarters of significant pain in cancer patients, with most of the remainder of cases consisting of sequelae of cancer therapy and, to a lesser extent, diagnostic procedures. A smaller proportion of pain problems results from general debility, chronic illness, and chronic disorders that predate and are not directly related to the diagnosis of cancer, such as degenerative joint disease or disc protrusion (premorbid chronic pain).

In addition to its etiology, cancer pain can be considered as emanating from a variety of pathophysiologic processes. Tumor-mediated pain may emanate from mechanisms that

TABLE 32–6. **Methods of Classifying Cancer Pain**

Method	Example	Clinical Significance
General etiology	Tumor-related pain Treatment-related pain Procedure-related pain Debility and chronic illness Premorbid chronic pain	Broadest of all classification schema. Determination of general etiology aids the clinician in formulating a rational treatment plan that takes into account the patient's prognosis for survival and the natural longitudinal course of the painful condition. Recognition of the broad underlying cause of pain is useful in determining what resources are best applied for management.
Chronicity	Acute Chronic	Relative acuity/chronicity helps determine the degree to which pain should be regarded as a diagnostic sign that may signal new underlying pathology. Acute pain may be more likely to respond to treatment directed at its source. Patients with chronic pain may require additional interdisciplinary resources to help manage depression and suffering, and to facilitate rehabilitation.
Severity or intensity	Mild, moderate, severe Visual Analogue Scale faces 0–10 numerical score	Usual determinant of the potency of prescribed analgesic (NSAID for mild pain, "weak" opioid for moderate pain, "strong" opioid for severe pain). Regular measurement is required to gauge treatment outcome.
Pathophysiology	Somatic nociceptive Visceral nociceptive Neuropathic	By helping target the source of pain, more specific treatment may be offered (e.g., sympathetic block for visceral nociceptive pain). The presence of neuropathic pain, which is typically less opioid responsive than nociceptive pain, is an important feature because adjuvant analgesics (antidepressants, anticonvulsants, oral local anesthetics) may play a relatively more important role.
Syndromal presentation	Plexopathy, cord compression, postsurgical syndromes, etc.	Recognition may provide valuable information about etiology, prognosis, and optimal treatment.
Disease stage	Newly diagnosed or recurrent disease, curable vs. terminal disease, etc.	May suggest specific treatment options and may predict response to therapy, e.g.: Patients in active treatment may exhibit high pain thresholds and may be reluctant to report pain, whereas pain control is usually a high priority for patients with terminal disease.
Patient characteristic	Anxiety, distant/recent history of alcohol or drug use, etc.	Special features may help determine need for multimodal therapy.
Temporal features	Constant, intermittent, mixed, breakthrough pain	Helps determine optimal schedule for prescribing analgesic drugs (p.r.n. vs. around-the-clock, vs. around-the-clock + p.r.n.)
Responsivity	Highly opioid responsive, moderately opioid responsive, poorly opioid responsive	Empiric responsivity to opioids, adjuvants, and other modalities helps determine the best treatment strategy in a given patient.

NSAID = nonsteroidal anti-inflammatory drug; p.r.n. = as needed.

include inflammation, edema, or necrosis of pain-sensitive tissues, or impingement on neighboring structures. Specific mechanisms include invasion of bone or soft tissues, obstruction of lymphatic and vascular channels, mesenteric torsion, distention of a hollow viscus, capsular stretch of a solid viscus, and involvement of nervous system structures. The underlying pathologic processes and events that appear to initiate and maintain pain (Table 32–8) are typically inferred by the patient's clinical presentation and the results of diagnostic imaging studies. Although it is often the case that more than one mechanism is operant, it remains useful to determine the predominant mechanism in order to plan treatment directed at the source of pain.

TABLE 32–7. **Classification of Cancer Pain by General Etiology**

- Pain due to direct effects of tumor progression (e.g., compression or ischemia of pain-sensitive structures)
- Pain due to cancer treatment (e.g., osteoradionecrosis, chemotherapy-induced neuropathy, postmastectomy syndrome)
- Pain due to diagnostic procedures (e.g., venipuncture, lumbar puncture, bone marrow biopsy)
- Pain due to chronic illness and debility (e.g., muscle spasm from prolonged bed rest, decubitus ulcers)
- Premorbid chronic pain (e.g., chronic radiculitis, osteoarthritis)

TABLE 32–8. **Classification of Cancer Pain by Its Underlying Pathophysiology**

- Tumor invasion or compression of pain-sensitive structures (e.g., periosteum, nerve, muscle)
- Reflex neural activity arising from nerve invasion or compression (neuropathic pain with wind-up)
- Pressure and obstruction of lymphatics and vessels
- Localized edema and inflammation
- Distention, stretch, or abnormal contraction (reflex spasm) of hollow viscera
- Stretch of the capsule surrounding solid viscera
- Ischemia or necrosis of smooth muscle of hollow viscera
- Chemical irritation of the serosal or mucosal surfaces of hollow viscera
- Distention, traction, or torsion of mesenteric and vascular attachments of viscera

Tumor-Mediated Versus Treatment-Related Pain

The incidence of pain due to cancer therapy is naturally greater in communities in which antineoplastic therapy is administered aggressively, and conversely, the incidence of pain as a result of tumor progression is typically greater in rural or less-developed regions in which cancer treatment is prescribed less intensively, either because patients initially present with advanced disease that is beyond treatment or because limited resources preclude comprehensive treatment. Pain that is progressively severe or that spreads, especially to anatomically unrelated areas, is more likely to be directly related to tumoral activity than to cancer treatment.

Pain related to cancer treatment typically has mixed neuropathic and musculoskeletal features, is more likely to remain localized to the same region, and, although it may wax and wane, its severity is less likely to steadily mount than when symptoms are the result of tumor progression. Because evidence of tissue damage may be absent, treatment-related pain is often poorly understood and is more likely to be undertreated, especially in the cancer survivor who is in remission. Despite survivorship, significant pain may persist indefinitely, particularly with tumors associated with intensive treatment (e.g., head and neck), but also after more apparently innocuous therapies such as mastectomy[24] or chemotherapy.[25, 26] Various pain syndromes (see later discussion) have been described both for tumor-mediated[27] and treatment-related[28] pain (Table 32–9) that are unique to the cancer population and that are characterized by more discrete clinical features.

Pain Resulting from Diagnostic Procedures

Although pain resulting from cancer or its treatment is typically chronic and ongoing, pain related to diagnostic procedures is acute and transient in nature. Pain as a result of diagnostic procedures is an especially important consideration in children because routine procedures (e.g., venipuncture, lumbar puncture, bone marrow aspiration, biopsy) that are often viewed as innocuous by adults are a major source of distress in children.[29] Distress and pain produce similar behavioral responses in children and thus may be difficult to distinguish.[30] Unfortunately, the signifi-

TABLE 32–9. **Examples of Cancer Pain Syndromes**

Bone invasion	Presentation is variable; usually constant, often greatest at night and with movement or weight bearing; often a dull ache or deep, intense pain; may be associated with referred pain, muscle spasm, or, when there is nerve compression, paroxysms of stabbing pain
Vertebral body invasion	Often presents as severe, localized, dull, steady, aching pain; often exacerbated by recumbency, sitting, movement, and local pressure; may be relieved by standing; localized midline tenderness may be present; associated nerve compression may produce radiating dermatomal pain and corresponding neurologic changes; may be associated with epidural–spinal cord compression
Base of skull metastases	Numerous specific syndromes described (middle fossa syndrome, jugular foramen syndrome, clivus metastases, orbital metastases, parasellar metastases, sphenoid sinus metastases, occipital condyle invasion, odontoid fractures); usually present with headache and a spectrum of neurologic findings, especially involving cranial nerves; usually a late finding; may be difficult to diagnose radiographically
Nerve invasion	Typically a constant, burning dysesthetic pain, often with an intermittent lancinating, electrical component; may be associated with neurologic deficit or diffuse hyperesthesia and localized paresthesia; muscle weakness and atrophy may be present in mixed or motor nerve syndromes
Leptomeningeal metastases, meningeal carcinomatosis	Most common with primary malignancies of breast and lung, lymphoma, and leukemia; headache is most common presenting complaint; characteristically unrelenting, may be associated with nausea, vomiting, nuchal rigidity, and mental status changes; associated neurologic abnormalities may include seizures, cranial nerve deficits, papilledema, hemiparesis, ataxia and cauda equina syndrome; diagnosis confirmed with lumbar puncture
Spinal cord compression	Pain almost always precedes neurologic changes; urgent radiologic work-up required for rapid progression of neurologic deficit, particularly motor weakness, or incontinence; early treatment may limit neurologic morbidity
Cervical plexopathy	May result from local invasion by head and neck cancers or pressure from enlarged nodes; symptoms primarily sensory, experienced as aching preauricular, postauricular, or neck pain
Brachial plexopathy	Most commonly due to upper lobe lung cancer (Pancoast's syndrome), breast cancer, or lymphoma; pain is an early symptom, usually preceding neurologic findings; usually diffuse aching in shoulder girdle, radiating down arm, often to the elbow and medial (ulnar) aspect of the hand; Horner's syndrome, dysesthesias, progressive atrophy, and neurologic impairment (weakness and numbness) may occur; must differentiate from radiation fibrosis, which characteristically is less severe, less often associated with motor changes, tends to involve the upper trunks, and may be associated with lymphedema
Lumbosacral plexopathy	May be due to local soft tissue invasion or compression; pain is usually presenting sign; may be referred to lower back, abdomen, buttocks, or lower extremity
Celiac plexopathy	Usually relentless, boring, midepigastric aching pain radiating to midback; often relieved by fetal position and worse with recumbency
Chemotherapy-induced polyneuropathy	Most common with vincristine, vinblastine, and cisplatin; may include jaw pain, claudication, and dysesthetic pain in the hands or feet
Postsurgical syndromes	Most common after mastectomy, thoracotomy, radical neck dissection, nephrectomy, and amputation; usually aching, shooting, or tingling in distribution of peripheral nerves (intercostal brachial and intercostal cervical plexus, etc.) with or without skin hypersensitivity

cance and even the existence of procedure-related pain are often not considered as a result of busy hospital routines, outmoded beliefs that children do not appreciate or remember pain, and insufficient resources. Treatment with standard pharmacologic and behavioral approaches, especially using parents as coaches, is usually effective but requires proactive, systematic application, usually in a programmatic context.[31] Effective management is especially important from the start to avoid anticipatory distress in children, especially when repeated painful diagnostic procedures are planned.

Premorbid Chronic Pain

Patients with pre-existing chronic pain resulting from traumatic, degenerative, or idiopathic causes comprise a smaller proportion of consultations for pain control. Assessment and management of these patients may be more complex because of the presence of psychological adaptation and established pain behaviors.[32]

CHRONICITY OF PAIN: ACUTE VERSUS CHRONIC PAIN

Acute pain is frequently associated with signs of sympathetic hyperactivity and heightened distress. It often is manifest at the onset of disease, and although analgesics may be required on a transient basis, symptoms may resolve as antitumor therapy progresses.[33] In contrast, assessment and management of patients with chronic pain tend to be more complex. With time, biologic and behavioral adjustment to symptoms occurs and associated signs of tachycardia, hypertension, and diaphoresis are often absent. Various pain behaviors (alterations in facial expression, gait, posture, and mood) may be observed, and may persist throughout treatment.[34] Premorbid chronic nonmalignant pain that precedes the diagnosis of cancer can complicate management. Pain due to cancer *per se* usually signals tumor progression with actual injury to tissue, and, as a result, response to intervention is relatively predictable. In contrast, chronic nonmalignant pain, even in the cancer patient, is more often an ingrained behavior and personality feature that may be associated with drug-seeking behavior, symptom magnification, and pain on the basis of depression, and thus symptoms may persist despite intervention.[35, 36]

Mechanism

A mechanistic classification based on inferred pathophysiology of pain that distinguishes among nociceptive (somatic and visceral) and neuropathic pain has become increasingly well accepted (Table 32–10).[37] Common clinical characteristics and shared responsivity to various therapeutic interventions have been observed for each type of pain, and hence consideration of this classification is useful when formulating an initial treatment approach. Cancer pain, especially when advanced, usually involves multiple sensory pathophysiologic mechanisms (mixed pain) that interact with related characterologic and environmental components (affective, cognitive, and behavioral), the sum of which contributes to a complex experience that defies simple categorization or management per a simple routine.

Nociceptive Pain

Nociceptive and neuropathic pain refer to broad categories of painful conditions, distinguished from each other based on their inferred mechanisms. Nociceptive pain is subdivided into somatic nociceptive pain and visceral nociceptive pain. Each type of pain is characteristically described by patients in similar terms and tends to respond similarly to various therapeutic interventions.[38]

Nociceptive pain is a result of an injury or insult to nonneurologic structures, and occurs in the presence of a fundamentally intact nervous system, that is, under conditions of normal peripheral and central nervous system function. Characteristically, pain appears to be proportional to and commensurate with the underlying tissue injury. Noxious stimuli result in transmission of impulses along classical pain pathways. Symptoms consist of sensations to which most people have a familiar frame of reference from previous painful experiences (e.g., trauma, surgery, and childbirth), and are characteristically described with adjectives or descriptors that are traditionally associated with pain. Nociceptive pain typically responds favorably and predictably to treatment with nonsteroidal anti-inflammatory drugs (NSAIDs) and the opioids in a graded fashion that is relatively proportional to dose, and favorable responses to treatment with adjuvant analgesics are unlikely. When appropriate, nociceptive pain is often amenable to relief by interruption of proximal pathways by neural blockade or surgery, at least temporarily.

SOMATIC NOCICEPTIVE PAIN

Nociceptive pain can be further subdivided into somatic nociceptive pain and visceral nociceptive pain. Somatic nociceptive pain occurs as a result of ongoing activation of cutaneous and deep nociceptors in somatic tissues (skin, muscle, bone, joint, tendon, and other connective tissues). These nociceptors are activated by mechanical, thermal, and chemical stimuli.[39] Pain may be acute or chronic in nature, is typically well localized, and is often characterized as aching, dull, sharp, or gnawing (see Table 32–10).

VISCERAL NOCICEPTIVE PAIN

Visceral nociceptive pain arises from injury to internal organs (thorax, abdomen, pelvis). Although it is insensitive to simple manipulation, cutting, and burning, visceral pain is elicited as a result of distention, stretch, abnormal contraction or reflex spasm, ischemia or necrosis of smooth muscle, chemical irritation of serosal or mucosal surfaces of hollow viscera, stretch of the capsular investment of solid viscera and distention, and traction or torsion of mesenteric and vascular attachments. Visceral injury often produces referred pain, defined as pain and hyperalgesia (hypersensitivity) that is localized to superficial or deep tissues, or to both, often distant from the source of pathology (e.g., back pain secondary to pancreatic cancer, right shoulder pain secondary to diaphragmatic irritation). In contrast to somatically mediated pain, visceral pain is characteristically described as vague in distribution and quality, and is often deep, dull, aching, dragging, squeezing, or pressure-like. When acute, it may be paroxysmal and colicky, and can be associated with nausea, vomiting, diaphoresis, and alterations in blood pressure and heart rate.

TABLE 32–10. **Classification of Pain by Its Underlying Mechanism**

Type of Pain	Common Clinical Features	Responsivity: Opioids and NSAIDs	Responsivity: Adjuvants	Responsivity: Neural Blockade
Somatic nociceptive	Constant, well-localized; dull, sharp, aching, throbbing, gnawing Examples: bone metastases, skin infiltration, muscle spasm	(+++)	(−)	(++)
Visceral nociceptive	Constant or paroxysmal; vague in distribution and quality; deep, dull, aching, dragging, squeezing, or pressure-like; acute: may be colicky; associated with nausea, vomiting, diaphoresis, and alterations in vital signs Examples: liver metastases, bowel or ureteral obstruction, pancreatic cancer	(++)	(−)	(++)
Neuropathic	When constant: burning, tingling, numbing, pressing, squeezing, and/or itching When paroxysmal: shooting, stabbing, lancinating, electrical, jolting, shock-like Examples: herpes zoster, postmastectomy or postthoracotomy pain, brachial or lumbosacral plexopathy, phantom limb pain, spinal cord injury, diabetic neuropathy, leptomeningeal metastases	(+)	(++)	(+)
Mixed	Various features from above, depending on predominant mechanism(s)	Variable	Variable	Variable

Neuropathic Pain

In contrast to nociceptive pain, neuropathic pain occurs as a consequence of neural injury and abnormal or pathologic transmission, processing, and integration. Peripheral or central nervous system injury results in aberrant somatosensory processing, and the resulting pain appears to be self-sustaining and poorly correlated with degree of apparent tissue injury. Neuropathic pain is often associated with objective neurologic signs or subjective reports of altered sensation, and especially alterations in sensory threshold, including anesthesia and allodynia (pain in response to a stimulus that usually does not provoke pain, e.g., a light stroke). Patients report experiences that are distinct from ordinary, familiar sensations of pain (e.g, burning, tingling, itching, numbness), considered together under the rubric *dysesthesias* (Latin for *bad feeling*). Pain is often diffuse and may be accompanied by exaggerated skeletal muscle and autonomic responses.

Neuropathic pain may be relatively constant and unrelenting (so-called tonic pain); predominantly intermittent, spontaneous, and shocklike or lancinating; or commonly a mix of tonic dysesthesia with superimposed electrical spikes. As a rule, neuropathic pain is more difficult to treat than nociceptive pain because it tends to be less responsive than nociceptive pain to opioids administered in routine doses, and typically requires the addition of adjuvant analgesics, including antidepressants and anticonvulsants (see Table 32–10). Examples of neuropathic pain include phantom limb pain, spinal cord injury, postherpetic neuralgia, and neuropathy due to chemotherapy or diabetes.

Idiopathic or Psychogenic Pain

Great controversy surrounds labeling a pain syndrome as wholly psychogenic in origin. It is fundamental to the subjective nature of pain and is now well accepted that patients' psychological states contribute significantly to complaints of pain and suffering. The presence of psychological influences on pain report or evidence for a placebo response should in no way be regarded as detracting from the authenticity of a complaint of pain. It is often difficult to ascertain the degree to which psychological disturbances are sequelae of chronic pain or constitute a more primary disorder that is expressed as pain. Regardless, symptoms and their associated distress are real to the patient, independent of the degree to which psychological factors are involved in their maintenance, and thus should always be taken seriously. Although it is essential that the clinician maintains a willingness to believe the patient's report of pain and investigates its cause, the presence of anxiety or depression should be carefully assessed so that appropriate supportive care or pharmacotherapy, or both, can be instituted.

Pain Intensity and Self-Report

Classification of cancer pain based on its intensity has considerable practical relevance. Because self-report remains the gold standard for assessing pain intensity, providing patients with the tools for assessing and reporting changes in pain intensity is a key patient education goal. Patients should be familiarized with a suitable measure of pain intensity on their first encounter, which should then be applied consistently from visit to visit. The use of a simple self-report scale empowers patients by providing a simple means for them to rapidly communicate volumes about a complex personal experience that is not otherwise readily accessible to an observer. In the absence of a shared language or tool for communicating changes in subjective symptoms, it is unreasonable for the clinician to expect to otherwise gauge outcome and the need to appropriately modify ongoing therapy.

Especially for unstable pain, patients may be instructed in the use of a pain diary to document changes in pain intensity between visits. The consistent use of a single schema for measuring pain intensity aids in the reliable assessment of patients' progress and, in addition, serves as a basis for interpatient comparison when data are being gathered for research purposes.

Any inclination to rely on measures other than self-report (observation, reports of family members and nurses, changes in vital signs or radiographs) except as adjunctive tools should be rejected because numerous studies have demonstrated the superiority of self-report.[40, 41] The particular self-report tool instituted is probably less important than a commitment to use an appropriate method consistently for a given patient. Most clinics have adopted a 0 to 10 scale (0 = no pain, 10 = the worst pain the patient can imagine), administered either verbally or with pen and paper. Patients are ideally asked for a numeric rating of their pain at present and over the previous week, with a best, worst, and on average.[42] In its written form, such a tool is referred to as a visual analogue scale. The prevailing convention involves the use of an uncalibrated horizontal line that is 10 cm in length and is anchored at its extremes with descriptors indicating *no pain* and *the most severe pain imaginable*.

A dynamic numeric rating is a somewhat abstract concept, and difficulties arise particularly in the very young or very old patient, as well as in the presence of factors that impair concentration such as severe pain or distress, debility resulting from chronic illness, and the effects of anesthetic or analgesic drugs. Novel tools have been developed for special indications, especially age-specific techniques used in pediatric populations. These techniques include pain thermometers, color scales, and sketches of faces that depict a continuum of changing expressions.[43]

Clinical Significance of Pain Intensity Ratings

Classification of cancer pain based on its intensity determines where the patient is likely to fall along the World Health Organization (WHO)–endorsed analgesic ladder,[12, 44] an effective but almost deceptively simple schema that has been incorporated into guidelines adopted by other expert bodies.[5–7, 22] The ladder employs a primary strategy of matching analgesic potency with pain intensity (NSAIDs for mild pain and various opioids for moderate to severe pain) and, secondarily, recommends selecting drugs based on the presumed mechanisms of pain (NSAIDs and opioids for nociceptive pain and adjuvants for neuropathic pain). Pain severity serves as the main determinant for determining the level at which the ladder is accessed, and thus whether treatment is rendered with a nonopioid analgesic, a so-called weak opioid, or a so-called strong/potent opioid. Recently, the terms *opioid conventionally used to treat moderate pain* and *opioid conventionally used to treat severe pain* have been advocated in preference to *weak* and *strong* opioids.

Consistently high pain scores should obviously alert the clinician to the urgent need for aggressive intervention. With the exception of the adjuvant analgesics, the dose-response relationship of drugs used in the ladder is tightly linked; when necessary, patients should be moved briskly through its tiers to avoid unnecessary delays in achieving pain relief. A determination of whether a drug of adequate potency and dose has been initially prescribed can usually be made with the administration of just a few doses, or at most after a few days. The WHO treatment hierarchy can be accessed at any level: Patients presenting initially with severe pain can be managed from the start with low doses of potent opioids.

Temporal Pattern of Pain

Pain may be constant and unremitting, in which case it is most amenable to an around-the-clock (a-t-c) dosing schedule, contingent on time rather than symptoms. This approach to management endeavors to prevent pain rather than treat it retroactively, and is best accomplished by the optimal use of long-acting oral or transdermal analgesics or, when indicated, a continuous parenteral infusion.

Despite establishing an effective preventive schedule, *breakthrough pain* is still a common phenomenon that must be anticipated and addressed. Breakthrough pain[45] refers to intermittent exacerbations of pain that can occur spontaneously or in relation to specific activity against a background of chronic unremitting pain. Breakthrough pain that is related to a specific activity, such as eating, bowel movements, socializing, or walking, is referred to as incident pain.[46] Breakthrough pain may also be idiopathic or related to the a-t-c dosing regimen (end-of-dose failure), in which case it usually occurs predictably near the end of a dosing interval, has a more gradual onset, and is more likely to be persistent. The incidence and severity of end-of-dose failure usually correlate with the adequacy of a-t-c dosing regimens prescribed for the management of basal pain, and this type of breakthrough pain is best countered by modifying the dose or schedule of long-acting a-t-c opioids. Idiopathic and incident types of breakthrough pain are best managed by supplementing the preventive regimen with analgesics characterized by rapid onset and short duration. Once a pattern of incident pain is established, breakthrough doses, rescue doses, or escape doses of analgesics can be administered in anticipation of the pain-provoking activity.[47] When treatment with an infusion (subcutaneous, intravenous, epidural) has been elected, the addition of patient-controlled analgesia, which permits patients to administer a preset amount of narcotic at preset intervals, is an effective means to manage breakthrough and incident pain.

Pain that is intermittent and unpredictable in onset represents a further challenge to management. Around-the-clock dosing is likely to be unsatisfactory because analgesia is often inadequate during painful episodes, and sedation usually supervenes during pain-free intervals. Pain that occurs intermittently is usually best managed by the *pro re nata* (p.r.n.) administration of an appropriately potent analgesic of rapid onset and short duration (e.g., morphine, hydromorphone, oxycodone, oral transmucosal fentanyl citrate). When intermittent pain is well localized, there may be a role for nerve blocks as well.

Patient and Disease Characteristics

The concept that assessment should include attention to disease-specific and person-specific factors that contribute to the meaning of pain is well accepted,[33] although formal schemata have not been detailed or validated. Neither assessment nor treatment should be strictly limited to a disease-specific focus. Optimally, the clinician's focus is on a human being who, in addition to cancer and pain, has thoughts, feelings, previous experiences, and memories that influence report and response. For example, the optimal approach to providing treatment for a patient who has observed a loved one die with unrelieved pain will necessarily differ from that needed for a patient who has observed family members' experiences with drug abuse. A classification scheme based on stage of disease and patient characteristics that may help predict patients' response to pain is summarized in Table 32–11.[33]

Syndromal Presentation

The importance of classifying cancer pain based on its syndromal presentation has become increasingly appreciated.[13, 27, 48] The clinical recognition of cancer pain syndromes is based on the clinician's knowledge of their clinical presentation and a careful history, physical examination, and review of diagnostic studies. Although an exhaustive description of known cancer pain syndromes is beyond the scope of this text, brief descriptions follow.

BONE METASTASES

Skeletal metastases are clinically evident in one third of cancer patients and are present in two thirds of cancer patients at autopsy,[49] and thus it is not surprising that infiltration of bone is the most common cause of cancer pain. Neoplasms with the greatest propensity to metastasize to bone include multiple myeloma, breast cancer, prostate cancer, and lung cancer.

Because up to 50% decalcification must be present before osseous lesions are visible on plain roentgenograms, scintigraphy (radioisotope scanning) is the diagnostic imaging technique of choice, except in the case of primary bone tumors, thyroid cancer, and multiple myeloma. Although they are ordinarily more sensitive than plain films, scintigrams are not highly specific; therefore, findings must be interpreted in the context of clinical findings and other studies. A biochemical mechanism has been advocated to explain much of the pain associated with osseous invasion, which would help explain why 20% to 25% of patients with even very large bone metastases are asymptomatic, whereas sometimes even very small lesions produce severe pain. Osseous metastases elaborate prostaglandin E_2, which, it is hypothesized, contributes to pain by sensitization of peripheral nociceptors. NSAIDs and steroids are postulated to be effective in the treatment of painful bony metastases on the basis of their activity to inhibit the cyclooxygenase pathway of arachidonic acid breakdown and thus decrease the formation of prostaglandin E_2. As deposits enlarge, stretching of the periosteum, pathologic fracture, and perineural invasion contribute to pain, and requirements for more potent analgesics increase. It has also been suggested that pain is more closely correlated with the rate of expansion of bony lesions than with their absolute size[50] or size *per se*. External beam radiotherapy has long been successfully employed to relieve pain emanating from bony metastases. More recently, radionuclides (e.g., strontium-89, samarium) have been used to treat pain in specific settings (after conventional radiotherapy has been maximized), especially in the presence of diffuse metastases, and in patients with hormone-dependent cancers (i.e., breast and prostate cancer). Hormonal therapy (e.g., chemotherapy, orchiectomy, hypophysectomy) is also often effective in reducing bony pain in patients with hormone-dependent disease, although the estrogen agent tamoxifen may increase pain transiently before it is relieved in a proportion of patients (tamoxifen flare).[51] Metastases to the skull, sternum, and upper limb tend not to be painful. When

TABLE 32–11. **Classification of Cancer Pain by Stage of Disease and Patient Characteristics**

Acute cancer-related pain	Biologic "red flag" signifying need to simultaneously investigate cause and rapidly institute treatment
Related to diagnosis or treatment	Patients tend to be hopeful May readily endure pain, often without seeking treatment
Recurrent pain	Identification with recrudescence of disease Psychological effects potentially devastating
Chronic cancer-related pain	Behavioral adaptation/maladaptation, pharmacologic tolerance, and physical dependence may be established
Associated with treatment	Overriding concern is re-establishment of functional lifestyle
Associated with progression	Hopelessness and helplessness often predominate
Pre-existing chronic pain	Pain behavior established; may require intensive intervention and support; accurate diagnosis essential
Dying patients	Adequacy of treatment has great impact on patient and family; Assure comfort at all reasonable costs
History of drug abuse	Evaluation and management are often complicated by legitimate concerns that pain treatment may result in maintenance or recrudescence of aberrant drug use; by the same token, a significant risk of undertreatment of pain exists as a consequence of such concerns
Distant history of abuse	Patient may be reluctant to use opioids due to fear of readdiction and criticism of peers and family
Ongoing methadone maintenance	May complicate pharmacologic management; requires coordination
Active drug abuse	Most challenging; interdisciplinary/multimodal management helpful; coordinate support services (e.g., rehabilitation, social work)
Pediatrics	Pain, anxiety, and distress evoke equivalent responses
Preverbal children	Pain expressed by crying, grimacing, and facial expressions
Toddlers	Tend to regress
Adolescents	Tend to withdraw

investigating pain that is thought to emanate from bony deposits, the clinician should consider imaging adjacent structures to exclude referred pain, as in the case of knee pain associated with metastatic involvement of the hip.

EPIDURAL SPINAL CORD COMPRESSION

Epidural spinal cord compression is a critically important clinical entity that all practitioners should be capable of recognizing. Onset is almost always heralded by pain, usually well in advance of discrete neurologic findings, and, therefore, a diagnosis should be considered in all at-risk patients who present with new onset or rapidly changing back pain.[52, 53] Early recognition and intervention may limit neurologic morbidity. Pain may be localized to the midline of the spine or associated with a radicular pattern of weakness and tingling. It tends to be dull, steady, and aching, increasing gradually over time, and often is exacerbated with recumbency or straining. Rapid progression of neurologic deficit, particularly of motor weakness or incontinence, signals progressive epidural–spinal cord compression and warrants urgent intervention. Magnetic resonance imaging has all but replaced computed tomography as the study of first choice, and treatment planning often involves collaboration of a neurosurgeon, radiologist, and radiation oncologist.[54, 55]

NEURAL INVASION

Invasion or compression of somatic nerves by tumor is generally associated with constant, burning dysesthetic pain, often with a superimposed intermittent stabbing component. Diffuse hyperesthesia and localized paresthesia are common, and muscle weakness and atrophy may be present if a mixed or motor nerve is involved in the affected structure. Pain attributable to nerve compression by tumor was diagnosed in 34%, 40%, 20%, and 31% of patients referred to an anesthesiology-pain service, tertiary care center, neurology service, and hospice, respectively.[56–59]

BRACHIAL AND LUMBOSACRAL PLEXOPATHY

Brachial plexus invasion (Pancoast's or superior sulcus syndrome) is associated most commonly with carcinoma of the lung (primary or metastatic) or breast, and lymphoma.[60] Differentiating brachial plexus abnormalities resulting from radiation fibrosis versus tumor invasion can be difficult because clinical findings are similar. Horner's syndrome and severe pain and weakness in the C8 to T1 (lower plexus) distribution are more commonly associated with tumor invasion, whereas lymphadenopathy and weakness of shoulder abduction and arm flexor (upper plexus) are more commonly encountered after radiation injury.[27] Work-up of suspected brachial plexopathy includes magnetic resonance imaging, nerve conduction studies, and, if epidural extension is suspected, consideration of spinal studies.

Lumbosacral plexopathy resulting from invasion of local soft tissue by tumor, lymphadenopathy, or compression from bony metastases occurs most commonly in association with tumors of the rectum, cervix, and breast, and with sarcoma and lymphoma. Involvement of the lumbar plexus characteristically produces radicular lower extremity pain that is usually described as aching or pressure-like. Pain is the presenting symptom in most patients, about half of whom go on to develop significant weakness and numbness within weeks or months of the initial appearance of pain.[61] Reflex asymmetry and mild sensory and motor changes are relatively early findings, whereas impotence and incontinence are infrequent findings. Suspected plexopathy must be differentiated from cord compression, cauda equina, and leptomeningeal metastases. Computed tomography investigations of the pelvis and lumbar spine and diagnostic nerve blocks are helpful to corroborate clinical findings.

Invasion of the sacral plexus is most often associated with severe constant lower backache, often progressing to perineal sensory loss and bowel or bladder dysfunction. Plain films, tomography, and scintigrams frequently demonstrate bony invasion of the sacral plates. Symptom control is most important in these settings because constant pain likely leads patients to become immobilized, depressed, and subject to increased risks of venous thrombosis, decubiti, and infection.

CRANIAL NEURALGIAS AND ASSOCIATED OROFACIAL PAIN

Although the responsivity of pain from head and neck tumors to routine analgesics is a subject of some controversy,[62, 63] pain in this setting can be extremely challenging for many reasons, not the least of which relates to the depression and impairment that often accompany treatment of these tumors.[64] New pain or an exacerbation after a long interval of stable symptoms should always raise the suspicion of recurrence, even when not clinically apparent.[65]

The head and neck are richly innervated by contributions from cranial nerves V, VII, IX, and X and the upper cervical nerves. Pain commonly emanates from bony and soft tissue growths that may impinge on cranial nerves and their branches. Specific etiologies for pain include soft tissue ulceration, infection, compression from adenopathy or tumor, mucositis, bony erosion, and nerve invasion.[62] Analgesia may be difficult to achieve because of the erosive character of many tumors and the ineffectiveness of physiologic splinting; physiologic splinting is an ordinarily protective reflex that is overridden by the pain that accompanies the relatively involuntary motion produced by swallowing, eating, coughing, talking, and other movements of the head. When cranial nerves and their branches are involved, symptoms may mimic trigeminal or glossopharyngeal neuralgia, with baseline dysesthetic pain and superimposed sudden, severe shocklike lancinating pain radiating to the receptive field of the affected division or divisions. Glossopharyngeal and intermedium neuralgias produce similar symptoms, but with pain more localized to the throat and ear, respectively.

If the tumor is unresectable, early consideration should be given to palliative radiotherapy. Depending on its underlying mechanism, pain may be responsive to treatment with steroids, NSAIDs, opioids, and anticonvulsants or antidepressants. Refractory pain may warrant empiric treatment with antibiotics because infection may be masked by bone marrow failure or sequestration.[66] Neurolytic blocks, neurosurgery, and intraventricular opioids are often successful for pain that is otherwise intractable.[67]

LEPTOMENINGEAL METASTASES/MENINGEAL CARCINOMATOSIS

Diffuse infiltration of the meninges by tumor has the potential to produce protean signs and symptoms, and as a result, a high index of suspicion is required to make an accurate diagnosis.[68, 69] This condition is most common in patients with primary malignancies of the breast and lung, lymphoma, and leukemia. About 40% of patients have headache or back pain as a result of traction on the pain-sensitive structures (meninges, cranial spinal nerves), or raised intracranial pressure, or both. The most common presenting complaint is headache, which is characteristically unrelenting and may be associated with nausea, vomiting, nuchal rigidity, and mental status changes. Other neurologic abnormalities that may develop include seizures, cranial nerve palsies, papilledema, hemiparesis, ataxia, and cauda equina syndrome. Diagnosis is confirmed by lumbar puncture and cerebrospinal fluid analysis, which identifies malignant cells, and may also be remarkable for an increased opening pressure, raised protein, and decreased glucose. Computed tomography, magnetic resonance imaging with contrast, and myelograms are helpful to evaluate the extent of disease. The natural history of patients with clinically evident leptomeningeal metastases is gradual decline and death over 4 to 8 weeks, although survival may be extended to 6 months or more when treatment with radiotherapy or intrathecal methotrexate, or both, is instituted.[69] Steroids may be useful in the management of associated headache.[70]

HEADACHE

Headache is a major but not invariable symptom of intracranial neoplasm,[71] present in 60% of patients in one survey, half of whom classified headache as their primary complaint.[72] Its pattern is indistinctive.[73] Patients typically describe pain that is steady, deep, dull and aching, and is rarely rhythmic or throbbing. It is usually intermittent and may be worse in the morning, with coughing or straining. Characteristically, the intensity of pain is only moderate, rarely awakening patients from sleep, and is generally less than that which is typically described in so-called benign headache syndromes. Symptoms often respond to simple measures including recumbency, the administration of aspirin or steroids,[74] and the application of cold packs. Symptoms often improve when radiotherapy is applied to treat the underlying malignancy.[75]

Cerebral tissue per se is insensitive to noxious stimuli, and thus headache is mediated by indirect mechanisms, with pain referred from adjacent pain-sensitive structures such as the venous sinuses and their tributaries; dural and cerebral arteries; the dura (especially at the base of the brain); cranial nerves V, IX, and X; and the upper three cervical nerves. Mechanisms include traction, displacement, and dilation of veins and arteries, inflammation near pain-sensitive structures, and direct pressure on cranial and cervical nerves. Reflex contraction of the cervical muscles is a common finding with headache in general, and it accompanies headache of neoplastic origin in a high proportion of cases. Although it is an important diagnostic sign of raised intracranial pressure (along with nausea, vomiting, mental status changes, and papilledema), headache may be absent, particularly when elevations in pressure are gradual or chronic.

Pain Treatment

Antineoplastic Treatment

Ideally, cancer pain is managed by direct treatment of its underlying cause. Once elucidated, the pathologic process responsible for pain can often be altered with surgical extirpation, external beam radiotherapy (targeted fractionated or single-dose therapy, hemibody or total body irradiation),[76–78] radionuclides (e.g., strontium-89, samarium–153),[79, 80] chemotherapy,[81] hormonal treatment,[82] and even whole-body hyperthermia.[83] Many patients are pleased to realize prompt and significant pain relief when their cancer responds to antitumor therapy. This is especially true for lymphoma treated with various chemotherapies and painful bone metastases that often respond promptly and dramatically to local irradiation, which, in some settings, can be administered in a single, nonfractionated dose.[84] Nevertheless, the majority of patients require some form of primary analgesic therapy while awaiting a tumoricidal response or because antitumor therapy has been maximized or is no longer applicable. Even when the goal of cancer cure has been abandoned, further antitumor therapy should be considered when new symptoms arise, or a change in the pain treatment strategy is planned. For rapid palliation of symptoms, as opposed to cure, radiotherapy is generally the most applicable of these modalities. It is important to recognize, however, that palliative antitumor measures have definite limitations with regard to efficacy, patient acceptance, and adverse effects, especially in patients with advanced disease. Finally, the decision to pursue antitumor therapy does not imply that analgesic drugs and other supportive therapy should be discontinued.

Pharmacologic Management

Until recently, most knowledge gleaned about opioid pharmacology was derived from single-dose or limited-dose studies conducted in the presence of either experimentally induced or acute pain. In a construct that recognizes chronic and acute pain as distinct disorders, there is limited justification for applying knowledge gained from one setting to the other uncritically. The inadequate scientific basis for prescribing practices is compounded by firmly held beliefs regarding the dangers of opioid therapy.[85] Such beliefs are now widely understood to be based more on cultural bias than medical considerations.[86–88] Recognition of these deficiencies has engendered an almost unparalleled scientific activism to dispel myths surrounding the treatment of pain with drugs and improve the plight of symptomatic cancer patients. Guidelines released by the WHO,[12, 44] American Pain Society,[6] American Society of Clinical Oncology,[7] the American Society of Anesthesiologists,[22] and the U.S. Government Agency for Health Care Policy Research[5] stress the importance of opioid therapy and articulate the need to overcome exaggerated concerns about its risks.

Oral analgesics are the mainstay of therapy for patients with cancer pain. An estimated 70% to 90% of patients can be rendered relatively free of pain when straightforward guideline-based principles of pharmacologic management are applied in a thorough, careful manner.[5, 6, 12, 89] Treatment is effective in adults and children across different cultures and in patients who are ambulatory or debilitated. The analgesia that is associated with systemically administered medications is titratable and suitable for pain that is multifocal or progressive, or both. Effects and side effects are reversible, and widespread implementation does not depend on sophisticated technology or scarce resources.[20, 90] The WHO has developed a three-step ladder approach to cancer pain management that relies exclusively on the administration of oral agents (Fig. 32–1), and this approach is usually effective.[12, 15] For example, in a prospective evaluation of the WHO method, Zech and associates observed good results in 76% of 2118 cancer patients treated over a 10-year interval.[89]

Although pain can be managed in most patients with oral agents alone, even through the terminal stages of illness, a small but important proportion of patients require alternative forms of therapy.[91] The role of more interventional forms of analgesia, ranging from parenteral analgesics to neural blockade and central nervous system (CNS) opioid therapy, remains poorly defined, although it is widely recognized that the judicious application of such approaches is essential when more conservative therapies produce inadequate results.

Noninvasive routes (e.g., oral, transdermal, transmucosal) should be maintained as long as possible for reasons that include simplicity, maintenance of independence and mobility, convenience, and cost. Treatment has been markedly simplified by the introduction of controlled-release preparations of oral opioids (e.g., MS Contin, Oramorph, Kadian, OxyContin), novel noninvasive approaches (e.g., transdermal fentanyl, oral transmucosal fentanyl citrate), and most importantly, the widespread acceptance of guideline-based therapies.

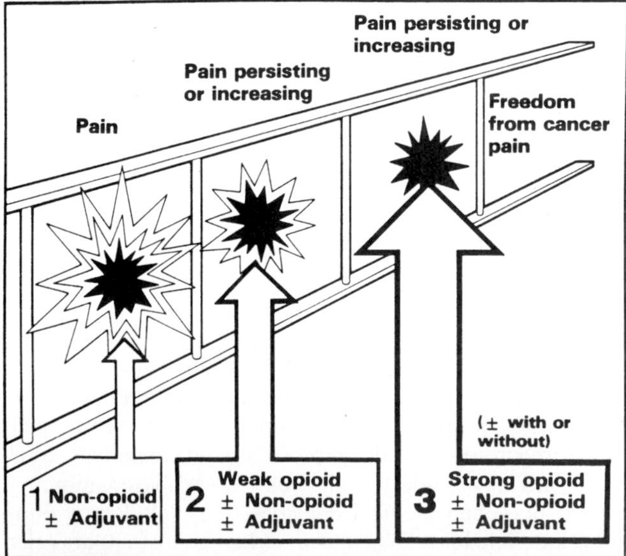

Figure 32–1. The World Health Organization's analgesic ladder is the nearly universally accepted methodology for selecting analgesics based primarily on intensity of pain and secondarily on pain analgesics of mild, moderate, and high potency—selected based on the presence of mild, moderate, or severe pain. At each step there is consideration for adding an adjuvant analgesic (e.g., tricyclic antidepressant, anticonvulsant) if neuropathic pain is thought to be present. Even with reliance on the oral route, this method produces durable pain relief in 70% to 90% of patients, independent of practice setting and cultural milieu.

NONSTEROIDAL ANTI-INFLAMMATORY DRUGS

Regular (a-t-c) administration of an NSAID is an appropriate starting point as the sole treatment for mild pain, and an NSAID combined with an opioid analgesic may be considered for moderate to severe pain.[92] Although they are potentially effective in all settings, NSAIDs are particularly effective for pain of inflammatory and bony metastatic origin, by virtue of interference with prostaglandin synthesis.[93] Potential benefits need to be balanced against potential toxicity (e.g., gastrointestinal [GI], genitourinary, CNS, and hematologic toxicities and masking of fever),[94] considerations that are especially pertinent in the context of recent antitumor therapy and advanced age.[95] Consider avoiding NSAIDs altogether or instituting prophylaxis in patients with bone marrow depression or those who are predisposed to developing gastropathy. If prophylaxis is indicated, misoprostol appears to be the most effective protective regimen.[96] The nonacetylated salicylates (sodium salicylate, choline magnesium trisalicylate) are associated with a favorable toxicity profile in that they fail to interfere with platelet aggregation, are rarely associated with GI bleeding, and are well tolerated in asthmatic patients.[97, 98] A parenteral formulation of ketorolac has been shown to be equianalgesic to low doses of morphine in some settings, but is associated with the same range of potential side effects as oral NSAIDs.[99]

In contrast to the opioid analgesics, NSAIDs are associated with a ceiling effect above which dose escalations produce toxicity but no greater analgesia. However, the ceiling dose for a given drug differs from patient to patient, allowing some potential for dose titration.[100] Regular (as opposed to intermittent) use promotes both anti-inflammatory and analgesic effects. Despite their apparent heterogeneity, the NSAIDs are, in most respects, clinically indistinguishable.[101] Selection is based on the patient's previous experience, minor differences in toxicity, clinician experience, schedule, and cost.[94] When efficacy is poor, the clinician may consider rotating to another NSAID, usually from a distinct biochemical class.[100]

WEAK OPIOIDS

When NSAIDs provide insufficient relief, are contraindicated, or are poorly tolerated, or when pain is severe at presentation, the addition or substitution of a weak opioid (i.e., codeine, hydrocodone, dihydrocodeine, oxycodone preparations) is recommended as an analgesic of intermediate potency.[6] Usually formulated as combination products, these agents are weak only insofar as the inclusion of aspirin, acetaminophen, or ibuprofen results in a ceiling dose above which the incidence of toxicity increases.[102] The nomenclature *opioids conventionally used to treat moderate pain* is now endorsed in preference to *weak opioids*, because when equianalgesic dosing is applied, the potency of the opioid per se is not a clinically important

TABLE 32–12. **Comparison of "Potent" Opioid Agonists Used in Cancer Pain Management**

Generic Name	Trade Name	Route	Equivalent Dose	Duration (Avg Range)
Morphine	Various	IM	10 mg	3–4 hr
	MSIR, etc.	Oral	20–30 mg	3–4 hr
	Various	Rectal	5 mg	4 hr
Controlled-release morphine	MS Contin	Oral	30 mg	8–12hr
	Oramorph SR	Oral	30 mg	8–12 hr
	Kadian	Oral	30 mg	12–24 hr
Hydromorphone	Dilaudid	Oral	7.5 mg	3–4 hr
		IM	1.5 mg	3–4 hr
Oxymorphone	Numorphan	IM	1 mg	3–6 hr
		Rectal	5–10 mg	4–6 hr
Meperidine	Demerol	Oral	300 mg	3–6 hr
		IM	75 mg	3–4 hr
Heroin	Diamorphine	IM	5 mg	4–5 hr
		Oral	60 mg	
Methadone	Dolophine	IM	20 mg	4–8 hr
		Oral	10 mg	4–8 hr
Levorphanol	Levo-Dromoran	IM	2 mg	4–8 hr
		Oral	2 mg	4–8 hr
Oxycodone	Various	Oral	30 mg	3–6 hr
Controlled-release oxycodone	OxyContin	Oral	30 mg	12 hr
Transdermal fentanyl	Duragesic	TD	See Table 32–13	72 hr

IM = intramuscular; TD = transdermal.

distinguishing feature of this class of drugs. For example, a sole-entity preparation of oxycodone is now available that, when prescribed in sufficient doses, is effective for even severe pain[103, 104] because the ceiling effect imposed by the aspirin or acetaminophen is absent. Likewise, fentanyl, though up to 100 times more potent than parenteral morphine, is rendered clinically useful by using a dosing schedule in a microgram rather than milligram range.

Although the weak opioids are appropriate for mild or intermittent pain, practitioners often rely excessively on these agents, frequently continuing their use after they are no longer effective in an ill-advised attempt to avoid prescribing more potent opioids that are also more highly regulated.[86] Propoxyphene is rarely appropriate for the management of cancer pain because of its low potency,[105] and codeine is considerably emetogenic and constipating relative to its analgesic potency.[106] Oxycodone, now available not only as a combination product (e.g., Percocet, Percodan), but also as a sole-entity preparation[103, 104] (e.g., Roxicodone) and in a slow-release formulation (OxyContin),[107] is considerably more potent than codeine and may be the most useful drug in this class. The potency of hydrocodone and dihydrocodeine preparations (e.g., Lortab, Vicodin) is between that of codeine and oxycodone.[108] These agents have the perceived advantage of not requiring triplicate prescriptions (DEA Class C-III vs. C-II), although the clinician must be cautious not to exceed the usual recommended dose of acetaminophen (4 g/day) as opioid requirements increase.

POTENT OPIOIDS

When combinations of codeine-like drugs and NSAIDs provide insufficient analgesia, or when pain is severe at presentation, therapy should progress to include more potent opioid analgesics in a ladder fashion (see Fig. 32–1).[12] Morphine, hydromorphone, transdermal fentanyl, and oxycodone are appropriate first-line agents for the institution of basal analgesia (Tables 32–12 and 32–13), whereas methadone and levorphanol are generally considered second-line agents (see following discussion). Less potent analgesics should not be summarily excluded because NSAIDs may provide additive or synergistic analgesia and codeine-like preparations may be useful for breakthrough or incident pain. Opioids should initially be introduced in low doses because the early development of side effects negatively influences compliance, but they should be rapidly titrated to effect. Pretreatment counseling is important to convert the common but unrealistic expectation that pain be eliminated to one of achieving the best balance possible between comfort and adverse effects.

MORPHINE

Morphine remains the standard of reference to which other analgesics are compared. Despite widespread use and ex-

TABLE 32–13. **Dosage Equivalency for Transdermal Fentanyl**

Oral Morphine (mg/24 hr)	IM Morphine (mg/24 hr)	Transdermal Fentanyl (μg/hr)
45–134	8–22	25
135–224	23–37	50
225–314	38–52	75
315–404	53–67	100
405–494	68–82	125
495–584	83–97	150
585–674	98–112	175
675–764	113–127	200
765–854	128–142	225
855–944	143–157	250
945–1034	158–172	275
1035–1124	173–187	300

tensive research, misconceptions about the use of morphine for chronic pain management continue to interfere with its optimal use (see Table 32–1).[86]

Morphine is readily absorbed from the GI tract and is metabolized in the liver. With chronic use, about one third of the orally administered dose ultimately exerts an analgesic effect (oral bioavailability of 3:1). This bioavailability is in contrast to the 6:1 parenteral-to-oral ratio determined from single-dose studies for acute pain. Because parenterally administered drug is not subject to this first-pass effect, clinicians may incorrectly perceive parenterally administered opioids as more effective than opioids administered orally. Research has focused on the role of morphine metabolites, once thought to be inactive. Morphine-3-glucuronide has been postulated to antagonize opioid analgesia, although morphine-6-glucuronide appears to possess potent analgesic properties, and may induce persistent nausea and sedation, especially in the presence of altered renal function.[109, 110] Although the clinical relevance of these metabolites is currently uncertain, persistent nausea or sedation during morphine therapy should warrant consideration of switching to an alternate opioid.

Morphine is available in a variety of formulations and is appropriate for administration by a variety of routes. The most important distinctions are between (1) immediate-release preparations (e.g., Roxanol), which have a short latency to effect (about 30 minutes), a short duration (2–4 hours), and are usually administered every 3 to 4 hours, and (2) controlled-release preparations (e.g., MS Contin, Oramorph), which have a longer latency to effect and duration, and, as a result, are usually administered every 12 or sometimes 8 hours. New controlled-release preparations include a capsular form that may be suitable for once daily administration, and an every-12-hours rectal suppository.[111, 112]

ALTERNATIVE POTENT OPIOIDS

Hydromorphone (Dilaudid) is available in a variety of formulations and can be administered by the oral, rectal, subcutaneous, and intravenous routes. It is seven to eight times more potent than morphine when administered parenterally, and when delivered enterally, is about four times as potent as oral morphine (parenteral-to-oral dose ratio of about 5:1). Administered by either route, its latency to effect and duration are relatively short (about 30 minutes and 2–4 hours, respectively). The main uses of hydromorphone are for subcutaneous infusions (in view of its solubility of up to 200 mg/mL), oral breakthrough dosing, and patients who are intolerant to morphine. Despite an unfortunate reputation for street abuse, hydromorphone represents an excellent alternative to morphine in most settings.

Methadone and, to a lesser extent, levorphanol are usually reserved for refractory pain because their half-lives are long and unpredictable, introducing the potential for accumulation, especially in the presence of advanced age and altered renal function.[113–115] Most charts describe methadone as equipotent with morphine when administered intramuscularly, and slightly more potent when administered orally, although newer data suggest that potency may be significantly greater over time as a result of accumulation. Although it is extremely inexpensive, this advantage is offset by a long and variable half-life (13–51 hours) that may lead to drug accumulation, especially in patients who are elderly or who have renal failure. Treatment may best be initiated by parenteral p.r.n. administration until a steady state is achieved, following which the interval between a-t-c administration may vary between 4 hours and 12 hours. Levorphanol (Levo-Dromoran) resembles methadone, in that as a result of its relatively long half-life (11 hours), accumulation may occur. Dosing intervals may vary from 4 to 8 or even 12 hours, and, as a result, the same precautions described for methadone apply to its use.[116] A parenteral dose of 2 mg and an oral dose of 4 mg are usually equianalgesic to 10 mg of parenteral morphine.

Practical Use of Oral Opioids

SCHEDULE

Most patients require simultaneous treatment with two different formulations of an opioid: a long-acting (basal) analgesic administered a-t-c and a short-acting analgesic administered p.r.n. This schema is analogous to the treatment of diabetes mellitus with long-acting (NPH) and short-acting (regular) formulations of insulin concurrently. A predominantly time-contingent (a-t-c) schedule for the administration of analgesics is generally preferred to symptom-contingent (p.r.n.) administration. With prolonged p.r.n. administration, patterns of anticipation and memory of pain become established and may contribute to suffering, even during periods of adequate analgesia.[117]

BASAL (AROUND-THE-CLOCK) ANALGESIA

Compliance and overall quality of analgesia are enhanced by the regular administration of a long-acting opioid analgesic for basal pain control, supplemented by a short-acting opioid analgesic administered p.r.n. (escape doses or rescue doses) for breakthrough and incident pain. This strategy promotes consistent therapeutic plasma levels and avoids roller coaster or sine wave kinetics and dynamics, characterized by alternating bouts of pain and toxicity (Fig. 32–2). If analgesics are withheld until pain becomes severe, sympathetic arousal occurs and even potent analgesics may be ineffective.[6] Prolonged p.r.n. administration may lead to the establishment of a pattern of anticipation and memory of pain that predisposes to persistent suffering even after a more regular administration of analgesics has been instituted (see Fig. 32–2).[117] Preferred basal analgesics include controlled-release morphine and oxycodone preparations[107, 118] that are available in a wide range of doses (but cannot be broken, crushed, or chewed) and transdermal fentanyl.[119, 120] Transdermal fentanyl (Fig. 32–3) is best reserved for the management of relatively stable basal pain. When these agents are poorly tolerated, methadone or levorphanol may be prescribed with careful monitoring, particularly in the presence of altered renal function and advanced age, to avoid accumulation and overdose, risks that are greatest during the initiation of treatment.[113]

SUPPLEMENTAL ANALGESIA WITH ESCAPE OR RESCUE DOSES

In addition to the aforementioned regimen, potent short-acting opioids with minimal potential for accumulation (immediate-release morphine, hydromorphone, oxycodone)

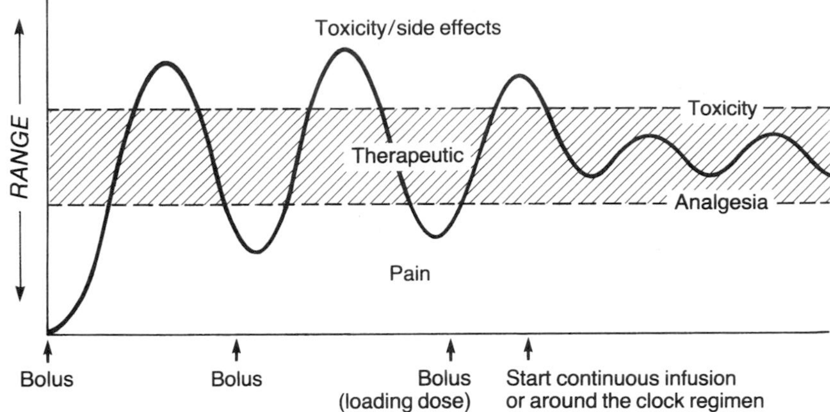

Figure 32–2. The ranges of blood levels of an analgesic achieved over time with various dosing regimens. The lowest sector corresponds to subtherapeutic blood levels and the presence of pain, and the uppermost sector corresponds to toxicity and side effects. The goal of clinical practice is to maintain blood levels within the middle section (therapeutic window) for as much time as possible. Symptom-contingent (p.r.n.) administration is associated with the potential for undesirable alternating bouts of toxicity and pain. Note the transition to time-contingent administration (continuous infusion, controlled-release tablets, or transdermal fentanyl), which minimizes so-called "roller coaster" or "sine wave" kinetics. Treating pain with analgesics is analogous to treating diabetes in that the therapeutic window is characterized by considerable interindividual, and over time, intraindividual variability versus treatment of an infection or seizure disorder (conditions that are characterized by predictable and more universally applicable target blood levels). (From Bruera E, Ripamonti C: Alternate routes of administration of opioids for the management of cancer pain. In: Patt RB [ed]: Cancer Pain, pp 162–167. Philadelphia, J. B. Lippincott Co., 1993.)

are generally made available on an as-needed basis, usually at intervals of 2 to 4 hours for exacerbations of pain (breakthrough pain).[45] The dose of p.r.n. analgesic is usually empirically derived by giving the equivalent of 10% of the sum of long-acting analgesics administered over 24 hours. For example, the patient taking 100 mg of controlled-release morphine every 12 hours should be started at about 20 mg of immediate-release morphine sulfate every 3 to 4 hours, after which the ideal dose is found through titration. Rescue doses are often prescribed in a range (i.e., 1–3 tablets every 3–4 hours), depending on the severity of each episode of breakthrough pain. Patients should be instructed to maintain careful records that accurately reflect their analgesic use.[121] When rescue doses are consistently needed more than two or three times over a 12-hour period, the dose of the basal, long-acting analgesic should be increased. Breakthrough pain that is predictably triggered by a specific event or activity is referred to as incident pain, which, if prevalent, is a signal that patients should be instructed to take their p.r.n. (rescue) dose in anticipation of the pain-provoking activity.[47] A formulation of oral transmucosal fentanyl citrate (Fig. 32–4) has been introduced that promises to produce meaningful relief of breakthrough pain within 5 minutes of initiating consumption, an onset that mimics IV administration, despite its noninvasive character.[122–124]

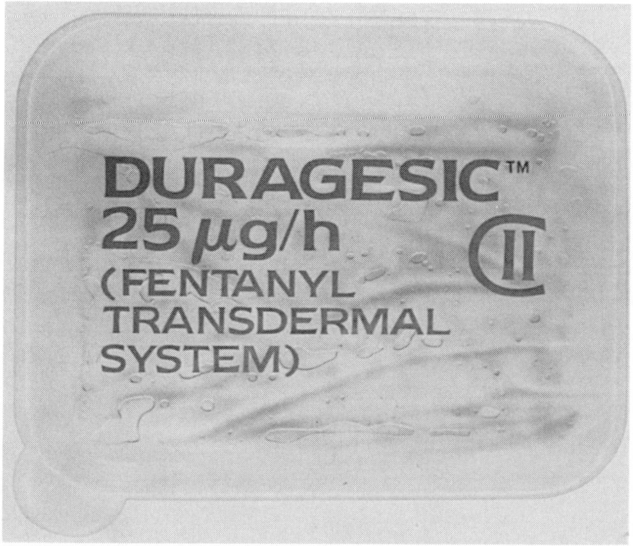

Figure 32–3. Transdermal fentanyl system. Patches are designed to deliver doses of 25, 50, 75, or 100 μg per hour of the potent opioid fentanyl. Once a steady state is achieved (12 to 24 hours), the device's drug reservoir and rate-controlling membrane ensure maintenance of relatively consistent blood levels of fentanyl for a 72-hour interval.

Initiating Therapy

Because dose response and side effects vary widely based on a number of physiologic and behavioral factors (e.g.,

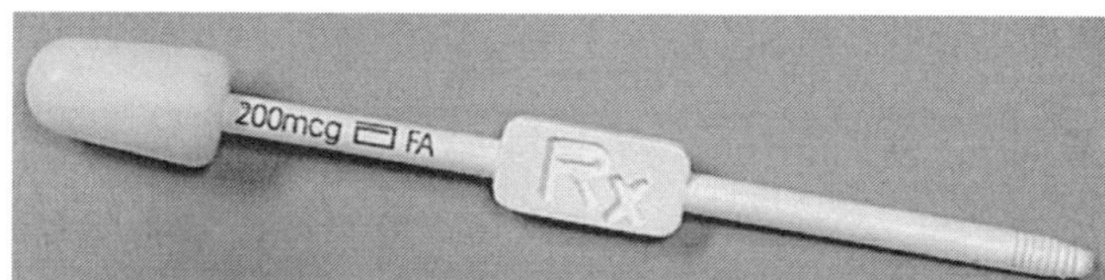

Figure 32–4. Oral trasmucosal fentanyl citrate. Approved for analgesia in the setting of painful procedures, this novel drug delivery system is now also approved for the rapid management of breakthrough pain in cancer patients. Clinical trials indicate that meaningful pain relief is generally noted 5 minutes after patients begin consuming a lozenge.

age, previous drug history, extent of disease),[125, 126] therapy should be individualized to suit the patient's needs. Effective doses often exceed guidelines recommended in standard texts, which, for the most part, are derived from experience with acute or postoperative pain in opioid-naive patients.

Treatment with oral morphine can be started several ways. In cases of severe pain, it may be desirable to initiate therapy with parenteral morphine that can later be converted to an oral drug regimen using a 3:1 ratio. More commonly, immediate-release oral morphine is administered every 3 to 4 hours to determine opioid requirements, following which the sum of the daily dose is halved and administered as a controlled-release preparation and supplemented by rescue doses of immediate-release morphine, each aliquot of which should equal 1/6 to 1/10 of the 24-hour dose. Alternatively, treatment can be initiated with an empirically selected dose of controlled-release morphine, supplemented by appropriate doses of immediate-release morphine. Regardless of the regimen that is selected, low starting doses with rapid upward titration are preferred to limit the frequency of side effects and enhance compliance.

DOSE TITRATION

The correct dose of morphine (or a morphine-line drug) for the management of cancer pain is the dose that effectively relieves the pain without inducing intolerable side effects. Daily doses of morphine required to adequately relieve cancer pain may vary from 60 to 3000 mg in divided doses.[127] There is no ceiling effect for morphine; that is, an increase in the dose always produces a concomitant increase in pain relief. The starting dose is gradually and steadily titrated upward until either pain control is achieved or side effects occur. If dose increases result in worsening side effects and only small increments in analgesia, the pain syndrome may be relatively opioid resistant (e.g., neuropathic pain or movement-related incident pain).[12, 128] Relatively opioid-resistant pain may require alternative therapeutic approaches.

INDIVIDUALIZATION

As mentioned earlier, pharmacologic therapy should be individualized in light of the specific characteristics and needs of each patient.[129] Dose response and side effects vary widely based on various physiologic and behavioral factors (e.g., age, previous drug history, extent of disease).[125, 126] Effective doses in the presence of chronic pain often dramatically exceed guidelines recommended in standard texts (10 mg intramuscularly, 30 mg orally), which usually are derived from experience with acute or postoperative pain in opioid-naive individuals.[130]

DOSING GUIDELINES

The correct dose of an opioid for the management of cancer pain is that which effectively relieves pain without inducing unacceptable side effects.[5, 7, 128] The starting dose is gradually and steadily titrated upwards until either pain control is achieved or side effects occur. If side effects ensue before adequate pain relief is established, they are treated aggressively in an algorithmic fashion, or by some other strategy (e.g., opioid rotation, anesthetic interventions).

SIDE EFFECTS

Treatment with the opioids may be associated with side effects, although in many cases these effects are transient and usually manageable. Prompt identification, assessment, and management of side effects is a cornerstone of treatment. Adverse effects are often perceived as barriers to the provision of analgesics in doses required to relieve pain effectively (dose-limiting side effects). Most drug-related side effects can be effectively relieved with careful management, but the same attention and skill required to tailor a pain management program need to be applied to selecting and titrating drugs to minimize the impact of side effects. Patient education is essential to ensure the best outcome and to avoid confusion between manageable side effects and allergy.[131] Patients should be encouraged to report problems as they occur.

Opioid-induced constipation is sufficiently common that it should almost universally be treated prophylactically. Usually a combined mild stimulant and softener is prescribed when opioid therapy commences, along with instructions for a sliding scale regimen that provides progressively stronger cathartics until a regular bowel habit ensues.[132, 133] An osmotic agent (e.g., lactulose) is the usual second-line agent of choice for refractory constipation. The evaluating clinician should remain alert for the presence of bowel obstruction as well as fecal impaction, which may present as spurious diarrhea as a result of the leakage of liquid stool around a distal fecal plug. Impaction is confirmed by manual rectal examination, and its occurrence leaves no other alternative than manual disimpaction, which is time consuming, unpleasant, and usually requires strong analgesics. Finally, unrecognized constipation can contribute to nausea and vomiting.

Opioid-mediated nausea and sedation occur in up to half of patients first exposed to an opioid and after a dose increase.[134, 135] These symptoms usually resolve spontaneously with continued opioid use, and thus patients should be reassured and encouraged to adhere to their prescribed regimen of analgesics. Patients who are not routinely apprised of these features mistake side effects for allergy. For nausea or vomiting, or both, a major tranquilizer (e.g., prochlorperazine, chlorpromazine) administered orally or rectally is the usual first-line agent of choice, especially when cost is a consideration.[133, 136] A properistaltic agent (e.g., metoclopramide) is appropriate when gastric stasis is suggested by nausea, bloating, and early satiety.[137] Scopolamine is particularly useful for nausea that is vertiginous in nature (i.e., amplified by ambulation).[134] Commonly used as an adjunct to emetic chemotherapies, ondansetron (Zofran) and similar agents can be considered for refractory nausea, but are usually avoided because of cost. Dronabinol, an oral agent containing active elements of marijuana and corticosteroids, is another alternative for refractory nausea, as is the combination of agents that act by distinct mechanisms.[138]

Like nausea, drowsiness and sedation occur commonly when opioid therapy is commenced or escalated, but usually resolve spontaneously with continued use. Sedation that fails to improve with time can often be managed effectively with a psychostimulant, such as methylphenidate or dextroamphetamine.[139] Methylphenidate is usually started in doses of 10 mg on awakening and 5 mg at noon, but may require titration, especially over time. The stimulants appear to enhance analgesia,[140] and are also associated with potent antidepressant actions that, in contrast to classic antidepressants, take effect almost immediately. Other than jitteriness, side effects are infrequent, although caution should be exercised in the presence of brain metastasis, psychotic disorders, hyperactive delirium, and tachyarrhythmias. Anorexia appears not to be a practical problem and, in fact, patients have anecdotally been observed to experience paradoxical weight gain, presumably as a result of increased wakefulness. Both methylphenidate and dextroamphetamine have relatively short half-lives, so sleep is typically not disturbed, and, should it be necessary, both agents are available in extended-release formulations.

REFRACTORY SIDE EFFECTS

When side effects are refractory to pharmacoreversal, consideration should be given to a trial of a similar, alternative opioid because side effects are often idiosyncratic and may not be triggered by agents that are in other respects similar.[128, 141] If indicated, the addition of a nonopioid adjuvant analgesic can be considered that, if successful, may serve to reduce side effects by an opioid-sparing effect.[142] Finally, in patients with amenable pain syndromes, the presence of refractory side effects is an indication to consider other more invasive therapeutic modalities, such as nerve blocks or spinal opioid therapy.[10]

REASSESSMENT

Once an acceptable drug regimen has been established, adequacy should be periodically reassessed.[5] Patients are often reluctant to spontaneously request more potent analgesics because of fear of addiction. Increased drug requirements related to progression of disease and attendant pain, as well as the development of tolerance, should be anticipated. Although tolerance is now viewed as a less vexing problem than in the past, when it occurs, it is most frequently manifested by decreased duration of analgesic effect.

EDUCATION AND ADDICTION POTENTIAL

Patient and family education is essential and is ideally accomplished through the combined efforts of physicians, nurses, and pharmacists. Patients commonly maintain deeply rooted fears of addiction that are culturally reinforced, regrettably often by their physicians. Distinctions between addiction (psychological dependence), physical dependence, and tolerance should be explained.[143] Tolerance, that is, the need for increasing dosages over time to maintain a desired effect, and physical dependence, that is, a state characterized by the onset of characteristic withdrawal symptoms when a drug is precipitously stopped or a specific antagonist is administered, are biophysiologic phenomena that are inevitable and should thus be regarded as pharmacologic effects (Table 32–14). They are unrelated to addiction and need not impede analgesic therapy. Because tolerance develops for most side effects as well as for analgesia, doses can usually be increased to counter tolerance; should opioid therapy become unnecessary, patients are generally able to discontinue use without problems when a gradual tapering off is instituted.[144]

Addiction is a psychobehavioral phenomenon with possi-

TABLE 32–14. **Contemporary Description of Phenomena Historically Associated with Addiction**

Phenomenon	Etiology	Definition	Incidence	Management
Physical dependence	Physiologic, pharmacologic	Withdrawal if opioids abruptly stopped or naloxone administered	Almost invariable	Avoid by gradual tapering
Tolerance[1]	Physiologic, pharmacologic	Increased dose required to achieve analgesia[2]	Almost invariable	Re-establish analgesia with upward titration
Addiction (psychological dependence)	Psychological, possible genetic influences	Overwhelming use, nonmedical use, use despite presence or threat of physiologic or psychological harm	Rare (<1%)	Identify and institute multidisciplinary management
Withdrawal (abstinence syndrome)	Physiologic, pharmacologic	Characteristic signs and symptoms[3]	Almost invariable	Avoid, reverse with opioids
Pseudo-addiction	Behavioral	Iatrogenic syndrome of apparent drug-seeking behavior that evolves as a consequence of undertreatment; arises as a consequence of well-meaning but ill-informed clinicians' concerns that dosing to effect will produce addiction	Regrettably common	Counter with education and more liberal prescribing habits

[1]Although inevitable to some degree, current thinking posits this phenomenon as considerably less severe than previously thought, recognizing instead that dose increases in cancer patients are most likely due to disease progression.

[2]Tolerance develops for most adverse effects as well, especially nausea and sedation, but slowly if at all to constipation and miosis.

[3]Characteristic signs and symptoms include lacrimation, diaphoresis, rhinorrhea, pupillary dilation, gooseflesh, muscle tremor, nausea and vomiting, abdominal cramping, diarrhea, raised heart rate, respiratory rate and blood pressure, chills, hyperthermia, flushing, yawning, restlessness, irritability, anorexia, disturbed sleep, and generalized body aches.

ble genetic influences characterized by (1) overwhelming drug use, (2) nonmedical drug use, and (3) continued use despite the presence or threat of physiologic or psychological harm. In contrast to tolerance and physical dependence, which are inevitable with chronic use, addiction is an infrequent outcome of medical treatment except in patients with a previous history of drug abuse who are at increased risks of both developing aberrant drug use and undertreatment.[145]

Adjuvant Analgesics

Selected patients will benefit from treatment with agents from among this heterogeneous classification. In general, these agents are mechanism specific and should be used based on a specific indication.

ROUTES OF ADMINISTRATION

ORAL ADMINISTRATION

When possible, analgesics should be administered orally or by a similarly noninvasive route (transdermal, rectal, oral transmucosal) to promote independence and mobility and for ease of titration.[5, 12] In the presence of a functional, intact GI system, once the dose is adjusted to account for a hepatic first-pass effect, oral administration provides analgesia that is as effective as parenteral (but not spinal) administration. Other more invasive routes should be considered only for specific indications. Ultimately, however, it appears that between one third and two thirds of patients benefit from at least the transient use of an alternate route at some time before death.[92, 146]

TRANSDERMAL ADMINISTRATION

Transdermal fentanyl is associated with advantages similar to those cited for oral administration except that, as a result of its pharmacokinetics, it is best reserved for patients with stable pain and should not be relied on in the presence of rapidly changing dose requirements.[119, 120] Although its use can be maintained in the presence of alimentary tract dysfunction, it need not be reserved specifically for this setting. It is particularly useful in patients with otherwise poor compliance, may be associated with high levels of patient acceptance, and may produce less constipation than oral opioids.

Once treatment is established, steady plasma levels of fentanyl are maintained for 72 hours following a single application of a 25-, 50-, 75-, or 100-μg/h patch.[147] The surface area of the patch is directly proportional to the administered dose of fentanyl, and patches can be combined to arrive at the desired dose. The system's rate-controlling membrane regulates drug release at a slower rate than average skin flux, thus ensuring that the delivery system, rather than the skin, is the main determinant of absorption. Of factors with the potential to influence the rate of absorption of transdermal fentanyl, temperature is most important, and, as a result, patients should be warned against applying heating pads or the like.[148] Although low levels of fentanyl can be detected in the blood stream just 1 hour after administration, because of the relative impermeability of the epidermis, a consistent, near-peak level is not obtained for a period of 12 to 18 hours after treatment is initiated. Patients need to be cautioned that pain relief accrues over the first day of treatment and should be provided with rescue doses of short-acting analgesics during this interval. In addition, as a result of the formation of a subcutaneous depot of drug, effects persist for 12 to 18 hours following removal of the patch, so that adverse effects may require prolonged treatment. Although the transdermal fentanyl system was originally studied predominantly in the perioperative setting, its ultimate approval was limited to the management of chronic pain. Conversion schemes are conservative, so that up to half of patients dosed according to the product's package insert require rapid upward titration. Because of the lag between dose and response, transdermal fentanyl analgesia is best suited for patients with relatively stable dose requirements and is particularly useful when the oral route is contraindicated.

RECTAL ADMINISTRATION

When the oral and transdermal routes are inappropriate, rectal administration is reliable for short-term use[149] except in the presence of diarrhea, fistulae, or other anatomic abnormalities. Rectal administration is usually avoided in older children and in the presence of conditions that increase pain when patients are positioned for suppository insertion. Morphine and hydromorphone are available in rectal preparations, and oxymorphone hydrochloride (Numorphan) rectal suppositories provide 4 to 6 hours of potent analgesia.[150] Rectal methadone has been shown to be safe and effective, but must be compounded by a manufacturing pharmacist.[151]

PARENTERAL ADMINISTRATION

With the growth of the hospice and home care movement, there has been increasing acceptance of chronic parenteral opioid administration by means of continuous subcutaneous or intravenous infusions administered by a portable pump, with or without a patient-controlled analgesia feature. When equianalgesic conversion is accounted for, there is no evidence that parenteral administration is associated with superior analgesia, and, as a result, conversion should be reserved for specific indications, such as titration for a pain emergency or alimentary tract failure (xerostomia, dysphagia, malabsorption, obstruction, vomiting, coma).[152]

CONTINUOUS SUBCUTANEOUS AND INTRAVENOUS INFUSIONS

Because of its reduced nursing requirements, the continuous subcutaneous infusion (CSCI) of opioids currently represents the route of choice for chronic home-based administration, unless permanent intravenous (IV) access has already been established.[151, 153] A variety of commercially available infusion pumps are portable, battery driven, inexpensively leased, and equipped with alarm systems.

To initiate a CSCI, the 24-hour dose of parenteral drug is summed. If the patient's drug regimen includes oral analgesics, conversion tables are used (see Tables 32–12 and 32–13) to calculate the equianalgesic parenteral dose of opioid (usually morphine or hydromorphone). The total daily dose of parenteral drug is divided by 24, and the pump is set accordingly. Tissue irritation is minimized when volumes under 1 to 2 mL are prescribed, a practice that is facilitated by ordering an appropriately concentrated formulation of the opioid. The pump's tubing is primed with drug and it is attached to a 27-g pediatric butterfly needle, which is inserted subcutaneously and taped flush with the patient's skin. Any subcutaneous site can be used, although the infraclavicular fossa and chest wall are frequently selected to facilitate easy ambulation. The infusion site is checked twice daily for signs of irritation, and is changed weekly or as needed.[154]

Absorption of subcutaneously administered opioids is rapid, and steady-state plasma levels are generally approached within 1 hour.[155] Most parenteral opioids are suitable for CSCI, although morphine and hydromorphone are used most commonly, and meperidine, methadone, and pentazocine should be avoided as a result of their potential for tissue irritation. Physician orders should provide for rescue doses of drug adequate to counter incomplete analgesia (usually a subcutaneous bolus injection equal to the hourly dose administered every 30 to 60 min, p.r.n.), and, at the end of 24 hours, the infusion is increased by the sum of the recorded rescue doses. If analgesia is adequate but side effects are prominent (usually oversedation), the infusion rate may be halved and titrated upwards, as needed.

More sophisticated hospice programs routinely infuse combinations of opioids, antiemetics, and steroids simultaneously without side effects and difficulties.[156] Novel subcutaneous applications include continuous infusions of ketamine[157] and lidocaine[158] for refractory neuropathic cancer pain syndromes, and the development of a hydromorphone pellet that, when implanted, provides continuous pain relief for periods of up to 4 weeks.[159]

Alternate Drugs Including Tramadol

Clinicians should maintain familiarity with the pharmacologic profiles of a variety of opioids (see Tables 32–12 and 32–13) and should consider drug rotation when a favorable balance between comfort and side effects cannot be achieved with a given regimen. When converting between drugs or routes, half to two thirds of the calculated equianalgesic dose of the new drug is usually recommended as a starting dose,[5, 6] which is then titrated rapidly, as needed.

Despite a unique mechanism that involves weak μ-agonist activity, as well as inhibition of norepinephrine and serotonin reuptake, the synthetic codeine analogue tramadol has, at best, a moderate role in the management of cancer pain. Although it may be used as an alternative to codeine or hydrocodone, it is unclear whether tramadol possesses any particular advantages, and it appears to be less satisfactory than morphine for the management of severe pain. Higher doses are associated with a ceiling effect and side effects that include dizziness, nausea, dry mouth, and sedation. However, abuse potential may be lower than that of classic opioid analgesics.

Drugs to Avoid

The chronic administration of meperidine, especially by the oral route, is contraindicated.[5, 6, 22] Administered chronically, all opioids may produce some degree of myoclonus, but the accumulation of normeperidine, a metabolite, may lead to frank seizure activity, especially when renal function is impaired.[160, 161]

Agonist-antagonist and partial agonist opioids should generally be avoided for a variety of reasons, the most important of which is the presence of a ceiling.[162] With the usual exception of buprenorphine, these agents may precipitate withdrawal, and their administration complicates the eventual, usually inevitable, transition to pure agonist agents. Pentazocine (Talwin), the only of these agents widely available orally, is associated with a high incidence of hallucinations and confusion, and buprenorphine is not easily or reliably reversed by naloxone.

Brompton's cocktail, one of the first preparations of an oral opioid to gain clinical acceptance, is now used only infrequently. Developed at Brompton's Chest Hospital in the United Kingdom, it consisted of a mixture of morphine hydrochloride (or heroin), cocaine hydrochloride, alcohol, syrup and chloroform water. In blinded trials, it has not been shown to produce analgesia that is superior to an oral opioid administered alone,[163] and its use should be discouraged because of the problems associated with titrating fixed-dose combinations. Likewise, no advantage has been demonstrated for treatment with heroin,[164] although it is still sometimes used in the United Kingdom and Canada, predominantly for subcutaneous infusions by virtue of its high solubility.

Alternative Therapies

Adequate pain relief cannot always be achieved through pharmacologic means alone. Initial screening should identify patients in whom behavioral or psychological modalities may be employed successfully. When careful trials of pharmacologic therapy have failed, consideration should be given to alternative modalities including additional antitumor therapy, neural blockade, CNS opioids, neurosurgical options, and, rarely, electrical stimulation.

Adjuvant Analgesics

The term *adjuvant analgesic* is used to refer to a heterogeneous group of medications originally developed for purposes other than relief of pain that have been observed to promote analgesia in specific clinical settings. Although a large variety of drugs are purported to possess adjuvant properties, only a limited number have been shown to reliably relieve pain in controlled or partially controlled trials. Patients with cancer pain may benefit from the addition of (1) corticosteroids; (2) selected, usually tricyclic, antidepressants; (3) anticonvulsants; (4) amphetamines; and, more rarely, (5) *N*-methyl D-aspartate (NMDA) antagonists; (6) alpha-adrenergic antagonists; (7) antihistamines; and (8) phenothiazines. Interestingly, not every agent belonging to each class appears to possess analgesic properties, and even those agents with confirmed analgesic properties are applicable only for specific types of pain; even then, pain relief does not accrue in all potential candidates.

The adjuvant analgesics differ from opioid analgesics in important general ways. Opioids are all-purpose analgesics in that, independent of the clinical condition being treated, if administered in an adequate dose, they always elicit some degree of pain relief. Although admittedly, some conditions appear to be less opioid responsive than others, the clinician can still count on achieving some degree of analgesia if an opioid is administered in a sufficient dose. Regrettably, in less opioid-responsive conditions, escalating side effects may eclipse the utility of analgesia, rendering therapy unacceptable. In contrast, responses to adjuvant analgesics are more binary in nature in that, depending on the nature of the clinical condition being treated (and perhaps other more obscure variables), treatment may or may not elicit pain relief. It happens that most currently recognized adjuvants are most likely to be effective for various types of neuropathic pain. A second fundamental difference relates to the dose-response relationship. Even in conditions in which adjuvants are clearly effective, the nature of the dose-response relationship is fundamentally different from that of the opioids. The relationship between dose and response is usually relatively linear for opioids, even though, depending on the responsivity of the pain, the slope of the line describing the dose-response relationship may be shallow or steep. In contrast, even should an adjuvant produce a desirable effect, there is no certainty that raising the dose will enhance analgesia, or that if a positive response occurs, it will be proportionate or replicable. These features of the adjuvants dictate the development of novel study methodologies.[165]

ANTIDEPRESSANTS

The efficacy of selected antidepressants as analgesics, independent of their effects on mood and nighttime sleep, has been demonstrated initially in noncancer models,[166–168] and, more recently, in cancer patients as well.[141, 169, 170] Because analgesia is characteristically induced with doses generally considered insufficient to relieve depression, there is an argument for a direct, independent, underlying mechanism of effect. In addition, although onset is not immediate, analgesia is generally established more rapidly than are antidepressant effects (typically 3 to 7 days vs. 14 to 21 days). The operant mechanism for antidepressant-mediated analgesia presumably relates to increased circulating pools of norepinephrine and serotonin induced by reductions in the postsynaptic uptake of these neurotransmitters. The most compelling indication for tricyclic antidepressant (TCA) therapy remains variants of neuropathic pain (e.g., postherpetic neuralgia, central pain, diabetic neuropathy), although more recent trials have demonstrated efficacy for disorders that include headache, arthritis, chronic lower back pain, and psychogenic pain.

Amitriptyline and, to a lesser extent, imipramine remain the most extensively studied of these agents, and, as a result, are the usual first choices of academically based pain specialists. Although these agents are usually relatively innocuous, side effects are especially prominent. Because amitriptyline and imipramine are, respectively, metabolized to nortriptyline and desipramine, agents with superior side effect profiles, many authorities, especially in private practice, advocate the latter two agents as drugs of first choice. Data from controlled clinical trials support the use of amitriptyline, nortriptyline, desipramine, imipramine, doxepin, maprotiline, and clomipramine. Trazadone, though sedating and thus potentially helpful for sleep disturbances, appears to be of limited value as an analgesic. Interestingly, despite their efficacy for depression and generally favorable side effect profiles, the newer selective serotonin reuptake inhibitors (SSRIs) such as fluoxetine (Prozac), paroxetine (Paxil), and sertraline (Zoloft) appear to be less effective for treating pain than the heterocyclic antidepressants. Obviously, in cases in which pain is a secondary manifestation of depression, the SSRIs and other antidepressants, administered in therapeutic doses, may be beneficial.

The main indication for treatment with the heterocyclic antidepressants is neuropathic pain that is relatively constant and unrelenting, and is not predominantly intermittent, lancinating, jabbing, or shocklike. Neuropathic pain of the latter (paroxysmal) type may also be treated effectively with TCAs, but is often first treated with an anticonvulsant. As noted, TCAs also have been used successfully in headache and other syndromes, and thus a trial in nearly any cancer pain syndrome that has not responded favorably to primary analgesics is justified.

Usually, amitriptyline, nortriptyline, or desipramine is started in doses of 10 to 25 mg nightly and is gradually titrated upwards, usually to a range of 50 to 125 mg and occasionally higher, until toxicity occurs or analgesia is established. Dry mouth, constipation, drowsiness, and dysphoria are the most prominent of a wide range of potential side effects, although more serious, usually anticholinergic side effects may occur (e.g., urinary retention, cardiac dysrhythmias). Unlike the side effects of opioid therapy, the development of tolerance is less robust, and side effects are less readily reversible; as a result, if side effects are more prominent than analgesia, the offending agent is usually discontinued, and a pharmacologic analogue or a drug from another class is usually started. Although they are not as reliably analgesic as the TCAs, the newer SSRIs may be preferred for (1) the fragile elderly, (2) patients predisposed to developing serious anticholinergic side effects, (3) patients for whom multiple trials of tricyclics have failed as a result of side effects, and (4) patients for whom depression is a prominent comorbidity. Usual starting doses of the SSRIs are the same as those suggested for the management of depression (fluoxetine 20 mg, paroxetine 20 mg, sertraline 50 mg), administered as a single morning dose to take advantage of their propensity to mildly stimulate activity. Interestingly, although these agents are not considered as reliable for analgesia as the heterocyclic antidepressants, paroxetine has been reported to be effective for refractory pruritus in patients with advanced cancer.[171]

ANTICONVULSANTS AND BACLOFEN

Based on ample but predominantly anecdotal reports on the efficacy of carbamazepine for the nonsurgical treatment of trigeminal neuralgia (tic douloureux),[172] carbamazepine, phenytoin, valproate, clonazepam, and most recently gabapentin, alone or in combination with the TCAs, have been used successfully to treat pain of neuropathic origin.[173–175] Most authorities consider them as drugs of first choice for neuropathic pain that resembles classic trigeminal neuralgia (i.e., predominantly paroxysmal, jabbing, shocklike pain). Anticonvulsants are also usually considered a second-line therapy for relatively steady, constant neuropathic pain when TCAs are poorly tolerated or have been ineffective or only partially effective.[38] Anticonvulsants relieve pain in these settings as a result of their ability to dampen ectopic foci of electrical activity and spontaneous discharge from injured nerves, in a manner analogous to their salutary effects in seizure disorders.

Carbamazepine therapy has been most thoroughly documented, and thus, in the absence of contraindications, it is usually considered the drug of first choice. The most toxic of the anticonvulsants used to treat pain, carbamazepine is associated with idiosyncratic hepatotoxicity (rare) and bone marrow depression (incidence of up to 2%), and thus is avoided in patients with liver metastases, bone marrow depletion, or those receiving cytotoxic therapy. Used chronically, carbamazepine therapy requires monitoring of complete blood count and liver function tests every 2 to 3 months. Ataxia, confusion, dizziness, and nausea are relatively common with upward dose titration, and therefore carbamazepine is also best avoided in the fragile elderly, especially combined with other psychotropic agents. Clonazepam, in doses of 0.5 mg b.i.d., is often well tolerated in patients who have experienced or are at risk for side effects with carbamazepine, phenytoin, and valproate. Carbamazepine is usually started at 100 mg b.i.d, and titrated upwards toward 300 to 400 mg q.i.d., while awaiting an analgesic response or toxicity.

Failure of one anticonvulsant does not appear to predict outcome for trials of an alternate agent. Gabapentin[176] is a new anticonvulsant that, according to anecdote, may be highly efficacious for neuropathic pain, especially when lancinating, although controlled trials have not yet been reported. Trials of gabapentin for neuropathic pain, in doses commencing at 100 mg t.i.d. and ranging to 300 q.i.d., have become almost ubiquitous, largely because serious side effects are infrequent. Although felbamate, another new anticonvulsant, is known to interact with the NMDA receptor, its use is probably only rarely warranted as a result of concerns regarding the development of aplastic anemia.[177]

Although it is a γ-aminobutyric acid agonist and not an anticonvulsant, baclofen, with or without carbamazepine, has been reported to be effective for lancinating, ticlike neuropathic pain. Baclofen is usually started at a dose of 5 mg b.i.d. or t.i.d., and may be titrated up to 30 to 90 mg/day as tolerated.[38] The other main role for baclofen in pain management is as an intrathecal infusion for spasticity resulting especially from spinal cord injury and multiple sclerosis.[178]

ORAL LOCAL ANESTHETICS

Based on historical accounts of transient relief of pain after IV infusions of local anesthetics, oral (and rectal) analogues already in use as antiarrhythmics have been exploited for relief of neuropathic pain.[179, 180] The agent of choice from this group is mexiletine, which is usually regarded as a second- or third-line agent for continuous or intermittent neuropathic pain disorders. The oral local anesthetics block sodium channels and relieve pain by mechanisms similar to those at work in anticonvulsant-mediated analgesia. Mexiletine is usually started in doses of 150 mg/day, and is titrated upwards to a maximum dose of 300 mg t.i.d. Up to 40% of patients may discontinue therapy due to side effects, the most common of which are nausea and vomiting.

AMPHETAMINES

The most accepted use for amphetamines in palliative care is as a means to reverse opioid-mediated sedation.[46, 138] A 1992 report even suggests durable improvements in cognitive function in cancer patients receiving opioids.[181] In addition to these primary effects, research suggests that dextroamphetamine and methylphenidate (Ritalin) possess analgesic properties[139] and are excellent antidepressants. Unlike classic antidepressants, their effect on mood is usually apparent with the first dose. Furthermore, before the introduction of SSRIs, methylphenidate had developed an excellent record of safety in geriatric patients with refractory depression, and their safe use has been reported in adolescent cancer patients receiving opioid therapy.[182] Arrhythmias are almost nonexistent, and, instead of inducing anorexia, these agents typically have a paradoxical effect of increasing appetite by enhancing alertness. Nervousness and agitation are the most common adverse effects and usually respond to dose reductions. Agitated delirium may occur in patients with coexisting psychiatric disorders, brain metastases, or metabolic disturbances, all of which are relative contraindications for use. Methylphenidate is typically started in doses of 10 mg on awakening and 5 mg with the noontime meal, after which titration to effect is instituted. Because of its short half-life, patients are usually able to sleep well at night,[183] especially if they have become more active as a result of increased alertness. Dextroamphetamine can be administered on a similar schedule, and extended-release formulations are available for both agents.

CORTICOSTEROIDS

The efficacy of corticosteroids as treatment for acute pain resulting from raised intracranial pressure and spinal cord compression is well established. In addition, these agents have been administered empirically for a variety of cancer pain syndromes with good results.[184, 185] Pain relief is presumably related to reduced peritumoral edema and inflammation, with consequent relief of pressure and traction on nerves and other pain-sensitive structures, although beneficial effects on mood, appetite, and weight also may indirectly contribute to improved subjective pain reports. Improvements in pain are often rapid and dramatic, but usually depend on continued administration. Although results may be maintained in a proportion of patients, benefits are often short lived, plateauing in a few weeks, presumably due to the replacement of edema by tumor growth in patients with aggressive disease. A trial of oral steroids may be beneficial in any patient with pain that appears to be predominantly due to spread of bulky tumor (e.g., selected patients with pelvic, rectal, esophageal, or hepatic tumor deposits or invasion of the brachial and lumbosacral plexus).

Dexamethasone is the usual drug of choice because it possesses less potent mineralocorticoid effects. Although a variety of side effects and complications can occur as a result of even acute steroid administration (e.g., diabetes mellitus, psychosis), serious problems usually arise only from chronic use. As a result, when a trial produces beneficial results, it is reasonable to maintain use, without tapering, in the presence of progressive cancer.[186] Although most patients note improvements in mood when steroid therapy is commenced, a small proportion experience dysphoria and even florid psychosis. Interestingly, the occurrence of such an episode does not appear to predict similar reactions on re-exposure. The optimal dose of steroids, both for oncologic emergencies (e.g., raised intracranial pressure, cord compression) and chronic pain, is not known. For oncologic emergencies, 100 mg IV dexamethasone is administered initially in some institutions, followed by IV maintenance. The large bolus dose produces severe but transient perineal burning (like ants in the pants) due to an unknown mechanism. For the management of nonemergent pain, an oral dose of 2 to 6 mg dexamethasone q.i.d. or t.i.d. is common.

N-METHYL D-ASPARTATE ANTAGONISTS

The NMDA receptor has recently been described and implicated in the transmission of pain.[187] Although research on various agents with antagonist activity at the NMDA receptor is under way, ketamine, a partial NMDA antagonist, is the only agent currently available that appears to mediate pain by this nonopioid mechanism.[188] Long used as an IV anesthetic agent, subanesthetic doses have been administered for prolonged periods with fair success in a small number of patients with refractory neuropathic cancer pain.[156, 189] Because of side effects and the risk of complications, ketamine infusion should be regarded as a treatment of desperation, reserved for rare use, until additional experience has been reported.

ALPHA-2 ADRENERGIC ANTAGONISTS

The centrally acting antihypertensive clonidine has been observed to promote analgesia for neuropathic pain when administered near the neuroaxis. Epidural administration has recently received Food and Drug Administration approval, and trials of intrathecal clonidine are under way. In a prospective, randomized study of 38 patients with severe cancer pain that had persisted despite large doses of spinal opioids, the addition of epidural clonidine was associated with significant improvement in 45% of patients overall and in 56% of patients with neuropathic pain.[190] Hypotension during the initiation of treatment and rebound hypertension during withdrawal are the main potential risks of treatment.

BISPHOSPHONATES

Whereas the primary indication for the bisphosphonates remains the management of symptomatic hypercalcemia, important roles for these agents are emerging for the prevention of skeletal complications of cancer. Nearly all of the bisphosphonates have been implicated in the reduction of phenomena that include osseous metastases, pain emanating from established bone metastases, osteoporosis, pathologic fracture, and immobility. Most studies demonstrating efficacy have been conducted in patients with multiple myeloma and metastatic breast and prostate cancer. Etidronate appears to be relatively ineffective for treating pain, whereas monthly IV injections of pamidronate appear to be the most reliable approach to inducing analgesia.[191, 192] The utility of oral pamidronate is unfortunately hampered by poor bioavailability and adverse effects, including GI toxicity, renal impairment, anemia, and electrolyte abnormalities. In one report, a series of five daily IV injections of olpadronate was observed to dramatically reduce bone pain for a period of 4 to 6 weeks, beyond which analgesia persisted only in patients maintained on oral therapy.[193] A trial of clodronate, administered as 600 to 1500 mg IV in 500 mL normal saline over 3 hours every 1 to 2 weeks, is an alternate regimen that has been shown to be effective for the management of painful bone metastases.

OTHER PURPORTED ADJUVANTS

Despite an absence of data from controlled trials, antihistamines, benzodiazepines, and antipsychotics have been used, mostly historically, in efforts to enhance analgesia. Although these agents have clear roles for primary indications other than pain (e.g., anxiolysis, antiemesis, etc.), with few exceptions, they are not reliably associated with analgesia, and thus should not be relied on as substitutes for opioid analgesics.[194, 195]

In contrast to other neuroleptics, methotrimeprazine reliably produced dose-related analgesia that was comparable to the opioid-mediated analgesia, but it recently has been withdrawn from the marketplace. Although clinical lore has perpetuated the hypothesis that the butyrophenones have utility as primary or adjuvant analgesics, these beliefs have been confirmed neither by controlled trials[196] nor survey data.[197] Proponents advocate trials for rectal tenesmus, bladder tenesmus, neuropathic pain, and whenever suffering or psychological distress is prominent.

A careful review of the literature reveals insufficient evidence to support the contention that the benzodiazepines have meaningful analgesic properties in most clinical circumstances.[193] Although treatment with the benzodiazepines may reduce complaints of pain, this result appears to be an indirect effect related to their psychotropic properties rather than true analgesia. Thus, the use of benzodiazepines should be discouraged except in extremely specific settings. Clinical experience suggests a potential role for short-term use to manage acute muscle spasm, as an anxiolytic when stress appears to influence reports of pain, and for lancinating neuropathic pain as a part of sequential trials, in which case clonazepam and alprazolam are the agents of choice. They should probably not be considered as first-line choices even for the above-mentioned indications because potential benefits are often eclipsed by the potential for the development of cognitive impairment, physical and psychological dependence, worsening depression, the risk of overdose, and other side effects.

Anesthetic and Neurosurgical Management

Although effective control of cancer pain can be achieved in a high proportion of patients with rigorously applied pharmacologic treatment, 10% to 30% of patients may require more aggressive management, ranging from the parenteral and spinal administration of opioids to neurodestructive procedures.

Nerve Blocks

Neural blockade involves the interruption of local pain pathways and has the potential advantage of relieving pain with less reliance on systemic medications, thereby minimizing attendant side effects.[9] Traditionally, such techniques have been considered either late in the course of a cancer diagnosis or as an exclusive alternative to systemic analgesics. Contemporary views recognize that selected patients benefit from early implementation of neural blockade, and that optimal control of symptoms requires careful integration of regional and systemic approaches.[5] Neural blockade is best regarded as a component of a therapeutic matrix that includes antitumor therapy, various pharmacologic strategies, and behavioral and psychiatric approaches, ideally implemented in a multidisciplinary setting.[10]

Neural blockade is a valuable method of relieving pain due to cancer in well-selected patients. Local anesthetic blocks temporarily interrupt fibers transmitting pain and are valuable diagnostic tools, whereas the injection of alcohol and phenol often provides lasting relief of oncologic pain. Abdominal and pelvic pain are particularly amenable to management with neural blockade. Celiac plexus block and superior hypogastric plexus block, when performed for abdominal and pelvic pain, respectively, are sufficiently safe and effective, and should be considered early in the course of treatment.

Local Anesthetic Blocks

The injection of local anesthetics in the vicinity of a nerve or nerve plexus (as is commonly practiced for dentistry) has a well-confirmed role for the management of nonmalignant pain, but its therapeutic role in cancer pain is limited. The main utility of local or temporary blocks in the setting of cancer pain is for diagnostic purposes, to confirm the anatomic pathways of pain transmission, for prognostic purposes, and to predict the efficacy and morbidity of more permanent or neurolytic blockade carried out with alcohol or phenol. Therapeutic trigger point blocks with local anesthesia are, however, occasionally carried out when muscle spasm is prominent, and they represent a technique that can be readily mastered by the general physician and administered at the bedside. Another relatively noninvasive approach may be helpful in patients with pain due to active herpes zoster or acute or subacute postherpetic neuralgia, who may benefit from the subcutaneous injection of a mixture of local anesthetic and steroid beneath the most sensitive areas of skin.

Neurolytic Blocks

Because cancer pain tends to be constant, unremitting, and progressive, treatment goals are for pain relief of at least moderate duration, so the nerves involved in pain transmission must actually be destroyed. In diagnosed cancer, pain no longer serves a warning function. The symptoms come to actually assume the role of disease, and it is appropriate that they be eliminated, even if further tissue is damaged in the process. Like analgesic neurosurgery, even neurolytic or destructive blocks are impermanent as a result of regrowth of neural tissue and the plasticity or adaptability of the nervous system, but effects tend to average 6 months, a duration that is generally sufficient for most patients.[9]

Neighboring nerves are usually injected because the sensory fields often overlap. Local anesthetic is injected before the definitive neurolytic procedure to confirm that pain relief follows and that the resulting sensation of numbness is well tolerated. Most patients gratefully exchange unremitting pain for numbness, but occasionally the numbness is experienced as an unpleasant, dysesthetic sensation that can be profoundly disturbing. Because alcohol and phenol produce indiscriminate destruction of neural tissue, nerves that transmit motor impulses to the limbs should not be injected unless movement is already compromised, either by tumor invasion or severe pain, and procedures are generally performed under radiologic guidance to limit the risk of neurologic morbidity.

Nerve blocks can be performed at various levels, including at the peripheral and cranial nerves, the exiting nerve roots within the subarachnoid or epidural space, and at the sympathetic ganglia.[198, 199] Alcohol celiac plexus block is of particular value for pain due to pancreatic cancer and other intra-abdominal neoplasms, and is associated with an extremely low incidence of serious complications.[200]

Neurosurgical Options

Most of the numerous neurosurgical approaches that have been developed over the years for managing pain have been abandoned because of their invasiveness, the need for specialized training, and the greater availability of effective conservative therapies.[201] The main exception, percutaneous cordotomy, is highly effective, not too demanding of a patient's limited reserves and, because open surgery is avoided, involves little recuperative time.[202] A needle introduced below the mastoid in the semi-awake patient is subject to highly controlled heating, and by generating a thermal lesion in the cord's lateral spinothalamic tract, offers relief of unilateral truncal and lower limb pain. Although it is associated with a somewhat higher incidence of complications, midline myelotomy is also still occasionally performed for refractory pelvic and lower extremity pain.[203] After laminectomy, an operating microscope is employed to aid sectioning the cord along its midline commissure where the decussating sensory fibers are interrupted, theoretically leaving motor fibers undisturbed.

Intraspinal Opioids

The introduction and evolution of intraspinal opioid therapy, a logical outgrowth of the discovery of opioid receptors, have dramatically altered contemporary cancer pain management over a remarkably short period of time.[204, 205] Intraspinal opioid therapy is considered for patients unable to achieve adequate comfort with the application of standard pharmacologic interventions, or when side effects prevail. Unlike destructive nerve blocks, cost-effective screening can be performed and, as with treatment using systemic opioids, effects are titratable and reversible. Side effects and complications occur in only a modest proportion of patients, and various drug delivery systems have been developed, increasing the feasibility of long-term use.

The benefits of intraspinal anesthesia (the administration of local anesthetics into the epidural or intrathecal space) are well known for patients with acute pain related to labor, surgery, and postoperative recovery. In general, this approach to pain relief is not applicable for patients with chronic cancer pain because its effects are nonselective;

reduction in pain is accompanied by motor weakness, sensory anesthesia, and interference with sympathetic activity, which can cause hypotension, precluding home use. In contrast, intraspinal analgesia is achieved by the epidural or intrathecal administration of an opioid. Pain transmitted by A-delta and C fibers, which corresponds to most oncologic pain, typically is dramatically relieved, but in a highly selective fashion, with an absence of motor, sensory, and sympathetic effects, making this modality highly adaptable to the home care environment.[206]

The principle underlying CNS opioid therapy is that, by introducing minute quantities of opioid drugs in close proximity to their receptors (substantia gelatinosa of the spinal cord), high local concentrations are achieved. As a result, in properly selected patients, analgesia is often superior to that achieved when opioids are administered by other routes, and because the absolute amount of drug administered is reduced, side effects are minimized.[207–209] Not uncommonly, opioid-induced cognitive failure and so-called narcotic bowel syndrome (pseudo-obstruction) are reversed in conjunction with marked improvements in comfort at much lower overall doses.

The CNS can be accessed via intrathecal, epidural, or intraventricular approaches, although an intraventricular route is used much less frequently, primarily for intractable head and neck pain, and then usually when an access device (e.g., Ommaya reservoir) is already in place.[210, 211] The institution of intraspinal opiate therapy requires the participation of an anesthesiologist or neurosurgeon familiar with techniques of screening, implantation, and maintenance, as well as a home care system that is adaptable and innovative. Perhaps the most important aspect of intraspinal opioid therapy is its reversibility, and the reliability and simplicity of advance screening measures for its efficacy. Screening generally can be accomplished on an outpatient basis by observing the patient's response to morphine, administered through a temporary epidural catheter that is inserted percutaneously. This procedure is simple and associated with minimal discomfort, and is generally well tolerated even in ill patients. If improved pain control and reduced side effects are sufficiently profound to warrant more prolonged therapy, temporary catheters usually are replaced with a so-called permanent implanted catheter (modified Hickman-Broviac catheter)[212] or a fully implanted, computer-controlled pump (because of concerns about infection and catheter migration). When cost is an overriding concern, or death is imminent, implantation at the bedside may be a reasonable option.[213, 214]

Although complications such as cord compression, epidural abscess, meningitis, and device failure have been reported, they are surprisingly infrequent.[215, 216] Whereas side effects (respiratory depression, nausea and vomiting, pruritus, urinary retention, dysphoria) are common in opioid-naive individuals treated for acute pain, they are rare in cancer patients chronically exposed to opioids.

Electrical Stimulation

Overall, modalities involving the application of electrical stimulation to various levels of the nervous system have few indications in the management of cancer pain. Transcutaneous electrical nerve stimulation is a noninvasive means of reducing pain that involves the application of low-voltage electrical stimulation over a painful site by means of a portable beeper-sized power source attached to ECG electrodes. Transcutaneous electrical nerve stimulation is most often used as an adjunct to other more reliably effective modalities because it rarely relieves pain entirely, and it appears to be partially dependent on the placebo response.[217] Although it is shown to relieve cancer pain effectively by promoting the release of endogenous opioid peptides,[218] deep brain stimulation, recently approved for the management of Parkinsonian tremor, is currently considered investigational for this application. Spinal cord stimulation, which involves the surgical implantation of electrodes near spinal cord segments involved in modulating painful signals, is increasingly accepted for the management of chronic nonmalignant pain, though it is not currently recommended for the management of cancer pain.[219]

Summary

Regrettably, chronic and acute pain occur in a high percentage of cancer patients. If pain is inadequately addressed by the clinician, it and other distressing symptoms may interfere with primary antitumor therapy and markedly detract from the quality of life of patients, family members, and care providers. Although a strong focus on pain control is important, independent of disease stage, it is a special priority in patients with advanced disease who are no longer candidates for potentially curative therapy.

Although it is rarely eliminated altogether, pain can be controlled in the vast majority of patients, usually with the careful application of straightforward pharmacologic measures, combined with diagnostic acumen and conscientious follow-up. In the small but significant proportion of patients whose pain is not readily controlled with noninvasive analgesics, a variety of alternative measures are available that, when selected carefully, are also associated with a high degree of success. An increasingly large cadre of clinicians has come to recognize that, far from an exercise in futility, caring for patients with advanced, irreversible illness can represent a highly satisfying endeavor that is usually met with considerable success. Thus, no patient should ever wish for death as a result of inadequate control of pain or other symptoms, and clinicians need never communicate overtly or indirectly that "there is nothing more that can be done." Comprehensive cancer care is best regarded as a continuum that commences with prevention and early detection, focuses intensely on curative therapy, and is ideally rendered complete by a seamless transition to palliation and attention to quality of life.

REFERENCES

1. Pickett M, Cooley ME, Gordon DB: Palliative care: past, present, and future perspectives. Semin Oncol Nurs 1998; 14:86.
2. Burge F: The epidemiology of palliative care in cancer. J Palliat Care 1992; 8:18.
3. Brescia FJ: Pain management issues as part of the comprehensive care of the cancer patient. Semin Oncol 1993; 20(suppl A):48.
4. MacDonald N: Cancer centres: Their role in palliative care. J Palliat Care 1992; 8:38.
5. Management of Cancer Pain Guideline Panel: Management of Can-

cer Pain: Clinical Practice Guideline No. 9. Rockville, MD, AHCPR Publication No. 94-0592, March 1994.
6. American Pain Society: Principles of Analgesic Use in the Treatment of Acute Pain and Chronic Cancer Pain, 3rd ed. Skokie, IL, American Pain Society, 1992.
7. Cancer pain assessment and treatment curriculum guidelines. J Clin Oncol 1992; 10:1976.
8. Patt RB: Anesthetic procedures for the control of cancer pain. In: Arbit E (ed): Management of Cancer Related Pain, p 381. Mount Kisco, Futura, 1993.
9. Patt RB, Jain S: The outcomes movement and neurolytic blockade for cancer pain management. Pain Digest 1995; 5:268.
10. Patt RB, Jain S: Therapeutic decision making for invasive procedures. In: Patt RB (ed): Cancer Pain, p 275. Philadelphia, Lippincott, 1993.
11. Cleeland CS, Gonin R, Hatfield AK, et al: Pain and its treatment in outpatients with metastatic cancer. N Engl J Med 1994; 330:592.
12. World Health Organization: Cancer Pain Relief. Geneva, WHO, 1986.
13. Portenoy RK: Cancer pain: Epidemiology and syndromes. Cancer 1989; 63:2307.
14. Ventafridda V, De Conno FD: Status of cancer pain and palliative care worldwide. J Pain Symptom Manage 1996; 12:79.
15. Jadad AR, Browman GP: The WHO analgesic ladder for cancer pain management: stepping up the quality of its evaluation. JAMA 1995; 274:1870.
16. Cleeland CS: Barriers to the management of cancer pain. Oncology 1987; 12(suppl):19.
17. Dubner R: Pain and hyperalgesia following tissue injury: new mechanisms and new treatments. Pain 1991; 44:213.
18. Merskey H: Classification of chronic pain. Pain 1986; 3(suppl):1.
19. Cherny NI, Coyle N, Foley KM: Suffering in the advanced cancer patient: a definition and taxonomy. J Palliat Care 1994; 10:57.
20. Ersek M, Ferrell BR: Providing relief from cancer pain by assisting in the search for meaning. J Palliat Care 1994; 10:15.
21. Ferrell BR, Dean G: The meaning of cancer pain. Semin Oncol Nurs 1995; 11:17.
22. Practice guidelines for cancer pain management: a report by the American Society of Anesthesiologists Task Force on Pain Management, Cancer Pain Section. Anesthesiology 1996; 84:1243.
23. Rowlingson J, Hammill RJ, Patt RB: Assessment of the patient with oncologic pain. In: Patt R (ed): Cancer Pain, p 23. Philadelphia, Lippincott, 1993.
24. Tasmuth T, Kataja M, Blomqvist C, et al: Treatment-related factors predisposing to chronic pain in patients with breast cancer—a multivariate approach. Acta Oncol 1997; 36:625.
25. McCarthy GM, Skillings JR: Jaw and other orofacial pain in patients receiving vincristine for the treatment of cancer. Oral Surg Oral Med Oral Pathol 1992; 74:299.
26. Tanner KD, Reichling DB, Levine JD: Nociceptor hyper-responsiveness during vincristine-induced painful peripheral neuropathy in the rat. J Neurosci 1998; 18:6480.
27. Patt RB: Cancer pain syndromes. In: Patt RB (ed): Cancer Pain, p 3. Philadelphia, Lippincott, 1993.
28. Campa JA, Payne R: Pain syndromes due to cancer. In: Patt RB (ed): Cancer Pain, p 41. Philadelphia, Lippincott, 1993.
29. Broome ME, Rehwaldt M, Fogg L: Relationships between cognitive behavioral techniques, temperament, observed distress, and pain reports in children and adolescents during lumbar puncture. J Pediatr Nurs 1998; 13:48.
30. Harris CV, Bradlyn AS, Ritchey AK, et al: Individual differences in pediatric cancer patients' reactions to invasive medical procedures: a repeated measures analysis. Pediatr Hematol Oncol 1994; 11:293.
31. McCarthy AM, Cool VA, Petersen M, et al: Cognitive behavioral pain and anxiety interventions in pediatric oncology centers and bone marrow transplant units. J Pediatr Oncol Nurs 1996; 13:3.
32. Reddy SK, Weinstein SM: Medical decision-making in a patient with a history of cancer and chronic non-malignant pain. Clin J Pain 1995; 11:242.
33. Foley KM: Treatment of cancer pain. N Engl J Med 1985; 313:84.
34. Keefe FJ, Dunsmore J: Pain behavior: Concepts and controversies. American Pain Society Journal 1992; 1:92.
35. Gamsa A: The role of psychological factors in chronic pain. I. A half century of study. Pain 1994; 57:5.
36. Gamsa A: The role of psychological factors in chronic pain. II. A critical appraisal. Pain 1994; 57:17.
37. Martin LA, Hagen NA: Neuropathic pain in cancer patients: mechanisms, syndromes, and clinical controversies. J Pain Symptom Manage 1997; 14:99.
38. Portenoy RK, Kanner RM: Nonopioid and adjuvant analgesics. In: Portenoy RK, Kanner RM (eds): Pain Management: Theory and Practice, p 219. Philadelphia, F.A. Davis, 1996.
39. Payne R: Cancer pain: Anatomy, physiology and pharmacology. Cancer 1989; 63(suppl):2266.
40. Grossman SA, Sheidler VR, Swedeen K, et al: Correlation of patient and caregiver ratings of cancer pain. J Pain Symptom Manage 1991; 6:53.
41. O'Brien J, Francis A: The use of next-of-kin to estimate pain in cancer patients. Pain 1988; 35:171.
42. Cleeland CS, Ryan KM: Pain assessment: global use of the Brief Pain Inventory. Ann Acad Med Singapore 1994; 23:129.
43. Beyer JE, Wells N: Assessment of cancer pain in children, p 57. In: Patt RB (ed): Cancer Pain. Philadelphia, Lippincott, 1993.
44. WHO Expert Committee: Cancer Pain Relief and Palliative Care. Geneva, WHO, 1990.
45. Patt RB, Ellison NM: Breakthrough pain in cancer patients: characteristics, prevalence, and treatment. Oncology 1998; 12:1035.
46. Bruera E, Fainsinger R, MacEachern T, et al: The use of methylphenidate in patients with incident cancer pain receiving regular opiates. A preliminary report. Pain 1992; 50:75.
47. Rogers AG: How to manage incident pain. J Pain Symptom Manage 1987; 2:99.
48. Foley KM: Cancer pain syndromes. J Pain Symptom Manage 1987; 2:S13.
49. Enneking WF, Conrad EU III: Common bone tumors. Clin Symp 1989; 41:1.
50. Akakura K, Akimoto S, Shimazaki J: Pain caused by bone metastasis in endocrine-therapy-refractory prostate cancer. J Cancer Res Clin Oncol 1996; 122:633.
51. DeVita VT Jr, Hellman S, Rosenberg SA (eds): Cancer: Principles and Practice of Oncology, 5th ed, p 1604. Philadelphia, Lippincott, 1997.
52. Bryne TN: Spinal cord compression from epidural metastases. N Engl J Med 1992; 327:614.
53. Sorensen S, Borgesen SE, Rohde K, et al: Metastatic epidural spinal cord compression. Cancer 1990; 65:1502.
54. Maranzano E, Latini P, Checcaglini F, et al: Radiation therapy of spinal cord compression caused by breast cancer: report of a prospective trial. Int J Radiat Oncol Biol Phys 1992; 24:301.
55. Ingham J, Beveridge A, Cooney NJ: The management of spinal cord compression in patients with advanced malignancy. J Pain Symptom Manage 1993; 8:1.
56. Grond S, Zech D, Diefenbach C, et al: Assessment of cancer pain: a prospective evaluation in 2266 cancer pain patients referred to a pain service. Pain 1996; 64:107.
57. Patchell RA, Posner JB: Neurologic complications of systemic cancer. Neurol Clin 1985; 3:729.
58. Gilbert MR, Grossman SA: Incidence and nature of neurologic problems in patients with solid tumors. Am J Med 1986; 81:951.
59. Twycross RG, Lack SA: Symptom Control in Far Advanced Cancer: Pain Relief. London, Pitman, 1983.
60. Kori SH, Foley KM, Posner JB: Brachial plexus lesions in patients with cancer: 100 cases. Neurology 1981; 31:45.
61. Jaekle KA, Young DF, Foley KM: The natural history of lumbosacral plexopathy in cancer. Neurology 1985; 35:8.
62. Vecht CJ, Hoff AM, Kansen PJ, et al: Types and causes of pain in cancer of the head and neck. Cancer 1992; 70:178.
63. Grond S, Zech D, Lynch J, et al: Validation of World Health Organization guidelines for pain relief in head and neck cancer. A prospective study. Ann Otol Rhinol Laryngol 1993; 102:342.
64. Bjordal K, Kaasa S: Psychological distress in head and neck cancer patients 7–11 years after curative treatment. Br J Cancer 1995; 71:592.
65. Wong JK, Wood RE, McLean M: Pain preceding recurrent head and neck cancer. J Orofac Pain 1998; 12:52.
66. Bruera E, MacDonald RN: Intractable pain in patients with advanced head and neck tumors: a possible role for local infection. Cancer Treat Rep 1986; 70:691.
67. Patt RB, Jain S: Management of a patient with osteoradionecrosis of the mandible with nerve blocks. J Pain Symptom Manage 1990; 5:59.

68. Wasserstrom WR, Glass JP, Posner JB: Diagnosis and treatment of leptomeningeal metastases from solid tumor: experience with 90 patients. Cancer 1982; 49:759.
69. Glass JP, Foley KM: Carcinomatous meningitis. In: Harris JR, Hellman S, Henderson IC, et al (eds): Breast Diseases, 2nd ed, p 700. Philadelphia, Lippincott, 1987.
70. Elliot K, Foley KM: Neurologic pain syndromes in patients with cancer. Crit Care Clin 1990; 6:393.
71. Kunkle EC, Hernandez RR, Wolff HG: Studies on headache: the mechanisms and significance of headache associated with brain tumor. Bull NY Acad Med 1942; 18:400.
72. Rushton JG, Rooke ED: Brain tumor headache. Headache 1962; 2:147.
73. Zimm S, Wampler GL, Stablein D, et al: Intracerebral metastases in solid tumor patients: natural history and results of treatment. Cancer 1981; 48:384.
74. Gutin PH: Corticosteroid therapy in patients with brain tumors. National Cancer Institute Monograph 1977; 46:151.
75. Black P: Brain metastasis: current status and recommended guidelines for management. Neurosurgery 1979; 5:617.
76. Hoskin PJ: Radiotherapy in the management of bone pain. Clin Orthop 1995; 312:105.
77. Salazar OM, Da Motta NW, Bridgman SM, et al: Fractionated half-body irradiation for pain palliation in widely metastatic cancers: Comparison with single dose. Int J Radiat Oncol Biol Phys 1996; 36:49.
78. Needham PR, Mithal NP, Hoskin PJ: Radiotherapy for bone pain. J R Soc Med 1994; 87:503.
79. Baziotis N, Yakoumakis E, Zissimopoulos A, et al: Strontium-89 chloride in the treatment of bone metastases from breast cancer. Oncology 1998; 55:377.
80. Serafini AN, Houston SJ, Resche I, et al: Palliation of pain associated with metastatic bone cancer using samarium-153 lexidronam: a double-blind placebo-controlled clinical trial. J Clin Oncol 1998; 16:1574.
81. Estes NC, Morphis JG, Hornback NB, et al: Intraarterial chemotherapy and hyperthermia for pain control in patients with recurrent rectal cancer. Am J Surg 1986; 152:597.
82. Mellette SJ: Management of malignant disease metastatic to the bone by hormonal alterations. Clin Orthop 1970; 73:73.
83. Faithfull NS, Reinhold HS, Van Den Berg AP, et al: The effectiveness and safety of whole body hyperthermia as a pain treatment in advanced malignancy. In: Erdmann W, Oyama T, Pernak MJ (eds): The Pain Clinic I: Proceedings of the First International Symposium, Delft, The Netherlands, May 31–June 2, 1984. Utrecht, VNU Science Press, 1985.
84. Price P, Hoskin PJ, Easton D, et al: Prospective randomized trial of single and multifraction radiotherapy schedules in the treatment of painful bone metastasis. Clin Oncol 1989; 1:56.
85. Cleeland CS: Documenting barriers to cancer pain management. In: Chapman CR, Foley KM (eds): Current and Emerging Issues in Cancer Pain: Research and Practice, p 321. New York, Raven Press, 1993.
86. Hill CS: Oral opioid analgesics. In: Patt RB (ed): Cancer Pain, p 129. Philadelphia, Lippincott, 1993.
87. Portenoy RK: Inadequate outcome of opioid therapy for cancer pain: influences on practitioners and patients. In: Patt RB (ed): Cancer Pain, p 119. Philadelphia, Lippincott, 1993.
88. Hill CS Jr: Relationship among cultural, educational, and regulatory agency influences on optimum cancer pain treatment. J Pain Symptom Manage 1990; 5(suppl):S37.
89. Zech DFJ, Grong S, Lynch J, et al: Validation of the World Health Organization guidelines for cancer pain relief: a 10-year prospective study. Pain 1996; 63:65.
90. Ventafridda V, De Conno FD: Status of cancer pain and palliative care worldwide. J Pain Symptom Manage 1996; 12:79.
91. Coyle N, Adelhardt J, Foley KM, et al: Character of terminal illness in the advanced cancer patient: pain and other symptoms during the last four weeks of life. J Pain Symptom Manage 1990; 5:83.
92. Stambaugh J: Role of nonsteroidal anti-inflammatory drugs. In: Patt RB (ed): Cancer Pain, p 105. Philadelphia, Lippincott, 1993.
93. Pace V: Use of nonsteroidal anti-inflammatory drugs in cancer. Palliat Med 1995; 9:273.
94. Eisenberg E, Berkey CS, Carr DB, et al: Efficacy and safety of nonsteroidal anti-inflammatory drugs for cancer pain: a meta-analysis. J Clin Oncol 1994; 12:2756.
95. Schlegel SI, Paulus HE: Nonsteroidal and analgesic use in the elderly. Clin Rheum Dis 1986; 12:245.
96. Valentini M, Cannizzaro R, Poletti M, et al: Nonsteroidal antiinflammatory drugs for cancer pain: comparison between misoprostol and ranitidine in prevention of upper gastrointestinal damage. J Clin Oncol 1995; 13:2637.
97. Rothwell KG: Efficacy and safety of a non-acetylated salicylate, choline magnesium trisalicylate in the treatment of rheumatoid arthritis. J Int Med Res 1983; 11:343.
98. Leonards JR, Levy G: Gastrointestinal blood loss from aspirin and sodium salicylate tablets in man. Clin Pharmacol Ther 1973; 14:62.
99. Buckley MMT, Brogden RN: Ketorolac: a review of its pharmacodynamic and pharmacokinetic properties and therapeutic potential. Drugs 1990; 39:86.
100. Portenoy R: Drug therapy for cancer pain. Am J Hosp Palliat Care 1990; 7:10.
101. Yalcin S, Gullu IH, Tekuzman G, et al: A comparison of two nonsteroidal antiinflammatory drugs (diflunisal versus dipyrone) in the treatment of moderate to severe cancer pain: a randomized crossover study. Am J Clin Oncol 1998; 21:185.
102. Dhaliwal HS, Sloan P, Arkinstall WW, et al: Randomized evaluation of controlled-release codeine and placebo in chronic cancer pain. J Pain Symptom Manage 1995; 10:612.
103. Kalso E, Vainio A: Morphine and oxycodone hydrochloride in the management of cancer pain. Clin Pharmacol Ther 1990; 47:639.
104. Glare PA, Walsh TD: Dose-ranging study of oxycodone for chronic pain in advanced cancer. J Clin Oncol 1993; 11:973.
105. Li Wan Po A, Zhang WY: Systematic overview of co-proxamol to assess analgesic effects of addition of dextropropoxyphene to paracetamol. Br Med J 1997; 315:1565.
106. Minotti V, De Angelis V, Righetti E, et al: Double-blind evaluation of short-term analgesic efficacy of orally administered diclofenac, diclofenac plus codeine, and diclofenac plus imipramine in chronic cancer pain. Pain 1998; 74:133.
107. Heiskanen T, Kalso E: Controlled-release oxycodone and morphine in cancer related pain. Pain 1997; 73:37.
108. Hopkinson JH III: Vicodin: a new analgesic: clinical evaluation of efficacy and safety of repeated doses. Current Therapeutic Research, Clinical and Experimental 1978; 24:633.
109. Portenoy RK, Foley KM, Stulman J, et al: Plasma morphine and morphine-6-glucuronide during chronic morphine therapy for cancer pain: plasma profiles, steady-state concentrations and the consequences of renal failure. Pain 1991; 47:13.
110. Portenoy RK, Thaler HT, Inturrisi CE, et al: The metabolite morphine-6-glucuronide contributes to the analgesia produced by morphine infusion in patients with pain and normal renal function. Clin Pharmacol Ther 1992; 51:422.
111. Broomhead A, Kerr R, Tester W, et al: Comparison of a once-a-day sustained-release morphine formulation with standard oral morphine treatment for cancer pain. J Pain Symptom Manage 1997; 14:63.
112. Bruera E, Fainsinger R, Spachynski K, et al: Clinical efficacy and safety of a novel controlled-release morphine suppository and subcutaneous morphine in cancer pain: a randomized evaluation. J Clin Oncol 1995; 13:1520.
113. Ettinger DS, Vitale PJ, Trump DL: Important clinical pharmacologic considerations in the use of methadone in cancer patients. Cancer Treat Rep 1979; 63:457.
114. Ripamonti C, De Conno F, Groff L, et al: Equianalgesic dose/ratio between methadone and other opioid agonists in cancer pain: comparison of two clinical experiences. Ann Oncol 1998; 9:79.
115. Lawlor PG, Turner KS, Hanson J, et al: Dose ratio between morphine and methadone in patients with cancer pain: a retrospective study. Cancer 1998; 82:1167.
116. Dixon R: Pharmacokinetics of levorphanol. Advances in Pain Research Therapy 1986; 8:217.
117. Paalzow LK: Pharmacokinetic aspects of optimal pain treatment. Acta Anaesthesiol Scand Suppl 1982; 74:37.
118. Warfield CA: Controlled-release morphine tablets in patients with chronic cancer pain: a narrative review of controlled clinical trials. Cancer 1998; 82:2299.
119. Sloan PA, Moulin DE, Hays H: A clinical evaluation of transdermal therapeutic system fentanyl for the treatment of cancer pain. J Pain Symptom Manage 1998; 16:102.
120. Jeal W, Benfield P: Transdermal fentanyl. A review of its pharmacological properties and therapeutic efficacy in pain control. Drugs 1997; 53:109.

121. Forest P: The use of a pain diary in patients with advanced cancer of the prostate. Urologic Nursing 1993; 13:17.
122. Fine PG, Marcus M, De Boer AJ, et al: An open label study of oral transmucosal fentanyl citrate (OTFC) for the treatment of breakthrough cancer pain. Pain 1991; 45:149.
123. Farrar JT, Cleary J, Rauck R, et al: Oral transmucosal fentanyl citrate: randomized, double-blinded, placebo-controlled trial for treatment of breakthrough pain in cancer patients. J Natl Cancer Inst 1998; 90:611.
124. Christie JM, Simmonds M, Patt R, et al: Dose titration, multicenter study of oral transmucosal fentanyl citrate for the treatment of breakthrough pain in cancer patients using transdermal fentanyl for persistent pain. J Clin Oncol 1998; 16:2238.
125. Kaiko RF, Wallenstein SL, Rogers AG, et al: Sources of variation in analgesic responses in cancer patients with chronic pain receiving morphine. Pain 1983; 15:191.
126. Cleeland CS, Tearnan BH: Behavioral control of cancer pain. In: Holzman AD, Turk DC (eds): Pain Management, p 193. New York, Pergamon Press, 1986.
127. Ventafridda V, Tambutini M, Carceni A, et al: A validation study of the WHO method for cancer pain relief. Cancer 1987; 59:850.
128. McQuay HJ: Pharmacological treatment of neuralgic and neuropathic pain. Cancer Surv 1988; 7:141.
129. Galer BS, Coyle N, Pasternak GW, et al: Individual variability in the response to different opioids: report of five cases. Pain 1992; 49:87.
130. Hanks GW, Forbes K: Co-proxamol is effective in chronic pain. BMJ 1998; 316:1980.
131. Ellison NM: Opioid analgesics: toxicities and their treatment. In: Patt RB (ed): Cancer Pain, p 185. Philadelphia, Lippincott, 1993.
132. Cameron JC: Constipation related to narcotic therapy. A protocol for nurses and patients. Cancer Nurs 1992; 15:372.
133. Glare P, Lickiss JN: Unrecognized constipation in patients with advanced cancer: a recipe for therapeutic disaster. J Pain Symptom Manage 1992; 7:369.
134. Baines M: Nausea and vomiting in the patient with advanced cancer. J Pain Symptom Manage 1988; 3:81.
135. Ferris FD, Kerr IG, Sone M, et al: Transdermal scopolamine use in the control of narcotic-induced nausea. J Pain Symptom Manage 1991; 6:389.
136. Frytak S, Moertel CG: Management of nausea and vomiting in the cancer patient. JAMA 1981; 245:393.
137. Bruera E, Seifert L, Watanabe S, et al: Chronic nausea in advanced cancer patients: a retrospective assessment of a metoclopramide-based antiemetic regimen. J Pain Symptom Manage 1996; 11:147.
138. Cubeddu LX, Pendergrass K, Ryan T, et al: Efficacy of oral ondansetron, a selective antagonist of 5-HT3 receptors, in the treatment of nausea and vomiting associated with cyclophosphamide-based chemotherapies. Ondansetron Study Group. Am J Clin Oncol 1994; 17:137.
139. Bruera E, Chadwick S, Brenneis C, et al: Methylphenidate associated with narcotics for the treatment of cancer pain. Cancer Treat Rep 1987; 71:67.
140. Forrest WH Jr, Brown BM Jr, Brown CR: Dextroamphetamine with morphine for the treatment of postoperative pain. N Engl J Med 1977; 13:712.
141. Fitzgibbon DR, Ready LB: Intravenous high-dose methadone administered by patient controlled analgesia and continuous infusion for the treatment of cancer pain refractory to high-dose morphine. Pain 1997; 73:259.
142. Bryson HM, Wilde MI: Amitriptyline. A review of its pharmacological properties and therapeutic use in chronic pain states. Drugs Aging 1996; 8:459.
143. Portenoy RK: Opioid therapy for chronic nonmalignant pain: a review of the critical issues. J Pain Symptom Manage 1996; 11:203.
144. Zenz M, Strumpf M, Tryba M: Long-term oral opioid therapy in patients with chronic nonmalignant pain. J Pain Symptom Manage 1992; 7:69.
145. Porter J, Jick H: Addiction rare in patients treated with narcotics. N Engl J Med 1980; 302:123.
146. Bruera E: Subcutaneous administration of opioids in the management of cancer pain. Recent Advances in Pain Research 1990; 16:203.
147. Portenoy RK, Southam MA, Gupta SK, et al: Transdermal fentanyl for cancer pain. Repeated dose pharmacokinetics. Anesthesiology 1993; 78:36.
148. Rose PG, Macfee MS, Boswell MV: Fentanyl transdermal system overdose secondary to cutaneous hyperthermia. Anesth Analg 1993; 77:390.
149. De Conno F, Ripamonti C, Saita L, et al: Role of rectal route in treating cancer pain: a randomized crossover clinical trial of oral versus rectal morphine administration in opioid-naive cancer patients with pain. J Clin Oncol 1995; 13:1004.
150. Cole L, Hanning CD: Review of the rectal use of opioids. J Pain Symptom Manage 1990; 5:118.
151. Ripamonti C, Zecca E, Brunelli C, et al: Rectal methadone in cancer patients with pain. A preliminary clinical and pharmacokinetic study. Ann Oncol 1995; 6:841.
152. Bruera E, Ripamonti C: Alternate routes of administration of narcotics. In: Patt RB (ed): Cancer Pain, p 16. Philadelphia, Lippincott, 1993.
153. Nelson KA, Glare PA, Walsh D, et al: A prospective, within-patient, crossover study of continuous intravenous and subcutaneous morphine for chronic cancer pain. J Pain Symptom Manage 1997; 13:262.
154. Bruera E, MacEachern T, MacMillan K, et al: Local tolerance to subcutaneous infusions of high concentrations of hydromorphone: a prospective study. J Pain Symptom Manage 1993; 8:201.
155. Nahata MC, Miser AW, Miser JS, et al: Analgesic plasma concentrations of morphine in children with terminal malignancy receiving a continuous subcutaneous infusion of morphine sulfate to control severe pain. Pain 1987; 18:109.
156. Ottesen S, Monrad L: Morphine-antiemetic mixtures for continuous subcutaneous infusion in terminal cancer. Tidsskr Nor Laegeforen 1992; 112:1817.
157. Mercadante S, Lodi F, Sapio M, et al: Long-term ketamine subcutaneous continuous infusion in neuropathic cancer pain. J Pain Symptom Manage 1995; 10:564.
158. Devulder JE, Ghys L, Dhondt W, et al: Neuropathic pain in a cancer patient responding to subcutaneously administered lignocaine. Clin J Pain 1993; 9:220.
159. Lesser GJ, Grossman SA, Leong KW, et al: In vitro and in vivo studies of subcutaneous hydromorphone implants designed for the treatment of cancer pain. Pain 1996; 65:265.
160. Kaiko RF, Foley KM, Grabinski PY, et al: Central nervous system excitatory effects of meperidine in cancer patients. Ann Neurol 1983; 13:180.
161. Szeto HH, Inturrusi CE, Houde R, et al: Accumulation of normeperidine, an active metabolite of meperidine, in patients with renal failure or cancer. Ann Intern Med 1977; 86:738.
162. Bono AV, Cuffari S: Effectiveness and tolerance of tramadol in cancer pain. A comparative study with respect to buprenorphine. Drugs 1997; 53(suppl 2):40.
163. Twycross RG: The brompton cocktail. Advances in Pain Research Therapy 1979; 2:291.
164. Twycross RG: The measurement of pain in terminal carcinoma. J Int Med Res 1976; 4:58.
165. Byas-Smith MG, Max MB, Muir J, et al: Transdermal clonidine compared to placebo in painful diabetic neuropathy using a two-stage 'enriched enrollment' design. Pain 1995; 60:267.
166. Kishore-Kumar R, Max MB, Schafer SC, et al: Desipramine relieves post-herpetic neuralgia. Clin Pharmacol Ther 1990; 47:305.
167. Panerai AE, Monza G, Mouilia P, et al: A randomized, within-patient, crossover, placebo-controlled trial on the efficacy and tolerability of the tricyclic antidepressants chlorimipramine and nortriptyline in central pain. Acta Neurol Scand 1990; 82:34.
168. Sindrup SH, Gram LF, Skjold T, et al: Clomipramine vs desipramine vs placebo in the treatment of diabetic neuropathy symptoms: a double-blind cross-over study. Br J Clin Pharmacol 1990; 30:683.
169. Eija K, Tiina T, Pertti NJ: Amitriptyline effectively relieves neuropathic pain following treatment of breast cancer. Pain 1996; 64:293.
170. Holland JC, Romano SJ, Heiligenstein JH, et al: A controlled trial of fluoxetine and desipramine in depressed women with advanced cancer. Psychooncol 1998; 7:291.
171. Zylicz Z, Smits C, Krajnik M: Paroxetine for pruritus in advanced cancer. J Pain Symptom Manage 1998; 16:121.
172. Sweet WH: Treatment of trigeminal neuralgia (tic douloureux). N Engl J Med 1986; 315:174.
173. McQuay H, Carroll D, Jadad AR, et al: Anticonvulsant drugs for management of pain: a systematic review. BMJ 1995; 311:1047.
174. Yajnik S, Singh GP, Singh G, et al: Phenytoin as a coanalgesic in cancer pain. J Pain Symptom Manage 1992; 7:209.

175. Chang VT: Intravenous phenytoin in the management of crescendo pelvic cancer-related pain. J Pain Symptom Manage 1997; 13:238.
176. Rosner H, Rubin L: Gabapentin adjunctive therapy in neuropathic pain states. Clin J Pain 1996; 12:56.
177. Rho JM, Donevan SD, Rogawski MA: Mechanisms of the anticonvulsant felbamate: opposing effects on N-methyl-D-aspartate and gamma aminobutyric acid-A receptors. Ann Neurol 1994; 35:229.
178. Ordia JI, Fischer E, Adamski E, et al: Chronic intrathecal delivery of baclofen by a programmable pump for the treatment of severe spasticity. J Neurosurg 1996; 85:452.
179. Dejgard A, Petersen P, Kastrup J: Mexiletine for treatment of chronic painful diabetic neuropathy. Lancet 1988; 1(8575):9.
180. Lindstrom P, Lindblom U: The analgesic effect of tocainide in trigeminal neuralgia. Pain 1987; 28:45.
181. Bruera E, Miller MJ, MacMillan K, et al: Neuropsychological effects of methylphenidate in patients receiving a continuous infusion of narcotics for cancer pain. Pain 1992; 48:163.
182. Yee JD, Berde CB: Dextroamphetamine or methylphenidate as adjuvants to opioid analgesia for adolescents with cancer. J Pain Symptom Manage 1994; 9:122.
183. Wilwerding MB, Loprinzi CL, Mailliard JA, et al: A randomized, crossover evaluation of methylphenidate in cancer patients receiving strong narcotics. Support Care Cancer 1995; 3:135.
184. Watanabe S, Bruera E: Corticosteroids as adjuvant analgesics. J Pain Symptom Manage 1994; 9:442.
185. Twycross R: The risks and benefits of corticosteroids in advanced cancer. Drug Saf 1994; 11:163.
186. Bruera E, Roca E, Cedaro L, et al: Action of oral methylprednisolone in terminal cancer patients: a prospective randomized double-blind study. Cancer Treat Rep 1985; 69:751.
187. Pud D, Eisenberg E, Spitzer A, et al: The NMDA receptor antagonist amantadine reduces surgical neuropathic pain in cancer patients: a double blind, randomized, placebo controlled trial. Pain 1998; 75:349.
188. Mercadante S: Ketamine in cancer pain: an update. Palliat Med 1996; 10:225.
189. Yang CY, Wong CS, Chang JY, et al: Intrathecal ketamine reduces morphine requirements in patients with terminal cancer pain. Can J Anaesth 1996; 43:379.
190. Eisenach JC, DuPen S, Dubois M, et al: Epidural clonidine analgesia for intractable cancer pain. Pain 1995; 61:391.
191. Diener KM: Bisphosphonates for controlling pain from metastatic bone disease. Am J Health Syst Pharm 1996; 53:1917.
192. Harvey HA, Lipton A: The role of bisphosphonates in the treatment of bone metastases—the U.S. experience. Support Care Cancer 1996; 4:213.
193. Pelger RC, Hamdy NA, Zwinderman AH, et al: Effects of the bisphosphonate olpadronate in patients with carcinoma of the prostate metastatic to the skeleton. Bone 1998; 22:403.
194. Patt RB, Reddy S: The benzodiazepines as adjuvant analgesics. J Pain Symptom Manage 1994; 9:510.
195. Patt RB, Proper G, Reddy S: The neuroleptics as adjuvant analgesics. J Pain Symptom Manage 1994; 9:446.
196. Judkins KC, Harmer M: Haloperidol as an adjunct analgesic in the management of postoperative pain. Anaesthesia 1982; 37:1118.
197. Hanks GW, Thomas PJ, Trueman T, et al: The myth of haloperidol potentiation. Lancet 1983; 2(8348):523.
198. Patt RB: Peripheral neurolysis and the management of cancer pain. Pain Digest 1992; 2:30.
199. Patt RB, Reddy S: Spinal neurolysis for cancer pain: indications and recent results. Ann Acad Med Singapore 1994; 23:216.
200. Patt RB, Reddy SK, Black RG: Neural blockade for abdominopelvic pain of oncologic origin. Cancer Bull 1995; 47:52.
201. Patt RB: Pain therapy. In: Frost EAM (ed): Clinical Anesthesia in Neurosurgery, 2nd ed, p 347. Boston, Butterworth-Heinemann, 1991.
202. Sanders M, Zuurmond W: Safety of unilateral and bilateral percutaneous cervical cordotomy in 80 terminally ill cancer patients. J Clin Oncol 1995; 13:1509.
203. Watling CJ, Payne R, Allen RR, et al: Commissural myelotomy for intractable cancer pain: report of two cases. Clin J Pain 1996; 12:151.
204. Chiang JS, Dai CT, Patt RB: Intraspinal opioid therapy for intractable cancer pain. Cancer Bull 1995; 47:61.
205. Krames ES: Intrathecal infusional therapies for intractable pain: patient management guidelines. J Pain Symptom Manage 1993; 8:36.
206. Gestin Y, Vainio A, Pegurier AM: Long-term intrathecal infusion of morphine in the home care of patients with advanced cancer. Acta Anaesthesiol Scand 1997; 41:12.
207. Schultheiss R, Schramm J, Neidhardt J: Dose changes in long- and medium-term intrathecal morphine therapy of cancer pain. Neurosurgery 1992; 31:664.
208. Sjoberg M, Nitescu P, Appelgren L, et al: Long-term intrathecal morphine and bupivacaine in patients with refractory cancer pain. Results from a morphine:bupivacaine dose regimen of 0.5:4.75 mg/ml. Anesthesiology 1994; 80:284.
209. van Dongen RT, Crul BJ, De Bock M: Long-term intrathecal infusion of morphine and morphine/bupivacaine mixtures in the treatment of cancer pain: a retrospective analysis of 51 cases. Pain 1993; 55:119.
210. Karavelis A, Foroglou G, Selviaridis P, et al: Intraventricular administration of morphine for control of intractable cancer pain in 90 patients. Neurosurgery 1996; 39:57.
211. Appelgren L, Janson M, Nitescu P, et al: Continuous intracisternal and high cervical intrathecal bupivacaine analgesia in refractory head and neck pain. Anesthesiol 1996; 84:256.
212. DuPen SL, Peterson DG, Bogosian AC, et al: A new permanent exteriorized epidural catheter for narcotic self-administration to control cancer pain. Cancer 1987; 59:986.
213. Hassenbusch SJ, Paice JA, Patt RB, et al: Clinical realities and economic considerations: economics of intrathecal therapy. J Pain Symptom Manage 1997; 14:S36.
214. Mercadante S: Intrathecal morphine and bupivacaine in advanced cancer pain patients implanted at home. J Pain Symptom Manage 1994; 9:201.
215. Blount JP, Remley KB, Yue SK, et al: Intrathecal granuloma complicating chronic spinal infusion of morphine. Report of three cases. J Neurosurg 1996; 84:272.
216. Sjoberg M, Karlsson PA, Nordborg C, et al: Neuropathologic findings after long-term intrathecal infusion of morphine and bupivacaine for pain treatment in cancer patients. Anesthesiology 1992; 76:173.
217. Ventafridda V, Sganzerla EP, Fochi C, et al: Transcutaneous nerve stimulation in cancer pain. Advances in Pain Research Therapy 1979; 2:509.
218. Young RF, Brechner T: Electrical stimulation of the brain for relief of intractable pain due to cancer. Cancer 1986; 57:1266.
219. Meglio M, Cioni B: Personal experience with spinal cord stimulation in chronic pain management. Appl Neurophysiol 1982; 45:195.

33 *Palliative Care*

PORTER STOREY, MD, FACP, Hospice and Palliative Medicine

Comforter, where, where is your comforting?
GERARD MANLEY HOPKINS

Perspective

According to the World Health Organization:

"Palliative care is the active total care of patients whose disease is not responsive to curative treatment. Control of pain, of other symptoms, and of psychological, social and spiritual problems is paramount. The goal of palliative care is achievement of the best possible quality of life for patients and their families (relatives or other key people). Many aspects of palliative care are also applicable earlier in the course of the illness, in conjunction with anticancer treatment.

"Palliative care:

- affirms life and regards dying as a normal process
- neither hastens nor postpones death
- provides relief from pain and other distressing symptoms
- integrates the psychological and spiritual aspects of patient care
- offers a support system to help patients live as actively as possible until death
- offers a support system to help the family cope during the patient's illness and in their own bereavement

"Radiotherapy, chemotherapy and surgery have a place in palliative care provided that the symptomatic benefits of treatment clearly outweigh the disadvantages. Investigative procedures are kept to a minimum. Palliative care has its origins in the hospice movement."[1]

In 1987, palliative medicine was recognized as a specialty in Britain, and in 1996, certification examinations were first offered by the American Board of Hospice and Palliative Medicine. This field is enjoying rapid growth, in part because the array of modern palliative care interventions can be so effective and so appreciated by patients and family.

Control of Distressing Symptoms

Pain

Pain, the most distressing of symptoms associated with palliative care, is discussed in detail in Chapter 32, Cancer Pain Management.

Dyspnea

Dyspnea or "breathlessness" can be defined as an uncomfortable awareness of breathing. Estimates of the prevalence of dyspnea in terminally ill patients vary from 12% to 74%.[2] Dyspnea is most common in patients with lung cancer, and it tends to worsen as death approaches. Like pain, dyspnea is highly feared and has a complex pathophysiology. It is affected by physical, social, psychological, and spiritual factors (Table 33–1), and a careful evaluation and team approach are essential.[3] Note that *all* of the factors listed in Table 33–1 are potentially reversible.

Iatrogenic complications frequently exacerbate dyspnea. Excessive doses of inhaled adrenergic agents or oral theophylline often cause a jittery feeling that increases anxiety and dyspnea.[4] Intravenous and tube feedings can cause volume overload, increased secretions, aspiration pneumonia (up to 56% in one series[5]), and increased metabolic demands for oxygen. Telling the family the patient will probably suffocate or telling the patient "there is nothing more I can do for you," increases fear, hopelessness, and family stress.

Physicians and hospice or palliative care teams can do a great deal to relieve dyspnea:

- A careful assessment not only helps identify reversible causes, it convinces the patient and family that a competent professional is there to help.
- Modification of the environment can be of assistance. A fan, an open window, or a hospital bed to allow sleeping upright may be enormously helpful.
- Remember to prevent and treat decubitus ulcers early

TABLE 33–1. **Reversible Causes of Dyspnea in Cancer Patients**

Physical	Psychological
Bronchospasm	Anxiety
Pneumonitis	Anticipating grief
Volume overload	Medication compliance
Heart failure	Fears of addiction or dependency
Secretion management	**Spiritual**
Anemia	Anguish
Effusions	Hopelessness
Social	Meaninglessness
Anger	Crisis of faith
Isolation	
Financial stress	
Caregiver burnout	

because an upright posture can increase the pressure on the buttocks and make turning difficult.

The other complication to remember to prevent is aspiration. If swallowing is more difficult, recommend pureed or very soft foods and thicken liquids with cornstarch. Tube feedings may need to be changed from continuous to bolus feeding so that gastric emptying can be assessed before each feeding.

The mainstay of the pharmacologic treatment of nonspecific cancer dyspnea is carefully titrated opioid analgesics. Studies have demonstrated that opioids are effective for the dyspnea of cancer and chronic obstructive pulmonary disease (COPD) and are remarkably safe.[6, 7] Opioids not only alleviate the sensation of dyspnea, they increase exercise tolerance.[8] A series of 20 cancer patients who had severe dyspnea despite oxygen therapy were given 2.5 times their regular dose of morphine (or 5 mg subcutaneously [SC] if not on any analgesic).[9] There was a marked improvement in the level of dyspnea (19 of 20 patients), but no change in respiratory rate or effort, oxygen saturation, or $PaCO_2$. Thus, it seems clear that both pain and dyspnea counteract the respiratory-depressant effects of opioid analgesics.

Dose titration is the key to a safe and effective use of opioids for dyspnea. If codeine or hydrocodone taken every 4 hours does not provide relief, the patient should receive a strong opioid, such as oxycodone, morphine, or hydromorphone, on a regular schedule. Breakthrough dyspnea should be treated aggressively with an additional 4-hourly dose of an immediate-release, strong opioid. Side effects such as constipation should be prevented with laxatives, and sedation can be alleviated by starting with low doses or by reducing the dose of benzodiazepines or other sedative medications, or both.

If swallowing is difficult or the patient is in severe distress, begin an intravenous (IV) or SC infusion of morphine or hydromorphone with boluses equal to twice the hourly rate, as necessary, for breakthrough dyspnea.[10] If needed, midazolam can be added to the infusion for anxiety and glycopyrrolate for troublesome secretions.[11] Nebulized morphine is also effective in some cancer patients with dyspnea[12] and can increase exercise endurance.[13]

Anorexia

Anorexia and cachexia are among the most common symptoms caused by advanced cancer in most series. Anorexia is extremely common and distressing to patients and families because progressive weight loss is often associated with deteriorating health and approaching death.

A careful history and physical examination often reveal potentially reversible factors that may be causing or exacerbating the anorexia (Table 33–2). A thorough evaluation also establishes a relationship between the physician and patient so that deeper issues can be shared. Anorexia may cause the patient or family distress because of erroneous information about how much time is left. This distress can be exacerbated if the family accuses the patient of willing his or her own death by refusing food, as sometimes occurs. In addition, well-meaning dietary advice like "make sure and get him to drink six cans of supplement per day or he will lose weight" increases guilt and fear.

TABLE 33–2. **Reversible Causes of Anorexia in Cancer Patients**

Physical	Psychological
Pain	Depression
Nausea	Anxiety
Candidiasis	"Purification" diets
Constipation	Fear of death
Peptic ulcers	
	Spiritual
Social	Hopelessness
Power struggles at mealtime	Meaninglessness
No one to prepare food	Abandonment by religious community
Pressure to eat	Inability to give or receive
	Forgiveness
	Guilt

The issue of artificial feeding often arises. A gastrostomy tube is certainly indicated for physically active, hungry patients who cannot swallow as a result of disease in the oropharynx or esophagus. In most other cases, it is important to review with patients and families the effects of artificial feeding of advanced cancer patients. There is now conclusive evidence that parenteral nutrition makes chemotherapy patients *die faster.*[14] When families understand how nutrition-dependent cancer growth is, and how unhelpful forced or tube feedings can be, they are usually willing to channel their concerns for the patient into more constructive avenues.

If underlying problems cannot be eliminated (see Table 33–2) and lack of appetite is a real concern to the patient, appetite stimulants should be considered. If the patient has bronchospasm, bone pain, or fevers, a glucocorticoid (e.g. prednisone 20 mg qAM, or dexamethasone 2 mg b.i.d.) may be the drug of choice. Megestrol has been proven effective if given in large doses (480–800 mg/d).[15] Nausea and fluid retention are occasional problematic side effects.

The most important intervention is giving your time and attention to the patient's and family's concerns. Usually, the gradual, gentle, repeated provision of information and expert care alleviates the anxiety and fear. At this time, the question changes from "How can we keep her from starving to death?" to "How will we be most helpful in the time she has left?"

Restlessness or Delirium

Up to 85% of advanced cancer patients experience agitation, restlessness, or delirium. Control of this distressing symptom is essential if patients are to remain comfortable in the place of their choosing and families are to cope and remember the final days as peaceful. *The Diagnostic and Statistical Manual of Mental Disorders*, 4th edition (DSM-IV), criteria for delirium are listed in Table 33–3.[16] Sometimes, this syndrome is better characterized as *cognitive failure, terminal restlessness, or confusion.*[17] Remember that a delirium may be superimposed on an underlying dementia in elderly or cognitively impaired patients.

A careful evaluation of the patient's physical condition and medication list can reveal reversible causes of delirium (Table 33–4). If practical, reduce sedative medications and consider treating infections or initiating steroid or radiation

TABLE 33–3. **DSM-IV Criteria for Delirium**

- Disturbance of consciousness with reduced ability to focus, sustain, or shift attention.
- Change in cognition (such as memory deficit, disorientation, language disturbance, or perceptual disturbances) that is not better accounted for by dementia.
- Disturbance develops over a short period of time (usually hours to days) and tends to fluctuate during the course of the day.
- Evidence from history, physical, or laboratory findings indicates the disturbance is caused by the direct physiological consequences of a general medical condition.

Modified from American Psychiatric Association: Diagnostic and Statistical Manual of Mental Disorders, 4th ed. Washington, DC, APA, 1996.

therapy if brain metastases are suspected. Some authors recommend a trial of rehydration by hypodermoclysis if the patient is dehydrated and confused.[18] Unfortunately, these efforts to reverse delirium are usually not successful in advanced cancer patients; in one series, only 18% of patients improved with these measures.[19] Therefore, the benefit-burden ratio of these interventions should be considered carefully.

A neuroleptic can calm the patient and improve mentation, for example, haloperidol (1–2 mg orally [PO] or SC hourly until calm, and then every 4–6 hours). A sedating phenothiazine, such as thioridazine or chlorpromazine (25–50 mg PO, rectally [PR], or IV hourly until calm and then every 4–6 hours), can also be quite effective. If even high doses of the above agents are not adequate, the addition of lorazepam (0.5–2 mg PO or sublingually [SL] every 4 hours) or midazolam (2–60 mg/d by SC or IV infusion) can provide much needed rest.[20]

Environment is important. A night light or large clock can alleviate disorientation, and moving the bed next to a wall with a high-backed chair on the other side, or even putting the mattress on the floor, can prevent disastrous falls. Helping the family organize into shifts or hiring sitters can ensure needed hands-on care. Respite care in the home or inpatient facility may be essential.

Explaining to families what is happening also is essential. Sometimes the patient's "symbolic language" can be reinterpreted as they develop a "nearing-death awareness."[21] It is usually helpful to explain the common, expected nature of the syndrome so that families understand that their loved one has not "gone crazy."

TABLE 33–4. **Some Reversible Causes of Delirium in Cancer Patients**

Drugs	**Organ Failure**
Hypnotics	Renal failure
Sedatives	Hepatic failure
Antidepressants	Heart failure
Excess opioids	Brain metastasis
Electrolyte Abnormalities	**Infection**
Hypercalcemia	Sepsis
Hyperglycemia	Pneumonia
Hypoxia	Urinary tract
	Abscess

Psychosocial and Spiritual Needs

Elisabeth Kübler-Ross wrote of the denial, anger, bargaining, depression, and acceptance she observed in patients that she saw near the end of life.[22] Exacerbation of physical symptoms and family stress is common as everyone struggles to cope. A great deal can be done to help, and meticulous attention to physical care and symptom control is essential. "Any group concerned with service to the dying should be talking about smoothing sheets, rubbing bottoms, relieving constipation, and sitting up at night. Counseling a dying person who is lying in a wet bed is ineffective. Such concerns loom large in the lives of critically ill patients and must be of importance to the physician if the physician is to treat the whole person."[23]

Skillful counseling can help the patient cope with anxiety and grief and make good choices. Social workers and therapists can create a sense of safe passage through this difficult time in life.[24] Facilitating life review can assist patients in finding meaning and coherence in their life story and resolving inner and family conflicts.[25] Guided imagery is a powerful technique that can dramatically increase coping and relieve subconscious turmoil.[26]

There are roles for both progressive muscle relaxation techniques and medication (e.g., alprazolam 0.5 mg PO t.i.d.[27]) in the treatment of anxious and depressed cancer patients. Skillful interdisciplinary teams can successfully foster hope in terminally ill patients with such strategies as increasing interpersonal connectedness, lightheartedness, courage, serenity, attainable goals, uplifting memories, and affirmations of worth.[28]

Burnout Prevention in Health Care Professionals

Health care managers can prevent exhaustion in dedicated palliative care professionals by providing manageable workloads, training, support, and adequate vacation time. Physicians should be on the lookout, in themselves and in colleagues, for such warning signs as insomnia, muscle tension, loss of libido, accidents, anger, loss of mood management, power struggles, distancing friends, or depersonalizing patients.[29] Healthy approaches to stress include increased self-awareness and self-care, sharing feelings and responsibilities, and developing a personal philosophy.[30] Ultimately, we learn to cope with our powerlessness in the face of death and still convey the essential message of palliative care:

> *You matter because you are you.*
> *You matter to the last moment of your life, and*
> *We will do all we can*
> *Not only to help you die peacefully, but*
> *To live, until you die.*
>
> CICELY SAUNDERS[31]

REFERENCES

1. World Health Organization: Technical Report Series—804. Cancer Pain Relief and Palliative Care, p 11. Geneva, World Health Organization, 1990.
2. Ahmedzai S: Palliation of respiratory symptoms. In: Doyle D, Hanks

GWC, MacDonald N (eds): Oxford Textbook of Palliative Medicine, pp 349–378. New York, Oxford University Press, 1993.
3. Storey P, Knight CF: Unipac Five: Caring for the Terminally Ill: Communication and Teamwork. American Academy of Hospice and Palliative Medicine. Dubuque, Kendall Hunt, 1998.
4. Swaminathan S, Paton JY, Ward SL, et al: Theophylline does not increase ventilatory responses to hypercapnia or hypoxia. Am Rev Respir Dis 1992; 146:1398–1401.
5. Crocon JO, Silverstone FA, Grover M, et al: Tube feeding in elderly patients indications, benefits, and complications. Arch Intern Med 1988; 148:429–433.
6. Bruera E, MacEachern T, Ripamonti C, et al: Subcutaneous morphine for dyspnea in cancer patients. Ann Intern Med 1993; 119:906–907.
7. Ripamonti C: Management of dyspnea in advanced cancer patients. Support Care Cancer 1999; 7:233–243.
8. Light RW, Stansbury DW, Webster JS: Effect of 30 mg of morphine alone or with promethazine or prochlorperazine on the exercise capacity of patients with COPD. Chest 1996; 109:975–981.
9. Bruera E, Macmillan K, Pather J, et al: Effects of morphine on the dyspnea of terminal cancer patients. J Pain Symptom Manage 1990; 5:341–344.
10. Storey, P, Hill HH, St Louis RH, et al: Subcutaneous infusions for control of cancer symptoms. J Pain Symptom Manage 1990; 5:33–41.
11. Bottomley DM, Hanks GW: Subcutaneous midazolam in palliative care. J Pain Symptom Manage 1990; 5:259–261.
12. Zeppetella G: Nebulized morphine in the palliation of dyspnea. Palliat Med 1997; 11:267–275.
13. Young, IH, Daviskas E, Keena VA: Effect of low dose nebulized morphine on exercise endurance in patients with chronic lung disease. Thorax 1989; 44:387–390.
14. American College of Physicians: Parenteral nutrition in patients receiving cancer chemotherapy (position paper). Ann Intern Med 1989; 110:734–738.
15. Bruera E, Macmillan K, Kuehn N, et al.: A controlled trial of megestrol acetate on appetite, caloric intake, nutritional status, and other symptoms in patients with advanced cancer. Cancer 1990; 66:1279–1282.
16. American Psychiatric Association: Diagnostic and Statistical Manual of Mental Disorders, 4th ed. Washington, DC, APA, 1996.
17. Breitbart W, Bruera E, Chochinor H, et al: Neuropsychiatric syndrome and psychological symptoms in patients with advanced cancer. J Pain Symptom Manage 1995; 10:131–141.
18. Fainsinger R, Bruera E: The management of dehydration in terminally ill patients. J Palliat Care 1994; 10:55–59.
19. Bruera E, Miller L, McMillion J, et al: Cognitive failure in patients with terminal cancer; a prospective study. J Pain Symptom Manage 1992; 7:192–195.
20. Storey P, Knight CF: Unipac Four: Management of Selected Nonpain Symptoms in the Terminally Ill, pp 55–60. Gainesville, American Academy of Hospice and Palliative Medicine, 1996.
21. Callanan M, Kelly P: Final Gifts: Understanding the Special Awareness, Needs, and Communications of the Dying. New York, Bantam, 1992.
22. Kübler-Ross E: On Death and Dying. New York, Macmillan, 1969.
23. Lack SA: The hospice concept—the adult with advanced cancer. Proceedings of the American Cancer Society's National Conference on Human Values and Cancer, Chicago, Sept 7–9, 1977.
24. Rusnack B, Scaefer SM, Moxley D: Hospice: social work's response to a new form of social caring. Soc Work Health Care 1990; 15:95–119.
25. Lichter I, Mooney J, Boyd M: Biography as therapy. Palliat Med 1993; 7:133–137.
26. Kearney M: Mortally Wounded: Stories of Soul, Pain, Death, and Healing. New York, Scribner, 1996.
27. Holland JC, Morrow GR, Schmale A, et al: A randomized trial of alprazolam versus progressive muscle relaxation in cancer patients with anxiety and depressive symptoms. J Clin Oncol 1991; 9:1004–1011.
28. Herth K: Fostering hope in terminally ill people. J Adv Nurs 1990; 15:1250–1259.
29. Vachon MLS: Occupational Stress in the Care of the Critically Ill, the Dying, and the Bereaved. New York, Hemisphere, 1987.
30. Quill TC, Williamson PR: Healthy approaches to physician stress. Arch Intern Med 1990; 150:1847–1861.
31. Saunders C: On dying well. Cambridge Review 1984; 49–52.

34 Late Effects of Cancer Treatment: Radiation and Chemotherapy Toxicity

PHILIP RUBIN, MD, Radiation Oncology
JACQUELINE P. WILLIAMS, PHD, Radiation Oncology
FRANK T. SLOVICK, MD, Medical Oncology

The problems of cancer therapy are in vivo problems that involve dynamic and interacting components of organized tissues, organs, and systems of the body . . . In the final analysis, the decision as to the specifics of a treatment schedule is a mixture of prevailing attitudes and ideas, as well as anecdotal events in practice.

ADAPTED FROM RUBIN AND CASARETT[1]

Perspective

Much of the mystery and fear surrounding cancer therapy evolves from concerns regarding the potential for late injury that can occur after the treatment has been completed; this is particularly true for radiation. A substantial body of clinical experience and pathologic data have established the progression, over time, of tissue injury triggered by a dose or course of radiation therapy. The sequence of events that occurs at a cellular level ultimately expresses itself in the form of structural and functional tissue or organ impairment. Therefore, depending on how vital the organ is, severe morbidity or even mortality can result. The radiation dose effect or dose response in a normal tissue needs to be evaluated with respect to time. A so-called time-course paradigm[2] (Fig. 34–1A) has been postulated in most normal tissues as a sequence of clinical events based on a series of histopathologic alterations following irradiation. Interestingly, a similar schema can also be applied to chemotherapy (Fig. 34–1B).

Rapid advances in radiation oncology, biology, and physics have led to an accumulation of information on the interactions of radiation with other therapeutic modalities (e.g., chemotherapy biologic response modifiers)[3–5]; these have impacted on our understanding of normal tissue toxicities. Radiation doses and chemotherapeutic regimens customarily deemed to be safe may no longer be so, because when they are combined with another modality, such doses can lead to severe late effects in different vital organs. Thus, previously defined radiation tolerance doses (TD_5 and TD_{50}) remain as valuable guides, but their applicability may have changed. Additional factors that are now relevant to defining tolerance doses include the type of therapy, the host, and the tumor, and an emphasis must often be placed on the *volume* of the organ irradiated, in addition to the *dose*. Mathematic models, such as nominal standard dose, tumor dose fractionation, and cumulative radiation effect, have been supplanted by the linear quadratic equation using α/β ratios and were presented earlier in Chapter 6, Principles of Radiation Oncology and Cancer Radiotherapy.

With the introduction of molecular biologic observations and techniques, new concepts of radiation and chemotherapeutic responses are emerging.[6, 7] For instance, one insight into the radiosensitivity and chemosensitivity of both tumors and normal tissues is an increased understanding of the importance of the immediate release of cytokines and chemokines following injury. Increasingly, the cytogenetics of post-therapy events are being uncovered and are providing markers to predict or monitor for later effects or tumor regression.[8, 9] Similar parallel concepts are emerging for both radiotherapeutic and chemotherapeutic response in tumors and normal tissues, and in many cases, cytokines are being used in combination with radiation and chemotherapy to improve treatment outcome.[10, 11]

In years past, it was believed that a major difference between radiation and chemotherapy was the absence of late effects after exposure to drugs; therefore, the major concern with regard to tolerance of chemotherapy regimens was in the acute and subacute toxicities of the chemotherapy. However, this difference was illusory, resulting from a paucity of data on the late toxicities of chemotherapy. The increasing documentation of late somatic changes in organs attributable to chemotherapy alone has dispelled the view that there are few late effects associated with the prolonged use of drugs. In fact, seemingly safe cyclic doses of chemotherapy can result in severe and life-threatening toxicities in a variety of organs.[12–14]

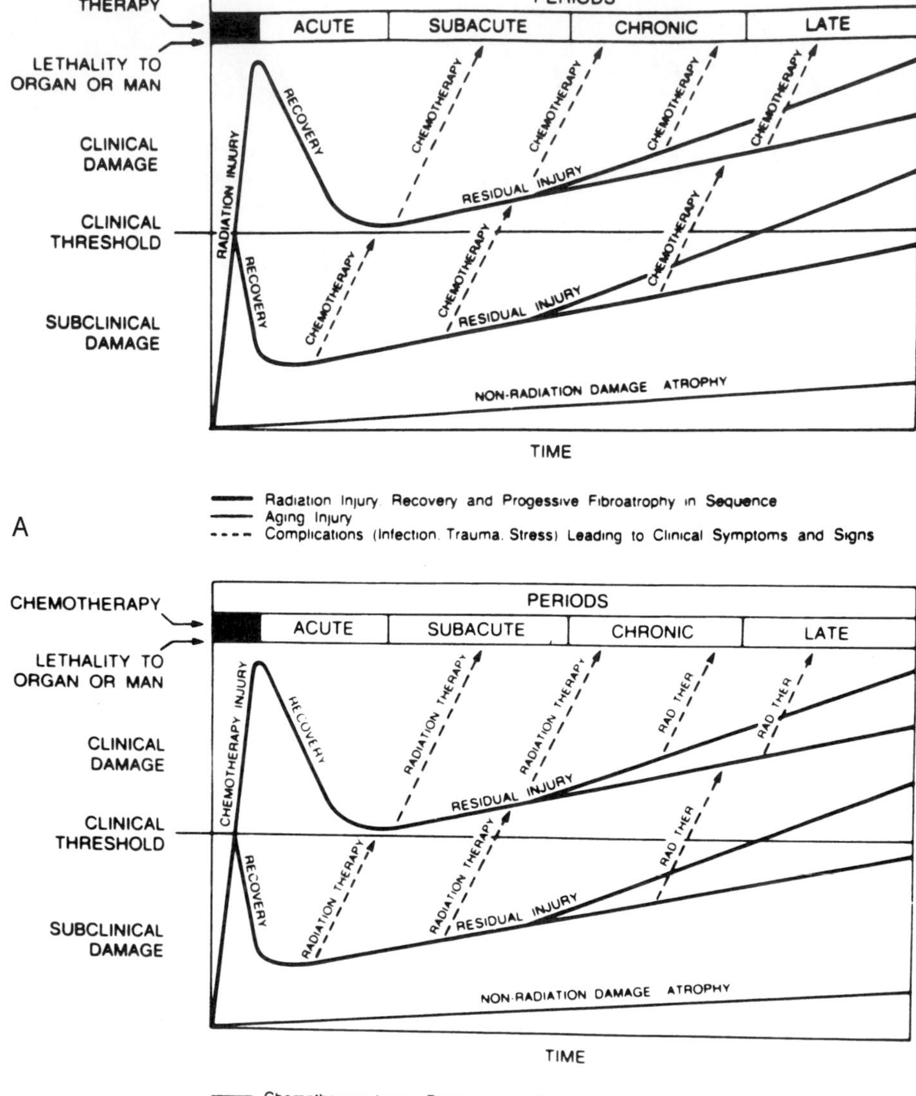

Figure 34–1. The clinicopathologic course of events following irradiation can be complicated by the addition of chemotherapy. Similarly, chemotherapy can result in a parallel set of events. (A) Classically, when radiation therapy precedes chemotherapy, the introduction of the second mode can lead to expression of subclinical damage or, when injury is present, to death. (B) The same is true if chemotherapy precedes radiation therapy. (Modified from Rubin P, Casarett GW: Clinical Radiation Pathology, pp 1–37. Philadelphia, W.B. Saunders, 1968, with permission.)

Late Effects in Normal Tissues and Molecular Biology

Our group has helped to pioneer the use of increasingly sophisticated molecular biologic methods to assess and analyze late effects in normal tissue (LENT). In so doing, we have extended the paradigm of the clinical pathologic course of events following irradiation or chemotherapy from target cells per se to include and emphasize the intercellular communication. In our current paradigm, during the course of LENT induction, the so-called cytokine cascade[15] can be considered to involve four basic cell components in tissues or organs—the parenchymal cell, the inflammatory cell, the endothelial cell, and the interstitial cell. These are illustrated in Figure 34–2A, as are a few of the proinflammatory and profibrotic cytokines that are thought to be expressed concurrently.

An intercellular conversation is initiated at the moment of irradiation, when injury to cell components occurs (e.g., membrane, cytoplasmic body, or DNA), which leads to altered gene expression. This reaction is often in the form of an immediate release of cytokine mRNA; in time, this reaction may provoke a series of downstream events through cell signaling, which is illustrated in Figure 34–2B. Through signal transduction, the receptor cells are activated; such activation may result in as little as additional or sequential cytokine expression or it can lead to proliferation or production of extracellular matrix proteins, depending on the species of receptor cell. In the specific case of the receptor cell being a fibroblast, activation of the collagen gene, which has been seen within 24 hours of injury,[16] can persist for days, weeks, or even months. This extended persistence may continue until the pathologic or clinical expression of injury is manifested.[15]

Using a mixture of molecular biologic techniques and *in vivo/in vitro* assays, a number of in-field effects can be appreciated. The release of cytokines occurs shortly after

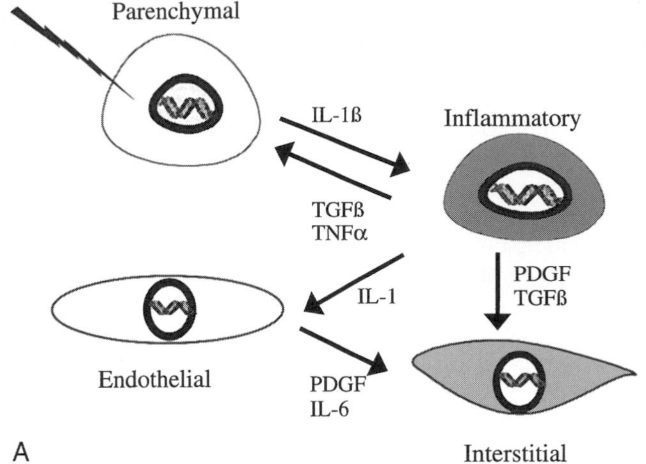

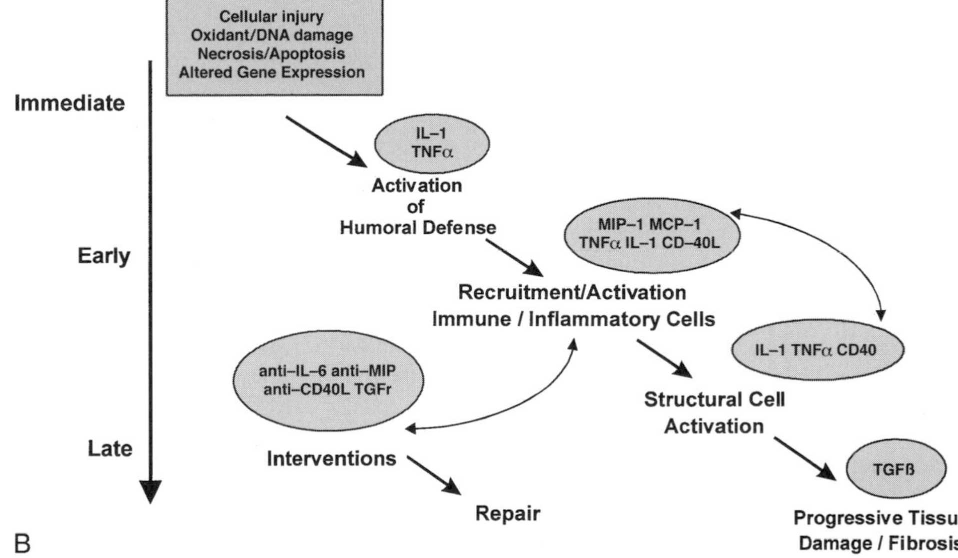

Figure 34-2. (A) Suggested chain of events beginning with the initial injury to the primary target cell—the parenchymal cell—and culminating in activation of the interstitial cells (e.g., fibroblasts) to lay down extracellular matrix. (B) Hypothetical pathway indicating the chain of events from initial injury to the final late effect (e.g., fibrosis). (A, From Rubin P, Finkelstein JN, Williams JP: Paradigm shifts in the radiation pathophysiology of late effects in normal tissues, molecular vs classic concepts. In: Tobias JS, Thomas PRM [eds]: Current Radiology Oncology, 3rd ed, pp 1–26. London, Arnold, 1998, with permission.)

irradiation and persists until the pathologic and clinical expression of late effects, and there is an arbitrary temporal division of cytokine expression:

- immediate: first 24 hours after injury
- early: days to ~ 8 weeks postinjury
- late: three to 6 months postinjury

This scenario can be seen to correlate and give further credence to the postulated shape of the clinical pathologic course of events (see Fig. 34–1). The potential to use cytokines to alter the therapeutic ratio favorably is of great interest to clinicians in the protocol design of new clinical trials.[10, 17]

General Concepts of Radiosensitivity and Chemosensitivity

Radiation Sensitivity

Cellular Radiosensitivity

The sequential changes that occur in tissue following irradiation are based on the mitotic behavior of component cells and their potential for either staying in cycle or differentiating.[18] However, the original descriptions used to illustrate cellular radiation sensitivity have been reinterpreted into cellular kinetic terminology.[19] The vegetative and differentiating intermitotic cells described by Cowdry[20] have been supplanted by undifferentiated and committed stem cells. The basic tenet of this concept is that cellular radiosensitivity is directly related to mitotic behavior, whereas the severity of radiation changes relates to the mitotic potential of the cell. The dividing or cycling cell (undifferentiated or committed stem cell) is more vulnerable to radiation than the nondividing cell, particularly if it is a functional mature cell or a reverting mature cell. That is, radiation cell death is expressed as a mitotically linked death and, with few exceptions, occurs only when the cell divides.

Cell Cycle Correlation to Radiosensitivity

The radiosensitivity of cells is based on their progression through the cell cycle. Undifferentiated stem cells are mainly a reserve compartment with only a small percentage moving from G_0 to G_1. In bone marrow, these cells constitute less than 1% of all cells in the reserve pool. Committed stem cells are programmed to differentiate and form the largest percentage of cycling cells from G_1 to S to G_2M. Reverting mature cells proliferate slowly and are generally found in G_0 to G_1; the length of G_1 increases as a function of increasing cell cycle time. Functional mature cells are found in G_0 and have no potential for division (e.g., neurons). Proliferating cells are more radiosensitive than quiescent cells, particularly when they are in early S phase and G_2M.

Organization of Tissues According to Cell Renewal

The parenchymal cell compartments of the various organs in the body can be considered to be either rapid or slow renewal systems. The epithelial tissues that line mucosal surfaces in the upper aerodigestive passages, gastrointestinal (GI) tract, urinary system, and bone marrow are examples of rapid renewal tissues. These tissues tend to have uncommitted or committed stem cell compartments that rapidly proliferate and differentiate. Slow renewal tissues are characterized by a parenchymal cell compartment that turns over slowly, but often has the capacity to respond by reverting to a stem cell and regenerating or repopulating the lost parenchymal cells. Examples of tissues that are conditionally proliferative include liver after partial resection, bone following fracture, microcirculation in wound healing, endocrine glands following increased trophic hormone stimulus, and bone marrow (protected areas) following irradiation of a large segment. Many adult organs have little or no capacity to restore their parenchymal cells, that is, proliferation occurs primarily early in life and is fixed. Examples of this type of tissue or organ are the central nervous system (CNS), heart, kidney, and muscle, in which lost cells are replaced by fibrosis.

Chemosensitivity

Drug Action as Phase or Cycle Specific

Cell cycle kinetics have been classically used to describe the response of cells to chemotherapeutic agents.[21, 22] Drug action has been defined either as *phase* or *cycle* specific, referring to cell killing either in S phase or elsewhere in the cycle. The expression of cell lethality at the time of mitosis in rapidly proliferating tissues appears clinically as an acute injury; the cells that are most vulnerable are the actively cycling or dividing stem cells that are targeted by M-specific agents, for example, vincristine, vinblastine, and etoposide. This situation contrasts with those cells in G_0 or prolonged G_1 that are protected, particularly from S phase–specific drugs, for example, methotrexate, fluorouracil, and hydroxyurea. The relationship between cell kill, dosage of the cytotoxic agents, and the proliferation rate is such that rapidly proliferating cells are more sensitive than slowly proliferating cells, and cell killing is an exponential function of drug dose.

It was thought that cells that are postmitotic are insensitive to drugs and that their tissues are correspondingly resistant to late effects. It is now known that this idea may apply to tumor effects but not necessarily to normal tissues. The vulnerability of cells to drugs is dependent upon the cell's capacity to absorb, concentrate, or metabolize the agents or their derivatives and, therefore, may be independent of cell mitotic behavior and maturation.

Drug Action on Stem Cell Depletion

The dose-limiting organ appears as a function of drug targeting in a specific tissue. The experimental evidence of Botnick and colleagues[23] showed that in a variety of tissues, despite the normal appearance of regenerated cells and tissues after chemotherapy insult, some of their proliferative reserve capacity had been lost. Because the proliferation capacity of a tissue is affected by time, drug toxicity varies relative to the patient's age.[24]

The term *stem cell senescence* has been introduced to describe the concept of depletion of stem cell reserve or loss of normal mitotic potential of reserve stem cells. Radiation acts in a similar fashion on these cells, and both drugs and radiation can induce accelerated aging that results from stem cell senescence.[25, 26]

Gonadal Effects

The late effects of chemotherapeutic agents on gonads must be considered, not only in terms of their effects on fertility but also their possible induction of premature failure creating endocrine deficiency states. Awareness of this possibility is important so that hormone replacement therapy can be offered to the patient, if it is appropriate. This effect has been most closely studied in young patients treated for Hodgkin's disease, in whom certain combinations of drugs used for advanced disease (e.g., MOPP*, MVPP†, and COPP‡) have been observed to produce a very high rate of infertility in men while not affecting testosterone production, libido, or potency.[27–29] By contrast, women receiving the same combinations of agents do not necessarily become infertile, but an early menopause with its attendant consequences is commonly produced.[30, 31] For this and other reasons, alternative combinations of drugs that are equally as effective against the disease (e.g., ABVD§) but do not appear to have similar effects on the gonads, have become the treatment of choice.

A similar effect in fertility and gonadal failure is observed in adult patients receiving high-dose therapy with stem cell transplantation.[32, 33] The treatment of advanced testicular cancer with chemotherapy does not appear to affect fertility, although certains aspects of the surgical management of the disease often impact potency and may cause ejaculatory dysfunction.[34–36] A major concern of the use of alkylating agents in the adjuvant treatment of premenopausal women with breast cancer has been the induction of premature ovarian failure. Reported rates are variable, but these are clearly higher with increased cumulative doses of alkylating agents as well as increasing age at the time of administration. Most studies have observed that, following adjuvant CMF|| therapy,[37, 38] 60% to 90% of

*Mechlorethamine, Oncovin (vincristine), procarbazine, prednisone.
†Mechlorethamine, vinblastine, procarbazine, prednisone.
‡Cyclophosphamide, Oncovin (vincristine), procarbazine, prednisone.
§Adriamycin (doxorubicin), bleomycin, vinblastine, decarbazine.
||Cyclophosphamide, methotrexate, 5-fluorouracil.

women treated at age 40 or older experience premature menopause. This can be particularly troubling because estrogen replacement therapy remains to be proved safe for patients with breast cancer.[39]

Chemoresistance and Radiation Resistance

Mechanisms of Drug Resistance

The concept of drug resistance[40–42] in tumors has been thoroughly explored and can be either primary or acquired, with the acquisition of drug resistance representing an adaptive change by a tumor cell. The mechanisms that lead to drug resistance are generally considered to be

- insufficient drug uptake by a cancer cell
- insufficient activation of a drug
- increased inactivation of a drug
- increased activation of a target enzyme
- decreased requirement for a specific metabolic product
- increased use of an alternative biochemical pathway—salvage
- rapid repair of a drug-induced lesion
- spontaneous mutation into drug-resistant cells, as expressed in the Coldman and Goldie hypothesis[43]

Multidrug (pleiotropic) resistance (MDR),[44] which is found in cells in response to a number of agents, has been associated with increased rates of drug removal. Various classes of drugs associated with the development of drug resistance, such as the vinca alkaloids, anthracyclines, and topoisomerase inhibitors, have different sites of action within the cell. Therefore, the mode of resistance development varies between drug classes, although many have been associated with high levels of an integral membrane-linked protein, P-glycoprotein (Pgp).[45, 46] The *MDR1* gene is found *in vitro* to be overexpressed in drug-resistant phenotypes and encodes for Pgp, which functions as an efflux drug pump.[47] The association between *MDR1* and Pgp led to a search for increased levels of Pgp as a marker for nonresponsive tumors; unfortunately, a similar *MDR1*-Pgp expression has been described in normal tissue.[44] The normal tissue distribution of Pgp includes brain capillary endothelial cells, proximal tubules of the kidney, adrenals, columnar epithelial cells of the intestine, normal blood cells of bone marrow, and biliary canaliculi of the liver. This expression in normal tissues complicates new efforts to circumvent Pgp-associated multidrug resistance. Therefore, in developing molecular methods to assay for gene products such as *MDR1*-Pgp in clinical biopsy specimens, the assay must be capable of distinguishing tumor from normal tissue, as well as being sensitive and specific. Although *MDR1*-Pgp expression has proved to be of prognostic value in acute leukemias, multiple myeloma, and malignant lymphomas, other agents, such as multidrug resistance protein and lipoprotein receptor–related protein, may also prove to be useful for different classes of drugs and, perhaps, different normal tissues.

Mechanisms of Radiation Resistance: Intrinsic and Extrinsic Factors

The major determinants of cell survival curves relate to the shoulder (D_q) and slope (D_0) and refer to the intrinsic radiosensitivity. The wider the shoulder and the shallower the slope, the more radioresistant the cell. To review this subject, the reader should see Chapter 5, Basic Principles of Radiobiology. Extrinsic factors, such as oxygenation, pH level, and (as alluded to previously) cell cycle, affect the radioresistance of a cell. Poorly oxygenated or hypoxic cells and cells in late S or early G_1 phase are more resistant to irradiation. The ability of cells to repair radiation injury is important, and both sublethal repair and potentially lethal repair capacities also determine a cell's radioresistance.

Radioresistance is a relative term in that all tissues, if exposed to doses beyond tolerance, will ultimately become necrotic because of parenchymal or vascular cell damage. The higher the fractional and total dose and the shorter the time of exposure, the more rapid the onset of tissue necrosis, with increasing numbers of cellular compartments being destroyed. In this regard, there is always a dose-limiting tissue in the radiation field and, most universally, it is the vasculoconnective tissue component. Although direct parenchymal cellular depletion of an organ occurs after irradiation, it is often the fine arteriocapillary circulation that either rapidly occludes and infarcts leading to necrosis or a slower sclerosis that triggers fibrosis. Both processes lead to a histochemical barrier, blocking transport of vital metabolities and, in turn, contributing to parenchymal cell depletion, hypoplasia, and eventual late effects. The distribution of many of the late radiation lesions reflects primarily vascular injury and is dose related,[48] and it cannot be explained simply as an indirect effect of parenchymal cell loss, resulting in underlying vascular injury. Devastating late effects as a result of this process can occur in both rapidly and slowly proliferating normal tissues without a clinically recognizable acute phase.

Clonogenic Tumor and Stem Cell Depletion

Whereas all forms of radiation are additive when they are delivered to the same tissue volume, combinations of agents are not, particularly when they are chosen to avoid overlapping toxicity in specific organs. Nonetheless, cell killing by drugs is similar to that developed for radiation therapy in that it is based on first-order kinetics or exponential cell kill.

An assumption is made that active drugs provide a degree of tumor cell log kill. In most multidrug regimens, the number of tumor cells is progressively reduced as the induction, consolidation, and maintenance phases of regimens are completed. If the tumor clonogenic cells are reduced to zero, then a cure results. If drug resistance appears, then the tumor can recur; the early or late reappearance of a tumor is often a function of the time at which drug resistance develops. Parallels between the phases of drug treatment and the radiation therapy regimen can be drawn: the radiation boost field and boost dose may be compared to the consolidation phase. In the current practice of radiation treatment, there is no equivalent to the prolonged and cyclical maintenance dose schedules found in chemotherapy.

When the concept of stem cell depletion is applied to normal tissues, similar sets of events can be expected. For the cancer treatment to be successful, a differential degree of tumor and normal tissue cell kill must occur. Either an extremely large number of stem cells must exist in the normal tissue or a greater capacity to repair and repopulate vital parenchyma must exist compared with tumors. As drug therapy or radiation regimens deplete the stem cells, reversible or irreversible injury occurs. A major conceptual difference between tumors and normal tissue is that there is no known radioresistance or chemoresistance seen in normal tissue.

Host Response

Although it is difficult to establish the genetic role of the host (patient heterogeneity) in radiation reactions, it has long been recognized as a factor in radiation treatment to account for differences in late effects in normal tissues. Host differences have been studied by a variety of investigators, for instance, through the use of fibroblast assays,[49, 50] and considerable data exist to show a wide variation in the response of individual patients to the same dose-fractionation schedules. For instance, Turesson and Notter, in a long-term study of breast cancer patients, documented large variations in telangiectasia expression in patients treated in a similar fashion.[51, 52]

In the laboratory, we have postulated and shown that apparent differences in tolerance to the development of pulmonary fibrosis demonstrated between strains of mice may be due to their cytokine expression following exposure to radiation.[16, 53] Our colleagues, Baecher-Allan and coworkers, and other investigators[54–56] have demonstrated strain-dependent variations in cytokine expression in bleomycin-induced lung fibrosis, and a similar correlation was shown with the severity of injury. This evidence strongly suggests that both radiation therapy and chemotherapy share common cytokine pathways; this may explain the so-called *recall phenomenon* and other unexpected toxicities associated with combined-modality therapy, when seemingly safe doses of each individual mode are used.[57, 58] In addition, it suggests that a demonstrated sensitivity or resistance to therapy—radiation or chemotherapy—may have a genetic basis and, therefore, predictive assays could be used to improve or prevent late effects.[59, 60]

Time-Course Paradigm

Clinical Pathologic Course of Events

The expression of injury after irradiation allows for identification of an early or acute injury, which is often reparable, and a later component, which is irreparable. The classically described mechanisms of action[1] have been presented both as a parenchymal cell loss and injury and alteration of the vasculoconnective tissue. The initial recovery at the tissue level is predominantly due to parenchymal cellular repopulation, but a later depletion of stem cell populations is a function of cell cycle time and kinetics, that is, fast versus slow renewal systems.[61] The progressive component is arteriocapillary fibrosis, which predominates in the late irreparable injury and accentuates cellular depletion in the parenchyma.

Rubin and Casarett have presented a clinical pathologic course for most normal tissues and organs[2] based on documented histopathophysiologic events in humans and *in vivo* in laboratory animals. The course of events was illustrated in terms of subclinical and clinical damage with a threshold that may be expressed as a radiation tolerance dose (see Fig. 34–1A). A similar clinical pathologic course was postulated following chemotherapy administration (see Fig. 34–1B). Precise quantification of pathophysiologic injury is often difficult to define and needs a solution in order to provide the data that can be clinically useful. The search for predictive biochemical, metabolic, or physiologic parameters in terms of early events following irradiation or chemotherapy (or both) is a major focus of research, and it is hoped that it can be used to monitor for more permanent pathologic damage that will occur, or is occurring, on a subclinical level.

The clinical pathologic course of events following radiation exposure can be complicated by the addition of chemotherapy. Depending on which mode of treatment is employed first, the evidence suggests that both will leave residual injury when large enough doses of either agent are used. This injury results in a subclinical residuum that may be uncovered by the subsequent use of a seemingly safe dose of the alternate therapy. Thus, classically, when radiation therapy precedes chemotherapy (see Fig. 34–1A), the introduction of a new drug can lead to the expression of subclinical damage; when frank injury is already present, increased morbidity or even fatality can result. The same is true of chemotherapy preceding radiation therapy (see Fig. 34–1B). In addition to complications (dashed lines) caused only by the addition of the second mode, associated infection, trauma, or stress can exacerbate the situation.

Combined Effects of Drugs and Radiation

There has been a tendency to refer to clinical drug-radiation reactions as *recall phenomena* or *enhancements* of radiation injury. However, there is evidence in the literature that many chemotherapeutic agents are either affecting different target cell populations or similar cell populations through entirely different pathophysiologic mechanisms. Radiation acts both on the microcirculatory systems and parenchymal cells of tissues and organs, whereas chemotherapy acts predominantly on the cellular parenchymal component.[62] In rapid renewal systems, the same stem cell population is affected and the increased acute toxicity of both modes when used in combination may be reduced by applying them sequentially. In slow renewal tissues, effects are often a result of actions on entirely different target cell populations in the same organ system, resulting in an additive pathophysiologic effect, particularly when they are administered concurrently.[63, 64]

There is a need to be aware of the syndromes secondary to all modes of cancer treatment so that they are not confused with recurrent or metastatic disease. The late effect syndromes occur at different times from tumor progression, and their time course of expression needs to be appreciated for their clinical recognition. In the pediatric setting, the many proliferating tissues are even more vulnerable than those in adults, in whom many normal organs are in a mature steady state with slow cell renewal kinetics.

Tolerance of Organs

Dose-Time-Volume Factors

Dose-limiting organs and tissues in radiation oncology have been defined according to their tolerance doses (Table 34–1).[65] The minimal tolerance dose ($TD_{5/5}$) and the maximal tissue tolerance dose ($TD_{50/5}$) refer to severe to life-threatening complications occurring in 5% and 50% of patients within 5 years of therapeutic radiation treatment. However, in this era of multimodality, there are many factors that affect our concepts of radiosensitivity. The rapid advances of radiation oncology and the related sciences of radiation biology and radiation physics and accumulating information on interactions with other therapeutic modalities (e.g., chemotherapy or biologic response modifiers) impact our understanding of normal tissue toxicities. Thus, although previously defined radiation tolerance doses (TD_5 and TD_{50}) remain as valuable guides, their applicability has changed. Radiation doses customarily deemed to be safe may no longer be so. When combined with another therapy, such doses can lead to severe late effects with regard to different vital organs. Factors relevant to defining tolerance doses include those from therapy, the host, and the tumor.

General Therapy Factors

- *Dose:* There is no absolute or fixed dose that ablates a normal tissue because the $TD_{5/5}$ and $TD_{50/5}$ are dependent on dose, time, and volume factors.
- *Fractionation:* The radiation fraction dose, the interval between fractions, and the overall duration of therapy are major determinants of both early and late effects.[66] The time to expression of the effect is related to the cell kinetics of different subpopulations within a tissue organ. With alternate fractionation regimens under investigation, the $TD_{5/5}$ and $TD_{50/5}$ will shift for different organs. Hyperfractionation, accelerated fractionation, and hypofractionation have different effects on tolerance doses.
- *Volume:* A major factor in determining a tolerance dose is whether the whole or part of an organ is exposed to radiation. With more widespread use of large fields, for example, total body irradiation (TBI) and hemibody irradiation (HBI), compared with very defined or small fields, for example, intraoperative radiation therapy and stereotactic radiosurgery, single or brief radiation exposures with various dose rates to different volumes will create a new set of normal tissue toxicities.[48]
- *Chemotherapy:* Of the various modalities, the addition of chemotherapy and the timing of its delivery relative to irradiation have a major impact on organ sensitivity.[67, 68] The use of an agent may dramatically affect either the same cells or different cell subpopulations, leading to lower threshold doses for organ injury. The widespread use of drugs is the most common factor altering the tolerance dose concepts of normal tissues.
- *Innovations:* The new modalities, radiosensitizers and radioprotectors, and immunologic and biologic responses modifiers, including gene therapy, may each or all alter late effects.

TABLE 34–1. **Parameters of Therapy: Tolerance Doses ($TD_{5/5}$–$TD_{50/5}$)**

Single Dose (Gy)		Fractionated Dose (Gy)	
Lymphoid	2–20	Testes	1–2
Bone marrow	2–10	Ovary	6–10
Ovary	2–6	Eye (lens)	6–12
Testes	2–10	Kidney	20–30
Eye (lens)	2–10	Thyroid	20–40
Mucosa	5–20	Lung	23–28
Lung	7–10	Skin	30–40
GI	5–10	Liver	35–40
Colorectal	10–20	Bone marrow	40–50
Kidney	10–20	Heart	43–50
Heart	18–20	GI	50–55
Vasculoconnective tissue	10–20	Vasculoconnective tissue	50–60
Liver	15–20	Spinal cord	50–60
Skin	15–20	Brain	55–70
Peripheral nerve	15–20	Peripheral nerve	65–77
Spinal cord	15–20	Mucosa	65–77
Brain	15–25	Bone and cartilage	>70
Bone and cartilage	>30	Muscle	>70
Muscle	>70		

From Rubin P: Law and order of radiation sensitivity. Absolute versus relative. In: Vaeth JM, Meyer JL (eds): Frontiers of Radiation Therapy and Oncology, 23rd ed, p 7. Basel, Karger, 1989, with permission.

The concept of an optimal radiation dose that provides maximal curability and minimal toxicity is the basis of varying fractionation schedules.[66, 69] Strandqvist lines or isoeffect plots based on varying dose-time regimens suggest that an optimal zone can be found, yielding a favorable therapeutic ratio.[70] Although these lines were originally drawn with parallel slopes, it became apparent to many investigators that tumors respond differently to normal tissues, and a divergence in isoeffect slopes occurs.[71] The importance of the volume of normal tissue in the field[72] and dose-time factors needs to be stressed when considering tolerance of normal tissue or organs. In re-examining and revising the tolerance doses for different vital dose-limiting tissues and organs, the volume factor is even more relevant today in view of the increasing use of TBI and HBI, in which whole organ systems are exposed. More time-concentrated schedules are in use, varying from single exposures to short, intense fractionation schedules. Another modality—intraoperative radiation therapy—has led to the use of large, single doses to large tissue volumes and has provided new insights into tolerance doses.[48, 73]

At present, the prescribed tolerance dose is, at best, a calculated estimate of the TD_5 and TD_{50} based on recorded human and animal data. The complication probability of either 5% (TD_5) or 50% (TD_{50}) assumes uniform irradiation of all or part of an organ, conventional fractionation schedules (1.8–2.0 Gy per fraction and five fractions per week), relatively normal organ function as a baseline, no adjuvant drugs or surgical manipulations, and age ranges that exclude children and the elderly (Table 34–2). In ordering the organ radiosensitivity according to dose level, a variety of factors are considered, including the end point chosen (late rather than acute effects), the use of single or fractionated regimens, and the volume of the organs. Because the literature is not always complete or precise, extrapolation is inevitably involved when using either clinical or experi-

TABLE 34–2. **Parameters of Therapy: Tolerance Doses TD_5–TD_{50}**

Target Cell	Complication End Point	Dose Range (Gy)* TD_5–TD_{50}
Range: 2–10 Gy		
Testes/spermatogonia	Sterility	1–2
Lymphoid tissue/lymphocytes	Lymphopenia	2–10
Diseased bone marrow (CLL or multiple myeloma)	Severe leukopenia and thrombocytopenia	3–5
Ovary/oocytes	Sterility	6–10
Range: 10–20 Gy		
Lens	Cataract	6–12
Bone marrow stem cells	Acute aplasia	15–20
Range: 20–30 Gy		
Lung—type II cells, vasculoconnective tissue	Pneumonitis/fibrosis	20–30
Kidney—glomeruli	Arterionephrosclerosis	23–28
Range: 30–40 Gy		
Bone marrow	Hypoplasia	25–35
Liver—central veins	Radiation hepatitis	35–40
Range: 40–50 Gy		
Heart (whole)	Pericarditis and pancarditis	43–50
Bone marrow microenvironments, sinuses	Permanent aplasia	45–50
Range: 50–60 Gy		
GI organ	Infarction necrosis	50–55
Spinal cord	Myelopathy	50–60
Brain	Encephalopathy	50–60
Heart (partial)	Cardiomyopathy	55–65
Range: >60–70 Gy		
Mucosa	Ulcer	65–75
Rectum	Ulcer	65–75
Bladder	Ulcer	65–75
Mature bones	Fracture	65–75

CCL = chronic lymphocytic leukemia.
*Doses are given as the total fractionated dose to whole or partial organs.
From Rubin P: Law and order of radiation sensitivity. Absolute versus relative. In: Vaeth JM, Meyer JL (eds): Frontiers of Radiation Therapy and Oncology, 23rd ed, p 7. Basel, Karger, 1989, with permission.

mental animal data. The dose levels are rounded off rather than recorded precisely to one or two decimals, as is occasionally reported. Such accuracy can be as misleading as the general estimates of tolerance doses offered.

Specific Organ Tolerances: Dose-Limiting Tissues

Most organs systems are composed of many cell subpopulations (20 to 40 or more), each performing an important activity. Therefore, organ tolerance is determined by the radiosensitivity of relevant stem cell subpopulations that may not always be proliferating or dividing[19]; the most radiosensitive, vital cell population determines organ tolerance and organ failure. Just as the degree of importance held by an irradiated organ determines the survival of an organism, the functional capacity of cells is often distinct from their regenerative capacity, permitting organ physiology to be preserved in the face of injury and allowing for recovery or repair from the insult.

LENT syndromes at each organ site are not random events but are specific entities that occur at certain times and are expressed in a recognizable fashion and often can be ameliorated. A LENT paradigm is presented in diagrammatic form for each organ site.

Bone Marrow

Clinical Syndromes

Bone marrow (Fig. 34–3) is a major dose-limiting organ, particularly when irradiation and chemotherapy are combined.[74] The effects of chemotherapy on bone marrow are reflected in peripheral blood counts, with the nadir occurring 2 to 3 weeks after treatment. In contrast, the effects of radiation therapy are more varied, as the compensatory mechanisms for regeneration are both dose dependent and volume dependent. Recovery is related to the degree of initial response and generally begins with a regeneration of depleted stem cells. If large volumes of bone marrow have been irradiated, a hypoplastic marrow can persist and may become aplastic. Aplastic marrow also can result from infiltration of the marrow, and this scenario should be suspected if the depression in blood count does not occur at a predictable time, or if only a limited volume of the bone marrow has been irradiated.

The acute sequelae of marrow toxicity are well known. They have been detailed elsewhere[74] and are illustrated in Figure 34–4.[75] The neutropenia seen in the first week results from a combination of cessation in production and the rapid turnover of these cells. This combination is followed by thrombocytopenia at 2 to 3 weeks and by anemia

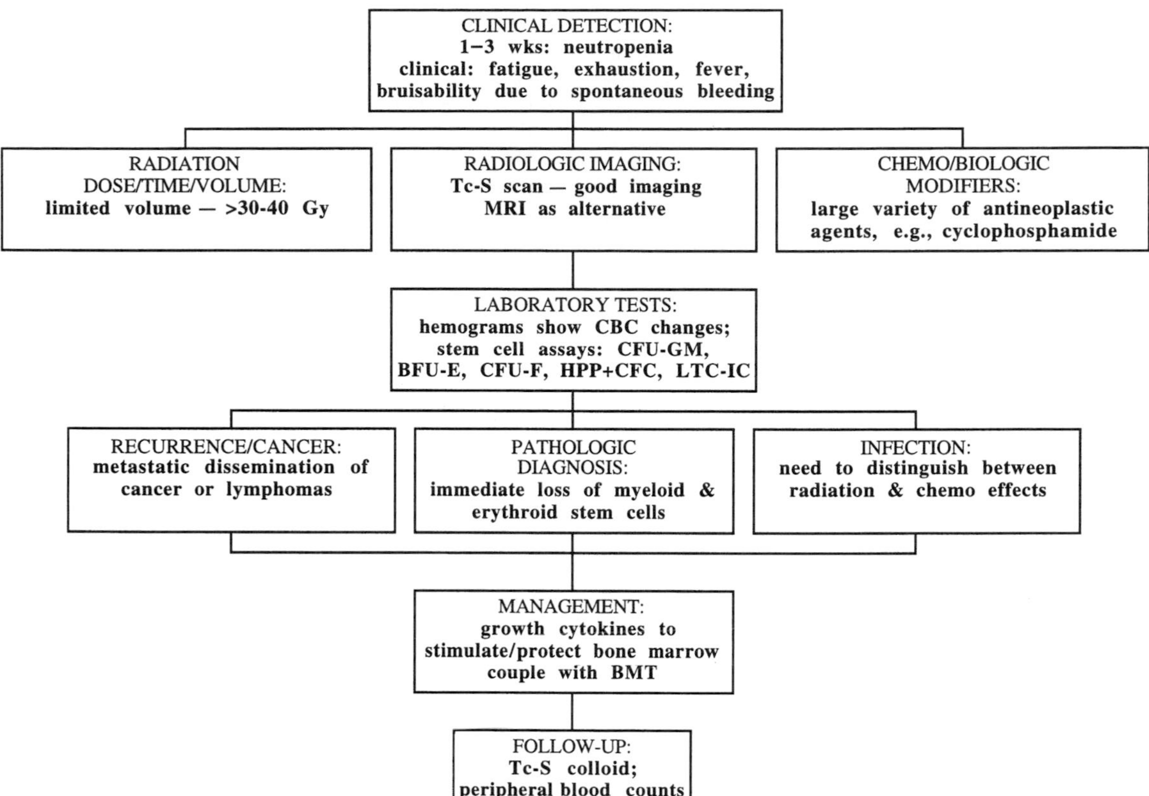

Figure 34–3. LENT diagram for bone marrow.

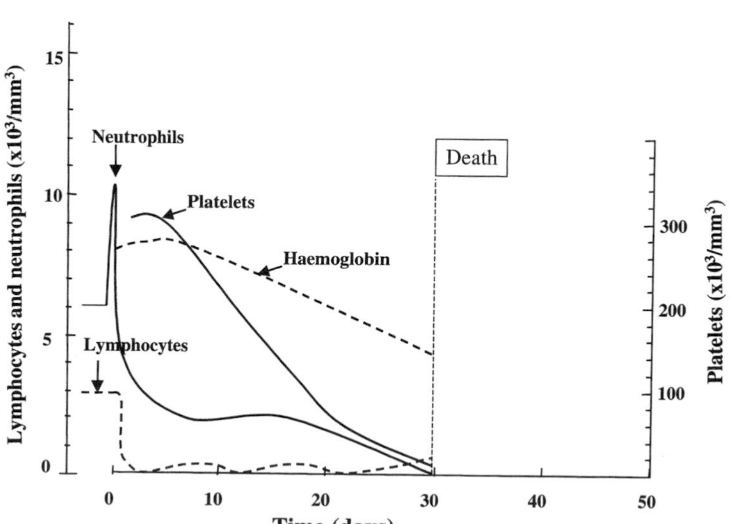

Figure 34–4. Expected hematologic response in a human following a single total body dose of 4.5 Gy. (From Andrews GA: Radiation accidents and their management. Radiat Res 1967; 7[suppl]:390–397, with permission.)

at 2 to 3 months. It has been shown that depression of a hematopoietic cell lineage translates into potential or observed difficulties for the patient, although the definitions of granulocytopenia, thrombocytopenia, and anemia are somewhat arbitrary in nature:

- *Granulocytopenia* is considered to be an absolute granulocyte count of 500/mm^3 or less, and it places a patient at risk for infection.[76] Declining counts between 500 and 1000/mm^3 as a consequence of antineoplastic therapy are considered by most oncologists to represent neutropenia.
- *Thrombocytopenia* is a platelet count less than 175,000/mm^3, although the symptoms of bruising, petechiae, and mucosal bleeding rarely occur at greater than 100,000/mm^3, and infrequently at greater than 20,000/mm^3.[77, 78] Intracranial hemorrhage is particularly rare, with most episodes occurring at counts less than 5000/mm^3.
- *Anemia* requiring red blood cell transfusion is more difficult to define because a variety of clinical judgments may be in operation.

The management of patients with chronic bone marrow toxicity includes, in addition to hematopoietic stem cell transplantation techniques, the administration of blood products (erythrocyte, platelet, and granulocyte transfusions), apheresis with peripheral blood stem cell transfusion, and the administration of growth factors.[74, 79, 80]

Pathophysiology

Elements of blood and bone marrow respond to radiation by progressively decreasing in numbers because of the destruction of radiosensitive precursor cells. The bone marrow compartment is defined by the composition of its various cell components together with the renewal ability of each stem cell population. The refinement of assay systems for progenitor cells, such as CFU-GM*, BFU-E†, CFU-Blast‡, and CFU-GEMM§, allows for the study of different cell lineages, whereas the assay for connective tissue stroma (CFU-F‖) gives an insight into the microenvironment essential for normal hematopoiesis. In addition, cell-sorting techniques give a rapid assessment of progenitor cells in the marrow or blood. However, it must be emphasized that none of these techniques specifically measures stem cells.[74] In the clinic, *in vitro* assays that measure colonies in long-term cultures may eventually provide a means to quantify primitive stem cells in humans.

Deciphering the interactions between cells has allowed us to have an insight into the dramatic sequence of bone marrow responses to radiation. In addition, some chemotherapeutic agents have been shown to act through similar cellular and molecular pathways to radiation; therefore, the combined use of these modalities in chemoradiation schedules sets up a competition for bone marrow compartments.[81, 82] The use of cytokines and other stimulating factors is beginning to gain wider use to improve bone marrow transplantation.[11, 81, 83] However, each chemotherapeutic agent modality has a so-called price tag for its use.

*Granulocyte-macrophage colony-forming unit.
†Erythroid burst-forming unit.
‡Blast cell colony-forming unit.
§Granulocyte-erythroid-monocyte-megakaryocyte–colony-forming unit.
‖Fibroblast colony-forming unit.

Radiation Effects

Bone marrow is one of the most radiosensitive organs (Fig. 34–5), responding to total body doses of 1.5 Gy to 7.5 Gy with a rapid depletion of vital stem cells within 1 week of exposure (see Fig. 34–4).[84, 85] Death usually occurs as a result of granulocytopenia and thrombocytopenia that predispose the patient to overwhelming infection and hemorrhage. Radiation doses of 3 to 5 Gy result in a lethal dose ($LD_{50/100}$), with a shorter interval to death resulting from 7.5 to 10.5 Gy. However, following bone marrow transplants, doses of 7.5 to 10.5 Gy are well tolerated because the microvasculature of the marrow allows for implantation and proliferation of transferred stem cells.

Fractionated radiation doses to the whole bone marrow organ are used in clinical schedules for treatment of certain leukemias, multiple myelomas, and non-Hodgkin's lymphoma, and in the form of TBI for bone marrow transplant. In non-Hodgkin's lymphoma, high-dose TBI schedules are frequently well tolerated, with 0.1 to 0.15 Gy being given twice weekly for 5 weeks. Cycles of treatment may be given monthly and can lead to total doses as high as 3 to 4.5 Gy; nonetheless, severe to life-threatening hematologic toxicity still may sometimes occur. Because of the possibility of severe thrombocytopenia, a process of dose titration is essential, and treatment should be withheld if the platelet count falls below 100,000/mm^3. Of note, patients with multiple myeloma and chronic lymphocytic leukemia appear to exhibit more hematologic sensitivity to TBI than those with normal bone marrow, and death has resulted after modest doses.[86, 87]

TBI is widely used in bone marrow transplantation. Thomas pioneered the use of TBI using telecobalt units to deliver very low dose rates (0.05 Gy per minute),[88] but more recently the widespread use of single-exposure TBI

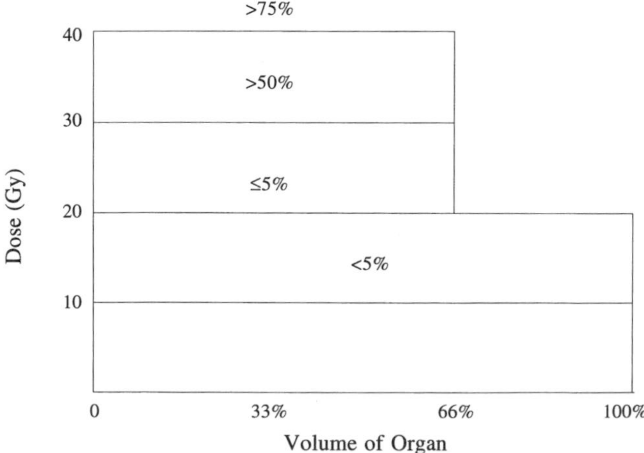

Figure 34–5. Dose-volume histogram for in-field bone marrow hypoplasia, illustrating the relationship between volume and tolerance doses. A different dose-volume histogram would be required for other end points, for example, peripheral cell count suppression.

techniques has been supplemented by safer fractionated schedules using both high and low dose rates. Total doses range from 5 to 10 Gy, fraction size varies from 1.2 to 4.0 Gy, and dose rates extend from 0.025 to 0.05 Gy per minute. These fractionation schedules, in conjunction with lung shields, are designed to protect against lung toxicity but they are not designed to be of therapeutic advantage in bone marrow ablation.

The regenerative activity of the bone marrow compartment is more volume dependent than dose dependent, which may be explained by dividing the volume effects into three arbitrary categories.[89] When less than 10% to 15% of bone marrow volume is irradiated, permanent ablation of bone marrow occurs with fractionated doses greater than 30 Gy and single doses of 20 Gy in the affected volume. The protected bone marrow is able to compensate by accelerating its rate of hematopoiesis, and there is localized regeneration. When 25% to 50% of bone marrow is exposed to radiation, permanent ablation occurs at similar dose levels to the above-mentioned levels, and all of the nonirradiated marrow becomes activated, remaining in a state of prolonged stimulus. However, there is a failure to regenerate bone marrow in-field, best demonstrated in patients with Hodgkin's disease after mantle treatment to doses of 30 to 40 Gy.[90, 91] When a larger volume of bone marrow is irradiated (>50%), the paradoxical phenomenon of in-field regeneration is seen 2 to 5 years later, and there is extension of bone marrow into previously quiescent long bones within 1 to 2 years.[92]

Chemotherapy Effects

Some antineoplastic drugs can induce long-term damage in the hematopoietic system; typical observations are listed in Table 34–3.[92, 93] Both acute and long-term effects that parallel radiation effects have been documented,[74] with changes in the cellular marrow seen within the first 48 hours. However, alterations in peripheral blood counts are not apparent for 1 to 3 weeks, reflecting the kinetics of cell maturation and the life span of mature peripheral blood cells (1 to 2 days for granulocytes, 10 to 20 days for platelets, and 120 days for erythrocytes). The precise mechanism of the action of drug-induced myelosuppression is not well defined; bone marrow that appears to be functioning normally following chemotherapy has demonstrated limited reserve when challenged by additional therapy.

In addition to the long-term suppression of blood counts that can occur with many chemotherapeutic agents, it has been observed with increasing frequency that certain drugs, when given alone or in combination, may contribute to the development of secondary acute myeloid leukemia (AML) or myelodysplastic syndromes (MDS).[94, 95] This has been observed, at least in part, because of the success of chemotherapy in producing long-term survival in diseases previously considered to be incurable, such as advanced Hodgkin's disease, other malignant lymphomas, childhood acute leukemias, and metastatic germ cell tumors. Unfortunately, it is also seen with the increasing use of alkylating agents in the adjuvant therapy for early-stage breast and other cancers, although with less frequency.[96, 97]

Secondary acute leukemias tend to occur in one of two distinct syndromes. With the use of alkylating agents, such as cyclophosphamide, melphalan, or nitrogen mustard, secondary leukemias are most frequently seen at 4 to 8 years after the onset of therapy, and they are often preceded by an MDS. Alkylating agent-induced secondary AML or MDS is usually of the M-1 or M-2 phenotype (French-American-British classification), and it is associated with abnormalities of chromosome 5 (del-5 or 5q−), 7 (del-7 or 7q−), or 8 (trisomy 8) in 80% to 90% of cases.[94, 95, 98–100] This abnormality may be seen in 10% or more of patients with Hodgkin's disease who are treated with the MOPP combination, as well as in 5% to 10% of patients treated with melphalan for myeloma who survive to 5 years.[101] The relative risk of secondary AML or MDS is lower in patients treated with cyclophosphamide-based adjuvant therapy for breast cancer or with CHOP* chemotherapy for non-Hodgkin's lymphoma, but the incidence is still 2 to 3 times greater than that of untreated age-matched controls.[96, 97] In most studies, the incidence has been greater in patients treated at an older age and with higher cumulative doses of alkylating agents.

The second form of secondary AML has been reported in patients treated with topoisomerase II inhibitors.[102–106] In patients treated with etoposide or teniposide for testicular cancers, childhood acute lymphoblastic leukemia, or small cell lung cancer, AML can occur and is typically of the M-4 or M-5 phenotype, and it is characterized by balanced translocations involving chromosome 11 (11q23) or 21 (21q22). This syndrome often occurs with a much shorter latency period than with the alkylating agents (2 to 4 years), is rarely preceded by MDS, and may respond to chemotherapy with the same results as *de novo* AML. A similar secondary AML has been reported in patients receiving doxorubicin, epirubicin, or mitoxantrone in conjunction with alkylating agents, such as cisplatin and cyclophosphamide.[104, 107] There have also been a few reported cases of typical acute promyelocytic leukemia with the t15,17 translocation in patients receiving topoisomerase II inhibitors.[108]

Finally, there have been some recent reports of a high frequency of secondary MDS or AML following high-dose therapy with autologous bone marrow or peripheral blood stem cell transplantation for lymphomas or breast cancer.[109–113] In these cases, the morphologic and cytogenetic features are characteristic of alkylating agent–induced secondary leukemias, but the latency period is often shorter. It continues to be controversial as to whether this syndrome is due to the preparative chemotherapy administered before the transplant or to chemotherapy given earlier in the course of the disease, but in many cases, the condition has proved to be very refractory to therapy.[114]

Combined Modalities

An explanation for the poor tolerance of the irradiated bone marrow organ to chemotherapy may include not only the ablation or suppression of certain segments but also the increased sensitivity of a hyperactive, unexposed marrow. With a greater proportion of bone marrow stem cells cycling in the unexposed segment owing to a compensatory mechanism, these cells will be more chemosensitive. Be-

*Cyclophosphamide, doxorubicin, Oncovin (vincristine), prednisone.

TABLE 34–3. **Agents Causing Long-Term Damage to the Hematopoietic System**

Malignancy	Drugs (dose, schedule)	Parameter	Type of Damage	Permanence of Damage
Gastric	Mitomycin C	Blood count	Thrombocytopenia	Longlasting, reversible
	Nitrosoureas	Blood count	Neutropenia, thrombocytopenia	Longlasting
	BCNU	GM-CFU in peripheral blood	Almost complete disappearance	Longlasting
		GM-CFU in bone marrow	Reduction, severe	Longlasting after regeneration of peripheral blood granulocytes
Brain	MeCCNU (120 mg/m² q 3 wks)	Blood count	Severe myelosuppression	Longlasting
Breast	L-Phenylalanine mustard	Bone marrow granulocyte reserve	Hypocellular marrow with reduced PMN reserve	8–21 mos after cessation of chemotherapy
	Doxorubicin (50 mg/m²) + cyclophosphamide (500 mg/m²) × 6 q 4 wk	Peripheral blood granulocytes	Decrease	6–8 mos after chemotherapy
		GM-CFU in bone marrow	Delayed regeneration and reduced numbers	55 days after chemotherapy
		GM-CFU in peripheral blood	Reduced	For at least 5 yrs after chemotherapy
	Cyclophosphamide + methotrexate + 5-FU	GM-CFU in peripheral blood	Reduced	More than 1 yr
Small cell lung	Doxorubicin + cyclophosphamide + vincristine q 3 wks	GM-CFU in bone marrow	Delayed regeneration	No long-term follow-up

BCNU = carmustine; q = every; MeCCNU = lomustine; 5-FU = 5-fluorouracil; GM-CFU = granulocyte-macrophage colony-forming unit; PMN = polymorphonuclear leukocytes.

From Mauch P, Constine L, Greenberger J, et al: Hematopoietic stem cell compartment: acute and late effects of radiation therapy and chemotherapy. Int J Radiat Oncol Biol Phys 1995; 31:1319–1339, with permission from Elsevier Science; modified from Lohrmann H, Schreml W: Long-term hemopoietic damage after cytotoxic drug therapy for solid tumors. In: Testa N, Gale R (eds): Hematopoiesis: Long-Term Effects of Chemotherapy and Radiation, p 325. New York, Marcel Dekker, 1968.

cause the temporal sequencing of modalities affects tolerance, courses of chemotherapy can render the subsequent delivery of full courses of radiation difficult because of a lack of marrow reserve. For instance, although MOPP therapy is well tolerated subsequent to total nodal irradiation (TNI), the poor tolerance of TNI following MOPP in advanced Hodgkin's disease requires modification of the radiation dose to lower values. Nonetheless, despite dose-limiting toxicity, many different agents, for example, cyclophosphamide, busulfan, etoposide, and melphalan, are often combined with TBI to enhance its effects, and long-term damage to the stem cell compartment has been found.[115–117] The simultaneous administration of chemotherapy and radiation therapy may, in some situations, be better tolerated than sequential courses that trigger compensatory mechanisms; however, the potential effects, both acute and long-term, may be much more complicated than expected. Reviews of TBI and chemotherapy regimens indicate that there is reduced long-term toxicity to the bone marrow when irradiation is omitted.[116, 118]

Total Body Irradiation

TBI in the clinical setting, along with the incidental low dose and dose rate exposures received during space travel, has stimulated an interest in the biologic effects of TBI. The various lethal syndromes that follow high-intensity irradiation are related to the doses received by entire, specific sensitive organs as a consequence of the different threshold dose levels existing for irreversible injury to the stem cell populations. Once exceeded, the result is loss of the organ's functional integrity coupled with an inability to repopulate or repair.[19]

The classic radiation lethality syndromes relating to bone marrow, GI tract, and CNS failure each have a tolerance dose and time course to fatality.[2] Therefore, when the whole body is irradiated with single exposures, death occurs within minutes to months as a function of dose and the organ system affected. Damage to other organs, which does not directly lead to death, contributes qualitatively or quantitatively to the syndrome. The prominent acute syndromes and modes of death after single-dose TBI are, in the order of occurrence and increasing threshold doses, the CNS syndrome, the GI syndrome, and the hematopoietic syndrome. Animal data available on these syndromes are generally consistent with observations in humans. For example, hematopoietic death occurs in 50% of humans in 30 to 60 days following single doses of 2.4 to 7.5 Gy.[119] In animal models, the hematopoietic $LD_{50/30-60}$ is 6 to 7 Gy in rodents, 6 Gy in rabbits, 2.5 Gy in pigs and goats, and 6 Gy in the macaque monkey. For any particular organ-related syndrome, the actual threshold dose may not be clinically relevant because the adverse effects resulting from injury to another organ system may predominate. Thus, when the dose is at the threshold for the CNS syndrome, it is far above the threshold for the GI and hematopoietic syndromes.

Clear differences exist in the time lines of pathology development following loss of relevant cells that lead to functional impairment in the determining organs. Thus, the CNS syndrome becomes apparent within a few minutes to hours after irradiation and continues to express itself during the early parts of the latent periods for the GI and hematopoietic syndromes. Similarly, when the dose permits survival of the patient through the period of the CNS syndrome but exceeds the threshold for the GI syndrome, this syndrome becomes apparent during the latent period for the hematopoietic syndrome. It should be noted that the median acute lethal dose ($LD_{50/60}$) for humans for brief, intensive TBI is not precisely known, nor is the influence of age or sex. However, this dose has been estimated to be between 3 and 5 Gy, with death being associated primarily with the hematopoietic and GI syndromes.

Central Nervous System—Brain

Clinical Syndromes

The initial response of the CNS (Fig. 34–6) to irradiation is frequently seen as increased intracranial pressure owing to radiation edema.[120] However, this is a complex event to analyze, because tumor-associated cerebral edema may exist before radiation treatment. Severe manifestations of infarction and gliosis appear in the subacute period, seen as brain necrosis or as Brown-Séquard syndrome when there is transection of the cord. In the chronic clinical period, children exhibit neurobehavioral deficits following cranial irradiation.[121, 122] It must be noted that pre-existing hydrocephalus, owing to posterior fossa tumors, also causes cerebral atrophy and poor mentation independent of, although augmenting, the radiation effect. Repeated courses of radiation may exceed tolerance, further obliterating the vasculature and increasing the risk of brain necrosis.

Although the onset of symptoms can be as early as 6 months after treatment, the peak time of presentation is 1 to 2 years. Radiation necrosis occurs in 1% to 5% of patients after 55- to 60-Gy doses, fractionated over 6 weeks; above this rather narrow dose range, the likelihood increases substantially. In one of the few prospective studies, Marks and colleagues[123] reported a 5% incidence of radiation necrosis in patients treated with 54 Gy or more in 1.8-Gy to 2-Gy fractions; 75% of the cases of radiation necrosis were apparent by 3 years. This condition is often progressive and fatal, and surgical debulking is performed when possible; corticosteroids may offer transient relief. Reducing the volume of the radiation field is presumed to decrease the risk for radiation necrosis, although this may not be true in children. On computed tomography (CT) scan, radiation necrosis is sometimes seen as a mass lesion with surrounding edema, but this is rare; angiography shows areas of avascularity, compared with the neovascularity apparent in a recurrent tumor. Magnetic resonance imaging (MRI) permits identification of a spectrum of radiation changes with great sensitivity.[124, 125] However, differentiation of radiation necrosis from recurrent tumor generally requires pathologic documentation; metabolic positron emission tomography (PET) scans may be helpful.

Headache and other expressions of increased intracranial pressure are frequently present, in addition to focal deficits. Focal necrosis after concentrated intensive irradiation is usually seen as an MRI change earlier than 6 months, with

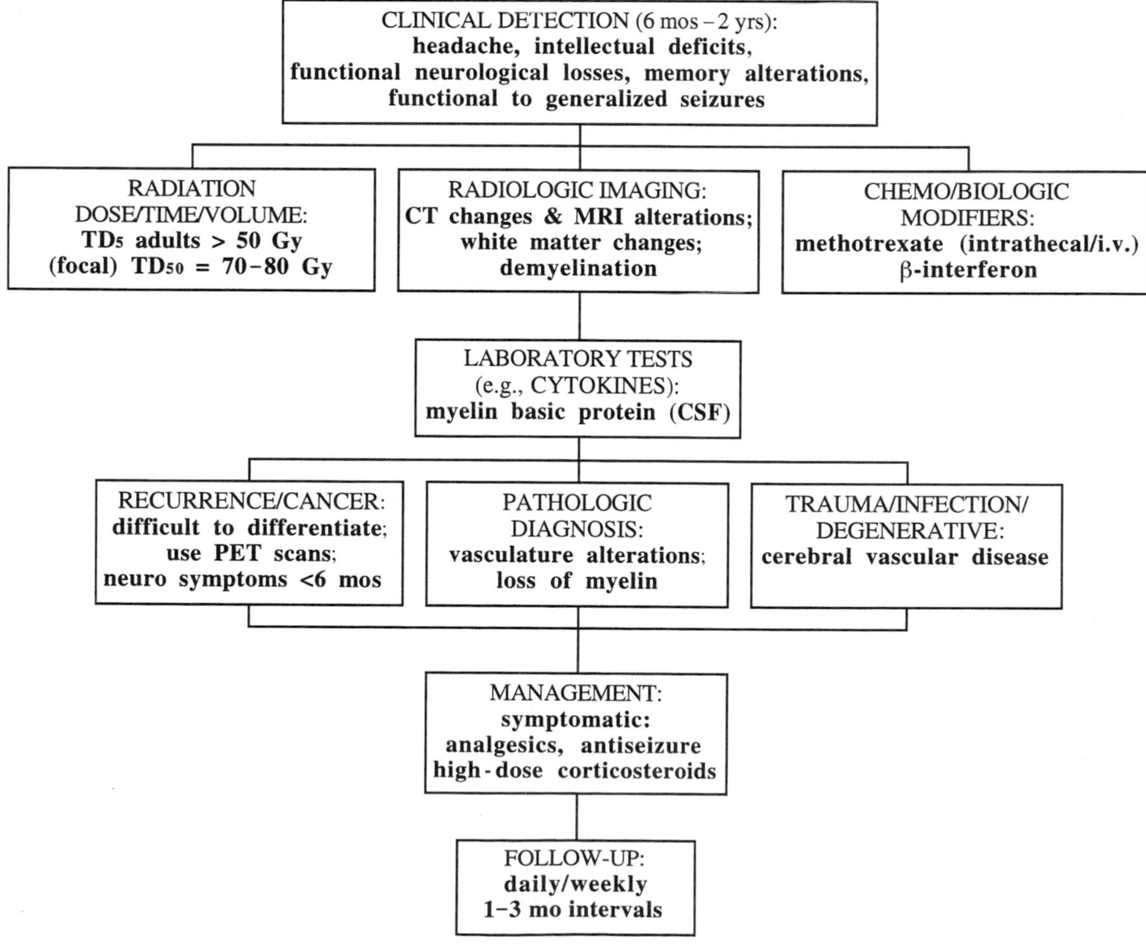

Figure 34–6. LENT diagram for the brain.

the persistence of subacute to chronic necrosis. Depending on whether neoplastic control is obtained, MRI alterations with focal edema and necrosis can appear in 2 to 4 weeks with stereotactic radiosurgery[126, 127] or interstitial implants,[128] and they can persist for months to years.

The clinical features of leukoencephalopathy—a condition characterized by multiple noninflammatory necrotic foci in the white matter, with demyelination and reactive astrocytosis—are lethargy, seizures, spasticity, paresis, and ataxia. This condition is seen following chemotherapy, as well as following greater than 20-Gy whole brain irradiation (a prophylaxis for CNS leukemia). Fifty percent of patients with established CNS leukemia or lymphoma will be affected following doses of more than 35 Gy or intrathecal methotrexate of 150 mg.

Pathophysiology

In their mature state, neurons and neuroganglions are considered to be some of the most resistant cells in the human body because they are fixed, postmitotic cells. Therefore, the vulnerable portions of the CNS are the proliferating cells, such as the oligodendrocytes that produce myelin, and the fine vasculature, which along with astrocytes constitutes the interstitium in the brain. Most radiation injuries reflect events occurring in the vasculoconnective tissue stroma (Fig. 34–7);[129] however, because the vasculature response varies, the CNS radiation pathology literature has become the classic chicken-or-the-egg argument. Careful studies of late effects in the brain by Brady[130] and in the spinal cord by van der Kogel and associates[131] confirmed the critical nature of damage to the interstitium and vasculature as the major targets of radiation injury in the CNS. In the first weeks following irradiation, early demyelinating changes are generally limited to scattered astrocytic or microglial reactions. Subsequently, neural tissue begins to break down, with the appearance of regions of myelin destruction, proliferative and degenerative changes in glial cells, and vascular changes, such as endothelial cell loss, proliferation, capillary occlusion, degeneration, and hemorrhagic exudates.

The three most commonly proposed target cells for CNS radiation damage may act alone or in combination. Damage to individual *nerve fibers* can be demonstrated quantitatively as early as 2 weeks after irradiation using electron microscopy, preceding most vascular damage[132]; however, changes in vessels have been observed as early as 24 hours postirradiation.[133] *Oligodendrocytes*, responsible for maintaining myelin, show a decrease in numbers within weeks following irradiation. Effects on myelin synthesis and maintenance may be especially important in childhood, because myelogenesis is most active in the first year of life. *Endothelial cells* are essential for patency of the microcirculation; these cells are radiosensitive, and damage is expressed as cell death or endothelial hyperplasia. Since endothelial cell turnover is slow, injury based on these cells occurs over a prolonged interval. An immunologic response to glial cell antigens may also contribute to CNS injury.

As discussed previously, there has been an identification of cytokines released immediately following CNS irradiation in animal models. Proinflammatory and profibrotic cytokines have been found in the CNS tissues within the first 24 hours following irradiation.[134, 135] Building on the multicellular paradigm, the underlying mechanism for demyelination becomes an interplay between the endothelial cell, the oligodendrocyte, the astrocyte, and the microglia. One scenario could be that following disruption of the endothelium,[136] an infiltration of lymphocytes initiates the expression of immunologic mechanisms that drive the pathogenesis of encephalopathy and myelopathy.[137–139]

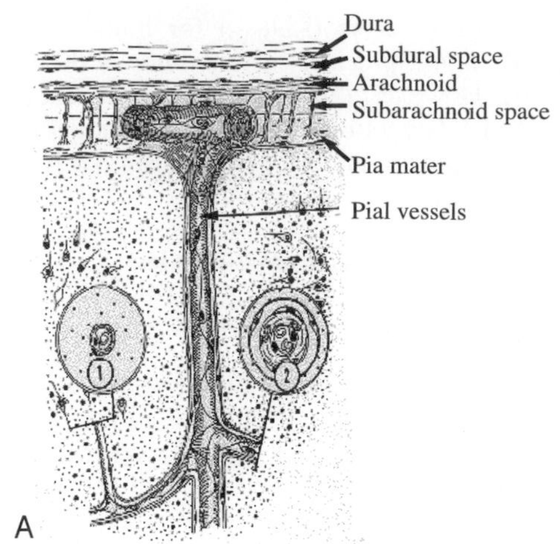

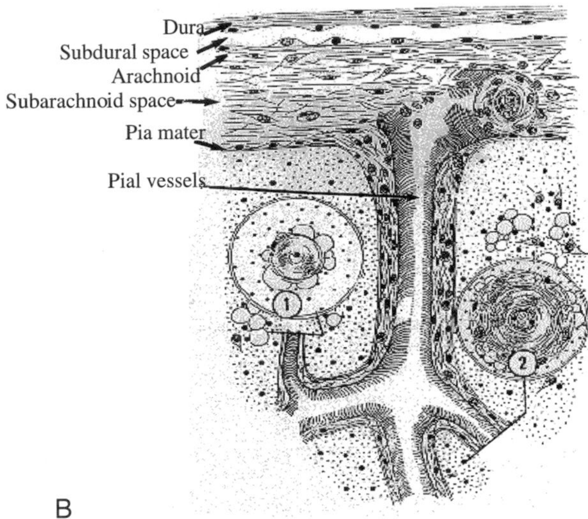

Figure 34–7. (A) Unirradiated cerebral cortex and (B) delayed radiation encephalopathy. (A) Certain fundamental structures within the cerebral cortex are identified. The pial vessels invaginate the connective tissue elements to form the Virchow-Robin spaces (cross section 2). The close contiguity of the microvasculature to the brain parenchyma is seen in insert 1. (B) The delayed encephalopathies are primarily in response to progressive vascular sclerosis. All ramifications of the pial vessels can demonstrate the effects of irradiation. Of prominence is connective tissue proliferation in the Virchow-Robin space (2), which, in conjunction with endothelial proliferation, compresses the lumen of the pial vessels. The developing circulatory compromise results in a relative ischemia in the dependent parenchyma, which reacts first with demyelination and then focal necrosis. (From White DC: An Atlas of Radiation Histopathology, p 213. Oak Ridge, U.S. Energy Research & Development Administration, 1975, with permission.)

Radiation Effects

The incidence of brain necrosis following single-dose radiation has been studied in animal models[132] and has been found to be strictly dependent on the volume of brain exposed, with necrosis occurring between 21 and 50 Gy to maximal volumes. Clinical data indicate that total doses of 45 to 55 Gy to the brain result in a 5% incidence of severe complications within 5 years (Fig. 34–8),[140] with 75% of cases occurring within 3 years.[141] Clinical data for single-dose radiation are sparse, but when Hindo and coworkers[142] used single doses of 10 Gy in patients with brain metastases, 7% of patients died within 48 hours. The importance of fraction size, in addition to total dose and time, has been stressed in determining tolerance to radiation.

Chemotherapy Effects

Owing to the blood-brain barrier, the role of drugs in the CNS has tended to be restricted to adjuvant therapy. Nonetheless, the number of chemotherapeutic agents associated with acute and late toxicities is increasing (Table 34–4).[122, 143–145] Entities such as acute and chronic encephalopathy, necrotizing leukoencephalopathy, acute cerebellar syndromes, and peripheral neuropathies reflect both drug and radiation toxicities. Of note is the vulnerability of the CNS of children and their overall lack of improvement following chemotherapy.[146, 147]

Combined Modalities

The most recognized example of adverse combined radiation and drug effects involves methotrexate (Fig. 34–9).[148–150] Large doses of methotrexate alone can lead to leukoencephalopathy; however, this complication is seen most often when the drug is given intrathecally or in high doses intravenously combined with whole brain irradiation. It had been assumed that most drugs would not cause CNS late effects because of their inability to cross the blood-brain barrier. However, because radiation alters and increases capillary permeability,[151] a combined-modality regimen may lead to systemically administered drugs entering

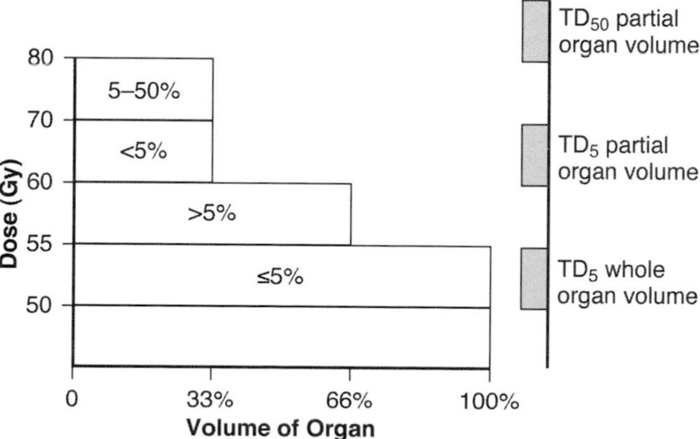

Figure 34–8. Dose-volume histogram for late effects seen in the brain, illustrating the relationship between volume and tolerance doses. The right y-axis indicates the tolerance dose ranges for the TD_5 for whole brain irradiation, as well as the TD_5 and TD_{50} for partial organ volume (POV) irradiation. (Modified from Rubin P, Constine LS, Williams JP: Late effects of cancer treatment: radiation and drug toxicity. In: Perez CA, Brady LW [eds]: Principles and Practice of Radiation Oncology, 3rd ed, pp 155–211. Philadelphia, Lippincott-Raven, 1997.)

TABLE 34–4. **Antineoplastic Drugs Associated with Cerebral Encephalopathy**

Antimetabolites
High-dose methotrexate
5-Fluorouracil (with allopurinol)
Cytosine arabinoside (ara-C)
Fludarabine
PALA (*N*-[phosphonacetyl]-L-aspartate)
Alkylating Agents
Cisplatin
Ifosfamide
BCNU (carmustine)
Spiromustine
Plant Alkyloids
Vincristine (associated with inappropriate antidiuretic hormone secretion)
High-Dose Regimens Used in Bone Marrow Transplantation
Nitrogen mustard
Etoposide
Procarbazine
Miscellaneous
Mitotane
Misonidazole
L-asparaginase
Hexamethylmelamine
Interleukin-2

From Kagan AR: Nervous system toxicity. In: Madhu JJ, Flam MS, Legha SS, et al (eds): Chemoradiation: An Integrated Approach to Cancer Treatment, p 582. Philadelphia, Lea & Febiger, 1993, with permission.

the brain.[152, 153] In addition, damage to the vascular choroid plexus can affect methotrexate clearance, decreasing turnover, thereby leading to higher drug concentrations. Therefore, combination therapy sequencing for brain neoplasms should be approached with caution.[154] For example, a 1998 study employing a combination of high-dose systemic methotrexate with intrathecal methotrexate followed by whole brain irradiation for primary CNS lymphoma has observed a high rate of severe leukoencephalopathy in patients older than 60 years of age.[155]

The increasing use of combined-modality therapy (e.g., the conditioning regimens for bone marrow transplantations) has led to an awareness of risk factors in the pediatric population.[156–158] An alertness must be maintained for signs of developmental difficulties, and attempts should be made at all times to minimize the radiation treatment fields in children.

Central Nervous System—Spinal Cord

Clinical Syndromes

Both transient and irreversible syndromes form the spectrum of radiation injuries to the spinal cord (Fig. 34–10).[120, 159] Transient myelopathy is the most common syndrome, seen 2 to 4 months following irradiation. Lhermitte's sign has been described frequently after 40 to 45 Gy mantle irradiation for Hodgkin's disease, and it appears as a shocklike sensation along the spine and tingling or pain in the hands from neck flexion or stretching of the arms.[160] The mechanism is presumably a transient demyelination. Very occa-

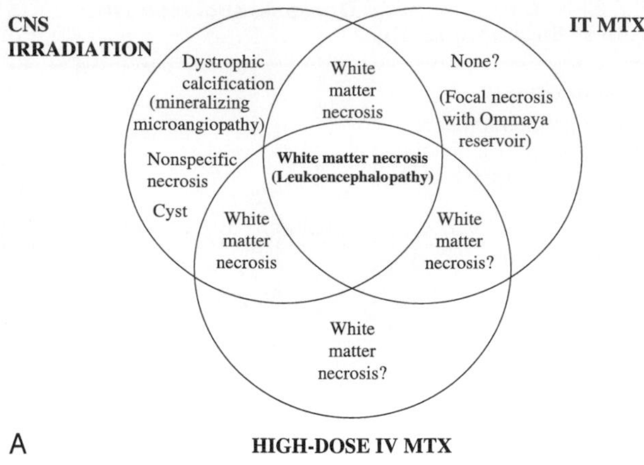

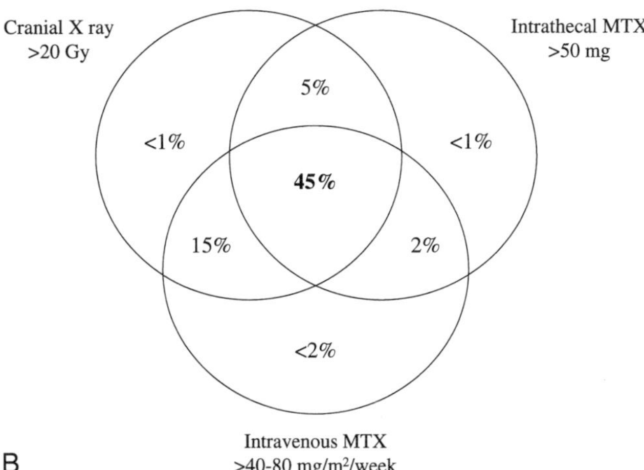

Figure 34–9. Encephalopathies are induced by both irradiation and chemotherapy and can be acute and chronic. (A) A Venn diagram illustrates the pathophysiology of delayed neurotoxic sequelae seen months to years later associated with CNS irradiation, intrathecal methotrexate, and high-dose intravenous methotrexate, alone or in combination. (B) Incidence is greatest for all modes combined. In this Venn diagram, the incidence is very low when either irradiation or chemotherapy is administered alone, but it increases considerably (up to 45%) when combined. The mechanism is believed to be attributable to alteration of the blood-brain barrier by irradiation, followed by direct entry of methotrexate into the CNS, causing diffuse necrosis and damage. (From Evans A, Bleyer A, Kaplan R, et al: Central nervous system workshop. Cancer Clin Trials 1981; 4[suppl]:31–35, with permission.)

sionally, rapidly evolving permanent paralysis is seen, possibly resulting from an acute infarction of the cord.

Chronic progressive radiation myelitis is rare. Intramedullary vascular damage that progresses to hemorrhagic necrosis or infarction is the likely mechanism, although extensive demyelination that progresses to white matter necrosis is an alternative explanation. Initial symptoms are usually paresthesias and sensory changes, starting 9 to 15 months following therapy and progressing over the subsequent year. Diagnosis of myelitis rests on supportive information: the lesion must be within the irradiated volume, and recurrent or metastatic tumor must be ruled out. In addition, the cerebrospinal fluid protein levels may be elevated; myelography can demonstrate cord swelling or atrophy, with MRI and CT scan providing additional supportive information.

Radiation Effects

A variety of data on the tolerances of the spinal cord to irradiation is available from studies on animals and patients. Reviews from both Leith and coworkers[161] and van der Kogel[132] found that the estimated radiation dose needed to produce spinal cord paralysis in 50% of rats ranged from 19 to 25 Gy. This range is larger when the dose is fractionated, but the applicability of such data to humans is not clear. The role played by cytokine expression in spinal cord injury, again, is of interest.[162]

Our concepts of spinal cord tolerance have changed (Fig. 34–11). The most widely observed clinical dose limits are 45 Gy in 22 to 25 fractions of 1.8 to 2.0 Gy, and the TD_5 of 50 Gy is recommended for segments smaller than 10 cm. However, Marcus and Million[163] have shown an incidence of radiation myelitis of less than or equal to 0.2% at 45 Gy; therefore, the true TD_5 is probably in the range of 57 to 61 Gy.[164] Worth noting is the increased risk of myelitis following use of a continuous hyperfractionated accelerated radiation treatment[165] that suggests a 6-hour interval between treatments is insufficient to allow for significant repair. Shortening the interval between treatments from 24 hours to 6 to 8 hours reduces spinal cord tolerance by 10% to 15%. Of additional note is the continuing work by van der Kogel and associates on spinal cord tolerance, which has demonstrated its dependence on dose rate in their animal model.[166, 167]

Chemotherapy and Combined Modalities

See "Central Nervous System—Brain" for the available data.

Gastrointestinal Tract

The length and complexity of the GI tract (esophagus, stomach, small and large intestines, concluding in the rectum and anus) span a variety of anatomic settings (Fig. 34–12). The spectrum of syndromes ranges from dramatic (arteriolar infarction, necrosis with perforation and fistulas) to subtle (dysmotility, dyspepsia, or unexplained bouts of diarrhea) presentations. Highlights of four major sites (esophagus, stomach, intestine, and rectum) are presented, and the LENT workshop and its publications[168] offer updated data.

Clinical Syndromes

The published Subjective, Objective, Management, and Analytic (SOMA) scales[168] provide a brief overview of the common symptoms, signs, and management of GI toxicity by the major anatomic GI sites.

Esophagus

Dysphagia is the most common symptom and reflects esophageal peristaltic dysfunction, seen 3 to 6 months postirradiation.[169, 170] Ulceration may occur with higher doses, particularly following intraluminal brachytherapy techniques.[171, 172]

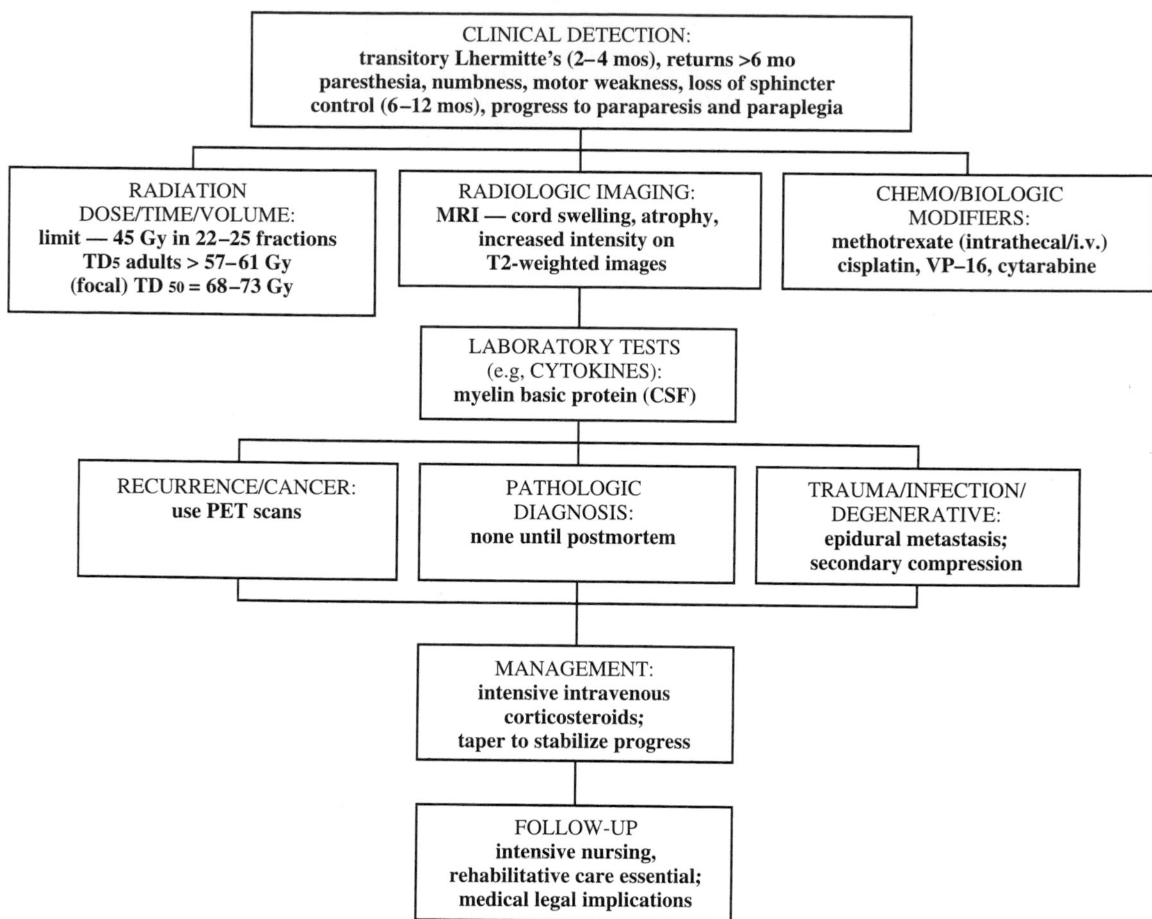

Figure 34–10. LENT diagram for the spinal cord.

Stomach

After modest doses of 15 to 20 Gy, the radiosensitivity of the gastric mucosa is evident in the early depression of hydrochloric acid and pepsin secretion. Suppression continues for a long time in many cases, yet complete recovery of function can take place within 1 year of therapy. However, at levels of 50 Gy or higher, cellular and functional recovery are never complete, and the chances of developing a radiation ulcer are high; this scenario may lead to hemorrhage and perforation, which can be fatal.

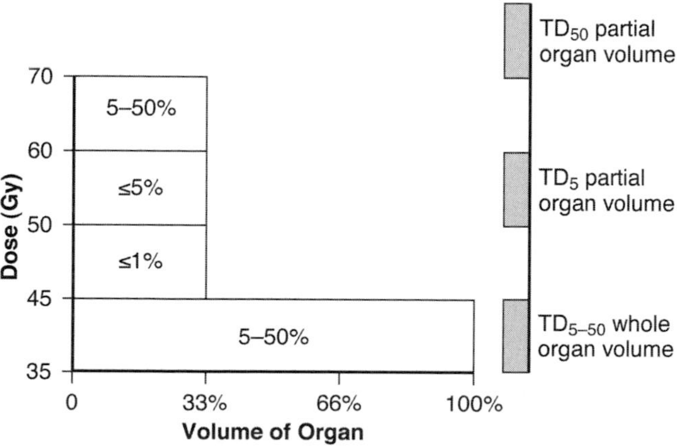

Figure 34–11. Dose-volume histogram for late effects seen in the spinal cord, illustrating the relationship between volume and tolerance doses. The right y-axis indicates the tolerance dose ranges for the TD_{5-50} for whole organ irradiation, as well as the TD_5 and TD_{50} for partial organ volume (POV) irradiation. (Modified from Rubin P, Constine LS, Williams JP: Late effects of cancer treatment: radiation and drug toxicity. In: Perez CA, Brady LW [eds]: Principles and Practice of Radiation Oncology, 3rd ed, pp 155–211. Philadelphia, Lippincott-Raven, 1997.)

Small Intestine

The small intestine is another radiosensitive section, demonstrating an early onset of fat malabsorption and hypermotility after modest doses of radiation. With higher doses, the clinical threshold is crossed, resulting in diarrhea and leakage of albumin into the bowel. If an obliterative arteritis develops, the risk of infarction and perforation remains despite recovery. The underlying lesion is one of ulceration and segmental enteritis, leading to stenosis of the bowel lumen with varying degrees of obstruction during the chronic period.

Colorectum

The colon and rectum are less radiosensitive than the small intestine. At levels of 10 to 20 Gy, the initial reaction of hypermotility rapidly disappears. However, if constipation is a later complication, roughage can traumatize the bowel surface mucosa. Higher doses may cause painless rectal

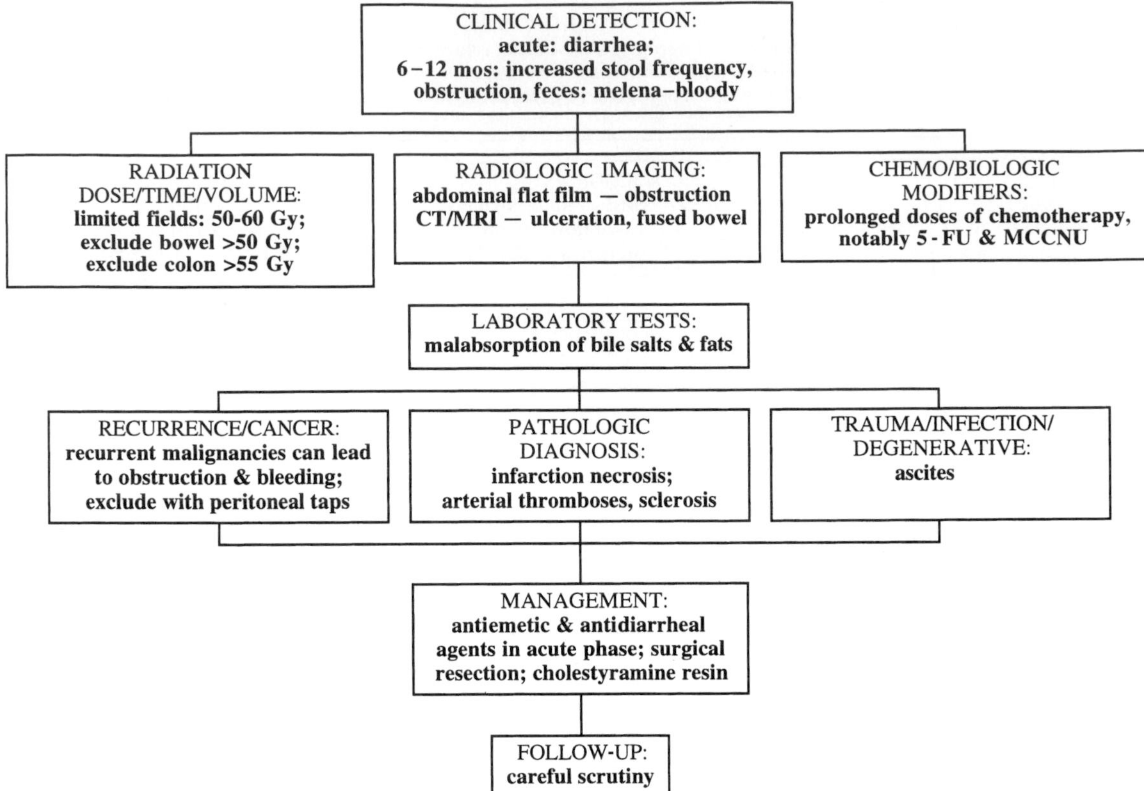

Figure 34–12. LENT diagram for the gastrointestinal tract.

bleeding at 6 to 12 months; this is rarely fatal. Segmental colitis, proctitis, and rectal strictures are major concerns; fortunately, severe bowel injury is not common, owing to improved radiation techniques and monitoring.

Pathophysiology

Progressive endoarteritis is the critical radiation lesion for late effects in the alimentary tract, resulting in either ulceration and infarction necrosis or an increasing slow fibrosis and stricture of bowel with either a rapid obliteration of vessels or a gradual narrowing of the fine vasculature, respectively (Fig. 34–13). The association of obliterative endoarteritis with zones of necrosis and perforation indicate an infarction necrosis of the supply vessels as an essential mechanism. Even months to years after irradiation, surgical handling of the bowel can interfere with a tenuous blood supply and precipitate alterations in hemodynamics; these factors may lead to repeated infarction necrosis, which often results in death.

The mucosa of the GI tract is a rapid renewal system with dramatic changes appearing within 7 to 14 days of injury; regenerating foci of epithelial cells occur within zones of complete denudation. Unlike the acute mucosal loss and gradual return of regenerative epithelial clonogenic clusters in bowel crypts after irradiation, late ulceration is spotty and focal. Mucosal surfaces are intact, with endoarteritis as an underlying defect, requiring an event such as surgical handling or trauma to result in a clinical manifestation.

Radiation Effects

Esophagus

A review of late effects by Emami and associates calculated the $TD_{5/5}$ for strictures or ulceration as 60 Gy for a third of the esophagus, and 55 Gy when the whole esophagus is treated.[173] Supplemental intraluminal brachytherapy as a boost following external beam irradiation can also lead to ulceration and perforation; a 90% rate of ulceration occurred when a single fraction of 20 Gy given intraluminally supplemented a fractionated 60 Gy dose.[174] A comprehensive review of the tolerance doses in the literature has been compiled by Coia and associates.[168]

Stomach

Retrospective studies of patients receiving 50 Gy doses to large fields have listed the primary gastric late effect as pyloric ulceration or irregular contractions of the antrum.[175] The LENT review[168] tabulated the major gastric complications according to dose: a 20% incidence of gastritis occurred in the 40 to 50 Gy range; gastric ulcers occurred in 15% of patients receiving doses of 50 Gy or higher; and perforated ulcers occurred in patients following 45 to 50 Gy, in 10% following 50 to 60 Gy, and in 16% at doses of higher than 60 Gy. These results may be because of direct radiation effects or indirect effects following transient alterations in the blood supply.[176]

Small Intestine

The terminal ileum has the greatest frequency of radiation-induced symptoms because of its high rate of epithelial

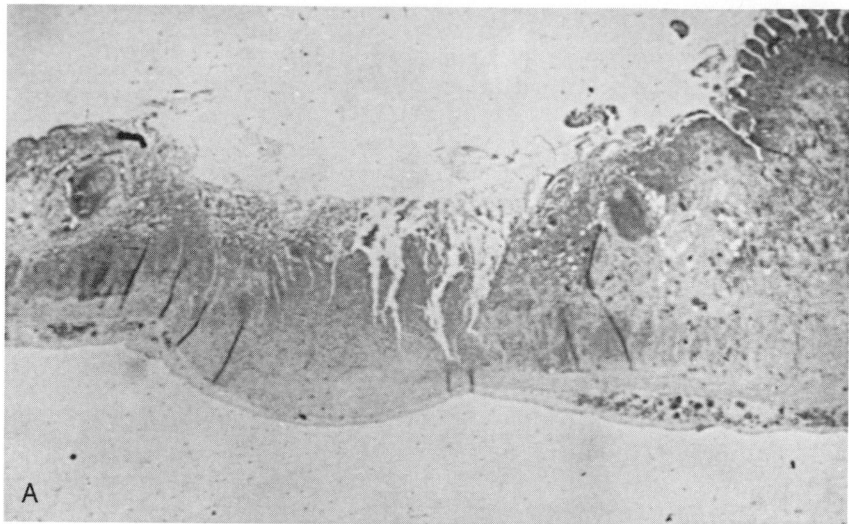

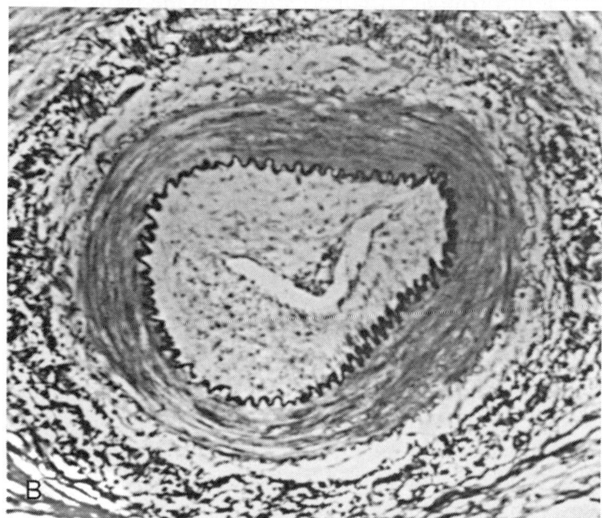

Figure 34–13. Radiation pathology of subacute clinical period: radiation ulcer of the small intestine. (A) Section of a region of small bowel with ulceration 6 months after radiation therapy (about 60 Gy; low magnification). (B) Cross section of a small artery underlying the ulcer shown in A, showing obstruction of the lumen by marked endothelial proliferation (endarteritis obliterans) and other changes in the arterial wall (high magnification). (From Rubin P, Casarett GW: Clinical Radiation Pathology, pp 193–240. Philadelphia, W.B. Saunders Co., 1968, with permission.)

cell turnover[19]; cell replacement in the crypts and villi occurs every 3 to 6 days. Pathologic changes include a cessation of mitosis, crypt cell pyknosis, fragmentation, and swelling and vacuolation of the cells in the enteric mucosa. After 6 to 8 hours, mucosal cells demonstrate a transient proliferation with a burst of atypical mitoses and, over the next 48 hours, cell loss without renewal is progressive with shortening of the crypts and villi. Subsequently, the villi show progressive denudation, resulting in a loss of protein and electrolytes. After low doses, recovery with a chronic reaction may ensue; the submucosa is most severely affected. Collagen and bizarre fibroblasts replace fatty tissue and vascular lesions occur. Delayed effects may take 10 or more years to develop.

There is a large volume of literature dealing with small bowel tolerance, in particular from patients with cervical cancer. The evidence indicates that 50 Gy is the threshold dose, but there is a steep dose-response curve using daily conventional fractions at 1.8 to 2.0 Gy. The incidence of small bowel injury was 15% to 25% if para-aortic radiation doses of 50 to 55 Gy were added to pelvic irradiation[177]; however, more recent studies have shown that 45 to 50 Gy is well tolerated.[178, 179] Perez and coworkers found a 1% incidence of small bowel toxicity with a pelvic sidewall dose of 50 Gy or less, and a 5% incidence at higher than 70 Gy.[180] In addition, a report by Eifel and colleagues, in a long-term follow-up study of patients with cervical cancer (20 years), illustrated an increased incidence in the complication rate over time.[181] This is particularly true of older patients.[182]

Colorectum

Kummermehr and Trott[183] have studied changes in the rat rectum following single doses of radiation and found that doses higher than 20 Gy caused severe proctitis in 50% of animals within 40 to 200 days; 24.5 Gy in two fractions caused similar changes. However, although these changes were volume dependent, the degree of dependency and the threshold values varied according to the criteria studied.[184]

Clinically, tolerance in the colorectal region is considered to be higher than in the small intestine and, again, is highly volume dependent.[185] Two excellent sources of data exist: patients with cervical cancer receiving external radiation and brachytherapy, and patients with cancer of the prostate also exposed to both external and internal sources. The incidence of severe proctitis in cancer of the cervix is dose dependent: less than 4% with doses of 80 Gy or lower, 7% to 8% for 80 to 95 Gy, and 13% for 95 Gy or higher.[180] In prostate cancer, the incidence is 5% for 60 to 70 Gy, and with dose escalation to 75 Gy, severe rectal bleeding occurs in 15% to 20% of patients with proton and photon beams.[186, 187] Rectal shielding has become more critical because improved techniques (e.g., three-dimensional dynamic conformal therapy) have allowed for dose escalation up to 80 Gy for patients with prostate cancer.[188, 189] With respect to volume, less than a third of the circumference is essential, but the smaller the circumference, the better tolerated are the higher doses (Fig. 34–14). Dosimetric considerations of the critical organs can lead to improved results.[190]

Chemotherapy Effects

Chemotherapy alone does not appear to produce significant late GI complications with any frequency, despite the well-documented acute toxicity caused by a long list of agents (Table 34–5).[191] Drugs, such as 5-fluorouracil (5-FU), produce diarrhea and, occasionally, small bowel toxicity.[192] More severe late effects, such as GI bleeding, generally have been seen only in combined-modality therapy, which has led to severe acute complications, particularly in the small bowel.[193, 194]

Esophagus

Toxicities associated with induction courses of chemotherapy alone are generally hematologic in nature, although incidences of mucositis have been reported[195, 196] and can be dose limiting.[197] Acute radiation effects, for example, esophagitis, are enhanced by agents such as cisplatin, 5-FU, mitomycin C, doxorubicin, and carboplatin, with the most severe esophageal toxicities occurring when concurrent chemotherapy is applied with hyperfractionated radiation.[198] The simultaneous delivery of agents by infusion and radiation doses of 60 Gy or higher raises the incidence of esophagitis and late benign stricture to 11%,[199] with doxorubicin being of particular concern, especially in children.[200]

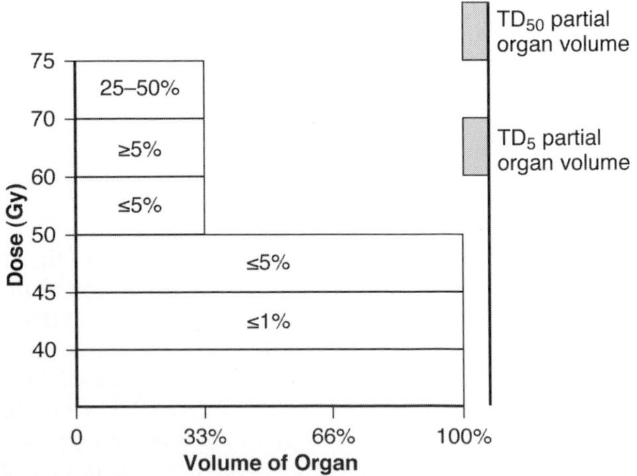

Figure 34–14. Dose-volume histogram for late effects seen in the gastrointestinal tract, illustrating the relationship between volume and tolerance doses. The right y-axis indicates the tolerance dose ranges for the TD_5 and TD_{50} for partial organ volume (POV) irradiation. (Modified from Rubin P, Constine LS, Williams JP: Late effects of cancer treatment: radiation and drug toxicity. In: Perez CA, Brady LW [eds]: Principles and Practice of Radiation Oncology, 3rd ed, pp 155–211. Philadelphia, Lippincott-Raven, 1997.)

TABLE 34–5. **Gastrointestinal Chemotoxic Agents and Their Late Effects**

Agent	Late Effect
5-Fluorouracil	Enteritis
5-Fluorouracil + mitomycin C (+ RT)	Late benign esophageal stricture
5-Fluorouracil + MeCCNU (+ RT)	Fistulas, perforation
Actinomycin D (+ RT)	Enteritis
Bleomycin (+ RT)	Esophagitis
Cisplatin (+ RT)	Enteritis
Cyclophosphamide (+ RT)	Esophagitis
Doxorubicin (+ RT)	Esophagitis
Methotrexate	Enteritis
Procarbazine	Enteritis

RT = radiation therapy.
Modified from Rubin P: The Franz Buschke Lecture: Late effects of chemotherapy and radiation therapy: a new hypothesis. Int J Radiat Oncol Biol Phys 1984; 10:5–34, with permission from Elsevier Science.

Stomach

There is little information to support increased toxicity from chemoradiation therapy. In pancreatic cancers, the use of agents such as doxorubicin and mitomycin C in combination with radiation has been well tolerated.[168] Since most radiation oncology protocols avoid doses higher than 45 to 50 Gy, gastric late effect toxicity is uncommon.

Small Intestine

Most of the evidence suggests that 5-FU infusion as a bolus, with radiation doses ranging from 45 to 50 Gy, is well tolerated with few reports of late toxicity. However, administering the chemotherapy concurrently frequently enhances the risk for intestinal complications.[201]

Colorectum

The absence of predictive parameters for late intestinal events was demonstrated in the catastrophic complications that occurred in a carefully piloted Eastern Cooperative Oncology Group (ECOG) study using split-course radiation (60 Gy in 10 weeks: 20 Gy in 2-week courses ×3 with 2-week rest intervals) and adjuvant 5-FU, and maintenance chemotherapy (5-FU and MeCCNU [semustine]) for 1 year.[202] Although no undue acute toxicity occurred with the administration of either radiation therapy or chemotherapy, late fistulization and necrosis occurred in 29% of patients 6 months to 2 years after all therapy ceased. Generally, 5-FU alone added to 45 to 50 Gy is well tolerated, but the addition of mitomycin C raises grade III toxicity to 25%,[203] and a similar addition of cisplatin in cancer of the cervix leads to an 18% large bowel complication rate.[204]

Heart

Clinical Syndromes

The heart is a highly complex organ (Fig. 34–15). The list of injuries it may exhibit includes acute pericarditis, delayed pericarditis that can present abruptly or as chronic pericardial effusion, pancarditis including pericardial and myocardial fibrosis, myopathy in the absence of significant pericardial disease, and coronary artery disease (CAD).[205–210] Among Hodgkin's disease survivors, three separate series of long-term follow-up have supported an increased relative risk for CAD of three times the normal control population.[211–213] The real concern with respect to cardiac late effects is in young pediatric patients,[214] especially girls or women younger than 20 years of age, in whom the highest incidence is found and the relative risk rises to 40%.[215, 216] However, utilizing ERNA (equilibrium radionuclide angiocardiography) and MUGA (multigated angiography) scans, asymptomatic Hodgkin's disease patients treated with cardiac shields at 35 Gy have shown minimal to no significant abnormalities in long-term follow-up (10 years' average).[217]

Chronic effusive-constrictive pericarditis develops in 10% to 15% of patients and may require pericardiectomy. Constriction can present 5 to 50 years following irradiation, with no antecedent acute disease.[218, 219] Cardiomyopathy is highly potentiated by doxorubicin, but it can occur in its absence. Right ventricular end-diastolic function has been shown to be reduced by up to 25% in asymptomatic patients, whereas ejection fractions may be decreased by up to 35%.[207]

Pathophysiology

Typical radiation changes in the human heart are experimentally reproducible in rabbits and other models.[220–222] The hallmarks are seen clinically as a pericardial effusion and pathologically as fibrosis. When the myocardium is involved, diffuse interstitial fibrosis occurs, which follows the pattern of septa in the myocardium (Fig. 34–16A). Worth noting is that following radiation doses in the normal therapeutic range, direct damage to myocytes in both humans and animals is not evident.

The coronary arteries are large enough to avoid being the focus of radiation lesions, and coronary thrombosis is a relatively infrequent occurrence that is found in less than 5% of patients treated. However, following a variety of radiation schedules, a serial sacrifice of rabbits yielded a predictable and identifiable sequence of lesions in the myocardial microvasculature.[223] Fajardo and Stewart hypothesized that radiation insult results in latent damage to the capillary endothelial cells, which is ultimately manifested as severe alterations in myocardial capillaries, cyto-

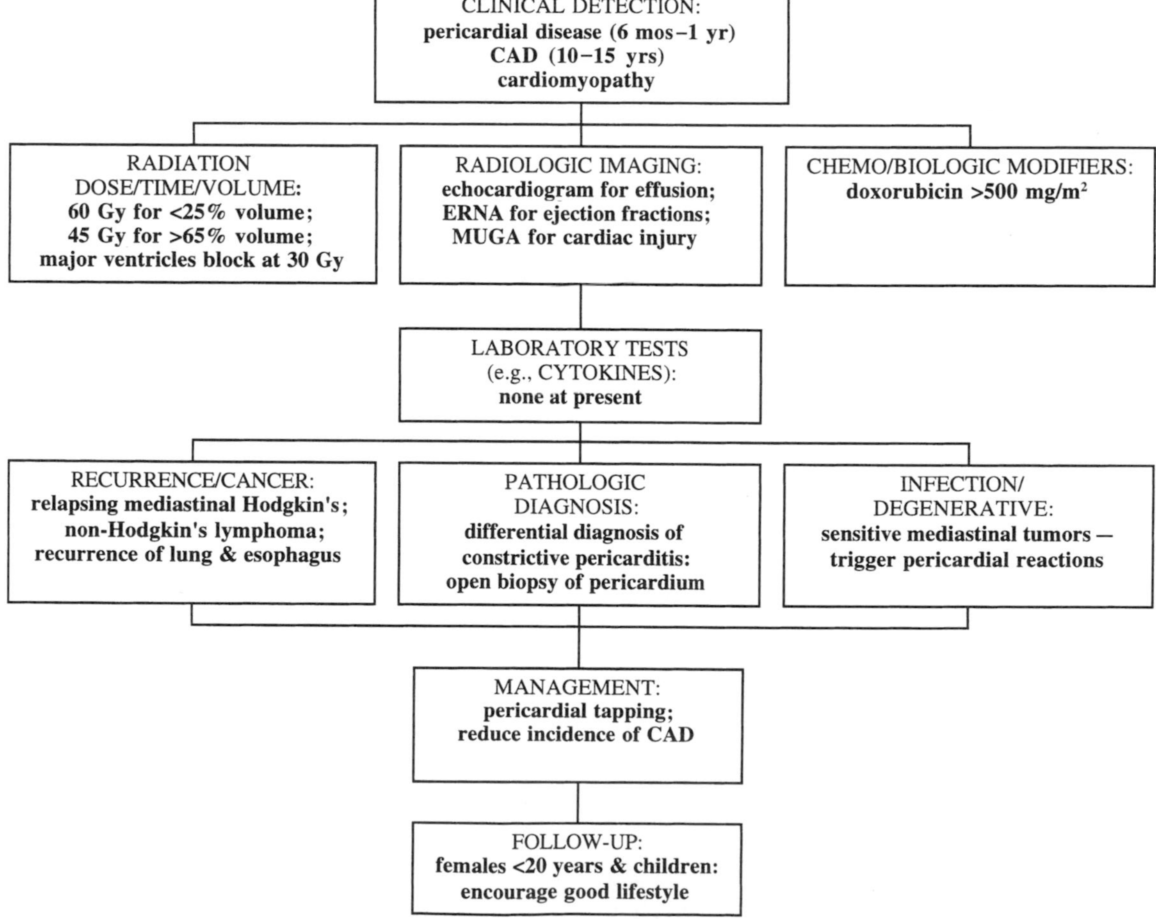

Figure 34–15. LENT diagram for the heart.

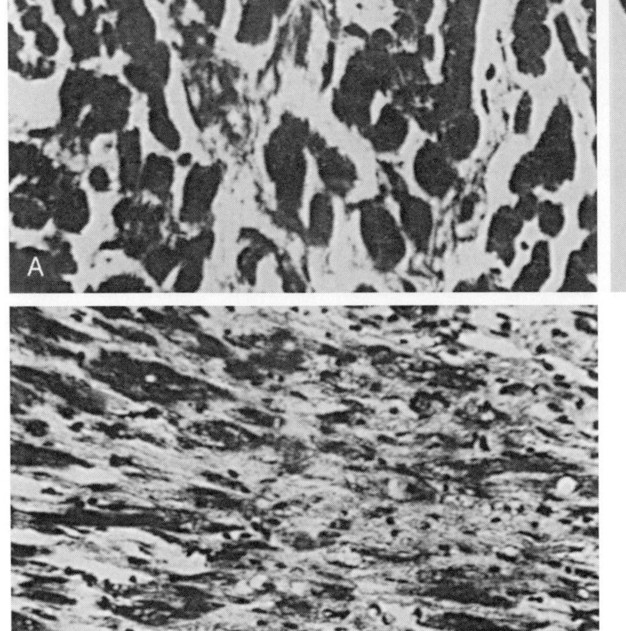

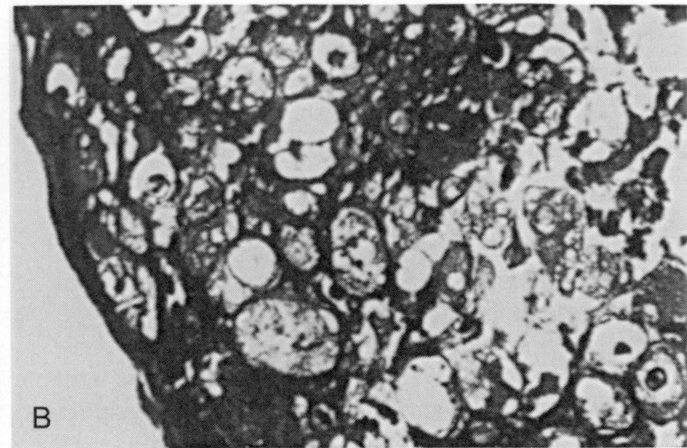

Figure 34–16. Pathologic late effects in the heart. (A) Radiation therapy effects. The myocardium or cardiac myocytes are normal in appearance, with increased fibrosis in the interstitium and capillary and arterial narrowing. (B) Chemotherapy effects. The effect of doxorubicin is dramatic, with vacuolization localized to the cardiac myocytes. The interstitium is normal in appearance, showing vascular sparing despite dramatic cellular changes. (C) Chemoradiation effects. Combined radiation and chemotherapy induce damage in both the vascular connective tissue stroma and the cardiac myocyte. (A, From Fajardo LF, Stewart JR: Experimental radiation-induced heart disease. I. Light microscopic studies. Am J Pathol 1970; 59:299, with permission. Copyright © 1970 American Society for Investigative Pathology. B and C, From Fajardo LF, Eltringham JR, Stewart JR: Combined cardiotoxicity of adriamycin and x-radiation. Lab Invest 1976; 34:86, with permission.)

plasmic swelling, thrombosis, and rupture of the walls.[220] Also, quantitative studies have shown that the ratio of capillaries to myocytes is reduced by approximately 50% over nonirradiated controls at 120 to 540 days. A compensatory burst of endothelial cell proliferation occurs and cells die in mitosis. The resulting reduction in capillaries leads to ischemia and, in turn, myocardial fibrosis. A reduction in capillary size has been shown in experimental animals, with focal loss of endothelial cell alkaline phosphatase and 5′nucleotidase in irradiated hearts.[224, 225] Enzyme activity is decreased and associated with foci of myocardial degeneration.

Radiation Effects

Experimental studies in a rabbit model[220] showed that single radiation doses of 18 to 20 Gy or fractionated doses of 54 Gy (4.5 Gy × 12) caused pericarditis in all animals, whereas doses lower than 18 Gy (single doses) caused no damage. The relevance of radiation dose to cardiac sequelae is underscored by differences in incidence following different radiation techniques. Thus, among patients treated for Hodgkin's disease, less than 5% develop pericarditis following equally weighted radiation doses of lower than 40 Gy, whereas a 30% incidence is seen following anteriorly weighted techniques using the same doses.[226] α/β ratios, based on animal studies in dogs and rabbits for myocardial and pericardial injury, have been calculated at approximately 3 Gy for the capillary component,[227, 228] and there is clear evidence that increasing the dose per fraction increases the risk of CAD. Volume factors have been correlated with dose and they share an inverse relationship, leading to cardiac damage (Fig. 34–17).[205]

Chemotherapy Effects

Chemotherapeutic injury, which has been best studied and documented for the anthracyclines (e.g., doxorubicin), leads to direct cytotoxicity of the cardiomyocytes (see

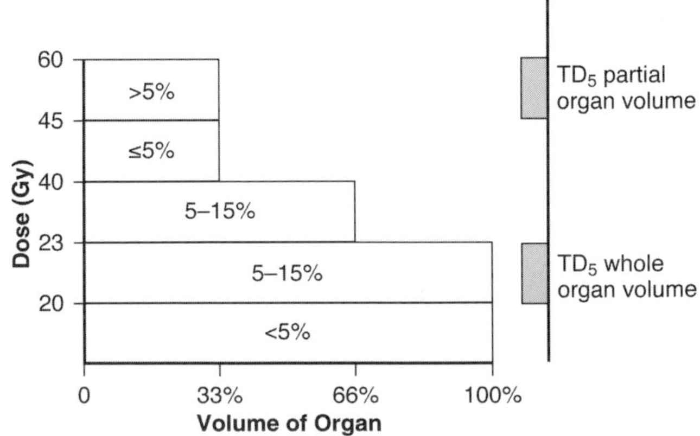

Figure 34–17. Dose-volume histogram for late effects seen in the heart, illustrating the relationship between volume and tolerance doses. The right y-axis indicates the tolerance dose ranges for the TD_5 for whole organ (heart) irradiation, as well as the TD_5 for partial organ volume (POV) irradiation. (Modified from Rubin P, Constine LS, Williams JP: Late effects of cancer treatment: radiation and drug toxicity. In: Perez CA, Brady LW [eds]: Principles and Practice of Radiation Oncology, 3rd ed, pp 155–211. Philadelphia, Lippincott-Raven, 1997.)

Fig. 34–16B).[229–231] No clinical manifestations are expected from low doses of doxorubicin, although microscopic changes on endocardial biopsy have been detected. The exact molecular lesion for doxorubicin is believed to be interference with myocardial DNA-dependent RNA synthesis at the mitochondrial level, which affects functional and structural proteins.[230, 232] This is expressed as direct damage to myocytes, and large diffuse patches of replacement fibrosis appear.

The use of dexrazoxane to prevent or delay anthracycline-induced cardiomyopathy has been the subject of much investigation, and its recommended use is summarized in the practice guidelines from the American Society of Clinical Oncology.[233] However, there continues to be some concern over enhanced myelotoxicity with dexrazoxane as compared with placebo, as well as possible decreases in tumor response rates.

A long list of other agents associated with late cardiomyopathy exists (Table 34–6). Many drugs cause myocardial damage through various mechanisms, including direct toxic damage and hypersensitivity. Histopathologically, the usual underlying lesion is the damaged myocyte, characterized either by loss of contractile elements (myofibrillar degeneration) or by sarcotubular vacuolization within myocytes. In patients who are at high risk, careful monitoring of left ventricular ejection fraction should be considered.[205, 207] Accelerated risks are seen in the elderly population with doxorubicin,[234] and some concerns now are being voiced with respect to high-dose chemotherapy regimens in the child and adolescent populations.[235, 236]

It has been observed that the combination of doxorubicin with paclitaxel, a highly active drug in the treatment of metastatic breast cancer, is associated with a high risk of cardiac toxicity with congestive heart failure.[237, 238] It has been suggested that this syndrome is due to an enhancement of doxorubicin toxicity related to a pharmacokinetic interface in the doxorubicin elimination by paclitaxel. Subsequent studies that have increased the time interval between the administration of the two drugs or have limited the total doxorubicin dose to 360 mg/m^2 have resulted in much lower cardiac toxicity.[239, 240] Sequential administration of doxorubicin and paclitaxel similarly reduces cardiac toxicity,[241] and there does not appear to be any additive effects when doxorubicin is given in conjunction with docetaxel (Taxotere).[240, 242]

A high risk of cardiac toxicity has been observed when doxorubicin is given in conjunction with trastuzumab (Herceptin) for breast cancer.[243] Trastuzumab does not appear to have a high risk of cardiac toxicity when administered as a single agent, but there is significant additive toxicity with doxorubicin when administered to patients previously untreated with anthracyclines. Similar additive toxicity is not seen when trastuzumab is administered in conjunction with paclitaxel to patients previously treated with doxorubicin, but careful clinical as well as functional monitoring of cardiac functioning is indicated during its use.[244] The mechanism by which trastuzumab may induce cardiac toxicity or increase anthracycline-induced toxicity remains to be investigated.

Cardiac toxicity has also proved to be a significant problem with certain types of high-dose chemotherapy when given as preparative regimens before stem cell transplantation.[245, 246] For instance, this is the dose-limiting toxicity for cyclophosphamide in the bone marrow transplant setting, and there appears to be a potential additive toxicity when this agent is administered in conjunction with cytosine arabinoside in high doses.[247–249] In addition, a severe, although usually reversible, depression of cardiac function associated with malignant arrhythmias has been reported following the use of high-dose ifosfamide,[250] and myocardial ischemia has been reported in patients receiving infusions of high-dose carmustine in a similar setting.[251]

TABLE 34–6. **Cardiac Chemotoxic Agents and Their Late Effects**

Agent	Late Effect
Antimetabolites	
5-Fluorouracil	Vasospasm with angina; arrhythmias, myocardial infarction, and left ventricular failure are less common
Alkylating Agents	
Cyclophosphamide (high dose)	Congestive heart failure from hemorrhagic myocarditis; transmural hemorrhage; and coronary artery vasculitis
Cisplatin	Raynaud's syndrome; angina pectoris
Ifosfamide (high dose)	Congestive heart failure with ventricular arrhythmias
Antibiotics	
Anthracyclines (e.g., doxorubicin)	Congestive heart failure; cardiomyopathy; ECG changes; pericarditis-myocarditis; acute hypertensive reactions
Bleomycin	Raynaud's syndrome
Pentostatin	Aortic stenosis; arterial anomaly; cardiomegaly; myocardial infarction
Mitotic Inhibitors	
Etoposide	Hypotension; hypertension
Vincristine	Raynaud's syndrome; cardiotoxicity
Vinblastine	Raynaud's syndrome; hypertension; myocardial infarction
Miscellaneous	
Paclitaxel	Hypotension; bradycardia; abnormal ECG; myocardial infarction; arrhythmia; severe A-V block
Procarbazine	Hypotension; tachycardia; syncope
Paclitaxel + doxorubicin	Enhanced cardiomyopathy
Trastuzumab + doxorubicin	Possible cardiotoxicity

ECG = electrocardiogram; A-V = atrioventricular.
Modified from Frishman WH, Sung HM, Yee HC, et al: Cardiovascular toxicity with cancer chemotherapy. Curr Problems Cardiol 1996; 21:225–286, with permission.

Combined Modalities

The effect of combining radiation and chemotherapy demonstrates additive effects through actions on two different populations of cells. For instance, doxorubicin appears not to affect endothelial cells directly, whereas radiation's primary target *is* the endothelial cell, affecting the fine vasculoconnective stroma of the myocardium.[220] The histopathologic and ultrastructural changes from doxorubicin alone, radiation alone, and radiation and doxorubicin together dramatically demonstrate the independent and additive effects of the two modes (see Figs. 34–16A, B, and C). In an intensive study by Eltringham and coworkers,[252] an additive effect was found using different fractionation schedules with doxorubicin. The histopathology showed both myocardial damage and interstitial fibrosis when both modalities were used. On the basis of dose and treatment interval, a radiation dose of 1 Gy was considered to be equivalent to a dose of 10 mg/m^2 of doxorubicin; the threshold dose of 450 to 500 mg/m^2 for doxorubicin paralleled the 45 to 50 Gy dose for radiation therapy. Recall of subthreshold radiation injury was time independent; doxorubicin administered 5 to 10 years after radiation therapy may still produce cardiac decompensation.

Kidney

Clinical Syndromes

Different periods in the progression of renal dysfunction following irradiation have been defined (Fig. 34–18).[2, 253, 254] The acute period (up to 6 months) is rarely symptomatic, although a decreased glomerular filtration rate may be present. More conventional measurements (blood urea nitrogen, serum creatinine and clearance) are not altered. From 6 to 12 months, the signs and symptoms include dyspnea on exertion, headaches, anemia, hypertension, elevated blood urea level, and urinary abnormalities. During this period, death may occur from chronic uremia or left ventricular failure, pulmonary edema, or pleural effusion, with or without hepatic congestion. During the later chronic period, dose-related benign or malignant hypertension may be seen. Chronic radiation nephropathy may not be diagnosed until 10 to 14 years following therapy[253, 255]; a contracted renal size (mild atrophy) is seen on intravenous pyelogram. When there is severe chronic nephropathy, death can result.

Pathophysiology

The major focus of change is in the arteriolar-glomerular region rather than the tubular epithelium, with the cortical rather than the medullary tubules being involved; this involvement usually follows vascular alterations (Fig. 34–19). In a classic study by Glatstein and colleagues,[256] radiation-induced lesions were shown to occur as a progressive replacement of capillary walls leading to glomerular sclerosis, followed by tubular atrophy. Larger arteries were not

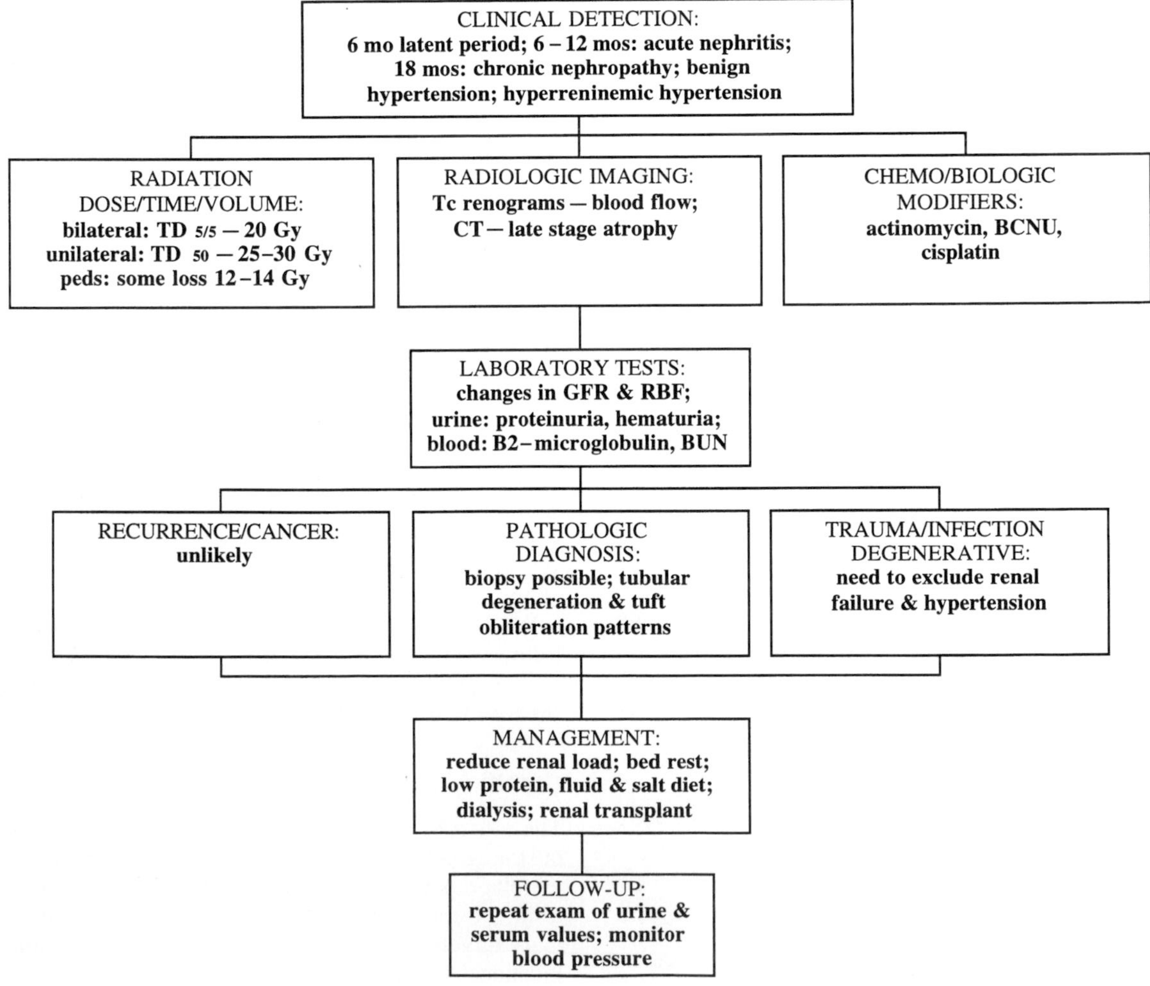

Figure 34–18. LENT diagram for the kidney.

Figure 34–19. The radiation response in the renal parenchyma. The responsive cell types are in the endothelium and epithelium. There is fibrinoid and hyaline accumulation associated with endothelial swelling in the afferent arterioles, which may spread beneath the glomerular capillary endothelium. The basement membrane thickens. Vascular compromise promotes thromboses, possibly leading to infarct. The tubular epithelium presents a variable picture, but there is some degree of interstitial fibrosis. As the vascular compromise develops, larger vessels may be affected, with focal necrosis and accumulations of foamy histiocytes. (From White DC: An Atlas of Radiation Histopathology, p 177. Oak Ridge, U.S. Energy Research & Development Administration, 1975, with permission.)

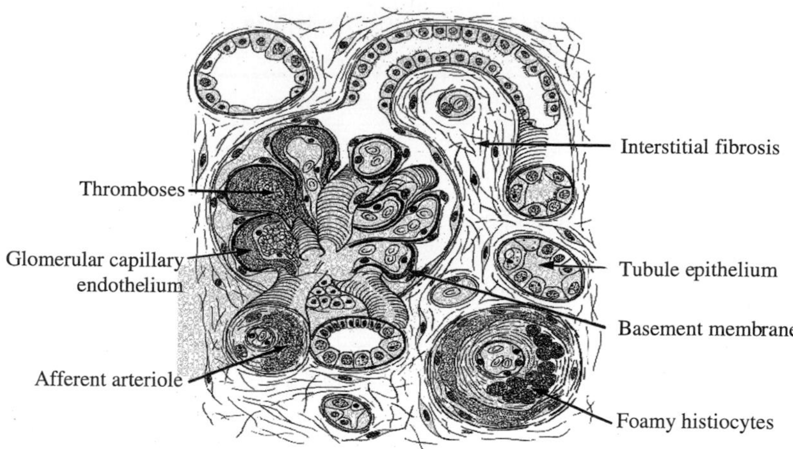

affected, although blood flow was reduced significantly and was still variable 2 to 3 months after irradiation. The evidence suggests that a functional lesion occurs in the glomerular capillaries, preceding tubular depletion. However, both elements are affected according to Hoopes and coworkers,[257, 258] who proposed that multiple target sites exist for radiation, offering the best explanation for the observed clinical syndromes. The pathologic mechanisms remain undefined at present, although damage to the vascular tissue plays a major role in the observed effects.[259–261]

Radiation Effects

The sensitivity of kidneys to radiation-induced injury makes these organs dose limiting in the treatment of nearby tumors.[255, 260, 262] In humans, dose-response data following high single-dose exposure to both kidneys are scarce; microscopically, both glomerulosclerosis and fibrinoid degeneration are evident. Toxicity is both dose and volume related.[253, 254, 263]

Glatstein and colleagues[256] showed that single radiation doses of higher than 19 Gy to both kidneys in mice caused renal failure and death, whereas 11 Gy allowed a 90% survival rate. Fractionated doses of 10 to 20 Gy induce a decrease in glomerular filtration rate and a suppression of tubular excretory capacity up to 12 months following therapy, although the blood urea and maximum urinary concentrating ability remain normal. Overall, kidney failure following fractionated radiation has been calculated to have a $TD_{5/5}$ of 23 Gy (5% incidence at 5 years) and a $TD_{50/5}$ of 28 Gy (50% incidence at 5 years) (Fig. 34–20).[253]

Pediatric renal tolerance to radiation is somewhat lower than tolerance in adults, but it is surprisingly close compared with most other organs. Twelve to 14 Gy given to infants led to chemical alterations in a limited number of patients according to Peschel and associates,[264] whereas Sagerman and coworkers[265] demonstrated delayed growth arrest in developing kidneys following 20 to 30 Gy unilateral irradiation. Overall, case studies in combination with data from the National Wilms' Study have shown that a threshold of 14 Gy can be deemed relatively safe in pediatric patients.[253, 266]

Chemotherapy Effects

Chemotherapy-induced acute renal dysfunction is dose related and generally reversible.[267] As seen in the heart, the late effects in the kidney induced by drugs are different from radiation effects. For agents such as cisplatin, ifosfamide, and high-dose methotrexate, the target cells are the renal tubular cells, in contrast to the fine microcirculation for irradiation (Table 34–7).[268] The major clinical expression of chemotherapy injury is renal failure, reflected as a decrease in creatinine clearance; combinations with other nontoxic agents can induce an additive effect, for example, with Taxol.[269] Pediatric patients are particularly sensitive and can demonstrate subclinical tubular toxicity as well as glomerular dysfunction.[270, 271]

A cancer-related hemolytic-uremic syndrome, characterized by microangiopathic hemolytic anemia, thrombocytopenia, and renal insufficiency associated with the deposition of platelets and fibrin in renal glomeruli, has been

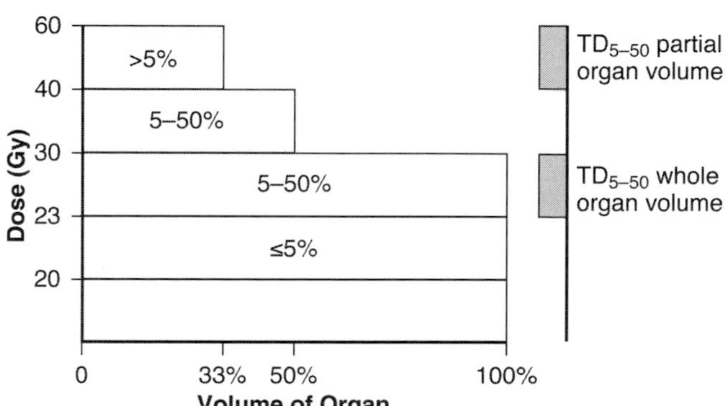

Figure 34–20. Dose-volume histogram for late effects seen in the kidney, illustrating the relationship between volume and tolerance doses. The right y-axis indicates the tolerance dose ranges for the TD_{5-50} for whole organ (kidney) irradiation, as well as the TD_{5-50} for partial organ volume (POV) irradiation. These figures apply to one as well as both kidneys, although following whole single kidney irradiation, compensatory changes will be observed in the contralateral organ. (Modified from Rubin P, Constine LS, Williams JP: Late effects of cancer treatment: radiation and drug toxicity. In: Perez CA, Brady LW [eds]: Principles and Practice of Radiation Oncology, 3rd ed, pp 155–211. Philadelphia, Lippincott-Raven, 1997.)

TABLE 34–7. **Renal Chemotoxic Agents, Their Site of Injury, and Their Late Effects**

Agent	Site of Injury	Late Effect
Cisplatin	Distal tubule	Hypomagnesemia
Ifosfamide	Proximal tubule	Fanconi's syndrome + rickets
Nitrosoureas (streptozotocin)	Glomerulus and proximal tubule	Often delayed
Methotrexate	Tubule	
Mitomycin C	Glomerulus	Hemolytic-uremic syndrome

Modified from Neglia JP, Nesbit ME Jr: Care and treatment of long-term survivors of childhood cancer. Cancer 1993; 71:3386–3391, with permission.

reported with mitomycin C[272–274] and, more recently, with gemcitabine.[275] This syndrome is frequently irreversible, despite treatment with plasmapheresis, as well as other measures employed in the therapy of idiopathic hemolytic-uremic syndrome.[276] With mitomycin C, this syndrome appears to be more common following high cumulative doses of the drug, but it may occur unpredictably after as little as 20 mg of the drug.

Amifostine, formerly known as WR-2721, is a naturally occurring thiol that has been approved for use in the prevention of cisplatin-induced renal toxicity,[277] but it appears to have other chemoprotective effects as well. Guidelines for its use were the subject of a review published in 1998.[234] It is important that it has not been shown to affect tumor responses to chemotherapy, but it does have the potential to increase the nausea and vomiting associated with cisplatin usage. The most clinically relevant toxicity associated with amifostine is hypotension,[278] which may occur anytime during infusion, so careful monitoring of the patient throughout its administration is advisable.

Combined Modalities

When combined therapy is used, additive or enhanced effects can occur; irradiation produces glomerulosclerosis and thickening of the fine afferent arterioles, and such lesions tend to precede the recognition of tubular cell injury. The effects of combining chemotherapy and radiation therapy have been described for patients with Wilms' tumor and appear as an enhancement of radiation changes.[279, 280] Agents used in the treatment of Wilms' tumor, such as dactinomycin, vincristine, cyclophosphamide, and doxorubicin, lead to little injury when combined without irradiation; however, these same combinations can induce an early appearance of lesions when administered with nontoxic radiation doses. Of particular concern are the pediatric patients requiring bone marrow transplantation, in which up to 20% of survivors suffer late-onset renal failure (Table 34–8).[262, 281–283] Sequencing chemoradiation is therefore topical and challenging; in rodent models, investigators have found that the most toxic sequence occurs when chemotherapy (e.g., cisplatin) is given before rather than after radiation therapy.[284, 285]

Liver

Clinical Syndromes

The mature liver (Fig. 34–21) was once considered to be resistant to the direct cytocidal actions of radiation because relatively large doses of radiation are required to cause marked acute inflammation in the liver, so that the acute clinical period appears to be silent.[286] However, it has now been realized that the liver is radiosensitive,[287] and it suffers progressive damage in the fine vasculature secondary to alterations in nonparenchymal cell populations.[288] This damage eventually leads to clinically significant degeneration late in or after the acute clinical period, depending on radiation dose and rate of progression of damage. Following high doses, a series of pathologic changes occurs, such as hyperemia, dilatation and congestion of sinusoids, and veno-occlusive lesions, appearing as early as 2 to 6 months after irradiation.[2, 289] The patient can develop anicteric ascites,[287] and there is an increase in hepatic size and a rise in alkaline phosphatase levels. This syndrome, known as radiation hepatitis or hepatopathy, may ultimately lead to hepatic fibrosis.[290]

Hepatic veno-occlusive disease (VOD) is an increasingly common occurrence in the setting of allogeneic bone marrow transplantation.[291, 292] In contrast to radiation hepatitis, which is expressed months after irradiation, the onset of symptoms typically occurs 1 to 2 weeks after TBI. Jaundice occurs in a large percentage of these patients,[293] in addition to weight gain, ascites, and hepatomegaly,[292] with lesions apparent in specific acinar zones as well as sublobular central venules.[288, 294] It must be noted that other causes of hepatitis need to be excluded, such as hepatic vein occlu-

TABLE 34–8. **Nephropathy after Bone Marrow Transplantation**

Author	Age Group	Primary Disease	Irradiation Technique	Preparatory Chemotherapy*	No. Affected/ No. Treated
Guinan et al[282]	Children	ALL (autologous)	12–14 Gy/6–8 fx	VM-26, cytosine arabinoside, cyclophosphamide	9/28
	Children	Neuroblastoma	12–14 Gy/6–8 fx	VM-26, melphalan, cisplatin, cyclophosphamide	7/11
Lawton et al[283]	Adults	Leukemia and lymphoma	14 Gy/9 fx t.i.d. (1.56 Gy/fx) 14 patients; 7.2 Gy/4 fx (b.i.d. × 2 days)	Various	14/103

ALL = acute lymphoblastic leukemia; fx = fractions; t.i.d. = three times per day; b.i.d. = twice per day; VM-26 = teniposide.
*Almost all of the patients were treated with several chemotherapeutic agents, including cisplatin.
From Cassady JR: Clinical radiation nephropathy. Int J Radiat Oncol Biol Phys 1995; 31:1249–1256, with permission from Elsevier Science.

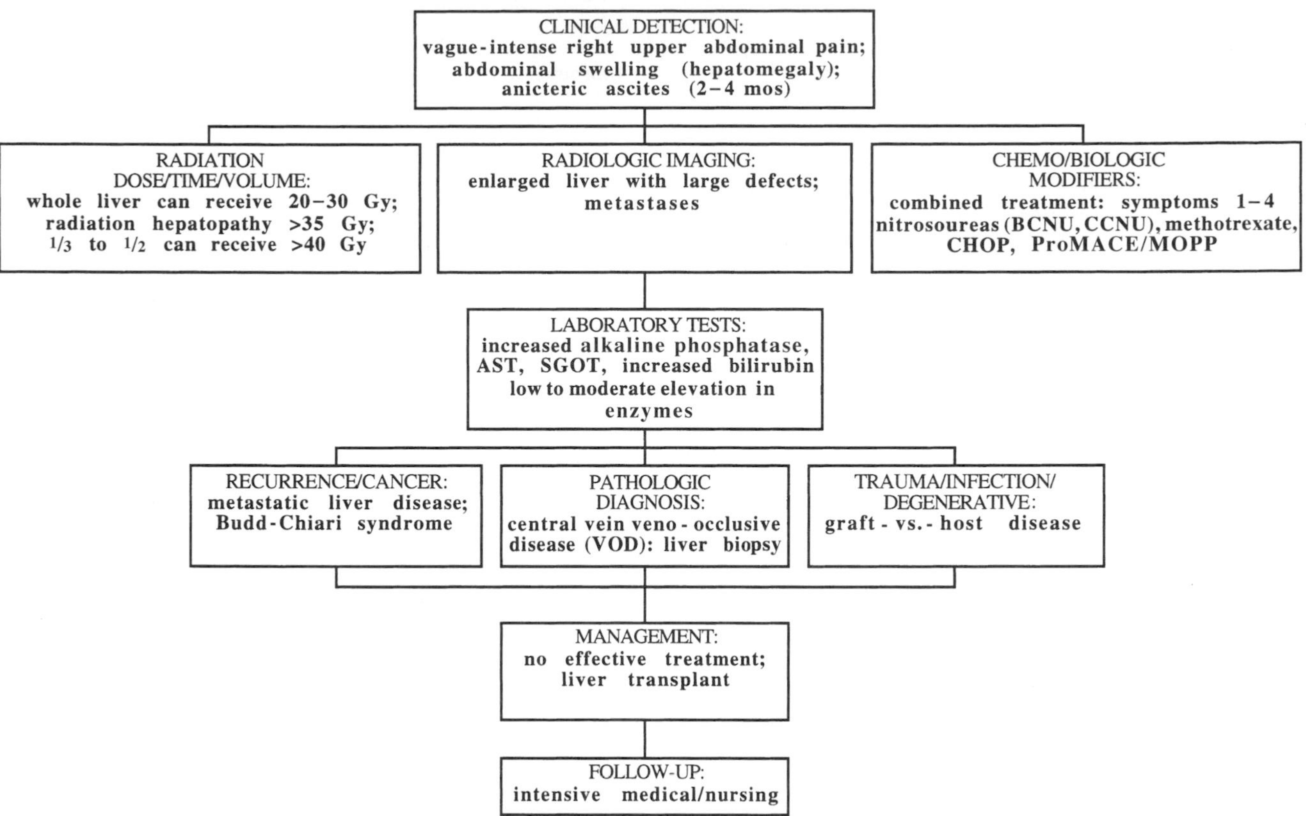

CLINICAL DETECTION:
vague-intense right upper abdominal pain; abdominal swelling (hepatomegaly); anicteric ascites (2–4 mos)
RADIATION DOSE/TIME/VOLUME:
whole liver can receive 20–30 Gy; radiation hepatopathy >35 Gy; 1/3 to 1/2 can receive >40 Gy
RADIOLOGIC IMAGING:
enlarged liver with large defects; metastases
CHEMO/BIOLOGIC MODIFIERS:
combined treatment: symptoms 1–4 nitrosoureas (BCNU, CCNU), methotrexate, CHOP, ProMACE/MOPP
LABORATORY TESTS:
increased alkaline phosphatase, AST, SGOT, increased bilirubin low to moderate elevation in enzymes
RECURRENCE/CANCER:
metastatic liver disease; Budd-Chiari syndrome
PATHOLOGIC DIAGNOSIS:
central vein veno-occlusive disease (VOD): liver biopsy
TRAUMA/INFECTION/ DEGENERATIVE:
graft-vs.-host disease
MANAGEMENT:
no effective treatment; liver transplant
FOLLOW-UP:
intensive medical/nursing

Figure 34–21. LENT diagram for the liver.

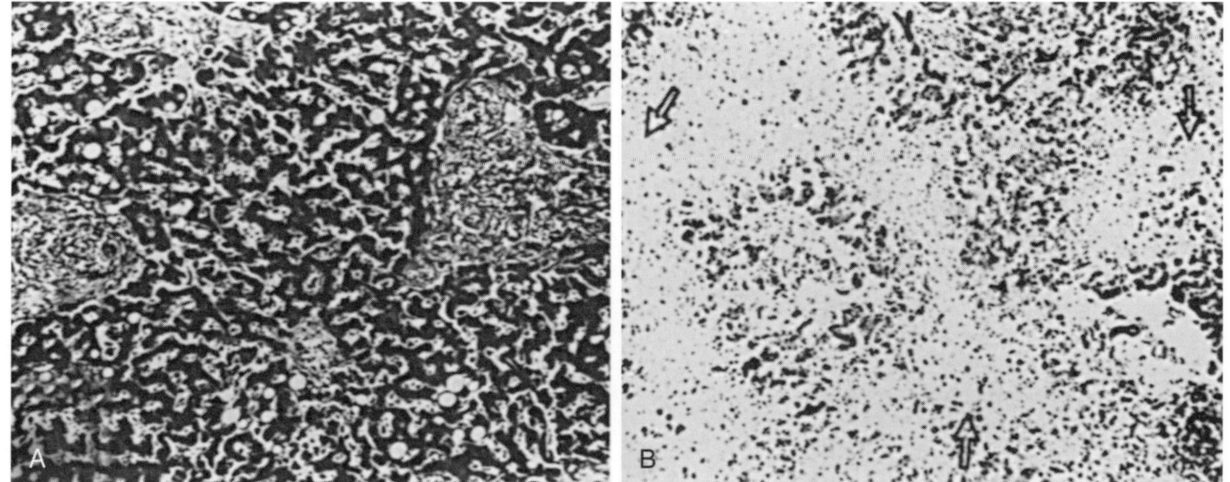

Figure 34–22. Hepatic late effects. (A) Chronic radiation hepatitis, showing scattered islands of fibrosis surrounding the central lobular veins and secondary atrophy of the surrounding hepatocytes. The rest of the lobule appears normal. (B) Chemotherapy (methotrexate) produces a diffuse necrosis of hepatocytes and fatty replacement, with zones of hepatic cell viability surrounding the central portal veins. (From Minow RA, Stern MH, Casey JH, et al: Clinicopathologic correlation of liver damage in patients treated with 6-mercaptopurine and adriamycin. Cancer 1976; 38:1524–1528. Copyright © 1976 American Cancer Society. Reprinted with permission of Wiley-Liss, Inc., a subsidiary of John Wiley & Sons, Inc.)

sion as a result of metastatic retroperitoneal nodes, viral hepatitis, intra-abdominal sepsis, or interstitial infarction.

Pathophysiology

The basic lesion of radiation hepatitis is injury to the endothelial cells of the central vein[289]; this results in retrograde congestion, leading to secondary alterations in surrounding hepatocytes (Fig. 34–22).[295, 296] Severe acute hepatic changes often progress to fibrosis and liver failure.[290] The pathogenesis of VOD is still obscure, owing to the difficulty of inducing a radiation hepatopathy in animals. A canine model of chemoradiation VOD has been developed; however, because of the combination mode of induction, it is difficult to separate the roles played by the individual therapies.[297] Nonetheless, although the etiology of the initiation of thrombi postirradiation is not known, there is substantial evidence that the cytokine transforming growth factor–β (TGFβ) plays a key role in their induction.[298–300]

Radiation Effects

Reviews of the literature[173, 301] have suggested a threshold dose for whole liver irradiation at approximately 20 Gy, with tolerance estimated as a function of both the volume[302] and dose; tolerance dose levels can be lowered in combination regimens.[303] VOD is an increasingly common and severe complication of TBI administered in preparation for bone marrow transplantation and can occur following single doses as low as 7.5 Gy.[304] Tefft and associates,[305] studying changes in liver function in children older than 5 years of age, observed that fractionated radiation doses of less than 25 Gy caused abnormal results in liver function tests and radionuclide scans in approximately 50% of patients, doses of 25 to 35 Gy caused abnormalities in 63%, and doses of higher than 35 Gy were highly toxic to 86% of patients (Fig. 34–23). These effects are more pronounced if the right side of the abdomen is treated compared with the left.[306] However, such results are decreasing in number because of improved technologies, in particular the increasing use of conformal beam therapy.[307]

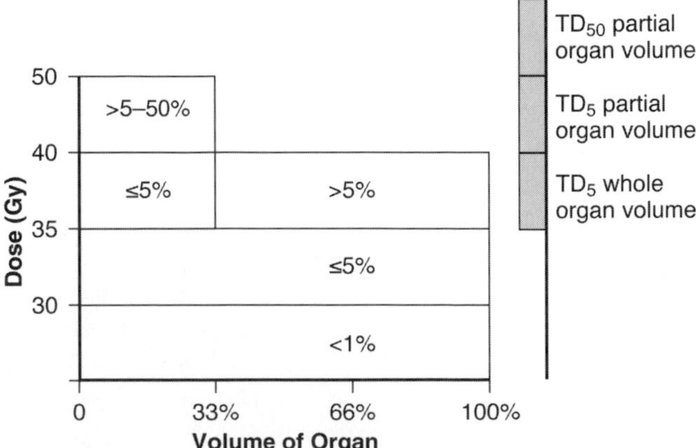

Figure 34–23. Dose-volume histogram for late effects seen in the liver, illustrating the relationship between volume and tolerance doses. There is a time factor in the tolerance range for whole liver irradiation, i.e., if 20 Gy is given in 1 week rather than over 2–3 weeks, there is high incidence of organ failure. The right y-axis indicates the tolerance dose ranges for the TD_5 for whole organ (liver) irradiation, as well as the TD_5 and TD_{50} for partial organ volume (POV) irradiation. (Modified from Rubin P, Constine LS, Williams JP: Late effects of cancer treatment: radiation and drug toxicity. In: Perez CA, Brady LW [eds]: Principles and Practice of Radiation Oncology, 3rd ed, pp 155–211. Philadelphia, Lippincott-Raven, 1997.)

TABLE 34–9. **Hepatic Chemotoxic Agents and Their Late Effects**

Agent	Late Effect
Antimetabolites	
5-Fluorouracil (infusion)	Chemical hepatitis (elevations in liver enzymes) or stricture of intra- or extrahepatic bile ducts; sclerosis
6-Mercaptopurine	Jaundice; bland cholestasis; necrosis
Cytosine arabinoside	Elevations in liver enzymes; cholestasis
Methotrexate	Elevations in liver enzymes; fibrosis; cirrhosis
Alkylating Agents	
Chlorambucil	Jaundice; fibrosis; cirrhosis
Busulfan	Cholestasis
Nitrosoureas	
BCNU (carmustine)	Elevated liver enzymes
Streptozotocin	Elevated liver enzymes
Miscellaneous	
Dactinomycin + vincristine	Veno-occlusive disease

Modified from King PD, Perry MC: Hepatotoxicity of chemotherapeutic and oncologic agents. Gastroenterol Clin North Am 1995; 24:969–990.

Chemotherapy Effects

The spectrum of hepatotoxic changes resulting from chemotherapy includes a direct parenchymal cell injury with fatty replacement, diffuse hepatocellular necrosis, as well as vascular lesions, including VOD similar to that seen in radiation injury (Table 34–9).[308] Such lesions have been seen following the use of a number of antineoplastic drugs, alone or in combination, for example, doxorubicin.[286, 309] In general, alkylating agents, such as the nitrosoureas, produce only a mild toxicity, although occasionally, severe damage that mimics radiation injury is reported.[310] 5-FU can be given intra-arterially for colorectal carcinoma; this agent has offered a higher response rate but at the cost of increased liver toxicity.[311] In some cases, combinations of agents have proven to be more toxic than single agents,[308] particularly in children,[312] with anecdotal cases of severe to life-threatening liver toxicity.[286, 313]

Combined Modalities

VOD was, at one time, infrequent and linked to the absorption of toxic agents or radiation. With the intensification of protocols in the setting of bone marrow transplantation, aggressive chemotherapy with TBI has proven additive for untoward effects in liver, kidney, and lung.[293, 294] Some studies have supported the view that radiation in a conditioning regimen is an independent factor in producing

VOD[314, 315]; however, radiation may alter liver pathophysiology,[316] affecting the liver's ability to metabolize agents, which has led to some agents (e.g., actinomycin D and vincristine) having longer half-lives in patients receiving liver irradiation, causing greater dysfunction and heightened marrow suppression.

As mentioned previously, TGFβ has been implicated in liver toxicity and has been shown by Anscher and associates to act as a predictor of risk in patients undergoing bone marrow transplantion.[298, 299] These investigators demonstrated that patients with pretransplant values greater than two deviations above the norm had a 90% probability of developing VOD. The rise in plasma TGFβ after induction chemotherapy also correlated to a patient's risk.

Lung

Clinical Syndromes

The lung is one of the most sensitive organs to cancer treatment, and radiation has long been known to induce dramatic effects, both early and late (Fig. 34–24).[317–319] The sequence of morphologic changes in the lung has been well documented.[320–322] Two distinct, delayed injuries occur following irradiation: the pneumonitic and fibrotic phases.[323] Acute pneumonitis occurs 1 to 3 months after irradiation and is seen following exposure to single doses exceeding 7.5 Gy; there is a steep dose response to 10 Gy, resulting in high lethality.[324] The role of vascular injury is an important aspect of interstitial fibrosis and occurs 2 to 4 months following irradiation; potentiation may occur with reirradiation.[325]

There are numerous pulmonary function parameters: pulmonary ventilation tests, nuclear medical techniques for aeration and blood flow, diffusion capacities, bronchoalveolar lavage for surfactant release and other factors,[326] and biopsy analyses. Radiographic studies, including CT scan and MRI, differentiate normal from abnormal irradiated tissues in the intact organ, although work by Marks and associates[327, 328] supports single photon emission computed tomography perfusion imaging as the most sensitive procedure. Symptoms are generally minimal if fibrosis is limited to less than 50% of one lung, leading to a disparity between clinical symptoms and radiographic findings. Risk factors include a smoking history and comorbid lung disease.[329]

Pathophysiology

The first observable event in the sequence toward pulmonary late effects, seen within minutes to hours after lung irradiation, is an immediate observable injury to the alveolar type II cell[330] and release of surfactant.[331] In the next phase, occurring between 1 and 3 months, type II pneumo-

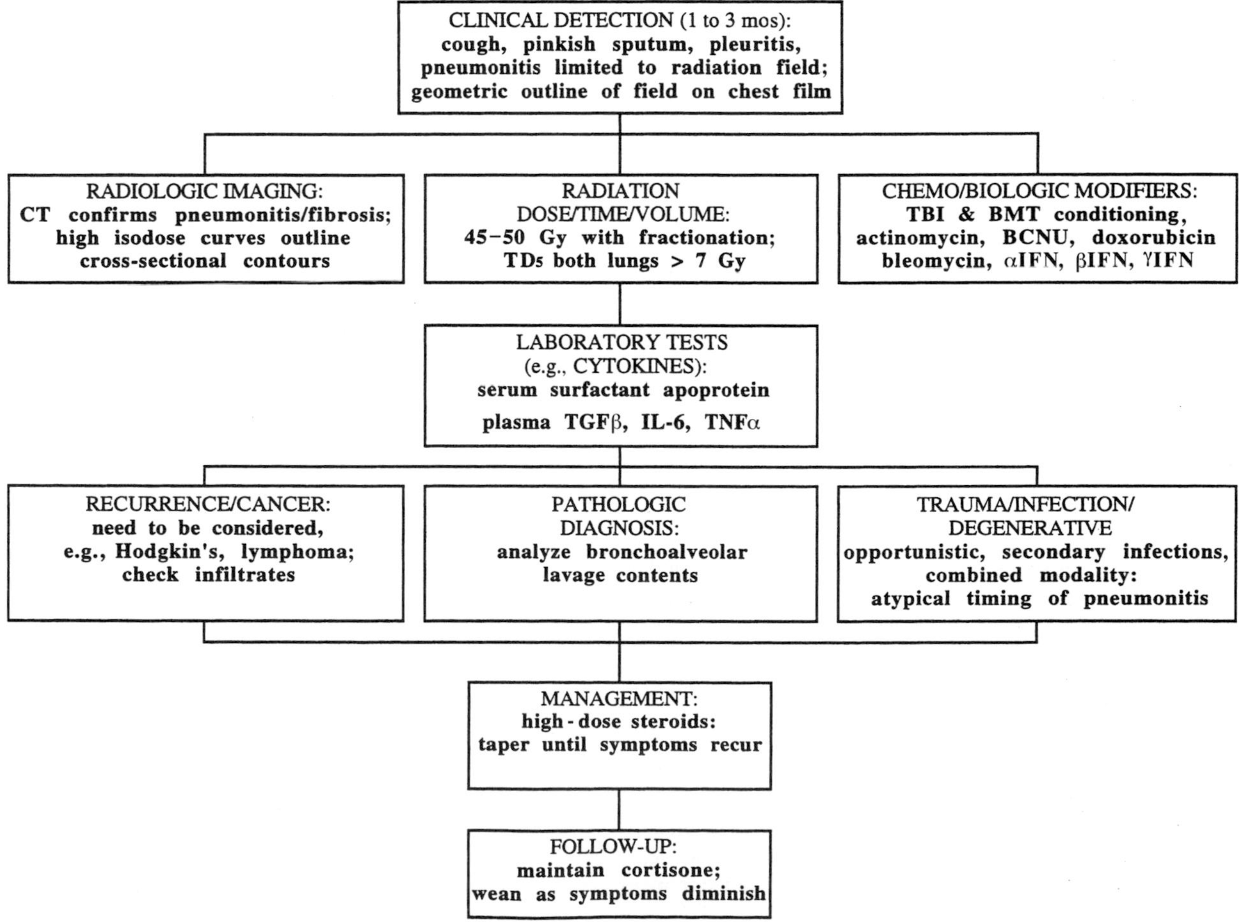

Figure 34–24. LENT diagram for the lung.

TABLE 34–10. **Ultrastructural Changes in the Lung After Radiation Therapy**

		Dose (Gy)			
Event	**Time**	***0***	***5***	***9***	***13***
Type II cell degranulation; surfactant release	1 hr–7 days	—	—	—	+
Loss of basal laminar proteoglycans	1 hr–7 days	—	±	+	+ +
Loss of alveolar macrophages	7 days	—	—	±	+
Surfactant recovery	4 wks	—	—	—	+
Replacement of laminar proteoglycans	4–12 wks	—	±	±	+
Radiation pneumonitis	12–30 wks	—	—	—	+
Peak in soluble fibronectin	12–30 wks	—	±	±	+ +
Fibrosis	30–60 wks	—	±	+	+
Peak in insoluble fibronectin	30–60 wks	—	+	+	+ +
Increased laminin	12–60 wks	—	±	+	+ +

Modified from Penney DP: Ultrastructural organization of the distal lung and potential target cells of ionizing radiation. Paper presented at: International Conference on New Biology of Lung and Lung Injury and Their Implications for Oncology; 1987; Porvoo, Finland.

cytes proliferate, and there is compensatory hypertrophy of lamellar bodies. The late fibrotic phase begins at 3 to 6 months, and it is recognized by sclerotic changes in the alveolar wall and extensive endothelial damage, with loss and replacement of some capillaries. Eventually, there is replacement of alveolar spaces and fibrosis, with loss of function.[317]

Sequential ultrastructural studies[319, 332] have identified the dramatic sequence of events starting with type II pneumocyte changes at 1 to 7 days, and alveolar macrophage numbers decreasing at 1 to 3 weeks. Endothelial cell changes are seen in alveolar capillaries within 5 days of irradiation, leading to platelet thrombi and luminal obstruction (Table 34–10)[333]; the fibroblast population increases at 2 to 6 months. Decreased pulmonary blood flow occurs months later and reflects the ongoing recanalization.

Over the past decade, our group has propounded a new paradigm to better explain the multicellular interaction seen in the lung.[15] There is an accumulation of supportive clinical data; for example, Anscher and associates have identified elevated TGFβ levels to be predictive for both lethal pneumonitis and hepatic VOD in patients undergoing bone marrow transplantation.[299, 334, 335] Similar cytokine cascades occur with chemotherapeutic agents, biologic response modifiers, surgery, and infection, providing an explanation for combined-modality additive effects[336] and a molecular rationale for their use as predictors.[337]

Radiation Effects

In mice, the single-dose survival curves are very steep, and increases in the dose of only 2 Gy can institute a change from an LD_{10} to an LD_{90}.[338] The dose range for radiation-induced pneumonitis is strain dependent, but it is usually about 12 Gy for a 5% incidence, 15 Gy for a 50% incidence, and 17 Gy for a 90% incidence following a single, high dose rate exposure. The relatively high radiosensitivity of the lung has been noted in fractionated radiation exposures as a component of TBI in bone marrow transplant programs, and it has been found that the dose-response relationship is shifted to the right for protracted low dose rate radiation. The relevance of dose rate has been examined by a number of investigators.[339, 340]

Fractionated radiation dramatically improves tolerance in both experimental and clinical settings. Wara and coworkers[341] demonstrated in a mouse model that the $LD_{50/160}$ changed from 13.65 Gy (single fraction) to 38.2 Gy (10 fractions) for a dose modification factor of 2.79. From clinical data, the dose modification factor for single versus fractionated doses is 3.2 in humans, demonstrating a considerable increase in tolerance for fractionated doses.[317] Of note, the degree of fibrosis is a function of the dose fraction size, as well as the total dose and total time for delivery.[336]

Different experiences are recorded regarding the incidence of pneumonopathy in patients treated for lung or breast cancer, and a specific range of injurious doses has not been identified. Patients with lung cancer may have pulmonary abnormalities resulting from changes produced by the cancer itself,[342] although assessment with CT scan provides sharper end points for the recognition of fibrosis. The total dose for the induction of fibrosis is 40 Gy and increases to 50 Gy for pneumonopathy (Fig. 34–25). Again,

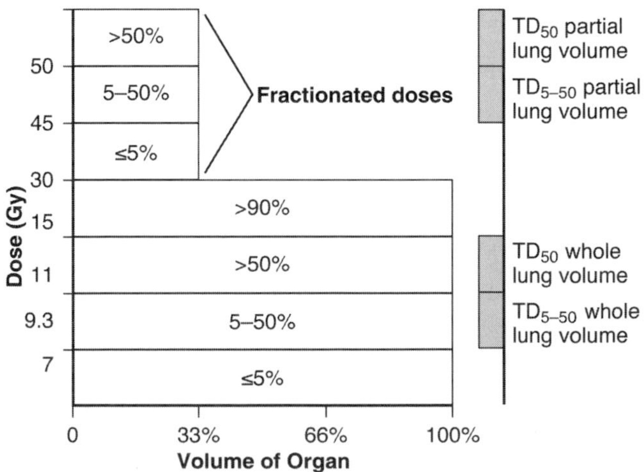

Figure 34–25. Dose-volume histogram for late effects seen in the lung, illustrating the relationship between volume and tolerance doses. The right y-axis indicates the tolerance dose ranges for the TD_5 and TD_{50} for whole organ (lungs) irradiation, as well as the TD_5 and TD_{50} for partial organ volume (POV) irradiation. (Modified from Rubin P, Constine LS, Williams JP: Late effects of cancer treatment: radiation and drug toxicity. In: Perez CA, Brady LW [eds]: Principles and Practice of Radiation Oncology, 3rd ed, pp 155–211. Philadelphia, Lippincott-Raven, 1997.)

late effects are being systematically reduced with improved methods.[343]

Chemotherapy Effects

Dose-response data for radiation and known toxic agents are being recorded in both animals and humans, and an increasing number of chemotherapeutic agents are known to cause pulmonary damage, producing a constellation of lesions (Table 34–11).[344] The most commonly reported agents to produce pulmonary toxicity are bleomycin[345, 346] and cyclophosphamide.[347, 348] With bleomycin, the initial lesions are seen in the capillary endothelium, with increasing permeability and interstitial edema,[349, 350] followed by swelling and necrosis of the alveolar type I cell.[350] The presence of capillary blistering following bleomycin and endothelial cell proliferation may indicate the ability of this agent to damage the microvasculature directly. A steep rise in pulmonary damage with bleomycin occurs with cumulative doses between 400 and 500 units; irradiation after bleomycin can heighten damage and add to lethality.

Alkylating agents, such as cyclophosphamide and ifosfamide, induce a similar form of interstitial pneumonitis, which may or may not be dose related.[351, 352] Nitrosoureas, BCNU in particular, induce a similar clinicopathologic profile to bleomycin, with fibrosis predominating. Antimetabolites, such as methotrexate and mercaptopurine, can cause desquamative interstitial pneumonitis and eosinophilic pneumonitis, although recovery is common on discontinuation of treatment, and fibrosis is unusual. In children, combination drug therapy can induce toxicity equal to radiation alone.[12, 353]

TABLE 34–11. **Pulmonary Chemotoxic Agents and Their Late Effects**

Agent	Late Effect
Antimetabolites	
Methotrexate	Pleural effusion; pneumonitis; occasional fibrosis
Alkylating Agents	
Chlorambucil	Acute alveolitis; interstitial pneumonitis
Busulfan	Pleural effusion; pneumonitis
Cyclophosphamide	Pleural effusion; interstitial pneumonitis
Nitrosoureas	
BCNU (carmustine)	Acute or late pneumonitis
Antibiotics	
Bleomycin	Pleural effusion; acute or late pneumonitis; fibrosis
Mitomycin	Acute alveolitis
Doxorubicin (+ radiation)	Accelerates radiation pneumonitis
Alkaloids	
Etoposide	Accelerates radiation pneumonitis
Miscellaneous	
Taxol	Hypersensitivity pneumonitis

Modified from McDonald S, Garrow G, Rubin P: Pulmonary complications of cancer therapy. In: Abeloff MD, Armitage JO, Lichter AS, et al (eds): Clinical Oncology, 2nd ed, pp 1023–1046. New York, Churchill Livingstone, 2000.

Combined Modalities

The combination of irradiation and chemotherapy can produce an intensified response and the recall phenomenon that appears when drugs are used after irradiation or in combination therapy.[354] This is exacerbated by radiation factors such as fraction size and total dose[355] and by the patient's age.[356] Actinomycin D, when used with radiation therapy for pulmonary metastases in Wilms' tumor, was found to produce lethal radiation pneumonitis following radiation doses within tolerance.[357, 358] More recently, it has been shown that bleomycin and the nitrosoureas alone can produce severe pneumonopathies, heighten radiation reactions, and lead to increased mortality when the two modalities are combined.[359]

As has been previously described, there is an increasing number of toxicities associated with bone marrow transplantation; pulmonary complications occur in 40% to 60% of patients. Late effects in the lung can be correlated to both chemotherapy-related and radiation therapy–related toxicity as well as graft-versus-host disease.[360–362]

Uniform Toxicity Scoring

To conclude on an important pragmatic note, there is a need to develop a uniform toxicity scoring for late effects. The introduction of multimodal management to cancer treatment has resulted in discipline-related differences in reporting toxicity. The radiation oncologist, in contrast to the medical oncologist, tends to be more aware of the importance of late effects after the acute phase of the reaction has been managed. However, chemotherapy produces late effects similar to those for irradiation, and although these complications are being increasingly documented in the literature, the focus remains on relatively acute and subacute effects. As a result, two different scoring and grading systems for toxicity have emerged: the radiation scores have been oriented toward specific pathologic lesions, whereas chemotherapy grades reflect functional and physiologic changes. Toxicity reporting of multiagent chemotherapy combinations and their interaction with radiation effects has stimulated national cooperative groups to form committees to assess acute effects and develop appropriate scoring and grading systems.

A recommendation for a uniform system is the desired end product based on consensus criteria. Following a conference on toxicity held in Baltimore, a subcommittee composed of representatives from several cooperative groups and the National Cancer Institute (NCI) was formed. Many of their recommendations were put into effect in the Common Toxicity Criteria, first distributed in 1988 by NCI, and some of the recommendations and conclusions made by the committee are summarized here.[363]

1. There is a need for uniform toxicity scoring, both for acute and late effects, but particularly with regard to late effects in vital organs.
2. The toxicity scale should consist of five grades: mild, moderate, severe, life-threatening, and fatal. The emphasis should be on grades three, four, and five, with

consideration for both peak grade and peak time in developing an appropriate index.
3. In addition to the major modalities of radiation therapy and chemotherapy, which are known to produce such late toxicities, the effects of host cofactors, other modalities, and recurrent tumor need to be carefully considered.
4. End points need to be clearly defined in terms of somatic and genetic effects and second malignant tumors with appropriate time scales set, preferably longer than 6 months following initiation of treatment. There is a need for a working committee on late effects representing all major modalities consisting of radiation, medical, and surgical oncologists, depending on the site.
5. Protocols for longitudinal studies of key dose-limiting normal tissues and organs, using appropriate standard diagnostic laboratory and imaging tests, need to be developed. These should include CT, MRI, and PET scans.
6. Actuarial risk reporting and recall of long-term survivors should be done initially in selected patient cohorts, namely survivors beyond 2 years. For malignancies in which a 50% survival rate has been considered most appropriate for such studies, this requirement may be too stringent; instead, the assessment of adverse effects should be done in all survivors beyond 2 years. This idea is particularly true for highly fatal cancers for which intensive regimens of combined modalities are being used.
7. Publications should routinely present therapeutic ratios and use standard toxicity and late effects scoring along with tumor response rates.

LENT formed the theme for an NCI conference held in San Francisco in July 1992 and, subsequently, the RTOG and EORTC, working in full cooperation, have simultaneously published the LENT scoring system in the *International Journal of Radiation Oncology, Biology and Physics,*[364] and *Radiotherapy and Oncology.*[365] These issues introduced the scoring systems that are based on the concept of grading according to four categories: Subjective, Objective, Management, and Analytic (SOMA). They also provided comprehensive reviews of late effects organized by organ or anatomic site. Whereas studies for interventions to modify acute effects and prevent late effects is the desired end result, these scales will allow for more accurate measures of improvement and will be a future area of development.

REFERENCES

1. Rubin P, Casarett GW: Clinical Radiation Pathology. Philadelphia, W.B. Saunders Co., 1968.
2. Casarett GW: Similarities and contrasts between radiation and time pathology. In: Strehler B (ed): Advances in Gerontological Research, p 109. New York, Academic Press, 1964.
3. Lichter AS, Abeloff MD, Armitage JO, et al: Multimodality therapy. In: Abeloff MD, Armitage JO, Lichter AS, et al (eds): Clinical Oncology, pp 307–314. New York, Churchill Livingstone, 1995.
4. John MJ: Radiotherapy and chemotherapy. In: Leibel SA, Phillips TL (eds): Textbook of Radiation Oncology, pp 69–89. Philadelphia, W.B. Saunders Co., 1998.
5. Bleyer WA: Chemoradiotherapy interactions in the central nervous system. Med Pediatr Oncol 1998; 31 (suppl 1):10–16.
6. Rubin P, Finkelstein JN, Williams JP: Paradigm shifts in the radiation pathophysiology of late effects in normal tissues: molecular vs classic concepts. In: Tobias JS, Thomas PRM (eds): Current Radiation Oncology, 3rd ed, pp 1–26. London, Arnold, 1998.
7. Cortner J, Vande Woude GF: Essentials of molecular biology. In: De Vita VT Jr, Hellman S, Rosenberg SA (eds): Cancer. Principles & Practice of Oncology, 5th ed, pp 3–33. Philadelphia, Lippincott-Raven, 1997.
8. Coleman CN, Harris JR: Current scientific issues related to clinical radiation oncology. Radiat Res 1998; 150:125–133.
9. Stone HB, Dewey WC, Wallace SS, et al: Molecular biology to radiation oncology: a model for translational research? Opportunities in basic and translational research. Radiat Res 1998; 150:134–147.
10. Fridman WH, Tartour E: The use of cytokines in the treatment of solid tumours. Hematol Cell Ther 1997; 39:105–108.
11. Shpall EJ: The utilization of cytokines in stem cell mobilization strategies. Bone Marrow Transplant 1999; 23 (suppl):S13–S19.
12. Fauroux B, Clement A, Tournier G: Pulmonary toxicity of drugs and thoracic irradiation in children. Rev Mal Respir 1996; 13:235–242.
13. Gardner RV: Long term hematopoietic damage after chemotherapy and cytokine. Front Biosci 1999; 4:47–57.
14. Hoekman K, Van der Vijgh WJ, Vermorken JB: Clinical and preclinical modulation of chemotherapy-induced toxicity in patients with cancer. Drugs 1999; 57:133–155.
15. Rubin P, Johnston CJ, Williams JP, et al: A perpetual cascade of cytokines postirradiation leads to pulmonary fibrosis. Int J Radiat Oncol Biol Phys 1995; 33:99–109.
16. Johnston CJ, Piedboeuf B, Rubin P, et al: Early and persistent alterations in the expression of interleukin-1 alpha, interleukin-1 beta and tumor necrosis factor alpha mRNA levels in fibrosis-resistant and sensitive mice after thoracic irradiation. Radiat Res 1996; 145:762–767.
17. Holyoake TL: Cytokines at the research-clinical interface: potential applications. Blood Rev 1996; 10:189–200.
18. Rubin P: The Franz Buschke lecture: late effects of chemotherapy and radiation therapy: a new hypothesis. Int J Radiat Oncol Biol Phys 1984; 10:5–34.
19. Hall EJ (ed): Radiobiology for the Radiologist, 4th ed. Philadelphia, J.B. Lippincott Co., 1994.
20. Cowdry EV (ed): Textbook of Histology, 4th ed. Philadelphia, Lea & Febiger, 1950.
21. Hill BT: Cancer chemotherapy. The relevance of certain concepts of cell cycle kinetics. Biochim Biophys Acta 1978; 516:389–417.
22. Hochhauser D: Modulation of chemosensitivity through altered expression of cell cycle regulatory genes in cancer. Anticancer Drugs 1997; 8:903–910.
23. Botnick LE, Hannon ECM, Hellman S: Late effects of cytotoxic agents on the normal tissue of mice. Front Radiat Ther Oncol 1979; 13:36–47.
24. Sundman-Engberg B, Tidefelt U, Paul C: Toxicity of cytostatic drugs to normal bone marrow cells in vitro. Cancer Chemother Pharmacol 1998; 42:17–23.
25. Peters LJ: Radiation therapy tolerance limits. For one or for all? Cancer 1996; 77:2379–2385.
26. Offner F, Kerre T, De Smedt M, et al: Bone marrow CD34 cells generate fewer T cells in vitro with increasing age and following chemotherapy. Br J Haematol 1999; 104:801–808.
27. King DJ, Ratcliffe MA, Dawson AA, et al: Fertility in young men and women after treatment for lymphoma: a study of a population. J Clin Pathol 1985; 38:1247–1251.
28. Kreuser ED, Xiros N, Hetzel WD, et al: Reproductive and endocrine gonadal capacity in patients treated with COPP chemotherapy for Hodgkin's disease. J Cancer Res Clin Oncol 1987; 113:260–266.
29. Marmor D, Duyck F: Male reproductive potential after MOPP therapy for Hodgkin's disease: a long-term survey. Andrologia 1995; 27:99–106.
30. Byrne J, Fears TR, Gail MH, et al: Early menopause in long-term survivors of cancer during adolescence. Am J Obstet Gynecol 1992; 166:788–793.
31. Chiarelli AM, Marrett LD, Darlington G: Early menopause and infertility in females after treatment for childhood cancer diagnosed in 1964–1988 in Ontario, Canada. Am J Epidemiol 1999; 150:245–254.
32. Chatterjee R, Goldstone AH: Gonadal damage and effects on fertility in adult patients with haematological malignancy undergoing stem cell transplantation. Bone Marrow Transplant 1996; 17:5–11.

33. Watson M, Wheatley K, Harrison GA, et al: Severe adverse impact on sexual functioning and fertility of bone marrow transplantation, either allogeneic or autologous, compared with consolidation chemotherapy alone. Cancer 1999; 86:1231–1239.
34. Brenner J, Vugrin D, Whitmore WF: Effect of treatment on fertility and sexual function in males with metastatic nonseminomatous germ cell tumors of testis. Am J Clin Oncol 1985; 8:178–182.
35. Lampe H, Horwich A, Norman A, et al: Fertility after chemotherapy for testicular germ cell cancers. J Clin Oncol 1997; 15:239–245.
36. Hartmann JT, Albrecht C, Schmoll H-J, et al: Long-term effects on sexual function and fertility after treatment of testicular cancer. Br J Cancer 1999; 80:801–807.
37. Chapman RM, Sutcliffe SB, Malpas JS: Cytotoxic-induced ovarian failure in women with Hodgkin's disease. JAMA 1979; 242:1877–1881.
38. Bines J, Oleske DM, Cobleigh MA: Ovarian function in premenopausal women treated with adjuvant chemotherapy for breast cancer. J Clin Oncol 1996; 14:1718–1729.
39. O'Brien M, Montes A, Powles TJ: Hormone-replacement therapy as treatment of breast cancer—a phase II study of Org OD 14 (tibilone). Br J Cancer 1996; 73:1086–1088.
40. Zhang K, Mack P, Wong KP: Glutathione-related mechanisms in cellular resistance to anticancer drugs. Int J Oncol 1998; 12:871–882.
41. Sonneveld P: Drug resistance in multiple myeloma. Pathol Biol 1999; 47:182–187.
42. Nishio K, Nakamura T, Koh Y, et al: Drug resistance in lung cancer. Curr Opin Oncol 1999; 11:109–115.
43. Coldman AJ, Goldie JH: Factors affecting the development of permanent drug resistance and its impact upon neoadjuvant chemotherapy. Recent Results Cancer Res 1986; 103:69–78.
44. Beck WT, Dalton WS: Mechanisms of drug resistance. In: DeVita VT Jr, Hellman S, Rosenberg SA (eds): Cancer. Principles & Practice of Oncology, 5th ed, pp 498–512. Philadelphia, Lippincott-Raven, 1997.
45. Shapiro AB, Fox K, Lee P, et al: Functional intracellular P-glycoprotein. Int J Cancer 1998; 76:857–864.
46. Bradshaw DM, Arceci RJ: Clinical relevance of transmembrane drug efflux as a mechanism of multidrug resistance. J Clin Oncol 1998; 16:3674–3690.
47. Shustik C, Dalton W, Gros P: P-glycoprotein–mediated multidrug resistance in tumor cells: biochemistry, clinical relevance and modulation. Mol Aspects Med 1995; 16:1–78.
48. Dubois JB: Late effects of intraoperative radiotherapy. Cancer Radiother 1997; 1:817–822.
49. Geara FB, Peters LJ, Ang KK, et al: Prospective comparison of in vitro normal cell radiosensitivity and normal tissue reactions in radiotherapy patients. Int J Radiat Oncol Biol Phys 1993; 27:1173–1179.
50. Brock WA, Tucker SL, Geara FB, et al: Fibroblast radiosensitivity versus acute and late normal skin responses in patients treated for breast cancer. Int J Radiat Oncol Biol Phys 1995; 32:1371–1379.
51. Turesson I, Notter G: The influence of fraction size in radiotherapy on the late normal tissue reaction—I: Comparison of the effects of daily and once-a-week fractionation on human skin. Int J Radiat Oncol Biol Phys 1984; 10:593–598.
52. Turesson I, Notter G: The influence of fraction size in radiotherapy on the late normal tissue reaction—II: Comparison of the effects of daily and twice-a-week fractionation on human skin. Int J Radiat Oncol Biol Phys 1984; 10:599–606.
53. Johnston CJ, Piedboeuf B, Baggs R, et al: Differences in correlation of mRNA gene expression in mice sensitive and resistant to radiation-induced pulmonary fibrosis. Radiat Res 1995; 142:197–203.
54. Schrier DJ, Kunkel RG, Phan SH: The role of strain variation in murine bleomycin-induced pulmonary fibrosis. Am Rev Respir Dis 1983; 127:63–66.
55. Hoyt DG, Lazo JS: Alterations in pulmonary mRNA encoding procollagens, fibronectin and transforming growth factor–beta precede bleomycin-induced pulmonary fibrosis in mice. J Pharmacol Exp Ther 1988; 246:765–771.
56. Baecher-Allan CM, Barth RK: PCR analysis of cytokine induction profiles associated with mouse strain variation in susceptibility to pulmonary fibrosis. Region Immunol 1993; 5: 207–217.
57. Moni J, Nori D: The pitfalls and complications of radiation therapy for esophageal carcinoma. Chest Surg Clin N Am 1997; 7:565–584.
58. Brizel DM: Future directions in toxicity prevention. Semin Radiat Oncol 1998; 8:17–20.
59. Tucker SL, Geara FB, Peters LJ, et al: How much could the radiotherapy dose be altered for individual patients based on a predictive assay of normal-tissue radiosensitivity? Radiother Oncol 1996; 38:103–113.
60. Budach W, Classen J, Belka C, et al: Clinical impact of predictive assays for acute and late radiation morbidity. Strahlenther Onkol 1998; 174 (suppl):20–24.
61. Withers HR, McBride WH: Biologic basis of radiation therapy. In: Perez CA, Brady LW (eds): Principles and Practice of Radiation Oncology, 3rd ed, pp 79–118. Philadelphia, Lippincott-Raven, 1998.
62. Fu KK: Biological basis for the interaction of chemotherapeutic agents and radiation therapy. Cancer 1985; 55:2123–2130.
63. Aisner J, Hiponia D, Conley B, et al: Combined modalities in the treatment of head and neck cancers. Semin Oncol 1995; 22:28–34.
64. Dubey AK, Recht A, Come S, et al: Why and how to combine chemotherapy and radiation therapy in breast cancer patients. Recent Results Cancer Res 1998; 152:247–254.
65. Rubin P: Law and order of radiation sensitivity. Absolute versus relative. In: Vaeth JM, Meyer JL (eds): Frontiers of Radiation Therapy and Oncology, 23rd ed, pp 7–40. Basel, Karger, 1989.
66. Hendry JH, Mackay RI, Roberts SA, et al: Outstanding issues in radiation dose-fractionation studies. Int J Radiat Biol 1998; 73:383–394.
67. Tordiglione M, Kalli M, Vavassori V, et al: Combined modality treatment for esophageal cancer. Tumori 1998; 84:252–258.
68. Kleinberg L, Grossman S, Piantadosi S, et al: The effects of sequential versus concurrent chemotherapy and radiotherapy on survival and toxicity in patients with newly diagnosed high-grade astrocytoma. Int J Radiat Oncol Biol Phys 1999; 44:535–543.
69. Ellis F: Is NSD-TDF useful to radiotherapy? Int J Radiat Oncol Biol Phys 1985; 11:1685–1697.
70. Strandqvist M: Studien uber die Kumulative Wirkung der Rontgenstrahlen bei Fraktionierung. Acta Radiol 1944; 55 (suppl):1–300.
71. Lyman JT: Normal tissue complication probabilities: variable dose per fraction. Int J Radiat Oncol Biol Phys 1992; 22:247–250.
72. Lyman JT: Complication probability as assessed from dose-volume histograms. Radiat Res 1985; 8 (suppl):S13–S19.
73. Johnstone PA, Sindelar WF, Kinsella TJ: Experimental and clinical studies of intraoperative radiation therapy. Curr Probl Cancer 1994; 18:249–290.
74. Mauch P, Constine L, Greenberger J, et al: Hematopoietic stem cell compartment: acute and late effects of radiation therapy and chemotherapy. Int J Radiat Oncol Biol Phys 1995; 31:1319–1339.
75. Andrews GA: Radiation accidents and their management. Radiat Res 1967; 7 (suppl):390–397.
76. van der Meer JW, Vogels MT, Netea MG, et al: Proinflammatory cytokines and treatment of disease. Ann NY Acad Sci 1998; 856:243–251.
77. Eisen D, Essell J: Drug-induced thrombocytopenia presenting with isolated oral lesions: report of two cases. Cutis 1998; 62:193–195.
78. Jih DM, Werth VP: Thrombocytopenia after a single test dose of methotrexate. J Am Acad Dermatol 1998; 39:349–351.
79. Gordon MS, Nemunaitis J, Hoffman R, et al: A phase I trial of recombinant human interleukin-6 in patients with myelodysplastic syndromes and thrombocytopenia. Blood 1995; 85:3066–3076.
80. Sundman-Engberg B, Tidefelt U, Paul C: Effect of cytokines on the toxicity of cytostatic drugs on leukemic cells in vitro and in vivo. Eur J Haematol 1996; 56:1–6.
81. Mauch P, Lamont C, Neben TY, et al: Hematopoietic stem cells in the blood after stem cell factor and interleukin-11 administration: evidence for different mechanisms of mobilization. Blood 1995; 86:4674–4680.
82. Freedman A, Neuberg D, Mauch P, et al: Cyclophosphamide, doxorubicin, vincristine, prednisone dose intensification with granulocyte colony-stimulating factor markedly depletes stem cell reserve for autologous bone marrow transplantation. Blood 1997; 90:4996–5001.
83. Robak T: Cytokines in the treatment of blood diseases. Acta Haematol Pol 1995; 26:72–78.
84. Tubiana M, Frindel E, Croizat H, et al: Effects of radiations on bone marrow. Pathol Biol (Paris) 1979; 27:326–334.
85. Coquard R: Late effects of ionizing radiations on the bone marrow. Cancer Radiother 1997; 1:792–800.

86. Molica S, De Rossi G, Luciani M, et al: Prognostic features and therapeutical approaches in B-cell chronic lymphocytic leukemia: an update. Haematologica 1995; 80:176–193.
87. Ketterer N, Sonet A, Dumontet C, et al: Toxicities after peripheral blood progenitor cell transplantation for lymphoid malignancies: analysis of 300 cases in a single institution. Bone Marrow Transplant 1999; 23:1309–1315.
88. Thomas ED, Storb R, Buckner CD: Total body irradiation in preparation for bone marrow engraftment. Transplant Proc 1976; 8:591–593.
89. Rubin P, Elbadawi NA, Thomson RA, et al: Bone marrow regeneration from cortex following segmental fractionated irradiation. Int J Radiat Oncol Biol Phys 1977; 2:27–38.
90. Parmentier C, Morardet N, Tubiana M: Late effects on human bone marrow after extended field radiotherapy. Int J Radiat Oncol Biol Phys 1983; 9:1303–1311.
91. Pierga JY, Follezou JY, Chelfi M, et al: Immediate hematological tolerance of extended irradiations after chemotherapy. Apropos of 78 cases of Hodgkin's disease stage III and IV without marrow involvement treated at the Gustave-Roussy Institute. Bull Cancer 1991; 78:921–929.
92. Rubin P, Constine LS, Scarantino CW: The paradoxes in patterns and mechanism of bone marrow regeneration after irradiation. 2. Total body irradiation. Radiother Oncol 1984; 2:227–233.
93. Lohrmann H, Schreml W: Long-term hemopoietic damage after cytotoxic drug therapy for solid tumors. In: Testa N, Gale R (eds): Hematopoiesis: Long-Term Effects of Chemotherapy and Radiation, p 325. New York, Marcel Dekker, 1988.
94. Hoyle CF, de Bastos M, Wheatley K, et al: AML associated with previous cytotoxic therapy, MDS or myeloproliferative disorders: results from the MRC's 9th AML trial. Br J Haematol 1989; 72:45–53.
95. Levine EG, Bloomfield CD: Leukemias and myelodysplastic syndromes secondary to drug, radiation, and environmental exposure. Semin Oncol 1992; 19:47–84.
96. Curtis RE, Boice JD, Stovall M, et al: Risk of leukemia after chemotherapy and radiation treatment for breast cancer. N Engl J Med 1992; 326:1745–1751.
97. Tallman MS, Gray R, Bennett JM, et al: Leukemogenic potential of adjuvant chemotherapy for early-stage breast cancer: The Eastern Cooperative Oncology Group experience. J Clin Oncol 1995; 13:1557–1563.
98. Iurlo A, Mecucci C, Van Orshoven A, et al: Cytogenetic and clinical investigations in 76 cases with therapy-related leukemia and myelodysplastic syndrome. Cancer Genet Cytogenet 1989; 43:227–241.
99. Groupe Français de Cytogénétique Hématologique (GFCH): Acute leukemia treated with intensive chemotherapy in patients with a history of previous chemo- and/or radiotherapy: prognostic significance of karyotype and preceding myelodysplastic syndrome. Leukemia 1994; 8:87–91.
100. Heim S: Cytogenetic findings in primary and secondary MDS. Leuk Res 1992; 16:43–46.
101. Kollmannsberger C, Hartmann JT, Kanz L, et al: Risk of secondary myeloid leukemia and myelodysplastic syndrome following standard-dose chemotherapy or high-dose chemotherapy with stem cell support in patients with potentially curable malignancies. J Cancer Res Clin Oncol 1998; 124:207–214.
102. Pui C-H, Behm FG, Raimondi SC, et al: Secondary acute myeloid leukemia in children treated for acute lymphoid leukemia. N Engl J Med 1989; 321:136–142.
103. Pedersen-Bjergaard J, Philip P, Larsen SO, et al: Chromosome aberrations and prognostic factors in therapy-related myelodysplasia and acute nonlymphocytic leukemia. Blood 1990; 76:1083–1091.
104. Pedersen-Bjergaard J, Sigsgaard TC, Nielsen D, et al: Acute monocytic or myelomonocytic leukemia with balanced chromosome translocations to band 11q23 after therapy with 4-epi-doxorubicin and cisplatin or cyclophosphamide for breast cancer. J Clin Oncol 1992; 10:1444–1451.
105. Pedersen-Bjergaard J, Pedersen M, Roulston D, et al: Different genetic pathways in leukemogenesis for patients presenting with therapy-related myelodysplasia and therapy-related acute myeloid leukemia. Blood 1995; 9:3542–3552.
106. Felix CA, Hosler MR, Winick NJ, et al: *ALL-1* gene rearrangements in DNA topoisomerase II inhibitor-related leukemia in children. Blood 1995; 85:3250–3256.
107. Sandoval C, Pui C-H, Bowman LC, et al: Secondary acute myeloid leukemia in children previously treated with alkylating agents, intercalating topoisomerase II inhibitors, and irradiation. J Clin Oncol 1993; 11:1039–1045.
108. Detourmignies L, Castaigne S, Stoppa AM, et al: Therapy-related acute promyelocytic leukemia: a report on 16 cases. J Clin Oncol 1992; 10:1430–1435.
109. Chan T, Juneja S, Wolf M, et al: Secondary myelodysplastic syndrome following bone marrow transplantation: report of two cases. Bone Marrow Transplant 1994; 13:145–148.
110. Miller JS, Arthur DC, Litz CE, et al: Myelodysplastic syndrome after autologous bone marrow transplantation: an additional late complication of curative cancer therapy. Blood 1994; 83:3780–3786.
111. Roman-Unfer S, Bitran JD, Hanauer S, et al: Acute myeloid leukemia and myelodysplasia following intensive chemotherapy for breast cancer. Bone Marrow Transplant 1995; 16:163–168.
112. Laughlin MJ, McGaughey DS, Crews JR, et al: Secondary myelodysplasia and acute leukemia in breast cancer patients after autologous bone marrow transplant. J Clin Oncol 1998; 16:1008–1012.
113. Sobecks RM, Le Beau MM, Anastasi J, et al: Myelodysplasia and acute leukemia following high-dose chemotherapy and autologous bone marrow or peripheral blood stem cell transplantation. Bone Marrow Transplant 1999; 23:1161–1165.
114. Friedberg JW, Neuberg D, Stone RM, et al: Outcome in patients with myelodysplastic syndrome after autologous bone marrow transplantation for non-Hodgkin's lymphoma. J Clin Oncol 1999; 17:3128–3135.
115. Horstmann M, Kroschke G, Stockschlader M, et al: Early toxicity of intensified conditioning with etoposide combined with total body irradiation/cyclophosphamide or busulfan/cyclophosphamide in children undergoing autologous or allogeneic bone marrow transplantation. Pediatr Hematol Oncol 1996; 13:45–53.
116. Kroger N, Hoffknecht M, Hanel M, et al: Busulfan, cyclophosphamide and etoposide as high-dose conditioning therapy in patients with malignant lymphoma and prior dose-limiting radiation therapy. Bone Marrow Transplant 1998; 21:1171–1175.
117. Mounier N, Gisselbrecht C: Conditioning regimens before transplantation in patients with aggressive non-Hodgkin's lymphoma. Ann Oncol 1998; 9(suppl 1):S15–S21.
118. Santos GW: Preparative regimens: chemotherapy versus chemoradiotherapy. A historical perspective. Ann NY Acad Sci 1995; 770:1–7.
119. Bond VP, Fludner TM, Archambeau JO: Mammalian Radiation Lethality. New York, Academic Press, 1965.
120. Schultheiss TE, Kun LE, Ang KK, et al: Radiation response of the central nervous system. Int J Radiat Oncol Biol Phys 1995; 31:1093–1112.
121. Chou RH, Wong GB, Kramer JH, et al: Toxicities of total-body irradiation for pediatric bone marrow transplantation. Int J Radiat Oncol Biol Phys 1996; 34:843–851.
122. Anderson V, Godber T, Smibert E, et al: Neurobehavioural sequelae following cranial irradiation and chemotherapy in children: an analysis of risk factors. Pediatr Rehabilitation 1997; 1:63–76.
123. Marks JE, Baglan RJ, Prassad SC, et al: Cerebral radionecrosis: incidence and risk in relation to dose, time, fractionation and volume. Int J Radiat Oncol Biol Phys 1981; 7:243–252.
124. Constine LS, Konski A, Ekholm S, et al: Adverse effects of brain irradiation correlated with MR and CT imaging. Int J Radiat Oncol Biol Phys 1988; 15:319–330.
125. Wang PY, Shen WC, Jan JS: Serial MRI changes in radiation myelopathy. Neuroradiology 1995; 37:374–377.
126. Loeffler JS, Siddon RL, Wen PY, et al: Stereotactic radiosurgery of the brain using a standard linear accelerator: a study of early and late effects. Radiother Oncol 1990; 17:311–321.
127. Flickinger JC, Kondziolka D, Pollock BE, et al: Complications from arteriovenous malformation radiosurgery: multivariate analysis and risk modeling. Int J Radiat Oncol Biol Phys 1997; 38:485–490.
128. Ostertag CB: Brachytherapy—interstitial implant radiosurgery. Acta Neurochir Suppl (Wein) 1993; 58:79–84.
129. White DC: An Atlas of Radiation Histopathology. Oak Ridge, U.S. Energy Research & Development Administration, 1975.
130. Brady LW: Conference on long term normal tissue effects of cancer treatment. Cancer Clinical Trials 1981; 4 (suppl 7):7–71.
131. van der Kogel AJ: Radiation-induced damage in the central nervous system: an interpretation of target cell responses. Br J Cancer 1986; 7(suppl):207–217.

132. van der Kogel AJ: Central nervous system radiation injury in small animal models. In: Gutin PH, Leibel SA, Sheline GE (eds): Radiation Injury to the Nervous System, pp 91–111. New York, Raven Press, 1991.
133. Acker JC, Marks LB, Spencer DP, et al: Serial in vivo observations of cerebral vasculature after treatment with a large single fraction of radiation. Radiat Res 1998; 149:350–359.
134. Hong JH, Chiang CS, Campbell IL, et al: Induction of acute phase gene expression by brain irradiation. Int J Radiat Oncol Biol Phys 1995; 33:619–626.
135. Olschowka JA, Kyrkanides S, Harvey BK, et al: ICAM-1 induction in the mouse CNS following irradiation. Brain Behav Immun 1997; 11:273–285.
136. Schultheiss TE, Stephens LC, Maor MH: Analysis of the histopathology of radiation myelopathy. Int J Radiat Oncol Biol Phys 1988; 14:27–32.
137. Schultheiss TE, Stephens LC: Permanent radiation myelopathy. Br J Radiol 1992; 65:737–753.
138. Licinio J: Central nervous system cytokines and their relevance for neurotoxicity and apoptosis. J Neural Transm 1997; 49(suppl):169–175.
139. Ledeen RW, Chakraborty G: Cytokines, signal transduction, and inflammatory demyelination: review and hypothesis. Neurochem Res 1998; 23:277–289.
140. Rubin P, Constine LS, Williams JP: Late effects of cancer treatment: Radiation and drug toxicity. In: Perez CA, Brady LW (eds): Principles and Practice of Radiation Oncology, 3rd ed, pp 155–211. Philadelphia, Lippincott-Raven, 1997.
141. Sheline GE, Wara WM, Smith V: Therapeutic irradiation and brain injury. Int J Radiat Oncol Biol Phys 1980; 6:1215–1228.
142. Hindo WA, DeTrana FA, Lee MS, et al: Large dose increment irradiation in treatment of cerebral metastases. Cancer 1970; 26:138–141.
143. Marks LB, Cuthbertson D, Friedman HS: Hematologic toxicity during craniospinal irradiation: the impact of prior chemotherapy. Med Pediatr Oncol 1995; 25:45–51.
144. Watterson J, Toogood I, Nieder M, et al: Excessive spinal cord toxicity from intensive central nervous system–directed therapies. Cancer 1994; 74:3034–3041.
145. Kagan AR: Nervous system toxicity. In: Madhu JJ, Flam MS, Legha SS, et al (eds): Chemoradiation: An Integrated Approach to Cancer Treatment, pp 582–590. Philadelphia, Lea & Febiger, 1993.
146. Allen JC, Siffert J: Contemporary chemotherapy issues for children with brainstem gliomas. Pediatr Neurosurg 1996; 24:98–102.
147. Prassopoulos P, Cavouras D, Evlogias N, et al: Brain atrophy in children undergoing systemic chemotherapy for extracranial solid tumors. Med Pediatr Oncol 1997; 28:228–233.
148. Bleyer WA: Neurologic sequelae of methotrexate and ionizing radiation: a new classification. Cancer Treat Rep 1981; 65 (suppl)1:89–98.
149. Bernaldez-Rios R, Villasis-Keever MA, Beltran-Adame G, et al: Neurological and psychological sequelae in children with acute lymphoblastic leukemia who had received radiotherapy and intrathecal methotrexate. Gac Med Mex 1998; 134:153–159.
150. Evans AE, Bleyer A, Kaplan R, et al: Central nervous system workshop. Cancer Clin Trials 1981; 4 (suppl):31–35.
151. Rubin P, Gash DM, Hansen JT, et al: Disruption of the blood-brain barrier as the primary effect of CNS irradiation. Radiother Oncol 1994; 31:51–60.
152. Williams JA, Roman-Goldstein S, Crossen JR, et al: Preirradiation osmotic blood-brain barrier disruption plus combination chemotherapy in gliomas: quantitation of tumor response to assess chemosensitivity. Adv Exp Med Biol 1993; 331:273–284.
153. Qin D, Ma J, Xiao J, et al: Effect of brain irradiation on blood-CSF barrier permeability of chemotherapeutic agents. Am J Clin Oncol 1997; 20:263–265.
154. Remsen LG, McCormick CI, Sexton G, et al: Long-term toxicity and neuropathology associated with the sequencing of cranial irradiation and enhanced chemotherapy delivery. Neurosurgery 1997; 40:1034–1040.
155. Abrey LE, DeAngelis LM, Yahalom J: Long-term survival in primary CNS lymphoma. J Clin Oncol 1998; 16:859–863.
156. Silber JH, Radcliffe J, Peckham V, et al: Whole-brain irradiation and decline in intelligence: the influence of dose and age on IQ score. J Clin Oncol 1992; 10:1390–1396.
157. Moore IM: Central nervous system toxicity of cancer therapy in children. J Pediatr Oncol Nurs 1995; 12:203–210.
158. Smedler AC, Nilsson C, Bolme P: Total body irradiation: a neuropsychological risk factor in pediatric bone marrow transplant recipients. Acta Paediatr 1995; 84:325–330.
159. Rampling R, Symonds P: Radiation myelopathy. Curr Opin Neurol 1998; 11:627–632.
160. Jones AM: Transient radiation myelopathy (with reference to Lhermitte's sign of electrical paresthesia). Br J Radiol 1964; 37:727–744.
161. Leith JT, DeWyngaert JK, Glicksman AS: Radiation myelopathy in the rat: an interpretation of dose effect relationships. Int J Radiat Oncol Biol Phys 1981; 7:1673–1677.
162. Gillen C, Jander S, Stoll G: Sequential expression of mRNA for proinflammatory cytokines and interleukin-10 in the rat peripheral nervous system: comparison between immune-mediated demyelination and Wallerian degeneration. J Neurosci Res 1998; 51:489–496.
163. Marcus RB Jr, Million RR: The incidence of myelitis after irradiation of the cervical spinal cord. Int J Radiat Oncol Biol Phys 1990; 19:3–8.
164. Schultheiss TE: Spinal cord radiation "tolerance": doctrine versus data. Int J Radiat Oncol Biol Phys 1990; 19:219–221.
165. Saunders MI, Dische S, Grosch EJ, et al: Experience with CHART. Int J Radiat Oncol Biol Phys 1991; 21:871–878.
166. Landuyt W, Fowler J, Ruifrok A, et al: Kinetics of repair in the spinal cord of the rat. Radiother Oncol 1997; 45:55–62.
167. Pop LA, van der Plas M, Ruifrok AC, et al: Tolerance of rat spinal cord to continuous interstitial irradiation. Int J Radiat Oncol Biol Phys 1998; 40:681–689.
168. Coia LR, Myerson RJ, Tepper JE: Late effects of radiation therapy on the gastrointestinal tract. Int J Radiat Oncol Biol Phys 1995; 31:1213–1236.
169. Collazzo LA, Levine MS, Rubesin SE, et al: Acute radiation esophagitis: radiographic findings. Am J Radiol 1997; 169:1067–1070.
170. Zimmermann FB, Geinitz H, Feldmann HJ: Therapy and prophylaxis of acute and late radiation-induced sequelae of the esophagus. Strahlenther Onkol 1998; 174 (suppl 3):78–81.
171. Sur M, Sur R, Cooper K, et al: Morphologic alterations in esophageal squamous cell carcinoma after preoperative high dose rate intraluminal brachytherapy. Cancer 1996; 77:2200–2205.
172. Taal BG, Aleman BM, Koning CC, et al: High dose rate brachytherapy before external beam irradiation in inoperable oesophageal cancer. Br J Cancer 1996; 74:1452–1457.
173. Emami B, Lyman J, Brown A, et al: Tolerance of normal tissue to therapeutic irradiation. Int J Radiat Oncol Biol Phys 1991; 21:109–122.
174. Hishikawa Y, Izumi M, Kurisu K, et al: Esophageal ulceration following high-dose-rate intraluminal brachytherapy for esophageal cancer. Radiother Oncol 1993; 28:252–254.
175. Goldstein HM, Rogers LF, Fletcher GH, et al: Radiological manifestations of radiation-induced injury to the normal upper gastrointestinal tract. Radiology 1975; 117:135–140.
176. Schultz-Hector S, Brechenmacher P, Dorr W, et al: Complications of combined intraoperative radiation (IORT) and external radiation (ERT) of the upper abdomen: an experimental model. Radiother Oncol 1996; 38:205–214.
177. Potish RA, Jones TK Jr, Levitt SH: Factors predisposing to radiation-related small-bowel damage. Radiology 1979; 132:479–482.
178. Pilepich MV, Krall JM, Sause WT, et al: Correlation of radiotherapeutic parameters and treatment-related morbidity in carcinoma of the prostate—analysis of RTOG study 75–06. Int J Radiat Oncol Biol Phys 1987; 13:351–357.
179. Munzenrider JE, Doppke KP, Brown AP, et al: Three-dimensional treatment planning for para-aortic node irradiation in patients with cervical cancer. Int J Radiat Oncol Biol Phys 1991; 21:229–242.
180. Perez CA, Fox S, Lockett MA, et al: Impact of dose in outcome of irradiation alone in carcinoma of the uterine cervix: analysis of two different methods. Int J Radiat Oncol Biol Phys 1991; 21:885–898.
181. Eifel PJ, Levenback C, Wharton JT, et al: Time course and incidence of late complications in patients treated with radiation therapy for FIGO stage IB carcinoma of the uterine cervix. Int J Radiat Oncol Biol Phys 1995; 32:1289–1300.
182. Huguenin P, Glanzmann C, Lutolf UM: Acute toxicity of curative radiotherapy in elderly patients. Strahlenther Onkol 1996; 172:658–663.
183. Kummermehr J, Trott KR: Chronic radiation damage in the rat

rectum: an analysis of the influences of fractionation, time and volume. Radiother Oncol 1994; 33:91–92.
184. Trott KR, Tamou S, Sassy T, et al: The effect of irradiated volume on the chronic radiation damage of the rat large bowel. Strahlenther Onkol 1995; 171:326–331.
185. Frykholm GJ, Isacsson U, Nygard K, et al: Preoperative radiotherapy in rectal carcinoma—aspects of acute adverse effects and radiation technique. Int J Radiat Oncol Biol Phys 1996; 35:1039–1048.
186. Shipley WU, Verhey LJ, Munzenrider JE, et al: Advanced prostate cancer: the results of a randomized comparative trial of high dose irradiation boosting with conformal protons compared with conventional dose irradiation using photons alone. Int J Radiat Oncol Biol Phys 1995; 32:3–12.
187. Teshima T, Hanks GE, Hanlon AL, et al: Rectal bleeding after conformal 3D treatment of prostate cancer: time to occurrence, response to treatment and duration of morbidity. Int J Radiat Oncol Biol Phys 1997; 39:77–83.
188. Horwitz EM, Hanlon AL, Hanks GE: Update on the treatment of prostate cancer with external beam irradiation. Prostate 1998; 37:195–206.
189. Hanks GE, Hanlon AL, Schultheiss TE, et al: Dose escalation with 3D conformal treatment: five year outcomes, treatment optimization, and future directions. Int J Radiat Oncol Biol Phys 1998; 41:501–510.
190. Pourquier H, Dubois JB, Delard R: Radiation therapy of cervical cancer with dosimetric prevention of late pelvic complications. Bull Cancer Radiother 1996; 83:135–143.
191. Mitchell EP: Gastrointestinal toxicity of chemotherapeutic agents. Semin Oncol 1992; 19:566–579.
192. Fata F, Ron IG, Kemeny N, et al: 5-fluorouracil-induced small bowel toxicity in patients with colorectal carcinoma. Cancer 1999; 86:1129–1134.
193. Minsky BD, Conti JA, Huang Y, et al: Relationship of acute gastrointestinal toxicity and the volume of irradiated small bowel in patients receiving combined modality therapy for rectal cancer. J Clin Oncol 1995; 13:1409–1416.
194. Bosset JF, Meneveau N, Pavy JJ: Late intestinal complications of adjuvant radiotherapy of rectal cancers. Cancer Radiother 1997; 1:770–774.
195. Calais G, Dorval E, Louisot P, et al: Radiotherapy with high dose rate brachytherapy boost and concomitant chemotherapy for Stages IIB and III esophageal carcinoma: results of a pilot study. Int J Radiat Oncol Biol Phys 1997; 38:769–775.
196. Hoffman PC, Haraf DJ, Ferguson MK, et al: Induction chemotherapy, surgery, and concomitant chemoradiotherapy for carcinoma of the esophagus: a long-term analysis. Ann Oncol 1998; 9:647–651.
197. Somlo G, Doroshow JH, Forman SJ, et al: High-dose doxorubicin, etoposide, and cyclophosphamide with stem cell reinfusion in patients with metastatic or high-risk primary breast cancer. City of Hope Bone Marrow Oncology Team. Cancer 1994; 73:1678–1685.
198. Byhardt RW, Scott C, Sause WT, et al: Response, toxicity, failure patterns, and survival in five Radiation Therapy Oncology Group (RTOG) trials of sequential and/or concurrent chemotherapy and radiotherapy for locally advanced non–small-cell carcinoma of the lung. Int J Radiat Oncol Biol Phys 1998; 42:469–478.
199. Coia LR, Engstrom PF, Paul AR, et al: Long-term results of infusional 5-FU, mitomycin-C and radiation as primary management of esophageal carcinoma. Int J Radiat Oncol Biol Phys 1991; 20:29–36.
200. Mahboubi S, Silber JH: Radiation-induced esophageal strictures in children with cancer. Eur Radiol 1997; 7:119–122.
201. Varveris H, Delakas D, Anezinis P, et al: Concurrent platinum and docetaxel chemotherapy and external radical radiotherapy in patients with invasive transitional cell bladder carcinoma. A preliminary report of tolerance and local control. Anticancer Res 1997; 17:4771–4780.
202. Danjoux CE, Catton GE: Delayed complications in colo-rectal carcinoma treated by combination radiotherapy and 5-fluorouracil— Eastern Cooperative Oncology Group (ECOG) pilot study. Int J Radiat Oncol Biol Phys 1979; 5:311–315.
203. Cummings BJ, Keane TJ, O'Sullivan B, et al: Epidermoid anal cancer: treatment by radiation alone or by radiation and 5-fluorouracil with and without mitomycin C. Int J Radiat Oncol Biol Phys 1991; 21:1115–1125.
204. Grigsby PW, Perez CA: Efficacy of 5-fluorouracil by continuous infusion and other agents as radiopotentiators for gynecologic malignancies. In: Rotman M, Rosenthal CJ (eds): Medical Radiology Series: Concomitant Continuous Infusion Chemotherapy and Radiation, p 259. Berlin, Springer-Verlag, 1991.
205. Stewart JR, Fajardo LF, Gillette SM, et al: Radiation injury to the heart. Int J Radiat Oncol Biol Phys 1995; 31:1205–1211.
206. Loire R, Saint-Pierre A: Radiation-induced pericarditis. Long-term outcome. 45 cases with thoracotomy and biopsy. Presse Medicale 1990; 19:1931–1936.
207. Aronow H, Kim M, Rubenfire M: Silent ischemic cardiomyopathy and left coronary ostial stenosis secondary to radiation therapy. Clin Cardiol 1996; 19:260–262.
208. Veeragandham RS, Goldin MD: Surgical management of radiation-induced heart disease. Ann Thorac Surg 1998; 65:1014–1019.
209. Grenier MA, Lipshultz SE: Epidemiology of anthracycline cardiotoxicity in children and adults. Semin Oncol 1998; 25 (suppl):72–85.
210. Selvaratnam G, Philips RH, Mohamed AK: Cardiotoxicity of cytotoxic chemotherapy and its prevention. Adverse Drug React Toxicol Rev 1999; 18:61–105.
211. Cosset JM, Henry-Amar M, Pellae-Cosset B, et al: Pericarditis and myocardial infarctions after Hodgkin's disease therapy. Int J Radiat Oncol Biol Phys 1991; 21:447–449.
212. Boivin JF, Hutchison GB, Lubin JH, et al: Coronary artery disease mortality in patients treated for Hodgkin's disease. Cancer 1992; 69:1241–1247.
213. Hancock SL, Tucker MA, Hoppe RT: Factors affecting late mortality from heart disease after treatment of Hodgkin's disease. JAMA 1993; 270:1949–1955.
214. Leandro J, Dyck J, Poppe D, et al: Cardiac dysfunction late after cardiotoxic therapy for childhood cancer. Am J Cardiol 1994; 74:1152–1156.
215. Hancock SL, Donaldson SS, Hoppe RT: Cardiac disease following treatment of Hodgkin's disease in children and adolescents. J Clin Oncol 1993; 11:1208–1215.
216. King V, Constine LS, Clark D, et al: Symptomatic coronary artery disease after mantle irradiation for Hodgkin's disease. Int J Radiat Oncol Biol Phys 1996; 36:881–889.
217. Constine LS, Schwartz RG, Savage DE, et al: Cardiac function, perfusion and morbidity in irradiated long-term survivors of Hodgkin's disease. Int J Radiat Oncol Biol Phys 1997; 39:897–906.
218. Karram T, Rinkevitch D, Markiewicz W: Poor outcome in radiation-induced constrictive pericarditis. Int J Radiat Oncol Biol Phys 1993; 25:329–331.
219. Kane GC, Edie RN, Mannion JD: Delayed appearance of effusive-constrictive pericarditis after radiation for Hodgkin lymphoma. Ann Intern Med 1996; 124:534–535.
220. Fajardo LF, Stewart JR: Pathogenesis of radiation-induced myocardial fibrosis. Lab Invest 1973; 29:244–257.
221. Gillette SM, Gillette EL, Shida T, et al: Late radiation response of canine mediastinal tissues. Radiother Oncol 1992; 23:41–52.
222. Schultz-Hector S: Radiation-induced heart disease: review of experimental data on dose response and pathogenesis. Int J Radiat Biol 1992; 61:149–160.
223. Fajardo LF, Stewart JR: Experimental radiation-induced heart disease. I. Light microscopic studies. Am J Pathol 1970; 59:299–316.
224. Lauk S: Endothelial alkaline phosphatase activity loss as an early stage in the development of radiation-induced heart disease in rats. Radiat Res 1987; 110:118–128.
225. Schultz-Hector S, Balz K: Radiation-induced loss of endothelial alkaline phosphatase activity and development of myocardial degeneration. An ultrastructural study. Lab Invest 1994; 71:252–260.
226. Applefeld MM: Radiation-induced cardiac disease. Am Heart J 1996; 131:1235–1236.
227. Gillette EL, McChesney SL, Hoopes PJ: Isoeffect curves for radiation-induced cardiomyopathy in the dog. Int J Radiat Oncol Biol Phys 1985; 11:2091–2097.
228. Schultz-Hector S, Sund M, Thames HD: Fractionation response and repair kinetics of radiation-induced heart failure in the rat. Radiother Oncol 1992; 23:33–40.
229. Frishman WH, Sung HM, Yee HC, et al: Cardiovascular toxicity with cancer chemotherapy. Curr Probl Cardiol 1996; 21:225–286.
230. Jeyaseelan R, Poizat C, Wu HY, et al: Molecular mechanisms of doxorubicin-induced cardiomyopathy. Selective suppression of Reiske iron-sulfur protein, ADP/ATP translocase, and phosphofructokinase genes is associated with ATP depletion in rat cardiomyocytes. J Biol Chem 1997; 272:5828–5832.

231. Mott MG: Anthracycline cardiotoxicity and its prevention. Ann NY Acad Sci 1997; 824:221–228.
232. Solem LE, Heller LJ, Wallace KB: Dose-dependent increase in sensitivity to calcium-induced mitochondrial dysfunction and cardiomyocyte cell injury by doxorubicin. J Mol Cell Cardiol 1996; 28:1023–1032.
233. Hensley ML, Schuchter LM, Lindley C, et al: American Society of Clinical Oncology clinical practice guidelines for the use of chemotherapy and radiotherapy protectants. J Clin Oncol 1999; 17:3333–3355.
234. Sekine I, Fukuda H, Kunitoh H, et al: Cancer chemotherapy in the elderly. Jpn J Clin Oncol 1998; 28:463–473.
235. Pihkala J, Saarinen UM, Lundstrom U, et al: Myocardial function in children and adolescents after therapy with anthracyclines and chest irradiation. Eur J Cancer 1996; 32A:97–103.
236. Davies HA, Wales JK: The effects of chemotherapy on the long-term survivors of malignancy. Br J Hosp Med 1997; 57:215–218.
237. Martin M, Lluch A, Ojeda B, et al: Paclitaxel plus doxorubicin in metastatic breast cancer: preliminary analysis of cardiotoxicity. Semin Oncol 1997; 24(suppl):S26–S30.
238. Kaufman PA: Paclitaxel and anthracycline combination chemotherapy for metastatic breast cancer. Semin Oncol 1999; 26 (suppl):S39–S46.
239. Hortobagyi GN, Willey J, Rahman Z, et al: Prospective assessment of cardiac toxicity during a randomized phase II trial of doxorubicin and paclitaxel in metastatic breast cancer. Semin Oncol 1997; 24 (suppl):S65–S68.
240. Sparano JA: Doxorubicin/taxane combinations: cardiac toxicity and pharmacokinetics. Semin Oncol 1999; 26 (suppl):14–19.
241. Hudis C, Riccio L, Seidman A, et al: Lack of increased cardiac toxicity with sequential doxorubicin and paclitaxel. Cancer Invest 1998; 16:67–71.
242. Nabholtz J-M, Tonkin K, Smylie M, et al: Review of docetaxel and doxorubicin-based combinations in the management of breast cancer: from metastatic to adjuvant setting. Semin Oncol 1999; 26 (suppl):10–16.
243. Slamon D, Leyland-Jones B, Shak S, et al: Addition of herceptin (humanized anti-HER2 antibody) to first line chemotherapy for HER2 overexpressing metastatic breast cancer (HER2+/MBC) markedly increases anticancer activity: a randomized, multinational controlled phase III trial. [Abstract]. Proceedings of the American Society of Clinical Oncology 1998; 17:377.
244. Ewer MS, Gibbs HR, Swafford J, et al: Cardiotoxicity in patients receiving trastuzumab (Herceptin): primary toxicity, synergistic or sequential stress, or surveillance artifact? Semin Oncol 1999; 26 (suppl):96–101.
245. Thomas ED: High-dose therapy and bone marrow transplantation. Semin Oncol 1985; 12:15–20.
246. Ayash LJ, Wright JE, Tretyakov O, et al: Cyclophosphamide pharmacokinetics: correlation with cardiac toxicity and tumor response. J Clin Oncol 1992; 10:995–1000.
247. Trigg ME, Finlay JL, Bozdech M, et al: Fatal cardiac toxicity in bone marrow transplant patients receiving cytosine arabinoside, cyclophosphamide, and total body irradiation. Cancer 1987; 59:38–42.
248. Ratanatharathorn V, Karanes C, Lum LG, et al: Allogenic bone marrow transplantation in high-risk myeloid disorders using busulfan, cytosine arabinoside and cyclophosphamide (BAC). Bone Marrow Transplant 1992; 9:49–55.
249. van Besien K, Tabocoff J, Rodriguez M, et al: High-dose chemotherapy with BEAC regimen and autologous bone marrow transplantation for intermediate grade and immunoblastic lymphoma: durable complete remissions, but a high rate of regimen-related toxicity. Bone Marrow Transplant 1995; 15:549–555.
250. Quezado ZMN, Wilson WH, Cunnion RE, et al: High-dose ifosfamide is associated with severe, reversible cardiac dysfunction. Ann Intern Med 1993; 118:31–36.
251. Kanj SS, Sharara AI, Shpall EJ, et al: Myocardial ischemia associated with high-dose carmustine infusion. Cancer 1991; 68:1910–1912.
252. Eltringham JR, Fajardo LF, Stewart JR: Adriamycin cardiomyopathy: enhanced cardiac damage in rabbits with combined drug and cardiac irradiation. Radiology 1975; 115:471–472.
253. Cassady JR: Clinical radiation nephropathy. Int J Radiat Oncol Biol Phys 1995; 31:1249–1256.
254. Krochak RJ, Baker DG: Radiation nephritis. Clinical manifestations and pathophysiologic mechanisms. Urology 1986; 27:389–393.
255. Beauvois S, Van Houtte P: Late effects of radiations on the kidney. Cancer Radiother 1997; 1:760–763.
256. Glatstein E, Fajardo LF, Brown JM: Radiation injury in the mouse kidney—I. Sequential light microscopic study. Int J Radiat Oncol Biol Phys 1977; 2:933–943.
257. Hoopes PJ, Gillette EL, Benjamin SA: The pathogenesis of radiation nephropathy in the dog. Radiat Res 1985; 104:406–419.
258. Hoopes PJ, Gillette EL, Cloran JA, et al: Radiation nephropathy in the dog. Br J Cancer 1986; 7 (suppl):273–276.
259. Rezvani M, Hopewell JW, Robbins ME: Initiation of non-neoplastic late effects: the role of endothelium and connective tissue. Stem Cells 1995; 13 (suppl 1):248–256.
260. Robbins ME, Bonsib SM: Radiation nephropathy: a review. Scanning Microsc 1995; 9:535–560.
261. Judas L, Bentzen SM, Stewart FA: Progression rate of radiation damage to the mouse kidney: a quantitative analysis of experimental data using a simple mathematical model of the nephron. Int J Radiat Biol 1997; 72:461–473.
262. Cohen EP, Lawton CA, Moulder JE: Bone marrow transplant nephropathy: radiation nephritis revisited. Nephron 1995; 70:217–222.
263. Stewart FA: Radiation nephropathy after abdominal irradiation or total-body irradiation. Radiat Res 1995; 143:235–237.
264. Peschel RE, Chen M, Seashore J: The treatment of massive hepatomegaly in stage IV-S neuroblastoma. Int J Radiat Oncol Biol Phys 1981; 7:549–553.
265. Sagerman RH, Berdon WE, Baker DH: Renal atrophy without hypertension following abdominal irradiation in infants and children. Ann Radiol 1969; 12:278–284.
266. Green DM, D'Angio GJ, Beckwith JB, et al: Wilms tumor. CA Cancer J Clin 1996; 46:46–63.
267. Agaliotis DP, Ballester OF, Mattox T, et al: Nephrotoxicity of high-dose ifosfamide/carboplatin/etoposide in adults undergoing autologous stem cell transplantation. Am J Med Sci 1997; 314:292–298.
268. Neglia JP, Nesbit ME Jr: Care and treatment of long-term survivors of childhood cancer. Cancer 1993; 71:3386–3391.
269. Merouani A, Davidson SA, Schrier RW: Increased nephrotoxicity of combination taxol and cisplatin chemotherapy in gynecologic cancers as compared to cisplatin alone. Am J Nephrol 1997; 17:53–58.
270. Cachat F, Guignard JP: The kidney in children under chemotherapy. Rev Med Suisse Romande 1996; 116:985–993.
271. Skinner R, Pearson AD, English MW, et al: Cisplatin dose rate as a risk factor for nephrotoxicity in children. Br J Cancer 1998; 77:1677–1682.
272. Lesesne JB, Rothschild N, Erickson B, et al: Cancer-associated hemolytic-uremic syndrome: analysis of 85 cases from a national registry. J Clin Oncol 1989; 7:781–789.
273. Schiebe ME, Hoffmann W, Belka C, et al: Mitomycin C-related hemolytic uremic syndrome in cancer patients. Anticancer Drugs 1998; 9:433–435.
274. Gordon LI, Kwaan HC: Thrombotic microangiography manifesting as thrombotic thrombocytopenic purpura/hemolytic uremic syndrome in the cancer patient. Semin Thromb Hemost 1999; 25:217–221.
275. Fung MC, Storniolo AM, Nguyen B, et al: A review of hemolytic uremic syndrome in patients treated with gemcitabine therapy. Cancer 1999; 85:2023–2032.
276. Chow S, Roscoe J, Cattran DC: Plasmapheresis and antiplatelet agents in the treatment of the hemolytic uremic syndrome secondary to mitomycin. Am J Kidney Dis 1986; 7:407–412.
277. Capizzi RL: Amifostine reduces the incidence of cumulative nephrotoxicity from cisplatin: laboratory and clinical aspects. Semin Oncol 1999; 26 (suppl):72–81.
278. Ryan SV, Carrithers SL, Parkinson SJ, et al: Hypotensive mechanisms of amifostine. J Clin Pharmacol 1996; 36:365–373.
279. Breslow NE, Takashima JR, Whitton JA, et al: Second malignant neoplasms following treatment for Wilms' tumor: a report from the National Wilms' Tumor Study Group. J Clin Oncol 1995; 13:1851–1859.
280. Smith GR, Thomas PR, Ritchey M, et al: Long-term renal function in patients with irradiated bilateral Wilms' tumor. National Wilms' Tumor Study Group. Am J Clin Oncol 1998; 21:58–63.
281. Oyama Y, Komatsuda A, Imai H, et al: Late onset bone marrow transplant nephropathy. Intern Med 1996; 35:489–493.

282. Guinan EC, Tarbell NJ, Niemeyer CM, et al: Intravascular hemolysis and renal insufficiency after bone marrow transplantation. Blood 1988; 72:451–455.
283. Lawton CA, Cohen EP, Barber-Derus SW, et al: Late renal dysfunction in adult survivors of bone marrow transplantation. Cancer 1991; 67:2795–2800.
284. Moulder JE, Fish BL: Influence of nephrotoxic drugs on the late renal toxicity associated with bone marrow transplant conditioning regimens. Int J Radiat Oncol Biol Phys 1991; 20:333–337.
285. Stewart FA, Bartelink H, van der Voet GB, et al: Renal damage in mice after sequential cisplatin and irradiation: the influence of prior irradiation on platinum elimination. Radiother Oncol 1991; 21:277–281.
286. Lawrence TS, Robertson JM, Anscher MS, et al: Hepatic toxicity resulting from cancer treatment. Int J Radiat Oncol Biol Phys 1995; 31:1237–1248.
287. Mornex F, Gerard F, Ramuz O, et al: Late effects of radiations on the liver. Cancer Radiother 1997; 1:753–759.
288. Geraci JP, Mariano MS: Radiation hepatology of the rat: parenchymal and nonparenchymal cell injury. Radiat Res 1993; 136:205–213.
289. Sempoux C, Horsmans Y, Geubel A, et al: Severe radiation-induced liver disease following localized radiation therapy for biliopancreatic carcinoma: activation of hepatic stellate cells as an early event. Hepatology 1997; 26:128–134.
290. Hebard DW, Jackson KL, Christensen GM: The chronological development of late radiation injury in the liver of the rat. Radiat Res 1980; 81:441–454.
291. Tabbara IA: Allogeneic bone marrow transplantation: acute and late complications. Anticancer Res 1996; 16:1019–1026.
292. Baron F, Deprez M, Beguin Y: The veno-occlusive disease of the liver. Haematologica 1997; 82:718–725.
293. Wasserheit C, Acaba L, Gulati S: Abnormal liver function in patients undergoing autologous bone marrow transplantation for hematological malignancies. Cancer Invest 1995; 13:347–354.
294. Faioni EM, Mannucci PM: Venocclusive disease of the liver after bone marrow transplantation: the role of hemostasis. Leuk Lymphoma 1997; 25:233–245.
295. Lewin K, Millis RR: Human radiation hepatitis. A morphologic study with emphasis on the late changes. Arch Pathol 1973; 96:21–26.
296. Minow RA, Stern MH, Casey JH, et al: Clinicopathologic correlation of liver damage in patients treated with 6-mercaptopurine and adriamycin. Cancer 1976; 38:1524–1528.
297. Shulman HM, Luk K, Deeg HJ, et al: Induction of hepatic veno-occlusive disease in dogs. Am J Pathol 1987; 126:114–125.
298. Anscher MS, Crocker IR, Jirtle RL: Transforming growth factor-beta 1 expression in irradiated liver. Radiat Res 1990; 122:77–85.
299. Anscher MS, Peters WP, Reisenbichler H, et al: Transforming growth factor-β as a predictor of liver and lung fibrosis after autologous bone marrow transplantation for advanced breast cancer. N Engl J Med 1993; 328:1592–1598.
300. Murase T, Anscher MS, Petros WP, et al: Changes in plasma transforming growth factor beta in response to high-dose chemotherapy for stage II breast cancer: possible implications for the prevention of hepatic veno-occlusive disease and pulmonary drug toxicity. Bone Marrow Transplant 1995; 15:173–178.
301. Jirtle RL, Anscher MS, Alati T: Radiation sensitivity of the liver. Adv Radiat Biol 1990; 14:269–311.
302. Jackson A, Ten Haken RK, Robertson JM, et al: Analysis of clinical complication data for radiation hepatitis using a parallel architecture model. Int J Radiat Oncol Biol Phys 1995; 31:883–891.
303. Evans DB, Abbruzzese JL, Cleary KR, et al: Preoperative chemoradiation for adenocarcinoma of the pancreas: excessive toxicity of prophylactic hepatic irradiation. Int J Radiat Oncol Biol Phys 1995; 33:913–918.
304. Woods WG, Dehner LP, Nesbit ME, et al: Fatal veno-occlusive disease of the liver following high dose chemotherapy, irradiation and bone marrow transplantation. Am J Med 1980; 68:285–290.
305. Tefft M, Mitus A, Das L, et al: Irradiation of the liver in children: review of experience in the acute and chronic phases, and in the intact normal and partially resected. Am J Roentgenol Radium Ther Nucl Med 1970; 108:365–385.
306. Thomas PR, Tefft M, D'Angio GJ, et al: Acute toxicities associated with radiation in the second National Wilms' Tumor Study. J Clin Oncol 1988; 6:1694–1698.
307. Yamasaki SA, Marn CS, Francis IR, et al: High-dose localized radiation therapy for treatment of hepatic malignant tumors: CT findings and their relation to radiation hepatitis. AJR Am J Roentgenol 1995; 165:79–84.
308. King PD, Perry MC: Hepatotoxicity of chemotherapeutic and oncologic agents. Gastroenterol Clin North Am 1995; 24:969–990.
309. Bagchi D, Bagchi M, Hassoun EA, et al: Adriamycin-induced hepatic and myocardial lipid peroxidation and DNA damage, and enhanced excretion of urinary lipid metabolites in rats. Toxicology 1995; 95:1–9.
310. Paolucci G, Rosito P, Di Caro A: Late data in pediatric oncology. Pediatr Med Chir 1990; 12:323–327.
311. Arai K, Kitamura M, Miyashita K, et al: Bile duct necrosis and hepatic necrosis following hepatic arterial infusion chemotherapy. Gan To Kagaku Ryoho 1991; 18:1856–1859.
312. Bisogno G, de Kraker J, Weirich A, et al: Veno-occlusive disease of the liver in children treated for Wilms tumor. Med Pediatr Oncol 1997; 29:245–251.
313. Pickles T, Graham P, Syndikus I, et al: Tolerance of nicotinamide and carbogen with radiation therapy for glioblastoma. Radiother Oncol 1996; 40:245–247.
314. Ganem G, Saint-Marc Girardin MF, Kuentz M, et al: Venocclusive disease of the liver after allogeneic bone marrow transplantation in man. Int J Radiat Oncol Biol Phys 1988; 14:879–884.
315. Piedbois P, Ganem G, Cordonnier C, et al: Interstitial pneumonitis and venocclusive disease of the liver after bone marrow transplantation. Radiother Oncol 1990; 18(suppl):125–127.
316. Johnson FL, Balis FM: Hepatopathy following irradiation and chemotherapy for Wilms' tumor. Am J Pediatr Hematol Oncol 1982; 4:217–221.
317. McDonald S, Rubin P, Phillips TL, et al: Injury to the lung from cancer therapy: clinical syndromes, measurable endpoints, and potential scoring systems. Int J Radiat Oncol Biol Phys 1995; 31:1187–1203.
318. Travis EL, Harley RA, Fenn JO, et al: Pathologic changes in the lung following single and multi-fraction irradiation. Int J Radiat Oncol Biol Phys 1977; 2:475–490.
319. Penney DP, Siemann DW, Rubin P, et al: Morphologic changes reflecting early and late effects of irradiation of the distal lung of the mouse: a review. Scanning Elect Microsc 1982; 413–425.
320. Davis SD, Yankelevitz DF, Henschke CI: Radiation effects on the lung: clinical features, pathology, and imaging findings. AJR Am J Roentgenol 1992; 159:1157–1164.
321. Guzzon A, Milani F, Spagnoli I, et al: Radiobiologic and pathologic characteristics of the irradiated lung and roentgenographic aspects. Tumori 1993; 79:1–8.
322. Marks LB: The pulmonary effects of thoracic irradiation. Oncology 1994; 8:89–106.
323. Herrmann T, Knorr A: Radiogenic lung reactions. Pathogenesis—prevention—therapy. Strahlenther Onkol 1995; 171:490–498.
324. Morgan GW, Breit SN: Radiation and the lung: a reevaluation of the mechanisms mediating pulmonary injury. Int J Radiat Oncol Biol Phys 1995; 31:361–369.
325. Kramer MR, Estenne M, Berkman N, et al: Radiation-induced pulmonary veno-occlusive disease. Chest 1993; 104:1282–1284.
326. Rubin P, Finkelstein JN, Siemann DW, et al: Predictive biochemical assays for late radiation effects. Int J Radiat Oncol Biol Phys 1986; 12:469–476.
327. Marks LB, Spencer DP, Bentel GC, et al: The utility of SPECT lung perfusion scans in minimizing and assessing the physiologic consequences of thoracic irradiation. Int J Radiat Oncol Biol Phys 1993; 26:659–668.
328. Marks LB, Munley MT, Spencer DP, et al: Quantification of radiation-induced regional lung injury with perfusion imaging. Int J Radiat Oncol Biol Phys 1997; 38:399–409.
329. Monson JM, Stark P, Reilly JJ, et al: Clinical radiation pneumonitis and radiographic changes after thoracic radiation therapy for lung carcinoma. Cancer 1998; 82:842–850.
330. Penney DP, Rubin P: Specific early fine structural changes in the lung irradiation. Int J Radiat Oncol Biol Phys 1977; 2:1123–1132.
331. Rubin P, Shapiro DL, Finkelstein JN, et al: The early release of surfactant following lung irradiation of alveolar type II cells. Int J Radiat Oncol Biol Phys 1980; 6:75–77.
332. Phillips TL: An ultrastructural study of the development of radiation injury in the lung. Radiology 1966; 87:49–54.

333. Penney DP: Ultrastructural organization of the distal lung and potential target cells of ionizing radiation. Paper presented at: International Conference on New Biology of Lung and Lung Injury and Their Implications for Oncology; 1987; Porvoo, Finland.
334. Anscher MS, Kong FM, Jirtle RL: The relevance of transforming growth factor beta 1 in pulmonary injury after radiation therapy. Lung Cancer 1998; 19:109–120.
335. Anscher MS, Murase T, Prescott DM, et al: Changes in plasma TGF beta levels during pulmonary radiotherapy as a predictor of the risk of developing radiation pneumonitis. Int J Radiat Oncol Biol Phys 1994; 30:671–676.
336. Girinsky T, Cosset JM: Pulmonary and cardiac late effects of ionizing radiations alone or combined with chemotherapy. Cancer Radiother 1997; 1:735–743.
337. Marks LB, Munley MT, Bentel GC, et al: Physical and biological predictors of changes in whole-lung function following thoracic irradiation. Int J Radiat Oncol Biol Phys 1997; 39:563–570.
338. Siemann DW, Hill RP, Penney DP: Early and late pulmonary toxicity in mice evaluated 180 and 420 days following localized lung irradiation. Radiat Res 1982; 89:396–407.
339. Down JD, Easton DF, Steel GG: Repair in the mouse lung during low dose-rate irradiation. Radiother Oncol 1986; 6:29–42.
340. Safwat A, Bentzen SM, Nielsen OS, et al: Repair capacity of mouse lung after total body irradiation alone or combined with cyclophosphamide. Radiother Oncol 1996; 40:249–257.
341. Wara WM, Phillips TL, Margolis LW, et al: Radiation pneumonitis: a new approach to the derivation of time-dose factors. Cancer 1973; 32:547–552.
342. Choi NC: Prospective prediction of postradiotherapy pulmonary function with regional pulmonary function data: promise and pitfalls. Int J Radiat Oncol Biol Phys 1988; 15:245–247.
343. Mohan R, Wang X, Jackson A: Optimization of 3-D conformal radiation treatment plans. Front Radiat Ther Oncol 1996; 29:86–103.
344. McDonald S, Garrow G, Rubin P: Pulmonary complications of cancer therapy. In: Abeloff MD, Armitage JO, Lichter AS, et al (eds): Clinical Oncology, 2nd ed, pp 1023–1046. New York, Churchill Livingstone, 2000.
345. Comis RL: Bleomycin pulmonary toxicity: current status and future directions. Semin Oncol 1992; 19:64–70.
346. Simpson AB, Paul J, Graham J, et al: Fatal bleomycin pulmonary toxicity in the west of Scotland 1991–95: a review of patients with germ cell tumours. Br J Cancer 1998; 78:1061–1066.
347. Kachel DL, Martin WJ: Cyclophosphamide-induced lung toxicity: mechanism of endothelial cell injury. J Pharmacol Exp Ther 1994; 268:42–46.
348. Sole A, Cordero PJ, Vera F: Pulmonary toxicity due to cyclophosphamide. Arch Bronconeumol 1999; 35:196–197.
349. Cooper JA, Zitnik R, Matthay RA: Mechanisms of drug-induced pulmonary disease. Ann Rev Med 1988; 39:395–404.
350. Hay J, Shahriar S, Laurent G: Mechanisms of bleomycin-induced lung damage. Arch Toxicol 1991; 65:81–94.
351. Baker W, Fistel SJ, Jones RV, et al: Interstitial pneumonitis associated with ifosfamide therapy. Cancer 1990; 65:2217–2221.
352. Lin AY, Flower CM, Chen MC, et al: Interstitial pneumonitis as a late complication of high dose therapy with cyclophosphamide/thiotepa and peripheral blood progenitor cell rescue for carcinoma of the breast. Clin Oncol 1998; 10:65.
353. Nysom K, Holm K, Hertz H, et al: Risk factors for reduced pulmonary function after malignant lymphoma in childhood. Med Pediatr Oncol 1998; 30:240–248.
354. Cohen IJ, Loven D, Schoenfeld T, et al: Dactinomycin potentiation of radiation pneumonitis: a forgotten interaction. Pediatr Hematol Oncol 1991; 8:187–192.
355. Roach M, Gandara DR, Yuo HS, et al: Radiation pneumonitis following combined modality therapy for lung cancer: analysis of prognostic factors. J Clin Oncol 1995; 13:2606–2612.
356. Bossi G, Cerveri I, Volpini E, et al: Long-term pulmonary sequelae after treatment of childhood Hodgkin's disease. Ann Oncol 1997; 8 (suppl 1):19–24.
357. Littman P, Meadows AT, Polgar G, et al: Pulmonary function in survivors of Wilm's tumor. Patterns of impairment. Cancer 1976; 37:2773–2776.
358. Jenkin RD, Jeffs RD, Stephens CA, et al: Wilms' tumour: adjuvant treatment with actinomycin D and vincristine. Can Med Assoc J 1976; 115:136–140.
359. Rosenow EC III, Limper AH: Drug-induced pulmonary disease. Semin Respir Infect 1995; 10:86–95.
360. Girinsky T, Socie G, Ammarguellat H, et al: Consequences of two different doses to the lungs during a single dose of total body irradiation: results of a randomized study on 85 patients. Int J Radiat Oncol Biol Phys 1994; 30:821–824.
361. Philit F, Cordonnier C, Michallet M, et al: Lung complications of hematopoietic stem cell transplantation. Rev Mal Respir 1996; 13:S71–S84.
362. Wilczynski SW, Erasmus JJ, Petros WP, et al: Delayed pulmonary toxicity syndrome following high-dose chemotherapy and bone marrow transplantation for breast cancer. Am J Crit Care Med 1998; 157:565–573.
363. Rubin P, Wasserman TH: International Clinical Trials in Radiation Oncology. The late effects of toxicity scoring. Int J Radiat Oncol Biol Phys 1988; 14 (suppl):S29–S38.
364. Rubin P: Special issue: Late Effects of Normal Tissues (LENT) Consensus Conference, including RTOG/EORTC SOMA scales. San Francisco, California, August 26–28, 1992. Int J Radiat Oncol Biol Phys 1995; 31:1035–1360.
365. Overgaard J, Bartelink H: Late Effects Consensus Conference: RTOG/EORTC. Radiother Oncol 1995; 35:1–82.

Glossary of Drug Terms

Nonproprietary Name	Trade Name
Acetaminophen	Tylenol
Acetylsalicylic acid	Aspirin
Allopurinol	Zyloprim
Alprazolam	Xanax
Aminoglutethimide	Cytadren
Amitriptyline	Elavil
Amphotericin B	Fungizone
Amsacrine	
Anastrozole	Arimidex
Azathioprine	Imuran
BCNU	BiCNU
Bicalutamide	Casodex
Bleomycin	Blenoxane
BudR	Bromodeoxyuridine
Bupropion	Wellbutrin
Buspirone	BuSpar
Busulfan	Myleran
Carbamazepine	
Carboplatin	Paraplatin
Carmustine	BiCNU
Chlorambucil	Leukeran
Chlordiazepoxide	Librium
Chlorpromazine	Thorazine, Promapar
Cis-diamminedichloroplatinum II	Platinol
Cisplatin	Platinol
Citalopram	Celexa
Cladribine	Leustatin
Clomipramine	
Clonazepam	
Clorazepate	
Codeine (with ASA)	
Conjugated estrogens	Premarin
Corticosteroids	
Cyclohexylchloroethyl nitrosourea	
Cyclophosphamide	Cytoxan, Neosar
Cyproheptadine	Periactin
Cytarabine	Cytosar-U
Cytosine arabinoside (Ara-C)	Cytosar-U
Dacarbazine	DTIC
Dactinomycin	Cosmegen
D-amphetamine	Dexedrine
Daunorubicin	Cerubidine
Deoxycoformycin	Nipent
Desipramine	Norpramin
Dexamethasone	Decadron, Hexadrol
Dexrazoxane	Zinecard
Diazepam	
Diethylstilbestrol	DES
Dinitrochlorobenzene	DNCB
Docetaxel	Taxotere
Doxepin	Sinequan

Nonproprietary Name	Trade Name
Doxorubicin	Adriamycin
Doxorubicin, liposomal	Doxil
Erythropoietin	Epogen, Procrit
Estramustine phosphate	Emcyt, Estracyte
Ethinyl estradiol	Estinyl
Etidronate disodium	Didronel
Etoposide	VePesid
Fludarabine	Fludara
Fluorouracil (5-FU)	Adrucil, Efudex
Fluoxetine	Prozac
Fluoxymesterone	Halotestin
Flutamide	Eulexin
Folinic Acid	Leucovorin
Gabapentin	Neurontin
Gallium nitrate	Ganite
G-CSF, filgrastim	Neupogen
Gemcitabine	Gemzar
GM-CSF	Leukine
Goserelin	Zoladex
Haloperidol	Haldol
Hexamethylmelamine, altretamine	Hexalen
Hydrocodone	Lorcet, Lortab
Hydromorphine	Dilaudid
Hydroxyprogesterone caproate	Delalutin
Hydroxyurea	Hydrea
Hydroxyzine	
Idarubicin	Idamycin
Ifosfamide	Ifex
Imipramine	Tofranil
Interferon alfa-2	Roferon-A, Intron-A, Alferon
Interleukin-2	Proleukin
Irinotecan	Camptosar
Lanreotide	
L-Asparaginase (*E. coli*)	Elspar
Letrozole	
Leucovorin	
Leuprolide	Lupron
Levamisole	Ergamisol
Lidocaine	Xylocaine
Lomustine	CeeNu
Lorazepam	
Mechlorethamine	Mustargen
Medroxyprogesterone acetate	Depo-Provera
Megestrol acetate	Megace
Melphalan	Alkeran
Meperidine	Demerol
Mercaptopurine	Purinethol
Mesna	Mesnex
Methadone	Dolophine
Methenamine	Cystamin, Cystogen
Methotrexate	Methotrexate
Methotrimeprazine, levomepromazine	
Methoxsalen	Oxsoralen
Methyl CCNU	Semustine
Methylphenidate	Ritalin

Nonproprietary Name	Trade Name
Methylprednisolone	Medrol
Metoclopramide	Reglan
Midazolam	Versed
Mirtazapine	Remeron
Misonidazole	
Mitomycin C	Mutamycin
Mitotane	Lysodren
Mitoxantrone	Novantrone
Morphine	
Nefazodone	Serzone
Nilutamide	Nilandron
Nortriptyline	Pamelor
Nystatin	Mycostatin
Octreotide acetate	Sandostatin
Ondansetron	Zofran
Oxazepam	
Oxycodone	Percocet, Percodan
Paclitaxel	Taxol
PALA, N-phosphonoacetyl-L-aspartate	
Pamidronate disodium	Aredia
Paroxetine	Paxil
Pemoline	Cylert
Pentostatin	Nipent
Phenytoin	Dilantin
Plicamycin	Mithracin
Porfimer sodium	Photofrin
Prednisone	Deltasone, Orasone
Procarbazine	Matulane
Pyrimethamine	Daraprim
Quinacrine	Atabrine
Rituximab	Rituxan
Sertraline	Zoloft
Spiromustine	
Streptozotocin	Zanosar
Tamoxifen	Nolvadex
Teniposide	Vumon
Tetracycline	Achromycin, Sumycin
Thioguanine	Thioguanine
Thioridazine	
Topotecan	Hycamtin
Toremifene	Fareston
Trastuzumab	Herceptin
Trazodone	Desyrel
Tretinoin	Vesanoid
Triethylenemelamine	Tretamine
Triethylenethiophosphoramide	Thiotepa
Valproate	Depacon
Venlafaxine	Effexor
Vinblastine	Velban
Vincristine	Oncovin
Vinorelbine	Navelbine
Zinc oxide	Calamine preparation

Index

Note: Page numbers in *italics* refer to illustrations; page numbers followed by t refer to tables.